Handbook of SPEECH-LANGUAGE PATHOLOGY AND AUDIOLOGY

Norman J. Lass, Ph.D.

Professor
Department of Speech Pathology and Audiology
West Virginia University
Morgantown, West Virginia

Leija V. McReynolds, Ph.D.

Professor
Department of Hearing and Speech
University of Kansas Medical Center
Kansas City, Kansas

Jerry L. Northern, Ph.D.

Professor
Department of Otolaryngology
Head, Audiology Division, University Hospital
University of Colorado Health Sciences Center
Denver, Colorado

David E. Yoder, Ph.D.

Professor and Chair
Department of Medical Allied Health Professions
University of North Carolina School of Medicine
Chapel Hill, North Carolina

1988
B.C. Decker Inc • Toronto • Philadelphia

Publisher

B.C. Decker Inc
3228 South Service Road
Burlington, Ontario L7N 3H8

B.C. Decker Inc
320 Walnut Street
Suite 400
Philadelphia, Pennsylvania 19106

Sales and Distribution

United States and Possessions	**The C.V. Mosby Company** 11830 Westline Industrial Drive St. Louis, Missouri 63146
Canada	**The C.V. Mosby Company, Ltd.** 5240 Finch Avenue East, Unit No. 1 Scarborough, Ontario M1S 4P2
United Kingdom, Europe and the Middle East	**Blackwell Scientific Publications, Ltd.** Osney Mead, Oxford OX2 OEL, England
Australia	**Harcourt Brace Jovanovich** 30–52 Smidmore Street Marrickville, N.S.W. 2204 Australia
Japan	**Igaku-Shoin Ltd.** Tokyo International P.O. Box 5063 1–28–36 Hongo, Bunkyo-ku, Tokyo 113, Japan
Asia	**Info-Med Ltd.** 802–3 Ruttonjee House 11 Duddell Street Central Hong Kong
South Africa	**Libriger Book Distributors** Warehouse Number 8 "Die Ou Looiery" Tannery Road Hamilton, Bloemfontein 9300
South America (non-stock list representative only)	**Inter-Book Marketing Services** Rua das Palmeriras, 32 Apto. 701 222–70 Rio de Janeiro RJ, Brazil

Handbook of Speech-Language Pathology and Audiology ISBN 1-55664-037-4

Library of Congress catalog card number: 87-72670

10 9 8 7 6 5 4 3 2 1

CONTRIBUTORS

JAMES H. ABBS, Ph.D.
Professor, Departments of Neurology and Neurophysiology, University of Wisconsin, Madison, Wisconsin
Neurophysiologic Processes of Speech Movement Control

RICHARD A. ALTSCHULER, Ph.D.
Adjunct Associate Professor, Department of Anatomy and Cell Biology and Associate Research Scientist, Department of Otorhinolaryngology, Kresge Hearing Research Institute, University of Michigan Medical School, Ann Arbor, Michigan
Neuroanatomic Bases of Hearing and Speech

JOHN M. BAUMGARTNER, Ph.D.
Assistant Professor, Section of Communicative Disorders and Sciences, Rush Medical College of Rush University; Attending Staff, Rush-Presbyterian-St. Luke's Medical Center, Chicago, Illinois
Stuttering in the Adult

FRED H. BESS, Ph.D.
Professor and Director, Division of Hearing and Speech Sciences, Vanderbilt University School of Medicine; Director, Bill Wilkerson Hearing and Speech Center, Nashville, Tennessee
Basic Hearing Measurement

SARAH W. BLACKSTONE, Ph.D.
Project Director, Implementation Strategies for Improving the Use of Communication Aids in Schools Serving Handicapped Children, American Speech-Language-Hearing Association, Rockville, Maryland
Augmentative Communication

WAYNE G. BODENHEMIER, Ph.D.
Clinical Instructor in Otolaryngology, University of Colorado Health Sciences Center School of Medicine; Executive Director, The Center for Hearing, Speech and Language, Denver, Colorado
Industrial Hearing Conservation

KATHRYN E. BRIGHT, Ph.D.
Assistant Professor, Department of Communication Disorders and Speech Science, University of Colorado, Boulder, Colorado
Hearing and Immittance Screening

E. LUCINDA CASSATT-JAMES, M.A.
Project Manager, Implementation Strategies for Improving the Use of Communication Aids in Schools Serving Handicapped Children, American Speech-Language-Hearing Association, Rockville, Maryland
Augmentative Communication

ROBIN S. CHAPMAN, Ph.D.
Professor, Department of Communicative Disorders and Section Head, Language Processes, Waisman Center on Mental Retardation and Human Development, University of Wisconsin, Madison, Wisconsin
Language Acquisition in the Child

DEE R. CHILD, M.S.
Clinical Instructor, Department of Communicative Disorders, Utah State University, Logan, Utah
Voice Disorders in the Child

PHIL J. CONNELL, Ph.D.
Associate Professor, Speech and Language Pathology Program, Department of Communication Sciences and Disorders, Northwestern University, Evanston, Illinois
A Clinical Science Approach to Treatment

JAMES R. CURRAN, M.S.
Research Audiologist, Starkey Laboratories, Inc., Minneapolis, Minnesota
Hearing Aids

ALLAN O. DIEFENDORF, Ph.D.
Associate Professor, Department of Audiology and Speech Pathology, University of Tennessee, Knoxville, Tennessee
Pediatric Audiology

MARION P. DOWNS, M.A., D.H.S.
Professor Emerita, Department of Otolaryngology, University of Colorado Health Sciences Center School of Medicine, Denver, Colorado
Early Identification of Hearing Loss

JUDITH FELSON DUCHAN, Ph.D.
Professor, Department of Communicative Disorders and Sciences, State University of New York, Buffalo, New York
Assessment Principles and Procedures

GERALD M. ENGLISH, M.D., F.A.C.S.
Clinical Professor, Department of Otolaryngology, University of Colorado Health Sciences Center School of Medicine, Denver, Colorado
Medical and Surgical Treatment of Hearing Loss

DONALD G. FERGUSON, Ed.D.
Professor, Department of Curriculum and Instruction, New Mexico State University, Las Cruces, New Mexico
Education of the Hearing Impaired Learner

KATHERINE PIKE GERKIN, M.A.
Clinical Instructor, Department of Otolaryngology, Audiology Division, University of Colorado Health Sciences Center School of Medicine, Denver, Colorado
Early Identification of Hearing Loss

JUDITH A. GIERUT, Ph.D.
National Institutes of Health Postdoctoral Fellow, Speech Research Laboratory, Department of Psychology, Indiana University, Bloomington, Indiana
Speech Perception

ARTHUR M. GUILFORD, Ph.D.
Professor and Director, Speech-Language Pathology, Department of Communicology, University of South Florida, Tampa, Florida
Language Disorders in the Adolescent

THOMAS W. GUYETTE, Ph.D.
Assistant Professor, Section of Communicative Disorders and Sciences, Rush Medical College of Rush University; Assistant Scientist, Rush-Presbyterian-St. Luke's Medical Center, Chicago, Illinois
Stuttering in the Adult

JAMES W. HALL III, Ph.D.
Associate Professor and Chief of Audiology, Department of Otolaryngology-Head and Neck Surgery, University of Texas Medical School; Director of Audiology, Hermann Hospital, Houston, Texas
Acoustic Immittance Measurements in Clinical Audiology

NATALIE L. HEDBERG, Ph.D.
Professor, Department of Communication Disorders and Speech Science, University of Colorado, Boulder, Colorado
Auditory Linguistic Processing

M. N. HEGDE, Ph.D.
Professor, Department of Communicative Disorders, California State University, Fresno, California
Principles of Management and Remediation

LINDA J. HESKETH, M.S.
Clinical Instructor, Department of Communicative Disorders, University of Wisconsin, Madison, Wisconsin
Speech and Language Disorders Related to Hearing Impairment

DOIN E. HICKS, Ed.D.
Professor, Department of Administration, Gallaudet University, Washington, D.C.
Education of the Hearing Impaired Learner

RAYMOND H. HULL, Ph.D.
Professor, Department of Communication Disorders and Audiology, College of Health and Human Services, University of Northern Colorado, Greeley, Colorado
Aural Rehabilitation in the Adult

JAMES F. JERGER, Ph.D.
Professor and Chief, Audiology and Speech Pathology, Department of Otorhinolaryngology and Communicative Sciences, Baylor College of Medicine; Director of Audiology and Speech Pathology, The Neurosensory Center, Houston, Texas
Acoustic Immittance Measurements in Clinical Audiology

THOMAS S. JOHNSON, Ph.D.
Professor and Head, Department of Communicative Disorders, Utah State University, Logan, Utah
Voice Disorders in the Child

JUDITH R. JOHNSTON, Ph.D.
Associate Professor, Department of Speech and Hearing Sciences, Indiana University, Bloomington, Indiana
Specific Language Disorders in the Child

JOEL C. KAHANE, Ph.D.
Associate Professor, Department of Audiology and Speech Pathology, Memphis State University, Memphis, Tennessee
Anatomy and Physiology of the Organs of the Peripheral Speech Mechanism

KEVIN P. KEARNS, Ph.D.
Adjunct Assistant Professor, Departments of Neurology and Psychiatry and Behavioral Sciences, Chicago Medical School; Chief, Audiology and Speech Pathology, Veterans Administration Medical Center, North Chicago, Illinois
Motor Speech Disorders: The Dysarthrias and Apraxia of Speech

ROBERT W. KEITH, Ph.D.
Professor, Department of Otolaryngology and Maxillofacial Surgery, Associate Professor, Department of Environmental Health, and Professor, Communication Disorders, Department of Communication, University of Cincinnati College of Medicine, Cincinnati, Ohio
Central Auditory Tests

JESSE G. KENNEDY III, Ph.D.
Professor, Department of Communicative Disorders, University of Wisconsin, Madison, Wisconsin
Basic Neurophysiologic Mechanisms Underlying Oral Communication

DAVID P. KUEHN, Ph.D.
Associate Professor, Department of Speech and Hearing Science, University of Illinois at Urbana-Champaign, Champaign, Illinois
Acoustics of Speech

CHARLES R. LARSON, Ph.D.
Associate Professor, Speech and Language Pathology, Department of Communication Sciences and Disorders, Northwestern University, Evanston, Illinois
Neuroanatomic Bases of Hearing and Speech

VICKI LORD LARSON, Ph.D.
Professor, Department of Communication Disorders, University of Wisconsin, Eau Claire, Wisconsin
Microcomputer Use in Assessment and Intervention with Speech and Language Disorders

NORMAN J. LASS, Ph.D.
Professor, Department of Speech Pathology and Audiology, West Virginia University; Joint Appointment, Professor, Department of Otolaryngology—Head and Neck Surgery, West Virginia University School of Medicine, Morgantown, West Virginia
Acoustics of Speech

MARGARET L. LEMME, Ph.D.
Associate Professor, Department of Speech Communication, University of Denver; Assistant Clinical Professor, Department of Physical Medicine and Rehabilitation, Health Sciences Center, Denver, Colorado
Auditory Linguistic Processing

DAVID M. LIPSCOMB, Ph.D.
Professor, Department of Audiology and Speech Pathology, University of Tennessee, Knoxville, Tennessee
Anatomy and Physiology of the Hearing Mechanism

LAURA K. McFARLANE LUNDE, M.A.
Neurosensory Laboratory Director, Denver Ear Institute, Denver, Colorado
Auditory Brain Stem Response and Electrocochleography

MALCOLM R. McNEIL, Ph.D.
Professor, Department of Communicative Disorders, University of Wisconsin; Consultant, Speech Pathology and Audiology Service, Veterans Administration Hospital, Madison, Wisconsin
Aphasia in the Adult

LEIJA V. McREYNOLDS, Ph.D.
Professor, Department of Hearing and Speech, University of Kansas Medical Center, Kansas City, Kansas
Articulation Disorders of Unknown Etiology
A Clinical Science Approach to Treatment

DIANNE J. MECKLENBURG, Ph.D.
Director of Clinical Studies, Cochlear Corporation, Englewood, Colorado
Cochlear Implants

MARY ROSS MORAN, Ph.D.
Associate Professor, Department of Special Education, University of Kansas Medical Center, Kansas City, Kansas
Reading and Writing Disorders in the Learning Disabled Student

MARIANA NEWTON, Ph.D.
Associate Professor, Department of Communication and Theater, University of North Carolina, Greensboro, North Carolina
Communication Disorders in the Aging

JERRY L. NORTHERN, Ph.D.
Professor, Department of Otolaryngology and Head, Audiology Division, University Hospital, University of Colorado Health Sciences Center, Denver, Colorado
Audiologic Manifestations

MARY JOE OSBERGER, Ph.D.
Assistant Professor, Department of Communicative Disorders, University of Wisconsin, Madison, Wisconsin
Speech and Language Disorders Related to Hearing Impairment

SALLY J. PETERSON-FALZONE, Ph.D.
Clinical Professor, Center for Craniofacial Anomalies, University of California, San Francisco, California
Speech Disorders Related to Craniofacial Structural Defects: Part 1
Speech Disorders Related to Craniofacial Structural Defects: Part 2

GLENN S. PFAU, Ph.D.
Professor, Department of Foundations, Gallaudet University, Washington, D.C.
Education of the Hearing Impaired Learner

BRYAN E. PFINGST, Ph.D.
Associate Professor, Department of Otolaryngology and Adjunct Associate Professor, Department of Psychology, University of Michigan Medical School, Ann Arbor, Michigan
Neuroanatomic Bases of Hearing and Speech

DAVID B. PISONI, Ph.D.
Professor and Director, Speech Research Laboratory, Department of Psychology, Indiana University, Bloomington, Indiana
Speech Perception

BARRY M. PRIZANT, Ph.D.
Assistant Professor, Division of Child and Adolescent Psychiatry, Department of Psychiatry and Human Behavior, Brown University Program in Medicine, Providence; Director, Communication Disorders Department, Emma Pendleton Bradley Hospital, Riverside and Staff Appointment, Department of Psychiatry, Women and Infants Hospital of Rhode Island, Providence, Rhode Island
Communication Problems in the Autistic Client

CHARLES G. REED, Ph.D.
Chief, Speech Pathology Section, Audiology and Speech Pathology Service, Veterans Administration Medical Center, San Francisco, California
Voice Disorders in the Adult

ALICE RICHARDSON, Ph.D.
Director, Speech and Hearing Center, Program in Communication Disorders, Department of Speech Communication, University of Texas, Austin, Texas
Language Delay in the Child

JOANNE ROBBINS, Ph.D.
Associate Scientist, Department of Neurology and Co-Director, Neurodysphagia Clinic, Center for Health Sciences, University of Wisconsin, Madison, Wisconsin
Dysphagia and Disorders of Speech

JACKSON ROUSH, Ph.D.
Instructor, Department of Otolaryngology, Harvard Medical School; Director, Hearing Aid Center, Massachusetts Eye and Ear Infirmary, Boston, Massachusetts
Hearing and Immittance Screening

JAY W. SANDERS, Ph.D.
Professor, Division of Hearing and Speech Sciences, Vanderbilt University School of Medicine; Research Associate, Bill Wilkerson Hearing and Speech Center, Nashville, Tennessee
Diagnostic Audiology

RUTH S. SARGENT, M.A.
Clinical Audiologist, Colorado Otolaryngology Professional Corporation, Englewood, Colorado
Medical and Surgical Treatment of Hearing Loss

JON K. SHALLOP, Ph.D.
Executive Director, Denver Ear Institute; Associate Clinical Professor, University of Colorado Health Sciences Center, Denver, Colorado
Cochlear Implants

JUNE E. SHOUP, Ph.D.
Associate Professor, Department of Communication Arts and Sciences, University of Southern California; Director, Speech Science Research Laboratory, Los Angeles, California
Acoustics of Speech

NINA N. SIMMONS, M.S.
Chief, Department of Speech Pathology, Touro Infirmary, New Orleans, Louisiana
Motor Speech Disorders: The Dysarthrias and Apraxia of Speech

STEVEN J. STALLER, Ph.D.
Director, Denver Ear Institute; Adjunct Assistant Professor, Department of Communication Disorders, University of Colorado, Boulder and Clinical Instructor, Department of Otolaryngology, University of Colorado Health Sciences Center School of Medicine, Denver, Colorado
Auditory Brain Stem Response and Electrocochleography

SYLVIA STEINER, Ph.D.
Professor, Department of Communication Disorders, University of Wisconsin, Eau Claire, Wisconsin
Microcomputer Use in Assessment and Intervention with Speech and Language Disorders

ORLANDO L. TAYLOR, Ph.D.
Dean and Professor, Department of Communications Arts and Sciences, School of Communications, Howard University, Washington, D.C.
Speech and Language Differences and Disorders of Multicultural Populations

CYNTHIA K. THOMPSON, Ph.D.
Speech Pathology Research Scientist, Veterans Administration Medical Center (Atlanta), Decatur, Georgia
Articulation Disorders in the Child with Neurogenic Pathology

JOHN D. TONKOVICH, Ph.D.
Director, Speech-Language Pathology Department, Rehabilitation Institute, Inc., Detroit, Michigan
Speech and Language Disorders Associated with Various Neuropathologies

ANNE VAN KLEECK, Ph.D.
Associate Professor, Department of Speech Communication, University of Texas, Austin, Texas
Language Delay in the Child

FRANCISCO VILLARRUEL, M.S.
Research Assistant, Waisman Center on Mental Retardation and Human Development, University of Wisconsin, Madison, Wisconsin
Effective Communication for the Severely Handicapped Child

MERYL J. WALL, Ph.D.
Associate Professor and Chairperson, Department of Speech Arts and Communicative Disorders, Adelphi University, Garden City, New York
Dysfluency in the Child

DONALD W. WARREN, D.D.S., Ph.D.
Kenan Professor and Director, Oral Facial and Communicative Disorders Program, Schools of Dentistry and Medicine and Dental Research Center, University of North Carolina; Attending Dentist, Hospital Dental Service, North Carolina Memorial Hospital, Chapel Hill, North Carolina
Aerodynamics of Speech

KENNETH L. WATKIN, Ph.D.
Associate Professor, Department of Biomedical Engineering, McGill University, Faculty of Medicine, Montreal, Quebec, Canada
Neuroanatomic Bases of Hearing and Speech

GARY WEISMER, Ph.D.
Associate Professor, Department of Communicative Disorders, University of Wisconsin, Madison, Wisconsin
Speech Production

DAVID E. YODER, Ph.D.
Professor and Chair, Department of Medical Allied Health Professions, University of North Carolina School of Medicine, Chapel Hill, North Carolina
Effective Communication for the Severely Handicapped Child

JANET M. ZARNOCH, M.A.
Director, Department of Speech Pathology and Audiology, St. Francis Hospital, Jersey City, New Jersey
Audiologic Manifestations

PREFACE

The *Handbook of Speech-Language Pathology and Audiology* is intended to serve as a comprehensive sourcebook containing under one cover contemporary information on the processes and pathologies of speech, language, and hearing. Because it provides in-depth coverage of topics by contemporary scholars, it can serve as both a textbook for numerous courses and as a reference source for graduate students and professionals in speech-language pathology, audiology, and speech and hearing sciences. The *Handbook* should also prove useful to students and professionals in related disciplines, including medicine, dentistry, nursing, education, special education, psychology, linguistics, and social work. The emphasis throughout the entire volume is on comprehensive coverage of contemporary information and approaches based on current research findings.

The book is divided into three sections: Normal Processes, Speech and Language Disorders, and Hearing Disorders. The Speech and Language Disorders section has six major divisions: Assessment and Intervention Principles, Articulation Disorders, Fluency Disorders, Language Disorders, Voice Disorders, and Special Populations and Communication. The Hearing Disorders section has two major divisions: Assessment and Rehabilitation of the Hearing Impaired.

We are indebted to many individuals, including the authors of the fifty-two chapters in the book. In addition to their expertise and skillful writing, they have been exceptionally cooperative and patient throughout the various stages of the book's development. We also wish to express our gratitude to the dedicated staff of B. C. Decker Inc: Agnes McIvor for her assistance, persistence, and perseverance in reminding editors and authors of their obligations and deadlines, and for her cooperative attitude that allowed us to progress toward completion of this book; Shireen Jeejeebhoy for her excellent editorial work; Dennis Boyes for his creative design of the book cover; and the entire production and editorial staff for their careful handling of the book. Our very special thanks are extended to Brian Decker, the publisher. His guidance, patience, and overall publishing experience have been invaluable to us throughout all stages of the *Handbook's* development. Without such a conscientious and ambitious staff, this project might well have remained merely a good idea among ivory-towered academics. And finally, to our colleagues who have expressed a real need for such a contemporary handbook and who have offered us the reassurance, encouragement, sympathy, and reminders necessary to bring this book to completion, we express our sincere appreciation.

Norman J. Lass
Leija V. McReynolds
Jerry L. Northern
David E. Yoder

CONTENTS

Section 1
NORMAL PROCESSES

Norman J. Lass

Section 2
SPEECH AND LANGUAGE DISORDERS

Leija V. McReynolds
David E. Yoder

Assessment and Intervention Principles

Articulation Disorders

Fluency Disorders

Language Disorders

Voice Disorders

Special Populations and Communication

Section 3
HEARING DISORDERS

Jerry L. Northern

Assessment

Rehabilitation of the Hearing Impaired

Section 1
NORMAL PROCESSES

Norman J. Lass, Ph.D.

1 Anatomy and Physiology of the Organs of the Peripheral Speech Mechanism

Joel C. Kahane, Ph.D.

The speech mechanism—does one exist? No single organ is designed expressly for speech production in the same way that some structures are especially adapted for hearing, respiration, mastication, or deglutition. Negus maintained that speech was *overlaid* upon other more vegetative functions.[1] This implies that humans adapt the organs whose primary biologic functions center around life-sustaining functions for the purposes of producing speech.

The mechanisms by which man marshalls these physiologic capabilities are still not fully understood; however, insights have been gained, and these are discussed by several authors in Chapters 4, 5, 7, and 8 of this book. Information basic to an understanding of the biomechanics of the speech mechanism must evolve from an understanding of the organs that compose it.

This chapter attempts to provide this information. I assume that the reader already has had an introduction to the anatomy and physiology of the speech mechanism. This chapter examines the respiratory system, larynx, supralaryngeal airways, and the major articulators in terms of (1) postnatal developmental morphology, so as to provide an understanding of those structural or functional changes that may differentiate varying levels of performance; (2) anatomy, to identify salient biologic and mechanical properties of each organ and system; and (3) nonspeech functions, to highlight the range of physiologic behaviors performed by these organs.

The anticipated benefit of this approach is a perspective that enables one to be a more knowledgeable observer of speech function. This ability is essential, for as DuBrul wrote,

> It is quite true that in speaking the lungs, respiratory diaphragm, and muscles of the belly wall and larynx twitter, but all animals have these parts, and only one of them can speak . . . I suspect that the difficulty in discovering the source of speech has been in not knowing where to look.[2]

THE RESPIRATORY SYSTEM

The respiratory system is composed of several diverse organs, beginning in the nose and ending in the alveoli of the lungs. It also has a complex musculoskeletal framework, which is centrally involved in the mechanical process of external respiration. The anatomic bases and functional roles of the aforementioned structures are described in the following section.

Postnatal Developmental Changes in Anatomy and Function

Although the respiratory system is capable of supporting life at birth, it is not completely structurally mature. The infant's and child's breathing mechanism exhibits differences in the breathing rate and the locus of breathing movements from that of older children and adults. These important differences in postnatal maturation of the respiratory system are described next.[3–5]

Tracheobronchial Tree

The morphology of the tracheobronchial tree in the newborn has been studied extensively.[3] The trachea in the newborn is approximately one-third its adult size, the bronchi one-half their adult size, and the bronchioles only one-quarter of their adult size. By age 4, 19 percent of the adult complement of alveoli are present as are more than one-half of the adult complement of terminal airways.[4] The bronchioles and alveoli reach their adult number and size by age 8; however, the lung continues to grow into adulthood through increases in the size of existing respiratory units. Growth changes in the chest, lungs, and airways are well correlated with increases in height and age.[6] Lung volumes (an index of lung growth) are greater in the male than in the female. In young children (shorter than 150 cm), the chest grows more rapidly than the lungs. In older children (taller than 150 cm), growth of the chest and lungs proceeds at fairly equal rates.

Thoracic Skeleton

The shape and morphology of the thorax change from birth to adulthood. These changes result from the development of upright posture and because of changes in respiratory needs.

At birth and through age 2, the ribs extend horizontally from the vertebral column and are largely cartilagenous. This results in a large vertebrosternal (anteroposterior) dimension that gives the thorax a rounded shape. As the ribs become more curved and inclined posteriorly, the anteroposterior dimension of the thorax diminishes relative to the increasing transverse dimension. This modeling results from muscle forces that develop to keep the body erect, which is required for walking. As the infant and child begin to balance themselves on their lower limbs, a curvature develops in the lumbar region of the vertebral column, and the ribs incline dorsally near their attachment to the vertebral column. These morphologic changes facilitate balancing of the trunk in the upright posture by permitting structures in the thorax to become aligned alongside and dorsal to the vertebral column. After age 2, the ribs become progressively more angled, and by age 7 they have assumed adult relationships.[7]

The contour of the infant's ribs does not enable the infant to significantly increase the size of the thoracic cavity during breathing. Subsequent changes in the shape of the ribs associated with strengthening of the respiratory muscles enables the chest wall to play a greater role in respiratory function with increasing age.[7]

Functional Changes

From a functional standpoint, developmental differences also occur in respiratory functioning.[8] For example, the frequency of breathing progressively decreases with age.[7] The infant takes 60 to 70 breaths per minute as compared to only 16 to 18 breaths per minute in the adult.

During infancy and for most of the first year of life, movements of the thoracic wall are minimal, whereas those of the diaphragm predominate. This arrangement causes the abdomen to move rhythmically in and out during respiration. After age 6 to 8 months and continuing to age 5 to 7 years, a mixed pattern of breathing exists that involves both abdominal and chest wall movements. After age 7, thoracic wall movements predominate.[8]

These changes in respiratory function may be attributed to several factors that include better control of the respiratory apparatus and more efficient use of oxygen (O_2) and to larger lung capacities, which permit greater intake and utilization of air.

Anatomy and Physiology

The respiratory system is conventionally subdivided into upper and lower respiratory tracts. These are distinguished upon the basis of the anatomic structures composing each and upon the different roles that each plays in the process of respiration. The following discussion examines these structures and the biomechanics of the chest wall and lungs during respiration.

The Upper Respiratory Tract

The upper respiratory tract (Fig. 1–1) is composed of the nasal cavities, oral cavity, pharynx, and larynx. As distinguished from the lower respiratory tract, which serves an exclusively respiratory function, the organs composing the upper respiratory tract serve several functions in addition to respiration. These functions are associated with mastication, deglutition, phonation, and resonation. The following discussion reviews the special contributions of each of these organs to respiration.

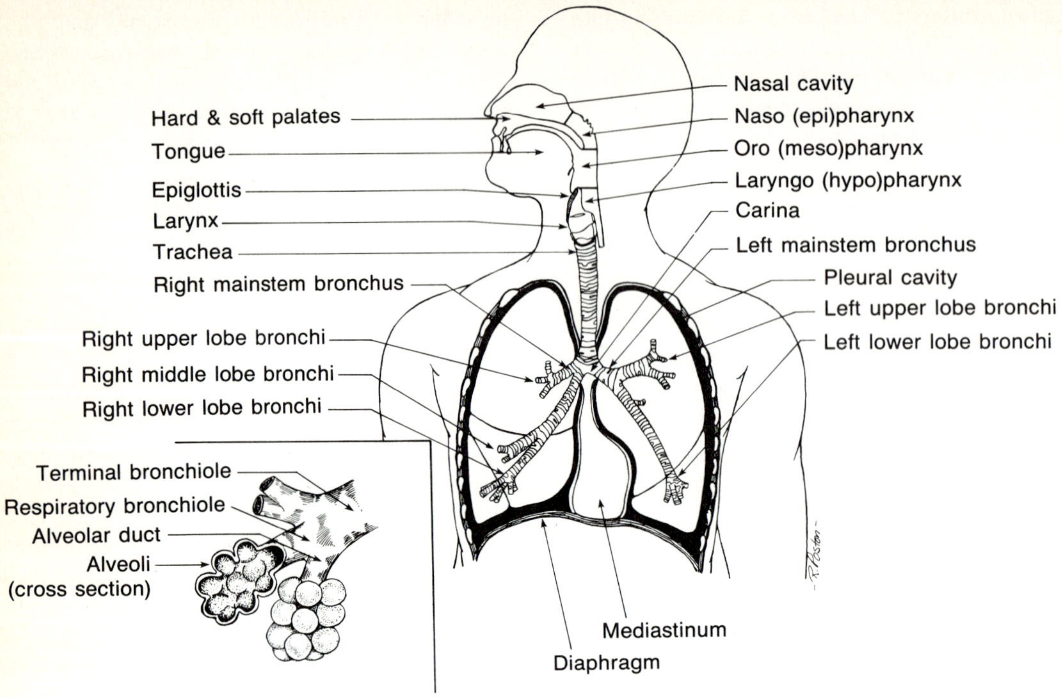

Figure 1–1 Schema of the respiratory system. Inset is a schematic drawing of the anatomy of the terminal portions of the bronchial tree that are not illustrated in the larger figure. (Adapted from Grant JB. Atlas of anatomy. 6th ed. Baltimore: Williams & Wilkins, 1972.)

Nasal Cavities. The nose is not simply a passive conduit through which air passes from the atmosphere into the pharynx; it is a highly specialized organ that performs three important respiratory functions: humidification, warming of inspired air, and protection of the upper airways. Anatomic specializations in the nasal cavities make these functions possible. The hair or vibrissae in the vestibule of the nose filter large particles from the inspired air. A rich blood supply located beneath the surface epithelium warms and moisturizes the inspired air. Respiratory epithelium containing goblet (mucous) cells lines all of the nasal cavity except the roof and anterior one-third. These glands produce a blanket of mucous that entraps airborne dirt, thus preventing it from entering the lungs. The cilia of the respiratory epithelium move the mucous blanket out of the nose and into the pharynx where it is swallowed or expectorated. The conchae or turbinates increase the surface area across which inspired air passes and facilitates the aforementioned process.[6,9,10]

Humidification or moisturizing of the air is important since rapid exchange of O_2 at the alveolar membrane requires that air be completely saturated with moisture. This humidification is accomplished in the nasal cavity when air passes over the nasal epithelium (especially the conchae), where it picks up moisture from the epithelial surface. The moisture is obtained from fluids that are drawn out from the underlying blood vessels.[5,6]

Warming of inspired air serves two important functions. It increases the capacity of air to hold moisture, and it minimizes reflex constriction of the smooth muscles in the walls of the bronchioles. This constriction may occur in response to cold air that passes through the terminal passages of the bronchial tree.[9] However, air is usually warmed as it passes over the epithelial surfaces of the nasal conchae and septum by heat, which is derived from the rich blood supply located immediately below the epithelial surfaces.[5,9]

Protection of the upper airways by the nasal cavities is accomplished in several ways. In addition to the filtering processes served by the vibrissae (hairs) in the vestibule of the nose and the mucous blanket, the mucous produced in the nose plays an important role in protecting the upper respiratory tract from infection. This protection is accomplished by immunoglobulin A (IgA), which is contained in the mucous secretions and which is produced in the glands and mucosal plasma cells in the nasal cavity.[5]

The foregoing discussion demonstrates that the nose plays a central role in preparing the air for efficient gaseous exchange. Recently, data from several investigators have shown that the nose may directly influence pulmonary function.[11–13] These authors found that various types of nasal or nasopharyngeal obstruction caused measurable changes in pulmonary function, including decreased lung volumes and flow rates that returned to normal levels when the obstructions were removed. Further research is needed to explore these nasopulmonary relationships.

The Pharynx. The pharynx plays a relatively passive role in respiration compared to the other structures in the upper airway. The nasopharynx serves a purely respiratory function and, in this respect, is specialized from the rest of the pharynx. Its physical dimensions are fixed as a result of the bony framework to which its walls are attached. As a consequence, the nasopharyngeal airway is always patent. Its walls are lined with respiratory epithelium that is continuous with that of the nasal cavity.[14,15]

The more caudal portions of the pharynx (oro- and laryngopharyngeal regions) serve as relatively passive conduits during respiration, although that oropharyngeal volume[16] may be enlarged through extension of the neck when respiratory needs increase. Oropharyngeal volume is not decreased in flexion of the neck because of coordinated anterior movements of the tongue and the hyoid bone.[17]

The Larynx. The larynx plays an essential role in respiration. The action of the laryngeal muscles controls the size of the rima glottidis—the inlet through which inspired air enters the lower respiratory tract. The larynx also protects the lower airway from becoming obstructed by food and other materials through reflexive closure and the cough reflex.[17,18]

Respiratory movements of the larynx are cyclical, rhythmic oscillations during respiration, which were first described by Garcia and Czermak.[19,20] Many investigators, using a variety of methods, have since described specific characteristics of respiratory movements of the larynx.[17,21–29] However, investigators still disagree on several points: Are these movements active or passive? Are they present in all degrees of respiratory activity or only during respiration more strenuous than the tidal breathing? What intrinsic laryngeal muscles are active during respiration? Inspiratory movements of the larynx have been shown to consist of a descent of the larynx and trachea posteriorly and to the left; an increase in the size of the rima glottidis; a lateral movement of the vocal processes; and an increase in the size of the laryngeal aditus and vestibule. Expiratory movements of the larynx reverse the effects of inspiration.[21,23,29]

The force behind these laryngeal movements was thought to result from active contraction of the sternothyroid and sternohyoid muscles, respectively.[21] Several investigators maintain that the movements are passive reactions to changes in intrathoracic pressure.[23,24,29] The latter viewpoint appears to be reasonable in that it requires the least expenditure of energy. One author asserted that respiratory movements of the larynx result from purely nonmuscular forces and that the enlargement of the laryngeal cavity is caused by unfolding of the soft tissues of the larynx;[29] elastic recoil of these stretched tissues returns the larynx to its resting state.

The central role of the larynx in respiration is to maintain a patent glottal airway. The rima glottidis is the most constricted portion of the laryngeal area. It represents a 75 percent reduction of the laryngeal airway,[30] having a cross-sectional area of 50 to 70 mm as compared to approximately 200 mm for the supra- and infraglottal areas located immediately above and below it. The size and shape of the glottal aperture is changed dramatically during respiration as evidenced in differences between normal tidal breathing (Fig. 1–2*A*) and forced inspiration (Fig. 1–2*B*). Recent data on laryngorespiratory function have revealed that the size of the glottis is systematically related to the volume of inspired air[27] and to the rate of airflow into the lungs.[28] The glottis enlarges with greater volume of inspired air and when the rate of airflow increases. Thus, during quiet breathing, the size of the rima glottidis changes little, but as respiratory demands increase, the vocal folds are moved progressively more laterally.

Researchers still do not agree completely as to the precise role of the intrinsic laryngeal muscles during respiration. The posterior cricoarytenoid muscle has long been thought of as the sole abductor and respiratory muscle of the larynx.[2,14,15,31–35] However, data from electromyographic studies suggest that reinterpretation may be necessary.[35–38] These data showed that posterior cricoarytenoid muscle activity during inspiration was inhibited or not always active during tidal or quiet inspiration. Much intersubject variability was found. This muscle has been found to be extremely active during forced inspiration when greater than resting volumes of air were required.[37,38]

The intrinsic laryngeal muscles show different extents of activity during respiration. Laryngeal

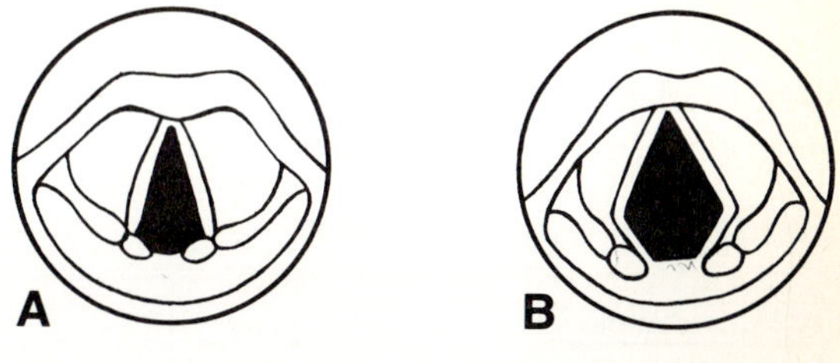

Figure 1–2 Laryngoscopic appearance of the rima glottidis during, *A*, quiet respiration and *B*, forced respiration.

muscles have been found to exhibit significantly greater electrical activity during quiet and forced expiration.[35] Related to this finding is that cricothyroid and lateral and posterior cricoarytenoid muscle activity is greatest in expiration. Other reports are less specific and simply address the fact that all intrinsic laryngeal muscles show increased activity during both phases of respiration.[39,40]

One can see that a wide variety of opinions exists about the roles of the specific laryngeal muscles during respiration. This variety may be due to the difficulties in isolating these muscles for recording purposes and their action with respiratory activity. Further research is clearly needed. Perhaps a fruitful approach would be to study the sensorimotor feedback loops in the larynx, as discussed by Wyke.[40]

The Lower Respiratory Tract

The lower respiratory tract consists of all the airways below the larynx. These are collectively referred to as the tracheobronchial tree and are illustrated in Figure 1–1. The special anatomic properties and respiratory functions of each component are discussed in the next two sections.

The Trachea. The trachea is composed of 16 to 20 C-shaped hyaline cartilage rings, which extend from about the level of the sixth cervical vertebra, immediately below the cricoid cartilage, to the level of the fourth thoracic vertebra where the trachea bifurcates (the carina), giving rise to a right and a left mainstem bronchus. The trachea is about 10 to 12 cm in length and 1.4 to 2.0 cm in width. The average cross-sectional area during quiet breathing is 1.5 cm^2. As shown in cross-section in Figure 1–3, the C-shaped tracheal cartilages are enclosed dorsally by fibroelastic tissue and smooth muscle fibers. The smooth muscle fibers form the trachealis muscle, which is composed of superficial fibers running longitudinally and deep fibers running transversely. The

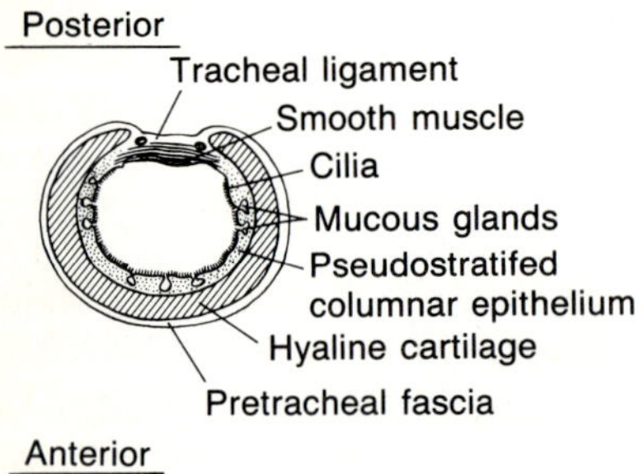

Figure 1–3 Cross-section of the human treachea. (From Becker RF, Wilson JW, Gehweiler JG. Anatomical basis of medical practice. Baltimore: Williams & Wilkins, 1971:456.)

trachea is lined with typical respiratory epithelium containing mucous cells and cilia that beat in a rostral direction (i.e., away from the lower airways).[30,41]

The trachea is not completely passive during respiration. The cartilagenous rings and smooth muscles of the trachea provide rigidity to the walls of the airways, insuring its patency. This support is important because without it, the changing pressures in the thorax would modify the tracheal airway. This modification is especially true in the case of inspiratory forces, which would cause the walls of an unsupported trachea to collapse. Some authors have maintained that the tracheal muscle further assists in maintaining the tracheal airway by resisting compression from the resting esophagus, which is immediately dorsal to it.[10] When one swallows, however, respiration momentarily ceases, and the dorsal region of the trachea gives way inwardly to allow the bolus of food to pass down the esophagus. During inspiration, the tracheal muscle relaxes, permitting the natural elasticity of the tracheal cartilages to expand the tracheal lumen. During expiration, especially forced expiration, the tracheal muscle contracts, firming up the dorsal wall of the trachea and bracing it against expiratory forces.

The Bronchial Tree. The bronchial tree consists of all the passageways below the trachea bifurcation. At this point, the trachea divides into a right and a left mainstem bronchus, which enter each lung, respectively, at the root (hilus). The right bronchus is 2 to 3 cm long and contains six to eight C-shaped cartilages, whereas the left bronchus is 4 to 5 cm long and contains nine to twelve cartilages. Each bronchus subdivides into smaller branches (primary bronchi), which enter each lobe of the lung (three in the right lung and two in the left lung). The bronchi undergo repeated dichotomous subdivisions (see Fig. 1–1) that increase the total cross-sectional area from 2.33 cm^2 in the mainstem bronchi to 11,800 cm^2 in the alveolar duct and between 43 to 80 m^2 in the alveoli.[42] Thus, although the diameter of any one passage decreases with each subsequent subdivision, the surface area of the bronchial tree increases geometrically, resulting in an enormous increase in sites for gaseous exchange in the alveoli.

The walls of air passages of the bronchial tree progressively lose their cartilaginous support. Bèginning with the bronchioles (which have approximately 1 mm diameters), the walls of the air passages are composed of smooth muscles around which are elastic and collagenous fibers. These provide a great deal of the elastic recoil in the lungs during expiration. Through nervous system and hormonal control of the smooth muscular walls, the diameter of these airways may be dilated or constricted, thus regulating the amount and rate of airflow into the alveolar sacs where oxygen (O_2) and carbon dioxide (CO_2) are exchanged with the blood. In contrast, the larger air passages, which are surrounded by cartilage, have relatively stable dimensions and serve largely as passive conduits for airflow into and out of the lungs.[42]

The Lungs and the Pleural Membranes. The lungs are two cone-shaped structures in the thoracic cavity on either side of the mediastinum (see Fig. 1–1). The base of each lung rests on the diaphragm, and the apex extends superiorly into the root of the neck. The bronchi, blood and lymph vessels, and nerves enter and leave the lung through the root or hilus. They are supported by connective tissue called the stroma of the lung. The stroma should be distinguished from the parenchyma, which is concerned with the exchange of O_2 and CO_2 with the pulmonary blood vessels. The lungs are highly distensible, light, and spongy. Each lung is freely suspended in the thoracic cavity and is attached only at the root by an underfolding of the pleural membranes called the "pulmonary fold" or "ligament."[14,15]

The right lung is shorter and broader than the left, owing to its position over the liver. It has upper, middle, and lower lobes. The left lung, longer and narrower than the right because of its relationship to the heart, is divided into upper and lower lobes. Forty-five percent of total gaseous exchange (volume) is taken in by the right lung, whereas 55 percent of total gaseous exchange is taken in by the left lung.[41]

Each lung is interconnected with the parietal pleura of the thoracic cage at only one point—the root. There are no direct connections between the lungs and thorax; however, the two expand and contract as a unit. This linkage is facilitated by minute amounts of fluid in the pleural space, which allow the lungs to slide over the inner surfaces of the thoracic wall.[14,15] The functional significance of this pleural linkage is discussed in the next section.

The basic structural and functional unit of the lung is the primary lobule or lung unit (see Fig. 1–1, inset). It consists of a respiratory bronchiole, alveolar ducts, alveolar sacs, and alveoli plus blood and lymph vessels and nerves. These primary lobules or lung units are the smallest subdivisions of each segmental bronchus (see Fig. 1–1). Each segmental bronchus, together with the portion of the lung that it supplies, is called a "bronchopulmonary segment." There are ten bronchopulmonary segments in the right lung and eight in the left.[41]

When the lungs expand during inhalation, dramatic changes occur in the elastic and collagenous fibers that surround the respiratory bronchioles, alveolar ducts, and mouths of the alveoli. These changes endow the lungs with their innate elasticity. Investigators using histologic methods found that elastic and collagenous fibers encircle the primary lobule in a helical fashion.[43] Uncoiling the elastic and collagenous fibers, in a process that twists and stretches these fibers, expands or dilates the terminal air passages. As the lungs expand, the fibers uncoil and become stretched while the respiratory bronchioles and alveolar ducts expand, allowing the inspired air to reach the alveoli. During expiration, the recoil forces stored in the stretched fibers restore them to their unstretched state. As a result, air is pushed out of the terminal air spaces and into the main conducting tubes where muscular and nonmuscular forces (from pleural linkage) help to drive the air rostrally into the upper airways and atmosphere.

Pleural Linkage

The lungs and thoracic cavity are lined by a serous membrane called the "pleura." The two pleurae form a double-walled sac consisting of two layers that are continuous only at the root of the lung (Fig. 1–4). An outer layer, the parietal pleura, lines the thoracic cavity and lies against the endothoracic fascia; an inner layer, the visceral pleura, is tightly adherent to the outer surface of the lung. The two pleurae are separated from each other by the narrow fluid-filled pleural space; the fluid between the pleural surfaces reduces surface tension and friction between the membranes and permits the lungs to move freely past the pleural lining of the thorax as they inflate and deflate during respiration.[6,14,15]

This arrangement, called the "pleural linkage," allows forces from the chest wall to be directly transmitted to the lungs, thereby enabling them to expand in accordance with changes in the thoracic cage (chest wall). This expansion occurs because the chest wall and the lungs are in a state of dynamic tension. The resting volume of the lungs is maintained at a higher level than would be the case in the unrestrained state (i.e., completely collapsed), whereas the resting volume of the rib cage is maintained at a lower level than it would assume in the unrestrained state (i.e., fully expanded). Thus, normally, the lungs are slightly stretched, and the chest wall is slightly compressed. The resting state of the respiratory system is a compromise between the opposing natural tendencies of the lungs and those of the rib cage. This state of dynamic equilibrium produces a resting pressure force that is capable of driving the respiratory system without muscular effort and within a restricted range of lung volumes. But it must be augmented by muscular effort at specified lung volumes for certain tasks, such as speech, in order to drive the larynx.[15]

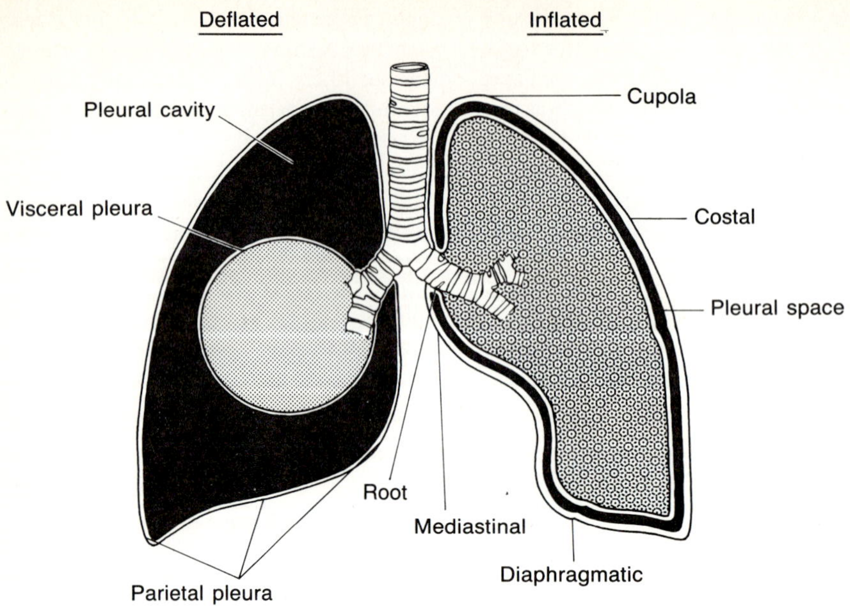

Figure 1–4 Schema of the pleural membranes. (Adapted from Grant JB. Atlas of anatomy. 6th ed. Baltimore: Williams & Wilkins, 1972.)

Morphology of the Thoracic Skeleton and Biomechanics of Rib Motion

The human thoracic skeleton is cone-shaped, narrow superiorly, and wide inferiorly. The superior aperture—the thoracic inlet—is bounded by the first thoracic vertebra and costal arch and the manubrium sterni. The cupula of each lung passes through the thoracic inlet and rests in the root of the neck. The lower aperture of the thorax is much larger than its counterpart superiorly. It is bounded by the diaphragm at its base, the costal cartilages of ribs seven, eight, nine, and ten laterally, and the xiphoid process anteriorly.[14,15]

The bony thorax consists of 12 thoracic vertebrae, 12 ribs, and the sternum. The ribs encircle the thorax; all of them attach to the vertebral column via the vertebrocostal joint. The upper seven ribs attach to the sternum through the costosternal joints.

The ribs have a downward inclination—the ventral ends are located caudal to the dorsal (vertebral) ends. Ribs one to seven increase in length rostrocaudally and exhibit progressively larger curvatures. Ribs eight to twelve decrease in length and become shorter without an appreciable change in curvature. The dorsoventral slope of the ribs becomes more oblique from rib one to rib nine, and the distance between the tubercle and angle increases from rib two to rib ten.[14,15]

Ribs are named for their relationship to the sternum and are numbered from one to twelve rostrocaudally. The first seven pairs are called the vertebrosternal (true) ribs because they attach directly to the sternum via the costosternal joint. The next lower three pairs of ribs (eight to ten) are called vertebrochondral (false) ribs because they do not directly attach to the sternum, but attach to each cartilagenous portion of the rib immediately above it. The last two pairs of ribs (11 and 12) are called vertebral (floating) ribs because they do not attach to the sternum.[14,15]

With the exceptions of ribs one, eleven, and twelve, the head of each rib articulates with the transverse process of the vertebrae immediately above and below it and onto the interposing articular disc by three different ligaments (Fig. 1–5). A similar arrangement holds for the articular facets on the transverse processes of each vertebra and rib, respectively. The articular facets on the transverse process of ribs two to seven (vertebrosternal) are concave, whereas the articular facets of the corresponding ribs are convex (Fig. 1–6). Since these ribs are elevated, each rotates around an axis that runs through the head of the rib and the tubercle. This rotation causes the sternum to be thrust forward (Fig. 1–7*A*), which increases the anteroposterior dimension of the thorax, and the shaft of the ribs also moves outwardly so that the transverse dimension of the thorax is also increased (see Fig. 1–7*A*). The costal cartilages of these ribs twist as the upper ribs are elevated. The torque that develops plays an important role in the reestablishment of the thoracic dimensions during expiration.[44]

Movements of the lower ribs (eight to ten) are

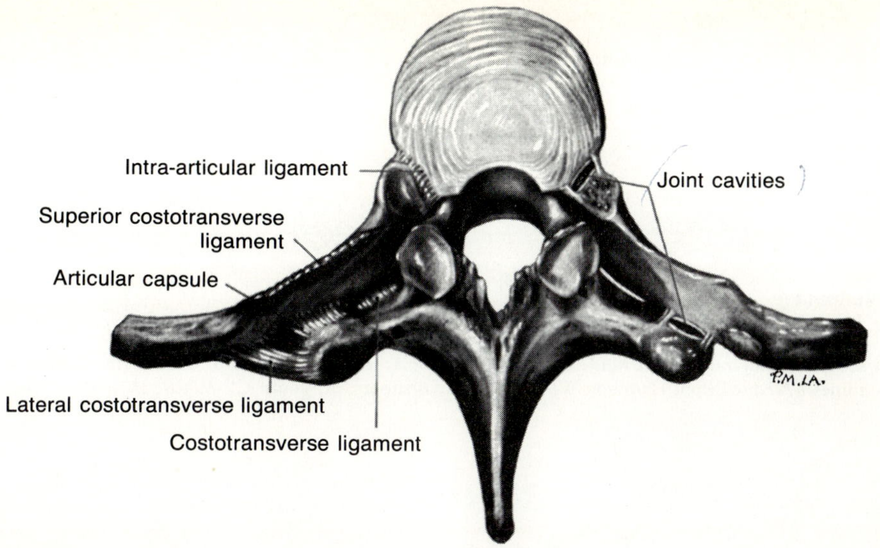

Figure 1–5 The superior aspect of the costovertebral joints. (From Williams PL, Warwick R. Gray's anatomy. 35the British ed. Philadelphia: WB Saunders, 1973:451.)

different from those of the upper ribs because of differences in the structure of the costovertebral joints. The articular facets on the transverse processes of the vertebrae and heads of the ribs are flat. They are located on the superior surface of the rib and are oriented obliquely (see Fig. 1–6*B*). This arrangement allows the ribs to *slide* upward and backward and downward and forward and results in an increase in the transverse dimension of the lower thorax (see Fig. 1–7*B*). This increase is important because it permits the abdominal contents to be relocated after they have become displaced by the descent of the diaphragm. Movement of the costosternal joint formed by the costal cartilages of ribs one to seven permits some slight mediolateral gliding, which may assist in increasing the transverse dimension of the upper thorax.[44]

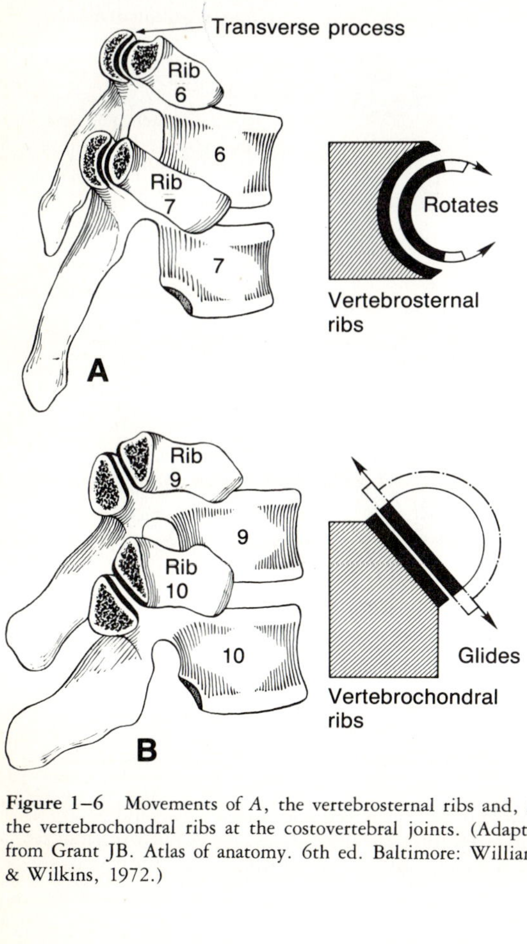

Figure 1–6 Movements of *A*, the vertebrosternal ribs and, *B*, the vertebrochondral ribs at the costovertebral joints. (Adapted from Grant JB. Atlas of anatomy. 6th ed. Baltimore: Williams & Wilkins, 1972.)

The Respiratory Muscles

The activity of the respiratory muscles is discussed in detail in several sources.[44,45] The following description of respiratory muscle activity concerns only those muscles that have been shown to be most consistently involved in respiratory activity. Figure 1–8 illustrates the topography of the respiratory muscles in the thorax and abdomen.

Inspiratory Muscles. The muscles most consistently mentioned in the literature as serving an inspiratory function are the diaphragm, the external intercostal, and the interchondral portion of the internal intercostal muscles. The scalene and sternocleidomastoid muscles also have been shown to be active under certain circumstances, as have the pectoralis major and pectoralis minor muscles to a lesser extent. The role of each of the respiratory muscles is briefly discussed.

Diaphragm. Many have noted that the diaphragm is the primary muscle of inspiration.[45–48]

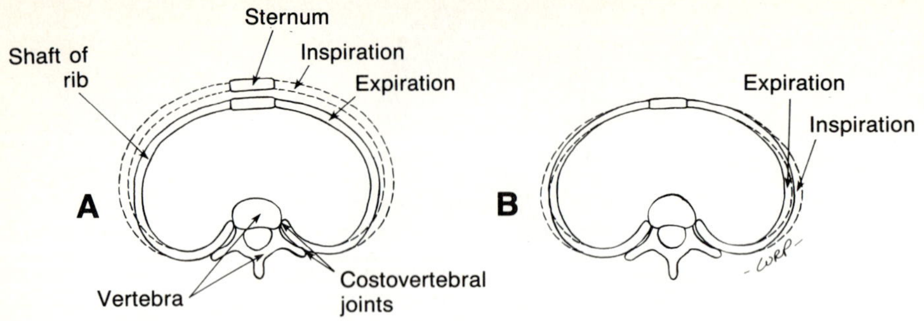

Figure 1-7 Transverse sections through the thorax illustrating movements of *A*, the upper ribs, and *B*, lower ribs. Inspiratory changes indicated by interrupted lines. (Adapted from Hamilton WJ. Textbook of anatomy. St. Louis: CV Mosby, 1976:57.)

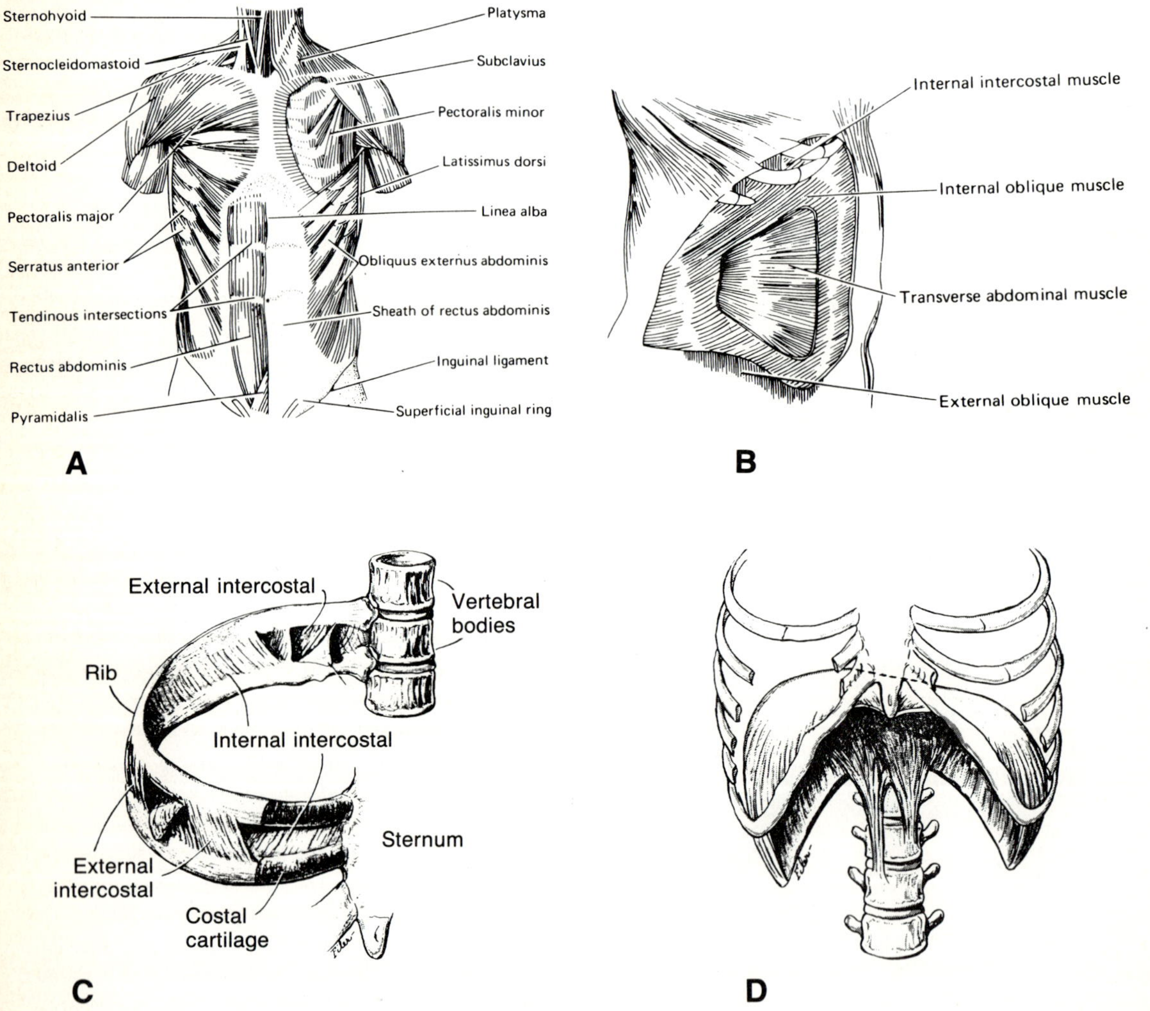

Figure 1-8 Respiratory muscles. *A*, Abdominal and thoracic muscles viewed ventrally (p 181). *B*, Layering of abdominal muscles (p 182). (From Kaplan H. Anatomy and physiology of speech. 2nd ed. New York: McGraw Hill, 1971.) *C*, Internal and external intercostal muscles (p 62). *D*, The diaphragm (p 71). (From Dickson D, Maue-Dickson W. Human vocal anatomy. Springfield, IL: CC Thomas, 1970.)

Activity of this muscle increases the vertical dimension of the thorax. The diaphragm moves about 1.5 cm during quiet breathing, and 6 to 7 cm during deep breathing.[48] About 350 ml of air is taken in per centimeter movement of the diaphragm, which is innervated by the phrenic nerve.[14,15]

External Intercostal and Interchondral Portion of the Internal Intercostal Muscles. As early as 1748, Hamberger proposed that the external intercostals and the interchondral portion of the internal intercostal muscles were active during inspiration.[49] Subsequent electromyographic research has confirmed Hamberger's hypothesis.[50–52] The external intercostal and the internal intercostal muscles have been found to be active during both quiet and effortful inspiration; particularly in the fifth to ninth intercostal spaces.[51] The intercostal muscles constitute a substantial inspiratory muscle group, second only in importance to the diaphragm. The external and internal intercostal nerves innervate the respective intercostal muscles.[14,15]

Sternocleidomastoid and Scalene Muscles. The scalene and sternocleidomastoid muscles have been shown to play significant roles in inspiration as accessory muscles;[53] the sternocleidomastoid muscles have been regarded as the most important accessory inspiratory muscles.[53] They assist in elevating the sternum and increase the anteroposterior dimension of the thorax. They are not active during quiet inspiration, but are during deep breathing. The sternocleidomastoids always contract at the end of maximum inspiration, when lung volumes are in the order of 70 to 80 percent of vital capacity.[53]

The scalene muscles have been found to be most active at higher lung volumes.[53] They do not play a role in quiet breathing nor in increased normal breathing, but are active in forced expiratory efforts, such as coughing, where they may help to support the apices of the lungs. Others found that the scalenes become active when pulmonary ventilation is above 40 L per minute. The sternocleidomastoid muscles are innervated by the spinal accessory nerve (eleventh cervical nerve), and the scalene muscles are innervated by the third and fourth cervical nerves.[14,15]

Pectoralis Major and Pectoralis Minor. These muscles have been found to be active only during forced breathing.[51,53] They exhibit similar patterns of activity, and both are innervated by the anterior and medial thoracic nerves.[14,15]

Expiratory Muscles. The abdominal muscles and the internal intercostal muscles have been shown to be muscles of expiration. Their respective roles in expiration are described briefly.

The Abdominal Muscles. The abdominal muscles (internal oblique, external oblique, rectus abdominis, and transversus abdominis) are the most important muscles of expiration.[44,54] These muscles lower the ribs and compress the abdominal viscera, thereby reducing the size of the thorax and increasing intrathoracic pressure. Intrathoracic pressures greater than 20 cm H_2O above atmospheric pressure result from abdominal muscle activity. The abdominal muscles are innervated by a variety of nerves. The rectus abdominis and transversus abdominis muscles are innervated by the lower six intercostal nerves and branches from the iliohypogastric and ilioinguinal nerves. The external and internal abdominal oblique muscles are innervated by the lower six thoracic and upper two lumbar nerves.[14,15]

Internal Intercostals. Electromyography of the intercostal muscles has shown that the interosseus portions of the internal intercostal muscles are not active during expiration and probably do not play a significant role in normal quiet respiration.[51] This finding does not support Hamberger's hypothesis; the results suggest that the major role of the internal intercostal muscles was to prevent the intercostal spaces from collapsing or bulging out as a result of changes in intrathoracic pressure during breathing.

THE LARYNX

The following discussion reviews salient aspects of the structure and function of the human larynx. Attention is given to those relationships that are central to an understanding of the myriad functions to which this organ contributes.

Postnatal Developmental Morphology

The infant's larynx is not simply a miniature of the adult's: it differs from its adult counterpart in size, consistency of tissues, position in the neck, and shape.[55] The cartilages are smaller, but the subcutaneous tissues and mucous membranes are more pliable than in the adult. The hyoid bone and thyroid cartilage are close together and the glottal aperture is small in the infant.[56] In infancy and childhood (Fig. 1–9), the membranous portion of the vocal folds is short and thickened, and the vocal processes assume a proportionally larger portion of the length of the glottis than in the adult. Consequently, the vocal folds in infancy and childhood are stabilized more posteriorly than in older children and adults, and the length of their vibrating mass is reduced.[56]

The shape of the infraglottal region of the infant's and child's larynx is also different from that of the adult.[1,55,57] In the infant and child,[1] the infraglottal area is funnel shaped (Fig. 1–10*A*) and the cricoid lamina is tilted posteriorly, serving as an ex-

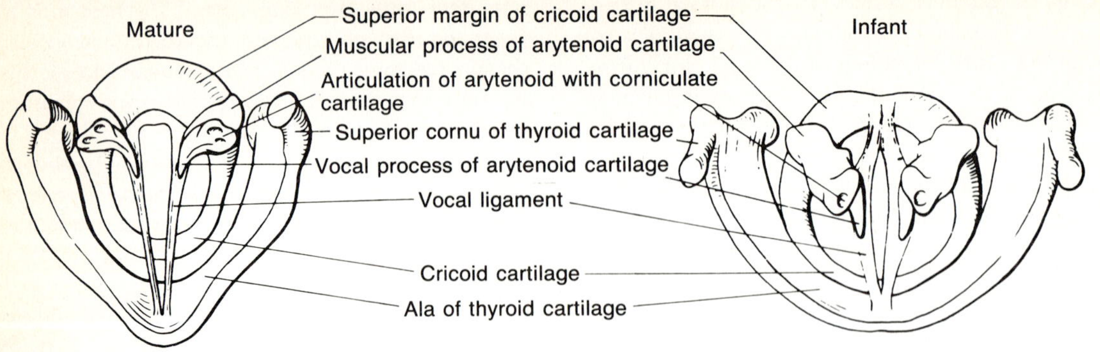

Figure 1–9 Superior view of the laryngeal skeleton in the adult (left) and infant (right). For demonstration of proportions, these schemas are made dimensionally equivalent at the external diameter of the cricoid cartilage in the midline. (From Bosma J. Anatomic and physiologic development of the speech apparatus. In: Tower DB, ed. The nervous system, Vol. 3. Human communication and its disorders. New York: Raven Press, 1975:469.)

pansion of the trachea and thereby assisting in respiration. The funnel shape becomes reduced by mid-childhood and disappears by adulthood (Fig. 1–10*B*) when the shape of the infraglottal region is tubular.

As a consequence of vertical growth of the pharynx and cervical vertebral column, the larynx becomes positioned more caudally in the neck.[57–59] In infancy, the larynx is located at a level between the first and second cervical vertebrae. It descends during childhood and, after puberty, assumes its adult position, with the cricoid cartilage at the level of the sixth cervical vertebra.

Laryngeal cartilages and the vocal folds increase in size postnatally. During the first 3 years of life, the larynx undergoes rapid and significant growth, after which there is a period of slow steady growth until puberty, when development once again accelerates.[2,57,60] Gedgowd reported that the male prepubertal larynx was larger than the female's,[57] but others found no significant morphologic differences between male and female larynges.[51,61] This morphologic congruence is illustrated in Figure 1–11*A*. In the pubertal male, the laryngeal cartilages and the vocal folds are significantly larger than pubertal female counterparts (Fig. 1–11*B*),[61] and, in addition, the male larynx undergoes significantly more growth than the female larynx from prepuberty to puberty. During this time, the male vocal folds undergo over twice the growth of the female vocal folds, and both reach adult length by puberty.

Growth of the larynx cannot be viewed independently of growth of the entire body. Laryngeal

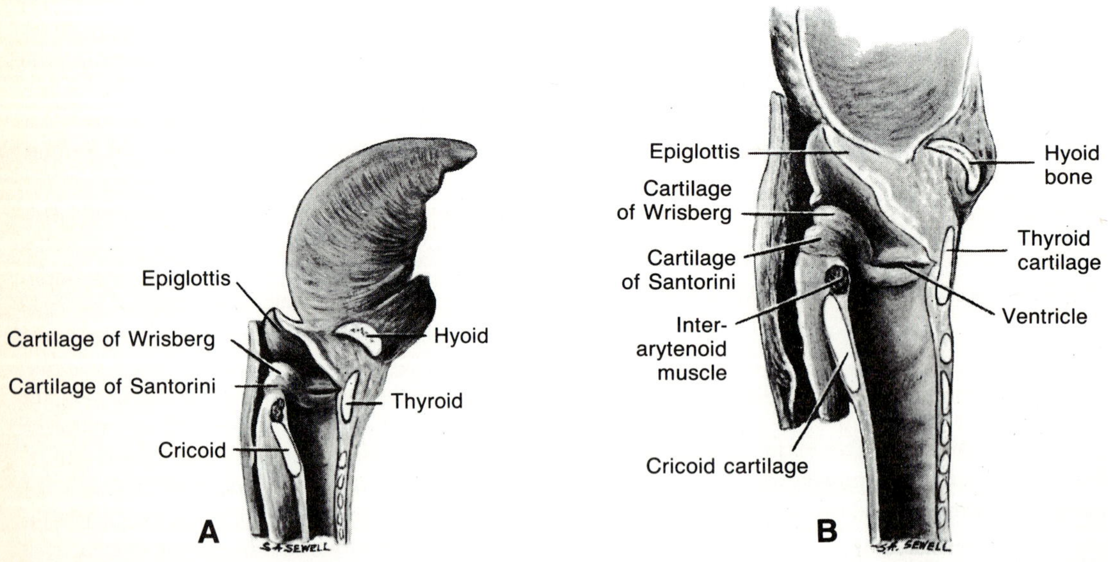

Figure 1–10 Midsagittal sections of, *A*, a 6-month-old and, *B*, a 6.5-year-old male larynx. Note the funnel shape of the infraglottal region in, *A*, the infant, which virtually disappears in, *B*, the child, resulting in a more tubular-shaped infraglottal region. (From Negus VE. The comparative anatomy and physiology of the larynx. New York: Hafner, 1949:179, 180.)

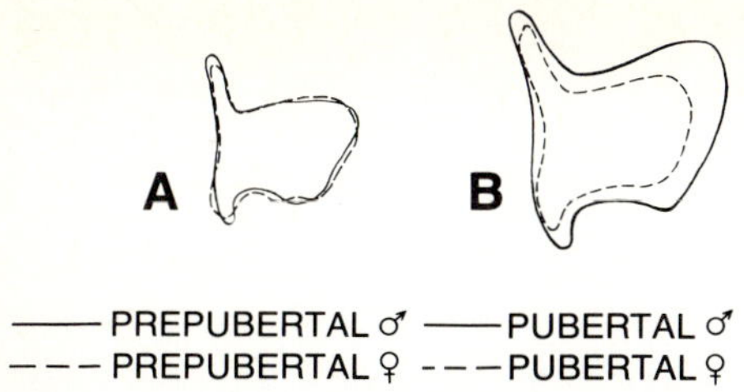

Figure 1-11 Typical morphology of, *A*, prepubertal and, *B*, pubertal thyroid cartilages (actual size) made from composite photographic reconstructions. (After Kahane JC. A morphological study of the human prepubertal and pubertal larynx. Am J Anat 1978; 151:11.)

growth has been shown to be related to growth in body height during infancy,[58] throughout childhood,[59] and during the circumpubertal period.[62] Thus growth of the larynx is not laryngeal-specific, but is under the same influences as those that control general somatic growth.

The foregoing discussion underscores the fact that the structure of the newborn larynx is not a miniature of the adult's. A number of dramatic structural changes occur before the larynx reaches its adult size; these must be taken into account in all considerations of postnatal vocal capacities.

The adult larynx is not immune to change. In fact, the adult larynx undergoes significant changes that result in a decrease in vocal efficiency. These age-related changes are referred to as involutionary. Data indicate that these changes are greater in the male than in the female.[63,64] Although more research is needed to fully identify the characteristics and functional significance of involutional changes in the larynx, it has been well established that the laryngeal cartilages become stiffer and that connective tissues undergo appreciable change. The latter likely affect the resiliency, recoil, and vibratory characteristics of the vocal folds. As such, they influence the fundamental frequency and some aspects of voice quality of older speakers.

Laryngeal Cartilages

The laryngeal skeleton is composed of four major cartilages. These are the thyroid, cricoid, a pair of arytenoids, and the epiglottis. Two pairs of smaller laryngeal cartilages exist but do not contribute to the laryngeal skeleton. The corniculate cartilages sit on top of the apices of the arytenoids, whereas the small kernel-shaped cuneiform cartilages are embedded into the aryepiglottic folds. The relationship among these cartilages is shown in Figure 1–12. With the exception of the epiglottis, which is composed of elastic cartilage, all other laryngeal cartilages are composed of hyaline cartilage. These cartilages surround the laryngeal cavity and protect the airway leading into the trachea. In addition, the cartilages serve as points of attachment for some muscles of the pharynx (inferior constrictor muscle of the pharynx and palatopharyngeal muscle) and the neck (sternothyroid and thyrohyoid) and for the intrinsic muscles of the larynx.[14,15,65]

The thyroid cartilage is the largest cartilage. (see Fig. 1–12*A*). It is V-shaped and formed from two plates (laminae) joined at the midline along all but the uppermost area, where a notch exists. The fused area is called the "thyroid eminence." The angulation of the thyroid eminence becomes more pronounced after adolescence, particularly in the male. Posteriorly, two pairs of projections extend from each lamina. The upper pair, the superior cornua (or horns), links the larynx to the hyoid bone via the thyrohyoid ligament. The lower pair, the inferior cornua (or horns), articulates with the cricoid cartilage at the cricothyroid joint.

The cricoid cartilage is shaped like a signet ring and sits on top of the first ring of the trachea (see Fig. 1–12*B*). It is composed of a thin ring of cartilage, the arch, which forms the anterior and lateral aspects of the cartilage. The arch is widest at its junction with a thickened plate, the lamina (plate), located posteriorly. The arch and the lamina enclose a space called the "cricoid lumen," which forms much of the laryngeal cavity below the vocal folds. The cricoid cartilage contains two pairs of articular facets that form portions of the two diarthrodial (movable) joints in the larynx. The facets located along the superior rim of the cartilage at the junction of the arch and lamina are called the "cricoarytenoid articular facets." The other pair of articular facets, located in the midportion of the arch posteriorly, are called the "cricothyroid articular facets." The joints associated with these structures are described in detail in a subsequent section.

The arytenoid cartilages are paired, pyramidal-shaped, and highly symmetrical (see Fig. 1–12*C*). Each arytenoid cartilage contains a mass of cartilage, which, in turn, contains three processes. The vocal process projects anteriorly, and the vocal ligament and vocal muscle fibers attach to it. The muscular process projects laterally and is the site of attachment of several intrinsic muscles. On its undersurface, it contains an articular facet that joins a counterpart on the cricoid cartilage to form the cricoarytenoid joint. The apex projects superiorly. The cuneiform cartilage sits on it and is a point of attachment for the aryepiglottic fold.

The epiglottis is shaped like a leaf and is flexible because of its elastic cartilage composition (see

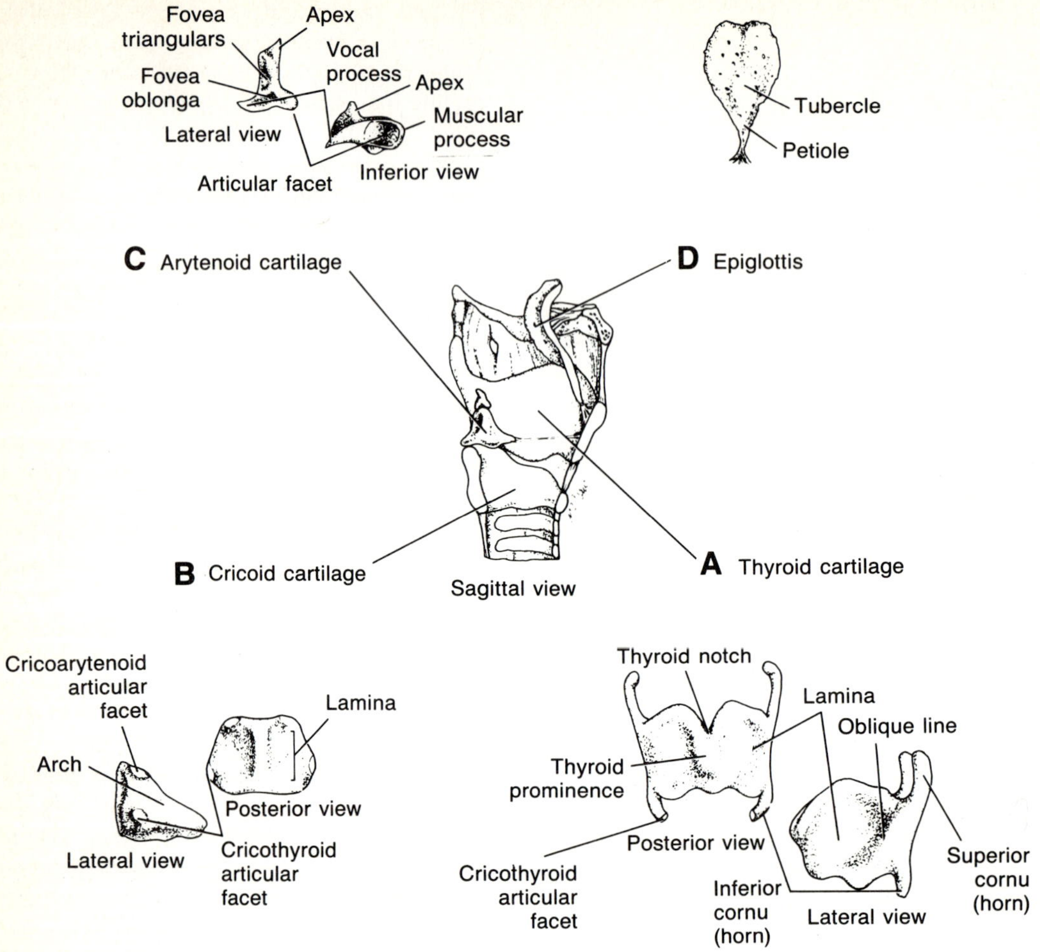

Figure 1–12 Laryngeal cartilages. The central figure in sagittal section shows the major articulated cartilages. The figures set to the sides, *A, B, C,* and *D,* show details of the individual cartilages.

Fig. 1–12*D*). It contains many glands and has a few scattered tastebuds. The epiglottis attaches anteriorly to the deep surface of the thyroid cartilage and extends vertically above the hyoid bone. There, it interconnects with the base of the tongue by fibroelastic bands of tissue called the "glossoepiglottic folds." This relationship is discussed more fully in the section on the tongue. The epiglottis is important because of the protection it affords the laryngeal airway during swallowing. Owing to its flexibility, the epiglottis is pushed backward by the tongue so that it covers the entrance into the laryngeal cavity, preventing food from entering the larynx and obstructing respiration.

The Functional Anatomy of the Cricothyroid and Cricoarytenoid Joints

The larynx has two pairs of movable (diarthrotic) joints: the cricothyroid and cricoarytenoid joints. They are morphologically specialized and serve different functions, which are described next.

The Cricothyroid Joint

The cricothyroid joint is a bilateral movable joint. It is formed by joining articular facets on the inferior cornua of the thyroid cartilage with those on the arch of the cricoid cartilage (Fig. 1–13*A*). The morphology of the articular cartilages has been studied extensively.[66] They have been found to exhibit great morphologic variability in size, shape, and the composition of the articular surfaces. The articular surfaces are surrounded by a synovial membrane and joint capsule and are kept in functional alignment by the anterior, posterior, and lateral cricothyroid (ceratocricoid) ligaments.[67] Of these, the posterior ligaments are most consistent in structure, clearly the most substantial. The cricothyroid joint ligaments limit the extent of excessive movements

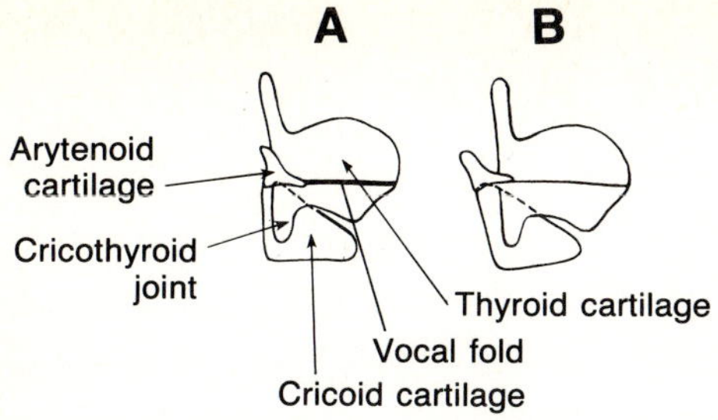

Figure 1–13 Diagram illustrating functional morphology of the cricothyroid joint. *A*, Orientation of the thyroid and cricoid cartilages at rest. *B*, Changes in orientation of the thyroid and cricoid cartilages through rotatory movement at the joint. Note the lengthening of the vocal folds and posterior tilting of the cricoid lamina that result.

at the cricothyroid joint, while providing mechanical stability to the joint during normal activity.

The primary motion at the cricothyroid joint is rotation through a horizontal axis that runs through the center of the joint (see Fig. 1–13*B*). Sliding motion at the joint is unlikely because of the shape and orientation of the articular facets that mitigate against it and because of the restraints imposed on anterior movements of the thyroid cartilage by the cricothyroid ligaments.[67]

Contraction of the cricothyroid muscles approximates the cricoid and thyroid cartilages; it displaces the superior aspect of the cricoid lamina and the arytenoid cartilages posteriorly and lengthens the vocal folds. This increases the tension or elasticity within the vocal folds and reduces mass per unit area. The rate of vibration increases (as does the fundamental frequency), and the listener perceives an increase in pitch.[67]

The Cricoarytenoid Joint

The cricoarytenoid joint is *central* to laryngeal functioning.[17,68] The movements of the vocal folds, changes in the rima glottidis, and alterations in glottal resistance are dependent on its function. Indeed, the maintenance of an adequate airway during respiration is dependent upon the structural and functional integrity of this joint.

Careful anatomic and physiologic studies of the cricoarytenoid joint have clarified its functional morphology.[25,69,70] These studies have shown that *rotation* about a vertical axis through the joint was untenable on anatomic grounds.[20,71] Despite the conclusiveness of these studies, many authors of modern textbooks of anatomy still describe motion of this joint as rotatory. Correction of this misconception is essential for proper understanding of the normal function and pathology of the vocal mechanism.

Gross Morphology. The cricoarytenoid joint is a bilateral and highly symmetrical articulation[66] formed by the articular facets of the cricoid and arytenoid cartilages. Each joint is surrounded by a fibroelastic joint capsule and synovial membrane. The arytenoid cartilages are anchored posteriorly by the small dense posterior cricoarytenoid ligament. The joint attaches to the medial surface of the arytenoid cartilages and to the cricoid cartilage just below the cricoarytenoid facets. This ligament prevents excessive anterior displacement of the arytenoid cartilages during movement.

The dimensions of the adult cricoarytenoid facets on the arytenoid and cricoid cartilages have been reported.[66,68] Figure 1–14 illustrates the relationship of the axes of the cricoarytenoid joint's articular facet to one another. The articular facets of the cricoid cartilage are located posteriorly on the superolateral surface of the cricoid lamina near the junction of the arch to the lamina. They are oval-shaped and convex, with the longitudinal axis running in a dorsomediocranial to ventrolaterocaudal direction and the transverse (short) axis running from posterolateral to anteromedial. The longitudinal axes intersect at a 60-degree angle.[66,68]

The articular facets of the arytenoid cartilages are found on the undersurface of the muscular process of the arytenoid cartilages. The facets are slightly ovoid and concave, with the transverse dimension exceeding the longitudinal dimension. As illustrated in Figure 1–14, when the arytenoids are at rest, the transverse axis of the articular facet (running posterolateral to anteromedial) is at right angles to the longitudinal axis of the cricoid articular facet. The transverse axis of the arytenoid articular facet is longer than the width of the cricoid articular facet with which it articulates. The longitudinal axis of the arytenoid facet is parallel and shorter than the longitudinal axis of the cricoid facet (see Fig. 1–14).[66]

Biomechanics. Based on the morphology of the articular facets of the cricoarytenoid joint, two principal movements are possible—sliding (gliding or linear translation) along the longitudinal axis of the cricoid facet and rocking around this axis (i.e., across the transverse dimension of the articular facet).[68] Sliding (Fig. 1–15) occurs along the longitudinal axis of the cricoid facet and permits a maximal movement of approximately 2 mm in the dorsomediocranial to ventrolaterocaudal direction. This sliding may result in some shortening or lengthening of the vocal folds, but is inadequate to cause sufficient adduction for sound production.

The principal movement of the cricoarytenoid joint is a rocking of the arytenoid cartilages around the longitudinal axes of the cricoid facet (see Fig. 1–15). Rotation of the cricoarytenoid joint around

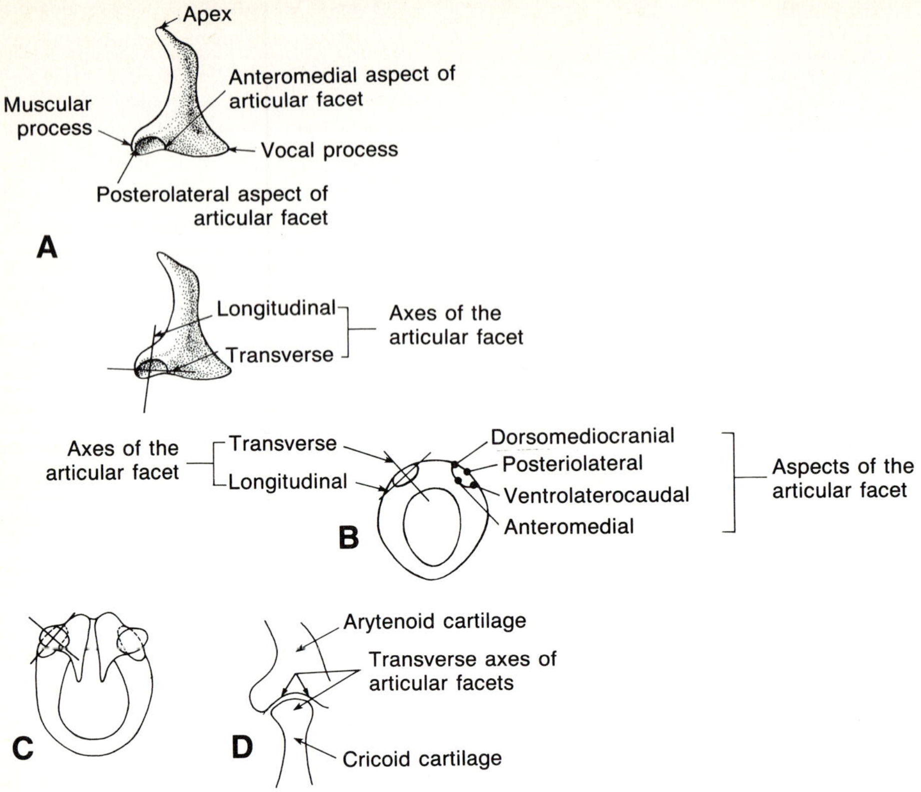

Figure 1–14 The articular facets of, *A*, the arytenoid and, *B*, the cricoid cartilages, illustrating their axes and anatomic boundaries. *C*, Superior view of the cricoarytenoid articulation illustrating the relationship of the cricoid and arytenoid facets to each other. Note the right angle relationship of the transverse axes of the arytenoid facets to the longitudinal axes of the cricoid facets. *D*, Sagittal section through the cricoarytenoid joint showing the relationships between articular surfaces of the joint.

a vertical axis through the arytenoid cartilage has been shown to be anatomically impossible.[68,69] The range of movement is approximately 35 degrees and is sufficient to bring the vocal folds together for sound production. During adduction, the arytenoid cartilages rock forward medially and downward (anteromediocaudally), bringing the vocal folds toward the midline while narrowing or closing the rima glottidis. During abduction, the arytenoid cartilages rock backward and outward (posterolaterocranially) along the transverse dimension of the cricoid facet, drawing the vocal processes backward, outward, and upward. This action draws the vocal folds away from the midline and enlarges the rima glottidis. The distance of the vocal process from the axis of the joint (the longitudinal axis of the cricoid facet) provides sufficient leverage for the muscles to open and close the rima glottidis.[68,71]

Movements of the arytenoid cartilages are complex and result in simultaneous displacements of parts of the cartilages in the horizontal, vertical, and depth planes.[71,72] Mechanoreceptors have been found in the cricoarytenoid joints.[40,68,73–76] Investigators have hypothesized that these mechanoreceptors play roles in

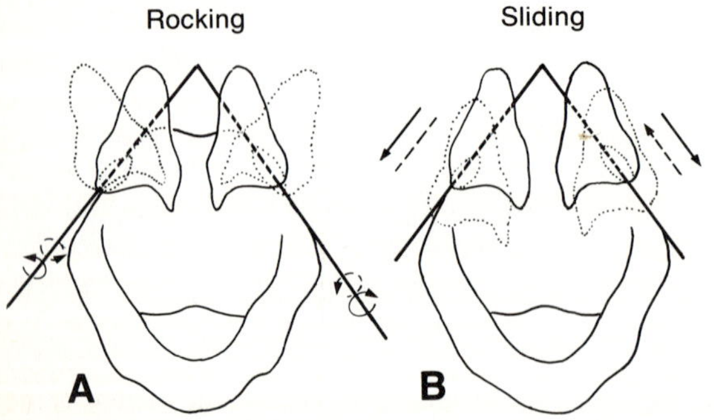

Figure 1–15 Two types of movement in the cricoarytenoid joint: *A*, rocking of the arytenoid cartilages during abduction (dotted line) and abduction (solid line) and, *B*, sliding of the arytenoid cartilages. (From Sonnesson B. Die funktionelle Anatomie des Cricoarytenoidgelenkes. A Anat Entwicklungsgesch 1959; 121:292–303.)

regulating the movement of the arytenoid cartilages as well as in modulating tension in the intrinsic laryngeal muscles during sound production. The neuroanatomic and neurophysiologic mechanisms involved must be better defined because they offer great promise for understanding neurologic control of the larynx.

The Laryngeal Cavity

The laryngeal cavity is a tubular passageway that connects the upper airway of the pharynx with the trachea (Fig. 1–16). The walls of the laryngeal cavity are lined with epithelium and reinforced with fibroelastic tissues. The laryngeal cavity is relatively straight except at its midpoint, where two pairs of longitudinally-coursing folds—the vestibular and true vocal folds—border an outpocket called the "laryngeal ventricle" (ventricle of Morgagni). The area above the vestibular folds is called the "supraglottal region"; the area between the vestibular and true vocal folds is called the "glottal region," and the portion of the cavity below the true vocal folds is called the "infraglottal region." The walls of the supraglottal and infraglottal regions and the ventricle are lined with respiratory (pseudostratified ciliated columnar)

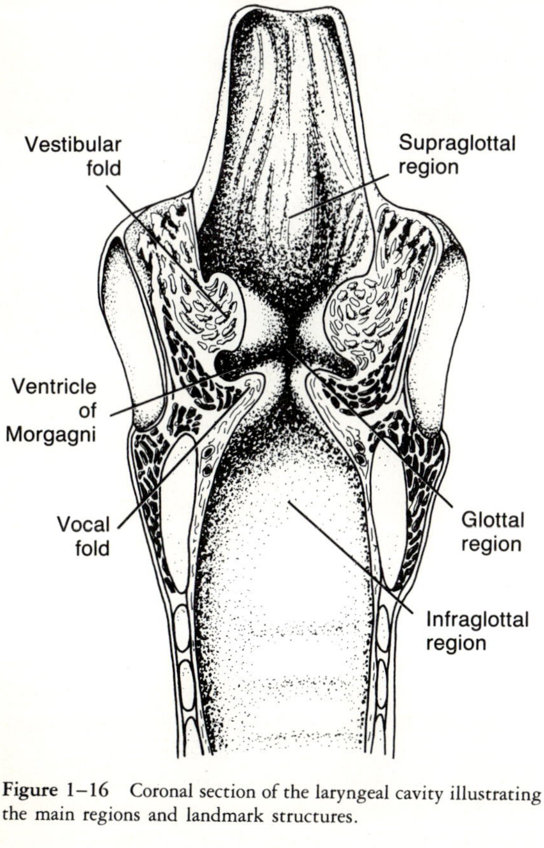

Figure 1–16 Coronal section of the laryngeal cavity illustrating the main regions and landmark structures.

epithelium. The medial or contacting surfaces of the vestibular and true vocal folds are covered by stratified squamous epithelium. This epithelium is designed to resist shearing forces caused by the rubbing together and tight approximation of the epithelial surfaces during such activities as vocal fold vibration or the tight approximation at the medial surfaces of the folds during effort closure (i.e., during swallowing or lifting or when developing intraabdominal pressures such as during defecation and urination). The shape of the laryngeal cavity changes during respiration and vocalization through movements of the vocal folds and displacement and elastic recoil of the fibroelastic tissue in the walls of the laryngeal cavity.[14,15,29]

Muscular Forces

The muscles of the larynx are conventionally divided into intrinsic and extrinsic groups on the basis of anatomic and functional differences. The gross anatomy of these muscles is well described in atlases[77] and anatomy textbooks.[14,15,65,78] The reader is referred to these sources for more detail.

Intrinsic Laryngeal Muscles

The intrinsic laryngeal muscles share several things in common. They are all branchiomeric muscles, that is, they are derived from branchial arch mesoderm and have origins and insertions from and onto the cartilages of the laryngeal skeleton from whence they take their names. For example, the cricothyroid originates from the cricoid cartilage and inserts onto the thyroid cartilage. The intrinsic muscles are small and delicate; they are richly innervated[72] and are among the fastest contracting muscles in the body.[35] Figure 1–17 illustrates the relationship among the intrinsic laryngeal muscles in the larynx. These properties enable them to function in the discrete manner required for respiratory and phonatory adjustments. Innervation of the intrinsic laryngeal muscles is through the superior laryngeal branch of the tenth cranial nerve (supplying the cricothyroid muscle) and the inferior laryngeal branch of the tenth cranial nerve (all other muscles).[14,15]

Although specific functions are conventionally assigned to each intrinsic laryngeal muscle (Table 1–1), it is certain that they work synergistically. As a group they change the relationship of the laryngeal cartilages to each other, alter the size and shape of the rima glottidis through abduction and adduction

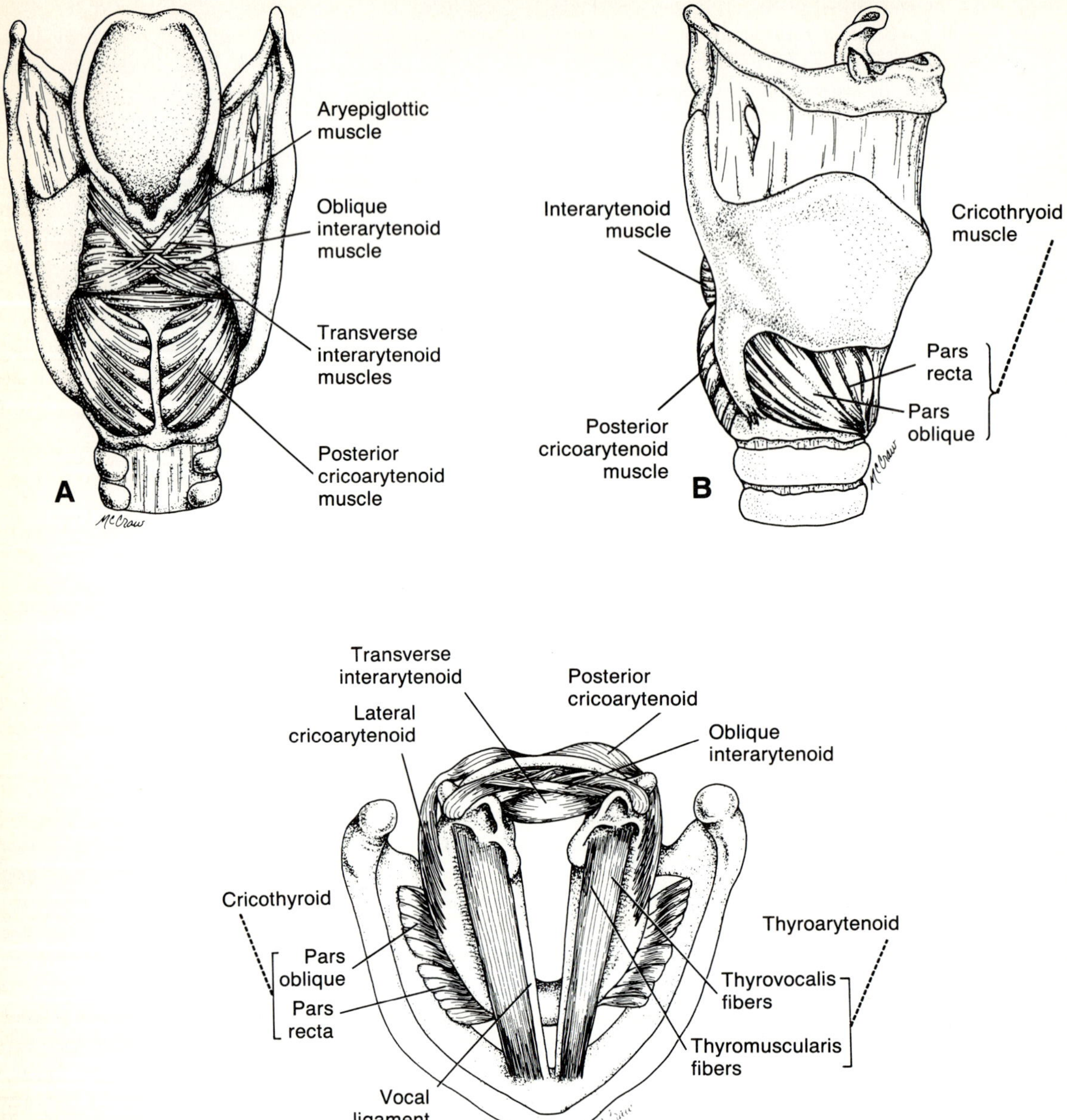

Figure 1–17 Intrinsic laryngeal muscles as viewed, *A*, posteriorly, *B*, laterally, and *C*, superiorly.

of the vocal folds, modify the physical properties of the vocal folds (i.e., length, tension, and mass per unit area), and influence glottal resistance.[30,65,79]

Quantitative data on the length, width, cross-sectional area, fiber diameter, and weight of the intrinsic laryngeal muscles have been reported.[35] Unfortunately, however, in these analyses, little information was provided about the sample size used or any sex differences.

Other properties of the human intrinsic laryngeal muscles have been determined through histochemical studies.[80–82] Results from these studies have identified specific metabolic properties of the laryngeal muscles that make them particularly well suited for the rapid and continuous activity associated with phonation, respiration, and other biologic activities.

Of all the intrinsic laryngeal muscles, the thyroarytenoid muscle has been most extensively studied because it is so much a part of the human vocal fold.[70] It is widely accepted today that the fibers of the thyroarytenoid muscle course anteroposteriorly from the thyroid to the arytenoid cartilages and do

TABLE 1–1 A Functional Classification of the Intrinsic and Extrinsic Laryngeal Muscles Shown to Directly Affect Phonatory Function

Muscle	*Function*
Intrinsic group	
Cricothyroid	Lengthens and tenses the vocal folds
Lateral cricothyroid	Adducts the vocal folds; narrows the rima glottidis
Posterior cricoarytenoid	Abducts the vocal folds; widens the rima glottidis
Interarytenoids (transverse arytenoids and oblique arytenoids)	Adducts vocal folds, particularly the posterior region
Thyroarytenoid	
Thyrovocalis portion	Shortens vocal folds and increases tension
Thyromuscularis portion	Adducts vocal folds and reduces tension
Extrinsic group	
Sternothyroid	Lowers thyroid cartilage; lowers larynx
Thyrohyoid	Raises thyroid cartilage; raises larynx; lowers hyoid bone.

not insert into the vocal ligament. However, they are intertwined with fibers of the conus elasticus. Several investigators have reported that the thyroarytenoid muscle may be anatomically divided into a medial bundle, thyrovocal muscle, and a lateral bundle, thyromuscular muscle which were thought to have different functions. The thyrovocal muscle was thought to control tension in the vocal fold, and the thyromuscular muscle to function in sphincteric closure.[70] However, these distinctions in the functional morphology of the thyroarytenoid muscle have not been supported by extensive anatomic and histologic examination.[70] Fibers from the thyroarytenoid muscle have been found to be well organized into a superior and an inferior group. The superior fibers run horizontally and parallel to the vocal ligament and insert onto the inferior and lateral aspect of the vocal process. The inferior fibers course laterally and posterosuperiorly to insert into the fovea oblonga of the arytenoid cartilage and its inferior margin. Superior fibers could not be separated from inferior ones. Thus one should regard the thyroarytenoid muscle as a single structure.

When the vocal folds are adducted (Fig. 1–18*A*), the thyroarytenoid muscle is twisted such that the superior fibers are horizontal and oriented in the sagittal plane, while the inferior fibers are twisted in the lateral direction. When the vocal folds are abducted (Fig. 1–18*B*), they become untwisted, and the horizontal fibers change orientation and come to lay in between the sagittal and horizontal planes. The hithertofore twisted morphology of the thyroarytenoid muscle may have led former anatomists astray in their descriptions of the muscle.[70]

Extrinsic Laryngeal Muscles

The extrinsic laryngeal muscles are divided into suprahyoid and infrahyoid groups. They are innervated by several nerves: trigeminal, facial, hypoglossal, and ansa cervicalis. For further information, consult Chapter 3 in this volume. These large muscles move the hyoid bone and/or larynx as a whole in the neck. The suprahyoid muscles (consisting of the anterior and posterior digastric, mylohyoid, geniohyoid, and stylohyoid muscles) are located between the skull and/or mandible and the hyoid bone. These muscles may open or retract the mandible when the hyoid bone is stabilized or elevate the hyoid bone and larynx during swallowing. The infrahyoid muscles or strap muscles (Fig. 1–19) consist of a deep layer (sternothyroid and thyrohyoid muscles), which may be considered as a single muscle, and a superficial layer of muscles (sternohyoid and omohyoid muscles).[14,15]

Therefore, the infrahyoid muscles extend from the sternum, scapula, and manubrium to the hyoid bone and either lower the hyoid bone and larynx or stabilize the hyoid bone (see Fig. 1–19). The deep strap muscles can work independently of the superficial muscles. Infra- and suprahyoid muscle activity in singers has been shown to play roles in the control of pitch during singing by helping to regulate length

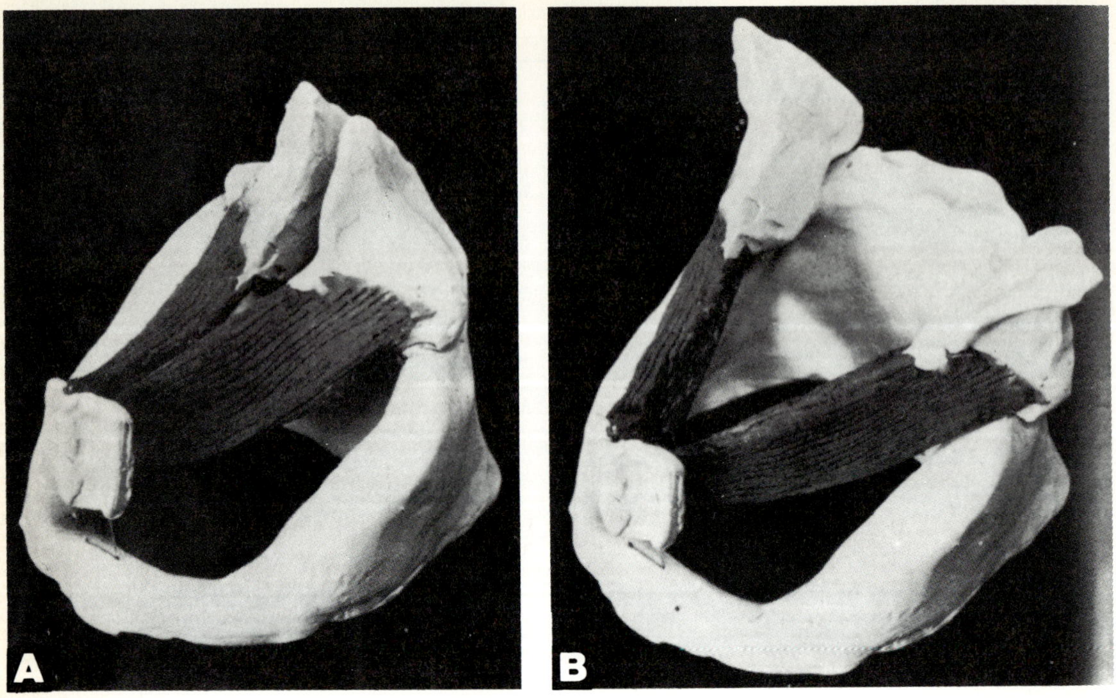

Figure 1–18 Changes in the topography of the thyroarytenoid muscles during, *A*, adduction, *B*, abduction of the vocal folds. (From Sonnesson B. On the anatomy and vibratory pattern of the human vocal folds. Acta Otolaryngol [Suppl] (Stockh) 1960; 156:1.)

and tension of the vocal folds.[81,83,84] Shipp has shown that sternothyroid and thyrohyoid muscles function differentially during high-pitch and low-pitch vocalization.[85] When pitch is lowered, the larynx assumes a lower position in the neck, sternohyoid muscle activity predominates, and thyrohyoid muscle activity is inhibited. When pitch is raised, the larynx is elevated, thyrohyoid muscle activity predominates, and sternohyoid muscle activity is inhibited.

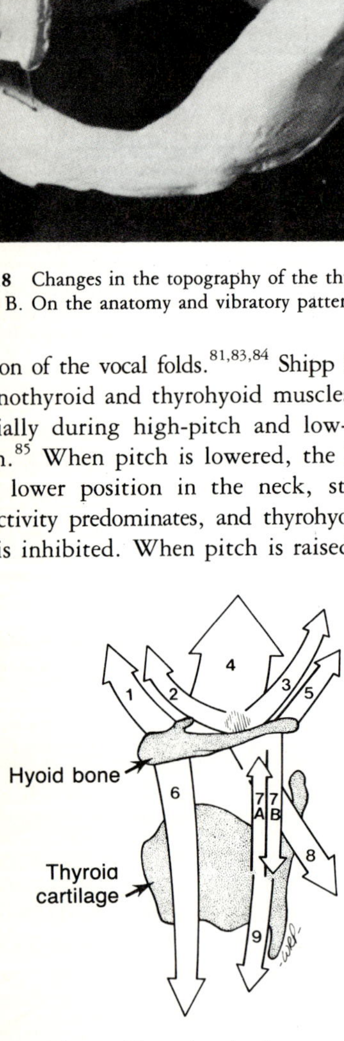

Figure 1–19 Diagram illustrating the force vectors of the suprahyoid and infrahyoid muscles (i.e., extrinsic muscles of the larynx). Note that the thyrohyoid muscle may elevate the thyroid cartilage and also lower the hyoid bone. Force vectors: 1, geniohyoid muscle; 2, anterior digastric muscle; 3, posterior digastric muscle; 4, mylohyoid muscle; 5, stylohyoid muscle; 6, sternohyoid muscle; 7A, thyrohyoid muscle (as elevator of thyroid cartilage); 7B, thyrohyoid muscle (as depressor of hyoid bone); 8, omohyoid muscle; 9, sternothyroid muscle.

The Structure of the Human Vocal Folds

The conventional light microscopic appearance of the human vocal folds is illustrated in Figure 1–20*A*. Histologically, the vocal folds consist of the mucosa (epithelium and submucosal connective tissue) and muscle fibers from the medial aspect of the vocal portion of the thyroarytenoid muscle. The vibrating portion of the vocal folds on the medial surface is lined by stratified squamous epithelium. There are no glands or large blood vessels located here that would create great resistance to vocal fold vibration. The densest portion of the lamina propria is the vocal ligament.[86,87]

Recent studies using the electron microscope on the human vocal folds have substantially enhanced speech-language pathologists' understanding of its ultrastructure.[86,87] The vocal folds have been found to be composed of three layers of tissue that are differentiated on the basis of structure and mechanical properties. These layers, oriented from the free surface of the vocal fold inwardly, are the cover, transition, and body, respectively. Each layer increases in stiffness in that order.

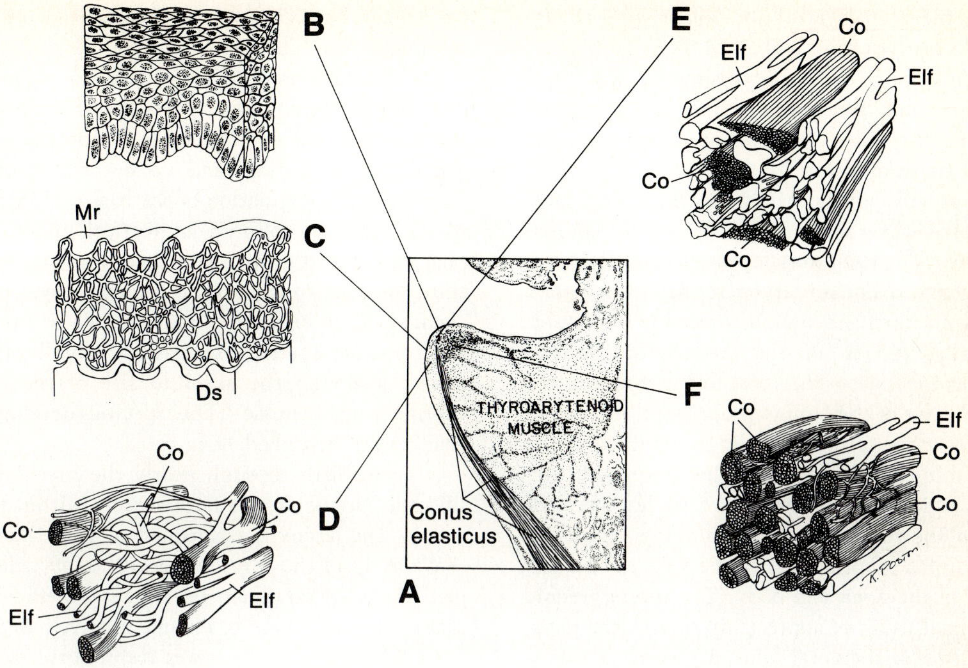

Figure 1–20 Composite figure illustrating the ultrastructure of the human vocal folds. See text for details. Abbreviations: Co = collagenous fibers; Elf = elastic fibers; Mr = microridges; Ds = desmosomes. (From Hirano M. Phonosurgery, basic and clinical investigations. Otologia Fukuoka 1975; 21:247, 249, 250, 251.)

Cover

The epithelium and superficial layers of the lamina propria form the cover of the vocal fold. The squamous epithelium on the medial (vibrating) edges of the vocal folds (see Fig. 1–20*B*) is eight layers thick. It is well suited to protect the delicate connective tissues of the vocal folds from the abrasion caused by contact of the medial margins of the vocal folds during phonation, sphincteric closure, and the flow of air into and out of the lungs. The structure of these epithelial cells, and indeed their layering, is fairly complex. The upper and lower surfaces of each epithelial cell (see Fig. 1–20*C*) are interconnected by minute cellular projections called tonofilaments. The separation of these layers in each cell and between cell layers provides a potential shearing force that may serve as an independent or accessory source of vibration during sound production. The superficial layer of the lamina propria (see Fig. 1–20*D*) corresponds to Reinke's space. It contains sparse amounts of large and small collagenous fibers as well as elastic fibers that are intertwined into a loosely arranged network.[86,87]

Transition Layer

The intermediate and deep layers of the lamina propria compose the transition layer of the vocal fold, and together form the vocal ligament. This layer measures approximately 0.8 mm. The intermediate layer is deep to the superficial layer of the lamina propria and consists largely of interlacing elastic fibers (see Fig. 1–20*E*). The deep layer is largely composed of densely packed collagenous fibers (see Fig. 1–20*F*) that run parallel from the deep surface of the thyroid cartilage to the vocal process of each arytenoid cartilage. The intermediate and deep layers of the lamina propria are intimately related, and their fibers are difficult to distinguish from each other. However, the outer layer is readily distinguishable from the superficial layer of the lamina propria. The density of elastic and collagenous fibers in the vocal ligament provides it with resiliency and extensibility. These are important physical properties that enable the vocal ligament to provide longitudinal stability to the vocal folds and enable it to be responsive to intrinsic laryngeal muscles, mechanical forces produced by particularly those of the thyroarytenoid muscle.[86,87]

Body

The thyrovocal portion of the thyroarytenoid muscle (if it really exists) composes the body of the vocal fold. It is intimately associated with the vocal ligament and the conus elasticus, which terminates rostrally in the deep layer of the lamina propria. Fibers from the deep layer of the lamina propria are interspersed between muscle fibers of the vocal muscle, effectively making the vocal ligament, the vocal musculature, and the conus elasticus a single functional unit that is highly efficient in transmitting subglottal pressure forces.[86,87]

The specific effect of each intrinsic laryngeal muscle on the cover and body of the vocal folds has been studied.[86,87] Each muscle was electrically stimulated in excised human larynges; the investigators found that the intrinsic muscles affect the vocal folds differentially. Action of the cricothyroid muscle stretches and elongates the vocal folds, thinning the superficial layer of the lamina propria and increasing the stiffness of the cover and body; this stiffness causes the vocal folds to vibrate at a higher frequency. Activity of the lateral cricoarytenoid muscle causes adduction of the vocal folds with thinning of the superficial lamina propria (edge of the folds) and slight stiffening of the cover and body. The interarytenoid muscles usually do not appreciably change the physical properties of the vocal folds. However, the posterior cricoarytenoid muscle thins the superficial layer of the lamina propria as it abducts the vocal folds. The vocal muscle tenses, shortens, and adducts the vocal folds. In this process, the body of the vocal fold stiffens, the superficial lamina propria thickens and the cover slackens.[86,87]

The specific role and contributions of the aforementioned changes in cover and body of the vocal folds during sound production are discussed by Weismer in Chapter 8 of this book.

THE PHARYNX

The pharyngeal cavities serve essential roles in respiration, deglutition, and resonation. This section chronicles significant postnatal developmental changes in the morphology of the pharynx and relates these changes to the formation of a functioning vocal tract and to maturation in the respiratory function of the supralaryngeal airways. In addition, essential morphologic and physiologic properties of the pharynx are described.

Postnatal Developmental Morphology of the Supralaryngeal Airway

Recent studies have provided data that document developmental changes in the supralaryngeal airways from birth to maturity.[88–90] These associated postnatal changes are related to the growth of the tongue and larynx and to establishment of the unique spatial relationships for the development of the vocal tract. Measurements of lateral head roentgenograms and casts of supralaryngeal airways of cadavers have revealed that postnatal changes in the shape of the supralaryngeal airway (and vocal tract) result from changes in the angulation of the basicranium relative to the vertebral column, to vertical growth of the pharynx, and to growth and descent of the posterior third of the tongue. The salient developmental changes occur between birth and age 5. After this time, mature spatial relationships have been established, although the absolute size of the pharynx continues to increase. The specific developmental changes are described next.

From birth through nearly the first 2 years of life, the tongue at rest lays entirely within the oral cavity. The larynx is positioned high in the neck so that the tip of the epiglottis and the soft palate contact. Such an arrangement allows for efficient respiration because there is a single relatively linear path from the nose into the lower respiratory tract. This path is highly efficient in that there is little airway resistance since it is of fairly uniform diameter and not tortuous. Consequently, there is no supralaryngeal airway or vocal tract. This anatomic arrangement is a special adaptation during infancy to allow the child to be nourished without interfering with his breathing.[88,89,91] This arrangement is accomplished by the interlocking of the nasopharynx and larynx (Fig. 1–21*A*) such that food passes laterally through the oral fauces over the pyriform sinuses and into the esophagus while air passes directly into the larynx.

Between 18 to 24 months, the posterior one-third of the tongue begins its descent into the pharyngeal cavity. No longer is it consistently positioned within the oral cavity. At the same time, the larynx begins to assume a more caudal position in the neck as a result of growth of the pharynx and cervical region. The upper airway begins to become more angulated (see Fig. 1–21*B*) and is being modified from a single tube into a double-tubed system that will serve separate respiratory and swallowing functions. Interlocking of the soft palate and the epiglottis still occurs, but less frequently and most often during swallowing and never during vocalization or crying.[90]

By age 4, the posterior one-third of the tongue has permanently descended into the pharynx, and the larynx has become positioned caudally so that the interlocking of the two structures is no longer possible. A two-tubed system (respiratory and deglutitory) has been established as has a vocal tract that the child uses effectively as a resonator during speech.[89]

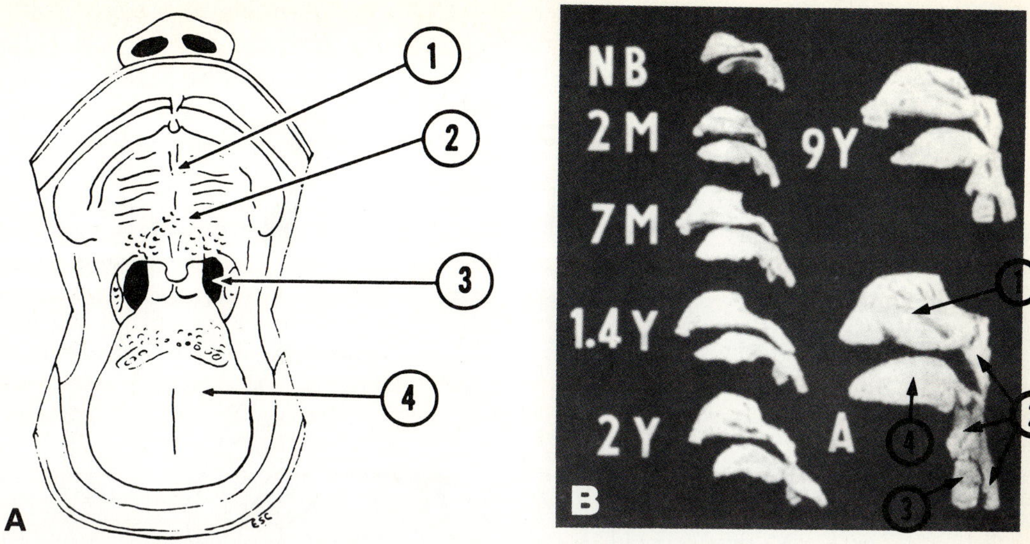

Figure 1–21 *A*, Intraoral view of newborn illustrating a possible mechanism for interlocking of the larynx and nasopharynx. 1, hard palate; 2, epiglottis (broken line) behind soft palate; 3, passageway through which milk can pass simultaneously during respiration; 4, tongue. *B*, Silicone rubber coats of human airways illustrating changing morphology in the newborn (NB), at 2 months (2M), 7 months (7M), 1.4 years (1.4Y), 2 years (2Y), 9 years (9Y), and adult (A). 1, nasal cavity; 2, pharynx; 3, larynx; 4, oral cavity. (From Laitman J, Crelin ES. Postnatal development of the basicranium and vocal tract region in man. In: Bosma JF, ed. Symposium of development of the basicranium. Washington, DC: Department of Health, Education and Welfare, 1976:206.)

After age 5 (see Fig. 1–21*B*), the mature configuration of the upper airway has been established: the posterior one-third of the tongue becomes located more caudally in the pharynx, as does the larynx, and the supraglottal airway is greatly expanded. Although this arrangement decreases respiratory efficiency in an absolute sense, it is better suited for human existence.[92] The increased and modified shape of the supralaryngeal region allows for (1) enlargement of the tongue and development of the flexibility needed for speech production and for manipulation and swallowing of large boluses of food; and (2) the development of a larger supralaryngeal airway that is important for resonance during speech.

Quantitative data on overall growth of the pharynx is limited,[91,93,94] as is detailed information on the growth of the nasopharynx.[94] However, some trends are apparent: the pharynx undergoes small amounts of growth anteroposteriorly, and its greatest growth is in the vertical dimension.

Before puberty, there are no significant differences in the length of the pharynx. The length of the nasal opening of the pharyngeal cavity is significantly larger in the male than in the female at all ages. Growth is continuous through age 16 in both sexes, although it is greater in males than in females.[94]

Growth of the Pharyngeal Tonsils (Adenoids)

There is great interest in growth and development of the nasopharynx and the pharyngeal tonsils (adenoids) because of their potential effects on velopharyngeal competence during speech. Changes in the physical dimensions of the nasopharynx must be considered in association with growth of the adenoids.

The adenoids extend from the roof of the nasopharynx (inferior to the body of the sphenoid bone and the basilar portion of the occipital bone) to the level of the soft palate—approximately in the same plane with the tubercle of the atlas. At its superior attachment, the adenoids may extend anteriorly into the regions of the posterior choanae and may even attach to the posterosuperior aspect of the vomer bone. In the midsagittal plane, the adenoid is convex, bulging anteriorly toward the soft palate.[14,15]

Investigators have reported from cadaveric studies that growth of the adenoids is similar to lymphatic tissue elsewhere in the body.[95] The adenoids increase rapidly in size during infancy and childhood and continue to grow at a slower rate until puberty, when they achieve their maximum size. After this time, they gradually atrophy or involute.[96]

Growth of the adenoid follows a predictable

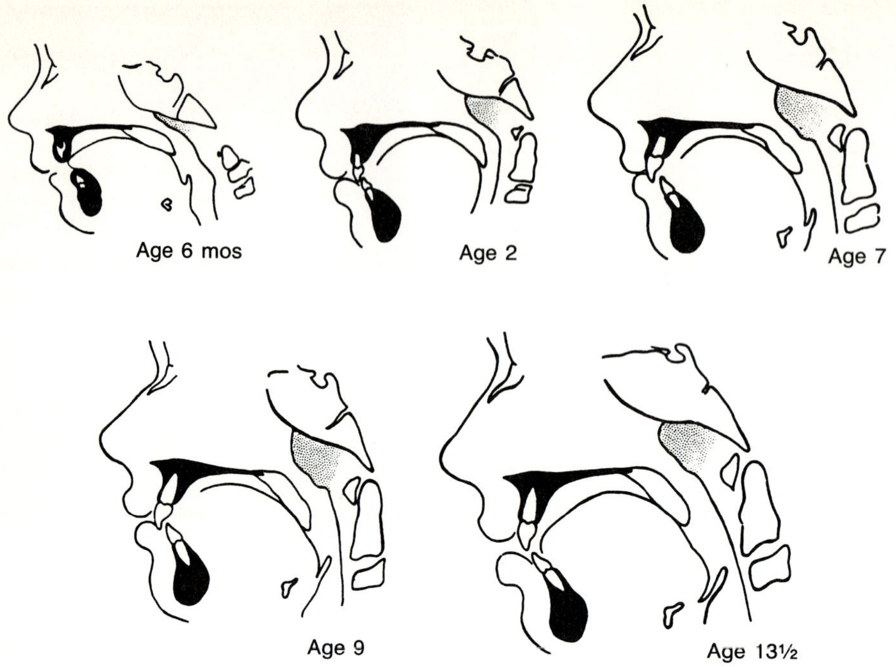

Figure 1–22 Longitudinal cephalometric tracings of an individual from infancy to peak adenoid growth at adolescence (stippled area represents adenoidal tissue as well as soft tissue contiguous to cranial base). (From Subtelny JD, Koepp-Baker H. The significance of adenoid tissue in velopharyngeal function. Plast Reconstr Surg 1956; 17:235.)

pattern (Fig. 1–22).[97] The adenoids are noticeable by 6 months to 1 year of age and are slightly convex on the roof of the nasopharynx. By 2 years of age, they are well developed and occupy nearly one-half of the nasopharyngeal area. Growth has progressed in a downward and forward direction primarily and continues this way until peak growth is attained between 9 to 15 years of age. After age 15, the adenoids begin to atrophy or involute. This atrophy occurs in a superoposterior fashion so that the distance between the posterior or nasal surface of the velum and the posterior pharyngeal wall gradually increases; the velum usually accommodates readily to this process. By age 25, the adenoids usually have completely atrophied.

Growth of the Nasopharynx

Little research exists on growth of the nasopharynx,[93,94] and reports disagree. One investigator reported that there was little growth of the anteroposterior dimension (depth) of the nasopharynx from 3 months to 16 years of age.[93] In the male, this amounted to 3.8 mm, whereas in the female it was only 2.6 mm. These data were not supported by another report in which lateral cephalometry was used to study 30 subjects, age 3 months to 18 years.[94] Results indicated that the nasopharynx underwent greater growth than previously reported. The mean increase in the anteroposterior dimension of the nasopharynx from 3 months to 18 years was approximately 10 mm.[94] Most of the actual growth appears to take place within the first 12 years of life. Further increases in the anteroposterior dimension of the nasopharynx from age 12 to 17 probably result from involution of the adenoids and from forward and downward growth of the mandible and midface rather than from actual growth of the nasopharynx. The vertical dimension of the nasopharynx increases by approximately 15 mm from 3 months to 18 years (13.3 mm to 28.1 mm), and the most rapid increase occurs during the first 18 months of life. This dimension increases steadily by approximately 0.5 to 1.0 mm per year up to age 15 years, when growth plateaus. No sex differences were reported.[94]

Anatomy

There is virtually no disagreement among anatomists about the morphology of the pharynx and its musculature.[14,15,65,97,98]

Muscles

The pharynx is a muscular membranous tube that extends from the base of the skull (pharyngeal

TABLE 1–2 Mean Dimensions of the Adult Human Pharynx (standard deviation in parentheses)

Shape		*Length*				*Width**	*Volume*[30]
		Pediatric[93] *7.5 yr (cm)*	*10.5 yr (cm)*	*14.0 yr (cm)*	*Adult* (cm)*	*Adult (cm)*	*Adult (ml)*
Inverted Cone (widest rostrally and tapering caudally)	Male	7.3 (4.4)	8.3 (4.8)	9.7 (5.3)	12.0 (no sex difference data)	Superiorly = 4.0 Inferiorly = 2.5	Nasopharynx = 30 Oropharynx = 30 Laryngopharynx = 20
	Female	7.2 (4.2)	8.2 (4.2)	9.4 (5.09)			

*From Zemlin S. Speech and hearing science: anatomy and physiology. Englewood Cliffs, NJ: Prentice-Hall, 1981:320.

tubercle) to the inferior border of the cricoid cartilage. It is funnel- or cone-shaped, having its widest diameter superiorly and its most narrow dimension inferiorly. The average physical dimensions of the human pharynx are summarized in Table 1–2. The pharyngeal musculature is not homogeneous, but complexly organized. It is innervated by a network of nerve fibers called the "pharyngeal plexus," which derive from the glossopharyngeal (ninth cranial nerve) and vagus (tenth cranial nerve) nerves.

The muscles of the pharynx are arranged into inner and outer layers (Fig. 1–23). The superior, middle, and inferior constrictor muscles are in the outer layer. The stylopharyngeal, palatopharyngeal, and salpingopharyngeal muscles form the inner layer. Fibers from the aforementioned muscles pierce and intermingle with those of the pharyngeal constrictors, which are the principle muscles of the pharynx.

The muscles in the outer layer constrict the pharynx during swallowing and gagging, whereas those in the inner layer share the common function of elevating the pharynx during swallowing. In addition, the stylopharyngeal muscle also has been shown to help dilate the pharynx, and the palatopharyngeal muscle to constrict the faucial pillars.

The bulk of the pharynx is formed by three muscles—superior, middle, and inferior pharyngeal constrictor muscles. They extend rostrocaudally (see Fig. 1–23) from the base of the skull to the inferior margin of the cricoid cartilage and are partially overlapping. These muscles fan out anterolaterally from the midline (pharyngeal raphe) and form the lateral walls of the pharynx. The posterior pharyngeal wall is formed by the midline union of the pharyngeal muscles; the anterior wall is incomplete and communicates with the nasal cavity (posterior choanae), oral cavity (oral isthmus), and the laryngeal aditus.

The wall of the pharynx is composed of four layers that are functionally specialized. From inward out, they are the (1) mucous membrane, (2) muscular wall, (3) pharyngeal raphe and buccopharyngeal fascia, and (4) loose areolar tissue.

The mucous membrane (and epithelium) cushions the pharyngeal muscles against pressures from ingested materials, serves as an inner lining for the digestive tube, and provides lubrication to the pharyngeal surfaces to facilitate the transport of swallowed material. The muscular layer is self-explanatory. The pharyngeal raphe is a tendinous zone at midline to which both halves of each pharyngeal constrictor are joined. The loose areolar tissue permits the pharyngeal musculature to move easily upward and downward past the vertebral column during peristalsis (swallowing).

Divisions

The pharynx is conventionally subdivided into three regions on the basis of the openings in its anterior wall. Each of these regions encloses important structures, which are summarized in Table 1–3. The uppermost portion of the pharynx (see Fig. 1–1) above the soft palate is called the "epi-" or "nasopharynx." The middle portion of the pharynx, between the soft palate and tip of the epiglottis, is called the

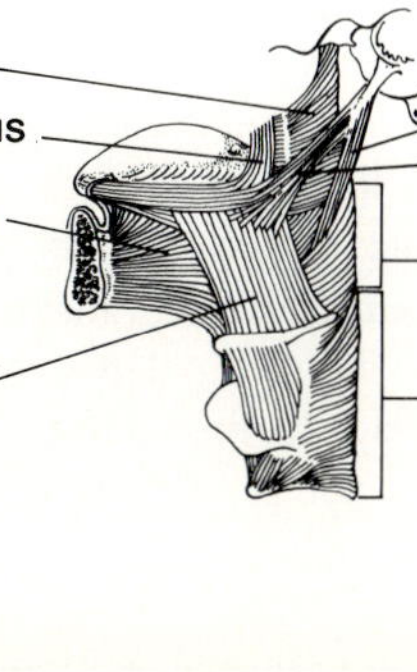

Figure 1–23 Schematic illustration of the topographic arrangement of the pharyngeal musculature and extrinsic tongue musculature. (After Heartwell CM, Rahn AO. Syllabus of complete dentures. 2nd ed. Philadelphia: Lea & Febiger, 1974:12.)

TABLE 1–3 Anatomic Divisions of the Human Pharynx with Associated Structures

Pharyngeal region	*Function*	*Boundaries*	*Associated structures*
Nasopharynx	Purely respiratory	Superior = superior margin of choanae to pharyngeal tubercle Posterior = superior pharyngeal constrictor extending from tubercle to level of 1st cervical vertebrae (C1) Inferior = soft palate Lateral = lateral pharyngeal wall (superior pharyngeal constrictor) Anterior = posterior chonae	Eustachian tube orifice; torus tubarius; fossa of Rosenmueller; salpingopharyngeal fold; pharyngeal tonsils; posterior choanae; soft palate
Oropharynx	Swallowing Respiration	Superior = soft palate Posterior = middle pharyngeal constrictor (C2–C4) Inferior = tip of epiglottis Lateral = lateral pharyngeal wall (middle pharyngeal constrictor) Anterior = faucial isthmus and pharyngeal portion of tongue	Uvula; anterior and posterior faucial pillars; palatine tonsils; pharyngeal portion of the tongue; medial and lateral glossoepiglottic folds; valleculae
Laryngopharynx	Swallowing Respiration	Superior = epiglottis below tip Posterior = inferior pharyngeal constrictor extending from C5–C6 Inferior = cricopharyngeal sphincter Lateral = lateral pharyngeal wall (inferior pharyngeal constrictor) Anterior = aditus laryngeus	Larynx; pyriform sinuses; upper esophageal sphincter

"meso-" or "oropharynx." The lowermost portion of the pharynx, between the epiglottis and the lower border of the cricoid cartilage, is called the "hypo-" or "laryngopharynx."

Physiology

The pharynx is involved in a number of varied and important biologic functions. The nasopharynx is almost exclusively involved in respiration; however, it also facilitates aeration and drainage of the middle ear via the eustachian tube and drainage of the nasal cavities and sinuses, and it serves as a resonator during speech.

The oropharynx and hypopharynx serve both respiratory and digestive system functions. They are usually open and serve as airways, except during swallowing (and vomiting). Respiratory functions have previously been noted. Peristalsis is the primary motor activity of the pharynx; it is an involuntary motor act initiated by trigger zones in the posterior pharyngeal walls,[99] which results in a rhythmic, sequential contraction of the pharyngeal musculature that is temporally sequenced and proceeds in a rostrocaudal fashion. This pharyngeal activity creates a positive pressure force that drives the bolus of food caudally into the esophagus where esophageal peristalsis delivers the bolus into the stomach. The interested reader is directed to reviews on this subject.[100,101]

THE SOFT PALATE AND THE VELOPHARYNGEAL MECHANISM

The velopharyngeal mechanism is complex structurally and physiologically. This section reviews the salient aspects of the morphology of this mechanism from the viewpoint of developmental and gross anatomy. The physiology of the mechanism is described in terms of the contribution that the velum and pharyngeal walls make to velopharyngeal valving in speech and nonspeech tasks.

Postnatal Developmental Morphology of the Soft Palate

Postnatal growth of the normal human soft palate has not been studied extensively. Growth of the soft palate from age 3 months to 18 years has been studied in a longitudinal fashion, with lateral cephalograms used to measure its resting length, thickness, and angulation.[94] Data from this study has shown that the soft palate increases in length from approximately 20 mm at age 3 months to approximately 35 mm at age 18 years. However, during this same time, it only increased 6 to 9 mm in thickness. The velum remained about one-third longer in length than the depth of the nasopharynx. The extent and rate of growth of the soft palate was not significantly different for males and females. The greatest growth occurred during the first 2 years of life, after which growth leveled off until after age 4 to 5 years when steady increases occurred in the length through age 18 years.

The angle of inclination of the resting soft palate changes as a function of age. In infancy and young childhood, the contour of the soft palate approximates the roof of the nasopharynx. With increasing age, the angulation of the soft palate changes, assuming a more vertical position that ultimately, in adulthood, parallels the posterior pharyngeal wall. These morphologic changes have been attributed to the forward and downward growth of the facial skeleton and to the vertical growth of the pharynx.[93,94]

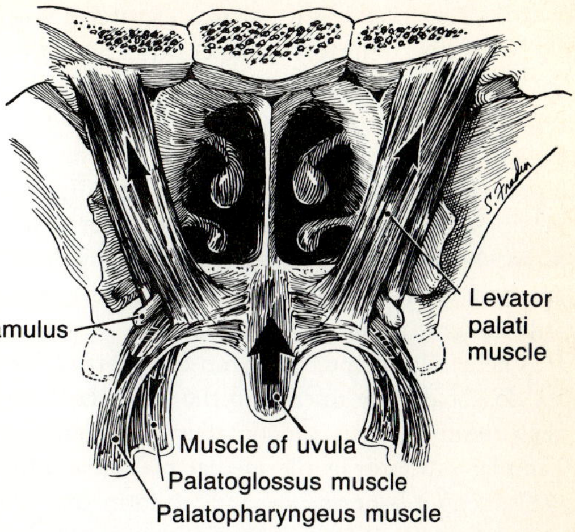

Figure 1–24 Schematic illustration of the topography of the soft palate muscles and their resultant effects on raising, lowering, and shortening the velum. (From Silverman S. Oral physiology. St. Louis: CV Mosby, 1961:371.)

Anatomy of the Soft Palate

The morphology of the soft palate is briefly reviewed in terms of its histology and gross anatomy.

Histology

The soft palate is a muscular structure that originates from the posterior border of the hard palate via an aponeurotic sheath called the "palatine aponeurosis" and extends posteriorly, terminating in the uvula. It consists of several layers. Beneath the oral and nasal epithelial surfaces are connective tissue layers that contain a highly dense capillary network. Deep to this layer is connective tissue that is heavily invested by glands; the muscles of the soft palate are sandwiched between the glandular layers. Because the epithelium on the oral surface of the soft palate is thinner than it is on the hard palate and because the underlying layer of capillaries is extensive, the soft palate has a deeper reddish color than the hard palate. The soft palate is highly mobile because of its muscular structure and strong because of the connective tissue elements. Details on the muscular anatomy of the soft palate are described next.[14,15]

Muscles

The soft palate, or velum, consists of five pairs of muscles: tensor veli palatini, levator veli palatini, uvulae, palatoglossus, and palatopharyngeus (see Fig. 1–24). Several investigators have shown that the superior fibers of the superior constrictor muscle also enter the velum.[102–104] Except for tensor veli palatini, which is innervated by the trigeminal nerve (fifth cranial nerve), all other velar muscles are innervated by the pharyngeal plexus (ninth and tenth cranial nerves). Muscle fibers of the superior constrictor are extensively interwoven with those of the levator veli palatini;[103] however, they insert into the soft palate at a point below the level of the hard palate. The topographic arrangement of the velar muscles and their force vectors are illustrated in Figures 1–24 and 1–25. Details on the points of attachment of these muscles may be found in several sources.[65,105,106.]

The muscles of the soft palate influence the movement of the soft palate in several ways (see Fig.

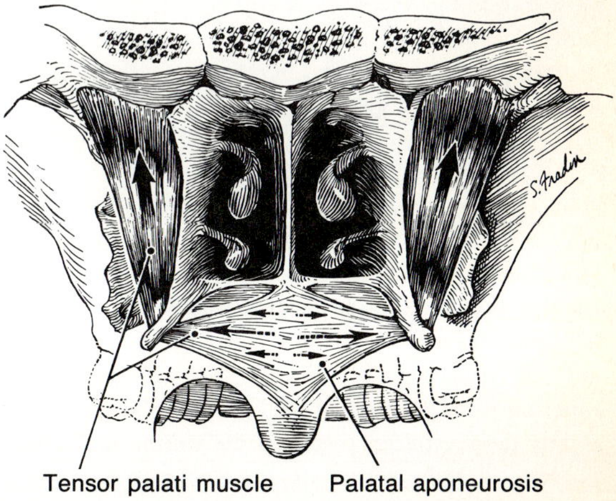

Figure 1–25 The effects of tensor veli palatini muscle activity on tensing of the palatine aponeurosis. (From Silverman S. Oral physiology. St Louis: CV Mosby, 1961:371.)

1–24). The levator veli palatini elevates and draws the velum posteriorly and superiorly. Both the palatoglossus and palatopharyngeus lower the velum, but in somewhat different ways. Palatoglossus lowers and draws the velum anteriorly, whereas the palatopharyngeus lowers the velum vertically. Tensor veli palatini has been described in older textbooks as an elevator and/or tensor of the soft palate. The anatomy of this muscle is complex, and anatomists still disagree about its structure.[104,107,108] However, it is generally accepted that muscle fibers of the tensor do not directly insert into the soft palate. Rather, they terminate in a tendon that wraps around the hamular processes of the medial pterygoid plates of the sphenoid bone and expands to form the palatine aponeurosis (see Fig. 1–25). Contraction of the tensor veli palatini muscle was thought to elevate and tense the anterior region of the soft palate, as drawn in Figure 1–25. Moreover, physiology studies have shown unequivocally that the tensor dilates the eustachian tube.[109,110] Earlier electromyographic studies indicate that the tensor is constantly active during swallowing (when the eustachian tube is opened),[105] and recent anatomic studies have reinforced this functional role.[107,108] The role of the tensor veli palatini in velopharyngeal function per se appears to be limited at best, if present at all. Until recently, the uvulae has been thought to play no significant functional role in velopharyngeal closure. However, results from anatomic studies of the uvulae have shown it to be highly complex.[111,112] Its morphology suggests that this muscle aids in contouring and adding bulk to the dorsal surface of the soft palate in the region of the velum, which makes contact with the posterior pharyngeal wall. The role of the superior constrictor muscle fibers in velopharyngeal function is described in regard to pharyngeal wall activity later in this section.

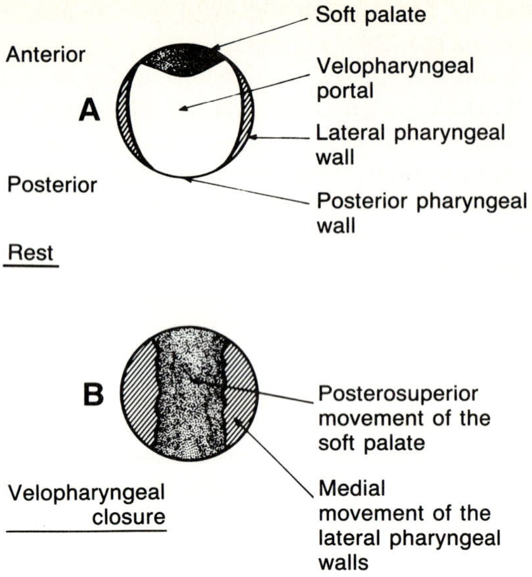

Figure 1–26 Diagrammatic representation of the velopharyngeal portal as viewed superiorly from the nasopharynx, during *A*, rest and *B*, velopharyngeal closure. Note that during velopharyngeal closure, the lateral pharyngeal walls (shaded regions) move medially and abut the lateral margins of the posterosuperiorly displaced soft palate (stippled area). Both velar and lateral pharyngeal wall movements are required to close off the velopharyngeal portal.

Physiology of the Velopharyngeal Mechanism

The basic mechanics of velopharyngeal closure have been well documented by means of multiview and base view cineflouroscopy[113] and nasoendoscopy.[114] These methods have permitted investigators to simultaneously study the activity of the velum and the pharyngeal walls during velopharyngeal function for a variety of tasks. Both techniques have clearly demonstrated that *both* the velum and lateral pharyngeal walls contribute to closure of the velopharyngeal portal. The effects of the convergence of the velum and pharyngeal walls are illustrated in Figure 1–26, which is a schema of the portal as it might appear in base view cinefluoroscopy or through nasopharyngoscopy.

One can see that as the velum is elevated and moves posteriorly, its mass closes off a large portion of the nasopharynx, but not all of it. The mesial movements of the lateral pharyngeal walls cause them to abut the lateral margins of the velum and to close off the lateral recesses of the nasopharyngeal airway. Thus *both* velar and lateral pharyngeal wall movements are necessary to close off the nasopharyngeal portal and to separate the oral from the nasal cavities. This closure is needed during swallowing, blowing, production of vowels and nonnasal consonants, and during vomiting in order to prevent gastric contents from entering the nasopharynx. Closure of the nasal cavity during sucking and puffing can be accomplished without velar activity through tongue action, which elevates the velum and helps it occlude the nasopharyngeal portal.[115]

Several aspects of velopharyngeal valving deserve further discussion. These include (1) the role(s) of the posterior pharyngeal wall and Passavant's bar in normal velopharyngeal closure; (2) special characteristics of velar activity during speech; (3) muscles responsible for lateral pharyngeal wall movements; and (4) differences in velopharyngeal closure for different tasks.

General Characteristics of Velar Movement

Activity of the velum during velopharyngeal valving has been studied extensively during speech production. Several investigators have noted differences in velar function during nonspeech valving. These are discussed separately later in this chapter. However, regardless of the task, the velum elevates posterosuperiorly and makes contact with the posterior pharyngeal wall.

Calnan was the first to systematically study what region (area) of the velum made contact with the posterior pharyngeal wall.[116] He noted that the middle third of the velum made contact with the posterior pharyngeal wall. Investigators, using more refined measurement techniques, found that as a rule, the third quadrant of the velum as measured from the hard palate posteriorly, contacted the posterior pharyngeal wall during velopharyngeal closure for speech.[117] This region did not correspond to the levator eminence, which is located just anterior to the site of closure.

The level of contact of the velum to the posterior pharyngeal wall has been shown to change as a function of age.[116,118] In childhood, before age 9, the velum contacts the posterior pharyngeal wall high in the nasopharynx.[118] However, with increasing age, the velum contacts the posterior pharyngeal wall at progressively lower levels. In the adult, velar contact occurs at the level of the hard palate. Differences in the site of velopharyngeal valving during childhood and adolescence is thought to result from the downward and forward growth of the facial skeleton, which alters the relative position of the hard palate to the posterior pharyngeal wall.[118]

Several investigators have studied sex differences in velar function during speech in adult male and female subjects.[119–121] Some found no significant differences between the extent of velar movement, the amount of velar contact to the posterior pharyngeal wall, and the height of velar elevation in male and female adult subjects.[119,120] However, other investigators, using lateral cinefluorography to make numerous measurements of the velopharyngeal mechanism during speech, found significant sex differences in several areas of velar functioning:[122]

1. In the male, the velum approximated the posterior pharyngeal wall at an acute angle (69.7 degrees); whereas in the female, the velum approximated the posterior pharyngeal wall at almost a right angle (88.1 degrees).
2. The height of velar elevation was greater in the male (10.05 mm) than in the female (5.90 mm).
3. The extent of velar contact (i.e., vertical span) to the posterior pharyngeal wall during velopharyngeal closure was significantly less in the male (5.70 mm) than in the female (9.50 mm).
4. The inferior point of contact in velopharyngeal closure in the male was at or above the palatal plane, whereas in the female it was usually below the palatal plane.
5. The mean length of the velum during speech was greater in the male (47.8 mm) than the female (41.0 mm).

These differences in adult male and female velopharyngeal function underscore the need to consider the influences of sex differences in studies of normal velopharyngeal function and in the clinical assessment of this mechanism.

Posterior and Lateral Pharyngeal Wall Activity During Velopharyngeal Closure

The posterior and lateral walls of the nasopharynx are formed by the superior pharyngeal constrictor muscle. Historically, some authors reported that both the posterior and lateral pharyngeal walls were active in normal velopharyngeal closure. However, in the last 20 years, researchers have shown that the posterior and lateral pharyngeal walls do not share equal roles in velopharyngeal function.

Posterior Pharyngeal Wall Activity. Passavant was the first to describe forward displacement of the posterior pharyngeal wall during velopharyngeal closure for speech.[123] He observed this displacement in a speaker with cleft palate during speech and maintained that it was an essential part of velopharyngeal closure that was obscured in persons with intact palates. Passavant maintained that anterior displacement of the posterior pharyngeal wall was caused by contraction of fibers of the superior constrictor muscle, which are attached to the lateral pterygoid plates of the sphenoid bone. This displacement resulted in a horizontal cross-roll that extended from midline to the eustachian tube orifices bilaterally.

Several investigators using cineradiography have shown that anterior displacement of the posterior pharyngeal wall rarely accompanied velopharyngeal closure.[117,120,124–126] When displacement was noted, it was limited and not thought to contribute significantly to velopharyngeal closure.

Much has been written about the structure and function of Passavant's bar.[116,117,120,124,127–132] The major objections to the functional role of Passavant's bar in normal velopharyngeal function are that (1) it occurred at a level too low in the nasopharynx to effectively participate in velopharyngeal closure; (2)

it is observed frequently in effortful velopharyngeal closure, such as during swallowing, gagging, and blowing, but it is not usually present during speech; and (3) its inconsistent and variable shape suggests that it is not an essential component of the velopharyngeal mechanism.

The frequent appearance of Passavant's bar in patients with cleft palate and those with velopharyngeal insufficiency suggests that it is a compensatory mechanism employed by these speakers to improve valving for speech. However, it is not an essential component of normal velopharyngeal mechanism for speech.

Lateral Pharyngeal Wall Activity. Lateral pharyngeal wall movement during normal velopharyngeal valving has been described by many investigators,[113,119,121,132–139] who agree on several points: (1) the predominant direction of movement is medial, (2) movement is extensive, and (3) the primary site of motion or displacement of the lateral pharyngeal wall is at the level of the hard palate. However, researchers disagree about which muscle causes the movement of the lateral pharyngeal walls—the levator veli palatini or the superior pharyngeal constrictor muscles.

The superior fibers of the superior constrictor muscle have been shown to enter the velum and were thought by some to be responsible for lateral pharyngeal wall movement.[102,103,140] Objections to this position have been raised based upon the attachments of this muscle and the course of muscle fibers within the lateral pharyngeal walls.[104] Fibers enter the soft palate below the level of the hard palate. Excluding the attachment of the superior constrictor to the pharyngeal raphe, the other muscle attachments are anterior to the soft palate, that is, the lateral pterygoid plates of the sphenoid bone, the maxillary tuberosity, and the pterygomandibular raphe. Thus contraction of muscle fibers of the superior constrictor muscle would most likely result in an anteromedial movement of the walls rather than a posteromedial motion, which is observed during velopharyngeal closure in speech. The precise role of the superior fibers of the superior constrictor muscle has not yet been determined. However, the superior constrictor muscle's anatomic structure has led investigators to conclude that contraction of its fibers results in the formation of Passavant's bar.

The results of several anatomic studies have supported the contention that the levator veli palatini not only elevates and draws the velum posteriorly but also causes lateral pharyngeal wall movement.[104,141,142] The muscle fibers of the levator veli palatini descend toward the soft palate at approximately a 45-degree angle from their attachment to the temporal bone superiorly. The fibers of this muscle have been found to cross inferiorly to the eustachian tube and laterally to the torus tubarios.[104] Thus contraction of the levator muscle fibers may move the torus tubarius in a medial and posterior direction, which would correspond to the direction of lateral pharyngeal wall movements during speech. These inferences about lateral pharyngeal wall movement based on anatomic data appear to be supported from physiologic studies. Data from frontal and baseview cineflouroscopy showed that the major site of movement of the lateral pharyngeal walls occurs above the palatal plane and that it often continues rostrally to the height of the levator eminence.[126] This structure has been defined as the point of insertion of the levator muscles.[143,144] Motion of the torus tubarius begins at the level of the hard palate and usually terminates just inferior to the superior aspect of the levator eminence and sometimes also above it. The movement of the lateral pharyngeal walls (and torus tubarius) was in a medial and posterior direction regardless of the task. This movement probably resulted from action of the levator veli palatini for two reasons: (1) the muscle courses laterally to the torus tubarius, and (2) contraction of the levator would result in a medioposterior displacement of the torus tubarius.

Variations in Velopharyngeal Valving According to Task

Studies have been conducted by many investigators to assess variations in velopharyngeal valving for speech, blowing, puffing, sucking, gagging, and swallowing.[115,116,126,134,135,139,145] However, differences have been found among these tasks, and complete descriptions and universal agreement are still lacking.

More recent data[139] from an extensive study employing synchronous lateral and frontal cinefluorography appear to support a dichotomous classification of velopharyngeal valving first proposed 35 years ago.[134] Data from the most recent study (1975) revealed that velopharyngeal closure for speech, blowing, and whistling were similar and that as a group were significantly different from velopharyngeal closure for swallowing and gagging.[139] Speech, blowing, and whistling—pneumatic tasks—share the common characteristic of requiring control and/or development of intraoral pressure. Swallowing and gagging—nonpneumatic tasks—do not. Significant differences in velar height, lateral pharyngeal movement, and the degree of contact of the lateral pharyngeal walls were found between pneumatic and nonpneumatic tasks. These are illustrated in Figure 1–27. No significant differences were found among activities within each group. Velar height, lateral pharyngeal wall movement, and the extent of contact of the medially-displaced lateral pharyngeal walls were significantly greater for nonpneumatic tasks than for pneumatic ones.

Lateral pharyngeal wall movement in pneumatic tasks was characterized by shelf-like contact at the level of the hard palate. In contrast, lateral pharyngeal wall movement in nonpneumatic tasks involves extensive pharyngeal wall contact above and below the hard palate.[139]

It has also been reported that during reflexive swallowing, the lateral pharyngeal walls do not approximate in the upper portion of the oropharynx, such that in frontal view the lateral pharyngeal walls exhibit a "Y" configuration. This finding suggests that during reflex swallowing (as compared to voluntary swallowing) there is no contraction of the uppermost fibers of the superior constrictor muscle.[139] Therefore it appears that lateral pharyngeal wall movement in pneumatic and nonpneumatic tasks is caused by different degrees of superior constrictor muscle activity. The shelf-like configurations of the lateral pharyngeal walls during pneumatic tasks are thought to result from the contraction of the uppermost fibers of the superior constrictor, and the extensive vertical approximation of the lateral pharyngeal wall during nonpneumatic tasks is thought to result in complete contraction of the superior constrictor muscle.

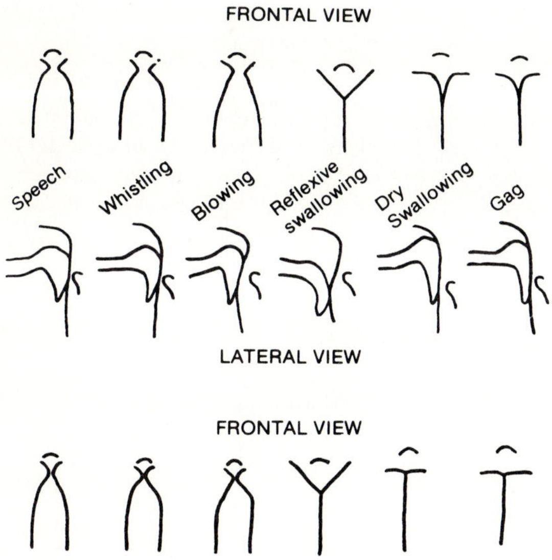

Figure 1–27 Tracings of frontal and lateral views during speech, whistling, blowing, reflexive swallowing, dry swallow, and gagging. (From Shprintzen RJ, Lencione RM, McCall GN, and Skolnick ML. A three-dimensional cinefluoroscopic analysis of velopharyngeal closure during speech and nonspeech activities in normals. Cleft Palate J 1974; 11:412.)

THE ORAL CAVITY

The oral cavity is the site of a wide range of activities, which include chewing, swallowing, respiration, digestion, and, of course, speech. The oral cavity can be divided into two parts: the vestibule and the oral cavity (cavum oris).

The Vestibule

The vestibule is a mucous membrane-lined trough that is bounded externally by the lips and cheeks and internally by the alveolar process and teeth of the maxilla and mandible, respectively (Fig. 1–28). Anteriorly it is referred to as the labial vestibule and laterally as the buccal vestibule. The mucous membrane of the vestibule is derived from reflections of the mucosa of the lip and cheek and is usually uniformly pink in color.

In the labial vestibule, a prominent fold of tissue, the labial frenulum, extends from the inner surface of each lip to the alveolar process. In the buccal vestibule, the mucosa is tightly adherent to the buccinator muscle so that movements of the cheek (through contraction of the buccinator muscle) do not dislodge the mucosa over the cutting edges of the teeth and cause the cheek to become bitten during chewing.

Small yellow dots are normally seen on the cheek mucosa near the corner of the mouth. These are called "Fordyce's spots" and are rudimentary sebaceous glands.

Oral Cavity Proper

The oral cavity or cavum oris is the area located between the alveolar arches. It is bounded anteriorly and laterally by the alveolar arches, superiorly by the hard and soft palates, inferiorly by the mylohyoid muscle, and posteriorly by the anterior faucial pillar. Figure 1–28 is a schema of the structure of the oral cavity. The oral cavity is highly vascularized and richly innervated by the trigeminal nerve (fifth cranial nerve). It contains a wide variety of sensory endings that provide significant feedback to the central nervous

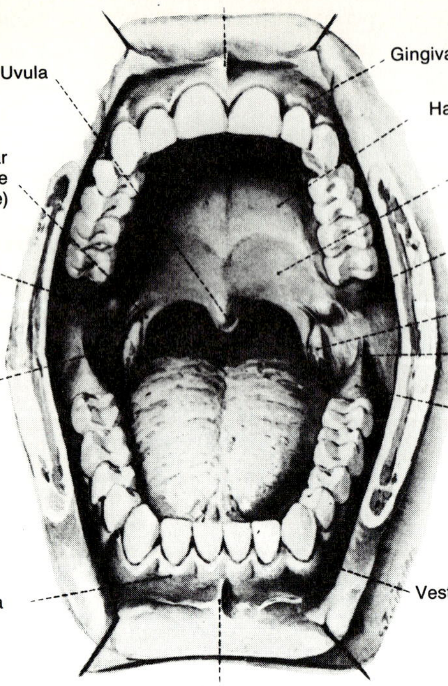

Figure 1–28 Anatomy of the vestibule and oral cavity. (From Massler M, Schour I. Atlas of the mouth. 2nd ed. Chicago: American Dental Association, 1958: plate 1.)

system regarding pain, touch, and pressure.[146] This information is used for monitoring purposes and for influencing motor actions.

Anterior and Lateral Boundaries

The alveolar arches separate the oral cavity proper from the vestibule. They are formed from the bone of the maxilla and the mandible and contain openings (sockets) for the roots of the teeth. The teeth are anchored into the alveolar bone by periodontal ligaments. The mucosa lining the alveolar processes is called the "gingiva." Projections of gingiva between the teeth are called "interdental papillae." Laterally, the gingiva becomes continuous with the mucosa of the vestibule.[15,65,147]

Figure 1–29 shows the position and type of each tooth within the alveolar processes (dental arch) of a normal child and adult. Each human is born with two sets of teeth. The first set to erupt is called the "deciduous" or "primary teeth." Ten deciduous teeth are found in each dental arch. Over a 4- to 6-year period, beginning at about age 6 years, each deciduous tooth is replaced by a permanent tooth. Additional permanent teeth are also added to make the normal adult complement: 32 teeth, 16 in each dental arch. Four bicuspids (two on each side) and two molars (one on each side) are added to each dental arch (see Fig. 1–29).[15,65]

Superior Boundary

The roof or superior boundary of the oral cavity is formed by the hard and soft palates. They are covered by two different types of mucosa that are well adapted to different types of mechanical forces.[147] The hard palate and the gingiva are covered by a thicker, more resilient type of mucosa called "masticatory mucosa." This mucosa is needed to handle the constant movement of food across these surfaces during mastication and the oral preparatory phases of swallowing. The mucosa in the anterior portion of the hard palate contains transverse folds, called the "palatine rugae." Just posterior to the central incisor teeth is an upraising of mucosa called the "incisive papilla." A narrow, sharp-edged ridge, called

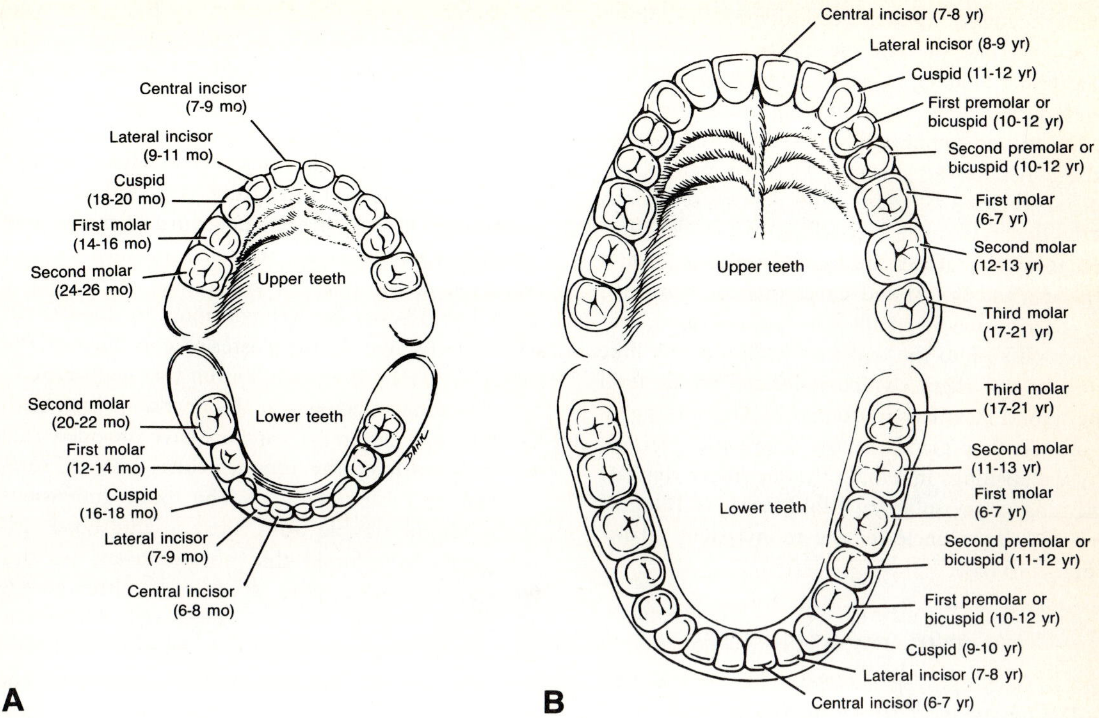

Figure 1-29 Dentition and their eruption times in *A*, the normal child and, *B*, the adult. (From Tortora GJ, Anagnostakos NP. Principles of anatomy and physiology. 4th ed. New York: Harper & Row, 1984.)

the "median palatine raphe," extends from it along the length of the hard palate. It is covered by mucosa, and its prominence varies from individual to individual. The soft palate is the mobile portion of the roof of the oral cavity owing to the muscles that act on it and make up a substantial portion of its structure. The most conspicuous portion of it in the oral cavity is a small pendulous portion at midline called the "uvula." It is the most distal portion of the soft palate and is composed largely of fat and glandular tissue. The mucosa of the soft palate is smooth and spongy due to the large number of glands that it contains. The lining mucosa is well suited for a mobile structure like the velum, because it is able to adapt to the changing shape of the soft palate and still provide protection to its delicate tissues.[15,65,14]

Inferior Boundary

The floor of the oral cavity is formed by the broad, flat mylohyoid muscle. It is lined by a thin, delicate lining mucosa. The tongue is intimately associated with the floor of the mouth, and its structure and function are discussed in a separate section.[15,65,147]

Posterior Boundary

The posterior boundary of the oral cavity is formed by an arch of tissue called the "anterior faucial pillar." It is covered by mucosa and contains the palatoglossus muscle, some fat, and connective tissue. Posterior and medial to it is a second arch, the posterior faucial pillar. It contains the palatopharyngeal muscle as well as some fat and connective tissue. Between the faucial pillars is a crypt that contains the palatine tonsil.[15,65,147]

Salivary Glands

Although not directly a part of the oral cavity, the salivary glands are important to oral functioning and maintaining the health of the oral mucosa. Saliva is a fluid composed mostly of water and containing enzymes, carbohydrates, and proteinaceous substances. Perhaps the most important function of saliva is in providing an adhesive medium for food particles, enabling them to be formed into a bolus and thus readily swallowed. Saliva also contains enzymes that are important for the initial breakdown of carbohydrates in food and it is important for lubrication of the oral mucosa. Saliva facilitates movement of food within the oral cavity and aids movements of the tongue across mucosal surfaces. In addition salivary secretions prevent the mucosa from drying out and from becoming damaged by mechanical forces incurred during swallowing, chewing, and speech.[148]

The parotid, sublingual, and submaxillary glands are the major salivary glands. They are paired, located outside the oral cavity, and deposit secretions into the oral cavity via ducts (Fig. 1–30). Smaller, scattered salivary glands are located in the hard and soft palates and buccal and labial mucosa; however, their contribution is small. The parotid gland introduces saliva into the oral cavity via a nipple-like opening in the cheek, which is located at the level of the second maxillary molar tooth. The sublingual and submaxillary glands deposit saliva into the oral cavity via openings in a fold of tissue under the base of the tongue (the sublingual fold for the sublingual gland and the caruncle for the submaxillary gland; see Fig. 1–31*B*).[148]

THE TONGUE

The tongue is an extraordinarily versatile organ that is important in mastication, deglutition, taste, and speech. Its structure and function are complex and highly specialized. The review that follows attempts to highlight these salient relationships.

Postnatal Developmental Morphology

The two significant postnatal changes in the morphology of the tongue relate to the caudal positioning of the posterior one-third of the tongue into the oropharynx and to growth of the physical dimensions of the tongue that increase its size.[149–152]

During the first 2 years of life, the entire tongue is contained within the oral cavity. However, beginning at 2 years of age, there is a gradual retropositioning of the posterior one-third of the tongue towards the oropharynx that accompanies vertical expansion of the pharynx and caudal displacement of the hyoid bone. Growth continues in this fashion such that by age 4, the posterior one-third of the tongue is contained entirely within the oropharynx.[89]

The tongue increases in all dimensions from birth to adulthood. Several researchers have provided data on the growth of the tongue; their data are summarized in Table1–4.[149–152] The mean dimensions of the tongue double from birth to adulthood. Investigators have found that no significant sex differences exist in neonates or adults,[149] although the adult male tongue is slightly larger than the female counterpart. Further research is required to determine the specific dimensions of the human tongue at all ages and to correlate these data with measurements of intermaxillary, intermandibular, and hard palate dimensions.

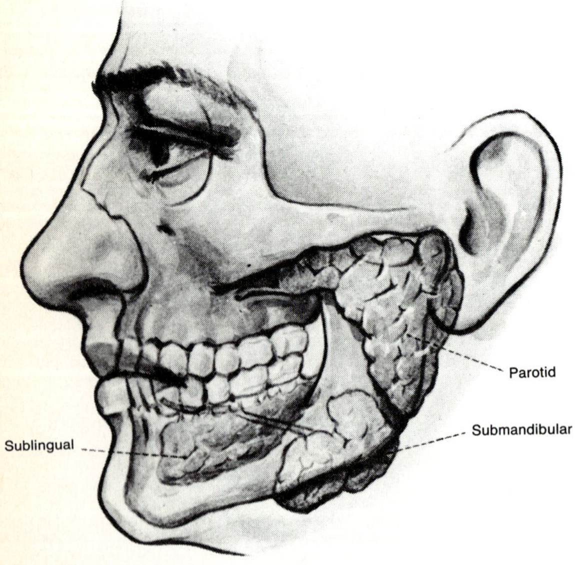

Figure 1-30 The relationship of the salivary glands to the oral cavity. (From Massler M, Schour I. Atlas of the mouth. 2nd ed. Chicago: American Dental Association, 1958: plate 52.)

Anatomy

The surface morphology of the tongue endows it with special properties as does the morphology of the intrinsic and extrinsic lingual muscles. The following discussion examines both of these important anatomic characteristics of the tongue.

Surface Morphology

The dorsal surface of the tongue (Fig. 1–31*A*) is anatomically divided into an anterior two-thirds (blade) and a posterior one-third (root) by a V-shaped fissure called the "sulcus terminalis." This structure terminates in a pit called the "foramen cecum linguae." A longitudinal furrow, the dosal or median sulcus, separates the anterior two-thirds of the tongue into right and left halves. The region anterior to the sulcus terminalis encompassess approximately two-thirds of the length and area of the tongue. It is contained entirely within the oral cavity and is highly mobile. Its surface is characterized by epithelial upraisings—the lingual papillae—which are specialized for mastication and especially for taste. Phoneticians, linguists, and speech-language pathologists functionally subdivide the dorsum of the tongue

TABLE 1–4 Physical Dimensions of the Human Tongue

					Data	
Author(s)	*Region of tongue*	*Subjects*	*Age*	*Measurements*	*Mean (SD) (mm)*	*Mean (SD) (mm)*
		Cadavers:			Neonate	Adult
Hopkin (1967)[149]	Dorsum	32 neonates (160 ♂, 16 ♀)	birth–15 days	Length (distance from epiglottis to apex)	39.91 (4.25)	79.83 (7.57)
		30 adults (14 ♂, 16 ♀)	29–85 yr	Breadth (widest part of tongue)	25.43 (2.58)	51.90 (4.24)
				Thickness (thickness of free edge at widest point	8.76 (0.98)	16.13 (2.51)
		Cephalograms:			Children	Adult
Vig and Cohen (1974)[150]	Dorsum	36 children 26 adults	not stated	Tongue area (vallecula at hyoid bone to menton)	23.2 (±2.7) cm^2	30.4 (±2.5) cm^2
		Live subjects:			Children	
Fletcher and Daly (1974)[151]	Sublingual region at midline	28 ♂ 28 ♀	1 mo–5 yr	Total length at midline from orifice of submandibular duct to apex of tongue	<1 yr	21.9 (4.7)
					1–2 yr	28.2 (3.6)
					3–5 yr	31.7 (5.1)
Fletcher (1978)[152]	Sublingual region at midline	30 ♂ 30 ♀	6–13 yr	Same as above	6–7 yr	31.8 (3.43)
					8–9 yr	32.3 (4.93)
					10–11 yr	35.5 (4.41)
					12–13 yr	41.4 (3.33)

into four regions based on the relationship of the dorsum of the tongue to the roof of the oral cavity. Thus the apex or tip is closest to the teeth; the blade is beneath the alveolar ridge; the front is beneath the hard palate; and the back is beneath the soft palate.[65]

In the child after age 4 years and in the adult, the posterior one-third of the tongue, or root, lies within the pharynx and is relatively immobile. It is covered by masses of lymphatic tissue that are collectively called the "lingual tonsils." The root of the tongue is attached to the epiglottis by membranous bands called the "median" and "lateral glossoepiglottic folds." They enclose depressions called the "valleculae."[14,15]

The roughened appearance of the anterior two-thirds of the tongue—the papillary portion—results from four types of papillae, which differ in shape, color, and function. Thread-like projections—filiform papillae—are found on the apex of the tongue, and their toughened outer surface is well suited for mastication. Round, red, mushroom-shaped projections—fungiform papillae—contain only a few taste buds and are scattered between the filiform papillae in the apex on the lateral margin of the tongue. These papillae in the apex are sensitive to sweet taste, whereas those at the lateral margins are sensitive to salty taste. In front of the sulcus terminalis are eight to ten circular upraisings that are surrounded by a narrow mucosal fold or trench. These are called the "circumvallate papillae." They contain numerous tastebuds (in the mucosal folds) and are sensitive to bitter substances.[14,15,153]

The epithelium covering the tongue is thin and highly vascularized, giving the surface a reddish color. It is also highly innervated by sensory nerves and is sensitive to pain, temperature, and touch (trigeminal nerve or fifth cranial nerve) and to taste in the anterior two-thirds (facial nerve or seventh cranial nerve) and posterior one-third (glossopharyngeal nerve or ninth cranial nerve) of the tongue.[14,15,153]

The ventral or undersurface of the tongue (Fig. 1–31*B*) is covered by a delicate lining membrane that is found on other epithelial surfaces in the oral cavity that are unexposed to abrasion. It is smooth in appearance compared to the dorsum of the tongue and contains a midline mucosal fold, called the "lingual frenulum," which extends along the undersurface for a variable distance and attaches the tongue to the floor of the mouth. This structure is not functionally significant and is only of clinical interest when it is short and restricts movement of the tongue, resulting in a condition called "ankyloglossia."[154–156] On either side of the base of the frenulum, two mucosal folds (sublingual folds) bulge upward from the floor of the mouth. The sublingual folds contain a series of small openings through which saliva passes into the oral cavity from the sublingual

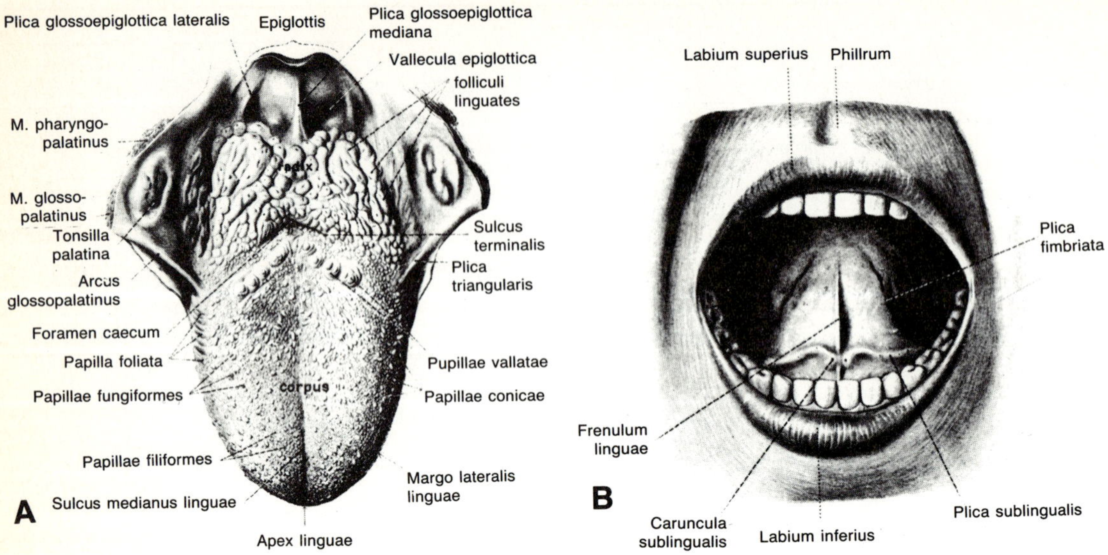

Figure 1–31 *A*, The dorsum of the tongue and *B*, the undersurface of the tongue. (From Sobatta J. Lehmanns med Atlanten Deskriptive Anatomie, Band III. Munich: JF Lehmanns, Verlag, 1922.)

glands. At the end of each sublingual fold is a dilation called the "caruncle," which is the aperture for salivary secretions from the submaxillary gland. On either side of the frenulum is a scalloped mucosal fold called the "plica fimbriata"—the fibriated fold. It runs lateral to the frenulum in an anteromedial to posterolateral direction.[14,15]

Quantitative data (see Table 1–4) on sublingual dimensions are only available for children age 1 month to 13 years.[151,152] The data indicate no significant sex differences.

Muscles

There have been several comprehensive studies of the morphology of the human tongue.[157–163] However, confusion still exists about the fine details of fiber orientation and direction and about the pattern of muscle fibers within the body of the tongue. This confusion may result from normal anatomic variations; vaguely defined measurement points used by investigators; lack of stringent controls for age, sex, and race; and/or the different research methods employed. Detailed discussion of these issues and the detailed anatomy of the lingual musculature is beyond the scope of this chapter. The interested reader is encouraged to examine the sources cited by Barnwell.[162,163]

The tongue is composed of a highly complex connective tissue support system[158] that serves as a scaffolding for the tongue, thus serving three major functions: (1) separating various muscle groups from each other; (2) providing various points of attachment for the intrinsic muscles; and (3) containing blood vessels and nerves that perfuse and innervate the tongue. This framework plays an important role in the biomechanics of specific tongue muscles.[158]

A functional classification of the lingual musculature, derived from several sources, is found in Table 1–5. The muscles of the tongue may be anatomically and functionally divided into intrinsic and extrinsic groups. These muscle groupings are not entirely anatomically distinct. Fibers from the intrinsic and extrinsic muscles are freely interwoven with each other, and only through careful dissection and microscopic study can the fibers be systematically differentiated. Except for the palatoglossus, which is innervated by the vagus nerve (tenth cranial nerve) through the plexus pharyngeus, all other intrinsic and extrinsic tongue muscles are innervated by the hypoglossal nerve (twelfth cranial nerve).[14,15]

The intrinsic muscles of the tongue both originate from and insert into the body of the tongue. They consist of four pairs of muscles and one unpaired (superior longitudinal) muscle and are named for the direction in which they course in the tongue: longitudinally, vertically, and transversely (Fig. 1–32). Direct stimulation of individual lingual muscles is technically difficult to accomplish. Information on

TABLE 1–5 Functional Classification of the Intrinsic and Extrinsic Muscles of the Tongue

Muscle	*Function*
Intrinsic group	
Superior longitudinal	Shortens tongue; turns tongue tip and sides upwards; makes dorsum concave
Inferior longitudinal	Shortens tongue; lowers tongue tip and sides
Transverse	Narrows tongue and increases its height
Vertical	Flattens tongue and widens it
Extrinsic group	
Styloglossus	Retracts and elevates tongue
Genioglossus	
anterior fibers	Retract and depress tip
intermediate fibers	Draw tongue forward and may lower middle of tongue
posterior fibers	Draw tongue forward
Hyglossus	Lowers the tongue and may help draw it backward
Styloglossus	Elevates and retracts tongue
Palatoglossus	Elevates back of tongue

the activity and biomechanics of the intrinsic muscles is therefore largely based on inference from gross anatomic studies and, to a lesser extent, from histologic studies.[14,15]

The actions of the intrinsic tongue muscles are visually described as if they occurred independently. However, it is more likely that they occur in combination with other reciprocally innervated intrinsic muscles and in combination with specific extrinsic muscles. As a group, the intrinsic tongue muscles alter the shape of the tongue dorsum by such actions as narrowing and flattening the blade and lifting or lowering the tongue tip. These maneuvers are important for the precise movments involved in speech production.

All extrinsic tongue muscles (see Fig. 1–33) are paired and have at least one attachment onto a structure external to the tongue such as the mandible (genioglossus), hyoid bone (hyoglossus), styloid process (styloglossus), and soft palate (palatoglossus). These muscles move the entire tongue within the oral cavity, protrude it outside the oral cavity, and alter the shape of the tongue to a limited extent. Thus protrusion, retraction, lateralization, elevation, and depression of the entire tongue, or large regions like the posterior portion of the dorsum or lateral margin, are made possible by differential activities of the extrinsic lingual muscles.[14,15]

Nonspeech Functions

The tongue is unquestionably the most important articulator for speech; however, it also plays essential roles in mastication and swallowing. In mastication, which involves a specific sequence of movements, its role is extensive and includes specific morphologic adjustments in order to receive the ingested food, position it on to the cutting edges of the teeth, and mix the food with saliva into a bolus preparatory to swallowing.[164]

The oral phase of swallowing has been studied by numerous investigators, and excellent descriptions of the process can be found in several sources.[164–167] The tongue's role in the oral stage of swallowing is to serve as a propulsive force that ejects the bolus from the oral cavity in a manner aptly described as akin to toothpaste being squeezed out of its tube.[165] The delicately sequenced action of the tongue, soft palate, faucial pillars, facial muscles, and mandible make this extraordinarily complex behavior appear deceivingly simple. It is not, and it is worthy of serious study by students of orofacial physiology.

THE TEMPOROMANDIBULAR JOINT AND THE CRANIOMANDIBULAR MUSCULATURE

The movement of the mandible is made possible by a uniquely structured joint and through the action of the muscles that attach to the mandible. The structural and functional relationships of this muscloskeletal unit are described in this section.

Postnatal Developmental Morphology

At birth, the temporomandibular joint (TMJ) is almost completely dependent on its joint capsule

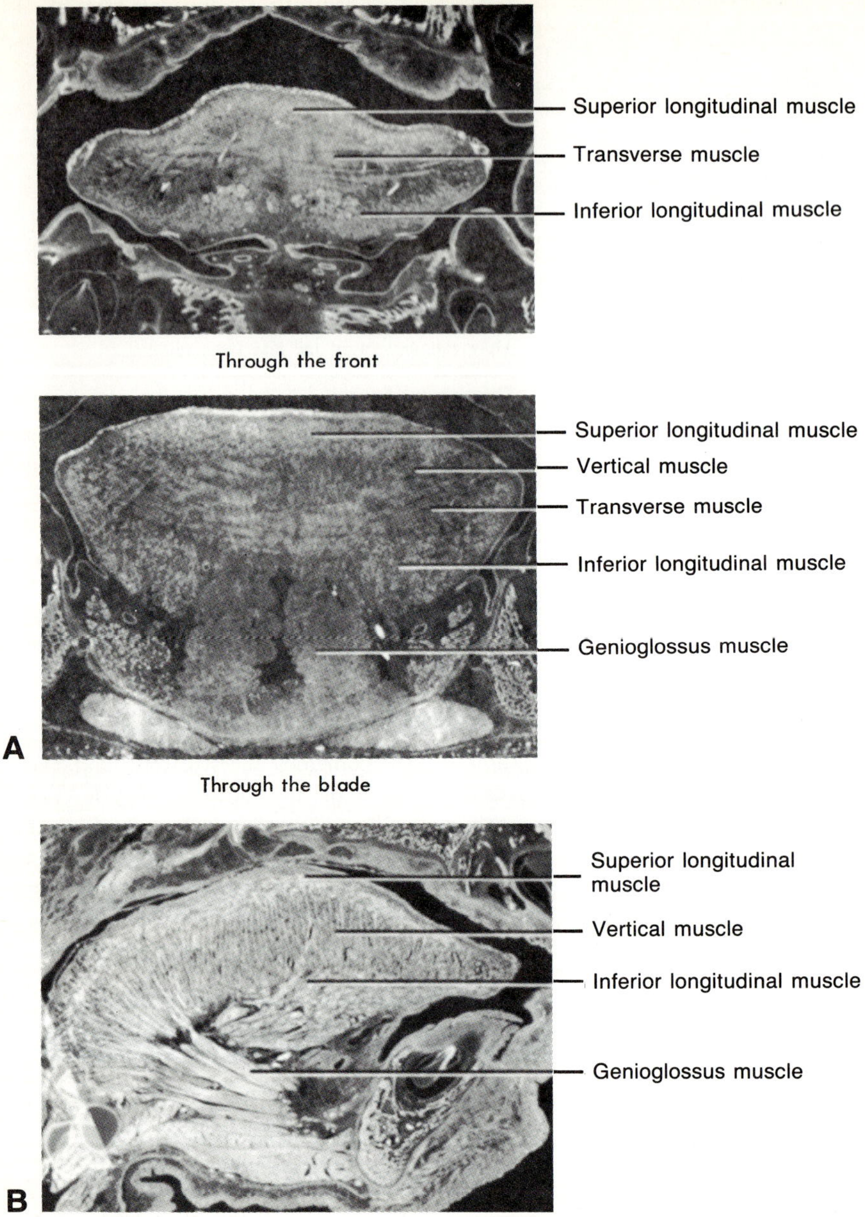

Figure 1–32 *A*, Frontal and *B*, parasagittal sections through a 5-month human fetal tongue. (From Zemlin W. Speech and hearing science: anatomy and physiology. Englewood Cliffs, NJ: Prentice-Hall, 1981:322.)

for stability. The TMJ is not structurally mature at birth;[168] the articular fossa is flat (compared to its concave adult shape), and no articular eminence exists. Only after the eruption of primary dentition does the articular eminence begin to develop and the articular fossa deepens. By 10 to 12 years of age, mature structural relationships are attained. These changes in the TMJ are the result of increased functional demands associated with mastication and deglutition and of changes in the shape and angulation of the cranial base.

The craniomandibular muscles, in addition to their obvious role as movers of the mandible, are involved in several postnatal changes in orofacial structure and function. The TMJ and the mandibular muscle activity become more prominent with the appearance of primary dentition and eating of solid foods.[169] During infancy, these muscles take a secondary role to facial muscle activity, which predominates. Craniomandibular muscles also play a central role in the postnatal development of the mandible.[170] Investigators have determined that the activity of the medial pterygoid muscle determines the ultimate form of the gonion and that the temporalis muscle activity determines the morphology of the coronoid process.

Anatomy of the Temporomandibular Joint

The TMJ is unique among articulations in the human body. The anatomy and functional role of each component of the TMJ are described in the following discussion.

Unique Properties

The TMJ is highly specialized and differs from other movable joints in several important ways:

1. The articular surfaces of the joint are not covered by hyaline cartilage.
2. An articular disc is interposed between the articular surfaces; it functionally divides the joint into an upper component that functions as an arthrodial (sliding) joint and a lower component that functions as a ginglymoid (rotatory) joint.
3. The upper (arthrodial) joint cavity is distinguished from other joints in the body by the absence of a layer of bone.
4. The lower (ginglymoid) joint is distinguished from other joints in not containing a fixed articular bone.
5. The function of the temporomandibular articulation is dependent on the coordinated activity or coupling of right and left joints; thus the TMJ is really a bilateral articulation in which both joints may be active to an equal extent, undergoing similar types of movements, or in which one condyle may be active while the other is passively translated in space or is fixed.
6. The movements of the TMJ are not dictated by the configuration of the articular fossa as is characteristic of most movable joints; it is governed by the coordinated action of the craniomandibular muscles, which exert forces on various parts of the mandible.
7. The position of the mandible and the position of the structural components of the TMJ are influenced by the presence, position, and form of contacting teeth in the upper and lower arches.

Components

Each TMJ is composed of a mandibular condyle, an articular fossa and eminence, an articular disc with a joint capsule, and associated ligaments. The anatomy of each of these components and their contribution to TMJ function are described next.

Mandibular Condyle. The mandibular condyle is a superiorly projecting process from the neck of the mandible. It projects 15 to 20 mm lateromedially and 8 to 10 mm anteroposteriorly. The lateromedial axis of the condyle is highly convex, whereas the anteroposterior axis is only slightly convex. Only the anterosuperior part of the condyle serves as the articulalting surface of the joint; the posterior portion is nonfunctional.[153]

Articular Fossa and Articular Eminence. The articular fossa and articular eminence are parts of the temporal bone (Fig. 1–33). The articular (glenoid) fossa is a concave depression on the anteroinferior aspect of the squamous portion of the tem-

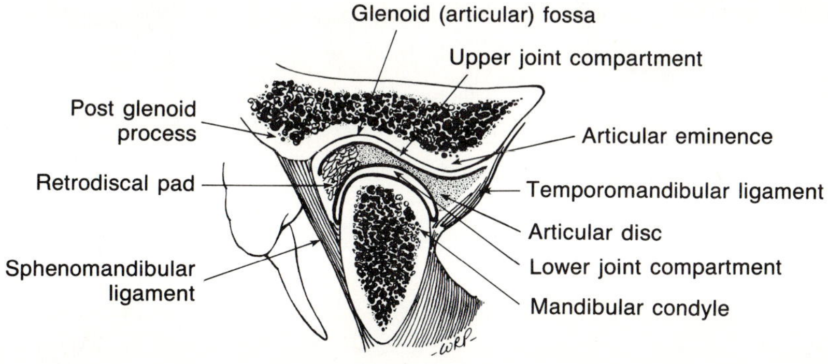

Figure 1–33 Diagram of a sagittal section through the temporomandibular joint. (After Silverman S. Oral physiology. St Louis: CV Mosby, 1961:320.)

poral bone. It is bound anteriorly by a convex prominence of bone called the "articular eminence" and posteriorly by a conical projection called the "post glenoid process." The roof of the fossa is thin, suggesting that it is a functionally insignificant part of the joint. There are upraisings laterally and medially that restrict excessive movement and dislocation of the condyle in these directions. The medial articular lip is always more substantial structurally.[153]

The articular tubercle or eminence is the anterior boundary of the articular fossa and serves an essential functional role. It is a transverse elevation of bone (5 to 15 mm in height) at the root of the zygomatic process of the temporal bone (see Fig. 1–33), and is highly convex anteroposteriorly and slightly concave lateromedially. The anterior border is indistinct, and there is no anterior slope. The surface of the articular tubercle is covered with hyaline cartilage, attesting to its functional role in joint action.[153]

Articular Disc. Interposed between the mandibular condyle and articular fossa is the miniscus or articular disc (see Fig. 1–33). It is an avascular biconcave disc composed of fibrocartilage, which is thickest along the periphery and which thins toward the center. The thickness of the disc appears to be correlated with the thickness of the articular eminence. The upper surface is convex, approximating the shape of the glenoid fossa. The lower surface is concave and approximates the contour of the head of the mandibular condyle. Anteriorly, the disc is fused with the ligament of the lateral pterygoid muscle. Posteriorly, it blends with a thick layer of loose vascularized connective tissue called the "retrodiscal pad," which is attached to the joint capsule and is freely movable. Laterally and medially, the disc is attached to the margins of the condyle. This anatomic feature insures that the disc and mandibular condyle move in unison.[14,15,153]

Articular Capsule and Ligaments. The TMJ is surrounded by a joint capsule, which is composed of fibrous tissue extending from the anterior, medial, and lateral surfaces of the articular tubercle and from the anterior surface of the post glenoid process. (Fig. 1–34). A synovial membrane attaches to the anterior and posterior aspects of the retrodiscal pad. The fibers of the joint capsule are placed less densely and attached more loosely anteriorly, posteriorly, and medially than laterally where the fibers are densely packed and reinforced. These lateral fibers are called the "temporomandibular ligament" and they serve the important role of limiting retrusive movements of the mandible, thus averting damage to vascular and neural structures contained in the retrodiscal area.[153]

The temporomandibular ligament has an inner or horizontal band of fibers, which courses from the anterolateral aspect of the disc to the lateral aspect of the condyle, and a vertical or outer band of fibers, which courses from the articular tubercle to the neck of the condyle (Fig. 1–34). The sphenomandibular and the stylomandibular ligaments, often called accessory ligaments of the TMJ, serve no support or physiologic function.[153]

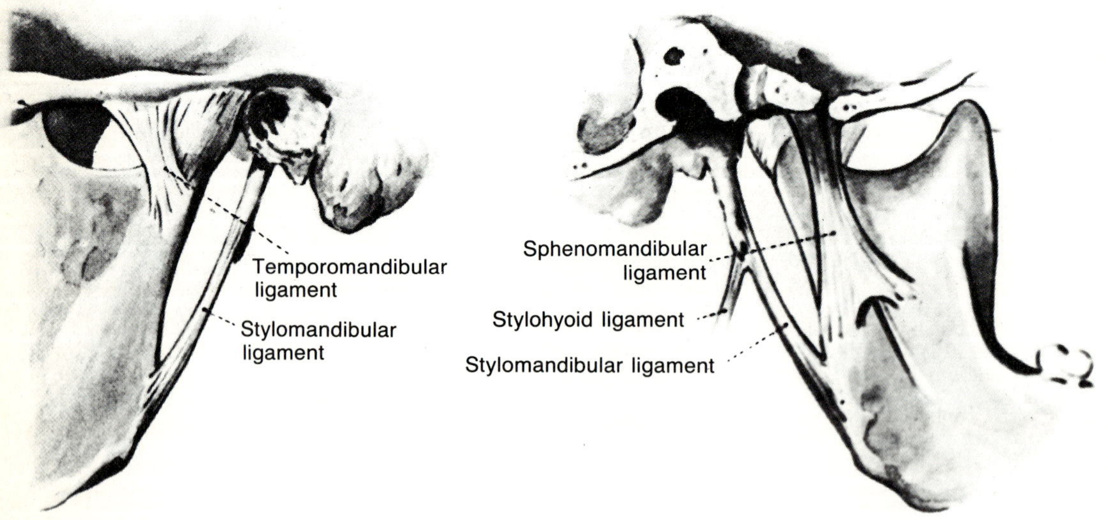

Figure 1-34 Ligaments of the tempormandibular joint. (From Massler M, Schour I. Atlas of the mouth, 2nd ed. Chicago: American Dental Association, 1958: plate 36.)

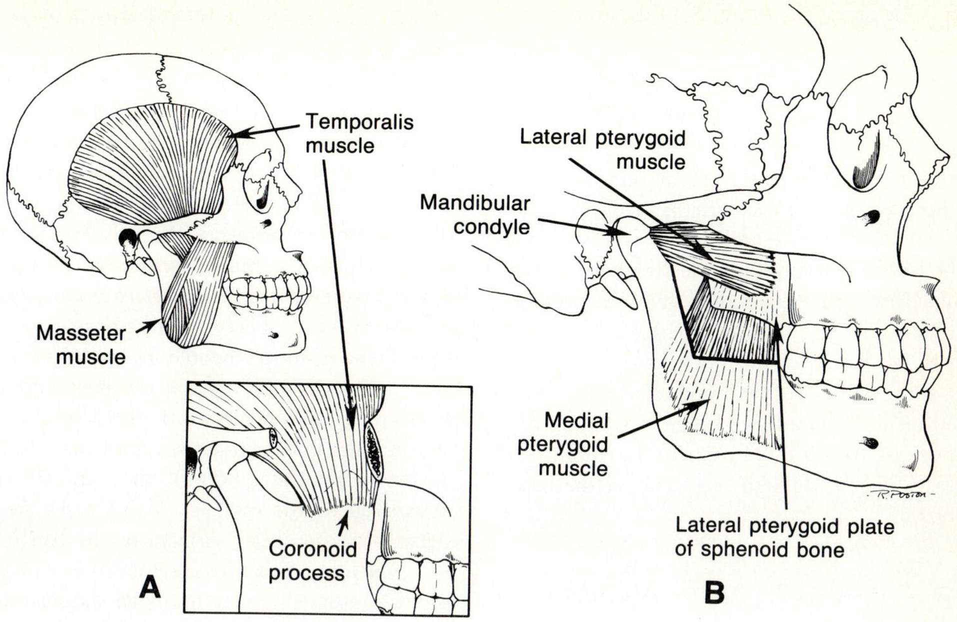

Figure 1–35 The craniomandibular (masticatory) muscles. *A*, Temporalis and masseter muscles. *B*, Lateral and medial pterygoid muscles. (After Basmajian JV. Primary anatomy, 5th ed. Baltimore: Williams & Wilkins, 1970:137.)

Craniomandibular Muscles

Five pairs of muscles move the mandible: the temporalis, the masseter, the medial (internal) pterygoid and lateral (external) pterygoid muscles, and the anterior digastric muscles. They are all innervated by the mandibular branch of the trigeminal nerve (fifth cranial nerve). All of the aforementioned muscles, except the anterior digastrics, are referred to as the muscles of mastication. Their relationship to the mandible is illustrated in Figure 1–35. The craniomandibular muscles elevate, depress, lateralize, protrude, and retrude the mandible (Table 1–6).

Physiology of the Movements of the Temporomandibular Joint

Movements of the mandible are made possible by action of the TMJ. These movements may be classified into basic and functional movements. Each class of movement illustrates different properties and functional relationships of the TMJ. These are summarized in the following discussion.

TABLE 1–6 Functional Movements of the Temporomandibular Joint and Associated Activity of Craniomandibular Muscles

Action	*Upper (U)/Lower (L) Joint(s)*	*Type of Movement*	*Muscles (Prime Movers)*
Opening	U + L	Sliding and hinge	Lateral pterygoid (inferior head); anterior digastric
Closing	U + L	Sliding and hinge	Medial pterygoid; masseter; temporalis; lateral pterygoid (superior head)
Protrusion	U	Sliding	Lateral pterygoid (inferior head)
Retrusion	U	Sliding	Temporalis (horizontal fibers); masseter (deep fibers)
Lateralization	U + L (side of deviation)	Sliding and hinge	Ipsilateral horizontal fibers of temporalis; lateral pterygoid
	U (contralateral side)	Sliding	Medial pterygoid

Basic Movements of the Mandible

Sliding and rotation are the basic movements of the mandible. Changes in the intra-articular relationships of the TMJ are illustrated in Figure 1–36. Sliding or transilatory movement occurs in the upper compartment near the articular disc and the glenoid fossa. The condyle and disc move as a unit because the lateral pterygoid muscle attaches to both the articular disc and the condyle and because the disc is attached to the condyle medially and laterally. This results in a sliding forward of these structures in unison along the posterior aspect of the articular eminence. Rotatory or hinge movement occurs in the articular disc. Movement is through a transverse axis passing through the center of the head of the condyle.[65,153]

Functional Movements of the Mandible

Functional movements of the mandible result from a combination of sliding and hinge movements of the TMJ, which are initiated by activity of the craniomandibular muscles (see Table 1–6). Action of these muscles on the TMJ result in opening, closing, protrusive, retrusive, and lateral movements of the mandible.[153]

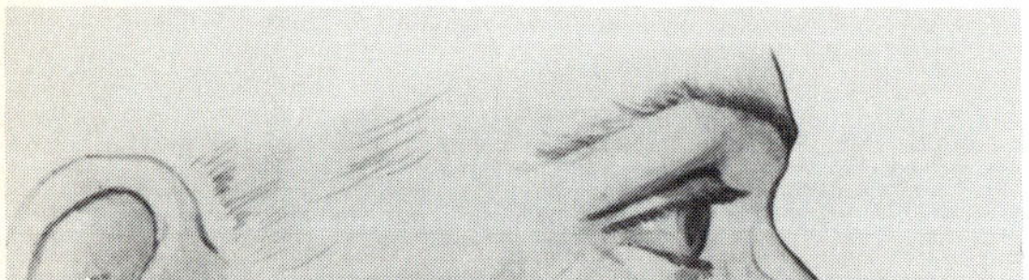

Figure 1-36 Anatomic and spatial relationships of the temporomandibular joint during opening and closing movements. (From Massler M, Schour I. Atlas of the mouth, 2nd ed. Chicago: American Dental Association, 1958: plate 37.)

Opening. The opening movement of the mandible is initiated by sliding activity caused by bilateral contraction of the medial pterygoid muscles, which fix the condyles against the posterior aspect of the articular eminence (Fig. 1–36). Immediately following this, a hinge movement occurs through action of the anterior digastric muscles, which lowers the mandible below its rest position. The hinge movement is supplemented by a sliding movement that draws the head of the condyle downward and forward across the surface of the articular eminence as the condyle continues to rotate about a transverse axis through the center of the condyle. This maneuver opens the mouth and increases the distance between the occlusal surfaces of the teeth.[153]

Closing. The closing movement of the mandible is initiated largely from the sliding motion that draws the condylar head backward and upward along the articular eminence (see Fig. 1–36). This closing movement is accomplished by contraction of several muscles: the masseter, the medial pterygoid, and the posterior fibers of the temporalis. The initial sliding (backward) movement of the mandible closes the mouth to approximately two-thirds of its maximal opening. Therefore, a combination of sliding and hinge (rotatory) movements raise the mandible to its rest position.[153]

Protrusion and Retrusion. Protrusion and retrusion of the mandible are largely a transilatory or sliding maneuver that occurs in the upper compartment of the joint. This maneuver requires symmetrical activity in both the right and left joints. The condyle and disc move as a single unit. Protrusion is effected by only one muscle—the lateral pterygoid—which attaches into the articular disc and condyle and exerts a linear force in that direction. Retrusion occurs from differential contraction of the posterior fibers of the temporalis and deep fibers of the masseter and through contraction of the geniohyoid muscles.[143]

Lateral. Lateral movements (or shifts) of the mandible result from differential or complimentary action of the left and right TMJs and mandibular muscles. The lateral movement of the mandible occurs when one condyle and one disc on the same side are pulled forward, downward, and medially to the base of the articular eminence while the contralateral (resting) condyle undergoes limited movement and rotates around a vertical axis. The resting condyle moves slightly forward and outward (Bennett's movement) while the contralateral condyle is undergoing the extensive movement described previously. The extent of movement of the resting condyle is limited by the temporomandibular ligaments.[153]

THE FACIAL MUSCLES

The facial muscles play essential roles in such diverse activities as speech, facial expression, swallowing and in helping to maintain normal occlusion and proper alignment of the teeth. These functions and other aspects of facial muscle activity are discussed in this section.

Postnatal Developmental Morphology

At birth, the facial muscles are more well developed than most other striated muscles in the body. This early development underlies their essential role in feeding of the infant and child during the first 12 to 18 months of life. By 18 to 24 months, the child develops a mature (somatic) swallowing pattern in which the masticatory muscles rather than the facial muscles are the predominant forces during feeding.[169] This transition in oral muscle function coincides with the eruption of the primary dentition and with the eating of solid foods. These changes in oral morphology require controlled movement of the jaw in order to provide efficient biting, tearing, and grinding, which are essential for effective mastication and deglutition.

External Features of the Face

Before a discussion is launched into the specifics of the facial musculature, it is helpful to review the external features of the face that are changed by the actions of the facial muscles. Figure 1–37 illustrates typical features of the adult face. The face can be roughly divided into upper, middle, and lower thirds. The length of the nose greatly affects this spatial relationship.

Lips

The lips are of particular importance to a normal appearance; a furrow in the skin around the lips adds greatly to the esthetics of this area.

The upper lip is separated from the cheek by

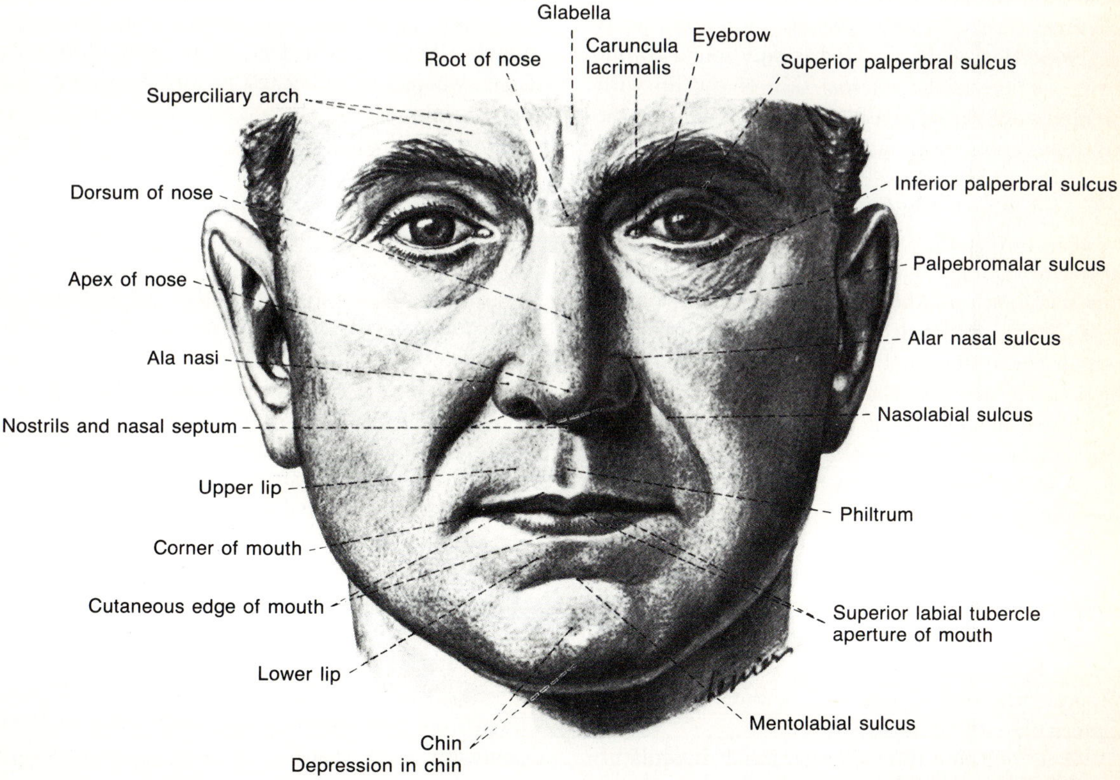

Figure 1–37 External landmarks of the face. (From Figge FHJ, ed. Atlas of human anatomy, Vol. 2. New York: Hafner Press, 1974.)

a deep groove, the nasolabial groove. It starts at the wing of the nose and extends inferolaterally, terminating some distance from the corner of the mouth. The upper lip is characterized by a midline groove of variable depth called the "philtrum." The lower lip is separated from the chin by the sharp and deep labiomental groove. Its depth depends on several factors among which are the thickness of the lip, the prominence of the chin, and the age of the individual.

The lip is divided anatomically into three regions: the skin of the external area, the vermillion border, and the mucous membrane of the vestibule.[148] The epithelium on the outside and the mucosa on the inside of the lips are tightly adherent to the connective tissue covering the muscular portion of the lips. This arrangement causes the skin and mucosa to follow the movements of the musculature of the lip without much folding.

Although there is regional specialization in the epithelium of the lip, it is supported by a connective tissue layer (dermis) that varies in thickness and in the amount of hair follicles as well as the glandular and vascular tissues present. Beneath the dermis is a muscular layer containing the orbicularis oris fibers. The skin on the exterior surface of the lip most distant from the mouth opening is thin, but able to withstand abrasive forces. It contains thin hairs and ducts of sweat and sebaceous glands but is rather deficient in blood vessels. The vermillion border is the red portion of the lips and is only found in humans; it connects the external skin of the lip with the mucosa of the vestibule. The epithelium in the vermillion is thin and translucent and takes on a red color because of the diffuse network of capillaries found in the subepithelial layers that are visible through it. The epithelium is lacking in glands and so is subject to drying out and becoming chafed. A distinct transition exists between the vermillion and the mucosa of the vestibule; the latter is a lighter pink in color and is devoid of hair follicles, having much the same composition as the mucosa of the cheek.[148]

There are important characteristics of the lip that are related to the shape of the vermillon border. In the middle of the vermillon of the upper lip is a protrusion called the "tubercle." Above it, the vermillian border dips slightly on both sides, forming a Cupid's bow. A slight indentation corresponding to the tubercle is found in the lower lip. These are the distinctive features of the lips. Conditions such as cleft lip or traumatic scarring not only result in physical deformity to this region, but also produce appreciable esthetic disturbances.[153]

The following discussion on facial musculature examines the nature of the muscles that cause movements in the face.

Anatomy of the Facial Musculature

There are several unique features of the facial muscles that differentiate them from other striated muscles in the body. In addition, the facial muscles exhibit a high degree of heterogeneity in structure and function. These aspects and others of the facial musculature are reviewed in the following discussion.

Unique Properties

The facial muscles are unique among the striated muscles of the body in several ways.

1. They are organized into flat sheets, which are located superficially, in close proximity to the skin from which they are difficult to separate out. Thus contraction of the facial musculature directly changes the contour and shape of the facial skin, which is necessary to order to show emotion and facial gestures.[14,15,153]
2. The muscle fibers course through a layer of adipose tissue on their way toward insertion into the facial skin or mucous membrane. One end of the muscle fiber is attached either to bone or to deep fascia, whereas the other inserts into the skin or mucous membrane.[14,15,153]
3. Facial muscles lack fascial sheaths and typical tendinous attachments found in most other striated muscle fibers. Facial muscle fibers insert into the skin or mucous membrane by thin, isolated fibers, which are continuations of the connective tissue sheaths surrounding individual fiber bundles.[98] This arrangement may facilitate the discrete action of muscle fibers on the skin and enhance the coordinated action of isolated fascicles within a muscle and between contiguous muscles.[171]
4. There is great inter- and intrasubject variability in the size and shape of facial muscles, which is usually the rule and not the exception.[98,172,173] Variability is most notable in muscles inferior to the oral opening.[173] The morphologic variability is attributed to differences in the number of muscle fibers, the space between fascicles, and the variation in the architecture of the muscle.
5. Nerves innervating facial muscles approach them from their deep surface rather than more superficially as is customarily seen in other striated

muscles. The facial muscles are also richly innervated, allowing them to perform refined and subtle movements.[14,15,153]

Regional Specialization

The facial muscles can be divided into four distinct groups based on function and topography. The muscles surrounding the eyes (orbicularis oculi, corrugator supercilii, and procerus) belong to the ocular group. Muscles related to nasal function (nasalis, compressor naris, dilator naris, and depressor septi nasi) compose the nasal group. Muscles of the external ear (anterior auricular, superior auricular, and posterior auricular muscles) and of the scalp (frontal and occipital bellies of the occipitofrontal muscle) form the auricular and epicranial groups, respectively. The remaining muscles insert into the region surrounding the opening into the mouth—the rima oris. These are referred to as the oral group or the perioral muscles. The following section describes perioral muscles because they are most important in speech and other oral functions.[14,15,153]

Perioral Muscles

The anatomy of the perioral muscles is described in standard anatomy texts and in detailed anatomic studies.[172–174] All of the facial muscles are innervated by the facial nerve (seventh cranial nerve). The topographic arrangement of facial muscles as they approach the rima oris is illustrated in Figure 1–38. The muscles insert into the perioral area from several directions. Most of the perioral muscles converge at the angle of the mouth into a tendinous band called the "modiolus" before inserting into the skin or mucous membrane overlying the orbicularis oris. Once these muscles insert into this region, their fibers become intertwined to form the bulk of the upper and lower lips, and they become arranged into superficial and deep layers (Fig. 1–39).

Fibers that insert superficially into the skin or mucous membrane of the lip become extensively interlaced and oriented in various directions. This arrangement provides the lips with great mobility. Fibers in the deep layer course elliptically around the oral opening, permitting them to contribute to sphincteric closure of the lips.

The perioral muscles are usually assigned specific functions (Table 1–7) based on convention, anatomic inference from points of attachment, and from the direction of coursing muscle fibers. It is certain that such classifications are not based completely on physiologic data, which are scarce. Quantitative data on the length, breadth, and angulation of the perioral musculature have only recently been reported.[173] There have been few physiologic investigations of the specific functions of the perioral muscles.[174–177] The buccinator muscle has been studied electromyographically during several activities,[178,179] but data from these studies do not alter the basic functions hithertofore assigned to these muscles. Rather, the variability of performance and circumstances that result in maximal activity of the muscle are more clearly understood.

The orbicularis oris muscle is not directly attached to bone. The deep layer, primarily formed by the buccinator muscle, is reinforced superiorly by the musculi incisivi labii superioris, which attaches to the maxilla, and inferiorly by the musculi incisivi

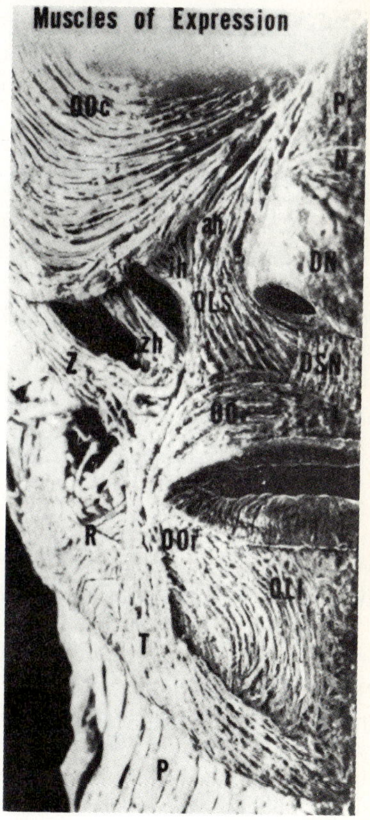

Figure 1–38 Dissection of the perioral musculature. Abbreviations: OOc = orbicularis oculi; Pr = procerus; N = nasalis; QLS = levator labi superioris; (levator anguli oris is not shown, but is deep to QLS); zh = zygomaticus minor; ih = infraorbital part of levator labii superioris; ah = levator labii superioris alaeque nasi; DN = dialtor naris; DSN = depressor septi nasi; Z = zygomaticus major; R = risorius; OOr = orbicularis oris; T = depressor anguli oris; QLI = depressor labii inferioris; P = platysma. (From Martone AL. Anatomy of facial expression and its prosthetic significance. J Prosthet Dent 1962; 12:1020.)

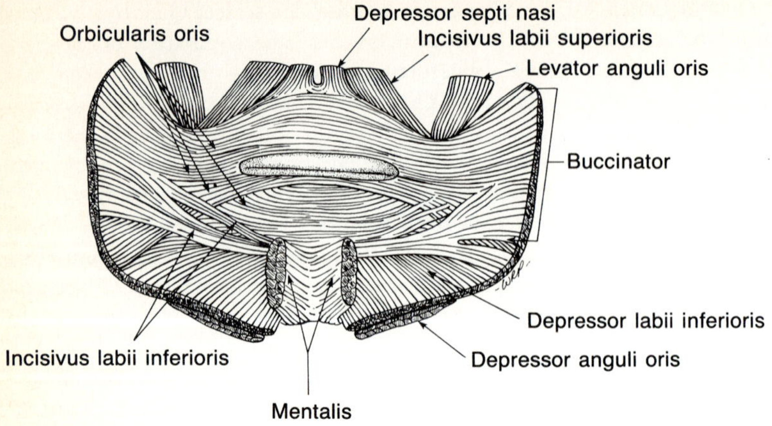

Figure 1–39 Deep and superficial layers of perioral muscles as viewed from behind. (After Sobatta J. Lehmanns Med Atlanten Deskriptive Anatomie, Band III. Munich: JF Lehmanns, Verlag, 1922.)

TABLE 1–7 Functional Classification of the Perioral Musculature

Muscle	*Action*
Zygomaticus minor Levator labii superioris Levator labii superioris alaquae nasi	Elevate upper lip near midline and lateral third of lip near philtrum
Depressor labii inferioris	Lowers upper lip and draws it slightly laterally
Levator anguli oris Zygomaticus minor	Elevate corner of mouth and lateral aspect of lower lip
Depressor anguli oris Platysma	Lower corner of mouth; lower lateral aspect of upper lip
Mentalis	Protrude lower lip
Orbicularis oris Buccinator	Protrude upper lip
Buccinator (fibers lateral to the modiolus) Zygomaticus major Risorius	Retract corner of mouth
Buccinator (deep fibers) Orbicularis oris	Compress lips

labii inferioris, which interconnects it to the mandible. The majority of the perioral muscle fibers are confined to one side and do not encircle the rima oris continuously. Muscle fibers interlace with their counterparts from the other side at midline. In the upper lip, this interlacing of muscle fibers occurs in the region of the philtrum where they attach onto the tendinous strip extending from the base of the nasal septum. In the lower lip, this reinforcement occurs near midline through interdigitation with fibers of the depressor labii inferioris.[14,15,172]

The sphincter function of the orbicularis oris is achieved through the interlacing of muscle fibers from the buccinator muscles, depressor anguli oris, and levator anguli oris. These fibers converge at the angle of the mouth (i.e., the modiolus) and then insert into the labial region in a complex fashion (Fig. 1–40). The upper fibers of the buccinator muscle be-

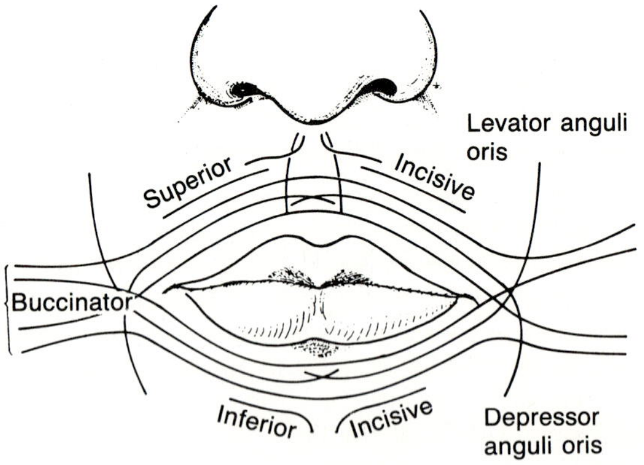

Figure 1–40 Diagram of decussating fibers of circumoral musculature, which illustrate their potential sphincter (purse-string) function. (From Graber TM. Craniofacial and dentitional development. In: Falkner F. Human development. Philadelphia: WB Saunders, 1966:563.)

come inserted into the mucous membrane of the upper lip, and the lower fibers insert into the mucous membrane of the lower lip. The central fibers decussate at the modiolus with the upper fibers inserting into the lower lip and the lower fibers inserting into the upper lip. The main bundle of fibers of the depressor anguli oris insert into the upper lip with a small number inserting into the lower lip. Similarly, the major bundle of fibers of the levator anguli oris insert into the upper lip with a small number inserting into the lower lip. Similarly, the major bundle of fibers of the levator anguli oris insert into the lower lip with a smaller number of fibers inserting into the upper lip. Contraction of the superior and inferior anguli oris in concert with the buccinator muscle and the orbicularis oris compresses the lips in a purse-string fashion, forming a firm seal during swallowing and sucking. Although the orbicularis oris is not a single anatomic entity, it should be considered a functional entity.[170] This notion is challenged by electromyographic data from several investigators who have shown that orbicularis oris superioris and orbicularis oris inferioris function differentially and in a complex fashion and so should be considered as separate muscles.[153,177,179,180]

The Potential Role of Facial Muscle Activity in Triggering Jaw Movements

In light of the intimate relationship between facial muscle activity and movement of the mandible during mastication and speech, it is tempting to search for a common physiologic basis for this association. It has been suggested that activation of certain functional groupings of facial muscles may serve to trigger craniomandibular (jaw) muscle activity and to coordinate jaw movements within certain facial muscle activities.[172] Such integration would be helpful in the articulation of speech sounds and during swallowing.

As an example of how this might work, Martone noted that there is anatomic continuity between the levator anguli oris (caninus) and the depressor anguli (triangularis).[172] This continuity occurs through the functional linkage of the muscles at the modiolus. If both muscles are viewed as a single anatomic unit, the vertically coursing muscle fibers may be thought of as having a fixed point of attachment on the maxilla and insertion onto the mobile mandible. When both muscles contract, as occurs in swallowing, their modioli become fixed, and a force vector is generated cranially toward the more stable point of attachment on the maxilla. This may result in elevating the mandible or may serve to facilitate the positioning of the mandible to permit contact of labial surfaces. Contraction of the buccinator muscles, which have attachments on the mandible and maxilla in the molar region, may exert a force on the mandible that stimulates or triggers its elevation.[172] Other investigators have also reported that the buccinator muscle contributes to mandibular movements.[178] Investigators have explained these actions as sympathetic and not prime action. More research is needed to examine how the facial muscles may influence the positioning of the mandible.

Neuroanatomic data from several sources support the possibility that facial muscle activation may influence jaw muscle activity and consequently jaw movement.[180–182] These investigators report the presence of direct interconnections between some fibers of the motor division of the trigeminal nerve (innervating mandibular muscles) and the facial nerve (innervating facial muscles). These anastomoses provide avenues for the transmission of proprioception from facial muscles via branches from the trigeminal nerve and for efferent signals from the facial nerve to be transmitted along the mandibular branch of the trigeminal nerve. Thus efferent signals originating in the motor nucleus of the facial nerve may in some way facilitate reciprocal activation of the mandibular muscles. These neuroanatomic relationships require detailed study, but suggest the possibility that the facial muscles may have a more direct role in controlling or influencing jaw movement than has previously been thought.

DIRECTIONS FOR FUTURE RESEARCH

This chapter has reviewed the anatomy and physiology of the organs that compose the peripheral speech mechanism. Although much is known about the structure and function of these organs, there are several areas for future research that are needed in order to gain a better understanding of their roles as speech organs per se.

More detailed information is required about the structural and physiologic changes in the speech mechanisms of children and adolescents. Such data would be invaluable in (1) updating textbooks of anatomy and physiology of the speech mechanism whose descriptions are based on adult morphology and function, and (2) providing clinicians with indices for objective measurement and observation of the functional morphology of the peripheral speech mechanism. Future research on the effects of aging on the peripheral speech mechanism is vitally necessary because little information is available.[183]

Quantitative studies need to be undertaken to specify biomechanical properties or organs of the speech mechanism. Data are needed that document the volume, cross-sectional area, course, and distribution of muscle fibers within all the organs of the peripheral speech mechanism, especially the tongue and the perioral and palatopharyngeal regions. Histochemistry of these various muscle groups would be helpful in identification of the basic biologic properties of these structures. Efforts must be made to specify morphologic differences based on sex and race. These are largely unavailable at present. Moreover, additional research is needed to describe the distribution of and physical properties of connective tissues—particularly elastic and collagenous fibers within the organs of the speech mechanism. These data are essential in order to understand the viscoelastic properties of these structures, the effects of certain tissue interfaces on movement, and their contributions to the displacement of tissues within an organ.

One of the primary benefits of this detailed information is its application in computer modeling of the entire speech mechanism, specific organs therein, and the larynx. Such computer simulation would enable investigators to study the contribution of specific structural or physiologic properties of the speech mechanism to speech or phonatory output.

Further research into the functional morphology of the speech mechanism is warranted. This research must be done on human subjects whenever possible. Infrahuman organisms, no matter how closely related phylogenetically, do *not* have comparable speech mechanisms. Inferences about speech and/or phonatory functions in humans from nonhuman subjects appear to be questionable and also fraught with serious limitations.

The intricacies of the structures forming the peripheral speech mechanism are formidable indeed. However, ultimately, these factors will not determine the success of future research endeavors; initiative, persistence, and creativity will determine them.

SUMMARY

My goal in this chapter has been to review the anatomy and physiology of the organs of the peripheral speech mechanism. In so doing, I have described salient structural and functional properties of the respiratory system, larynx, supralaryngeal airways and the oral and facial regions. Sometimes this has been done without specific regard to speech production, as this is discussed in detail by Weismer (Chapter 8, *Speech Production*) in this volume. My efforts in this chapter have been directed toward providing information about the structure and biologic properties of those organs that are *united in function* during the production of speech and voice. It is my hope that the speech-language pathologist, armed with this information, will develop a fuller appreciation of the processes that amazingly become marshalled during human speech production.

REFERENCES

1. Negus VE. The comparative anatomy and physiology of the larynx. New York: Hafner, 1949.
2. DuBrul L. The evolution of the speech apparatus. Springfield, IL: CC Thomas, 1958.
3. Engel S. Lung structure. Springfield, IL: CC Thomas, 1962.
4. Dunnhil MS. Postnatal growth of the lung. Thorax 1962; 17:329–333.
5. Abramson M, Harker LA. Physiology of the nose. In: Bernstein L, ed. Symposium on nasal cavities. Otolaryngol Clin North Am 1973; 6(3):623–635.
6. Bouhuys A. The physiology of breathing. New York: Grune & Stratton, 1977.
7. Eichorn DH. Physiological development. In: Mussen PH, ed. Carmichael's manual of child psychology. Vol. 1. 3rd ed. New York: John Wiley & Sons, 1970:157.
8. Peiper A. Cerebral function in infancy and childhood. New York: Consultants Bureau, 1963.
9. Comroe JH Jr. Physiology of respiration. Chicago Year Book Medical Publishers, 1965:122.
10. Steen EB, Montague A. Anatomy and physiology. Vol. 2. New York: Barnes & Noble, 1964.
11. Noonan JA. Reversible cor pulmonale due to hypertrophied tonsils and adenoids (abstract). Trans Am Pediatr Soc 1965; 48:202.
12. Ogura JH, Togawa K, Danimkoehler D, Nelson JR, Kawasaki M. Nasal obstruction and the mechanics of breathing. Arch Otolaryngol 1966; 83:135–150.
13. Luke MJ, Mehrizi A, Folger GM, Rowe RO. Chronic nasopharyngeal obstruction causing cor pulmonale. Pediatrics 1966; 37:762–768.
14. Woodburne RT. Essentials of human anatomy. 4th ed. New York: Oxford University Press, 1969.
15. Gray H. Anatomy of the human body. 29th ed. Philadelphia: Lea & Febiger, 1973.
16. Bosma JF. Physiology of the mouth, pharynx and esophagus. In: Paparella MM, Shumrick DA, eds. Otolaryngology. Philadelphia: WB Saunders, 1973:356.
17. Pressman JJ. Physiology of the vocal cords in phonation and respiration. Arch Otolaryngol 1942; 35:355–398.
18. Von Leden H, Isshiki N. An analysis of coughing at the level of the larynx. Arch Otolaryngol 1965; 81:616–625.
19. Garcia M. Observations on the human voice. Proc Soc Lond 1855; 7:300–420.
20. Czermak JN. On the laryngoscope and its employment in physiology and medicine. London: New Sydenham Society, 1861.
21. Rosenthal J. Die Physiologic der Atembewegungen und der Innervation derselben. In: Hermann L, ed. Handbuch der Physiologic. Vol. 4. Leipzig: FCW Fogel, 1882:163.
22. French TR. On a perfected method of photographing the larynx. NY Med J 1884; 40:653–656.
23. Dessy G. Movimenti respiratori del laringe in condizioni normali e pathologiche. Riv Pathol Clin Tuberc 1938; 12:791–806.

24. Fink BR, Basek M, Epanchin V. The mechanism of opening of the human larynx. Laryngoscope 1956; 66:410–425.
25. Von Leden H, Moore GP. The larynx and voice: the function of the normal larynx. Arch Otolaryngol 1957; 66:735–736.
26. Ardran GM, Kemp FH. The mechanism of the larynx part 1: the movements of the arytenoid and cricoid cartilages. Br J Radiol 1966; 39:641–654.
27. Stanescu DC, Pattijn J, Clement J, Van de Woestijne KP. Glottis opening and airway resistance. J Appl Physiol 1972; 32:460–466.
28. Clement J, Stanescu DC, Van de Woestijne KP. Glottis opening and effort-dependent part of the isovolume pressure-flow curves. J Appl Physiol 1973; 34:18–22.
29. Fink BR. The human larynx. New York: Raven Press, 1975.
30. Judson LSV, Weaver AT. Voice science. 2nd ed. New York: Appleton-Century-Crofts, 1965.
31. Schech P. Experimentelle Untersuchungen über die Funktion der Nerven und Muskeln des Kehlkopfes. F Biol 1873 9:258–296.
32. Ruhlmann A. Untersuchungen über das Zusammenwirkei der Muskela bei einigen haufiger vorkommenden, Kehl kopfstellungen. Sitzungsber Kaiserlich Akad Wiss, Math not Cl. 1874; 69:257–308.
33. Bosworth FH. Paralyses of the recurrent laryngeal nerve NY State J Med 1880; 3:460.
34. Green JH, Neil E. Respiratory function of laryngeal muscles, J Physiol 1955; 129:134–141.
35. Faaborg-Andersen K. Electromyographic investigation intrinsic laryngeal muscles in humans. Acta Physiol Scai [Suppl] 1957; 41:9–148.
36. Dedo HH. The paralyzed larynx: an electromyographic study in dogs and humans. Laryngoscope 1970; 80:1455–1517.
37. Kotby MN, Haugen LK. Critical evaluation of the action of the posterior cricoarytenoid muscle utilizing direct EMG study. Acta Otolaryngol (Stockh) 1970; 70:260–268.
38. Kotby MN, Haugen LK. Attempts at evaluation of the function of various laryngeal muscles in the light of muscle and nerve stimulation experiments in man. Acta Otolaryngol (Stockh) 1970; 70:419–427.
39. Weddel A, Feinstein B, Pattle RE. The electrical activity of voluntary muscle in man under normal and pathological conditions. Brain 1944; 67:178–272.
40. Wyke BD. Respiratory activity of the intrinsic laryngeal muscles: an experimental study. In: Wyke BD, ed. Ventilatory and phonatory control systems. New York: Oxford University Press, 1974:408.
41. Sackner MA. Pulmonary structure and pathology. In: Kline J, ed. Biological foundations of biomedical engineering. Boston: Little, Brown and Company, 1976:231.
42. Weibel FR. Morphometry of the human lung. Berlin: Springer-Verlag, 1963.
43. Pierce JA, Ebert RV. Fibrous network of the lung and its change with age. Thorax 1965; 20:469–476.
44. Basmajian JV. Primary anatomy. 5th ed. Philadelphia: WB Saunders, 1970.
45. Rankin J, Dempsey JA. Respiratory muscles and the mechanisms of breathing. Am J Phys Med 1967; 46:198–244.
46. Tozikane T, Kawamata K, Tokizane H. Electromyographic studies on the human respiratory muscles. Jpn J Physiol 1952; 2:232–247.
47. Wade OL, Gilson JC. The effect of posture on diaphragmatic movement and vital capacity in normal subjects with a note on spirometry as an aid in determining radiological chest volumes. Thorax 1951; 6:103–126.
48. Wade OL. Movements of the thoracic cage and diaphragm in respiration. J Physiol 1954; 124:193–212.
49. Hamberger GE. Dissertatio de Respirationis Mechanisms et Usu genuino. Jena, 1748. In: Agostoni E. Action of respiratory muscles. In: Fenn WO, Rahn H, eds. Handbook of physiology. Vol. 3. Baltimore: American Physiological Society, 1964:357.
50. Bronk DW, Ferguson LK. The nervous control of intercostal respiration. Am J Physiol 1935; 110:700–707.
51. Campbell EJM. An electromyographic examination of the role of the intercostal muscles in breathing in man. J Physiol 1955; 129:12–26.
52. Anderson FM, Lindsley DB. Action potentials from intercostal muscles before and after unilateral pneumectomy. J Lab Clin Med 1935; 20:623–628.
53. Roper AJ, Thompson WT Jr., Shapiro W, Patterson JL. Scalene and sternomastoid muscle function. J Appl Physiol 1966; 21:497–502.
54. Campbell EJM, Green JH. The behavior of the abdominal muscles and the intra-abdominal pressure during quiet breathing and increased pulmonary ventilation: a study in man. J Physiol 1955; 127:423–426.
55. Wilson TG. Some observations on the anatomy of the infantile larynx. Acta otolaryngol (Stockh) 1953; 43:95–99.
56. Bosma JF. Anatomic and physiologic development of the speech apparatus. In: Tower DB, ed. The nervous system. Vol. 3. Human communication and its disorders. New York: Raven Press, 1975:469.
57. Gedgowd VA. Anatomical peculiarities of the respiratory organs in children. Doctoral Dissertation, St. Petersburg. Translated by Polevoy S, 1900.
58. Noback GJ. The developmental topography of the larynx, trachea and lungs in the fetus, newborn, infant and child. Am J Dis Child 1923; 26:515–533.
59. Roche AF, Barkla DH. The level of the larynx during childhood. Am Otol Rhinol Laryngol 1965; 74:645–654.
60. Klock LE Jr. The growth and development of the human larynx from birth to adolescence. Masters Thesis, University of Washington, School of Medicine, 1968.
61. Kahane JC. A morphological study of the human prepubertal and pubertal larynx. Am J Anat 1978; 151:11–20.
62. Kahane JC. Growth of the human prepubertal and pubertal larynx. J Speech Hear Res 1982; 25:446–455.
63. Kahane JC. Postnatal development and aging of the human larynx. Semin Speech Lang 1983; 4 (3):189–203.
64. Kahane JC. A survey of age related changes in the connective tissues of the human adult larynx. In: Abbs J, Bless DM, eds. Vocal fold physiology. San Diego: Chapter College Hill Press, 1983:44.
65. Zemlin W. Speech and hearing science. Englewood Cliffs, NJ: Prentice-Hall, 1981.
66. Maue WM. Cartilages, ligaments and articulations of the adult human larynx. Doctoral Dissertation, University of Pittsburgh, 1970.
67. Mayet A, Mundnich K. Beitrag sur. Anatomic und zur Function des M. cricothyroideus and der Cricothyreordgelenke. Acta Anat (Basel) 1958; 33:273–288.
68. Von Leden H, Moore P. The mechanics of the cricoarytenoid joints. Arch Otolaryngol (Stockh) 1961; 73:541–550.
69. Snell CARD. On the function of the crico-arytenoid joints in the movements of the vocal cords. Proc K Ned Akad Wet 1959; 50:1370–1381.
70. Sonesson B. On the anatomy and vibratory pattern of the human vocal folds. Acta Otolaryngol (Stockh) [Suppl] 1960; 156:1–76.
71. Frable MA. Computation of motion at the cricoarytenoid joints. Arch Otolaryngol (Stockh) 1961; 73:551–555.
72. Baken R, Isshiki N. Arytenoid displacement by simulated intrinsic muscle contraction. Folia Phoniatr (Basel) 1977; 29:206–216.
73. Kirchner JA, Wyke B. Articular reflex mechanisms in the larynx. Ann Otol Rhinol Laryngol 1961; 74:749–768.
74. Kirchner JA, Wyke B. Electromyographic analysis of laryngeal articular reflexes. Nature 1964; 203:1243–1245.
75. Kirchner JA, Suzuki M. Laryngeal reflexes and voice pro-

duction. Ann NY Acad Sci 1968; 55:98–109.
76. Wyke BD. Recent advances in the neurology of phonation: phonatory reflex mechanisms in the larynx. Br J Disord Commun 1967; 2:2–14.
77. Kahane JC, Folkins JW. Atlas of speech and hearing anatomy. Columbus: CE Merrill, 1984.
78. Dickson DR, Maue WM. Human vocal anatomy. Springfield, IL: CC Thomas, 1970.
79. Faaborg-Andersen K, Sonninen A. The function of the intrinsic laryngeal muscles at different pitches. Acta Otolaryngol (Stockh) 1960; 51:89–93.
80. Matzelt D, Vosteen KH. Electroenoptische und enzymatische Untersuchungen an menschlicher Kehlkopfmuskulatur. Arch Ohr Nas Kehlk Heilk 1963; 181:447–457.
81. Ganz, H. The metabolism of laryngeal muscles. Arch Otolaryngol 1971; 94:97–107.
82. Teig E, Dahl HA, Thorkelsen H. Actomyosin ATPase activity of human laryngeal muscles. Acta Otolaryngol (Stockh) 1978; 85:272–281.
83. Sonninen AA. The role of the external laryngeal muscles in length-adjustment of the vocal cords in singing. Acta Otolaryngol (Stockh) [Suppl] 1956; 130:1–102.
84. Sonninen AA. The external frame function in the control of pitch in the human voice. Ann NY Acad Sci 1968; 155:68–89.
85. Shipp T. Vertical laryngeal position during continuous and discrete vocal frequency change. J Speech Hear Res 1975; 18:707–718.
86. Hirano M. Morphological structure of the vocal cord as a vibrator and its variations. Folia Phoniatr (Basel) 1974; 26:89–94.
87. Hirano M. Phonosurgery, basic and clinical investigations. Otologia Fukuoka 1975; 21:239–440.
88. Crelin FS. Functional anatomy of the newborn. New Haven: Yale University Press, 1973.
89. Laitman J, Crelin FS. Postnatal development of the basicranium and vocal tract region in man. In: Bosma JF ed. Symposium on development of the basicranium. Washington: U.S. Dept of Health Education and Welfare, 1976:206.
90. Sasaki CT, Levine PA, Laitman JT, Crehn ES. Postnatal descent of the epiglottis in man. Arch Otolaryngol 1972; 103:169–171.
91. Crelin FS. Development of the upper respiratory system. Ciba Clin Symp 1976; 28:3–26.
92. Kirchner JA. Pressman and Keleman's physiology of the larynx. Minneapolis: American Academy of Ophthalmology and Otolaryngology, 1970.
93. Castelli WA, Ramirez PC, Nasjleti CF. Linear growth study of the pharyngeal cavity. J Dent Res 1973; 52:1245–1248.
94. Subtelny JD. Width of the nasopharynx and related anatomical structures in normal and unoperated cleft palate children. Am J Ortholaryngol 1955; 41:889–909.
95. Scammon RE. Measurement of man, Minnesota sigma xi lectures. Minneapolis: University of Minnesota Press, 1930.
96. Subtelny JD, Koepp Baker H. The significance of adenoid tissue in velopharyngeal function. Plast Reconstr Surg 1956; 17:235–250.
97. Hamilton WJ. Textbook of anatomy. St. Louis: CV Mosby, 1976.
98. White ER, Basmajian JV. Electromyography of lip muscles and their role in trumpet playing. J Appl Physiol 1973; 36:892–897.
99. Hightower NC. Swallowing and esophageal motility. Am J Digestive Dis 1958; 3:562–583.
100. Doty RW, Bosma JF. An electromyographic analysis of reflex deglutition. J Neurophysic 1956; 19:44–60.
101. Cohen BR, Wolf BS. Cineradiographic and intraluminal pressure correlations in the pharynx and esophagus. Handbook of physiology 6. Am Physiol Soc 1965; 4(6):1841–1859.
102. Whillis J. A note on the muscles of the palate and the superior constrictor. J Anat 1930; 65:92–95.
103. Harrington RM. Pterygopharyngeus and its relationship to M. palatopharyngeus. Laryngoscope 1945; 55:499–508.
104. Dickson DR, Dickson WM. Velopharyngeal anatomy. J Speech Hear Res 1972; 15:372–381.
105. Fritzell B. The velopharyngeal muscles in speech. Acta Otolaryngol (Stockh) [Suppl] 1969; 250:5–81.
106. Kriens O. Anatomy of the velopharyngeal area in cleft palate. Clin Plast Surg 1975; 2:261–283.
107. Rood SR. A functional anatomic study of the muscles related to the eustachian tube. Doctoral dissertation, University of Pittsburgh, 1972.
108. Rood SR, Doyle WJ. Morphology of tensor veli palatini, tensor tympani and dilator tubae muscles. Ann Otol Rhinol Laryngol 1978; 87:202–210.
109. Rich AR. The innervation of the tensor veli palatini and levator veli palatini muscles. Johns Hopkins Hosp Bull 1920; 355:305–310.
110. Rich AR. A physiological study of the eustachian tube and its related muscles. Johns Hopkins Hosp Bull 1920; 352:206–214.
111. Azzan NA, Kuehn DP. The morphology of musculus uvulae. Cleft Palate J 1977; 14:78–87.
112. Langdon HL, Kuebler K. The longitudinal fibromuscular component of the soft palate in the fifteen-week human fetus: musculus uvulae and palatine raphe. Cleft Palate J 1978; 15:337–348.
113. Skolnick ML. Video velopharyngography in patients with nasal speech with emphasis on lateral pharyngeal motion in velopharyngeal closure. Radiology 1969; 93:747–755.
114. Pigott RW. The nasendoscopic appearance of the normal velopharyngeal mechanism. Plast Reconstr Surg 1969; 43:19–24.
115. Moll KL. A cinefluorographic study of velopharyngeal function in normals during various activities. Cleft Palate J 1970; 7:652–662.
116. Calnan JS. Movements of the soft palate. Br J Plast Surg 1953; 5:286–296.
117. Graber TM, Bzoch KR, Aoba R. A functional study of the palatal and pharyngeal structures. Angle Orthodont 1959; 29:30–40.
118. Aram A, Subtelny JD. Velopharyngeal function and cleft palate prostheses. J Prosthet Dent 1959; 9:149–158.
119. Bjork L. Velopharyngeal function in connected speech. Acta Radio (Stockh) [Suppl] 1961; 202:5–94.
120. Bjork L, Nylen B. The function of the soft palate during connected speech. Acta Chir Scand 1963; 26:434–444.
121. McKerns D, Bzoch K. Variations in velopharyngeal valving: the factor of sex. Cleft Palate J 1970; 7:652–662.
122. Ardran GM, Kemp FH. A radiographic study of movements of the tongue in swallowing. Dent Pract 1955; 5:252–264.
123. Passavant G. Ueber die Verschliessung des Schlundes beim Sprechen. Arch F Pathol Anat Physiol 1869; 46:1–31.
124. Hagerty RF, Hill MJ. Pharyngeal wall and palatal movement in postoperative cleft palates and normals. J Speech Hear Res 1960; 3:59–66.
125. Warren D, Hofmann FA. A cineradiographic study of velopharyngeal closure. Plast Reconstr Surg 1961; 38:656–659.
126. Lavorato AS. Normal lateral pharyngeal wall motion during velopharyngeal functioning. Doctoral dissertation. University of Pittsburgh, 1975.
127. Townshend RH. The formation of Passavant's bar. J Laryngol Otol 1940; 55:154–165.
128. Bosma JF. Deglutition: pharyngeal stage. Physiol Rev 1957; 37:275–300.
129. Calnan JS. The error of Gustav Passavant. Plast Reconstr Surg 1954; 13:275–289.
130. Calnan JS. Diagnosis, prognosis and treatment of "pala-

topharyngeal-incompetence" with special reference to radiographic investigations. Br J Plast Surg 1956; 8:265–282.
131. Calnan J. Modern views on Passavants ridge. Br J Plast Surg 1957; 10:89–113.
132. Carpenter M, Morris H. A preliminary study of Passavant's pad. Cleft Palate J 1968; 5:61–72.
133. Perlman HB. Mouth of the eustachian tube—action during swallowing and phonation. Arch Otolarynol 1951; 53:353–369.
134. Bloomer HH. Observations on palatopharyngeal movements in speech and deglutition. J Speech Hear Dis 1953; 18:230–246.
135. Astley R. The movements of the lateral walls of the nasopharynx: a cineradiographic study. J Laryngol Otol 1958; 72:325–328.
136. Skolnick ML. Videofluoroscopic examination of the velopharyngeal portal during phonation in lateral and base projection—a new technique for studying the mechanics of closure. Cleft Palate J 1970; 7:803–816.
137. Hoopes JE, Dellon AL, Fabrikant JI, Edgerton MT Jr, Soliman AM. Cineradiographic definition of the functional anatomy and pathophysiology of the velopharynx. Cleft Palate J 1970; 7:443–454.
138. Dickson DR. Normal and cleft palate anatomy. Cleft Palate J 1972; 9:280–293.
139. Shprintzen RJ. A three-dimensional cinefluoroscopic analysis of velopharyngeal closure during speech and nonspeech activities in normals. Doctoral dissertation, Syracuse University, 1973.
140. Harrington R. A study of the mechanism of velopharyngeal closure. J Speech Hear Dis 1944; 9:325–345.
141. Bosma JF. A correlated study of the anatomy and motor activity of the upper pharynx by cadaver dissection and cinematic study of patients after maxillofacial surgery. Ann Otol Rhinol Laryng 1953; 62:51–72.
142. Ruding R. Cleft palate. Anatomic and surgical considerations. Plast Reconstr Surg 1964; 33:132–147.
143. Green R. The radiology of speech defects. Radiography 1961; 27:331–338.
144. Westlake H, Rutherford D. Cleft palate. Englewood Cliffs, NJ: Prentice-Hall, 1966:61.
145. Falkson R. The functions of the soft palate and pharynx. Virchows Arch 1880; 79:477.
146. Grossman RG, Hattis BF. Oral mucosal sensory innervation and sensory experiences: a review. In: Bosma J, ed. Oral sensation and perception. Springfield, IL: CC Thomas, 1967:5.
147. Squire C, Johnson NW, Hoops RM. Human oral mucosa: development, structure and function. London: Blackwell Scientific Publications, 1976.
148. Provenza V. Oral mucosa. In: Provenza V. Histology. Philadelphia: Lippincott, 1964:361.
149. Hopkin GB. Neonatal and adult tongue dimensions. Angle Orthodont 1967; 37:132–133.
150. Vig P, Cohen A. The size of the tongue and the intermaxillary space. Angle Orthod 1974; 44:25–28.
151. Fletcher SG, Daly DA. Sublingual dimensions in infants and young children. Arch Otolaryngol 1974; 99:292–296.
152. Fletcher SG. Diagnosing speech disorders from cleft palate. New York: Grune & Stratton, 1978.
153. Sicher H, DuBrul L. Oral anatomy. 5th ed. St. Louis: CV Mosby, 1970.
154. Whitman CL, Rankow RM. Diagnosis and management of ankyloglossia. Am J Orthod 1961; 47:423–428.
155. Fletcher SG, Meldrum JR. Lingual function and relative length of the lingual frenulum. J Speech Hear Res 1968; 11:382–390.
156. Catlin FI, DeHaan V. Tongue-tie. Arch Otolaryngol 1971; 94:548–557.
157. Gibbons JW. The human tongue. Br J Dent SC Lond 1898; 41:869–879.
158. Abd-El-Malek S. Observations on the morphology of the human tongue. J Anat 1939; 73:201–210.
159. Strong LH. Muscle fibers of the tongue functional in consonant production. Anat Rec 1956; 126:61–79.
160. Hill KC. The musculature of the tongue. UCLA Work Papers Phonet 1964; 1:22.
161. Doran GA, Bagget M. The genioglossus muscle: a reassessment of its anatomy in some mammals, including man. Acta Anat 1972; 83:403–410.
162. Barnwell YM. The morphology of musculus styloglossus in fifteen-week human fetuses. Int J Oral Myol 1977; 3:8–46.
163. Barnwell YM. Human lingual and musculature: an historical review. Int J Oral Myol 1976; 2:31–41.
164. Abd-El-Malek S. The past played by the tongue in mastication and deglutition. J Anat 1955; 89:250–254.
165. Whillis J. Movements of the tongue in swallowing. J Anat 1946; 80:115–116.
166. Shelton RL, Bosma JF, Sheets BV. Tongue, hyoid and larynx displacement in swallow and phonation. J Appl Physiol 1960; 15:283–288.
167. Wildman AJ, Fletcher SG, Cox B. Patterns of deglutition. Angle Orthod 1964; 34:132–141.
168. Scott JH. Growth changes in the glenoid fossa. Dent Pract Dent Rec 1955; 6:117–120.
169. Graber TM. Craniofacial and dentitional development. In: Falkner F, ed. Human development. Philadelphia: WB Saunders, 1966:510.
170. Scott JH. The analysis of facial growth from fetal life to adulthood. Angle Orthod 1963; 33:110–113.
171. Martone AL, Edwards LF. Anatomy of the mouth and related structures. Part 2. J Prosthet Dent 1962; 12:4–27.
172. Martone AL. Anatomy of facial expression and its prosthetic significance. J Prosthet Dent 1962; 12:1020–1042.
173. Kennedy JC, Abbs JH. Anatomical studies of the perioral major system: foundations for studies in speech physiology. In: Lass NJ, ed. Speech and language: advances in basic research and practice. Vol. 1. New York: Academic Press, 1979:211.
174. Lightoller GS. Facial muscles—the modiolus and muscles surrounding the rima oris with some remarks about the panniculus adiposus. J Anat 1925; 60:1–85.
175. Schlossberg L, Harris SC. An electromyographic investigation of the functioning perioral and suprahyoid musculature in normal occlusion and class I and division I dysplasia cases (abstr.). Am J Orthod 1956; 42:153.
176. Jacob PP, Haridos R, Ammal PJ. An electromyographic study of the behavior of orticularis oris and mentalis muscle. Indian J Med Res 1971; 59:311–320.
177. Basmajian JV, White ER. Neuromuscular control of trumpeters' lips. Nature 1973; 241:70.
178. Blanton PL, Biggs WL, Perkins RC. Electromyographic analysis of the buccinator muscle. J Dent Res 1970; 49:389–394.
179. Basmajian JV. Muscles alive. 4th ed. Baltimore: Williams & Wilkins, 1978.
180. Bowden REM, Mahran ZY, Groding MR. Communications between the facial and trigeminal nerves in certain mammals. Proc Zool Soc Lond 1960; 135:587–611.
181. Conley JJ. Accessory neuromotor pathways to the face. Trans Am Acad Ophthalmol Otolaryngol 1964; 68:1064–1067.
182. Baumel JJ. Trigeminal-facial nerve communicators. Arch Otolaryngol 1974; 99:34–44.
183. Kahane JC. Anatomical and physiological changes in the aging peripheral speech mechanism. In: Beasley DS, Davis GA, eds. Speech, language and hearing and the aging process. New York: Grune & Stratton, 1982:21.

2 Anatomy and Physiology of the Hearing Mechanism*

David M. Lipscomb, Ph.D.

The mystery of the majesty of creation is abundantly evident in the structure and function of the ear. Originating as a simple extension of pressure sensitivity in primitive sea creatures, the hearing mechanism has become so complex in its operation that clinicians have scarcely begun to understand the vast capabilities inherent in this sensory apparatus.

The ear began as a small precursor to the inner ear and underwent myriad modifications and expansion to become the highly functional unit it is in mammals today. Each alteration in structure was occasioned by a distinct need for the modification. To the extent possible, those reasons for structural refinement will be itemized.

IN THE BEGINNING

The most primitive sensory structure considered to be the first "ear" bore absolutely no resemblance to the ear as we normally think of it. Rather, a refinement in the anterior portion of the lateral line organ of primitive fish yielded increased sensation of pressure waves borne via the water to the fish. As this extension of sensation developed, the sensory structures moved subcutaneously and ultimately located inside the head on either side. Along with this step came a sequence of changes in form. No longer was the early otolabyrinthine organ a loosely organized grouping of scattered cells; the developing labyrinth began to take on a distinct organization, and the sensory receptors modified so that specific responses to stimulation could occur (Fig. 2–1). Essentially, pressure waves, propagated through the water, transmitted freely to the fluid-filled labyrinths where a very slight alteration in pressure could be translated (encoded) into neurologic events and carried to the central nervous system (CNS).

With relocation of the special sensory area to a place beneath the surface of the head, the tissue lying between the water bearing the pressure waves and the rudimentary ear exerted an *attenuation* (reduction in the transmission of sound waves). Essentially, outer head tissues served as a barrier to the sound. Eventually, this difficulty was overcome as a result of a further development. Some fishes, as their bodies underwent improvements, began to possess a sac that could be inflated or deflated as a means of buoyancy control. This new device, the swimbladder, was greatly larger than the labyrinths. Therefore, with its greater surface area to receive waterborne vibration (pressure waves) and proximity to the dorsal fin for additional sound wave collection, the swimbladder provided the first truly distant pressure sense. The lateral line organ was strictly limited to sensing pressure variation in its immediate vicinity, and early labyrinths were little more sensitive to pressure waves originating from a distance than was the lateral line organ. Now with the swimbladder to serve as a collector for fluid-borne vibrations, another vital accessory was developed, the Weberian ossicles (Fig. 2–2). This network of bones carried vibrations collected by the swimbladder to the skull region and, hence, to the labyrinth. Thus the first somewhat complex auditory mechanism was

*The organization of this chapter differs from most treatments by discussing ear tissues from inner to outer components because that is the sequence of their development.

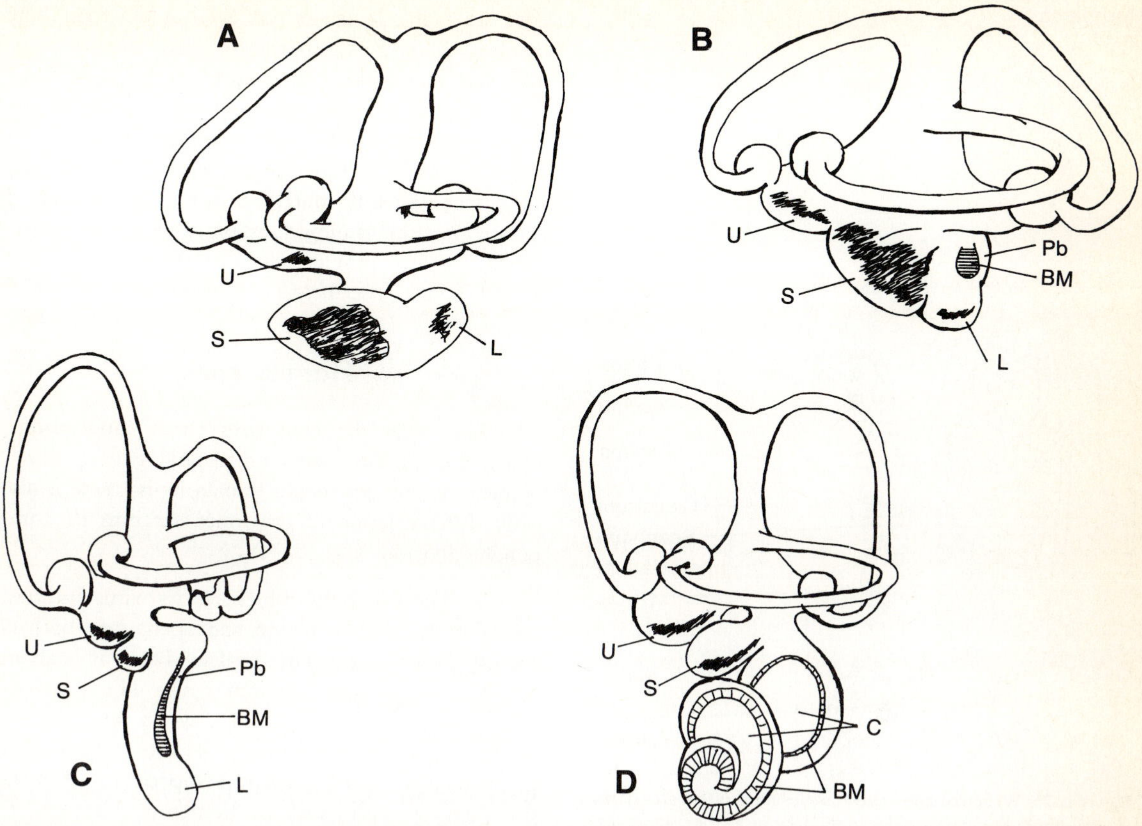

Figure 2–1 Inner ear structure of four representative vertebrates ranging from primitive to more sophisticated systems: *A* fish, *B* turtle, *C* bird, and *D* mammal. The greatest variation occurs in the auditory portion beginning as a small lagena and developing into a coiled cochlea. U = utricle, S = saccule, L = lagena, BM = basilar membrane, Pb = basilar papilla, C = cochlea. (Redrawn by Gail Lipscomb after Wersäll J, Flock Å. Functional anatomy of the vestibular and lateral line organ. In: Neff WD, ed. Contributions to sensory physiology. Vol 1. New York: Academic Press, 1965:40.[1])

formed, with sound being collected first by the dorsal fin of the fish and directed to the swimbladder (which also served as a collector of the oscillating pressure waves). The vibratory energy was then carried via the Weberian ossicles to the labyrinths. At this stage, even the foregoing refinements yielded no more than a crude sense of hearing—probably little more than the detection of the presence of sound pressure waves. The major limiting feature was the relatively unsophisticated analyzer located in a small part of the labyrinth. This analyzer, the lagena, is the historical forerunner of the cochlea, a structure that will be discussed in great detail in the next section. At this point in the history of hearing development, the labyrinth contained primarily a sense of balance and functioned with the developing visual capabilities to keep the fish in a desired orientation. At first, the lagena was simply a small "wart" on the labyrinth with only a few sensory cells. To this day, not much is understood about the lagena, but it is presumed to have been the earliest representative of an auditory response and analyzing region, as is suggested in Figure 2–1 *B*, *C*, and *D*.

THE INNER EAR

In fishes, few additional developments or refinements have occurred in the hearing mechanism beyond those just described. Further expansion of the ear awaited a most significant stage in animal evolution: the escape from a total hydrous environment to land. The amphibian ear manifests the widest variety of inner ear structure forms of any family known. There are so many nuances in the structure from one representative specie to another, that Dr. E. Glen Wever suggests that the amphibian ear appears to have been Nature's laboratory for the further improvement of the inner ear.

Amphibian, Reptile, and Bird Ears

Regardless of the form it took, the amphibian inner ear had some common components with reptile and aviary structures, which allowed for more adequate response to acoustic stimuli in a much more analytic manner than was possible in the simple fish lagena.

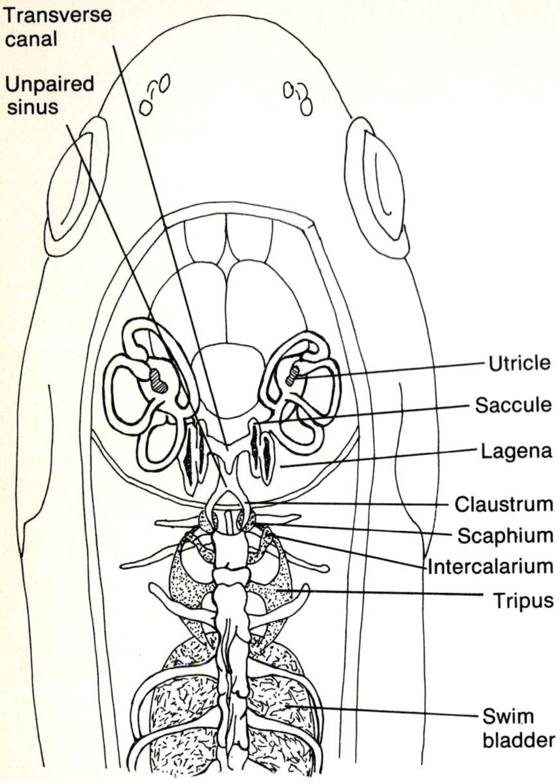

Figure 2-2 Weberian apparatus (ossicles) of the fish are shown in gray. From the swimbladder to the labyrinth, they are tripus, intercalarium, scaphium, and claustrum. (Redrawn by Gail Lipscomb after van Bergeijk WA. The evolution of vertebrate hearing. In: Neff WD, ed. Contributions to sensory physiology. Vol 2. New York: Academic Press, 1965:23.[2])

Further refinements in the inner ear occurred in the aviary and reptilian forms (Figs. 2–1 and 2–3); sensory cells are topped with groups of tiny hairs (cilia) projecting from the upper surface of the cell. For this reason, the auditory sensory cells are commonly called hair cells. Since the magnitude of displacement caused by the pressure waves set up in the inner ear is so small (sometimes submolecular in dimension), some means is necessary to provide a mechanical stimulation of the sensory hair cells. Therefore, rather than have the cilia wave in the fluid disturbance set up by pressure waves, a more direct mechanical linkage was provided. When pressure waves occurred in the inner ear, the support membrane for the hair cells (called the "basilar membrane") was caused to move up and down. This movement, of course, carried with it the superstructure containing the sensory hair cells, which along with their supporting cells are termed the "organ of Corti." Resting on top of the cilia is a finger-like projection, which somewhat resists the up and down motion because of its mass and inertia. The end result is the exertion of pressure along the entire length of interlinked tissues. The most flexible region in this tissue chain is located at the cilia; therefore the cilia are bent. It is not yet well understood how bending the cilia is important to the ultimate stimulation of nerves associated with the hair cells, but in all auditory mechanisms from the simplest to the very complex mammal ear, it appears to be an essential mechanical function in hearing. Ciliary displacement probably contributes to the generation of certain electrophysiologic responses in the inner ear, which, in turn, provide adequate stimulation of the nerves to carry the message to the CNS.

Human Ear

The inner ear comprises three subdivisions, which differentiated early on in phylogenetic development. In the developing human fetus, there is also early differentiation of the inner ear into its component divisions (Fig. 2–4):

1. The vestibule, which, as its name implies, serves as the middle region and opens into both of the other areas. Somewhat oval in shape, it is about 5.5 mm across and 3.0 mm deep. The vestibule contains the utricle and saccule, two of the five parts of the balance or labyrinthine sensory organs. The inner (medial) wall and the top (superior) wall of the vestibule are perforated in numerous locations to permit the transmission of nerve fibers from the sensory portions of the vestibular end organs, including nerve fibers from the region of the semicircular canals. The posterior aspect of the medial wall contains a small opening, the vestibular aqueduct, which transmits a small vein and contains a tubular prolongation of the membranous system, the endolymph duct. This duct terminates in a small bulb just outside the petrous bone at the level of the dura mater, adjacent to the brain. The endolymph duct is the only contact the inner ear membranous system has outside its boundaries.

2. The semicircular canals open from the vestibule in the posterior dimension. These canals contain three receptor organs (cristae), the remaining sensory end-organs for balance. Each canal is located in one of the body planes (sagittal, coronal, and transverse) so that motion in any or a combination of the planes can be sensed. Unequal in length, each canal describes the greater part of a circle. They measure approximately 0.8 mm in diameter, and at one end, there is an enlargement, the ampulla, which is more than twice the diameter of the rest of the canal. The superior semicircular canal is 15 to 20 mm in length and cuts a vertical direction from side to side (coronal plane). Its most lateral extremity is ampullated and opens into the superior portion of the posterior wall of the vestibule. The opposite end joins with the nonampullated end of the posterior

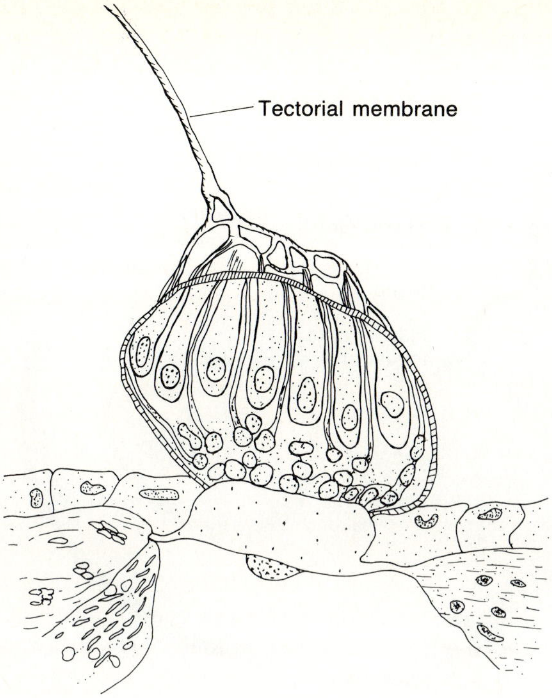

Figure 2-3 Representative lizard auditory papilla (Gecko, gecko) magnified 500×. (Redrawn by Gail Lipscomb after Wever EG. The tectorial membrane of the lizard ear: types of structure. J Morpol 1967; 122:313.[3])

semicircular canal and forms the crus commune, a common opening into the upper and medial part of the vestibule. The posterior semicircular canal is also vertical in direction, but in the front-to-back plane (sagittal). It is the longest of the three canals, measuring 18 to 22 mm. The superior nonampullated end is part of the crus commune just described, and the ampullated end enters the vestibule on its posterior wall. The lateral or horizontal canal, as its name suggests, lies in the horizontal plane and is the shortest of the three, being 12 to 15 mm in length. The ampullated end of the horizontal canal opens into the vestibule at its posterior superior margin immediately lateral to the location of the ampullated end of the superior canal. The nonampullated end connects to the posterior medial wall of the vestibule.

3. The cochlear portion of the osseous labyrinth, located in the anterior aspect of the inner ear, is similar in configuration to a snail shell viewed from within. The apex (capula) of the cochlea is oriented toward the front and side (anterolateral). Consisting of a single 0.3-mm diameter tube, the cochlear canal has a spiral course winding around a central core, the modiolus, for approximately $2^2/_3$ turns. This canal has three openings: (1) the elliptical opening into the vestibule; (2) the membrane-covered round window at the base of the cochlea; and (3) the cochlear aqueduct, a tiny funnel-shaped canal that opens into the anterior surface of the petrous bone, through which cerebrospinal fluid can enter the perilymphatic spaces of the inner ear from the subarachnoid cavity in the vicinity of the brain.

The inner ear is a membranous system within a bony cavity. The prism-shaped petrous bone encasing the inner ear region is actually hollowed out to provide chambers in which are located sensory receptors and their associated tissues. The inner ear is made up of two interrelated labyrinth systems, the osseous and membranous labyrinths. These two systems bear the same general configuration, but differ in embryologic development and in histologic architecture. Figure 2–4 is actually a fanciful rendition of the outer shell of the inner ear if one carefully removed all but the portion of the petrous bone closest to the fluid-filled cavities. This outer shell, the bony or osseous labyrinth, provides structural support as well as form for the inner ear. Three geographic regions (vestibule, semicircular canals, and cochlea) can readily be identified in Figure 2–4. Contained within the osseous labyrinth and in direct contact with the periosteum-lined walls is a clear fluid, perilymph. Also located inside the osseous labyrinth and maintaining something of the same shape is the membranous labyrinth (Fig. 2–5). This system can also be considered in three parts, as was the osseous labyrinth. The fluid contained within the boundaries of the membranous labyrinth, endolymph, is also a clear liquid, but it has a chemical composition quite different from perilymph.

The schematized illustration of a bisected cochlea at the midmodiolar point points out a number of the structures visible to the unaided eye (Fig. 2–6). Projecting into the cochlear canal is a bony ledge, the osseous spiral lamina, named thus because it consists of two thin sheets of bone joined (laminated) at the outer lip of the projection. That outer lip is perforated along its length to allow nerve fibers from the membranous portion of the cochlea to be transmitted into the modiolus, wherein they make up the auditory portion of the statoacoustic nerve (cranial nerve VIII). The outer lip of the osseous spiral lamina has perforations (habenula perforada) spaced side by side, giving it the appearance of the edge of a harmonica. Of importance to cochlear architecture is the fact that the osseous spiral lamina partially divides the cochlear canal into two major divisions (scalae). This division is completed by the basilar membrane, which will be discussed in detail later. The bony cochlea (otic capsule) has a number of shape and size variations in mammals, but the general organization is consistent throughout the mammalian forms. In humans, the otic capsule stands only about 5 mm high and is 9 mm across at the base. The

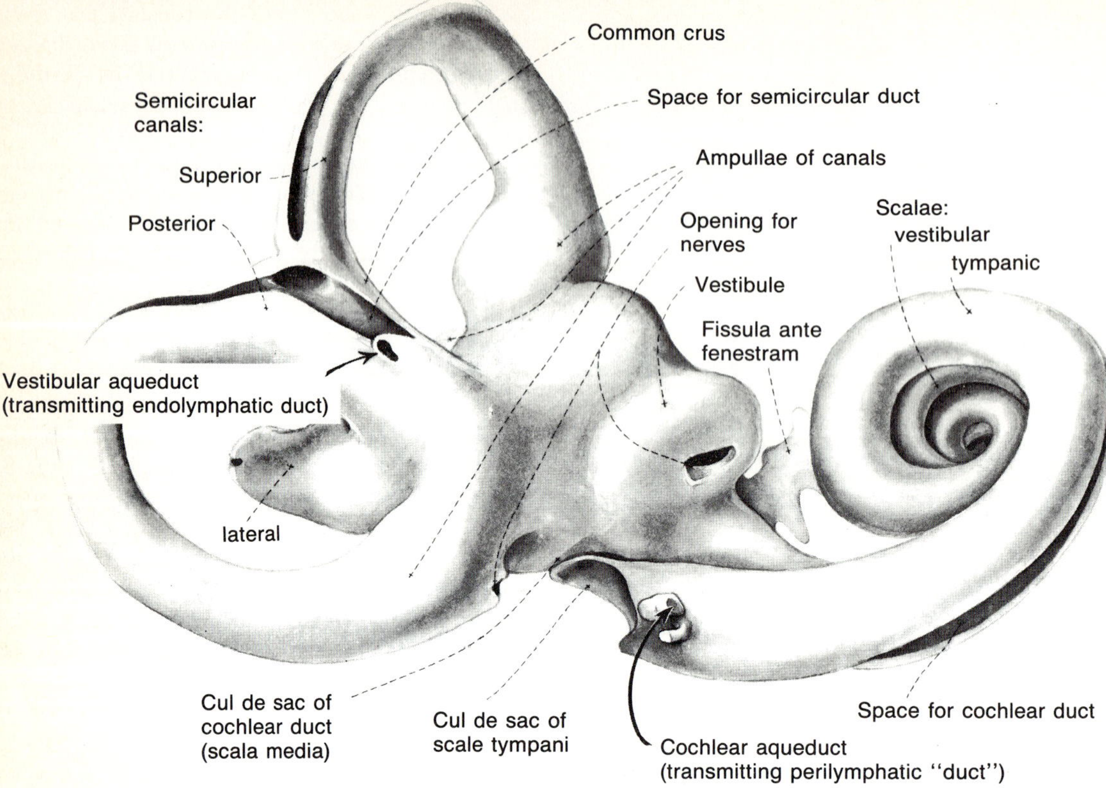

Figure 2–4 Osseous labyrinth as seen from the medial aspect. See text for details of anatomic structures and landmarks. (From Anson BJ, Donaldson JA. Surgical anatomy of the temporal bone and ear. 2nd ed. Philadelphia: WB Saunders, 1973:278.[4])

modiolus opens at the base of the cochlea into a short bony canal, the internal auditory meatus or canal. Fibers of the statoacoustic nerve (cranial nerve VIII) pass through this canal and on to the higher centers, as will be detailed in Chapter 3.

The inferior margin of the cochlear portion of the membranous labyrinth, the basilar membrane, consists of two areas. The innermost part is thin and serves to support the complex of sensory cells and supportive tissue of the end-organ of hearing, the organ of Corti. The outer extremity of the basilar membrane, which attaches to the bony outer wall, fans out to a thick, striated tissue, the spiral ligament. At its inner margin, the basilar membrane is affixed to the lip of the osseous spiral lamina.

Also visible at this level of magnification is another partition, the vestibular or Reissner's membrane, which rises from soft tissue atop the osseous spiral lamina and attaches at the upper crest of the spiral ligament. With this structure, the three major subdivisions of the cochlear canal are complete. The uppermost chamber, the perilymph-filled scala vestibuli, is so named because it opens into the vestibule. Terminating at the round window, sometimes called the secondary tympanic membrane, is the lower chamber, the scala tympani, also containing perilymph. The scala media is the cochlear portion of the membranous labyrinth and contains endolymph. This chamber is a blind duct, beginning at the base of the cochlea with a narrow communication with the vestibular membranous system and terminating at the helicotrema, where the vestibular and basilar membranes join to close off the scala at the apex.

Other portions of the membranous labyrinth are important as the locations of sensory end-organs for numerous vestibular (balance) sense functions. In the vestibule itself are situated two membranous sacs, the utricle and the saccule. The utricle is the larger one, oblong in form, and is located in the posterosuperior region of the vestibular cavity. The saccule is shaped more like a globe and lies near the middle of the vestibule, close to the oval window, an important landmark to be discussed in detail later. These two sacs communicate by means of the utriculosaccular duct, which leads from the anterior wall of the utricle and joins with the tube leaving the posterior wall of the saccule. This forms an elongation, the endolymphatic duct, which terminates in a blind sac at the level of the dura mater. From the inferior border of the saccule, a short tube, the canalis reuniens of Hensen, passes downward and opens into the scala

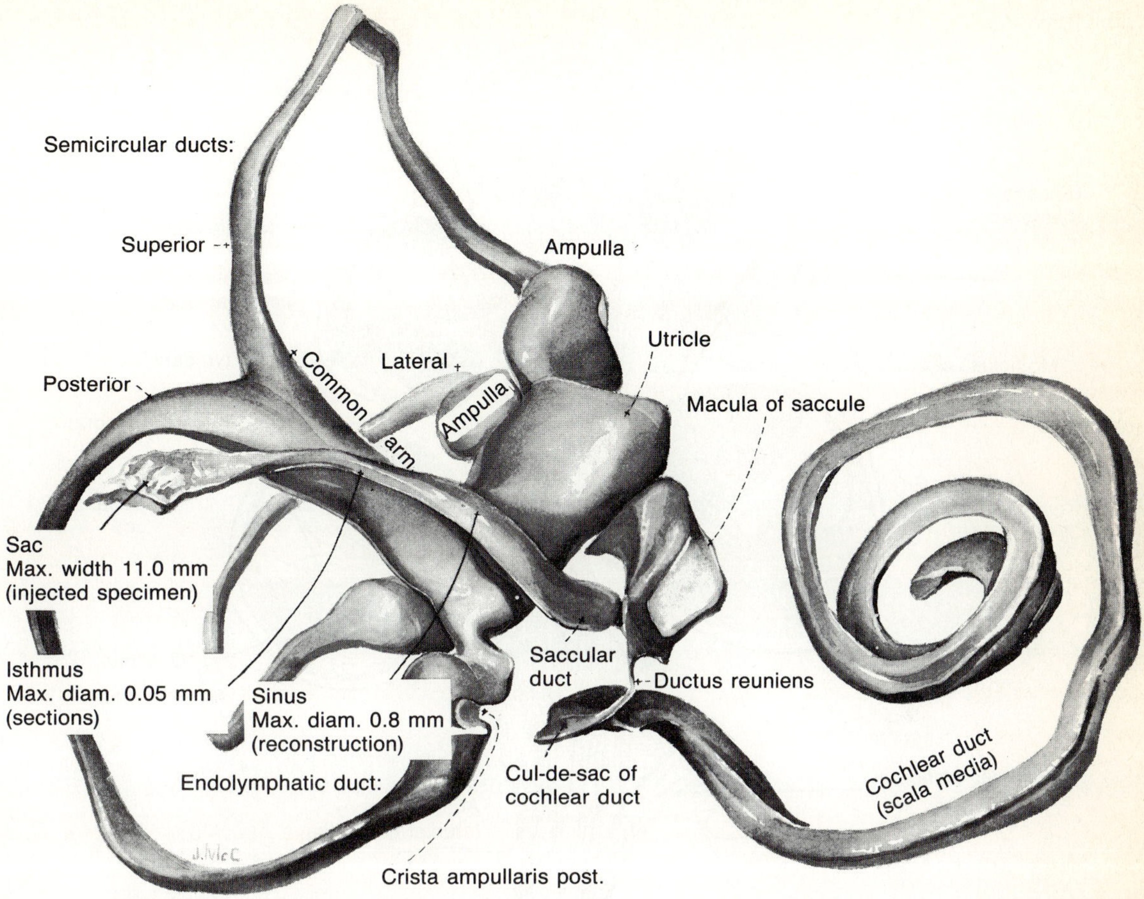

Figure 2–5 Membranous labyrinth of the left ear. See text for discussion. (From Anson BJ, Donaldson JA. Surgical anatomy of the temporal bone and ear. 2nd ed. Philadelphia: WB Saunders, 1973:276.[4])

media. This duct tends to become obliterated in adults, thus separating the cochlear and vestibular portions of the membranous labyrinth.

Thickened portions of the utricle and saccule are the maculae, containing cells that sense deviation from either the vertical (saccule) or horizontal (utricle) orientation. Cristae in the ampullated ends of the semicircular canals are found in the thickened membranous portion of each canal (Fig. 2–7). Status information provided by these sensory centers includes acceleration, deceleration, and rotation. Long cilia rising from the top surfaces of sensory cells in the cristae are embedded in a gelatinous matrix that moves with endolymphatic fluid motion. When endolymphatic fluid is disturbed and presses on the crest, the cilia bend, giving rise to stimulation of the sensory hair cells and a resultant neural impulse. Depending upon the force exerted and the direction of the pressure, differential information is provided to the CNS and is perceived as motion. Since each of the three canals is located in one of the anatomic body planes, acceleration, deceleration, or rotation creates a disturbance in one or more of the semicircular canals and activates the appropriate cristae. One can see that a complex series of nerve impulses is set up according to the type and direction of stimulation. The CNS processes the various clues sent by these sensory receptors so that we know when we change direction or speed.

Utilizing the mass of a group of calcium carbonate granules (otoconia), the maculae of the utricle and saccule operate in a somewhat different fashion than the cristae (Fig. 2–8). With the macula for the saccule located in the vertical plane and the macula for the utricle in the horizontal plane, these two regions are differentially sensitive to "tilting" from either of the two planes. The base of the macula is rather firmly affixed in place, whereas the calcium carbonate granules are located in a gelatinous matrix and are somewhat more free to move. When the body is tilted in one direction or another, a differential pressure is set up at either end of the macular region, causing a momentary variation in distance between the otoconia of one end and the otoconia of the other end of the structure. The variation in distance results in a variation in nerve firing pattern

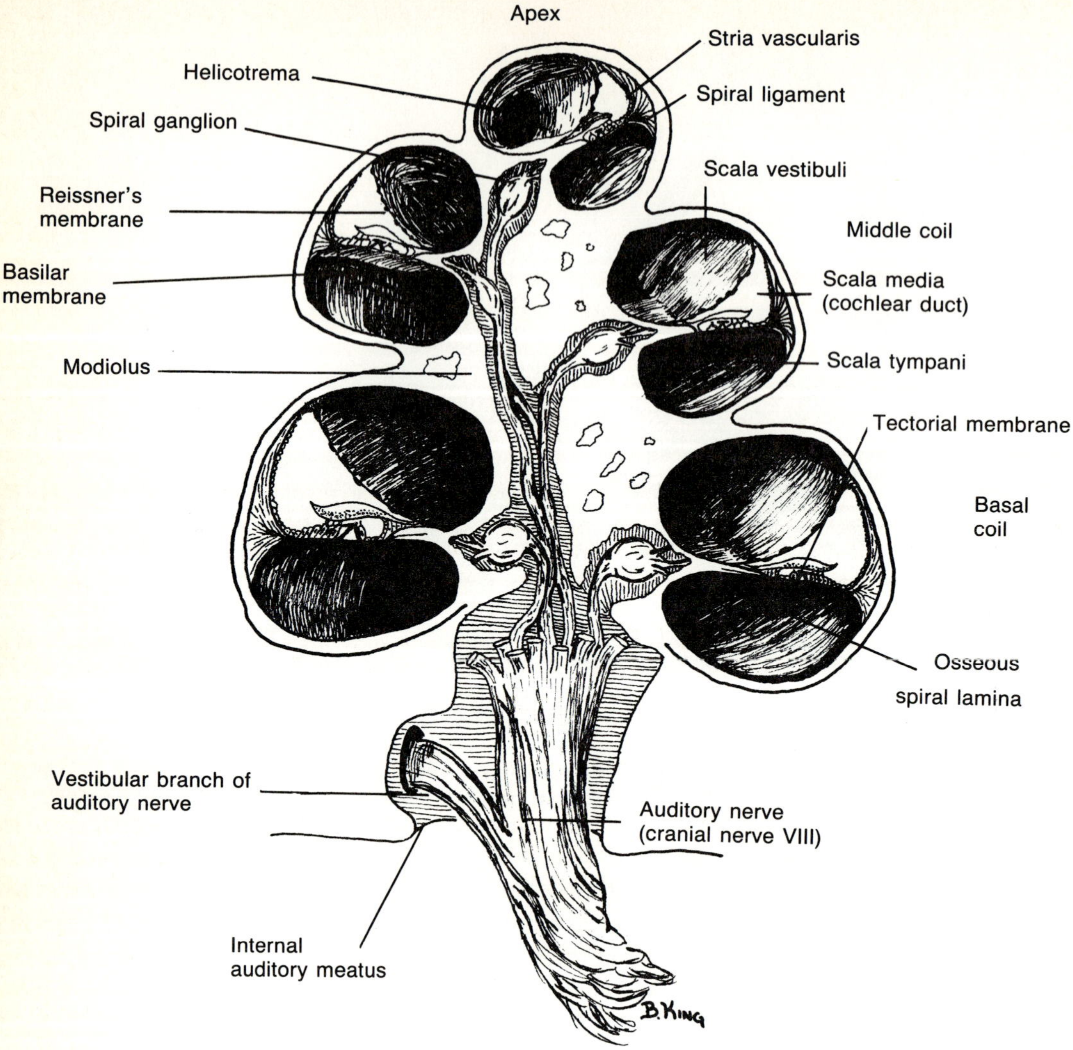

Figure 2–6 Midmodiolar bisection of the human cochlea shown in schematic form. See text for description.

that is peculiar to the particular type of motion. Again, a complex set of neural signals is sent for the CNS to interpret into a cue about the type and form of movement.

The five sensory regions in the vestibule and semicircular canals work in concert to provide a constantly changing pattern of encoded signals to the CNS in order to keep us aware of variations in status or orientation in our environment. Without the high development of this system, upright posture would be limiting and much less refined. It is because of the inclusion of nerve fibers from this region that the most accurate name for the eighth cranial nerve is "statoacoustic," since both status and auditory information are transmitted along its fibers.

The remainder of this section will concentrate on the details of the cochlea and its sensory area, the organ of Corti. Looking at an enlargement of one part of the cochlear canal (Fig. 2–9) as if it were being seen at about 100 times magnification, a number of the larger structures are readily observed. However, finer details of the organ of Corti are not visible until the magnification reaches 400 times or better.

Set on a flexible base, the basilar membrane, the auditory end-organ consists of numerous interrelated components. Providing the skeletal framework for the structure are two rows of rodlike bodies, the inner and outer rods or the pillars of Corti. The bases of the rods rest on the basilar membrane. The bases of the inner pillars are located somewhat distant from the bases of the outer pillars. They incline toward each other, and their heads come in contact to enclose between them and the basilar membrane a triangular tunnel, the tunnel of Corti, containing a fluid called "cortilymph" and nerve fi-

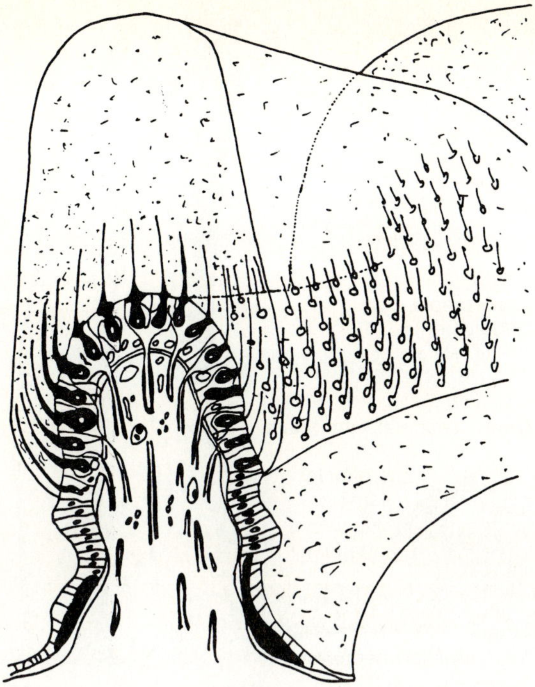

Figure 2–7 Schematic representation of the crista of a semicircular canal. See text for description. (From Lipscomb DM. An introduction to the laboratory study of the ear. Springfield, IL: CC Thomas, 1974:22.[5])

bers, the radial tunnel fibers. There are about 6,000 inner rods and 4,000 outer rods. The outer rods are longer and more obliquely set than are the inner rods. Convex heads of outer rods fit into the concavity of the head of adjacent inner rods to form a strong bond. Phalangeal processes, thin flattened projections of the head plate of outer pillars, are directed toward the outer wall and join with the phalangeal processes arising from Deiters' cells to form the reticular lamina. The top (cuticular) surfaces of the outer hair cells are interjected between phalangeal processes and present a solid surface that cannot be penetrated by endolymphatic fluid. Separation of fluids is very important, since endolymph is high in potassium and would seriously disrupt the normal function of hair cells and nerve fibers should it come into contact with them. Therefore the fluid in direct contact with sensory hair cells throughout the region immediately below the reticular membrane is perilymph or something similar in composition. Perilymph is low in potassium and high in sodium; thus it provides a proper fluid environment for the cells and neural tissue.

Located on either side of the pillars are the two types of sensory hair cells. Immediately above the lip of the osseous spiral lamina is a single row of inner hair cells. Situated at about the midpoint of the basilar membrane toward the outer wall from the osseous spiral lamina lip are the more numerous outer hair cells. To these highly specialized epithelial cells is ascribed the vital function of converting fluid-borne pressure waves within the cochlea into neural impulses that are carried to the CNS. For a number of reasons, the two groups of cells are best considered to be separate from each other:

1. Inner hair cells are considered to be the more primitive of the two cell groups.
2. Nearly 95 percent of all afferent (sensory) nerve fibers of the acoustic portion of cranial nerve VIII serve the 3,500 to 4,000 inner hair cells, resulting in sizeable *divergence* of neural activity; the approximately 12,000 outer hair cells have to share the remaining 5 percent of the afferent nerve fibers, resulting in considerable neural *convergence.* Thus, one nerve fiber (neuron) communicates with several outer hair cells via considerable branching of the nerve endings. More about this feature will be presented in Chapter 3.
3. Cytoarchitecture (cell shape) for the two types of cells is disparate. Inner hair cells are somewhat pear-shaped, whereas outer hair cells are longer and column-shaped.
4. Inner hair cells are arranged in a well-kept single row, whereas outer hair cells are, in the human, rather loosely organized into about three rows at the basal end and four rows at the apical end of the organ of Corti. The spacing between the outer hair cells is irregular in the human, whereas they are geometrically proportioned better in lower mammals.
5. The three rows of about 60 cilia atop the inner hair cells are arranged in a slight crescent formation, whereas the three rows of 100 to 200 cilia projecting from the cuticular surface of outer hair cells form into a "W" configuration that opens toward the modiolus (Fig. 2–10). Note that the cilia are arranged in three rows with varying height for each row.
6. Inner hair cells are held rigidly in place by the inner pillar cells and supportive cells, whereas

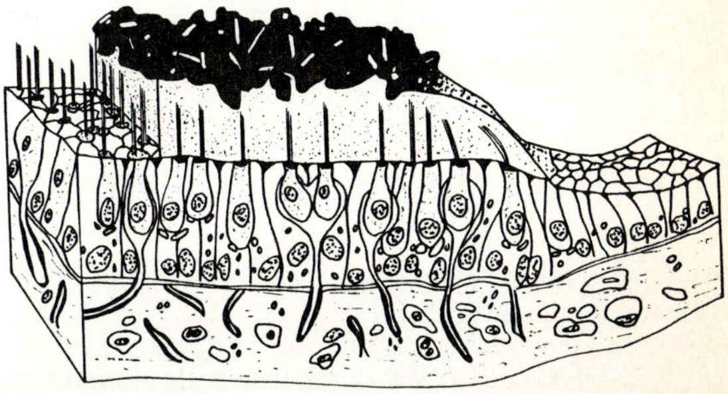

Figure 2-8 Schematic view of a macula. See text for description. (From Lipscomb DM. An introduction to the laboratory study of the ear. Springfield, IL: CC Thomas, 1974:21.[5])

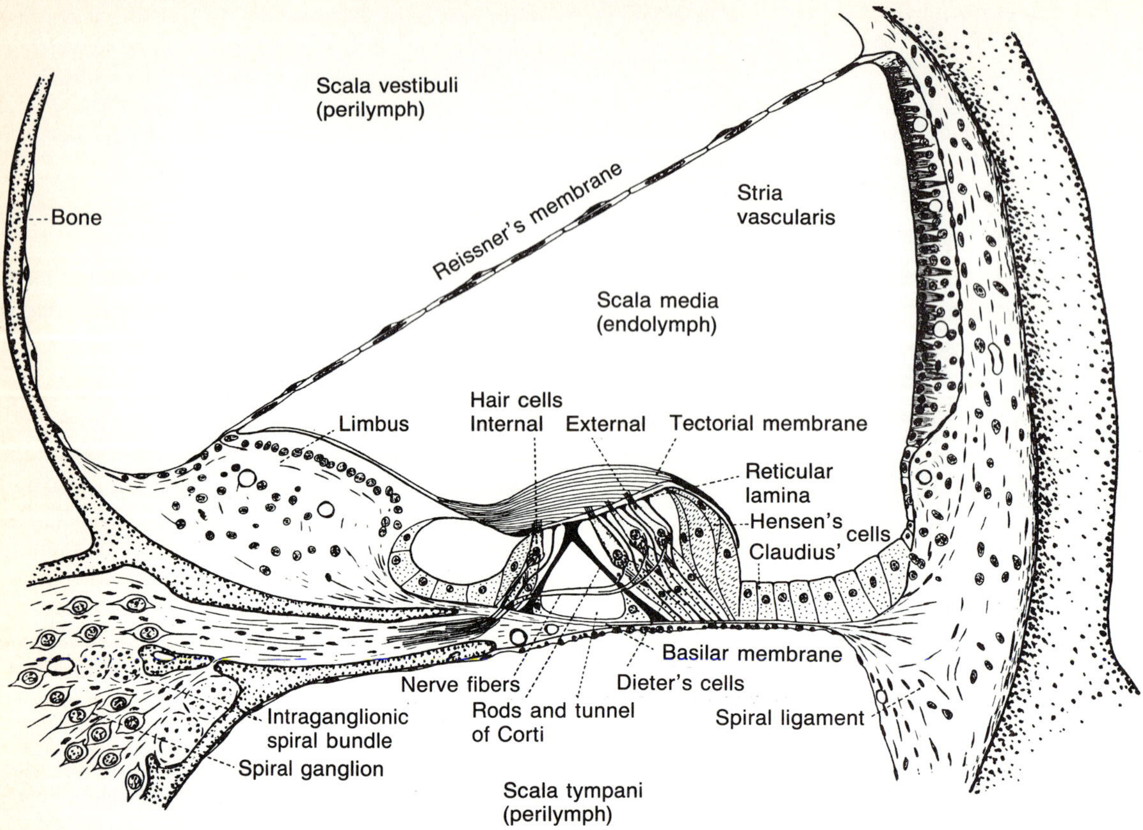

Figure 2–9 Structures contained in the scala media shown schematically as if they were enlarged approximately 100 ×. (From Davis H, et al. Acoustic trauma in the guinea pig. J Acoust Soc Am 1953; 25:1180–1189.[6])

the outer hair cells are more free-standing, with attachments only to the reticular membrane at the top and to a Deiters' cell on the bottom.

7. Because of their relative location on the basilar membrane, the outer hair cells are subject to more mechanical activity. Therefore, they are probably more sensitive to lower levels of sound stimulation than are the inner hair cells. In fact, studies indicate that the outer hair cells are more sensitive by a factor of about 30 dB.

8. The tops of the longest cilia of outer hair cells are firmly rooted in the underside of the tectorial membrane, but the cilia of inner hair cells are not attached to the tectorial membrane. In fact, they are protected from the tectorial membrane by trabeculae that act as spanners between Hensen's stripe and the cuticular surface of the inner hair cells.

9. Nerve connections of outer hair cells are restricted to the bottom of the cell, whereas inner hair cells have nerve connections over most of the lower two-thirds of the cell.

Just how inner and outer hair cells respond to pressure waves in the scala media is not yet clear. Further, the exact mechanism for differential cilia movement is not well understood. Structural differences suggest that physical principles associated with

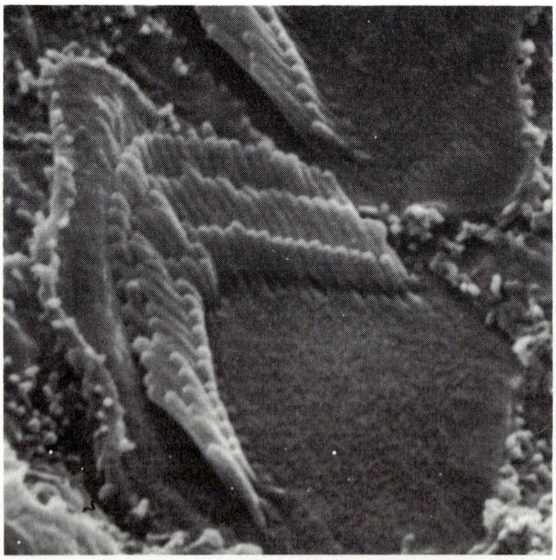

Figure 2–10 Scanning electron photomicrograph of outer hair cilia (12,000 ×). The hairs are situated in three rows of varying height forming a "W" shape. The taller row lies toward the outer wall.

mechanical displacement of cilia are different for the two groups of sensory hair cells. Still another area of inadequate knowledge involves the mechanism for exciting the hair cells by ciliary bending. The complex analytic function the cochlea is designed to accomplish leads to the conclusion that these two cell types perform complementary functions in increasing refinement of the encoded messages sent to the CNS.

In addition to the sensory cells, numerous other undifferentiated supportive cells are present in the organ of Corti. Toward the modiolus from the inner hair cells making up the limbus region are interdental cells and inner sulcus cells separated by a depression termed the "inner sulcus." It is the inner sulcus cells that serve to hold the inner hair cells in place between them and the inner pillar cells. Directly beneath and directly supporting the outer hair cells are Deiters' cells. Next to the Deiters' cells toward the outer wall are Hensen's cells, and, finally, atop the basilar membrane from the Hensen's cells to the basilar crest are Claudius' cells.

Hovering over the entire organ of Corti is the delicate and extremely flexible tectorial membrane. This membrane is affixed to the superior surface of the limbus at its inner edge and to the Hensen's cells at the outside by the marginal net. On the underside of the tectorial membrane is a clear band, Hensen's stripe, immediately above but not touching the cilia of the inner hair cells, and Hardesty's membrane is located over the outer hair cells in direct physical contact with the tallest cilia of the outer hair cells.

The tectorial membrane is of immense functional importance to the organ of Corti. Because its point of attachment to the limbus differs from that of the basilar membrane, up and down deflection of the basilar membrane caused by pressure waves in the cochlea results in a shearing motion of the tectorial membrane relative to the top surface of the outer hair cells. The resultant deflection of outer hair cell cilia triggers nerve impulses (Fig. 2–11). The shearing motion, of course, does not explain how inner hair cells initiate impulses, but it does provide a mechanical basis for the exquisite sensitivity of the outer hair cells to extremely small magnitude basilar membrane motion. Inner hair cell stimulation must be explained in some other fashion. Perhaps small eddy currents set up in the space between the reticular and tectorial membranes move the inner hair cell cilia sufficiently to initiate their action when pressure waves reach a somewhat higher magnitude. Differential modes of hair cell stimulation are felt by some to be the cause of the approximately 30-dB greater sensitivity of outer hair cells.

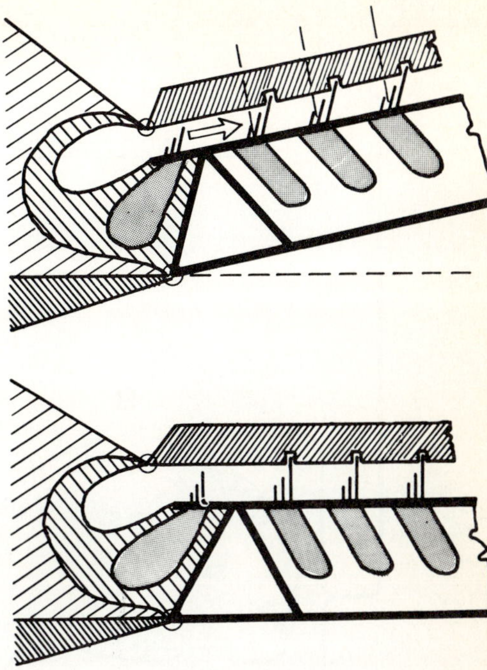

Figure 2–11 Relationshp between the tectorial membrane and the cilia of the outer hair cells. At rest (lower illustration), the cilia stand perpendicular to the cuticular surface of the cell. When pressure waves move the basilar membrane, a "shearing" force acts to alter the angle of the cilia with respect to the cuticular surface. Note that the cilia of the inner hair cells are shown to bend, not from tectorial membrane attachment, but from fluid motion. (From Dallos P, Ryan A. Physiology of the inner ear. In: Northern JL, ed. Hearing disorders. Boston: Little, Brown, 1976:95.[7])

Cochlear Blood Supply

Long overlooked in most discussions of inner ear anatomy is the vital role of the cochlear vascular system. In its function, the cochlea employs a number of principles in addition to mechanical deflection of the basilar membrane and resultant bending of cilia of sensory hair cells. Cell physiology maintains the vital chemical balances necessary for normal function. Metabolic activity results in electrophysiologic charging of parts of the structure critical to their ultimate contribution to the hearing process. Metabolic activity is almost entirely due to the extremely rich vascular organization in the cochlea.

Access to blood for the cochlea is extremely limited in that there is only one arterial entrance from the heart and a single venous exit returning the blood to the heart (Fig. 2–12*A*). Blood enters the cochlea through arterial links, beginning with a junction of the subclavian artery into the left and right vertebral arteries, which become the basal artery. It in turn throws off a branch, the inferior anterior cerebral artery, which then sends off a smaller

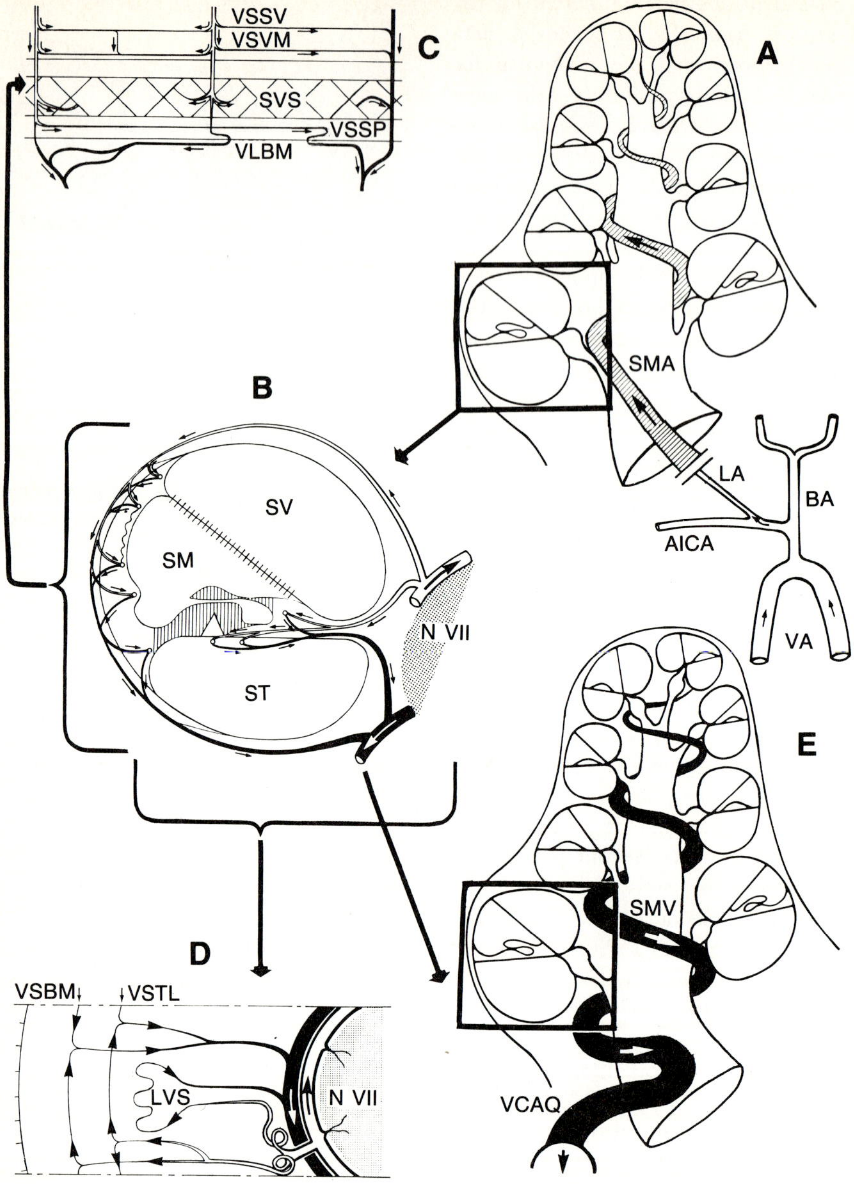

Figure 2–12 Composite schematic diagram of cochlear blood supply: *A*, Arterial system. *B*, Vessels of the cochlear canal. *C*, Stria vascularis on the outer wall. *D*, Vascular system of the limbus serving the organ of Corti. *E*, Venous system. See text for description of the course of blood through the cochlear region. (From Axelsson A. The vascular anatomy of the cochlea in the guinea pig and in man. Acta Otolaryngol 1968; Suppl. 243:107.[8])

aqueduct, the labyrinthine artery, entering the inner ear through the internal auditory meatus (the same passageway that carries the statoacoustic nerve and the facial nerve). In the internal auditory meatus, the anterior vestibular artery ramifies to the vestibule and semicircular canals. Another branching takes place inside the internal auditory meatus, which sends off an arterial link, the vestibular-cochlear artery, to the basal region of the cochlea. Interestingly, the base of the cochlea has a seemingly independent blood supply system, which may be a clue to its more primitive origins. The remaining channel in the most lateral portion of the internal auditory meatus is the spiral modiolar artery, which coils inside the modiolar core of the cochlea all the way to the apex, periodically giving off radiating arterioles either to the outer wall or to the limbus region (Fig. 2–12*B*).

For all practical purposes, there are two independent vascular systems within the cochlear canal. Radiating arterioles follow the outer wall of the scala vestibuli and supply blood to a dense capillary network, the stria vascularis (Fig. 2–12*C*). Also, radiating arterioles are given off to the region of the limbus, as shown in Figure 2–12*D*. The arteriole thins down to two capillaries at the lip region of the osseous spiral lamina—the vein of the tympanic lip and the vein of the basilar membrane. Apparently, the two systems have differing physiologic mandates. The stria vascularis, with its high metabolic activity, not only influences chemical and oxygen (O_2) balances of the endolymphatic fluid, but it also creates a high (+80 mv) charge on the stria that is complemented by an equivalent negative charge in the organ of Corti. The vascular supply of the limbus region serves the O_2 needs of the organ of Corti.

From both of these regions, collecting venules carry blood back to the base of the cochlea. The vein of the scala tympani collects blood from the stria vascularis and carries it along the wall of the scala tympani, where it unites with the descending spiral modiolar vein (Fig. 2–12*E*). The vein of the scala vestibuli, providing the egress for blood in the limbus region, also enters the spiral modiolar vein, which forms the vein of the cochlear aqueduct at the base of the cochlea. Ultimately, the venous drainage system empties into the jugular vein for the return trip to the heart, thereby completing an intricate vascular cycle.

The vascular tree of the cochlea is not only intricate and functional, but it is also impressive when viewed alone (Fig. 2–13). This observation is made possible by injecting a liquid latex solution into the vascular channels, thereby replacing the blood. When the latex hardens, the temporal bone is placed in a strong acid that oxidizes all the tissue structures, leaving the latex matrix showing the outline of the cochlear vascular system.

Cochlear Mechanics

Exactly how the complex cochlear mechanism converts fluid pressure waves into neural code is still partly shrouded in mystery because the anatomic parts are so tiny and because they have been inaccessible due to the dense bony protection afforded them. Much of our understanding of the mechanism has been advanced with the use of representative models. A key concept involves the comprehension that cochlear fluid is incompressible. Thus, pressure exerted at one point of the column of fluid contained in the cochlear walls is transferred instantaneously to other points.

The elliptical opening of the scala vestibuli into the vestibule and the termination of the scala tympani at the round window are effectively at opposite ends of a column of fluid. The most common route for acoustic pressure waves is into the oval window, an opening into the vestibule in close proximity to the origin of the scala vestibuli. Conceptually, a pressure wave initiated by forcing the oval window inward would at the same time have the effect of pushing the round window membrane outward (Fig. 2–14). This sets up so-called traveling waves on the basilar membrane, which reach an instantaneous crest according to the frequency of the stimulating sound (Fig. 2–15). In the laws of physics, the wave length of a sound is defined as the distance a pressure wave travels during completion of one cycle (Hertz). If we consider the human audible frequency range to be from about 20 Hz to 20,000 Hz, the human ear is responsive to sounds with wavelengths ranging from about 17.2 m for the low-frequency limit to around 1.7 cm at the high-frequency end of the audible spectrum. Since the length of the basilar membrane is only approximately 3.2 cm, obviously some type of analogue must be utilized by the cochlea. This is accomplished by the frequency-displacement transformation, which, simply stated, is an analogous representation along the basilar membrane for the various frequencies audible to the human being. High frequencies are represented by the base of the basilar membrane, and, with decreasing frequency of the sound stimulus, the place of the crest of the traveling waves moves increasingly toward the apical end. As distortion of the basilar membrane occurs at differing locations according to the frequency content of sound stimuli, hair cell activity is greatest at the point of the traveling wave crest; increasingly less toward the base of the cochlea, since the amount of basilar membrane displacement is smaller; and nonexistent at locations apical to the crest of the traveling wave. Thus, frequency information according to "places" stimulated is encoded by the organ of Corti and sent to the brain for further refinement and the step we call perception. In this manner, the cochlea serves as an analyzer, leaving the higher centers free to elaborate on the importance of the stimulus in perceptual function.

Of course, sound has another important dimension, amplitude, which is ultimately perceived as loudness. With increasing amplitude, the sound stimulus exerts more force on the auditory mechanism, resulting in an elevated magnitude of the fluid-borne pressure waves in the cochlea. This greater force in the traveling wave displaces the basilar membrane more, and the crest of the traveling wave rises to a greater amplitude. Thus the spread of effect is increased, stimulating a larger number of sensory receptors and encoding an additional message to the CNS that more nerves are firing; therefore the stimulation is of a higher magnitude.

The resolving capabilities of the cochlea are impressive when one understands that it is possible to detect approximately 280 changes in the amplitude of a stimulus from the softest sound audible to the most intense sound that can be withstood. Further,

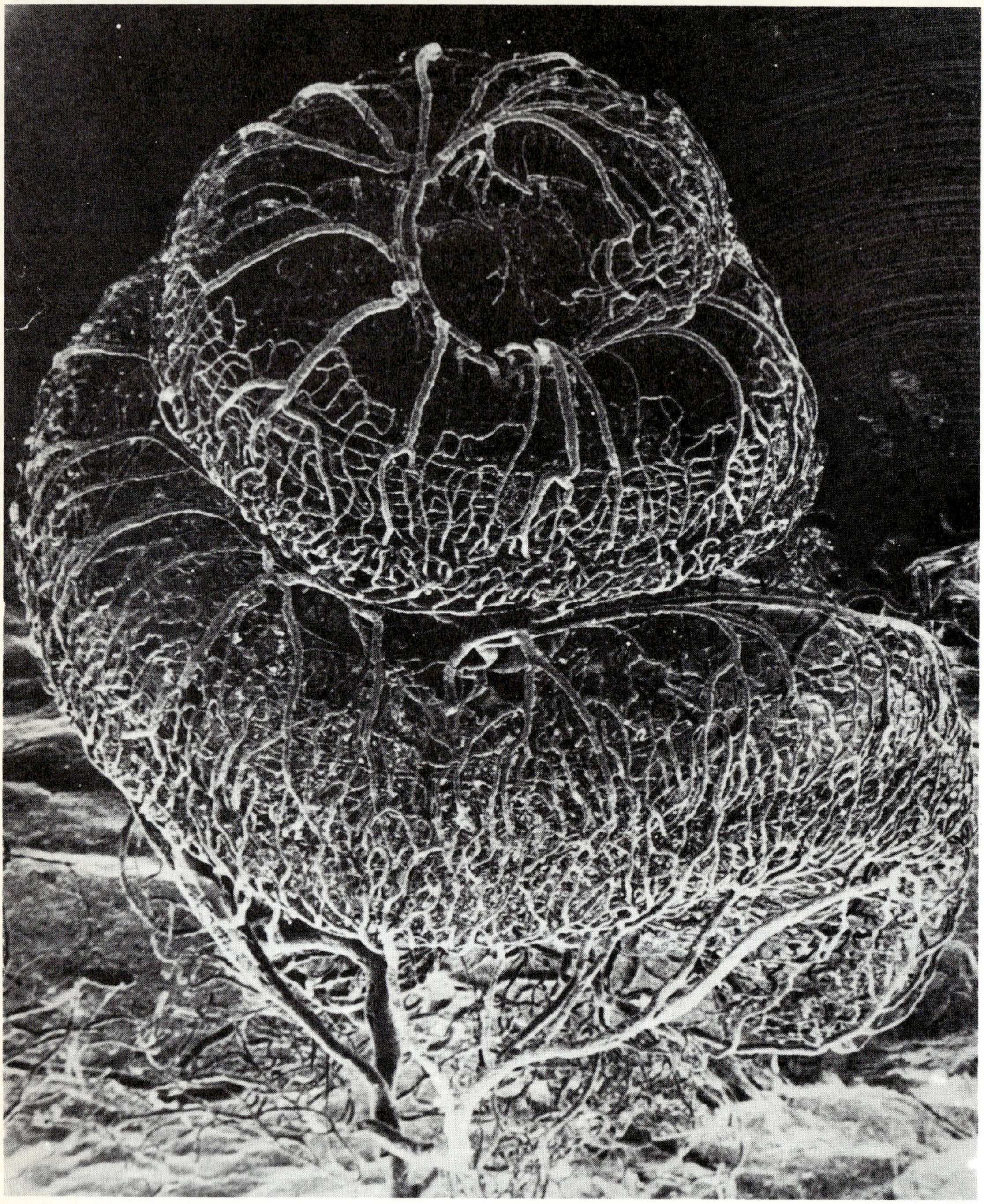

Figure 2-13 Vascular "tree" of the rat cochlea. This is a low magnification scanning electron photomicrograph of tissue prepared by injecting latex into the vascular system. After the latex solidified, all the cochlear tissue was dissolved in acid to reveal only latex-filled vascular channels. (Photo provided by Dr. Jack Vernon, Kresge Hearing Reseach Laboratory, Portland Oregon.)

1,400 pitch changes can be detected when one sweeps through the audible frequency range. In combination, this means the normal human ear can distinguish nearly 400,000 discrete intensity and frequency combinations—a truly remarkable achievement for such a tiny structure.

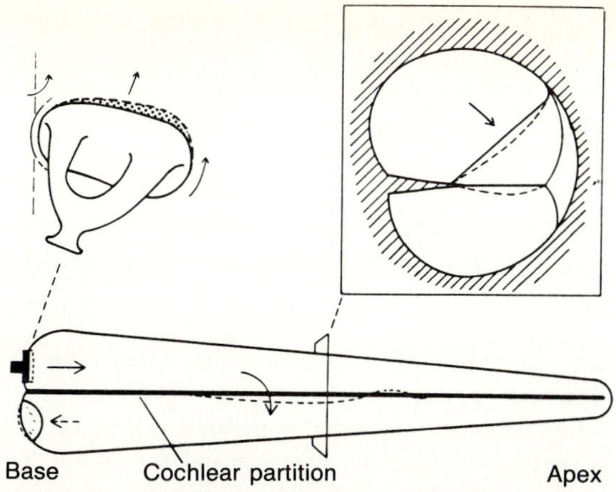

Figure 2–14 Diagram of the pneumatic relationship between the oval and round windows. Stapes displacement sets up fluid pressure waves in the cochlea, disturbing the scala media. Round window motion compensates for the fluid displacement, allowing for specific stimulation of places along the basilar membrane according to the frequency and amplitude characteristics of the stimulus. (From Durrant JD, Lovrinic JH. Bases of hearing science. Baltimore: Williams & Wilkins, 1977:91.[9])

Hearing Theory

Hearing theory dates back to early pronouncements by Empedocles in the fifth century B.C. He perceived correctly that sound was carried through air in the environment, but he speculated incorrectly that its perception depended upon an "internal air" that was implanted for the purpose of giving meaning to acoustic signals. Later, Plato furthered the discussion of the implanted air hypothesis, suggesting that it was implanted during uterine development. For over 2,000 years, the implanted air concept was the basis of hearing theory, until more was known about anatomy and the discussions of Galen in about A.D. 175 shed more light of understanding upon the function of the auditory mechanism. However, little progress was made until civilization emerged from the Dark Ages and scientific inquiry in the sixteenth century initiated modern hearing theory with the discovery and description of the middle ear mechanism. Hearing theory can be summarized by discussing four principles that characterize most of the features considered in theoretical concepts of auditory function.

Resonance Theory. Expanding upon the early considerations by Bauhin in 1605 and Du Verney in 1683, Helmholtz during the middle of the last century postulated that frequency resolution was the result of stimulation of tuned transverse fibers along the basilar membrane. A sound with its characteristic frequency would activate the fiber tuned to that pitch, signaling to the sensory cells and ultimately the nerve fibers the physical attribute of the sound.

It should be noted that Helmholtz was an astute observer of the mechanical and physical properties of the ear, and some of his measurements have stood the test of time. However, although he accomplished some of the primary early work on the subject of resonance (Helmholtz resonators are still used to illustrate the concept in classrooms today), he overlooked an important physical principle inherent in resonance. For a string to resonate, it must be free to vibrate independently. This concept can best be illustrated by plucking a guitar string and then touching it with the hand. Motion stops as soon as contact is made with the string. Owing to a high degree of damping by cochlear tissue, fibers in the basilar membrane are anything but free to move independently, and so the resonance concept could not be maintained and Helmholtz's resonance theory has been rejected.

Frequency Theory. Prior to the increase in knowledge of physiologic capabilities and limitations of nerve fibers, a series of theorists proposed that the inner ear serves simply as a transducer, a component that converts one form of energy into another form. Sound stimulating the inner ear was simply changed into neural impulses of the same frequency and carried to the brain for analysis and per-

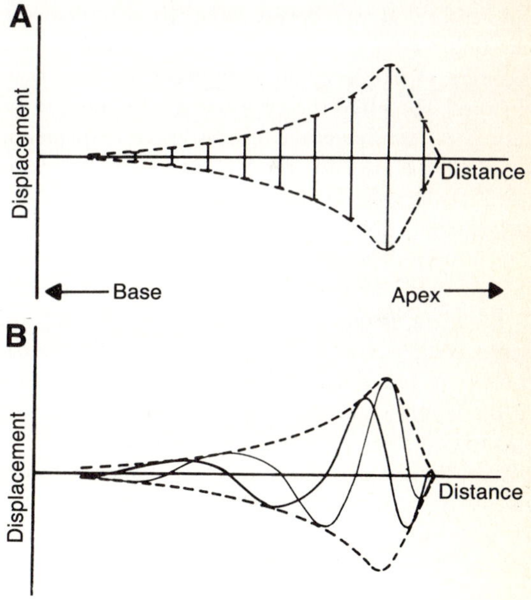

Figure 2–15 Highly simplified diagram of the traveling wave action in the cochlea along the basilar membrane. *A*, Basilar membrane envelope displacement (peak to peak) is shown. The envelope is drawn by connecting points of membrane excursion (marked by vertical lines) with a smoothed line. *B*, Two instantaneous waves shown as the membrane reaches its maximum displacement. The waves are confined to the envelope described in *A*. Note: this illustration is schematic in that the amount of displacement is greatly amplified. In reality, these wave motions are molecular dimensions. (From Durrant JD, Lovrinc JH. Bases of hearing science. Baltimore: Williams & Wilkins, 1977:92.[9])

ception. These theorists, most notably Rutherford in 1880, were not privy to the later findings that there is a decided limit on the speed at which nerves can fire. This limit is imposed by the absolute refractory period, a waiting time until the nerve can again be stimulated to fire. Since the absolute refractory period is in the 1-msec domain, a nerve cannot possibly fire more than approximately 1,000 times per second. Therefore, the frequency theory that suggested that a 10,000 Hz signal would set up nerve impulses at the same rate had to be scrapped. However, the frequency *principle* can still be put to good use for frequencies below the firing rate limit for nerves.

Place Theory. Taking a clue from the work of Helmholtz, several theorists suggested that although independent vibration of single basilar membrane fibers was not feasible, there still could be some resonance-type response resulting in a *place* of maximum stimulation. Numerous attempts were made to explain this concept, but it took the outstanding modeling and measurements of a Hungarian telephone engineer, who had immigrated to America, to provide the definitions of the place principle. George von Békésy, the only Nobel Prize laureate in the field of audiology, worked out a complex but believable series of explanations in the first half of this century. It was Békésy who best described the traveling wave and the way it results in differential encoding of frequency and amplitude by the organ of Corti. The place theory leaves a good deal to be desired for considerations of the lower frequencies, but the place principle cannot be disputed as an integral component in the understanding of auditory physiology.

Volley Theory. Wever proposed that, although single nerve fibers could not fire as rapidly as the many frequencies stimulate them, groups of nerves could fire in *volleys,* setting up in the statoacoustic nerve sequential neural impulses analogous to the frequency of the stimulus. Thus, he inserted this volley principle into his volley theory, a tripartite suggestion. First, the volley theory recognizes that the frequency principle can hold for sounds of lower frequency, perhaps up to 500 to 800 Hz. Then, employing the volley principle, Wever suggested that the frequency principle could be extended up to 5,000 Hz. For frequencies above 5,000 Hz, the place principle is employed. Thus, Wever has combined the best parts of three principles to develop his volley theory, a plausible description of the means whereby the inner ear analyzes and encodes messages for the CNS.

THE MIDDLE EAR

Developmental History

In primitive ears, an inner ear struture was all that was necessary to provide response to fluid-borne sound signals. Further, simple inner ears were adequate to serve the simple CNS capabilities of these creatures. With the migration out of the water and onto land, however, the inner ear needed help to deal with a different acoustic environment. Suddenly, there was a sizeable impedance mismatch between the fluid of the inner ear and the air in the environment. The mechanical impedance of air is about 41.5 mechanical ohms, whereas the impedance of the perilymphatic fluid is in the range of 140,000 mechanical ohms. Therefore, with such an impedance mismatch, considerable loss in the transmission of acoustic pressure waves to the cochlea occurred. This loss is due to the reflection of about 99.9 percent of the sound pressure by the surface of the perilymph, resulting in approximately a 35-dB *transmission* loss. Thus early amphibian-type animals probably had severely reduced auditory function, a physiologic feature that needed improvement if they were to survive in the hostile world around them. Hearing is the only distant 360-degree warning sense humans have. Vision is limited to the amount one can turn the head and affords only a little more than 180 degrees in any given field. Taction (touch) is a 360-degree sense, but it serves poorly for warning, since it can often only report "it's got me." And so a magnificent addition to the auditory mechanism developed with the middle ear mechanism, which ultimately served to closely match the impedance of air to that of the inner ear fluids.

Interestingly, middle ear development was closely associated with changes in lower jaw structure. The first middle ear structure to develop was the quadrate bone, a precursor of the present stapes. This flattened, roughly square bone served as an interface between the outer air and the inner ear by collecting the sound pressure waves over its surface and concentrating them at the point of attachment, a forerunner of the oval window. The early quadrate structure was very simple. It was large and took up all the available space for any middle ear structure, precluding the refinement necessary to improve the impedance matching. Later changes in the mandibular and maxillary structure allowed for reduction in size of the quadrate and improved design with a fragile but functional articuloquadrate joint. It was imperative that the mass of the quadrate be eliminated, because mass impairs transfer of higher frequency energy. Therefore early middle ear structures were largely low-frequency receptors, because the quadrate-like structures just could not be moved well by high-frequency sound. Improvement was slow in coming because the huge mastication musculature required considerable space, leaving only a small amount of room for the emerging middle ear. When the size of mastication muscles diminished, then a more efficient middle ear mechanism had space in which to develop.

Located immediately lateral to the inner ear region, the middle ear cavity (tympanic cavity) is an irregularly configured air-filled compartment with approximately 2 ml volume capacity. Its anteroposterior and superior-inferior dimensions are about 15 mm each. The medial-lateral dimension ranges between 2 and 6 mm.

To introduce the middle ear cavity, a schematic representation of its six sides is provided in Figure 2–16. For illustrative purposes, this simplified drawing discounts the fact that the cavity is not truly a cube. Dominating the lateral wall of the cavity is the tympanic membrane. On the anterior wall is located the opening of a tube connecting the middle ear and nasopharynx (eustachian tube). The medial wall is also the lateral wall of the inner ear and contains several important landmarks: the oval window; the round window niche; the promontory with the tympanic plexus, a group of canals containing nerve fibers on its surface; the pyramidal eminence of the stapedius muscle; the canal for the tensor tympani muscle; and the prominence of the facial canal, which houses the facial nerve (cranial nerve VII). The mastoid antrum, an entrance into a system of interconnected mastoid cells, comprises the posterior wall of the middle ear cavity. The superior wall is a thin dense layer of bone, the tegmen tympani, which

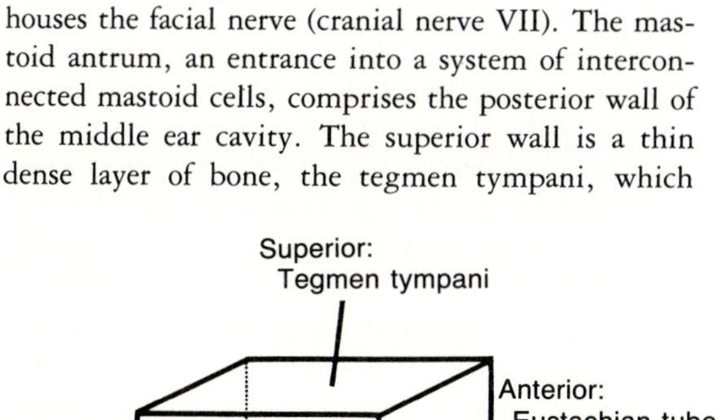

Figure 2-16 Schematic of the middle ear cavity boundaries as if the space were a cube. See text for details. (From Lipscomb DM. Mechanisms of the middle ear. In: Northern JL. Hearing disorders. Boston: Little, Brown, 1976:79.[10])

separates the middle ear cavity from the brain cavity. Finally, the jugular wall is the inferior margin that lies immediately above the jugular bulb and consists of a thin bony plate, the fundus tympani. All of the middle ear cavity is lined with mucous membrane, a delicate continuation of the lining of the throat, mouth, and nasal cavities.

Middle Ear Structures

The three densest and tiniest bones in the body make up an interconnected mechanical system that serves to transmit sound pressure across the middle ear cavity. These bones, the end result of the evolutionary process previously described, are termed the malleus, incus, and stapes (Fig. 2–17). The malleus is firmly attached to the tympanic membrane, and the footplate of the stapes is held in place in the oval window. Also in this region, the two smallest muscles of the body attach to the ossicular chain. The tendon of the tensor tympani muscle emerges from its canal and crosses the middle ear cavity to insert into the manubrium of the malleus. Arising from its pyramid-shaped orifice, the tendon of the stapedius muscle attaches to the neck region of the stapes. Innervating the tensor muscle is a branch of the cranial nerve V, the trigeminal nerve. The stapedius muscle is innervated by the stapedial branch of the facial nerve (cranial nerve VII). Mastoid cells, located posterior to the middle ear cavity, provide a pneumatic space. Mastoid cells are resonant cavities, slightly affecting the overall frequency response of the ear.

On the anterior portion of the cavity, the eustachian tube provides the only communication between the middle ear and the outside world by allowing the ingress and egress of air. It is the eustachian tube function that one experiences when the ears "pop" during a change in altitude. The middle ear end of the eustachian tube is patent (always open), and the other extremity, located on the posterior wall of the nasopharynx directly on a line posterior to the nostrils, is normally collapsed, thus reducing the opportunity for foreign particles to make their way into the middle ear cavity. In addition to its pneumatic function, the eustachian tube also serves as a drainage canal for fluid that might develop in the middle ear because of some disturbance in that cavity.

A fascinating component of the middle ear is the tympanic membrane, a pearl gray, three-layered, cone-shaped membrane whose function is to collect the acoustic pressure waves and direct them to the ossicular chain. The outer layer of the tympanic membrane is a continuation of the epithelial tissue (skin) lining the outer ear canal. In the middle layer are arranged radial and circular fibers increasing the

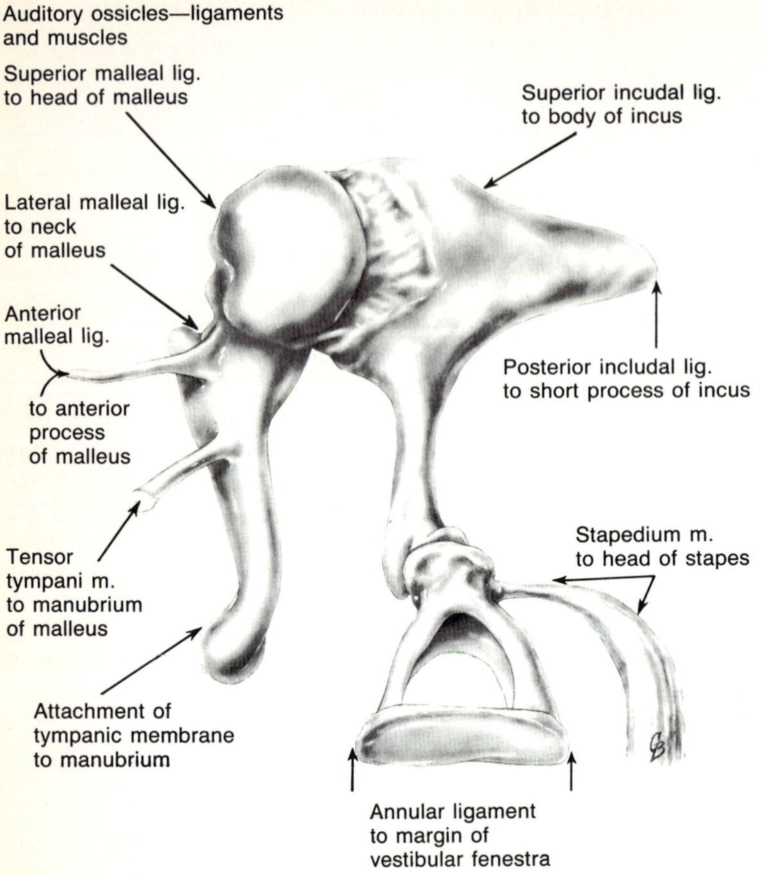

Figure 2–17 Ossicular chain and muscles of the middle ear. See text for description. (From Anson BJ, Donaldson JA. Surgical anatomy of the temporal bone and ear. 2nd ed. Philadelphia: WB Saunders, 1973:245.[4])

tensile strength of the membrane. These fibers, similar in appearance to a spider web, are absent in the superior portion of the membrane, an area termed Shrapnell's membrane (pars flaccida).

The innermost layer of the tympanic membrane is the mucous lining, a continuation of the lining of the rest of the middle ear cavity. Since mucus is a soft tissue with little tensile strength, the malleus is rigidly affixed to the middle, fibrous layer of the membrane and the mucus is draped over the handle (manubrium) of the malleus.

Although the tympanic membrane is only about 0.07 mm thick with an average area of 63 mm, it has an amazing degree of strength as well as extraordinary sensitivity to airborne sound. When one considers the extremes of energy experienced throughout the dynamic range of hearing, the tympanic membrane design is immensely impressive. Considering that from the average threshold of hearing (0 dB) to the pain threshold (140 dB) there is a growth of exerted energy of 100 trillion to one, a construction is required that can withstand such a range of pressure variation and still maintain remarkable sensitivity. At threshold levels of hearing, the tympanic membrane moves only about 40 millionths of a cm, yet it responds to sound. That dimension is less than one one-hundredth the width of the hydrogen molecule, the smallest one known. Thus the ear, partly owing to the great sensitivity of the tympanic membrane, is capable of operating in submolecular dimensions.

Other landmarks on the tympanic membrane include the umbo, the deepest depression of the cone adjacent to the tip of the manubrium; the attic, located at the superior margin of the tympanic membrane; and the malleolar prominence, a small bump caused by the lateral process of the malleus. Around the circumference of the membrane is a thickened edge, the fibrous annulus or tympanic ring, which is seated in a groove, the tympanic sulcus, to further anchor the tympanic membrane in place. Visible through the partially translucent membrane is the manubrium, a landmark termed the "malleolar stria."

Functional Correlates of the Middle Ear

Although each of the structures will be discussed somewhat independently of other components of the middle ear, one must remember that they all combine to function as a system to provide the necessary transformations for which the middle ear was intended.

Tympanic Membrane

To augment its role as a sound collector, the orientation of the tympanic membrane is such that it lies in a plane nearly perpendicular to the direction of sound in the external ear canal. The manubrium of the malleus increases the total area without enlarging its circumference by holding the tympanic membrane in a cone-shaped position, which also has the effect of maintaining appropriate tension on the structure. If the membrane is too tightly stretched, it does not move readily and sound energy is reflected from its surface. If, however, the membrane becomes flaccid, it moves so readily that energy is absorbed and not efficiently passed on to the ossicular chain. Sound pressure at threshold is only 0.0002 millionths of barometric pressure (0.0002 μbar). The pattern with which the membrane moves has been found to be less piston-like and more segmental (Fig. 2–18). Except during very high-level sound stimulation when the membrane does move more as a unit, tympanic membrane motion is greatest in the inferior portion of the surface of the membrane and becomes increasingly smaller toward the outer and superior regions. Thus the tympanic membrane responds effectively to sound over only about two-thirds of its surface.

Ossicular Chain

The benefits of the ossicular chain could be largely negated by the mass of the bones if it were not for the suspension system which holds it in place. With the need for rigid attachment to prevent their breaking away and for flexibility for energy-transferring motion, the ossicles are differentially suspended by attachments to the upper and lateral margins of the middle ear as well as by muscle attachments and interconnections between the bones themselves. With the support provided, the ossicles move around finely aligned axes, allowing them to work with a high degree of efficiency. Each of the three bones is suspended differently, depending upon its size and location. The malleus, a club-shaped structure, weighs about 25 mg. Being comparatively large, the malleus is suspended from above to reduce the influence of its mass on the transmission capabilities of the ossicular chain. To direct its motion, other attachments are the ligamentous strands to the lateral and anterior walls of the middle ear; the attachment of the tensor muscle; and its articulation with the second bone in the chain, the incus. Shaped differently, but weighing about the same as the malleus, the incus is also suspended from above and projects a long crus or leg downward to articulate with the tiniest of the three bones, the stapes at the tip or the lenticular process. The stapes, bearing a real resemblance to a stirrup, is not suspended in the same manner as the other two ossicular bones; it is held in the oval window by an annular ligament around the entire circumference of the stapes footplate. The stapes is further held by its articulation with the incus, the incudostapedius joint and by the stapedius muscle. The mass of the stapes is only about one-tenth that of the other two ossicles, partly because it is constructed with hollow arches (crura), an architectural form known in gothic style architecture to be a strong yet light formation. If the stapes were not so built, its mass would mediate against transmission of high-frequency energy.

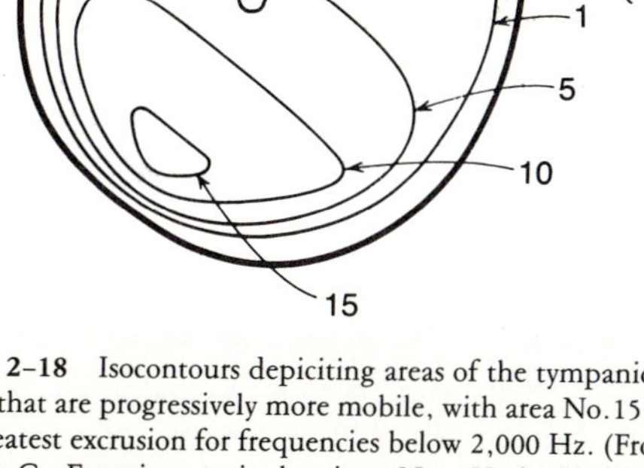

Figure 2–18 Isocontours depiciting areas of the tympanic membrane that are progressively more mobile, with area No.15 having the greatest excrusion for frequencies below 2,000 Hz. (From von Békésy G. Experiments in hearing. New York: McGraw-Hill, 1960:101.[11])

Ossicular motion varies as a function of the frequency and intensity of the sound directed along the structures. With the exertion of positive acoustic pressure on the tympanic membrane, the inward motion of the tympanic membrane is transferred to an inward movement of the manubrium of the malleus, concurrently displacing the head of the malleus lateralward. This displacement pulls the body of the incus lateralward as well and, because of restrictions in direction of movement afforded by the suspension system of the incus, forces the long process of the incus medialward, thus pushing the anterior portion of the footplate of the stapes into the oval window and setting up a positive pressure wave in the fluid of the inner ear. The anterior portion of the annular ligament is thinner than the posterior portion, allowing for greater mobility of the anterior edge of the footplate. At higher intensities of signal strength, ossicular movement is modified such that the entire stapes footplate is pressed into the window in piston-like form. Then, at an even higher intensity, the stapes footplate motion is modified again to somewhat reduce the total pressure delivered to the cochlea. Freedom for the stapes to displace cochlear fluid depends upon free movement of the round window. During the negative phase of the sound pressure wave, all motion just described is reversed, with the end result being the withdrawing of the footplate of the stapes and the medial movement of the round window membrane. In sum, for low- and medium-amplitude sound waves, the ossicular chain efficiently transports the energy into the inner ear. This efficiency declines when higher amplitude sounds occur, thus providing some degree of protection of the cochlear structures from high-level sound.

Middle Ear Muscles

The effect of contraction by the tensor tympani muscle is to displace the manubrium of the malleus and tympanic membrane medially. This medial displacement increases tension on the middle ear mechanism and can reduce the responsivity of the mechanism slightly, predominantly in the frequencies below 2,000 Hz. Being the larger of the two middle ear muscles, the tensor is about 25 mm in length, with a cross-sectional area of around 5 mm^2. In its normal, uncontracted state, the tensor muscle exerts a slight pull of about 0.5 g just by being affixed to the malleus. With contraction, of course, this pull increases, affecting the total compliance of the ossicular chain. The effective force of the stapedius muscle is in the opposite direction to that exerted by the tensor; thus the two muscles can be considered to be antagonistic to each other. Being considerably smaller, only 6- to 7-mm long with a cross-sectional area of 5 mm^2, the total force of which the stapedius muscle is capable is less than that of the tensor. However, its location magnifies the effect of the force it is capable of exerting. With contraction, the stapedius forces the ossicular chain in a direction opposite to that described by the stimulation with a positive pressure wave in that the result of stapedius contraction is to move the tympanic membrane lateralward. Since its action is directly upon the stapes itself by lifting the footplate out of the oval window, a given contractile force of the stapedius muscle can have a stronger effect on stapes motion than can the tensor muscle contracting with the same amount of force.

Middle ear muscle contractions can be voluntarily initiated by some people or they can be triggered by certain forms of stimulation. Tensor contractions result from tickling the face or directing a jet of air into the ear canal, thereby stimulating regions served by cranial nerve V. Forcing the eyelids closed in a severe squint and clenching teeth can produce a "rushing" sound, indicating that the tensor muscle has contracted. Firm pressure on the eyeball, although not recommended, can initiate the tensor reflex. Using high-level sound is the most predictable means of causing a stapedius muscle reflex because of a neurologic reflex arc between the cochlea, centers in the brain stem, and the facial nerve (cranial nerve VII). This process and its clinical significance are discussed in detail in Chapters 3 and 40.

The impact of middle ear muscle contraction is to reduce the efficiency of the transmission mechanism and to serve a limited protective function against possible damage to cochlear tissues in the wake of high-level sound stimulation. It must be remembered that this protective function is limited at best and can be of consequence only for frequencies below 2,000 Hz. The limitation is due to the fact that muscle contraction produces an increase in stiffness of the ossicular chain. Stiffness has the effect of reducing low-frequency energy transmission only; therefore higher frequencies overcome the stiffness readily, thereby circumventing any protective characteristic of the middle ear muscles.

Contribution of the Middle Ear

There are two major contributors to the almost unbelievable acoustic sensitivity of the ear: (1) shearing motion in the organ of Corti, which has already been described; and (2) middle ear transformer function. A shortcoming in the auditory structures of early land-dwelling creatures was a poor interface between air in the environment and fluid in the inner ear, resulting in the impedance mismatch previously described. Impedance, the degree to which a structure opposes a driving force directed against it, is a critical area in the understanding of auditory function. Regardless of the physical phenomenon involved, impedance is a combination of three factors that have different names depending upon the physical properties being considered. In acoustic terms, these three components are acoustic resistance, acoustic mass, and acoustic compliance.

Acoustic Resistance

Resistance is the opposition offered by the responding mechanism, which is analogous to mechanical friction. It reduces transfer of energy independent of the frequency characteristics of the driving force. In other words, resistance impedes sound transmission to an equal degree for all frequencies.

Acoustic Mass

Inertia, the direct result of object or structure weight (mass), also opposes energy transfer. The effect of mass grows with frequency and so is dependent upon frequency. Mass is less effective in opposing low-frequency sound transmission, but becomes more of a factor with higher frequency stimulation. It is for this reason that it was pointed out that the design of the stapes to make it very light reduced opposition to transfer of higher frequency sound.

Acoustic Compliance (Stiffness)

The name of this third component connotes that it has something to do with the ability of a structure to *comply* with a driving force. A stiff (noncompliant) response mechanism discourages the transfer of energy. Energy transfer can also be reduced if the mechanism is overly compliant, but for a different reason. The latter situation is the result of energy absorption caused by inadequate coupling to the mechanism. A noncompliant mechanism exerts a barrier effect, causing an inordinate amount of the driving force to be reflected. Acoustic compliance is also dependent upon frequency, having a greater effect in the lower frequencies. Therefore, as was stated earlier, when middle ear muscles contract, increasing ossicular chain stiffness, the effect is to reduce transmission of low frequencies much more than high frequencies.

These three components combine to equal the total impedance of a given response system. In some cases, the system is compliance dominated, whereas other conditions lead to mass domination with resultant alterations in frequency transmission characteristics. If the middle ear has become inordinately stiff, as in the case of otosclerosis, then the effect is a loss of hearing predominantly in the low frequencies. Since acoustic mass and acoustic compliance differentially affect transmission of certain frequencies, their combined presence can sometimes offset each other, leaving only acoustic resistance as the impeding factor. In all physical entities, there is a *natural* frequency, that is, a frequency at which mass and compliance interact to cancel each other, resulting in somewhat better energy transfer at that frequency. For the normal human ear, the natural frequency is in the 800 to 1,000 Hz frequency region.

The Middle Ear Transformer

Structural design of the middle ear fosters an effective amplification of the force exerted against the tympanic membrane. This is accomplished by two factors: by the areal relationship between the tympanic membrane and the footplate of the stapes and by the ossicles serving as a mechanical lever.

Areal Relationship. In humans, the overall area of the tympanic membrane exceeds that of the footplate of the stapes by a factor of approximately 21:1. Consider that only two-thirds of the tympanic membrane surface is mobile, the effective ratio becomes 14:1. Calculations have shown that a 14:1 ratio results in a magnification of footplate force by about 23 dB, which means that the collective capacity of the tympanic membrane is channeled to the stapes with an overall force gain of 23 dB. It would seem that greater force transfer could be achieved by enlarging the effective areal ratio to 30:1 or more. For this to occur, the tympanic membrane would necessarily be enlarged to greater than twice its size, yielding approximately only a 3-dB improvement in transfer. Further, a tympanic membrane that large would be difficult to damp (terminate movement upon cessation of the driving force). Thus an undesirable side effect would be a ringing, the continued movement of a response mechanism although the stimulation has ceased. This condition would cause rapidly occurring sounds to run together and become much less comprehensible. It would occasion an acoustic experience akin to trying to play the Minute Waltz on a piano while holding the sustain pedal down throughout the entire piece.

Lever Action. The manubrium of the malleus is 1.3 times as long as the long process of the incus; and so a slight lever advantage of 1.3:1 occurs as a result of the relative size and location of the two larger structures in the ossicular chain. Translated into quantified sound values, the lever action of the chain results in a further 2.5-dB advantage, which would not be realized if the lever did not exist.

These two factors in the transformer function are additive, resulting in a total transfer value of slightly over 25 dB. This additional auditory sensitivity was a significant force in the development of hearing and probably contributed to the ultimate emergence of Homo sapiens. The ear introduced a previously unknown ability, the reception of sound originating from a distance. Smaller creatures could be alerted to the presence of danger at an earlier time, which certainly fostered preservation and, hence, proliferation of many species. To the extent that we understand anthropology, our distant ancestors apparently sprang from creatures that were not as large as the predators from whom the prehumans needed protection. Therefore we humans can probably thank the ear, and most specifically the middle ear, for our existence.

Normal Requirements

Two conditions must be met in order for the middle ear to function normally: (1) air pressure must be equivalent on both sides of the tympanic membrane, a responsibility of the eustachian tube, and (2) mobility of the moving parts must be maintained. Stapes motion should be free of inhibiting influences such as adhesions, calcium deposits, accumulated fluid, and debris. The round window membrane cannot operate normally unless it is free to complete its normal back-and-forth motion in response to stapes movement.

A Secondary Pathway

Human hearing depends almost entirely on sound delivered to the tympanic membrane and transmitted along the air conduction pathway described previously. There is a secondary pathway, termed "bone conduction," which follows an alternate route and provides direct stimulation to the inner ear region. In order for bone conduction to occur, the skull itself must be set into vibration. Vibratory energy enters the cochlea in addition to or instead of following the ossicular chain. Three modes of bone conduction exist.

Compressional Mode. Alternating pressure waves, if sufficiently intense, cause the skull to pulse in and out in synchrony with the stimulus. The alternate compression and decompression of the cochlear and labyrinthine walls result in pressure waves in the cochlear canal the same as if the stapes had been forced in and out of the oval window. In bone conduction, the round window membrane moves to serve the same pressure relief function it maintains in air conduction. Regardless of how the pressure waves are introduced into the cochlea, the organ of Corti can and will respond to the disturbance. Therefore the compressional mode of bone conduction is effective in stimulating the cochlea once the force behind the sound sets the skull in vibration. Although its contribution is somewhat greater at high frequencies, the compressional mode is considered to occur at most frequencies.

Inertial Mode. The ossicular chain is not directly stimulated by skull vibrations, since the tissue in its suspension system serves to isolate the ossicles from the skull. When vibrations occur involving the skull as a whole, the ossicular chain begins to vibrate, but lags in its movement because of structure inertia and the isolation afforded by the suspension system. Therefore the footplate of the stapes moves in and out of the oval window, not because tympanic membrane movement directs it to do so, but because the skull, and specifically the temporal bone, vibrates around the stapes. The effect is the same. Pressure waves are set up in the fluid of the inner ear. The contribution of the inertial mode is predominantly in the low frequencies where there is time for the lagging motion of the ossicular chain to have an impact. As the frequency of stimulating sound increases, there is insufficient time for the interaction between the stapes and oval window to occur, and this mode fades from effective participation.

Osseotympanic Mode. The external ear canal is located in close proximity to the temporomandibular joint. The point of attachment of the lower jaw also serves an isolating function, causing skull vibrations transmitted to the lower jaw to be delayed, which introduces another type of inertial factor. In this case, the lagging movement of the lower jaw causes it to "bump" the temporal bone alternately in synchrony with the frequency of the driving sound stimulus, setting up a string of stimulus synchronous "clicks" in the external ear canal. Since all forms of energy choose to take the path of least resistance, the "clicks" simply exit the open ear canal and have no effect, unless the external ear canal is not open. With canal blockage, the path of least resistance becomes the air conduction pathway for sound, and so the "clicks" are directed against the tympanic membrane and follow the ossicular chain. This mode, greatest for low frequencies, is the least contributive since the external canal is normally open. When the ear canal is blocked, a distinct change in the sound of one's voice occurs owing to the insertion of the osseotympanic mode into the auditory experience.

Depending upon the condition in effect, all three modes operate when stimulation reaches a level that can cause skull vibration. Interaction between the modes depends upon the frequency of the stimulating sound.

THE EXTERNAL EAR

The final stage in ear development came very late. In fact, the external ear is chiefly an attribute of mammals. Amphibian ears, such as that of the frog, possess a simple middle ear with the columella. The tympanic membrane is located directly on the side of the head. Gradually, with other modifications in form, the tympanic membrane moved inward and a canal began to form, which provided the access for sound to the auditory mechanism. Birds, for example, also have a columella in the middle ear with a fairly long ear canal, sometimes reaching a length of 1 cm. Only mammals have developed the external earflap.

External Ear Structure

The external ear can be considered in two parts. (1) The earlier developed external auditory meatus or canal emerged as the auditory structures, particularly the middle ear, were relocated deeper into the skull. As dependence upon hearing increased, it apparently became necessary to afford the auditory apparatus more protection; hence a pathway was created to direct acoustic signals to the well-protected ear. (2) The auricle or pinna is a convoluted, irregularly shaped flap of skin with some cartilaginous support found only in land-dwelling mammals. The pinna has historically been considered to be of relatively little value to the sense of hearing. However, recent investigations have indicated that the pinna does make some rather significant contributions to our refined sense of hearing.

The External Canal

In humans, the external canal attains a length in adulthood of approximately 2.5 cm with a diameter of about 0.7 cm. The shape and course of the canal is highly variable. A curious design has developed that affords both protection from air-borne foreign objects and access for sound. The course of the external meatus follows a tortuous "S"-shape from its opening to its medial terminal point at the tympanic membrane. Particles in the air and small insects are thus presented with a type of obstacle course. In addition, the outer third of the canal contains hairs that tend to filter out unwanted substances by causing them to adhere to the surface of the hairs. Also located in the skin of the outer third of the canal are ceruminous and sebaceous glands, which secrete a bitter tasting, brown, wax-like substance—cerumen—commonly called "earwax." This sticky material is toxic to small insects that sometimes find their way into the canal. It usually precludes the deep penetration by the insect. Being a mild adhesive, the cerumen coats the hairs in the canal, rendering them more effective in trapping foreign particles, which, if allowed to reach the tympanic membrane, could cause discomfort or could even damage the membrane.

The entire canal is lined with epithelial tissue, a continuation of the covering of the auricle. Beginning at the center of the tympanic membrane, there is a systematic migration of epithelial cells toward the opening of the canal. In time, this migratory activity, serving like a slow-moving conveyer belt, deposits the old, dirty cerumen outside the ear. Excessive probing in the ear canal undercuts the function of this migration.

The Auricle

Although the external earflap has some distinguishing geographic regions, its variability in shape and size is highly individualized in humans and in animals. No two persons have identical auricles, a factor that has caused criminologists to seriously consider using the auricle for identification purposes along with or in place of fingerprints.

Major landmarks and geographic areas on the auricle are shown in Figure 2–19. The concha is the deepest depression in the auricle, located near the center below the midpoint and is the expanded opening of the external meatus. A curved rim, the helix, describes the outer portion of the superior and posterior portion of the earflap. Since the helix is slightly doubled over in a loose roll, it, along with the extended portion of the auricle, serves as a cushioning for each side of the head in the event of trauma. The protective function is rather minimal, but, conceivably, it can mean the difference between a skull fracture and a nasty bruise. Anteriorly, the helix descends into the region of the concha and divides it into two areas, the cymba to the rear and the cavitus adjacent to the canal opening.

A second ridge, the antihelix, is located just toward the concha from the helix. Mentioned earlier, the tragus hovers over the canal opening and partially occludes the canal from the anterior side. The area bordering the lower opening into the concha, the antitragus, is highly variable in size from one individual to another. Often indistinguishable is Darwin's tubercle (tuberculum auriculae), a small flattened area on the posterior margin of the helix. Finally, the lobule or earlap is a fleshy, fat-filled globe that descends below the area of the concha and has little apparent function other than serving as a place to locate decorative jewelry.

A newly discovered value of the auricle is its aid in auditory localization. When sound originates on the midline directly in front of or directly behind an individual, acoustic pressure waves arrive at the two ears at the same instant. That temporal relationship is interpreted as being a midline sound origin by the CNS, which integrates information from both ears. If a source is displaced to one side, then the times of arrival at the ears are different because sound requires a fraction of a second longer to arrive

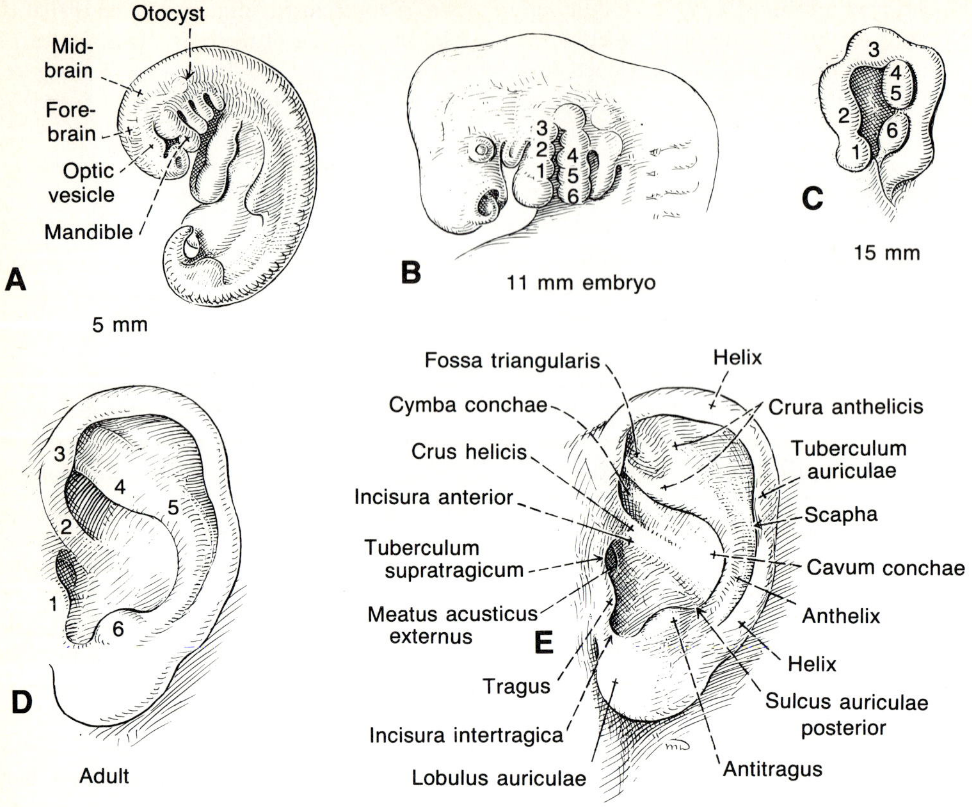

Figure 2–19 Structures and landmarks of the auricle. (From Anson BJ, Donaldson JA. Surgical anatomy of the temporal bone and ear. Philadelphia: WB Saunders, 1973:31.[4])

at the more distant ear and is slightly lower in level because it has to work past the partial barrier effect of the head. In this case, the CNS has learned to interpret the location of sound origin as being toward the side. Studies in psychophysics have indicated that humans can localize sound to one side or another with amazing facility. This aspect of sound localization is primarily due to the temporal (time of arrival at each ear) and intensive (relative level of the sound striking the two ears) parameters. These parameters offer little assistance in distinguishing whether sound originated from the front or behind. Further, there is still inadequate information as to the origin of the sound away from the horizontal plane of the head (above or below). Looking at the numerous creases of the auricle and understanding that the CNS is capable of resolving time and amplitude differences of remarkably little magnitude, it can then be discerned that regardless of the direction from which a sound occurs, the reflective surface for the sound presented by the auricle is different. This reflective surface, it is felt, contributes the information necessary for the auditory mechanism to use so that accurate determination of location of the sound source can be made within the entire spherical environment served by the ear. In effect, the extremely accurate localization of which humans are capable relies in large part upon the configuration of the auricle. When humans are confused about the precise orientation of a sound source, that confusion is more than likely a result of quirks within the auditory environment rather than a breakdown of the system itself, that is, unusual reflecting surfaces confusing the direction to the source.

SUMMARY

It is awesome to review the known capacity of the ear in distinguishing the presence of sound and in differentiating among a wide range of acoustic signals according to their meaningfulness. As you have seen, this immensely complex interactive group of specialized tissues did not simply spring instantaneously into being. Millions of years were spent using considerable experimentation and countless forms to achieve the highly sensitive and functional auditory mechanism we have studied here (Fig. 2–20).

A major theme throughout the development of hearing is the economy of creation. The ear takes up surprisingly little space, an economy that keeps the

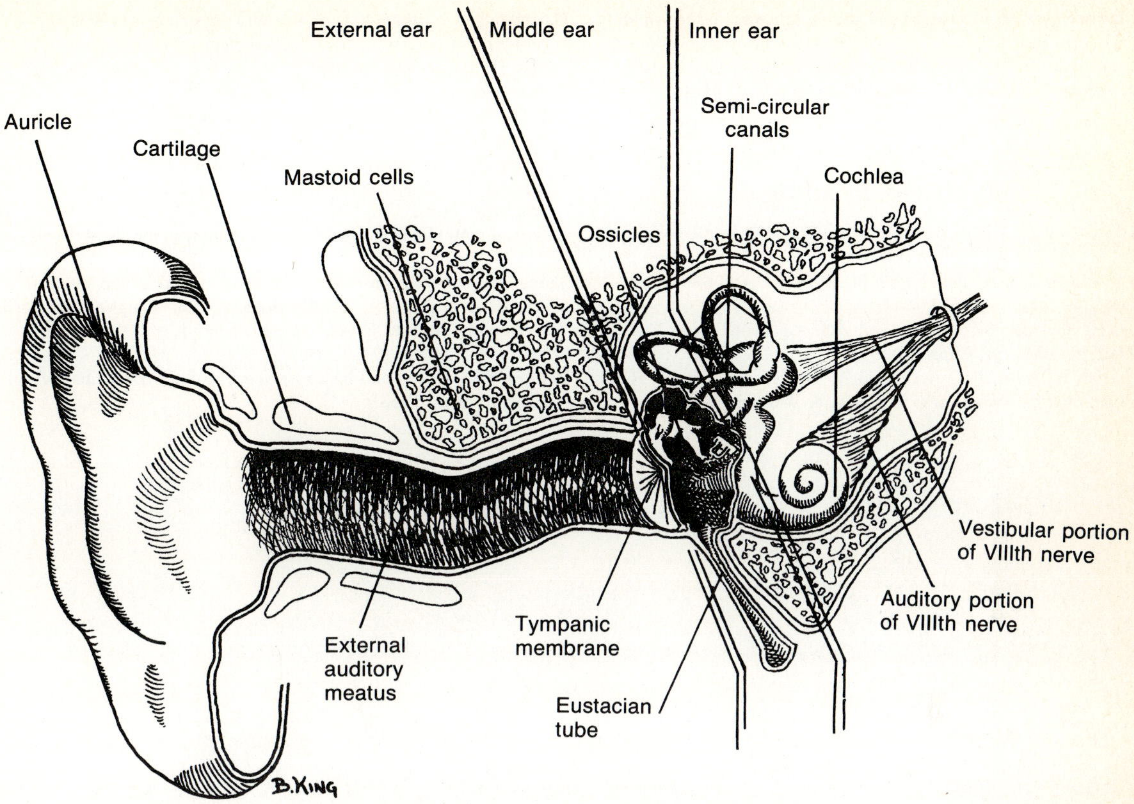

Figure 2–20 The ear in semidiagrammatic form.

head no larger than necessary. Throughout the progressive stages of development, ear forms were provided that adequately served but did not outperform the CNS, an economy that precluded expanding ability beyond the point of diminishing returns. Redundancy in auditory signals has been matched by redundancy inherent in auditory function to economize on transfer of the information content of each stimulus. The developing inner ear took on an increasing role as an analyzer, leaving the CNS free to develop greater perceptual skills, an economy in neural organization. Providing the simplest structure that could accomplish a given task has been the policy in the design of the auditory mechanism throughout the range of structure variations, an economy in tissue acquisition and usage. No special anatomic, biochemical, mechanical, or architectural principles were invented to serve audition. The ear was designed by means of existing principles according to the most economical method in order to employ each principle or set of principles. In sum, the design and structure of the ear are so complete and so intelligent that to conceive or to manufacture a system of the size and complexity of the ear that even comes close to the quality of performance we take for granted in our hearing sense is an impossibility.

REFERENCES

1. Wersäll J, Flock Å. Functional anatomy of the vestibular and lateral line organ. In: Neff WD, ed. Contributions to sensory physiology. Vol. 1. New York: Academic Press, 1965:39.
2. van Bergeijk WA. The evolution of vertebrate hearing. In: Neff WD, ed. Contributions to sensory physiology. Vol. 2. New York: Academic Press, 1967:1.
3. Wever EG. The tectorial membrane of the lizard ear: types of structure. J Morphol 1967; 122:307–320.
4. Anson BJ, Donaldson JA. Surgical anatomy of the temporal bone and ear. 2nd ed. Philadelphia: WB Saunders, 1973.
5. Lipscomb DM. An introduction to the laboratory study of the ear. Springfield, IL: CC Thomas, 1974.
6. Davis H, Benson RW, Covell WP, Fernandez C, Goldstein R, Tatsuki J, Legouix JP, McAuliffe DR, Tasaki I. Acoustic trauma in the guinea pig. J Acoust Soc Am 1953; 25:1180–1189.
7. Dallos P, Ryan A. Physiology of the inner ear. In: Northern JL, ed. Hearing disorders. Boston: Little, Brown, 1976:89.
8. Axelsson A. The vascular anatomy of the cochlea in the guinea pig and in man. Acta Otolaryngol [Suppl] (Stockh) 1968; 243:1–134.
9. Durrant JD, Lovrinic JH. Bases of hearing science. Baltimore: Williams & Wilkins, 1977.

Acknowledgements. I am indebted to Dr. Henry L. Witter for his numerous suggestions and critical review of the text of this chapter.

10. Lipscomb DM. Mechanisms of the middle ear. In: Northern JL, ed. Hearing disorders, Boston: Little, Brown 1976:78.
11. Békésy, G von. Experiments in hearing. Translated and edited by EG Wever. New York: McGraw-Hill, 1960.

Suggested Reading

Bredberg G. Cellular pattern and nerve supply of the human organ of Corti. Acta Otolaryngol Suppl (Stockh) 1968; 236:1–135.

Davis H, Silverman SR. Hearing and deafness. 3rd ed. New York: Holt, Rinehart, & Winston, 1970.

Engström H, Ades HW, Andersson A. Structural pattern of the organ of corti. New York: Williams & Wilkins, 1966.

Gallagher JC. Histology of the human temporal bone. Washington: Armed Forces Institute of Pathology, 1967.

Harris JD. Anatomy and physiology of the peripheral hearing mechanism. New York: Bobbs-Merrill, 1974.

Lim DJ. Fine morphology of the tectorial membrane. Arch Otolaryngol 1972; 96:199–215.

Naunton RF. The measurement of hearing by bone conduction. In: Jerger J, ed. Modern developments in audiology. New York: Academic Press, 1963:1.

Polyak SL, McHugh G, Judd DK. The human ear. New York: TH McKenna, 1946.

Tumarkin A. Evolution of the auditory conducting apparatus in terrestrial vertebrates. In: De Reuck AVS, Knight J, eds. Hearing mechanisms in vertebrates. London: J. and A. Churchill, 1970:18.

Zemlin WR. Speech and hearing science. Englewood Cliffs, NJ: Prentice-Hall, 1968.

3 Neuroanatomic Bases of Hearing and Speech

Bryan E. Pfingst, Ph.D.
Richard A. Altschuler, Ph.D.
Kenneth L. Watkin, Ph.D.
Charles R. Larson, Ph.D.

Human speech perception and production involve the interaction of the peripheral transduction and articulatory structures with a sophisticated nervous system. This chapter presents the anatomy of the nervous system as it relates to hearing and speech production. An understanding of the nervous system is necessary for those studying the physiology of hearing, speech production, and neurologic disorders affecting speech, language, and hearing.

The nervous system may be divided into two components, the central nervous system (CNS) and the peripheral nervous system (PNS). The CNS includes the brain and spinal cord, and the PNS includes sensory receptors and nerves lying outside the CNS. These nerves carry information from receptors in the ear and the articulators to the CNS via afferent pathways, and information from the CNS to the effector organs and muscles via efferent pathways.

For ease of understanding, the brain may be organized into anatomic regions. Starting from the periphery, the brain and spinal cord meet at the caudal edge of the medulla oblongata (Fig. 3–1). The medulla (myelencephalon) extends to the caudal border of the pons, and the pons (metencephalon) extends rostrally to the caudal edge of the midbrain region (mesencephalon), which contains the nuclei forming the inferior and superior colliculi. The midbrain can be divided into two parts by the cerebral aqueduct, the dorsal portion called the "roof" or "tectum," and the ventral portion called the "cerebral peduncle." The cerebral peduncle can, in turn, be divided into a ventral portion termed the "crus cerebri" and a dorsal portion, just ventral to the cerebral aqueduct, called the "tegmentum." The major portion of the inferior colliculus is located in the tectum, but there are tegmental divisions of the inferior colliculus as well.

Rostral to the midbrain region lies the diencephalon, consisting of the hypothalamus, thalamus, and adjacent structures. The thalamus is the major relay nucleus to the cerebral cortex for all sensory systems, with the possible exception of olfaction. It consists of a number of sensory and motor relay nuclei in close proximity, situated next to the midline. The thalamus is bordered dorsally by cortical fibers and the tail of the caudate nucleus, and laterally it is surrounded by fibers of the cerebral hemispheres. Each of the nuclear groups in the thalamus is involved in a specific sensory or motor function and is heavily connected by afferent and efferent fibers with a specific area of the cerebral cortex (Fig. 3–2).

The medulla, pons, mesencephalon, and diencephalon are collectively known as the brain stem. Dorsal to the brain stem lies the cerebellum, which, along with the pons, constitutes the metencephalon. Rostral to the brain stem lies the telencephalon, which consists of the cerebral cortex and the corpus striatum (basal ganglia).

The cerebral cortex (Fig. 3–3) is a highly convoluted structure that almost completely envelopes and obscures other areas of the brain. The fissures or folds of the cortex are known as sulci, and the rounded portions are called gyri. The patterns of sulci and gyri differ somewhat from brain to brain, but certain characteristic features of the gyri are found in most normal brains.

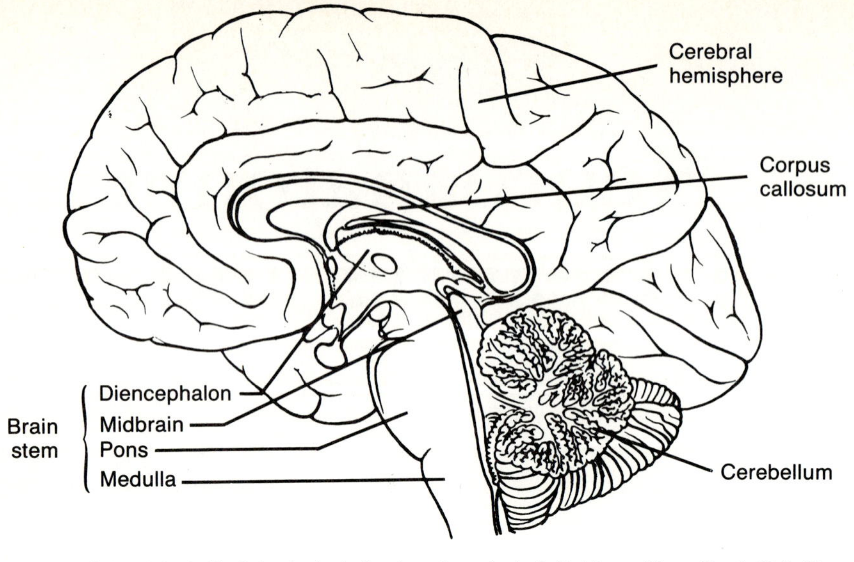

Figure 3–1 Median view of the right half of the brain indicating the principal divisions. (From Reed GM, Sheppard VF. Basic structures of the head and neck. Philadelphia: WB Saunders, 1976:175.)

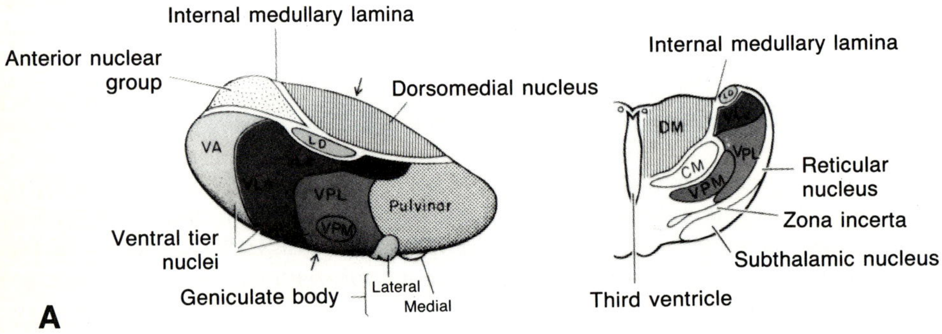

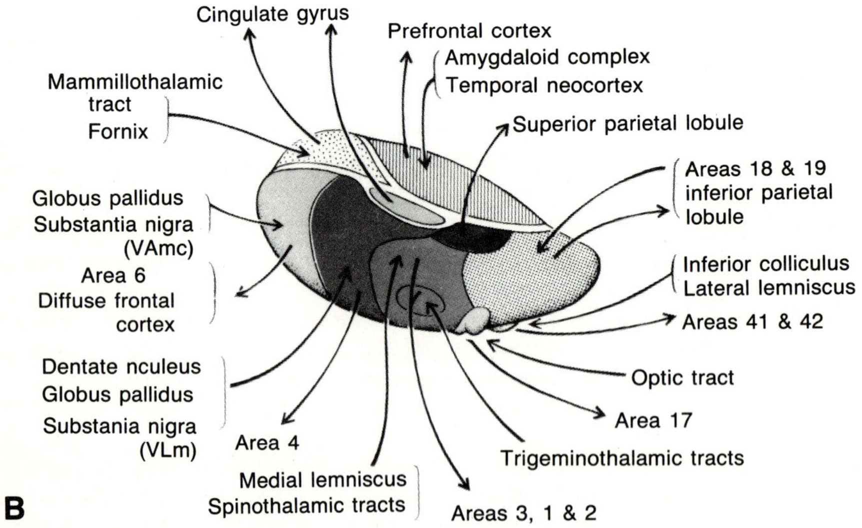

Figure 3–2 Schematic diagrams of the major thalamic nuclei. *A*, An oblique dorsolateral view of the thalamus and its major subdivisions is shown on the left. A transverse section of the thalamus at level of arrows is shown on the right and indicates (1) the relationships between VPM and VPL and (2) the location of CM with respect to the internal medullary lamina of the thalamus. *B*, The principal afferent and efferent projections of particular thalamic subdivisions are indicated (see Fig. 3–24 for a map of the projection areas). Although most cortical areas project fibers back to the thalamic nuclei from which fibers are received, not all of these are shown. (From Carpenter MB. Human neuroanatomy. Baltimore: Williams & Wilkins, 1983:508.)

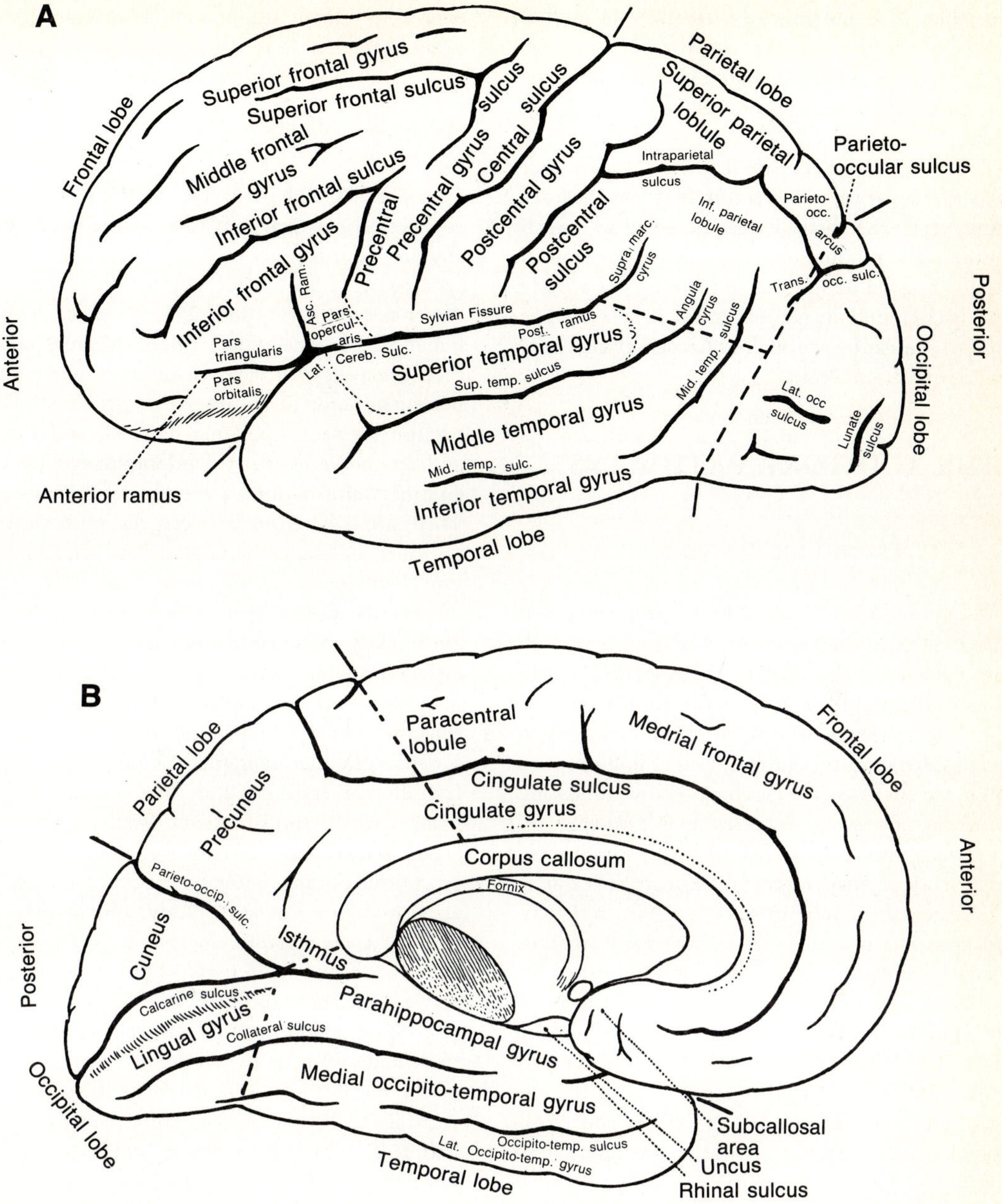

Figure 3–3 *A*, Lateral and *B*, medial views of the human cerebral cortex indicating principal sulci and gyri and four of the five major divisions (lobes). The frontal lobe extends from the anterior boundary of the brain posteriorly to the central sulcus and Sylvian fissure. The parietal lobe is bounded anteriorly by the central sulcus, inferiorly by the Sylvian fissure, and posteriorly by the parieto-occipital line (indicated by the dashed line extending from the parieto-occipital fissure to the shallow depression on the ventral surface of the cortex). The temporal lobe is bounded by the Sylvian fissure, the ventral surface of the cortex, the parieto-occipital line, and the dashed line in *A* drawn from the Sylvian fissure to the parieto-occipital line. The occipital lobe extends from the parieto-occipital line to the posterior surface of the brain. The fifth lobe, the insula, lies within the Sylvian fissure (see Fig. 3–17*B*) and is not visible in these drawings. (From Warwick R, Williams PL, eds. Gray's anatomy. 35th Br ed. Philadelphia: WB Saunders, 1973; 923, 927.)

The cortex comprises layers of cell bodies and fibers (1.5 to 4.5 mm thick) overlying massive fiber tracts. The cell bodies are unmyelinated and thus gray in appearance; the fibers make connections between the gray matter and other cortical and subcortical areas.

The cerebral cortex is divided into two halves or hemispheres, right and left, by the deep longitudinal fissure running along the midline of the brain; the hemispheres are connected by a band of fibers called the "corpus callosum" (see Figs. 3–1 and 3–3*B*). Each hemisphere comprises five lobes: frontal, occipital, temporal, parietal, and insular (see Fig. 3–3). The fifth lobe, the insula, is hidden in a surface view, but one may see it by parting the Sylvian fissure (see Fig. 3–17*B*). If the brain is bisected in the midline, it is possible to visualize the medial surface of the cortex (see Fig. 3–3*B*). Many of the gyri that are viewed from the lateral surface continue onto the medial surface, where additional gyri and sulci are also apparent.

This chapter will be divided into three major sections in which we will describe first the auditory pathways, then the cortical areas involved in speech perception and production, and finally the motor pathways involved in speech production. For a more general background in neuroanatomy, the reader is referred to standard texts such as Crosby et al,[1] Brodal,[2] Carpenter,[3] or Peele.[3a]

THE AUDITORY PATHWAYS

Ascending Systems

Communication involves both production and receptive (hearing) processes. In this section we will discuss the anatomy of neural structures involved in hearing by beginning at the input to the nervous system, the connection between the sensory organ (organ of Corti) and the auditory nerve, and progress through the brain to the cerebral cortex, following the pathway of nervous impulses related to the processing of acoustic stimuli. We will then discuss descending auditory pathways and auditory reflex arcs.

The neural pathway from the cochlea to the auditory cortex is complex, involving many neurons and many synapses. Tonotopicity is established by the spectral analyzer in the cochlea (see Chapter 2) and maintained throughout the auditory pathway in a series of orderly cochleotopic maps. The central auditory system involves divergence and convergence of pathways, binaural interactions, and crossing of information from one side of the brain stem to the other. These complexities allow for detailed and intricate processing of information, and a system that has built-in redundancy and is therefore resistant to disruption by small lesions.

The primary nuclei and fiber tracts composing the auditory pathway are listed in Table 3–1 and are depicted in the context of related structures in Figures 3–4, 3–5, and 3–6. In the next sections, we will examine the structure of each station along the auditory pathway in more detail.

Much of what is known about the anatomy and physiology of the central auditory pathways derives from work on experimental research animals, particularly rodents, cats, and monkeys. The nervous system of the monkey most closely resembles the human nervous system. In describing the auditory pathways, we will concentrate whenever possible on data from human and nonhuman primates, with occasional references to other mammals.

Auditory Nerve

The first synapse in the auditory pathway is the connection between hair cells of the organ of Corti and the auditory nerve (Fig. 3–7). Inner hair cells synapse with the major population of afferent auditory nerve fibers (comprising 95 percent of the afferent fibers), the type I fibers, whereas outer hair cells synapse with type II auditory nerve fibers (5 percent of afferent auditory nerve fibers).[4] The connection between the inner hair cell and the type I auditory nerve fiber is the important one for sending auditory information to the central nervous system. There are differences between the synaptic contacts on inner and outer hair cells. The synapse between type I afferents and the inner hair cells is marked by pre- and postsynaptic membrane densities, which are thicker postsynaptically,[5] and a presynaptic specialization which usually consists of a synaptic body or synaptic bar surrounded by synaptic vesicles.[6] The synaptic cleft is 20 nm in humans,[7] often containing a dense granular material. Outer hair cells receive few afferent endings, and these are not marked by many synaptic specializations. Postsynaptically, a few layers of membrane density are present; whereas presynaptically, scarce, clear synaptic vesicles, only rarely associated with a synaptic body, are present.[6] On the basis of their synaptic morphology, the inner hair cell synapses with afferents would appear to be more active than those of outer hair cells.

Spiral ganglion cells, the cell bodies of the primary auditory neurons, are located in the central core of the cochlea, the modiolus, in Rosenthal's canal, surrounded by the osseous spiral lamina (Figs. 3–7 and 3–8). This group of ganglion cells spirals along with the cochlea for $2^1/_2$ turns in humans (thereby acquiring the name "the spiral ganglion"). The spiral ganglion contains 30,000 to 40,000 neurons in the human,[8,9] 25,000 to 30,000 in the monkey, and 50,000 to 60,000 in the cat.[10] The number of spiral ganglion cells in the human declines with age at a rate of about 2,000 fibers per decade.[11] The two populations of auditory nerve fibers have different types of cell bodies, called "type I and type II spiral ganglion cells" (Fig. 3–9).[12,13] Type I spiral ganglion cells are larger than type II cells, bipolar in shape, with an abundance of rough endoplasmic reticulum in the cytoplasm. Type II spiral ganglion cells (which constitute only 5 to 10 percent of spiral ganglion cells) are pseudomonopolar in shape and contain abundant neurofilaments in their cytoplasm. Type II cells are evenly distributed along the length

TABLE 3–1 Structures of the Auditory Pathway

- AN—Auditory portion of eighth cranial nerve (auditory nerve)
- CN—Cochlear nuclei
    - AVCN—Anteroventral cochlear nucleus
    - PVCN—Posteroventral cochlear nucleus
    - DCN—Dorsal cochlear nucleus
- AS—Acoustic striae
    - SM—Stria of Monakow (dorsal acoustic stria)
    - SH—Stria of Held (intermediate acoustic stria)
    - TB—Trapezoid body (ventral acoustic stria)
        - NTB—Nucleus of the trapezoid body
- SOC—Superior olivary complex
    - LSO—Lateral superior olive (S-segment)
    - MSO—Medial superior olive (accessory nucleus)
    - DPO—Dorsal periolivary nucleus (retroolivary cell group)
    - MPO—Medial preolivary nucleus
    - LPO—Lateral preolivary nucleus
- OCB—Olivocochlear bundle
- LL—Lateral lemniscus
    - LLV—Ventral nucleus of the lateral lemniscus
    - LLD—Dorsal nucleus of the lateral lemniscus
        - CP—Commissure of Probst (commissure of the lateral lemniscus)
- IC—Inferior colliculus
    - ICC—Central nucleus of the inferior colliculus
    - PC—Paracentral nuclei
    - CX—Cortex of inferior colliculus
    - TA—Tegmental areas
    - CIC—Commissure of the inferior colliculus
- BIC—Brachium of the inferior colliculus
- MGN—Medial geniculate nucleus
    - MGP—Principal division
        - MGV—Ventral division
            - PO—Pars ovoidea
            - PL—Pars lateralis
        - MGD—Dorsal division
    - MGM—Magnocellular division (medial division)
- AR—Auditory radiation to cortex
- AC—Auditory cortex

MONKEY		CAT
AI—Koniocortex	Primary auditory cortex	AI—Koniocortex
		AII—Area AII
L—Lateral area CM—Caudomedial area RL—Rostrolateral area	Belt areas	EP—Ectosylvian posterior area INS—Insular area AIII—Area AIII

of the cochlear spiral, singly or in small clusters, often in the periphery of the ganglion.[14]

Each spiral ganglion cell sends a peripheral process to hair cells and a central process to the cochlear nucleus (to be described). The peripheral processes of type I spiral ganglion cells are myelinated fibers (2 to 3 μm in diameter) that lose their myelin sheath as they exit the osseous spiral lamina through small holes in the bone termed "habenulae perforatae" (see Fig. 3–7). They follow a rather direct radial path from the soma in the spiral ganglion to the inner hair cells and so are termed "inner radial fibers." In humans and monkeys, the peripheral process may branch just prior to reaching the inner hair cell bases and contact more than one (although rarely more than two or three) inner hair cells.[7] In cats (at least in the second turn of the cat cochlea), each peripheral process contacts just one inner hair cell,[15]

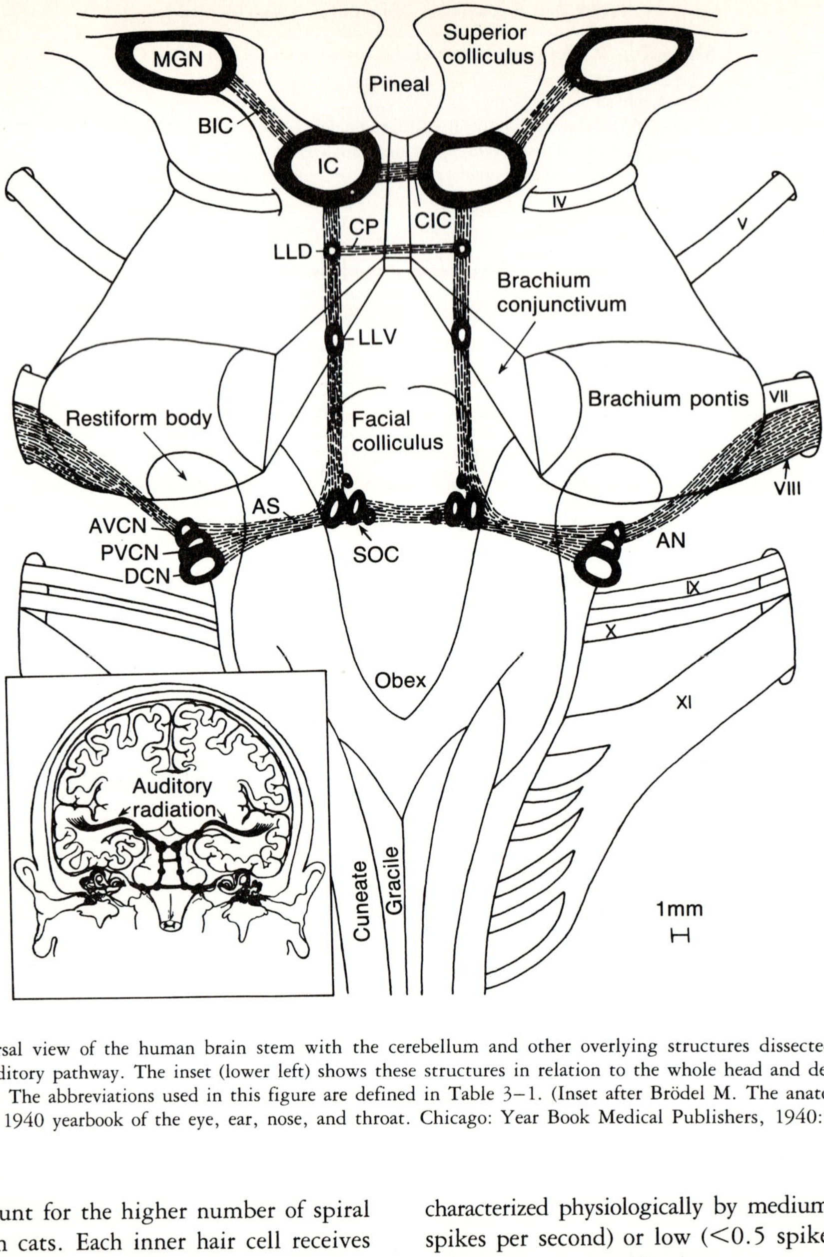

Figure 3–4 A dorsal view of the human brain stem with the cerebellum and other overlying structures dissected away to reveal structures in the auditory pathway. The inset (lower left) shows these structures in relation to the whole head and depicts the cochlea and auditory cortex. The abbreviations used in this figure are defined in Table 3–1. (Inset after Brödel M. The anatomy of the organ of hearing. In: The 1940 yearbook of the eye, ear, nose, and throat. Chicago: Year Book Medical Publishers, 1940:338.)

which may account for the higher number of spiral ganglion cells in cats. Each inner hair cell receives the peripheral processes of 10 to 20 spiral ganglion cells.[16]

Type I auditory nerve fibers can be subdivided into two or three classes based on their anatomic and physiologic properties.[17–19] Roughly 61 percent of the type I radial afferent fibers are larger in diameter, synapse on the pillar side of the inner hair cells, are rich in mitochondria, and are characterized physiologically by high spontaneous discharge rates (>18 spikes per second), low thresholds, and small dynamic ranges (30 to 50 dB). Smaller diameter fibers comprise the remaining 39 percent of radial afferent fibers, synapse on the modiolar side of the inner hair cell, have fewer mitochondria, and are characterized physiologically by medium (0.5 to 18.0 spikes per second) or low (<0.5 spikes per second) spontaneous rates. The low spontaneous-rate fibers have the highest thresholds and the largest dynamic ranges (up to 70 to 80 dB), but comprise only about 16 percent of auditory nerve fibers.

The peripheral processes of type II spiral ganglion cells are thin (approximately 0.5 μm in diameter) and unmyelinated. They travel along with the radial afferent peripheral processes of type I cells through the osseous spiral lamina, exit through the habenulae perforatae, and spiral for varying distances, usually in an apical direction, before crossing the base of the tunnel of Corti. In the region of outer hair cell bases, they course spirally to form the outer spiral fibers, which branch extensively and innervate

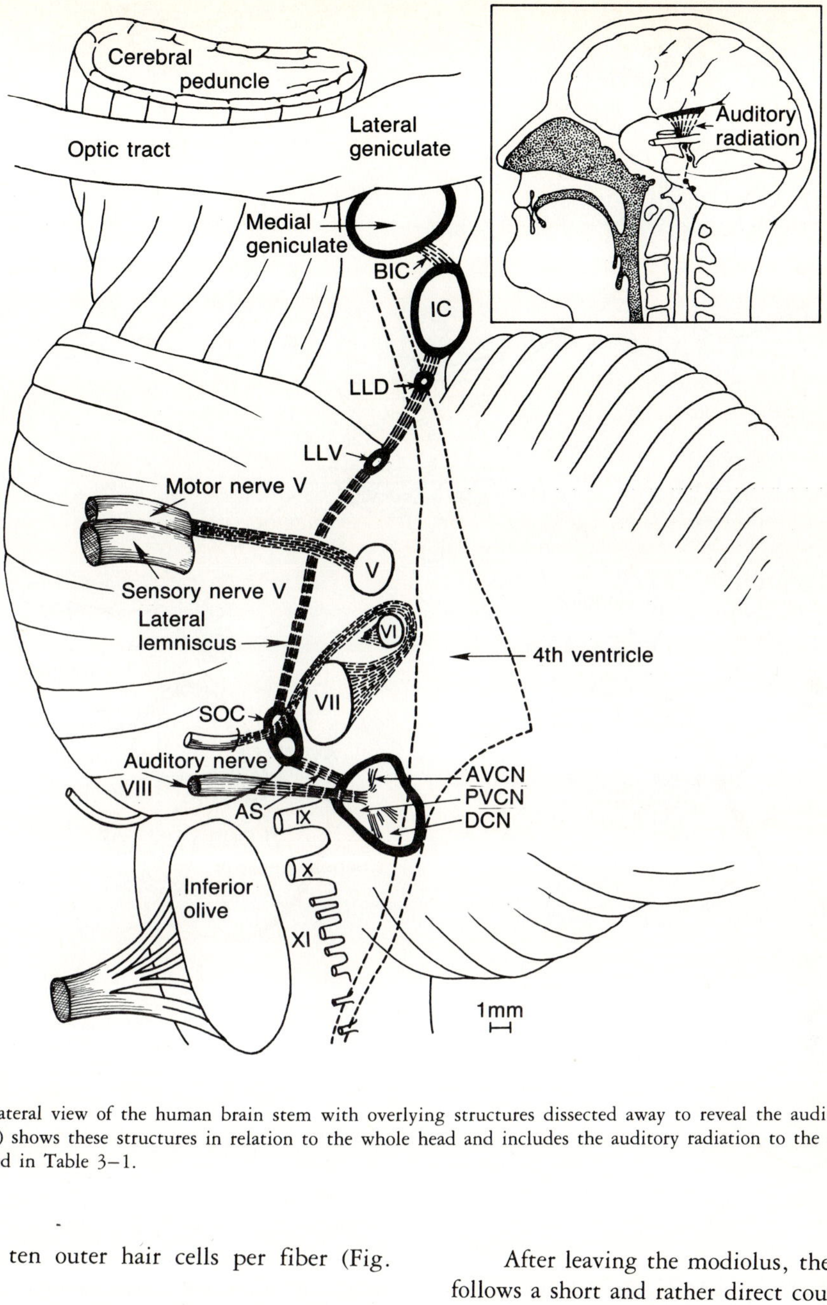

Figure 3–5 A lateral view of the human brain stem with overlying structures dissected away to reveal the auditory pathway. The inset (upper right) shows these structures in relation to the whole head and includes the auditory radiation to the cortex. The abbreviations are defined in Table 3–1.

approximately ten outer hair cells per fiber (Fig. 3–7).[4]

The central processes of the spiral ganglion cells project through the modiolus in the center of the cochlea and proceed through the internal auditory meatus to the brain stem, carrying information from the hair cells to the cochlear nuclei. Fibers innervating the cochlea are tuned with best frequencies corresponding to the region innervated. As these fibers pass from the cochlea through the internal auditory meatus (see Figs. 3–8 and 3–10), they tend to spiral so that apical (low-frequency) fibers lie at the center of the nerve and basal (high-frequency) fibers are on the outside.[20–22]

After leaving the modiolus, the auditory nerve follows a short and rather direct course to the brain stem, where it enters and immediately terminates in the cochlear nuclear complex. The eighth nerve is the second shortest of the cranial nerves (next to the olfactory nerve); it ranges in length from 16 to 19 mm in the adult human.[23]

Cochlear Nucleus

All central processes of the auditory nerve terminate in the ipsilateral cochlear nucleus, which is located on the lateral and dorsal surfaces of the brain

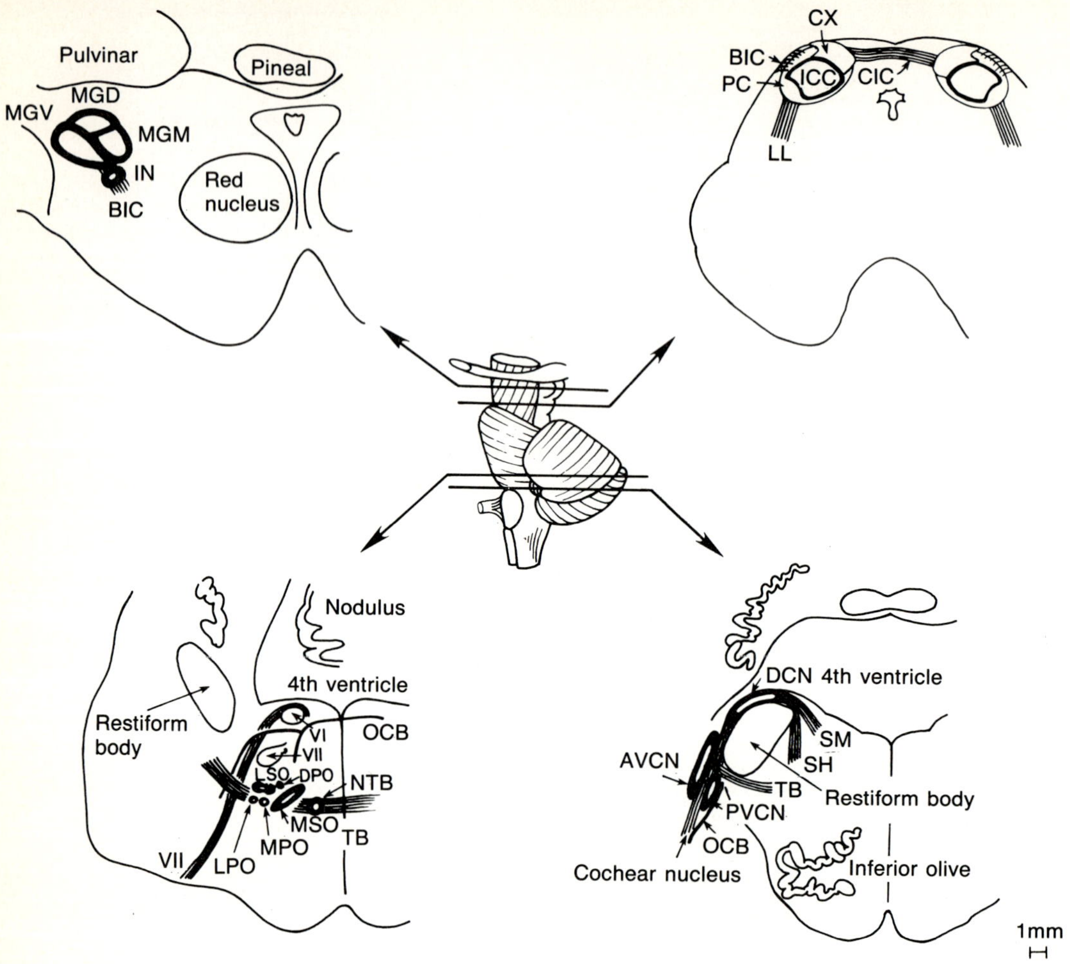

Figure 3–6 Four cross-sections of the human brain stem taken at the levels indicated in the center diagram. All four sections are oriented with the anterior portion toward the bottom of the page and the posterior portion toward the top. More detailed drawings and photographs of human brain stem sections may be found in many standard anatomy texts such as Villiger,[290] Riley,[289] Crosby et al,[1] Peele,[3a] and Carpenter.[3] The abbreviations are defined in Table 3–1.

stem partially surrounding the inferior cerebellar peduncle (the restiform body) at the level where the medulla and pons meet (see Figs. 3–4 and 3–6). The cochlear nucleus can be divided into the dorsal cochlear nucleus and the ventral cochlear nucleus. The ventral cochlear nucleus can, in turn, be subdivided by the bifurcation of the auditory nerve into anterior and posterior subdivisions: the anteroventral cochlear nucleus and posteroventral cochlear nucleus.

Across mammalian species, the ventral cochlear nuclei tend to be similar,[24] but the composition of the dorsal cochlear nucleus differs. Cell types found in the dorsal cochlear nucleus of the cat are not present in human and nonhuman primates, and the laminar structure seen in lower mammals is lost in higher primates.[25,26]

The auditory nerve enters the brain stem in the rostral medulla, not far from the medullary pontine junction. As the auditory nerve enters the cochlear nucleus it bifurcates, with one branch ascending to the anteroventral cochlear nucleus and the other branch descending to the posteroventral cochlear nucleus and the dorsal cochlear nucleus (Fig. 3–10).[27–29] Ascending branches are generally shorter and thicker than descending ones. Each of the branches gives rise to terminals on several cells in specific tonotopic regions of the anteroventral, posteroventral, or dorsal cochlear nucleus, according to the best frequency of the auditory nerve fiber.[22,30,31] For example, fibers connected to apically located inner hair cells (low frequency) bifurcate ventrolaterally, and ascending fibers terminate on cells in the rostroventral antero-

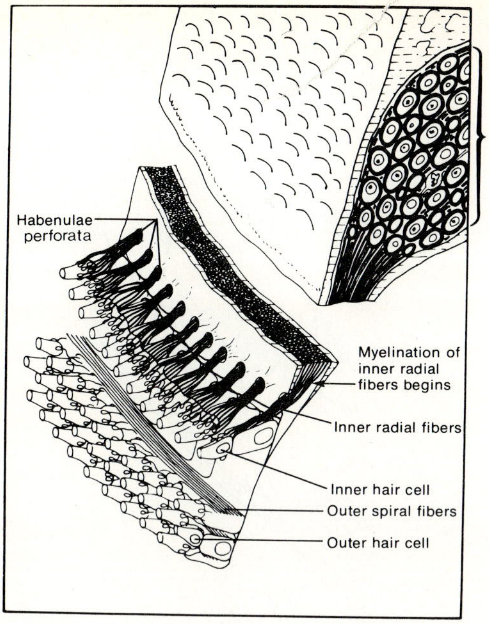

Figure 3-7 Schematic illustration of the innervation of inner and outer hair cells by peripheral processes of the auditory nerve. For orientation of this section in relation to the rest of the cochlea, see Figure 3-8. (After Spoendlin H. Innervation densities of the cochlea. Acta Otolaryngol (Stockh) 1972; 73:246.)

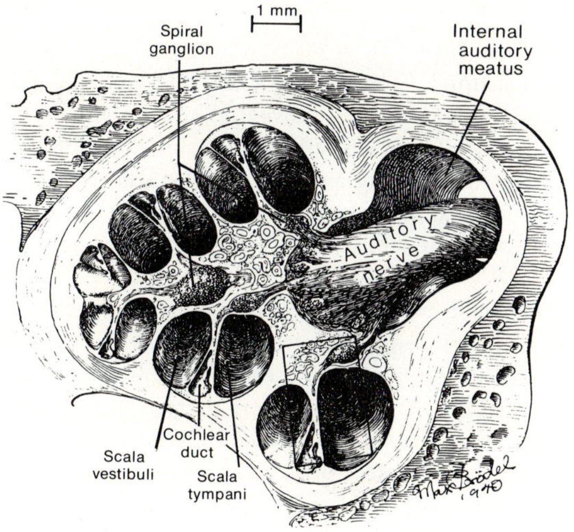

Figure 3-8 Schematic illustration of a cross-section of a left human cochlea. The area enclosed by the box in the basal turn is illustrated in greater detail in Figure 3-7. (After Brödel M. The anatomy of the organ of hearing. In: The 1940 year-book of the eye, ear, nose, and throat. Chicago: Year Book Medical Publishers 1940:338.

ventral cochlear nucleus; whereas fibers from more basally located inner hair cells bifurcate more dorsomedially, and ascending fibers terminate on cells in the dorsocaudal anteroventral cochlear nucleus.

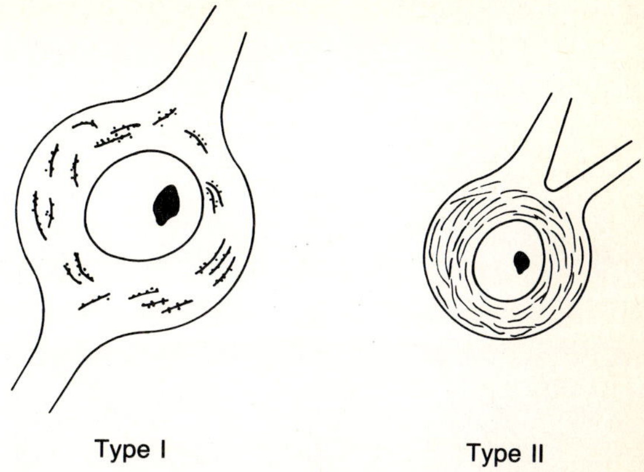

Figure 3-9 Schematic representation of the larger myelinated type I, and the smaller, unmyelinated type II spiral ganglion cells. (From Schwartz AM. Auditory nerve and spiral ganglion cells: morphology and organization. In: Altschuler RA, Hoffman DJ, Bobbin RP, eds. Neurobiology of hearing: the cochlea. New York: Raven Press, 1986:272.)

Each auditory nerve fiber innervates many cells in each tonotopic area. Most cells receive input from many auditory nerve fibers except in the rostral anteroventral cochlear nucleus where spherical bushy cells receive input from only a few, sometimes only one, auditory nerve fiber. In addition, many interneurons are present in the cochlear nucleus, particularly in the dorsal cochlear nucleus, which send projections to other neurons in the nucleus. The number of nerve cells in the cochlear nucleus is large compared to the number of incoming auditory nerve fibers. In the monkey, for example, there are an estimated 88,000 cochlear nucleus cells[32] compared to 30,000 incoming auditory nerve fibers.[10]

The cochlear nucleus is an obligatory synapse in the auditory pathway, meaning that all auditory nerve fibers synapse there. The auditory pathway after the cochlear nucleus changes from a single channel to a multichannel system of parallel ascending pathways. There is a divergence into many distinct pathways mediated by the different projections of the different cochlear nucleus neurons. The ventral and dorsal cochlear nuclei differ considerably in the cell types, innervation, and projections, and are consequently also marked by differences in their physiology. In the following paragraphs, we will discuss the major projection neurons of the cochlear nucleus. This discussion will exclude the many interneurons, mostly small cells, which undoubtedly have a major role in the transformation and processing of auditory information within the cochlear nucleus. Fibers leaving the cochlear nucleus form three major stria (see Fig. 3-6): the ventral acoustic stria (trapezoid body), intermediate acoustic stria (stria of Held), and dorsal acoustic stria (stria of Monakow).

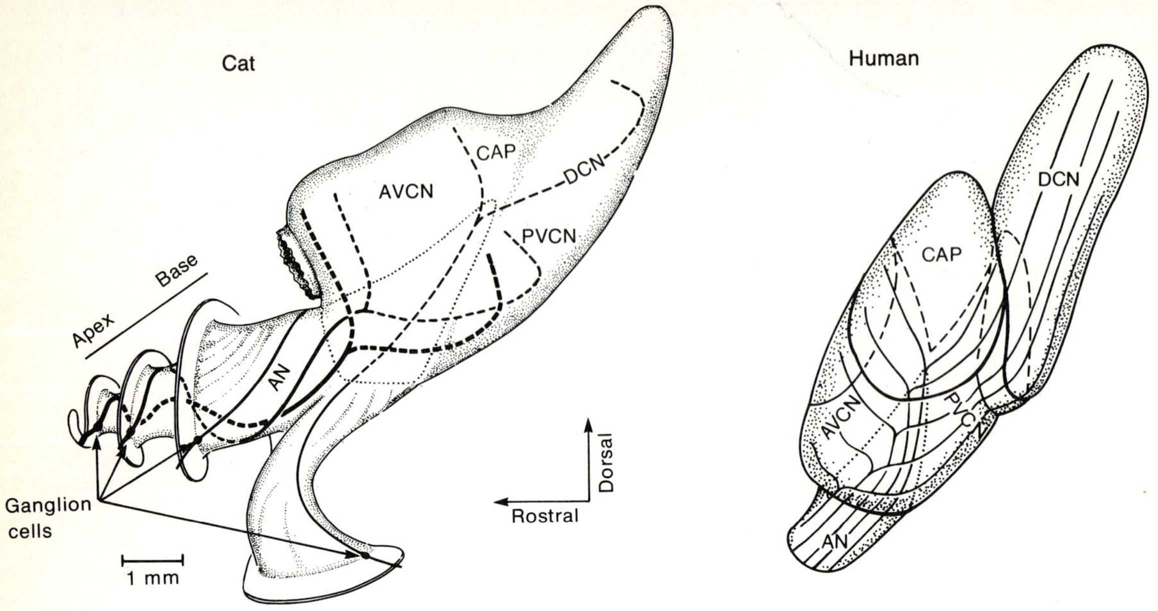

Figure 3–10 Diagrammatic illustration of the projections of auditory nerve fibers into the cochlear nuclei of the cat and the human. For the cat, the cochlea is also illustrated. The PVCN is buried within the nucleus in this view. Note that in the human, the direction of axons passing through the DCN is different than in the cat and other mammals. The cap region of the AVCN, containing small cells that seem to project only within the cochlear nucleus, is especially large in the human. For definitions of abbreviations, see Table 3–1. (After Arnesen AR, Osen KK. The cochlear nerve in the cat topography, cochleotopy, and fiber spectrum. J Comp Neurol 1978; 178:673. Moore JK, Osen KK. The cochlear nuclei in man. Amer J Anat 1979; 15:7.)

Spherical Bushy Cells. These cells[33–36] (Fig. 3–11), located in the rostral region of the anteroventral cochlear nucleus, are spherical in shape and receive much of their input on their somas in the form of one to three large synapses called end bulbs of Held.[37,38] Their response properties are termed "primary-like" in that they closely mimic those of the auditory nerve fibers.[39,40] These cells project via the ventral acoustic stria to the ipsilateral lateral superior olivary nucleus and to both ipsi- and contralateral medial superior olivary nuclei. It is also possible that a subpopulation of these cells projects to the contralateral nucleus of the lateral lemniscus.

Globular Bushy Cells. These cells (Fig. 3–11), located in the caudal anteroventral cochlear nucleus and the most rostral posteroventral cochlear nucleus, are similar to spherical bushy cells, with a similar though more irregular spherical shape and with a sparser, coarser, and more elongated pattern of dendrites.[34–36] They also receive much of their input through large synaptic terminals on their soma, and their response properties are also believed to closely mimic those of the auditory nerve fibers that they receive, except for a slight notch (brief quiet period). Their response is therefore termed "notch-primary-like." These cells project primarily via the ventral acoustic stria to the contralateral medial nucleus of the trapezoid body with collaterals to periolivary nuclei.

Octopus Cells. These cells (Fig. 3–11), located in the caudal posteroventral cochlear nucleus, are also similar to the spherical bushy and globular bushy cells in having a spherical shape and receiving much of their input on their soma, but they have their own characteristic pattern of dendritic arborization.[34–36,41,42] As opposed to the spherical bushy and globular bushy cells that receive large input from relatively few auditory nerve fibers, octopus cells receive input from many different auditory nerve fibers. These cells have an onset pattern of response with a brief response followed by relative quiet.[39] Octopus cells project bilaterally through the intermediate acoustic stria to the periolivary nuclei and may also project to the inferior colliculus and nuclei of the lateral lemniscus.

Multipolar Stellate Cells. These cells (Fig. 3–11) are a heterogeneous group of cells that often have an oval shape, receive most of their input on their dendrites, and are scattered throughout the ventral cochlear nucleus.[27,34–36,41] Their physiologic response properties are often characterized as chopper responses, meaning that they respond to an auditory stimulus with a variable number of sharp peaks of activity.[39,43] Since this is a heterogeneous group of

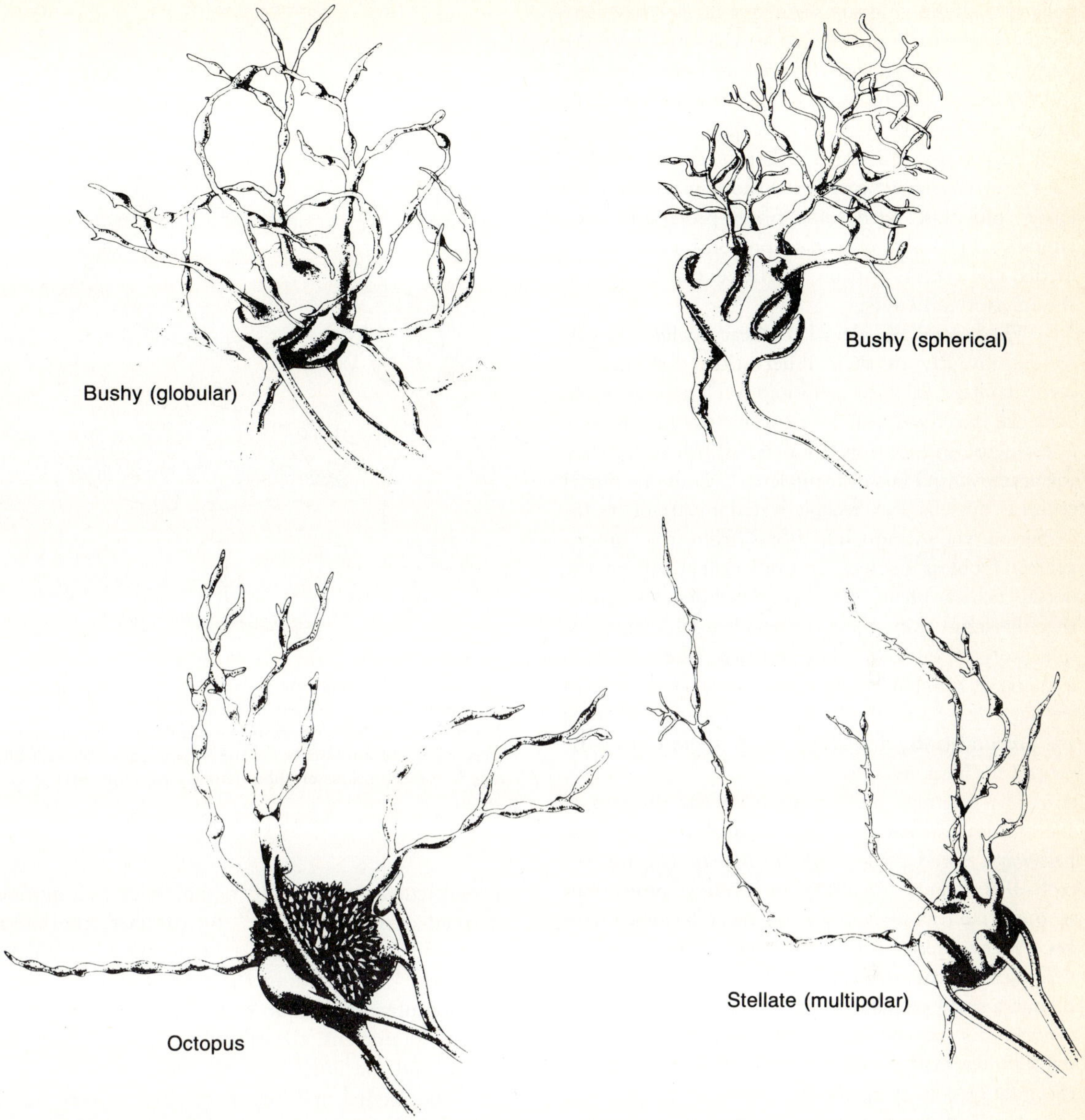

Figure 3–11 Schematic representation of principal cell types of the cochlear nucleus, including inputs from auditory nerve fibers. (From Caspary DM. Cochlear nuclei: functional neuropharmacology of the principal cell types. In: Altschuler RA, Hoffman DW, Bobbin RP, eds. Neurobiology of hearing: the cochlea. New York: Raven Press, 1986:303.)

cells, they likely do not all share the same projection pattern. However, there is a major projection of multipolar stellate cells of the anteroventral cochlear nucleus directly to the contralateral inferior colliculus, with a smaller projection to the ipsilateral inferior colliculus. Other multipolar stellate cells may project to the superior olivary complex, whereas some in the posteroventral cochlear nucleus may project to the cerebellum.

Giant Cells. These cells are the only class of projection neurons that are present in both the dorsal and ventral cochlear nucleus, although they are represented more in the deep layers of the dorsal cochlear nucleus.[34–36] Their response properties have not been well characterized. Giant cells project both to the contralateral cochlear nucleus and to the inferior colliculus.

In lower mammals, the dorsal cochlear nucleus is characterized by a laminar cytoarchitecture, formed by a layer of fusiform cells, dividing a superficial molecular layer from a deep layer. In the human, the molecular layer is vestigial, and the same laminar arrangement is therefore not seen.[26]

Fusiform Cells. These cells have a triangular-shaped soma with the tip oriented superficially, except in the human where cells considered homologous to fusiform cells are seen, but do not have any regular orientation orthogonal to the surface of the nucleus.[34–36] Input is distributed on both the soma and dendrites. The response property of fusiform cells is termed "pauser" in that it is quiet initially and then builds up.[44] Fusiform cells project via the dorsal acoustic stria, primarily to the contralateral inferior colliculus, with some fibers projecting ipsilaterally. The fibers terminate predominantly in the medial and central portions of the central nucleus of the inferior colliculus.

The ventral and dorsal cochlear nuclei may differ significantly in their innervation pattern and, consequently, in their physiology. There is some evidence that the dorsal cochlear nucleus may receive a less dense innervation from the eighth nerve than the anteroventral cochlear nucleus.[45] Thus the dorsal cochlear nucleus may receive a major part of its innervation via intranuclear fibers from the anteroventral cochlear nucleus or from other cells in the dorsal cochlear nuclei. Physiologic evidence suggests that the input from these intranuclear fibers may be inhibitory in nature.[46,47] Intranuclear fibers are particularly prominent in the dorsal cochlear nucleus in the cat, whereas in the human the intrinsic neurons are predominantly found in a cap region over the ventral cochlear nucleus.[48]

The different projections from the neurons of the cochlear nucleus give rise to separate ascending pathways, some projecting directly to the inferior colliculus, others synapsing or sending projections to other nuclei on their way to the inferior colliculus. At the inferior colliculus, there is largely a convergence of the multiple auditory pathways, although a small proportion may pass through to higher centers in some species.[49] The auditory brain stem nuclei interposed between the cochlear nucleus and the inferior colliculus are the nuclei of the superior olivary complex (consisting of lateral and medial nuclei of the superior olive, nuclei of the trapezoid body, and periolivary nuclei) and the nuclei of the lateral lemniscus. These have many interconnections as well as projections to the inferior colliculus.

Superior Olivary Complex

The superior olivary complex is a collection of six nuclei located in the caudal- to mid-pons (Fig. 3–12). The largest nuclei in this group are the lateral superior olive, or S-segment, and the medial superior olive, or accessory nucleus. Both nuclei contain an orderly tonotopic map.[50,51] In the adult human, the medial superior olive comprises an average of 11,500 cells. The lateral superior olive is smaller, containing about 4,000 cells, and is rather

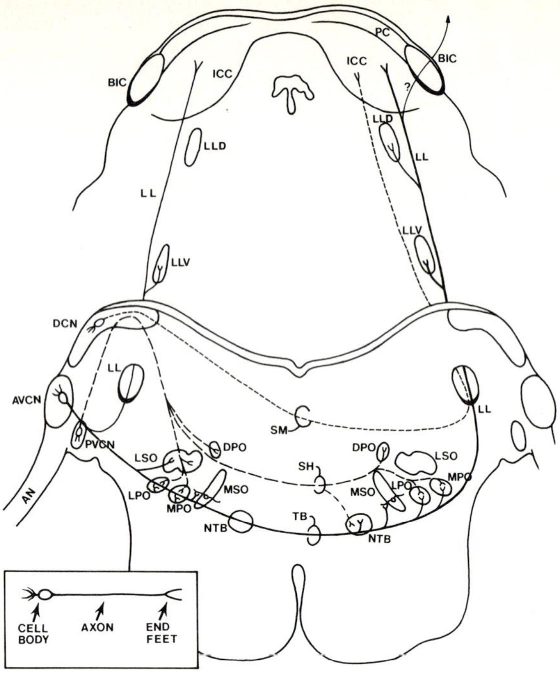

Figure 3–12 A diagrammatic view of the brain stem illustrating some projections of the left cochlear nucleus. Only projections demonstrated in higher primates (as described by Strominger,[291] Strominger and Strominger,[292] and Strominger et al[49]) are illustrated. For definitions of abbreviations, see Table 3–1.

inconspicuous owing to its organization as a number of small clusters of cells.[52] By contrast, the lateral superior olive in the cat is a prominant S-shaped structure.[53] Surrounding the medial and the lateral superior olives are four smaller nuclei: the dorsal periolivary nucleus, the medial and lateral preolivary nuclei, and the nucleus of the trapezoid body.

The medial and lateral superior olivary nuclei are of particular interest with regard to binaural interaction. These nuclei receive direct orderly projections from the anteroventral cochlear nuclei on either side of the brain. For example, fibers from the left cochlear nucleus project to the left half of the medial superior olive and fibers from the right cochlear nucleus project to the right half (Fig. 3–13). Both projections are ordered cochleotopically so that corresponding regions of the two cochleae are represented together on the same medial superior olivary neurons. This is the first point along the auditory pathway at which there is an opportunity for interaction of input from the two ears. It is, in fact, an optimal location for such interaction. Recall that the fibers of the eighth nerve are short and make secure synapses with cells in the anteroventral cochlear nucleus, and that the pathway from the anteroventral cochlear nucleus to the medial superior olive is short

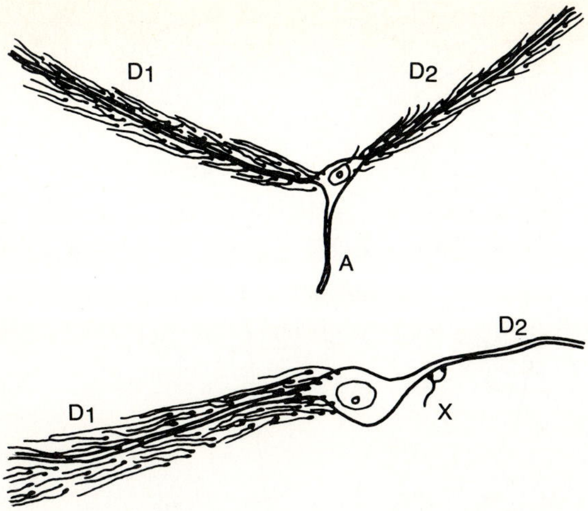

Figure 3–13 Schematic illustration of the results of an experiment by Stotler.[57] The top drawing shows a normal cell from the medial superior olive. The lower drawing shows the appearance of such a cell after destruction of the right cochlear nucleus. This result indicates that most of the endings on dendrite D2 came from the right cochlear nucleus and those on D1 came from the left, which suggests that cells in the medial superior olive receive equal inputs from the two ears and in a highly organized fashion. (From Stotler WA. An experimental study of the cells and connections of the superior olivary complex of the cat. J Comp Neurol 1953:405.)

and well-ordered. Thus it is reasonable to expect that precise temporal information important for sound localization and other binaurally dependent processes would be well preserved at this level of the auditory pathway. Indeed, electrophysiologic studies have indicated that the medial superior olive is involved in detecting differences in time of arrival of signals at the two ears,[54] whereas the lateral superior olive is involved in analysis of internal differences in intensity and spectrum.[55,56]

The medial and the lateral superior olives and possibly other superior olivary nuclei send ipsilateral projections to the inferior colliculus and probably to the nuclei of the lateral lemniscus. In addition, the lateral superior olive has projections to the contralateral inferior colliculus (see Fig. 3–12).[57]

Lateral Lemniscus

The lateral lemniscus is the fiber tract containing projections from the cochlear nuclei and superior olivary nuclei to the inferior colliculus (see Figs. 3–4, 3–5, and 3–12). Within the lateral lemniscus are two auditory nuclei, the dorsal and ventral nuclei of the lateral lemniscus (see Fig. 3–12). Both contain orderly tonotopic maps with low frequencies rostral and high frequencies more caudal.[58] These nuclei receive input from the cochlear nuclei and the superior olivary complex and project primarily to the central nucleus of the ipsilateral inferior colliculus. The ventral nucleus of the lateral lemniscus also sends a projection contralaterally through the commissure of Probst (see Fig. 3–4) to the contralateral dorsal nucleus of the lateral lemniscus and to the contralateral inferior colliculus.[59] However, many of the fibers in the lateral lemniscus do not synapse at these nuclei, but rather bypass them and synapse at the inferior colliculus. In the human, the ventral nucleus of the lateral lemniscus is vestigial.[48]

Inferior Colliculus

The inferior colliculus, located in midbrain, has both tectal and tegmental divisions. The inferior colliculus is the second obligatory synapse in the auditory pathway, receiving second-order fibers from the cochlear nucleus as well as higher-order fibers from interposed relay nuclei in the superior olivary complex and lateral lemniscus.[59–62] It is the point at which the divergent parallel ascending pathways from the cochlear nucleus converge. The inferior colliculus represents a great expansion in number of cells as compared to nuclei lower in the auditory pathway; in the monkey, it comprises approximately 392,000 cells.[32]

The inferior colliculus can be divided into several nuclei, characterized by different cell types. The largest and most extensively studied portion is the central nucleus of the inferior colliculus (Fig. 3–14). The central nucleus is characterized by laminae formed by the dendrites of the principal cells and the terminal fibers of ascending auditory pathways.[63–67] The central nucleus is organized tonotopically with low-frequency cells found dorsally and high-frequency cells ventrally.[68–70] Layers of cells tuned to a particular frequency correspond roughly to the laminae described previously.[65]

The central nucleus of the inferior colliculus has four subdivisions based on four distinct configurations of laminar organization: the central, medial, lateral, and ventral divisions (see Fig. 3–14).[65] There is evidence that multiple tonotopic maps may exist in the central nucleus, perhaps corresponding to these divisions. In all divisions, there are alternating bands of coarse and fine fibers ascending from caudal levels of the auditory system.[65] A four-layer cortex overlies the central nucleus, and there are paracentral nuclei scattered around the central nucleus: the commissural, dorsomedial, rostral pole, lateral, and ventro-

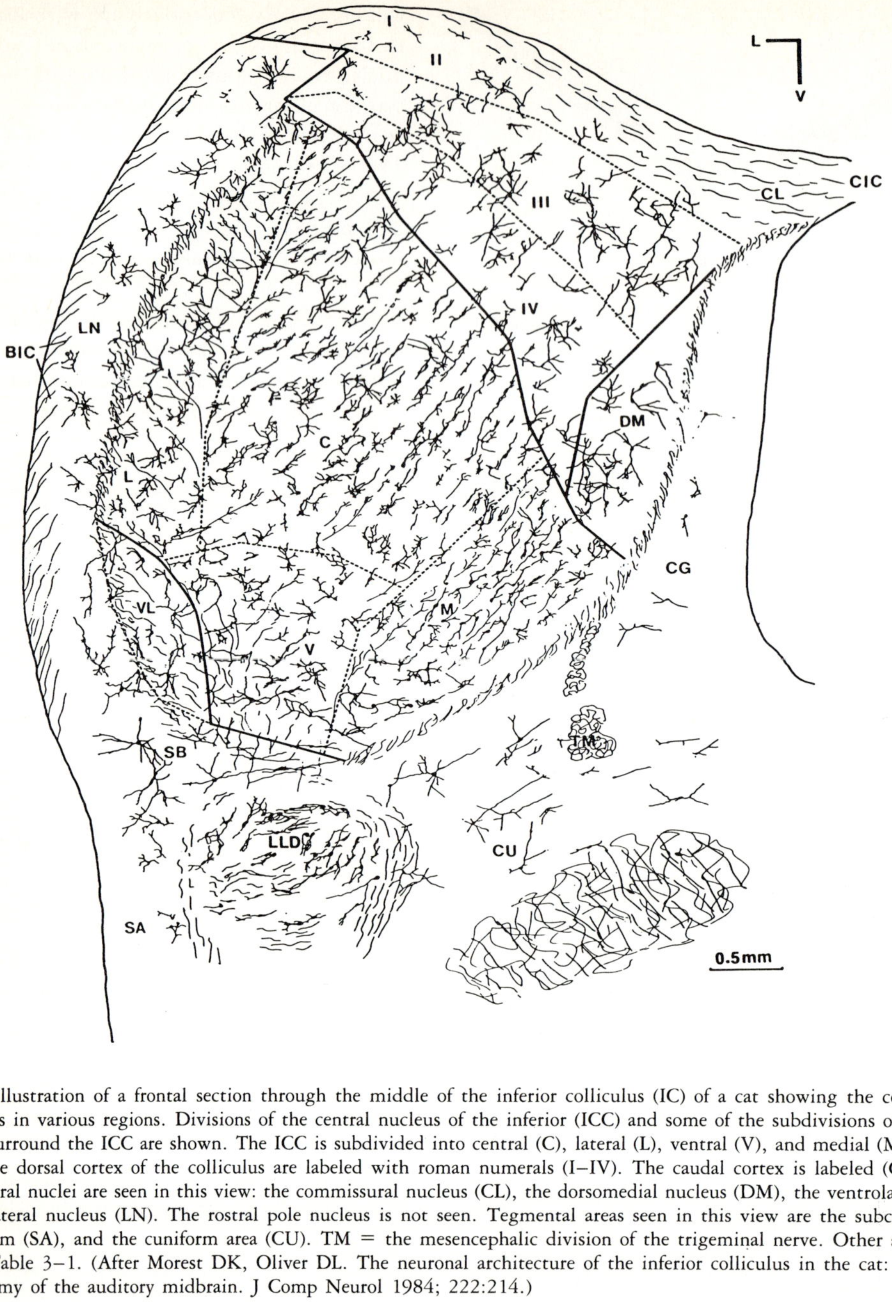

Figure 3–14 Illustration of a frontal section through the middle of the inferior colliculus (IC) of a cat showing the cell types and their orientations in various regions. Divisions of the central nucleus of the inferior (ICC) and some of the subdivisions of the inferior colliculus that surround the ICC are shown. The ICC is subdivided into central (C), lateral (L), ventral (V), and medial (M) parts. The four layers of the dorsal cortex of the colliculus are labeled with roman numerals (I–IV). The caudal cortex is labeled (CG). Four of the five paracentral nuclei are seen in this view: the commissural nucleus (CL), the dorsomedial nucleus (DM), the ventrolateral nucleus (VL), and the lateral nucleus (LN). The rostral pole nucleus is not seen. Tegmental areas seen in this view are the subcollicular area (SB), the sagulum (SA), and the cuniform area (CU). TM = the mesencephalic division of the trigeminal nerve. Other abbreviations are defined in Table 3–1. (After Morest DK, Oliver DL. The neuronal architecture of the inferior colliculus in the cat: defining the functional anatomy of the auditory midbrain. J Comp Neurol 1984; 222:214.)

lateral nuclei (see Fig. 3–14). Located in the tegmental portion of the inferior colliculus are the pericollicular nuclei, the nucleus of the brachium of the inferior colliculus, and the sagulum. Although the tectal nuclei of the inferior colliculus (central nucleus and paracentral) receive predominantly auditory inputs, the tegmental nuclei receive a wide variety of inputs in addition to auditory (e.g., somatosensory).[55,71,72] Therefore the inferior colliculus provides not only convergence of the auditory pathways, but also opportunity for interactions with other modalities.

The primary ascending projection of the inferior colliculus is to the ipsilateral medial geniculate nucleus in the thalamus, via the brachium of the inferior colliculus.[73] A minor projection goes through the commissure of the inferior colliculus to the contralateral inferior colliculus and thalamus. The inferior colliculus also sends descending projections, which will be discussed in a later section on Descending Systems.

Medial Geniculate Nucleus

The next major synapse in the auditory pathway is the medial geniculate nucleus, located in the thalamus. The thalamus is the major relay station to the cerebral cortex for all sensory systems, with the possible exception of olfaction (see Fig. 3–3). The medial geniculate nucleus can be divided into several parts (Fig. 3–15): a ventral division (previously termed "pars principalis"), a medial division (previously termed "pars magnocellularis"), and a dorsal division.[74,75] Each of these divisions sends projections to the auditory cortex. The ventral division contains neurons with dendritic fields forming laminae, similar to the inferior colliculus. The ventral nucleus can be subdivided into a pars lateralis, where the laminae are arranged parallel to the lateral margin of the geniculate, and a pars ovoidea, with the laminae in a coiled configuration.[74-76] Tonotopic maps have been described in both subdivisions. In the pars lateralis, cells tuned to high frequencies are located dorsorostromedially in the nucleus, whereas cells tuned to low frequencies have

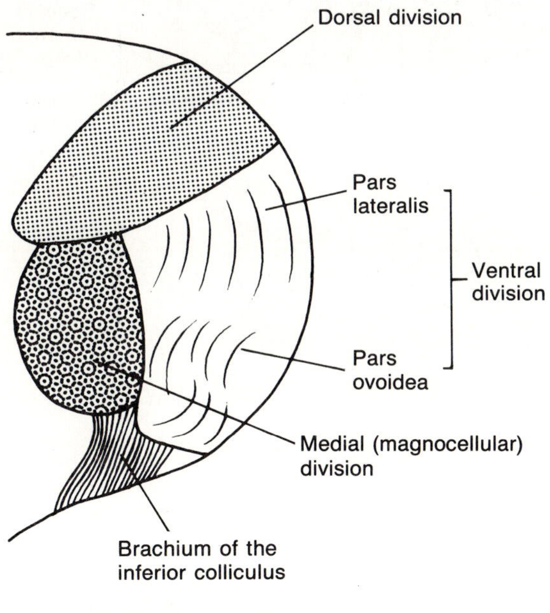

Figure 3–15 Schema illustrating the divisions of the medial geniculate body based on Morest.[74,78] The laminar arrangement of the two parts of the ventral division is indicated. In the older parcellation of Rose and Woolsey,[81] the dorsal division and the anterior two-thirds of the ventral division were known as the principal division. Also included in Morest's dorsal division is the lateral part of the posterior cell group described by Rose and Woolsey.

a more ventrocaudolateral location.[77] Isofrequency laminae resemble morphologically-derived laminae.[76,78] The tonotopic mapping in pars ovoidea is less well-defined, perhaps due to the twisted laminar arrangement. Neurons show frequency selectivity, but sequences of best frequencies encountered are less regular than in pars lateralis.[79] However, there is a low-to-high gradient of best frequencies that runs from lateral to medial.[76] In the monkey, the lateral division contains about 364,000 cells, whereas the medial division contains about 58,000 cells.[32]

The ventral division of the medial geniculate body is the major relay to the primary auditory cortex and receives its input primarily from the central nucleus of the inferior colliculus. Incoming fibers from the colliculus run in layers parallel to the dendritic laminae of the ventral division. The projection from the ventral division to the primary auditory cortex is orderly. In the monkey, the anterior parts of the ventral division project to the posterior auditory cortex, whereas the middle ventral division fibers project to the anterior cortex; the medial portion of the ventral division connects to the medial auditory cortex, and the lateral portion projects laterally.[80]

In the cat, the anterior parts of the ventral division project to anterior cortical area AI and the middle portion of the ventral division projects posteriorly in AI.[81] In addition to this orderly projection from medial geniculate to cortex, there is also evidence of a more diffuse projection.[82]

The medial and dorsal divisions of the medial geniculate body (see Fig. 3–15) are involved in more diffuse pathways to the auditory cortex. The medial division receives auditory projections from the inferior colliculus, but it also receives input from several nonauditory sensory pathways. The medial division projects to secondary auditory cortical fields that surround the primary auditory cortex (see Figs. 3–17 and 3–18). The dorsal division of the medial geniculate body receives no direct input from the central nucleus of the inferior colliculus. Its auditory input is probably from the paracentral nuclei of the inferior colliculus[83] and from other medial geniculate areas. It also receives a number of nonauditory sensory inputs. The most posterior parts of the ventral division of the medial geniculate body, as well as parts of the dorsal division, project to an area anterior to the primary auditory cortex in the monkey (see Fig. 3–17)[80] and to the insular-temporal cortex in the cat (see Fig. 3–18).[84]

Two types of cortical projections from the medial geniculate body have been described (Fig. 3–16). Sustaining projections are fibers that bifurcate, innervating two or more cortical regions. A lesion in one region results in retrograde degeneration of

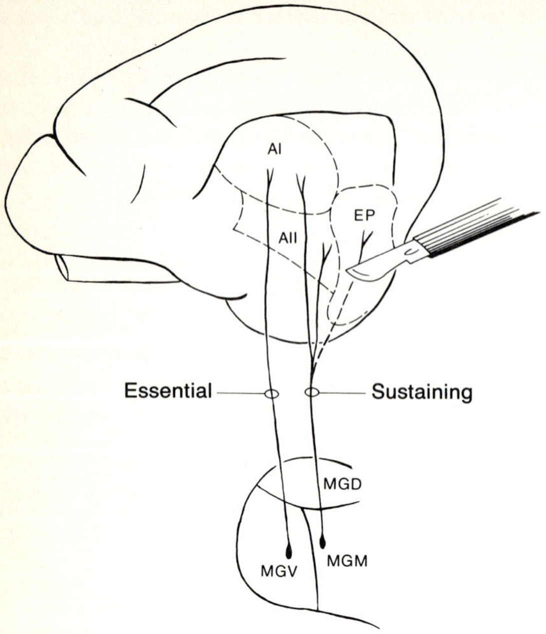

Figure 3–16 A schematic drawing illustrating the concept of essential and sustaining projections from the medial geniculate nucleus to the auditory cortex in the cat as defined by Rose and Woolsey.[85] Essential projections project to only one cortical area, whereas sustaining projections bifurcate and project to two or more cortical areas. If a lesion is made involving only one branch of the sustaining projection (in this example, the branch innervating cortical area EP), retrograde degeneration progresses only to the point of the bifurcation, leaving the remaining axon and the cell body in the medial geniculate nucleus intact. Only by lesioning all three cortical areas, AI, AII, and EP, would degeneration be seen in the neuron in the medial geniculate. If the essential projection to area AI were damaged, however, degeneration would progress all the way down the axon to the cell body in the medial geniculate. For definitions of abbreviations, see Table 3–1.

the fiber only to the point of the bifurcation, leaving the cell body and other projections intact. Essential projections are fibers that innervate only a single cortical area.[81,85]

In addition to the medial geniculate nucleus, the lateral posterior complex in the thalamus also receives auditory input, is tonotopically organized, and has an orderly projection to the auditory cortex.[86]

Auditory Cortex

The auditory cortex in the human[87,88] and in many nonhuman primates[89,90,97] is located primarily on the superior, medial, and lateral surfaces of the superior temporal gyrus and so is buried, for the most part, within the Sylvian fissure (Fig. 3–17). This cortex is estimated to contain over 10 million nerve cells.[32] In the cat (Fig. 3–18), the auditory

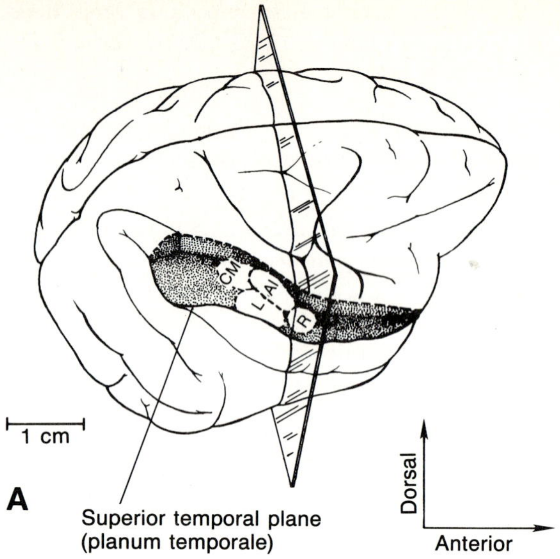

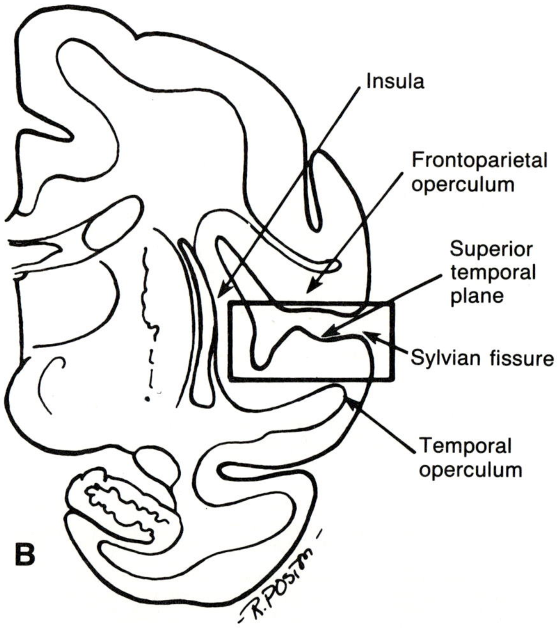

Figure 3–17 Illustration of the brain of a rhesus monkey showing the location of the auditory cortex. The location in man is similar. *A*, In this view, the frontal and parietal lobes are drawn as transparent so that the superior surface of the superior temporal gyrus can be seen. Various auditory fields as determined by electrophysiological mapping studies of Merzenich and Brugge[89] are indicated. AI is the primary auditory cortex. CM, L, and R are secondary (belt) auditory cortical areas (see Table 3–1). The brain is sectioned by a glass plate in a frontal plane to indicate the anteroposterior location of *B*. *B*, Frontal section of the brain made in the plane indicated in *A*. Only the right hemisphere is shown. The box around the temporal operculum indicates the location of Figure 3–19.

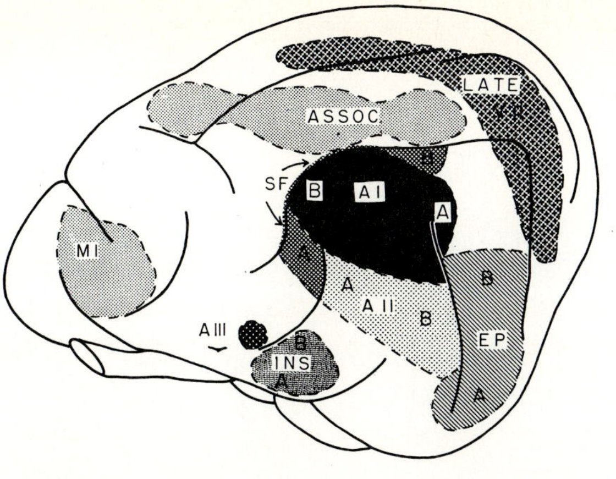

Figure 3-18 Lateral view of the cat brain showing the classic auditory fields. AI is the primary auditory cortex; AII, EP, INS, and SF are the surrounding secondary (belt) auditory cortical fields. Within each of these fields there is an orderly representation of frequencies, with low frequencies (cochlea apex) represented in the area marked A and high frequencies (cochlear base) represented in the area marked B. Area SF is buried in part in the suprasylvian sulcus. Auditory evoked responses are also found in area AIII, area MI (motor cortex), and association cortex. Long latency responses are found in parts of the visual cortex (here labeled LATE). Recently some slight revisions in this map have been proposed on the basis of single unit studies (see Knight,[293] Reale and Imig,[294] Clarey and Irvine.[295]). (From Woolsey CN. Organization of cortical auditory systems: a review and a synthesis. In: Rasmussen GL, Windle WF, eds. Neural mechanisms of the auditory and vestibular systems. Springfield, IL: CC Thomas, 1960:179.)

cortex represents a large area mostly on the lateral surface of the brain.[91]

The auditory cortex may be divided into several distinct areas on the basis of the cell patterns and the arrangement of incoming myelinated fibers (cytoarchitecture and myeloarchitecture).[81,88,92] These architectonic maps correspond roughly to maps based on characteristics of the cortical cells as determined electrophysiologically. The different cortical areas shown in Figures 3–17 and 3–18 are based on the electrophysiologic criteria, primarily the tonotopic organization of the cortex. Each of the areas represented is characterized either by an orderly arrangement of cells tuned to specific frequencies of stimulation or by clustering of cells with some other unique response properties.

The primary auditory cortex, also known as area AI or auditory koniocortex, is the most easily identified of the auditory cortical areas. Architectonically (Fig. 3–19), it is characterized by a dense concentration of cells in layers II, III, and IV, a sparsely populated layer V, and a dense layer VI. Layers III and IV are characterized by an orderly columnar arrangement of cell bodies, giving this area an appearance that von Economo described as a rain shower formation.[92–96]

A complete frequency representation is found in area AI; in the monkey, low frequencies are represented anteriorly and high frequencies posteriorly,[89,90,97] and, in the cat, the organization is reversed.[98]

Figure 3–20 shows a map of the auditory cortex in the owl monkey. The numbers shown on the surface of the cortex indicate the approximate best frequencies of neurons found in penetrations made perpendicular to the surface at the points indicated. It is generally the case that all neurons encountered in a penetration made perpendicular to the cortical surface are tuned to approximately the same fre-

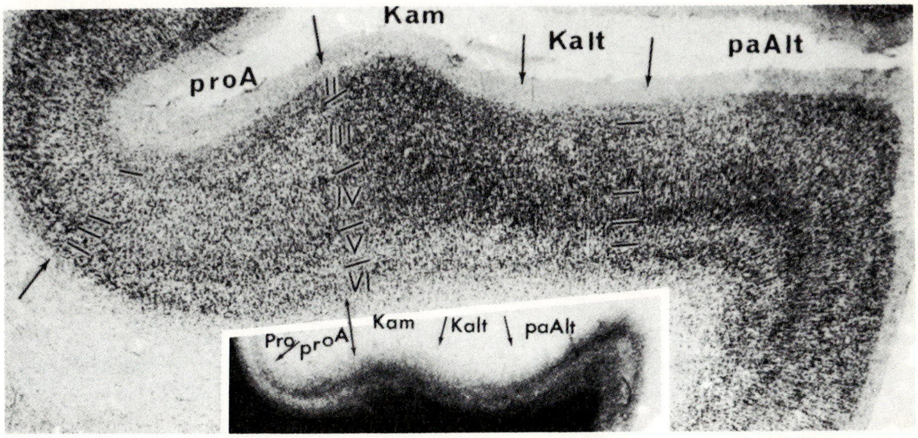

Figure 3-19 A frontal section through the auditory cortex of a rhesus monkey taken at the level indicated by the box in Figure 3–17*B*. Roman numerals indicate cell layers. The primary auditory cortex is designated by the letters Kam and Kalt; Pro A and pa Alt are belt areas. In the inset, incoming fibers are stained to show differences in the fiber pattern in the primary auditory cortex as opposed to the surrounding belt areas. (From Pandya DN, Sanides F. Architecture parcellation of the temporal operculum in rhesus monkey and its projection pattern. Z Anat Entwicki-Gesch 1973; 139:127.)

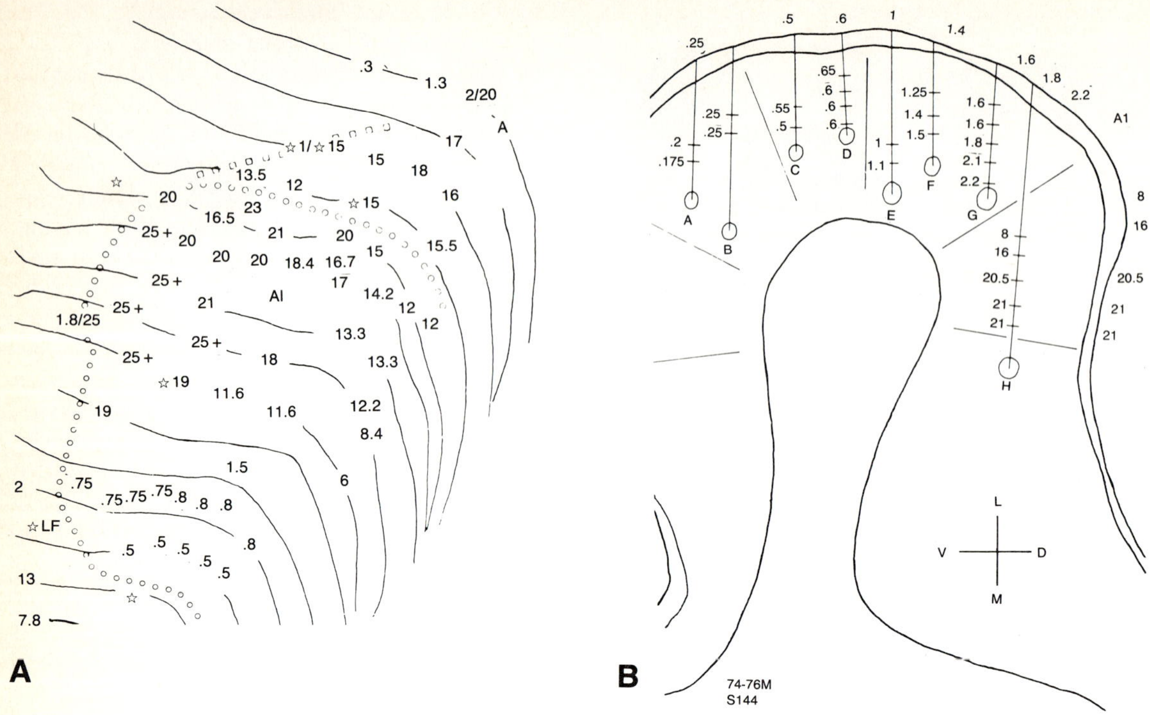

Figure 3–20 Two views of the primary auditory cortex (AI) in the owl monkey showing the tonotopic arrangement of cells as determined by microelectrode recordings. *A,* Surface view of the superior temporal gyrus indicating the best frequencies (in kHz) of neurons encountered in vertical penetrations at various locations. *B,* A frontal section of the auditory cortex showing the best frequencies of neurons encountered in single penetrations. The vertical line indicates the path followed by the microelectrode and the cross-hatches indicate the levels at which the best frequencies of single neurons or clusters of neurons were measured. The best frequencies in kHz are indicated by the numbers to the left of each hatchmark. The circle at the bottom of each vertical penetration indicates the location of a lesion which was used later to construct this map. (From Imig TJ, Ruggero MA, Kitzes LM, Javel E, Brugge JF. Organization of auditory cortex in the owl monkey (*Aotus trivirgatus*). J Comp Neurol 1977; 171:117, 119.)

quency (Fig. 3–20*B*). Notice also that the same frequency tends to be represented in a lateral strip across the cortex. This tendency suggests that the cortex is composed of parallel sheets of neurons having similar frequency-tuning characteristics.

Superimposed on this tonotopic map may be several other organizations of cells according to their tuning characteristics. For example, Imig and Adrian found, in the primary auditory cortex of the cat, columns of cells in which all of the neurons were characterized by the degree to which one ear or the other dominated the response properties of the cell.[99] These columns tended to fall in elongated patches oriented perpendicular to the isofrequency strips. Schreiner and Cynader found that bandwidth of neurons increased as the sampling electrode moved from area AI into area AII in the cat.[100] Tunturi presented evidence for an orderly arrangement of information about stimulus intensity in the dog auditory cortex, but this has not been found in other species.[101]

There is some controversy as to the tightness of organization of the auditory cortex in this regard. Although it is probably true that the orderly cochleotopic arrangement found throughout the auditory pathway is preserved to some degree at the cortex, there is also evidence that this organization has degenerated somewhat by the time the cortical level is reached or that a more diffuse projection is mixed with the cochleotopic projection.[82,97,102,103]

Area AI is surrounded by a number of other cortical areas, each with its own cytoarchitectonic, myeloarchitectonic, and electrophysiologic characteristics (see Figs. 3–17 and 3–18). In the monkey, area AI is surrounded by several fields that are architectonically distinct and are tonotopically organized (e.g., areas L and RL). In addition, there are areas (e.g., area CM) in which the cells are broadly tuned and in which to specify a best frequency is difficult.[89,97] The relative location of these auditory belt areas varies from species to species.

There is some evidence that the area surrounding area AI represents a phylogenetically older cortex.[92] According to this view, the cortex developed as a series of rings in which newer cortex appearing at the center of the ring displaced phylogenetically older tissue laterally. The last, or latest, step in this process was the growth of a highly specialized core of koniocortex corresponding to area AI. In its broadest interpretation, this evolutionary hypothesis leads to a consideration that the development of specifically organized primary sensory cortical areas was a prerequisite to the evolution of higher intelligence.[104] The primary auditory cortex then may be viewed as one of the most advanced organizations of neural tissue.

The primary auditory cortex in the monkey sends projections to the surrounding belt areas (with the exception of the rostral area), terminating in layer IV.[92] In the cat, area AI projects to area AII and EP, and there is a light projection to the insular-temporal region.[105,106] Projections to area AII are predominantly from layers III and IV, with lighter projections from the other layers.[107] These connections between cortical fields are precisely organized tonotopically; that is, cells tend to connect with other cells with the same best frequency.[108]

Area AI also sends a topographic projection through the corpus callosum to layer III and to a lesser extent to other layers in contralateral area AI.[109,110] In this case, the strongest connections are between cells that are excited by both ears. Neurons that are excited by one ear and inhibited by the other make relatively sparse interhemispheric connections.[111] The auditory belt areas are all interconnected by reciprocal projections, but send only minor projections to layers I and II of area AI. In addition, the auditory belt areas also project to a number of nonauditory cortical areas: to the prefrontal and premotor cortex in the frontal lobe, to the parietal lobe, and to the cingulate gyrus.[112] The primary auditory cortex sends major descending projections to the medial geniculate body and the inferior colliculus as described in the next section.

Descending Systems

The ascending auditory pathways are influenced and modulated throughout their course by the descending auditory pathways. These descending pathways parallel the ascending ones and terminate in most of the auditory nuclei previously mentioned.

The primary auditory cortex sends major descending projections to the ventral division of the medial geniculate body and the central nucleus of the inferior colliculus.[110,113–116] In both nuclei, these descending fibers run parallel to, and terminate in, layers parallel to the laminae. Other thalamic nuclei, including the dorsal and medial divisions of the medial geniculate body (MGB) and the posterior thalamic nuclei, receive descending projections as well.[113] The medial geniculate body and the inferior colliculus, in turn, send descending projections to lower auditory nuclei.

An important distinction between ascending and descending auditory pathways, which otherwise parallel each other, is that although there is an ascending projection from the cochlea to the cochlear nucleus, there is no descending projection from the cochlear nucleus to the cochlea. The projection from the auditory brain stem to the cochlea has its origin in the superior olivary complex. Therefore the final descending connection is the superior olivary complex to the cochlea (as well as the superior olivary complex to the cochlear nucleus).

The superior olivary complex to cochlea connection has classically been called the "olivocochlear bundle." Although originally divided into crossed and uncrossed components,[117,118] these have recently been reclassified into a medial and lateral system, based on studies in the cat, rat, and guinea pig (Fig. 3–21).[119–121] Neurons in the lateral olivocochlear system have their cells of origin in or close to the lateral superior olivary nucleus and project predominantly to the ipsilateral cochlea, terminating almost exclusively beneath inner hair cells on the peripheral processes of eighth nerve fibers. Neurons of the medial olivocochlear system are located in more medially located olivary nuclei. In the monkey, these are ventral to the medial superior olive and project predominantly to the contralateral cochlea (a ratio of 3:2 contra- to ipsilateral in monkey)[122] and terminate mainly beneath outer hair cells, largely on outer hair cell bases. It is likely that most olivocochlear neurons, in both medial and lateral systems, are excited by the side that they innervate.[123]

Just as there is a tonotopic organization of afferents, there is also a tonotopic organization of olivocochlear efferents. For the lateral olivocochlear system in the cat, the most lateral cells innervate the apical cochlea and the more medial cells the more basal cochlea. For the medial olivocochlear system, the more dorsally located the cells of origin the more basal their projection to the cochlea.[119,123]

Reflex Pathways

There are two muscles in the middle ear, the stapedius muscle and the tensor tympani muscle, which are each attached to one of the small bones of the middle ear, termed ossicles. The stapedius muscle receives innervation from the facial nerve (seventh cranial nerve) and inserts into the stapes. The tensor tympani muscle is innervated by a branch of the mandibular division of the trigeminal nerve

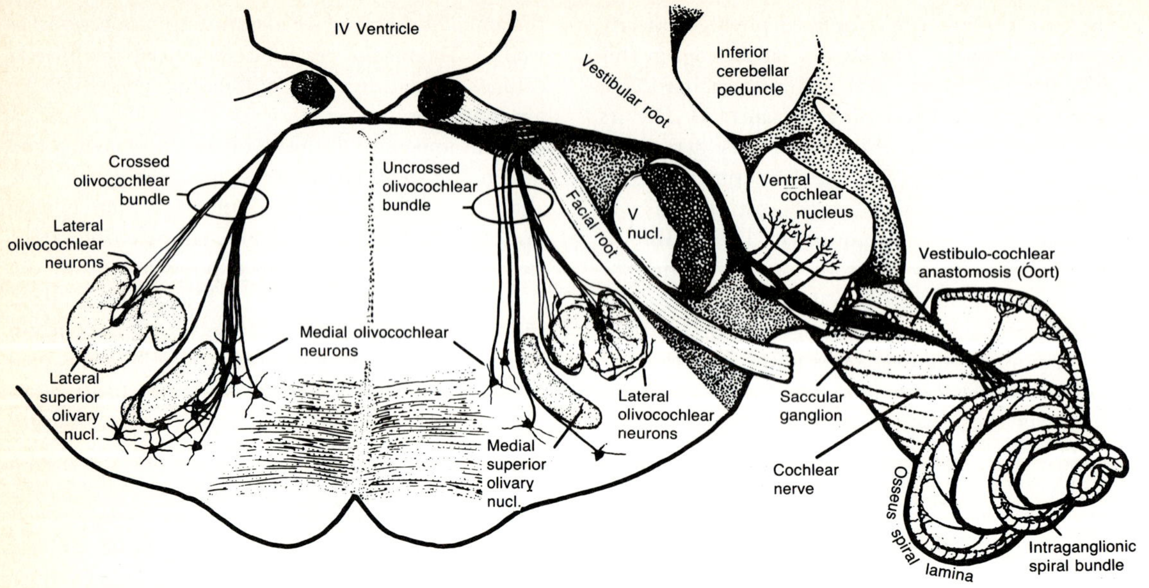

Figure 3-21 A drawing summarizing the origins, course, and distribution of the OCB to the left cochlea of the cat, as would be seen from the front. (After Rasmussen GL. Efferent fibers of the cochlear nerve and cochlear nucleus. In: Rasmussen GL, Windle WF, eds. Neural mechanisms of the auditory and vestibular systems. Springfield, IL: CC Thomas, 1960:105.) Note that some uncrossed medial OC axons course closer to the midline than indicated here. (From Warr WB et al. Organization of the efferent fibers: the lateral and medial systems. In: Altschuler RA, Hoffman DW, Bobbin RP, eds. Neurobiology of hearing: the cochlea. New York: Raven Press, 1986:339.)

(fifth cranial nerve) and attaches to the manubrium of the malleus. In both cases, the contraction of these muscles is involuntary, the result of activation of reflex pathways. Contraction of middle ear muscles is bilateral even when elicited by stimulation to only one ear. The threshold for activation of tensor tympani is higher than for stapedius, and in both cases is well above the threshold for hearing in man. The reflex is generally elicited by loud sounds; its function is protection from damage to the inner ear. In both cases, the reflex arc involves four neurons (Fig. 3–22). For the stapedius reflex, the response involves (1) the auditory nerve (eighth cranial nerve) activating (2) neurons in the cochlear nucleus that, in turn, project to and activate (3) neurons in the superior olivary complex, which project to and activate (4) neurons in the nearby nucleus of the seventh nerve, which innervate the stapedius muscle and result in its contraction, thereby pulling the stapes away from the oval window and so reducing the transmission of sound impulses. For the tensor tympani reflex, elements one to three are the same, but the neurons of the superior olivary complex instead activate neurons of the motor nucleus of the fifth nerve, which innervate the tensor tympani, causing its contraction and resulting in reduced sound transmission in the middle ear.[124] The reader should note that the pathways described here were demonstrated in the rabbit. There may be variations in this pathway in other species.[125]

CORTICAL AREAS INVOLVED IN SPEECH PERCEPTION AND PRODUCTION

We will now review the areas of the brain involved in speech production and perception, beginning with the cortical areas, then proceeding to subcortical areas, and finally describing the peripheral motor pathways.

Both speech perception and speech production, as learned, voluntary motor behaviors, involve several regions of the human cerebral cortex. Our knowledge of the role of the human cortex in speech has been derived through direct electrical stimulation of cortical structures during surgical procedures, through examination of speech behavior matched with radiographic images of the brain or images of the brain reflecting its metabolic functioning during speech production and perception, and through speech disorders resulting from damage to more or less specific regions of the cortex.

Before considering specific cortical areas involved in speech and language, we will overview the cortex as a whole, adding some details to the brief description given in the introduction to this chapter. Some authors have correlated cytoarchitectonically distinct areas of cortex with functionally defined areas.[126] Although there have been many proposed frameworks that subdivide the cerebral cortex regionally, there appear to be two dominant schemes.

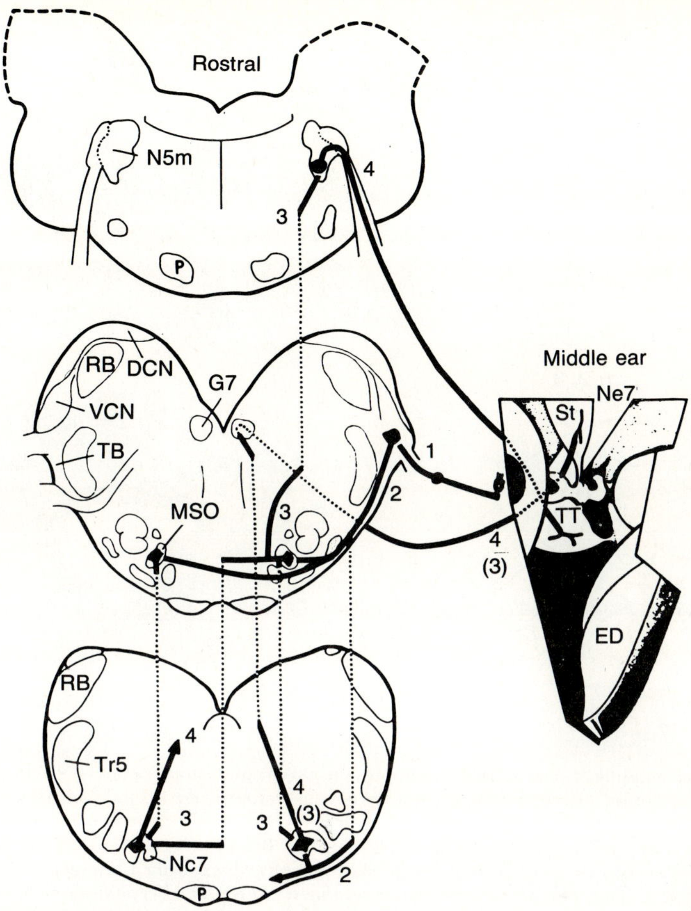

Figure 3–22 Neuronal organization of the acoustic stapedius (St) and tensor tympani (TT) reflexes as shown in three transverse sections through the rabbit brain stem. The middle ear is shown schematically in posterior view. Solid lines represent nerve tracts. Dotted lines show the connections between the sections. Stapedius reflex: the first neuron (1), the primary auditory neuron from the hair cells to the cochlear nucleus, has contact with the second order neuron (2) in the ventral cochlear nucleus (VCN). The second neuron (2) passes through the trapezoidal body (TB) and has contact directly with the ipsilateral stapedius motoneurons in the motor nucleus of the seventh cranial nerve (Nc7). Via interneurons (3) in, or near, the medial superior olive (MSO), it relays to the ipsilateral and contralateral Nc7. The motoneuron (3 or 4) follows the facial nerve to the stapedius muscle in the middle ear. The tensor tympani reflex: the first order (1) and the second order (2) neurons follow the same course as for the stapedius reflex. There are no direct connections from second order neuron to the motor nucleus of the fifth cranial nerve (N 5 m). The motoneuron (4) follows the mandibular branch of the trigeminal nerve to the tensor tympani (TT) in the middle ear. ED is the eardrum, P is pyramidal tract, RB restiform body, DCN dorsal cochlear nucleus, G 7 internal geniculum of the seventh nerve, Tr 5 spinal trigeminal tract, cochlear nucleus, Tr 5 spinal trigeminal tract, Ne 7 seventh nerve. (From Borg E. On the neuronal organization of the acoustic middle ear reflex. A physiological and anatomical study. Brain Res 1973; 49:116.)

The first scheme focuses on the anatomically unique properties of specific cerebral cortex locations. A wide variety of cortical maps has been produced. Exner prepared a complex map with over a hundred subdivisions.[127] More widely accepted cortical maps with fewer subdivisions were prepared by Brodmann in 1909[128] and von Economo in 1929.[93] Currently, the Brodmann map (Fig. 3–23*A*) is the most widely accepted. The second scheme focuses on the functional patterns of shared regions of the cerebral cortex.[129] Based upon the work of Broca,[130] Abbie,[131] Filimonoff,[132] Yakovlev,[133] and Sanides,[134] this approach divides the cerebral cortex into typologically and architectonically distinct regions whose structural complexity and differentiation increase gradually. A comparison of the locations associated with Brodmann's map of the cerebral cortex and the cortical mantle subtypes described in Mesulam[129] is illustrated in Figure 3–23*B*.

The Cortical Speech Areas

Two primary cortical areas are known to be major speech centers. These areas are named after the men who first described them, Paul Broca and Carl Wer-

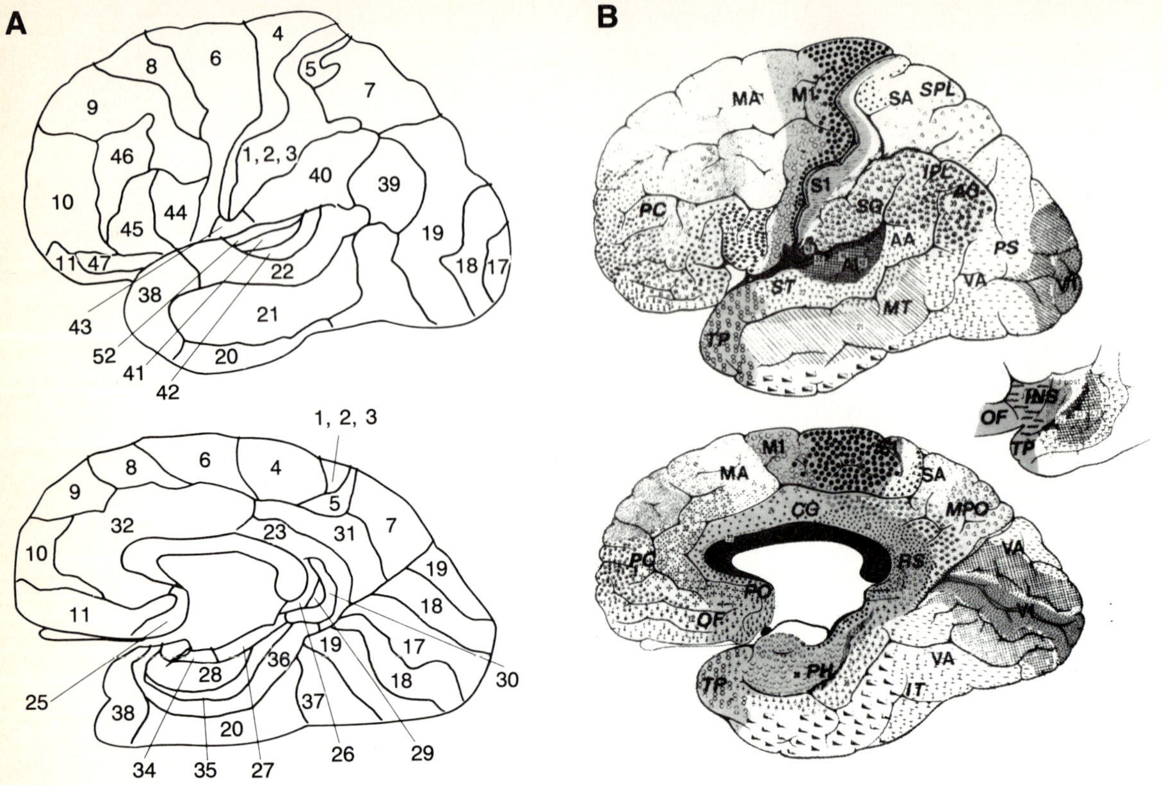

Figure 3-23 *A*, Neocortical quiltwork of areas or fields was mapped in 1909 by the German neurologist Korbinian Brodmann; his scheme is the one now favored for neocortical parcellation. In it the primary visual cortex is area 17; the primary auditory cortex (largely hidden on the upper face of the temporal lobe in the Sylvian fissure—see Fig. 3–17) is area 41; the primary somatic sensory cortex is areas 1, 2, and 3; the motor cortex is area 4. The speech areas are harder to place. Broca's area, not far from the motor cortex, is more or less coextensive with area 44. Wernicke's area, not far from the primary auditory cortex, is the convergence of three of Brodmann's areas: 22, 39, and 40. The cortical level for control of eye movement is even more elusive. The electrical stimulation of three areas—8, 19, and 22—can cause the eyes to turn in unison toward the contralateral side of the visual world. (From Nauta WJH, Freirtag M. Fundamental neuroanatomy. New York: WH Freeman, 1986:301.) *B*, Distribution of functional zones in relationship to Brodmann's map of the human brain. The boundaries are not intended to be precise. Much of this information is based on experimental evidence obtained from laboratory animals and needs to be confirmed in the human brain. Abbreviations: AA = auditory association cortex; AG = angular gyrus; AI = primary auditory cortex; CG = cingulate cortex; INS = insula; IPL = inferior parietal lobule; IT = inferior temporal gyrus; MA = motor association cortex; MPO = medial parieto-occipital area; MT = middle temporal gyrus; MI = primary motor area; OF = orbitofrontal region; PC = prefrontal cortex; PH = parahippocampal region; PO = parolfactory area; PS = peristriate cortex; RS = retrosplenial area; SA = somatosensory association cortex; SG = supramarginal gyrus; SPL = superior parietal lobule; ST = superior temporal gyrus; SI = supramarginal gyrus; SPL = superior parietal lobule; ST = superior temporal gyrus; SI = primary somatosensory area; TP = temporopolar cortex; VA = visual association cortex; V1 = primary visual cortex. (From Mesulam M-M. Principles of behavioral neurology. Philadelphia: FA Davis, 1985:12.)

nicke. In discussing Wernicke's and Broca's areas, we are referring to these topographic areas only in a statistical sense. That is, these areas are generally found in the location indicated in Figure 3–24, but in no two individuals can one expect to find exactly the same cortical area related to speech control. One should also remember that these areas have been located by surgical intervention in patients with known neural pathology or by postmortem examination of patients with pathologic conditions. Thus the investigations have used a population that is, at onset, abnormal. Nevertheless, the great number of cases that have been reviewed and the general agreement among them lead to the conclusion that these areas of the cortex are involved in speech control.[135]

The discoveries of Broca and Wernicke that damage to the left hemisphere resulted in aphasia led to acceptance of the concept of a dominant hemisphere for speech and language. The left hemisphere is usually the dominant hemisphere for these functions, but in a few left-handed individuals, the right hemisphere may dominate.[135–140] In support of the behavioral data on left cerebral dominance for speech production are anatomic differences in the left and right hemispheres. The planum temporale on the superior surface of the temporal lobe has been found in both adults and in newborn infants to be longer in the left hemisphere than in the right.[141–144]

Although the role of the left hemisphere in speech and language has received considerable atten-

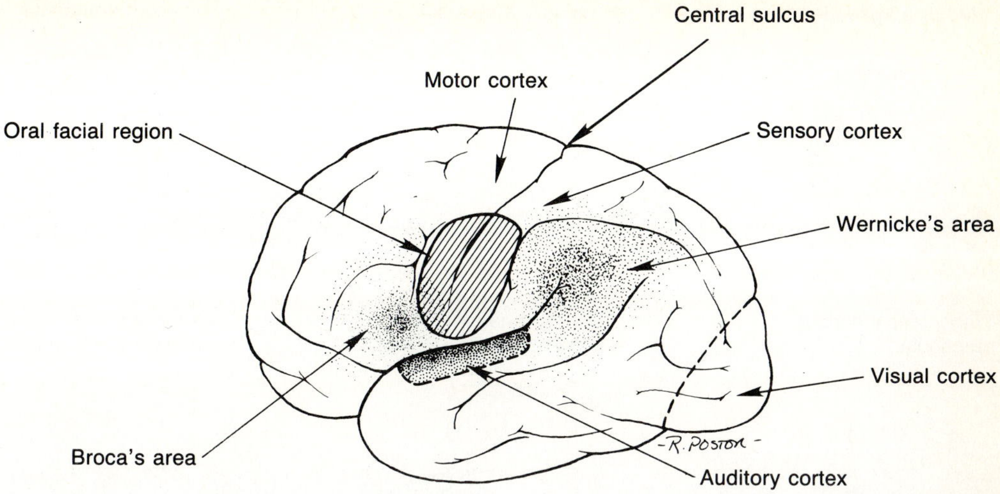

Figure 3–24 Lateral view of the human cerebral cortex indicating some important functional areas. Broca's and Wernicke's speech areas are indicated by stippling: the denser the stippling, the greater the relationship to speech mechanisms (see text for more detail). The auditory cortex, indicated by hatch marks, is mostly buried within the Sylvian fissure (see Fig. 3–17). The more lateral areas of the sensorimotor cortex are related to structures involved in speech production.

tion, recent research has emphasized the role of the right hemisphere and suggests that both hemispheres play an important role in speech and language.[145–150] Studies of the perception of speech intonation revealed a distinct left ear (right hemisphere) advantage.[151,152] More recently, regional cerebral blood flow studies have suggested that the right and left hemispheres are active during speech production and perception.[146,148] Electrophysiologic studies of cortical activity also suggest that the right hemisphere is active during speech. In a series of studies, Ross and his colleagues demonstrated that the right hemisphere was dominant in organizing the affective prosodic components of speech and gestural behavior and that the right hemisphere is organized functionally and anatomically like the left hemisphere (see Fig. 3–25).[149,150,153–155]

Speech Perception

A broad range of the perisylvian cortex in the frontal, temporal, and parietal lobes plays an important part in speech perception. Kimura, using verbally presented stimuli, reported that both temporal lobes take part in the elaboration of activity at the auditory receiving area of the same side.[156] Kimura also emphasized that the left temporal lobe is particularly important in the perception of verbal or speech stimuli. Using stimulation mapping techniques, Ojemann and Mateer have found in the left hemisphere that the precentral gyrus, Broca's and Wernicke's areas, and the superior temporal gyrus are involved in both sequential oral-motor movements and perception of speech sounds.[157] These investigators found that a specific point of stimulation interfered with both motor and perceptual events. It is noteworthy that oral-motor control extends posteriorly from Broca's area and the motor cortex. It is also of interest with regard to theories of speech perception that a motor act and speech perception were anatomically related.

The use of dichotically presented stimuli has been useful in the identification of the behavioral functions of the cerebral cortex. Interhemispheric connections appear to play an important role in speech perception. The presentation of speech stimuli dichotically has shown that distinct hemispheric roles exist. In particular, there is a right ear advantage (REA) for verbal or speech stimuli and a left ear advantage (LEA) for nonspeech materials. This effect is reversed for individuals who are known to have right hemisphere language dominance.[156] The stimuli producing these effects did not have to be meaningful. That is, backward speech and nonsense syllables also produced a REA. However, not all speech sounds produce the equivalent REA. Stop consonants produce the strongest REA, whereas liquids (/r/,/l/) produce a weaker REA.[158,159] Vowel sounds have not produced any significant REA. These results have been attributed to the functional prepotency of the contralateral pathway from the right ear to the language-dominant left hemisphere following the model reported in Kimura.[156] More recently, Musiek et al have reported on the perceptual pro-

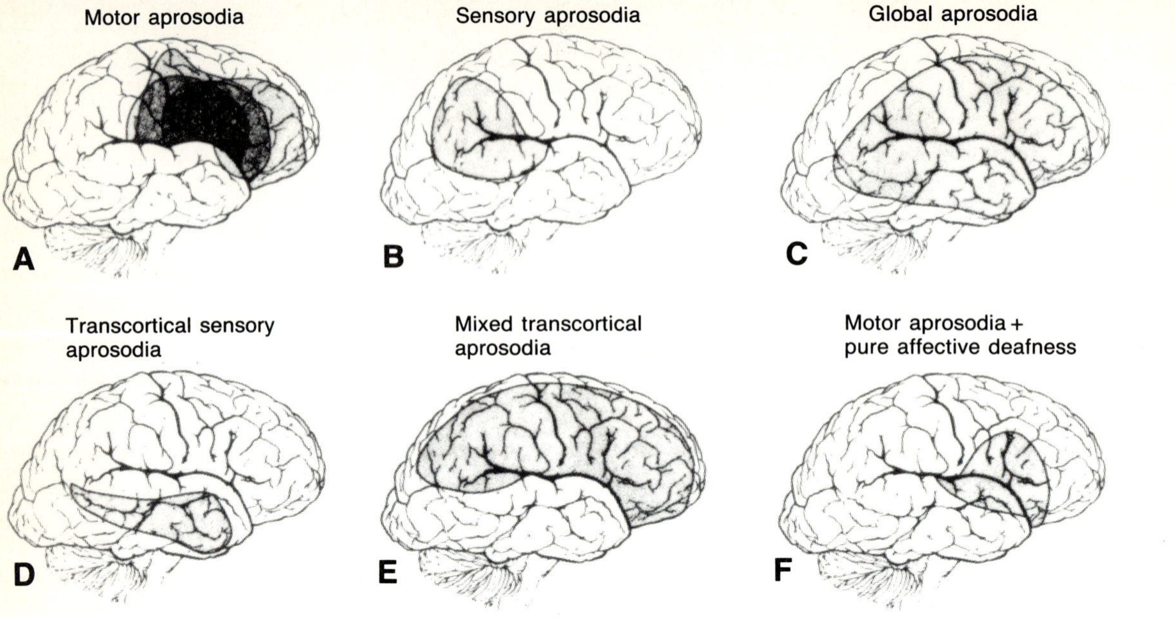

Figure 3–25 Right lateral brain templates showing the distribution of infarctions on CT scans.[149] Since the clustering of affective-prosodic deficits appeared similar to the clustering of linguistic deficits observed in patients with left brain damage, the same modifiers as those used in aphasias were supplied for classification purposes. (From Ross ED. Modulation of affect and nonverbal communication by the right hemisphere. In: Mesulam M-M, ed. Principles of behavioral neurology. Philadelphia: FA Davis, 1985:245.)

cessing of individuals before and after two-stage callossotomy.[160] After the first operation (sectioning of the posterior half of the corpus callosum), the dichotic tests revealed a decrease in left ear scores, and this decrease was attributed to suppression of ipsilateral auditory pathways. Musiek and colleagues also reported improved right-ear performance, which they attributed to a reduction of central auditory competition.[160] Thus the posterior portion of the corpus callosum is involved in auditory processing, including speech, which is consistent with neuroanatomic studies in monkeys.[161]

MOTOR PATHWAYS RELATED TO SPEECH PRODUCTION

Motor Cortex

Primary Motor Cortex

The primary motor area (M1) is located in the precentral gyrus and is a part of the idiotypic cortex (see Fig. 3–23). Identification of the region has involved several different types of information. Electrical stimulation of the cortex has been used in the identification of primary motor regions. The threshold for eliciting movement upon electrical stimulation is lowest in the M1 region when compared to other motor regions. The appearance of large pyramidal cells (Betz's cells) within its fifth layer is often used to identify the region. The greatest density of neurons comprising the corticospinal and corticobulbar fibers originate in M1. There are no sharp boundaries between the areas of the motor cortex. The distinction between M1 and the premotor cortex is the subject of controversy. Some researchers equate M1 with only Brodmann area 4, whereas others include area 4 and the posterior half of area 6 as a part of M1.[129] Projections from the different regions of the thalamic nuclei have been used to determine the line of demarcation of M1 from AI (Area 3a) below the central sulcus.[162]

The primary motor cortex is subdivided into several areas organized in an inverted manner. Electrical stimulation of the superior region results in movements of the lower extremity. Stimulation of the medial regions results in movements of the upper extremity, whereas stimulation of the inferior regions results in movements of the face, tongue, and jaw. A common representation of the primary motor region with the associated body parts is provided in Figure 3–26.

Supplementary Motor Cortex

Along with the primary motor area of the cortex (M1), the supplementary motor area (M2) is involved in motor control and speech. M2 is located on the medial surface of the left hemisphere just an-

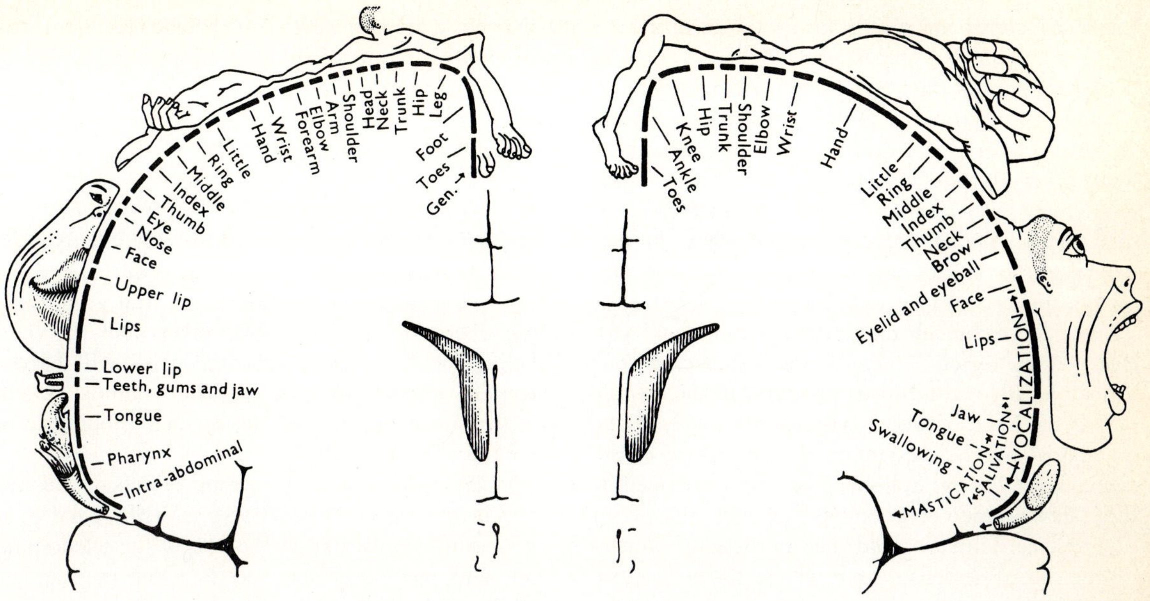

Figure 3–26 Schematic illustration of functional areas of the somatosensory cortex of man as first described by Penfield and Rasmussen.[296] The motor representation is shown on the right side of the figure and the sensory representation is shown on the left. The homunculi in these figures indicate the relatively large areas of sensory and motor cortices devoted to the head and face region (see text). (Reprinted with permission by the MacMillan Publishing Company. From Penfield and Rasmussen. The cerebral cortex of man. New York: MacMillan, 1950. Copyright 1950 by MacMillan Publishing Co., renewed 1978 by Theodore Rasmussen.)

terior to M1 (Area 4) (see Fig. 3–23). Early studies noted that when the supplementary motor area was stimulated, it arrested speech production.[135] Studies on the organization of the supplementary motor area suggest that it may be organized in a topographic manner[163,164] and may be involved in motor planning.[148]

Premotor Cortex

The premotor cortex has a more granular appearance than the primary motor cortex, and provides cortical inputs to the primary motor cortex. Although this area contributes a substantial number of fibers to the corticospinal and corticobulbar systems, the density of these fibers is less than that observed in the primary motor cortex.[165] To elicit movement, the threshold of stimulation of the premotor cortex is higher than in the primary motor area. Fibers from the premotor cortex project to the reticular formation either directly or via the basal ganglia. Some authors consider anterior area 6, the supplementary motor region (M2), posterior area 8, and area 44 (a segment of Broca's region) as the motor association cortex (see Fig. 3–25).[129]

Sensorimotor Cortex

Primary Somatosensory Cortex. The primary somatosensory cortex, S1 (see Fig. 3–23*B*), is in the postcentral gyrus. This area receives projections from the ventroposterior thalamic nucleus, which serves as a relay for ascending somatosensory pathways. In each hemisphere, the body is somatotopically mapped onto S1. The somatotopical mapping of the primary somatosensory cortex is similar to the primary motor cortex. The homunculi in Figure 3–26 also apply to S1. In addition, most S1 areas have callosal connections with homologous parts of S1 in the opposite hemisphere.

Secondary Sensorimotor Area. The secondary sensorimotor areas are traditionally identified as A2, M2, S2, and V2. A2 is just medial to A1 (see Fig. 3–23*B*). S2 is in the parietal operculum adjacent to the dorsal insula. V2 is located in the peristriate cortex. M2 is located on the medial surface of the hemisphere anterior to M1. M2 was discussed earlier because of its role in speech production, especially in motor planning.[135,148] However, the physiology and role in speech production, speech perception, and language of the other areas (A2,S2,V2) are not understood fully.

Cortical Motor Output

Pyramidal Pathway

Traditionally, the output from the cerebral cortex has been described as consisting of two different pathways. One pathway originates primarily from the motor cortex and travels without interruption to the brain stem and spinal cord (Fig. 3–27). This pathway is called the "pyramidal system." The fibers in this system originate from cortical areas 1,2,3,4,5 and 7, and other areas as well. Some of these fibers originate from the giant Betz's cells, which are located only in area 4. From the cortex, fibers pass toward the internal capsule, which is located lateral to the caudate nucleus and thalamus and medial to the lenticular nucleus (Fig. 3–27). Fibers then proceed down through the cerebral peduncle and into the pontine region. Fibers to the spinal cord continue caudally and form the pyramids in the medulla. At the lower border of the medulla, many of the pyramidal fibers decussate to the other side of the spinal cord. In the midbrain, pontine, and medullary areas, some corticobulbar fibers branch off to the reticular formation and then to the motor nuclei of the cranial nervous system, whereas others course directly to lower motor neurons of some cranial nerves. The corticobulbar fibers have bilateral, ipsilateral, and some contralateral projections to the cranial motor nuclei and sensory relay nuclei.[3,166] The pyramidal system is extremely important for speech production; a lesion involving the pyramidal system may result in paralysis of the speech muscles.

Extrapyramidal Pathway

The other major pathway from the cerebral cortex is called the "extrapyramidal tract." This is an extremely complicated system that is difficult to define and involves several different nuclear groups and the fibers joining them, the cortex, and the cerebellum. Each of these subcomponents will be described. Abnormalities of the extrapyramidal system may result in speech pathologies such as observed in parkinsonian patients.[167]

Basal Ganglia. One group of subcortical nuclei in the extrapyramidal system is the basal ganglia, which is situated at the base of the telencephalon and mesencephalon and includes the caudate nucleus, putamen, and the globus pallidus (see Fig. 3–28). Other extrapyramidal nuclear groups are the subthalamic nuclei, substantia nigra, zona incerta, red nucleus, and deep tegmental nucleus. The relationship between the nuclear groups of the extra-

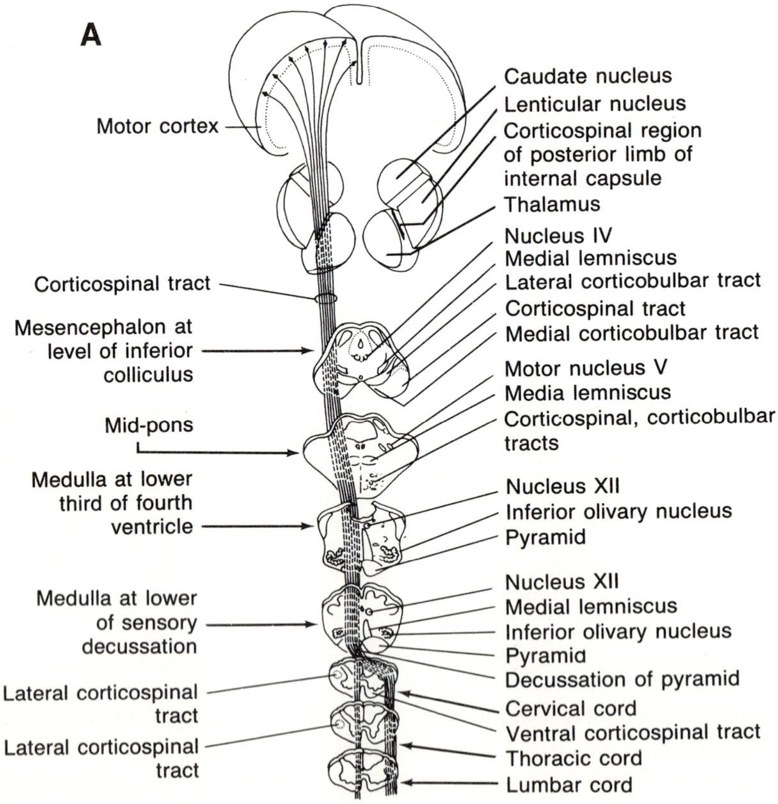

Figure 3–27 Illustration of the pathways of the pyramidal tract fibers (*A* is corticospinal and *B* is corticobulbar) as they descend from the cerebral cortex through the corona radiata and internal capsule into the brain stem and down to the spinal cord. The levels as well as principal anatomical features along the pathways are labeled. (From House EL, Pansky B. A functional approach to neuroanatomy. New York: McGraw-Hill, 1967:394, 395.)

pyramidal system is illustrated schematically in Figure 3–28.

The circuitry involved in the basal ganglia and extrapyramidal system may be summarized in the following way. In primates, the putamen and the caudate nucleus are referred to as the striatum and are separated by the internal capsule. Wide areas of the cerebral cortex, including areas 4 and 6, project to the putamen and caudate nucleus of the basal ganglia. The globus pallidus, which is ventromedial to the putamen, is divided by the medial medullary lamina into an external and internal segment (lateral and medial, respectively). Striatum axons terminate in both segments of the globus pallidus. The internal segment of the globus pallidus and the pars reticulata of the substantia nigra are the major output nuclei for the motor components of the basal ganglia and project to several thalamic nuclei and other nuclei involved in motor control.[129,168–171] The extrapyramidal system influences motor control by a complex network of feedback circuits that ultimately project back to the cerebral cortex, deep tegmental nucleus, reticular nuclei, or the red nucleus. The red nucleus, deep tegmental nucleus, and cerebral cortex project to interneurons in the reticular formation, which, in turn, send fibers to the motor and sensory nuclei of the brain stem.[3,172,173]

Thalamus. Research on humans has implicated certain thalamic nuclei in speech control. The techniques of this research have utilized analysis of speech and postmortem examination of individuals with accidental or experimentally induced alteration of normal thalamic function. Evidence obtained with these methods indicates that the pulvinar[135,174] and ventral lateral nucleus[175–177] are involved in speech control (see Fig. 3–2).

Cerebellar and basal ganglia outputs supply three systems of subcortical afferents to the ventrolateral thalamus, which form parallel pathways to the motor and premotor cortex.[178] One pathway begins in the caudal portion of the deep cerebellar nuclei and, via thalamic area X (near area DM), influences the arcuate premotor area, and a second pathway, originating in the pars reticulata of the substantia nigra and the internal segment of the globus pallidus, influences the supplementary motor cortex. The third pathway originates in the rostral portions of the deep cerebellar nuclei and influences the motor cortex via

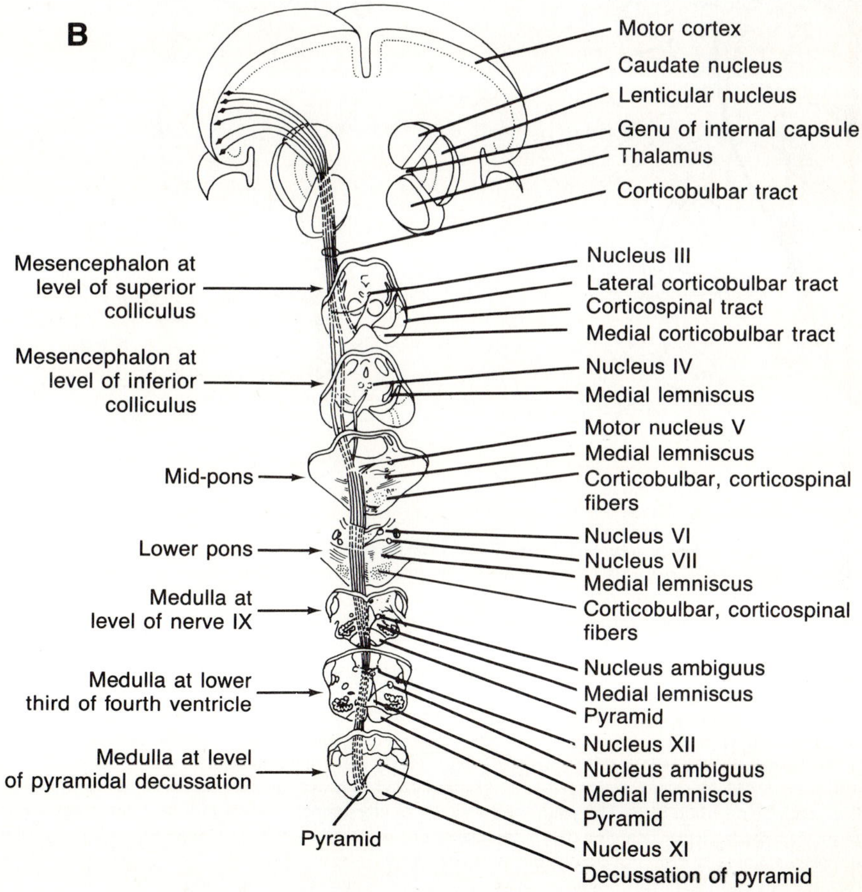

Figure 3–27 Continued

the pars oralis of the ventrolateral thalamus.[170] These thalamic nuclei are part of larger subcortical networks that are important for motor control in general and for speech in particular.

Since sensory information from the orofacial region may be used in speech control, it is important to consider thalamic sensory mechanisms that may be used in speech. Evidence obtained from animal investigations indicates that sensory information from the orofacial region projects to the nucleus ventralis posteromedialis of the thalamus.[179–184] From the ventralis posteromedialis, sensory information projects to the somatosensory cortex[185,186] and back from the cortex to the ventralis posteromedialis.[187] Although the thalamocortical connections may be specific, evidence obtained from animals indicates that thalamic projections to the cortex may be more diffuse than previously thought.[188]

Cerebellum. The cerebellum lies dorsal to the brain stem and inferior to the occipital lobe of the cerebral cortex and is an area of the brain important for motor control.[198] Damage to the cerebellum frequently results in abnormal speech called "ataxic dysarthria."[189–191]

The cerebellum is smaller than the cerebral cortex; however, in structure it is, in many ways, similar to the cerebral cortex. Like the cerebral cortex, the cerebellar cortex is folded; the grooves are known as fissures, and the folded portions are called folia. The cerebellar cortex is composed of layers of cell bodies on the surface that extend down into the depths of the fissures. Deep to the surface layer of cell bodies is the white matter of the cerebellum, which is composed of fiber tracts to and from the cerebellar cortex. In the central region of the cerebellum are four bilateral nuclei. The most medial is the fastigial nucleus; lateral to this are the globose and emboliform nuclei, and the most lateral nucleus is the dentate.

Figure 3–29*A* is a schematic illustration of the surface of the cerebellum laid out flat. The phylogenetically newest regions and the largest lateral expansions of the cerebellar cortex are the simplex (VI) lobe and crura I and II (VII) of the semilunar lobes.

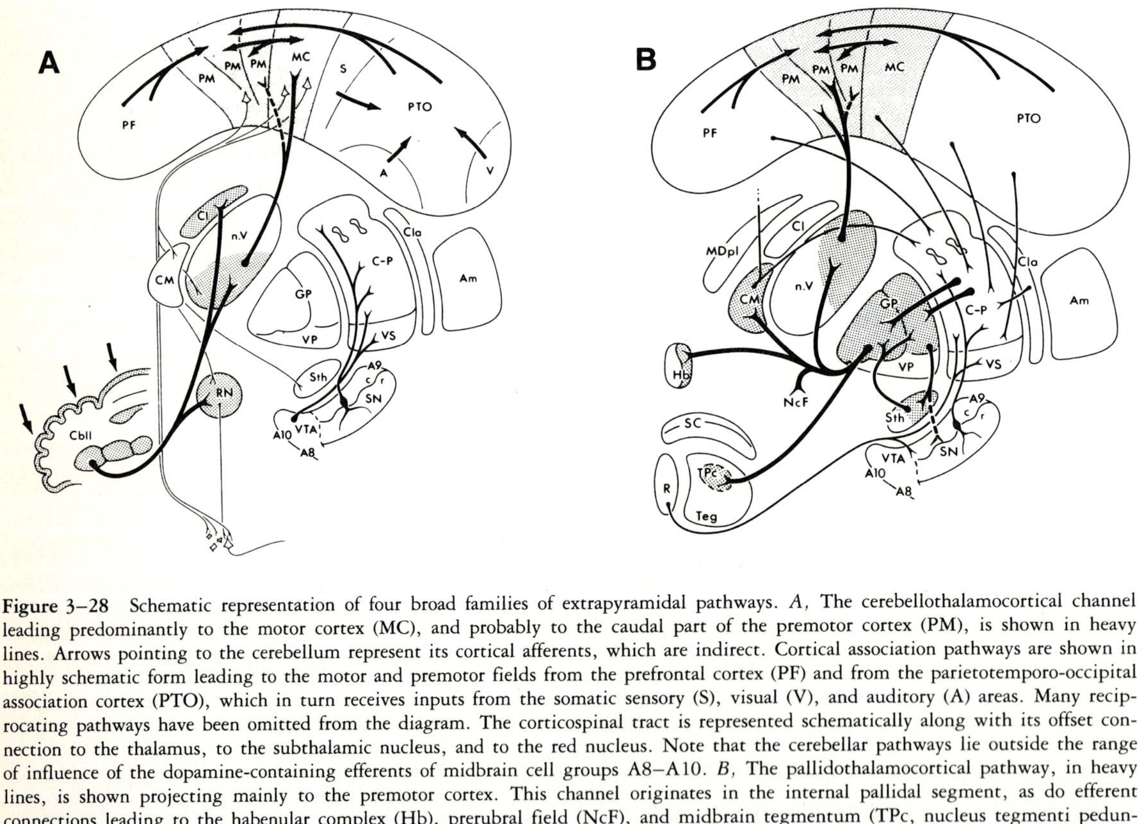

Figure 3–28 Schematic representation of four broad families of extrapyramidal pathways. *A,* The cerebellothalamocortical channel leading predominantly to the motor cortex (MC), and probably to the caudal part of the premotor cortex (PM), is shown in heavy lines. Arrows pointing to the cerebellum represent its cortical afferents, which are indirect. Cortical association pathways are shown in highly schematic form leading to the motor and premotor fields from the prefrontal cortex (PF) and from the parietotemporo-occipital association cortex (PTO), which in turn receives inputs from the somatic sensory (S), visual (V), and auditory (A) areas. Many reciprocating pathways have been omitted from the diagram. The corticospinal tract is represented schematically along with its offset connection to the thalamus, to the subthalamic nucleus, and to the red nucleus. Note that the cerebellar pathways lie outside the range of influence of the dopamine-containing efferents of midbrain cell groups A8–A10. *B,* The pallidothalamocortical pathway, in heavy lines, is shown projecting mainly to the premotor cortex. This channel originates in the internal pallidal segment, as do efferent connections leading to the habenular complex (Hb), prerubral field (NcF), and midbrain tegmentum (TPc, nucleus tegmenti pedunculopontinus pars compacta or "pedunculopontine nucleus"). Also indicated in heavy lines are inputs to the pallidum from the striatum (C-P), and the pallidosubthalamopallido loop. The main inputs to the caudoputamen, shown in finer lines, originate in the neocortex, the thalamic center median-parafascicular complex (CM), the claustrum (Cla), the serotonin-containing dorsal raphe nucleus (R), and the midbrain dopamine-containing nuclei, principally the substantia nigra pars compacta (c, A9). Distinctions between afferents innervating the caudate nucleus and the putamen are not indicated.[297,298] The projection from the ventral tegmental area to the ventral caudoputamen is indicated in *A* and *D*.

In higher primates and the human, the greatly expanded VI and VII lobes are believed by several investigators to be important for manual dexterity and speech control.[189] Indeed, sensory information from the tongue, face, jaws, larynx, and auditory system projects to the medial regions of these lobes.[192–196] Thus the integration of auditory information and other forms of sensory feedback by the cerebellum could possibly be important for speech control.

The cerebellum has a uniformity of structure that has made it a popular topic for anatomists and physiologists for many years. There are two main types of afferent fibers that enter the cerebellum and terminate in its cortex. Climbing fibers originate from the contralateral inferior olive, pass through the inferior cerebellar peduncle (the restiform body) (Fig. 3–29*B*), and terminate around the large Purkinje's cells in the cerebellar cortex. Mossy fibers originate from the reticular and pontine nuclei, the vestibular complex, and the spinal cord and pass through the middle, inferior, and superior cerebellar peduncles (see Fig. 3–29*B*) to terminate in the cerebellar cortex. There are five major cell types in the cerebellar cortex, and their interactions are summarized in Figure 3–30. The only output of the cerebellar cortex is via the Purkinje's cell's axon, which projects to the cerebellar nuclei and vestibular nuclei. The cerebellar nuclei then send their axons out to the cerebellum primarily via the superior cerebellar peduncles (see Fig. 3–29*B*).[197–200]

Cerebellar projections from the fastigial nucleus, both crossed and uncrossed, arch over the superior cerebellar peduncle, and some of the fibers exit the cerebellum via the superior cerebellar peduncle,[1] whereas most fibers exit via the juxtarestiform body (a fiber bundle just medial to the main restiform body). These cerebellar efferent fibers terminate in the vestibular nuclei,[1,3] thalamus,[201] and the ventral tegmentum (for example, the substantia nigra).[202] Fibers from the globose, emboliform, and dentate nuclei traverse the superior cerebellar peduncle and either go through the red nucleus on their way to the ventral lateral nucleus of the thalamus or terminate in the red nucleus (Fig. 3–29*C*). Within

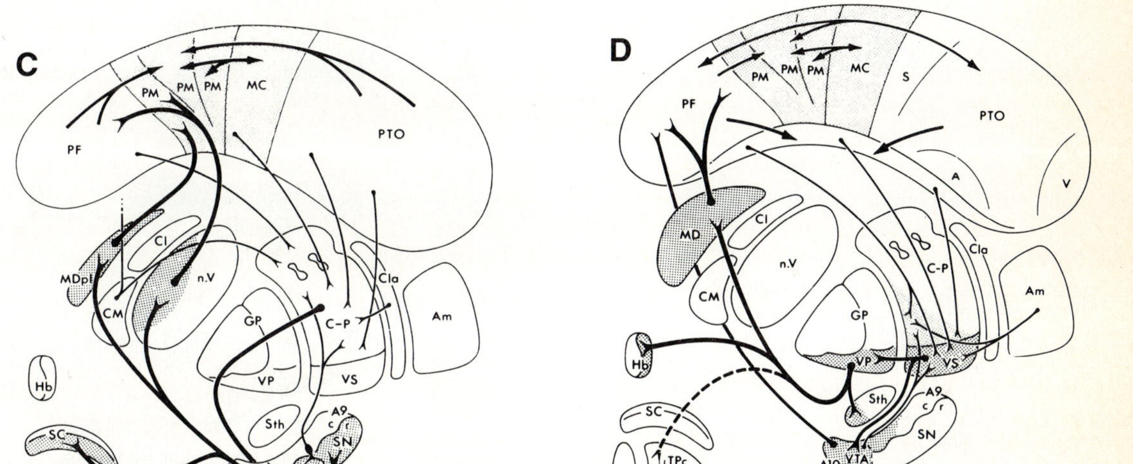

Figure 3-28 Continued *C*, The nigrothalamocortical pathways carried over the medial part of the ventral thalamic complex and the paralamellar part of the mediodorsal nucleus (MDpl) are shown in heavy lines. Also shown in heavy lines are the strionigral pathway and the nigral efferents terminating in the deep layers of the superior colliculus and in the midbrain tegmentum, especially in the TPc nucleus. *D*, The pathways linking the ventral pallidum (VP) with the prefrontal cortex (and with subcortical sites) are shown in heavy lines. The main inputs to the ventral pallidum originate in the ventral striatum (VS), which in turn receives input from the ventral tegmental area (VTA, A10) and A8 dopamine-containing cell groups of the midbrain, from the amygdala (AM) and from regions of prelimbic and limbic cortex, which themselves receive inputs from prefrontal (PF) and posterior (PTO) association cortex. Note the direct corticipetal dopamine system paralleling the indirect striopallidothalamocortical pathway that leads through the mediodorsal nucleus. Abbreviations: A = auditory cortex; AM = amygdaloid complex, A8, A9 and A10-cell groups A8,m A9, A10 of Dahlström and Fuxe; CbII = cerebellum; CI = nucleus centralis lateralis of thalamus; Cla = claustrum; CM = center median-parafascicular complex of thalamus; C-P = caudoputamen (caudate nucleus and putamen); GP = globus pallidus; Hb = habenular complex; MC = motor cortex; MD = mediodorsal nucleus of the thalamus; MDpI = paralamellar part of the thalamic mediodorsal nucleus; NcF = nucleus campi Foreli; n.V, nucleus ventralis of thalamus; PF = prefrontal cortex; PM = premotor cortical fields; PTO = parietotemporooccipital association cortex; R = raphe nuclei (especially dorsal raphe nucleus); RN = red nucleus; S = somatic sensory cortex; SC = superior colliculus; SNc = substantia nigra pars compacta; SNr = substantia nigra pars reticulata; Sth = subthalamic nucleus; Teg = midbrain tegmentum; TPc = nucleus tegmenti pedunculopontinus or "pedunculopontine" nucleus; V = visual cortex; VP = ventral pallidum; VS = ventral striatum; VTA = ventral tegmental area (cell group A10). (From Graybiel AM. Neurochemically specified substances in the basal ganglia. In: Symposium on functions of the basal ganglia. London: Pitman (Ciba Foundation), 1984:114).

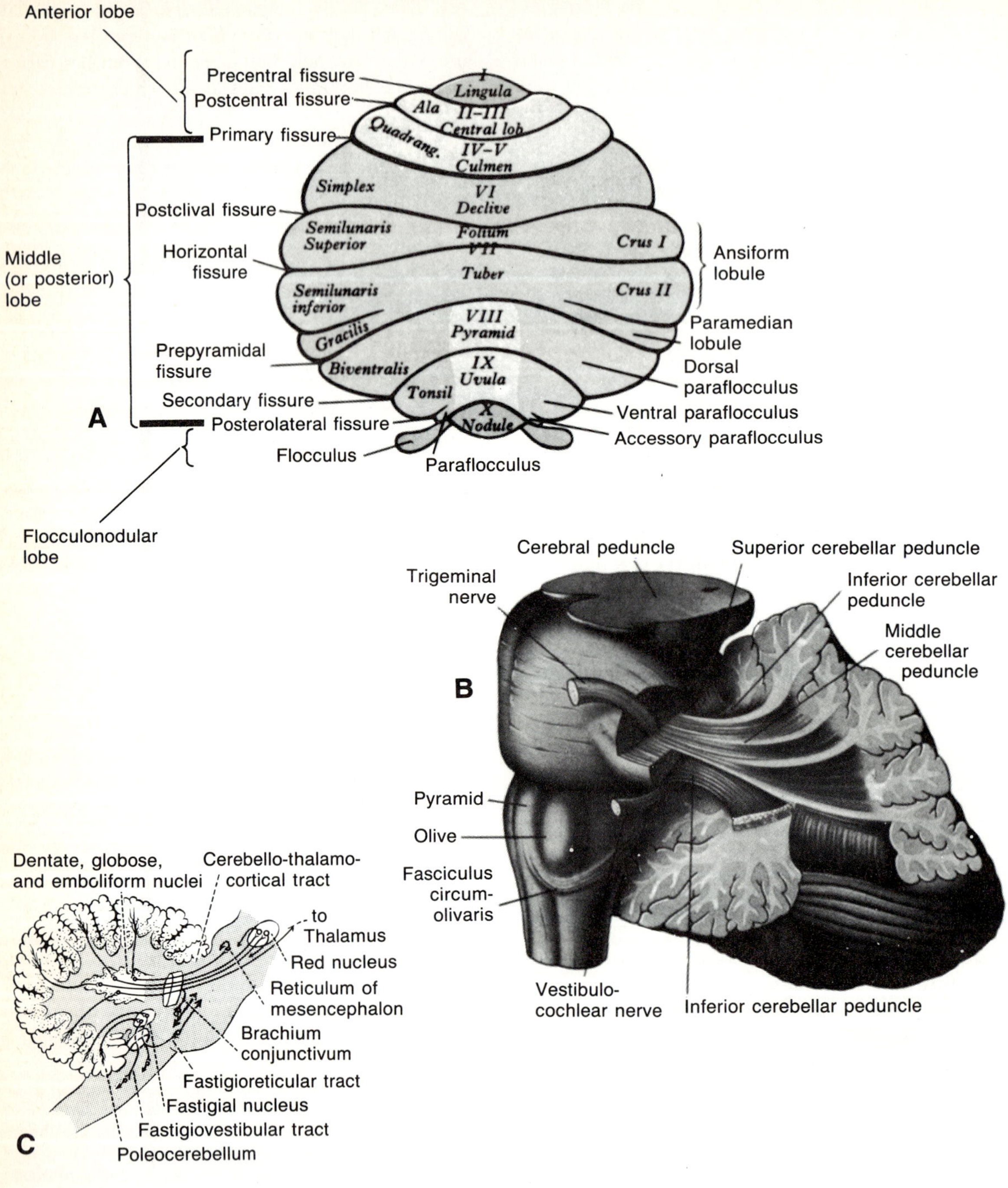

Figure 3–29 *A*, Lobar and lobular structure of the cerebellum. Nomenclature for the human is shown on the left and that for other mammals on the right. Abbreviations: Lob. ant. and post = lobi anterior and posterior; Li = lingula; L.c. = lobulus centralis; Cu. = culmen; De. = declive; F.v. = folium vermis; T.v. = tuber vermis; P. = pyramis; U. = uvula; N. = nodulus; Lob. quadrang. ant. and post. = lobulus quadrangularis, pars anterior, and pars posterior; Lob. semilum. sup. and inf. = lobuli semilunaris superior and inferior; Lob. gracil. = lobulus gracilis; Lob. bivent. = lobulus biventer; Paraflocc. ac. = paraflocculus accessorius; Flocc. = flocculus; Fiss. praec. = fissura precentralis; Fiss. praecul. = fissura preculminatus; Fiss. prim. = fissura prima; F. sup. ant. = anterior superior fissure; Fiss. sup. post. = posterior superior fissure; Fiss. intercrur. = intercrural fissure; F. horizont. = great horizontal fissure; Fiss. ansoparamed. = ansoparamedian fissure; F. inf. post. = posterior inferior fissure; Fiss. parafl. = parafloccular fissure; F. inf. ant. = anterior inferior fissure; Fiss. intraparaflocc. = intraparafloccular fissure; F. retrotons. = retronsillar fissure; Fiss. po. lat. = fissura posterolateralis. (From Warwick R, Williams PL, eds. Gray's anatomy. 35th Br ed. Philadelphia: WB Saunders, 1973:874.) *B*, Partial dissection of the brain stem and cerebellum to reveal the three cerebellar penducles. For further explanation, see the text. (From Warwick R, Williams PL, eds. Gray's anatomy. 35th Br ed. Philadelphia: WB Saunders, 1973:859.) *C*, Schematic diagram of the route of the principal fiber projections from the cerebellar nuclei. Additional projections from the fastigial nucleus are described in the text. (From Guyton AC. Organ physiology: structure and function of the nervous system. Philadelphia: WB Saunders, 1976:165.)

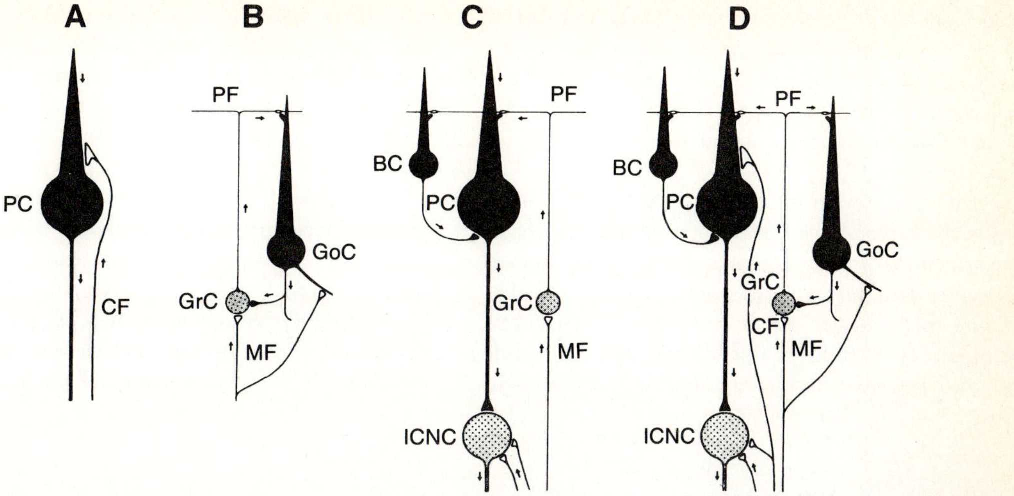

Figure 3–30 Schematic representation of the neuronal connections in the cerebellar cortex. Starting from the left (*A* to *C*) are shown individual elements of the total circuit, and on the right (*D*) is shown the composite circuit. Black cells have an output that inhibits cells with which they make synaptic contact, whereas white cells have an excitatory influence on postsynaptic cells. Abbreviations: PC = Purkinje cell; CF = climbing fiber; GrC = granule cell; GoC = Golgi cell; MF = mossy fiber; PF = parallel fiber; BC = basket cell; ICNC = intercerebellar nuclear cell. Arrows show direction of travel of neural impulses. (From Eccles JC, Ito M, Szentagothai J. The cerebellum as a neuronal machine. Berlin: Springer-Verlag, 1967.)

the red nucleus, fibers from the emboliform and globose nuclei end primarily in the magnocellular division, and the dentate nucleus fibers end in the parvocellular division.[201,203] From the red nucleus, projections are sent to the motor neurons for the muscles of speech production, that is, the trigeminal and facial nuclei.[204–206]

Brain Stem

The brain stem, which lies between the cerebrum and the spinal cord, is composed of the diencephalon, midbrain, pons, and medulla oblongata (see Fig. 3–1). The cerebellum is joined to the three brain stem units by three cerebellar peduncles, the superior peduncle, the middle peduncle, and the inferior peduncle, which join the midbrain, pons, and medulla, respectively. Much of the reticular formation is found in the brain stem.

The brain stem nuclear groups (Fig. 3–31) provide the final common path for nerve signals being sent from the CNS to the muscles regulated by cranial nerves. In addition, some of these nuclei also provide the relays, or synaptic connections, for incoming sensory information to the CNS.

Trigeminal System

The trigeminal system is the largest of the brain stem nuclear groups. There are four major nuclei in this system: the motor nucleus, chief sensory nucleus, spinal nucleus, and the mesencephalic nucleus of the trigeminal (fifth) nerve.

The motor nucleus of the trigeminal is an oval group of neurons situated in the dorsal lateral pontine area of the brain stem just medial to the chief sensory nucleus of the trigeminal (Fig. 3–31B). The motor neurons innervating the temporal muscle occupy the most dorsal lateral position, with the medial pterygoid and masseter muscle motor neurons lying more ventral. Ventromedially in the motor nucleus are found the motor neurons for the anterior belly of the digastric and mylohyoid muscles.[207–210] The axons of these motor neurons pass out of the brain stem, forming the motor root, and then join the mandibular branch of the trigeminal nerve.

The chief sensory nucleus is located just lateral to the motor nucleus and extends slightly rostrally and caudally (Fig. 3–32). Caudally, the chief sensory nucleus merges with the spinal nucleus of the fifth cranial nerve. The latter is a long group of cell bodies that extends down into the upper reaches of the cervical spinal cord. Incoming primary afferent fibers enter the brain stem, and some of the fibers bifurcate, sending branches to the chief sensory and spinal nuclei.[3] Within the chief sensory and spinal nuclei of the trigeminal, the incoming fibers synapse with the second-order sensory neurons.

There is a dorsoventral as well as a mediolateral organization of the chief sensory and spinal nuclei. Cells representing higher positions on the face and head are located dorsally.[211–214] The mesencephalic nucleus of the trigeminal nerve is dorsal and rostral to the motor nucleus and adjacent to the fourth ventricle.[215] However, unlike other sensory cells, the cell bodies of masticatory muscle spindles and some periodontal receptors are found within the CNS in this nucleus.

As is true with other brain stem nuclei, there are both direct and indirect corticobulbar fibers to the trigeminal motor nucleus.[1] Direct fibers branch off the corticobulbar in the pontine region and distribute bilaterally to the motor nucleus of the trigeminal nerve. Indirect fibers leave the corticobulbar tract and distribute in the midbrain tegmentum reticular formation.[205] From the reticular formation, fibers project to the ipsilateral and contralateral trigeminal motor nuclei.[205,216] In addition, fibers from the cortex also have been traced to the red nucleus and to interneurons surrounding the trigeminal nuclei.[205]

The spinal and chief sensory nuclei of the trigeminal have three main ascending projection systems. The largest projection (ventral secondary ascending tract) crosses the midline, intermingles with fibers of the dorsal medial lemniscus, and ascends to the medial region of the nucleus ventralis posteromedialis.[179,183,184] The second and smaller projection

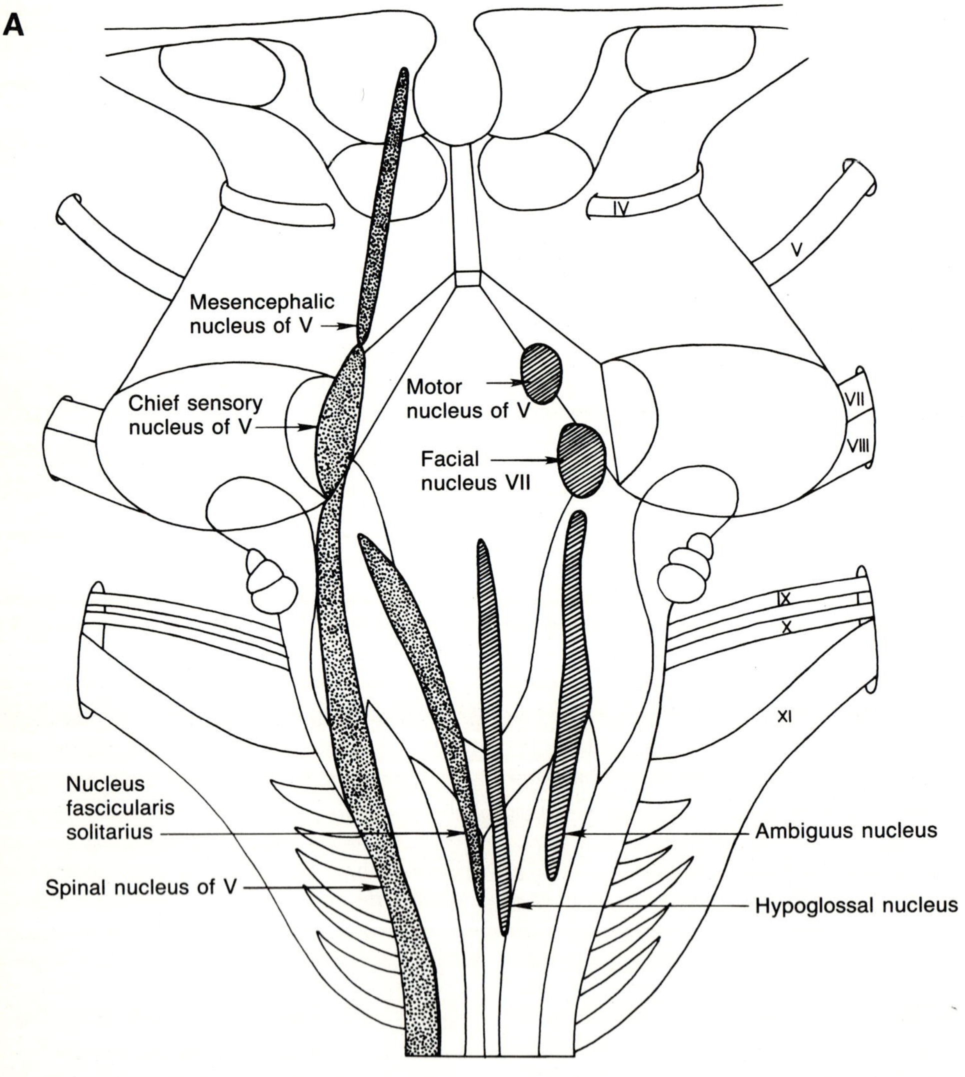

Figure 3–31 *A*, Diagrammatic representation of a dorsal view of the principal sensory and motor nuclei of the brain stem, which are important for speech motor control. The shaded nuclei are sensory, and the hatched areas are motor nuclei. Roman numerals refer to cranial nerves IV, V, VI, VIII, IX, X and XI.

(dorsal secondary ascending tract) remains ipsilateral as it ascends through the tegmentum of the reticular formation to terminate in the dorsal medial region of the nucleus ventralis posteromedialis.[179,183,184] The third projection connects pontine reticular formation cells with cells in the contralateral motor nucleus of the trigeminal nerve.[183,184] This midbrain decussation is believed to be important for bilateral control of trigeminally innervated structures. From the ventralis posteromedialis of the thalamus, projections reach pre- and postcentral gyri of the cerebral cortex.[185,186]

Facial Nucleus

The facial complex provides sensory innervation for taste, part of the external auditory meatus, and the auricle; it also supplies motor fibers for the face and lips.[215] This nucleus (see Fig. 3–32) lies in the lower third of the pontine region medial to the spinal tract of the trigeminal nerve.[3] Cells in the dorsal and medial parts of the facial nucleus innervate muscles in the dorsal and posterior head regions, such as the orbicularis oculi and posterior auricular, and ventrolaterally located cells, of which

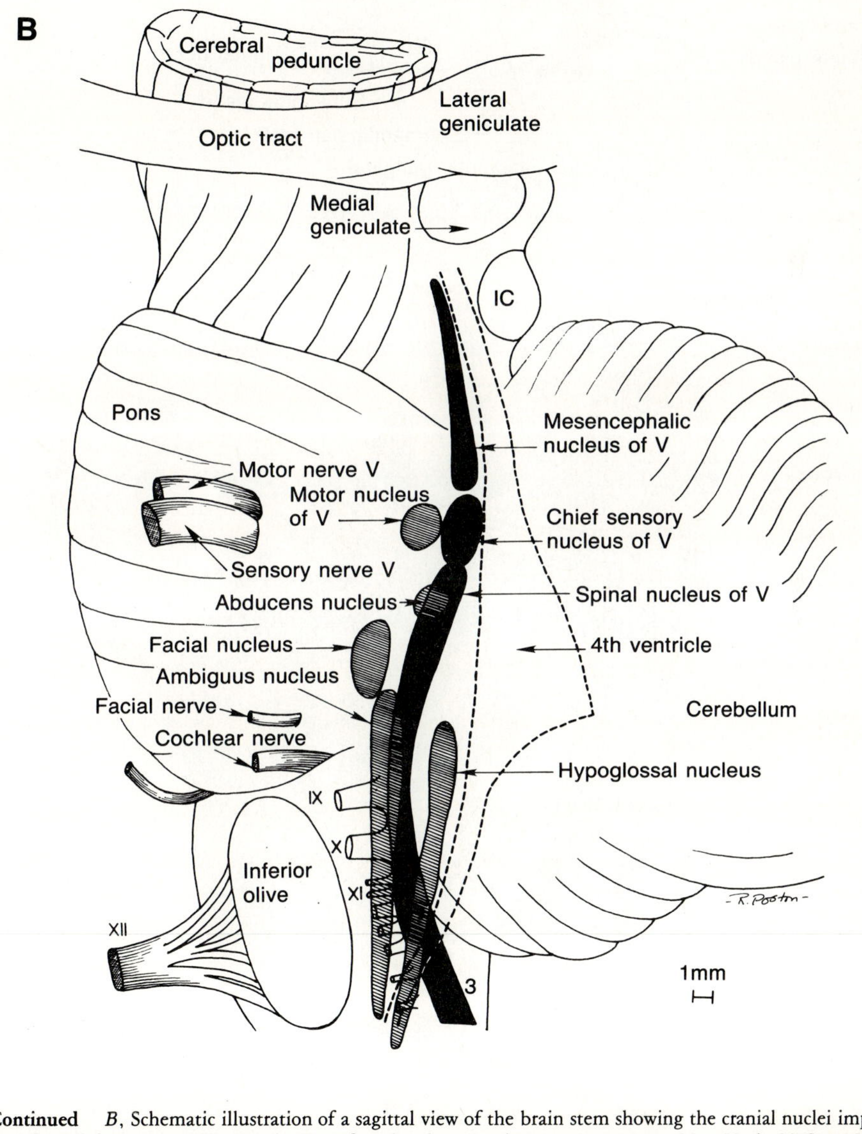

Figure 3-31 Continued *B*, Schematic illustration of a sagittal view of the brain stem showing the cranial nuclei important for speech motor control. (Adapted from House EL, Pansky B. A functional approach to neuroanatomy. New York: McGraw-Hill, 1967; Crosby EC, Humphrey T, Lauer EW. Correlative anatomy of the nervous system. New York: Macmillan, 1962; Carpenter MB. Human neuroanatomy. Baltimore: Williams & Wilkins, 1983; Warwick R, Williams PL, eds. Gray's anatomy. 35th Br ed. Philadelphia: WB Saunders, 1973).

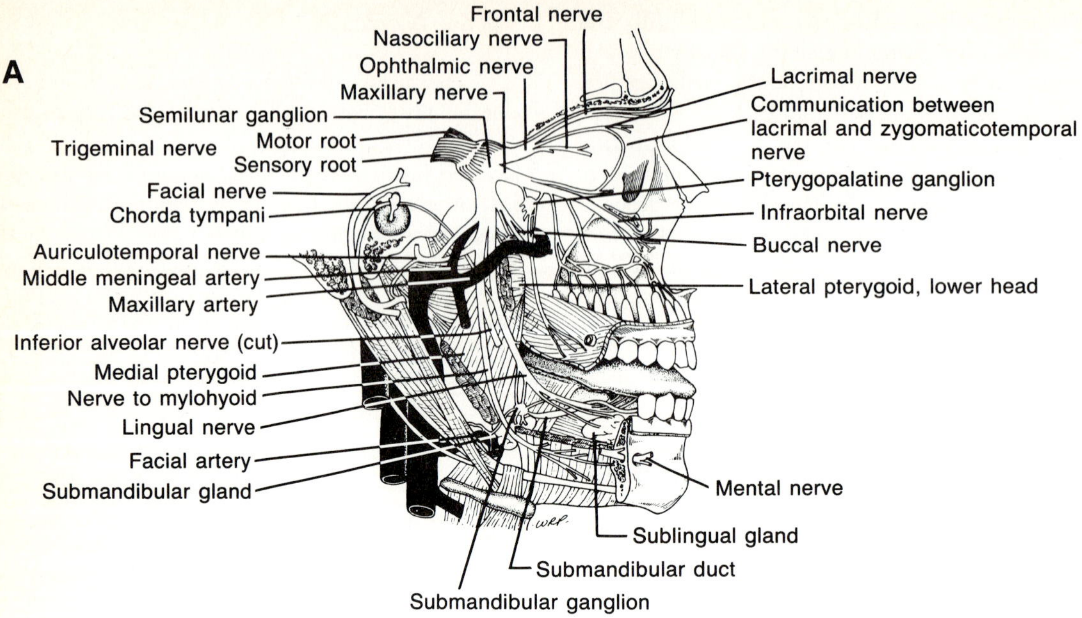

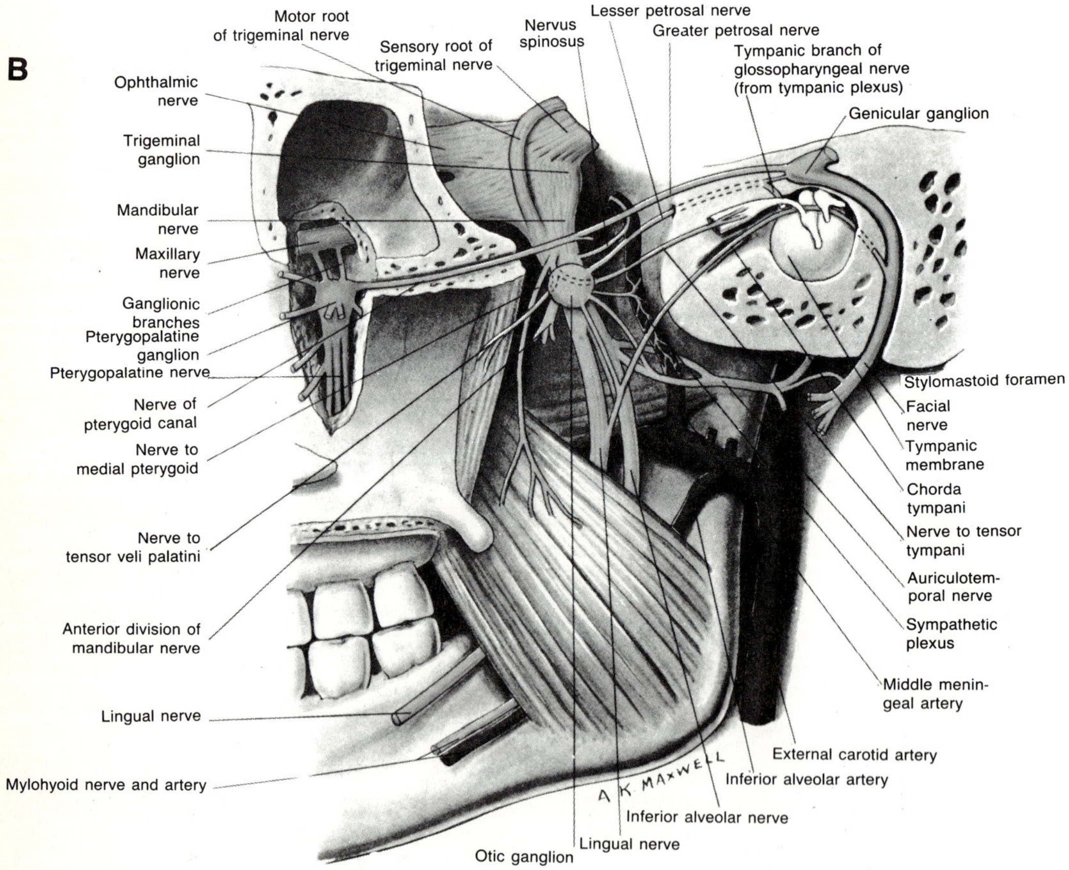

Figure 3–32 *A*, Partial dissection of the right side of the face to reveal some of the major components of the trigeminal nerve. *B*, Medial view of trigeminal and pterygopalatine ganglia. Distribution of some branches of the trigeminal nerve is shown, as is the route of the facial nerve through the temporal bone.

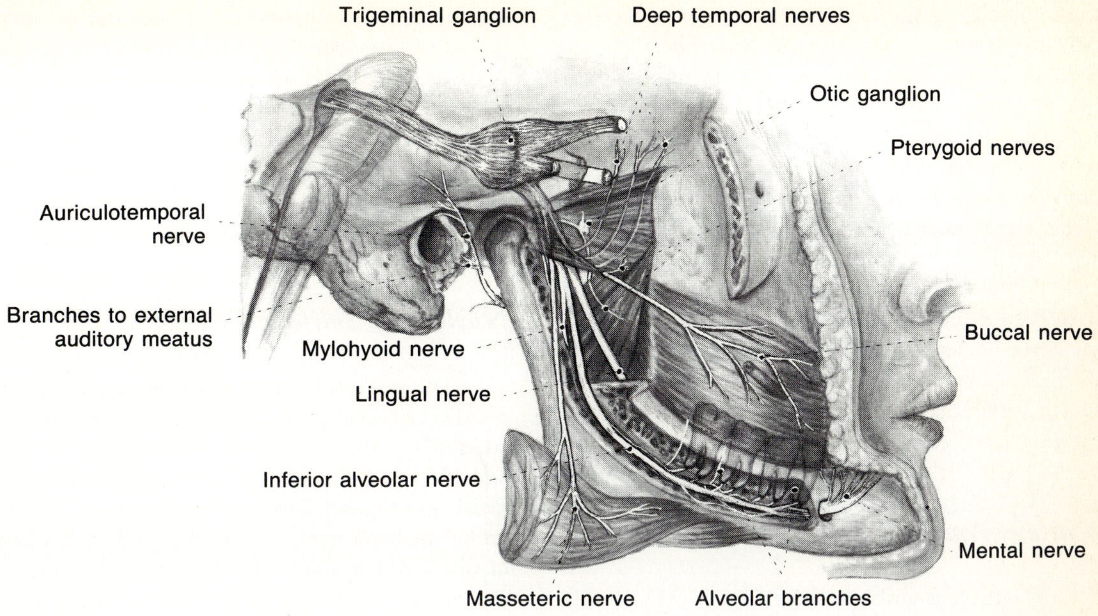

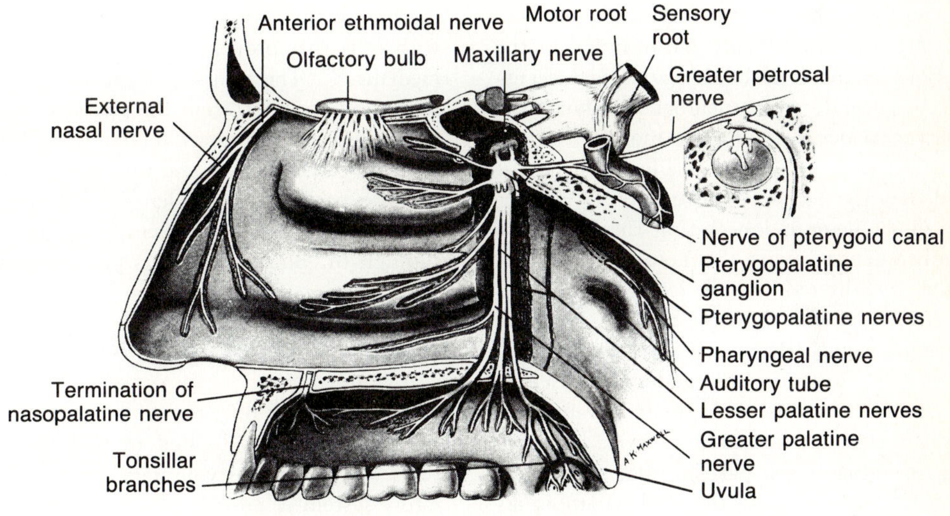

Figure 3-32 Continued *C*, Further dissection of the right face to reveal trigeminal distributions to the muscles of mastication as well as termination of the buccal nerve. *D*, The complete distribution of the pterygopalatine nerves from the pterygopalatine ganglion is shown. (*A*, *B*, and *D* from Warwick R, Williams PL, eds. Gray's anatomy. 35th Br ed. Philadelphia: WB Saunders 1973:1005, 1006, 1008. *C* from Langman J, Woerdeman MW. Atlas of medical anatomy. Philadelphia: WB Saunders, 1978:453.)

there are a great many in the human, innervate the buccal and labial muscles of speech such as the orbicularis oris muscles.[217–219] The fibers from the facial nucleus pass rostrally, medially, and dorsally around the abducens nucleus and then pass out of the brain stem in the ventrolateral area of the pons. The bend of the fibers around the abducens nucleus is known as the genu of the facial nerve.

There is a variety of input to the facial nucleus from other neural areas. In the cat, the cerebral cortex projects mainly contralaterally to the facial nucleus via interneurons, possibly located in the spinal trigeminal nucleus.[220] However, in the human, corticobulbar fibers project both directly and indirectly to the facial nucleus. The dorsal part of the facial nucleus, which innervates upper areas of the face, receives ipsilateral and contralateral direct projections. The ventrolateral facial nucleus, which innervates muscles of speech lower in the face, receives only contralateral direct corticobulbar fibers.[1,221,222] Indirect fibers to the facial nucleus are relayed from the corticobulbar tract through interneurons in the reticular formation. Analysis of facial and perioral reflexes in the human indicates a multisynaptic pathway from the trigeminal sensory nuclei to the facial motor nucleus.[223] One synapse is located in the trigeminal sensory nuclei and another in the facial nucleus.[224] Other inputs to the facial nucleus have been demonstrated to arise from the hypoglossal nerve,[225] lateral reticular formation,[216] fastigial nucleus of the cerebellum, spinal cord rostral to the fourth cervical segment (C-4), ventral periaqueductal gray, and red nucleus.[204,206]

Nucleus Ambiguus

The nucleus ambiguus (see Fig. 3–31) gets its name from the fact that it supplies motor fibers to the ninth (glossopharyngeal), tenth (vagus), and eleventh (accessory) cranial nerves.[215,226] The nucleus ambiguus extends about 10 mm from the upper border of the medulla just caudally and in line with the facial nucleus to the level of the pyramidal decussation.[227] In general, motor neurons supplying the glossopharyngeal nerve occupy the most rostral extent of the nucleus, followed caudally by the vagus nerve and then the accessory nerve.[1,3]

The motor neurons innervating the larynx are functionally organized, with the motor neurons supplying the cricothyroid muscle located most rostrally, followed by the abductor muscle, posterior cricoarytenoid, and then the adductor muscles.[1,221,222,228,229] However, the adductor muscle is represented more ventrally.[230] In the most caudal region of the nucleus are the motor neurons innervating the uvula, levator veli palatini, and pharyngeal constrictor.[231] Fibers leaving the nucleus ambiguus exit the brain stem in a line on the lateral side of the medulla between the olive and inferior cerebellar peduncle.[231]

The inputs to the nucleus ambiguus are varied and reflect pathways involved in voluntary control of the larynx and pharynx for speech as well as for involuntary reflex mechanisms. Inputs to the nucleus from the cortex are probably both direct and indirect.[1,185,232–234] The anterior cingulate gyrus may also indirectly project to the nucleus ambiguus, since damage to the cingulate affects phonation.[235,236] Direct inputs to the nucleus ambiguus have also been traced from the midbrain periaqueductal gray.[237,238] The periaqueductal gray is important in vocal control since its stimulation elicits vocalization and the activity of its neurons has been shown to be related to laryngeal muscle activity and vocalization.[239,240]

From the analysis of brain stem reflexes and acute experiments on animals, inputs to the nucleus ambiguus from the nucleus of solitary fasciculus,[241,242] hypoglossal nucleus,[243,244] and spinal nucleus of the fifth nerve[245] have been determined.

Nucleus of Solitary Fasciculus

The nucleus of the solitary fasciculus (see Fig. 3–31) is situated in the dorsal part of the brain stem adjacent to the dorsal motor nucleus of the vagus and the vestibular nuclei.[3] Afferent fibers from the facial, glossopharyngeal, and vagus nerves, upon entering the brain stem, turn sharply and form a bundle of fibers which gives off a branch to the nucleus of the solitary tract. The vagus afferents carry sensory information from the larynx.[246–248] Some laryngeal afferents bifurcate, sending one fiber to the solitary tract and the other to a site just rostral to the motor nucleus of the fifth cranial nerve where it synapses with cells that project to nucleus ventralis posteromedialis.[249] The glossopharyngeal afferents carry sensory information from the pharynx.[3] Cells in the nucleus solitarius project to the nucleus ambiguus; the hypoglossal, facial, and fifth motor nerve nuclei; and the parabrachial nuclei.[242,250] Projections ultimately reach the somatosensory cortex, probably through the nucleus ventralis posteromedialis.[172]

Central Mechanisms of Respiration

The control of automatic, metabolic breathing (see Fig. 3–31) is located in bulbopontine structures,[251–254] whereas voluntary control of the respiratory system is provided by the cortex, other forebrain structures,[238] and the cerebellum.[255,256] Some of these cortical pathways involve the pyramidal system,[257] but extrapyramidal pathways are also involved. Cortical areas involved in respiratory control are the same sites involved in speech control plus the anterior cingulate gyrus, ventromedial temporal lobe, posterior orbital cortex, and anterior insular cortex.[258,259]

Located throughout the reticular formation, but concentrated primarily near the nucleus of solitary fasciculus and nucleus ambiguus, are interneurons for respiratory activity. These cells lie intermingled with cells of a variety of other functions and are not grouped into discrete nuclei.[260] Fibers from these cells project down to the ventral portion of the cervical spinal cord where they excite the phrenic motor neurons, which innervate the diaphragm.

In addition to the motor aspects of respiration, there are well-known afferent influences on respiratory activity. Vagal afferent fibers from the respiratory system enter the medulla and terminate in the caudal region of the nucleus of solitary fasciculus.[258]

Hypoglossal Nucleus

The hypoglossal nucleus (see Fig. 3–31) supplies the motor innervation for the tongue and lies near the midline, just ventral to the fourth ventricle. It is approximately 18 mm long and extends through most of the medulla.[3] The fibers emerge from the nucleus, passing ventrally and exiting the brain stem in the anterolateral sulcus.

The specific interconnections between the hypoglossal nucleus and other areas of the brain are poorly understood. Evidence from reflex analysis suggests that the trigeminal system projects to the hypoglossal nucleus,[261–263] and projections from other neural areas such as the cerebral cortex may reach the hypoglossal nucleus through interneurons that project from the lateral reticular formation.[216]

Peripheral Motor Pathways

We shall now discuss the peripheral courses of the nerves that innervate the speech articulators and their sensory receptors. Unless otherwise indicated, information from this section has been obtained from Garrison,[264] Goss,[231] and Mathers.[265]

Trigeminal Nerve

The trigeminal, the largest cranial nerve (see Fig. 3–32), at its exit from the brain stem is composed of two parts, the sensory and motor roots. Both roots pass anteriorly in the posterior cranial fossa to reach the trigeminal ganglion, where the cell bodies from the sensory root are located. From the ganglion, the ophthalmic, maxillary, and mandibular branches of the trigeminal emerge. The ophthalmic branch has little relevance for speech and therefore will not be discussed in this chapter.

The maxillary nerve (see Fig. 3–32) provides sensory innervation to the midfacial region and comprises several branches. The zygomatic nerve branches off from the maxillary nerve and then divides into two smaller branches. The zygomaticotemporal branch supplies the skin on the side of the forehead (see Fig. 3–32) and the zygomaticofacial branch supplies sensory innervation to the skin of the cheek (see Fig. 3–32).

The pterygopalatine nerves branch off the maxillary nerve in the pterygopalatine fossa (see Fig. 3–32). The greater palatine branch supplies sensory innervation to the hard palate mucous membrane, gums, and part of the soft palate, and the lesser palatine branch supplies innervation for the soft palate, uvula, and pharyngeal tonsils. The pharyngeal branch of the pterygopalatine nerve supplies innervation to the nasal portion of the pharynx.

The superior and anterior superior alveolar nerves innervate the teeth and floor of the nasal cavity (see Fig. 3–32), and the posterior superior alveolar branch sends terminals to the teeth, gums, and mucous membrane of the cheek. The infraorbital nerve passes through the infraorbital canal beneath the orbit and emerges into the front of the face through the infraorbital foramen (see Figs. 3–32 and 3–33). After exiting the foramen, this nerve rapidly branches out into many fine filaments, forming a plexus; communicating rami are made with the facial nerve in this plexus. The infraorbital nerve innervates the upper lip as well as the skin and mucous membrane in the region of the upper lip.

Understanding of the sensory receptors of the maxillary branch is limited. Largely on the basis of animal research, it is known that the areas of densest sensory innervation are along the rugae of the hard palate, the junction of the hard and soft palates, the uvula, papilla, tip of the tongue,[266] and the perioral regions.[212] Since these same areas are important for speech articulation, they would likely be highly innervated in the human as well. In the perioral region, it is known that there are both rapidly and slowly adapting mechanoreceptors[212,213,267] and the receptive fields are smallest close to the lip.[212] Some of these receptors may be Golgi-Mazzoni corpuscles,[268] but that many muscle spindles are in the perioral region is doubtful.[269–272]

The mandibular branch (see Fig. 3–32) of the trigeminal is the largest of the three branches and has both motor and sensory components. The sensory field in general occupies the lower facial region and extends up to the temporal region. From the trigeminal ganglion, the mandibular nerve splits into two main trunks, anterior and posterior. Near the point of bifurcation the short medial pterygoid nerve passes through the otic ganglion and enters the medial pterygoid muscle. This branch also has two lesser branches, one of which supplies motor innervation to the musculus tensor veli palatini and the other to the tensor tympani (see Fig. 3–32).

The anterior division of the mandibular branch contains most of the motor nerves of the trigeminal (see Fig. 3–32). The masseter nerve enters the masseter muscle near its insertion on the zygomatic arch. The motor nerves to the temporal muscle are frequently divided into two main branches, one of which supplies the deep anterior temporal muscle and the other innervates the posterior temporal muscle. The motor nerve to the lateral pterygoid muscle enters that muscle after branching off the buccal nerve (see Fig. 3–32).

As was mentioned previously, the motor nerves to the muscles of mastication also carry proprioceptive fibers from receptors in the muscles. There is considerable anatomic[3,273,274] and physiologic[275–277] evidence for the presence of muscle spindles in the muscles of mastication, that is, masseter, temporal, and medial pterygoid muscles. There are also Golgi tendon organs in the temporal and masseter muscles.[274–278] The afferent fibers from these receptors may possibly pass through the sensory root with the cell bodies in the trigeminal ganglion,[279] but this is not certain.

The buccal nerve is variable in both its origin and pattern of distribution (see Figs. 3–32 and 3–33). It passes beneath and anterior to the anterior border of the masseter muscle, then ramifies over the buccinator, supplying sensory innervation to the skin, mucous membrane, and gums of the buccal area.

The posterior division of the mandibular branch has sensory and motor components, and the auriculotemporal branch supplies sensory innervation to the skin of the temporal region (see Figs. 3–32 and 3–33). A small branch of the auriculotemporal innervates the skin of the external auditory meatus and part of the tympanic membrane. There are small branches of this nerve, called the "articular branches," that enter the temporomandibular joint (TMJ). These branches may innervate the Golgi-Mazzoni corpuscles in the TMJ,[280] which would be important for sensing jaw position and movement during speech.

The lingual nerve splits off from the posterior division a short distance from the trigeminal ganglion, runs parallel to the inferior alveolar nerve and between the mandible and the medial pterygoid muscle, and across the superior constrictor muscle to the side of the tongue (see Fig. 3–32), where it proceeds to the tip of the tongue, running just under the mucosal surface on the under side. The lingual nerve supplies sensory innervation to the mucous membrane of the anterior two-thirds of the tongue. The sensory innervation of the mucosal surface of the tongue is composed of three main types of sensory endings (exclusive of taste buds), but these are only elaborations of the same basic type. The three types, nonmyelinated free nerve endings, semiorganized, and organized endings,[281] are found throughout the surface of the tongue, but are most abundant in the tongue tip followed by the posterior

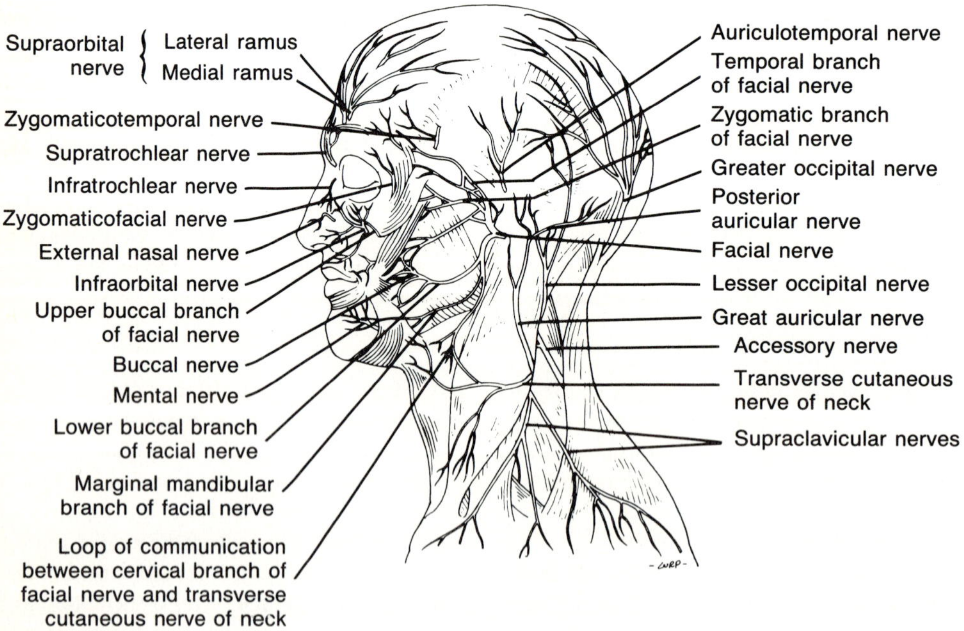

Figure 3–33 Distribution of the facial nerve of man to the muscles of speech and facial expression. Some cutaneous sensory branches of the trigeminal nerve, not shown in Figure 3–32, are also indicated here. For further descriptions see the text. (From Warwick R, Williams PL, eds. Gray's anatomy. 35th Br ed. Philadelphia: WB Saunders, 1973:1013.)

dorsal surface. Moreover, the medial region is less densely innervated than the lateral borders.[281]

The inferior alveolar nerve enters the mandibular canal in the mandibular foramen (see Fig. 3–32). The mylohyoid nerve leaves the inferior alveolar nerve at the point of entry into the mandibular canal and descends to the mylohyoid and anterior belly of the digastric muscles, which it innervates (see Fig. 3–32). Within the mandibular canal the inferior alveolar nerve ramifies into branches that supply innervation to the mandibular teeth (see Fig. 3–32). The mental nerve branches off within the canal, exits the mandible through the mental foramen on the anterior surface of the mandible, and supplies sensory information to the tissues of the lower lip and skin of the jaw (see Fig. 3–32). The same types of sensory ending that were discussed for the infraorbital nerve apply to the mental branch as well.

Facial Nerve

The facial, or seventh cranial, nerve (see Figs. 3–32*A* and *B* and 3–33) contains some sensory fibers and provides motor fibers to the face and lower jaw. It is composed of two roots, sensory and motor, which leave the CNS together. This nerve accompanies the acoustic nerve into the internal acoustic meatus before separating and entering the facial canal within the temporal bone. It travels in the facial canal along the wall of the middle ear and at one point makes an abrupt bend where the geniculate ganglion is located. This ganglion houses the cell bodies of the sensory fibers of the facial nerve.

The facial nerve emerges from the cranium at the stylomastoid foramen (see Fig. 3–33). Within the facial canal, one small motor branch is given off this main facial nerve to innervate the stapedius muscle of the middle ear. Another branch goes to the tympanic plexus, a network of nerve fibers formed by branches of the seventh, ninth, and tenth cranial nerves (Fig. 3–34). The chorda tympani nerve branches off the facial nerve in the middle ear and runs across the tympanic membrane before exiting the cranium, where it joins the lingual branch of the trigeminal nerve (see Figs. 3–32*A* and *B*). The chorda tympani travels with the lingual nerve to the tongue and supplies the tongue with sensory fibers for taste. The posterior auricular nerve leaves the main facial

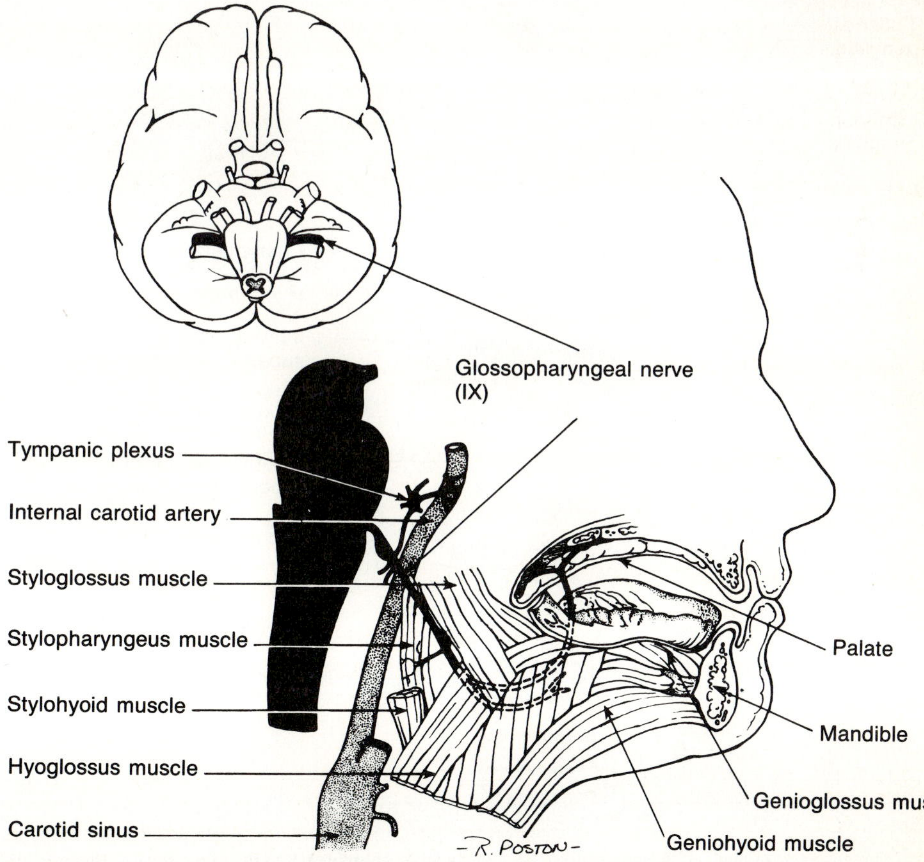

Figure 3–34 Distribution of the glossopharyngeal nerve to the palatal region of man. The only motor component of this nerve innervates the stylopharyngeus muscle. Other branches are sensory. For further description, see the text. (From Jacob SW, Francone CA. Structure and function in man. Philadelphia: WB Saunders 1982:2290.)

nerve just after its exit from the foramen and innervates the muscles of the occipital region and the posterior auricular muscles. Also diverting from the facial nerve near the stylomastoid foramen are nerves that innervate the posterior belly of the digastric and stylohyoid muscles.

From the foramen, the main facial nerve runs anteriorly through the parotid gland, and, at the posterior edge of the ramus of the mandible, it divides into the superior (temporofacial) and inferior (cervicofacial) branches (see Fig. 3–33). The temporal branches run superiorly to innervate the anterior and superior auricular, orbicularis oculi, frontal, and corrugator muscles. The zygomatic branch of the facial nerve runs anteriorly across the face and innervates portions of the orbicularis oculi and other facial muscles lateral and superior to the mouth.

The primary sources of innervation for the muscles of facial expression and speech are contributed by the buccal and mandibular branches of the facial nerve. The buccal nerve passes anteriorly but more inferiorly to the zygomatic branch and innervates the orbicularis oris superior, levator labii, buccinator, and zygomatic muscles, and the muscles of the side of the nose. The mandibular branch runs more inferiorly and anteriorly in the face and innervates the orbicularis oris inferior, depressor anguli oris, depressor labii, and mentalis muscles. The cervical branch of the facial nerve communicates with cervical nerves to innervate the platysma muscle of the neck, lower jaw, and chin.

Glossopharyngeal Nerve

The glossopharyngeal nerve (see Fig. 3–34) is both a motor and a sensory nerve. It exits the cranium through the jugular foramen along with the vagus nerve. The only motor branch of this nerve innervates the stylopharyngeal muscle. Other than

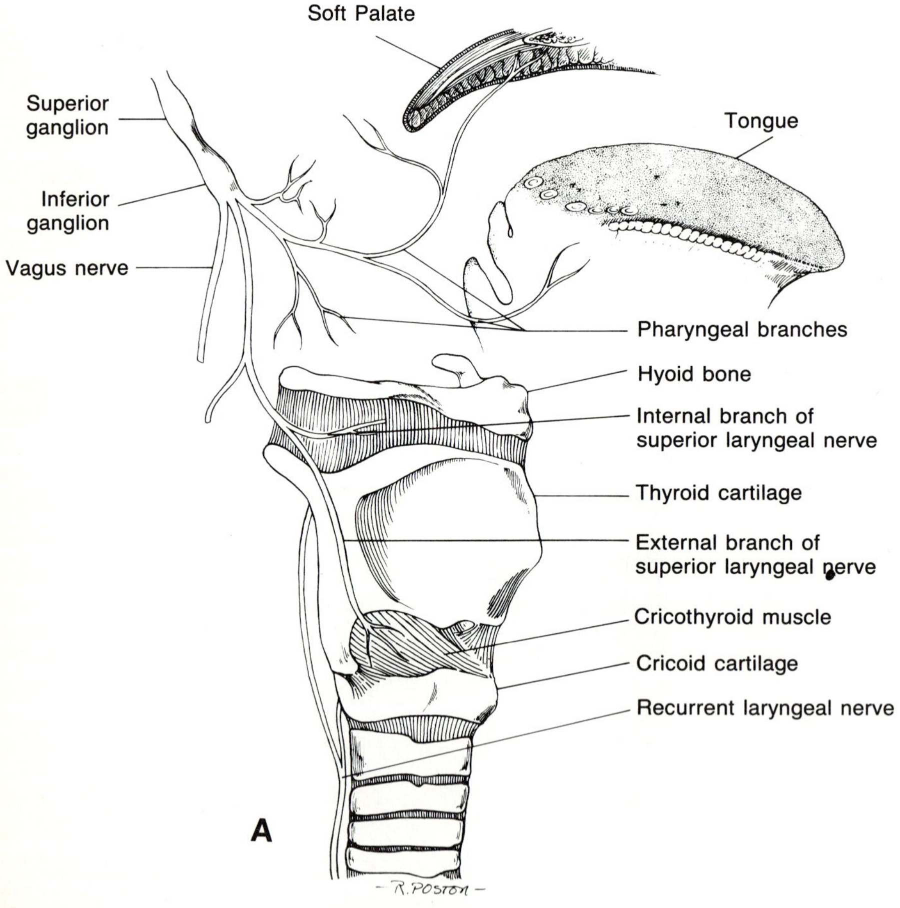

Figure 3-35 The vagus nerve of man. *A*, Schematic illustration of the main components of the vagus nerve to the head and neck region. Many of the motor fibers to the larynx through the external branch of the superior laryngeal nerve and the recurrent laryngeal nerve are thought to be part of the accessory (XI) nerve.

the visceral afferent fibers for taste and blood pressure, the glossopharyngeal nerve supplies sensory fibers for the ear and the mucous membrane of the pharynx. The tympanic branch goes to the tympanic plexus, and from the plexus sensory fibers are distributed to the oval and round windows and the tympanic membrane. The tonsillar branch supplies sensory fibers to the palatine tonsil, soft palate, and fauces, whereas the lingual branches innervate the mucous membrane of the posterior part of the tongue. Sensory innervation of the pharyngeal region likely involves the same types of receptors that are found in the anterior tongue.[281]

Vagus Nerve

The vagus nerve (Fig. 3–35) has many varied functions related to the cardiovascular and visceral activities of the thorax and abdomen which will not be described here. This nerve also supplies sensory fibers to the pharynx, larynx, soft palate, tympanic plexus, and trachea as well as motor fibers to the larynx and pharynx. It exits the cranium through the jugular foramen. Two ganglia are found on the vagus nerve: the superior (jugular) and inferior (nodose) ganglia, which contain the cell bodies for afferent fibers in the vagus nerve. Communications with

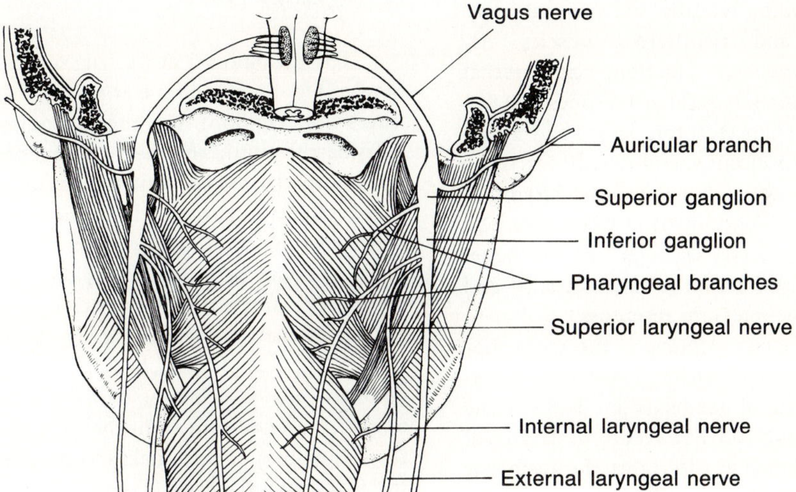

Figure 3-35 Continued *B*, A partial dissection of the posterior veiw of the muscles of the larynx and pharynx to reveal the distribution of the vagus branches to these muscles. The differing routes of the left and right recurrent laryngeal nerves are also shown. For further details, see text. (*B* after Langman J, Woerdeman MW. Atlas of medical anatomy. Philadelphia: WB Saunders, 1978:457.)

the hypoglossal, accessory, glossopharyngeal, and facial nerves are also made at these ganglia.[282] Communication with the accessory nerve will be included in this description since many functions of the accessory and vagus nerves pertaining to the larynx are duplicative.

Near the nodose ganglion, the superior laryngeal nerve leaves the vagus and travels caudally and medially to the thyroid cartilage. It bifurcates into an internal and external branch and then penetrates the pharyngeal constrictor muscle. The internal branch of the superior laryngeal nerve is purely sensory and supplies fibers to the mucous membrane of the epiglottis, base of the tongue, aryepiglottic folds, and the larynx down to the level of the vocal folds. After branching off the main superior laryngeal nerve, the external branch continues caudally and innervates the inferior constrictor and cricothyroid muscles. Although primarily motor in function, the external branch of the superior laryngeal nerve does contain some sensory fibers from receptors located in a diamond-shaped area of mucous membrane beneath the vocal folds on the anterior border of the larynx.[247] The sensory receptors found in the larynx are muscle spindles,[283–285] free nerve endings, subepithelial endings, fundiform and retiform corpuscles,[286] and nonspecified joint and pressure receptors.[247,287]

The recurrent laryngeal nerve is the main motor nerve of the larynx and sensory nerve for the trachea and lower laryngeal region (Fig. 3–35). The pathways for the right and left recurrent laryngeal nerves differ somewhat. On the right, the recurrent laryngeal nerve leaves the vagus at the base of the neck, passes under the subclavian artery, and then runs cranially alongside the trachea and esophagus. On the left side, it loops under the arch of the aorta, thus traveling farther caudally on the left side before turning cranially alongside the trachea. It then enters the larynx under the thyroid cartilage on the posterolateral side and supplies the motor fibers to all other muscles of the larynx except the cricothyroid. Some filaments are given off to supply motor fibers to the inferior constrictor muscle of the pharynx before the recurrent laryngeal nerve enters the larynx. The recurrent laryngeal nerve also supplies sensory fibers to the trachea, esophagus, and receptors located on the undersides of the vocal folds.[248]

Another group of sensory and motor fibers of the vagus nerve innervates the pharyngeal region through the pharyngeal branches (see Fig. 3–35). These branches arise just below the nodose ganglion and supply motor innervation to the middle constrictor muscle. Sensory fibers travel to the mucous membrane of the pharynx and soft palate, and the receptors in this vicinity are free nerve and subepithelial endings.

Accessory Nerve

As already mentioned, the accessory nerve, a motor nerve (see Fig. 3–35), travels with the vagus nerve through the jugular foramen and then joins the vagus just proximal to the nodose ganglion. Its fibers travel with the pharyngeal branches of the vagus to provide motor innervation to the pharyngeal muscles. In addition, other fibers travel with the laryngeal branches of the vagus to innervate the larynx. It is thought that perhaps most of the laryngeal motor fibers may actually be part of the accessory nerve.[226]

Hypoglossal Nerve

The hypoglossal nerve, the motor nerve for the tongue (Fig. 3–36), after exiting from the brain stem, leaves the cranium via the hypoglossal foramen. Outside the skull, this nerve forms communicating links with the closely situated vagus nerve. It then runs caudally and anteriorly to the level of the hyoid bone. At this point, the hypoglossal nerve turns cranially and runs between the mylohyoid and hyoglossus muscles anteriorly in the genioglossus muscle to the tip of the tongue. Along its route through the tongue, it gives off branches to the styloglossus, hyoglossus, genioglossus, and intrinsic muscles of the tongue. In its descent from the hypoglossal foramen, the hypoglossal nerve makes communications with the first cervical nerve. These cervical branches innervate the omohyoid, sternohyoid, sternothyroid, thyrohyoid, and geniohyoid muscles. In addition to carrying motor fibers to the tongue muscles, the hypoglossal nerve may contain some proprioceptive fibers, and the sensory fibers most probably arise from muscle spindles.[288]

Respiratory Nerves

The motor and sensory nerves that innervate the muscles of respiration are widespread, occupying a large part of the cervical and thoracic divisions of the spinal cord (Fig. 3–37). The phrenic nerve, which contains motor and sensory fibers for the diaphragm, originates primarily from the fourth cervical nerve. Further caudally, additional motor nerve rootlets also supply fibers to the phrenic nerve. This nerve passes through the middle of the thorax and adjacent to the heart on its caudal progression to the diaphragm muscle (Fig. 3–37*A*).

A large number of muscles, situated throughout the thorax and abdomen, are involved in res-

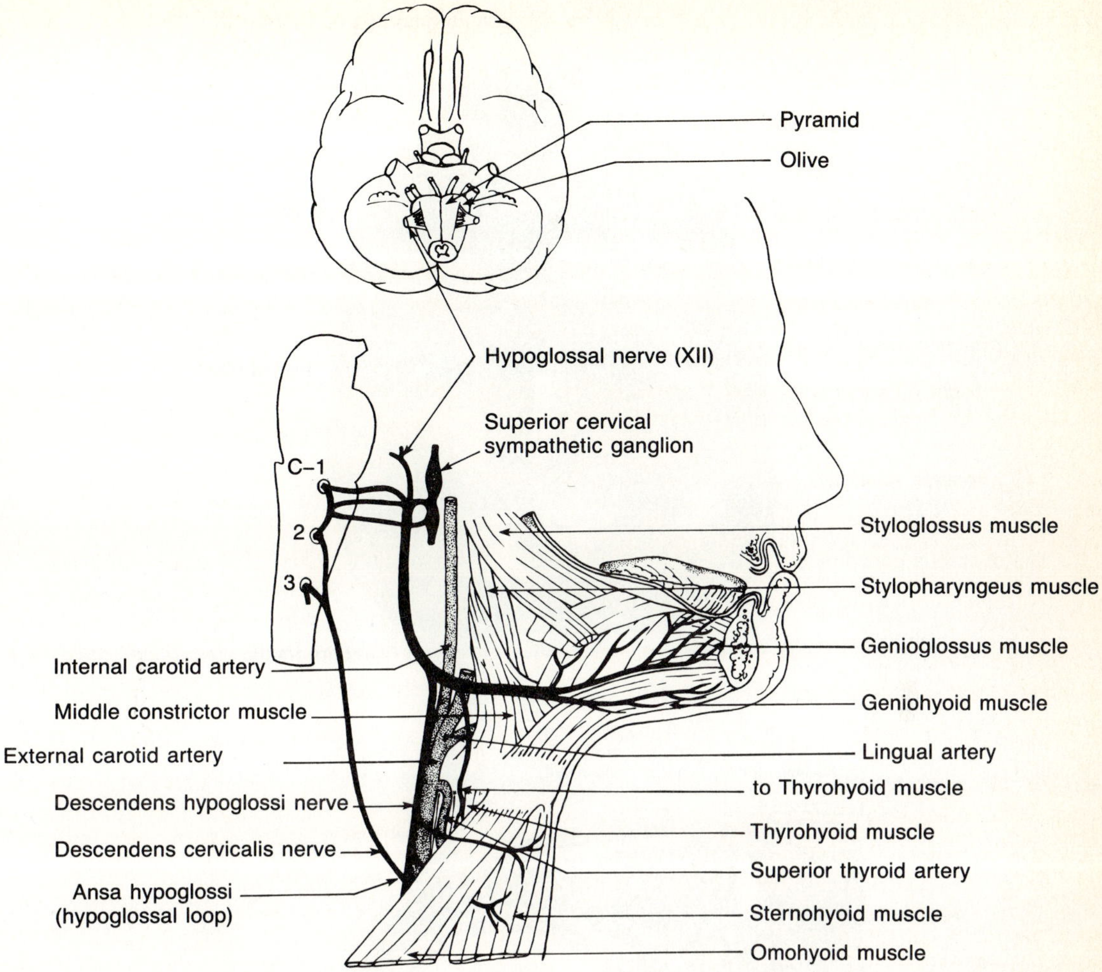

Figure 3–36 Distribution of the hypoglossal nerve of man to the muscles of the tongue. Communications with the cervical nerves are also shown along with their muscular terminations. (From Jacob SW, Francone CA. Structure and function in man. Philadelphia: WB Saunders 1982:293.)

piration. These muscles receive motor innervation from the cervical, thoracic, and lumbar nerves (Fig. 3–37*B*). As with all spinal nerves, the motor portions exit the spinal cord from the ventral roots. The cell bodies of these fibers lie in the ventral horn of the spinal gray column.

The sensory fibers from the respiratory muscles enter the spinal cord in the dorsal root with the cell bodies in the dorsal root ganglion. Upon entering the spinal cord in the dorsal column, the fibers may travel one or more segments of the cord before synapsing onto ascending fiber systems.

SUMMARY

The anatomic pathways involved in speech, language, and hearing are indeed complex. However, careful anatomic research has revealed a systematic organization of these pathways. In this chapter we have attempted to describe the neuroanatomic structures involved in speech, language, and hearing in an orderly fashion, but with enough detail to enable the reader to appreciate the details of the organization that exists at each level of the nervous system. We have also attempted to provide enough references so that the interested reader can pursue any particular topic in depth.

Within the complex anatomic organization of the nervous system, there are some relatively simple and direct pathways running parallel to more complex and diffuse pathways. This organization can be illustrated by considering the auditory pathway. On the one hand, there are rather direct pathways that allow for rapid and precise conveyance of information about the auditory environment from the pe-

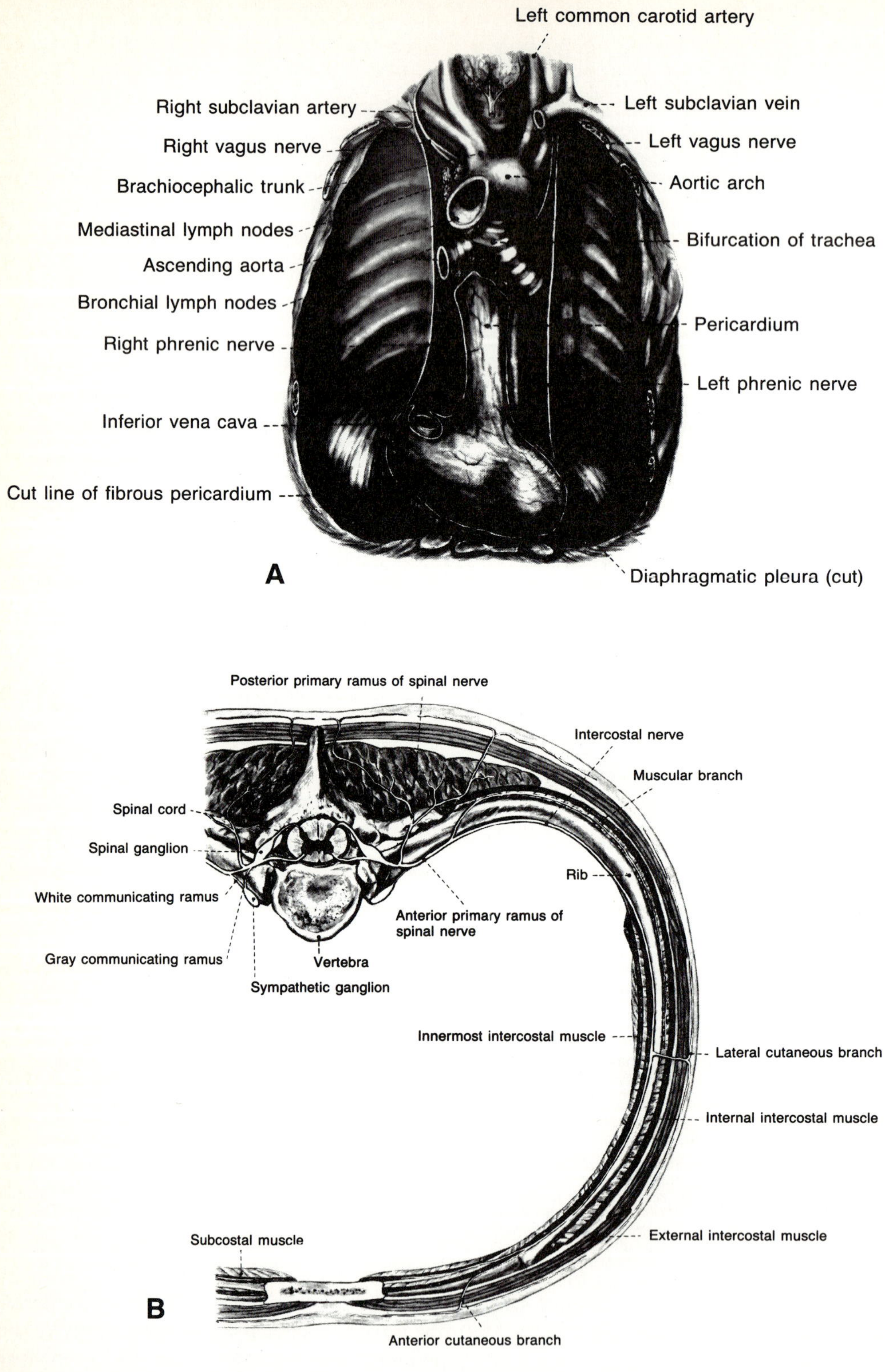

Figure 3–37 *A,* Distribution of primary nerves to muscles of respiration. The route of the phrenic nerve through the thorax to the diaphragm muscle is shown. In this dissection, the heart has been removed. Not shown in this view is the route of the phrenic nerve arising from the fourth cervical section of the spinal cord and passing down through the neck. *B,* A cut-away view of the chest wall to illustrate the pathway of a typical spinal nerve from the thoracic division of the spinal cord. The spinal cord, vertebra, ribs, and intercostal muscles are also shown. The routes of all 12 thoracic spinal nerves follow a similar pathway to that shown in this figure. (From Langman J, Woerdeman MW. Atlas of medical anatomy. Philadelphia: WB Saunders, 1978:20, 58.)

riphery to the auditory cortex. Some eighth nerve fibers make specific and secure contacts with cells in the anteroventral cochlear nucleus, and the axons of these cells project directly to superior olivary nuclei or to the inferior colliculus. From the inferior colliculus only one additional synapse, in the medial geniculate body, is required to reach the auditory cortex. On the other hand, there are also much more complex pathways in the auditory system, giving the opportunity for intricate processing of information. Each of the nuclei along the auditory pathway is composed of distinguishable divisions at each level. Furthermore, there is a variety of crossed and uncrossed pathways connecting the various auditory nuclei. Thus there are likely a number of channels of information of varying complexity proceeding along the auditory pathway, each involved in a separate function.

One must also recognize that each station in the auditory pathway receives not only afferent input from areas lower in the pathway, but also efferent input from higher centers. At most levels, efferents project to cells that are involved directly in afferent output; this arrangement holds for the hair cells as well as for cells in the cochlear nucleus, inferior colliculus, and medial geniculate body. Thus complex patterns of information processing and feedback control are possible.

The decoding of auditory information and the translation of sensory aspects of speech and language to speech production involve a broad area of the cerebral cortex and a number of parallel motor pathways, both simple and complex. Cortical areas involved include the parietal speech area (Wernicke's area), the superior temporal gyrus, the insula, the somatosensory cortex, the frontal speech area (Broca's area), and premotor areas. From the cerebral cortex, neural signals related to speech production are projected through the pyramidal tract directly to the brain stem regions that contain the motor nuclei responsible for control of the speech articulators. Cortical speech areas also project to the cerebellum and to subcortical nuclei involved in the extrapyramidal system. The importance of the latter areas in speech production is underscored by the variety of dysarthrias accompanying disease and injury to these regions. The complex extrapyramidal system processes information, which ultimately finds its way back either to the cerebral cortex, cerebellum, or the motor nuclei of the brain stem. From the brain stem nuclei, neural signals are sent to the respiratory, laryngeal, pharyngeal, palatal, lingual, mandibular, and labial muscles of the articulators. The aforementioned CNS structures insure that the neural signals sent to the muscles are coordinated in such a way as to produce intelligible speech.

Concurrently with the motor outflow from the brain to the muscles, a variety of sensory nerves feed data back to the brain for processing. This sensory information may be used to monitor the acoustic consequences of muscular contractions as well as the mechanical properties of the articulators.

The existence of these various channels in the sensory and motor pathways implies some degree of redundancy. This redundancy should make the pathways fairly resistant to disruptions by small lesions or other disturbances, and so may have some advantage for retaining function in the face of minor insults to pathways; however, its disadvantage is that small malignant defects are difficult to detect until they have grown to a dangerous proportion.

From this review, it is apparent that the neural structures involved in speech, language, and hearing are extensive, which is not surprising considering that speech, language, and hearing are perhaps the most sophisticated behaviors seen in man. Indeed, that we will find them to be even more intricate than they are currently perceived would not be surprising as we learn more about these precise and detailed systems.

Acknowledgement. This work was supported in part by NIH Grants NS21440 and NS24369. We express appreciation to Jane Rodgers, Cathy Thompson, Daniel Rai, and José Nuncio-Cantera for assistance in preparation of the manuscript.

REFERENCES

1. Crosby EC, Humphrey T, Lauer EW. Correlative anatomy of the nervous system. New York: Macmillan, 1962.
2. Brodal A. Neurological anatomy in relation to clinical medicine. London: Oxford University Press, 1981.
3. Carpenter MB. Human neuroanatomy. Baltimore: Williams & Wilkins, 1983.

3a. Peele TL. The neuroanatomic basis for clinical neurology. New York: McGraw-Hill, 1976.

4. Spoendlin H. Innervation densities of the cochlea. Acta Otolaryngol (Stockh) 1972; 73:235–248.
5. Saito K. Fine structure of the sensory epithelium of the guinea pig organ of Corti: afferent and efferent synapses of hair cells. J Ultrastruct Res 1980; 71:222–232.
6. Pujol R, Lenoir M. The four types of synapses in the organ of Corti. In: Altschuler RA, Hoffman DW, Bobbin RP, eds. Neurobiology of hearing: the cochlea. New York: Raven Press, 1986:161.
7. Nadol JB Jr. Serial section reconstruction of the neural poles of hair cells in the human organ of Corti. Inner hair cells. Laryngoscope 1983; 93:599–614.
8. Rasmussen, AT. Studies of the eighth cranial nerve of man. Laryngoscope 1940; 50:67–83.
9. Hinojosa R, Marion M. Histopathology of profound sensorineural deafness. Ann NY Acad Sci 1983; 405:459–484.
10. Gacek RR, Rasmussen GL. Fiber analysis of the statoacoustic nerve of guinea pig, cat, and monkey. Anat Rec 1961; 139:455–463.
11. Otte J, Schuknecht HF, Kerr AG. Ganglion cell populations in normal and pathological human cochleae. Impli-

cations for cochlear implantation. Laryngoscope 1978; 88:1231–1246.
12. Ota CY, Kimura RS. Ultrastructural study of the human spiral ganglion. Acta Otolaryngol (Stockh) 1980; 89:53–62.
13. Kimura RS, Ota CY, Takarashi T. Nerve fiber synapses on spiral ganglion cells in the human cochlea. Ann Otol Rhinol Laryngol 1979; 88:1–17.
14. Spoendlin H. Differentiation of cochlear afferent neurons. Acta Otolaryngol (Stockh) 1981; 91:451–456.
15. Liberman MC. Morphological differentiation among radial afferent fibers in the cat cochlea: an electron-microscopic study of serial sections. Hear Res 1980; 3:45–63.
16. Kimura RS. Differences in innervation of cochlear inner and outer hair cells. Abstr Midwinter Res Meet Assoc Res Otolaryngol 1978; 40–41.
17. Liberman MC. Auditory-nerve response from cats raised in a low-noise chamber. J Acoust Soc Am 1978; 63:442–455.
18. Liberman MC, Oliver ME. Morphometry of intracellularly labeled neurons of the auditory nerve: correlations with functional properties. J Comp Neurol 1984; 223(2):163–176.
19. Evans EF, Palmer AR. Relationship between the dynamic range of cochlear nerve fibers and their spontaneous activity. Exp Brain Res 1980; 40:115–118.
20. Arnesen AR, Osen KK. The cochlear nerve in the cat: topography, cochleotopy, and fiber spectrum. J Comp Neurol 1978; 178:661–678.
21. Arnesen AR, Osen KK, Mugnaini E. Temporal and spatial sequence of anterograde degeneration in the cochlear nerve fibers of the cat. A light microscopic study. J Comp Neurol 1978; 178:679–696.
22. Sando I. The anatomical interrelationships of the cochlear nerve fibers. Acta Otolaryngol (Stockh) 1965; 59:417–436.
23. Courville CB. The nervus acusticus. I. Applied anatomy of the VIIIth nerve and its environs, the cerebellopontile angle. Laryngoscope 1932; 42:415–431.
24. Bacsik RD, Strominger NL. The cytoarchitecture of the human anteroventral cochlear nucleus. J Comp Neurol 1973; 147:281–290.
25. Adams JC. Neuronal morphology in the human cochlear nucleus. Arch Otolaryngol 1986; 112:1253–1261.
26. Moore JK. The primate cochlear nuclei: loss of lamination as a phylogenetic process. J Comp Neurol 1980; 193:609–630.
27. Moore JK, Osen KK. The cochlear nuclei in man. Am J Anat 1979; 154:393–418.
28. Noda Y, Pirsig W. Anatomical projection of the cochlea to the cochlear nuclei of the guinea pig. Arch Otorhinolaryngol 1974; 208:107–120.
29. Fekete DM, Rouiller EM, Liberman MC, Ryugo DK. The central projection of intracellularly labeled auditory nerve fibers in the cat. J Comp Neurol 1984; 229:432–450.
30. Moskowitz N, Liu JC. Central projections of the spiral ganglion of the squirrel monkey. J Comp Neurol 1972; 144:335–344.
31. Rose JE, Galambos R, Hughes J. Microelectrode studies of the cochlear nuclei of the cat. Johns Hopkins Hosp Bull 1959; 104:211–251.
32. Chow KL. Numerical estimates of the auditory central nervous system of the rhesus monkey. J Comp Neurol 1951; 95:159–175.
33. Brawer JR, Morest DK, Kane EC. The neuronal architecture of the cochlear nucleus of the cat. J Comp Neurol 1974; 155:251–300.
34. Cant NB, Morest DK. The structural basis for stimulus coding in the cochlear nucleus of the rat. In: Berlin C, ed. Hearing science. San Diego: College-Hill Press, 1984:371.
35. Caspary DM. Cochlear nuclei: functional neuropharmacology of the principal cell types. In: Altschuler RA, Hoffman DW, Bobbin RP, eds. Neurobiology of hearing: the cochlea. New York: Raven Press, 1986:303.
36. Moore JK. Cochlear nucleus relations to auditory nerve. In: Altschuler RA, Hoffman DW, Bobbin RP, eds. Neurobiology of hearing: the cochlea. New York: Raven Press, 1986:283.
37. Lorente de No R. Anatomy of the eighth nerve. III. General plan of structure of the primary cochlear nuclei. Laryngoscope 1933; 43:327–350.
38. Ryugo DK, Fekete DM. Morphology of primary axosomatic endings in the anteroventral cochlear nucleus of the cat: a study of the endbulbs of Held. J Comp Neurol 1982; 210:239–257.
39. Rhode WS, Oertel D, Smith PH. Physiological response properties of cells labeled intracellularly with horseradish peroxidase in cat ventral cochlear nucleus. J Comp Neurol 1983; 213:448–463.
40. Pfeiffer RR. Classification of response patterns of spike discharge for units in the cochlear nucleus: tone burst stimulation. Exp Brain Res 1966; 1:220–235.
41. Harrison JM, Irving R. The anterior ventral cochlear nucleus. J Comp Neurol 1965; 124:15–42.
42. Osen KK. Cytoarchitecture of the cochlear nuclei in the cat. J Comp Neurol 1969; 136:453–484.
43. Rouiller EM, Ryugo DK. Intracellular marking of physiologically characterized cells in the ventral cochlear nucleus of the cat. J Comp Neurol 1984; 225:167–186.
44. Rhode WS, Smith PH, Oertel D. Physiological response properties of cells labeled intracellularly with horseradish peroxidase in cat dorsal cochlear nucleus. J Comp Neurol 1983; 213:426–447.
45. Harrison JM, Warr WB. A study of the cochlear nuclei and the ascending auditory pathways in the medulla. J Comp Neurol 1962; 119:341–380.
46. Evans EF, Nelson PG. On the functional relationship between the dorsal and ventral divisions of the cochlear nucleus of the cat. Exp Brain Res 1973; 17:428–442.
47. Young ED, Brownell WE. Responses to tones and noise of single cells in dorsal cochlear nucleus of unanesthetized cats. J Neurophysiol 1976; 39:282–300.
48. Moore JK. The human auditory brainstem: a comparative view. Hearing Res 1987; 29:1–32.
49. Strominger NL, Nelson LR, Dougherty WJ. Second order auditory pathways in the chimpanzee. J Comp Neurol 1977; 172:349–366.
50. Tsuchitani C, Boudreau JC. Single unit analysis of cat superior olive s segment with tonal stimuli. J Neurophysiol 1966; 29:684–697.
51. Goldberg JM, Brown PB. Functional organization of the dog superior olivary complex: an anatomical and electrophysiological study. J Neurophysiol 1968; 31:639–656.
52. Strominger NL, Hurwitz JL. Anatomical aspects of the superior olivary complex. J Comp Neurol 1976; 170:485–498.
53. Irving R, Harrison JM. The superior olivary complex and audition: a comparative study. J Comp Neurol 1967; 130:77–86.
54. Goldberg JM, Brown PB. Response of binaural neurons of dog superior olivary complex to dichotic tonal stimuli: some physiological mechanisms of sound localization. J Neurophysiol 1969; 32:613–636.
55. Boudreau JC, Tsuchitani C. Cat superior olive s-segment cell discharge to tonal stimuli. Contr Sensory Physiol 1970; 4:143–213.
56. Glendenning KK, Hutson KA, Nudo RJ, Masterton RB. Acoustic chiasm II. Anatomical bases of binaurality in lateral superior olive of cat. J Comp Neurol 1985; 232:261–285.
57. Stotler WA. An experimental study of the cells and connections of the superior olivary complex of the cat. J Comp Neurol 1953; 98:401–431.
58. Aitkin LM, Anderson DJ, Brugge JF. Tonotopic organi-

zation and discharge characteristics of single neurons in nuclei of the lateral lemniscus of the cat. J Neurophysiol 1970; 33:421–440.
59. Goldberg JM, Moore RY. Ascending projections of the lateral lemniscus in the cat and monkey. J Comp Neurol 1967; 129:143–156.
60. Adams JC. Ascending projections to the inferior colliculus. J Comp Neurol 1979; 183:519–538.
61. Brunso-Bechtold JK, Thompson GC, Masterton RB. HRP study of the organization of auditory afferents ascending to central nucleus of inferior colliculus in cat. J Comp Neurol 1981; 197:705–722.
62. Aitkin LM, Phillips SC. Is the inferior colliculus an obligatory relay in the cat auditory system? Neurosci Lett 1984; 44:259–264.
63. Geniec P, Morest DK. The neuronal architecture of the human posterior colliculus. A study with the golgi method. Acta Otolaryngol [Suppl] (Stockh) 1971; 295:1–33.
64. FitzPatrick KA. Cellular architecture and topographic organization of the inferior colliculus of the squirrel monkey. J Comp Neurol 1975; 164:185–208.
65. Oliver DL, Morest DK. The central nucleus of the inferior colliculus in the cat. J Comp Neurol 1984; 222:237–264.
66. Rockel AJ, Jones EG. The neuronal organization of the inferior colliculus of the adult cat. I. The central nucleus. J Comp Neurol 1973; 147:11–60.
67. Rockel AJ, Jones EG. The neuronal organization of the inferior colliculus of the adult cat. II. The pericentral nucleus. J Comp Neurol 1973; 149:301–334.
68. Merzenich MM, Reid MD. Representation of the cochlea within the inferior colliculus of the cat. Brain Res 1974; 77:397–415.
69. Roth GL, Aitkin LM, Anderson RA, Merzenich MM. Some features of the spatial organization of the central nucleus of the inferior colliculus of the cat. J Comp Neurol 1978; 182:661–680.
70. Webster WR, Serviere J, Crewther D, Crewther S. Isofrequency-frequency 2-DG contours in the inferior colliculus of the awake monkey. Exp Brain Res 1984; 56:425–437.
71. Moore RY, Goldberg JM. Ascending projections of the inferior colliculus in the cat. J Comp Neurol 1963; 121:109–136.
72. Moore RY, Goldberg JM. Projections of the inferior colliculus in the monkey. Exp Neurol 1966; 14:429–438.
73. Kudo M, Niimi K. Ascending projections of the inferior colliculus in the cat: an autoradiographic study. J Comp Neurol 1980; 191:545–556.
74. Morest DK. The neuronal architecture of the medial geniculate body of the cat. J Anat 1964; 98:611–630.
75. Morest DK. The laminar structure of the medial geniculate body of the cat. J Anat 1965; 99:143–160.
76. Imig TJ, Morel A. Organization of the thalamo-cortical auditory system in the cat. Ann Rev Neurosci 1983; 6:95–120.
77. Calford MB, Webster WR. Auditory representation within principal division of cat medial geniculate body: an electrophysiological study. J Neurophysiol 1981; 45:1013–1028.
78. Morest DK. The lateral tegmental system of the mid-brain and the medial geniculate body: study with golgi and nauta methods in cat. J Anat 1965; 99:611–634.
79. Aitkin LM, Webster WR. Medial geniculate body of the cat: organization and responses to tonal stimuli of neurons in ventral division. J Neurophysiol 1972; 32:365–380.
80. Mesulam M-M, Pandya DN. The projections of the medial geniculate complex within the sylvian fissure of the rhesus monkey. Brain Res 1973; 60:315–333.
81. Rose JE, Woolsey CN. The relations of thalamic connections, cellular structure and evocable electrical activity in the auditory region of the cat. J Comp Neurol 1949; 91:441–466.
82. Wilson ME, Craig BG. Projections from the medical geniculate body to the cerebral cortex in cat. Brain Res 1969; 13:462–475.
83. Calford MB, Aitkin LM. Ascending projections to the medial geniculate body of the cat: evidence for multiple, parallel auditory pathways through the thalamus. J Neurosci 1983; 3(11):2365–2380.
84. Diamond IT, Chow KL, Neff WD. Degeneration of caudal medial geniculate body following cortical lesions ventral to auditory area II in the cat. J Comp Neurol 1958; 109:349–362.
85. Rose JE, Woolsey CN. Cortical connections and functional organization of the thalamic auditory system of cat. In: Harlow HF, Woolsey DN, eds. Biological and biochemical bases of behavior. Madison, WI: University of Wisconsin Press, 1958:127.
86. Imig TJ, Morel A. Topographic and cytoarchitectonic organization of thalamic neurons related to their targets in low-, middle-, and high-frequency representations in cat auditory cortex. J Comp Neurol 1984; 227:511–539.
87. Celesia GG. Organization of auditory cortical areas in man. Brain 1976; 99:403–414.
88. Galaburda A, Sanides F. Cytoarchitectonic organization of the human auditory cortex. J Comp Neurol 1980; 190:597–610.
89. Merzenich MM, Brugge JF. Representation of the cochlear partition on the superior plane of the macaque monkey. Brain Res 1973; 50:275–296.
90. Imig TJ, Ruggero MA, Kitzes LM, Javel E, Brugge JF. Organization of auditory cortex in the owl monkey (Aotus trivirgatus). J Comp Neurol 1977; 171:111–128.
91. Woolsey CN. Organization of cortical auditory systems: a review and a synthesis. In: Rasmussen GL, Windle WF, eds. Neural mechanisms of the auditory and vestibular systems. Springfield, IL: CC Thomas, 1960:165.
92. Pandya DN, Sanides F. Architecture parcellation of the temporal operculum in rhesus monkey and its projection pattern. Z Anat Entwicki-Gesch 1973; 139:127–161.
93. von Economo C. The cytoarchitectonics of the human cerebral cortex. Translated by Parker S. London: Oxford University Press, 1929.
94. von Bonin G, Bailey P. The neocortex of macaca mulatta. Urbana: University of Illinois Press, 1947.
95. Rose JE. The cellular structure of the auditory region of the cat. J Comp Neurol 1949; 91:409–440.
96. Smith DE, Moskowitz N. Ultrastructure of layer IV of the primary auditory cortex of the squirrel monkey. Neuroscience 1979; 4:349–359.
97. Pfingst BE, O'Connor TA. Characteristics of neurons in auditory cortex of monkeys performing a simple auditory task. J Neurophysiol 1981; 45:139–155.
98. Merzenich MM, Knight PL, Roth GL. Representation of cochlea within primary auditory cortex in the cat. J Neurophysiol 1975; 38:231–249.
99. Imig TJ, Adrian HO. Binaural columns in the primary field (AI) of cat auditory cortex. Brain Res 1977; 138:241–257.
100. Schreiner CE, Cynader MS. Basic functional organization of second auditory cortical field (AII) of the cat. J Neurophysiol 1984; 51:1284–1305.
101. Tunturi AR. A difference in the representation of auditory signals for the left and right ears in the isofrequency-frequency contours of the right middle ectosylvian auditory cortex of the dog. Am J Physiol 1952; 168:712–722.
102. Evans EF, Ross HF, Whitfield IC. The spatial distribution of unit characteristic frequency in the primary auditory cortex of the cat. J Physiol 1965; 179:238–247.
103. Goldstein MH, Abeles M, Daly RL, McIntosh J. Functional architecture in cat primary auditory cortex: tonotopic organization. J Neurophysiol 1970; 33:188–197.
104. Diamond IT. The sensory neocortex. In: Neff WD, ed. Contributions to sensory physiology. New York: Academic Press, 1967:51.

105. Diamond IT, Jones EG, Powell TPS. Interhemispheric fiber connections of auditory cortex of the cat. Brain Res 1968; 11:177–193.
106. Diamond IT, Jones EG, Powell TPS. The association connections of auditory cortex of the cat. Brain Res 1968; 11:560–579.
107. Winguth SD, Winer JA. Corticocortical connections of cat primary auditory cortex (AI): laminar organization and identification of supragranular neurons projecting to area AII. J Comp Neurol 1986; 248:36–56.
108. Imig TJ, Reale RA. Patterns of cortico-cortical connections related to tonotopic maps in cat auditory cortex. J Comp Neurol 1980; 192:293–332.
109. Code RA, Winer JA. Columnar organization and reciprocity of commissural connections in cat primary auditory-cortex (AI). Hearing Res 1986; 23:205–222.
110. Kelly JP, Wong D. Laminar connections of the cat's auditory cortex. Brain Res 1981; 212:1–15.
111. Imig TJ, Brugge JF. Sources and terminations of callosal axons related to binaural and frequency maps in primary auditory cortex of the cat. J Comp Neurol 1978; 182:637–660.
112. Pandya DN, Hallett M, Mukherjee SK. Intra- and interhemispheric connections of the neocortical auditory system in the rhesus monkey. Brain Res 1969; 14:49–65.
113. Andersen RA, Knight PL, Merzenich MM. The thalamocortical and corticothalamic connections of the AI, AII, and the anterior auditory field (AAF) in the cat: EVI device for two largely segregated systems of connections. J Comp Neurol 1980; 194:663–701.
114. FitzPatrick KA, Imig TJ. Projections of auditory cortex upon the thalamus and midbrain in the owl monkey. J Comp Neurol 1978; 177:537–556.
115. Forbes BF, Moskowitz N. Projections of auditory responsive cortex in the squirrel monkey. Brain Res 1974; 67:239–254.
116. Diamond IT, Jones EG, Powell TPS. The projection of the auditory cortex upon the diencephalon and brainstem in the cat. Brain Res 1969; 15:305–340.
117. Rasmussen GL. Further observations of the efferent cochlear bundle. J Comp Neurol 1953; 99:61–74.
118. Rasmussen GL. Efferent fibers of the cochlear nerve and cochlear nucleus. In: Rasmussen GL, Windle WF, eds. Neural mechanisms of the auditory and vestibular systems. Springfield: CC Thomas, 1960:105.
119. Guinan JJ Jr, Warr WB, Norris BE. Tonotopic organization of the olivocochlear projections from the lateral and medial zones of the superior olivary complex. J Comp Neurol 1984; 226:21–27.
120. Warr WB, Guinan JJ Jr. Efferent innervation of the organ of corti: two separate systems. Brain Res 1979; 173:152–155.
121. White JS, Warr WB. The dual origins of the olivocochlear bundle in the albino rat. J Comp Neurol 1983; 219:203–214.
122. Strominger NL, Silver SM, Truscott TC, Goldstein JC. The cells of origin of the olivocochlear bundle in new and old world monkeys (abstr). Anat Rec 1981; 199:246.
123. Warr WB, Guinan JJ Jr, White JS. Organization of the efferent fibers: the lateral and medial systems. In: Altschuler RA, Hoffman DW, Bobbin RP, eds. Neurobiology of hearing: the cochlea. New York: Raven Press, 1986:333.
124. Borg E. On the neuronal organization of the acoustic middle ear reflex. A physiological and anatomical study. Brain Res 1973; 49:101–123.
125. Itoh K, Nomura S, Konishi A, Yasui Y, Sugimoto T, Mizuno N. A morphological evidence of direct connections from the cochlear nuclei to tensor tympani motoneurons in the cat: a possible afferent limb of the acoustic middle ear reflex pathways. Brain Res 1986; 375:214–219.
126. Phillips CG, Zeki S, Barlow HB. Localization of function in cerebral cortex architecture. Brain 1984; 107:327–362.
127. Exner S. Untersuchungen uber Localisation der functionen in der Grosshirnrinde des Menschen. Vienna: W Braumuller, 1881.
128. Brodmann K. Vergleichende Lokalisationlehre der Grosshirnrinde in ihren Prinzipien dargestellt auf Grund des Zellenbaues. Leipzig: JA Barth, 1909.
129. Mesulam M-M. Principles of behavioral neurology. Philadelphia: FA Davis, 1985.
130. Broca P. Anatome comparee des circonvolutions cerebrales: le grand lobe limbique dans la serie des mammiferes. Rev Anthropol 1878; 1:384–498.
131. Abbie AA. Cortical lamination in a polyprotodont marsupial, Perameles nasuta. J Comp Neurol 1942; 76:509–535.
132. Filimonoff IN. A rational subdivision of the cerebral cortex. Arch Neurol Psychiatr 1948; 58:296–311.
133. Yakovlev PI. Pathoarchitectonic studies of cerebral malformations. III. Arrhineencephalies (holotelencephalies). J Neuropathol Exp Neurol 1959; 18:22–55.
134. Sanides F. Functional architecture of motor and sensory cortices in primates in the light of a new concept of neocortex evolution. In: Noback CR, Montagna W, eds. The primate brain. New York: Appleton-Century-Crofts, 1970:137.
135. Penfield W, Roberts L. Speech and brain mechanisms. Princeton, NJ: Princeton University Press, 1959.
136. Lenneberg EH. Biological foundations of language. New York: John Wiley & Sons, 1967.
137. Kinsbourne M. The ontogeny of cerebral dominance. Ann NY Acad Sci 1975; 263:244–250.
138. Kimura D. Cerebral dominance for speech. In: Tower DB, ed. The nervous system. Vol 3. Human communication and its disorders. New York: Raven Press, 1975:365.
139. Luria AR. Traumatic aphasia. The Hague: Mouton, 1970.
140. Gazzaniga MS, Hillyard SA. Language and speech capacity of the right hemisphere. Neuropsychologia 1971; 9:273–280.
141. Geschwind N, Levitsky W. Human brain: left-right asymmetries in temporal speech region. Science 1968; 161:186–187.
142. Witelson SF, Pallie W. Left hemisphere specialization for language in the newborn. Brain 1973; 96:641–646.
143. Yeni-Komshian GH, Benson DA. Anatomical study of cerebral asymmetry in the temporal lobe of humans, chimpanzees, and rhesus monkeys. Science 1976; 92:387–389.
144. Seldon HL. Structure of human auditory cortex: I. Cytoarchitectonics and dendritic distributions. Brain Res 1981; 229:227–294.
145. Geschwind N, Galaburda AM, eds. Cerebral dominance: the biological foundations. Cambridge: Harvard University Press, 1984.
146. Ingvar DH. Functional landscapes in the cerebral cortex related to speech. In: Grillner S, Lindblom B, eds. Speech motor control. Oxford: Pergamon Press, 1981:61.
147. Duffy FH. Topographic display of evoked potentials: clinical applications of brain electrical activity mapping (BEAM). Ann NY Acad Sci 1982; 388:183–196.
148. Roland PE, Larsen B, Lassen NA, Skinhoj E. Supplementary motor area and other cortical areas in organization of voluntary movements in man. J Neurophysiol 1980; 43:118–136.
149. Ross ED. The aprosodias: functional-anatomic organization of the affective components of language in the right hemisphere. Arch Neurol 1981; 38:561–569.
150. Ross ED, Mesulam M-M. Dominant language functions of the right hemisphere: prosody and emotional gesturing. Arch Neurol 1979; 36:144–148.
151. Zurif EB. Language mechanisms: a neuropsychological perspective. Am Scientist 1980; 68:305–311.
152. Blumstein S, Cooper WD. Identification vs. discrimination of distinctive features in speech perception. Q J Exp Psych 1972; 24:207–214.

153. Ross ED. Modulation of affect and nonverbal communication by the right hemisphere. In: Mesulam M-M, ed. Principles of behavioral neurology. Philadelphia: FA Davis, 1985:239.
154. Ross ED, Harney JH, deLacoste C, Purdy P. How the brain integrates affective and propositional language into a unified brain function. Hypotheses based on clinicopathological correlations. Arch Neurol 1981; 38:745–748.
155. Ross ED, Holzapfel D, Freeman F. Assessment of affective behavior in brain damaged patients using quantitative acoustical-phonetic and gestural measurements (abstr). Neurology (Suppl. 2) 1983; 33:219–220.
156. Kimura D. Some effects of temporal lobe damage on auditory perception. Can J Psychol 1961; 15:157–165.
157. Ojemann GA, Mateer C. Human language cortex: localization of memory, syntax, and sequential motor-phoneme identification systems. Science 1979; 205:1401–1403.
158. Studdert-Kennedy M, Shankweiler D. Hemispheric specialization for speech perception. J Acoust Soc Am 1969; 48:579–594.
159. Cutting JE. Two left-hemisphere mechanisms in speech perception. Percept Psychophys 1974; 16:601–612.
160. Musiek FE, Reeves AG, Baran JA. Release from central auditory competition in the split-brain patient. Neurology 1985; 35(7):983–987.
161. Pandya D. The topography of the commissural fibers. In: Lepore F, Pitito M, Jasper H, eds. Two hemispheres, one brain. Functions of the corpus callosum. New York: Alan R Liss, 1986:47.
162. Evarts EV. Role of motor cortex in voluntary movements in primates. In: Brooks V, ed. Handbook of physiology. Vol. II. Motor control. Motor functioning. Philadelphia: American Physiological Society, 1981.
163. Damasio AR, Van Hoesen GW. Structure and function of the supplementary motor area (abstr). Neurology 1980; 30:359.
164. Wiesendanger M, Hummelsheim H, Bianchetti. Sensory input to the motor fields of the agranular frontal cortex: a comparison of the precentral, supplementary motor and premotor cortex. Behav Brain Res 1985; 18:89–94.
165. Wise SP, Strick PL. Anatomical and physiological organization of the nonprimary motor cortex. TINS 1984; 7:442–446.
166. Wiesendanger M. The pyramidal tract: its structure and function. In: Towe AL, Luschei ES, eds. Handbook of behavioral neurobiology. Vol. 5. Motor coordination. New York: Plenum Press, 1981:401.
167. Huncker CJ, Abbs JH, Barlow SM. The relationship between parkinsonian rigidity and hypokinesia in the orofacial system: a quantitative analysis. Neurology 1982; 32:755–761.
168. Anderson ME. The basal ganglia and movement. In: Towe AL, Luschei ES, eds. Handbook of behavioral neurobiology. Vol. 5. Motor coordination. New York: Plenum Press, 1981: 367.
169. Nauta WJH, Domesick VB. Afferent and efferent relationships of the basal ganglia. In: Evered D, O'Connor M, eds. Symposium on functions of the basal ganglia. London: Pitman (Ciba Foundation), 1984:3.
170. Strick PL. How do the basal ganglia and cerebellum gain access to the corticalmotor areas? Behav Brain Res 1985; 18:107–123.
171. Garcia-Rill E. The basal ganglia and the locomotor regions. Brain Res Rev 1986; 11:47–63.
172. House EL, Pansky B. A functional approach to neuroanatomy. New York: McGraw-Hill, 1967.
173. Nauta WJH, Freirtag M. Fundamental neuroanatomy. New York: WH Freeman, 1986.
174. Ojemann GA, Fedio P, van Buren JM. Anomia from pulvinar and subcortical parietal stimulation. Brain 1968; 91:99–116.
175. Ojemann GA. Language and the thalamus: object naming and recall during and after thalamic stimulation. Brain Lang 1975; 2:101–120.
176. Ojemann GA, Ward AA. Speech representation in ventrolateral thalamus. Brain 1971; 94:669–680.
177. Reynolds AF, Harris AB, Ojemann GA, Turner PT. Aphasia and left thalamic hemorrhage. J Neurosurg 1978; 48:570–574.
178. Tasker RR, Organ LW, Hawrylyshyn PA. The thalamus and midbrain of man. Springfield, IL: CC Thomas, 1982.
179. Carpenter MB, Hanna GR. Fiber projections from the spinal trigeminal nucleus in the cat. J Comp Neurol 1961; 117:117–131.
180. Bombardieri RA, Johnson JI Jr., Campos GB. Species differences in mechanosensory projections from the mouth to the ventrobasal thalamus. J Comp Neurol 1975; 163:41–64.
181. Hayward JN. Response of ventrobasal thalamic cells to hair displacement on the face of the waking monkey. J Physiol 1975; 250:385–407.
182. Loe PR, Whitsel BL, Dreyer DA, Metz CB. Body representation in ventrobasal thalamus of macaque: a single-unit analysis. J Neurophysiol 1977; 40:1339–1355.
183. Mizuno N. Projection fibers from the main sensory trigeminal nucleus and the supratrigeminal region. J Comp Neurol 1970; 139:457–472.
184. Smith RL. Axonal projection and connections of the principal sensory trigeminal nucleus in the monkey. J Comp Neurol 1975; 163:347–376.
185. O'Brien JH, Pimpaneau A, Albe-Fessard D. Evoked cortical responses to vagal, laryngeal and facial afferents in monkeys under chloralose anesthesia. EEG Clin Neurophysiol 1971; 31:7–20.
186. Dreyer DA, Loe PR, Metz DB, Whitsel BL. Representation of head and face in postcentral gyrus of the macaque. J Neurophysiol 1975; 38:714–733.
187. Kunzle H. Thalamic projections from the precentral motor cortex in *Macaca* fascicularis. Brain Res 1976; 105:253–267.
188. Kasdon DL, Jacobson S. The thalamic afferents to the inferior parietal lobule of the rhesus monkey. J Comp Neurol. 1978; 177:685–706.
189. Brown JR, Darley FL, Aronson AE. Ataxic dysarthria. Int J Neurol 1970; 7:302–318.
190. Holmes G. The symptoms of acute cerebellar injuries due to gunshot injuries. Brain 1917; 40:461–535.
191. Kent R, Netsell R. A case study of an ataxic dysarthric: cineradiographic and spectrographic observations. J Speech Hear Res 1975; 40:115–134.
192. Azzena GB, Desole C, Palmieri G. Cerebellar projections of the masticatory and extraocular muscle proprioception. Exp Neurol 1970; 27:151–161.
193. Bowman JP, Combs CM. Cerebellar responsiveness to stimulation of the lingual spindle afferent fibers in the hypoglossal nerve of the rhesus monkey. Exp Neurol 1969; 23:537–543.
194. Bortolami R, Callegari E, Lucchi ML. Anatomical relationship between mesencephalic trigeminal nucleus and cerebellum in the duck. Brain Res 1972; 47:317–329.
195. Lam RL, Ogura JH. An afferent representation of the larynx in the cerebellum. Laryngoscope 1952; 62:486–495.
196. Snider RS, Stowell A. Receiving areas of the tactile, auditory, and visual systems in the cerebellum. J Neurophysiol 1944; 7:331–357.
197. Eccles JC. The cerebellum as a computer: patterns in space and time. J Physiol 1973; 337:199–217.
198. Ito MI. The cerebellum and neural control. New York: Raven Press, 1984.
199. Llinas R, Hillman DE. Physiological and morphological organization of the cerebellar circuits in various vertebrates. In: Llinas R, ed. Neurobiology of cerebellar evolution and

development. Chicago: American Medical Association, 1969:43.
200. Llinas RR, Simpson JI. Cerebellar control of movement. In: Towe AL, Luschei ES, eds. Handbook of behavioral neurobiology. Vol. 5. Motor coordination. New York: Plenum Press, 1981:231.
201. Allen GI, Tsukahara N. Cerebrocerebellar communication systems. Physiol Rev 1974; 54:957–1006.
202. Snider RS, Maiti A, Snider SR. Cerebellar pathways to ventral midbrain and nigra. Exp Neurol 1976; 53:714–728.
203. Flumerfelt BA, Otabe S, Courville J. Distinct projections to the red nucleus from the dentate and interposed nuclei in the monkey. Brain Res 1973; 50:408–414.
204. Mizuno N, Mochizuki K, Akimoto C, Matsushima R, Nakamura Y. Rubrobulbar projections in the rabbit. A light and electron microscopic study. J Comp Neurol 1973; 147:267–280.
205. Mizuno N, Nakamura Y, Iwahori N. Central afferent fibers to trigeminal motor system. Bull Tokyo Med Dent Univ [Suppl] 1974; 21:18–21.
206. Panneton WM, Martin GF. Midbrain projections to the facial nucleus in the opossum. Brain Res 1978; 145:355–359.
207. Mizuno N, Konishi A, Sato M. Localization of masticatory motoneurons in the cat and rat by means of retrograde axonal transport of horseradish peroxidase. J Comp Neurol 1975; 164:105–116.
208. Landgren S, Olsson KA. Localization of evoked potentials in the digastric, masseteric, supra- and intertrigeminal subnuclei of the cat. Exp Brain Res 1976; 26:299–318.
209. Limwongse V, DeSantis M. Cell body locations and axonal pathways of neurons innervating muscles of mastication in the rat. Am J Anat 1977; 149:477–488.
210. Batini C, Buisseret-Delmas C, Corvisier J. Horseradish peroxidase localization of masticatory muscle motoneurons in cat. J Physiol (Paris) 1976; 72:301–309.
211. Grant G, Arvidsson J. Transganglionic degeneration in trigeminal primary sensory neurons. Brain Res 1975; 95:265–279.
212. Kerr FWL, Kruger L, Schwassman HO, Stern R. Somatotopic organization of mechanoreceptor units in the trigeminal nuclear complex of the macaque. J Comp Neurol 1968; 134:127–144.
213. Kirkpatrick DB, Kruger L. Physiological properties of neurons in the principal sensory trigeminal nucleus of the cat. Exp Neurol 1975; 48:664–690.
214. Kruger L, Michel F. A single neuron analysis of buccal cavity representation in the sensory trigeminal complex of the cat. Arch Oral Biol 1962; 7:491–503.
215. Craigmyle MBL. The mixed cranial nerves. New York: John Wiley & Sons, 1985.
216. Holstege G, Kuypers HGJM, Dekker JJ. The organization of the bulbar fibre connections to the trigeminal, facial, and hypoglossal motor nuclei. Brain 1977; 100:265–286.
217. Courville J. The nucleus of the facial nerve: the relation between cellular groups and peripheral branches of the nerve. Brain Res 1966; 1:338–354.
218. Provis J. The organization of the facial nucleus of the brush-tailed possum (*Trichosurus volpecula*). J Comp Neurol 1977; 172:177–188.
219. Radpour S. Organization of the facial nerve nucleus in the cat. Laryngoscope 1977; 87:557–574.
220. Tanaka T. Pyramidal activation of the facial nucleus in the cat. Brain Res 1976; 103:389–393.
221. Davis PJ, Nail BS. On the location and size of laryngeal motoneurons in the cat and rabbit. J Comp Neurol 1984; 230:13–32.
222. Yoshida Y, Mitsimasu T, Miyazaki T, Hirano M, Kanaseki T. Distribution of motoneurons in the brainstem of monkeys, innervating the larynx. Brain Res Bull 1984; 13:413–419.
223. McClean MD, Folkins JW, Larson CR. The role of the perioral reflex in lip motor control for speech. Brain Lang 1979; 7:42–61.
224. Tanaka T, Takeuchi Y, Nakano K. Cells of origin of the spino-facial pathway in the cat: a horseradish peroxidase study. Brain Res 1978; 142:580–585.
225. Tanaka T. Afferent projections in the hypoglossal nerve to the facial neurons of the cat. Brain Res 1975; 99:140–144.
226. Arnold GE. Vocal rehabilitation of paralytic dysphonia. Arch Otolaryngol 1957; 65:317–336.
227. Tomasch J, Ebnessajjade D. The human nucleus ambiguus. Anat Rec 1961; 141:247–252.
228. Furstenberg AC, Magielski JE. A motor pattern in the nucleus ambiguus. Its clinical significance. Ann Otol Rhinol Laryngol 1955; 64:788–793.
229. Lawn AM. The localization, in the nucleus ambiguus of the rabbit, of the cells of origin of motor nerve fibers in the glossopharyngeal nerve and various branches of the vagus nerve by means of retrograde degeneration. J Comp Neurol 1966; 127:293–306.
230. Gacek RR, Malmgren LT, Lyon MJ. Localization of adductor and abductor motor nerve fibers to the larynx. Ann Otol Rhinol Laryngol 1977; 86:1–7.
231. Goss CM, ed. Gray's anatomy of the human body. 29th Am ed. Philadelphia: Lea & Febiger, 1973.
232. Hast MH, Fischer JM, Wetzel AB, Thompson VE. Cortical motor representation of the laryngeal muscles in Macaca mulatta. Brain Res 1974; 73:229–240.
233. Hast MH, Milojevic B. The response of the vocal folds to electrical stimulation of the inferior frontal cortex of the squirrel monkey. Acta Otolaryngol 1966; 61:196–204.
234. Kirikae I, Hirose H, Kawamura S, Sawashima M, Kobayashi T. An experimental study of central motor innervation of the laryngeal muscles in the cat. Ann Otol Rhinol Laryngol 1962; 71:222–241.
235. Barris RW, Schuman HR. Bilateral anterior cingulate gyrus lesions. Neurology 1953; 3:44–52.
236. Sutton D, Larson C, Lindemann RC. Neocortical and limbic lesions effects on primate phonation. Brain Res 1974; 71:61–75.
237. Yoshida Y, Mitsumasu T, Hirano M, Kanaseki T. Afferent connections to the nucleus ambiguus in the brainstem of the cat; an HRP study. A paper presented at the fourth international conference on Vocal Fold Physiology, Yale University, New Haven, Connecticut, 1985.
238. Jürgens U, Pratt R. Role of the periaqueductal grey in vocal expression of emotion. Brain Res 1979; 167:367–378.
239. Larson CR. The midbrain periaqueductal gray: a brainstem structure involved in vocalization. J Speech Hear Res 1985; 28:241–249.
240. Larson CR, Kistler MK. The relationship of periaqueductal gray neurons to vocalization and laryngeal EMG in the behaving monkey. Exp Brain Res 1986; 63:596–606.
241. Dunker E, Rehren D von, Wachsmuth D. The vago-vagal reflex arc: some properties of its central part. Pflugers Arch 1972; 337:199–217.
242. Porter R. Unit response evoked in the medulla oblongata by vagus nerve stimulation. J Physiol 1963; 168:717–735.
243. Murakami Y, Kirchner JA. Electrophysiological properties of laryngeal reflex closure. Acta Otolaryngol (Stockh) 1971; 71:416–425.
244. Sauerland EK, Mizuno N. Hypoglossal nerve afferents: elicitation of a polysynaptic hypoglosso-laryngeal reflex. Brain Res 1968; 10:256–258.
245. Sessle BJ, Greenwood LF. Inputs to trigeminal brainstem neurones from facial, oral, tooth pulp, and pharyngolaryngeal tissues: I. Responses to innocuous and noxious stimuli. Brain Res 1976; 117:211–226.
246. Mårtensson A. Proprioceptive impulse patterns during contraction of intrinsic laryngeal muscles. Acta Physiol Scand 1964; 62:176–194.

247. Suzuki M, Kirchner JA. Afferent nerve fibers in the external branch of the superior laryngeal nerve in the cat. Ann Otol Rhinol Laryngol 1968; 77:1059–1070.
248. Suzuki M, Kirchner JA. Sensory fibers in the recurrent laryngeal nerve. Ann Otol Rhinol 1969; 78:21–31.
249. Car A, Jean A, Roman C. A pontine primary relay for ascending projections of the superior laryngeal nerve. Exp Brain Res 1975; 22:197–210.
250. Norgren R. Projections from the nucleus of the solitary tract in the rat. Neuroscience 1978; 3:207–218.
251. Cohen MI. Neurogenesis of respiratory rhythm in the mammal. Physiol Rev 1979; 59:1105–1173.
252. Cohen MI. Central determinants of respiratory rhythm. Ann Rev Physiol 1981; 43:91–104.
253. von Euler C. The functional organization of the respiratory phase switching mechanisms. Fed Proc 1977; 36:2375–2380.
254. von Euler C. Some aspects of speech breathing physiology. In: Grillner S, Lindblom B, eds. Speech motor control. Oxford: Pergamon Press, 1981:95.
255. Dow RS, Moruzzi G. The physiology and pathology of the cerebellum. Minneapolis: University of Minnesota Press, 1958.
256. Zentay PJ. Motor disorders of the central nervous system and their significance for speech. Part I. Cerebral and cerebellar dysarthrias. Laryngoscope 1937; 47:147–156.
257. Sears TA. Pathways of supra-spinal origin regulating the activity of respiratory motoneurons. In: Granit R, ed. Muscular afferents and motor control. Stockholm: Almquist and Wiksell, 1966:187.
258. Campbell EJM, Agonstini E, Newsom Davis J. The respiratory muscles. London: Lloyd-Luke, 1970.
259. Plum F. Cerebral control of breathing. In: Wyke B, ed. Ventilatory and phonatory control systems. London: Oxford University Press, 1974:208.
260. Cohen MI. Activity of respiratory control neurons in the brainstem. In: Wyke B, ed. Ventilatory and phonatory control systems. London: Oxford University Press, 1974:188.
261. Bratzlavsky M. Reflexes with intraoral afferents in human lip musculature. Exp Neurol 1972; 37:179–187.
262. Porter R. The synaptic basis of a bilateral lingual-hypoglossal reflex in cats. J Physiol 1967; 190:611–627.
263. Yamamoto T. Linguo-hypoglossal reflex: effects of mechanical, thermal, and taste stimuli. Brain Res 1975; 92:499–504.
264. Garrison DW. Cranial nerves: a systems approach. Springfield: CC Thomas, 1986.
265. Mathers, LH. The peripheral nervous system: structure, function and clinical correlations. Menlo Park: Addison-Wesley, 1985.
266. Vij S, Kanagasuntheram R, Krishnamurti A. Sensory nerve terminations in the oral tissues of some pongidae. Folia Primatol (Basel) 1973; 20:312–320.
267. Dubner R, Sumino R, Starkman S. Responses of facial cutaneous thermosensitive and mechanosensitive afferent fibers in the monkey to noxious heat stimulation. Adv Neurol 1974; 4:61–71.
268. Sakada S. Response of Golgi-Mazzoni corpuscles in the cat periostea to mechanical stimuli. In: Dubner R, Kawamura Y, eds. Oral-facial sensory and motor mechanisms. New York: Appleton-Century-Crofts, 1971:105.
269. Bowden R, Mahran Z. The functional significance of innervation of the muscle quadratus labii superioris of the rabbit, cat, and rat. J Anat 1956; 90:217–227.
270. Folkins JW, Larson CR. In search of a tonic vibration reflex in the human lip. Brain Res 1978; 151:409–412.
271. Hosokawa H. Proprioceptive innervation of striated muscles in the territory of cranial nerve. Tex Repr Biol Med 1961; 19:405–464.
272. Larson CR, Folkins JW, McClean MD, Muller E. Sensitivity of the human perioral reflex to parameters of mechanical stretch. Brain Res 1978; 146:159–164.
273. Kubota K, Masegi T. Oral sensory and proprioceptive innervation in the squirrel monkey. In: Proceedings of the third conference on experimental medical surgery in primates, Part II. Basel: Karger, 1972:182.
274. Lund JP, Richmond FJR, Touloumis C, Patry Y, Lamarre Y. The distribution of Golgi tendon organs and muscle spindles in masseter and temporalis muscles of the cat. Neuroscience 1978; 3:259–270.
275. Goodwin GM, Luschei ES. Discharge of spindle afferents from jaw closing muscles during chewing in alert monkeys. J Neurophysiol 1975; 38:560–571.
276. Harrison F, Corbin KB. The central pathway for the jaw jerk. Am J Physiol 1942; 135:439–445.
277. Lamarre Y, Lund JP. Load compensation in human masseter muscles. J Physiol 1975; 253:21–35.
278. Kawamura Y, Hamada T. Studies on morphology and functions of Golgi tendon organ of masticatory muscle in cat. Bull Tokyo Med Dent Univ [Suppl] 1974; 21:7–10.
279. Hufschmidt HJ, Spuler H. Mono- and polysynaptic reflex of the trigeminal muscles in human beings. J Neurol Neurosurg Psychiatr 1962; 25:332–335.
280. Kawamura Y, Abe K. Role of sensory information from temporomandibular joint. Bull Tokyo Med Dent Univ 1974; 21:78–82.
281. Marlow CD, Winkelmann RK, Gibilisco JA. General sensory innervation of the human tongue. Anat Rec 1965; 152:503–512.
282. Warwick R, Williams PL, eds. Gray's anatomy. 35th Br ed. Philadelphia: WB Saunders, 1973.
283. Larson C, Sutton D, Lindemann RC. Muscle spindles in nonhuman primate laryngeal muscles. Folia Primatol (Basel) 1974; 22:315–323.
284. Lucas-Keene MF. Muscle spindles in human laryngeal muscles. J Anat 1961; 95:25–29.
285. Paulsen K. Über Vorkommen und Zahl von Muskelspindeln in inneren Kehlkopfmuskeln des Menschen (*M. cricoarytenoideus dorsalis, M. cricothyroideus*). Z Zellforsch 1958; 48:349–355.
286. Konig WF, von Leden H. The peripheral nervous system of the human larynx. Arch Otolaryngol 1961; 73:21–34.
287. Sessle BJ. Presynaptic excitability changes induced in single laryngeal primary afferent fibers. Brain Res 1973; 53:333–342.
288. Cooper S. Muscle spindles in intrinsic muscles of human tongue. J Physiol 1953; 122:193–202.
289. Riley HA. An atlas of the basal ganglia, brainstem and spinal cord based on myelin-stained material. New York: Hafner, 1960.
290. Villiger ME. Brain and spinal cord. Translated by GA Piersol. Philadelphia: JB Lippincott, 1912.
291. Strominger NL. The origins, course, and distribution of the dorsal and intermediate acoustic striae in the rhesus monkey. J Comp Neurol 1973; 147:209–234.
292. Strominger NL, Strominger Al. Ascending brainstem projections of the anteroventral cochlea nucleus in the rhesus monkey. J Comp Neurol 1971; 143:217–242.
293. Knight PL. Representation of the cochlea within the anterior auditory field (AAF) of the cat. Brain Res 1977; 130:447–467.
294. Reale RA, Imig TJ. Tonotopic organization in auditory cortex of the cat. J Comp Neurol 1980; 192:265–292.
295. Clarey JC. Irvine DRF. Auditory response properties of neurons in the anterior ectosylvian sulcus of the cat. Brain Res 1986; 386:12–19.
296. Penfield W, Rasmussen T. The cerebral cortex of man. New York: Hafner, 1968.
297. Graybiel AM, Ragsdale CW Jr. Fiber connections of the basal ganglia. Prog Brain Res 1979; 51:239–283.
298. Graybiel AM, Ragsdale CW Jr. Biochemical anatomy of the striatum. In: Emson PC, ed. Chemical neuroanatomy. New York: Raven Press, 1983:427.

4 Basic Neurophysiologic Mechanisms Underlying Oral Communication

Jesse G. Kennedy III, Ph.D.

Within the last 20 years, scientists utilizing innovative investigative techniques have examined the physiologic aspects of the complex process of human communication with unprecedented detail and sophistication, accumulating a storehouse of information that is expanding at never-before-seen rates. As this data base expands, it becomes increasingly apparent that the ability to understand and utilize its information critically depends on a working knowledge of the basic mechanisms of the nervous system. The ability to tap into this data base is crucial both for the scientist interested primarily in research and for the modern clinician faced daily with subtly varying profiles of abnormally functioning systems.

It is the intent in this chapter to provide a cursory overview of basic neurophysiologic mechanisms, providing key concepts that may form the basis of further, more detailed study. An initial concept is concerned with identification of the basic functional unit of the nervous system, an issue that was surrounded by controversy for many years.[1,2]

In the late 1800s, the controversy surrounding the identification of the basic unit of the nervous system led to the formation of two opposing schools of thought. One school, influenced largely by Hans Held and Camillo Golgi, maintained that the axon membrane of one neuron directly contacted and pierced the membrane of another, thereby allowing both neurons to share a common cytoplasm.[3] By sharing a common cytoplasm, the entire nervous system became a continuous network or reticulum, a system devoid of intervening membrane barriers. This view of the organization of the nervous system as a continuous network became known as the "syncytium" or "continuity" theory. The opposing school, influenced mainly by Ramon y Cajal and contemporaries such as Sherrington, Forel, and His, maintained that although the neurons came in close proximity, they were physically isolated and did not share a common cytoplasm; instead, each neuron acted as an independent, autonomous unit.[3] This view of the organization of the nervous system as composed of individual neurons became known as the "neuronal" or "contact" theory. The ideas of the neuron theorists were summarized by Waldeyer in 1891 and provided the basis for delineation of the neuron doctrine,[2] a declaration of classic principles of the organization of the nervous system, stating that (1) each neuron is an independent outgrowth from a single primitive neural cell (a neuroblast); (2) neurons have a certain polarity, with information entering through the dendrites and the soma and exiting through the axon; (3) neurons are the basic functional units of the nervous system; and (4) neurons demonstrate physiologic and functional specificity. The controversy between the syncytium theorists and the neuron theorists was based on evidence derived from light microscopy and had to wait for the invention of the electron microscope before it was finally resolved in favor of Cajal's neuron theories.[4]

The identification of the neuron as the basic structural unit provides a logical point of entry for this study of the neurophysiology of a system as complex as the human nervous system. The discussion will begin with the physiology of a single neuron and culminate with the physiology of groups of neurons as they interact in a most basic unit of behavior: a reflex. In completing this task, a number of topics will be discussed including:

1. The basic unit of the nervous system: the neuron.
2. Fundamental neuronal integration: the synapse.
3. Principles of grouped neuron interactions.
4. The input to the system: sensory mechanisms.
5. The output of the system: motor mechanisms.
6. Interactions between system input and output: reflexes.

THE NEURON

The central nervous system is estimated to be composed of more than 10^{11} neurons, each, according to the neuron doctrine, acting as an independent functional entity. Each of these neurons reflects many of the functions of the nervous system as a whole; each neuron is capable of receiving information from multiple sources and processing it into integrated units of information that may then be transmitted long distances throughout the body in order to coordinate the operation of other neurons. Indeed, in many ways each neuron is a complete nervous system in microcosm.

This discussion of the neuron will initially examine the structural aspects of a neuron, delineating in detail its differentially permeable membrane. The special qualities of the neuron as an excitable cell will then be examined in both the resting and the active states.

Basic Neuronal Morphology

We will briefly review the basic features and then concentrate on the one feature which has characteristics that underlie most fundamentals of neuronal function. The neuron consists of (1) a dendritic zone, which is specialized for reception of impulses and includes numerous cytoplasmic extensions called "dendrites" that profusely branch and taper to be covered with fine dendritic spines (gemmules) on their distal terminations; (2) a soma (neuronal cell body, perikaryon), which regulates many of the metabolic and cell support funtions of the neuron; and (3) an axon, longer, thinner, and of more uniform diameter than dendrites, which arises from the axon hillock of the soma and may be either myelinated or unmyelinated as it transmits neural information impulses and metabolic nutrients away from the soma and to the axon terminal end-plates (terminal buttons, end-feet, telodendria) at its most distal extension. The neuron is enclosed by a plasma membrane that is differentially permeable, that is, a membrane that selectively allows some materials to pass while blocking the passage of other materials as it regulates the exchange of matter between the ion-rich fluids inside the neuron and the ion-rich fluids in the surrounding environment. The cell membrane is capable of undergoing rapid changes in its electrical properties when appropriately stimulated, a characteristic that places neurons in the special subcategory of living cells called "excitable cells." This special membrane is capable of changing its characteristics in response to the reception of special chemical neurotransmitters at circumscribed membrane locations; it can propagate electrical impulses the length of its axons, and the axon terminal membrane can respond with the release of chemical neurotransmitters.[5]

Many types of neurons are found throughout the nervous system, each varying in size, shape, and the characteristics of their projections. This extensive variability has led to the creation of a number of classification schemes designed to create order in the neuronal chaos. Classification schemes have been based on function: sensory, motor, or associative (intercalary, interneurons). In addition, neurons have been functionally classified by their influence, as being either excitatory or inhibitory. Classification schemes have also been based on structure, grouping neurons by the length of their axons and so producing groups such as Golgi type I neurons with long axons and Golgi type II neurons with short axons. Further structural classification schemes are based on the number of processes (Table 4–1). In light of the predominant nature of the multipolar neurons, this discussion will concentrate on myelinated Golgi type I multipolar neurons as the model neuron, realizing that most of the neurophysiologic principles discussed apply to the entire complement of neurons within vertebrate nervous systems.

The neuron cell membrane is approximately 75 to 100 Å (7.5 to 10 nm) thick and is composed of three layers: an internal layer interposed between two surface layers (Fig. 4–1). The internal membrane layer is a bimolecular layer composed of lipid tissues. Lipids are organic substances such as fatty acids, natural fats, and waxes. The surface membrane layers are composed of various protein complexes. This chemical configuration forms an effective barrier separating the fluids outside the cell (extracellular, interstitial) from the fluids inside the cell (intracellular) and allows storage of electrical charges much like an electrical capacitor (with the lipid layer acting as the dielectric).

Considered as a continuous, uninterrupted barrier, this membrane configuration demonstrates the basis for some aspects of membrane differential permeability. This structure would allow any material that may be dissolved in lipids (lipid-soluble organic ions) to pass, whereas material that was not dissolved by lipids (water-soluble inorganic ions such as sodium [Na^+], potassium [K^+], and chloride [Cl^-])

TABLE 4–1 Characteristic Neuron Configurations

<table>
<tr><th>Type</th><th>Schematic Configuration</th><th>Characteristics</th></tr>
<tr><td>Unipolar
(Pseudounipolar)</td><td>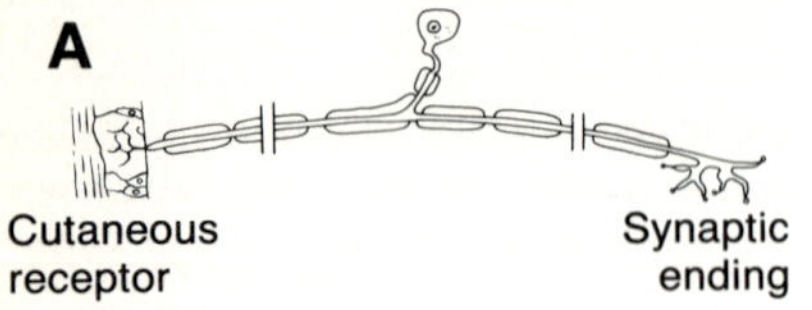
</td><td>Typically peripheral sensory receptor neurons found in the spinal ganglia and mesencephalic nucleus of the trigeminal nerve. Unipolar neurons are also found in the sensory ganglia of cranial nerves 5, 7, 9, and 10. These neurons are characterized by a single T-shaped process that may be divided into two parts: (1) a distal portion, which terminates in a sensory receptor, and (2) a proximal portion, which enters the central nervous system.</td></tr>
<tr><td>Bipolar</td><td>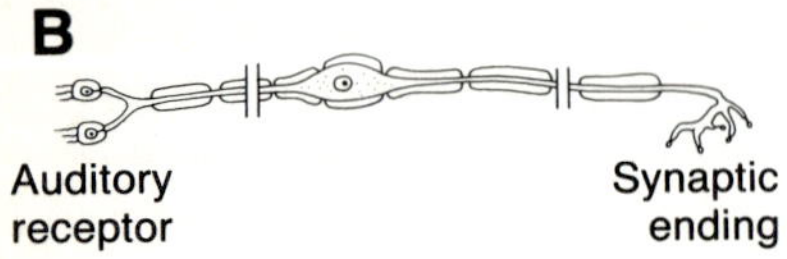
</td><td>Typically peripheral sensory receptor neurons that subserve audition and equilibrium in the cranial nervous system. These neurons have one dendrite and one axon.</td></tr>
<tr><td>Multipolar</td><td>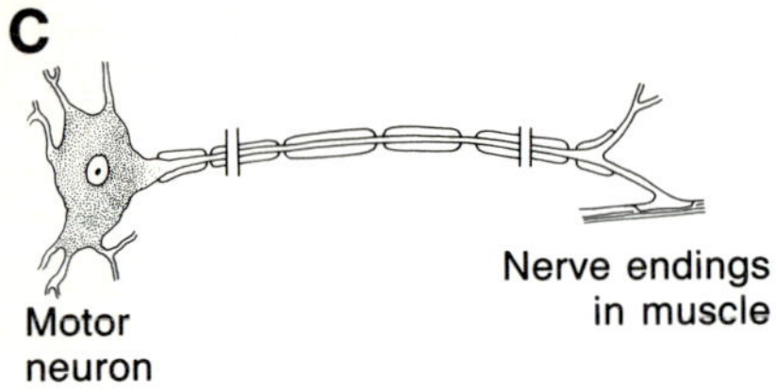

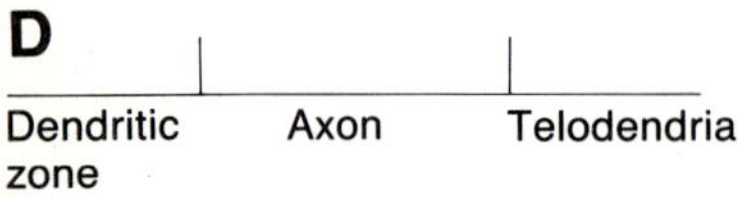
</td><td>The most numerous neuron form of the nervous system; these neurons have multiple dendrites and a single axon. They are observed in various specialized configurations.</td></tr>
</table>

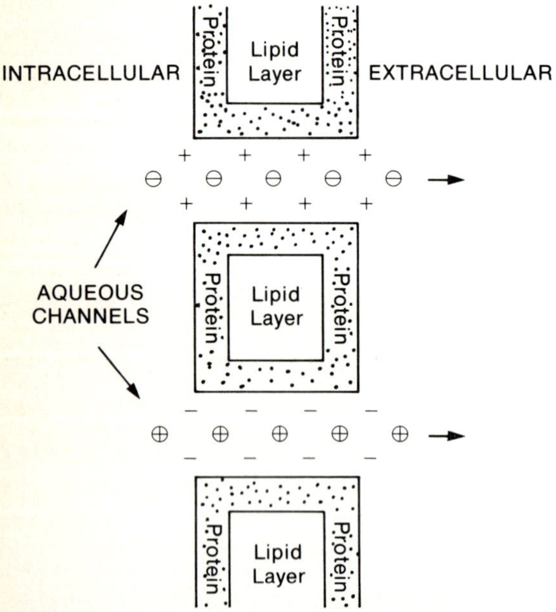

Figure 4–1 Schematic representation of a neuron membrane consisting of outer protein layers, an inner lipid layer, and aqueous channels for the transport of water-soluble substances. (After Eyzaguirre C, Fidone S. Physiology of the nervous system—an introductory text. 2nd ed. Chicago: Year Book Medical Publishers, 1975:8.)

could not pass through the membrane. However, as shown by radioactive tracing techniques, inorganic ions *do* pass through the membrane. The explanation of this apparent contradiction lies in the function of water-filled ion channels (pores) that interrupt the membrane continuity and selectively allow inorganic ions to penetrate. The effect of these ion channels is to make the membrane relatively impermeable to substances that must pass through the bimolecular layer (such as organic ions) and permeable to substances that pass through the ion channels (inorganic ions such as Na^+, Cl^-, and K^+). These channels demonstrate two operating characteristics: selectivity and gating. The selectivity of the channels is such that a single channel allows only one type of ion to pass through. Much like a key opening a lock, the gating mechanism of membrane channels regulates the opening of the channels by responding to either an electrical trigger or a chemical trigger (perhaps in the form of a neurotransmitter).[5]

The Resting Neuron

Many of the characteristics of resting cells may be revealed by utilization of a basic tool of the modern neurophysiologist, the microelectrode. A microelectrode (attached to a suitable display device) is carefully thrust through the cell membrane of a large neuron. Prior to penetration (when the electrode and its reference are in the same extracellular fluid), there is no electrical difference between the two, and the meter reads zero. As the microelectrode passes through the living cell membrane and into the intracellular fluid, the meter suddenly indicates −85 mv (actually, the magnitude depends on the type of cell, varying from −55 to −100 mv for nerve and skeletal muscle cells in warm-blooded animals).[6,7] This negative voltage indicates a potential electrical difference between the extracellular and intracellular environments as measured across the membrane; it is therefore labelled a "membrane potential," and, when it occurs in the resting cell, it is called a "resting potential." The origin of this electrical potential may be observed in the uneven distribution of positively charged ions (cations) on one surface of a membrane and negatively charged ions (anions) on the opposite surface. This condition allows the cell membrane to act as an electrical capacitor.

The explanation of the potential electrical difference across the cell membrane requires the description of two basic physiologic mechanisms that transport charged ions through membranes and that may thus lead to the imbalances that generate membrane potentials. The transport mechanisms include an *active* transport mechanism and a *passive* transport mechanism. The active transport mechanism is a chemical system located in the cell membrane that moves substances through the cell membrane much like a water pump; it may move fluids against a resistance such as gravity or osmotic pressure. In neurons, this active mechanism transports two to five Na^+ ions out of the neuron for each K^+ ion it brings in. In view of the ions it transports, this active mechanism is referred to as the sodium-potassium pump. On the other hand, the passive mechanism utilizes diffusion to transport ions through the membrane. Special characteristics of the membrane allow K^+ to diffuse through the membrane with ease, whereas Na^+ can diffuse only with difficulty. The effectiveness of the passive diffusion transport mechanism depends on differences in concentration of ions across the membrane (the concentration gradient) and differences in the electrical charge on the membrane (the electrical gradient). The magnitude of the membrane potential caused by these diffusional processes depends largely on the logarithmic relationship between the ion concentration inside a cell and the concentration outside the cell, a relationship described for single ions by the Nernst equation and for multiple ions by the Goldman (Goldman-Hodgkin-Katz) equation.[7] Both the sodium-potassium pump and ionic diffusion create and maintain imbalances in the ionic concentrations (and hence electrical charges) between the internal and external neuronal environments, imbalances that lead to the formation of the resting potential in a quiescent neuron.

The nature of the imbalances in ionic concentrations is schematically depicted in Figure 4–2. The principal ions involved include two cations, K^+ and Na^+, and two anions, Cl^- and large protein anions (A^-). The concentration differences for the individual ions may be observed readily. The concentration of positively charged K^+ ions *inside* the cell is approximately 40 times greater than that outside. Na^+ has an opposite concentration gradient, with positively charged ion concentrations approximately 12 times greater *outside* the cell than inside. The concentration of negatively charged Cl^- ions is roughly the reciprocal of K^+. Finally, negatively charged large A^- are locked in high concentration within the cell.[8]

By combining the ion transport mechanisms that produce and maintain the ion imbalances just described, a summary discussion of the mechanisms that contribute to the development of the resting potential may begin. Initially, in order to maintain ionic concentration, Na^+ is actively pumped out of the cell (to maintain its high concentration outside the cell), while simultaneously K^+ is actively pumped *into* the cell (to maintain its high concentration inside the cell). However, the sodium-potassium pump moves two to five Na^+ ions *out* for every K^+ ion *in,* resulting in more positive ions being transported *out* of the cell than are being pumped *into* the cell. The action of the ion pump is opposed by diffusion, with small amounts of Na^+ entering and K^+ readily exiting. As these mechanisms operate, high concentrations of large, nondiffusing, negatively charged A^- are trapped within the cell membrane. These

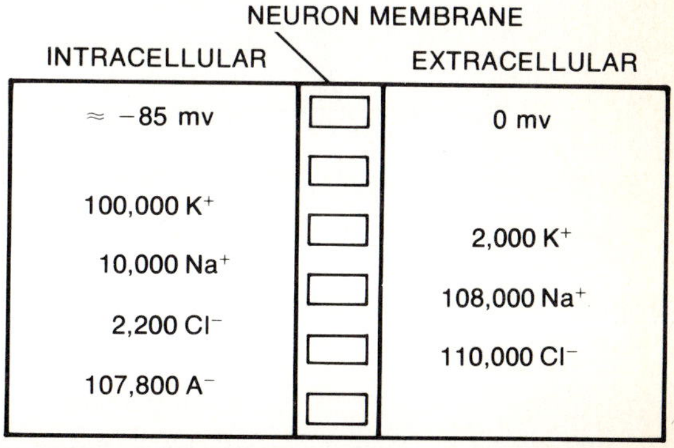

Figure 4–2 Chemical concentrations about a neuron membrane, demonstrating the number of ions in adjacent spaces 1μ × 1 μm × 1/1,000 μm. (After Schmidt R, ed. Fundamentals of neurophysiology. 2nd ed. New York: Springer-Verlag, 1978:22.)

conditions result in an excess of negative ions within the cell, which imparts a negative charge to the intracellular fluid, providing the genesis of the resting membrane potential.[4,9–11]

The Active Neuron

This brief discussion of the origin of the resting potential has indicated a number of basic principles characteristic of nervous system function. Perhaps the preeminent principles include (1) the observation that the electrical activity that forms the basis of nervous system operation is due largely to the differential distribution of ionic fluids across cell membranes and (2) the fact that these ionic imbalances are maintained primarily through active processes (the sodium-potassium pump) and secondarily through the passive process of ionic diffusion. When the cell begins to work, however, there is a reversal in the order: the passive process of ionic diffusion becomes of major importance and active processes take on secondary importance.

The resting potential serves as a prerequisite for neural function, a long-term reference maintained at a constant level of about −85 mv unless something occurs to change the permeability of the cell membrane to sodium. If the cell membrane permeability is sufficiently changed, the neuron begins to work and an extremely rapid sequence of events begins, a sequence lasting approximately two-thousandths of a second, during which the membrane potential may change from its −85 mv resting potential to a positive potential approaching +45 mv. This rapid change in the membrane potential of the working neuron is called an "action potential" (Fig. 4–3).

The events leading to the action potential involve changes in membrane permeability that lead to depolarization of the cell membrane potential. Dilation of the membrane channels for Na^+ produces a change in the permeability (conductance) of the membrane to Na^+ ions (the channels may be opened by electrical stimulation, application of chemicals, or mechanical damage), which, in turn, allows Na^+ ions to diffuse through the membrane. Because of the high extracellular and low intracellular concentrations of Na^+ ions, the ions flow *into* the cell, adding positive charges to the cell and making its −85 mv potential less negative (depolarization). If the membrane potential depolarizes to approximately −45 mv (a threshold value), the cell membrane charge becomes unstable and the rapid, all-or-none events of an action potential begin and continue in four discernible stages.[12] The first stage of the action potential is the opening of Na^+ channels, which creates a massive (perhaps 5,000-fold) increase in membrane conductance to Na^+. Because of the high extracellular Na^+ concentration, positive ions flow in, not only effectively neutralizing the normal electronegativity, but also reversing the polarity of the membrane to a reversal potential as high as +45 mv (which approaches the equilibrium constant for Na^+). The second event occurs after ap-

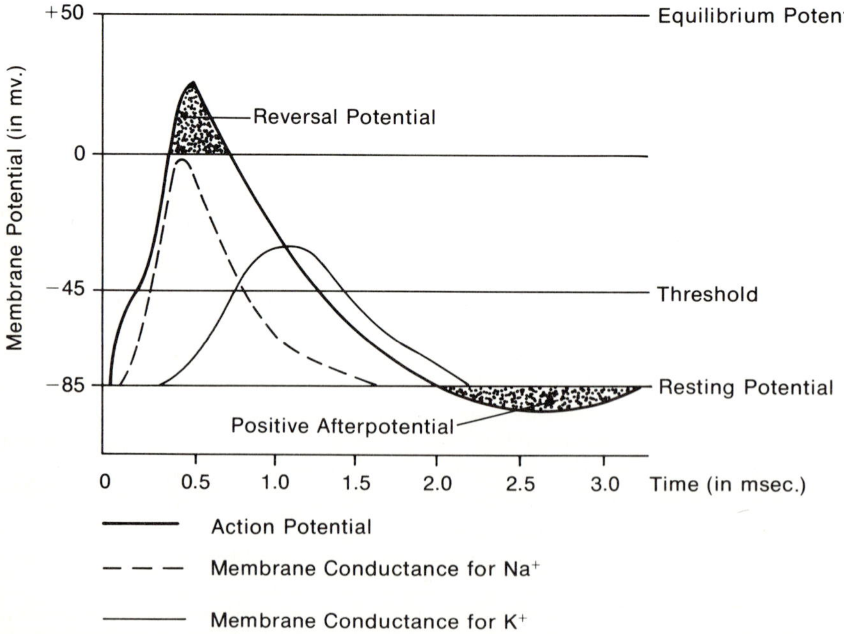

Figure 4–3 Schematic representation of an action potential and the changes in membrane conductance that occur. (After Eyzaguirre C, Fidone S. Physiology of the nervous system—an introductory text. 2nd ed. Chicago: Year Book Medical Publishers, 1975:18.)

proximately 0.5 msec and consists of a rapid increase in K^+ conductance as the Na^+ conductance returns to normal. The increase in K^+ conductance allows large numbers of positive K^+ ions to flow *out* of the cell along their concentration gradient, returning the membrane to its normal resting electronegativity. The K^+ ion conductance then returns to normal levels as the third event. The final stage of the action potential occurs as Na^+ is actively transported out of the cell, while K^+ is both actively and passively transported into the cell, thereby restoring the neuron to its normal resting state.[13,14]

Propagation of the Action Potential

The previous discussion has described the basis of excitation of the cell membrane. This section will discuss the actual task of the neuron and the muscle membrane: the propagation of electrical excitation.

Action potentials arise at the axon hillock of the nerve membrane and propagate toward both ends of the neuron membrane. The speed at which the wave of depolarization traverses the neural membrane (conduction velocity) depends on (1) fiber diameter (large nerves conduct faster than small nerves), (2) nerve temperature (warm nerves conduct faster than cold nerves), and (3) the presence or absence of insulating myelin. The presence or absence of myelin determines the mode of propagation of the neural impulse. Membranes without myelin transmit impulses via local circuit propagation. Myelinated neurons propagate impulses by saltatory propagation. Figure 4–4*A* demonstrates the characteristics of local circuit propagation in unmyelinated nerves. A distinctive feature is manifested in the eddy currents that occur in the leading edge of the wave of depolarization of the action potential. The eddy currents depolarize the adjacent segment, which, in turn, excites the next segment without a decrease in the amplitude of the neural impulse, electrotonically spreading the impulse to the termination of the membrane. Saltatory conduction in myelinated nerves is depicted in Figure 4–4*B*. A key to the understanding of saltatory conduction is that myelin (with high electrical resistance) does not run continuously along an axon; there are circumscribed unmyelinated areas, nodes of Ranvier. Membrane depolarization occurs only at the unmyelinated nodes, because of their low electrical resistance, and propagates down the membrane, rapidly "leaping" over the myelinated internodes.[12,15,16] The depolarization of the membrane occurs at widely spaced intervals; therefore saltatory propagation produces much higher conduction velocities than local circuit propagation, achieving velocities as high as 100 m per second (Table 4–2).

Characteristics of Excitation

Excitation describes the process by which action potentials are elicited. A number of factors describe the efficiency of the excitation process: accommodation, the excitability curve, and refractoriness.[6,17]

If a stimulus is applied to a nerve fiber and its magnitude is increased slowly, the voltage necessary to exceed threshold (and thereby elicit an action potential) increases. In this condition, the nerve has

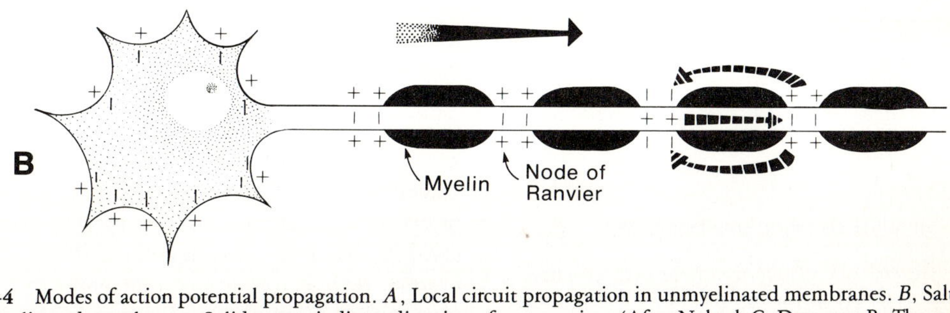

Figure 4–4 Modes of action potential propagation. *A*, Local circuit propagation in unmyelinated membranes. *B*, Saltatory propagation in myelinated membranes. Solid arrows indicate direction of propagation. (After Noback C, Demarest R. The nervous system—introduction and review. New York: McGraw-Hill, 1972:20.)

TABLE 4–2 Nerve Conduction Velocities

Erlanger/ Gasser Fiber Type		*Lloyd/Hunt Fiber Type*	*Function*	*Fiber Diameter (μm)*		*Conduction Velocity (m/sec)*	
A	α	Ia	Primary muscle spindle afferents (annulospiral endings), motor to skeletal muscles	12–20	(15)	70–120	(100)
	α	Ib	Golgi tendon organ afferents	12–20	(15)	70–120	(100)
	β	II	Secondary muscle spindle afferents (flower-spray), touch and pressure afferents	5–12	(8)	30–70	(50)
	γ	II	Efferent to muscle spindles	3–6	(5)	15–30	(20)
	δ	III	Cutaneous pain, temperature, and touch afferents, deep pressure in muscle	2–5	(3)	12–30	(15)
B		—	Preganglionic sympathetics	<3	(3)	3–15	(7)
C	dr	IV	Unmyelinated pain fibers	0.4–1.2	(0.5)	0.5–2	(1)
S		—	Postganglionic sympathetics	0.3–1.3	(0.5)	0.7–2.3	(1)

Abbreviations: dr = dorsal root fibers; S = sympathetic C fibers.
Figures in parentheses indicate average conduction velocities.

become accommodated to the increasing stimulus.[18] Accommodation may become so severe that it is impossible for the neuron to reach threshold.

In order for a stimulus to be effective in eliciting an action potential, it must fulfill certain amplitude and duration characteristics. Figure 4–5 relates these characteristics in the excitability curve (strength-duration curve).[7] As indicated, the duration of a stimulus is approximately inversely proportional to the amplitude needed to exceed threshold. For example, as the duration of a stimulus decreases, its amplitude must increase in order to effectively trigger an action potential.

Immediately following the reversal potential, a period of time occurs during which the membrane remains depolarized. During this time, the membrane is inexcitable; that is, it is difficult or impossible for a second stimulus to elicit an action potential. When this condition occurs, the nerve is said to be in its refractory period.[17] The initial stage of the refractory period is characterized by total inactivation of the Na^+ carrier mechanism, completely blocking the production of an action potential; therefore this stage is labelled the "absolute refractory period." The absolute refractory period constitutes the minimal time between action potentials and therefore provides an index of the maximum firing rate of a neuron. For example, a neuron with an absolute refractory period of 1 msec has a maximum firing rate of 1,000 Hz. Following the absolute refractory period, there is a period of only partial Na^+ inactivation during which a second action potential may be elicited with difficulty; this stage is called the "partial refractory period."

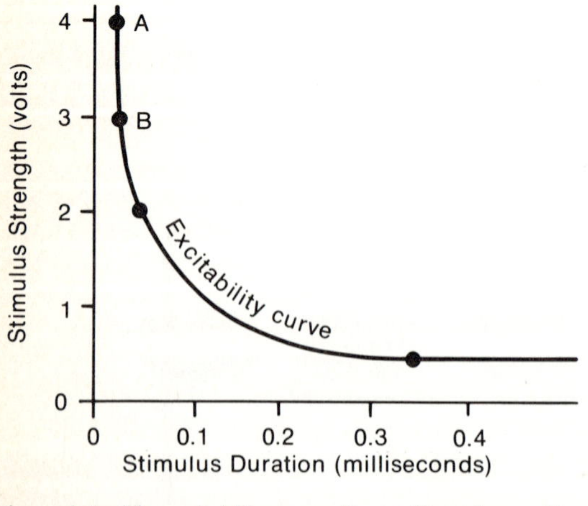

Figure 4–5 The excitability curve of a myelinated nerve fiber. (After Guyton A. Organ physiology—structure and function of the nervous system. 2nd ed. Philadelphia: WB Saunders, 1976:20.)

THE SYNAPSE

The discussion thus far has concentrated on the neuron as the basic functional unit of the nervous system; yet seldom does the excitation of a single neuron produce a desired response. Instead, the nervous system accomplishes its work through the interactions of large groups of neurons. Essential to the grouped neuron interactions of the nervous system is the interface between two neurons or between a neuron and a muscle.[17,19,20] This interface was labelled the "synapse" by Sir Charles Sherrington.[21,22] The functional significance of the synapse is manifested in its role as an integrator; the synapse takes multiple excitatory and inhibitory influences and averages their effects, thereby regulating transmission of neural information. The synapse has been implicated in the most complex of nervous system behaviors, such as learning and memory. In the study of synapses, examination of not only the structure and function of a single synapse occurring between two neurons (as characteristic of the central nervous system) but also the synapses that occur between neurons and muscles (as characteristic of the peripheral nervous system) is necessary.

Central Nervous System Synapses: Neuron to Neuron

Two basic types of synaptic transmission have been observed and labelled, by virtue of the synaptic stimulus, as either "electrical" (electronic) or "chemical" synapses.[18] At electrical synapses, the neuronal membranes are in direct juxtaposition, allowing electrical activity to produce bidirectional neuronal transmission. However, chemical synapses have an extracellular space between neurons and rely on chemicals called "neurotransmitters" for unidirectional, orthodromic neural transmission. Electrical synapses have been primarily documented in invertebrates, and much of their role in the vertebrate nervous system is yet to be discovered. The most widely studied vertebrate synapse is the chemical synapse; therefore discussion will concentrate on chemical synaptic mechanisms.[17]

A neuron-to-neuron synapse may occur between (1) axon and dendrite (axodendritic), (2) axon and soma (axosomatic), or (3) axon and axon (axoaxonal). The basic structures of a central synapse are shown in Figure 4–6. The presynaptic terminal (terminal knobs, boutons terminaux) houses two major structures within its membrane: mitochondria (which provide chemicals necessary for the synthesis of neurotransmitters) and synaptic vesicles (which contain specific amounts, or quanta, of neurotransmitters).

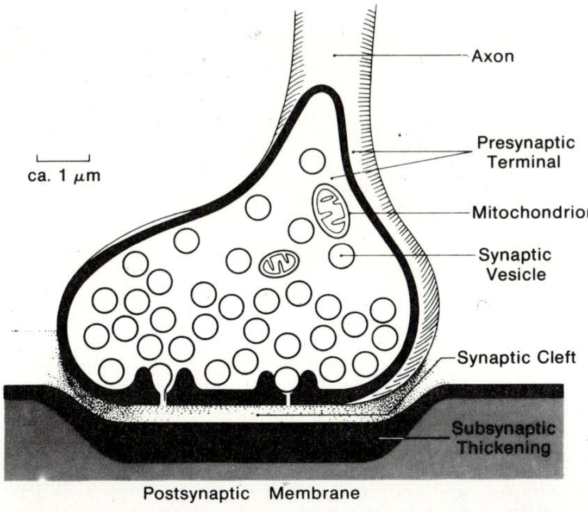

Figure 4–6 A schematic representation of a neuron-to-neuron chemical synapse as found in the central nervous system. (After Schmidt R, ed. Fundamentals of neurophysiology. 2nd ed. New York: Springer-Verlag, 1978:73.)

The presynaptic terminal membrane is separated from its receptor membrane by a synaptic cleft, 200 to 300 Å (20 to 30 nm) wide filled with as yet undescribed fibrous materials. The synaptic cleft separates the presynaptic membrane from the membrane to which the neural impulse is being transmitted, the subsynaptic portion of the postsynaptic membrane, which may be characterized by an area of membrane thickening.

The sequence of events involved in synaptic transmission begins with the nerve impulse surrounding the presynaptic terminal, producing membrane depolarization. The depolarization opens voltage-gated channels in the membrane and creates a brief increase in the concentration of positive ions within the presynaptic terminal. This transient increase in intracellular positive charges leads the synaptic vesicles to attach to the presynaptic membrane. The fused synaptic vesicles then discharge their quanta of neurotransmitters through the cell membrane into the synaptic cleft (exocytosis) and are quickly reclaimed to be refilled with neurotransmitters.[8] The released neurotransmitters rapidly cross the synaptic cleft to attach to chemically gated channels on the postsynaptic membrane, and much as a key opens the lock on a door, they effectively open the membrane channels. The resulting local, nonpropagated change in the postsynaptic membrane potential depends on the ion selectivity of the opened channels. If channels are opened that allow positively charged Na^+ ions to flow into the postsynaptic cell, the voltage change is in a positive (depolarizing) direction; this may, in turn, open more voltage-gated channels to allow greater flow of Na^+ ions, perhaps leading to the generation of an action potential. Such local, subthreshold depolarizing changes in the postsynaptic membrane are called "excitatory postsynaptic potentials" (EPSPs). If the opened membrane channels allow negatively charged ions (perhaps Cl^-) to flow into the cell, the net membrane potential changes in the negative (hyperpolarizing) direction, closing voltage-gated channels and opposing the generation of a nerve impulse in the postsynaptic nerve. This local hyperpolarizing potential change in the postsynaptic membrane is called an "inhibitory postsynaptic potential" (IPSP).

A single excitatory postsynaptic potential seldom leads to the generation of an action potential; the simultaneous activity of a number of EPSPs is necessary, all spreading electrotonically to the axon hillock in order to generate the action potential. As shown in Figure 4–7, the influences of multiple EPSPs combine in two ways in order to facilitate the creation of an action potential: temporally and spatially.[23] Temporal facilitation, as demonstrated in Figure 4–7*A*, consists of multiple successive

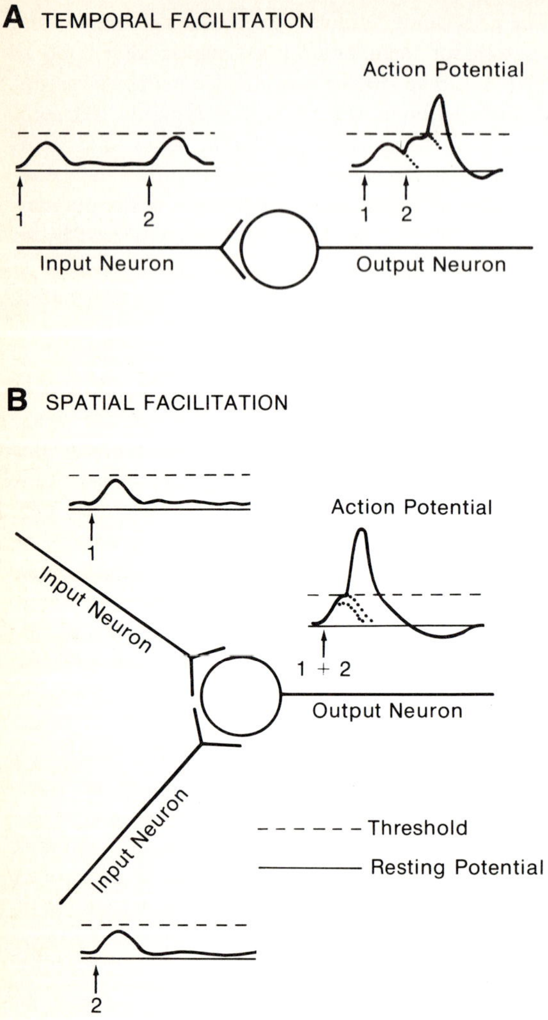

Figure 4–7 Facilitation. *A*, Temporal facilitation in which two subthreshold stimuli sum in time to create an action potential. *B*, Spatial facilitation in which two adjacent subthreshold stimuli sum to create an action potential. (After Schmidt R, ed. Fundamentals of neurophysiology. 2nd ed. New York: Springer-Verlag, 1978:109.)

subthreshold EPSPs, summing to exceed threshold because they occur in such rapid succession that before one EPSP fully decays another arrives, thus adding to the already existing depolarization. Figure 4–7*B* indicates the summation of two simultaneous subthreshold EPSPs due to the spatial proximity of their synapses, resulting in spatial facilitation.

In addition to the IPSP, a number of other synaptic mechanisms produce neuronal inhibition. For example, if the concentrations of K^+ and Cl^- ions are in exact equilibrium during the normal resting state of a neuron, then the opening of inhibitory membrane channels produces no outflow of positive ions. Without the outflow of positive ions, no IPSP is formed, yet inhibition occurs because the membrane is clamped at its resting potential. Another form of inhibition involves not the postsynaptic membrane, but the terminal end of an axon through a mechanism called presynaptic inhibition.[24,25] An example of presynaptic inhibition occurs when an inhibitory spinal interneuron synapses directly on an excitatory terminal end (Fig. 4–8). The inhibitory interneuron diffuses a neurotransmitter, partially depolarizing the excitatory terminal and decreasing the amount of excitatory neurotransmitter that the excitatory terminal may release; thus the interneuron effectively inhibits the normally excitatory synapse. Frequently observed as axoaxonal synapses, presynaptic inhibition has been observed in the peripheral sensory synapses and has been implicated in the process of sharpening the boundaries of sensory stimuli (contrast enhancement).[18]

Observation of the repetitive synaptic stimulation indicates two aspects of synaptic function that have significant consequences for nervous system function: synaptic fatigue and post-tetanic facilitation.[8] When a synapse is repetitively stimulated at a high rate, the discharge frequency of the postsynaptic neuron declines in synaptic fatigue. Synaptic fatigue functions to protect the nervous system from overstimulating itself. In this role, it has been implicated as a natural mechanism in subduing the excessive activity of an epileptic convulsion. If a synapse is repetitively stimulated for a period of time and then allowed to rest, the postsynaptic neuron becomes hypersensitive to stimuli, resulting in post-tetanic facilitation (post-tetanic potentiation), which may last for hours. Although the functional importance of post-tetanic facilitation is not yet understood fully, it is being investigated as a mechanism involved in learning and short-term memory. Significantly, long post-tetanic potentiations occur in a central nervous system structure highly involved in memory and learning: the hippocampus.

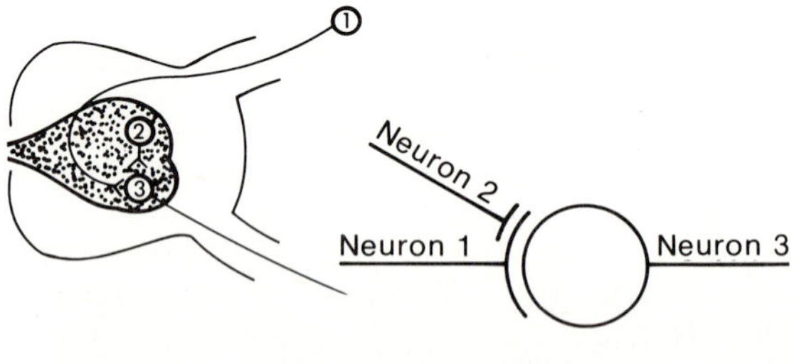

Figure 4–8 Presynaptic inhibition. Neuron 1 is presynaptic to neuron 3, and neuron 2 is presynaptic to neuron 1. If neuron 2 fires before neuron 1, the amount of neurotransmitter released by neuron 1 is reduced, with a consequent lowering of the amplitude of the EPSP elicited in neuron 3. (After Schmidt R, ed. Fundamentals of neurophysiology. 2nd ed. New York: Springer-Verlag, 1978:100.)

Peripheral Nervous System Synapses: Neuron to Muscle Fiber

In the periphery of the body, most synapses occur between a neuron and a muscle fiber; this synaptic configuration is called a "neuromuscular junction" (myoneural junction).[26] The morphology of neuromuscular junctions is shown in Figure 4–9. The presynaptic structure includes the motor end-plate, which invaginates the muscle fiber and is covered by insulating Schwann cells. The depression in which the end-plate resides is the synaptic gutter. Separating the end-plate from the muscle fiber, the synaptic cleft displays numerous folds of tissue that greatly increase the surface area on which neurotransmitters may act.

The events that occur at the peripheral neuromuscular junction are in many ways similar to those that occur at the central neuronal synapsè. In response to the depolarization of the presynaptic membrane by an action potential, quanta of neurotransmitters are released in the synaptic cleft. The action of the neurotransmitters on the subsynaptic membrane induces permeability changes that generate a membrane potential in the end-plate (Fig. 4–10). The potential generated is called the end-plate potential (EPP) and, like the EPSP of neuronal synapses, is local, may be graded in amplitude, and may be modified by the application of drugs. In contrast to the typically subthreshold EPSP, the EPP is normally suprathreshold, consistently leading to the generation of a propagated muscle action potential (MAP).[17,27]

Neurotransmitters of Synaptic Action

A key element in chemical synapses is the neurotransmitter. Unfortunately, relatively little is known about the characteristics or complement of neurotransmitters other than that each neuron secretes only one neurotransmitter according to Dale's principle.[28] However, some substances have been identified as excitatory neurotransmitters. Acetylcholine (ACh) has been identified confidently as an excitatory neurotransmitter at the peripheral neuromuscular junction and in autonomic ganglia. However, in central neuronal synapses, acetylcholine may sometimes function as an excitatory agent and at other times as an inhibitory agent. Other substances that appear to be excitatory agents in central nervous synapses include dopamine (acting as an adrenergic transmitter), norepinephrine, and serotonin. Two neural amino acids have been identified as apparent inhibitory neurotransmitters, gamma-aminobutyric acid (GABA) in the brain and glycine in the spinal cord.[29,30]

PRINCIPLES OF GROUPED NEURON INTERACTIONS

The function of the nervous system is to transmit and process information. The information is coded

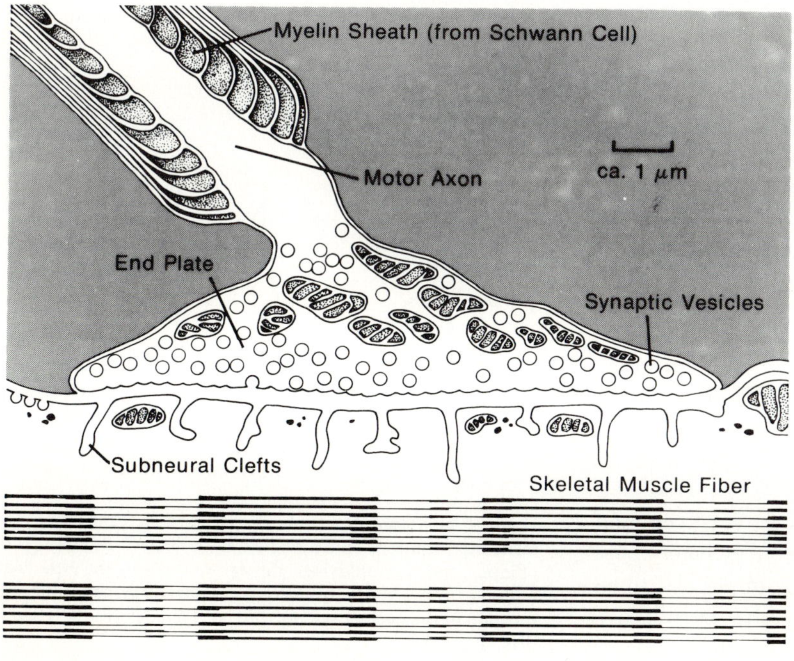

Figure 4–9 Schematic representation of a synapse between a neuron and a skeletal muscle fiber in the peripheral nervous system. (After Schmidt R, ed. Fundamentals of neurophysiology. 2nd ed. New York: Springer-Verlag, 1978:75.)

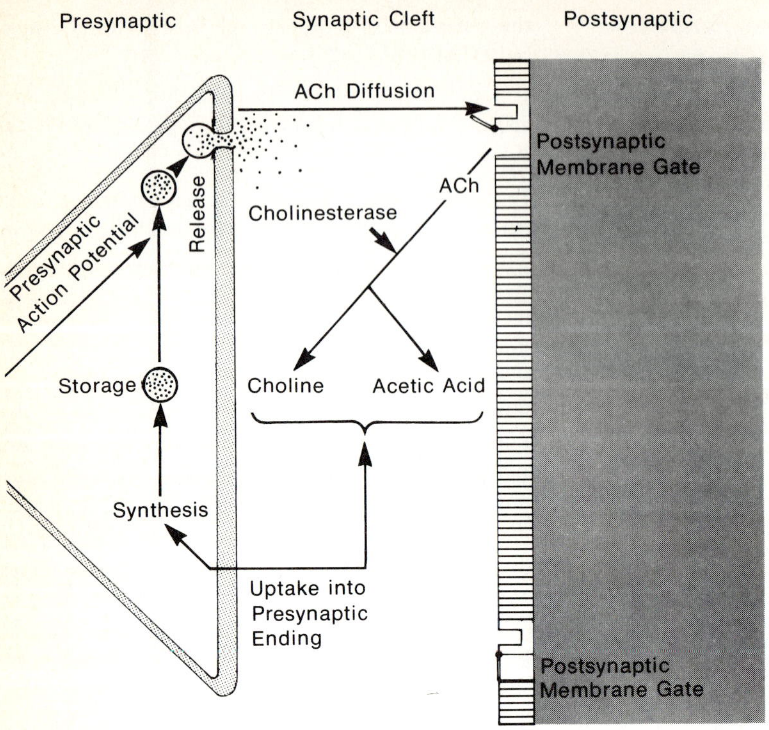

Figure 4–10 Chemical activity at a neuromuscular junction. (After Schmidt R, ed. Fundamentals of neurophysiology. 2nd ed. New York: Springer-Verlag, 1978:81.)

into individual, all-or-none neural impulses of constant amplitude and varying frequency. The transmission of information is encoded by varying the frequency of firing of neurons, leading to the characterization of the nervous system as a frequency modulated (FM) system.[7] It must be remembered that the functions of this system are carried out not by isolated neurons, but by complex groups of neurons combined into functional pools.[19,31]

Basic Organizational Principles

Convergence and divergence are perhaps the two most basic factors influencing information transfer in the nervous system. Figure 4–11*A* illustrates neuronal convergence, in which a single neuron is controlled by multiple, converging inputs. The multiple inputs may come from many different neurons or from a single source. An example of multiple source inputs is observed in the spinal interneuron, which receives inputs from (1) incoming sensory neurons, (2) intersegmental propriospinal tracts, and (3) descending upper motoneurons. The principle of convergence on motoneurons led Sherrington[21] to describe the lower motoneuron as the final common pathway on which all sensory, motor, excitatory, and inhibitory influences converge. Figure 4–11*B* illustrates the excitation of multiple pathways by a single neuron: divergence.

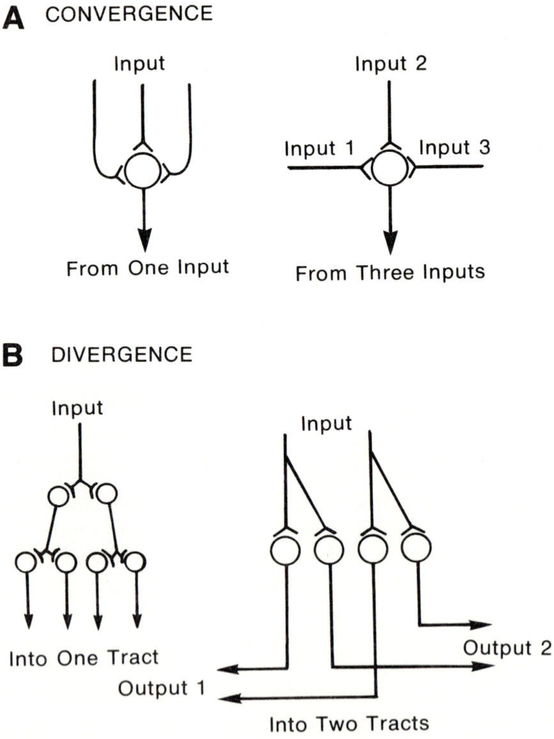

Figure 4–11 Multiple neuron interactions. *A*, Convergence of many input neurons onto a single output neuron. *B*, Divergence of input, either "amplifying" the signal or routing the input into multiple tracts. (After Guyton A. Organ physiology—structure and function of the nervous system. 2nd ed. Philadelphia: WB Saunders, 1976:77.)

Divergence may function to amplify the effect of a neural signal. Motoneurons present an example of divergent amplification in that a single neuron may innervate varying numbers of muscle fibers. The average divergence of a motoneuron can be calculated from the number of motoneurons entering a muscle: one neuron may innervate perhaps three muscle fibers in the precisely controlled perioral muscles, and, in the more powerful, less precisely controlled leg muscles, one neuron may innervate up to 1,900 muscle fibers.[10] Divergence may also function to provide information from one neuron to a number of different neuron tracts, as in sensory information that is relayed to many structures including the deep thalamic nuclei, specific areas of the cerebral cortex, and the cerebellum.

Spatial and temporal facilitation of single neurons has already been discussed, yet similar principles also apply to overlapping populations of neurons as demonstrated in Figure 4–12. Figure 4–12*A* demonstrates spatial facilitation in which the simultaneous excitation of two neurons may summate and excite a greater number of neurons than the firing of either neuron alone would cause. The phenomenon of occlusion is shown in Figure 4–12*B*. Occlusion occurs when the total response to multiple stimuli provides less excitation than the algebraic sum of the individual stimuli would produce.

Basic neuronal circuits exist that not only immediately modify neuron pools, as already discussed, but may also prolong the effects of stimulation, creating afterdischarge. The circuits involved in afterdischarge are shown in Figure 4–13. Figure 4–13*A* shows a parallel circuit, which may prolong neuronal discharge by multiple parallel paths of different delay.[32] Each parallel branch has a different number of synapses, each with a synaptic delay of approximately 0.5 msec. The varying number of synapses contributing to the transmission delays of each path slows each stimulus transmission by a different amount, causing each stimulus to arrive on the output neuron at slightly different intervals, thereby prolonging the neuronal discharge. Afterdischarge may also be initiated by reverberating neurons (Fig. 4–13*B*). The most basic reverberating circuit involves a neuron collateral that reflects back upon itself, forming a self-exciting positive feedback loop. The duration of reverberation in such a circuit depends on the resistance of each synapse to fatigue, with fatigue-resistant circuits reverberating for the longest time.

In addition to the excitatory circuitry discussed

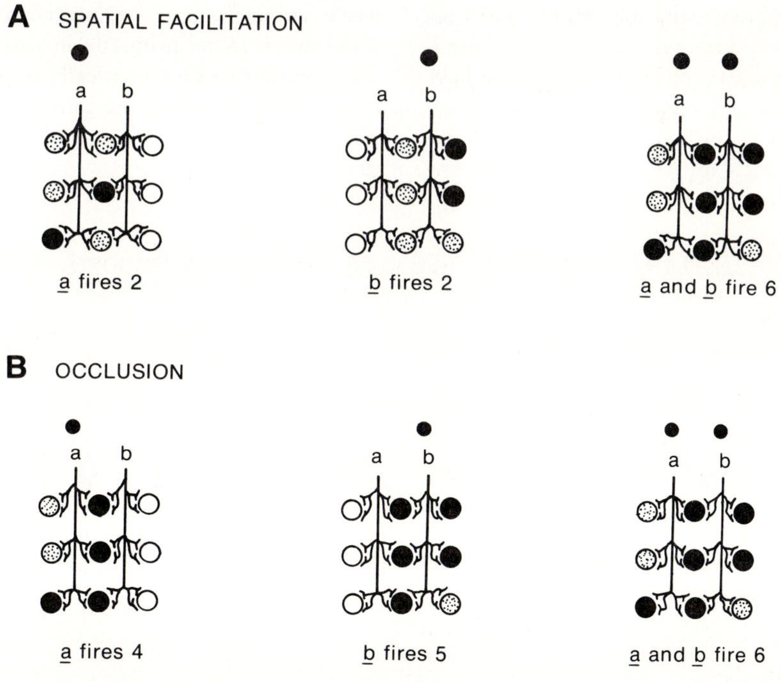

Figure 4–12 Facilitation and occlusion. *A*, Spatial facilitation occurs when simultaneous activation of both *a* and *b* produces a greater effect than the sum of excitation of either *a* or *b* activated alone. *B*, Occlusion occurs when simultaneous activation of both *a* and *b* produces a lesser effect than the sum of either *a* and *b* activated alone. Open circles = unexcited neurons; textured circles = subliminally excited neurons; closed circles = excited neurons. (After Schmidt R, ed. Fundamentals of neurophysiology. 2nd ed. New York: Springer-Verlag, 1978:110.)

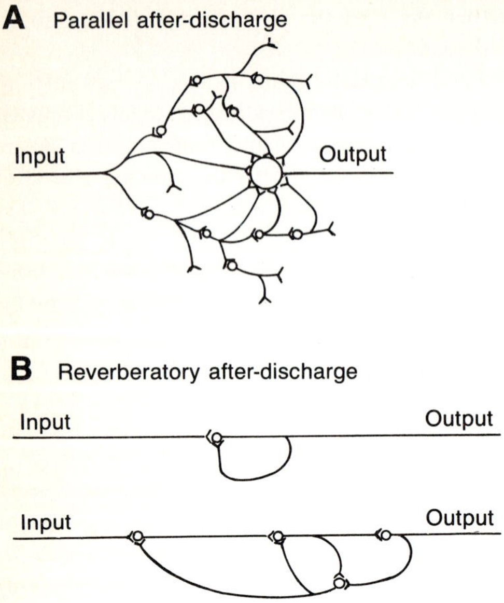

Figure 4-13 Neuron circuits capable of prolonging neuron discharge: *A*, parallel afterdischarge and, *B*, reverberatory afterdischarge. (After Guyton A. Organ physiology—structure and function of the nervous system. 2nd ed. Philadelphia: WB Saunders, 1976:80.)

previously, a number of neuronal circuits also exist that perform vital inhibitory functions, thus stabilizing the neuronal circuitry while protecting the nervous system from overexcitation. Figure 4–14 illustrates some basic inhibitory circuits of the central nervous system. As shown in Figure 4–14*A*, antagonist inhibition forms an inhibitory circuit common to the motor system.[25] Such a circuit might arise in the situation in which muscle spindles reflexively excite agonist muscles and inhibit antagonist muscles; hence an excitatory impulse to the flexor motoneuron inhibits the extensor motoneuron. When multiple parallel paths affect adjacent pathways (Fig. 4–14*A*), forward lateral inhibition occurs.[18] If, on the other hand, an inhibitory interneuron rejoins the original neuron at a more distant point, feedforward inhibition occurs. Feedforward inhibition is readily observed in the circuitry of the cerebellum. In both forward lateral and feedforward inhibition, the inhibitory stimulus arises from the input neuron.

Another inhibitory circuit of the central nervous system is shown in Figure 4–14*B*. In this circuit, the inhibitory interneurons reflect their influence back on the neural pathways by which they were stimulated. The inhibitory signals arise from motoneuron collaterals (within the spinal cord), which excite inhibitory interneurons in a negative feedback circuit, forming Renshaw inhibition.[24] This type of inhibition has been identified mainly in the ventral horns of the spinal cord and has yet to be functionally identified in the brain stem. Renshaw inhibition may be directed back to the cell of origin (feedback or self-inhibition) or may affect other cells (backward lateral inhibition).

Figure 4–14*C* indicates an inhibitory circuit that forms a special case of extensive backward lateral inhibition called "surround inhibition." This circuit utilizes collaterals to create an inhibited field, which surrounds an excited central core neuron. This inhibition is found primarily in sensory systems and may occur either presynaptically or postsynaptically, functionally increasing the contrast between the inhibited surround and the excited core in order to sharpen sensory input.

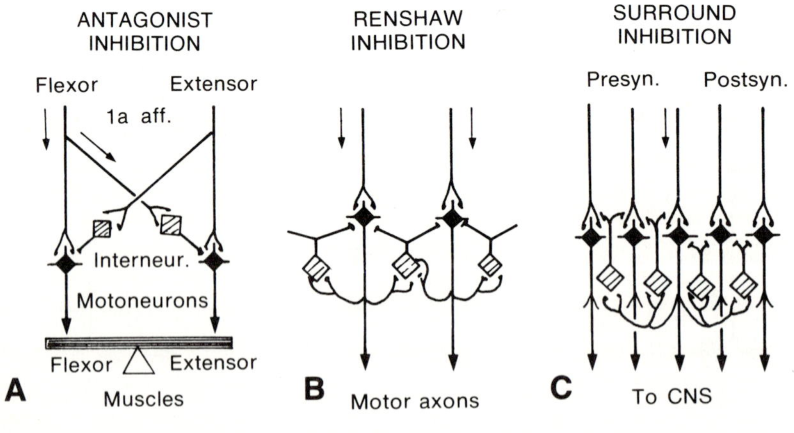

Figure 4-14 Inhibitory circuits. *A*, Antagonist inhibition in which an interneuron inhibits an antagonist motoneuron. *B*, Renshaw inhibition in which a motoneuron collateral activates an inhibitory interneuron, which reflects back upon the mononeuron of origin. *C*, Surround inhibition in which neuron collaterals activate an inhibitory interneuron, which inhibits surrounding neurons either pre- or postsynaptically. (After Schmidt R, ed. Fundamentals of neurophysiology. 2nd ed. New York: Springer-Verlag, 1978:112.)

THE SENSORY MECHANISM

In order for the body to maintain itself and interact with its surroundings, the nervous system requires a constantly updated stream of environmental information input to its processing center. The incoming information is changed (transduced) from its original modality (pressure, heat, light) into a neural impulse code by sensory receptors (sensory end-organs) and centripetally conducted to the processing centers along afferent neurons. The processing centers deal with environmental events that have already occurred, that is, past events, events delayed by at least the amount of transit time from the sensory receptors to the centers.[33,34]

Basic Characteristics

Multiple and diverse physiologic systems are coupled together to complete the communication process. The sensory receptors that provide input to the nervous system are as diverse as the systems they subserve. This discussion will concentrate on a group of receptors called "mechanoreceptors," which are capable of providing the nervous system with information on touch, movement, mechanical deformation of deep tissues, and hearing. Mechanoreceptors may be categorized further as being either encapsulated or unencapsulated, depending on the presence of a connective tissue covering. Basic characteristics of selected mechanoreceptors are provided in Table 4–3.

Although the sensory mechanism exhibits such great diversity, two general principles appear to apply to all receptors: differential sensitivity and adaptation. The concept of differential sensitivity originated in Johannes Muller's suggestion that different afferent nerves elicit different sensations because of "specific nerve energies." This statement proposes that a nerve fiber transmits only one modality of sensation regardless of how the nerve was stimulated.[35] The apparent reason for this theory lies in the observation that nerve tracts terminate at specific areas within the central nervous system, and the sensation felt is determined by the location of that termination.

Adaptation describes the response of nerves to continued stimulation.[8] Some receptors respond only to the application or removal of the stimulus. Receptors with this characteristic are considered to be rapidly adapting (rate, phasic, or movement) receptors. Other receptors continue to respond as long as the stimulus is applied. These receptors are considered to be slowly adapting (tonic) receptors. Rapidly adapting receptors, because of their movement sensitivities, are capable of providing a predictive function within the nervous system. The vestibular apparatus of the head provides an excellent example of the importance of the ability to predict the state of the body ahead of time. This apparatus is capable of indicating the velocity of head rotation as an individual turns a corner. By knowing the velocity of head movement, the nervous system can compute the number of degrees the body will turn in the next few seconds and consequently adjust the motion of the limbs to that future state, thereby avoiding the loss of balance.

Sensory Function

The basic function of the sensory mechanism is that of a transducer.[7] That is, the sensory mechanism functions to take energy in one form and to convert it into a form that may be used by the nervous system. For example, the unusable form might be pressure on the skin; the usable form is a coded series of nerve impulses with frequency characteristics that relate to the intensity of the pressure applied.

The process by which nerve endings fulfill their functions as transducers involves four stages. The first stage involves the application of an appropriate stimulus to a sensory end-organ, resulting in a change in the receptor membrane permeability. As a second state, this change in membrane permeability leads to a generator current within the receptor. The third stage occurs when the generator current induces a local membrane depolarization called the "generator potential" (receptor potential). The fourth stage occurs as the generator potential electrotonically spreads as a nonpropagating impulse, which, if suprathreshold, initiates a propagated action potential in the peripheral afferent fiber.

THE MOTOR APPARATUS

The output of the nervous system is directed at maintaining the internal environment of the body and acting upon the external environment. These activities are achieved largely through mechanical units capable of shortening and generating force in the form of muscles. The nervous system commands muscles to activate via centrifugal efferent pathways. As sensory mechanisms are involved in past events, the motor apparatus is involved in future events. Actual muscle contraction and structural movement lag behind the generation of the efferent motor command, creating a situation in which the motor commands

TABLE 4–3 Sensory Receptors: Mechanoreceptors

Type	*Location*	*Description*	*Innervation**	*Sensitivity*
Encapsulated Receptors				
Muscle spindle (neuromuscular spindle) 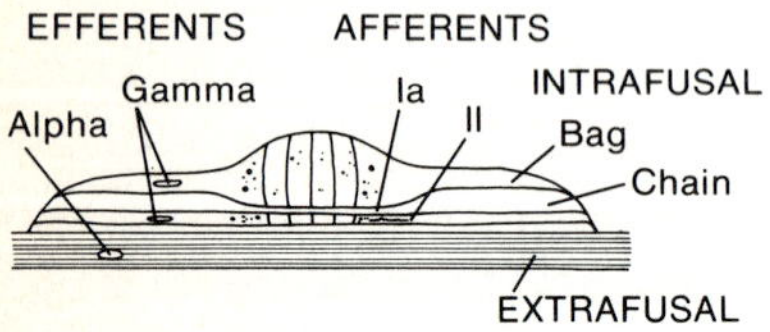	Muscles, often near musculotendinous junctions	Highly developed receptors connected in parallel to large extrafusal muscle fibers. Spindles consist of two types of small intrafusal muscle fibers: four to 11 uniform diameter nuclear chain fibers, and three to four nuclear bag fibers, which have a pronounced thickening halfway along their length.	Motor: Myelinated gamma motoneurons to intrafusal muscle fibers (15–30 m/sec) Sensory: Type Ia from the middle of both bag and chain fibers (70–120 m/sec) Type II from ends of most chain and some bag fibers (30–70 m/sec)	Muscle length, rate of change of muscle length (velocity of stretch)
Golgi tendon organs (neurotendinous endings) 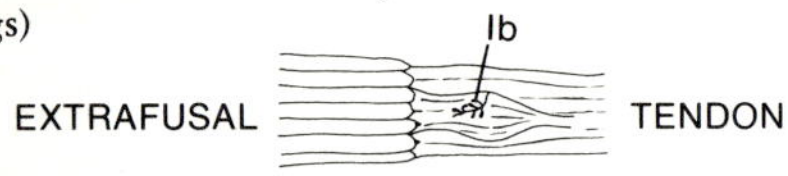	Muscle tendons and periosteum	Small tendon fascicles located in series with large extrafusal muscle fibers.	Type Ib myelinated sensory fibers (70–120 m/sec)	Muscle tension
Golgi type endings	Ligaments and joints	Large joint receptors, which resemble Golgi tendon organs.	Type II myelinated sensory fibers (30–70 m/sec)	Slowly adapting responses to the position of bones around a joint
Pacinian corpuscles 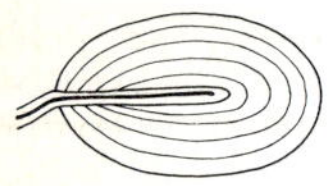	Deep skin and mucosa, connective tissue, periosteum, ligaments	The largest (3–4 mm in length) and most numerous encapsulated receptors, Pacinian corpuscles, have a single nerve fiber surrounded by a concentric laminated connective capsule that appears much like an onion.	Type II myelinated sensory fiber (30–70 m/sec)	Highly sensitive, rapidly adapting responses to vibration (150–300 Hz) and deep pressure
Golgi-Mazzoni corpuscles 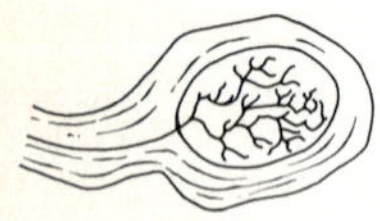	Fibrous capsules of joints, subcutaneous tissue, and tendon surfaces	Closely resemble small Pacinian corpuscles.	Type II myelinated sensory fiber (30–70 m/sec)	Rapidly adapting responses, signaling the velocity of joint movement, deep pressure, and tissue vibration
Ruffini end-organs 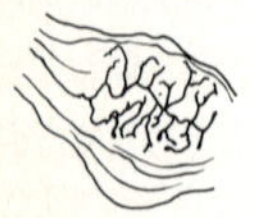	Joints, deep connective tissue, fascial sheaths	An oval end-organ formed by the extensive arborization of a myelinated nerve termination and surrounded by a connective tissue capsule.	Type II myelinated sensory fiber (30–70 m/sec)	Slowly adapting response to the direction and movement of joints, skin stretch, and indentation of the skin

TABLE 4–3 Continued

Type	*Location*	*Description*	*Innervation**	*Sensitivity*
Encapsulated Receptors				
Meissner's corpuscles (Meissner's tactile corpuscles)	Mucosa of tongue tip, alveolar ridge 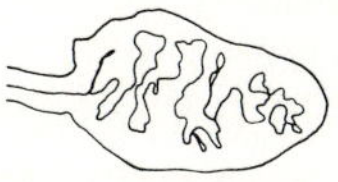	Small, oblong end-organs formed by the tangled looping of from one to four neurons.	Type II and perhaps Type III myelinated sensory fibers (12–70 m/sec)	Rapidly adapting tactile sensation subserving two-point discrimination
Krause end-bulbs (mucocutaneous end-organ)	Skin, synovial membranes of some joints, oral, labial, and lingual mucosa near mucocutaneous junction	Similar to Meissner's corpuscles, Krause end-bulbs have loops of unmyelinated fiber terminations forming a round ball.	Type III myelinated sensory fiber (12–30 m/sec)	Uncertain
Unencapsulated Receptors				
Merkel's discs 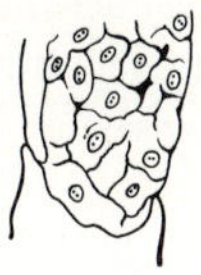	Deep skin layers, mucosa of alveolar ridge	Concave disc-like terminations of specialized epithelium found at the end of a branching nerve fiber. These may form "domes" in hairy skin or Merkel rete papilla in the alveolar ridge.	Type I myelinated sensory fiber (15–70 m/sec)	Slowly adapting tactile responses to vertical skin deformation
Free nerve endings 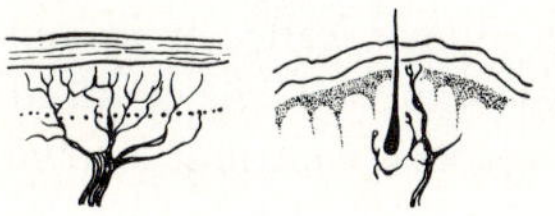	Mucosa, epidermis, muscle, connective tissue, and around the base of hair follicles	The most widely distributed nerve endings, this free form nerve ending is made up of fine neural fibrillae at the termination of neurons.	Small, myelinated or unmyelinated Type III and Type IV sensory fibers (0.5–30 m/sec)	Pain, temperature, diffuse touch, and hair movement

*Figures in parentheses represent the conduction velocity of the nerve in meters per second.

relate to events that have yet to occur.[6,17,36,37] Three conditions must be met for appropriate motor activity to occur: (1) information must be directed from sensory and motor cortices to appropriate motor neurons; (2) the nervous system must control the degree of contraction; and (3) contractions of many muscles must be coordinated.

Morphologic and Functional Characteristics

Histologically, there are three types of muscle: striated (somatic), unstriated (smooth, visceral), and cardiac. Of these three muscle types, this discussion will concentrate on striated muscles, which may be willfully controlled; they are classically considered voluntary muscles.

The structure of a striated skeletal muscle is shown in Figure 4–15. The fiber bundle illustrated is composed of numerous fibers, 10 to 80 μm in diameter, which generally run the full length of the muscle; the fibers terminate in collagenous connective tissue tendons. Each muscle fiber is innervated by a single motoneuron and contains several hundred contractile protein structures (myofibrils). Examination of a single myofibril indicates a number of cross-striations composed of alternating isotropic light bands (I bands) and anisotropic dark bands (A bands). In the middle of the I band is a dark strip called the "Z line" (Z disc). The area between two successive Z lines forms the functional unit of muscle contraction: the sarcomere. The light and dark bands of the myofibril are created by the overlapping of myofilaments. The A line is composed primarily of thick myosin myofilaments, which are overlapped by the ends of thin actin myofilaments. In the area of overlap, cross-bridges link both the actin

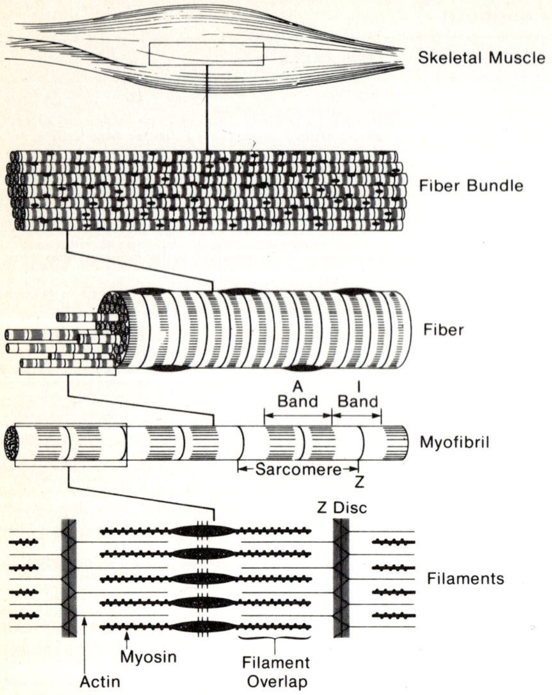

Figure 4-15 Schematic representations of the fine structure of skeletal muscle, increasing in detail from the whole muscle at the top to the muscle filaments at the bottom. (After Schmidt R, ed. Fundamentals of neurophysiology. 2nd ed. New York: Springer-Verlag, 1978:133.)

and myosin. The I line contains mainly actin myofilaments.

Muscle Contraction

Mechanism: Sliding Filament Theory

The generation of a suprathreshold EPP leads to the propagation of an all-or-none MAP both along the muscle surface and throughout the interior of the muscle fiber. This event leads to the contraction of the muscle (Fig. 4–16).

The resting muscle is shown in Figure 4–16*A*. In this state, the ends of two thin actin filaments overlap the ends of the thick myosin filament. Figure 4–16*B* illustrates the response of the muscle to depolarization. The configuration of the cross-bridges has changed, causing the thin actin filaments to slide past the myosin filaments (as indicated by the shortening of the I bands). This sliding mechanism draws the Z lines together, effectively shortening the sarcomere. The apparent sliding of the actin filaments past the myosin filaments led to the labelling of this mechanism as the "sliding filament theory" of muscle contraction.

Characteristics

The functional characteristics of muscle contraction have been investigated by allowing a muscle to contract auxotonically, isometrically, or isotonically.[18] During auxotonic contraction, the elastic attachment of the muscle to bone contributes to in-

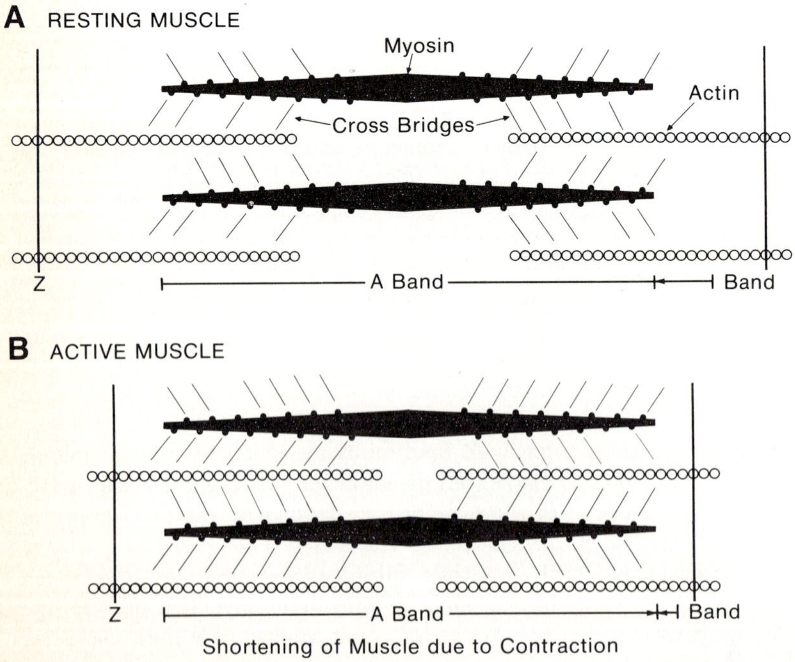

Figure 4-16 Schematic representation of the mechanism of muscle shortening, as observed in a single sarcomere in *A*, a resting muscle and *B*, an active muscle. (After Schmidt R, ed. Fundamentals of neurophysiology. 2nd ed. New York: Springer-Verlag, 1978:135.)

creasing contractile force as the muscle length decreases. During isometric conditions, the length of the muscle is held constant, theoretically not allowing myofibrils to slide past each other as the muscle develops contractile force. Isotonic conditions allow the length of the muscle to change as it contracts against a constant load. Isometric contractions are typically utilized in order to analyze the rapid events of single muscle impulses (twitches). Isotonic contractions are much slower than isometric, yet they allow analysis of muscle as it performs external work. These isometric and isotonic contractions actually represent two extremes of a contractile continuum, neither being utilized in a "pure" form during normal function. Auxotonic contractions approximate muscle function in situ.

Investigations utilizing isometric contractions have indicated the relationship between isolated muscle contraction and muscle fiber length. This relationship is shown in the length-tension curve of Figure 4–17. Note that a maximum contraction occurs only at the natural length of the muscle, its resting length. Owing to configurational characteristics of actin and myosin, the ability to generate contractile muscle force diminishes when the muscle is either longer or shorter than resting length, demonstrating an optimal operating length for muscle in vitro. Figure 4–18 utilizes information gathered during isotonic contractions to describe the relationship between the load on a muscle and its velocity of shortening as indicated by the force-velocity curve. The force-velocity curve indicates that as the load on a muscle increases, its maximum velocity of contraction is reduced; conversely, fast movements can be accomplished only with light loads.

If a single action potential activates a muscle held in an isometric condition, a single short duration peak of force develops in the form of a muscle

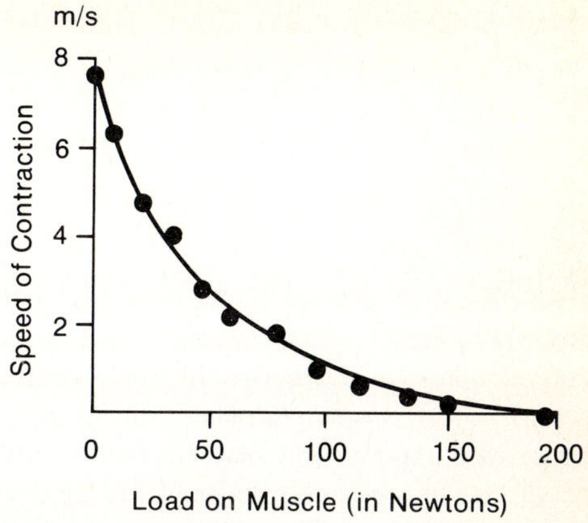

Figure 4–18 The relationship between the load on a muscle and the maximum speed at which a muscle can contract. (After Schmidt R, ed. Fundamentals of neurophysiology. 2nd ed. New York: Springer-Verlag, 1978:142.)

twitch. If repetitive stimuli are delivered to a muscle at intervals that do not allow the muscle to fully relax before the subsequent stimulus arrives, the contractile forces may add together in the process of summation. The relationship between stimulus rate and force development is illustrated in the twitch-tension curve of Figure 4–19. From this curve, it is apparent that increasing the frequency of stimulation produces a nonlinear increase in force, gradually smoothing the curve until individual twitches

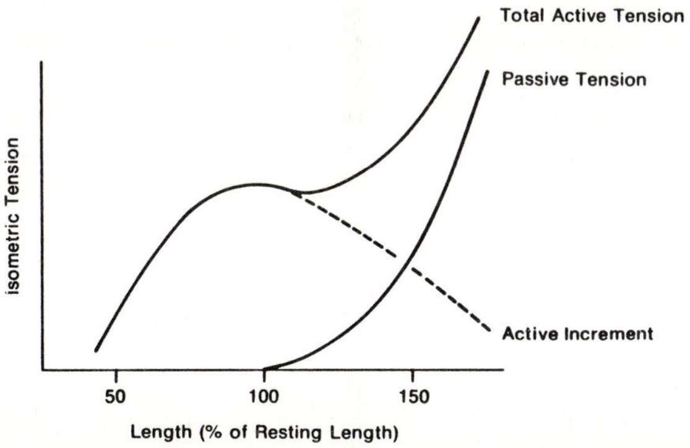

Figure 4–17 The relationship between muscle length and the ability to generate contractile force. (After Aidley D. The physiology of excitable cells. 2nd ed. London: Cambridge University Press, 1978:193.)

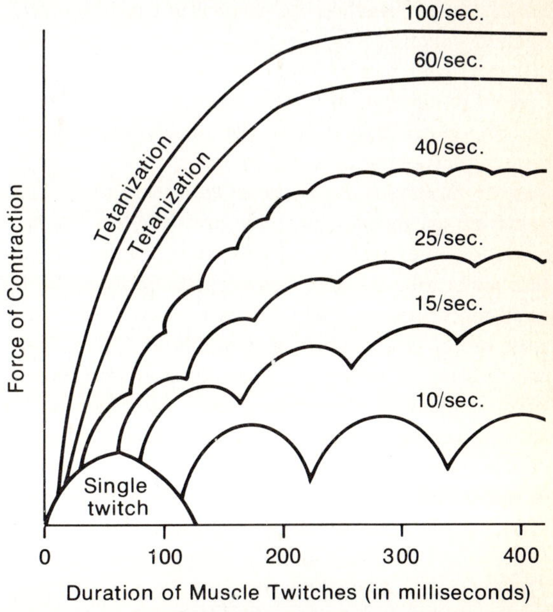

Figure 4–19 The relationship between the frequency at which a muscle is stimulated and the contractile force that is generated. (After Guyton A. Organ physiology—structure and function of the nervous system. 2nd ed. Philadelphia: WB Saunders, 1976:37.)

are no longer discernible and maximal contractile force is generated. This state of muscle contraction is called "tetany."

Regulation

As previously discussed, the motoneurons that synapse peripherally with muscle fibers undergo varying amounts of divergence. In finely controlled muscles like the perioral muscles and extrinsic eye muscles, each motoneuron may innervate only six muscle fibers. In the large muscles of the legs, which require less precision in the gradation of muscle force, each motoneuron may innervate up to 1,900 muscle fibers. These divergent structures form the basic element of control of muscle contraction: the motor unit. Each motor unit is composed of a single motoneuron and the muscle fibers innervated by it.[6,38]

The regulation of contraction of a muscle may be achieved by (1) varying the frequency at which motor units fire and/or (2) modulating the number of motor units that are simultaneously fired.

Control of muscle force by varying the frequency of motor unit firing is called "wave summation" (rate coding).[39] By examining the twitch-tension curve described earlier, it becomes apparent that increasing the frequency of firing increases, to a first approximation, muscle contractile force, an observation that forms the basis for gradation of muscle contraction via wave summation.

A second method for controlling muscle contraction involves varying the number of simultaneously firing motor units, a process called "multiple unit summation" (recruitment).[18,39] The basic underlying principle of multiple unit summation indicates that as more motor units fire, more muscle force is produced. A source of nonlinearity in the gradation of muscle force by multiple unit summation is observed in the diverse sizes of motor units that make up a muscle. Each muscle contains both small motor units, which generate small forces, and large motor units, which generate large forces. The nonlinearity of gradation occurs because of size-related preferential recruitment order of motor units as theorized by Henneman's size principle.[40] Small motor units have small motoneurons, and these are recruited first in accordance with the size principle. Large motor units with large motoneurons are recruited only at high levels of muscle contraction. This relation creates the situation in which small gradations in muscle force occur with recruitment in the weakly contracting muscle; and, as the overall muscle contraction level increases, so does the size of force gradations, thereby decreasing the precision with which the contractile force of a strongly contracting muscle may be regulated. Data indicate that the size principle might not be rigidly adhered to in the muscles innervated by the cranial nervous system.

Functional Classification of Muscles

In addition to being classified as striated, smooth, or cardiac, muscles may be categorized by various functional and metabolic elements.[41] An examination of the duration of muscle twitch contractions led to the categorization of muscles as being either phasic (fast, white) or tonic (slow, red) contracting muscles (Fig. 4–20). Phasic muscles typically show short contraction times and high levels of force generated, yet they fatigue rapidly (Fig. 4–20*A*). These muscles are best suited for the fast discontinuous movements such as those required by the eyes. But tonic muscles have long contraction times and characteristically develop less contractile force than phasic muscles (Fig. 4–20*B*). Tonic muscles are highly resistant to fatigue, well suiting them for tasks that involve prolonged work, such as supporting the body against gravity. Few muscles are exclusively phasic or tonic; most are combinations of these two types. Investigations by John Eccles and Arthur Buller indicate that motoneurons and muscle fibers have matching properties, such that innervating a slow muscle fiber with a fast motoneuron causes the slow muscle fiber to convert to a fast fiber.[42]

THE REFLEX

With completion of this brief description of neural input pathways (afferent pathways) and neural output pathways (efferent pathways), an examination of the interactions between these two pathways is possible.

For over 400 years, it has been observed that the application of an appropriate external stimulus to a specific location of the body (like tapping the patellar tendon of the knee) could elicit a time-locked response within the motor structures that affects that location (a jerking extension of the knee joint). These reactions represent the most basic interactions between sensory input pathways and motor output pathways, an interaction that produces the motor behaviors labelled "reflexes" by Unzer in 1771.[43] These behaviors have provided the basis for many classic studies of the control of movement because the motor reactions that are elicited are relatively stereotypical and are repeatable through the controlled application of the stimulus.[10,18,38,44,45]

Classic studies of reflexes have led to the for-

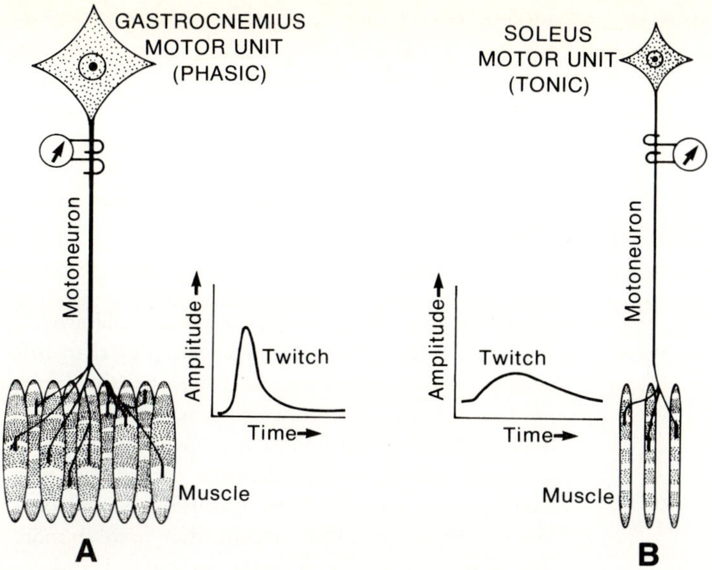

Figure 4–20 Phasic and tonic motor units. *A*, A phasic motor unit with a large number of muscle fibers per motoneuron and fast twitch characteristics. *B*, A tonic motor unit with fever muscle fibers and slower twitch characteristics. (After Eyzaguirre C, Fidone S. Physiology of the nervous system—an introductory text. 2nd ed. Chicago: Year Book Medical Publishers, 1975:215.)

mulation of many basic concepts of nervous system organization and function. Premier among these concepts is the premise that the regulation of a structure's function is based on sensory information, which originates in the structure being regulated. This concept of reflex regulation is basic to the study of the function of the "hard-wired" reflex arcs that both originate and terminate on the same structure. These studies have also led to the formulation of a concept that considers the basic behavioral unit of the nervous system to be the reflex and that all behaviors may be explained as hierarchical "chains" of coordinated, interactive reflexes of varying complexity.[46]

In light of the extensive study of reflexes and their apparent significance in nervous system function, it is paradoxical that a single, unambiguous, and straightforward definition has proved to be so elusive. The traditional definitions rely heavily upon the dichotomization of "involuntary" reflex behaviors and willed "voluntary" behaviors, providing a most Cartesian framework.[8] In conjunction with this dichotomy, reflexes are defined as behavioral units that are (1) based on "hard-wired" neuron circuits that are present before birth (having been observed in the 7-week embryo) and do not require learning; (2) predictable from the nature and magnitude of the stimulus; (3) triggered by, and time-locked to, external stimuli; (4) stereotypic; (5) utilized to regulate or protect the organism; (6) involuntary, unconscious, and automatic responses; and (7) observed with shorter time delays between stimulus and consequent motor reactions than are observed with "voluntary" reactions.

Reflexes in the Spinal Cord

Most traditional studies of reflexes have examined the behaviors that utilize neuronal structures contained primarily within the spinal cord. These spinal reflexes vary greatly in structural complexity, yet all contain three basic elements: (1) an afferent pathway that centripetally conducts sensory information from the peripheral sensory end-organs; (2) an integrating interconnection located within the central grey matter of the spinal cord; and (3) an efferent pathway that centrifugally conducts motor commands to the peripheral musculature. These elements may combine to form a reflex that is confined to a single level of the spinal cord (intrasegmental or segmental reflexes) or a reflex that spreads the influence of a sensory stimulus over multiple levels of the spinal cord (intersegmental reflexes).

Intrasegmental Reflexes

Intrasegmental spinal reflexes utilize structures of a single level of the spinal cord as defined by the entry of a dorsal sensory nerve root and the exit of a ventral motor nerve root.[47] The most basic of intrasegmental spinal reflexes is in the form of the monosynaptic reflex arc that involves only two neurons and a single synapse (Fig. 4–21). The afferent pathway of this reflex originates in a muscle spindle that is positioned in parallel with its surrounding extrafusal muscle fibers. The muscle spindle senses both static muscle length and dynamic changes in muscle length, increasing its discharge rate when the

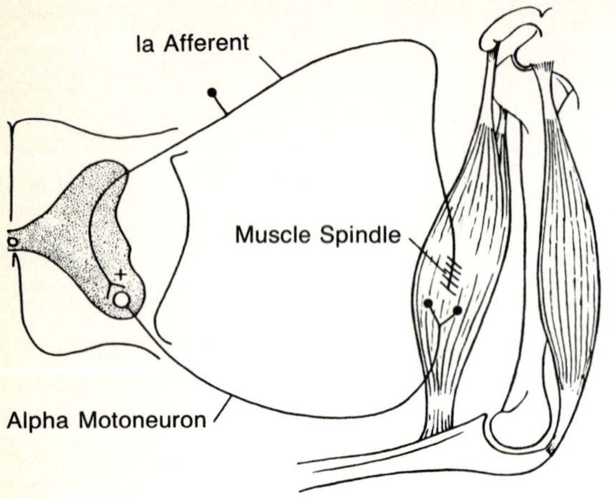

Figure 4–21 A monosynaptic two neuron reflex arc. (After Gardner E. Fundamentals of neurology—a psychophysiological approach. 6th ed. Philadelphia: WB Saunders, 1975:117.)

extrafusal muscle is stretched. This forms the basis for the reflex referred to as the stretch reflex (muscle spindle or myotatic reflex). This reflex is activated when the muscle spindle senses a change in muscle length, which is then encoded by the receptor and transmitted along Ia afferent fibers through the dorsal nerve root to the central grey matter of the spinal cord. Within the grey matter, the afferent fibers form a direct excitatory synapse on large alpha-motoneurons that innervate the muscle originally lengthened, causing the muscle to contract, thereby restoring it to its former length. Because the reflex arc requires that only a single synapse be traversed, and need not travel to the cerebral cortex, the time between the onset of the stimulus and the reaction of the muscle (reflex time) is much less than that required to voluntarily react to the stimulus. This reflex, because the receptors and effectors are located within the same structure, is referred to as an intrinsic reflex.

The intrinsic monosynaptic reflex just described provides the most simple illustration of a complete reflex arc of the nervous system. However, the majority of reflexes are more complex than this simple circuit; complexity increases by the interposition of varying numbers of additional neurons (interneurons or internuncial neurons) within the integrating interconnection between the afferent and efferent nerve roots. The interposition of additional neurons results in reflex circuits that involve more than a single synapse: polysynaptic reflexes.

A most basic intrinsic polysynaptic reflex is characterized by the tendon reflex (Ib, Golgi tendon organ, or inverse myotatic reflex).[48] The tendon reflex utilizes a Golgi tendon organ as its afferent end-organ (Fig. 4–22). This neural receptor is positioned in series with its extrafusal muscle and so is ideally suited to transduce tension within the muscle. As muscle tension increases, the Golgi tendon organ is stimulated (Fig. 4–22*A*), and the resulting neural impulses are centripetally conveyed along afferent nerve roots just smaller than those of the spindle reflex (neurons classified as Ib rather than Ia). Within the spinal cord, the Ib afferent forms an ex-

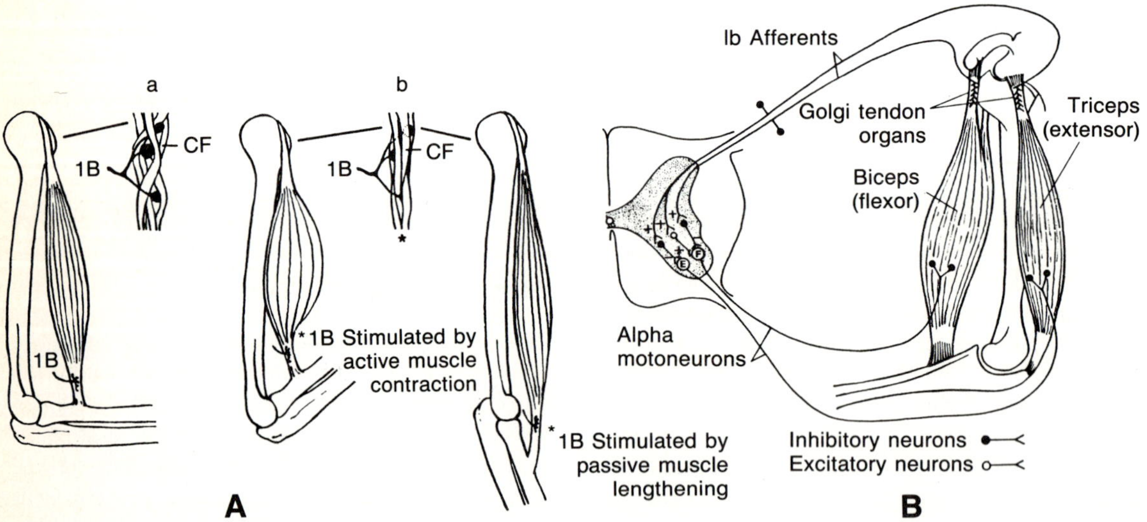

Figure 4–22 *A*, Excitation of 1b fibers by Golgi tendon organs. *a*, A relaxed muscle in which the collagenous fibers that make up the tendon are relaxed and the Golgi tendon organ is not activated. *b*, Either muscle contraction or muscle lengthening causes the collagenous fibers to compress the Golgi tendon organ, thus causing it to fire. *B*, Neural connections of the polysynaptic Golgi tendon organ reflex. Abbreviations: CF = collagenous fibers; + = excitatory synapse; – = inhibitory synapse; E = extensor motoneurons; F = flexor motoneurons. (*A*, after Werner J. Neuroscience—a clinical perspective. Philadelphia: WB Saunders, 1980:25. *B*, after Schmidt R, ed. Fundamentals of neurophysiology. 2nd ed. New York: Springer-Verlag, 1978:166.)

citatory synapse on an inhibitory interneuron. The activated inhibitory interneuron then synapses upon, and directly inhibits, the intrinsic anterior motoneuron of the muscle of origin (Fig. 4–22*B*).

Multiple (polysynaptic) synapses also vary in complexity; not always restricted to intrinsic circuits alone, these reflexes participate in circuits in which the sensory receptor is spatially separated from the effector in extrinsic configurations.

Examination of the transmission pathway of sensory impulses generated by muscle spindles has indicated the existence of an excitatory intrinsic monosynaptic pathway to the muscle of origin. This pathway is activated by stretching the muscle spindle, and the resulting reflex activates the homonymous muscle of origin, which, in turn, acts as a prime mover in the production of a movement (acting as an agonist muscle). Further examination of the transmission pathways from muscle spindles demonstrates the existence of a more complex, extrinsic polysynaptic pathway to the muscle that would oppose the movement (the antagonist muscle). This polysynaptic extrinsic pathway produces inhibition in the antagonist muscle through the excitation of an inhibitory interneuron. This circuit, as depicted in Figure 4–23, forms an interactive reflex network referred to as reciprocal antagonist inhibition (reciprocal or Sherrington's inhibition).[18] The utility of this network becomes clear by realizing that for a movement to occur not only must the agonist muscle be excited, but the antagonist muscle must be inhibited and relaxed simultaneously as well.

The effects of intrasegmental extrinsic polysynaptic spinal reflexes are not always restricted to the side of the body that is stimulated (ipsilateral effects); many reflexes involve activity on the side opposite that stimulated (contralateral effects). Figure 4–24 illustrates the components of a reflex network that may be activated upon painful stimulation of the foot (a nociceptive stimulation). This reflex network withdraws the injured foot by exciting the muscles that flex the knee (flexors) and inhibiting the muscles that extend the knee (extensors). The sensory impulse is simultaneously conveyed contralaterally across the midline by commissural interneurons within the central grey, which produce a reversed pattern of excitation and inhibition, inhibiting the flexors and exciting the extensors. This reflex action allows the opposite leg to support the entire weight of the body while the ipsilateral leg is withdrawn, forming the crossed extensor reflex.[49]

Intersegmental Reflexes

Thus far this basic discussion has concentrated on reflex networks that are restricted to a single segment of the spinal cord. However, afferent axons also

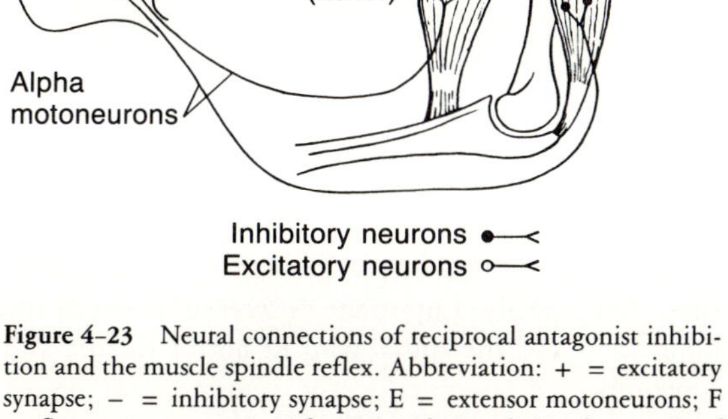

Figure 4-23 Neural connections of reciprocal antagonist inhibition and the muscle spindle reflex. Abbreviation: + = excitatory synapse; − = inhibitory synapse; E = extensor motoneurons; F = flexor motoneurons. (After Schmidt R, ed. Fundamentals of neurophysiology. 2nd ed. New York: Springer-Verlag, 1978:162.)

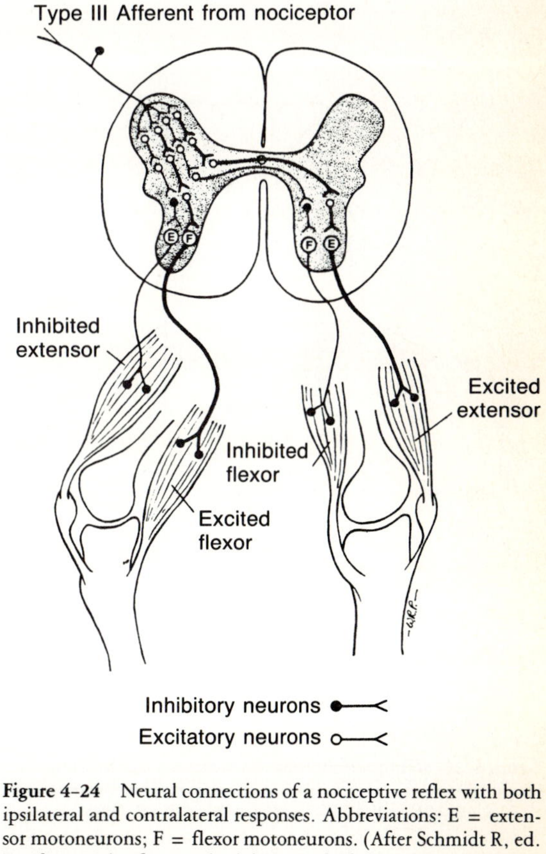

Figure 4-24 Neural connections of a nociceptive reflex with both ipsilateral and contralateral responses. Abbreviations: E = extensor motoneurons; F = flexor motoneurons. (After Schmidt R, ed. Fundamentals of neurophysiology. 2nd ed. New York: Springer-Verlag, 1978:170.)

synapse on central grey neurons that ascend and descend to terminate on different segments of the spinal cord: propriospinal neurons.[18] Propriospinal neurons constitute the majority of central grey matter neurons, transmitting the sensory information from an isolated stimulus across many spinal cord segments through bundles of axons that traverse the spinal cord white matter in propriospinal tracts. The more complex neuronal circuitry, which coordinates the action of these intersegmental reflex networks, functions both ipsilaterally and contralaterally (Fig. 4–25). Intersegmental reflexes may be observed in the production and regulation of such basic behaviors as the coordination that occurs between upper and lower limbs during locomotion.

Basic Characteristics

This most cursory examination suggests that not all spinal reflexes are as basic as the stretch reflex; they vary greatly in the behaviors they elicit and the complexity of the neuronal circuitry involved. Despite this variability and complexity, however, polysynaptic spinal reflexes appear to have a number of common functional characteristics.

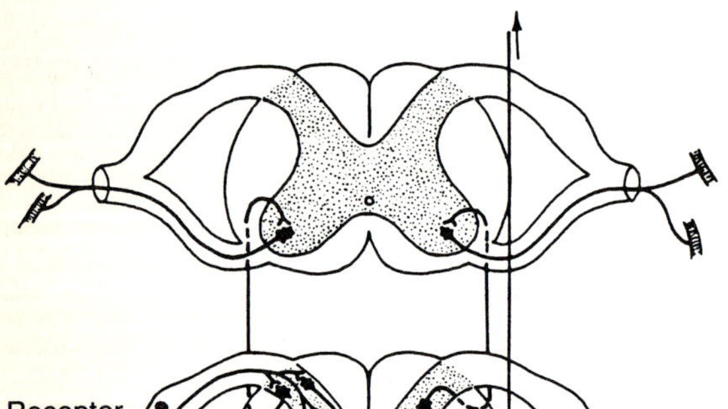

Figure 4–25 Neural connections by which the sensory impulses of a single sensory receptor may initiate ipsilateral, contralateral, and multisegmental responses. (After Gardner E. Fundamentals of neurology—a psychophysiological approach. 6th ed. Philadelphia: WB Saunders, 1975:121.)

Easily observed in flexor reflexes, reflex fatigue is characterized by a decrement in the amplitude of the reflex response during maintained application of the stimulus. This reflex characteristic is a central nervous system phenomenon created by progressive fatigue of synaptic transmission.

Primarily observed in crossed extension reflexes, reflex rebound describes the changes in reflex threshold that occur following removal of the stimulus. The reflex threshold is temporarily elevated in the agonist muscle following stimulus removal, making it difficult to elicit a second reflex of the same type. Conversely, however, reflex rebound lowers the threshold of the antagonist muscle, allowing antagonist reflex activity to be elicited with relative ease. The utility of reflex rebound is primarily manifested in behaviors that require rhythmic alternating movements, behaviors such as walking.

Manipulation of the duration and intensity of the stimulus yields further functional characteristics. Afterdischarge is observed in the persistence of reflex activity following removal of the stimulus. This characteristic is apparently due to activity in reverberating circuits, as described previously. The duration of afterdischarge relates proportionally to the intensity of the stimulus: strong stimuli evoke a long afterdischarge, and weak stimuli evoke little or no afterdischarge. In contrast to monosynaptic reflexes, stimulus intensity modifies the reflex time (the time between stimulation and reflex response) of polysynaptic reflexes. The location of the stimulus affects the response (local sign).[7] Spatial and temporal facilitation combines to decrease reflex time as stimulus intensity increases. Continued stimulation of the same place at the same intensity might attenuate the reflex even though the excitability of receptors, neurons, and muscles remains unchanged (habituation). The magnitude of the reflex response corresponds to the intensity of the stimulus, with the reflex response increasing as stimulus intensity increases. As the reflex response grows, previously uninvolved muscle groups may become involved in a reflex phenomenon called "spreading" (irradiation).

Brain Stem Reflexes

For the study of the largely brain stem-mediated motor behaviors of speech, the extensive historical examination of spinal reflexes yields information of less than optimal applicability. Although there are similarities, there are also important differences between the brain stem and the spinal cord in both structure and functions.[50–52] Structurally, the cranial nerves of the brain stem are not separated into distinct ventral and dorsal roots. The extensive sensory cortex representation of the speech mechanism receives its information from pathways that originate in a widely diverse array of highly specialized sensory end-organs positioned in dense arrays in the cutaneous, mucosal, muscular, and joint structures. The musculature of the area (demonstrated by the perioral and lingual musculature) interdigitates frequently with both adjacent muscles and the overlying cutaneous or mucosal layers. The motoneurons apparently lack axon collaterals, thereby precluding Renshaw inhibition. Functionally, the muscles innervated by the cranial nerves of the brain stem demonstrate few direct agonist and antagonist pairs. Few muscles of the laryngeal or supralaryngeal mechanisms are located in an environment in which gravitational influences are significant. Rather than operating in bilateral asymmetry (like the limbs in locomotion), the muscles of the speech mechanism typically operate in bilateral symmetry, with midline-justified synergy. Furthermore, cranial nerve nuclei may function as totally sensory, totally motor, or mixed function integrators.

In appreciation of the unique nature of the brain stem system, recent investigations have begun to elucidate the nature of brain stem-mediated reflexes, initially examining their involvement in such basic processes as mastication and more currently examining their involvement in such complex motor behaviors as speech. These pioneering examinations indicate the existence of reflex mechanisms similar to those of the spinal cord. Monosynaptic reflexes have been observed in the jaw-closing muscles, producing a reflex behavior called the jaw jerk. The sensory end-organ for this reflex is a muscle spindle that, sensing lengthening of the masseter muscle (perhaps induced by tapping the chin), conveys the sensory impulse centripetally along the motor root of the trigeminal nerve through the mesencephalic nucleus to synapse in the trigeminal motor nucleus. A monosynaptic connection within the trigeminal motor nucleus initiates a motor impulse that is centrifugally conveyed bilaterally along the motor trigeminal nerve to the homonymous masseter muscle.

The reflexes of the brain stem demonstrate reflex profiles in which polysynaptic pathways apparently dominate. Polysynaptic reflexes have been demonstrated within the tongue, in which stimulation of the mucosal surface leads to inhibitory responses in the extrinsic lingual muscles such as the genioglossus muscle. The perioral reflex, elicited by mechanical perturbation of the lips, elicits multiple responses in the orbicularis oris muscle, the shortest of which apparently traverses a polysynaptic pathway. Numerous polysynaptic brain stem reflexes have been identified: reflexes having complex responses that include both excitatory and inhibitory effects and reflexes with neuronal pathways yet to be delineated.

In view of the synergistic operation of the multiple and diverse structures that contribute motor equivalent behaviors to achieve the total vocal tract transfer function, perhaps it is most useful to consider the brain stem reflex pathways that interrelate the activity of spatially and temporally separated articulatory structures. Examples of the operation of such interrelated reflexes are obvious when one considers the interaction between lip and jaw when the jaw is blocked in a single position by the dental interposition of a pipe or, more subtly, the observation that one may continue to speak while continuously turning one's head from side to side. Preliminary investigations have partially documented the reflex interactions capable of producing some of these adjustments. A jaw-tongue reflex operates to retract the tongue (by activation of the extrinsic lingual musculature) when the mandible is lowered. Lip and jaw interactions have been documented in both masticatory activity and speechlike activities in which perturbation of the perioral structures modifies the activity of the jaw-closing muscles.

Reexamination of the Concept of Reflexes

This brief discussion began with the traditional concept that reflexes form the basic functional unit of motor behavior and offered traditional definitions of these behaviors. The traditional defining characteristics contend that reflexes are totally automatic motor responses, that they are time-locked to the application of the triggering stimulus, and that they are predictable from the nature and magnitude of the stimulus. Close examination of many of the motor behaviors that are referred to as "reflexes" indicates that some do not match these defining characteristics. The isolated automaticity, the "machine-like fatality," of behaviors is observed only in abnormal or pathologic conditions, such as decerebration of a cat. Reflexes as discussed do not occur or function in isolation; they are composite parts of highly integrated activities, inseparably organized so that most motoneurons and interneurons are involved in multiple reflex circuits. The afterdischarge characteristics of polysynaptic reflexes negate the time-locked relationship between stimuli and motor responses demanded by the traditional definition of reflex behaviors. Varying the magnitude of a suprathreshold stimulus does not always lead to correlated changes in the magnitude of the reflex response, an observation that violates the requisite proportionality between stimulus magnitude and response magnitude. In addition, owing to increased phylogenetic encephalization, each neuronal circuit that contributes to traditional reflex behaviors may be controlled by descending influences that originate in higher levels of the neuraxis. These descending influences may be as direct as the modification of muscle spindle excitability by the gamma motor system or as indirect as the modification of the excitability of lower motoneuron pools.

These incongruities have indicated the need to reexamine the traditional Cartesian dichotomy between involuntary reflex movements and voluntary movements. Initial hypotheses that attempt to explain the incongruities propose the existence of three categories of motor behavior: reflexive, triggered actions, and voluntary centrally patterned.[53] The term "reflex" is redefined to indicate local, highly differentiated, unconditional automatic motor reactions with the magnitude proportional to the stimulus intensity. The spatial requirements of reflex behaviors are specified through the activation of hard-wired neural connections, and the temporal features are continuously generated by afferent feedback sampled during the movement. The voluntary centrally patterned movements require both consciousness and decisionmaking, specifying the spatial and temporal movement requirements from "motor tapes" stored within the central nervous system. Intermediate between reflex and voluntary motor behaviors are triggered actions that comprise complex motor behaviors released by the application of external sensory stimuli and shaped by either previous instruction or intention (rather than stimulus parameters). Working within this proposed framework, it appears no longer profitable to force studies of movement into dichotomous either-or categories of voluntary versus involuntary action; perhaps the more appropriate examinations may be directed at delineating the mechanisms by which the central nervous system utilizes various blends of reflexes, triggered actions, and voluntary movements in optimally producing precise motor behaviors.[53]

Utility of Reflexes

In the face of the current reexamination of reflex behaviors, it is important to appreciate their utility in both research and clinical settings. Research has demonstrated the participation of reflex-like behaviors in all phases of motor control.[10,45,54,55] The apparent participation of the muscle spindle reflex may be to provide damping of structural movement by smoothing muscle contractions. Golgi tendon organ reflexes have been implicated in motor control feedback systems that regulate muscle tension rather than muscle length. Even if reflexes do not function as the basic unit of motor control, the study of brain stem reflexes provides information about the excitability of the brain stem. From this information, a profile of the mechanism by which the central nervous system controls lower motor neuron pools may emerge. Reflexes provide information about the learning of skilled motor activities. The afferent limb of reflex pathways is hypothesized to lay down memories of complex motor activities (sensory engrams), which may later be recalled in order to allow duplication of the motor activity without the reliance upon sensory feedback that was necessary during the learning period. The clinical examination of reflex profiles provides diagnostic information about the nature, extent, and location of neural lesions.

SUMMARY

This chapter has attempted to provide an overview of concepts thought to be crucial to the understanding of the basic functional mechanisms of the nervous system. The discussion began with the identification of the functional unit of the nervous system, the neuron. Synaptic connections between neurons were examined in order to better understand the interactions of grouped neurons. Description of sensory and motor systems formed the basis for the concluding discussion, which examined the sensory-motor interactions that result in basic motor behaviors. However, as an overview this chapter is incomplete; it is now necessary for each reader to complete the outline by supplying the details required to meet his or her special individual needs.

REFERENCES

1. van der Loos H. The history of the neuron. In: Hyden H, ed. The neuron. Amsterdam: Elsevier, 1967:1.
2. Shepherd G. The neuron doctrine: a revision of functional concepts. Yale J Biol Med 1972; 45:584–599.
3. Barr M, Kiernan J. The human nervous system: an anatomical viewpoint. 4th ed. Philadelphia: Harper and Row, 1983.
4. Mountcastle V, ed. Medical physiology. Vol. 1. St. Louis: CV Mosby, 1974.
5. Stevens C. The neuron. Sci Am 1979; 241:54–65.
6. Aidley D. The physiology of excitable cells. Cambridge: Cambridge University Press, 1971.
7. Eyzaguirre C, Fidone S. Physiology of the nervous system—An introductory text. 2nd ed. Chicago: Year Book Medical Publishers, 1975.
8. Kandel E, Schwartz J. Principles of neural science. New York: Elsevier/North-Holland, 1981.
9. Albers R. Biochemical aspects of active transport. Annu Rev Biochem 1967; 36:727–756.
10. Stein R. Peripheral control of movement. Physiol Rev 1974; 54:215–243.
11. Davies M. Functions of biological membranes. New York: Halsted Press, 1973.
12. Hodgkin A. The conduction of the nervous impulse. Springfield, IL: CC Thomas, 1964.

13. Woodbury J. Action potential. Properties of excitable membranes. In: Ruch T, Patton H, eds. Physiology and biophysics. Philadelphia: WB Saunders, 1966:28.
14. Brazier M. The electrical activity of the nervous system. Baltimore: Williams and Wilkins, 1968.
15. Bishop G. Natural history of the nerve impulse. Physiol Rev 1956; 36:376–399.
16. Morell P, Norton W. Myelin. Sci Am 1980; 242:88–118.
17. Katz G. Nerve, muscle, and synapse. New York: McGraw-Hill, 1966.
18. Schmidt R, Thews G. Human physiology. New York: Springer-Verlag, 1983.
19. Shepherd G. The synaptic organization of the brain: an introduction. New York: Oxford University Press, 1974.
20. Kuffler S, Nicholls J. From neuron to brain. Sunderland, MA: Sinauer Associates, 1976.
21. Sherrington C. The integrative action of the nervous system. New Haven: Yale University Press, 1906.
22. Willis W, Grossman R. Medical neurobiology. 3rd ed. St. Louis: CV Mosby, 1981.
23. Brock L, Coombs J, Eccles J. The recording of potentials from motoneurones with an intracellular electrode. J Physiol (Lond) 1952; 117:431–469.
24. Eccles J. The physiology of nerve cells. Baltimore: Johns Hopkins University Press, 1957.
25. Eccles J. The inhibitory pathways of the central nervous system. The Sherrington lectures IX. Springfield, IL: CC Thomas, 1969.
26. Zaimis E, ed. Neuromuscular junction. New York: Springer, 1976.
27. Nastuk W. Fundamental aspects of neuromuscular transmission. Ann NY Acad Sci 1966; 135:110–135.
28. Dale H, Feldberg W, Vogt M. Release of acetylcholine at voluntary motor nerve endings. J Physiol (Lond) 1936; 86:353–380.
29. Axelrod J. Neurotransmitters. Sci Am 1974; 230:58–71.
30. Krnjevic K. Chemical nature of synaptic transmission in vertebrates. Physiol Rev 1974; 54:418–540.
31. Bennett M, ed. Synaptic transmission and neuronal interaction. New York: Raven Press, 1975.
32. Guyton A. Organ physiology—structure and function of the nervous system. 2nd ed. Philadelphia: WB Saunders, 1976.
33. Adrian E. The basis of sensation. New York: Hafner, 1964.
34. Sinclair D. Cutaneous sensation. New York: Oxford University Press, 1967.
35. Boring E. Sensation and perception in the history of experimental psychology. New York: Appleton-Century-Crofts, 1942.
36. Tonomura Y, Oosawa F. Molecular mechanism of contraction. Annu Rev Biophys Bioeng 1972; 1:159–190.
37. Bourne G. The structure and function of muscle. New York: Academic Press, 1973.
38. Granit R. The basis of motor control. New York: Academic Press, 1970.
39. Carlson F, Wilkie D. Muscle physiology. Englewood Cliffs, NJ: Prentice-Hall, 1974.
40. Henneman E. Relation between size of neurons and their susceptibility to discharge. Science 1957; 126:1345–1347.
41. Henneman E, Olson C. Relations between structure and function in the design of skeletal muscles. J Physiol 1965; 28:581–598.
42. Buller A, Eccles J, Eccles R. Interactions between motoneurones and muscles in respect of the characteristic speeds of their responses. J Physiol (Lond) 1960; 150:417–439.
43. Fearing F. Reflex action. A study in the history of physiological psychology. Baltimore: Williams and Wilkins, 1930.
44. Matthews P. Mammalian muscle receptors and their central actions. London: Arnold, 1972.
45. Evarts E. Brain mechanisms in movement. Sci Am 1973; 229:96–103.
46. Easton T. On the normal use of reflexes. Am Sci 1972; 60:591–599.
47. Hunt C, Perl E. Spinal reflex mechanisms concerned with skeletal muscle. Physiol Rev 1960; 40:538–579.
48. Houk J, Henneman E. Responses of Golgi tendon organs to active contractions of the soleus muscle of the cat. J Neurophysiol 1967; 30:466–481.
49. Werner J. Neuroscience—a clinical perspective. Philadelphia: WB Saunders, 1980.
50. Seto H. Sensibility of the digestive organs. In: Seto H, ed. Studies on sensory innervation. Springfield, IL: CC Thomas, 1963:104.
51. Bratzlevsky M. Behavior of human brainstem reflexes in muscles with antagonist function. In: Shahani M, ed. The motor system: neurophysiology and muscle mechanics. Amsterdam: Elsevier, 1976:135.
52. Dubner R, Sessle B, Storey A. The neural basis of oral and facial function. New York: Plenum Press, 1978.
53. Evarts E, Bizzi E, Burke R, DeLong M, Thach W. Central control of movement. Neurosci Res Prog Bull 1972; 9:1–170.
54. Phillips C. Motor apparatus of the baboon's hand. Proc R Soc Biol 1969; 173:141–164.
55. Stelmach G, ed. Motor control: issues and trends. New York: Academic Press, 1976.

5 Neurophysiologic Processes of Speech Movement Control

James H. Abbs, Ph.D.

Well over 50 years ago, Nobel laureate Sir Charles Sherrington argued that "the crown of life is an action, not a thought . . . to move things is all mankind can do . . . whether in whispering a syllable or in felling a forest."[1] In modern society, perhaps no actions are any more important than the movements that underlie oral communication. Although Sherrington's perspective on the importance of motor actions is timeless, and especially on those for speech, neuroscientists' knowledge of these functions is in a state of great change. In general, the last two decades have been witness to startling advances in the understanding of how the brain generates and controls movements, including those for speech. In parallel, the influence of anticipation, learning, injury, experience, and environment on the neural functions of movement generation and control has similarly been illuminated. These advances, in no small part, have resulted from new interdisciplinary approaches to neural processes underlying all forms of movement, involving intensive collaboration among neuroanatomists, electrophysiologists, biochemists, psychologists, engineers, and computer scientists.

Until about 1965, most studies of neuromotor function were focused primarily on muscles innervated by spinal nerves and involved two major methods of investigation: (1) electrical stimulation of various parts of the nervous system and recording of evoked potentials in anesthetized, curarized, or decerebrate animals and (2) the qualitative observation of motor behaviors prior to and following the introduction of nervous system lesions. These kinds of studies provided a great deal of indirect information on the possible contribution of certain nervous system mechanisms to the control of movement. However, there were obvious limitations on inferences to neural mechanisms underlying voluntary motor control in the waking human or, in particular, to the control of the orofacial, laryngeal, and respiratory musculature for speech. Some knowledge of brain mechanisms for speech motor control and coordination has come from naturally occurring brain damage in humans. Although on the surface these human lesion data may seem fairly direct, detailed animal and human observations indicate quite clearly that behavioral deficits following lesions to a given part of the brain simply are not interpretable in relation to the function of that part; rather, these deficits reflect how the remaining parts of the brain function without the damaged region.[2–4]

As is apparent, stimulation techniques in anesthetized animals and analyses of lesion-related movement deficits in animals or in humans provide only remote perspectives on the neurobiology of movement control. Recent approaches, although focused primarily in animals, have been both more direct and more quantitative with substantial implications for human speech motor functions. As noted, the origins of these recent developments cannot be attributed directly to any particular discipline, but have been the result of converging ideas and approaches from several different scientific fields. In the middle 1960s, Evarts devised and demonstrated new methods that combined behavioral training methods and electrophysiologic recording techniques.[5,6] These procedures involved the careful training of monkeys to produce consistent goal-oriented movements and parallel recording (in those awake animals) of single pyramidal tract neurons during performance of the movements. With Evarts' methodology, it was thus possible to correlate single nerve cell activity within a portion of the brain with specific voluntary motor output variables, including muscle force, movement amplitude, and movement velocity, observed simultaneously. This basic methodology has been extended to many other portions of the central nervous system (CNS) in recent years, substantially increasing speech-language pathologists' understanding of the contributions that various masses of neural tissue make to motor behavior in waking organisms. Portions of the brain studied in this manner include the basal ganglia, deep cerebellar nuclei, premotor and supplementary motor cortices, somatic sensory cortex, and parietal cortex. These data have yielded consideration of voluntary motor control issues that simply could not be addressed previously.

In parallel with these behavioral approaches to motor neurophysiology, a number of life scientists began to employ the analysis and quantitative modeling techniques of engineering and cybernetics to test and extend their understanding of biologic motor control systems. The early applications of systems physiology to the study of motor control were influenced most clearly by the ideas of Wiener;[7] some of this history as well as some very interesting early studies are reviewed in a monograph by Stark.[8] These engineering techniques and approaches have also been utilized in some analyses of impaired motor control systems, providing increasingly sophisticated techniques for observing and characterizing functional properties of underlying neural mechanisms. The work of Houk and his colleagues in their studies of feedback control[9–17] and of the workers at Massachusetts Institute of Technology, particularly Bizzi and his associates in their analyses of arm movements,[18–24] are excellent examples of combining engineering analyses and motor physiology. As a result of these developments, workers with clinical interests have been able to use increasingly sophisticated analysis techniques for the study of movement disorders such as Parkinson's disease, spasticity, and cerebellar damage. Additionally, there has been a wealth of new neurophysiologic data upon which to extend the understanding of these motor control impairments. Given this recent history, where the only constant is change itself, a state-of-the-art review of the neural mechanisms underlying speech motor control is not meaningful unless it incorporates current perspectives in basic motor neurophysiology. Indeed, considerations of speech motor neurophysiology written prior to 1975 or even 1980 have been reduced primarily to historical value by these newer developments.

Even though techniques such as neural unit recording in awake animals or quantitative modeling of motor processes have not been utilized widely in the study of speech motor control for obvious reasons, the basic findings from such studies have helped substantially in highlighting the probable processes involved. For example, it has become increasingly apparent that to fully appreciate the function of the brain in speech movement control, the underlying biologic complexity must be identified or, at the least, realistically acknowledged. Unfortunately, for many years speech scientists' concepts have been blurred by somewhat oversimplistic concepts of the processes underlying speech production; to a degree, these oversimplistic concepts are reflected in the traditional "wedding cake" representation of the layers underlying speech production shown in Figure 5–1*A*. This representation includes the typical set of so-called linguistic, phonologic, phonetic, muscle contraction, movement, and acoustic processes. In certain respects, the scheme shown in Figure 5–1*A* is analogous to the oversimplified economic theories offered by members of certain political factions; such explanations appear to have great appeal because processes that were otherwise thought to be complicated are understood with ease. By contrast, Figure 5–1*B* provides a more realistic (and obviously more complicated) version of probable components of speech neuromotor control, which is drawn from both contemporary neurophysiology and parallel knowledge of speech production processes. Figure 5–1*B* is an attempt to illustrate the multiple nervous system transformations from motor goals to movements that have obligatory influences upon aerodynamically and acoustically significant vocal tract manipulations.

Despite the substantial increase in the degree of detail provided in Figure 5–1*B* (as compared to 5–1*A*), it remains simplified. Indeed, many of the single processes or individual steps shown in Figure 5–1*B* are comprised of several yet smaller elements that have been the focus of much effort in their own right. For example, the way that motoneuron signals activate muscle to generate force has alone been the subject of an estimated 100,000 published investigations.[25] However, rarely are any of the potential influences of muscle, the critical end-organ of all movement systems, considered even parenthetically in interpretations of speech motor patterns. The implicit assumption is that transforming motoneuron signals and muscle contraction into muscle force is simple and linear. As noted recently by Partridge and Benton in their classic analysis of these motoneuron to muscle force processes, "Deficiencies lie in both the formal models available and in defects in our understanding of the rules of the

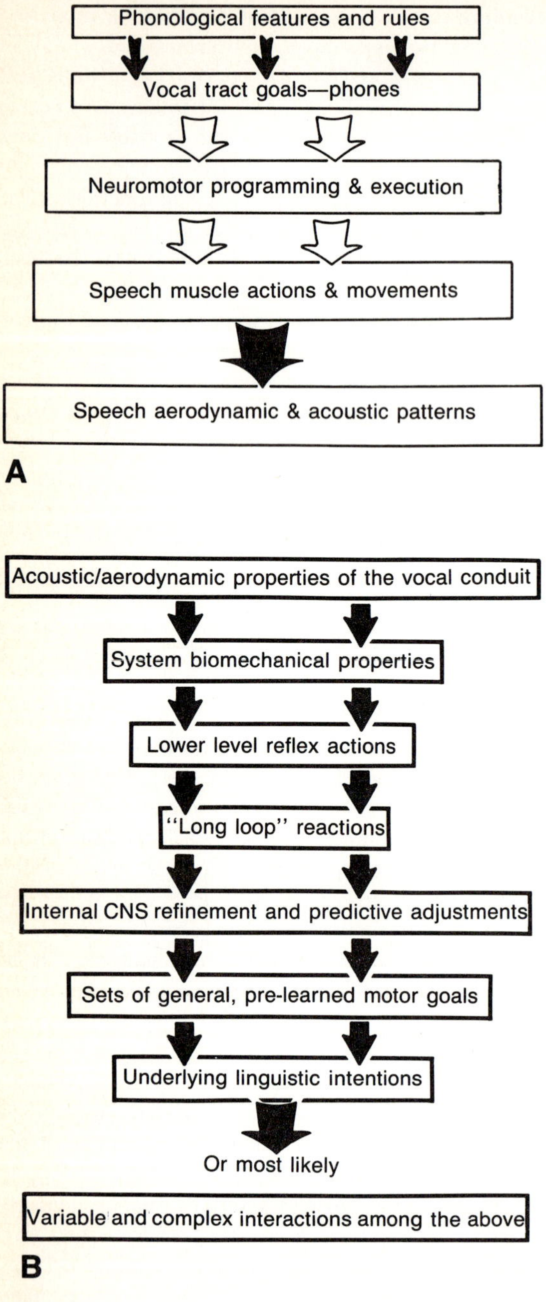

Figure 5–1 *A*, Typical representation of the levels of the speech production process; *B*, Alternate representation of the speech production process with inclusion of neural programming, sensorimotor correction, biomechanical properties, and reflex actions.

biological muscle as it responds to mechanical and neural actions" (p 47).[26] As is apparent, except under limited circumstances, an understanding of the seemingly simple relation between motoneuron firing patterns and resulting movement is rudimentary. However, without such an understanding, inferences from movement to nervous system actions, such as have been made in some interpretations of speech neural control, must be accomplished cautiously. The complex levels of motor programming and control identified in Figure 5–1*B* also highlight the importance of considering the undeniable contributions of such multiple biologic mechanisms to the relatively superficial events that one is able to observe at the speech production periphery. In other words, for any apparently significant normal or abnormal feature of the speech production output, be it perceptually, acoustically, aerodynamically, or electromyographically detected, one cannot, without being extremely careful, talk about its underlying nervous system origins.

One way to undertake the development of a neurobiologic understanding of speech motor control is to draw upon knowledge gained from studies of other motor systems. Although there may be some appeal in the time-worn platitudes suggesting that speech is one of the human's most complex acts, that speech production is not accomplished by a unique set of biologic processes is undeniable; rather, it is a motor action that shares underlying elements with other voluntary motor behavior in terms of muscle contractions, movements, biomechanics, motoneuron recruitment, and so on. As such, in the attempt to decipher nervous system function for speech production, acknowledging and understanding these common elements is important, thereby giving one at least an initial perspective on the complexities involved. The degree of imbalance in some current approaches to speech neurophysiology is reflected in the nearly exclusive use of acoustic, aerodynamic, or perceptual analyses to discern the movement patterns of the vocal organs, data that often and explicitly are used as a basis upon which to make subsequent inferences on function and dysfunction of the nervous system. Ironically, acoustic signals are commonly interpreted via models of vocal tract resonance that assume an oversimplified linear relation between vocal tract behavior and certain signal parameters. Paradoxically, little or no parallel consideration is given to the even more complex and nonlinear properties of muscle contraction, biomechanics, motor unit recruitment, and so on. This omission is striking particularly because, as noted previously, researchers have empirically demonstrated that determining moment-to-moment nervous system actions is exceedingly difficult even when the motor behaviors (movement and muscle activity) are observed directly.[26,27] Thus these neurophysiologic considerations bring into sharp focus the parallel ambiguity in discerning sensorimotor operation from the far less direct acoustic, aerodynamic, or transcriptional analyses. Attempting to understand nervous system function with techniques borrowed from experimental phonetics and descriptive linguistics is not only ineffective, it is unfortunate; more suitable techniques, procedures, and hypotheses have been forwarded in the area of human motor control for more than two decades.

COORDINATION: THE ESSENCE OF SPEECH MOTOR CONTROL

As a basis for the discussions that follow, exploration of the nature of what must be controlled is useful initially, namely, what are the objectives of speech motor actions. Figure 5–2 is a diagrammatic representation of the major ways in which respiratory, laryngeal, and upper airway movements are utilized to generate the acoustic signals that one recognizes as human speech. As is apparent, movements for speech are involved in several different functions. These include, as shown; (1) the manipulation of air volumes to create and control air pressures; (2) the generation of airway constrictions and occlusions across which these air pressures equalize to generate vibratory, turbulent, or plosive sound; and (3) the dynamic shaping and sizing of the upper airway cavities so as to provide the resonance or filtering of the acoustic signals to yield characteristic speech-related spectral properties. Even this partial and peripheral representation of the speech production process provides important perspectives on the requirements of neural control processes for speech movements. That is, for the most simple speech behavior, with only the contributions illustrated in Figure 5–2, the obviously critical features of this control are the temporal and spatial coordination among the movements that accomplish these three speech movement functions. For example, if the speech objective is to generate a voiceless stop consonant, the volumetric manipulation of the upper airway (reduction in volume), the oral airstream occlusion, and the associated abduction of the vocal folds must be controlled such that (1) each is initiated at the correct time in relation to the overall series of events (i.e., vocal fold abduction, oral cavity reduction, and occlusion) and the time required from the initiation to the completion of each action (e.g., movement time of the oral occlusion); (2) the magnitude of each is appropriate both absolutely and in terms of the magnitude of the other components of the overall gesture (i.e., the volumetric adjustment does not create intraoral air pressures that exceed the occlusion strength of the oral closure); and (3) the termination of each action is similarly sequenced appropriately with the other constituent actions (i.e., oral occlusion release and vocal fold adjustments).

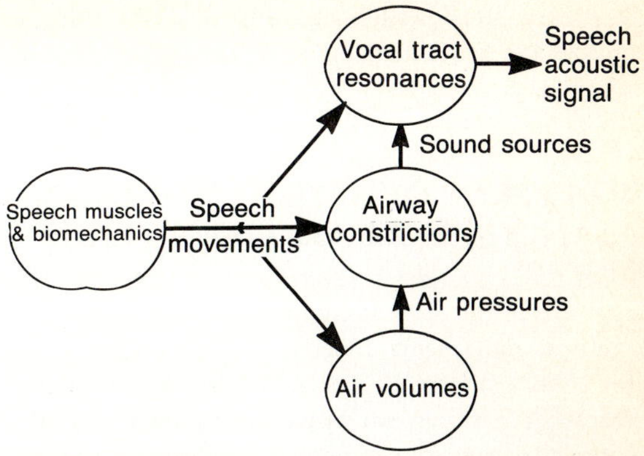

Figure 5–2 Graphic representation of the multiple ways that movements contribute to the peripheral generation of speech acoustic signals.

Obviously, even though the previous example is consistent with the common description of coordination among respiratory, laryngeal, and upper airway (articulatory) actions, it reflects only the most general level of this neural control problem. That is, at another level immediately upstream, each of the three vocal tract manipulations is in turn the result of multiple movements, which also must be coordinated with certain temporal and magnitude requirements. For example, one can consider oral occlusion as a single action in terms of its influence acoustically or aerodynamically. However, from the standpoint of neural control, such occlusions typically involve at least two if not three quasi-independent movements. Lingual stop sounds require jaw and tongue movements, at the least. If the occlusion is an anterior tongue tip articulation (/t/,/d/), three actions, the jaw, tongue body, and tongue tip movements must be controlled *and coordinated.* Similarly, with a labial stop sound, the upper lip, lower lip, and jaw are involved in oral occlusion. In addition to the multiple movements for oral occlusion, several movements and muscles contribute to the parallel changes in oral cavity size (i.e., tongue body forwarding, pharyngeal constriction, laryngeal elevation). The initiation times, magnitudes, and termination times of these submovements obviously must similarly be coordinated. At yet another level, one cannot ignore that each of these individual movements is accomplished by the coordinated actions of more than one muscle. Specifically, for jaw elevation, there are at least two if not three closing muscles and two opening muscles. Labial closing is accomplished similarly by several different muscles. These considerations lead one to dramatically expand the representation of muscle actions and movements in Figures 5–1*A* and 5–2. In particular, one must replace layers four and five of the representation shown in Figure 5–1*B* with something like the multiple muscle and movement model schematicized in Figure 5–3.

PATTERNS OF SPEECH MOVEMENT AND MUSCLE COORDINATION

Given the obvious complexity of organizing the multiple movements underlying a given speech motor action, intuitively one is led initially to expect that after learning, such patterns are relatively stereotypic, presumably being generated from some centrally stored representation of muscle contraction patterns. Such operations would reduce the need to generate the necessary output afresh with each iteration and thus relax the demands for otherwise fairly complex neurobiologic "hardware" and "software." Obviously, the principle of parsimony has been a strong factor in the initial popularity of such stereotypy, along with an attempt at making such theories conceptually tractable. Unfortunately, the patterns of multiple speech movements, even for repetitions of exactly the same phonetic sequence are almost never stereotypic. Specifically, if one examines the way in which multiple articulators contribute to a common acoustic or aerodynamic objective (like oral occlusion or opening) across multiple repetitions of that behavior in the same subject, one sees patterns such as those shown in Figure 5–4. The three trials of upper and lower lip movements shown in Figure 5–4 accomplish the same oral occlusion objective, but, as indicated, the contributions of their relative displacement covary from trial to trial. Figure 5–5 illustrates the movements of the upper lip, lower lip, and jaw superimposed for multiple repetitions of the word "sapapple." The degree of variability in these three speech movements for oral closure on the first "p" is apparent in the separation among the multiple superimposed traces. Interestingly, by comparison, the combined upper lip, lower lip, and jaw movement (the fourth trace) is much less variable across trials. Essentially, the kind of results shown in Figures 5–4 and 5–5 can only be due to the phenomenon that when one movement element (upper lip) is moved less for a given repetition, the other movements (the lower lip and/or jaw) are moved proportionately less. These data thus indicate that a flexible trade-off occurs among the multiple movements contributing to the oral opening and closing gesture. Quantitative analyses of the relative covariability among multiple speech movements lead to results such as that shown in Figure 5–6.

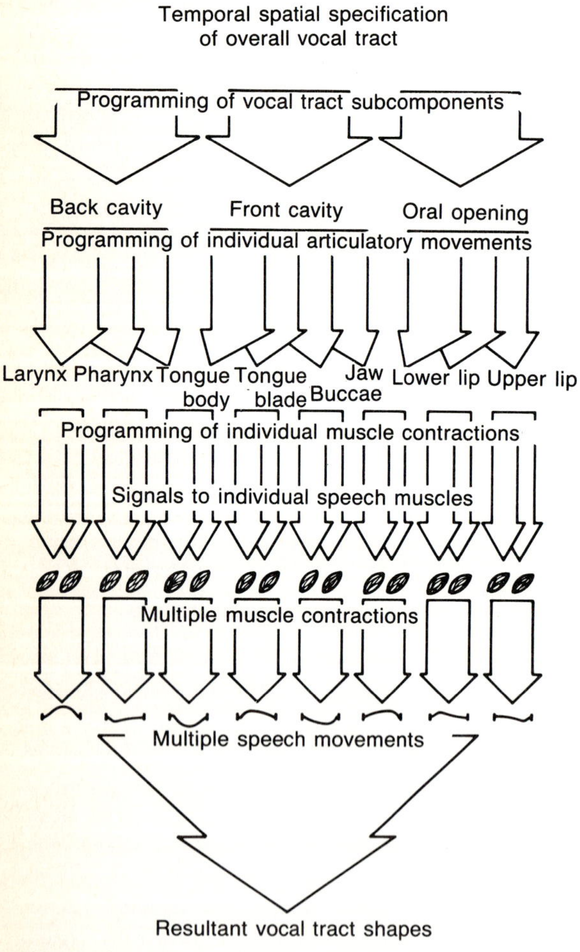

Figure 5-3 Schematic illustration of the hierarchy of peripheral muscle contractions, movements, and vocal tract shape and size manipulations that underlie speech production.

Observations of these kinds of movement patterns in speech were reported originally over a decade ago,[28] and although there were some methodologic concerns about the original analyses,[29] reconsideration[30] and subsequent observations[31] leave little doubt concerning their validity. Importantly, the phenomenon of multiple, errorless repetitions of an unrestrained motor task being accomplished with strikingly different combinations of the constituent kinematic and muscle actions has been recognized for over 50 years.[32–41] Parallel patterns have been observed for movements of the hand as well.[35,38,42,43] As Bernstein commented: "If we turn from the simplest and most repetitive actions to more complex and purposive movements, . . . such broad variations in the motor composition of movements become a universal rule" (p 133).[33] In describing these patterns in speech movements and in other motor behaviors, this phenomenon has been termed "motor equivalence," although the origin of the term is obscure.[28,31,35,36,38] However, it is apparent that the operation of motor equivalence, as demonstrated, in-

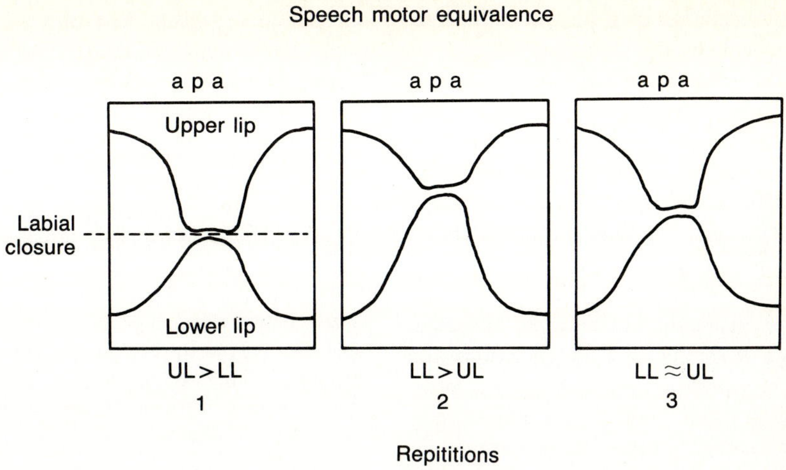

Figure 5–4 Upper and lower lip movements for three repetitions of the utterance /apa/. The trade-off between these two articulators for the three repetitions is obvious.

dicates that it is not viable to entertain concepts of stereotypic generation of multiple speech movements, possibly reflecting some learned, totally preplanned patterns. Rather, the nervous system generates the necessary set of muscle contractions and movements afresh for each repetition of a given speech production task. Based upon the perceived complexity of that generation process, one perspective is that such multiple, potentially redundant ways of generating the same speech motor end product is taxing upon the neural control hardware.[44] However, another perspective is that though such arguments, appeal to one's inherent discomfort with such complexity, they are based upon some premature assumptions of what is complicated to the nervous system.[45–47] Moreover, a number of investigators view the capability for accomplishing a given motor objective flexibly as a phenomenon that rather facilitates neural control of complex, natural movement [22,48,49] by providing the inherent ability to accommodate changes in the control requirements of the motor task due to unanticipated errors or fatigue. Indeed, it has been suggested that the learning of a given skilled motor behavior (such as speech) is likely to be facilitated by this flexibility.[48] Quantitative analyses of multimuscle, multimovement behaviors, such as hand actions for handwriting, indicate that this complexity

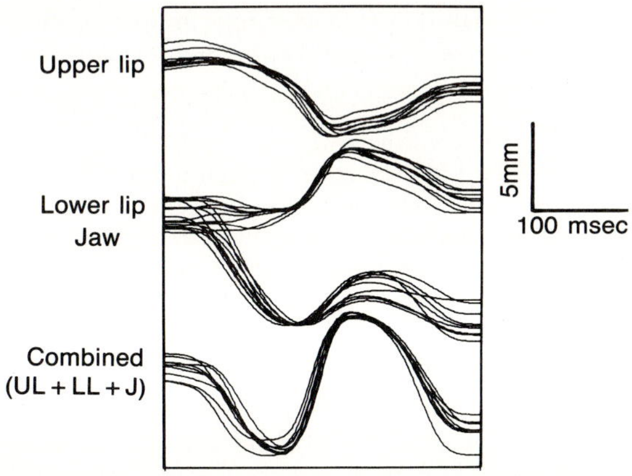

Figure 5–5 Multiple trials of upper lip, lower lip, and jaw movements for oral closure along with the combined upper lip + lower lip + jaw signal. Motor equivalence is illustrated by the relatively greater variability for each of the individual movements, compared to that for the combined movement.

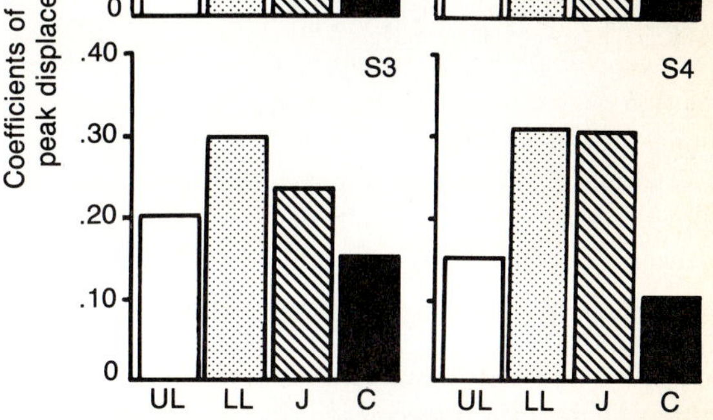

Figure 5–6 Magnitudes of the coefficient of variability of the upper lip (UL), lower lip (LL), jaw (J), and combined UL, LL, and J (C) for multiple repetitions of the oral closure for the utterance "sapapple." (Adapted from Gracco VL, Abbs JH. Variant and invariant characteristics of speech movement planning. Exp Brain Res 1986; 65:156–166.)

"serves not to complicate handwriting, but to provide a variety of orthogonal configurations" (p 39).[50]

In general, the observations of multimovement coordination, including that for speech, thus indicate that such behavior is flexibly accomplished by the nervous system, perhaps to ease what might be impossible, namely, achieving a given functionally significant goal in exactly the same way each time. The implications of this general principle of multimovement coordination for speech motor control are multiple. First, apparently, classifications of speech elements in terms of tongue or labial positions are not particularly meaningful inasmuch as the multimovement goals for this behavior are not stereotyped articulatory spatial targets as once argued.[51] Rather, the actual nervous system goals and presumably their underlying phonologic representation are any set of those movements that yields an acoustically or aerodynamically equivalent end product,[31,43,52] as should be obvious from Figure 5–4. This figure shows movements from multiple repetitions of /apa/, which are aerodynamically and acoustically indistinguishable, but vary significantly in the individual lip positions utilized for the /p/. Similarly, Riordan demonstrated labial protrusion and laryngeal lowering trade-offs in their joint contributions to the necessary vocal tract length for production of so-called rounded vowels.[53] Whereas the empirical data addressing this issue in speech, especially for movements of the tongue, are relatively rare, the lip, jaw, and larynx data that are available are consistent with findings in all other multimovement behaviors. Moreover, the early work on modeling the vocal tract,[54,55] even in two dimensions, illustrates the dramatic capability for comparable acoustic patterns to be generated with different vocal tract configurations. The phenomenon of motor equivalence flexibility, coupled with the vocal tract modeling data of Stevens and House,[54,55] also suggest the difficulty of attempting to discern articulatory movement patterns via analyses of the speech acoustic signal. Fundamentally, there is no unique relation between parameters of the speech acoustic signal and movements of the vocal tract. This lack of relationship is not to suggest that the acoustic signal is a useless global index of speech output, but rather that such analyses are limited for making inferences to underlying speech movement or neural control processes.

As noted at the outset of this section, coordination of multiple movements, including those for speech, seems to pose a major undertaking in the process of motor learning. This apparent problem is even more striking in the recognition of the fact that to learn a single pattern for each element of a given motor behavior is impossible. Rather, some abilities in the management and orchestration of the multiple movements apparently must develop. Interestingly, this is exactly the conclusion offered by Bernstein in his consideration of this issue. He notes,

> Coordination of movement is the process of mastering redundant degrees of freedom of the moving organ, in other words its conversion to a controllable system . . . and that fixation or reducing the degrees of freedom is not the normal process of learning . . . Elimination of the redundant degrees of freedom mentioned above is employed only as the most primitive and inconvenient method, and then only at the beginning of the mastery of the motor skill, being later displaced by more flexible, expedient and economic methods of overcoming this redundancy through the organization of the process as a whole (p 127).[33]

The flexible covariability observed among the constituent elements of natural multimovement gestures appears to provide insights on the underlying nervous system organization. As pointed out by several authors, such patterns presumably reflect a multilevel control process.[30,31,35,38,43] Specifically, due to the contrast between (1) the relative consistency with which overall vocal tract goals are achieved and (2) the variability of individual articulatory movements and muscle activity patterns, these two outputs would appear to be indicative of control processes at two different levels of the nervous system. One suggestion by many scientists over the last several years has been that while functionally significant motor objectives (perhaps corresponding to phonologic features) are specified at one level of the multimovement control process, the flexible achievement of those objectives is accomplished at subordinate levels via moment-to-moment flexible adjustments of the evolving speech motor output.[30,56–59] This interpretation is consistent with that of most investigators addressing this issue. For example, Lacquaniti and Soechting, in interpreting motor equivalence covariability among shoulder, elbow, and wrist movements, suggest that

> At higher levels the general structure of a motor act would be defined in abstract terms whose features are only those properties of the motor act that remain invariant under different levels of spatio-temporal transformations. At lower levels of organization, more contingent parameters of the movement (such as the muscles required and their pattern of activation) would be defined on the basis of the specific task demands (for instance the speed of execution) and of the current state of the environment and the muscular-skeletal apparatus (p 408).[35]

The recognition that control of speech motor behavior is implemented via a hierarchical process is not a revelation. However, the speech movement flexibility described previously provides some perspectives on the possible neurobiologic correlates of this hierarchy. Specifically, whereas the speech motor behavior is the result of multiple movements coordinated to yield certain net vocal tract configurations necessary for the manipulation of acoustic and aerodynamic signals, the pattern of those individual movements is flexible and changing, even with equivalent acoustic and aerodynamic results. This places interesting demands on the nervous system and leads one to posit a potential role of sensory processes in multimovement coordination. As will be apparent in the discussion that follows, such mechanisms appear to be prominently involved.

SPEECH MOVEMENT COORDINATION VIA SENSORIMOTOR LINKAGES

Many seemingly insolvable control problems associated with the flexible coordination of speech multimovement systems are tractable if sensory processes, providing moment-to-moment information on the status of the evolving movements, can be utilized to assure net movement contributions toward the common intended goals. This hypothesis has been favored particularly in the last several years, and increasing data support it. Demonstration of sensorimotor contributions to the flexible intermovement trade-offs that occur for multimovement coordination has come largely from the utilization of the unanticipated perturbation paradigm. This technique involves the introduction of unexpected errors in the movement of one of the speech articulators and the observation of whether or not that induced movement error yields functional neuromotor compensations.

Specifically, if one introduces an error in jaw movement during the course of a coordinated upper lip, lower lip, and jaw multimovement articulation (oral closure for /p/), there are at least three alternative results: (1) there are no movement or muscle activity responses to the induced error; (2) jaw movements and muscle activity are increased, with short latency adjustments to overcome the error; or (3) upper lip and lower lip movement and muscle adjustments occur along with those of the jaw. The first result implies that the pattern of upper lip, lower lip, and jaw movement is rigidly predetermined (preprogrammed); with such control, unanticipated errors in the evolving movement are not corrected, and perturbations yield corresponding errors in the final vocal tract goal. The second alternative suggests that when errors are introduced into a given movement, local afferent mechanisms provide information on those errors, and adjustments are made in the ongoing muscle activity to correct the induced movement error. If the error is corrected in this manner, the original pattern among the multiple movements is preserved and the speech motor objective is accomplished as predetermined. The third result, *which is the one observed in all such studies to date,* suggests that the nervous system monitors each individual constituent movement, processes that information in relation to the intended multimovement goal, and when errors are detected, distributes the corrections or adjustments among the movements in relation to that goal. This latter process, whereby errors in one constituent movement of a multimovement behavior yield corrections in all the contributing active elements, is a case where the intended goal is accomplished but *not* in any predetermined manner. This phenomenon appears to be an essential element in the neural coordination among multiple speech movements or in any multimovement behavior. Moreover, the distribution of magnitude adjustments among multiple constituent elements as a result of unanticipated inputs is rather unequivocal evidence for sensorimotor contributions to coordination.

The specific data supporting sensory contributions to coordination have come from several different experiments and enhance the general interpretations provided before. As illustrated in Figure 5–7, if one introduces unanticipated errors in the lip movement prior to or during that course of an upper lip, lower lip, and jaw movement, compensations are distributed across all three components of this action.[60–63] Similarly, if perturbations are introduced on the lower lip during an upper lip and lower lip articulatory action or an upper lip, lower lip, and jaw gesture, compensations are observed in all the contributing movements and associated muscles.[58,59,64] Comparable results are seen if perturbations are introduced on the upper lip rather than the lower lip. Multimovement compensations of this kind appear to reflect natural sensorimotor processes to the extent that they are seen in naive subjects the first time a perturbation is introduced; even if subjects are instructed to repress the compensation, they are unable to do so. These particular contributions of sensorimotor actions to coordination of multimovement behaviors are not only confined to speech motor control, but appear to be a general neural mechanism as well. A number of investigators have reported comparable compensatory patterns to unanticipated perturbations in coordinated finger, wrist, forearm, torso, head, and eye movements as well.[52]

Overall, these results indicate that one means by which the multimovement behaviors for speech are coupled flexibly to accomplish intended goals consistently with variable means is via the following processes: (1) moment-to-moment sensory monitor-

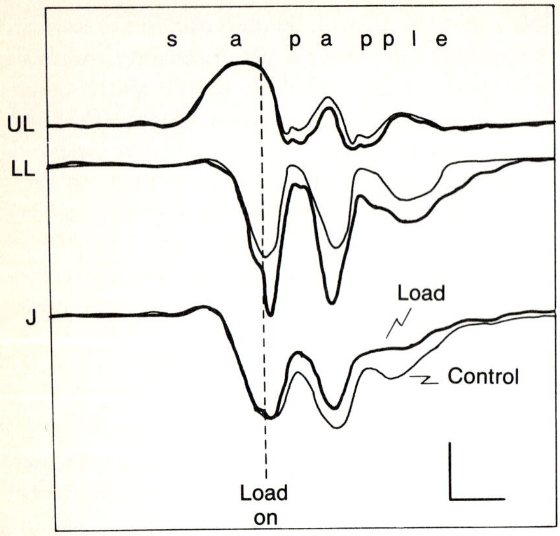

Figure 5–7 Upper lip, lower lip, and jaw movements for a control trial (thin line) for production of the utterance "sapapple," superimposed with a trial in which the lower lip has been loaded (thick line).

ing of the peripheral movement state; (2) integration of that information from multiple constituent movements as these might additively interact; (3) comparison of that integrated or processed information on the premovement state or the evolving movement in relation to expected progress toward the intended goal; and (4) appropriately graded and distributed adjustments of the multiple constituent elements so as to cancel discrepancies between current or predicted output and that intended goal. If one considers the alternative control scheme reflected in the classic tongue-position based descriptions of phonetic elements (namely, predetermined specification of each muscle contraction and articulatory movement) this more flexible system, involving sensory monitoring and adjustment, is appealing.

Additionally, from a teleonomic standpoint, the adaptive modification and adjustment of muscle and movement actions via sensorimotor actions are rational. For example, the orofacial system is critical to the multiple functions of chewing, swallowing, and breathing in addition to speech. Other less natural behaviors include holding cigarettes between the lips, chewing tobacco, and clenching a pipe between the teeth. Because many of these activities can (and must) be interweaved or overlapped without major interference or conscious compensation, a nervous system capability for on-line adaptive adjustment appears almost necessary. Such semiautomatic adaptation also seems likely in laryngeal and respiratory control for speech as well. Physiologic investigations of the laryngeal and respiratory systems, as well as consideration of peripheral anatomy, indicate that torso, head, and arm movements have significant influences upon specific muscle contractions required for speech. Trained singers are aware of these influences. However, in many circumstances, one has little difficulty in sustaining continuous and intelligible speech concurrently with vigorous body movements. Observing an aerobics teacher perform calisthenics and at the same time continuously coach and sooth the participating pupils is an obvious example of this phenomenon. In these and other similar cases (e.g., a vigorous university lecturer), one cannot help but be impressed with the human ability to produce continuous speech without major interference from the variable and extraneous movements associated with other concurrent functions. Possibly these multiple motor functions could be generated and preadjusted interactively in parallel, but such an organization is contradictory to the unanticipated perturbation findings that indicate sensorimotor contributions to unanticipated variations and the intractable motor prespecification that would be required to coordinate such multiple motor outputs.

The nature of sensorimotor contributions to multimovement coordination and control for speech has been expanded by other more recent perturbation studies as well. For example, recent observations suggest that sensory information contributes not only to the coordination of movement magnitude among multiple constituent elements, but also to the timing among these speech actions. One study was aimed at the role of sensory information in the timing of the laryngeal adduction and abduction patterns that are important for the linguistically significant distinctions between voiced and voiceless consonants. Specifically, Shaiman et al found that when perturbations were introduced on the lower lip, resulting in increased lower lip movement durations for bilabial voiceless stop consonant closure, laryngeal adduction and vibration cessation consistently were delayed in parallel.[65] The interpretation of this result is that sensory information associated with evolving movement in one part of the speech production system is utilized to ensure proper co-timing of movements in other parts of the system. And seemingly, despite some arguments to the contrary, temporal patterning among multiple speech motor actions is flexibly adjusted, depending on the state of the periphery and moment-to-moment variations in the evolving speech motor action. The other findings that speak to the importance of sensorimotor mechanisms in coordination of speech movements are data suggesting that the particular distribution of sensorimotor adjustments is task dependent. Specifically, as illustrated in Figure 5–8, if the lower lip is perturbed during an upper lip and lower lip gesture (/p/), compensations are seen (as noted) in both the upper and lower lips. By contrast, if the lower lip is perturbed during an /f/, upper lip compensatory actions are functionally absent.[66] Comparable results have been obtained in perturbations of the jaw during/z/ and /b/, yielding responses more or less confined to the tongue and lip, respectively.[62] In general, these latter results suggest that as part of the so-called program for a given multimovement speech motor action, particular sensorimotor processes are selected to contribute, while others are inhibited or gated out. Thus these results further imply that coordination of multiple speech movements is implemented by delegating the pathways and neural processes for the downstream motor execution, not by prespecification of the individual parameters of muscle contraction and movement. What may be prespecified is the final acoustic or aerodynamic speech objective; however, the particular pattern of movements and muscle contractions leading to the achievement of that objective apparently are determined by moment-to-moment sensorimotor actions.

The coordination among multiple constituent movements via task-dependent sensorimotor adjustments is clear and provides additional insight into possible neurobiologic correlates. To address this important issue in more detail, it is useful to examine the specific contributions of such sensory information and then subsequently determine whether or not one can correlate those different contributions with different neural centers.

MULTIPLE CONTRIBUTIONS OF SENSORIMOTOR PROCESSES TO SPEECH COORDINATION

The objective of identifying neurobiologic correlates of speech control and the evidence reviewed before leads one to a comment by Grillner in the conclusion to an extensive review of the neural mechanisms underlying locomotion.[67] He noted that "sterile discussion on entirely central versus basically reflex control belong to the past." As he suggested subsequently, such exercises need to be replaced by fruitful endeavors as to how sensory inputs actually contribute to movement. It is obviously important to concentrate on the detailed contributions of sensory information rather than to expend unnecessary energy on the defense or advocacy of extreme positions. The same is true, as apparent from the data reviewed before, in the understanding of speech motor control and the necessary multimovement coordination. Moreover, one avenue to address the issue of neurobiologic correlates of speech motor processes is to exploit the fact, revealed in perturbation experiments and other studies, that sensory processes contribute in several different ways to speech movement coordination. Fundamentally, from the recent studies described previously, one can distinguish several different contributions of sensorimotor actions. Two basic distinctions relate to (1) the movement and muscle distribution of the responses to the perturbation of a given movement and (2) the time-varying character of those responses. As detailed previously,[68] the distinctions among these different sensorimotor contributions provide insights for identifying correspondingly distinct sensorimotor pathways and neural control centers.

Autogenic Versus Nonautogenic Sensorimotor Actions

Figure 5–9 schematically illustrates the kinds of functional connections reflected in most of the perturbation experiments described previously. An unanticipated error is introduced on one movement in a multimovement speech action and compensatory responses are of two distinct kinds: autogenic and nonautogenic. Autogenic sensorimotor processes

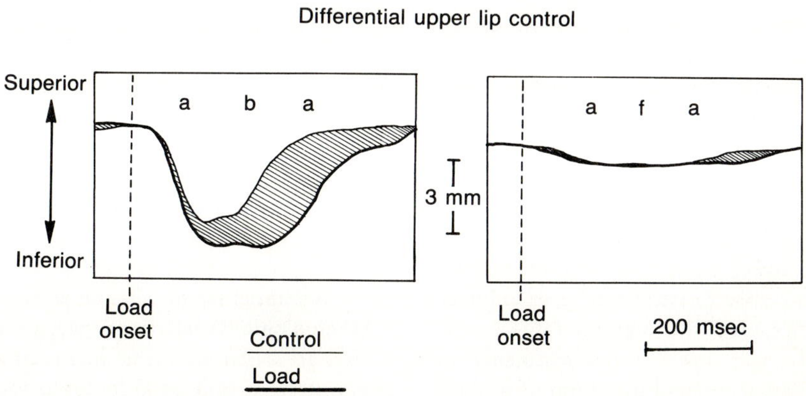

Figure 5–8 Illustration of the influence of lower lip perturbation on upper lip movement for /aba/ versus /afa/.

are ones in which the resulting compensation is of a form to correct the induced error at the same site where it was introduced. For example, when a perturbation is introduced on the lower lip, responses observed in lower lip muscles and movements are autogenic, reflecting a classic closed-loop feedback compensation; this is the kind of sensory control illustrated in most basic physiology or biology textbooks. Very often in a description of this kind of sensory regulatory process, muscle spindles are involved in detecting errors in intended muscle length and the associated autogenic compensatory responses are said to be generated to correct those muscle length errors. By contrast, for that same perturbation, if one observes responses in the muscles and movements of the upper lip and jaw, these are considered to be indicative of nonautogenic adjustments. Such distributed or remote autogenic responses do not correct the error at the site where it was introduced or detected; rather they act to cancel its influence on the combined output. Although this distinction initially may appear subtle, it has significant functional importance. Some investigators and control system modelers have viewed the autogenic sensorimotor process as the classic feedback controller, requiring comparisons between desired and intended goals as well as having the inherent time delays and instability associated with such nervous system functions.[48,58,69] In contrast, the nonautogenic processes (referred to by some as feedforward controllers)[48,58,70] have been characterized as having faster response times, higher stability, and greater flexiblity than autogenic sensorimotor actions. Importantly, there are data to support some of these claims, and the functional separability of autogenic and nonautogenic sensorimotor processes have been demonstrated empirically.[58,59]

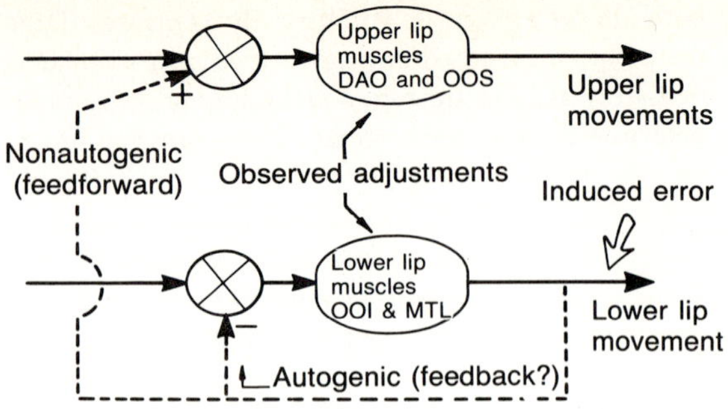

Figure 5-9 Schematic representation of the difference between autogenic and nonautogenic sensorimotor adjustments to lower lip perturbations.

change in movement (upper or lower lip) divided by the magnitude of induced perturbation displacement. In general, as shown in Figure 5-10, for lower lip perturbations introduced 0.0 to 50 msec prior to the onset of muscle activity for bilabial closure, the autogenic or lower lip responses had a consistently greater gain than the nonautogenic or upper lip responses. In a subsequent experiment, when perturbations were introduced on the upper lip, upper lip responses (autogenic) had a similarly greater gain than their lower lip (nonautogenic) counterparts. This shift in response locus not only documents the distinction between autogenic and nonautogenic, but also indicates that the early loads may be sampling the control process at a time when somatic sensory information is being utilized differently than for later loads.

In particular, early loads apparently result in an overall reorganization of the speech movement pattern. This reorganization might be considered as parallel to the parameter estimation period[71] that precedes initial movement execution. By contrast, compensations to later loads appear to reflect a different process, essentially an on-line shaping of the movement pattern. Thus the response pattern that one sees to early loads might be considered as indicative of how sensory information is utilized during so-called programming of the upcoming movement, whereas responses to later loads would reflect the utilization of such sensory information during movement execution.

Parameter Estimation Versus On-line Shaping

In most of the aforementioned speech perturbation experiments, to precisely time the onset of the load was impossible. As such, the objective was to distribute the loads somewhat uniformly over a 100 msec interval centered on the onset of musculus orbicularis oris inferior activity. Perhaps the most complete analyses of these time-varying functions have been undertaken in perturbation studies of the upper and lower lip movements for bilabial closure. Gracco and Abbs devised an index of compensatory movement responses that permitted direct comparison of upper and lower lip adjustments to perturbations.[59] This index took the form of a pseudogain function, specifically a ratio of the percentage

NEUROANATOMIC CORRELATES OF MULTIPLE SENSORIMOTOR CONTROL FUNCTIONS

Attempts in this chapter at identification of the neurobiologic correlates of speech sensorimotor processes are based upon the dual premises that sensory information is utilized in multiple ways and that these different processes, in turn, reflect the actions of different neural centers. Furthermore, this particular set of hypotheses is focused on the different ways in which sensory information can influence the motoneurons of the orofacial musculature; for simplicity and due to limited data, respiratory and laryngeal motor processes have been ignored.

Initially, since several studies have demonstrated that the primary influences do not have latencies consistent with brain stem–mediated reflex pathways,[58,72,73] it would appear that all such sensorimotor actions are funnelled via the pyramidal cells of the primary motor cortex.[48,56,57] These motor cortex cells appear to make monosynaptic connections with motoneurons of the facial, motor trigeminal, and hypoglossal nuclei; hence their role as the major CNS output upon which multiple converging sensory influences impinge to modify and shape speech motor output. Indeed, most voluntary motor behaviors have as their final common path the descending pathways from the motor cortex. Given these assumptions, Figure 5–11 provides a schematic overview of the different pathways over which orofacial sensory influences could access the primary motor cortex pyramidal cells. As has been advanced previously, it is possible to offer a theory of how these pathways might contribute differentially to motor programming and execution, as well as to how the parallel functions of autogenic versus nonautogenic adjustments are implemented.

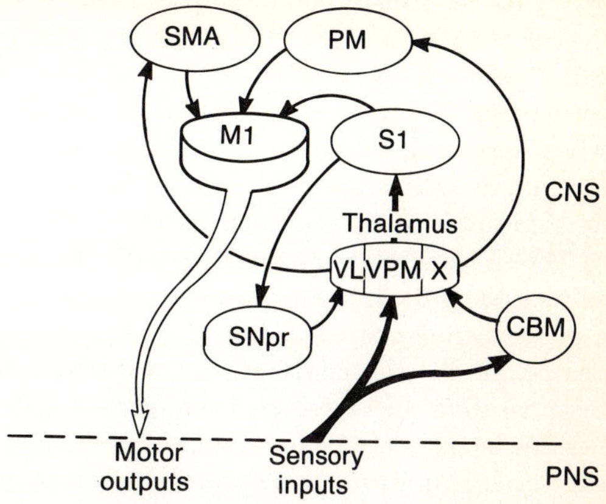

Figure 5–11 General illustration of the multiple sensorimotor pathways involved in the control of lip movements for speech. (Based upon a general model for such influences suggested by Gracco VL, Abbs JH. Programming and execution processes of speech movement control: potential neural correlates. In: Keller E, Gopnik M, eds. Symposium on motor and sensory language processes. Hillsdale, NJ: Erlbaum, 1987:163; Abbs JH. Invariance and variability in speech production: a distinction between linguistic intent and its neuromotor implementation. In: Perkell J, Klatt D, eds. Invariance and variability of speech process. Hillsdale, NJ: Erlbaum, 1986:202.)

Sensorimotor Pathways for Speech Motor Programming

Basically, it appears that certain sensorimotor pathways are preferentially involved in contributing to motor programming, whereas others contribute to motor execution. Obviously, specification of a complete separation between motor execution and motor programming (or preparation) is impossible, at least without new techniques for studying brain functions in human subjects. Indeed, attempting to identify what parts of the brain underlie motor programming or, for that matter, how to define motor programming is a task that deserves a chapter in itself. For the present discussion, the more modest goal is to identify the neural mechanisms associated with sensory monitoring of the state of the periphery as a basis for an upcoming movement; this function perhaps is better considered as one of premovement parameter estimation as a subset of a larger so-called motor programming process. By definition, this process obviously occurs prior to the implementation or initiation of a motor act. Referring to Figure 5–11, two brain centers have commonly been argued to contribute in this manner with several different forms of data to support such operation. These are the basal ganglia and the cerebellum.[74–79] Additionally, as reflected in Figure 5–11, recent data by Schell and Strick, along with their reinterpretation of some earlier results, indicate that the regions of the basal ganglia and cerebellum associated with orofacial function project to the supplementary motor and premotor cortices, respectively.[80] Furthermore, these and parallel observations suggest that although the basal ganglia and cerebellum have important influ-

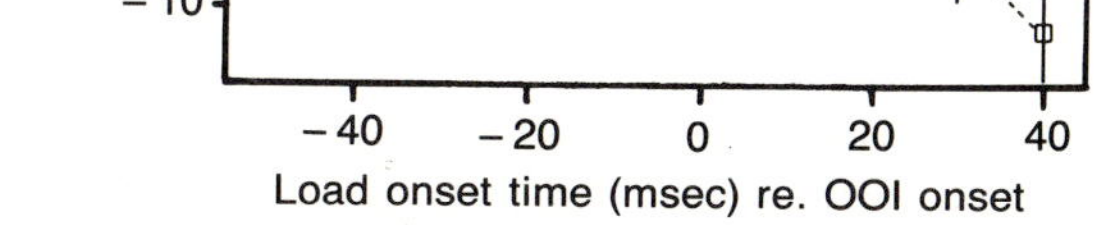

Figure 5-10 Differential adjustment (expressed as "relative gain") in upper and lower lip movements as a function of timing variations when lower lip perturbations are introduced. Load onset times are referenced to the onset of activity in Obicularis Oris Inferior (OOI). (Adapted from Gracco VL, Abbs JH. Dynamic control of the perioral system during speech: Kinematic analyses of autogenic and nonautogenic sensorimotor processes. J Neurophysiol 1985; 54:418.)

ences upon the primary motor cortex, these inputs are mediated via these secondary motor cortex regions.[81,82] Hence, as summarized in Figure 5–11, sensory projections to the cerebullum and basal ganglia are apparently involved in processes of motor programming and parameter estimation by virtue of influences upon areas of secondary motor cortices.

The sensory pathways to the basal ganglia, somewhat simplified, would include projections to the somatic sensory cortex and then, in turn, via the putamen, to the substantia nigra, pars reticulata. Projections from the substantia nigra, pars reticulata via the thalamus and then to the supplementary motor cortex and, in turn, to the primary motor cortex would complete the sensorimotor route. The executive role of the basal ganglia has been suggested numerous times,[77,83] and a higher-level function for the supplementary motor cortex has been concluded in several recent investigations.[84–87] The function of the basal ganglia and the supplementary motor cortex as serial centers implies that lesions to one or the other may result in similar impairments. Interestingly, reports of similar behavioral deficits for damage to the basal ganglia and the supplementary motor cortex, though rare, have been reported.[88–92]

The pathways are fairly direct for the cerebellar mediation of sensory information that might be utilized in the setting up of the system for motor execution. As illustrated in Figure 5–11, ascending projections include those from the trigeminal nuclei to the cerebellar cortex and on to the cerebellar nuclei.[93–97] The cerebellar cortex regions associated with orofacial function apparently project primarily to the caudal portions of the dentate deep cerebellar nucleus, from there to area X of the thalamus (with a notable lack of projections to the ventral lateral medial) and then, in turn, to the premotor area of the cerebral cortex. The available data (particularly those of Schell and Strick)[80] indicate clearly that the cerebellar influences associated with orofacial processes (via area X) do not project to primary motor cortex directly, but rather via the premotor cortex. Interestingly, recent reviews argue for a special role of the premotor cortex in orofacial coordination and control,[56,98] perhaps related to the hypothesized function of Broca's area in humans (Brodmann's area 44), as previously hypothesized. However, the important point is that this cortical region is similarly upstream or in an apparent executive position in relation to the primary motor cortex; hence it has a likely role in motor preparation or programming. Moreover, recent work suggesting the role of the premotor area in orofacial motor coordination and results of studies addressing breakdowns in speech movements in patients with such problems,[99] lend credence to the concept that the cerebellum and the premotor area are functioning in a serial fashion. Indeed, even some general analyses with acoustic techniques[100] have suggested a possible similarity between cerebellar dysarthria and apraxia of speech, the latter presumably related, at least in part, to anterolateral lesions of the premotor cortex.

Inasmuch as the utilization of sensory information from the orofacial region for the preparation of a motor action is not as time critical as moment-to-moment adjustments, short latencies perhaps are not absolutely necessary. However, peripheral sensory stimulation yields responses in the basal ganglia and the supplementary motor cortex with latencies ranging from 15 to 25 msec;[101,102] unfortunately data on monkeys are limited.

Sensorimotor Contributions to Speech Motor Execution

Once a movement is under way or at the least after muscle activity has been initiated, based upon data presented earlier, the sensory information appears to be utilized differently. Fortunately, the contribution of sensory information to the execution phase of movement is a more direct one, and the pathways almost certainly would involve projections to the somatic sensory cortex and, in turn, to the primary motor regions. Perhaps the most direct and short-latency transmission of sensory information from the orofacial region is via the trigeminothalamic projections, originating in the main sensory nucleus and nucleus suboralis of the trigeminal nerve. Information transmitted via this pathway carries all of the peripheral details, apparently with limited processing and minimal convergence,[103] to the ventral posteromedial nucleus of the thalamas.[104] Information via this pathway is, in turn, transmitted to the somatic sensory cortical areas 3b and 1.[105–107]

The latencies of responses in the somatic sensory cortex (in monkeys) are from 5 to 12 msec,[108] with only slightly longer pathways to the motor cortex of 7 to 14 msec. Assuming a descending cortical latency comparable to the ascending one, a direct pathway with a total response latency of 15 to 20 msec is not unreasonable. Obviously, short-lactency pathways by which to implement moment-to-moment adjustments of the evolving speech motor output are available via these cortical connections without relying upon brain stem connections. Interestingly, the classic transcortical pathway is thought to be involved primarily in autogenic or feedback corrections; other pathways would appear to be involved in the nonautogenic adjustments. A likely pathway for nonautogenic adjustments would appear to be via the somatic sensory cortex to the lateral premotor cortex (see Fig. 5–11). This anterolateral region of the cerebral cortex receives sensory input from the orofacial region, and, as shown by the work of Muakkassa and Strick,[82] is upstream from the primary motor cortex. Somatic sensory input is manifest in the lateral premotor area with latencies as short as 10 to 12 msec.[108,109] Additionally, both of these investigators found that this region of cortex is particularly responsive to more complex, multimovement (lip, tongue, larynx), goal-oriented stimuli than the primary motor cortex. Finally, it was shown that lesions of this lateral region had a differential influence upon orofacial movement coordination[110–112] as compared to the primary motor cortex. Obviously, such preferential responsiveness to complex somatic sensory stimuli and the differential influences of lesions upon coordination suggest a special role for this area in complex orofacial movements. Probably, that this area of cortex is part of Broca's region in humans is not coincidental, with clear importance in speech motor control.

SUMMARY

As noted at the outset of this chapter, recent advances have made it possible to consider the neural control of speech movements in relation to specific neural centers and specifically with regard to coordination of the muscle contractions and movements that must occur to yield this important human behavior. This comment is not to imply that the linguistic or information-processing models of speech generation are to be totally replaced. Rather, it is first important at this juncture to recognize that such models or theories are relevant primarily as abstract metaphors of the brain mechanisms for speech production. Second, rather than throwing out the proverbial baby, it will be at least partially useful to incorporate such phonetic unit-related concepts, such as forward coarticulation and seriation, into biologic models. A useful process will be to determine if one can identify the means by which these black box operations are implemented by the nervous system and their relations to processes of actual motor control. Such attempts are already under way,[56] but much remains to be done. One expects that important information will come as a result of cross-disciplinary studies in which scientists specializing in motor control will collaborate with colleagues in speech as a means to accelerate the already rapid growth in the area of motor control.

Aside from general implications for advances in speech-language pathologists' understanding of the neural processes underlying speech motor control and coordination, the considerations raised in this chapter have important implications for many disorders of speech. The directions from speech motor neurophysiology for disorders of speech production would appear to be important both for the way in which one conceptualizes the disorder processes as well as for the development of improved programs for assessment and treatment.

For example, in relation to individuals with speech neuromotor disorders, the implications seem self-evident, including

1. An increased need to exercise caution when drawing conclusions concerning speech motor aberrations based upon neurologic assessments that primarily focus upon distal musculature that is moved differently, is innervated differently (both in afferent and efferent mechanisms), and has different representations at all levels of the neuraxis when compared to the motor subsystems of the speech production mechanism, despite some potential overlap between these systems in their functional operation.
2. The need to refine the measures used to describe and study these populations, based upon the awareness that traditional observational techniques may not reveal nor permit optimally useful inferences to underlying mechanisms of motor control dysfunction; an example of the latter includes the limitations of electromyography, as noted previously, in discerning the details of higher-level programming and execution processes.
3. The apparent dependency between coordination of normal speech movements and possible sensory contributions to this process, which may be an important key to the apparent concurrence of deficiencies in these functions in individuals with brain damage, as well as suggesting directions for rehabilitation through reestablishment of control via the use of external afference (namely, biofeedback).
4. The movement and control requirements between the different subsystems of the speech production mechanism and within a particular subsystem for different speech elements, which create a circumstance wherein it would be unusual if upper motoneuron damage in a particular dysarthric individual did not yield substantial variation in motor impairment when contrasting the lips, tongue, jaw, or impairments within one of these subsystems for different speech elements (e.g., consonant versus vowel production).[113]

The implications of these variations for improving assessment and rehabilitation procedures with dysarthric populations are at the same time both promising and extremely challenging. However, what is apparent is that general views of the speech mechanism as a single neuromotor system (as in some neurologic reports in which a patient's symptoms are reported to include a dysarthria among other things) must be changed if more effective treatment is to result.

A final point that emerges from examination of normal speech motor control concerns the traditional labelling and concepts of speech production disorders in terms of etiologies. Although the fact that an individual with Parkinson's dysarthria has a motor control dysfunction is apparent, such unitary specification of etiology for a child with so-called phonologic deficiencies may simply be inappropriate. One can concede that articulation errors appear to occur in certain patterns related to features and/or rules hypothesized by one linguistic categorization scheme or another. However, to surmise from this observation that the etiology is linguistic or cognitive may be an oversimplification. For example, it would seem as plausible to suggest that this child simply may not have the normal capability to develop sensorimotor control and thus cannot *learn* the processes necessary for executing certain linguistic rule processes consistently. Indeed, if the modes of control and/or neural pathways involved in the generation of particular motor gestures are sensitive to experience, attention, and intentions, that children with speech articulation problems also manifest, in many cases, parallel learning, attention, and perceptual difficulties, is not surprising. These considerations may also be of value in demystifying some of the social and/or psychological and environmental variability in the quality of speech performance in populations like stutterers and some of the neurologically impaired. Perhaps future research will speak more directly to these issues.

These comments should not be interpreted to suggest that the bases of all speech production disorders are found in the study of motor control. However, it would seem critical to discard the almost Cartesian dualism that has guided our approach to speech problems in some populations. In so doing, speech-language pathologists need to temper their thinking with the knowledge that the neurophysiologic mechanisms of speech control cannot be separated functionally from the less well-understood neural processes involving motivation, attention, conceptualization, and sensory awareness, all of which have been implicated increasingly as influential factors in motor execution processes.

REFERENCES

1. Eccles JC, Gibson WC. Sherrington: his life and thought. Berlin: Springer, 1979.
2. Glassman RB. The logic of the lesion experiment and its role in the neural sciences. In: Finger S, ed. Recovery from brain damage: research and theory. New York: Plenum Press, 1978:3.
3. Jackson JH. Clinical and physiological localization of movements in the brain. Selected writings. Vol. 1. London: Churchill, 1875:37.
4. Marshall JF. Brain function: neural adaptations and recovery from injury. Annu Rev Psychol 1984; 35:277–308.
5. Evarts EV. Methods for recording activity of individual neurons in moving animals. In: Rushmer RF, ed. Methods in medical research. Chicago: Year Book Medical Publishers, 1966:241.
6. Evarts EV. Representation of movements and muscles by pyramidal tract neurons of the precentral motor cortex. In: Yahr MD, Purpura DP, eds. Neurophysiological basis of normal and abnormal motor activities. New York: Raven Press, 1967:215.
7. Wiener N. Cybernetics. New York: John Wiley & Sons, 1948.
8. Stark L. Neurological control systems: studies in bioengineering. In: Alt F, ed. Advances in bioengineering and instrumentation. New York: Plenum Press, 1968.
9. Crago PE, Houk JC, Hasan Z. Regulatory actions of human stretch reflex. J Neurophysiol 1976; 39:925–935.
10. Houk JC. The phylogeny of muscular control configurations. In: Drischel H, Dellmar P, eds. The third international symposium on biocybernetics proceedings. Vol. 4. Jena: Veb Gustav Fischer Verlag, 1972:125.
11. Houk JC. An assessment of stretch reflex function. Brain Res 1976; 44:303–314.
12. Houk JC. Participation of reflex mechanisms and reaction-time processes in the compensatory adjustments to mechanical disturbances. In: Desmedt JE, ed. Progress in clinical neurophysiology. Cerebral motor control in man: long loop mechanism. Vol. 4. Basel: Karger, 1978:193.
13. Houk JC, Henneman E. Feedback control of skeletal muscles. In: Mountcastle VB, ed. Brain Res 1967; 5:433–451.
14. Houk JC, Henneman E. Responses of Golgi tendon organs to active contractions of the soleus muscle of the cat. J Neurophysiol 1967; 30:466–481.
15. Houk JC, Rymer WZ. Neural control of muscle length and tension. In: Handbook of physiology: section 1. The nervous system. Vol. II. Motor control, part 2. Bethesda, MD: American Physiological Society, 1981:257.
16. Houk JC, Singer JJ, Goldman MR. An evaluation of length and force feedback to soleus muscles of decerebrate cats. J Neurophysiol 1970; 33:784–811.
17. Nichols TR, Houk JC. The improvement in linearity and the regulation of stiffness that results from the actions of the stretch reflex. J Neurophysiol 1976; 39:119–142.
18. Bizzi E, Accornero N, Chapple W, Hogan N. Posture control and trajectory formation during arm movement. J Neurosci 1984; 4:2738–2744.
19. Flash T, Hogan N. The coordination of arm movements: an experimentally confirmed mathematical model. J Neurosci 1985; 5:1688–1703.
20. Hogan N. Impedance control: an approach to manipulation. Proceedings of the American Control Conference. Presented at American Control Conference, San Diego, 1984, 304-313.
21. Hogan N. An organizing principle for a class of voluntary movements. J Neurosci 1984; 4:2745–2754.
22. Hogan N. The mechanics of multi-joint posture and movement control. Biol Cyber 1985; 52:315–331.
23. Hollerbach JM. Computers, brains and the control of movement. Trends Neurosci 1982; 5:189–192.
24. Hollerbach JM, Flash T. Dynamic interactions between limb segments during planar arm movement. Biol Cyber 1982; 44:67–77.
25. Partridge LD. A proposal for study of a static description of the motor control system. In: Shahani M, ed. The motor

system: neurophysiological and muscle mechanics. New York: Elsevier, 1972:363.

26. Partridge LD, Benton LA. Muscle, the motor. In: Brooks VB, ed. Handbook of physiology, section 1. The nervous system. Vol. II. Motor control, part 1. Bethesda, MD: American Physiological Society, 1981:43.
27. Alexander RM. Biomechanics of skeleton and tendons. In: Brooks VB, ed. Handbook of physiology, section 1. The nervous system. Vol. II. Motor control, part 1. Bethesda, MD: American Physiological Society, 1981:17.
28. Hughes OM, Abbs JH. Labial-mandibular coordination in the production of speech: implications for the operation of motor equivalence. Phonetica 1976; 33:199–221.
29. Sussman HM. Methodological problems in evaluating lip/jaw reciprocity as an index of motor equivalence. J Speech Hear Res 1980; 23:699–702.
30. Abbs JH. Speech motor equivalence: a need for a multilevel control model. Proceedings of the Ninth International Congress of Phonetics. Vol. II. Copenhagen, 1979:318–324.
31. Gracco VL, Abbs JH. Variant and invariant charcteristics of speech movement planning. Exp Brain Res 1986; 65:156-166.
32. Bernstein NA. On the construction of movements. Monograph (in Russian), Moscow, 1947.
33. Bernstein NA. The co-ordination and regulation of movements. Oxford: Pergamon Press, 1967.
34. Granit R. The purposive brain. Cambridge, MA: MIT Press, 1977.
35. Lacquaniti F, Soechting JF. Coordination of arm and wrist motion during a reaching task. J Neurosci 1982; 2:399–408.
36. Lashley KS. Basic neural mechanisms in behavior. Psychol Rev 1930; 37:1–24.
37. Lashley KS. The problem of serial order in behavior. In: Jeffress LA, ed. Cerebral mechanisms in behavior (the Hixon Symposium). New York: John Wiley & Sons, 1951:112.
38. Morasso P. Spatial control of arm movements. Exp Brain Res 1981; 42:223-227.
39. Paillard J. The patterning of skilled movements. In: Field J, Magoun H, Hall V, eds. Handbook of physiology, section 1. Neurophysiology. Vol. 3. Washington: American Physiology Society, 1960:1679.
40. Phillips CG. Cortical localization and sensorimotor processes at the "middle level" in primates. Hughlings Jackson Lecture, Proceedings of the Royal Society of Medicine 1973; 66:987-1002.
41. Phillips CG, Porter R. Corticospinal neurones: their role in movement. London: Academic Press, 1977.
42. Abend W, Bizzi E, Morasso P. Human arm trajectory formation. Brain 1982; 105:331–348.
43. Cole KJ, Abbs JH. Coordination of three-joint digit movements for rapid, finger-thumb grasp. J Neurophysiol 1986; 55:1407-1423.
44. Turvey MT, Shaw RE, Mace W. Issues in the theory of action: degrees of freedom, coordinative structures and coalitions. In: Requin J, ed. Attention and performance VII. Hillsdale, NJ: Erlbaum, 1978:557.
45. Hinton G. Some computational solutions to Bernstein's problems. In: Whiting TA, ed. Human motor actions-Bernstein reassessed. North-Holland: Elsevier, 1984:413.
46. Loeb GE. Finding common ground between robotics and physiology. Trends Neurosci 1983; 6:203–204.
47. Requin J, Semjen A, Bonnet M. Bernstein's purposive brain. In: Whiting HTA, ed. Human motor actions-Bernstein revisited. Amsterdam: North-Holland Publishing Company, 1984:467.
48. Abbs JH, Gracco VL, Cole KJ. Control of multimovement coordination: sensorimotor mechanisms in speech motor programming. J Motor Behav 1984; 16:195–232.
49. Fentress JC. The development of coordination. J Motor Behav 1984; 16:99–134.
50. Hollerbach JM. An oscillation theory of handwriting. Biol Cyber 1981; 39:139–156.
51. MacNeilage P. Motor control of serial ordering of speech. Psychol Rev 1970; 77:182–196.
52. Abbs JH, Cole KJ. Neural mechanisms of motor equivalence and goal achievement. In: Wise S, Evarts EV, eds. Higher brain functions: recent explorations of the brain's emergent properties. New York: John Wiley & Sons, 1987:15.
53. Riordan CJ. Control of vocal-tract length in speech. J Acoust Soc Am 1977; 62:998–1002.
54. Stevens KN, House AS. Development of a quantitative description of vowel articulation. J Acoust Soc Am 1955; 27:484–493.
55. Stevens KN, House AS. An acoustical theory of vowel production and some of its implications. J Speech Hear Res 1961; 4:303–320.
56. Abbs JH. Invariance and variability in speech production: a distinction between linguistic intent and its neuromotor implementation. In: Perkell J, Klatt D, eds. Invariance and variability of speech process. Hillsdale, NJ: Erlbaum, 1986:202.
57. Abbs JH, Cole KJ. Consideration of bulbar and suprabulbar afferent influences upon speech motor coordination and programming. In: Grillner S, Lindblom, B, Lubker J, Persson A, eds. Speech motor control. New York: Pergamon Press, 1982:159.
58. Abbs JH, Gracco VL. Control of complex motor gestures: orofacial muscle responses to load perturbations of the lip during speech. J Neurophysiol 1984; 52:705–723.
59. Gracco VL, Abbs JH. Dynamic control of the perioral system during speech: kinematic analyses of autogenic and nonautogenic sensorimotor processes. J Neurophysiol 1985; 54:418–432.
60. Folkins JW, Abbs JH. Lip and jaw motor control during speech: responses to resistive loading of the jaw. J Speech Hear Res 1975; 18:207–220.
61. Folkins J, Abbs JH. Additional observations on responses to resistive loading of the jaw. J Speech Hear Res 1976; 19:820–821.
62. Kelso JAS, Tuller B, Fowler CA. The functional specificity of articulatory control and coordination. J Acoust Soc Am 1982; 72:S103.
63. Kelso JAS, Tuller B, V–Bateson E, Fowler CA. Functionally specific articulatory cooperation following jaw perturbations during speech: evidence for coordinative structures. J Exp Psychol [Hum Percep] 1984; 10:812–832.
64. Abbs JH, Gracco VL. Kinematic evidence for differential control of speech movement temporal and magnitude parameters. Paper presented at the XXX International Union of Physiological Sciences, Vancouver, WA, 1986.
65. Shaiman S, Abbs JH, Gracco VL. Sensorimotor contributions to oral-laryngeal coordination for speech. Paper presented at the Society for Neuroscience Meeting, Dallas, 1985.
66. Abbs JH, Shaiman S, Gracco VL, Cole KJ. Task-dependent sensorimotor actions are inherent in speech motor programs. Paper presented at the Society for Neuroscience Meeting, Dallas, TX, 1985.
67. Grillner S. Locomotion in vertebrates—central mechanisms and reflex interaction. Physiol Rev 1975; 55:247–304.
68. Gracco VL, Abbs JH. Programming and execution processes of speech movement control: potential neural correlates. In: Keller E, Gopnik M, eds. Symposium on motor and sensory language processes. Hillsdale, NJ: Erlbaum, 1987:163.
69. Robinson DA. Control of eye movements. In: Brooks VB, ed. Handbook of physiology: section 1. The nervous system. Vol. II. Motor control, part 2. Bethesda, MD: American Physiological Society, 1981:1275.
70. Robinson DA. Key problems in the programming of movements: concluding session. Brain Res 1974; 71:549.
71. Arbib MA. Perceptual structures and distributed motor

control. In: Brookhart JM, Mountcastle VB, eds. Handbook of physiology, section 1. The nervous system. Vol. II. Motor control, part 2. Bethesda, MD: American Physiological Society, 1981:1449.
72. Abbs JH, Gracco VL. Motor control of multi-movement behaviors: orofacial muscle responses to load perturbations of the lips during speech. Soc Neurosci 1982; 8:282.
73. Gracco VL, Abbs JH. Compensatory response capabilities of the labial system in relation to variation in the onset of unanticipated loads. J Acoust Soc Am 1982; 71:S34.
74. Allen GI, Tsukahara N. Cerebrocerebellar communication systems. Physiol Rev 1974; 54:957–1005.
75. Brooks VB. Motor program revisited. In: Talbott RE, Humphrey DR, eds. Posture and movement: perspectives for integrating sensory and motor research on the mammalian nervous system. New York: Raven Press, 1979:13.
76. Brooks VB, Thach WT. Cerebellar control of posture and movement. In: Brookhart JM, Mountcastle VB, eds. Handbook of physiology: section 1. The nervous system. Vol. II. Motor control, part 2. Bethesda, MD: American Physiological Society, 1981:877.
77. DeLong MR, Georgopoulos AP. Motor functions of the basal ganglia. In: Brookhart JM, Mountcastle VB, eds. Handbook of physiology: section 1. The nervous system: volume II. Motor control, part 2. Bethesda, MD: American Physiological Society, 1981:1017.
78. Kemp JM, Powell TPS. The connections of the striatum and globus pallidus: synthesis and speculation. Philos Trans R Soc Lond [Biol] 1971; 262:441–457.
79. Paillard J. Introductory lecture: the functional labelling of neural codes. In: Massion J, Paillard J, Schultz W, Wiesendanger M, eds. Neural coding of motor performance. Berlin: Springer, 1983:1.
80. Schell GR, Strick PL. The origin of thalamic inputs to the arcuate premotor and supplementary motor areas. J Neurosci 1984; 4:539–560.
81. Matelli M, Camarda R, Glickstein M, Rizzolatti G. Interconnections within the postarcuate cortex (area 6) of the macaque monkey. Brain Res 1984; 310:388–392.
82. Muakkassa KF, Strick PL. Frontal lobe inputs to primate motor cortex: evidence for four somatotopically organized 'premotor' areas. Brain Res 1979; 177:176–182.
83. Marsden CD. The mysterious motor function of the basal ganglia: the Robert Wartenberg lecture. Neurol 1982; 32:514–539.
84. Brinkman C, Porter R. Supplementary motor area in the monkey: activity of neurons during performance of a learned motor task. J Neurophysiol 1979; 42:681–709.
85. Jurgens U. The efferent and afferent connections of the supplementary motor area. Brain Res 1984; 300:63–81.
86. Roland PE, Larsen B, Lassen NA, Shinhøj E. Supplementary motor area and other cortical areas in organization of voluntary movements in man. J Neurophysiol 1980; 43:118–136.
87. Tanji J. The neuronal activity in the supplementary motor area of primates. Trends Neurosciences 1984; 7:282–285.
88. Arseni C, Boetz MI. Speech disturbances caused by tumors of the supplementary motor area. Acta Psychiatr Neurol Scand 1961; 36:279–298.
89. Caplan LR, Zervas NT. Speech arrest in a dextral with a right mesial frontal astrocytoma. Arch Neurol 1978; 35:252–253.
90. Damasio AR, Van Hoesen GW. Structure and function of the supplementary motor area. Neurology 1980; 30:359.
91. Darley FL, Aronson AE, Brown JR. Motor speech disorders. Philadelphia: WB Saunders, 1975.
92. Masdeu JC, Schoene WC, Funkenstein H. Aphasia following infarction of the left supplementary motor area: a clinicopathologic study. Neurol 1978; 28:1220–1223.
93. Chan-Palay V. Cerebellar dentate nucleus: organization, cytology and transmitters. New York: Springer, 1977.
94. Cody FWJ, Richardson HC. Mossy and climbing fibre projections of trigeminal inputs to the cerebellar cortex in the cat. Brain Res 1978; 153:351–356.
95. Eller T, Chan-Palay V. Afferents to the cerebellar lateral nucleus: evidence from retrograde transport of horseradish peroxidase after pressure injections through micropipettes. J Comp Neurol 1979; 166:285–302.
96. Miles TS, Wiesendanger M. Climbing fibre inputs to cerebellar Purkinje cells from trigeminal cutaneous afferents and the S1 face area of the cerebral cortex in the cat. J Physiol 1975; 245:425–445.
97. Snider RS, Stowell A. Receiving areas of the tactile, auditory, and visual systems in the cerebellum. J Neurophysiol 1944; 7:331–357.
98. Abbs JH, Welt C. Structure and function of the lateral precentral cortex: significance for speech motor control. In: Daniloff RG, ed. Recent advances in speech science. San Diego: College-Hill Press, 1985:155.
99. Fromm D, Abbs JH, McNeil MR, Rosenbek JC. Simultaneous perceptual-physiological method for studying apraxia of speech. In: Brookshire R, ed. Proceedings of the Annual Clinical Aphasiology Conference. Minneapolis:BRK Publishers, 1982:155.
100. Kent RD, Rosenbek JC. Prosodic disturbance and neurologic lesion. Brain Lang 1982; 15:259–291.
101. Lemon RN. Functional properties of monkey motor cortex neurones receiving afferent input from the hand and fingers. J Physiol 1981; 311:497–519.
102. Schneider JS, Morse JR, Lidsky TI. Somatosensory information encoding in the globus pallidus of behaving cats. Exp Brain Res 1982; 46:311–314.
103. Darian-Smith I. Neural mechanisms of face sensation. Int Rev Neurobiol 1966; 9:301–395.
104. Smith RL. Axonal projections and connections of the principal sensory trigeminal nucleus in the monkey. J Comp Neurol 1975; 163:347–376.
105. Felleman DJ, Nelson RJ, Sur M, Kaas JH. Representations of the body surface in areas 3b and 1 of postcentral parietal cortex of cebus monkeys. Brain Res. 1983; 268:15–26.
106. Kaas KH, Nelson RJ, Sur M, Dykes RW, Merzenich MM. The somatotopic organization of the ventroposterior thalamus of the squirrel monkey, saimiri sciureus. J Comp Neurol 1984; 226:111–140.
107. Merzenich MM, Kaas JH, Sur M, Lin CS. Double representation of the body surface within cytoarchitectonic areas 3b and 1 in "S1" in the owl monkeys (Aotus trivirgatus). J Comp Neurol 1978; 181:41–47.
108. O'Brien JH, Pimpaneau A, Albe–Fessard D. Evoked cortical responses to vagal, laryngeal and facial afferents in monkeys under chloralose anaesthesia. Electroencephalogr Clin Neurophysiol 1971; 31:7–20.
109. Rizzolatti G, Scandolara C, Gentilucci M, Camarda R. Response properties and behavioral modulation of "mouth" neurons of the postarcuate cortex (area 6) in macaque monkeys. Brain Res 1981; 255:421–424.
110. Larson CR, Byrd KE, Garthwaite CR, Luschei ES. Alternations in the pattern of mastication after ablations of the lateral precentral cortex in rhesus macaques. Exp Neurol 1980; 70:638–651.
111. Luschei ES, Goodwin GM. Role of monkey precentral cortex in control of voluntary jaw movements. J Neurophysiol 1975; 38:146–157.
112. Watson C. The role of precentral gyrus in the control of facial movement in Macaca mulatta. Doctoral Dissertation, University of Chicago, 1975.
113. Barlow SM, Abbs JH. Orofacial fine motor control impairments in congenital spasticity: evidence against hypertonus-related performance deficits. Neurology 1984; 34:145–150.

6 Acoustics of Speech

June E. Shoup, Ph.D.
Norman J. Lass, Ph.D.
David P. Kuehn, Ph.D.

Speech has been described as "a continuously changing stream of sound."[1] The primary concern of this chapter is with the acoustic characteristics of speech production. However, since speech involves a continuously changing stream of acoustic energy, having a clear understanding of the nature of sound in general is important. Therefore, before we proceed with a detailed discussion of the acoustics of speech, a brief review of some basic concepts of acoustics—the study of sound—is in order to fully appreciate and understand speech acoustics. Emphasis will be directed toward those aspects of acoustics that are considered important for an understanding of the acoustics of speech production.

SOUND AND VIBRATION

Sound has been defined by Hoops as "a condition of disturbance of the particles of an elastic medium which is propagated in a wave outward in all directions from a vibrating body, and takes the form of displacement of the particles forward and backward from their positions of rest in the direction of the propagation of the wave" (p 5).[2] This definition reflects the need for the presence of certain elements in order for sound to exist. These elements include a source of energy, a vibrator, a transmitting medium and, in applying sound to human perception, a receiving mechanism.

All waves involve vibration, a to-and-fro movement of a body about its resting position. Vibrations may be periodic or aperiodic. A periodic vibration is one in which the vibration repeats itself in equal time intervals, whereas an aperiodic vibration is one in which the vibration does not repeat itself regularly. However, regardless of the type of vibration, some common components are necessary for the occurrence of all vibrations, including mass, elasticity, inertia, and a small damping factor.

Mass is any form of matter (solid, liquid, or gas) capable of vibratory motion. Elasticity is the tendency of an object to resume its original condition after some change has been introduced. Inertia is the property that causes a body in motion to remain in motion and a body at rest to remain at rest. The damping factor is any force that interferes with vibration and causes an energy loss to the system.

An example frequently employed to illustrate the concept of vibration is a spring-mass model, as shown in Figure 6–1. The figure shows a spring that is attached to a mass on one end and to a rigid point of attachment on the other end. The mass lies at rest on a surface across which it can move easily; in its normal resting position, the pointer attached to the mass lies at point B on the displacement scale.

If the mass is moved in the direction of point A on the scale (Fig. 6–2), the spring exerts a force on the mass that tends to move it back toward its original position of rest. The spring serves as a restoring force, a force tending to move the mass toward its resting position (elasticity). However, because of inertia, the mass, having been set in motion, continues beyond its rest position (point B) and moves toward point C on the scale, where the spring's restoring force opposes the mass's further motion in that direction. And again, the mass is moved by the spring's restoring force acting in the direction of the mass's resting position (point B), and it will pass through its resting position and move toward point C on the scale; the mass continues to move back and forth in this manner until energy loss in the system prevents its movement. The same result occurs if the mass is initially moved in the opposite direction, that is, toward point C on the displacement scale (Fig. 6–3). The spring exerts a force on the mass

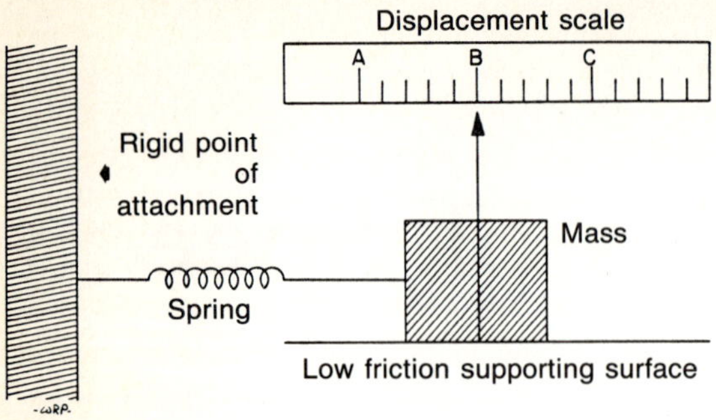

Figure 6–1 A spring-mass system employed to illustrate the concept of vibration. (From Denes P, Pinson EN. The speech chain. Garden City, NY: Anchor Press/Doubleday, 1973.)

that tends to move it back toward its original resting position (point B), with the mass moving beyond this position toward point A on the scale. The spring's restoring force opposes the mass's further motion in that direction and causes the mass to move toward its resting position (point B). The mass passes through its resting position and continues to move beyond it toward point A on the scale; it continues to move back and forth in this manner until energy loss in the system prevents it from doing so. This to-and-fro motion of the mass about its resting position is called "vibration" or "oscillation." Vibrations can occur if there is a small damping factor,

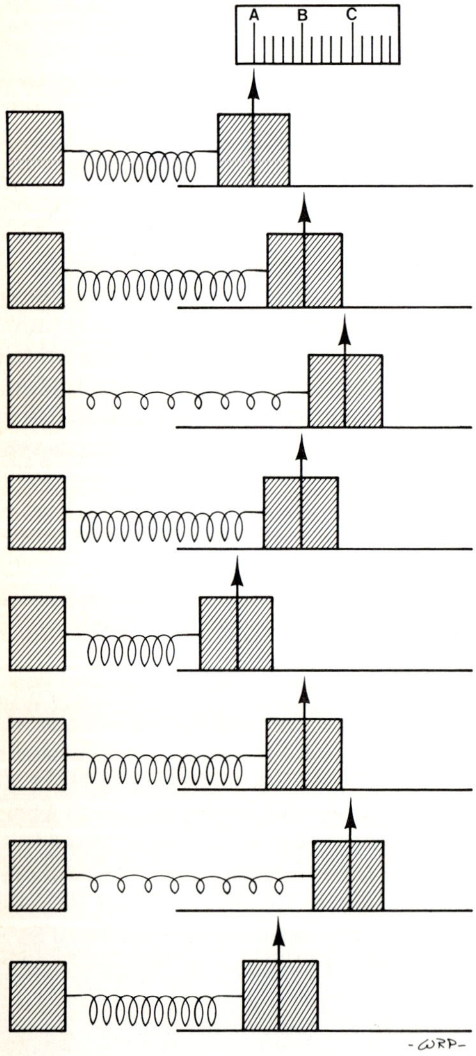

Figure 6–2 The effect of moving the mass in the direction of point A (on the displacement scale) on the spring-mass system.

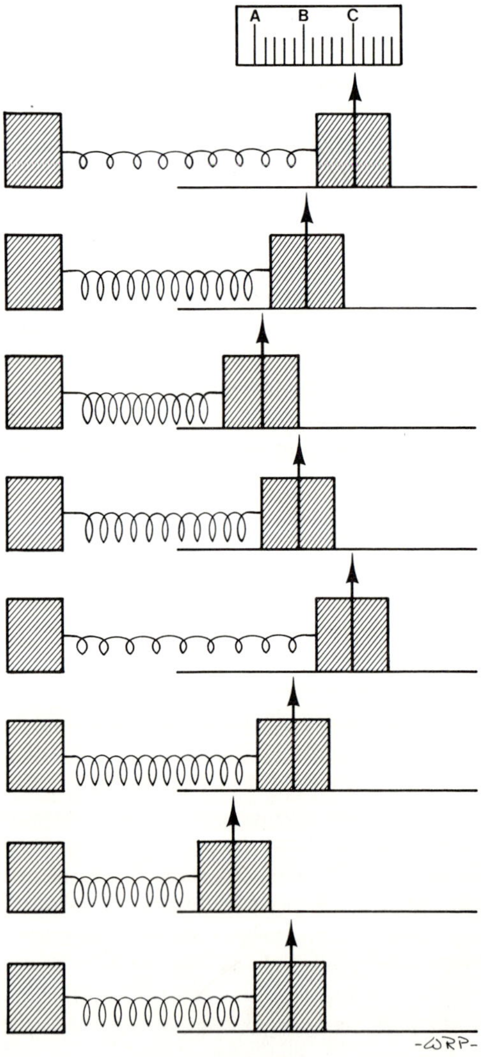

Figure 6–3 The effect of moving the mass in the direction of point C (on the displacement scale) on the spring-mass system.

that is, if the effect of interfering forces that cause energy losses to a vibrating system is small.

SOUND WAVES IN AIR

The previous spring-mass example can also be applied to an understanding of wave motion in air. Air consists of small particles called "molecules," and each molecule has an average stable, or resting, position from which it is displaced by the passage of a sound wave. The air molecules behave in a manner similar to small masses of matter connected by springs, as described previously in the spring-mass example. An illustration of their behavior is shown in Figures 6–4 and 6–5. If molecule A is displaced toward the right (Fig. 6–4), the spring between A and B is compressed, thus increasing the force on the spring between molecules B and C, C and D, and D and E, thereby causing the molecules to temporarily occupy positions closer to each other than is normal in their resting position. When molecules are nearer to each other, there is increased pressure, and a state of compression (or condensation) exists, as illustrated in Figure 6–4. Now, if molecule A is displaced toward the left (Fig. 6–5), the spring between molecules A and B is stretched and molecule B is also displaced toward the left, thus stretching temporarily the spring between molecules B and C, C and D, and D and E. When molecules are forced farther apart from each other, there is decreased pressure, and a state of expansion (or rarefaction) exists, as shown in Figure 6–5.

Every cycle of vibration involves a state (wave) of compression followed by a state (wave) of expansion of the air molecules. Furthermore, it is the disturbance (i.e., the vibration) that moves along the line of molecules, while the molecules move back and forth only about their fixed resting positions. Thus a sound wave is the movement (or propagation) of a disturbance through an elastic medium without permanent displacement of the particles themselves.

The kind of motion produced by a vibrating tuning fork is an example of simple harmonic motion, motion that can be described by a sine wave. A sine wave is an illustration of a sound wave with a certain pattern, as shown in Figure 6–6*A*; it is a graphic display of the sine function and can be constructed from certain trigonometric functions of right angles. However, it is also a graph of the pressure variations generated by a sound source that vibrates with simple harmonic motion (Fig. 6–6*B*). When the curve is above the line in the graph, a state of compression exists, and the height of the curve above the zero line corresponds to the amount of increased pressure at any instant in time. Below the zero line, the curve indicates a state of expansion. The zero line represents the atmospheric pressure that was present before the sound wave passed by or the average of all the different pressures that were present as the wave passed by.

In addition to representing a pressure curve, the sine wave also represents the movement of a single air particle at a given instant in time (Fig. 6–6*C*). When the curve is above the line, it means that the

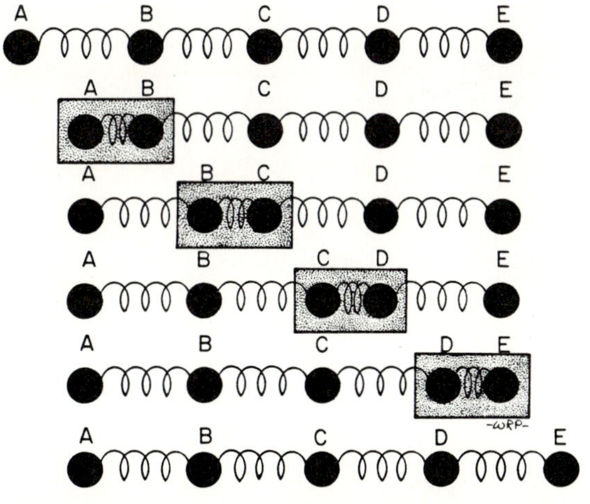

Figure 6–4 A schema of the propagation of a wave of compression (condensation) along the molecules of air, showing the molecules' positions at successive instants in time. (From Denes P, Pinson EN. The speech chain. Garden City, NY: Anchor Press/Doubleday, 1973.)

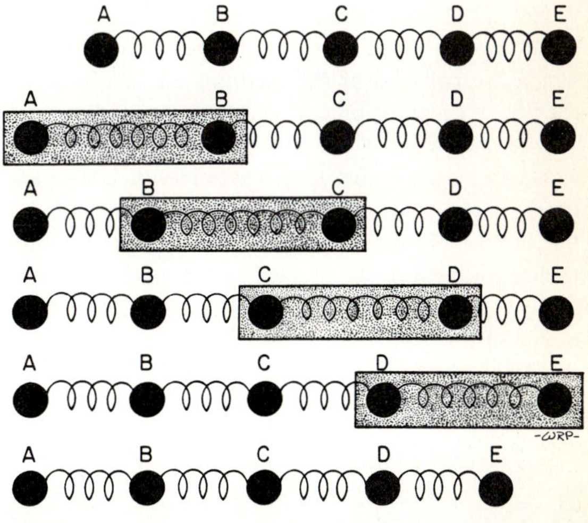

Figure 6–5 A schema of the propagation of a wave of expansion (rarefaction) along the molecules of air, showing the molecules' positions at successive instants in time. (From Denes P, Pinson EN. The speech chain. Garden City, NY: Anchor Press/Doubleday, 1973.)

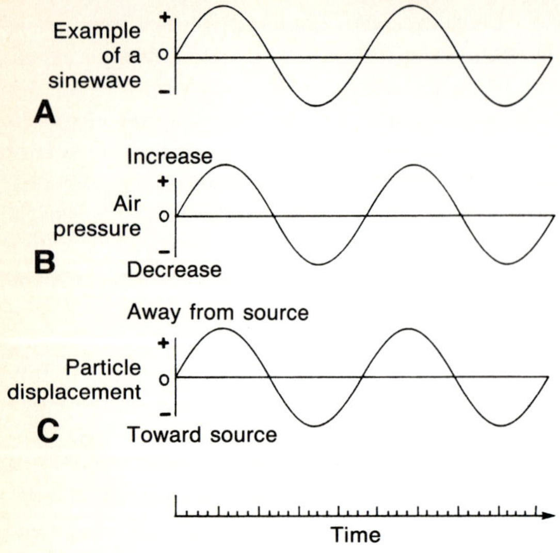

Figure 6-6 Sine waves. *A*, A sine wave as a graphic display of the sine function constructed from certain trigonometric functions of right angles. *B*, A sine wave as a graphic display of pressure variations generated by a sound source that vibrates with simple harmonic motion. *C*, A sine wave as a graphic display of the movement of an air molecule at a given instant in time.

particle at that instant in time is displaced from its resting position away from the sound source. When the curve is below the line, the air particle is displaced toward the source. The zero line represents the particle's resting position.

Thus the sine wave allows an opportunity to view the same event in different ways. We will use this sine wave in our discussion of the properties of sound waves in the next section. It should be noted here that sine waves, although used to illustrate sound waves, do not provide a true visual reproduction of sound waves. Sound waves are longitudinal waves in which the particles of the medium are displaced in the line of propagation of (i.e., in the same direction as) the movement of the wave itself. However, sine waves are actually transverse waves in which the particles of the medium are moving perpendicular to the line of propagation of the wave. We use sine waves to illustrate the properties of sound waves because they provide a more convenient visual explanation of the properties of sound waves than do longitudinal waves.

PROPERTIES OF SOUND WAVES

There are some properties common to all vibratory systems, including sound waves. In referring again to Figures 6–2 and 6–3, if the mass is displaced from its resting position (B) and vibrates, it moves back and forth between two positions (A and C) representing the extreme limits of its motion. The distance of the mass from position B (resting position) at any instant in time is called its "displacement," and its maximum displacement is called the "amplitude" of its vibration. Figure 6–7*A* illustrates the concept of amplitude in sine waves.

A "cycle" of vibration can be clearly defined by again referring to Figures 6–2 and 6–3. In Figure 6–2, it is the movement of the mass from position B to position A, back through position B to position C, and back again to position B. In Figure 6–3, it is the movement of the mass from position B to position C, back through position B to position A, and back again to position B. Figure 6–7*A* illustrates a cycle of vibration in sine waves. It is the movement of a particle from its position of rest to maximum displacement in one direction, back through its position of rest to maximum displacement in the opposite direction, and then back again to its original resting position.

"Phase" is the portion of a cycle that has been passed through up to a given instant in time and is usually measured in degrees of a circle (see Figs. 6–7*A* and 6–7*B*). "Wavelength" (λ) is the distance between points of identical phase in two adjacent cycles of a wave (see Fig. 6–7*A*).

The "frequency" of a vibration is the number of complete cycles that occur in 1 second of time. If 10 cycles occur in 1 second, the frequency of that

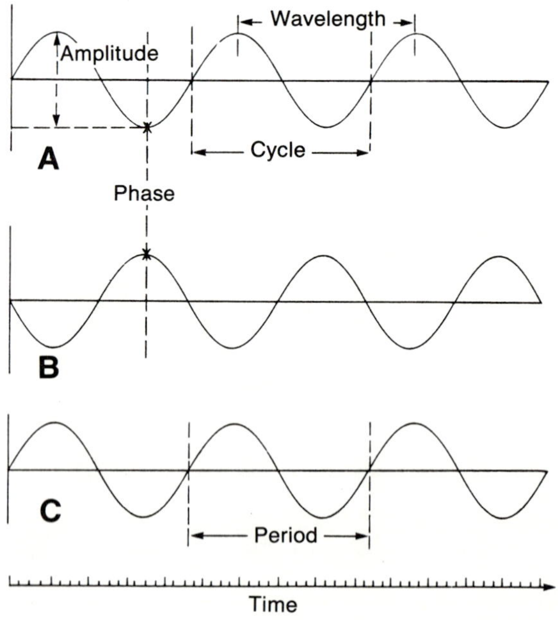

Figure 6-7 Sine curves illustrating the common properties of sound waves.

vibration is 10 cycles per second (cps) or Hertz (Hz); if 100 cycles occur in 1 second, then the frequency is 100 cycles per second (cps) or Hertz (Hz).

The time required to complete one cycle of vibration is referred to as the "period" of the vibration (see Fig. 6–7*C*). As frequency indicates the number of cycles per second, period represents the number of seconds per cycle. The relationship of period to frequency is expressed as follows:

$$T = \frac{1}{f}$$

where T = period and f = frequency. For example, if the frequency of a vibration is 10 cycles per second, its period is $^1/_{10}$ second; if its frequency is 100 cycles per second, its period is $^1/_{100}$ second.

The "velocity" of the wave is the speed at which the vibrations propagate through the medium. Velocity is related to three factors within the medium: elasticity, density, and temperature. The velocity of sound waves through air is 340 meters per second at room temperature.

In the illustrations of the properties of sound waves shown in Figure 6–7, the waves are shown as if they continue indefinitely. However, in reality, the waves' amplitudes of vibrations decrease because of energy losses in the vibrating system. The dying away of waves through a progressive decrease or decay in amplitude of the vibrations is called "damping," which is illustrated in Figure 6–8.

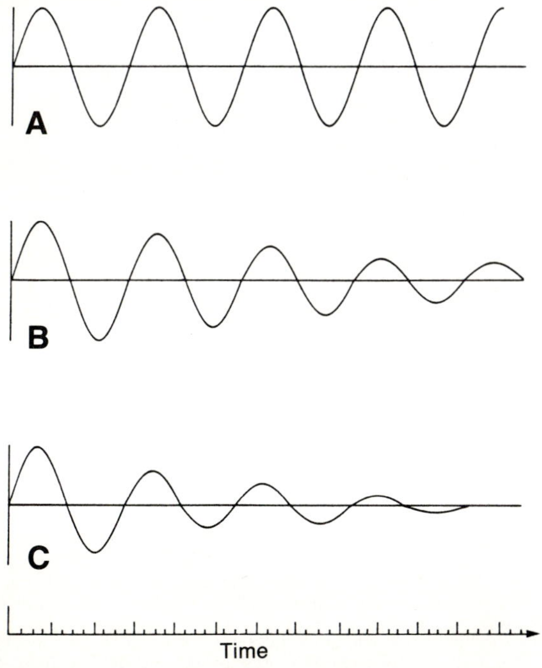

Figure 6–8 Examples of sound waves exhibiting *A*, no damping, *B*, light damping, and *C*, heavy damping.

COMPLEX WAVES

To this point the discussion of sound waves has included only simple waves, that is, waves produced by simple harmonic motion of the vibrator and containing only one frequency and one amplitude. Such waves are called "pure tones." However, in the real world, most sounds, including speech sounds, are not pure tones, but rather complex waves composed of numerous pure tones.

There are two types of complex waves: periodic and aperiodic. Complex periodic waves are produced by a vibrator's complex periodic motion, whereas complex aperiodic waves are the result of a vibrator's complex aperiodic motion. Complex waves can be broken down to be represented as the sum of numerous simple waves of differing frequencies, amplitudes, and phases, as shown in Figure 6–9.

The acoustic characteristics of complex waves can be described in terms of the respective frequencies and amplitudes of the simple waves that comprise them. These simple waves are referred to as the "components" of the complex waves, and they can be displayed conveniently in a "spectrum," a graphic representation of the frequencies and amplitudes of the components of a complex wave.

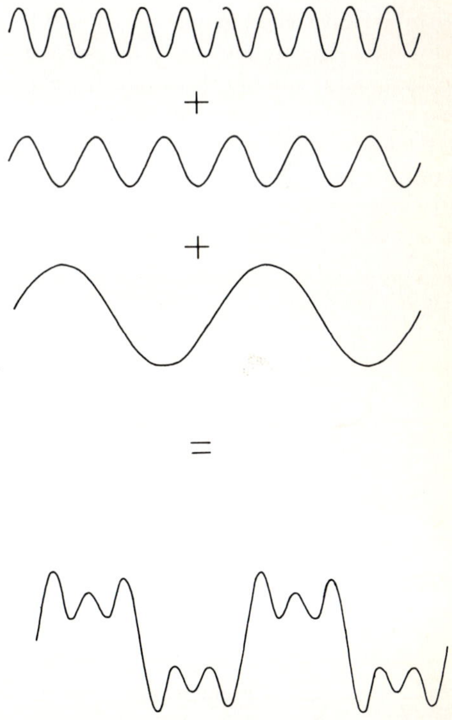

Figure 6–9 An illustration of the fact that complex waves are the sum of numerous simple waves. (From Denes P, Pinson EN. The speech chain. Garden City, NY: Anchor Press/Doubleday, 1973.)

There are two types of spectra, one for complex periodic waves and the other for complex aperiodic waves. For periodic waves, the spectrum contains the discrete frequency and relative amplitude of each component, as illustrated in Figure 6–10*A*; it is referred to as a "discrete" or "line spectrum." For aperiodic waves, the spectrum does not display discrete frequencies, but rather shows the energy present in the complex wave as a continuous, varying line, as illustrated in Figure 6–10*B*; this kind of spectrum is called a "continuous spectrum."

For periodic waves, a particular relationship exists among all the components' frequencies; the frequency of each component is an integral (whole-number) multiple of the frequency of the lowest component. The lowest component of a complex periodic wave is referred to as its "fundamental," and the frequency of this lowest component is called its "fundamental frequency." All components above the fundamental frequency are "harmonics," whole-number multiples of the fundamental frequency. The component whose frequency is twice the fundamental frequency is the second harmonic; the component that has a frequency that is three times the fundamental frequency is the third harmonic, and so on. For example, if the fundamental frequency of a complex periodic wave is 500 Hz, then its second harmonic is 1,000 Hz, its third harmonic is 1,500 Hz, its fourth harmonic 2,000 Hz, and so on. In Figure 6–10*A*, the fundamental frequency is 1,000 Hz and the harmonics that are present in the spectrum are the second, third, and fourth harmonics. However, unlike periodic waves, no systematic relationship between the lowest and higher components of the waves occurs in complex aperiodic waves. Spectrum analysis is important for future considerations of the acoustics of speech waves, since speech sound waves are composed of both periodic and aperiodic complex waveshapes. In fact, a common method for describing speech sound waves is through their spectra, and frequently these spectra are obtained by means of a sound spectrograph, an instrument that displays the spectra of sound waves.[3–5]

RESONANCE

Resonance is the phenomenon whereby a body (resonator), which has a natural tendency to vibrate at a certain frequency (its "natural" or "resonant frequency"), exhibits greater amplitudes of vibration when set into vibration by another body (driving system) whose frequency of vibration is identical, or similar, to the natural frequency of the first body (resonator).

The relevance of resonance for speech production is the case of cavity or acoustical resonance. The human vocal tract consists of several cavities capable of functioning as resonators, the most important of which are the pharyngeal, oral, and nasal cavities. The pharyngeal and oral cavities (independent of the nasal cavity) are sometimes referred to as the vocal tract, and they provide the primary transmission path for nonnasal speech sounds. The nasal cavity provides an alternative or additional pathway for nasalized speech sounds.

SINGLE HELMHOLTZ RESONATOR

To gain a better understanding of resonance as it pertains to speech, simulating the vocal cavities with simpler systems in which the acoustic properties can be determined with relative ease is helpful. Some of the early efforts in this regard were to model the vocal tract as a simple resonator of the

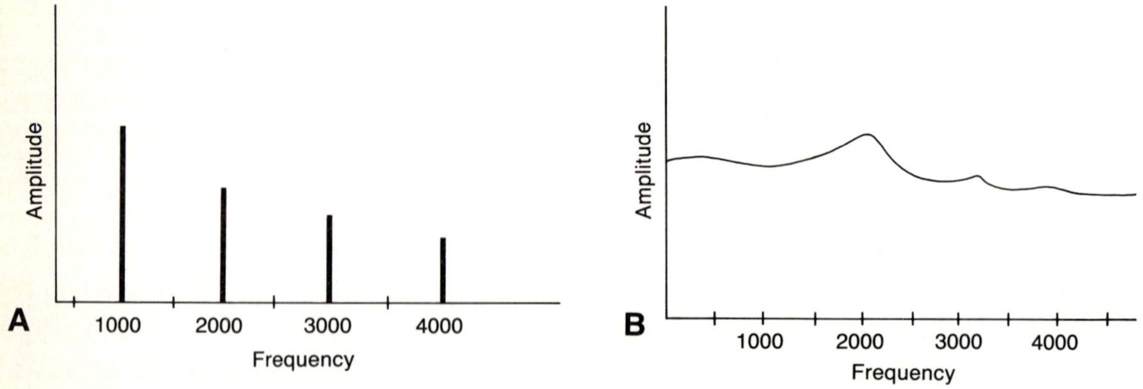

Figure 6–10 Spectra of complex waves. *A*, A discrete spectrum containing the frequencies and amplitudes of the sinusoidal components of a complex periodic wave. *B*, A continuous spectrum showing the energy present in a complex aperiodic wave as a continuous, varying line.

single Helmholtz type, like that shown in Figure 6–11*A*.[6] In these simulations, the vocal tract is viewed as a single chamber closed at the glottal end, not open to the nasal cavity, and open to the atmosphere through the interlabial channel.

The acoustic properties of a single Helmholtz resonator depend on the volume of the chamber and the dimensions of the channel leading to the atmosphere, but not on the exact shape of the chamber. These acoustic properties may be represented by the analogous electrical circuit shown in Figure 6–11*B*. In this circuit, C is a capacitive element that represents the vocal tract volume (V in Figure 6–11*A*). The larger the volume, the larger the capacitance. The inductive element, M, represents the mouth configuration. For this term, the smaller the area of the mouth opening (A in Figure 6–11*A*) and the longer the interlabial channel (L in Figure 6–11*A*), the greater the inductance. Given the appropriate values for C and M based on actual vocal tract dimensions, it is possible to obtain a resonance curve such as that shown in Figure 6–11*C*, the peak frequency of which corresponds to the resonant frequency of the particular vocal tract configuration. One may obtain such a resonance curve by applying a signal of constant amplitude at the input to the circuit of Figure 6–11*B*, initially starting at a low frequency and gradually increasing the frequency of the signal. The input signal is modified, resulting in an output that has a variable amplitude, depending on the frequency-selective resonant properties of the system. Each frequency component is attenuated relative to the peak component corresponding to the resonant frequency as shown in Figure 6–11*C*.

One may shift the resonant frequency along the frequency axis by changing C or M and analogously the associated dimensions of the acoustic system. Specifically, the resonant frequency is inversely proportional to changes in C and/or M. Stating this in terms of the acoustic system, the resonant frequency is lowered with (1) increases in volume (V) of the resonant chamber, (2) increases in the length (L) of the interlabial channel, and (3) decreases in the area (A) of the mouth opening. With increasing resonant frequency, the converse of these relationships is, of course, also true.

The sharpness of the peak in Figure 6–11*C* is determined by the length (L) and the area (A) of the Helmholtz resonator of Figure 6–11*A*. The smaller the area and the longer the neck, the sharper the tuning of the resonant peak. Tuning relates to the damping properties or dissipation of energy (represented by R in Figure 6–11*B*), which is inherent in any resonant system. Damping may be quantified in terms of the bandwidth of the resonance curve, which

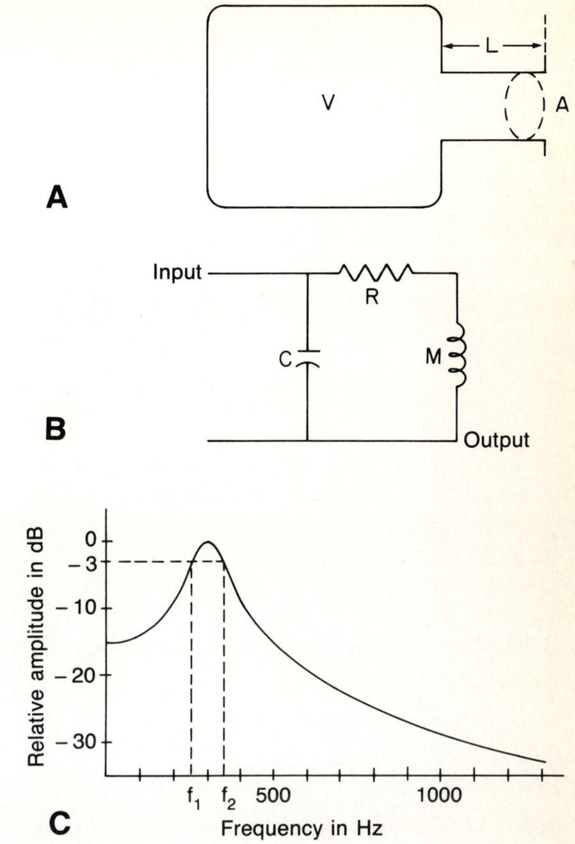

Figure 6–11 *A*, A single Helmholtz resonator. Abbreviations: V = the total volume of the vocal tract; L = the length of the interlabial channel; A = the area of the lip opening. *B*, The equivalent electrical circuit. Abbreviations: C (the capacitive element) = V; M (the inductive element) = L and A; R (the resistive element) = the dissipative energy losses. *C*, The typical resonance curve associated with the circuit in *B*. Abbreviations: f_1 and f_2 = resonance bandwidth. (After Stevens KN, House AS. An acoustical theory of vowel production and some of its implications. J Speech Hear Res 1961; 4:303.)

is usually specified as the half-power points or the width of the resonance curve 3 dB (or decibels, which is a measure of relative amplitude) below the peak (see Fig. 6–11*C*).

DOUBLE HELMHOLTZ RESONATOR

Unfortunately, for the sake of simplicity, the vocal tract configuration for most vowels and consonants is unlike that of a simple Helmholtz resonator primarily because, in the actual vocal tract, a constriction is imposed by the tongue in the resonant chamber. A more reasonable approximation to the vocal tract is a double Helmholtz resonator, as shown in Figure 6–12*A*. In this model, the pha-

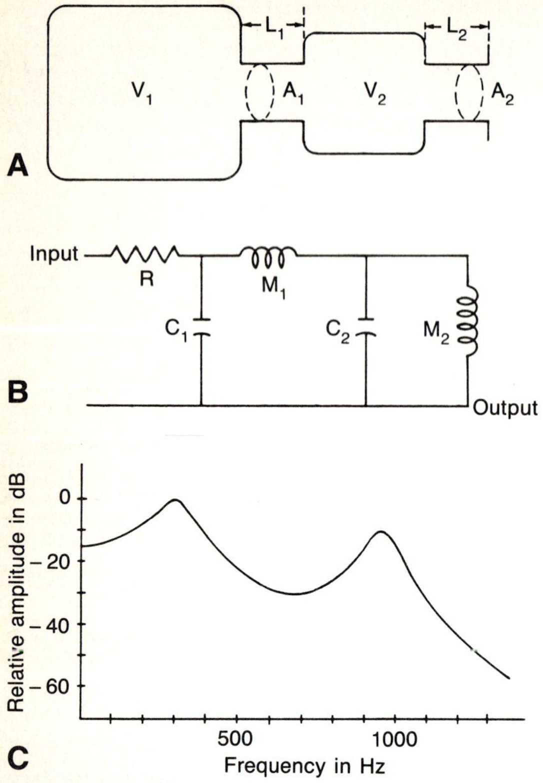

Figure 6–12 *A*, A double Helmholtz resonator. Abbreviations: V_1 = the volume of the pharyngeal cavity; V_2 = the volume of the oral cavity; L_1 = the length of the constriction between the tongue and palate; L_2 = the length of the interlabial channel; A_1 = the area of the constriction between the tongue and palate; A_2 = the area of the lip opening. *B*, The equivalent electrical circuit. Abbreviations: C_1, = V_1; C_2 = V_2; M = L_1; M_2 = the mouth opening; R = the dissipative element. *C*, The typical resonance curve associated with the circuit in *B*. (After Stevens KN, House AS. An acoustical theory of vowel production and some of its implications. J Speech Hear Res 1961; 4:303.)

ryngeal and oral cavities are represented by separate volumes connected to each other by a channel representing the constriction between the tongue and hard palate. The oral cavity volume opens to the atmosphere through the interlabial channel. An analogous electrical circuit is shown in Figure 6–12*B*, and a corresponding resonance curve in Figure 6–12*C*. One can see that two resonances are associated with a double Helmholtz resonator. Each resonant frequency depends on the volumes and constrictions of *both* resonator cavities, although each may be more closely associated with one cavity than the other. The greater the coupling between cavities (i.e., the greater the area A_1 in Figure 6–12*A*), the less the affiliation of one resonance with a particular cavity. This is an important consideration in terms of vocal tract resonances in that most vowels are produced with a considerable degree of acoustic coupling between the pharyngeal and oral cavities. The tongue does not closely approximate the hard palate, and so it is generally not valid to assign a resonant frequency exclusively to a particular cavity.[6,7]

A major disadvantage involved in modeling the vocal tract with single or double Helmholtz resonators is that only one resonance in a relatively low-frequency range can be validly determined for each resonator cavity because calculations require the assumption that the wavelength of the resonant frequency must be large compared to the dimensions of the corresponding resonator cavity. This assumption was maintained for the resonant system of Figure 6–12. However, it can be seen that the higher resonant frequency in the example shown is less than 1,000 Hz, and it is well known that speech is characterized by a wide spectrum of frequency components, including those considerably higher than 1,000 Hz. A multiple resonator of the Helmholtz type is not adequate in representing these higher-frequency components. Another major problem involved in modeling the vocal tract by single or compound Helmholtz resonators is that actual vocal tract constrictions, such as the lip area for low vowels or the separation between the oral and pharyngeal cavities for front vowels,[6] are often too large. In such cases, the vocal tract does not physically resemble the resonators of Figures 6–11*A* or 6–12*A*.

ACOUSTIC TRANSMISSION LINE

A more accurate approach to modeling the vocal tract is to treat it as a type of acoustic transmission line. Specifically, the vocal tract can be considered as a tube closed at one end and open at the other. The closed end corresponds to the glottis, which offers a high resistance to airflow when the vocal folds are adducted. The open end is the lip orifice.

The column of air enclosed in such a tube transmits sound waves in a characteristic fashion. A sound source applied to the closed end of the tube sets up a compressional wave that propagates along the whole length of the tube. Upon reaching the open end, a wave of rarefaction is reflected back to the closed end. The waves continue to be reflected back and forth between each end as long as a sound source is present. This establishes a pattern of standing waves similar to that associated with a vibrating string. Standing waves are characterized by nodes and antinodes, which correspond to points wherein vibration is minimal and maximal, respectively. The distribution of nodes and antinodes determines the modes of vibration or the natural (resonant) frequencies of the column of air. (For more comprehensive coverage of standing waves, see Backus.[8] Figure

6–13 shows standing wave patterns representing the first four modes of vibration of a column of air in a tube closed at one end and open at the other. A tracing of the vocal tract in a relatively unconstricted state is shown below each standing wave pattern. The positions of antinodes (A) are indicated within the tube and also at corresponding locations in the vocal tract. We should point out that a uniform tube exhibits the same standing wave pattern whether straight or curved, provided that no constrictions or expansions are introduced.

The longest portion of a standing wave that fits in a tube closed at one end and open at the other is one that has its node (minimal volume velocity vibration) at the closed end and its adjacent antinode (maximal volume velocity vibration) at the open end; it represents one-fourth of a complete standing wave. Therefore, the lowest mode of vibration or resonant frequency corresponds to a frequency whose wavelength is four times the length of the tube. For an unconstricted tube 17 cm long, which is the approximate length of the adult male voice tract, the lowest mode of vibration is 500 Hz. The higher modes of vibration also correspond to standing waves, each of which is progressively shorter relative to the length of the tube. The frequencies of these vibrational modes are odd-number multiples of the lowest. For the 17-cm tube, the second mode occurs at 1,500 Hz, the third at 2,500 Hz, and so on. Theoretically, an infinite number of resonances exists. In reference to vocal tract acoustics, the resonant frequencies are called "formants"; the lowest is the first formant (F_1), the next is the second formant (F_2), and so on.

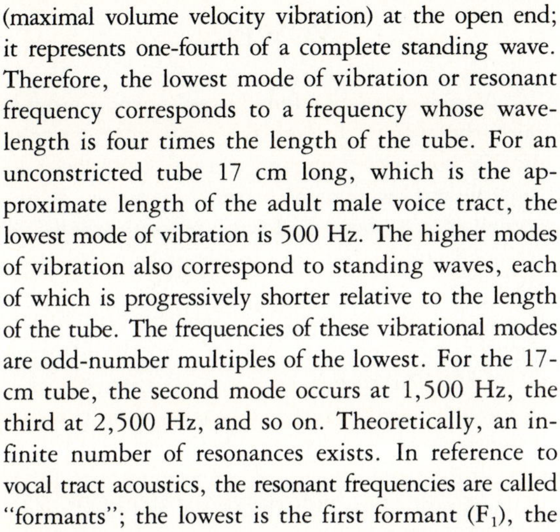

Figure 6–13 Volume velocity standing wave patterns for the first four modes of vibration of a column of air in a tube closed at one end and open at the other. The positions of volume velocity antinodes, A_x (where x = 1, 2, 3, or 4), are indicated within each tube and corresponding locations in a relatively unconstricted vocal tract. (From Fant G. Acoustic theory of speech production. The Hague: Mouton, 1960.)

The frequency of the lowest resonant mode and the spacing of higher resonant modes depend on the length and shape of the resonator tube. The longer the tube, the lower the first resonant mode and the smaller the spacing between higher resonant modes, provided the tube is not changed in shape. Constrictions and expansions along the tube (vocal tract) change the spacing among resonant frequencies. In relation to standing wave patterns, if a constriction occurs at an antinode (see Figure 6–13 for positions along the vocal tract), the corresponding resonant frequency is lowered, whereas a constriction at a node raises the corresponding resonant frequency.[6,9] For example, closure of the lips lowers all resonant frequencies (formants) because an antinode occurs at this location for each mode of vibration. A constriction in the middle of the oral cavity lowers F_3, which is necessary for the production of a perceptually acceptable /r/.

VOCAL TRACT TRANSFER FUNCTION

The distribution of resonances along the frequency scale is referred to as the transfer function of the vocal tract. In more exact terms, a transfer function describes the transmission properties of the vocal tract by forming a ratio between the output signal and input signal for each frequency component. A given transfer function is completely specified by the center frequency and bandwidth of each resonant mode. Formant bandwidths are related to vocal damping and are directly proportional to formant center frequencies.[10,11] That is, as formant frequencies increase, so do their bandwidths. The illustrations in Figures 6–11*C* and 6–12*C* represent transfer functions of the single and double Helmholtz resonators, respectively.

Vocal tract transfer functions have many resonant modes, theoretically an infinite number. However, only the first two or three are usually of interest acoustically and perceptually. The transfer function depends on the overall shape of the vocal tract and is unique for each vowel and consonant, except for voiced and voiceless pairs, which involve the same articulatory place of production and therefore the same vocal tract shape. All portions of the vocal tract contribute to the complete transfer function, but with varying degrees, depending on the exact configuration.[6]

The vocal tract transfer function may be simulated electronically by means of a series of electronic filters. Such a simulation is referred to as an electrical transmission line. An example is shown in Figure 6–14. Each filter section represents a short

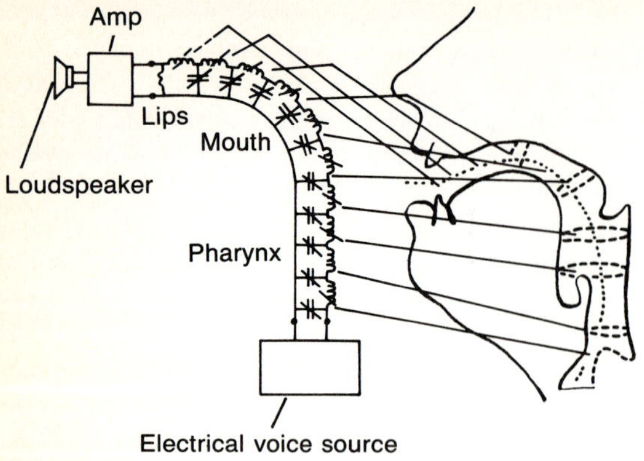

Figure 6–14 A simplified diagram of an electrical analogue of the vocal tract. (From Fant G. Acoustic analysis and synthesis of speech with applications to Swedish. Stockholm: The Royal Institute of Technology, 1959.)

segment of the vocal tract (e.g., 0.5 cm). The parameters of each filter are adjusted in accordance with the cross-sectional area of the corresponding vocal tract section that it represents. Such electrical analogue models of the vocal tract have been extremely useful in synthetic speech generation and continue to be used in formulating more accurate models of the acoustic behavior of the vocal tract. Not shown in Figure 6–14 are series and parallel resistances, which represent energy losses along the vocal tract. Such energy losses are important in the specification of damping properties of the vocal tract and therefore formant bandwidths. Wakita and Fant have dealt with these resistive elements in their transmission line model of the vocal tract.[11]

SOUND SOURCES

The vocal tract resonant system may be excited by a sound source *at* the larynx (that is, vocal fold vibration) or a sound source *within* the vocal tract itself. The laryngeal sound source is normally a periodic tone consisting of a fundamental frequency component and a series of higher harmonics (see Fig. 6–15*D*). The sound source produced within the vocal tract is an aperiodic noise of relatively long duration, such as that for /s/, or a transient, such as that associated with /p/. Regardless of the type of sound source, whether laryngeal or supralaryngeal, periodic or aperiodic, the resonant characteristics of the vocal tract acting as an acoustic filter modify the sound source. Frequency components in the source that correspond to the resonant frequencies of the vocal tract are allowed to vibrate relatively freely and other frequencies are suppressed. Therefore all speech sounds, including consonants as well as vowels, are characterized by concentrations of energy along the frequency scale corresponding to the resonant frequencies or formants of the vocal tract.

Figure 6–15 summarizes the acoustic filtering effect of the vocal tract transfer function imposed on the laryngeal (glottal) sound source. One can see that the spectrum of the sound radiated from the lips is markedly different from the spectrum of the sound entering the vocal tract (glottal spectrum). It is the set of varied spectra of sounds that can be formed by different configurations of the vocal tract, which we identify as the vowels and consonants of speech.

VOWELS

Vowels are often referred to as "open" sounds because the airflow through the vocal tract is not ordinarily constricted enough to cause turbulence and thus the airflow remains primarily laminar. With a normal speech power or driving pressure, the vowels are nonfrictional and are capable of being sustained for a considerable period of time. The speech wave is usually quasiperiodic for vowels, and, consequently, these speech sounds are normally identified as voiced. The speech wave can be aperiodic, such as for generating whispered vowels, but this condition is much less frequent than quasiperiodic. Although the nasal cavities are sometimes open for releasing vowels through both the oral and nasal cavities to form nasalized vowels, the great majority of vowels are produced with the transmission of air only through the laryngopharynx, the oropharynx, and the mouth, so that the vowels are normally referred to as "oral" speech sounds. It is important to realize that vowels tend to be primarily open, voiced, oral formations, but these terms do not define the concept of vowel; they simply describe the common properties associated with vowels. In the formation of larger units, such as the syllable, the vowel is the nucleus or central portion of the syllable. Thus vowels are of considerable importance in all languages and are essential for recognizing speech.

The acoustic identification or discrimination of vowel types is primarily by their first three resonances, called "formants." Figure 6–16 shows examples of formant structures for some rounded and unrounded oral vowels. The symbolization is based on that of the International Phonetic Association.[12] The first formant is lower for vowels articulated near the roof of the mouth, and it is higher for those formed further away from the roof. The second formant generally decreases from the front vowels, such as [i] and [I], through the midvowels, such as [e] and [ɛ], to the back ones, such as [u] and [U]. The

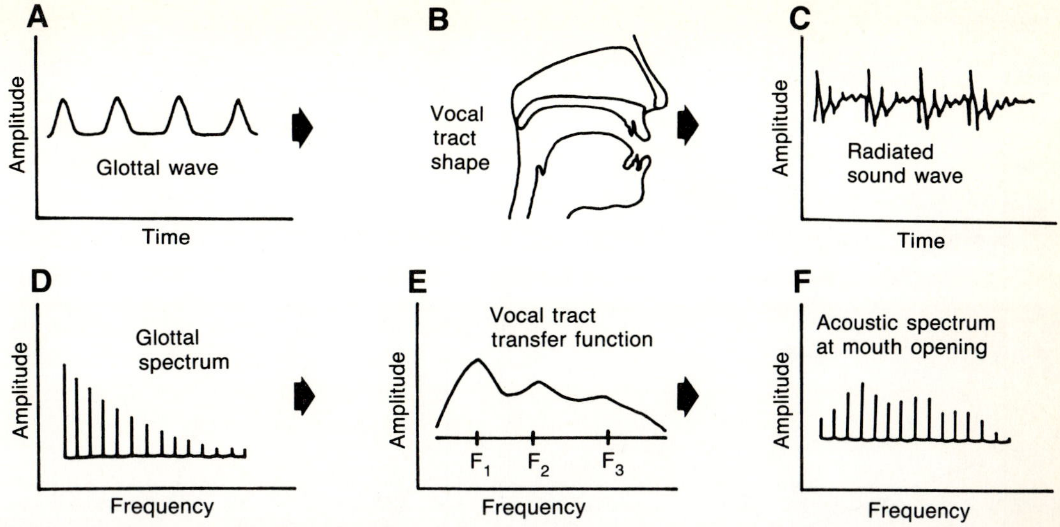

Figure 6–15 The effects of acoustic filtering provided by the vocal tract resonant system. *A*, The glottal source waveform. *B*, A schema of the vocal tract's resonant cavity. *C*, A modified sound wave. *D*, The glottal source spectrum. *E*, The vocal tract's transfer function. *F*, The modified sound spectrum. (After Minifie FD. Speech acoustics. In: Minifie FD, Hixon TJ, Williams F, eds. Normal aspects of speech, hearing, and language. Englewood Cliffs, NJ: Prentice-Hall, 1973.)

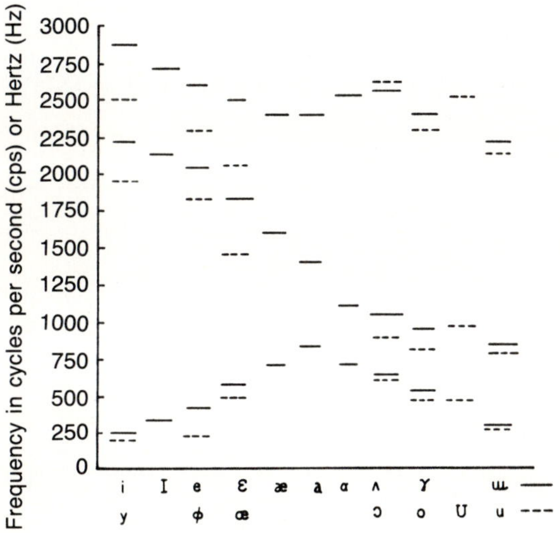

Figure 6-16 Examples of formant structures for some rounded and unrounded oral vowels.

third formant pattern is generally the inverse of the first formant, being higher for the high vowels and lower for the low ones. As can be seen by the dashed lines in the figure, rounding usually tends to lower the three formants from those of their unrounded counterparts.

As discussed earlier, the size of the vocal tract determines in large measure the range of formant frequencies for the various speech sound formations. The smaller the vocal tract, the higher the formant frequencies. Thus children have the highest formants; males have the lowest formants; females have formants in the middle range. These relationships are shown in Table 6–1, which is from the classic vowel study by Peterson and Barney.[13]

There is a general correlation between vowel formant bandwidth and vowel formant frequency. Table 6–2, which was taken from Dunn's thorough study of vowel bandwidths,[14] indicates the findings from different researchers. Although there are variations in the actual measures for the bandwidths of the formants, there is general agreement that bandwidth increases as formant frequency progresses from first to second to third.

In producing English vowels in isolation or in monosyllabic words, speakers tend to use certain patterns of fundamental frequency, duration, and speech power. Figure 6–17 shows the average fundamental frequency spoken by children (*A*), women (*B*), and men (*C*).[13] The fundamental frequency ranges are dependent upon the size of the larynx of the speaker; thus it is highest for children, next highest for women, and lowest for men. However, regardless of the speaker, high vowels, such as [i] and [u], tend to have a higher fundamental frequency than lower vowels, such as [a] and [ɔ]. This finding is attributed in part to the raising of the tongue, which results in a lengthening of the vocal folds for the higher vowels, thus generating a higher fundamental frequency.

Peterson and Lehiste studied the average duration of English vowels.[15] Figure 6–18 summarizes their results. The tense-lax oppositions of [i] and [I], [u] and [U], and so on, are shown in the patterns

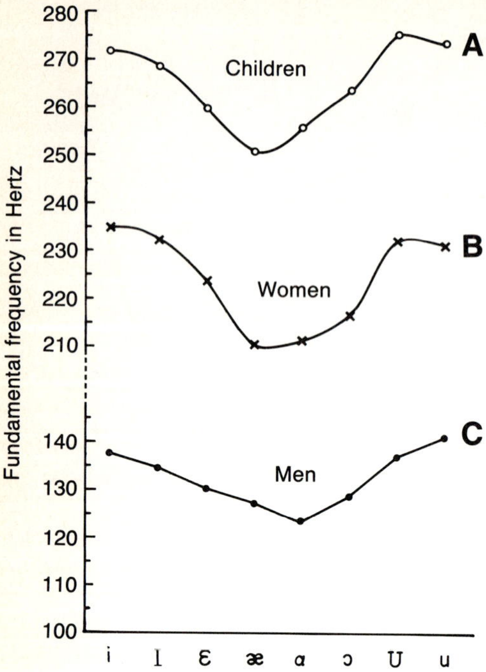

Figure 6–17 Average fundamental frequencies for eight English vowels spoken by *A*, children, *B*, women, and *C*, men. (After Peterson GE, Barney HL. Control methods used in a study of the vowels. J Acoust Soc Am 1952; 2:175.)

of longer durations for the tense vowels and shorter ones for the lax counterparts. Table 6–3 shows the findings of three investigators researching power or intensity of the English vowels. The high vowels tend

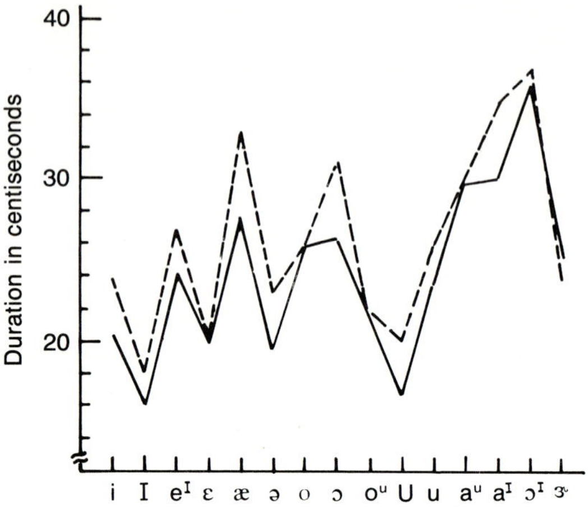

Figure 6–18 Average duration of syllable nuclei, measured from minimal pairs differing in the voicing of the final consonant. Abbreviations: The solid curve = a large set of CNC words spoken by GEP; the dotted curve = the values for 30 minimal pairs uttered by five speakers. (From Peterson GE, Lehiste I. Duration of syllable nuclei in English. J Acoust Soc Am 1960; 32:701.)

TABLE 6–1 Averages of Formant Frequencies in Hertz (Hz) of Vowels by 76 Speakers

		i	I	ɛ	æ	*a*	ɔ	U	*u*	ʌ	ɝ
Formant frequencies (Hz)											
F_1	M	270	390	530	660	730	570	440	300	640	490
	W	310	430	610	860	850	590	470	370	760	500
	Ch	370	530	690	1010	1030	680	560	430	850	560
F_2	M	2290	1990	1840	1720	1090	840	1020	870	1190	1350
	W	2790	2480	2330	2050	1220	920	1160	950	1400	1640
	Ch	3200	2730	2610	2320	1370	1060	1410	1170	1590	1820
F_3	M	3010	2550	2480	2410	2440	2410	2240	2240	2390	1690
	W	3310	3070	2990	2850	2810	2710	2680	2670	2780	1960
	Ch	3730	3600	3570	3320	3170	3180	3310	3260	3360	2160

Abbreviations: M = men; W = women; Ch = children.
From Peterson GE, Barney HL. Control methods used in a study of the vowels. J Acoust Soc Am 1952; 24:175.

TABLE 6–2 Vowel Formant Bandwidths*

	Year	*Number of Voices*	*Number of Vowels*	*First Formant*	*Second Formant*	*Third Formant*
Steinberg	1934	1	7	83	118	—
Lewis	1936	1	5	39	51	80
Lewis and Tuthill	1940	6	2	45	50	93
Tarnóczy	1943	—	4 to 9	110	190	260
Bogert	1953	33	10	130	150	185
van den Berg	1955	1	11	54	66	89
House and Stevens	1958	3	8	54	65	77
Dunn (spectrograms)	1961	20	10	50	64	115
Dunn (artificial larynx)	1961	2	12	47	75	106

*Average half-power bandwidths of three vowel formants (Hz).
From Dunn HK. Methods of measuring vowel formant bandwidths. J Acoust Soc Am 1961; 33:1737.

TABLE 6–3 Comparison of Three Power Studies of Vowels

Black		*Lehiste and Peterson (Relative Power in dB)*		*Fletcher (Power in mW)*	
o	3.71	ɔ	5.5	ɔ	45
a	3.69	*a*	5.1	*a*	41
æ	3.44	o	4.6	ʊ	26
ɔ	3.22	ɘ	4.6	æ	25
ɛ	3.12	æ	4.3	o	25
ɪ	2.86	ɛ	4.2	ɘ	24
u	2.56	e	3.5	u	23
ʊ	2.52	ʊ	3.3	e	23
ʌ	2.21	u	3.1	ɛ	22
e	1.77	ɪ	3.0	ɪ	20
i	0.00	i	0.0	i	20

Information assembled from Black JW. Relationships among fundamental frequencies, vocal sound pressure and rate of speaking. Lang Speech 1961; 4:196–199. Lehiste I, Peterson GE. Vowel amplitude and phonemic stress in American English. J Acoust Soc Am 1959; 31:428–435. Fletcher H. Speech and hearing in communications. New York: Van Nostrand, 1953.

to be less intense (i.e., produced with less power) than the low vowels.

As mentioned earlier, nasalization of vowel productions is one of the modifications that occurs when the nasal cavity is coupled to the vocal tract by lowering the soft palate. The timing of palatal movements relative to other articulatory events is important in providing the appropriate degree of nasal coupling in connected speech. Since the soft palate tends to move somewhat slower than other articulators,[16] it appears necessary that palatal movements begin well in advance of the corresponding speech segment.[17,18] Therefore nasal coupling is more pervasive in normal connected speech than would be suggested by the limited number of phonemes that require this feature.

The acoustic effects of nasal coupling are complex. The complete vocal tract transfer function depends on the resonance properties of the pharyngeal oral cavity, the nasal cavity, and the interaction between the two cavity systems. If the right and left nasal channels on each side of the nasal septum are perfectly symmetrical, they function acoustically as a single cavity system.[6] However, they are usually not symmetrical owing to deviation of the nasal septum and other factors. Therefore each nasal pathway contributes its own resonant frequencies. Moreover, the resonant characteristics of the nasal cavity may also depend on the further shunting effect of the maxillary and frontal sinuses, which communicate with the nasal cavity and function as additional resonant cavities.[19]

As pointed out by Curtis, interaction between the pharyngeal oral cavity and the nasal cavity is complexly related to the extent of acoustic coupling between them.[20] For nasalized vowels, the pharyngeal oral cavity is the primary acoustic resonator, and the nasal cavity is a side branch. The distribution of acoustic energy between the nasal cavity and the pharyngeal oral cavity depends not only on the size of the velopharyngeal opening, but also on the configuration of the pharyngeal oral cavity. Thus greater pharyngeal oral cavity constriction results in greater impedance in this channel, and relatively more energy is distributed to the nasal cavity. Since oral cavity impedance differs among vowels (because of different articulatory configurations), it follows that the effects of nasal coupling differ for each vowel even if the size of the velopharyngeal orifice is the same. This concept is important since it suggests that nasality does not involve a constant acoustic correlate that is merely superimposed on an otherwise nonnasal utterance.

House and Stevens studied the effect of various degrees of nasal coupling on vowel production using an electrical analogue of the vocal tract, such as that shown in Figure 6–14, with the addition of a simulated nasal channel.[21] The velopharyngeal opening size was varied electronically. Figure 6–19 shows the results of changing velopharyngeal orifice size for different vowels. Increasing nasal coupling has the effect of widening the bandwidth of formants (represented by peaks in the spectrum envelopes) and reducing formant amplitudes. These changes are related to the greater damping properties of the nasal cavity compared to the pharyngeal oral cavities. The nasal cavity consists of a convoluted configuration providing a relatively large surface area at any given cross-section, which accounts for the greater acoustic damping and wider bandwidths. The perceptual effects of indistinct spectral peaks produced by increased damping may be a lack of differentiation among different vowels.

Figure 6–19 shows that the same velopharyngeal orifice size may have widely differing effects, depending on the particular vowel that is produced. A vowel exhibiting large oral cavity impedance (e.g., /i/ and /u/) is influenced to a much greater extent than a vowel of small oral cavity impedance (e.g., /a/) by a velopharyngeal opening of the same size.

Theoretically, the addition of a side-branch resonator such as the nasal cavity introduces antiresonances in the transfer function of the complete resonator system. Asymmetries in the nasal channel also introduce antiresonances. Antiresonances have the opposite effect of resonances in that they produce spectral minima or valleys as opposed to spectral maxima or peaks. Similar to resonances, however, they are characterized by specific frequency locations and bandwidths. They may have the effect of par-

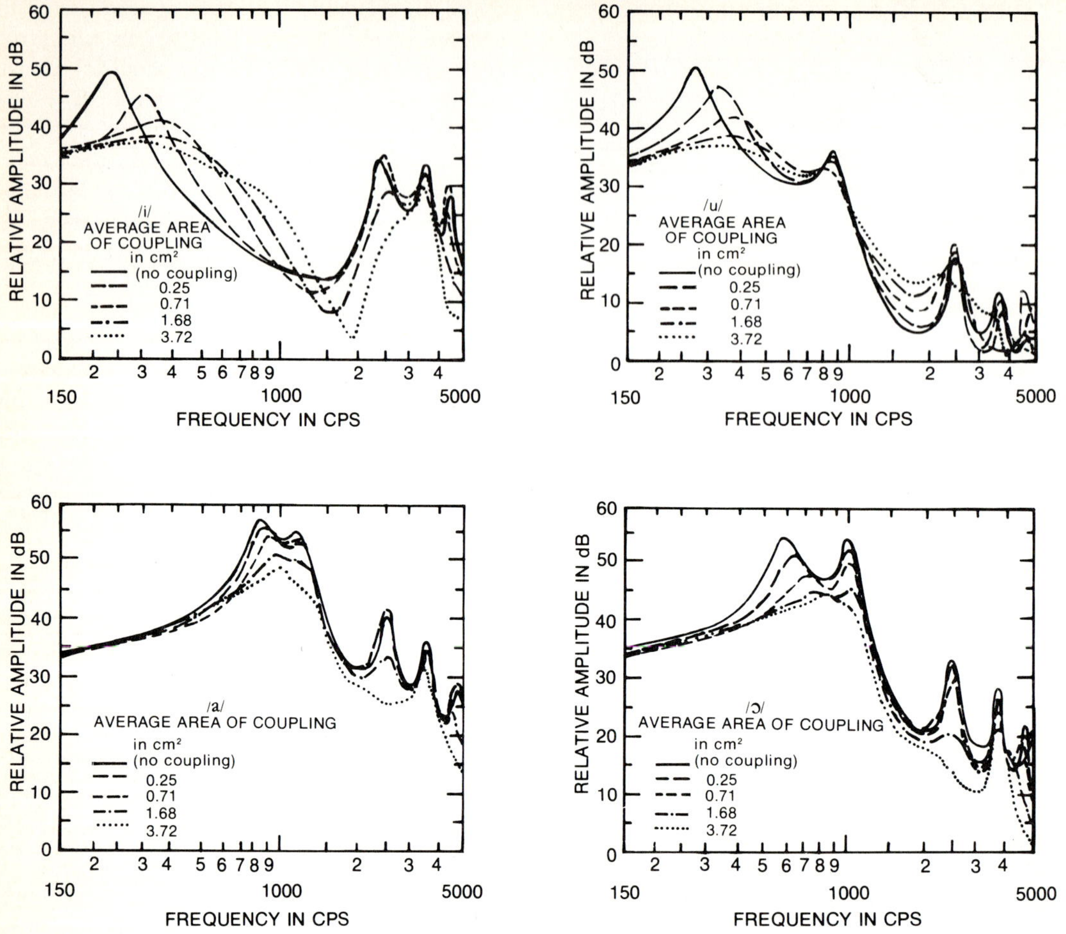

Figure 6–19 Spectrum envelopes showing the acoustic effects of varying degrees of nasal coupling associated with the vowels /i/, /u/, / a /, and / ɔ /. An electrical analogue of the vocal tract produced the vowels and simulated nasal coupling. (From Curtis JF. Acoustics of speech production and nasalization. In: Spriesterbach DC, Sherman D, eds. Cleft palate and communication. New York: Academic Press, 1968.)

tially cancelling a resonant mode in a nearby frequency location. Researchers have demonstrated on the basis of electric circuit theory that any antiresonance due to a shunting side branch is always paired with a resonance.[6] If the coupling of the side branch is small, the added resonance and antiresonance are close together in frequency, thereby cancelling each other and causing little or no effect on the acoustic spectrum. However, if the coupling is great (i.e., if the orifice area is large), the added resonance and antiresonance are well separated in frequency. In the case of nasal coupling, it is possible that the antiresonance may have the effect of partially cancelling the first formant of the uncoupled vocal tract,[6] which would reduce the amplitude of the first formant.

Hattori et al studied the acoustic characteristics of the nasalization of vowels and nasal consonants.[22] They indicated the main features of vowel nasalization to be an extra resonance at 250 Hz, an antiresonance at 500 Hz, and somewhat weak components between the formants of the vowels in the frequency region from 1,000 to 2,500 Hz. Some of these features are also found in nasal consonants, which will be discussed next.

NASAL CONSONANTS

In contrast to the previous discussion for nasalization of the vowels, the oral cavity is the occluded side branch for the nasal consonants, and the pharynx, coupled with the nasal cavity, represents the primary acoustic resonator. Because of the rather fixed shape of the pharynx and nasal cavity, the nasal consonants are characterized by fairly constant formant frequencies. The formants of the pharynx and nasal cavity are generally lower than those of the pharyngeal oral cavity because of the greater overall length of the former. The nasal consonants are differentiated according to place of articulation by various clues, including vowel transitions, second formant frequencies, and the frequency positions of the nasal antiresonances. In the last case, the frequency positions of nasal antiresonances depend on the length of the oral cavity side branch.[22,23] The longer the side branch, the lower the antiresonant frequency. For example, a characteristic antiresonant for /m/ is about 1,000 Hz, for /n/ approximately 3,500 Hz, and for /ŋ/ higher than 5,000 Hz. Discrimination of the nasals is also based on varying second formant frequencies,[24] with /m/ identified when this formant is at 1,300 Hz, /n/ at 1,800 Hz, and /ŋ/ at 2,000 Hz. Close agreement can be seen with Nakata who found the best judgements of synthesized nasals to be with second formants of 1,100 Hz for /m/, 1,700 Hz for /n/, and 2,300 Hz for /ŋ/.[25]

Vowel transitions have been identified through synthesis experiments at Haskins Laboratories as one of the most important cues for the discrimination of place of articulation of the nasal consonants.[26] Figure 6–20 shows the shape of the second formant transition patterns from the vowel /a/, which are necessary to obtain the correct identification of /m/, /n/, and /ŋ/. As can be noted, the second formant falls for /m/, rises slightly for /n/, and rises significantly for /ŋ/. This same phenomenon will be cited for the plosives /p/ and /b/, /t/ and /d/, and /k/ and /g/ in the next section. The importance of the vowel transitions was also shown by Malecot[27] in his tape-splicing experiments and by Nakata.[25]

Abramson et al found that the vowel environment affects the perception of nasal consonants.[28] Using a vocal tract analogue synthesizer, they varied nasal coupling by "lowering the velum" in equal increments, thus producing an acoustic continuum ranging from a clearly identifiable /d/ to a clearly identifiable /n/. Each of these acoustic stimuli was paired with the synthesized vowels /i/, /ʌ/, or

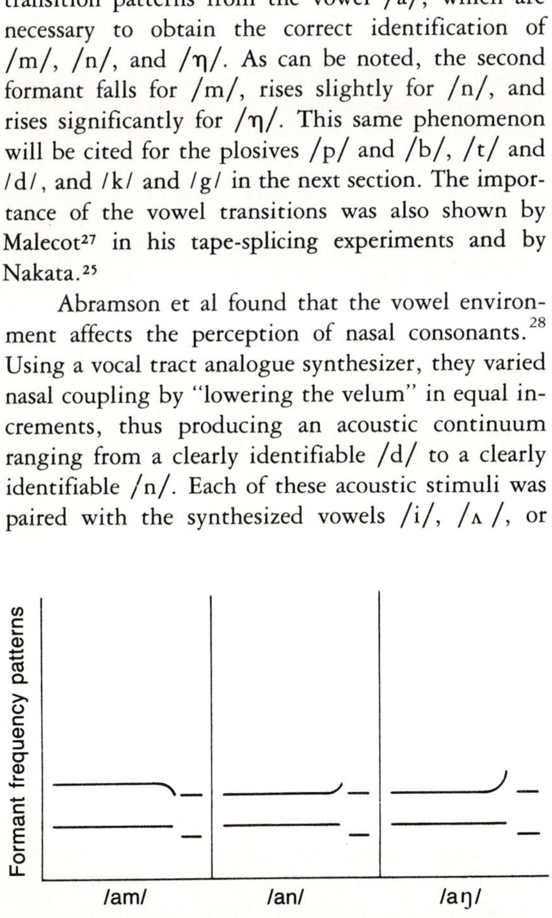

Figure 6–20 Second formant transition patterns from the vowel /a/ to the nasal consonants /m/, /n/, and /ŋ/.

/a/ following the consonant. They found that a low vowel environment (i.e., /a/) required a larger velopharyngeal port area to produce the percept of a nasal consonant. Conversely, in a high vowel environment (/i/) a smaller velopharyngeal port area led to the percept of a nasal consonant. These results are consistent with data concerning velar positions during connected speech. In a cineradiographic study, Kuehn found that during nasal consonant production, the velum is higher within a high vowel context than within a low vowel context.[16]

Most studies of the nasals have cited the differentiating cues to separate the places of articulation, but Fujimura investigated the nasals and reported three properties that they had in common: (1) a low first formant around 300 Hz, (2) high damping of the formants, and (3) high density of the formants in the frequency domain.[29] These results agree substantially with those of Hattori et al, who reported a general nasal resonance around 250 Hz for nasalized vowels and for nasal consonants.[22] The somewhat fixed size and shape of the nasal cavity, prominent in the production of nasal speech sounds, is the primary factor in the commonalities found in the resonance properties of both nasalized vowels and nasal consonants. The similarities in the acoustic features of nasal consonants that make place of articulation distinctions difficult to determine are somewhat parallel to those of the stop consonants, which will be discussed in the next section.

STOP CONSONANTS

The stop consonants are identified not only by the formant transitions to and from adjacent vowels (mentioned in the preceding section), but also by the burst of the stop releases and by the voice onset time. Stop consonants include plosives, implosives, clicks, and ejectives, all of which block or stop the airflow so that a burst is possible upon the release of the articulatory closure that forms the stop. Vowels and consonants other than stops are referred to as continuants because the acoustic pattern for the speech sound can be sustained and is of the same general type of waveform throughout. However, the acoustic pattern for a stop consonant changes during its production. At the time of the closure of a voiceless stop, such as /p/, /t/, or /k/, no sound is produced and, consequently, no acoustic speech wave is present, only silence. During the closure for voiced stops, such as /b/, /d/, or /g/, the vocal folds are vibrating and producing a quasiperiodic speech wave with a low first formant and possible, but weaker, higher formants. Following either the voiceless or the voiced closure, all stop consonants may have an acoustic impulse or burst at the moment of release of the closure. The concentration of energy in these bursts is an indicator of the place of articulation of the stop consonants.

Halle et al studied the acoustic properties of English plosives.[30] They reported that labial stops, such as /p/ and /b/, have their major concentration of energy for the bursts in the low frequencies, between 500 and 1,500 Hz. The bursts of alveolar stops, such as /t/ and /d/, were found to have a flat spectrum or one in which the frequencies above 4,000 Hz predominate. The palatal and velar stops found in the various productions of /k/ and /g/ showed bursts with primary concentrations of energy in the frequency range of 1,500 to 4,000 Hz. Although the spectral peaks for the velar stops were much lower in frequency than those for the palatal stops, the latter had a range from 2,000 to 4,000 Hz. Similar findings of burst cues were reported by investigators at Haskins Laboratories in a series of speech synthesis experiments.[31]

As mentioned previously, second formant transitions of adjacent vowels are also major indicators of place of articulation for the stop consonants. The synthetic speech experiments at Haskins Laboratories rather clearly defined the correlations between place of articulation and second formant transitions of the associated vowels.[31–35] Figure 6–21*A* indicates the formant frequency patterns for the voiceless English plosives, /p/, /t/, and /k/, preceding /a/, and Figure 6–21*B* shows their voiced counterparts, /b/, /d/, and /g/, preceding the same vowel. As can be seen, the second formant transition for labial stops rises to the following /a/, those for alveolar stops descend slightly, and those for palatal and velar stops descend more steeply.

There is a continued interest in determining the perceptual cues of stop consonants. In a series of listening tests with synthesized CV syllables, Blumstein and Stevens have shown that correct identifications can be made for stop place of articulations from the 10 to 20 msec of speech immediately following the onset of the syllable.[36] The decisions are reliable whether the second and higher formants are moving or not and whether an initial burst is present or not. The results of this study support the suggestion made by various investigators that spectral analysis of the speech signal provides uniquely different patterns that correspond to individual phonetic features, such as place of articulation.[37,38] Dorman and Raphael studied the effects of bursts, opening transitions, closing transitions, and the duration of the closure on judgements of place of articulation.[39] All of these cues were found to be influential.

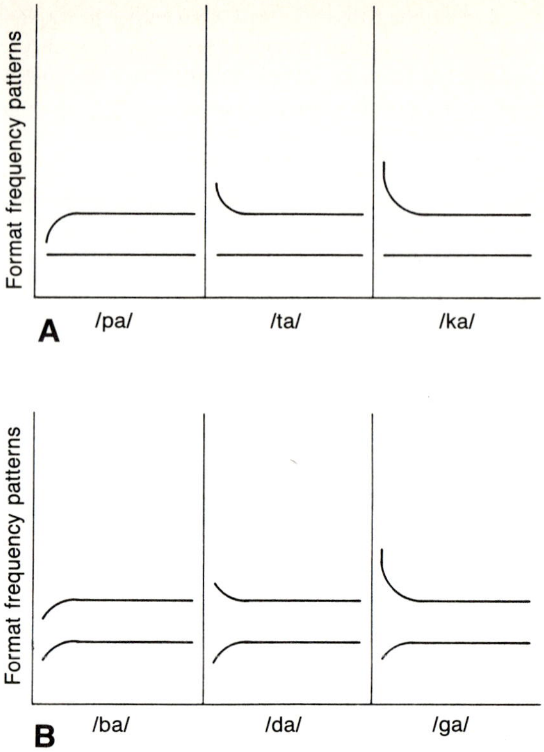

Figure 6–21 *A*, The formant frequency patterns for /a/ preceded by the voiceless English plosives /p/, /t/, and /k/. *B*, The formant frequency patterns for /a/ preceded by the voiced English plosives /b/, /d/, and /g/.

The perception of voiceless and voiced distinction among stops has been shown to be a function of many acoustic cues, including the length of time for the closure and the voice onset time in CV syllables. Lisker showed that silent closures of a duration less than 75 msec are identified as voiced stops, despite the absence of any vibration of the vocal folds during the closure.[40] He also found that intervals for the silent closures that were greater than 130 msec would be judged as voiceless stops. Lisker and Abramson reported that increases in voice onset time produced increases of voiceless identifications for the stops, and decision shifted from voiced to voiceless when the voice onset time was approximately 23 msec for labials, 37 msec for alveolars, and 42 msec for velars.[41,42] Studies by Massaro and Oden indicated the importance of voice onset time cues as well as second and third formant transitions for the judgements of voicing of stop consonants.[43]

Korean stops have a fortis and lenis distinction that is not found in English stops. A summary of the various studies that have been conducted on this distinction is presented by Dart.[44] Fortis stops are said to be unaspirated, whereas lenis stops are slightly aspirated in contrast to other ones that are heavily aspirated. Acoustic studies have indicated that fortis stops have a greater intensity and their fundamental frequency is higher than after corresponding lenis stops. Perceptually, fortis and lenis distinctions are difficult. The stop consonants are not unique in their difficulty in speech perception since the fricatives and sibiliants, which will be discussed in the next section, are similarly challenging.

FRICATIVES AND SIBILANTS

The types of speech sounds discussed thus far, vowels, nasals, and stops, normally have quasiperiodic speech waves produced by the vibration of the true vocal folds. In the aspiration of plosives and in the production of fricatives and sibilants, quasirandom speech waves result from the generation of turbulence at the place of constriction. There are two simultaneous sound sources, namely, the vibration of the vocal folds for the voicing and the noise produced at the place of articulation for voiced fricatives and sibilants. The primary acoustic cue for identifying the class of consonants known as fricatives and sibilants is the quasirandom speech wave that gives a broad-band continuous spectrum. There are also resonances and antiresonances, as well as vowel transitional cues, that help discriminate the individual fricatives and sibilants. Tarnóczy summarizes the literature on these consonants through the mid-1950s.[45]

Harris has indicated in perception studies that discrimination of the English fricatives and sibilants requires information from the transitions into following vowels as well as the noise portion of the speech sounds themselves.[46,47] Hughes and Halle developed objective identification criteria by measuring the density spectra of gated segments of fricatives and sibilants.[48] These were presented to listeners who had no difficulty in making voiced versus voiceless decisions based on the voicing cue of the quasiperiodicity of the speech wave, which was evident in the spectra as a very strong component below 700 Hz. In separating the /f/ and /v/, /s/ and /z/, and /ʃ/ and /ʒ/, it was found that the labials have no high-frequency peak below 10 kHz, and alveolars have peaks at consistently higher frequencies than the palatals.

Strevens has provided one of the most comprehensive studies of fricatives and sibilants.[49] The general broad-band spectra ranges that he found are shown in Figure 6–22. The cross bars indicate typical peaks of energy for the formants. Although certain patterns can be clearly seen (e.g., the high-frequency spectrum for /s/), considerable overlap occurs in the ranges of the spectra, and the formants are not as definitive as with vowels. In fact, the formants for /h/ are normally a function of the adjacent vowel, and thus a typical formant pattern is not appropriate for that fricative. The following acoustic properties were found for the fricatives and sibilants according to gross place of articulation: the front group, /ɸ/, /f/, /θ/, had the lowest relative intensity and the longest spectrum length, between 5,000 and 6,000 Hz; the mid group, /s/, /ʃ/, /ɝ/, had the highest relative intensity and the shortest spectrum length, between 3,000 and 4,000 Hz; the back group, /x/, /X/, /h/, had the medium relative intensity and the medium spectrum length, between 4,000 and 5,500 Hz. For nearly three decades of acoustic study of fricatives and sibilants, it has proven difficult to obtain the information-bearing cues that distinguish each fricative and sibilant from all the others. As a group, they are easily marked with their broad-band spectra, but individual identities within the group are not at all clear.

SONORANTS

The last consonants to be discussed are grouped under the heading sonorants, which is used to spec-

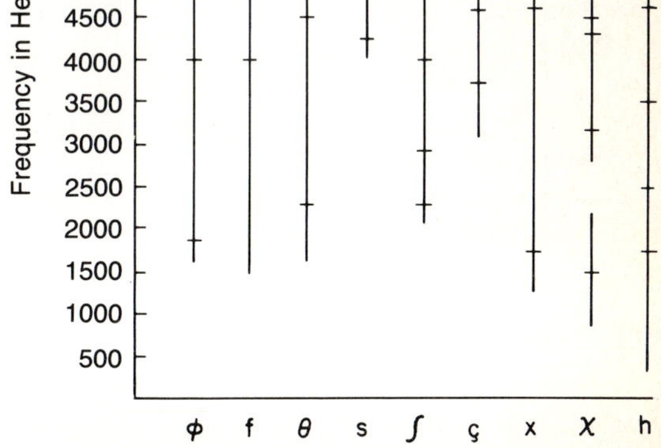

Figure 6–22 General broad-band spectra ranges from voiceless fricatives. (After Strevens P. Spectra of fricative noise in human speech. Lang Speech 1960; 3:32.)

ify that set of sounds produced with an airflow neither as laminar as that for vowels nor as turbulent as that for fricatives. The speech wave is usually quasiperiodic, but occasionally it may also be quasirandom from the frictional property associated with certain sonorant productions. The English sounds included in this sonorant grouping are semivowels, such as /w/ and /j/, laterals, such as /l/, and retroflexed consonants, such as /r/.

Semivowels /w/ and /j/ have acoustic properties similar to the vowels /u/ and /i/, respectively. The similarity of production can easily be seen in English words such as "woo" /wu/ and "ye" /ji/. That the formant structures of the semivowels and vowels are close to one another is not surprising. Lehiste published one of the most thorough studies on the acoustic properties of English sonorants.[50] A summary of her findings is presented succinctly in Figure 6–23. The similarities between the respective pairs of semivowels and vowels, /w/ and /j/ with /u/ and /i/, are seen if one compares the formant patterns of the semivowels in Figure 6–23 with those of the vowels in Figure 6–19. In general, the first two formants for the sonorants were lower in frequency than those for the corresponding vowels. In addition, the third formant for /w/ was sometimes weak or even missing. The third formant for /j/ was higher in frequency than for /i/. Durations

Figure 6-23 Formant patterns for sonorant consonants. (After Lehiste I. Acoustical characteristics of selected English consonants. Int J Am Ling 1964; 30:1.)

of the semivowels are of considerably shorter periods of time than those of the vowels. Because of this reduced duration for /w/ and /j/, in comparison with the often-stressed vowels of /u/ and /i/, the formant patterns for the sonorants are moving throughout while the vowels usually have some period of steady vowel formant structures.

The laterals shown in Figure 6–23 have interesting acoustic properties. The [l], which is not velarized and is normally in syllable initial position in English, has a second formant frequency that is dependent on the following vowel. This dependence is indicated in the figure by the double-headed arrow between second formant frequencies of approximately 800 Hz and those of nearly 1,400 Hz. The velarized lateral is usually in syllable final position and has a second formant frequency range which is lower than that for the nonvelarized counterpart. In contrast, the first formant for the velarized lateral is often higher in frequency than for the nonvelarized one. The syllabic lateral in English is produced with velarization and tends to have lower second and third formants than the nonsyllabic velarized laterals, as indicated by the double-headed arrows shown in Figure 6–23.

One of the most descriptive studies of the production of retroflexed consonants, such as the /r/ in English, was published by Delattre.[51] He showed that there are a number of physiological formations that produce a perceptually acceptable retroflexed sound. Despite these articulatory differences, there is a distinct acoustic cue for the retroflexed consonants, namely, an exceedingly low third-formant frequency. In her study of sonorants, Lehiste indicated that acoustic allophonic differences of /r/ were correlated to position in sound sequences (i.e., initial, medial, or final) rather than to the physiological formation differences.[50] As one can see in Figure 6–23, the initial /r/, shown by (I), has lower formant frequencies throughout than either the medial (M) or final (F) retroflexed sonorants. These latter two sounds have similar first formant frequencies, but the medial /r/ second-formant frequency range is lower than the final /r/ and, similarly, the third-formant frequency of the medial /r/ tends to be of a lower frequency than that of the final /r/. Similar to /l/, the adjacent vowels of middle and final retroflexed consonants influence their second-formant frequencies, as shown by the double-headed arrows for these sounds in Figure 6–23. In comparing the retroflexed consonant /r/ with the retroflexed vowel /ɝ/, Lehiste found the primary acoustic distinction to be a higher third formant for the retroflexed vowel.

Scientists have been as interested in the perception of sonorants as they have been in that of other consonants. Lisker studied the perception of sonorants in intervocalic position,[40] and O'Connor et al studied them in initial position.[52] In synthesis experiments, scientists showed that the second formant transitions can separate /w/ from /r-l/ from /j/, since they are low in origin for /w/, middle for /r-l/, and high for /j/. The third formant transition is used to distinguish between /r/ and /l/, since retroflexed sounds have such an unusually low third formant. The durations of the transitions were found to be important for perceiving sonorants as a class of sounds. It is necessary for the formant transitions to be shorter for sonorants than for vowels, but longer for sonorants than for stops and nasals.

SUMMARY

The complex waves of speech can be studied acoustically to obtain a better understanding of the structure of vowels and consonants. The fundamental frequency, formant frequencies, amplitudes of the frequencies, and, in the case of frication, the broadband spectra of speech sounds are all acoustic cues for identifying the individual units of articulation. In both analysis and synthesis, the formant frequencies are perhaps the single most important set of features for understanding the structure of speech sounds. Although much is now known about the acoustic properties of the vowels and consonants, much research is still needed to describe fully all of the individual sounds of speech.

REFERENCES

1. Borden GJ, Harris KS. Speech science primer: physiology, acoustics, and perception of speech. 2nd ed. Baltimore: Williams & Wilkins, 1984.
2. Hoops RA. Speech science: acoustics in speech. 2nd ed. Springfield, IL: CC Thomas, 1969.
3. Shoup JE, Pfeifer LL. Acoustic characteristics of speech sounds. In: Lass NJ, ed. Contemporary issues in experimental phonetics. New York: Academic Press, 1976:171.
4. Painter C. An introduction to instrumental phonetics. Baltimore: University Park Press, 1979.
5. Baker RJ. Clinical measurement of speech and voice. Boston: College-Hill Press, 1987.
6. Fant G. Acoustic theory of speech production. The Hague: Mouton, 1960.
7. Stevens KN, House AS. An acoustical theory of vowel production and some of its implications. J Speech Hear Res 1961; 4:303–320.
8. Backus J. The acoustical foundations of music. 2nd ed. New York: WW Norton, 1977.
9. Chiba T, Kajiyama M. The vowel—its nature and structure. Tokyo: Kaisekan Publishing, 1941.
10. House AS, Stevens KN. Estimation of formant bandwidths from measurement of transient response of the vocal tract. J Speech Hear Res 1958; 1:309–315.
11. Wakita H, Fant G. Toward a better vocal tract model. Royal Institute of Technology, Stockholm. Speech Transmiss Lab Q Prog Status Rep 1978; 1:9–27.
12. International Phonetic Association. The principles of the international phonetic association. London: Department of Phonetics, University College, 1966.
13. Peterson GE, Barney HL. Control methods used in a study of the vowels. J Acoust Soc Am 1952; 2:175–184.
14. Dunn HK. Methods of measuring vowel formant bandwidths. J Acoust Soc Am 1961; 33:1737–1746.
15. Peterson GE, Lehiste I. Duration of syllable nuclei in English. J Acoust Soc Am 1960; 32:693–703.
16. Kuehn DP. A cineradiographic investigation of velar movement variables in two normals. Cleft Palate J 1976; 13:33–103.
17. Kent RD, Carney PJ, Severeid L. Velar movement and timing: evaluation of a model for binary control. J Speech Hear Res 1974; 17:470–488.
18. Moll KL, Daniloff RG. Investigation of the timing of velar movements during speech. J Acoust Soc Am 1971; 50:678–684.
19. Lindquist-Gauffin J, Sundberg J. Acoustic properties of the nasal tract. Phonetica 1976; 33:161–168.
20. Curtis JF. Acoustics of speech production and nasalization. In: Spriesterbach DC, Sherman D, eds. Cleft palate and communication. New York: Academic Press, 1968.
21. House AS, Stevens KN. Analog studies of the nasalization of vowels. J Speech Hear Disord 1956; 21:218–232.
22. Hattori S, Yamamoto K, Fujimura O. Nasalization of vowels in relation to nasals. J Acoust Soc Am 1958; 30:267–274.
23. House AS. Analog studies of nasal consonants. J Speech Hear Disord 1957; 22:190–204.
24. Hecker MHL. Studies of nasal consonants with an articulatory speech synthesizer. J Acoust Soc Am 1962; 34:179–188.
25. Nakata K. Synthesis and perception of nasal consonants. J Acoust Soc Am 1959; 31:661–666.
26. Liberman AM, Delattre PC, Cooper FS, Gerstman LJ. The role of consonant vowel transitions in the perception of the stop and nasal consonants. In: Psychological monographs general and applied. Washington, DC: Herbert S Conrad, 1954:1.
27. Malecot A. Acoustic cues for nasal consonants: an experimental study involving a tape-splicing technique. Language 1956; 32:274–284.
28. Abramson AS, Nye PW, Henderson JB, Marshall CW. Vowel height and the perception of consonant nasality. J Acoust Soc Am 1981; 70:329–339.
29. Fujimura O. Analysis of nasal consonants. J Acoust Soc Am 1962; 34:1865–1875.
30. Halle M, Hughes GW, Radley J-PA. Acoustic properties of stop consonants. J Acoust Soc Am 1957; 29:107–116
31. Liberman AM. Some results of research in speech perception. J Acoust Soc Am 1957; 29:117–123.
32. Cooper FS, Delattre PC, Liberman AM, Borst JM, Gerstman LJ. Some experiments on the perception of synthetic speech sounds. J Acoust Soc Am 1952; 24:597–606.
33. Delattre PC, Liberman AM, Cooper FS. Acoustic loci and transitional cues for consonants. J Acoust Soc Am 1975; 27:769–773.
34. Harris KS, Hoffman HS, Liberman AM, Delattre PC, Cooper FS. Effect of third-formant transitions on the perception of the voiced stop consonants. J Acoust Soc Am 1958; 30:122–126.
35. Hoffman HS. Study of some cues on the perception of the voiced stop consonants. J Acoust Soc Am 1958; 30:1035–1041.
36. Blumstein SE, Stevens KN. Perceptual invariance and onset spectra for stop consonants in different vowel environments. J Acoust Soc Am 1980; 67:648–662.

37. Jakobson R, Fant CGM, Halle M. Preliminaries to speech analysis. Cambridge: MIT Press, 1963.
38. Zue V. Acoustic characteristics of stop consonants: a controlled study. Sc.D. Dissertation, Massachusetts Institute of Technology, 1976.
39. Dorman MF, Raphael LS. Distribution of acoustic cues for stop consonant place of articulation in VCV syllables. J Acoust Soc Am 1980; 67:1333–1335.
40. Lisker L. Closure duration and the intervocalic voiced-voiceless distinction in English. Language 1957; 33:42–49.
41. Lisker L, Abramson AS. A cross-language study of voicing of initial stops: acoustic measurements. Word 1964; 20:384–422.
42. Lisker L, Abramson AS. The voicing dimension: some experiments in comparative phonetics. Proceedings of the Sixth International Congress of Phonetic Resources, 1967. Prague: Academia Prague, 1970:563–567.
43. Massaro DW, Oden GC. Evaluation and intergration of acoustic features in speech perception. J Acoust Soc Am 1980; 67:996–1013.
44. Dart SN. An aerodynamic study of Korean stop consonants: measurement and modeling. J Acoust Soc Am 1987; 81:138–147.
45. Tarnóczy T. Die akustiche Struktur der stimmlosen Engelaute. Acta Ling 1954; 4:313–349.
46. Harris KS. Cues for the identification of the fricatives of American English. J Acoust Soc Am 1954; 26:952*A*.
47. Harris KS. Cues for the discrimination of American English fricatives in spoken syllables. Lang Speech 1958; 1:1–7.
48. Hughes GW, Halle M. Spectral properties of fricative consonants. J Acoust Soc Am 1956; 28:303–310.
49. Strevens P. Spectra of fricative noise in human speech. Lang Speech 1960; 3:32–49.
50. Lehiste I. Acoustical characteristics of selected English consonants. Int J Am Ling 1964; 30:1–97.
51. Delattre P. Comparing the phonetic features of English, German, Spanish, and French: an interim report. Heidelberg: Julius Groos Verlag, 1965.
52. O'Connor JD, Gerstman LJ, Liberman AM, Delattre PC, Cooper FS. Acoustic cues for the perception of initial /w, j, r, l/ in English. Word 1957; 13:24–43.

7 Aerodynamics of Speech

Donald W. Warren, D.D.S., Ph.D.

The generation of speech requires precise control of airflow along the respiratory tract. Changes in shape and size of the lower airway produce an air stream that is continuously modified by laryngeal and supralaryngeal structures. The activities of these structures are controlled by neural and chemical centers in the brain and by neural input from the periphery. The system is complex because the specialized aerodynamics of speech are superimposed on a highly regulated respiratory system. Moreover, the requirements of the body to maintain a proper chemical environment provide gross restraints on the availability of the respiratory system for speech purposes. This means that only a limited time interval is available for speech before the need to remove carbon dioxide (CO_2) and receive oxygen (O_2) prevails (Fig. 7–1).

MECHANICS OF AIRFLOW

Air flows from one region to another because of a difference in pressure between two areas.[1] When airflow is smooth and laminar (Fig. 7–2), the pressure required to move air is directly proportional to the viscosity of fluid:

$$P = k_1 \dot{V}$$

where P is pressure; k_1 is a constant that includes viscosity, length, and radius; and $\dot{V}$ is airflow.

However, flow is not always laminar because of the branching (irregular shape) of the respiratory tract. Eddying occurs at bifurcations or when the surface is rough or constricted. When airflow is turbulent (Fig. 7–3), the pressure necessary to produce a given amount of airflow varies with the square of flow:

$$P = k_2 \dot{V}^2$$

where k_2 relates to density, length, and radius. Thus density of the gas, rather than viscosity, becomes a factor. Turbulence occurs when the relationship of density × velocity × diameter to viscosity exceeds 2,000, which is Reynold's number.[2]

Constrictions that form along the vocal tract (i.e., the glottis during voicing) produce an orifice type of airflow. The resulting pressure drop is expressed as

$$P = \frac{d}{2K^2}\left[\frac{\dot{V}}{A}\right]^2$$

where A is the area, d is the density of air, and K is the discharge coefficient that depends upon the sharpness of the edge of the orifice and on Reynold's number. K has a value of 0.6 to 0.7 in the speech and breathing airflow range.[3] When air flows through a narrow orifice (Fig. 7–4), the gas molecules are accelerated and the rate of discharge through the orifice is proportional to the area (A) times the linear velocity of the fluid.

THE RESPIRATORY SYSTEM FOR BREATHING: THE GENERATION OF PRESSURES

Breathing, which is the movement of air into and out of the lungs, results from contractions of the respiratory muscles, which produce changes in the volume of the chest cage. The lungs fill the thoracic cavity, and its outer surface (visceral pleura) is in intimate contact with the inner surface of the thoracic cavity (parietal pleura). The two pleural layers are in apposition, separated only by a thin film of fluid, so that the lung slides freely within the cavity. Whenever the chest cage enlarges, the lungs also enlarge.[4]

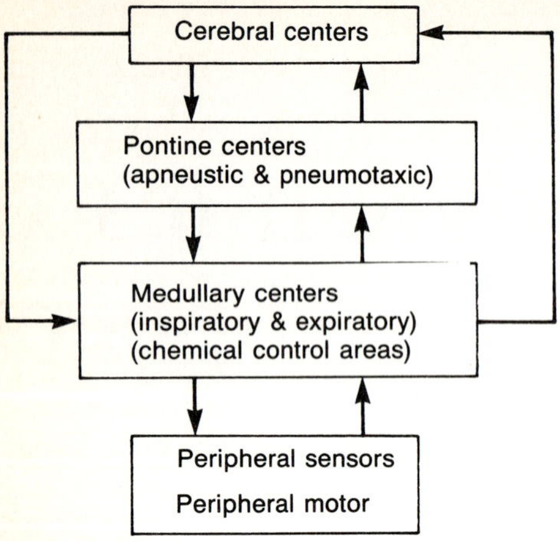

Figure 7–1 The control of speech aerodynamics involves a complicated feedback system that integrates information from various centers in the brain with data from the periphery.

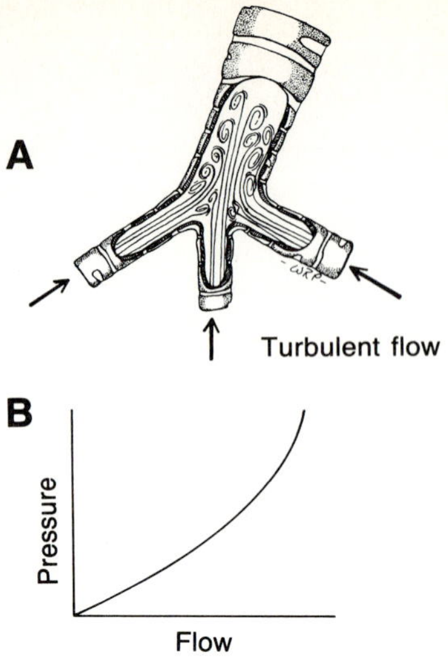

Figure 7-3 When airflow is turbulent *A*, eddying occurs and *B*, pressure is quadratically related to airflow.

At the end of expiration, when the respiratory muscles are relaxed, pressure within the lungs (pulmonary pressure) is atmospheric and there is no airflow. This is the resting level; at this point, a balance of elastic forces exists between the lungs and the chest wall (Fig. 7–5). Both the lungs and the chest wall contain considerable elastic tissue, and at resting position these pull in equal but opposite directions. Although the lungs and chest operate as a unit, the two have different resting positions when separated; that is, the lungs would collapse and the thoracic cavity would enlarge somewhat. Again, it is the pleural linkage that prevents this occurrence and allows a balance of elastic forces at rest position. However, when the diaghragm and the intercostal muscles contract during inspiration, the volume of the thoracic cage enlarges and the elastic forces of the two units change. When the diaphragm contracts, its dome moves downward into the abdomen, thus enlarging the thoracic cavity (Fig. 7–6). Simultaneously, the inspiratory intercostal muscles move the rib cage upward and outward, also increasing the volume of the thoracic cavity. This movement enlarges the volume of air within the lungs, pressure falls below atmospheric level, and air is drawn into the expanding lungs.[4]

Although inspiration is an active process involving muscle contractions, normal expiration is primarily a passive event.[4] The elasticity of stretched tissues and gravitational force tend to return the thorax to its resting position without any further expenditure of energy. The elastic elements that have been stretched during inspiration have a natural tendency

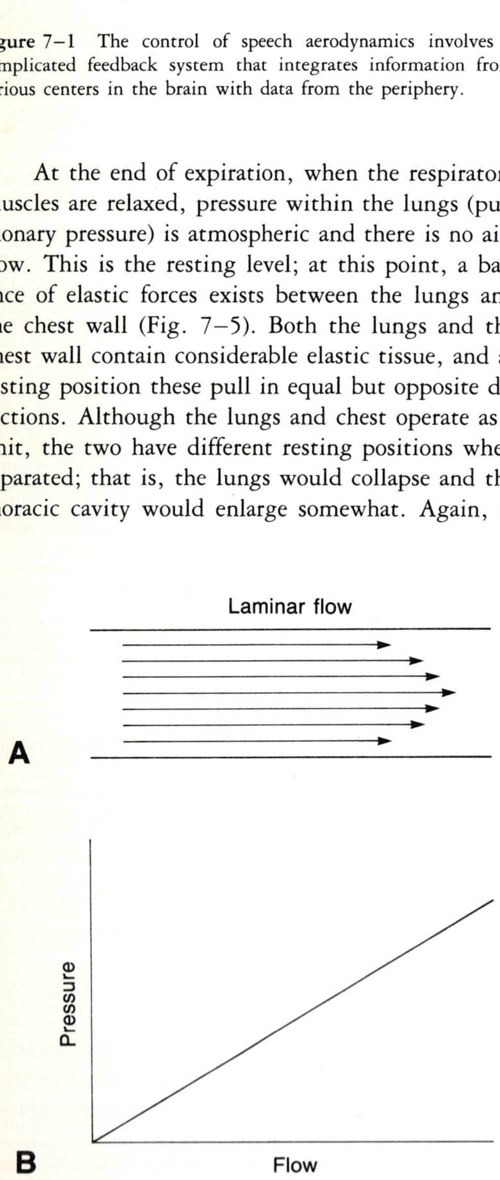

Figure 7–2 When airflow is laminar *A*, the lines of flow are smooth and *B*, pressure is linearly proportional to airflow.

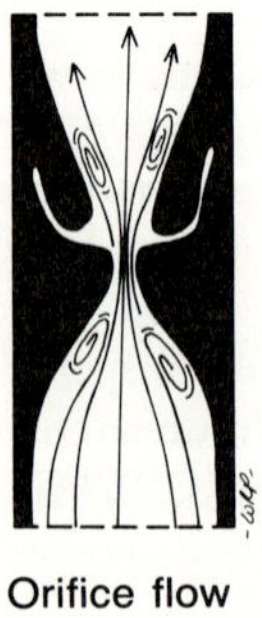

Figure 7–4 Constrictions along the vocal tract produce an orifice type of airflow.

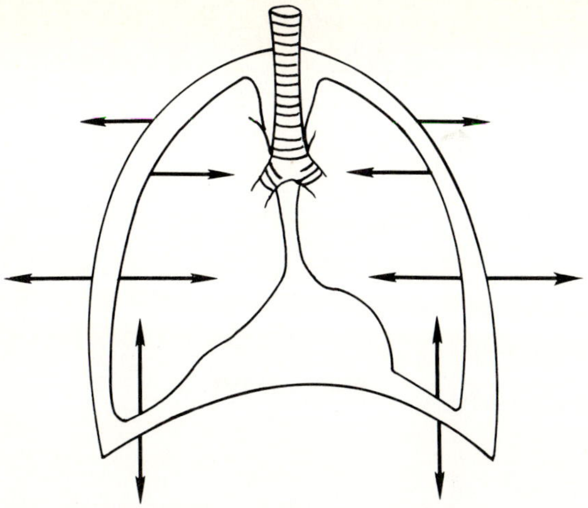

Figure 7-5 At resting level, a balance of elastic forces exists because the lung and chest wall pull in opposite directions. (From Warren DW. Aerodynamics of speech production. In: Lass NJ, ed. Contemporary issues in experimental phonetics. New York: Academic Press, 1976:105.)

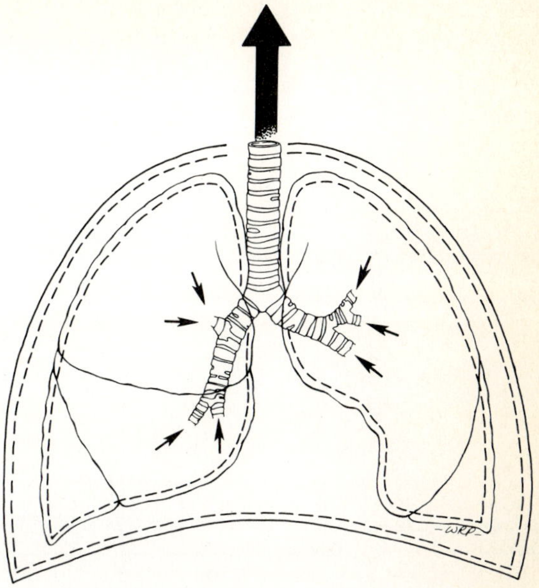

Figure 7–7 Recoil of the lungs and chest cage during expiration compresses the air in the lungs, and the resulting increase in pressure causes air to flow out.

to regain their original position after relaxation of the inspiratory muscles. As the thorax and lungs spring back to their original sizes, pulmonary air becomes temporarily compressed so that its pressure exceeds atmospheric pressure, and air flows from the lungs to the outside (Fig. 7–7).

The Work of Breathing

During inspiration, active muscle contraction provides the energy required to expand the thorax

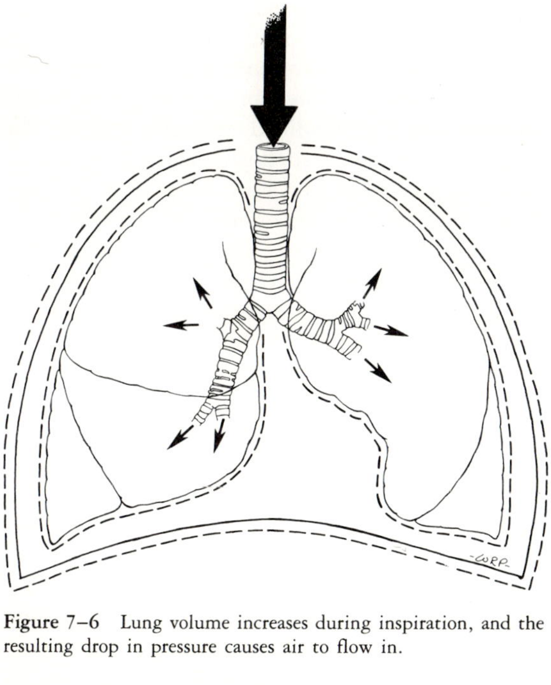

Figure 7–6 Lung volume increases during inspiration, and the resulting drop in pressure causes air to flow in.

and lungs. The primary forces that must be overcome include the elastic fibers in the tissues involved, airway resistance, and surface tension. The elastic behavior of the respiratory system is usually described in terms of its pressure-volume relationship; the elastic forces of the lungs and chest wall vary with lung volume.[5] The relaxation pressure curve is obtained by recording pulmonary pressure at different degrees of lung distention while airflow is obstructed at the mouth and all muscles are relaxed.[5] The pressure obtained at any lung volume is the result of the elastic forces of the lungs and chest wall. This is a measure of effort exerted previously in order to overcome the elasticity of the tissues involved. The curve illustrated in Figure 7–8 is the result of elastic recoil. At 60 percent of total lung capacity, the chest wall is at its natural size; and since its elastic fibers are not being stretched, they offer no recoil pressure. On the other hand, the elastic fibers in the lungs are being stretched so at that volume lung recoil pressure equals relaxation pressure. As inspiration continues, both the lungs and chest wall recoil when the muscles relax and the pressures are additive.[4]

During expiration when the muscles are relaxed and the lungs are deflated below resting level, a negative pressure develops. This negative pressure indicates the effort previously exerted to overcome the elastic resistance of the chest wall and lungs. Although the lungs would exert a positive pressure until they completely collapse, the lungs' pressure is more than counterbalanced by the chest wall, which

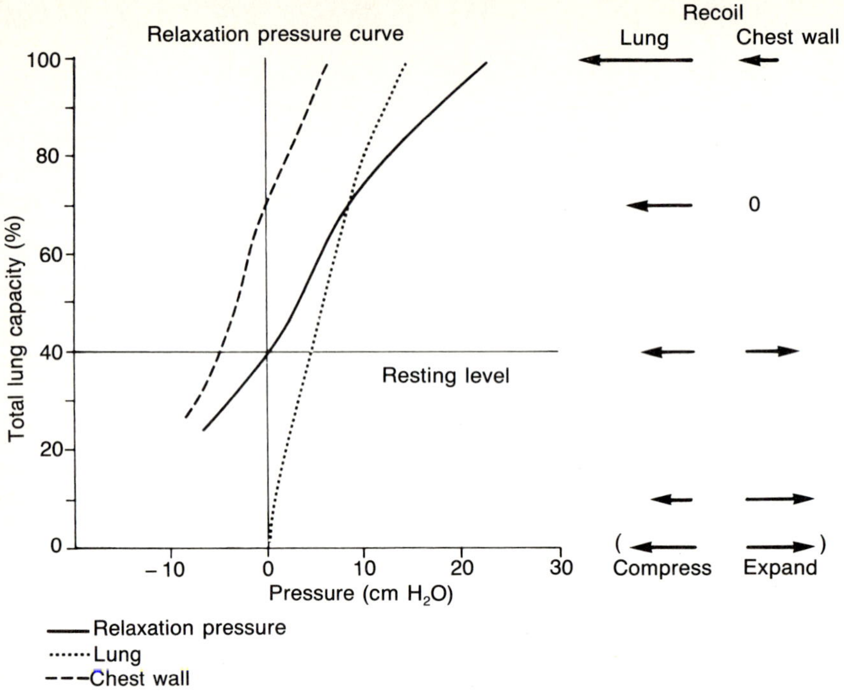

Figure 7-8 The relaxation pressure curve. The pressure at any lung volume is the result of elastic forces of the lung and chest wall. The curve is obtained by stopping airflow at various points of inspiration and expiration. (After Rahn H, Otis AB, Chadwick LE, Fenn WO. The pressure-volume diagram of the thorax and lung. Am J Physiol 1946; 146:161.)

exerts a greater negative pressure when it is smaller than its natural size.[4]

Most of the work involved in filling the lungs is used to overcome elastic recoil, and the energy required is stored during inspiration and utilized during expiration. The compliance of the respiratory system, or the degree of distensibility that occurs with the application of pressure, is an important factor in determining the amount of energy required to move air into and out of the lungs.[4]

The second factor determining the degree of work required for breathing is the magnitude of airway resistance. When the airway is open and airflow is mostly smooth (laminar), resistance is low. However, in disease states, increased respiratory secretions or obstuctions can increase resistance greatly. Airflow becomes more turbulent and greater effort is necessary to move air into and out of the lungs.

The third factor relates to a very special surface film that lines the alveoli of the lungs and produces surface tension. The fluid lining tends to shorten the surface and resist further stretching. Thus, inspiration would require additional energy to expand the alveolar sacs. Fortunately, a surface-active substance, surfactant, is present, which reduces surface tension. The recoil force of surface tension results in a pressure of about 20 cm H_2O when the lungs are fully inflated and about 2 cm H_2O at lower volumes.[2]

Maintenance of Airway Pressure for Speech

A constant pressure head must be maintained to power the speech mechanism. In spite of the complex interplay between muscular and nonmuscular forces, the actual generation of pressure in the lower airway and the air movement that results appear to be well controlled. Since speech occurs during the expiratory phase of breathing, normal expiratory pressure must be modified to some extent. The subglottal pressure head during normal expiratory breathing fluctuates between 10 cm H_2O and atmospheric, depending upon the phase of expiration (Fig. 7–9). However, the subglottal pressure head for speech is maintained at approximately 6 to 8 cm H_2O. Thus, expiratory forces must be modified so that an appropriate and consistent magnitude of subglottal pressure is generated during the speech process (Fig. 7–10). That is, in order to maintain a constant subglottal pressure, relaxation pressure resulting from the recoil of elastic fibers in the lungs and chest wall must be checked initially by active contraction of the inspiratory muscles.[6]

Similarly, as lung volume decreases, relaxation pressure falls and activation of the expiratory muscles is necessary at some stage to maintain the subglottal pressure head. Ladefoged et al observed elec-

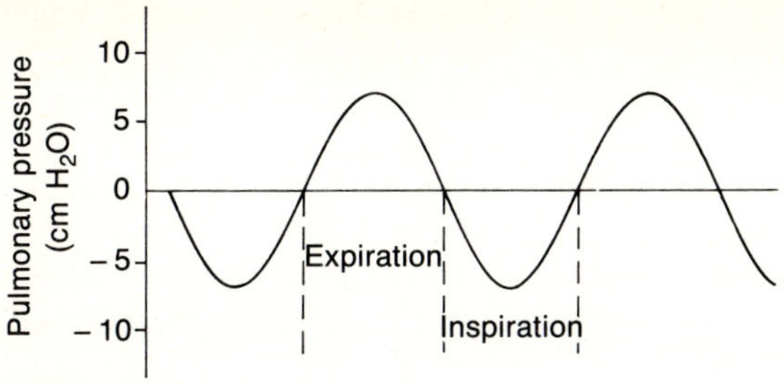

Figure 7–9 Pulmonary pressures during breathing. During inspiration pulmonary pressure is below atmospheric pressure and during expiration it is above atmospheric pressure.

tromyographically that the external intercostal muscles remain in action at the beginning of the utterance to check the descent of the rib cage and to counteract relaxation pressure (Fig. 7–11).[7] As lung volume decreases, external intercostal activity diminishes; it ceases completely when lung volume is slightly less than it is after a normal inspiration. At that point, relaxation pressure seems to be sufficient to provide the pressure head for the utterance. Expiratory muscle activity is then required to maintain pressure, with the internal intercostal muscles gradually increasing activity. Supplemental activity may occur in the later stage, with the external oblique, rectus abdominis, and latissimus dorsi contracting when lung volume is below resting level.[8] On the other hand, Hixon et al have emphasized the important role of the diaphragm in speech breathing.[9] They suggest that Ladefoged et al may not have adequately assessed speech breathing in their experiments because electromyographic sampling of muscle sites was limited.[7,9] Hixon, benefitting from more advanced technology, was able to analyze muscular effort more precisely and observed definite abdominal activity during speech production.[10]

Maintenance of a subglottal pressure head requires more than the checking or enhancement of elastic recoil forces. The sudden changes in respiratory load that occur when the upper airway closes or opens must be compensated for almost instantaneously if pressure is to be maintained at a near-constant level. Otherwise, sound intensity and fundamental frequency would be unstable. This poses a considerable error control problem that is not encountered in breathing. For example, phonation of the word /papa/ involves abrupt closure of the lips and impounding of air (Fig. 7–12). The subglottal pressure head is maintained by labial closure. The lips open for the vowel, and the vocal folds adduct to maintain the pressure head below. The flow of air from the lungs does not appreciably affect pulmonary pressure because the respiratory muscles adjust recoil forces. The lips close again for /p/ and the glottis opens. Once again the pressure head is sustained by closure of the oral port.

Undoubtedly, a complicated feedback system regulating pressure and airflow must be involved. Although there is some general information available, current models are still highly speculative. Warren has proposed that speech breathing conforms to

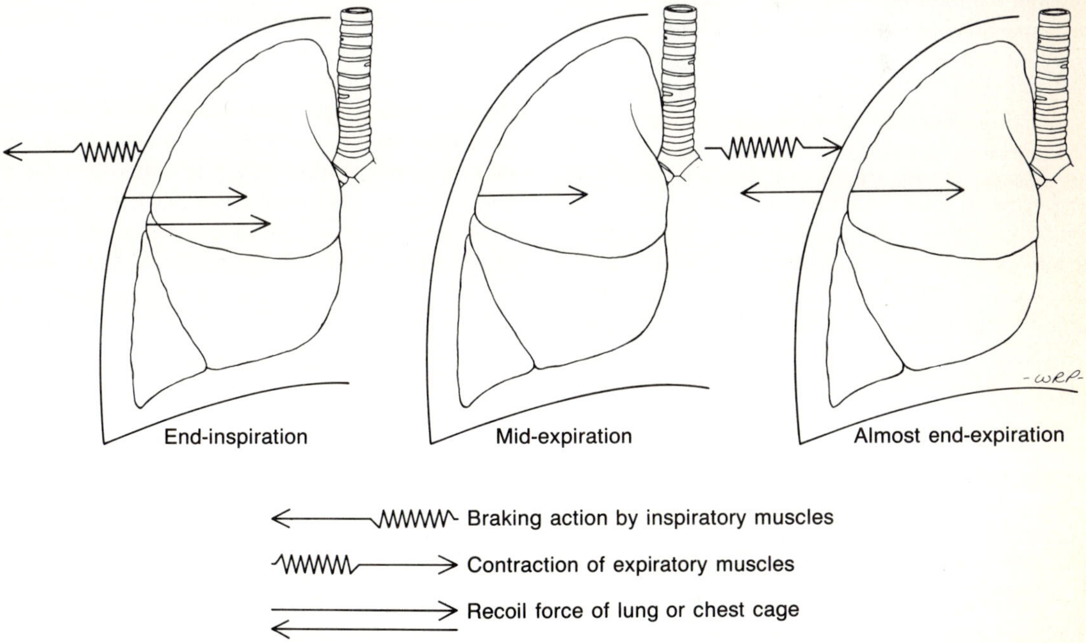

Figure 7–10 Subglottal pressure is maintained by the checking of elastic recoil at the beginning of expiration and the contraction of expiratory muscles near the end of expiration.

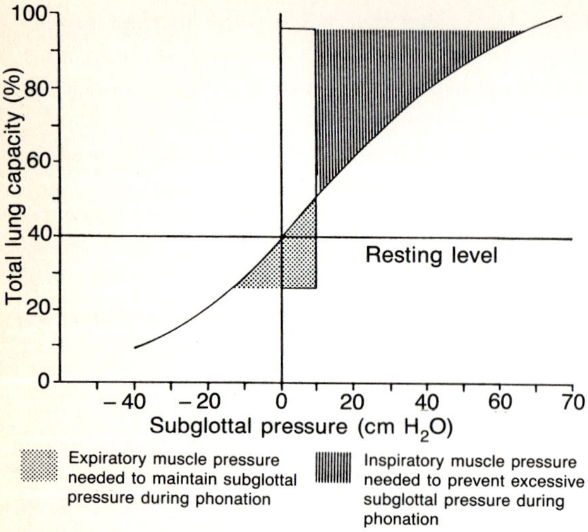

Figure 7-11 Lung volume and pressure relationships during speech. At high lung volumes, inspiratory muscle action is required to check recoil pressures and to prevent excessive subglottal pressure. At low lung volumes, expiratory muscle activity is required to maintain subglottal pressure for speech. (After Hixon T. Respiratory function in speech. In: Minifie F, Hixon T, Williams F, eds. Normal aspects of speech, hearing and language. Englewood Cliffs, NJ: Prentice-Hall, 1973:73.)

patterns characteristic of a regulating system.[11] I suggest that speech behaviors are manifestations of regulation and control strategies. In a typical regulating system (e.g., cardiovascular, temperature, body fluids, respiration), a physiologic parameter is said to be regulated if it remains relatively constant under different conditions. Response mechanisms or controls tend to keep such parameters constant; therefore the respiratory system is especially relevant since speech production represents modified respiratory performance. Although the regulated parameter in breathing is probably CO_2 concentration, maintaining breathing pressures, by controlling airway resistance and airflow, influences gas exchange and provides a stable CO_2 environment (Fig. 7–13).

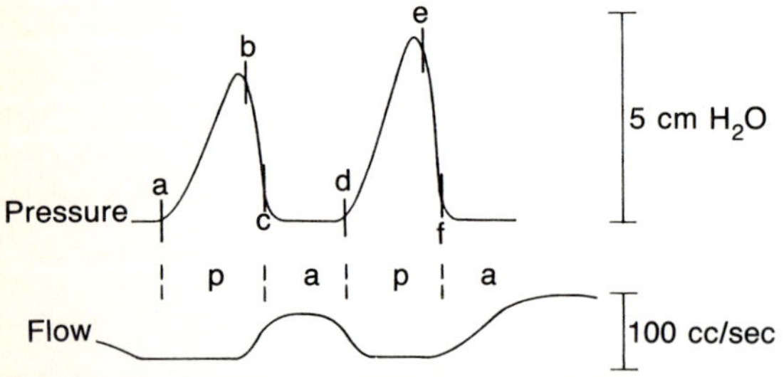

Figure 7-12 The constant subglottal pressure head is modulated into discrete patterns by the movement of upper airway structures. For example, in the word /papa/, the lips close at *a* and intraoral pressure builds to *b*. At that point, the lips part and pressure falls. Voicing for the vowel begins at *c*. At *d* the lips close again and pressure rises until the lips part at *e*. Voicing begins again at *f*. Airflow occurs during vowel production.

There is evidence that resistance in the respiratory airway is controlled for breathing purposes.[12] During expiration, the nasal valve is about 10 percent smaller than during inspiration.[13] In addition, the glottis adducts more strongly during the expiratory phase of breathing.[14] The additional resistances during expiration serve as an expiratory brake, thereby providing longer intervals for gas exchange at the alveoli.[15] Individuals appear to perceive differences in airway resistance during breathing and respond accordingly; for example, we mouth-breathe when our nasal airway seems obstructed.

Certain responses of the speech articulators are similar to those of the respiratory structures, and there appears to be control of resistances along the vocal tract during speech, somewhat paralleling the previously noted controls within the respiratory tract during breathing. The vocal tract is a tube containing oral, pharyngeal, and glottal structures capable of producing a variety of constrictions. The production of speech requires a relatively constant subglottal pressure, which serves as the energy source.[16–19] Intraoral pressures for consonants also appear to be fairly constant within subjects and seem to vary only according to consonant type or context.[20]

For speech aerodynamics, subglottal pressure is kept relatively constant by the checking or enhancement of elastic forces and by the compensation for sudden changes in respiratory load that occur with opening and closing of the upper airway. Precise control over the movement of upper airway structures and airflow tends to keep the subglottal pressure regulated.[21] Similar responses provide relatively stable intraoral pressures for consonants. Although the position of an articulatory structure varies according to phonetic context, overall resistance across the vocal tract remains fairly stable (Fig. 7–14). Thus, in normal speech, vocal fold resistance for a vowel is approximately 40 to 80 cm H_2O per liter per second,[21,22] but only 25 cm H_2O per liter per second for voiced fricatives. However, oral port resistance for fricatives is approximately 75 cm H_2O per liter per second, thus providing an overall resistance within

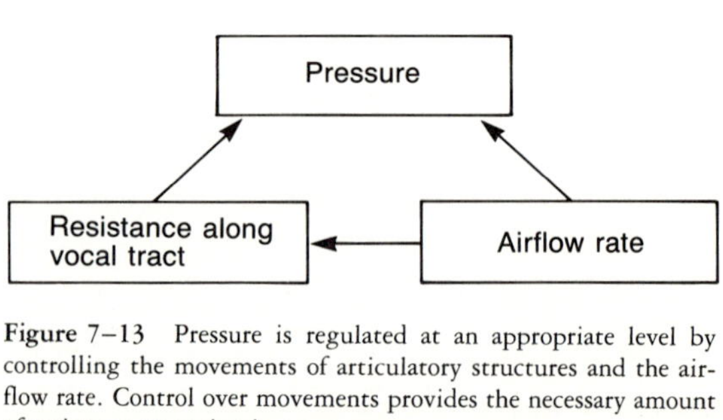

Figure 7-13 Pressure is regulated at an appropriate level by controlling the movements of articulatory structures and the airflow rate. Control over movements provides the necessary amount of resistance to maintain pressures.

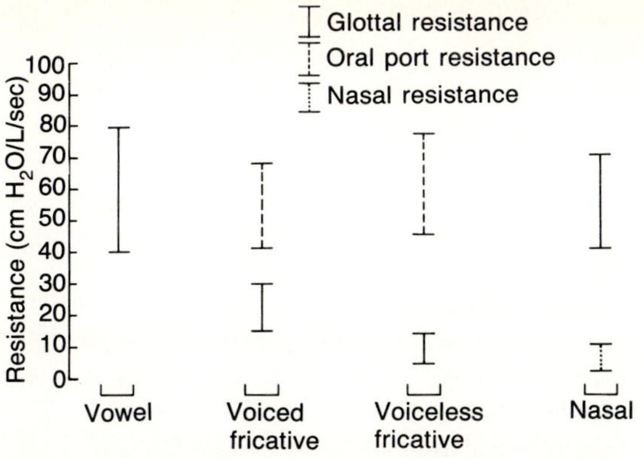

Figure 7–14 Resistance across the vocal tract is controlled to maintain pressures across consonant type. Approximate ranges are illustrated.

the airway similar in magnitude to that observed for vowels.[21]

Another example of stable resistance is glottal resistance for voiceless fricatives and plosives. The resistance for voiceless fricatives is approximately 10 cm H_2O per liter per second compared to about 6 cm H_2O per liter per second for voiceless plosives. On the other hand, resistance is infinite for plosives at the oral port and about 75 cm H_2O per liter per second for fricatives. Such interrelationships suggest that resistances of the speech structures may be synchronously controlled in a manner analogous to respiratory control.[21] A regulating system would prevent a rapid fall in subglottal pressure and would provide flexible, local energy sources throughout the vocal tract. The important point is that the same structures that modify airway resistance during breathing are also used as articulatory structures during speech. Sequenced breathing behavior presumably is programmed prior to birth and, therefore, is available for later use in speech.[14,23]

In any regulating system, there must be a relationship among input, processing, and output. Mechanisms to detect or identify change are necessary components if control factors are to operate. The presence of sensory receptors must be established, their location identified, and their sensitivity determined. The physiologic detection system does not have to respond to the variable being regulated; it can respond to some correlate or function related to it.[24]

Respiratory receptors have been found in the trachea,[25] in the larynx,[26] and in the nasopharynx of humans.[27] Intrathoracic receptors signal both volume and flow; extrathoracic receptors signal flow and upper airway resistance.[25] Similarly, laryngeal receptors sensing pressure, airflow, and contraction of muscles have been described.[25] There is also evidence that muscles in the upper airway play a functional role in instantaneous control of airflow and compensation for changes in airway resistance during breathing.[28,29] Remmers and Bartlett observed a "tracking" behavior, involving extrathoracic tracheal stretch receptors, in which the respiratory muscles during expiration compensated for changes in upper airway resistance.[12] The expiratory discharge of the receptors was determined by the relationship between upper airway resistance and instantaneous flow. This provides information useful for coordinating the activity of expiratory flow controllers. If this afferent information were compared centrally with that derived from intrathoracic pulmonary receptors, the relative magnitude of upper airway resistance could be estimated. Such information might allow adjustment of laryngeal resistance in response to changes in supralaryngeal pressures. Recent studies by England and Bartlett demonstrate that the larynx activity controls respiratory flow in humans by varying the degree of glottal adduction.[14] Thus, there appears to be a detection system for breathing that may, in some fashion, operate in speech as well.

Systematic study of a regulating system involves experiments that identify and describe the mechanisms of control. Evidence of a regulating system is obtained by studies that perturb the airway and introduce an error.

Bite blocks have been used to produce unnatural jaw openings as a means for assessing aerodynamic responses to sudden change in the vocal tract. Insertion of a bite block forces a speaker into compensatory maneuvers that can be evaluated quantitatively.[30–32] The results of these studies are similar, with the data clearly showing the remarkable adaptive behaviors of the speech structures. Although the vertical dimension was dramatically increased, oral port cross-sectional opening for fricatives showed little or no change. Whenever port size did increase slightly, airflow rate also increased and intraoral pressure was maintained. On the other hand, an increased frequency of misarticulations with each increase in vertical dimension was observed, in spite of the fact that port size did not change significantly.[30] These studies suggest that structural responses to sudden change successfully maintain a normal aerodynamic environment for speech, but the speech outcome, as judged by listeners, is compromised.

Putnam et al recently published some data on compensatory responses to bite-block and bleed-valve maneuvers.[33] Their findings support the hypothesis of regulation and control. When bite blocks were inserted, intraoral pressures were maintained at an appropriate level and airflow rate increased. Presumably, as in other bite-block studies, the tongue was manipulated to close the induced open bite, and these maneuvers resulted in maintenance of adequate oral port resistance. The increased airflow observed in their study also would have augmented port resistance.

Another segment of this interesting study involved the use of bleed tubes of different diameters during plosive consonant productions. The bleed device prevented lingual maneuvers as a compensatory response. The investigators found that airflow rate increased in a linear fashion as the size of the bleed tubes increased. Although pressure fell with increased opening, it was always maintained above 4 cm H_2O.

Putnam et al also observed another characteristic of aeromechanical integrity.[33] Airflow in the postconsonantal vowels exhibited remarkably stable patterns across bleed and block conditions. The investigators reported that

> ...this implies some accommodating adjustments in laryngeal airway resistance to normalize vowel flow in spite of the aeromechanical perturbations introduced during the preceding /p/ and /s/ segments....Such data lend credence to the attractive but inherently elusive hypothesis that vocal tract pressures are somehow monitored and airway resistances regulated.

One possible system is illustrated in Figure 7–15. It consists of a controller unit or computer coordinating center, sensors or receptors to transmit information, and effectors to power the system and produce articulatory movements.[34] The controller most certainly is in the brain, and presumably higher centers and the medulla are involved. Sensors may be located in the lung and along the vocal tract. The effectors are the respiratory muscles that power the pump, and the articulatory structures are the variable resistances that modulate the airstream. This hypothetical model is presented only for the purpose of demonstrating our limited knowledge. Receptors for sensing such parameters as pressure and airflow have not been identified, yet monitoring is necessary if errors are to be corrected. For example, in breathing, overinflation of the lung is prevented by receptors that transmit information about volume to the respiratory centers. However, breathing is a slow process in comparison to speech, and regulation of volume can be accomplished to a great extent by the alpha motor neuron system, although the gamma efferent system is available for rapid readjustments when required. More rapid and frequent adjustments of pressure and airflow would be necessary for speech. Gross muscle activity such as checking elastic recoil may be controlled by the alpha system, but changes in respiratory load in response to events in the upper airway require a faster response. The gamma efferent system may provide the rapid, sensitive adjustments needed to maintain a constant pressure head. In addition, simultaneous preprogramming for the respiratory muscles as well as for the articulators is also a possibility.

There is evidence that the brain prepares the articulators for the production of speech sounds well in advance.[35–41] An interval of preparation exists for a specific sound, and this interval presumably involves advanced neural input to the articulators. The same advanced programming may provide simultaneous input to the respiratory muscles to prepare for possible events such as transient back pressures. Indeed, coarticulation seems to be a reflection of advanced programming. The gamma loop and the small motor fiber system associated with it would still operate as a servo to drive the main muscle fibers, but their operating range would be smaller with preprogramming of the alpha system.

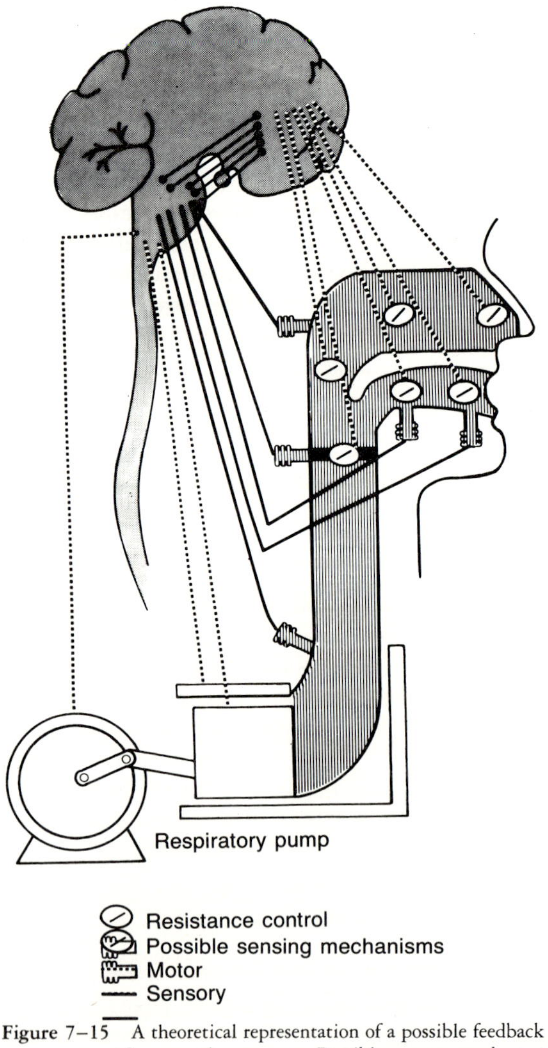

Figure 7–15 A theoretical representation of a possible feedback system to regulate speech pressures. Possible sensors send error messages to resistance controllers via the brain.

Although the hypothesis that speech aerodynamics follows regulation and control principles may be novel, it is much in line with modern theories of speech-motor control as described by Kelso et al[42] and Kelso and Tuller.[43] The speech-motor control theory is framed in such terms as "motor equivalence" and "coordinative structures." For segmental speech activities, the postulate is that functionally and anatomically distinct parts of the speech system are constrained to act together toward a common goal. Within this framework, the respiratory and articulatory systems are hypothesized to form a coordinative structure whose goal is to regulate speech pressures.

Lower Airway Dynamics

Airflow in the lower airway is influenced by the shape of the alveolar sacs, the bronchi, and the trachea.[44] The bronchi branch dichotomously, each giving rise to two bronchi. The length and diameter of the bronchi decrease with each generation in a regular fashion, and their total cross-sectional area increases with each generation. The area of the peripheral bronchi is about 1,000 times larger than that of the trachea. Since the mean velocity of the airstream varies inversely with the cross-sectional area, the velocity of airflow increases as it moves from the periphery upward (Fig. 7–16). Thus, airflow may increase in velocity from less than 0.1 cm per second in the small bronchi to 100 cm per second in the trachea.

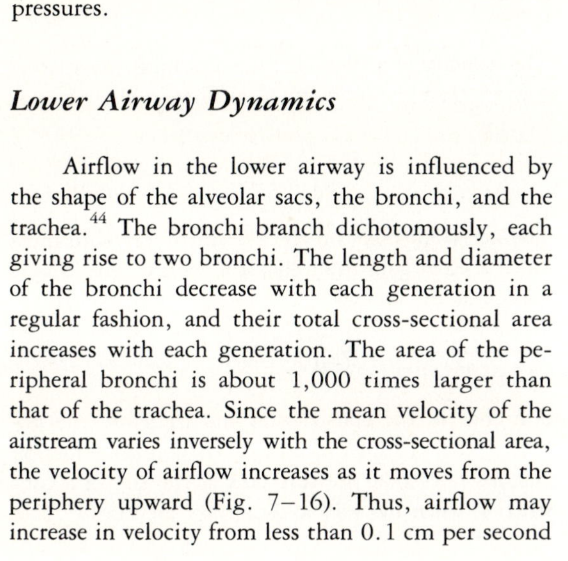

Figure 7–16 As cross-sectional area increases, velocity of airflow decreases. *A*, An illustration of the branching that occurs in the respiratory tract. *B*, An illustration to show that velocity decreases as cross-sectional area increases. (From Warren DW. Aerodynamics of speech production. In: Lass NJ, ed. Contemporary issues in experimental phoentics. New York: Academic Press, 1976:116.)

The subglottal pressure head appears to remain fairly stable throughout the production of speech.[16–19] Pressure is maintained by using the respiratory muscles to check elastic recoil and prevent an over-pressure or by using the muscles to compress the chest cage further to prevent an under-pressure as speech is being produced (Fig. 7–17).

The flow of air is also modulated by the glottis and the supraglottal constrictors (i.e., tongue, palate, nose, lips, and teeth) so that pressure is maintained over a period of time. The increase in subglottic pressure that occurs with increased loudness or stress apparently is due, in large part, to changes in activity of the respiratory muscles.[17] There is less external intercostal muscle suppression of elastic recoil at high lung volumes and greater internal intercostal augmentation at lower lung volumes. The result is higher subglottal pressure during stress or loud utterances. Normal conversational speech occurs at the midrange of total lung capacity.[18] The breathing cycle is modified by increasing the depth of inspiration and prolonging expiration. Approximately 25 percent of the total lung capacity is utilized and about 1.2 to 1.5 L of air is involved (Fig. 7–18).[45] In comparison, during quiet breathing approximately 0.5 L of air is moved with each inspiration or expiration, and this breathing uses only 10 to 15 percent of the total lung capacity.[4] Larger lung volumes, perhaps as great as 4 to 5 L, are used when loudness is increased; similarly, respiratory effort is lower when the utterance is softer than normal.[6,46,47]

Hixon observed that speakers usually initiate conversational speech at approximately 60 percent of vital capacity and continue speaking until about 35 percent of vital capacity.[48] As shown in Figure 7–11, relaxation pressures in the 60 to 35 percent range of vital capacity are not too far above or below the usual magnitude of subglottal pressure. Thus, only little respiratory muscle effort is required to maintain appropriate subglottal pressures.

Russell, using a new technique involving in-

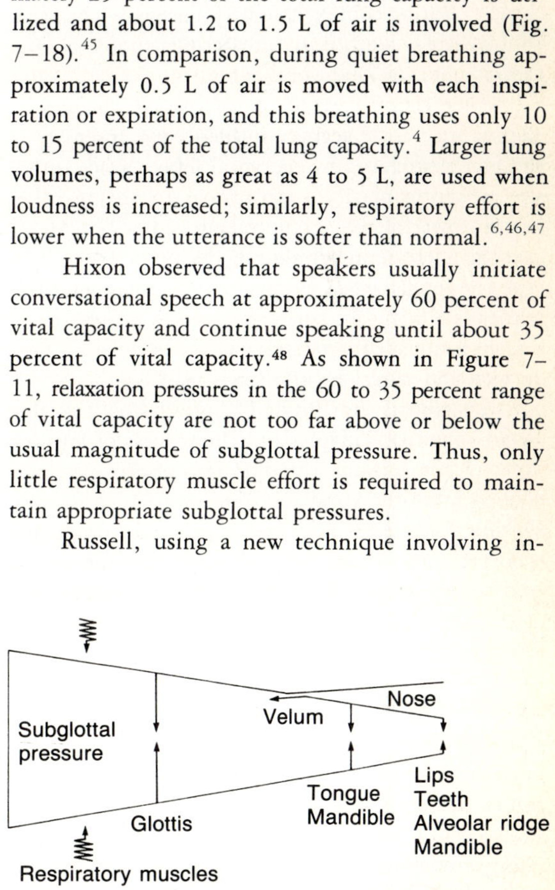

Figure 7–17 The subglottal pressure head is maintained by the respiratory muscles and by constrictions of upper airway articulators.

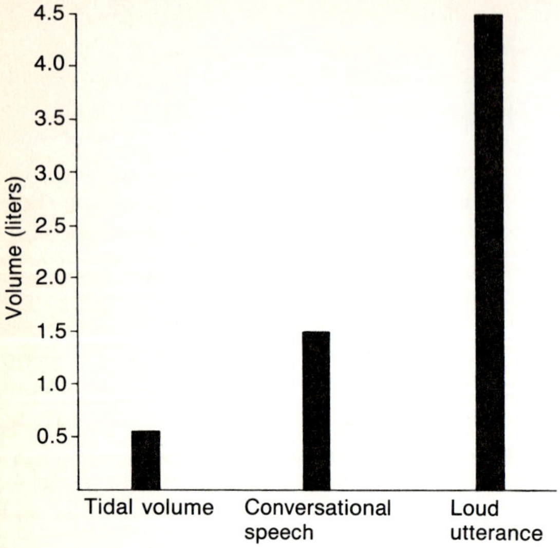

Figure 7–18 Comparison of lung volumes used during breathing, conversational speech, and loud utterances.

ductive plethysmography, compared respiratory behaviors of children and adults as a function of articulatory and intensity factors.[49] She observed that children and adults used similar percentages of vital capacity during comfortable vocal intensity, but that adults used a significantly greater percentage of vital capacity during loud vocal intensity.

There is also evidence that small changes in respiratory muscle activity influence the intensity of the sound produced by the vocal folds. Voice intensity is approximately proportional to the third or fourth power of the subglottal pressure.[50–52] Moreover, an increase in subglottal pressure also tends to raise the fundamental frequency.[51] Fundamental frequency is a dominant parameter used to denote stress, although other parameters, such as manner of production and duration, also have an effect.[53–55]

Laryngeal Activity. The glottis is the first major constrictor involved in the process of forming speech. Air passing through the glottis produces sounds when the vocal folds are properly adducted. During voicing the folds open and close, producing quasiperiodic airflow. The vibration-like movement of the folds results from aerodynamic, muscular, and elastic tissue forces which act in a complex way. The aerodynamic forces that are exerted on the vocal folds include subglottal air pressure, the Bernoulli force produced by negative pressure created transglottally by high velocity airflow, and supraglottal pressure produced by articulatory constrictions in the upper airway. The Bernoulli force is essentially the work-energy theorem for fluid flow. Although the effect of opening and closing the vocal folds is complex, the aerodynamic events that produce glottal movements can be described in the oversimplified terms of Bernoulli's principle.[56] Consider that airflow through the glottal constriction is steady, nonviscous, and incompressible (Fig. 7–19). The volume velocity of airflow across A_1 is equal to A_1v_1d, where d is the density of air, A_1 is the cross-sectional area of the trachea, and v_1 is the velocity of airflow. Assuming that airflow is uniform, the same mass of air must travel per unit of time through the constricted vocal folds so that

$$A_1v_1d = A_2v_2d$$

where A_2 is the cross-sectional area of the vocal folds and v_2 is the velocity of airflow at the glottis. Since the density, d, is constant,

$$A_1v_1 = A_2v_2$$

The velocity of airflow at the vocal folds is therefore greater than the velocity of airflow in the pharynx because

$$v_2 = \frac{A_1v_1}{A_2}$$

The net work done on the system by pressure must equal the net gain in mechanical energy. The kinetic energy of the airflow

$$\tfrac{1}{2}d\left[\frac{A_1v_1}{A_2}\right]^2$$

is higher in the constriction and therefore the potential energy must decrease. Bernoulli's equation demonstrates that pressure falls at the site of a constriction when the velocity of airflow increases.[56] That is,

$$\tfrac{1}{2}dv^2 + P = \text{constant}$$

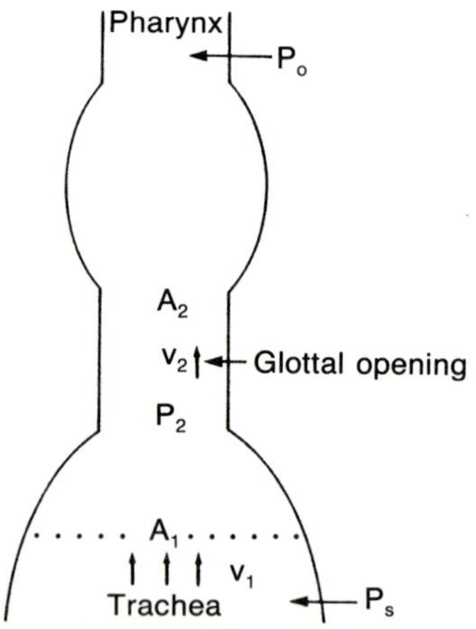

Figure 7–19 Schematic view of the vocal folds. Area A_2 is the cross-sectional area of the glottal constriction. P_2 and v_2 are the air pressure and particle velocity, respectively, at the glottal constriction. Area A_1 = the cross-sectional area of the trachea; v_1 = particle velocity; P_s = pressure in the trachea; and P_o = oral pressure or pressure in the mouth. (From Lieberman P. Vocal cord motion in man. In: Bouhuys A, ed. Sound production in man. Ann NY Acad Sci 1968; 155:29.)

The pressure at the glottal constriction may fall below atmospheric pressure, thereby drawing the folds together. Glottal tissue resistance then increases as the area of the constriction decreases, thus allowing the Bernoulli force to increase only up to a certain point.[57] This interaction of aerodynamic forces with muscle and elastic activity produces vocal fold vibrations which, in turn, provide the acoustic source for voicing.

It must be recognized that the previous discussion is only an idealized and simplified approximation of what actually occurs during voicing. The model described assumes laminar and incompressible airflow; however, although flow is probably incompressible, it is not always laminar or uniform. Similarly, the folds may not act symmetrically, and the static forces provided by the muscles and ligaments may not behave as idealized springs. Ishizaka and Matsudaira present a more complex model of vocal fold activity that accounts, to some extent, for vertical phase differences between the upper and lower parts of the folds.[58] They have shown that different pressures acting on the upper and lower parts of the folds cause a dragging effect and are responsible for the slight lag of the upper part of the folds behind the lower part.

Titze presented a configurational model of the glottis and vocal folds, which depicted the vocal folds in three dimensions.[59] His model describes the relation between vocal fold structure and vocal fold vibration more completely than the Ishizaka and Matsudaira two-mass model.[58] Scherer, Curtis, and Titze, using such models, suggest that existing pressure-flow equations for the larynx may be adequate approximations, but they lack sensitivity to glottal shape and to geometry to be applicable to a range of conditions associated with phonation.[60]

Although models of laryngeal function can be made complex, the outcome of tissue and aerodynamic coupling is still the same: the rapid closing and opening of the glottis mold airflow into a modulated stream that provides the basic source of speech.

The Effects of Glottal Activity on Air Pressure and Airflow. The vocal folds, like other articulatory structures, have a significant effect on pressure and airflow during speech.[61] The size of the glottal constriction affects the transglottal pressure loss, although articulatory changes occurring above the glottis also influence pressure at the folds. For example, opening the airway for vowels reduces supraglottal pressure almost to atmospheric pressure, while vocal constriction maintains subglottal pressure (Fig. 7–20). In comparison, the small oral port opening for fricatives raises intraoral pressure, while vocal fold constriction causes only a slight transglottal pressure drop. Plosives prior to voicing, on

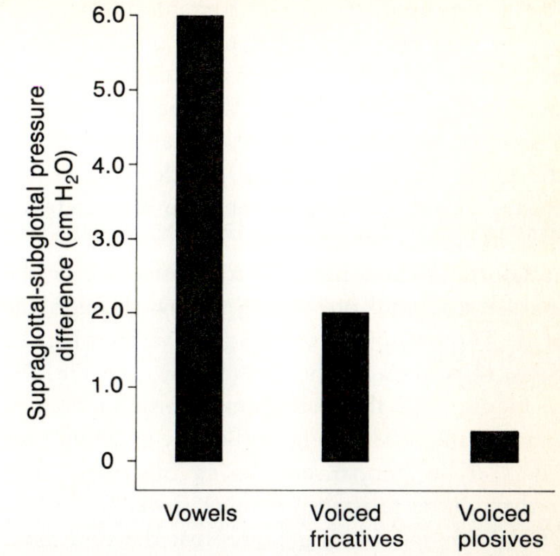

Figure 7–20 The supraglottal-subglottal pressure difference is influenced by the oral airway opening. Airway opening is largest for vowels, and the supraglottal pressure is nearly atmospheric under these circumstances. A closed oral airway for voiced plosives results in a small pressure drop. Voiced fricatives fall between vowels and plosives because the slight opening of the oral port helps to maintain airway pressure.

the other hand, have approximately equal supraglottal and subglottal pressures.

Glottal Activity During Stop Consonants. Voicing requires airflow across the vocal folds; to achieve this airflow in the closed system of stop consonants, a difference in pressure between the subglottal and supraglottal cavities must occur. Although in many instances voicing occurs on release of the plosive, there are times when it occurs during the stop phase of the consonant. Rothenberg has proposed three mechanisms for producing transglottal airflow during voiced stop productions:[62] (1) a passive, pressure-activated expansion of one or more walls of the supraglottal cavity; (2) a muscularly activated enlargement of the supraglottal cavity; and (3) nasal airflow through a slightly open palatal sphincter. A study by Lubker discounts nasal airflow and favors the active-expansion mechanism.[63] Perkell[64] and Kent and Moll[65] have demonstrated that voiced stops are produced with larger supraglottal volumes than their voiceless cognates. Further, the Kent and Moll data reveal that pharyngeal expansion occurs simultaneously with the depression of the hyoid bone, which is an active process. There is indirect evidence against passive enlargement of the oropharynx.

Rothenberg's study indicates that, considering the range of supraglottal cavity compliance, there are many instances in which the voiced interval of voiced alveolar plosives is too long and/or the voicing too strong to be maintained by passive expansion alone.[62] Similarly, if passive expansion did result from greater respiratory muscle activity during voicing, cognate differences in supraglottal pressure should occur; but they apparently do not.[19] Bell-Berti has proposed two modes of expanding the pharynx for voiced stops, each applying to a different group of muscles.[66] She presents evidence for an active mode, requiring increased muscle activity, and a passive mode, requiring suppression of muscle activity, to expand the pharynx.

Glottal Resistance. Glottal resistance is the ratio of transglottal pressure to airflow through the glottis. The magnitude of resistance varies with the cross-sectional area of the constriction (see Fig. 7–21). Figure 7–22 illustrates some approximations of glottal resistance according to the type of sound produced and, in comparison, during breathing. The fact that glottal resistance is much lower for voiced fricatives than for vowels indicates that the vocal folds do not adduct as much for fricatives as they do for vowels.[61] An estimate of vocal fold opening for vowels would be about 0.05 cm^2 and for fricatives about 0.10 to 0.15 cm^2. When the opening is larger than 0.50 cm^2, resistance is negligible. The volume rate of airflow used during sound production also affects glottal resistance (Fig. 7–23). Increased effort results in a higher resistance for a given amount of glottal opening. Similarly, adduction of the vocal folds has a considerable effect on respiratory volumes and the volume velocity of airflow.[67] Figures 7–24 and 7–25 illustrate that airflow rate is considerably higher and air volumes are much greater for voiceless sounds. This suggests that greater respiratory effort is required for voiceless consonant production. A comparison of volumes is made in Figure 7–26. However, it still is not known whether the differences arise simply as a result of vocal fold resistance or because greater respiratory effort is required to provide additional acoustic cues in the absence of a glottal sound source.

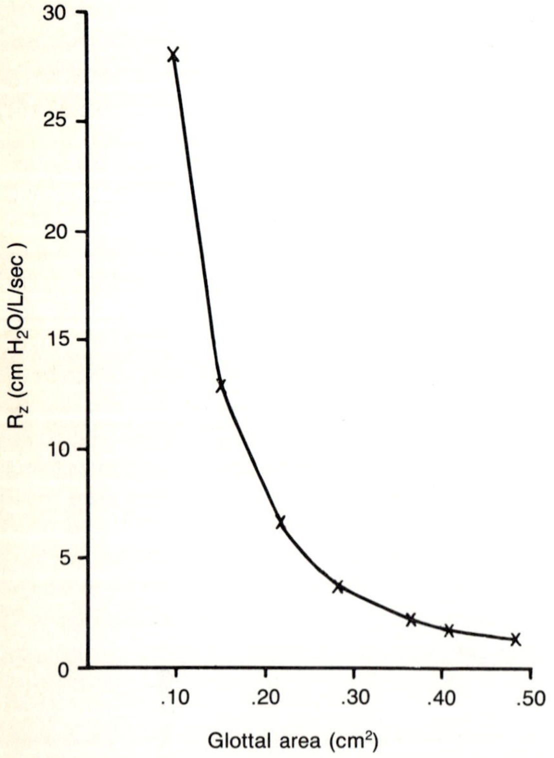

Figure 7-21 The relationship between glottal area and glottal resistance. (From Warren DW. Aerodynamics of speech production. In: Lass NJ, ed. Contemporary issues in experimental phonetics. New York: Academic Press, 1976:120.)

Whisper. The glottal chink is narrow but open during whisper, and resistance is approximately 4.0 to 6.0 cm H_2O per liter per second.[34] Respiratory effort is considerably increased, and this increased effort is reflected by increased airflow rates and greater intraoral pressures (Fig. 7–27). The time duration of sound production is also increased during whisper, and this probably accounts for much of the threefold increase in respiratory volumes used.[68] Presumably, increased time and effort are necessary to generate airflow turbulence and produce the sounds of whispered speech.

There is evidence that the unique glottal gestures associated with normally phonated voiceless and voiced stops are preserved, to some extent, in whisper. Weismer observed differences in peak flow for the release of voiceless versus voiced stops in whisper and differences in intraoral pressure slopes between the cognate pairs.[69]

Upper Airway Dynamics

Structures in the upper airway play an essential role in the speech process by modulating the airstream into precise patterns. The direction and velocity of air movement are controlled primarily by changes in airway size. These changes occur well in advance of the sounds to be produced and so influence the preceding segments of speech as well.[70]

Most speech activity is directed through the oral airway, and the resistance to airflow varies from less than 1.0 cm H_2O per liter per second for low vowels to an infinite resistance or complete obstruction in the case of plosives. Air actually flows more readily through the oral cavity than it does through the nasal cavity because resistance is approximately one-half, provided the tongue is not elevated to any great extent. That is, for low vowels, airflow would pass through the oral cavity even if the palatopharyngeal orifice were open. Whether air exits from the mouth or nose under these circumstances depends upon the relative amounts of resistance in each cavity. In normal situations, nasal airway resistance is between 1.0

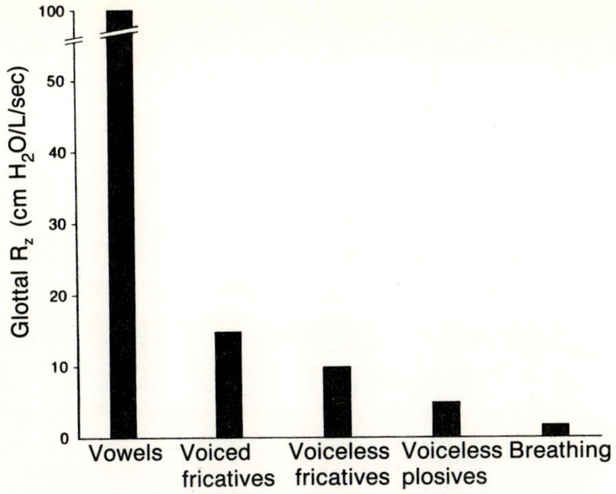

Figure 7–22 Approximate glottal resistances for vowels and consonants compared to breathing.

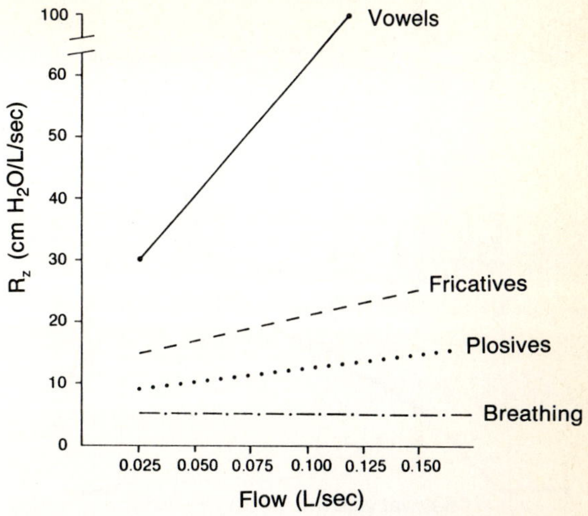

Figure 7–23 The relationship between glottal resistance and airflow rate for vowels, fricatives, plosives, and breathing. Resistance increases as effort increases. Glottal resistance is also influenced by the size of the oral airway opening.

and 3.0 cm H_2O per liter per second.[71] However, lip, tongue, and soft palate movement can modify resistance to airflow considerably and shunt airflow through the nose, as in nasal sounds.

Figure 7–28 illustrates the effect of size of the oral airway opening on velopharyngeal sphincter resistance at different degrees of velopharyngeal opening. It should be evident that in spite of an open velopharyngeal orifice, the nasal chamber, with its smaller cross-sectional area and higher resistance, receives substantial amounts of airflow only when the oral airway is constricted. This relationship between oral airway resistance and nasal airway resistance becomes very important in individuals with a cleft palate.[72]

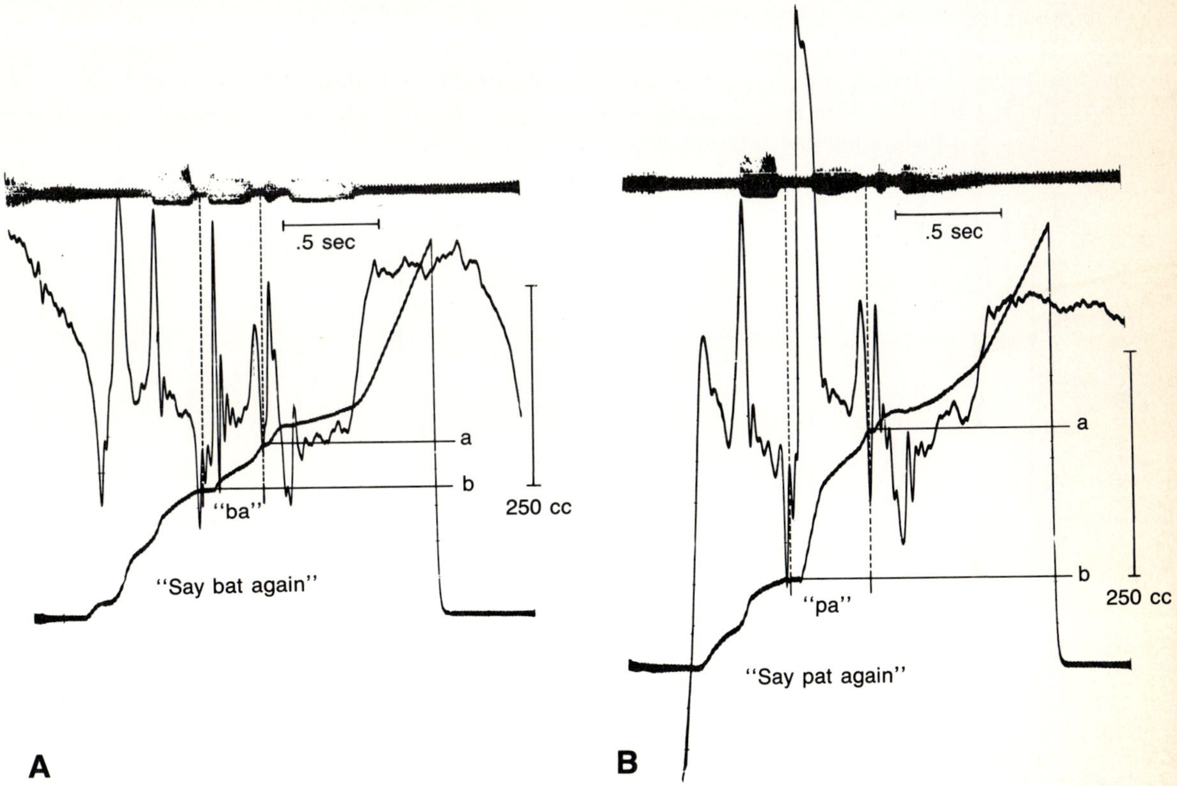

Figure 7–24 Typical sound wave, volume rate of airflow, and volume patterns for *A*, voiced and *B*, voiceless plosives. A higher rate of airflow and greater respiratory air volume for voiceless sounds are apparent. The distance between *a* and *b* represents the volume of air for the consonant-vowel.

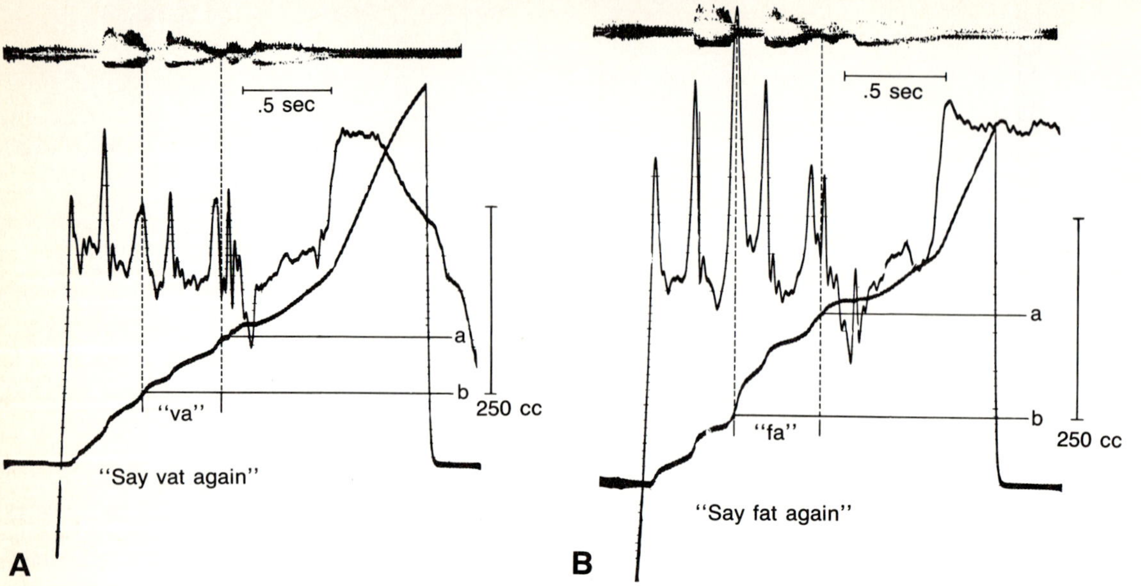

Figure 7–25 Typical sound wave volume rate of airflow, and volume patterns for *A*, voiced and *B*, voiceless fricatives. Voiceless fricatives exhibit higher rates of airflow and greater respiratory air volumes than their voiced counterparts.

Aerodynamics of Voiceless Plosives

Figure 7–29 illustrates the aerodynamic patterns of voiceless plosive production. The lips close the oral port and the soft palate seals the nasal port, while the glottis remains open (a). Intraoral pressure rises and the magnitude is determined by speech effort. This is usually 3 to 7 cm H_2O.[73] Supraglottal pressure usually equals subglottal pressure, but it can be slightly less. If, after initial release of air into the oral cavity, the vocal folds close until release of oral air pressure, a small pressure difference between the supraglottal and subglottal cavities can occur, especially if the oral cavity enlarges slightly. The approximate volume of air utilized for voiceless plosives is 80 ml, and pressure is impounded for approximately 125 msec. When the oral port opens (b), pressure falls rapidly. Voicing for the vowel begins at c.

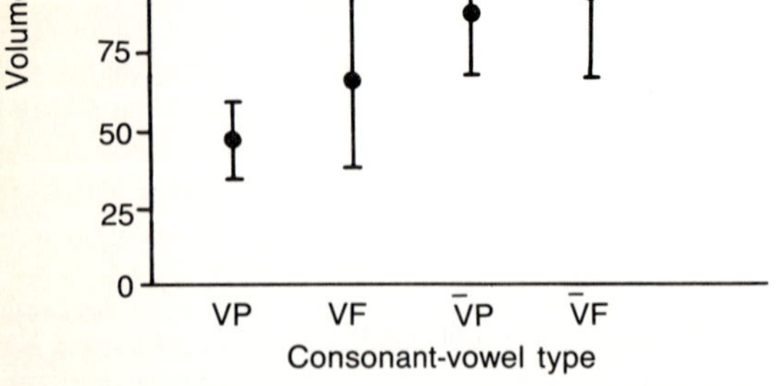

Figure 7–26 Respiratory air volume means and standard deviations for VP (voiced plosives), $\overline{VP}$ (voiceless plosives), VF (voiced fricatives), and $\overline{VF}$ (voiceless fricatives). (From Waren DW. Aerodynamics of speech production. In: Lass NJ, ed. Contemporary issues in experimental phonetics. New York: Academic Press, 1976:126.)

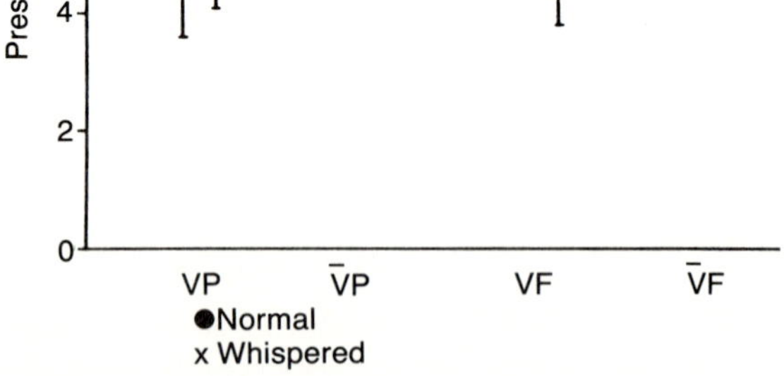

Figure 7–27 Comparison of mean intraoral pressures and standard deviations for conversational speech and whisper. VP = voiced plosives; $\overline{VP}$ = voiceless plosives; VF = voiced fricatives; and $\overline{VF}$ = voiceless fricatives. (From Warren DW Aerodynamics of speech production. In: Lass NJ, ed. Contemporary issues in experimental phonetics. New York: Academic Press, 1976:126.)

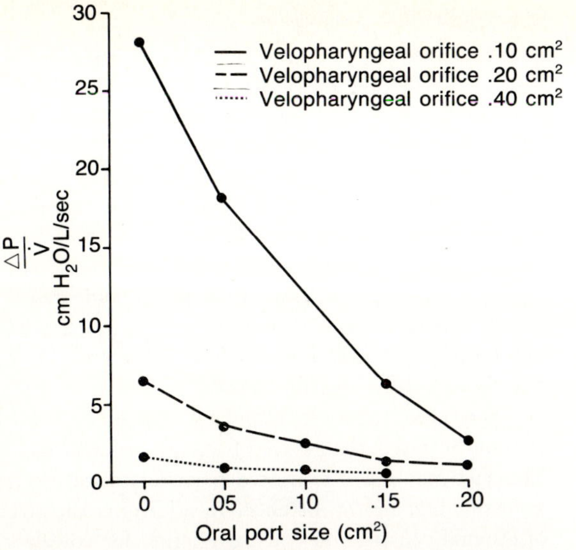

Figure 7–28 The relationship between velopharyngeal orifice resistance and oral port size at varying degrees of velopharyngeal closure. (From Warren DW. Aerodynamics of speech production. In: Lass NJ, ed. Contemporary issues in experimental phonetics. New York: Academic Press, 1976:132.)

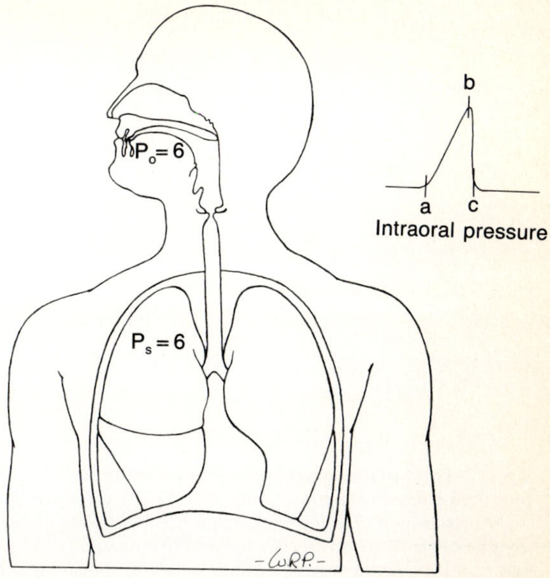

Figure 7–29 Aerodynamics of the voiceless plosive /p/. The lips close at *a* and pressure rises until *b* when the lips part. Voicing of the vowel begins at *c*. There is no airflow until the lips part. Subglottal pressure (P_s) is usually equal to intraoral pressure (P_o) during the impounding phase (*a* to *b*).

Aerodynamics of Voiced Plosives

The pressure profile of a voiced plosive depends to a great extent on when voicing begins. As noted earlier, voicing can occur only if a transglottal pressure drop is created. This is presumed to result from active enlargement of the supraglottal cavity during the stop phase. This increase in size causes supraglottal pressure to drop slightly below subglottal pressure, and the resulting airflow through the vocal folds initiates voicing. As shown in Figure 7–30, when voicing begins at the onset of the pressure rise, the shape and magnitude of the pressure pulse are altered. The pressure magnitude of voiceless sounds is between 3 and 5 cm H_2O, which is slightly lower than its voiceless counterpart.[74] Similarly, the airflow rate is lower for voiced plosives.[75] Usually about 50 ml of air is used, and air is impounded for approximately 125 msec. If voicing begins after pressure release, the peak pressure of voiced plosives may equal the peak pressure of voiceless plosives.

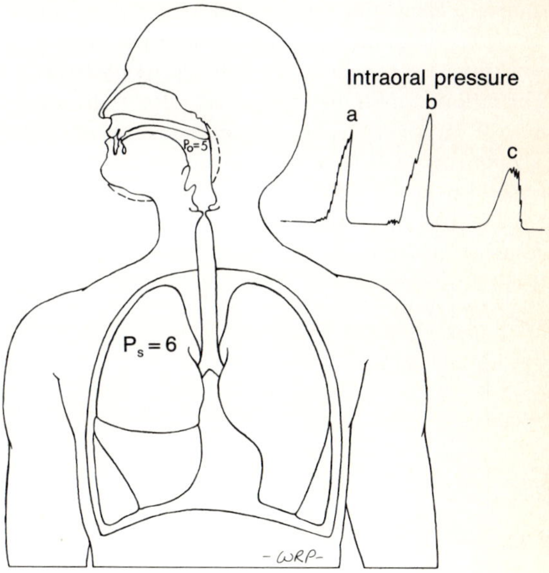

Figure 7–30 Aerodynamics of the voiced plosive /b/. The shape of the pressure pulse is determined by when voicing begins. In *a* voicing occurs throughout the pressure-rise phase. This usually lowers pressures to some degree. In *b* voicing occurs only during a portion of the pressure-rise interval, and usually pressure is higher. In *c* voicing occurs at pressure release. Whenever voicing occurs, a slight pressure difference between the supraglottal and subglottal cavities is present. For voicing to occur during the stop phase, intraoral volume must increase to create this pressure difference (broken lines). P_s = subglottal pressure; P_o = intraoral pressure.

Aerodynamics of Voiceless Fricatives

Figure 7–31 illustrates the pressure and airflow profiles of voiceless fricatives. Respiratory effort is greater for voiceless fricatives than for other consonants because of the need to maintain a pressure head behind an air leak.[76] The oral port opens slightly

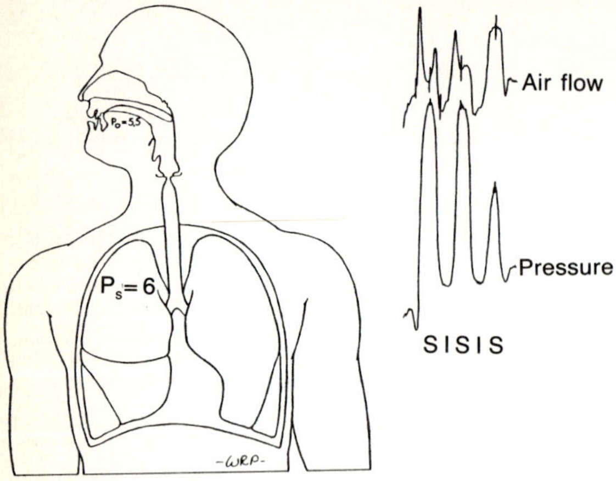

Figure 7–31 Aerodynamics of the voiceless fricative /s/. The airflow profile demonstrates two peaks with the dip corresponding to the pressure peak. The increased airflow rate during the pressure-rise phase and the increased airflow rate at the pressure-fall phase may maintain pressure magnitude duration during the closing and opening of the oral constriction. The pressure difference between the supraglottal and subglottal cavities is small. P_s = subglottal pressure; P_o = intraoral pressure.

(about 0.05 cm^2), and a pressure head of approximately 3 to 8 cm H_2O forces airflow through this constriction at a high velocity.[77] The turbulence created by this high-velocity airflow is the fricative sound source.[78] The volume of air used for a typical voiceless fricative production is approximately 100 ml, which is a larger volume than other consonants use.[76] The airflow profile has two peaks, also a characteristic of fricatives.[67] This phenomenon may relate to adjustments in airflow rate in order to maintain intraoral pressure over an adequate period of time.

Warren and Davis believe that airflow rate is adjusted to the size of the oral opening.[79] As Figure 7–32 illustrates, oral port opening may vary slightly as an individual produces a series of fricatives. The larger the opening, the greater the rate of the airflow used. This maintains intraoral pressure at a fairly consistent magnitude, as shown in Figure 7–33. Brown and McGlone reported such a consistency in intraoral pressures on consonant repetitions.[20] Thus, the dip in the airflow record may relate to reaching the maximum constriction of the oral port. However, pressure magnitude is reached prior to that point through increased airflow (first peak) and maintained during the initial reopening of the oral port (second peak) by increasing the rate of airflow. Flow rate then declines for the vowel.

Voiceless fricatives also have longer duration times (150 msec) than voiced fricatives or plosives.[80] This fact may relate to a need to generate sufficient acoustic cues for the listener. In addition, the size of the oral constriction is usually larger for voiceless fricatives than for their voiced counterparts.[81] Bilabial fricatives differ somewhat aerodynamically from linguoalveolar fricatives in that they often display some stop consonant characteristics, that is, almost no airflow at one point as a result of momentary but complete lip closure against the teeth.

Aerodynamics of Voiced Fricatives

Figure 7–34 illustrates the pressure and airflow profiles of voiced fricatives. Respiratory effort is less for these sounds than for their voiceless counterparts, possibly owing to less reliance on airflow turbulence for acoustic cues since sound is generated at the vocal folds. The shape and magnitude of the pressure pulse are influenced by the timing of voicing. Moreover, airflow rate is lower than for voiceless sounds, and the air volume used (about 75 ml)

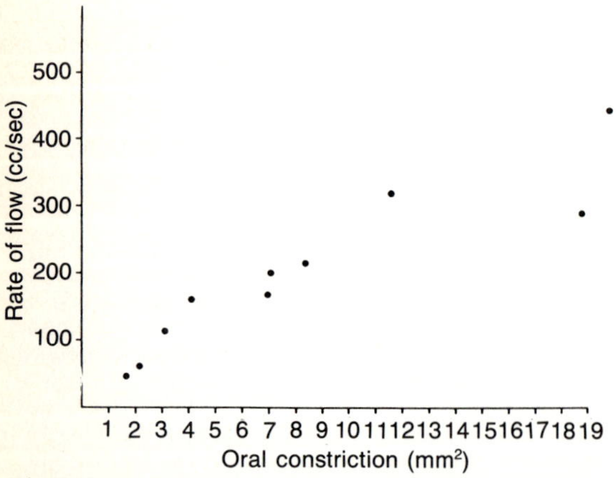

Figure 7–32 Airflow rate increases as the size of the oral opening increases for /s/. This tends to maintain intraoral pressure magnitude in spite of fluctuations in constriction size.

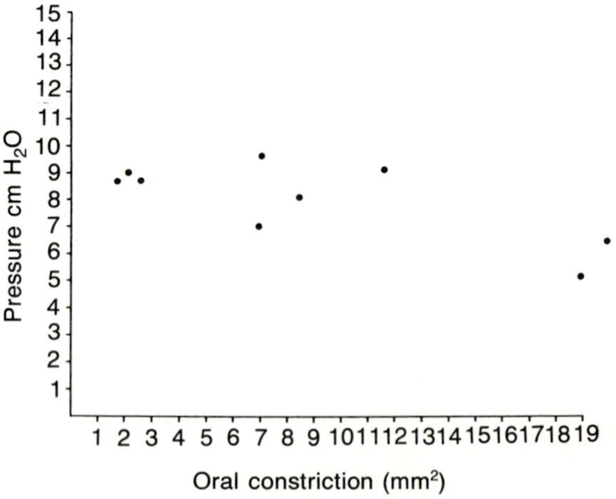

Figure 7–33 Intraoral pressure magnitude is maintained for /s/ over a range of oral port openings.

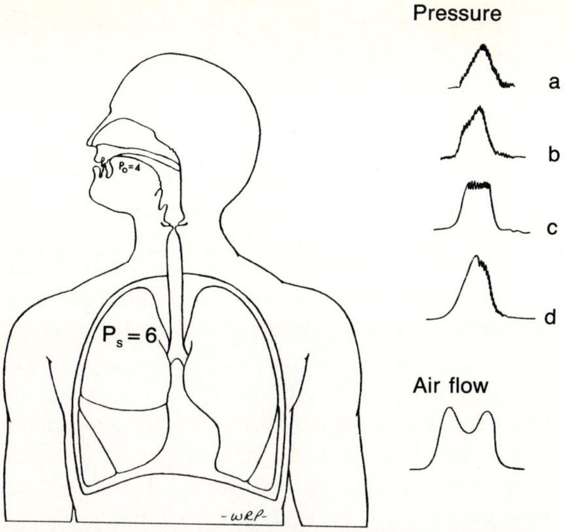

Figure 7–34 Aerodynamics of the voiced fricative /z/. The pressure gradient between subglottal (P_s) and supraglottal (P_o) pressure is larger because of vocal fold resistance. The shape and size of the pressure pulse depend upon when voicing begins. In *a* voicing occurs throughout; in *b* voicing occurs in the middle of the pressure-rise phase; in *c* voicing occurs at the peak; and in *d* voicing occurs at the release phase. Airflow demonstrates the twin peak phenomenon.

is less.[75,76] Oral port constriction is about 0.05 cm^2 but can range from 0.01 to about 0.15 cm^2. The duration of constriction for impounding air is approximately 125 msec.[80]

Aerodynamics of Vowels

Figure 7–35 illustrates the pressure and airflow profiles of vowels. Intraoral pressure is almost atmospheric for vowels since the oral airway is open. Approximately 50 to 70 ml of air are used in producing the vowel sound.[76] Airflow rate is low, as the vocal folds impede airflow to provide voicing as well as to maintain the subglottal pressure head. Glottal resistance is much greater for vowels than for voiced fricatives; this may be the result of an aerodynamic need rather than an acoustic one. That is, the glottis is the only valve protecting the subglottal pressure head during vowel productions; whereas for voiced fricatives, the oral port is constricted to about 0.05 cm^2. Thus, aerodynamically, the glottis does not need to close as much to maintain subglottal pressure.

The Effects of the Velopharyngeal Orifice

During the production of nonnasal sounds, the soft palate and pharyngeal walls form a valve that prevents airflow from entering the nasal cavity. Ordinarily in most individuals, closure is tight and complete. However, some normal speakers demonstrate very small openings at times: 0.02 to 0.03 cm^2.[70] In addition, the period of time that the orifice is open for nasal sounds varies among speakers. Figure 7–36 illustrates an opening sequence, and demonstrates that nasalization may occur two phonetic segments ahead of the nasal consonant. Similarly, the closing phase causes a portion of the plosive consonant to be nasalized. Nasal emission of air occurs during this entire interval. In the specific example shown, the velopharyngeal orifice opened well in advance and, in this instance, began as far back as at the voiceless /h/ in preparation for the nasal /m/. For example, the duration of the /m/ segment is 120 msec (compared to an opening interval of 284 msec) prior to the initiation of the sound. The orifice, therefore, was open 404 msec or nearly 3.5 times longer than the actual /m/ segment. When the velopharyngeal orifice is closed, pressure in the nasal cavity is at the atmospheric level during speech because of open communication with the outside. When it is open, as in the speech sample just cited, or in the case of a cleft palate, its effect on speech aerodynamics can be substantial.[70]

As indicated earlier, an intraoral pressure of 3 to 8 cm H_2O is normal for pressure consonants. If the velopharyngeal mechanism is open more than 0.2 cm^2 for nonnasal sounds, intraoral pressure cannot be maintained at this level unless the nasal cavity is obstructed[3] or respiratory effort is increased.[11] Actually, most speakers would demonstrate audible nasal emission and some hypernasality with openings

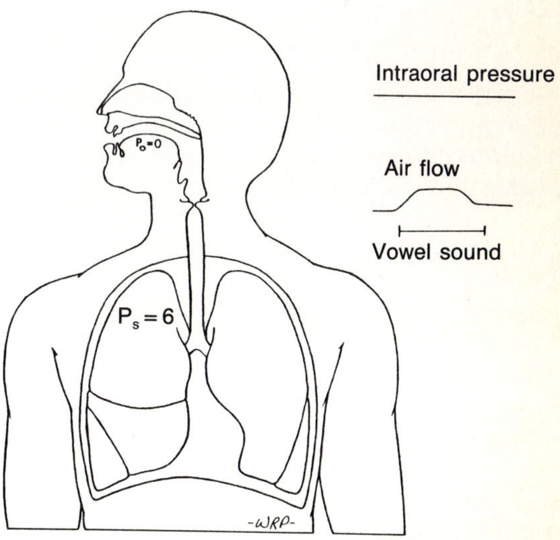

Figure 7–35 Aerodynamics of vowel production. Intraoral pressure (P_o) is atmospheric because the mouth is open. Airflow is fairly constant and, unlike fricatives and plosives, does not peak at release of the sound. P_s = subglottal pressure.

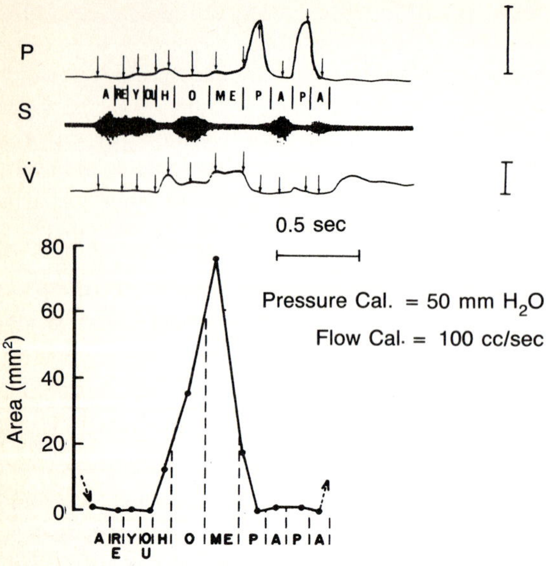

Figure 7-36 A typical intraoral pressure (P), sound (S), nasal airflow ($\dot{V}$), and velopharyngeal orifice area record of the sentence, "Are you home, papa?" Opening of the orifice occurs well in advance of the nasal consontant. This nasalizes the vowel and results in nasal emission of air prior to the nasal sound. (From Warren DW. Velopharyngeal orifice size and upper pharyngeal pressure-flow patterns in normal speech. Plast Reconstr Surg 1964; 33:148.)

between 0.1 and 0.2 cm^2. However, other structures in addition to the velum influence nasal airflow. The amount of oral airway opening, airway resistance of the nasal cavity, and oral cavity volume all influence pressure and airflow in an interactive way.[72,82] If the velopharyngeal mechanism is open during a pressure-consonant sound, the relationship between intraoral pressure and size of the opening can be described by the equation

$$P = k_3\left[\frac{\dot{V}}{A}\right]^2 + {}^1/_2(k_2\dot{V}_2 + k_1\dot{V})$$

For plosive sounds, A relates to the size of the velopharyngeal orifice; whereas for fricative sounds, A relates to the opening at the oral port as well. The portion of the equation

$$k_3\left[\frac{\dot{V}}{A}\right]^2$$

indicates an orifice type of airflow through the oral or nasal ports, and

$${}^1/_2(k_2\dot{V}^2 + k_1\dot{V})$$

indicates that flow through both chambers has laminar and turbulent components. If respiratory effort is increased, the laminar components are diminished and the equation changes to

$$P = k_3\left[\frac{\dot{V}}{A}\right]^2 + k_2\dot{V}^2$$

Nasal resonance is also modified if the palatal orifice is not open enough for nasal sounds.[83] Denasal voice quality results when the opening is small (possibly smaller than 0.20 cm^2) or the nasal airway infections, enlarged adenoids, or after treatment for is blocked. This may occur with upper respiratory cleft palate. Figure 7–37 indicates that the velopharyngeal sphincter not only must be opened an adequate amount for nasalization, but should begin to open at least with the vowel preceding the nasal consonant; otherwise, denasal voice quality results.

Warren proposed recently that compensatory speech behaviors associated with cleft palate may be manifestations of regulation and control strategies.[11] That is, in the presence of a velar deficit, aerodynamic performance rather than acoustic accuracy would receive priority in the speech-motor control program.

Figure 7–38 suggests possible control responses to velopharyngeal inadequacy. Greater respiratory muscle activity results in an increased airflow rate. Since resistance is dependent on flow, velar resistance would increase and, as a consequence, greater intraoral pressure would be achieved. Individuals with high nasal resistance would require less airflow to maintain intraoral pressure. Additionally, nasal resistance can be increased by the constriction of the nasal valve. This is the physiologic manifestation of the nasal grimace and could increase nasal resistance by 10 to 30 percent. As discussed before, the nasal valve normally constricts more during expiration than during inspiration, and this reflex associated with breathing is also available for speech function.[11]

High tongue carriage and the pharyngeal fricatives would also increase vocal tract resistance in

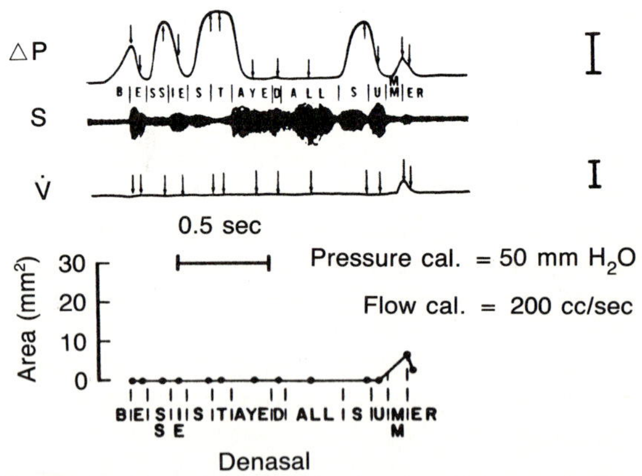

Figure 7-37 Denasal speech results when the velopharyngeal orifice does not open sufficiently and in advance of the nasal consonant. Nasal emission of air is diminished and the preceding vowel is not nasalized. ΔP = pressure difference between the nose and mouth; S = sound record; and $\dot{V}$ = airflow through the velopharyngeal orifice. (From Warren DW. Velopharyngeal orifice size and upper pharyngeal pressure-flow patterns in cleft palate speech: a preliminary study. Plast Reconstr Surg 1964; 34:15.)

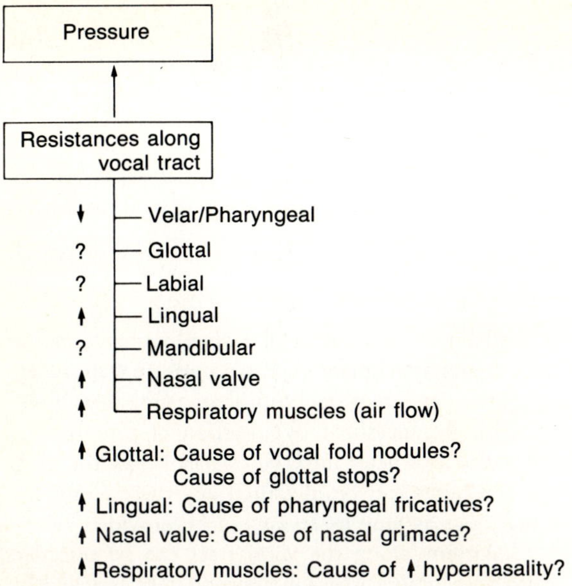

Figure 7–38 Proposed possible effects of velar resistance deficit resulting from velopharyngeal incompetence.

the presence of a velar deficit. Similarly, the glottis normally serves as an expiratory brake during breathing and adducts more during expiration than during inspiration. The glottal stop could be a more forceful manifestation of this reflex. The well-known Passavant's bar activity of the posterior pharyngeal wall may also be an airway response to a loss of resistance. The anterior movement of the muscle decreases cross-sectional size of the airway and so increases airway resistance. The point to be emphasized is that a speech regulating system would be dedicated to maintaining speech pressures, and many of the compensatory behaviors in cleft palate appear to fit the description of control responses.[11]

INSTRUMENTATION FOR AERODYNAMIC STUDIES

Manometry

Various manometric devices have been used to measure intraoral pressures during breathing and maximum expiratory efforts.[84] Most of these instruments are modifications of the U-tube manometer (Fig. 7-39). Their use has been limited because nonspeech tasks, such as maximum expiratory effort, may not reflect the capability of the speech mechanism. However, in some instances oral manometers are useful in providing a gross measure of the efficiency of the palatopharyngeal mechanism during blowing.

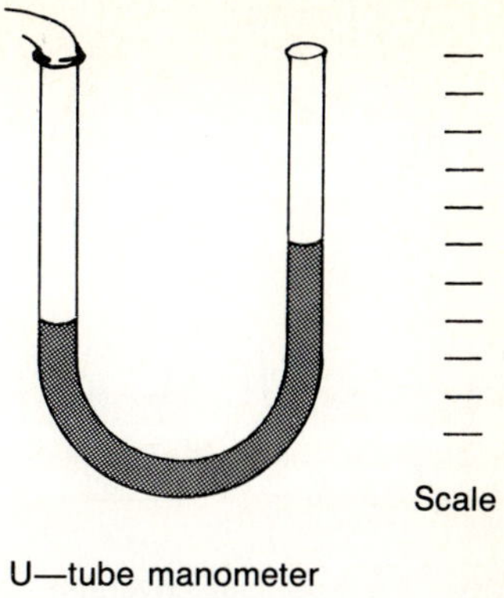

Figure 7–39 Manometry involves the displacement of a fluid by blowing or sucking. Measurement is made by reading the displacement scale.

Aerodynamic Devices

Instruments providing precise measurements of respiratory parameters associated with speech are currently available. These include flowmeters, which record volume rates of airflow, and pressure transducers, which record airway pressures within the vocal tract.[85]

Air Pressure Devices

Strain gauge transducers are the most commonly used devices for measuring pressure. Based on unbonded resistance strain gauge principles, the pressure-transducing element activates whenever pressure is applied to a diaphragm in the unit. Displacement of the diaphragm is transmitted to a Wheatstone bridge, and these changes in resistance unbalance the bridge in proportion to the applied pressure.

It is common practice to amplify the signal from transducers to provide power to drive galvanometers. However, the mechanical inertia of some direct writing galvanometers is so great that the frequency response is limited and amplification is required to provide any measurable response. Usually a carrier amplifier is used in combination with a strain gauge transducer. An oscillator supplies an alternating current, and the amplitude is continuously affected by the varying resistance of the Wheatstone bridge. The output of the transducer enters a capacitance-coupled amplifier, which amplifies the modulated carrier wave. Then the signals are rectified and the carrier wave is filtered out, leaving a direct current (DC) voltage that powers the recording instrument. Usually a small catheter is used to transmit the pressure to the transducer.[21]

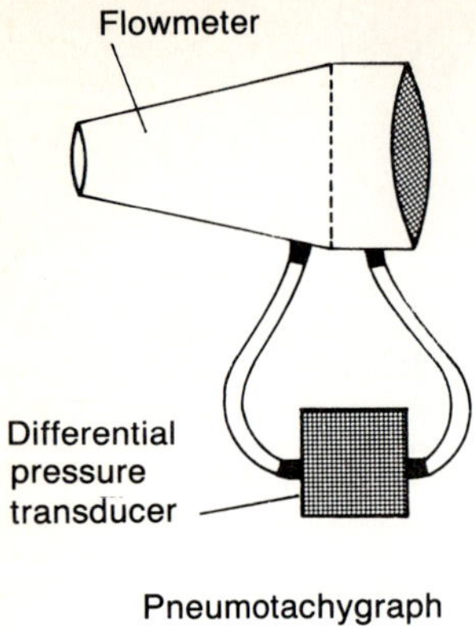

Figure 7–40 The pneumotachygraph consists of a flowmeter and a differential pressure transducer. As air flows across the mesh screen in the flowmeter, a pressure drop results and is recorded by the transducer. The pressure drop is proportional to the rate of airflow.

Airflow Devices

The most accepted instrument for measuring the volume rate of airflow is the heated pneumotachygraph, which consists of a flowmeter and a differential pressure transducer (Fig. 7–40). The device utilizes the principle that as air flows across a resistance, the resulting pressure drop is linearly related to the volume rate of airflow. In most cases, the resistance is a wire mesh screen that is heated to prevent condensation. A pressure tap is situated on each side of the screen, and both are connected to a sensitive differential pressure transducer. The pressure drop is converted to a voltage that is amplified and recorded either on tape or on a direct writing instrument. Both ingressive and egressive airflow can be measured.[21]

APPLICATION OF AERODYNAMIC TECHNIQUES

Pressure and airflow devices have been used in a variety of ways to measure the aerodynamics of speech production.[84] Intraoral pressure can be recorded by the placement of a small catheter in the mouth and attachment of it to a pressure transducer, amplifier, and recorder. Similarly, subglottal pressure can be measured by insertion of a needle attached to a catheter into the trachea below the glottis. Pressures can be measured anywhere along the vocal tract as long as access can be provided.

Airflow along the vocal tract can be recorded with a pneumotachygraph appropriately attached by tubing or a mask to the mouth, nose, or both (Fig. 7–41). Integration of airflow values over time provides a measure of air volumes used in speech.

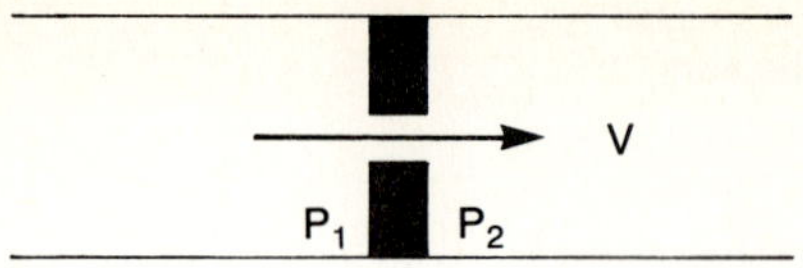

Figure 7–42 The area of a constriction of pipes can be calculated from measurements of airflow through the constriction ($\dot{V}$) and the pressure drop (from P_1 to P_2) across the constriction.

Aerodynamic techniques have been used to obtain important information about normal and abnormal speech production. The techniques usually involve the application of hydraulic principles.[34] Upper airway structures such as the tongue, teeth, lips, and palate form numerous constrictions that affect airflow and pressure. Hydraulic equations are used to estimate the size of these constrictions. The basis for such measurements can be explained by the analogy of air flowing through simple pipes (Fig. 7–42). The size of a constriction in a pipe can be calculated by the measurement of the airflow through the pipe ($\dot{V}$) and the pressure drop across the pipe (P_1 to P_2). The area of the constriction is then calculated from the equation

$$A = \frac{\dot{V}}{k\sqrt{\frac{2\Delta P}{d}}}$$

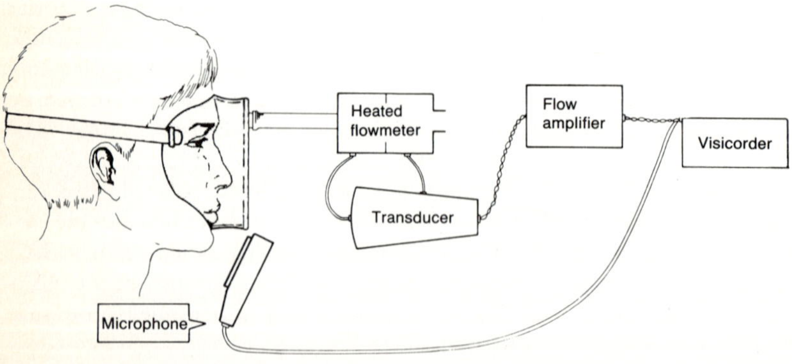

Figure 7–41 Airflow is measured by means of a face mask, pneumotachygraph, and recorder.

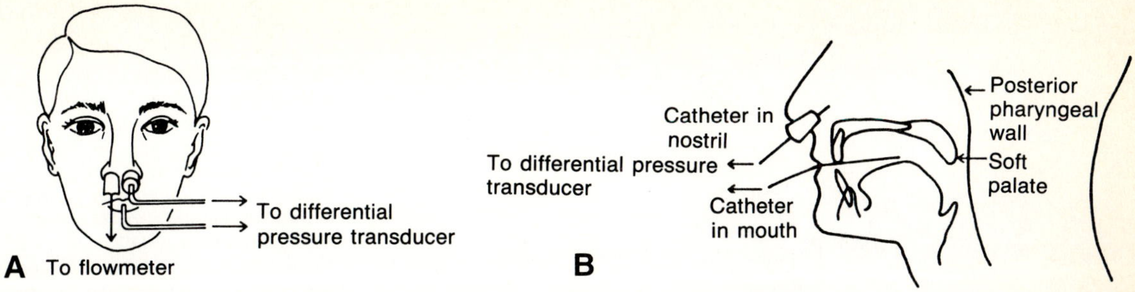

Figure 7–43 Catheters are placed above and below the orifice to measure the differential pressure. *A*, The catheter placed in the left nostril is secured by a cork, which plugs the nostril and creates a stagnant air column above the orifice. *B*, The second catheter is placed in the mouth. Both catheters are connected to a differential pressure transducer. The pneumotachygraph is connected to the right nostril and collects orifice airflow through the nose. (From Warren DW. Aerodynamics of speech production. In: Lass NJ, ed. Contemporary issues in experimental phonetics. New York: Academic Press, 1976:113.)

As Figure 7–43 illustrates, the size of articulatory constrictions can also be estimated in this manner.[34] Thus, if one wanted to measure the size of the velopharyngeal orifice, it would be necessary to record the pressure difference between the nose and the mouth and the volume rate of airflow through the nose during speech. This measurement is especially important in people with cleft palates. Similarly, the size of the oral opening during fricative productions can be estimated by the placement of catheters and a face mask in the positions illustrated in Figure 7–44.[81,86]

Upper airway structures also act as resistors to airflow. The equation

$$R = \frac{\Delta P}{\dot{V}}$$

(where R = resistance) can be used to estimate these resistances during speech.[71] For example, to calculate the magnitude of nasal resistance, the pressure drop across the nose and airflow through the nose would be measured as in Figure 7–45. Moreover, the same technique can be used to measure lingual, palatal, or oral port resistance during speech.

Resistance measurements can also be generated from area measurements. The actual relationship between nasal airway size and nasal resistance can be described in mathematical terms by means of an empirically devised conversion equation as follows:

$$R = 1.9 + \left(\frac{0.03 + 0.0009 \times \text{flow}}{A^2}\right)$$

Figure 7–46 illustrates inspiratory and expiratory breathing data from which measurements of resistance and area are generated.

SUMMARY

The speech process involves many complex behaviors that are controlled in precise ways. Generation of the airstream and its modification by artic-

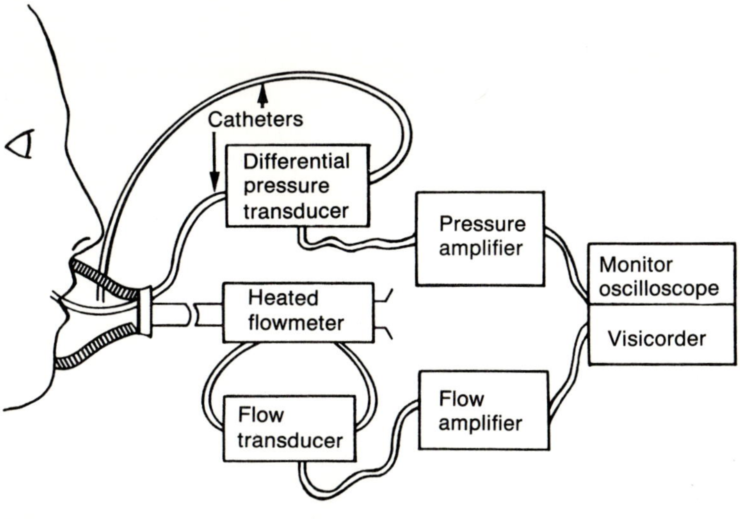

Figure 7-44 The catheters are placed on both sides of the oral constriction to measure oral port opening for fricatives. Airflow is collected in a face mask and goes to the pneumotachygraph. (From Smith HZ, Allen GD, Warren DW, Hall DJ. The consistency of the pressure-flow technique for assessing oral port size. J Acoust Soc Am 1978; 64:1203.)

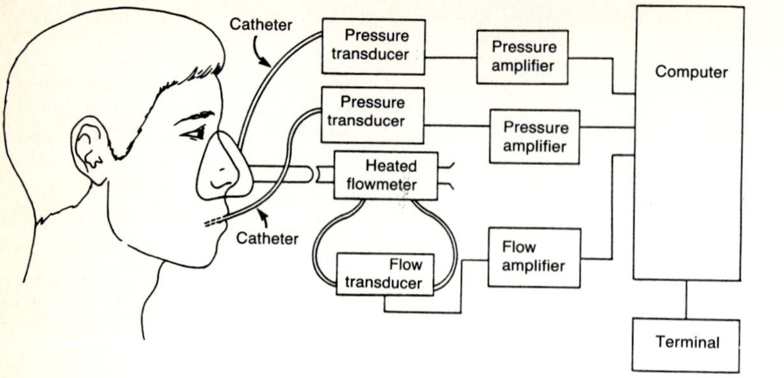

Figure 7–45 Nasal airway resistance is measured by recording the pressure drop across the structure and the airflow through it. A face mask is used to collect airflow from the nose. Closing the lips around the pressure catheter provides a measure of pressure across the nasal airway. (After Warren DW, Duany LF, Fischer ND. Nasal pathway resistance in normal and cleft lip and palate subjects. Cleft Palate J 1969; 6:134.)

ulators within the vocal tract require a high degree of integration and coordination at central and peripheral levels. Muscular and nonmuscular forces produce a fairly constant subglottal pressure head and at the same time allow changing supraglottal pressures. The resulting aerodynamic patterns generate the sounds that are perceived by the listener as speech.

REFERENCES

1. Mead J, Agostoni E. Dynamics of breathing. In: Fenn W, Rahn H, eds. Handbook of physiology. Respiration I. Washington, DC: American Physiological Society, 1964: 411.
2. Comroe JH. Physiology of respiration. Chicago: Year Book Medical Publishers, 1965:115.

Mean	OP	NP	DP	NF	Area	Resist
Nasin	−3.390	−1.621	−1.769	−705.196	−.584	3.856
Nasex	2.378	1.045	1.332	541.339	.516	3.847

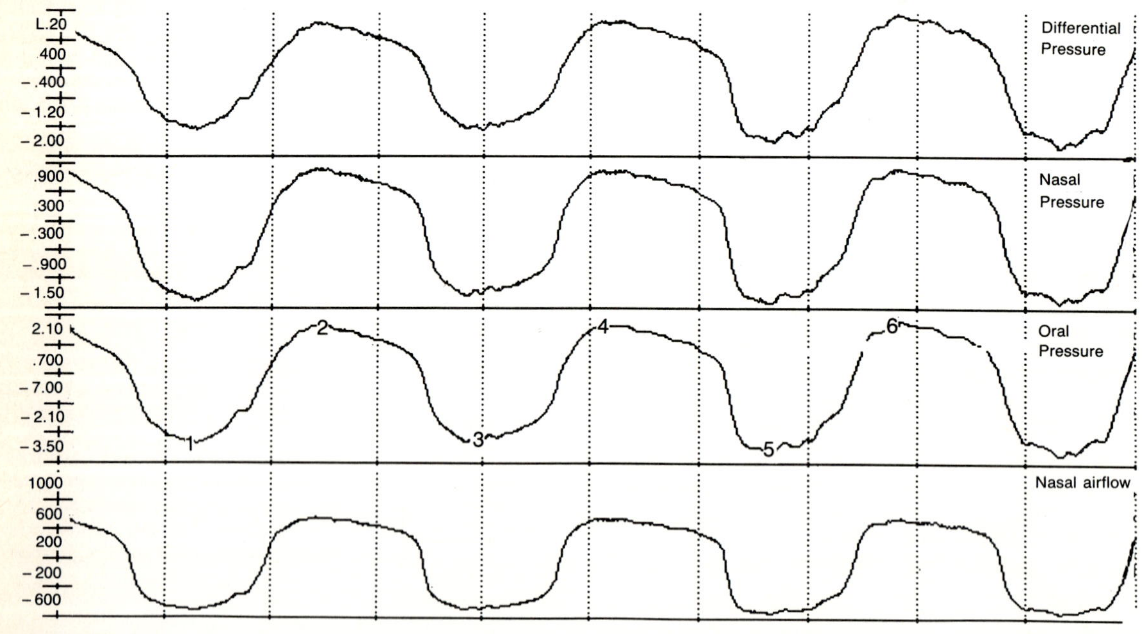

Figure 7–46 Resistance and area measurements can be generated from pressure-airflow data. The bottom record is nasal airflow; the record above the bottom one is oral pressure; the record below the top one is nasal pressure; and the top record is differential pressure. Mean data for pressures, airflow, area, and resistance are at the top. Numbers on oral pressure records, 1 to 6, denote where measurements were obtained.

3. Warren DW, DuBois AB. A pressure-flow technique for measuring velopharyngeal orifice area during continuous speech. Cleft Palate J 1964; 1:52–71.
4. Cherniack RM, Cherniack L. Respiration in health and disease. Philadelphia: WB Saunders, 1961.
5. Agostoni E, Mead J. Statics of the respiratory system. In: Fenn W, Rahn H, eds. Handbook of physiology. Respiration I. Washington, DC: American Physiological Society, 1964:387.
6. Hixon TJ. Respiratory function in speech. In: Minifie F, Hixon T, Williams F, eds. Normal aspects of speech, hearing, and language. Englewood Cliffs, NJ: Prentice-Hall, 1973:73.
7. Ladefoged P, Draper MH, Whitteridge D. Syllables and stress. Misc Phonetica 1958; 3:1–15.
8. Campbell EJM. The respiratory muscles. In: Bouhuys A, ed. Sound production in man. Ann NY Acad Sci 1968; 155:135–139.
9. Hixon TJ, Weismer G, Putnam HB. A tutorial requiem for the Edinburgh studies of speech breathing. Paper presented at the Annual Convention of the American Speech-Language-Hearing Association, 1979.
10. Weismer G. Speech breathing: contemporary views and findings. In: Daniloff RG, ed. Recent advances in speech sciences. San Diego: College-Hill Press, 1985:47.
11. Warren DW. Compensatory speech behaviors in individuals with cleft palate: a regulation/control phenomenon? Cleft Palate J 1986; 23:251–260.
12. Remmers JE, Bartlett D Jr. Reflex control of expiratory airflow and duration. J Appl Physiol 1977; 42:80–87.
13. Hairfield WM, Warren DW, Hinton VA, Seaton DL. Inspiratory and expiratory effects of nasal breathing. Cleft Palate J 1987; 24:183–189.
14. England SJ, Bartlett D Jr. Changes in respiratory movements of human vocal cords during hyperpnea. J Appl Physiol 1982; 52:780–785.
15. Gautier H, Remmers JE, Bartlett D Jr. Control duration of expiration. Respir Physiol 1973; 18:205–221.
16. Ladefoged P. Subglottal activity during speech. Proc Fourth Intl Congr Phonetic Sci, The Hague 1962;73–91.
17. Ladefoged P. Linguistic aspects of respiratory phenomena. In: Bouhuys A, ed. Sound production in man. Ann NY Acad Sci 1968; 155:141–151.
18. Mead J, Bouhuys A, Procter DF. Mechanisms generating subglottic pressure. In: Bouhuys A, ed. Sound production in man. Ann NY Acad Sci 1968; 155:177–181.
19. Netsell R. Subglottal and intraoral air pressures during the intervocalic /t/ and /d/. Phonetica 1969; 20:68–73.
20. Brown WS, McGlone RE. Constancy of intraoral air pressure. Folia Phoniatr 1969; 21:332–339.
21. Warren DW. Aerodynamics of speech. In: Lass NJ, McReynolds LV, Northern JL, Yoder DE, eds. Speech, language, and hearing. Vol. 1. Philadelphia: WB Saunders, 1982:219.
22. Smitheran R, Hixon TJ. A clinical method for estimating laryngeal airway resistance during vowel production. J Speech Hear Disord 1981; 46:138–147.
23. Warren DW, Hairfield WM, Hinton VA. The respiratory significance of the nasal grimace (abstr). Asha 1985; 27:82.
24. Brobeck JR. Exchange, control, and regulation. In: Brobeck JR, Yamamoto WS, eds. Physiological control and regulations. Philadelphia: WB Saunders, 1965:1.
25. Sant'Ambrogio G. Information arising from the tracheobronchial tree in mammals. Physiol Rev 1982; 62:531–569.
26. Sant'Ambrogio G, Matthew OP, Fisher JT, Sant'Ambrogio FB. Laryngeal receptors responding to transmural pressure, airflow and local muscle activity. Respir Physiol 1983; 54:317–330.
27. McBride B, Whitelaw WA. A physiological stimulus to upper airway receptors in humans. J Appl Physiol 1981; 51:1179–1189.
28. Cohen MI. Phrenic and recurrent laryngeal discharge patterns and the Hering-Breuer reflex. Am J Physiol 1975; 228:1489–1496.
29. Brouillette RT, Thach BT. Control of genioglossus muscle inspiratory activity. J Appl Physiol 1980; 49:801–808.
30. Warren DW, Nelson GR, Allen G. Effects of increased vertical dimension on size of constriction port and fricative sound intelligibility. J Acoust Soc Am 1980; 67:1828–1831.
31. Warren DW, Hall DJ, Davis J. Oral port constriction and pressure-flow relationships during sibilant productions. Folia Phoniatr 1981; 33:380–389.
32. Warren DW, Allen G, King HA. Physiologic and perceptual effects of induced anterior open bite. Folia Phoniatr 1984; 36:164–173.
33. Putnam AHB, Shelton RL, Kastner CV. Intraoral air pressure and oral air flow under different bleed and bite-block conditions. J Speech Hear Res 1986; 29:37–49.
34. Warren DW. Aerodynamics of speech production. In: Lass NJ, ed. Contemporary issues in experimental phonetics. New York: Academic Press, 1976:105.
35. Kozhevnikov VA, Chistovich LA. Speech: articulation and perception. Washington, DC: United States Department of Commerce, Joint Publications Research Service, 1965.
36. Ohman SEG. Coarticulation in VCV utterances: spectrographic measurements. J Acoust Soc Am 1966; 39:151–168.
37. Ohman SEG. Numerical model of coarticulation. J Acoust Soc Am 1967; 41:310–320.
38. Daniloff RG, Moll KL. Coarticulation of lip rounding. J Speech Hear Res 1968; 11:707–721.
39. Moll KL, Daniloff RG. Investigation of the timing of velar movements during speech. J Acoust Soc Am 1971; 50:678–684.
40. Daniloff RG, Hammerberg RE. On defining coarticulation. J Phonetics 1973; 1:239–248.
41. Kent RD, Minifie FD. Coarticulation in recent speech production models. J Phonetics 1977; 5:115–133.
42. Kelso JAS, Tuller B, Harris KS. A "dynamic pattern" perspective on the control and coordination of movement. In: MacNeilage P, ed. The production of speech. New York: Springer-Verlag, 1983:137.
43. Kelso JAS, Tuller B. Converging evidence in support of common dynamic principles for speech and movement. Am J Physiol (Regulatory, Integrative, and Comparative Physiology) 1984; 246:928–935.
44. Jaeger M, Matthys H. The pressure flow characteristics of the human airways. In: Bouhuys A, ed. Airway dynamics. Springfield, IL: CC Thomas, 1970:21.
45. Hixon TJ, Goldman MD, Mead J. Kinematics of chest wall during speech production: volume displacements of the rib cage, abdomen, and lung. J Speech Hear Res 1973; 16:78–115.
46. Ladefoged P, McKinney NP. Loudness, sound pressure and subglottal pressure in speech. J Acoust Soc Am 1963; 35:454–460.
47. Lieberman P. Intonation, perception, and language. Cambridge: MIT Press, 1967:230.
48. Hixon TJ. Speech breathing kinematics and mechanism inferences therefrom. In: Grillner S, Lindblom B, Lubker J, Persson A, eds. Speech motor control. New York: Pergamon Press, 1982:75.
49. Russell NK. Respiration during speech production in normal speaking adults and children. J Speech Hear Res 1987.
50. van den Berg JW. Direct and indirect determination of mean subglottic pressure. Folia Phoniatr 1956; 8:1–24.
51. Isshiki N. Regulatory mechanism of voice intensity variation. J Speech Hear Res 1964; 7:17–29.
52. Cavagna GA, Margaria R. An analysis of the mechanics of phonation. J Appl Physiol 1965; 20:301–307.
53. Fry DB. Duration and intensity as physical correlates of linguistic stress. J Acoust Soc Am 1955; 27:765–768.
54. Lieberman P. Some acoustic correlates of word stress in

American English. J Acoust Soc Am 1960; 32:451–454.
55. Brown WS, McGlone RE. Aerodynamic and acoustic study of stress in sentence productions. J Acoust Soc Am 1974; 56:971–974.
56. Lieberman P. Vocal cord motion in man. In: Bouhuys A, ed. Sound production in man. Ann NY Acad Sci 1968; 155:28–38.
57. van den Berg JW, Zantema JT, Doornenbal P. On the air resistance and the Bernoulli effect of the human larynx. J Acoust Soc Am 1957; 29:626–631.
58. Ishizaka K, Matsudaira M. Fluid mechanical consideration of vocal cord vibration. SCRL Monograph No. 8. Santa Barbara: Speech Communications Research Laboratory, 1972.
59. Titze IR. Parameterization of the glottal area, glottal flow, and vocal fold contact area. J Acoust Soc Am 1984; 75:570–580.
60. Scherer RC, Curtis JF, Titze IR. Pressure-flow relationships within static models of the larynx. J Acoust Soc Am (Suppl. 1) 1980; 68:S101.
61. Klatt DH, Stevens KN, Mead J. Studies of articulatory activity and airflow during speech. In: Bouhuys A, ed. Sound production in man. Ann NY Acad Sci 1968; 155:42–55.
62. Rothenberg M. The breath-stream dynamics of simple-released-plosive production. Bibl Phonetica 1968; 6:1–117.
63. Lubker JF. A consideration of transglottal airflow during stop consonant production. J Acoust Soc Am 1973; 53:212–215.
64. Perkell JA. Physiology of speech production: results and implications of a quantitative cineradiographic study. Cambridge: MIT Press, 1969.
65. Kent RD, Moll KL. Vocal-tract characteristics of the stop cognates. J Acoust Soc Am 1969; 46:1549–1555.
66. Bell-Berti F. Control of pharyngeal cavity size for English voiced and voiceless stops. J Acoust Soc Am 1975; 57:456–461.
67. Warren DW, Hall DJ. Glottal activity and intraoral pressure during stop consonant productions. Folia Phoniatr 1973; 25:121–129.
68. Warren DW, Hall DJ. Intraoral pressures in whispered speech: differences among voiced and voiceless consonants. Paper presented at the Annual Convention of the American Speech and Hearing Association, 1969.
69. Weismer G. Segmental gestures at the laryngeal level in whispered speech: evidence from an aerodynamic study. J Speech Hear Res 1980; 23:383–392.
70. Warren DW. Velopharyngeal orifice size and upper pharyngeal pressure-flow patterns in normal speech. Plast Reconstr Surg 1964; 33:148–162.
71. Warren DW, Duany LF, Fischer ND. Nasal pathway resistance in normal and cleft lip and palate subjects. Cleft Palate J 1969; 6:134–140.
72. Warren DW, Ryon WE. Oral port constriction, nasal resistance, and respiratory aspects of cleft palate speech: an analog study. Cleft Palate J 1967; 4:38–46.
73. Malecot A. An experimental study of force of articulation. Studia Linguist 1955; 9:35–44.
74. Arkebauer HJ, Hixon TJ, Hardy JC. Peak intraoral air pressures during speech. J Speech Hear Res 1967; 10:196–208.
75. Isshiki N, Ringel R. Airflow during the production of selected consonants. J Speech Hear Res 1964; 7:233–244.
76. Warren DW, Wood MT. Respiratory volumes in normal speech: a possible reason for intraoral pressure differences among voiced and voiceless consonants. J Acoust Soc Am 1969; 45:466–469.
77. Klechak TL, Bradley DP, Warren DW. Anterior open bite and oral port constriction. Angle Orthod 1976; 46:232–242.
78. Hixon TJ. Turbulent noise sources for speech. Folia Phoniatr 1966; 18:168–182.
79. Warren DW, Davis JD. Effects of oral structures on airway conductance during normal speech (abstr). J Dent Res 1977; 56:232.
80. Warren DW, Mackler SB. Duration of oral port constriction in normal and cleft palate speech. J Speech Hear Res 1968; 11:391–401.
81. Smith HZ, Allen GD, Warren DW, Hall DJ. The consistency of the pressure-flow technique for assessing oral port size. J Acoust Soc Am 1978; 64:1203–1206.
82. Warren DW, Devereux JL. An analog study of cleft palate speech. Cleft Palate J 1966; 3:103–114.
83. Warren DW. Velopharyngeal orifice size and upper pharyngeal pressure-flow patterns in cleft palate speech: a preliminary study. Plast Reconstr Surg 1964; 34:15–26.
84. Warren DW. The determination of velopharyngeal incompetence by aerodynamic and acoustical techniques. Clin Plast Surg 1975; 2:299–304.
85. Lubker JF. Aerodynamic and ultrasonic assessment techniques in speech-dentofacial research. In: Speech and the dentofacial complex: the state of the art. Asha Reports 1970; 5:207–223.
86. Claypoole WH, Warren DW, Bradley DP. The effect of cleft palate on oral port constriction during fricative productions. Cleft Palate J 1974; 11:95–104.

8 Speech Production

Gary Weismer, Ph.D.

The purpose of this chapter is to review what is known about respiratory, laryngeal, and supraglottal function for speech production. The emphasis throughout is on the actual data and theory of speech production, rather than on the technology of speech production research. Where the technology and interpretation of data are highly interdependent, some discussion is devoted to explanation of specific techniques. For the most part, however, the reader is encouraged to consult primary sources for details of research instrumentation and measurement strategies.[1]

Within each of the three major sections of the chapter, an effort is made to show how investigators have turned their attention from isolated muscular or structural events to an understanding of the concerted performance of a system. The view of each system as a "collective" is reflective of contemporary speech production research; future work will almost certainly explore the nature of *cross-system* collectives (i.e., respiratory and laryngeal or laryngeal and supraglottal collectives), a matter left essentially unaddressed in this chapter.

SPEECH BREATHING

Most investigators would agree that the main task of the respiratory system during speech production is to maintain a roughly constant subglottal pressure (Ps) for the duration of an utterance.[2,3] This task would seem to require fairly precise, ongoing control of the respiratory musculature, because the *nonmuscular* forces exerted by respiratory structures as well as the load against which the respiratory system works change constantly throughout an utterance.

The functional effect of the nonmuscular forces exerted by the respiratory system can be summarized by plotting the relaxation pressure (Pr) as a function of lung volume. Strictly speaking, Pr is the pressure measured inside the lungs when all muscles capable of producing compressions or expansions of the lungs are known to be inactive; the lung pressure measured under these circumstances must be attributable to recoil forces generated by stretched or compressed respiratory structures, and as such are viewed as "hard-wired" force-generating characteristics of the respiratory system.* In practice, Pr is measured by having subjects inhale or exhale to known lung volumes and then relax against a closed airway that includes a pressure-sensing tube connected to an appropriate transducer. The classic study of Pr in man was performed by Rahn, Otis, Chadwick, and Fenn,[4] whose results are plotted in Figure 8–1 as a continuous function of lung volume. Rahn et al sampled Pr at discrete points throughout lung volume, but the interpolation creating the continuous function is justified by the small lung volume increments between the sampled points.† The function shows that when lung volume is above the resting expiratory level (REL), or the point in lung volume typically reached at the end of rest exhalation, Pr is positive. The magnitude of this positive Pr increases with increasing lung volume above REL. Similarly, Pr is negative below REL and becomes increasingly more negative as lung volume decreases.[1,2,5]

Figure 8–2 shows a typical lung pressure (i.e., subglottal pressure) demand for a speech utterance that begins at 60 percent VC and ends at 30 percent VC; the shaded part of this pressure demand is the

* The nature of these "hard-wired" forces changes with age, health status, and so forth, but at a given point in time can be regarded as fixed.

† Because the Pr function is almost always displayed continuously, students are often confused about how the function is generated in the laboratory. As indicated in the text, the function is generated under static conditions (i.e., maintaining a lung volume by relaxing against a closed airway), but could be recorded continuously (down to REL) by having a subject inhale to nearly 100 percent vital capacity (VC) and then exhale through a slight resistance (such as pursed lips) while relaxing the respiratory muscles. The continuous recording of the negative part of the function (below Pr) would require that a subject exhale to nearly 0.0 percent VC and then inhale through a slight resistance.

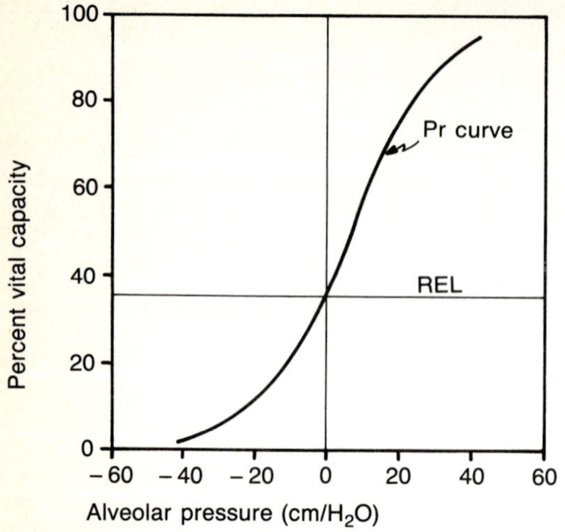

Figure 8–1 Alveolar relaxation pressure (Pr) as a function of lung volume. REL = resting expiratory level.

time history (i.e., volume history) of Pr that would be expected from the volume-pressure function displayed in Figure 8–1. Figure 8–2 shows clearly that as the utterance proceeds there is an increasing demand for a compressive effort by the respiratory musculature to maintain constant Ps. Therefore a primary issue for speech researchers has been to determine how the respiratory system accomplishes the task of balancing muscular effort against the volume-dependent (and so for speech, time-dependent changes in Pr. Many early studies of speech breathing[3,6] were focused on the particular muscles used to adjust the constantly changing Pr to the Ps demand. Figure 8–3 is a summary graphic of the findings of one of these studies, that published by Draper et al[3,6] was later reproduced in many textbooks (see Weismer's discussion[5]) as the accepted account of speech breathing physiology. This figure, which represents a schematized view of electromyographic (EMG) and aerodynamic activity associated with respiratory function for a counting task that spanned most of the VC, was used by Draper et al to make several major points. First, Draper et al argued that when Pr exceeded the Ps demand, inspiratory muscles were used to offset the excess recoil (the so-called "checking" action). Second, when Pr was less than the Ps demand, only the interni intercostales were used to augment the recoil effect. Third, when Pr equaled Ps demand, the respiratory musculature was "turned off" because the pressure requirements of the utterance could be satisfied by the recoil forces alone. Fourth, abdominal muscles were employed during speech only at very low lung volumes or for high-intensity speech.

Throughout the 1960s, a fair amount of speech breathing research[7–9] was devoted to issues similar to those studied by Draper et al.[3,6] Some of the conclusions reached by Draper et al were challenged on methodologic grounds (see Kunze[7] and Ladefoged's[10] response), but textbooks continued to describe speech breathing in the terms dictated by the schematic summary of Figure 8–3. In a series of studies performed in the late 1960s and early 1970s, Hixon and colleagues did not replicate the four features of the Draper et al view of speech breathing physiology.[11,12] Indeed, the publications based on Hixon's work demonstrated rather clearly that the view espoused by Draper et al was incorrect on all accounts. In a case such as this, one immediately looks to methodologic differences between the two sets of investigations to explain the differences in findings. When such a comparison is made of the Hixon et

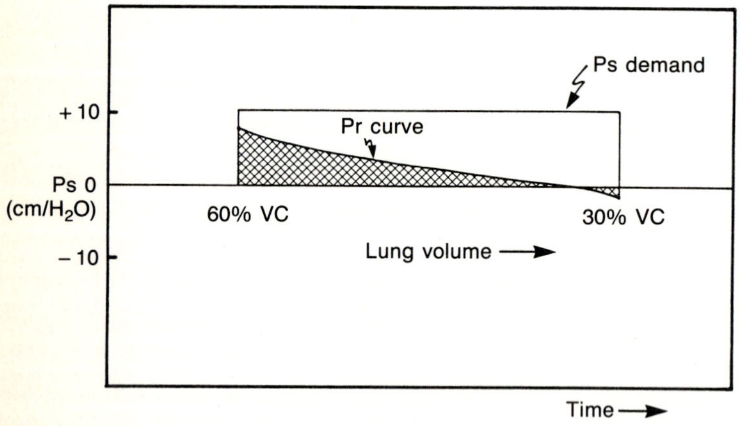

Figure 8–2 Schematic depiction of relaxation pressure available throughout a speech task initiated at 60 percent VC and ending at 30 percent VC. Ps = subglottal pressure. The *x*-axis is labeled as both *lung volume* and *time* because the decreasing lung volume associated with an utterance occurs over time.

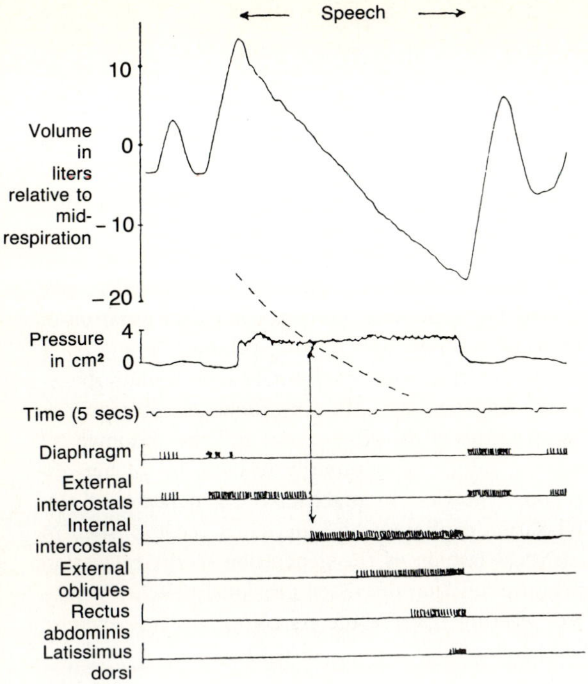

Figure 8–3 A schematic summary of the experimental results of Draper et al. The upper record shows lung volume throughout a counting task at normal loudness; the record immediately below shows the pressure measured by an esophageal balloon (solid line) and the relaxation pressure (dotted line). The bottom six lines show diagrammatic patterns of respiratory muscle activity throughout the counting task. (From Draper MH, Ladefoged P, Whitteridge D. Respiratory muscles in speech. J Speech Hear Res 1959; 2:20.)

al and Draper et al methods, the discrepancies become much less puzzling.

The Techniques and Their Implications

Draper et al, in attempting to represent the muscular activity of the respiratory system, sampled the EMG activity of only a few muscles (intercostales externi and interni, rectus abdominis, obliquus externus abdominis, latissimus dorsi, and the diaphragm) and only single locations within a muscle group.[3] From the perspective of obtaining information on selected muscle activity during speech breathing, such an approach might be reasonable. However, Draper et al used these selected muscles and sampling sites to draw global inferences concerning muscular force-generating capabilities of the respiratory system. For example, the single sampling sites in the intercostales externi and interni were taken as representative of the sheet-like intercostals as a whole, and the abdominal sites sampled were apparently regarded as adequate representations of abdominal muscular activity. However, a single sampling site within the intercostals (that is, within a given costal interspace) can provide only a poor representation of global intercostal activity because EMG activity within a given interspace is very much dependent on lung volume level.[13] The abdominal sites sampled by Draper et al are equally as problematic because the absence of an electrode pair in the musculus transversus abdominis (the deepest of the abdominal muscles and therefore the most difficult to sample electromyographically in a safe way) eliminates reasonable inferences concerning abdominal function in speech production. The potential impact of these EMG sampling problems on the Draper et al summary of speech breathing characteristics is easy to imagine: perhaps the observation that all respiratory muscles are turned off when Pr equals Ps demand reflects only the fact that lung volume thresholds for EMG activity were not exceeded for the particular spaces sampled by Draper et al, and perhaps the observed lack of abdominal activity is an artifact of not sampling from a muscle whose girdle-like structure makes it a likely candidate to produce efficient compressions of the abdominal contents.

The techniques used by Hixon et al do not provide insight into the function of particular respiratory muscles, but do provide indices of overall muscular efforts of the chest wall parts.[11,12] Following the lead of Mead and his colleagues,[14] Hixon et al defined the chest wall as consisting of two functional parts, the rib cage and the diaphragm-abdomen.

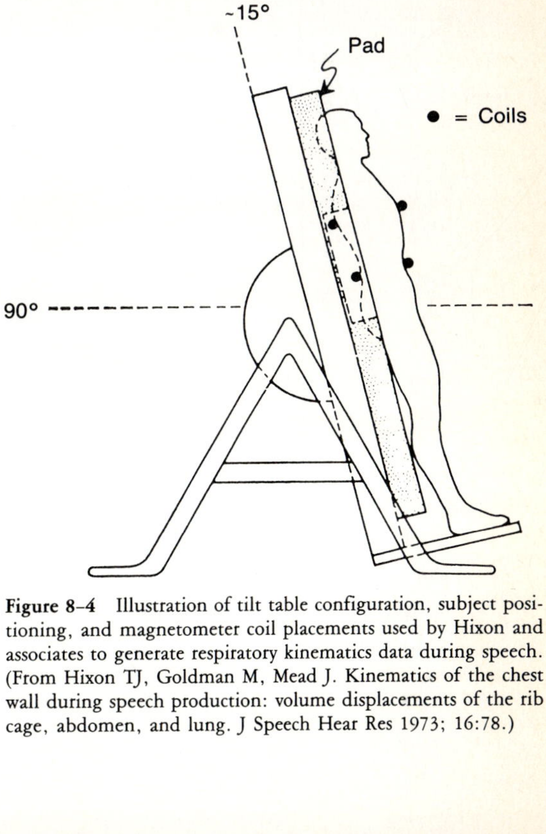

Figure 8–4 Illustration of tilt table configuration, subject positioning, and magnetometer coil placements used by Hixon and associates to generate respiratory kinematics data during speech. (From Hixon TJ, Goldman M, Mead J. Kinematics of the chest wall during speech production: volume displacements of the rib cage, abdomen, and lung. J Speech Hear Res 1973; 16:78.)

Movement of either of these parts, powered by muscular and nonmuscular (recoil) forces, can produce volume changes of the lungs. These movements can be transduced on the body surface by using magnetometers. As shown in Figure 8–4, the subject wears a magnetometer (coil) pair on the thorax and the abdomen; the distance between each pair induces a magnetic field, the strength of which is expressed as a voltage that is a linear function of the intercoil distance. It can be demonstrated that the measurement of a single anteroposterior distance on both the thoracic and abdominal surfaces is an adequate representation of the lung volume displacement outcomes of overall size changes (i.e., compression or expansion) of the rib cage and abdomen. When these distance changes are displayed in an x-y format (rib cage versus abdomen), the resulting motion-motion display provides a rich source of information on various aspects of speech breathing.

A motion-motion display that might be obtained for the utterance "Joe took father's shoe bench out and then he split it with an ax," spoken by a young adult male at a conversational level and on a single breath, is shown in Figure 8–5. Three major features of this chart must be identified before the tracings can be interpreted and reasons given for why Hixon et al's examination of such records suggested that the Draper et al view of speech breathing must be incorrect.

1. The series of open circles connected by the dotted line represent the relaxation configuration of the chest wall throughout lung volume. At any point along this relaxation configuration function, the x-y position represents the simultaneous anteroposterior distances of the rib cage (x) and the abdomen (y) when a subject is voluntarily relaxing his or her respiratory muscles. In practice, the generation of this relaxation configuration function is accomplished in identical fashion as the generation of the relaxation pressure function discussed previously. When a subject wearing magnetometers completes this exercise

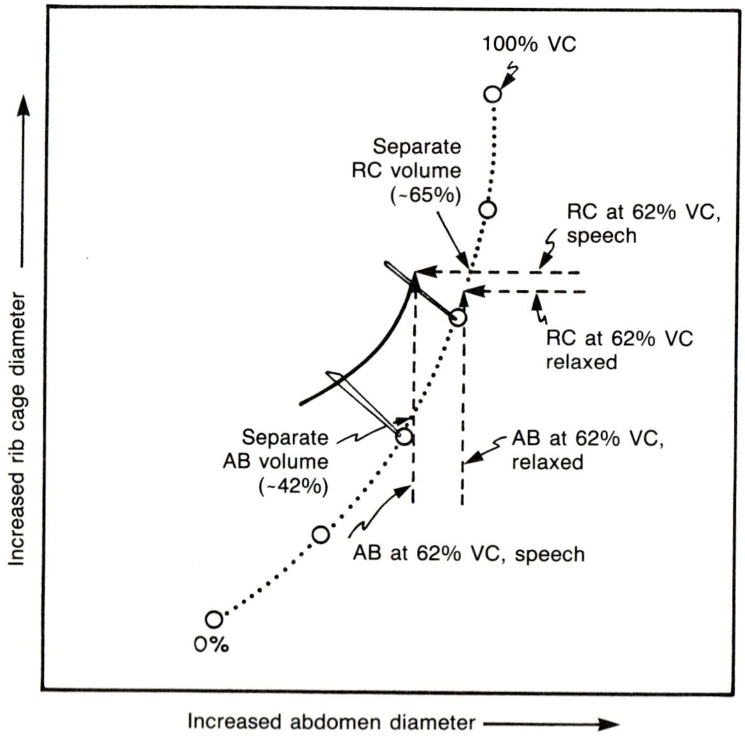

Figure 8–5 Hypothetical expiratory limb for speech utterance (heavy line) plotted with chest wall relaxation function (dotted line). Open circles on the relaxation function indicate consecutive 20 percent increments of lung volume; the nearly flattened loops extending from the 60 percent VC and 40 percent VC points are isovolume lines, as described in text. The horizontal dashed lines indicate the rib cage configuration at 62 percent VC (overall lung volume) for relaxation (bottom line) and speech (top line); the vertical dashed lines indicate the abdominal configuration at 62 percent for relaxation (right line) and speech (left line). The *separate* volumes of the two chest wall parts at utterance initiation can be estimated by determining where the horizontal (rib cage) and vertical (abdomen) projection lines from the beginning of the expiratory limb intersect the relaxation line. For rib cage this volume is approximately 65 percent VC, and for abdomen approximately 42 percent VC.

at successive points throughout the VC, the collection of x-y relaxation configurations provides a subject-specific calibration of chest wall shape *under the influence of recoil forces only*. Thus any deviation from this configuration during nonspeech or speech behaviors must be attributed to the addition of muscular forces to the prevailing recoil forces.

2. The nearly flattened loops extending diagonally (leftward and upward) from the 60 percent VC and functional residual capacity (FRC) (approximately 40 percent VC) markers on the relaxation configuration function are isovolume lines. The isovolume lines trace the range of chest wall shapes (rib cage versus abdomen diameters) that can be produced at a given lung volume. In practice, an isovolume line is generated by having a subject inhale or exhale to a particular percentage of the VC, voluntarily close off the respiratory system from the atmosphere by adducting the vocal folds (as one would do for lifting or defecating), and then slowly alternate between a protruding and retracting gesture of the ventral abdominal wall. The effect of this cyclic gesture is to shift volume displacement from the rib cage to the abdomen, then from the abdomen to the rib cage, when no volume is displaced from the lungs to the atmosphere. Thus, in Figure 8–5, leftward and upward tracings from the open circles represent the volume shift from the abdomen to the rib cage; the leftward movement represents a decreasing abdominal diameter (shift of volume from the abdomen) and the upward movement an increasing rib cage diameter (shift of volume to the rib cage). The isovolume line is an important factor in the interpretation of motion-motion diagrams because when the respiratory system is open to the atmosphere, as during speech, a variety of chest wall shapes may be used at a given lung volume to produce the same effect. Because a series of isovolume lines at selected epochs throughout lung volume provide a calibration of actual volume events against chest wall shapes, the volume history of a motion-motion pattern produced during speech can be specified precisely.*

3. The solid line extending from just above the 60 percent VC isovolume line to below the 40 percent VC isovolume line traces the motion-motion pathway for the rather long utterance identified above. Such pathways are usually called "expiratory limbs,"[11] and I will follow this terminology. This particular expiratory limb appears to begin around 63 to 65 percent VC and ends around 30 to 35 percent VC.

Hixon et al observed that in the upright posture expiratory limbs for conversational speech (1) always started well to the left of the relaxation configuration; (2) always involved rib cage sizes (diameters) that were larger than those observed at corresponding lung volumes in the relaxed state; (3) typically started around 60 percent VC for conversational level speech and ended around 35 to 40 percent VC; and (4) showed a fair degree of variation (i.e., absence of stereotypy) within and across subjects.[11]

A Contemporary Account of Speech Breathing

The observation that expiratory limbs typically begin to the left of the relaxation configuration and around 60 percent VC, and that rib cage size is greater during speech than during relaxation for corresponding lung volumes, is inconsistent with three aspects of the Draper et al[3,6] summary of speech breathing. First, the leftward displacement from the relaxation configuration indicates that the abdomen is compressed by muscular forces at the outset of an utterance; this compression apparently is maintained throughout most utterances because the motion-motion diagrams showed a constant or somewhat increasing leftward tracing throughout individual utterances. According to the Draper et al view,[6] leftward displacement from the relaxation configuration should occur only during loud speech or perhaps at the end of an utterance. Second, the observation that at the outset of an utterance abdominal diameter is smaller and rib cage diameter larger than the respective diameters at corresponding lung volumes in the relaxed configuration indicates that substantial respiratory muscular activity is associated with utterance onset. Yet when the lung volume for utterance onset is approximately 60 percent VC, as it was for many of the conversational limbs in the Hixon et al study,[11] the pressure in the lungs generated by recoil forces alone is similar to typical subglottal pressure demands for conversational speech (approximately 8 to 10 cm/H_2O). Draper et al argued that when Pr equals Ps demand, all respiratory muscles were "turned off," and the pressure requirement for

* Based on an analysis of A-P and transverse diameter changes of the rib cage during various respiratory maneuvers, McCool, Loring, and Mead concluded that certain maneuvers, especially those involving substantial rib cage elevation, result in distortion of rib cage shape.[15] In such cases, estimation of volume change from a single A-P diameter change on the rib cage is inappropriate. McCool et al point out that this problem can be avoided if inductance belts, rather than magnetometers, are used. The inductance belt is sensitive to circumferential change of a chest wall part and so avoids the problem of single-point estimation of rib-cage contribution to lung volume change. When magnetometers are used and A-P measures provide the estimate of volume change due to size change of the rib cage, McCool et al caution that isovolume maneuvers should be performed with a minimum of voluntary rib cage expansion.

the utterance was satisfied by recoil forces alone;[6] as lung volume decreased with the continuing utterance, more and more muscular effort would be needed to supplement the decreasing relaxation pressure. If this view of respiratory muscular activity during speech breathing is accurate, then motion-motion diagrams for conversational utterances should start close to the relaxation configuration and progressively deviate from that configuration as the utterance proceeds.* The motion-motion diagrams presented in Hixon et al, as indicated before, are not consistent with this expectation.[11] Third, the simultaneous leftward (abdomen compressed) and upward (rib cage expanded) tracings at utterance onset may not be consistent with the Draper et al[6] position that opposed muscular efforts do not occur during speech breathing.

Whereas the kinematics technique provides information on the displacements of the two chest wall parts relative to the relaxation configuration, an additional type of data was required to understand the global muscular forcing functions underlying the observed motions. The technique of respiratory dynamics[12] partially solves this problem by the study of air pressures related to compressive and expanding efforts by the chest wall parts. In brief, the technique involves swallowing two pressure-sensitive balloons connected to catheter tubing. One balloon is positioned in the esophagus at midchest level (above the diaphragm), and the other in the stomach at the level of the umbilicus (below the diaphragm). When the proximal ends of the tubes are connected to differential pressure transducers, pressure fluctuations in the chest (pleural pressure) and the abdominal cavities (abdominal pressure) caused by muscular and recoil forces are transmitted to the balloons and converted to voltages by the transducers.

Like the kinematics technique, the dynamics technique makes use of a comparison between a relaxation characteristic and measures taken during speech production. Relaxation pressure characteristics are generated throughout lung volume for pleural and abdominal pressures, and deviations from these characteristics during speech provide an index of the sign and magnitude of muscular effort. Hixon et al provide a detailed explanation of the dynamics technique and combine the motion-motion displays with dynamics analysis to show how the kinematics technique can be used to make strong inferences concerning the underlying muscular efforts of the chest wall parts.[12]

As mentioned previously, Hixon et al noticed a marked absence of stereotypy in speech breathing patterns.[11] The variability in chest wall kinematics for various speech tasks is exemplified in Figure 8–6, which shows data from three of the subjects studied by Hixon et al. In each of these motion-motion diagrams, the multiple expiratory limbs represent multiple utterances. In conversational speech, trajectories of the expiratory limbs vary radically from individual to individual; subject MG uses a relatively great amount of abdominal motion throughout his utterances, whereas subject AG begins his utterances with a fair amount of abdominal contribution to lung volume change, but then switches to a predominant rib cage contribution (concave limbs relative to the relaxation configuration). Even within a subject, the production of multiple utterances is associated with variable chest wall behavior; subject JB begins his utterances at widely varying lung volumes, and all subjects seem to produce utterances with varying amounts of abdominal compression (i.e., variable leftward displacement from the relaxation configuration). The effect on speech breathing of different speaking tasks seems to be minimal for chest wall configuration and perhaps somewhat greater for the amount of lung volume exchanged per limb. In other words, for a given subject, the general chest wall trajectories in any task seem to predict the trajectories in other tasks.

Effect of Subject Factors on Speech Breathing

In contemporary theories of motor behavior and control, researchers often attempt to explain variability in processes, rather than regard the variability as noise that confounds the identification of some prototype process. The variability observed in chest wall behavior across individuals may be related systematically to a number of factors, including age, sex, and body type. One might assume that speech breathing characteristics would vary across individuals differing in age because nonmuscular (recoil) and muscular characteristics of the respiratory system change throughout the lifespan. For example, the overall stiffness of the chest wall increases from infancy through old age,[16,17] and muscular strength increases with age in children[18] and probably decreases from young adulthood to old age. Two studies using the kinematics technique have examined aging effects on speech breathing. Russell and Stathopoulos reported that children tend to produce utterances that encroach on the FRC to a greater ex-

* Actually, if one adopted the strict interpretation of the Draper et al summary of speech breathing,[6] the expiratory limb that would be generated (reflecting all rib cage compression and no abdomen compression) would describe a highly improbable, if not impossible, sequence of chest wall configurations for an utterance having a roughly constant Ps.

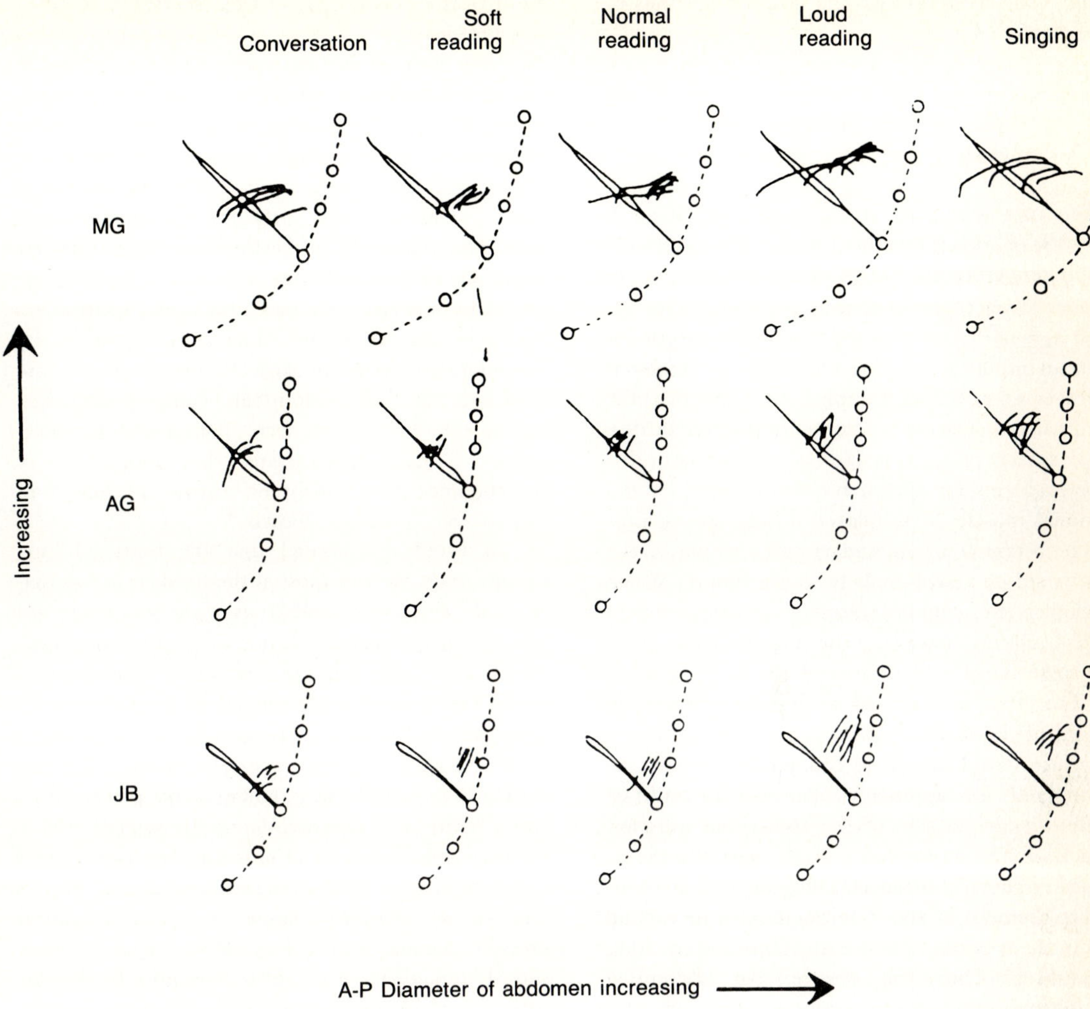

Figure 8–6 Motion-motion diagrams from three subjects performing conversation, soft, normal, loud reading, and singing tasks. (From Hixon TJ, Goldman M, Mead J. Kinematics of the chest wall during speech production: volume displacements of the rib cage, abdomen, and lung. J Speech Hear Res 1983; 16:78.)

tent than adults.[19] Hoit and Hixon demonstrated that elderly males use greater rib cage expansions than young adult males for speech and take more breaths per utterance than the young males.[20] These patterns may reflect compensation for age-related differences in laryngeal valving.

Stiffness of the chest wall may also vary across sex,[21] which might imply different patterns of chest wall function for speech in males and females. Hodge, Putnam, and Weismer reported that adult females tend to use chest wall shapes dominated by rib cage contribution to overall lung volume change;[22] three of the six males studied by Hixon et al showed clear tendencies to use major abdominal contributions to lung volume change during all or part of their expiratory limbs.[11] Hodge et al also noted that many of their female subjects encroached on FRC during conversational speech, an observation also made by Wilder[23] for adult females. The tendency for children and adult females to speak into the FRC is in contrast to the observation by Hixon et al[11] that adult males rarely go below the REL during conversational speech.

Variation in body type across subjects may partially explain some of the reported differences in speech breathing strategies both within and across studies. Hoit and Hixon have shown that among a small group of subjects, males of lean build (ectomorphs) used a predominant rib cage contribution to lung volume change for speech, whereas relatively greater abdominal compression was used by males of heavy build (endomorphs).[24] Males of average build (mesomorphs) used less homogeneous chest wall patterns for speech than either ectomorphs or endomorphs. Many of the subjects studied by Hoit and Hixon extended their expiratory limbs into the FRC, regardless of body type;[24] as noted previously, this finding is inconsistent with the original findings of Hixon et al.[11]

Speech Breathing and Biological Efficiency

Weismer attempted to summarize the Hixon et al[11,12] view of speech breathing within the framework of respiratory efficiency.[5] Many of the characteristics of Hixon et al's account of speech breathing were regarded as more efficient (i.e., maximum output for minimum input[25]) than the mechanisms suggested by Draper et al.[6] For example, the view that the abdominal musculature is essentially inactive during normal speech production creates at least two efficiency problems for speech breathing. First, if the abdominal muscles were relaxed during speech production, active (i.e., muscular) compression of the lungs would be vested entirely in the thorax. When the thoracic musculature exerts a compressive (expiratory) effort, however, the intrathoracic pressure—that is, pleural pressure—tends to be positive. The effect of this positive pleural pressure on the floor of the thoracic cavity—the diaphragm—is to displace it caudally if no counterforce resists the displacement. The appropriate counterforce could be supplied by contraction of the abdominal muscles; the lack of this counterforce would partially defeat the goal of thoracic muscular effort because the caudal displacement of the diaphragm acts to expand the lungs, whereas the overall objective is lung compression. Thus the presence of abdominal compression during speech production prevents wastage of the effort expended by thoracic musculature. The second efficiency problem due to inactive abdominal musculature also concerns diaphragmatic displacement caused by the positive pleural pressure. Inspiratory pauses between successive utterances are typically rapid and forceful, reflecting the need to increase lung volume by 20 to 30 percent of the VC while still "maintaining the floor." Because the diaphragm produces most, if not all, of the inspiratory muscular effort for refilling the lungs between utterances,[12] optimization of the contractile properties of the diaphragm for speech inspirations would seem desirable. Muscles typically produce the most efficient contractile efforts when the contractions are initiated at or near the physiologic rest length;[26] because the diaphragm is roughly at rest length when transmural pressure (pressure across the diaphragm) is near zero, any transmural pressure differential would tend to displace diaphragmatic muscle fibers from rest length (see footnote 1 in Weismer[5]).

The transmural pressure differential that would result during speech production if abdominal muscles were inactive would be fairly large at the critical instant preceding interutterance refills, because the end of an utterance typically occurs at lung volumes where the recoil forces are near zero and the demand for muscular effort is high. Abdominal contraction during speech production guarantees that the transmural pressure remains fairly low, thus maintaining diaphragmatic fibers at nearly optimal lengths for rapid, forceful contractions.

This discussion of how abdominal contraction makes speech breathing efficient is supported by the observation that virtually all normal speakers use some degree of abdominal compression during speech.[11,23,24,27] In fact, Baken and his colleagues[28–31] have demonstrated that compression of the abdomen is a consistent feature of chest wall preparation to initiate speech.*

Weismer also argued that the restricted lung volume range used by most of the speakers in the Hixon et al[11] study was a reflection of the respiratory system seeking an efficient solution to the problem of generating a constant subglottal pressure.[5] The speakers in the Hixon et al study tended to speak in the 60 to 40 percent VC range; a portion of the VC in which alveolar relaxation pressure varies between approximately 8 cm H_2O (approximately 60 percent VC) and 0.0 cm H_2O (approximately 40 percent VC).[11] Because typical subglottal pressures for speech are 8 to 10 cm H_2O,[34] utterances initiated around 60 percent VC would nearly match the typical subglottal pressure demand with the available relaxation pressure. Utterance onset would thus require little muscular effort to supplement the relaxation pressure and, as the utterance proceeds on a decreasing lung volume, only modest increments in muscular effort would be needed. By not continuing utterances past approximately 40 percent VC, or the point in lung volume where the relaxation pressure equals zero, speakers would not create a situation in which ex-

* Cavallo and Baken argue that the chest wall preparation gesture, in which the abdomen compresses and the rib cage expands, may often be characterized by the rib cage elevation gesture leading the abdominal compression gesture.[31] They continue this line of argument by suggesting that the rib cage elevation gesture is often, if not always, an active one. Two considerations lead to the conclusion that Cavallo and Baken misinterpreted their data. First, these authors seem to be unaware of work that shows how the anatomic linkages between the rib cage, diaphragm, and abdomen predict passive rib cage expansion following abdominal compression.[32,33] Second, if rib cage expansion did lead abdominal compression as the chest wall "set up" for speech, one would expect to hear a slight inspiratory "gasp" preceding phonation (that is, an inspiratory event following the prespeech inspiration) or see evidence of the brief, net expansion of the lungs. I have never seen a flow or volume record that would support the assertion that the rib cage elevation leads abdominal compression.

piratory muscular effort must be exerted against inspiratory recoil forces.

Although these considerations support the notion of a most efficient lung volume range for conversational speech, recent data suggest that Weismer's position[5] was stated too strongly. Examination of published motion-motion diagrams[11,23,24,27] indicates that many utterances encroach on FRC; obviously, the presumed loss of efficiency associated with speaking at lung volumes where relaxation pressures are negative is not too costly. Wilder reported that when female subjects read long, as compared to short, passages they typically do not adjust the starting lung volume, but rather use more of the FRC.[23] This may seem to be an inefficient strategy, but the use of high starting lung volumes for long utterances would also require that muscular forces (inspiratory) oppose recoil forces if speech intensity was to remain at normal levels. More work is needed to understand the interaction between chest wall configurations and the typical operating range for volume expenditure during speech.

An area in need of attention is the organization of speech breathing in connected discourse. Whereas several studies report data on conversational speech,[11,24] there is no in-depth analysis of the influence of, for example, grammatic structure or passage content on chest wall behavior. Grosjean and Collins have demonstrated that the location of major speech inspirations in reading is predictable from the grammatic structure,[35] but these results are not likely to provide much insight to speech breathing for spontaneous speech (see Goldman-Eisler[36]). In a recent study, Schönle and Conrad examined the locations of filled pauses (hesitation vowels) in spontaneous utterances and found a strong tendency for such pauses to occur near the beginning of expiratory limbs.[37] The filled pause is often interpreted as evidence of a planning mechanism, whereby a speaker holds his or her conversational turn with a phonatory filler while planning the next sequence of meaningful speech.[38] Schönle and Conrad regard the tendency for filled pauses to occur early in expiratory limbs as evidence of a motoric subroutine designed to prevent the respiratory system from resetting to vegetative breathing during periods of halting speech.[37] Their conclusion is that ". . . a straightforward account for the existence and distribution of hesitation vowels can be given on speech motor physiological grounds without need for psycholinguistic interpretations."[37] Schönle and Conrad's experiment was not designed to differentiate between a psycholinguistic and motor account of filled pauses, and so their conclusion should be regarded as an opinion rather than a logical interpretation of the results. However, the data on the distribution of filled pauses are important because they provide some preliminary insights to the organizational aspects of speech breathing.

LARYNGEAL FUNCTION IN SPEECH

The larynx consists of tiny structures that move minute distances during vocal fold vibration, yet the structures and movements are remarkably complex. In the last 10 years, there has been an explosion of research on laryngeal anatomy and physiology, much of which has been reported in the proceedings of a recurring conference.[39–42] This intense contemporary interest in vocal fold physiology derives in large part from Hirano's pioneering work on the gross anatomic, histologic, and mechanical characteristics of vocal fold tissue.[43–46] Hirano and his colleagues have described a layer structure of the vocal fold that is often referred to in a more general sense as the cover-body complex of the vocal fold. These anatomic investigations have led directly to a cover-body theory of vocal fold vibration, wherein certain vibratory phenomena can be explained in terms of variations in the mechanical properties of different vocal fold layers. Because the anatomical facts are so important to understanding the nature of vocal fold vibration, a brief review of Hirano's findings is provided here.

Prior to this review, however, a brief statement regarding voice registers is in order. Throughout this section, the terms "pulse," "modal," and "loft" register will be used. This terminology is consistent with that advocated by Hollien[47] and should be interpreted in the following physiologic sense. Modal register is typical of most phonation for conversational purposes and is characterized by vertical phase difference (see Cover-Body Complex section), a well-defined closed phase, and fairly large-amplitude, lateral excursions of the folds. Loft register typically (although not always) involves fundamental frequencies higher than those of the modal register and is characterized by the absence of vertical phase difference (due to high longitudinal tension on the vocal fold), a glottal cycle having a poorly defined or nonexistent closed phase, and minute amplitude excursions of the folds involving the medial edges only. Pulse register involves frequencies typically (but not always) below those of the modal register and is characterized by shortened, thick folds that may vibrate in a double-beat fashion and offer a high resistance to airflow. The pulse, modal, and loft registers are often referred to as the vocal fry, chest, and falsetto registers, respectively. The reader should consult Hollien for a rationale for the former terminology as well as information on the acoustic and perceptual correlates of registers.

Cover-Body Complex

Figure 8–7 shows a schema of a frontal section of the vocal fold, taken roughly at the middle of the membranous portion of the glottis. According to Hirano, the layer structure of the vocal fold consists of the cover, transition, and body;[43] details of the histologic structure of these layers are provided in Chapter 1, and so they will not be repeated here. The functional significance of this arrangement is that stiffness varies across the layers. More precisely, the stiffness of the cover is less than that of the transition, which, in turn, is less than that of the body. As pointed out by Hirano and Kakita, the layer-dependent variation in vocal fold stiffness explains why vocal fold vibration can be associated with such a wide range of tonal qualities.[46]

For the purposes of understanding the effect of laryngeal muscle contraction on the configuration of the vocal fold and the nature of vocal fold vibration, it has become customary to combine the cover and transition (i.e., the mucosa) and contrast its behavior to that of the body (i.e, the musculus vocalis). Hirano and Kakita have proposed that the action of three intrinsic laryngeal muscles—the cricothyroideus, lateral cricoarytenoideus, and posterior cricoarytenoideus—produces a stiffening of both the cover and body. Contraction of the musculus vocalis

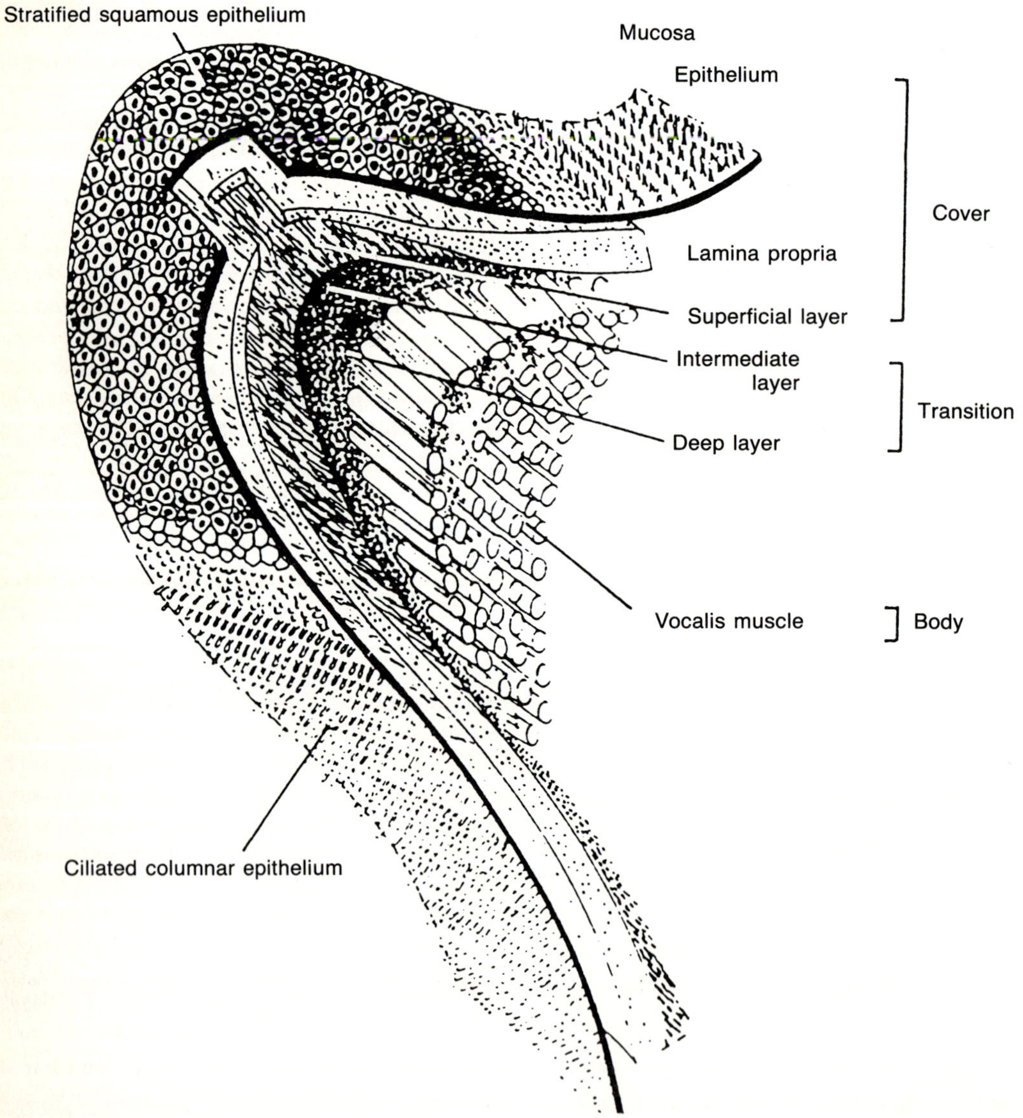

Figure 8–7 Schematic representation of the structure of the human vocal fold. (From Hirano M. Structure and vibratory behavior of the vocal folds. In: Sawashima M, Cooper FS, eds. Dynamic aspects of speech production. Tokyo: University of Tokyo Press, 1977:13.)

stiffens the body but slackens the cover, whereas contraction of the interarytenoideus may slacken both the body and cover.[46] The relative stiffness of the cover and body is determined by the overall pattern of contraction among the intrinsic laryngeal muscles. For example, the relationship of cover stiffness to body stiffness could, in principle, be varied in small degrees by adjusting the relative contraction strengths of the vocalis, cricothyroideus, and lateral cricoarytenoideus. Strong contraction of the vocalis, relative to the cricothyroideus and lateral cricoarytenoideus, should result in a relatively slack cover but stiff body. This type of contraction pattern would thus yield a fair amount of independence between cover and body movement during vocal fold vibration. In contrast, strong contraction of the musculus cricothyroideus coupled with moderate contractions of the vocalis and lateral cricoarytenoideus would stiffen both the cover and body and make the overall layer structure of the vocal fold move as a unit.

Hirano has summarized these observations by representing schematically a frontal section of a single vocal fold under different conditions of vocalis and cricothyroideus contraction (Fig. 8–8).[48] In each of the four frontal sections shown in Figure 8–8, the body is indicated by the hatched area and the more superficial cover by the unfilled area. Beneath each frontal section, strength of contraction for the vocalis and cricothyroideus is indicated qualitatively, and beneath this is the associated stiffness relationship between the cover and body. Figure 8–8*A* depicts the state of the vocal folds during soft phonation at low fundamental frequencies, wherein both the vocalis and cricothyroideus contract weakly. Here the aerodynamic and mechanical forces associated with vocal fold fibration deform the slack cover and body to a roughly equal degree (i.e., cover equals body). The vocal fold contour in Figure 8–8*A* is shown with two protuberances, which represent the upper and lower lip of the vocal fold. For certain modes of vibration, the folds are separated into upper and lower sections because of the vertical phase difference, wherein opening and closing movements occur at different times across the depth of contact between the folds.

The configuration of the vocal fold for loud phonation at medium values of fundamental frequency (120 to 140 Hz) is shown in Figure 8–8*B*. Because of the strong vocalis contraction and weaker cricothyroideus contraction, the body is very stiff while the cover is relatively slack. In this case, the stiff body is minimally involved in vibration; rather most of the vibratory motion is seen in the cover. Figure 8–8*C* shows a situation like that in Figure 8–8*B*, except here the difference between the strength of the vocalis and cricothryoideus contraction is not so great. Hirano and Kakita claim that this situation, where the body is slightly stiffer than the cover, is typical of most phonation in the modal register.[46] Under these circumstances, both the body and cover show deformations throughout the vibratory cycle with somewhat greater movement in the slacker cover.

Observation of vocal fold vibration via high-speed motion picture filming typically reveals wave-like motions of the folds for vocal fold configurations like those shown in Figure 8–8*A* to *C*. These motions, which are discussed in the section on Microaspects, reflect either the easy deformations of the cover and body (see Fig. 8–8*A*) or the motions of the cover relative to the body (see Fig. 8–8*B* and *C*). The wave-like motions are not observed often for

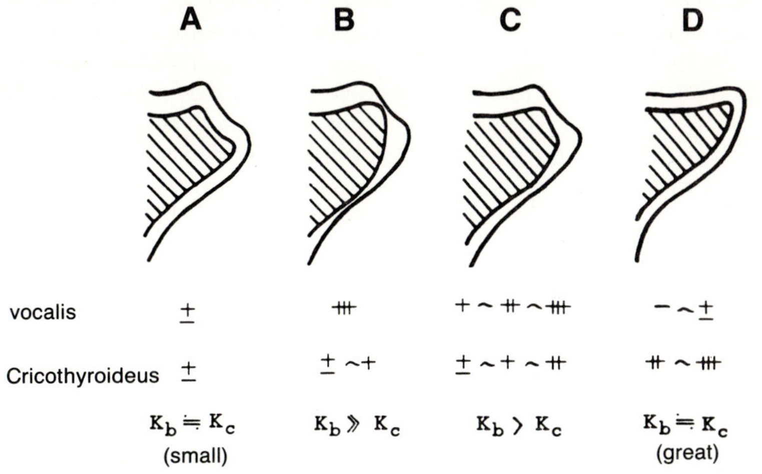

Figure 8–8 Schematic representation of vocal folds (frontal sections) showing effects of different levels of vocalis and cricothyroideus contraction on vocal fold shape during vibration. *Kb* = stiffness of body, *Kc* = stiffness of cover. (From Hirano M. Morphological structure of the vocal cord as a vibrator and its variations. Folia Phoniatr (Base) 1974; 26:86.)

vocal configurations like the one shown in Figure 8–8*D*, where the combination of strong cricothyroideus contraction and weak or absent vocalis contraction produces a uniform stiffening of the entire cover-body complex. This configuration is observed for phonation in the loft register; uniform stiffness of the cover-body complex results in small vocal fold movements that do not have wave-like characteristics.

Laryngeal Muscle Activity: EMG Data

Hirano's conceptualization of vocal fold configuration is in terms of the collective contraction pattern of the intrinsic laryngeal musculature and the effect of such patterns on the relative stiffness of the cover and body. Much of the available EMG data on laryngeal muscular activity during phonatory maneuvers (such as changing fundamental frequency or intensity) suggest some concerted activity to effect a particular adjustment in phonatory output. Table 8–1 contains some summary information from several studies[49–58] that have been concerned with laryngeal EMG and adjustment of fundamental frequency and/or phonatory intensity. This table is not meant to provide an exhaustive survey of laryngeal EMG studies, but rather a profile of work cited often in the area. Many factors that might have an effect on the pattern of muscular activity associated with an adjustment of phonatory output are variable across these studies. For example, the manner in which fundamental frequency or intensity adjustments are elicited from subjects is different across studies, as well as the strategies for processing and reducing the EMG signals. Moreover, the results summarized here may apply only to a specific register and, in some cases, may reflect idiosyncratic speaker characteristics. Another consideration in evaluating this set of results is that the various studies typically do *not* focus on the same set of muscles; the choice of which muscles to study seems to be a function of the investigators' biases, ease of electrode insertion, subjects' ability to tolerate multiple electrode insertions, or some combination of these factors.

An examination of Table 8–1 suggests that control of fundamental frequency derives from the action of three muscles, including the cricothyroideus, vocalis, and lateral cricoarytenoideus. Most investigators agree that the cricothyroideus is primarily responsible for increases in fundamental frequency, but the covariance of lateral cricoarytenoideus and vocalis activity with fundamental frequency is obvious in EMG records like the one shown in Figure 8–9. The precise balance of activity within this muscle "collective" is almost certainly variable depending on factors such as fundamental frequency range, register, and direction of fundamental frequency change.* With respect to the latter factor, whereas the mechanism of fundamental frequency *increase* has seemed to be relatively straightforward—at least in the general terms of the collective described before—the mechanism of fundamental frequency lowering has been more controversial.

Several studies show that decreases in fundamental frequency are associated with decreasing cricothyroideus activity and *increasing* activity of the sternohyoideus and sternothyroideus (strap). However, the precise role of the strap muscles in regulating fundamental frequency lowering is uncertain because the activity in these muscles does not precede the decrease in fundamental frequency.[50,57] Rather, it seems as if the strap muscle activity plays some kind of supplementary role in the control of fundamental frequency lowering.[59]

One must note here that some investigators have argued that primary control of fundamental frequency, at least in declarative-type utterances, is vested in the respiratory system. Lieberman demonstrated an apparent covariation between Ps and fundamental frequency contours during declarative utterances, and presented data indicating that ΔFO/ΔPs was large enough (approximately 20 Hz per cm H_2O) to implicate subglottal pressure as the primary control variable for fundamental frequency change.[60] Lieberman's position and other relevant studies have been reviewed by Ohala,[59] who concludes that the typical ΔFO/ΔPs is not large enough to explain fundamental frequency fluctuations in connected speech, which are sometimes as great as 100 Hz. According to Ohala, most studies have shown ΔFO/ΔPs to be approximately 2 to 4Hz per cm H_2O. If the latter relationship is accurate, Lieberman's hypothesis would seem to require huge Ps swings throughout utterances to produce typical fundamental frequency variation. The results of some recent experiments[49,61] seem to provide partial support for Lieberman's position, but this interpretation should be regarded cautiously because both studies used only a single speaker and employed relational (correlation) statistical analyses. It is possible, for example, that strong covariation could be observed between Ps and fundamental frequency with the Ps contour determined partly by the action of laryngeal muscles, rather than totally by respiratory forces. More

---

* Honda would argue that the muscle collective responsible for the control of fundamental frequency should include lingual muscles such as the genioglossus because his data show that laryngeal muscle activity for fundamental frequency increments depends on the activity pattern of various tongue muscles.[51]

TABLE 8–1 Selected EMG Data From Laryngeal Muscles*

	N *Males (M)/ Females (F)*	*Muscles*****	*Frequency Increase*	*Intensity Increase*
Shipp and McGlone[55]	14M	VOC	↑	
		CT	↑	
		PCA	↔	
		INT	↔	
Hirano, Ohala, Vennard[56]	5M/1F	VOC (N = 4)	↑ †	↑ †
		CT (N = 6)	↑	↔
		LCA (N = 6)	↑	↑
Collier[57]	1M	CT	↑ ‡	
		SH	§	
		ST	§	
		TH	↔	
Sapir et al[58]	2M	CT	↑	
Atkinson[49]	1M	VOC	↑ **	
		LCA	↑	
		SH	↓	
		CT	↑	
		ST	↓	
Erickson, Baer, and Harris[50]	4 (sex unknown)	CT	↓ ††	
		SH	↑	
Honda[51]		CT	↑ ‡‡	
		LCA	↑ §§	
		INT	↑	
Faaborg-Anderson[52]	25M	CT	↑	↔
	7F	VOC	↑	↔
		THY	↑	↔
		INT		No data
		PCA		No data
Gay, Hirose, Strome, Sawashima[53]	4M	VOC	↑ ***	↔ †††
	1F	CT	↑	↔
		LCA	↔	↔
		PCA	↔	↔
		INT	↔	↔
Simada and Hirose[54]	1M	LCA	↑	
		CT	↑	
		SH	↓	

*All studies used hook-wire electrodes, except Faaborg-Anderson, who used concentric, bipolar electrodes. An upward pointing arrow indicates that muscle activity increased for a frequency or intensity increase, whereas a downward pointing arrow indicates a decrease in muscle activity for a frequency or intensity increase. A horizontal arrow indicates no clear trend in muscle activity with frequency or intensity changes.

†Results somewhat different for model and loft registers or for different frequency.

‡Discusses CT relaxation and falling Fo.

§SH, ST sometimes associated with Fo lowering, but apparently not causally.

**Particular combination of muscles depends on Fo range—different laryngeal "modes" in different ranges.

††Data for Fo fall from high frequencies.

‡‡Data somewhat different for anterior and posterior parts of CT.

§§This relationship for vowel /i/, not for vowel /a/.

***These results similar for Fo changes at low and high intensities; data for modal register.

†††Some muscles show slight increases for increments of intensity, but authors argue such slight changes couldn't account for large phonatory intensity changes.

****Abbreviations: VOC = vocalis; CT = cricothyroideus; PCA = posterior cricoarytenoideus; INT = interarytenoideus; SH = sternohyoideus; ST = sternothyroideus; TH = thyrohyoideus; THY = thyroarytenoideus.

work is obviously needed to determine the relative contributions of laryngeal and respiratory forces to fundamental frequency control.

Laryngeal control of phonatory intensity has not been studied to the same degree as fundamental frequency, probably because of the recognition that intensity is controlled primarily by fluctuations in subglottal pressure. Phonatory intensity is related to subglottal pressure according to a power function, the exponent of which varies somewhat with vowel quality and ranges between 0.6 and 1.2.[62] Some authors have pointed out that in connected speech, fundamental frequency and intensity typically covary (e.g., with changes in lexical, contrastive, and emphatic stress),[49] and so the muscular and aerodynamic mechanisms underlying these changes should not be regarded as separable for speech production. Separating mechanisms of fundamental frequency and intensity control for singing is useful, but this will not be pursued in the current chapter (see Hollien and Schoenhard for a review[63]). The available EMG data indicate that vocalis and lateral cricoarytenoideus activity increase with phonatory intensity, although the increment in muscular activity may be small and therefore of questionable utility in controlling intensity (compare Gay et al[53] to Hirano, Ohala, and Vennard[56]). Additional experiments are needed to specify the role of laryngeal muscles in the control of both increases and decreases of phonatory intensity, especially as this role varies at different fundamental frequencies.

Vocal Fold Vibration

The discussion of vocal fold vibration will be divided into two sections. The first section will describe microaspects of vocal fold vibration, and the second section will summarize more global aspects of vibration. Microaspects of vocal fold vibration refer to the motions of different points on or within the cover-body complex; global aspects of vocal fold vibration refer to certain indices that describe regularities of the glottal area time function.

Microaspects

Early high-speed films of the vibrating vocal folds showed clearly a wave-like motion on the superior surface of the folds.[64] These waves seemed to be reflected back and forth between the medial and lateral boundaries of the vocal fold, and they did not necessarily mirror the movement of the main vocal fold mass. In contemporary terms, the superimposition of this wave motion on the motion of the vocal fold mass reflected a loose coupling between the cover and body (e.g., as in Fig. 8–8*C*). In recent years, investigators have been interested in characterizing more precisely the motions of the wave-like disturbance relative to the motions of the body. Because the movements of interest are so small (the maximum medial-to-lateral displacement of a vocal fold during phonation is approximately 1 mm, whereas the depth of contact between the vibrating vocal folds may range between 3 to 4 mm), special techniques and careful management of the measurement process are necessary to obtain useful information. Many of the experiments involve the use of excised human and animal larynges,[65] but some investigators have developed techniques that can be used in the phonating human.

Hirano, Kakita, Kawasaki, Gould, and Lambiase took high-speed motion pictures of a 22-year-old male phonating in the modal register at 128 Hz and used medial-to-lateral landmarks on the superior surface of the vocal fold to document motion during vibration.[66] Figure 8–10 shows some results from this study, in the form of displacement plots of selected measurement points as a function of film frame (interframe duration approximately 0.2 msec), for a single vibratory cycle. Four displacement plots are shown, one for the right vocal fold edge (*E* in the figure inset) and three for highly visible blood vessels on the vocal fold surface (1, 2, and 3 in the inset). The plotted displacement is actually the distance of each point from the edge of the left ventricular fold (V in the inset). The displacement plots clearly show that maximum excursion for these four points occurs at different times throughout the vibratory cycle. The vocal fold edge reaches maximum displacement first, followed by the next lateral

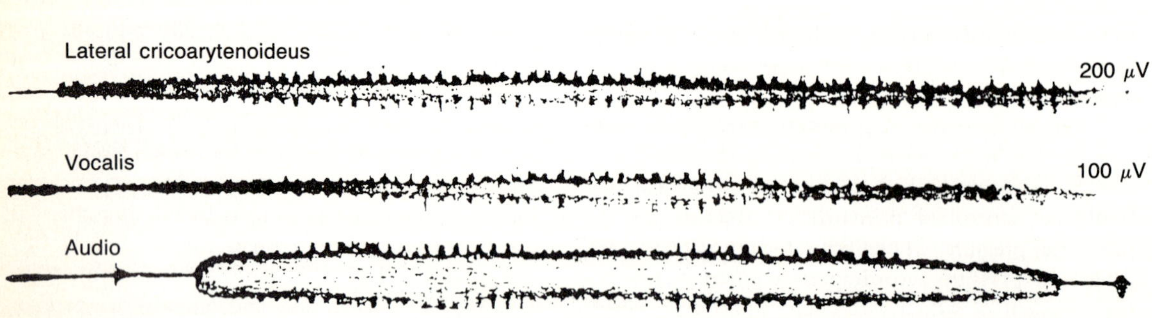

Figure 8-9 Fundamental frequency, cricothyroideus, lateral cricoarytenoideus, and vocalis EMG traces showing muscular activity during a glissando in modal register. (From Hirano M, Ohala HH, Vennard W. The function of the laryngeal muscles in regulating fundamental frequency and intensity of phonation. J Speech Hear Res 1969; 12:616.)

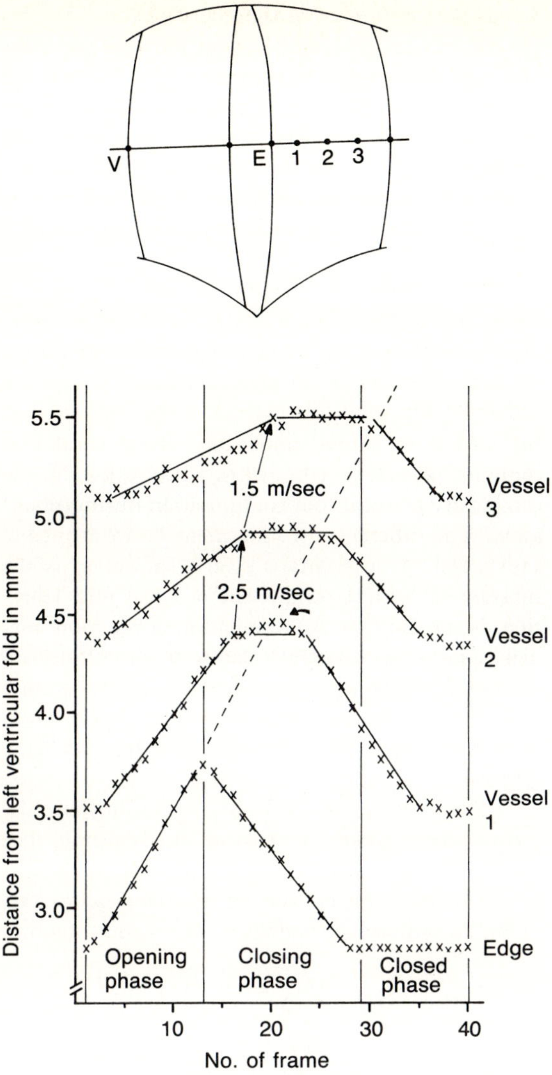

Figure 8-10 Lateral displacement throughout a single vibratory cycle of various medial-to-lateral points (shown in schematic superior view of vocal folds) on vocal fold. Note how displacement of more medial points leads displacement of more lateral points. (From Hirano M, Kakita Y, Ohmaru K, Kurita S. The structre of the vocal folds. In: Stevens KN, Hirano M, eds. Vocal fold physiology. Tokyo: University of Tokyo Press, 1981:33.)

point (vessel 1), then the next (vessel 2), and so forth. Hirano et al believe that the vibratory lag of lateral as compared to medial points reflects the delays associated with wave propagation through the cover.[66] For opening movements of the folds, the propagation speed through the tissue is not uniform, but seems to decrease as the measurement points become more lateral. Hirano suggests that the waves are caused by (1) air pressure acting on the inferior surface of the folds, (2) collision of the two folds, and (3) reflections from the lateral wall of the ventricle.[39] Hirano, Matsuo, Kakita, Kawasaki, and Kurita have shown that phase differences are also observed along the longitudinal extent of the vocal fold.[67] That is, points close to the anterior commissure reach maximum displacement at a different time than points close to the vocal process of the arytenoid cartilage (see Childers, Hicks, Moore, and Alsaka for a discussion of the horizontal phase difference[68]). Some of these horizontal phase differences may reflect the longitudinal variation in histologic characteristics of the cover, which has been reviewed by Hirano and Kakita.[46]

This work on point parameterization of the wavelike motion in the mediolateral and longitudinal dimensions illustrates several aspects of the complexity of vocal fold vibration. However, neither of the Hirano et al studies provided data on *vertical* motions of vocal fold tissue,[66,67] which cannot be resolved from high-speed motion pictures of the larynx. Studies using excised human and canine larynges[69–71] permit observations of both the vertical and horizontal components of vocal fold vibration. In the Japanese studies, small lead pellets were inserted at various locations in the vocal fold, and a combination of cineradiography (x-ray motion pictures) and stroboscopy* was used to track pellet motion throughout a vibratory cycle.[69,71] Figure 8–11 shows a frontal view of the vocal folds and the location of the pellets in the Saito et al study.[69] Pellet A is within the vocalis, pellet B is immediately below the surface of the free edge of the cover, and pellet C is within the cover but deeper and more lateral than pellet B. Motions of each of these pellets throughout a single vibratory cycle are shown in the lower part of Figure 8–11. Consideration of the three trajectories suggests that all pellets travel roughly elliptical paths throughout a vibratory cycle, but that the pellet closest to the midline of the glottis (B) travels in a more circular fashion than the other two pellets. The movements of both the vocalis pellet (A) and the lateral and deep cover pellet (C) describe relatively flattened ellipses, but the orientation of the long axis (major axis) of these two ellipses is different. These trajectories thus indicate that the greatest movement occurs at the free edge of the fold, and that this movement has significant components in both the medial to lateral (horizontal) and inferior to superior (vertical) dimensions. The movements of the deeper and more lateral cover pellets are not as great, but

* Stroboscopy is a technique that involves a continuous series of light pulses timed to coincide exactly or nearly exactly with some periodic event that is the object of study. In the case of vocal fold vibration, the timing relationship between the glottal period and the stroboscope period can be adjusted to "freeze" vocal fold position at a given phase of the cycle or to produce an apparent slow-motion movement of the folds. Stroboscopy allows an investigator to perform analyses similar to those associated with high-speed motion pictures, but without the need for the tedious frame-by-frame analysis.

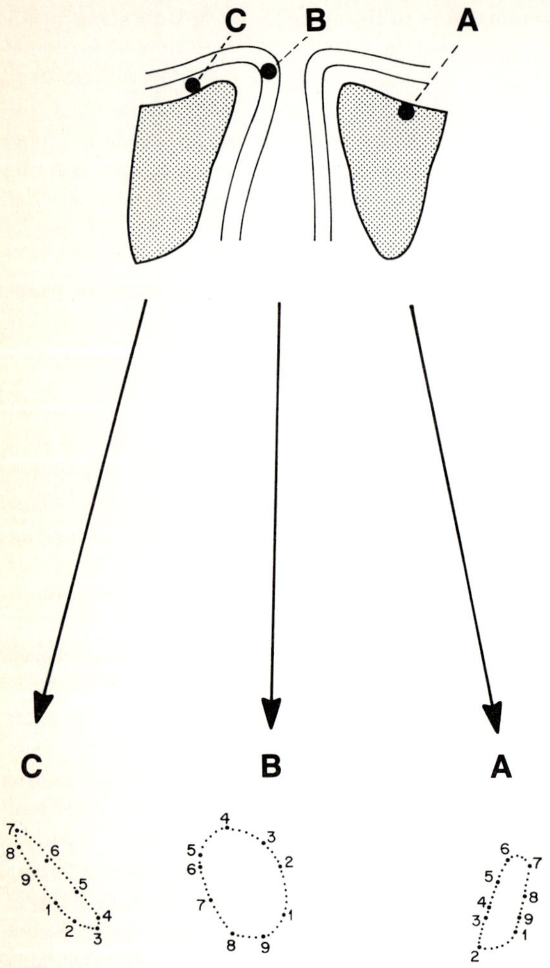

Figure 8–11 Location of lead pellets in frontal view of vocal fold tissue (top), and motion trajectories of the same pellets throughout a single cycle of vocal fold vibration (bottom). (From Saito S, Fukuda H, Isogai Y, Ono H. X-ray stroboscopy. In: Stevens KN, Hirano M, eds. Vocal fold physiology. Tokyo: University of Tokyo Press, 1981:95.)

also have significant horizontal and vertical components, whereas the movement of the vocalis pellet is largely in the vertical dimension. Baer's[70] observations on excised canine larynges are consistent with the findings of Saito et al.[69,71] Baer noted that vocal fold vibrations could be characterized partly as "displacement waves propagating in the superior direction" and partly as bulk deformations of the body.[70] The vibratory components due to bulk deformations can be distinguished from those due to displacement waves on the basis of speed of propagation between two tissue points, this speed being substantially greater in the case of bulk deformations.

Fukuda et al[71] used the same point parameterization approach as Saito et al,[69] but embedded a larger number of pellets along the vocal fold surface to obtain a more comprehensive description of vocal fold motions. Because the pellet locations ranged from the superolateral edge to the inferior part of the vocal fold, Fukuda et al were able to derive a vocal fold contour during a vibratory cycle by tracing through the multiple pellet positions at a given instant in time. When these contours are constructed for several time points throughout a glottal period, a plot such as the one in Figure 8–12 is obtained. This plot shows seven superimposed contours of a single vocal fold in the frontal plane, with contours 1 and 8 defining the beginning and end, respectively, of a single vibratory cycle (f_o = 200 Hz, medium intensity). Only two pellet locations are shown on these contours. Both pellets are on the superior surface of the vocal fold but are widely separated in the medial to lateral dimension. These vocal fold contours provide a compelling illustration of the complexity of vocal fold configuration during phonation. The difference in movement between medial and lateral tissue points is clearly shown, as is the substantial vertical component of vocal fold vibration. Note also how the orientation of the more medial tissue point changes relative to the glottis: in contour 1, the point is clearly on the superior surface of the vocal fold; whereas in contour 3, the point is on the medial edge of the fold in line with the airstream.

The contours in Figure 8–12 also illustrate the vertical phase difference of vocal fold vibration. The vertical phase difference, which is most prominent in the modal register, can be described as a mode of vibration in which the vocal folds open inferiorly

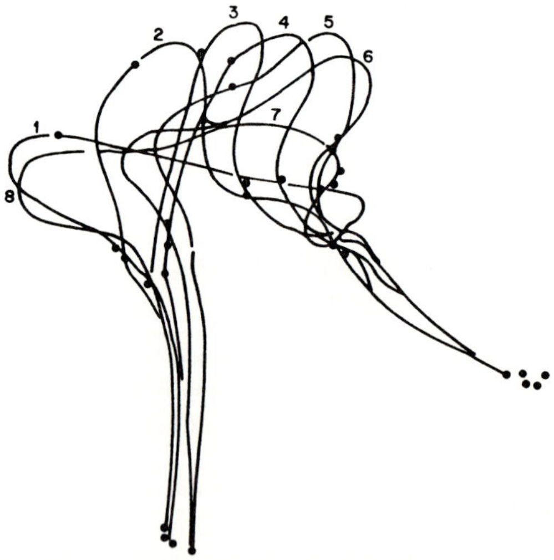

Figure 8–12 Superimposed vocal fold contours, frontal plane view, defining vocal fold shapes throughout a single cycle of vibration. The contours labeled "1" and "8" begin and end the cycle, respectively. Middle intensity phonation, FO = 200 Hz. (From Fukudo H, Saito S, Kitahara S, Isogai Y, Makino K, Tsuzuki T, Kowgawa N, Ono H. Vocal fold vibration in excised larynges used with an x-ray stroboscope and an ultra-high speed camera. In: Bless DM, Abbs JH, eds. Vocal fold physiology. San Diego: College-Hill Press, 1983:238.)

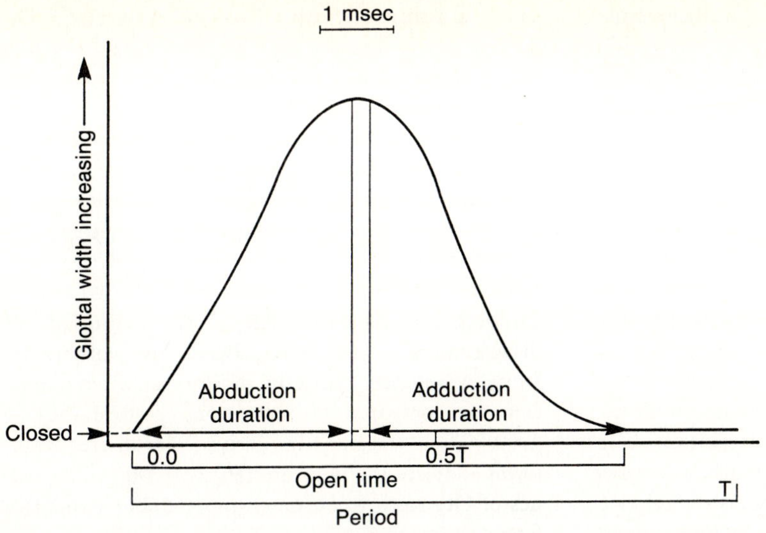

Figure 8–13 Glottal width function for one cycle of vocal fold vibration in the modal register. (After Timcke R, von Leden H, Moore P. Laryngeal vibrations: measurement of the glottic wave. Part I: the normal vibratory cycle. Arch Otolarygol 1958; 68:1.)

before they open superiorly and close inferiorly before they close superiorly (recall Baer's description of vocal fold vibration as a displacement wave propagating in the superior direction). Contour 2, which represents vocal fold configuration soon after the beginning of a glottal cycle, shows the inferior part of the vocal fold to be displaced more laterally than the superior part; contour 6, the vocal fold configuration near the end of a cycle (contour 8), clearly shows the more inferior portion of the vocal fold leading the superior part toward the midline closure position.

The contours and point trajectories shown in Figure 8–12 vary depending on voice fundamental frequency and intensity. Fukuda et al have reported that the complexity of vocal fold vibration (both in terms of contour shape and movement magnitude) seems to decrease at high fundamental frequency, but increase at high intensity.[71] Under all these phonatory conditions, however, the wave-like aspect of vocal fold vibration is obvious.

These vibratory characteristics of the vocal folds are obviously under significant influence of both aerodynamic and mechanical forces. A simplified description of the interaction of these forces in modal phonation can be derived from an extensive review published by Broad.[72] When the vocal folds are brought together in the phonation-ready position, they offer some resistance to being displaced laterally and superiorly. At some point, the positive subglottal pressure overcomes this resistance, and the folds are displaced away from the midline. An important point here is that the subglottal pressure is primarily effective on the *lower* part of the vocal fold tissue; thus movement of the lower part precedes movement of the upper part, which is eventually dragged laterally because of the mechanical connection with the lower part. The lower part of the folds reaches maximum lateral excursion first and begins to move medially because of the elastic characteristics of the tissue. At some point where the conduits between the lower and upper parts of the two folds have certain critical dimensions, Bernoulli's force (sucking action due to accelerated flow and thus negative pressure) assists the medial movement toward closure with the upper parts of the folds again being dragged along. The interaction of the aerodynamic and mechanical forces explains the vertical phase differences: aerodynamic forces control the lower part of the folds, which drags along the mechanically-linked upper part of the folds.

Global Aspects

In a series of classic papers, Timcke, von Leden, and Moore reported on vibratory phenomena associated with single cycles of vocal fold vibration in phonating humans.[73–75] The study of these vibratory patterns was made possible by the use of ultrahigh-speed cinematography, whereby the vibrating larynx was filmed at speeds of 3,000 to 5,000 frames per second. By advancing the exposed film frame by frame and taking measures of glottal width for each frame, Timcke et al were able to construct time functions showing the movements of the vocal folds in the horizontal plane (medial to lateral). Figure 8–13 shows one such function for phonation in the modal register at a medium intensity. In this figure, the continuous wave is the glottal width function for a single fold, with upward deflections indicating movement away from the midline; the point labeled "closed" on the ordinate represents vocal fold closure. Timcke et al quantified their observations using two primary measures, the speed quotient (SQ) and the open quotient (OQ). SQ was defined as the duration of the abduction gesture divided by the duration of the adduction gesture, whereas OQ was defined as the time during which the vocal folds were open divided by the duration of the entire period. Timcke et al found that SQ was typically less than unity, indicating a somewhat faster abduction, as compared to adduction, gesture;[73] at very high phonatory intensities, however, this relationship was reversed, yielding an SQ exceeding unity. Typical values of OQ in the modal register ranged between 0.64 and 0.88 with increasingly smaller values associated with greater phonatory intensities. The general asymmetries in the glottal width waveform implied by SQs less than 1.00, as well as the relative open time per glottal period suggested by OQs around 0.70, are also seen in glottal area functions published by Childers, Naik, Larar, Krishnamurthy, and Moore.[76]

Because the collection of ultrahigh speed film data is bothersome for the subject and the analysis of the films costly and tedious, only a limited amount of data of the kind reported by Timcke et al are available. In recent years, investigators have sought alternate techniques for studying the glottal waveform in human subjects. These techniques include photoglottography (PGG), electroglottography (EGG), and inverse filtering of the oral airflow or acoustic waveform. The PGG technique is implemented with a light source, usually positioned above the larynx, and a photodetector placed on the external neck surface at a level below the glottis. The time-varying glottal area admits to the subglottal space a varying amount of light, which is sensed by the photodetector and transduced to a voltage representation. Baer, Löfqvist, and McGarr have shown that PGG time functions during phonation provide good estimates of the actual glottal width functions derived from high-speed films.[77] In EGG, two electrodes are placed on the external neck surface, one over each thyroid laminae, and a current is supplied to one of the electrodes. The electrical impedance between the two electrodes depends on the tissue impedance in the current path, which is dependent on the amount of contact (surface area contact) between the vocal folds. With the source current held constant, the voltage across the electrodes varies as more or less tissue from the two folds comes into contact during vocal fold vibration. An excellent review of the EGG technique has been published by Childers and Krishnamurthy.[78] Finally, inverse filtering is a technique wherein the acoustic pressure waveform or oral airflow waveform is submitted to a filter that is the mirror image (the inverse) of the vocal tract transfer function associated with a phonated vowel.[79,80] The output of the inverse filter is theoretically the part of the speech signal not associated with vocal tract shape, that is, the glottal volume velocity.

Figure 8–14 shows simultaneously-obtained EGG signals and film-derived glottal area functions. Although there is some degree of similarity in the glottal waveshapes across the different methods described above, quantitative summaries of the functions are often in disagreement. As pointed out by Childers and Krishnamurthy,[78] the nature of the disagreement is that EGG, PGG, and volume velocity waveforms typically indicate a faster adduction, as compared to abduction, gesture ($SQ > 1.00$[79,81,82]), whereas film-derived glottal area waveforms indicate the opposite ($SQ < 1.00$[73,76]).* Values of OQ seem to be much more stable across different techniques.

The use of EGG, PGG, or inverse filtering to study the glottal waveform represents an attempt to avoid the tedious aspects of high-speed film analysis. However, the PGG and inverse filtering techniques have drawbacks that mitigate against their use in large-N studies† or clinical settings. PGG is invasive because it requires a light source (usually carried by a fiberscope) that is inserted through the nose and positioned above the glottis. Inverse filtering can be implemented with a variety of models of the vocal tract transfer function, all of which entail certain assumptions that are difficult to meet for a particular speaker or group of speakers. Because EGG is noninvasive and produces a signal that need not be decomposed (as in inverse filtering), it would seem to be the most likely candidate for collecting large amounts of glottal waveform data. Childers and his associates have performed many simultaneous analyses of film-derived glottal area and EGG functions.[83] These analyses show how the EGG waveform can be interpreted to give reliable information concerning global features of vocal fold vibration. Figure 8–15 provides a schematic illustration of an EGG waveform, together with a number code indicating the correspondence of a waveform feature with an event observed from high-speed films. The interpretation of EGG waveform features depicted in Figure 8–15

* Actually, Timcke et al had previously reviewed evidence that glottal area waveforms and volume velocity waveforms derived from inverse filtering yielded substantially different SQ values.[73]

† A major problem with many of the glottal waveform features is that only a few subjects are studied. This may explain, in part, some of the discrepancies in the findings of various studies. Large-N studies of glottal waveform features are necessary to determine statistical characteristics of measures such as SQ and OQ.

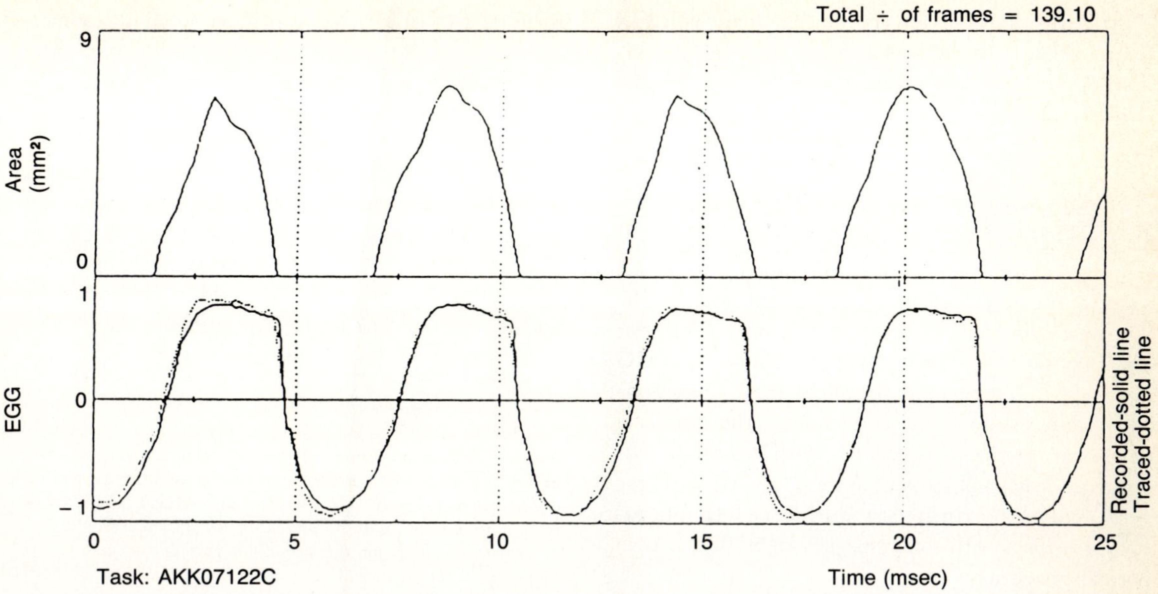

Figure 8–14 Simultaneously-obtained film-derived glottal areas (upper panel) and EGG (lower panel) waveforms (from Childers DG, Naik JM, Larar JN, Krishnamurthy AK, Moore GP. Electroglottography, speech, and ultra-high speed cinematography. In: Titze IR, Scherer RC, eds. Vocal fold physiology. Denver: Denver Center for the Performing Arts, 1985:202).

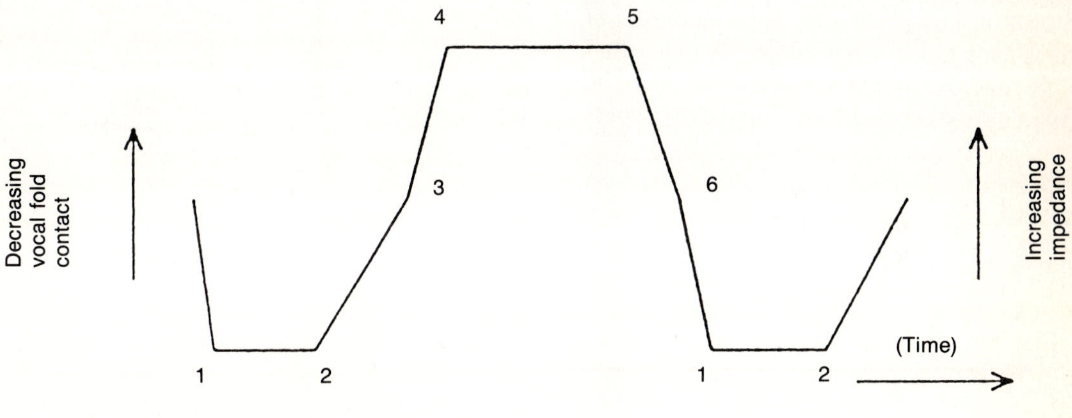

1–2 Vocal folds maximally closed. Maximum contact area.
2–3 Folds parting, usually from lower margins toward upper margins and posterior to anterior.
3 When this break point is present this usually corresponds to folds opening along upper margin.
3–4 Upper fold margins continue to open.
4–5 Folds apart, minimum contact area.
3–5 Open phase.
5 Folds in contact along lower margin. Glottal area zero.
5–6 Folds closing from lower to upper margin and from anterior to posterior.
6–1 Rapid increase in vocal fold contact.
5–2 Closed phase.

Figure 8–15 A schematic representation of an electroglottographic waveform, together with a key indicating how events along the waveform may be interpreted in terms of vocal fold vibration (from Childers DG, Hicks DM, Moore GP, Alsaka YA. A model for vocal fold vibratory motion, contact area, and the electroglottogram. J Acoust Soc Am 1986; 80:1309.)

is strictly valid only for the normal male voice in the modal register; irregular modes of vocal fold vibration make the interpretation of EGG signals particularly tenuous.[68]

Segmental Laryngeal Behavior

In addition to providing the source for vocalic sounds, the larynx plays an important role in the voicing distinction for obstruents (stops, fricatives, and affricatives). Early studies using a PGG approach[84–86] revealed a relatively slow abduction-adduction gesture of the vocal folds—the laryngeal devoicing gesture—associated with voiceless obstruents. Voiced obstruents were produced with the vocal folds approximated as during normal phonation or perhaps with somewhat less tight closure than normal phonation.

Hirose and his colleagues have investigated the phenomenon and mechanism of the laryngeal devoicing gesture,[87–89] which appears to be as follows. In a vowel-consonant-vowel (VCV) sequence, where C = voiceless aspirated stop, vocal fold vibration for the first vowel is stopped by the onset of the laryngeal devoicing gesture. This devoicing gesture, which involves a relatively slow lateral movement of the vocal folds from the closed glottis (phonation ready) position, is initiated simultaneously with the onset of supralaryngeal closure. The lateral movement of the vocal folds continues until the glottis is at least as wide as the maximum opening during phonatory cycles, whereupon an adduction gesture brings the folds back toward the midline to prepare for the phonation requirement of the following vowel.

The glottal area time function shown in Figure 8–16 illustrates the effect of the laryngeal devoicing gesture. The glottal area function is single peaked and shows little or no plateau at maximum opening, suggesting that the abduction-adduction gesture is executed in an integrated, immutable way.* The

* This is the position argued by myself in an earlier publication.[90] Important aspects of this argument are (1) the laryngeal devoicing gesture apparently retains its essential form of abduction-adduction even when the voiceless obstruent is in *utterance-initial* position (i.e., with no preceding vowel, which would seem to obviate the need for the abduction part of the gesture: see Lindqvist[85]); (2) the gesture does not seem amenable to voluntary control, other than in categorical ways;[91] and (3) there is no *phonetic* motivation to exert separate control over the abduction and adduction parts of the gesture.[90] Nevertheless, some writers apparently feel that abductory and adductory control strategies could be somewhat independent (e.g., Munhall and Ostry[92]): "The differences in the kinematic patterns of abduction and adduction perhaps result from differing functional roles of the opening and closing gestures. The timing of the abduction gesture appears to be related to the oral closure timing. The abduction movement must ensure that the glottal state can produce the appropriate aerodynamic conditions for consonant production. The adduction movement, on the other hand, is associated with bringing the laryngeal apparatus to a vowel production posture. The timing demands of these two roles are presumably different" (p 160).

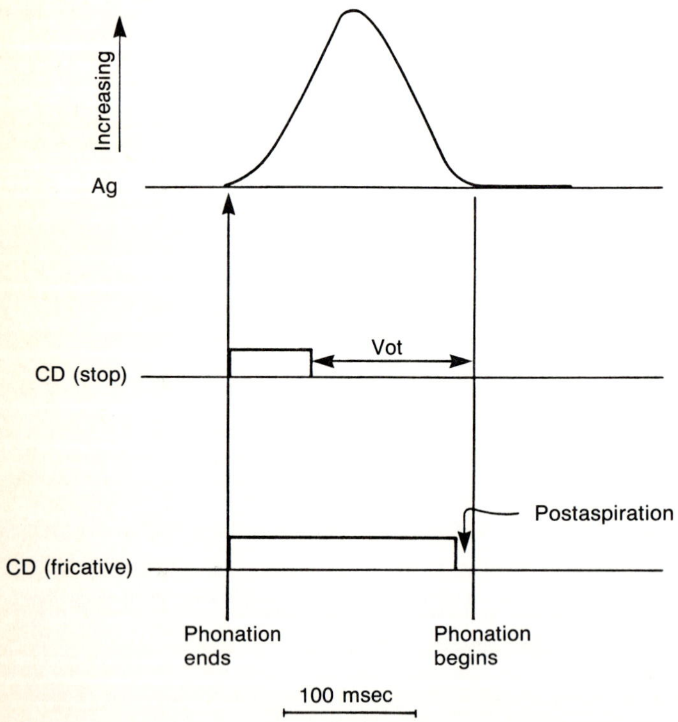

Figure 8–16 Diagram showing the time course of laryngeal and supraglottal events for production of voiceless stops and fricatives in American English. The top trace is glottal area function, and the middle and bottom traces show the duration of supraglottal constriction for stops and fricatives, respectively. See text for further details.

duration of the gesture, measured from the onset of abduction to the resumption of closed glottis conditions (between the vertical lines in Fig. 8–16), is highly variable across individuals, but probably averages around 150 msec for voiceless stops preceding a stressed vowel.

The presumed mechanism underlying the laryngeal devoicing gesture is illustrated in Figure 8–17. The four traces in this figure are, from top to bottom, glottal width (a glottal area function should appear similar to this), EMG for the interarytenoideus, EMG for cricoarytenoideus posterior, and an audio signal; the latter three traces are rectified and integrated versions of the original signals. Whereas the VCV sequence (/ise/) shown in Figure 8–17 was from a Japanese utterance, this basic pattern has been shown to occur in a variety of languages, including English.[89] Some 60 to 70 msec preceding the increase in glottal width, the interarytenoideus and the cricoarytenoideus posterior show sharp and opposite changes in EMG activity levels. This pattern of cricoarytenoideus posterior activation and interarytenoideus suppression, which initiates the laryngeal devoicing gesture, is reversed approximately 150 msec later as the vocal folds are prepared for phonation of the following vowel. For the most part, the time course of these activation and suppression patterns accounts well for the time course of the glottal width (or glottal area) function.

More recently, Löfqvist and his associates have studied the laryngeal devoicing gesture as it relates to the supraglottal gesture for obstruents.[93–95] These investigators have shown that the maximum glottal opening and peak velocity are greater for fricatives, than for stops. In addition, the time interval between the onset of the laryngeal devoicing gesture and the point of maximum glottal opening seems to be related directly to the duration of the *supraglottal* constriction, although the precise nature of the relationship is different for stops and fricatives (see also Munhall and Ostry[92]). And, as well, the essential form of the gesture depicted in Figure 8–17 is preserved for /s/ plus stop clusters, except when a word boundary intervenes between the members of the cluster; in this case, the glottal area function has a double-peaked profile. Although the significance of the latter observation is fairly obvious, there is not a good understanding of the glottal-supraglottal relationships reported by Löfqvist. The pervasiveness of obstruent voicing distinctions in languages of the world makes this an important area for future investigations.

SUPRAGLOTTAL FUNCTION IN SPEECH

Like research on laryngeal and respiratory function in speech production, the focus in research on supraglottal articulation has shifted somewhat over the past 10 years. Although speech researchers have recognized for many years that the articulators function together to create vocal tract shapes that produce acoustic events having linguistic significance, the aim of many researchers had been to describe the electromyographic and/or movement characteristics of single articulators.[96,97] Part of this approach might be attributed to technologic limitations, but much of it can be attributed to the complexity of designing analytic strategies that capture the important characteristics of a multidimensional profile of EMG and/or kinematic records. In other words, a goal in the study of supraglottal articulation is to describe the mapping between the articulatory ensemble and the vocal tract shape. The complexity of this goal can be highlighted by considering the following ba-

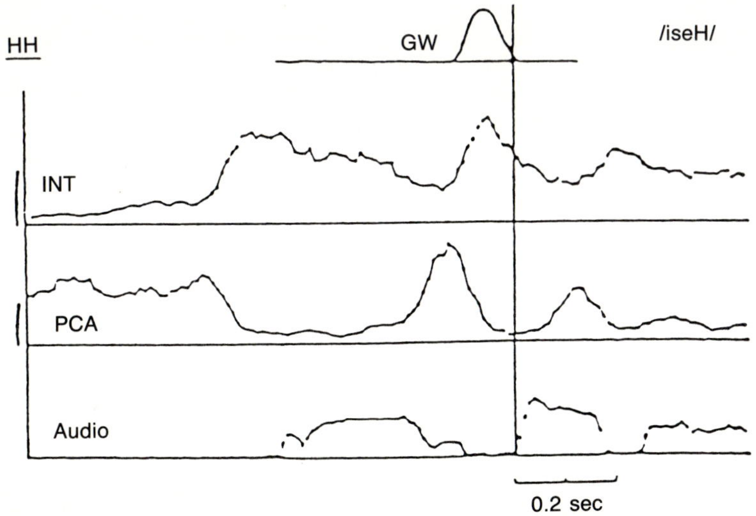

Figure 8–17 Simultaneous glottal width (GW), EMG (interarytenoideus [INT] and posterior cricoarytenoideus [PCA]) and audio events associated with an intervocalic, voiceless fricative. (Adapted from Sawashima M, Hirose H. Larygneal gestures in speech production. In: MacNeilage PF, ed. The production of speech. New York: Springer-Verlag, 1983:11.)

sic questions: How is the articulatory ensemble to be defined? More specifically, what are the relevant parameters of this definition; that is, should the definition be in EMG and/or kinematic terms, and which aspects of these signals (peaks or integrals for EMG; displacement, velocity, acceleration for kinematics) should be considered as critical?[98] How should components (articulators) of the ensemble be weighted—both in the spatial and temporal domains—in creating vocal tract shapes? And how does the weighting fluctuate with variations in phonetic requirements? To what extent can the components of the ensemble vary in producing a vocal tract shape? And is the observed variability lawful or stochastic? To what extent does the parameterization of the ensemble depend on speaker-specific anatomic characteristics?

Obviously, the experimental environment that would permit an investigator to answer these questions has not been available generally. The simultaneous collection of a sufficient number of signals to define the ensemble is technically complex, but feasible; the discovery of ensemble characteristics, followed by the development of pattern recognition and production schemes that can recognize and recreate future ensembles, is somewhat less likely to occur in the near future. One approach to the problem of constructing such ensembles is to reduce the descriptive dimensionality while maintaining descriptive adequacy. Most digital simulations of articulation[99–102] depend to some extent on this approach. Although these simulations have enjoyed a certain amount of success, the principles of their operation may or may not be relevant to an understanding of speech production as a *biologic* phenomenon.

The recent trend in speech production literature to understand linkages between structures emphasizes the need to undertake multidimensional analyses of articulatory behavior. Following reviews of vocal tract muscle activity and articulatory kinematics, the chapter is concluded by consideration of some contemporary theoretical issues in speech production, including that of articulatory linkages.

Vocal Tract Muscular Activity

Folkins and Kuehn have provided an excellent summary of articulatory EMG data, and so only a brief review will be offered here.[1] The majority of the research findings described next were obtained by means of hooked-wire electrodes; some investigators[103] argue that surface electrodes can be used effectively in the study of certain lip muscles.

In the velopharynx, the levator veli palatini is typically active for velar raising gestures, whereas velar lowering gestures are produced by relaxation of the levator veli palatini or possibly by contraction of the musculus palatoglossus, depending on the relative positions of the tongue and velum.[96,104–106] The palatopharyngeus seems to be active when the levator veli palatini is active (i.e., it plays an unknown role in velopharyngeal closure), but the tensor veli palatini does not appear to have a systematic activity pattern in speech production.

EMG findings for superior and middle pharyngeal constrictor function during speech have been inconsistent.[104,107] It is not clear if superior constrictor fibers located at the level of velopharyngeal closure are active in concert with the levator veli palatini to effect velopharyngeal closure for obstruents, although movement of the lateral pharyngeal walls at this level has been observed for stop consonant production.[107] Niimi's data[107] also seem to be consistent with Folkins and Kuehn's[1] suggestion that the upper and lower regions of the superior constrictor show different activity patterns during speech.

As described by Folkins and Kuehn, EMG data on the tongue musculature are both scant and difficult to interpret.[1] In the case of the intrinsic tongue muscles, the interdigitating matrix of fibers running in the inferior to superior, anterior to posterior, and transverse directions make it virtually impossible to specify the actions of individual muscles even when using sophisticated intramuscular electrode techniques. Textbooks report the action of each of the four intrinsic muscles of the tongue,[108,109] but the statements are based on the orientation of the muscles and their assumed suitability for shaping the tongue in accord with particular phonetic requirements.[110] More information is available on the EMG characteristics of the extrinsic muscles of the tongue. Alfonso, Honda, Baer, and Harris used hooked-wire electrodes to sample six sites in extrinsic tongue musculature.[111] In this study, the activity of the posterior fibers of the genioglossus seemed to have a primary role in raising the tongue for /i/, although simultaneous activity of genioglossus posterior, mylohyoideus, and geniohyoideus was often observed for certain raising gestures. The genioglossus seems to be involved in a variety of tongue gestures, judging from its activity pattern for a wide variety of speech sounds.[110] This muscle seems to be inactive for low-back vowel articulations. The hyoglossus and styloglossus were typically active for the lowering and retraction gesture required for /a/ production; the styloglossus has also been implicated as an important contributor to the raising and retraction gesture associated with /u/. Obviously, the remaining vowels would require various balances of force exerted by the ensemble of extrinsic muscles that can influence tongue position.

Some years ago, Perkell advanced a notion concerning the functional significance of the anatomic distinction between the intrinsic and extrinsic tongue muscles.[112] Specifically, the extrinsic muscles were thought to be responsible in large part for the gross positioning of the tongue primarily associated with vocalic sounds, whereas the intrinsic muscles created the more fine-grained shapings of the tongue required for consonant production. In this view, lingual articulation can be thought of as a slowly varying positioning gesture—akin to a continuous diphthong-like gesture—on which consonant shaping gestures are intermittently superimposed (for a good review of related evidence, see Fowler[113]). A more recent version of this theory of vowel production is that the exact nature of the forces used to modify tongue position within the vocal tract is not necessarily important. Modeling efforts[114] as well as x-ray microbeam data on variability of tongue position for the same vowel[115,116] suggest that a more qualitative representation of forces operating on the tongue may be sufficient to achieve the desired acoustic output of the vocal tract. In other words, speakers need only specify rather gross aspects of muscle forcing functions to move the tongue into a general region associated with a particular acoustic output.* Of course, the gross forcing functions must be constrained to some degree, and probably in accord with the acoustic requirements of vowel production. For example, Perkell and Nelson showed that variability of lingual fleshpoints for repeated productions of certain vowels was relatively limited in the dimension that determines vocal tract *constriction,* but not in the dimension along the long axis of the vocal tract.[116] An example of these data is shown in Figure 8–18. Perkell and Nelson suggest that the variability along the long axis of the vocal tract has a minimal effect on vowel acoustics and so can be relatively unconstrained.[116] Yet variability in the dimension of constriction is likely to affect the acoustic output of the vocal tract and so must be more closely controlled. A more refined theory of vowel articulation would have to explain how gross forcing functions of lingual muscles are distributed to achieve different degrees of control in different vocal tract dimensions. Similarly, such a theory would also need to account for a possible independence between dynamic tongue gestures of advancement and raising.[118]

As indicated by Folkins and Kuehn, muscular activity for jaw opening and closing has often been inferred from the anatomic orientation of muscle fibers relative to the mandible and its attachment at the temporomandibular joint.[1] However, various aspects of these inferences may not always apply to jaw activity during speech production, as demonstrated in several studies.[119,120] For example, Tuller et al sampled EMG data from a variety of muscles purported to open and close the jaw and found that the contribution of certain muscles to *nonspeech* gestures of jaw opening and closing was not necessarily predictive of the muscles' activity in speech.[119] Temporalis and masseter are typically described as jaw closers, but Tuller et al could not find evidence of consistent activity in these muscles for jaw elevation during speech production. If these muscles are only active during jaw movements characterized by large displacements and velocities,[1] then the speech sample used by Tuller et al may not have been sensitive enough to elicit closing-related activity. Pterygoideus medialis and the superior head of the pterygoideus lateralis seemed to be active during jaw closing, whereas the anterior belly of the digastricus and the inferior head of the pterygoideus lateralis were active for jaw opening. Folkins' data are essentially consistent with those of Tuller et al;[120] an interesting contribution of Folkins' work is his observation of large variability for jaw muscle activity during speech, both across subjects and within subjects for repetitions of the same utterance. Folkins argues that precise levels of activity among the jaw closers or openers are not critical.[120] Rather the attainment of desired movement patterns is critical; such patterns are accomplished by means of a variety of muscular activities. Thus a muscle like the anterior belly of the digastricus, the activity of which is typically thought to be associated with jaw opening, may show varying levels of activity across repetitions of the same utterance. The variation in the level of activity in a single muscle, even when more globally defined goals (e.g., movements) remain fairly constant, is further testimony to the need to conceptualize muscular activity of the vocal tract in ensemble terms.

Finally, the muscles that are thought to play some role in lip gestures during speech production include the orbicularis oris superior and inferior, mentalis, depressor anguli oris, buccinator, depressor labii inferior, and levator labii superior. As described by Folkins and Kuehn, the first five of these muscles (regarding the orbicularis oris superior and inferior as separate muscles) seem to be active for lip closing, whereas the depressor and levator labii su-

* The central thesis of the quantal theory of articulation[117] can be discerned here. Within certain regions of the vocal tract, variability in tongue position does not have much of an effect on the acoustic output of the vocal tract.

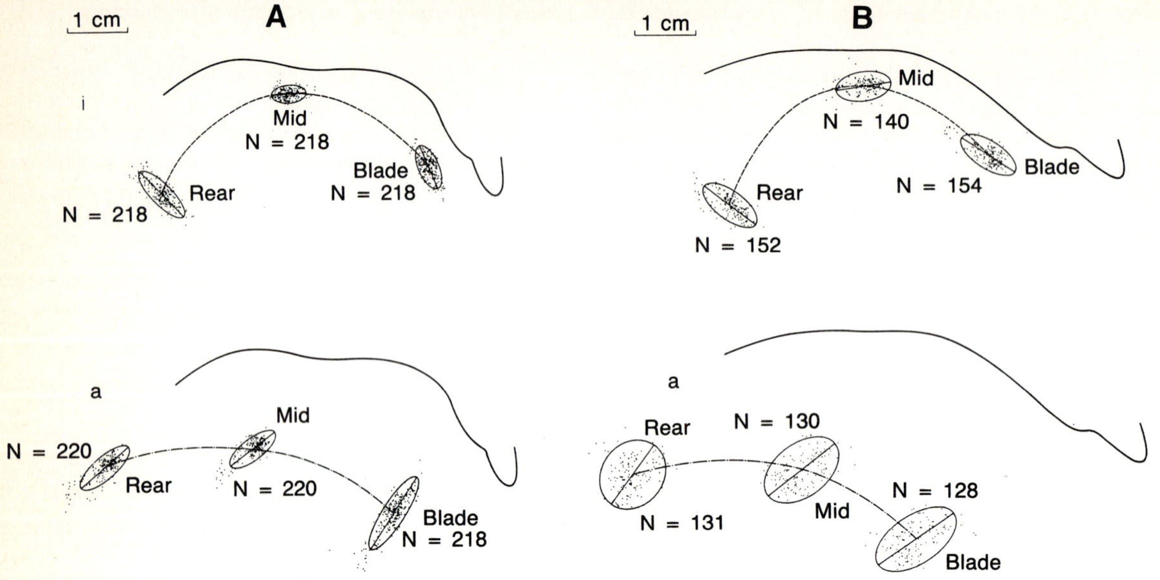

Figure 8–18 Scatterplots of variability of points on the tongue for repetitions of vowels /i/ (top plots) and /a/ (bottom plots) produced by two subjects (*A* and *B*). Each plotted point represents the *x-y* coordinate for a single vowel repetition, and the ellipses represent statistical approximations to the main axes of variability. See text for additional detail (from Perkell JS, Nelson WL. Variability in the production of the vowels /i/ and / æ /. J Acoust Soc Am 1985; 77:1889.)

perior are active for lip opening.[1] Lip rounding seems to be produced by activity of both the orbicularis oris superior and orbicularis oris inferior, and lip spreading possibly by the combined action of the depressor and levator anguli orii. However, Folkins and Kuehn have pointed out that these descriptions may not always hold because muscles designated as lip closers (e.g., the orbicularis oris inferior or the mentalis) may show some activity during lip opening.[1] The problem of EMG sampling of labial musculature has been treated more formally by Blair and Smith,[121] who argue that the complex interdigitization of muscle fibers in the region typically sampled for activity of the orbicularis oris inferior makes it impossible to isolate the activity of this muscle.[122] The anatomic issues discussed by Blair and Smith[121] suggest that the so-called compartmentalization of the orbicularis oris inferior activity reported by Abbs, Gracco, and Blair[123] was in fact a range of activity from *several* muscles whose fibers are intertwined in the orbicularis oris inferior sampling region.

EMG and Speech Production Research: Some Caveats

As suggested by this brief review, much valuable information concerning muscle activity of the upper articulators can be obtained using EMG techniques. However, the investigator who uses EMG techniques to study articulatory behavior, or the research consumer who wants to apply published research findings to theoretical or clinical efforts, must be aware of the limitations and vagaries of EMG techniques. First, as Blair and Smith have shown, even careful intramuscular insertion of hook-wire electrodes with minimal interelectrode distance (to minimize recording field) may not avoid an EMG recording that reflects activity from more than one muscle.[121] Although Blair and Smith make this case for EMG recording in the region of orbicularis oris inferior, this problem has been recognized for many years as the major obstacle to obtaining isolated EMG from the highly interdigitated, intrinsic muscles of the tongue. Even when a muscle is relatively free of fibers from other muscles, however, different electrode locations within the homogeneous muscle may not yield the same data. Cooper and Folkins,[124] following Lubker and May,[96] obtained simultaneous EMG recordings from a low, middle, and high location in the palatoglossus, a relatively simple muscle that seems to be involved in tongue raising for both vowels and consonants and perhaps in lowering of the velum for some subjects. Cooper and Folkins found that the recorded EMG activity during speech could vary quite a bit depending on electrode location and that the variation across electrode location may depend on utterance type or on the time at which the comparison was made within a single utterance. Figure 8–19 shows sample data from one of Cooper and Folkins' subjects who showed fairly large interlocation differences in EMG activity for

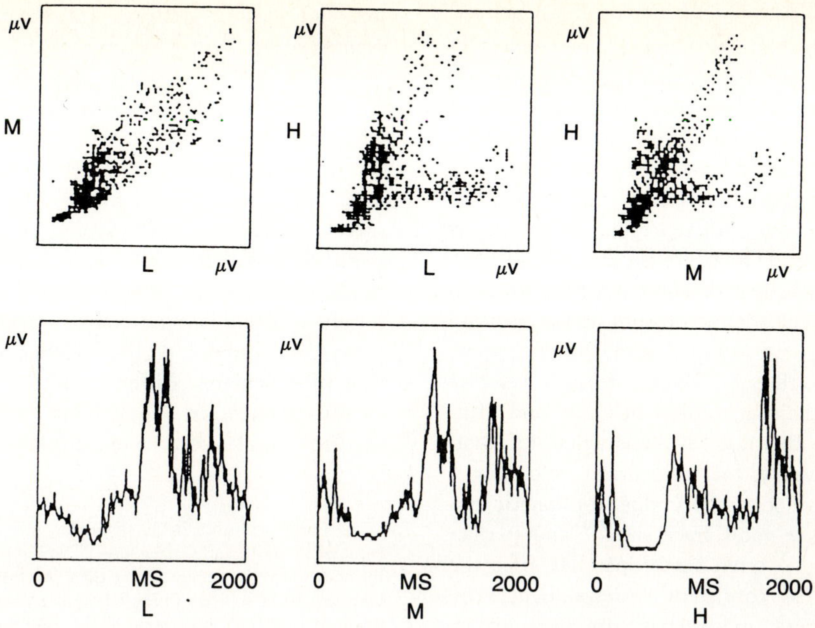

Figure 8–19 Pairwise correlations between EMG amplitudes (top plots) and simultaneously-recorded EMG waveforms (bottom plots) from three different electrode locations within palatoglossus muscle. The pairwise correlations are between all combinations of a low (L), medium (M), and high (H) location electrode in the muscle; if any electrode location was strictly representative of any other locations, the plots would all show straight line relationships. Similarly, the variation in the time history plots of the three electrode locations (bottom) shows that the activity from a particular electrode does not represent the activity from other electrodes (from Cooper DS, Folkins JW. Comparison of electromyographic signals from different electrode placements in the palatoglossus muscle. J Acoust Soc Am 1985; 78:1530.)

the utterance "dan." The bottom set of panels displays EMG waveforms for the three electrode locations, and the upper panels show scattergrams of microvolt values recorded every 2 msec for combinations of each pair of electrode locations. The differences in the waveforms at the three locations, plus the complex correlation patterns for electrode pairs,* suggest that it is not always prudent to take the activity from a single sampling site as a good representation of whole muscle activity. This result, together with points raised by Blair and Smith,[121] may explain the large intersubject differences in EMG that are often found in studies of articulation. It also points to the difficulty of relating EMG activity from a single muscle to structural movement[125] and strengthens the need for an ensemble of EMG data, both across and *within* muscles of interest.

* If the sampled activity from any location within a muscle was exactly representative of the sampled activity from any other location, the associated scattergram relating the activity at the two locations would show a straight line increasing in magnitude from left to right (r = 1.00).[121]

Articulatory Kinematics

Kinematic characteristics of the supraglottal articulators have been reported for the upper and lower lip, mandible, tongue, velum, and pharynx. It is not easy to provide concise summary statements for the kinematics of a particular articulator because speech samples, data collection techniques, and speakers vary widely across studies that have different purposes. Nevertheless, the available literature suggests that at least the following factors may exert a major influence on articulator displacements, velocities, accelerations, and gesture durations: syllable stress level, speaking rate, vocal tract dimensions of the speaker, gesture direction (opening or closing), and segment identity.

Table 8–2 summarizes selected kinematic data reported in the speech production literature.[126–132] The lack of a uniform organizational scheme for the different data sets reflects the variety of experimental designs and purposes noted before. Much of the variation in velocity values within and across studies may initially appear to be associated with factors such as stress, speaking rate, phonetic context, and so forth, but these relationships may be explained better by a general relationship between articulatory displacement and velocity. For example, Kelso et al report consistently lower velocities of the lower lip and jaw complex for unstressed, as compared to stressed, /ba/ repetitions, but this velocity difference is accompanied by similar differences in lower lip-jaw displacement (see also Ostry, Keller, and Parush[140]).[126] Similarly, the two subjects who reduce the lowering displacement of the tongue dorsum across speaking rate in the Ostry and Munhall study produce a corresponding reduction in tongue dorsum velocity; however, the remaining subject in Ostry and Munhall produced identical displacements for both speaking rates and virtually identical velocities.[127] Examination of velocity effects due to phonetic context,[129,139] speaker vocal tract size,[128] and perhaps even articulator,[128] often reveal parallel effects of displacement. Less consistent correspondences between displacement and velocity are seen for the comparison between opening and closing gestures.[126,129,130,132] This finding may be explained partly by the typically small differences between opening and closing gestures for the same phonetic events[139] (e.g., /ap/ versus /pa/).†

Although the general relationship between articulatory displacement and velocity has been known for some time,[135] its theoretical status has only recently been explored. Because the same correspondence has been shown for limb movements,[143,144] some speech researchers have adapted principles of limb motor control to the explanation component of speech production theories. Kelso et al[126] and Ostry and Munhall,[127] following Cooke,[144] argue that the velocity-displacement correspondence is a manifestation of articulator stiffness control by the central nervous system. In a particularly coherent account of this notion, Ostry and Munhall show that the

† One discrepancy in the displacement–velocity relationship is found in Smith and Gartenberg,[130] who reported greater lower lip and jaw velocities in adults than in children, even though both groups of subjects produced similar lower lip and jaw displacements. The interpretation of this finding is complicated by the results of a later study[142] in which kinematic details of the jaw were separated from those of the lower lip; whereas the jaw was faster for adults, as compared to children, the reverse was true for the lower lip.

TABLE 8–2 Selected Kinematic Data for Supraglottal Structures*

		Displacement	*Duration*	*Velocity*	*Comments*
Conversational	S1 O	14.6, 11.8	124, 112	229, 204	Source: Kelso et al[126] Speech: reiterant /ba/ repetitions. Kinematic data for combined lower lip and jaw. Technique: modified SELSPOT. O = opening (CV) gestures, C = closing (VC) gestures. First value in each cell = stressed syllable, second value = unstressed syllable.
	C	13.9, 12.1	92, 83	297, 265	
	S2 O	16.0, 12.6	140, 115	263, 239	
	C	16.0, 12.1	106, 85	322, 272	
Fast	S1 O	13.4, 10.4	103, 85	241, 216	
	C	13.0, 10.3	66, 65	348, 281	
	S2 O	14.9, 8.3	120, 81	241, 170	
	C	14.9, 8.2	87, 67	323, 202	
Conversational (slow)	S1	9.7	210	95.7	Source: Ostry and Munhall[127] Speech: Repeated /$\{^{k}_{g}\}$V/ pairs where V = /a/, /o/, and /u/. Kinematic data for lowering gesture of tongue dorsum, pooled across vowels and consonant voicing. Technique: ultrasound.
	S2	8.1	219	72.8	
	S3	9.4	184	98.5	
Fast	S1	7.9	171	82.6	
	S2	8.1	202	77.2	
	S3	7.2	148	87.2	
	Lower lip	12.2	80	166	Source: Kuehn and Moll[128] Speech: nonsense CV, VCVC sequences. Kinematic data for indicated structures pooled across 5 adults. Technique: lateral-view cineradiography and pellet-tracking.
Conversational	Tongue tip	14.2	83	196	
	Tongue dorsum	10.0	74	129	

TABLE 8–2 (Continued)

	Displacement	*Duration*	*Velocity*	*Acceleration*	*Comments*
S1 O	8, 6, 3	180, 144, 120	86, 69, 39		Source: Parush et al[129]
C	8, 6, 3	130, 140, 145	108, 78, 40		Speech: Symmetric VCVs, with V = /a/, /o/, and /u/, C = /k/, /g/. Kinematic data for tongue dorsum, apparently pooled across two consonants. The three values in each cell are for V = /a/, /o/, /u/, respectively.
Conversational S2 O	8, 7, 3	192, 149, 137	84, 83, 40		Technique: ultrasound.
C	8, 7, 4	183, 214, 140	83, 72, 46		
S3 O	8, 7, 3	167, 136, 140	89, 86, 43		
C	9, 8, 5	167, 165, 193	89, 84, 51		
Jaw and lower lip O	6.6, 13.4	No data	103, 162		Source: Smith and Gartenberg[130]
Conversational C	6.3, 6.2	No data	131, 160		Speech: CVC words in carrier, where C = /p/, /b/, /f/, V = /i/, /I/, /a/. Kinematic data pooled across three adults and consonants; velocity data reported here derived from published figures. First value in each cell = high vowel context, second value = low vowel context. Closing data for displacement are for VC gesture preceding initial C in target word, as a function of target-word vowel.
Jaw O	2.8, 8.0	No data	32, 86		Technique: strain-gauges mounted on beams; jaw beam attached to chin.
Lower Lip C	2.7, 2.4	No data	41, 70		
O	3.8, 5.4	No data	71, 76		
C	3.6, 3.8	No data	93, 92		
S1	0.3, 2.6	62, 311	6, 28	196, 686	Source: Nelson et al[131]
Opening S2	1.1, 6.6	74, 262	22, 69	490, 1275	Speech: continuous repetition of /sa/, from very slow to very fast. Kinematic data for jaw. First value in each cell is minimum, second value is maximum of three slow-to-fast trials.
S3	2.1, 15.7	53, 287	62, 272	1471, 8531	Technique: strain-gauge mounted on beam attached to tooth.
S1	0.2, 2.7	55, 227	3, 27	98, 1079	
Closing S2	1.0, 6.7	78, 414	17, 61	196, 2059	
S3	1.9, 16.6	67, 252	39, 203	784, 11473	
S1 O	4.7	96	49		Source: Kuehn[132].
C	7.9	124	70		Speech: VCNV and VNCV sequences (N = nasal) in carrier phrase. Kinematic data for velum. Opening gestures for VCNV sequences, closing gestures for VNCV sequences.
S2 O	7.1	97	96		Technique: lateral-view cineradiography and pellet-tracking.
C	9.3	109	104		

Additional kinematic data can be found in references 112, 133–141.

*Displacement values in mm; time values in msec; velocity values in mm/sec; acceleration data in mm/sec/sec.

ratio of maximum lowering velocity (tongue dorsum) to movement amplitude (Vmax/D), which serves as an estimate of stiffness, varies in an inverse, curvilinear way with movement duration (T).[127] Figure 8–20 illustrates this relationship for each of the three subjects studied by Ostry and Munhall,[127] who suggest that "Since systematic relationships between Vmax/D and T are present on a within condition basis, the patterns . . . presumably reflect the mechanisms by which the nervous system actually affects (sic) changes in movement duration. That is, the patterns do not appear to arise simply as a consequence of manipulating variables such as rate, vowel, or consonant" (p 654). In other words, the nervous system need not work out a variety of duration specifications for the various phenomena such as stress, rate, phonetic identity, and so forth; rather a specification of articulator stiffness alone dictates the movement duration. Articulators set at high stiffness produce movements of short duration, whereas more compliant settings result in movements of longer duration. The stiffness parameterization is not categorized according to movements associated with a given phenomenon (e.g., movements from a dorsal consonant to a high-front vowel, or movements associated with fast speaking rates), but seems to vary across movement duration in a continuous fashion.

For Ostry and Munhall, the function relating articulatory movement duration to stiffness offers an appealingly simple account of the systematic variability in articulatory kinematics;[127] moreover, this perspective on speech motor control is consistent with contemporary trends in general motor control theory, which is traditionally formulated to account for limb behavior. Kelso et al arrive at a similar conclusion, although their account provides a more explicit formulation of articulatory dynamics in terms of mass-spring behavior.[126] Kelso et al are also concerned more directly with an account of articulatory dynamics wherein time is not imposed on the movements (see next section and Nelson[145]).[126]

Theories of Speech Production: Central Issues

Coarticulation

Coarticulation is a term used to describe a phenomenon wherein the articulation of a given sound is affected by the identity of the surrounding context. Forward or right-to-left coarticulation implies that some aspect of the articulation of a sound is affected by the articulatory characteristics of a sound occurring later in a sequence; backward or left-to right coarticulation implies that some aspect of the articulation of a sound is affected by the articulatory characteristics of a sound that occurred previously in a sequence. Well-known examples of coarticulation are [stu], wherein the /s/ and /t/ are produced with the lip rounding required for the vowel /u/ (forward coarticulation), and [nou], wherein the velopharyngeal opening required for /n/ shows up to some degree for the vowel (backward coarticulation). This standard concept of coarticulation[146] requires, in a theoretical sense, that specific articulatory requirements be part of the specification of a language's phonemes. How these requirements might be specified—and if they should be specified at all—has been the subject of no small debate.[147]

Coarticulation is a pervasive phenomenon in speech production. Context-conditioned variability in speech production has been demonstrated in the pharynx,[148] velum[97,149] tongue[135] jaw,[119] and lips.[150] Moreover, coarticulatory phenomena can be observed at any level of analysis, as evidenced by EMG,[151,152] movement,[136] palatographic,[153] aerodynamic,[154] acoustic,[155–157] and perceptual[158] data.

A standard explanation for coarticulation is as follows.[146] As part of utterance formulation, a speaker chooses and arrays the appropriate phonemes in the proper ordinal sequence (i.e., in notional time; see Kent and Minifie[147]). Each phoneme has articulatory specifications, which are perhaps those that correspond to a context-less articulation (canonical form; see Daniloff and Hammarberg[146]) of the sound. On the one hand, forward coarticulation occurs when a scanning mechanism (Henke's look-ahead operator[159]) looks down the sequence and notes those articulatory requirements for upcoming phonemes that are compatible with the articulatory requirements of the currently executed phoneme. On the other hand, backward coarticulation is not a reflection of a planning mechanism, but rather is a manifestation of the inertial characteristics of the articulators. Typically, the domain of backward coarticulation effects is limited to adjacent or twice-removed phonemes, but under certain circumstances, forward coarticulation effects may span up to six phonemes. As discussed by Kent and Minifie in their comprehensive review of coarticulation,[147] there are variants on the theme summarized previously, but this is the understanding of coarticulatory phenomena that has dominated the field for many years.

Coproduction, Coordinative Structures, and Action Theory

In recent years, several investigators have questioned this standard view of coarticulation, mostly

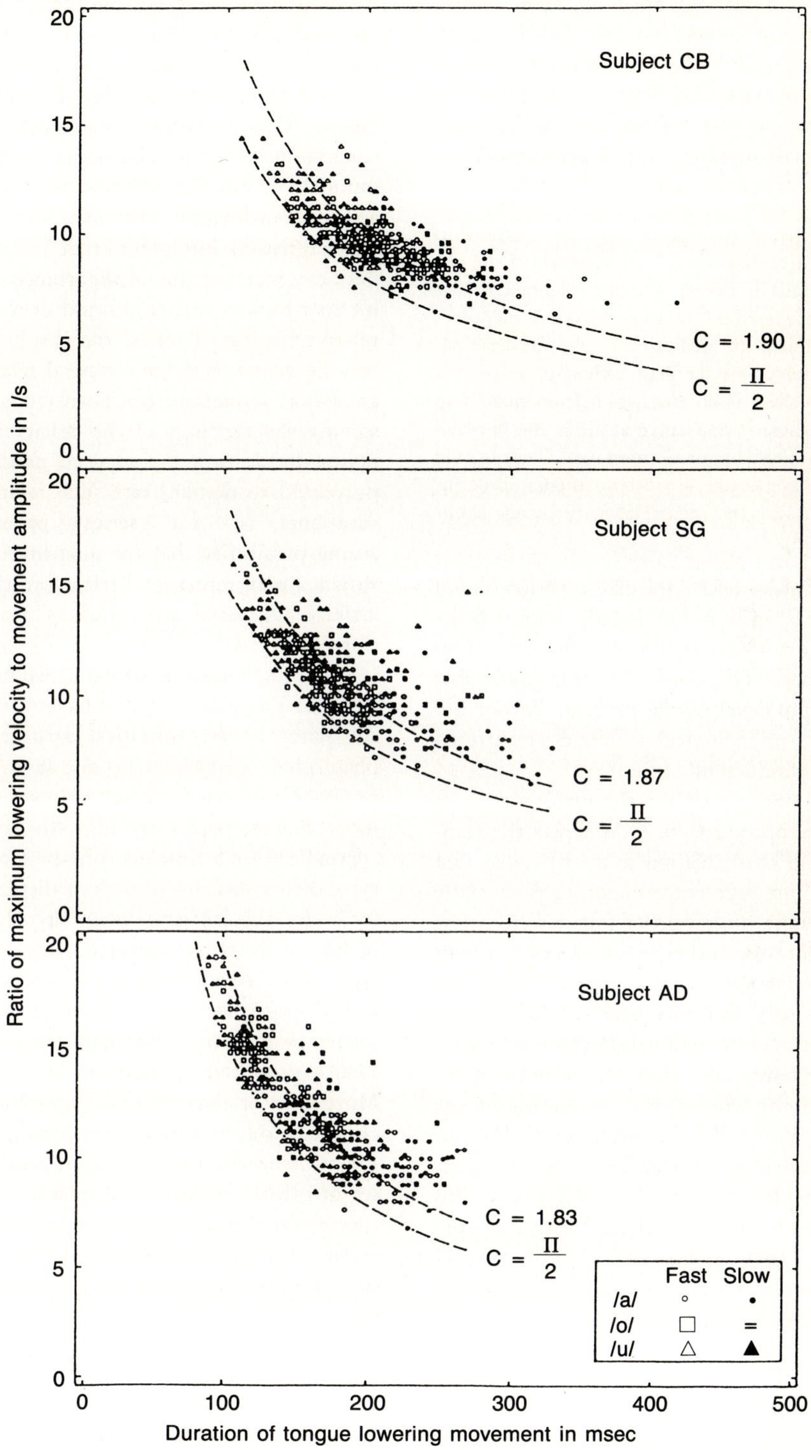

Figure 8-20 Relationship between maximum velocity/movement amplitude ration (*y*-axis) and duration of tongue lowering (*x*-axis) across three vowels (/a/, /o/, /u/) and two speaking rates (conversational and fast). Data are shown for three subjects. The dashed lines show best fit functions for relationship $V\max/D = C/T$ (top line in each panel) and functions where $C = \pi/2$, or a mass-spring system without damping (bottom line in each panel) (from Ostry DJ, Munhall KG. Control of rate and duration of speech movements. J Acoust Soc Am 1985; 77:640.)

because of a dissatisfaction with the need to invoke and reify the phoneme. The most explicit argument against theories that envision arrays of phonemes as a stage in producing speech has been advanced by Fowler.[160] Fowler argues that theories requiring a translation from mental activity (i.e., the phoneme array) to physical activity (observable articulatory behavior) are unparsimonious and therefore undesirable. Rather, she suggests that

> A different way of conceptualizing the relationship between plan and actualization . . . makes use of the observation that language forms, whether planned or actualized, are always realized in some physical medium. When they are planned, the medium . . . is at least neural; when they are uttered it is at least articulatory. In this conceptualization, there is no translation from mental to physical; indeed, there is no change at all at the 'mental' or cognitive level of the linguistic message. There is only a replication of the message across two media, brought about in whatever way that neural activity brings about motor activity (p 235).[161]

In other words, Fowler rejects the classic notion (found in many textbooks) of neatly arranged, discrete units at an organizational level of the speech production process being smashed together in an unrecognizable mess at the output level of the process. Fowler believes that ". . . phonological segments are uttered intact in speech production" (p 238).[161]

Fowler chooses to redefine the phenomenon of coarticulation as coproduction.[161] Whereas the standard conception of coarticulation seems to imply that the influence of one segment on another potentially involves a wholesale migration of features from one discrete time slot to another, coproduction allows that the component gestures of a segment may not occur simultaneously and may overlap with one or more component gestures of a neighboring segment. Moreover, these temporally complex patterns of coproduction are highly changeable, depending on the prevailing goal of the speech mechanism. Various articulatory gestures may be transiently linked to accomplish an articulatory goal, then unlinked as this goal expires and the next one arises. These goal-specific linkages, often called "coordinative structures,"[101,161] have been demonstrated for speech production behavior by Kelso, Tuller, Vatikiotis-Bateson, and Fowler.[162] When the jaw closing gesture for the final obstruent in /bæb/ and /bæz/ was perturbed, a relatively large and apparently compensatory displacement of the upper lip was observed for final /b/ but not /z/. EMG data from the intrinsic tongue muscles provided the complementary finding of apparently compensatory lingual adjustments for /z/ but not /b/ during jaw perturbation. Thus the linkages between articulators are functional, adapting themselves to the prevailing task requirements. Details of how these linkages (coordinative structures) are modified from moment to moment and how they may span adjacent goals (in standard terms, segments) have not been worked out.

As discussed by Kugler, Kelso, and Turvey,[163] Fowler,[161] and others, coordinative structures presumably have certain characteristics that make them uniquely adaptable to the control of action. For example, coordinative structures have certain variable characteristics, but others that are invariant. Much has been made of the unimportance of absolute time for coordinative structures and of the importance of relative timing. That is, the absolute rate of action may be varied, but the temporal relationships within an action sequence stay fairly constant, thus preserving the topology of the behavior.[163] Several experiments dealing with speech production behavior purported to demonstrate such relational, temporal invariants,[164–166] but a series of papers has raised the strong possibility that the quantitatively defined invariance may represent little more than a statistical artifact associated with various aspects of correlational analysis.[167–170]

Kelso, Vatikiotis-Bateson, Saltzman, and Kay[126] (see also Kelso et al[101–102]) have attempted to avoid the potential for statistical artifact by employing phase-plane analysis of lip and jaw movement. Figure 8–21 illustrates how a time history of movement characteristics can be redisplayed (and reconceptualized) in a timeless, phase-plane display.* The typical time-history records of displacement and velocity for the jaw and lower lip, shown at the left of Figure 8–21, are plotted point by point on the right in an x-y coordinate space where x = velocity and y = displacement. The multiple orbits shown in the jaw and lower lip phase planes are for repeated /ba/s, produced in the form of reiterant speech.[172] Movement of the jaw and lower lip from one /b/ closure to the next /b/ closure would describe a single orbit on the phase plane. Examination of either set of orbits reveals the displacement-velocity relationship reviewed before (i.e., as the top-to-bottom extent of an orbit increases, so does its width) and suggests a certain morphologic similarity across orbits of differing height and width.

Kelso et al attempt to circumvent the statistical problems associated with their relative timing analysis by using the cyclic nature of phase plane orbits to implement an analysis of the constancy of

---

* The claim that the phase-plane displays shown by Kelso et al[126] do not incorporate time explicitly has been questioned by Kent, who points out that the inclusion of velocity in the phase-plane provides a time aspect in the display.[171]

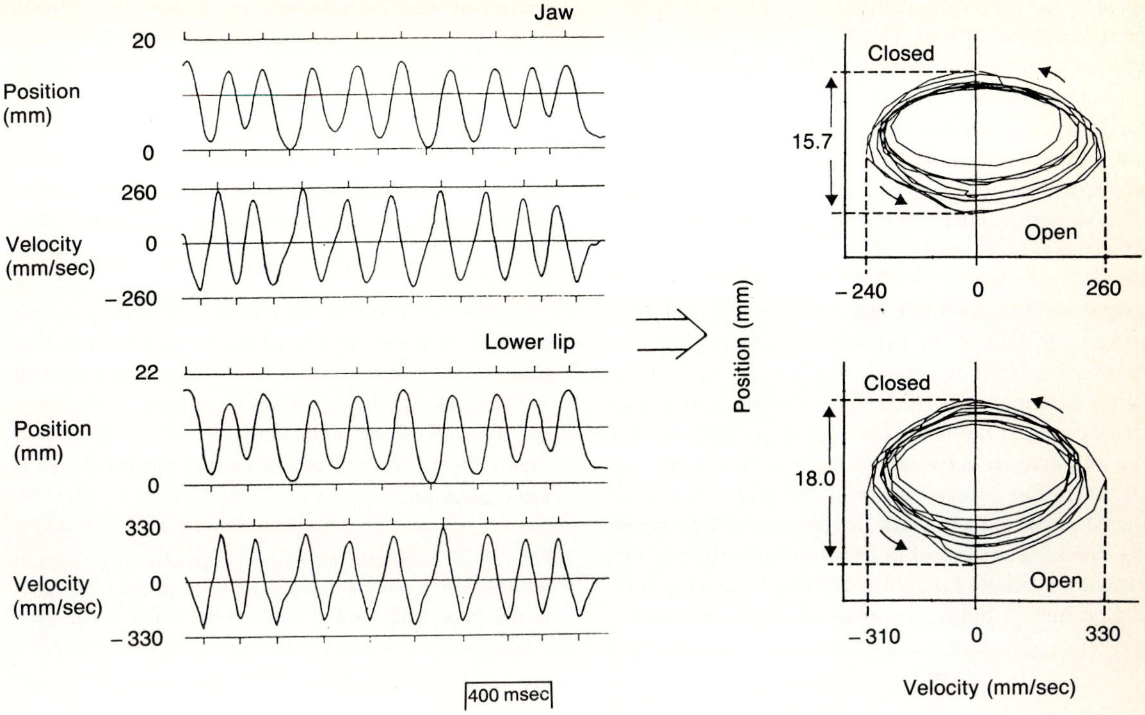

Figure 8–21 Position and velocity time histories for jaw and lower lip (left panels), and their mappings onto phase planes depicting position on the *y*-axis and velocity on the *x*-axis. The multiple orbits on the phase plane correspond to the multiple repetitions of /ba/, shown as the cyclic patterns in the time-history records (from Kelso JAS, Vatikiotis-Bateson E, Saltzman EL, Kay B. A qualitative dynamic analysis of reiterant speech production: phase portraits, kinematics, and dynamic modeling. J Acoust Soc Am 1985; 77:266.)

interarticulator phasing.[101,102] Using angular notation, Kelso et al identify on the jaw phase plane the onset of inferior upper lip movement to effect closure (or rounding) for medial /b/, /p/, and /w/ in CVCVC sequences. Statistical evaluation of the influence of stress and speaking rate on upper lip phasing in the jaw phase plane revealed no significant effects, suggesting a relational invariant under conditions where large changes occur in articulatory durations and displacements. Kelso et al regard the analysis scheme and results as important because

...once articulatory motions are represented geometrically on the phase plane, the phase angle serves to normalize duration across speaker, stress, speaking rate . . . these analyses potentially provide a grounding for so-called intrinsic timing theories of speech production[160,173] since neither absolute nor relative durations need be monitored or controlled extrinsically, and no time-keeping mechanisms or time controllers are required in this formulation (p 44).[101]

See also Kelso and Tuller.[174] Lubker attempted to replicate the findings of Kelso et al,[101] but could not demonstrate the phasing constancies described above.[175] For their part, Kelso et al claim that Lubker's analysis is not comparable to theirs because of his failure to normalize the units of analysis in the phase plane.[102] The reader is encouraged to examine the January 1986 issue of *Journal of Phonetics* for an in-depth presentation of the Kelso and colleagues position as well as the several objections to it.

Motor Equivalence

When a speaker produces the same phonetic sequence many times, the articulatory movements are not strictly stereotypical across repetitions. Rather small variations are observed in characteristics of the articulatory gestures (such as displacement, velocity, duration, and so on) needed to produce the phonetic sequence. This phenomenon—that there are many ways to achieve a single goal—has been called "motor equivalence" and has been taken to imply a subordination of the details of individual movements to the overall goal of an action.[176] Gracco and Abbs have presented data suggesting that even when the displacements or velocities of two articulators involved in a phonetic goal are plotted against one another, the across-repetition variability is large (Fig. 8–22) even though the phonetic goal (producing bilabial closure for the first /p/ in the sequence /sæpæpl/) is realized.[177] This result seems to be inconsistent—at least in a broad sense—with the constant phasing notion of Kelso et al.[101]

The subordination of individual movements to larger goals (whether they be goals defined at the vocal tract level, acoustic level, or some combination of the former and latter; see Perkell[178]) has also been demonstrated under conditions where normal speech movements are transiently or statically disturbed during articulation.[179–184] In the case of transient perturbations, corrective responses are typically observed not only in the perturbed structure, but also in nonperturbed structures involved in the articulatory gesture under study. For example, a transient disturbance to the lower lip–closing gesture for /b/ elicits corrective responses in both the lower and upper lips. The precise nature of the perturbation-induced response in the two lips appears to depend on the temporal relationship between perturbation onset and the onset of muscular activity for the lip-closing gesture.[181] Static disturbances in articulatory behavior, as may be achieved by fixing jaw position with various-sized bite blocks, result in some adjustment of upper and lower lip movement parameters but not in the eventual goal of closing the lips.[182] Because lip closure was found to occur at a variety of spatial locations with different-sized bite blocks, the notion of some relatively invariant space-coordinate system for articulatory goals[185] (see MacNeilage for additional counter evidence[186]) seems to be rejectable.

Most of these studies deal with the construct of goals to which individual movements are subordinated, but few authors have developed coherent notions about goals and shown how these can be tested in the laboratory (MacNeilage being a notable exception[185]). Perkell has described orosensory vocal tract goals as

> . . . the production-related correlates of distinctive features. The goals are determined by anatomical, sensory, neurological, and quantal-acoustic constraints. The goals

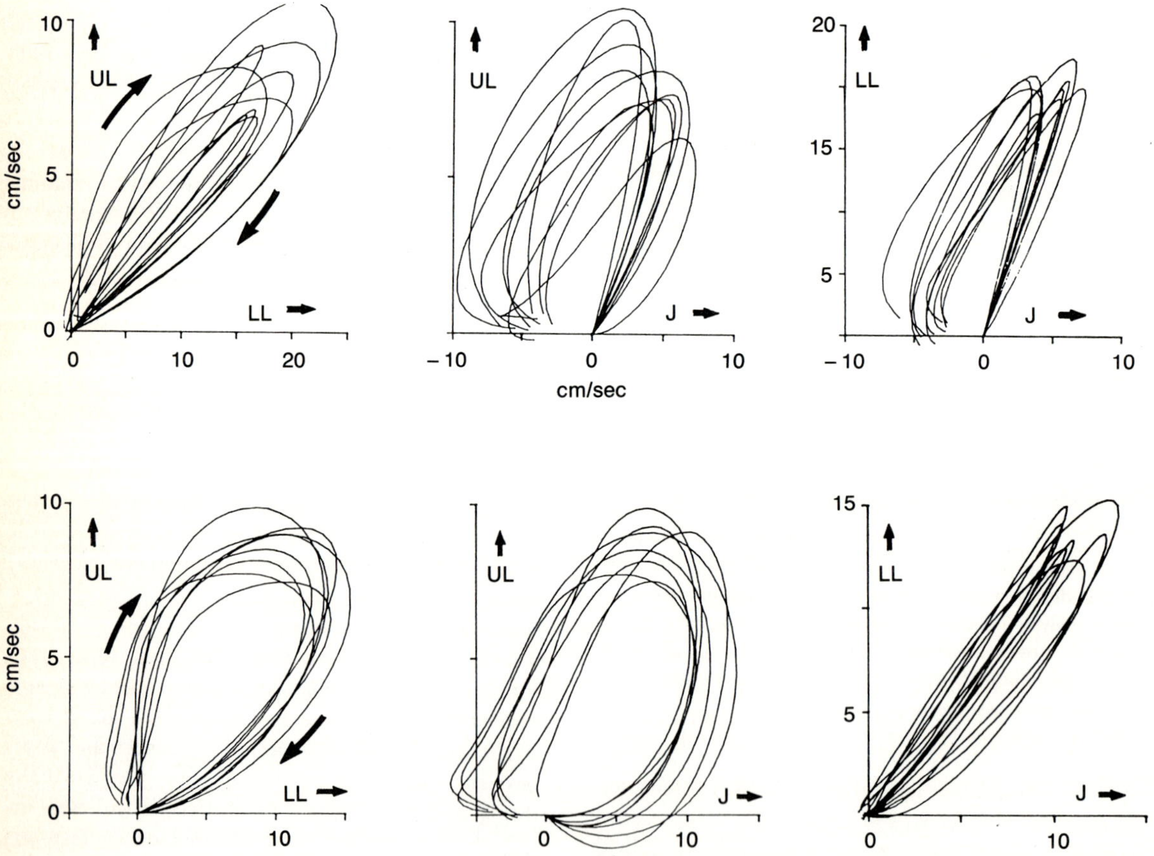

Figure 8–22 Instantaneous velocities of upper lip (UL) versus lower lip (LL) (left panels), UL versus jaw (J) (middle panels), and LL versus J (right panels) for two subjects (subject 1-top panels, subject 2-bottom panels) producing the first bilabial closing gesture in "sap apple." The long arrows in the left panels indicate the progression of motion, which is the same for all plots. Note the absence of stereotypy in the velocity-velocity displays (from Gracco VL, Abbs JH. Variant and invariant characteristics of speech movement. Exp Brain Res 1986; 65:156.)

may include patterns and forces of contact between articulators that oppose one another, levels of intraoral air pressure and air flow, and amounts of tension that muscles may develop (p 344).[178]

The inclusion of the many factors (such as aerodynamics, muscle sense, and so forth) that are part of the phenomenon of speech production is an attractive aspect of Perkell's concept of goals, but the inclusiveness also makes it difficult to formulate specific hypotheses to test the concept. Other candidates for vocal tract goals during speech production include aerodynamic resistance[187] (i.e., constriction magnitudes) and spectral or spectrotemporal characteristics of the speech waveform.[188,189]

Constancies and Building Blocks of Articulatory Behavior

Earlier in this section, I described the search for constancies in the relative timing of articulatory sequences and interarticulator phasing. Investigators have also been interested in the possibility that certain simple stereotypic articulatory movements may be variously combined to create more complex articulatory sequences. For example, Kent showed that the articulatory gestures for two VCVs (such as /aga/ and /ama/) could be superimposed and adjusted in time to match the gestures associated with a VCCV sequence (such as /agma/).[190] Moreover, a degree of stereotypy in vowel-to-consonant and consonant-to-vowel transitions may serve as a highly stable feature of these simple articulatory building blocks.[137,190–191] Kent's views on combining stereotypic articulatory movements to form complex articulatory sequences are consistent with the spirit of Fowler's notion of coproduction[161] wherein the boundaries between sounds do not involve discrete terminations and beginnings of articulatory gestures, but rather involve overlap of the sequential gestures.

The stability of articulatory transitions has been elevated to an axiom of speech production theory by Fujimura,[192] who has described an iceberg model of articulatory invariance. The iceberg pattern is a metaphor for an elementary gesture that can be varied temporally relative to the movements of other articulators. The temporal variation of the iceberg does not disturb the invariant and elemental characteristics of the pattern. The affinity of this concept to Kent's stereotypic articulatory movements should be obvious. Figure 8–23 illustrates movement data supporting the iceberg concept. Nine movement trajectories of a point on the tongue blade (x-ray microbeam data) for the [sɛ] sequence of the word "seven" are shown. These nine trajectories, derived from nine separate utterances in which factors such as rate and stress varied, have a central portion (the iceberg) that is remarkably similar in terms of distance covered and slope. Other motor control theorists have also argued that transition phenomena can represent highly stable anchor points for the assembly of fluent movement sequences.[191,193] The phenomenology and theoretical status of elemental articulatory gestures should be active areas of investigation as new techniques increase the feasibility of collection and analysis of large data bases for speech movements.

SUMMARY

Speech breathing is characterized by a stereotyped chest wall posture that is subtly modified throughout lung volume to achieve the subglottal pressure requirement of an utterance. The global characteristics of this posture are similar across speakers, although details of the chest wall configuration seem to be speaker-specific and are preserved across speaking tasks. This chest wall posture, or the inference of it, was not accounted for by the well-known work of Draper et al partly because of a method

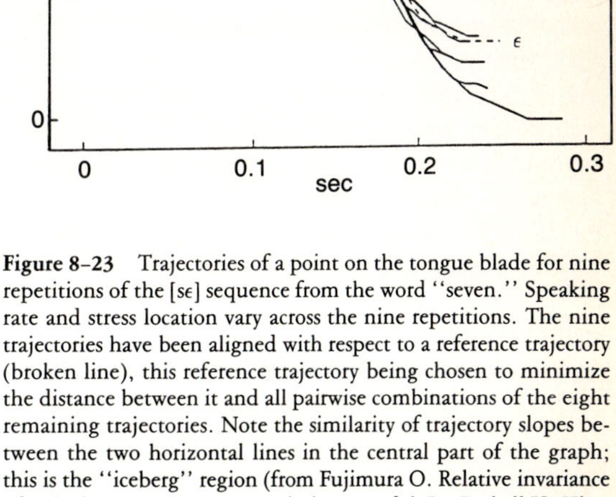

Figure 8–23 Trajectories of a point on the tongue blade for nine repetitions of the [sɛ] sequence from the word "seven." Speaking rate and stress location vary across the nine repetitions. The nine trajectories have been aligned with respect to a reference trajectory (broken line), this reference trajectory being chosen to minimize the distance between it and all pairwise combinations of the eight remaining trajectories. Note the similarity of trajectory slopes between the two horizontal lines in the central part of the graph; this is the "iceberg" region (from Fujimura O. Relative invariance of articulatory movements: an iceberg model. In: Perkell JS, Klatt DH, eds. Invariance and variability in speech processes. Hillsdale, NJ: Erlbaum, 1986:221.)

that focused on individual muscles rather than chest wall parts. The kinematics and dynamics techniques are logical methodologic solutions to the problems raised by speech production therories that stress the action of muscle groups or collectives, rather than the action of individual muscles or structures; such theories are considered toward the end of the chapter. Knowledge of the integration of speech breathing with overall language processes is meager, but some recently published works point to a future line of inquiry that can address this issue.

Vocal fold vibration involves highly complex movements that are predictable from the histologic structure of the tissue and from the forces imposed on the tissue. Mechanisms of frequency and intensity control, as well as the mode of vocal fold vibration, suggest that researchers should study the overall pattern of muscular activity in order to understand laryngeal control in speech. Advances have been made in noninvasive techniques for the study of vocal fold vibration, and refinement of these techniques should lead to a larger data base than has heretofore been available. The larynx serves an important role in segmental articulation, as evidenced by studies of the laryngeal devoicing gesture.

Contemporary work in the area of articulatory behavior focuses on the determination of articulator movement characteristics and the ways in which the movements are coordinated and assembled as cooperatives to achieve phonetic goals. Several theories of speech production have been described; no one theory emerges as an obvious choice, but several interesting directions for future study and evaluation of the existing theories are proposed.

In the last 30 years, tremendous advances in the understanding of speech production processes have been made. Many of these advances can be tied to technologic breakthroughs, but just as many are probably attributable to innovations in the conceptual domain. For example, the current understanding of laryngeal physiology is undoubtedly due to technologic advances in histologic and movement analysis, whereas the current view of articulatory behavior has more to do with conceptual developments. The contemporary view of respiratory function for speech probably reflects more of a combination of technologic and conceptual innovations, as described previously in the section on Speech Breathing. In my opinion, a careful review of the literature suggests the danger of allowing technology to drive the questions that one asks about the speech production process. The major unanswered questions about speech production—such as the manner in which the respiratory, laryngeal, and supraglottal structures are *co-controlled* as a superordinate coordinative structure—demand careful conceptual analysis to guide research efforts. This analysis should be informed by technologic issues, but must be equally informed by the extant body of speech physiology, acoustic, and linguistic data.

REFERENCES

1. Folkins JW, Kuehn DP. Speech production. In: Lass NJ, McReynolds LV, Northern JL, Yoder DE, eds. Speech, language, and hearing. Vol. 1. Normal processes. Philadelphia: WB Saunders, 1982:246.
2. Hixon TJ. Respiratory function in speech. In: Minifie FD, Hixon TJ, Williams F, eds. Normal aspects of speech, hearing, and language. Englewood Cliffs, NJ: Prentice-Hall, 1973:37.
3. Draper MH, Ladefoged P, Whitteridge D. Respiratory muscles in speech. J Speech Hear Res 1959; 2:16–27.
4. Rahn H, Otis AB, Chadwick LE, Fenn WO. The pressure volume diagram of the thorax and lung. Am J Physiol 1946; 146:161–178.
5. Weismer G. Speech breathing. In: Daniloff RG, ed. Speech science. San Diego: College-Hill Press, 1985:47.
6. Draper MH, Ladefoged P, Whitteridge D. Expiratory muscles and airflow during speech. Br Med J 1960; 18:1837–1843.
7. Kunze LH. Evaluation of methods of estimating sub-glottal air pressure. J Speech Hear Res 1964; 7:151–164.
8. Eblen RE Jr. Limitations on use of surface electromyography in studies of speech breathing. J Speech Hear Res 1963; 6:3–18.
9. Hoshiko MS. Sequence of action of breathing muscles during speech. J Speech Hear Res 1960; 3:291–297.
10. Ladefoged P. Comment on "Evaluation of methods of estimating sub-glottal air pressure." J Speech Hear Res 1964; 7:291.
11. Hixon TJ, Goldman M, Mead J. Kinematics of the chest wall during speech production: volume displacements of the rib cage, abdomen, and lung. J Speech Hear Res 1973; 16:78–115.
12. Hixon TJ, Mead J, Goldman MD. Dynamics of the chest wall during speech production: function of the thorax, rib cage, diaphragm, and abdomen. J Speech Hear Res 1976; 19:297–356.
13. Sears TA. Servo-control of the intercostal muscles. In: Desmedt JE, ed. New developments in electromyography and clinical neurophysiology. Basel: Karger, 1973:404.
14. Konno K, Mead J. Measurement of the separate volume changes of rib cage and abdomen during breathing. J Appl Physiol 1967; 22:407–422.
15. McCool FD, Loring SH, Mead J. Rib cage distortion during voluntary and involuntary breathing acts. J Appl Physiol 1985; 58:1703–1712.
16. DeTroyer A, Yernault JC, Englert M, Baran D, Paiva M. Evolution of intrathoracic airway mechanics during lung growth. J Appl Physiol 1978; 44:521–527.
17. Estenne M, Yernault JC, DeTroyer A. Rib cage and diaphragm-abdomen compliance in humans: effects of age and posture. J Appl Physiol 1985; 59:1842–1848.
18. Gaultier C, Zinman R. Maximal static pressure in healthy children. Respir Physiol 1983; 51:45–61.
19. Russell NK, Stathopoulos ET. Adult/child lung volume differences during speech production. J Speech Hear Res 1987; in press.
20. Hoit J, Hixon TJ. Age and speech breathing. J Speech Hear Res 1987; 30:351–366.

21. Fugl-Meyer A. Relative respiratory contributions of the rib cage and abdomen in males and females with special regard to posture. Respiration 1974; 31:240–251.
22. Hodge MM, Putnam AHB, Weismer G. Respiratory kinematics in adult female speakers. Paper presented at the American Speech-Language-Hearing Association Annual Convention, Detroit, MI, 1986.
23. Wilder CN. Chest wall preparation for phonation in female speakers. In: Bless DM, Abbs JH, eds. Vocal fold physiology. San Diego: College-Hill Press, 1983:109.
24. Hoit JD, Hixon TJ. Body type and speech breathing. J Speech Hear Res 1986; 29:313–324.
25. Daubenspeck JA. Influence of small mechanical loads on variability of breathing pattern. J Appl Physiol: Respir Environ Exerc Physiol 1981; 50:299–306.
26. Newsom Davis J. Introduction. In: Campbell EJM, Agostoni E, Newsom Davis J, eds. The respiratory muscles: mechanics and neural control. Philadelphia: WB Saunders, 1970:1.
27. Watson PJ, Hixon TJ. Respiratory kinematics in classical (opera) singers. J Speech Hear Res 1985; 28:104–122.
28. Baken RJ. Estimation of lung volume change from torso hemicircumferences. J Speech Hear Res 1977; 20:808–812.
29. Baken RJ, Cavallo SA. Prephonatory chest wall posturing. Folia Phoniatr (Basel) 1981; 33:193–203.
30. Baken RJ, Cavallo SA, Weissman KL. Chest wall movements prior to phonation. J Speech Hear Res 1979; 22:862–872.
31. Cavallo SA, Baken RJ. Prephonatory laryngeal and chest wall dynamics. J Speech Hear Res 1985; 28:79–87.
32. Mead J, Loring SH. Analysis of volume displacement and length changes of the diaphragm during breathing. J Appl Physiol: Respir Environ Exerc Physiol 1982; 53:750–755.
33. Loring SH, Mead J. Action of the diaphragm on the rib cage inferred from a force-balance analysis. J Appl Physiol: Respir Environ Exerc Physiol 1982; 53:756–760.
34. Lieberman P. Direct comparison of sub-glottal and esophageal pressure during speech. J Acoust Soc Am 1968; 43:1157–1164.
35. Grosjean F, Collins M. Breathing, pausing and reading. Phonetica 1979; 36:98–114.
36. Goldman Eisler F. Psycholinguistics: experiments in spontaneous speech. London: Academic Press, 1968.
37. Schönle PW, Conrad B. Hesitation vowels: a motor speech respiration hypothesis. Neurosci Lett 1985; 55:293–296.
38. Siegman AW. Cognition and hesitation in speech. In: Siegman AW, Feldstein S, eds. Of speech and time. Temporal speech patterns in interpersonal contexts. Hillsdale, NJ: Erlbaum, 1979:179.
39. Stevens KN, Hirano M. Vocal fold physiology. Tokyo: University of Tokyo Press, 1981.
40. Bless DM, Abbs JH, eds. Vocal fold physiology. San Diego: College-Hill Press, 1983.
41. Titze IR, Scherer RC. Vocal fold physiology: biomechanics, acoustics, and phonatory control. Denver: Denver Center for the Performing Arts, 1985.
42. Baer T, Sasaki C, Harris K. Laryngeal function in phonation and respiration. San Diego: College-Hill Press, 1987.
43. Hirano M. Structure and vibratory behavior of the vocal folds. In: Sawashima M, Cooper FS, eds. Dynamic aspects of speech production. Tokyo: University of Tokyo Press, 1977:13.
44. Hirano M, Kurita S, Nakashima T. The structure of the vocal folds. In: Stevens KN, Hirano M, eds. Vocal fold physiology. Tokyo: University of Tokyo Press, 1981:33.
45. Hirano M, Kakita Y, Ohmaru K, Kurita S. Structure and mechanical properties of the vocal fold. In: Lass NJ, ed. Speech and language: advances in basic research and practice. Vol. 7. New York: Academic Press, 1982:271.
46. Hirano M, Kakita Y. Cover-body theory of vocal fold vibration. In: Daniloff RG, ed. Speech science. San Diego: College-Hill Press, 1985:1.
47. Hollien H. On vocal registers. J Phonetics 1974; 2:125–143.
48. Hirano M. Morphological structure of the vocal cord as a vibrator and its variations. Folia Phoniatr (Basel) 1974; 26:89–94.
49. Atkinson JE. Correlation analysis of the physiological factors controlling fundamental voice frequency. J Acous Soc Am 1978; 63:211–222.
50. Erickson D, Baer T, Harris KS. The role of the strap muscles in pitch lowering. In: Bless DM, Abbs JH, eds. Vocal fold physiology. San Diego: College-Hill Press, 1983:279.
51. Honda K. Variability analysis of laryngeal muscle activities. In: Titze IR, Scherer RC, eds. Vocal fold physiology. San Diego: College-Hill Press, 1983:127.
52. Faaborg-Andersen K. Electromyographic investigation of intrinsic laryngeal muscles in humans. Acta Physiol Scand [Suppl] 1957; 41:140.
53. Gay T, Hirose H, Strome M, Sawashima M. Electromyography of the intrinsic laryngeal muscles during phonation. Ann Otol, Rhinol, Laryngol 1972; 81:401–409.
54. Simada Z, Hirose H. The function of the laryngeal muscles in respect to the word accent distinction. Ann Bull Res Inst Logoped and Phoniat 1970; 4:27–40.
55. Shipp T, McGlone RE. Laryngeal dynamics associated with voice frequency change. J Speech Hear Res 1971; 14:761–768.
56. Hirano M, Ohala JJ, Vennard W. The function of laryngeal muscles in regulating fundamental frequency and intensity of phonation. J Speech Hear Res 1969; 12:616–628.
57. Collier R. Physiological correlates of intonation patterns. J Acoust Soc Am 1975; 58:249–255.
58. Sapir S, McClean M, Luschei ES. Time relations between cricothyroid muscle activity and the voice fundamental frequency (FØ) during sinusoidal modulations of FØ. J Acoust Soc Am 1984; 75:1639–1641.
59. Ohala JJ. Production of tone. In: Fromkin VA, ed. Tone: a linguistic survey. New York: Academic Press, 1978:5.
60. Lieberman P. Intonation, perception, and language. Cambridge: MIT Press, 1967.
61. Gelfer CE, Harris KS, Collier R, Baer T. Is declination actively controlled? In: Titze IR, Scherer RC, eds. Vocal fold physiology: biomechanics, acoustics, and phonatory control. Denver: Denver Center for the Performing Arts, 1985:113.
62. Ladefoged P. Three areas of experimental phonetics. Oxford: Oxford University Press, 1967.
63. Hollien H, Schoenhard C. The riddle of the "middle" register. In: Titze IR, Scherer RC, eds. Vocal fold physiology: biomechanics, acoustics, and phonatory control. Denver: Denver Center for the Performing Arts, 1985:258.
64. Farnsworth DW. High-speed motion pictures of the human vocal cords. Bell Lab Rec 1940; 18:203–208.
65. van den Berg J, Tan TS. Results of experiments with human larynges. Pract Otorhinolaryngol 1959; 21:425–450.
66. Hirano M, Kakita Y, Kawasaki H, Gould WJ, Lambiase A. Data from high-speed motion picture studies. In: Stevens KN, Hirano M, eds. Vocal fold physiology. Tokyo: University of Tokyo Press, 1981:85.
67. Hirano M, Matsuo K, Kakita Y, Kawasaki H, Kurita S. Vibratory behavior versus the structure of the vocal fold. In: Titze IR, Scherer RC, eds. Vocal fold physiology: biomechanics, acoustics, and phonatory control. Denver: Denver Center for the Performing Arts, 1985:26.
68. Childers DG, Hicks DM, Moore GP, Alsaka YA. A model for vocal fold vibratory motion, contact area, and the electroglottogram. J Acoust Soc Am 1986; 80:1309–1320.
69. Saito S, Fukuda H, Isogai Y, Ono H. X-ray stroboscopy. In: Stevens KN, Hirano M, eds. Vocal fold physiology. Tokyo: University of Tokyo Press, 1981:95.
70. Baer T. Observation of vocal fold vibration: measurement of excised larynges. In: Stevens KN, Hirano M, eds. Vocal fold physiology. Tokyo: University of Tokyo Press, 1981:119.

71. Fukuda H, Saito S, Kitahara S, Isogai Y, Makino K, Tsuzuki T, Kogawa N, Ono H. Vocal fold vibration in excised larynges viewed with an X-ray stroboscope and an ultrahigh speed camera. In: Bless DM, Abbs JH, eds. Vocal fold physiology. San Diego: College-Hill Press, 1983:238.
72. Broad DJ. The new theories of vocal fold vibration. In: Lass NJ, ed. Speech and language: advances in basic research and practice. Vol. 2. New York: Academic Press, 1979:203.
73. Timcke R, von Leden H, Moore P. Laryngeal vibrations: measurements of the glottic wave. Part I: the normal vibratory cycle. Arch Otolaryngol 1958; 68:1–19.
74. Timcke R, von Leden H, Moore P. Laryngeal vibrations: measurements of the glottic wave. Part II: physiologic variations. Arch Otolaryngol 1959; 69:438–444.
75. von Leden H, Moore P, Timcke R. Laryngeal vibrations: measurements of the glottal wave. Part III: the pathologic larynx. Arch Otolaryngol 1960; 71:16–35.
76. Childers DG, Naik JM, Larar JN, Krishnamurthy AK, Moore GP. Electroglottography, speech, and ultra-high speed cinematography. In: Titze IR, Scherer RC, eds. Vocal fold physiology. Denver: Denver Center for the Performing Arts, 1985:202.
77. Baer T, Löfqvist A, McGarr NS. Laryngeal vibrations: a comparison between high-speed filming and glottographic techniques. J Acoust Soc Am 1983; 73:1304–1308.
78. Childers DG, Krishnamurthy AK. A critical review of electroglottography. CRC Crit Rev Biomed Eng 1985; 12:131–161.
79. Rothenberg M. A new inverse filtering technique for deriving the glottal airflow waveform during voicing. J Acoust Soc Am 1973; 53:1632–1645.
80. Fant G. The voice source-acoustic modeling. Speech Transmiss Lab Q Prog Status Rep 1982; 4:28–48.
81. Kelman AW. Vibratory pattern of the vocal folds. Folia Phoniatr (Basel) 1981; 33:73–99.
82. Baer T, Titze I, Yoshioka H. Multiple simultaneous measures of vocal fold activity. In: Bless DM, Abbs JH, eds. Vocal fold physiology. San Diego: College-Hill Press, 1983:229.
83. Childers DG, Smith AM, Moore GP. Relationships between electroglottograph, speech, and vocal cord contact. Folia Phoniatr (Basel) 1984; 36:105–118.
84. Benguerel AP, Hirose H, Sawashima M, Ushijima T. Laryngeal control in French stop production: a fiberscopic, acoustic, and electromyographic study. Folia Phoniatr (Basel) 1978; 30:175–198.
85. Lindqvist J. Laryngeal articulations studied on Swedish subjects. Speech Transmiss Lab Q Prog Status Rep 1972; 2–3:10–27.
86. Sawashima M, Abramson AS, Cooper FS, Lisker L. Observing laryngeal adjustments during running speech by use of a fiberoptics system. Phonetica 1970; 22:193–201.
87. Hirose H. Posterior cricoarytenoid as a speech muscle. Ann Otol Rhinol Laryngol 1976; 85:334–343.
88. Hirose H, Sawashima M. Function of the laryngeal muscles in speech. In: Stevens KN, Hirano M, eds. Vocal fold physiology. Tokyo: University of Tokyo Press, 1981:137.
89. Sawashima M, Hirose H. Laryngeal gestures in speech production. In: MacNeilage PF, ed. The production of speech. New York: Springer-Verlag, 1983:11.
90. Weismer G. Control of the voicing distinction for intervocalic stops and fricatives: some data and theoretical considerations. J Phonetics 1980; 8:417–428.
91. Löfqvist A, Baer T, Yoshioka H. Scaling of glottal opening. Phonetica 1981; 38:265–276.
92. Munhall KG, Ostry DJ. Ultrasonic measurement of laryngeal kinematics. In: Titze IR, Scherer RC, eds. Vocal fold physiology: biomechanics, acoustics, and phonatory control. Denver: Denver Center for the Performing Arts, 1985:145.
93. Löfqvist A. Interarticulator programming in stop production. J Phonetics 1980; 8:475–490.
94. Löfqvist A. Interarticulator programming in obstruent production. Phonetica 1981; 38:21–34.
95. Löfqvist A, Yoshioka H. Intrasegmental timing: laryngeal-oral coordination in voiceless consonant production. Speech Commun 1984; 3:279–289.
96. Lubker JF, May K. Palatoglossus function in normal speech production. Papers Inst Linguist (University of Stockholm) 1973; 17:17–26.
97. Kent RD, Carney PJ, Severeid LR. Velar movement and timing: evaluation of a model for binary control. J Speech Hear Res 1974; 17:470–488.
98. Stein RB. What muscle variable(s) does the nervous system control in limb movements. Behav Brain Sci 1982; 5:535–541.
99. Mermelstein P. Articulatory model for the study of speech production. J Acoust Soc Am 1973; 53:1070–1082.
100. Rubin P, Baer T, Mermelstein P. An articulatory synthesizer for perceptual research. J Acoust Soc Am 1981; 70:321–328.
101. Kelso JAS, Saltzman EL, Tuller B. The dynamical perspective on speech production: data and theory. J Phonetics 1986; 14:29–59.
102. Kelso JAS, Saltzman EL, Tuller B. Intentional contents, communicative context, and task dynamics: a reply to the commentators. J Phonetics 1986; 14:171–196.
103. Cole KJ, Konopacki RA, Abbs JH. A miniature electrode for surface electromyography during speech. J Acoust Soc Am 1983; 74:1362–1366.
104. Fritzell B. The velopharyngeal muscles in speech: an electromyographic and cineradiographic study. Acta Otolaryngol [Suppl] (Stockh) 1986; 250:1–81.
105. Bell-Berti F. An electromyographic study of velopharyngeal function in speech. J Speech Hear Res 1976; 19:225–240.
106. Seaver EJ, Kuehn DP. A cineradiographic investigation of velar positioning in nonnasal speech. Cleft Palate J 1980; 17:216–226.
107. Niimi S. Pharyngeal wall movement during speech. Annu Bull Res Inst Logoped Phoniatr 1979; 13:43–51.
108. Minifie FD, Hixon TJ, Williams F. Normal aspects of speech, hearing, and language. Englewood Cliffs, NJ: Prentice-Hall, 1973.
109. Zemlin WR. Speech and hearing science: anatomy and physiology. Englewood Cliffs, NJ: Prentice-Hall, 1968.
110. Miyawaki K, Hirose H, Ushijima T, Sawashima M. A preliminary report on the electromyographic study of the activity of lingual muscles. Annu Bull Res Inst Logoped Phoniatr 1975; 9:91–106.
111. Alfonso PJ, Honda K, Baer T, Harris KS. Multi-channel study of tongue EMG during vowel production (abstr). J Acoust Soc Am 1982; 71:554.
112. Perkell J. Physiology of speech production. Cambridge: MIT Press, 1969.
113. Fowler CA. Converging sources of evidence on spoken and perceived rhythms of speech: cyclic production of vowels in monosyllabic stress feet. J Exp Psychol [Gen] 1983; 112:386–412.
114. Fujimura O, Kakita Y. Remarks on quantitative description of the lingual articulation. In: Lindblom B, Öhman S, eds. Frontiers of speech communication research. London: Academic Press, 1979:17.
115. Perkell JS, Nelson WL. Articulatory targets and speech motor control: a study of vowel production. In: Grillner S, Lindblom B, Lubker J, and Persson A, eds. Speech motor control. Oxford: Pergamon Press, 1982:187.
116. Perkell JS, Nelson WL. Variability in the production of the vowels /i/ and /æ/. J Acoust Soc Am 1985; 77:1889–1895.
117. Stevens KN. The quantal nature of speech: evidence from

articulatory-acoustic data. In: Denes PB, Davis EE, eds. Human communication, a unified view. New York: McGraw-Hill, 1972:51.
118. Alfonso PJ, Baer T. Dynamics of vowel articulation. Lang Speech 1982; 25:151–173.
119. Tuller B, Harris KS, Gross B. Electromyographic study of the jaw muscles during speech. J Phonetics 1981; 9:175–188.
120. Folkins JW. Muscle activity for jaw closing during speech. J Speech Hear Res 1981; 24:601–615.
121. Blair C, Smith A. EMG recording in human lip muscles: can single muscles be isolated? J Speech Hear Res 1986; 29:256–266.
122. Blair C. Interdigitating muscle fibers throughout orbicularis oris inferior: preliminary observations. J Speech Hear Res 1986; 29:266–269.
123. Abbs JH, Gracco VL, Blair C. Functional muscle partitioning during voluntary movement: facial muscle activity for speech. Exp Neurol 1984; 85:469–479.
124. Cooper DS, Folkins JW. Comparison of electromyographic signals from different electrode placements in the palatoglossus muscle. J Acoust Soc Am 1985; 78:1530–1540.
125. Kuehn DP, Folkins JW, Cutting CB. Relationships between muscle activity and velar position. Cleft Palate J 1982; 19:25–35.
126. Kelso JAS, Vatikiotis-Bateson E, Saltzman EL, Kay B. A qualitative dynamic analysis of reiterant speech production: phase portraits, kinematics, and dynamic modeling. J Acoust Soc Am 1985; 77:266–280.
127. Ostry DJ, Munhall KG. Control of rate and duration of speech movements. J Acoust Soc Am 1985; 77:640–648.
128. Kuehn DP, Moll KL. A cineradiographic study of VC and CV articulatory velocities. J Phonetics 1976; 4:303–320.
129. Parush A, Ostry DJ, Munhall KG. A kinematic study of lingual coarticulation in VCV sequences. J Acoust Soc Am 1983; 74:1115–1125.
130. Smith BL, Gartenberg TE. Initial observations concerning developmental characteristics of labio-mandibular kinematics. J Acoust Soc Am 1984; 75:1599–1605.
131. Nelson WL, Perkell JS, Westbury JR. Mandible movements during increasingly rapid articulations of single syllables: preliminary observations. J Acoust Soc Am 1984; 75:945–951.
132. Kuehn DP. A cineradiographic investigation of velar movement variables in two normals. Cleft Palate J 1976; 13:88–103.
133. Kent RD. Some considerations in the cinefluorographic analysis of tongue movement during speech. Phonetica 1972; 26:16–32.
134. Kent RD, Netsell R. Effects of stress contrasts on certain articulatory parameters. Phonetica 1971; 23:23–44.
135. Kent RD, Moll KL. Cinefluorographic analysis of selected lingual consonants. J Speech Hear Res 1972; 15:453–473.
136. Kent RD, Moll KL. Tongue body articulation during vowel and diphthong gestures. Folia Phoniatr (Basel) 1972; 24:278–300.
137. Kent RD, Moll KL. Articulatory timing in selected consonant sequences. Brain Lang 1975; 2:304–323.
138. Abbs JH. The influence of the gamma motor system on jaw movements during speech: a theoretical framework and some preliminary observations. J Speech Hear Res 1973; 16:175–200.
139. Sussman HM, MacNeilage PF, Hanson RJ. Labial and mandibular dynamics during the production of bilabial consonants: preliminary observations. J Speech Hear Res 1973; 16:397–420.
140. Ostry DJ, Keller E, Parush A. Similarities in the control of the speech articulators and the limbs: kinematics of tongue dorsum movement in speech. J Exp Psychol [Hum Percept] 1983; 9:622–636.
141. Keller E, Ostry DJ. Computerized measurement of tongue dorsum movement with pulsed-echo ultrasound. J Acoust Soc Am 1983; 73:1309–1315.
142. Smith BL, McLean-Muse A. Articulatory movement characteristics of labial consonant productions by children and adults. J Acoust Soc Am 1986; 80:1321–1328.
143. Freund HJ, Büdingen HJ. The relationship between speed and amplitude of the fastest voluntary contractions of human arm muscles. Exp Brain Res 1978; 31:1–12.
144. Cooke JD. The organization of simple skilled movements. In: Stelmach GE, Requin J, eds. Tutorials in motor behavior. Amsterdam: North Holland, 1980:199.
145. Nelson WL. Physical principles for economies of skilled movements. Biol Cybern 1983; 46:135–147.
146. Daniloff RG, Hammarberg RE. On defining coarticulation. J Phonetics 1973; 1:239–248.
147. Kent RD, Minifie FD. Coarticulation in speech production models. J Phonetics 1977; 5:115–133.
148. Parush A, Ostry DJ. Superior lateral pharyngeal wall movements in speech. J Acoust Soc Am 1986; 80:749–756.
149. Moll KL, Daniloff RG. Investigation of the timing of velar movements during speech. J Acoust Soc Am 1971; 50:678–684.
150. Benguerel AP, Cowan HA. Coarticulation of upper lip protrusion in French. Phonetica 1974; 30:41–55.
151. MacNeilage PF, Declerk JL. On the motor control of coarticulation in CVC monosyllables. J Acoust Soc Am 1969; 45:1217–1233.
152. Sussman HM, Westbury JR. The effects of antagonistic gestures on temporal and amplitude parameters of anticipatory labial coarticulation. J Speech Hear Res 1981; 24:16–24.
153. Butcher A, Weiher E. An electropalatographic investigation of coarticulation in VCV sequences. J Phonetics 1976; 4:59–74.
154. Barry W, Kuenzel H. Co-articulatory airflow characteristics of intervocalic voiceless plosives. J Phonetics 1975; 3:263–288.
155. Öhman SEG. Coarticulation in VCV utterances: spectrographic measurements. J Acoust Soc Am 1966; 39:151–168.
156. Bladon RAW, Al-Bamerni A. Coarticulation resistance in English /l/. J Phonetics 1976; 4:137–150.
157. Recasens D. Coarticulatory patterns and degrees of coarticulatory resistance in Catalan CV sequences. Lang Speech 1985; 28:97–114.
158. Fowler CA. An event approach to the study of speech perception from a direct-realist perspective. J Phonetics 1986; 14:3–28.
159. Henke W. Dynamic articulatory model of speech production using computer simulation. Doctoral Dissertation. Cambridge, MA: Massachusetts Institute of Technology, 1966.
160. Fowler CA. Coarticulation and theories of extrinsic timing. J Phonetics 1980; 8:113–133.
161. Fowler CA. Current perspectives on language and speech production: a critical review. In: Daniloff RG, ed. Speech science. San Diego: College-Hill Press, 1985:193.
162. Kelso JAS, Tuller B, Vatikiotis-Bateson E, Fowler CA. Functionally specific articulatory cooperation following jaw perturbations during speech: evidence for coordinative structures. J Exp Psychol [Hum Percept] 1984; 10:812–832.
163. Kugler PN, Kelso JAS, Turvey MT. On the control and coordination of naturally developing systems. In: Kelso JAS, Clark JE, eds. The development of movement control and coordination. Chichester: John Wiley & Sons, 1982:5.
164. Tuller B, Kelso JAS, Harris KS. Interarticulator phasing as an index of temporal regularity in speech. J Exp Psychol [Hum Percept] 1982; 8:460–472.

165. Tuller B, Kelso JAS. The timing of articulatory gestures: evidence for relational invariants. J Acoust Soc Am 1984; 76:1030–1036.
166. Löfqvist A. Stability and change. J Phonetics 1986; 14:139–144.
167. Barry WJ. Some problems of interarticulator phasing as an index of temporal regularity in speech. J Exp Psychol [Hum Percept] 1983; 9:826–828.
168. Munhall KG. An examination of intra-articulator relative timing. J Acoust Soc Am 1985; 78:1548–1555.
169. Benoit C. Note on the use of correlations in speech timing. J Acoust Soc Am 1986; 80:1846–1849.
170. Gentner DR. Evidence against a central control model of timing in typing. J Exp Psychol [Hum Percept] 1982; 8:793–810.
171. Kent RD. Is a paradigm change needed? J Phonetics 1986; 14:111–115.
172. Liberman M, Streeter LA. Use of nonsense syllable mimicry in the study of prosodic phenomena. J Acoust Soc Am 1978; 63:231–233.
173. Fowler CA, Rubin P, Remez R, Turvey MT. Implications for speech of a general theory of action. In: Butterworth B, ed. Language production. New York: Academic Press, 1980:373.
174. Kelso JAS, Tuller B. Intrinsic time in speech production: theory, methodology, and preliminary observations. In: Keller E, Gopnik M, eds. Motor and sensory processes of language. Hillsdale, NJ: Erlbaum, 1987:203.
175. Lubker J. Articulatory timing and the concept of phase. J Phonetics 1986; 14:133–137.
176. Gracco VL, Abbs JH. Programming and execution processes of speech movement control: potential neural correlates. In: Keller E, Gopnik M, eds. Motor and sensory processes of language. Hillsdale, NJ: Erlbaum, 1987:163–201.
177. Gracco VL, Abbs JH. Variant and invariant characteristics of speech movements. Exp Brain Res 1986; 65:156–166.
178. Perkell JS. Phonetic features and the physiology of speech production. In: Butterworth B, ed. Language production. Vol. 1. Speech and talk. London: Academic Press, 1980:337.
179. Abbs JH, Gracco VL. Control of complex motor gestures: orofacial muscle responses to load perturbations of lip during speech. J Neurophysiol 1984; 51:705–723.
180. Abbs JH, Gracco VL, Cole KJ. Sensorimotor contributions to the coordination of multicomponent behaviors: evidence from recent studies of speech movement control. J Motor Behav 1984; 16:195–231.
181. Gracco VL, Abbs JH. Dynamic control of the perioral system during speech: kinematic analyses of autogenic and nonautogenic sensorimotor processes. J Neurophysiol 1985; 54:418–432.
182. Folkins JW, Canty JL. Movements of the upper and lower lips during speech: interactions between lips with the jaw fixed at different positions. J Speech Hear Res 1986; 29:348–356.
183. Folkins JW, Abbs JH. Lip and jaw motor control during speech: responses to resistive loading of the jaw. J Speech Hear Res 1975; 18:207–220.
184. Folkins J, Abbs JH. Additional observations on responses to resistive loading of the jaw. J Speech Hear Res 1976; 19:820–821.
185. MacNeilage PF. Motor control of serial ordering of speech. Psychol Rev 1970; 77:182–196.
186. MacNeilage PF. Speech production. Lang Speech 1980; 23:3–22.
187. Warren DW. Compensatory speech behaviors in cleft palate: a regulation/control phenomenon. Cleft Palate J 1986; 23:251–260.
188. Nearey TM. On the physical interpretation of vowel quality: cinefluorographic and acoustic evidence. J Phonetics 1980; 8:213–241.
189. Bladon RAW, Henton CG, Pickering JB. Towards an auditory theory of speaker normalization. Lang Commun 1984; 4:59–69.
190. Kent RD. The iceberg hypothesis: the temporal assembly of speech movements. In: Perkell JS, Klatt DH, eds. Invariance and variability in speech processes. Hillsdale, NJ: Erlbaum, 1986:234.
191. Kent RD. The segmental organization of speech. In: MacNeilage PF, ed. The production of speech. New York: Springer-Verlag, 1983:57.
192. Fujimura O. Relative invariance of articulatory movements: an iceberg model. In: Perkell JS, Klatt DH, eds. Invariance and variability in speech processes. Hillsdale, NJ: Erlbaum, 1986:226.
193. Shaffer LH. Rhythm and timing in skill. Psychol Rev 1982; 89:109–122.

9 Speech Perception

Judith A. Gierut, Ph.D.
David B. Pisoni, Ph.D.

Speech perception can be described most simply as the transformation of an acoustic signal transmitted from a speaker to an intended communicative message heard by a listener. For the listener, the perception of speech seems to be effortless and automatic. For the researcher, however, the perception of speech is an extremely complex and multifaceted problem. Insight into the basic process of speech perception requires an understanding of the various levels of speech analysis, beginning with an initial auditory analysis of the stimulus input and continuing to higher levels of linguistic analysis. The process of speech perception also requires a general understanding of human communication and thought. Given its scope, it is not surprising to find that many different disciplines have been involved in trying to understand the nature of speech perception including, for example, cognitive psychology, computer science, engineering, linguistics, and speech science. Despite these multidisciplinary interests, certain well-defined issues underlie the central body of speech perception research.

The primary and, perhaps, most difficult set of issues in speech perception relates to the lack of invariance, linearity, and segmentation of the speech signal.[1–4] The *invariance condition* states that a distinct set of acoustic features corresponds to each phoneme. This condition assumes that, when a given phoneme is used, the same acoustic cues are identifiable in the signal regardless of context. The *linearity condition* states that a specific sound corresponds to each phoneme in a spoken word. This condition assumes that units of sound corresponding to phonemes are discrete and that these units are ordered in a particular sequence. The *segmentation condition* states that the speech signal can be sliced (and recombined) into acoustically distinct, independent units corresponding to specific phonemes. Together, these three conditions suggest a one-to-one invariant mapping between the acoustic and phonemic properties of sounds in words that facilitates a listener's perception of speech. Over 40 years of research have revealed that speech does not conform to these basic conditions. Generally, phonemic elements in words are outnumbered by acoustic cues. In addition, acoustic properties of a given sound change and vary dramatically in different contexts. Finally, at a given point in the signal, overlapping information is present about the acoustic properties of a specific phoneme as well as preceding and following phonemes. How, then, are listeners able to perceive speech sounds when a serious gap in correspondence exists between the acoustic signal and the phonetic message?[1–4]

A second key issue involves intra- and intertalker normalization. Speakers vary their production of speech sounds in conversation by altering the rate, pitch, stress, or loudness of their voice. Speakers also vary production of sounds on the basis of certain sociolinguistic factors, such as the social status of the listener, mood or attitude, and affect. Moreover, across different speakers, production of sounds changes with age and sex; these variations are associated with vocal tracts of different shapes and sizes for males, females, and children. Sounds are also produced differently in different dialects. Despite these variations in sound production within and across speakers, listeners seem to have little difficulty perceiving an intended message. How are listeners able to ignore these irrelevant aspects of the speech signal on the one hand, but to attend to the relevant aspects of the signal associated with sounds and words on the other?[1–4]

A third major issue is associated with the internal representation of speech signals and the linguistic units to which they correspond. For the most part, researchers agree that speech is internally represented in some form for cognitive processing in both speech perception and production. However, the nature of this representation is cause for debate.

The representation of speech may lie at the sensory level as a neurogram, at a phonetic level as a spectrogram, at a phonemic level as a bundle of distinctive features, or at a lexical level as an acoustically-based morpheme. How do listeners represent speech input? Moreover, what is the basic unit or units of speech analysis and representation?[1–4]

Key issues of this type have dominated speech perception research for nearly four decades and constitute what has been called the "primary recognition problem," that is, how the form of a spoken word is recognized from acoustic information in the speech waveform.[5] Although not abandoning these basic problems, researchers have become increasingly interested in multiple sources of knowledge and the interaction of these sources in speech perception. How does experiential, conceptual, or linguistic knowledge or memory play a role in speech perception? How and when are these different knowledge sources tapped in perceptual processing? Researchers are no longer limiting their questions to those of bottom-up processing associated with information in the acoustic and phonetic codes, but are starting to explore questions of top-down processing associated with the important contributions of phonological, lexical, contextual, and memory codes.

In this chapter, we review both primary recognition problems and contemporary problems involving the role of various knowledge sources in speech perception. We limit our review to data from three distinct populations: adults, infants and children, and special populations, namely, children with phonological disorders and adults acquiring a second language. Our review of evidence from adult speech perception research serves as the foundation and motivation for examining related issues and problems in developing and special populations. We illustrate how these unique populations contribute to and challenge models of adult perception, thereby furthering the basic understanding of the nature and process of speech perception.

SPEECH PERCEPTION IN THE ADULT

Cues to the Perception of Stops

The earliest experimental studies of the primary recognition problem in speech perception were aimed at identifying properties in the acoustic signal that cued particular speech sounds. That is, was there any evidence in the acoustic signal that facilitated the perception of sounds such that a listener could perceive and identify sounds accurately and consistently despite speaker, contextual, or environmental variance?

The search for invariant acoustic correlates for phonemes has focused primarily on stop consonants. The first study examining cues to the perception of stops was conducted by Liberman, Delattre, and Cooper,[6] who used what were then novel procedures, namely, spectrographic analysis combined with speech synthesis techniques. Liberman et al observed spectrographically that the voiceless stops /p/, /t/, and /k/ could be distinguished by the frequency of the stop release burst. This cue was then manipulated synthetically and combined with a series of vowels to form consonant-vowel (CV) units. Adults who judged the synthetic CV tokens identified voiceless stops as a function of both the release burst frequency and the quality of the following vowel. For example, a release burst of a particular frequency was heard as /p/ before the vowels /i/ and /u/, but as /k/ before the vowel /a/. Listeners' percepts of stops thus differed relative to the following vowel and the frequency of the release burst.

In addition to frequency of the release burst and vowel context, formant transitions have also been shown to be important cues to stops.[7–8] Cooper et al demonstrated that variations in the first formant transition signalled voice and manner;[7] whereas variations in the second formant transition cued place of articulation. As with release burst frequency, formant transitions were reliable cues relative to the following vowel.

Subsequent studies have explored other various acoustic attributes as cues to the perception of stops. Over 16 such cues have been identified.[9] In the search for invariance, evidence of this type suggested that there was no simple one-to-one correspondence between the acoustic signal and the phonetic percept as was initially thought. However, a recent position suggests that invariant cues can be identified in the acoustic signal if the signal is examined properly. Two such approaches have been proposed, namely, those of Stevens and Blumstein and of Kewley-Port.

Stevens and Blumstein suggest that invariant cues in the acoustic signal are complex and require an integration of simple isolated cues.[10–12] They have targeted the overall shape of the onset spectrum as the invariant cue for stop consonants and have identified three general spectral patterns: diffuse-falling, diffuse-rising, and compact, as shown in Figure 9–1. The diffuse-falling pattern characterizes the bilabial stops /p/ and /b/, which have a low-frequency onset followed by a rise in spectral energy. The diffuse-rising pattern characterizes the alveolar stops /t/ and /d/, which have a high-frequency onset followed by a fall in spectral energy. The compact

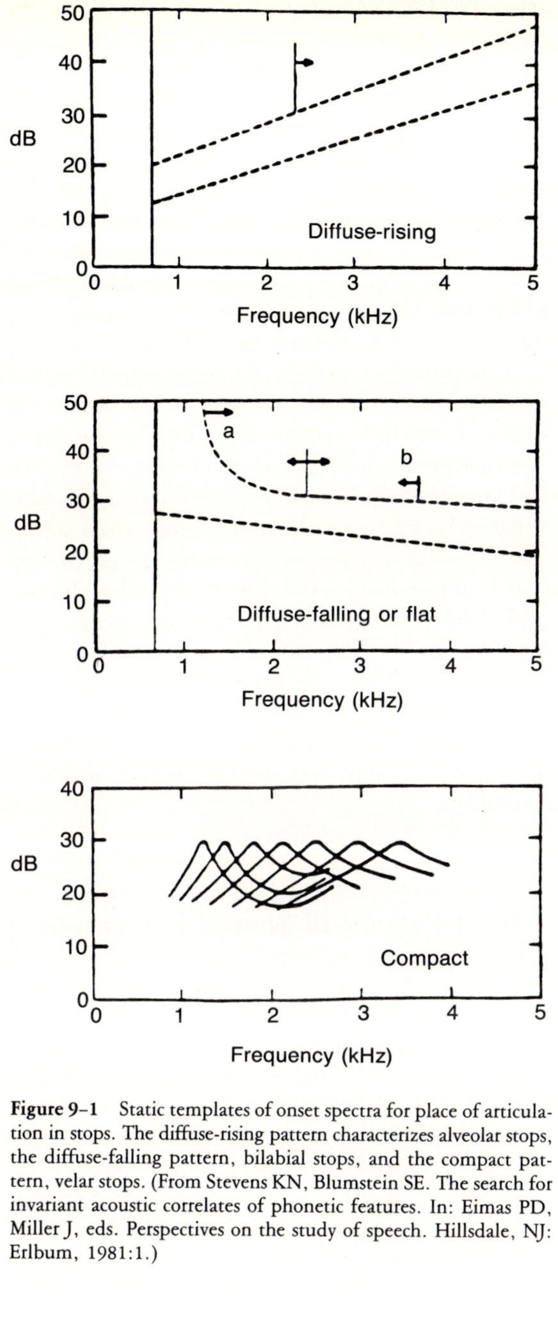

Figure 9–1 Static templates of onset spectra for place of articulation in stops. The diffuse-rising pattern characterizes alveolar stops, the diffuse-falling pattern, bilabial stops, and the compact pattern, velar stops. (From Stevens KN, Blumstein SE. The search for invariant acoustic correlates of phonetic features. In: Eimas PD, Miller J, eds. Perspectives on the study of speech. Hillsdale, NJ: Erlbum, 1981:1.)

pattern characterizes the velar stops /k/ and /g/, which have onset energy concentrated in the mid-frequencies followed by a spreading of energy to frequencies above and below the onset. These three different spectral patterns presumably correspond to distinctive phonetic features.[13–18] Moreover, the three spectral patterns are considered the primary cues to different places of articulation in stops; other properties, such as formant transitions, are viewed as secondary cues. In addition, the spectral characterization of stops is regarded as a type of static template that overrides contexual or speaker variability.

Experimental tests of the constancy of the spectral patterns have been conducted for both speech production and speech perception. In one production study, Blumstein and Stevens had adults utter CV and vowel-consonant (VC) syllables consisting of voiced and voiceless stops in combination with a series of vowels.[10] Acoustic analyses of the productions were then visually matched to static spectral templates by judges. For productions of stops in CV syllables, bilabials were matched to the appropriate template with 86 percent accuracy, alveolars with 81 percent accuracy, and velars with 85 percent accuracy. Correct matches of VC productions to the appropriate templates were much poorer.

Whether listeners actually used the primary spectral cues to perceive stops was also evaluated.[12] Synthetic /b/, /d/, and /g/ plus vowel stimuli that conformed to the three different spectral templates were generated and presented to adults for identification. Listeners not only judged these syllables appropriately, but they were able to identify different places of articulation in stops based on stimuli of very short durations (i.e., 10 to 20 msec). Moreover, the elimination of secondary cues, namely, formant transitions, did not influence the listeners' responses. However, more recent studies have indicated that secondary formant transitions do play an important role in stop perception and may even take priority over onset spectra.[19,20]

More recent research has focused on modifying and extending Stevens' and Blumstein's original characterization of onset spectra. Efforts have been directed toward examinations of the reliability and validity of spectral cues to stops across different languages[21,22] and across different phonetic contrasts.[21,23] Further research is needed to establish whether spectral cues remain invariant across different contexts and speakers. Moreover, the status of different acoustic cues as either primary or secondary in perception requires additional attention. The distinction, as originally proposed by Stevens and Blumstein to characterize the difference between invariant and context-dependent cues, may be misleading and potentially an incorrect approach to phonetic perception.

Kewley-Port advanced a different view of acoustic invariance.[24–27] Here, the focus was on dynamic changes in the acoustic signal and transformations of the signal in the peripheral auditory system. Unlike the linguistically-based distinctive feature approach of Stevens and Blumstein, Kewley-Port adopted a psychophysical approach to invariance. Within this approach, cues to stops were located in the distribution of spectral energy and the changes in energy over time. Changes in energy were analyzed by examining three-dimensional running spectral displays, following the earlier work of Searle and colleagues,[28,29] with frequency along the x-axis, amplitude along the y-axis, and time along the z-axis, as shown in Figure 9–2. Three time-varying invariant cues to stops were identified from these displays: (1) tilt of the spectrum at burst onset, (2) late onset of low-frequency energy, and (3) midfrequency peaks across time. Tilt of the spectrum at burst onset characterizes both bilabial and alveolar stops, as in Stevens and Blumstein,[10–12] with bilabials identified by a rising spectrum and alveolars by a falling spectrum. Late onset of low-frequency energy and mid-frequency peaks across time characterize velar stops.

To evaluate the validity of these proposed dynamic time-varying cues in stop identification, two production studies were conducted. In the first study, talkers were instructed to produce CV syllables composed of voiced stops and a series of vowels.[24] Running spectral displays were then made from the talkers' productions. Trained judges were able to visually identify stops from the displays using the three time-varying cues with 88 percent accuracy. In a second study that more closely approximated fluent speech, talkers produced both voiced and voiceless stops with vowels in CV syllables at different speaking rates: normal, fast, and slow.[30] In addition, the time-varying cues were slightly modified to more closely model the filtering properties and the sensitivity of the peripheral auditory system. Using the modified time-varying cues, judges visually examined running spectral displays in the identification of stops. On the average, productions were identified with 89 percent accuracy overall and with 90 percent, 83 percent, and 85 percent accuracy at normal, slow, and fast rates, respectively.

Perceptual evaluations of dynamic cues in running spectra were also conducted in a series of three experiments.[27] In the first experiment, listeners identified place of articulation in natural tokens of /b/, /d/, and /g/ plus vowel stimuli. Only the first 20 to 40 msec of these syllables were presented. Results indicated that place of articulation in stops was identified with 93 percent accuracy overall, confirming that invariant acoustic cues are located in the initial portion of the speech signal. The other two experiments specifically evaluated whether listeners use dynamic (as proposed by Kewley-Port[24–27]) versus static (as proposed by Stevens and Blumstein[10–12]) properties of the signal in speech perception. In both experiments, listeners identified stop place of articulation in CV stimuli. In the second experiment, synthetic stimuli were used; whereas in the third experiment, stimuli were generated using linear prediction. Both experiments showed that listeners more accurately identified place of articulation in stops using dynamic, rather than static, cues, lending support to the running spectra approach to invariance. However, these studies did not evaluate the three specific time-varying features proposed by Kewley-Port; this remains an area for future investigation. Thus the running spectra approach holds potential in the search for invariance in that it emphasizes the dynamic properties of speech and the role of the peripheral auditory system in speech perception.

Specialization of Speech Perception

A second line of research on the primary recognition problem grew out of early experimental work on categorical perception. *Categorical perception* refers to the perception of stimuli *within* a phonemic category as identical, but stimuli *across* a phonemic category as different. The finding that listeners per-

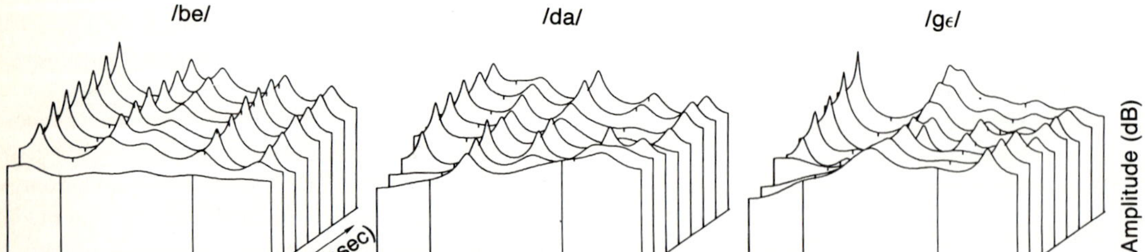

Figure 9–2 Dynamic running spectral displays of /be/, /da/ and /gɛ/. Frequency is represented along the x-axis, amplitude along the y-axis, and time (in 5 msec steps) along the z-axis. (After Kewley-Port D. Representation of spectral change as cues to place of articulation in stop consonants. Research on speech perception (technical report no.3). Bloomington, IN: Speech Research Laboratory, Department of Psychology, Indiana University, 1980.)

ceive sounds categorically was first reported in a study by Liberman, Harris, Hoffman, and Griffith.[31] In this study, listeners were instructed to discriminate and identify the speech stimuli /b/, /d/, and /g/ that varied along a continuum. Results indicated that the listeners' discrimination was no better than their identification, even though the distance between sounds on the continuum was equivalent acoustically. This finding was unusual and interesting since listeners appeared to perceive speech stimuli differently than nonspeech stimuli. In nonspeech experiments, listeners generally perceived stimuli continuously along a continuum.[32] That is, listeners discriminated acoustic stimuli from within the same category.

These results prompted a series of studies that examined whether perception of sounds other than stops was also categorical.[33] One particular study that deserves mention evaluated perception of vowels, namely, /ɪ/, /ɛ/, /æ/.[34] Results of this study indicated that adults perceived vowels continuously in much the same manner as perception of nonspeech stimuli.[35]

The fact that vowels were perceived continuously and consonants categorically led researchers to hypothesize about the nature of perceptual processing and the differences in perception of speech versus nonspeech. The strong hypothesis was that perception of speech requires a specialized mode of processing and that linguistically relevant stimuli are processed by a specific speech decoder.[36–40] The underlying assumption was that listeners have a basic knowledge of speech sounds and how sounds are articulated. Consonants are produced and, likewise, perceived categorically because their production requires a constriction at some point along the vocal tract, that is, discontinous production. But vowels are produced with an essentially open or uninterrupted vocal tract and consequently are perceived continuously. This intimate relationship between production and perception of sounds eventually developed into what is known as the motor theory of speech perception.[39,41]

Categorical Perception of Nonspeech Stimuli

Tests of the strong hypothesis that speech requires a specialized mode of processing have focused, in part, on the perception of nonspeech stimuli and comparisons between speech and nonspeech signals. The logic here was that if nonspeech stimuli were shown to be perceived categorically like speech stimuli, then a specialized linguistic mode of perception would not need to be posited.

Two studies have evaluated the perception of nonspeech stimuli approximating voice onset time, a cue to the perception of stop consonants.[42,43] In one study, Miller, Wier, Pastore, Kelly, and Dooling generated a series of stimuli varying along a noise-buzz continuum.[44] Aperiodic noise bursts simulated the burst frication in stops, whereas periodic buzzes modeled voicing. Subjects responded to the nonspeech noise-buzz stimuli categorically, discriminating two different categories. Pisoni also examined nonspeech stimuli resembling voice onset time.[45] However, in this study, stimuli were even less speech-like than those used by Miller et al, consisting only of two tones differing in relative onset time. Categorical perception of nonspeech sounds was again observed; moreover, the obtained discrimination functions closely resembled those reported by Lisker and Abramson[42,43] for perception of stops.

These data failed to provide support for the hypothesis that speech perception requires a specialized mode of processing. Instead these investigators proposed that categorical perception of certain sounds may be associated directly with the nature of the auditory system's sensitivity and processing capabilities.[35,44–51] This interpretation and supporting experimental results have recently come under criticism because only temporal and not spectral aspects of speech were examined.[33,52] In several recent studies, however, spectral as well as temporal cues have been manipulated, and similar findings have been observed.[53,54] The fact remains that obtained categorical perception results for both speech and nonspeech stimuli can adequately be accounted for by a general auditory processing model and do not require a specialization model.

In addition to studies examining nonspeech analogues of voice onset time in stops, there have been perception studies of other nonspeech stimuli. In particular, rise time in fricatives and affricates[55–59] and differences in speaking rate in production of stops and glides[54] have been simulated with nonspeech stimuli. These nonspeech studies have generated categorical perception results comparable to those using speech stimuli. Overall, research using nonspeech control stimuli suggests that the auditory system processes speech and other acoustic signals in a similar and unified way and that differences may be due to experience and methods employed.

Trading Relations

However, the specialization hypothesis has received some additional support from studies dealing with a phenomenon known as trading relations.[60]

Trading relations describe the way in which multiple acoustic cues are used to signal a single phonetic contrast. If a particular cue is masked in some way, other cues seem to engage the listener's attention, signalling the appropriate distinction. Thus trading relations assumes an equivalence among acoustic cues.

Trading relations among cues was first advanced as evidence in favor of specialization for two reasons.[60] First, in continuous speech, a listener is bombarded with a variety of spectral and temporal cues distributed over relatively long periods of time. The listener must integrate these cues over larger windows of time to perceive speech and to extract the linguistic message. Without a specialized processor, that this integration would actually occur was presumed unlikely. Second, trading relations do not occur for nonspeech sounds.[61,62]

Recently, however, this position has been modified.[63] Trading relations among cues have now been cited as merely specific instances of pattern mapping. Listeners learn specific patterns associated with speech sounds and then rely on trading relations among the cues in perception. As was the case for nonspeech data, a general model of auditory processing seemed to adequately account for the phenomenon of trading relations.

Although evidence in favor of a specialized linguistic mode of processing seems to be relatively sparse, there are data from studies of laterality, dichotic listening, and the integration of visual and auditory information (i.e., the McGurk effect) that lend support to speech specialization.[40,64–69] To date, however, the exact structure and function of a specialized linguistic processing mechanism and its integration with other cognitive abilities still remain topics of debate and continued basic research.

Speech Perception in Spoken Language Processing

Thus far, we have been concerned with problems associated with primary recognition, focusing on the perception of individual phonemes and the auditory analysis of sounds in syllables. Yet spoken language clearly involves more than just strings of sounds, and perception of spoken language involves much more than just analyses of the sensory information in the speech waveform. Listeners rely on a broader knowledge of language structure and function in perception and interpretation of a spoken message. They use their tacit knowledge of language to access and retrieve words stored in long-term memory from information contained in the acoustic signal. In this section, we turn our attention to several contemporary speech processing problems. Three of the many aspects of spoken language that influence speech perception will be examined: phonological rules and lexical, syntactic, and semantic information.

Phonological Rules

Both allophonic rules and phonotactic constraints affect the perception of speech. *Allophonic rules* describe systematic phonetic variations observed in the production of sounds. For example, speakers rarely say [du#ju#want#tu#goʊ] except, perhaps, in careful speech; instead, they are more likely to say [ʤə#wanə#goʊ]. Allophonic variation is predictable and rule-governed in such cases when speech is not exact. To perceive a spoken message, then, listeners likely rely on their tacit knowledge of allophonic rules of the language.

Experimental support for the use of allophonic information in speech perception has been provided primarily by Nakatani and colleagues.[70–73] The primary focus of this research has been on the identification of word boundaries, important for segmenting the beginnings and endings of words in sentences. Does the end of one word, the beginning of the next word, or a combination of both words signal a word boundary? Nakatani and Dukes used pairs of words involving identical phonetic but different lexical information to address this question.[70] Word pairs (e.g., "no notion"—"known ocean") were first recorded. Then that portion common to each word was excised and exchanged with the other word in the pair. The original version of the word pairs along with the spliced version were presented to adults for identification. The main finding was that word boundaries were cued in nearly all cases by the beginning of the second word; the only exceptions were words beginning or ending in /r/ or /l/. This difference is likely due to the fact that liquids have such varied and distinct allophones (e.g., "red" versus "fur" versus "weather" or "look" versus "cool").

The role of other allophonic rules in the segmentation of words has also been examined, including aspiration, gemination, stress, and vowel reduction.[71–73] Results of these studies provided further support for the claim that listeners rely on predictable allophonic variation and apparently use this information in speech perception.

Phonotactic constraints describe the permissible sounds and sound sequences in a language. In English, for example, the velar nasal /ŋ/ is permissible in intervocalic (e.g., "hanger") and word-final (e.g., "ring") positions, but is not used in word-initial position. Thus English has a phonotactic constraint allowing production of the velar nasal in postvocalic positions.

Massaro and Cohen examined the influence of English phonotactics on the perception of /r/ and /l/.[74] In this study, a CV continuum ranging from /ri/ to /li/ was constructed. Appended to the beginnings of these syllables were the sounds /s/, /t/, /p/, or /v/, resulting in pairs such as /sri/ versus /sli/ and /vri/ versus /vli/. The continua were played to adults for identification. As expected, listeners were influenced by the phonotactics of English in labelling the /ri/ to /li/ continuum. Specifically, in the /sri/ versus /sli/ pair, responses were biased in the direction of /l/ since this syllable involved a permissable sequence of sounds in English. In the /tri/ versus /tli/ pair, responses were shifted in the direction of /r/ for a similar reason. In the /pri/ versus /pli/ pair, responses were weighted equally since both sequences are permissable in English. Responses to the /vri/ versus /vli/ pair were also equivalent because both sequences are impermissible. These results demonstrate that higher-level phonological information about the phonotactics of language is used by listeners in the perception of speech sounds and sequences of speech sounds.

Lexical Information

Lexical knowledge has also been shown to be integral in the coding of acoustic information. Two different paradigms, phoneme restoration and phoneme monitoring, have been used to examine lexical effects in perception. *Phoneme restoration* is a procedure whereby a sound is excised from a word and replaced with a noise, such as a cough or a tone.[75] Listeners seem not to notice the missing sound, integrating segmental properties of words in speech. Samuel used the phoneme restoration paradigm in combination with varying degrees of lexical information.[76,77] Three main findings emerged from these studies: (1) restoration improved as word length increased; (2) restoration was better for high-frequency than low-frequency words; and (3) restoration was better for real words than acceptable nonwords. Lexical information thus seemed to influence the listeners' perception and integration of missing or degraded speech sounds.

The *phoneme monitoring* paradigm requires listeners to detect a specific sound in an utterance.[78] To execute this task, it was thought that listeners first processed an entire word and then sorted out individual segments.[79,80] However, recent research has shown that this may not be the case.[81,82] Presentations of words and nonwords in phoneme monitoring tasks have shown that listeners are able to monitor and perceive specific sounds in utterances consisting of nonwords. If perception and recognition of whole words were prerequisites to the perception of individual phonemes, then listeners should not have been able to monitor sounds in nonwords.

Together, the results of phoneme restoration and phoneme monitoring experiments highlight the importance of lexical information in the perception of speech. These results illustrate the complexity of and interaction between top-down lexical knowledge and the bottom-up analysis of the sensory input.

Syntactic and Semantic Information

Gating is one experimental paradigm that has been used to demonstrate the role of syntactic information in speech perception.[83–86] Gating is a measure that determines how much acoustic information must be present in the signal before a word can be recognized. For instance, in a gating experiment conducted by Salasoo and Pisoni, a word in a sentence was replaced with noise.[85] The sentence was then heard by a listener over successive trials. On each trial, the noise was replaced in systematic increments with relevant acoustic information from the original word. The listener responded as soon as the gated word was recognized. Salasoo and Pisoni used the gating paradigm with normal and semantically anomalous sentences.[85] Results indicated that less acoustic information was needed to recognize words in normal sentences than in semantically anomalous sentences, suggesting that listeners used context and linguistic information to facilitate perception. Similar results were obtained for gated words presented in isolation versus a sentence context. As more top-down information about language is brought to bear on perception, less bottom-up sensory information is necessary from the speech waveform.

Studies involving other experimental paradigms have shown comparable effects.[87–92] For example, listeners' identification of words in noise presented in isolation was not as good as identification of the same words embedded in sentences. In addition, identification of words in noise presented in grammatical sentences was better than in either anomalous or ungrammatical sentences. Finally, other types of higher-level linguistic information have been shown to play an important role in speech perception, including prosody, lexical access, and word recognition.[93]

Models of Speech Perception

The goal of a model of speech perception is to be sufficiently global to account for relevant data, but specific enough to be testable and falsifiable. Given the complexity of speech perception, it is not surprising that relatively few comprehensive models have been proposed. The earliest models of speech perception, such as Fant's auditory theory,[94,95] analysis-by-synthesis,[96–98] or motor theory,[39] emphasized explanatory accounts of limited perceptual phenomena rather than integrated accounts of perceptual processing. Three contemporary models of speech perception—motor theory revised, fuzzy logical model, and TRACE—are reviewed in this section. These models were selected specifically to illustrate (1) a renewed interest in a biological basis of speech perception, (2) an integration of feature and phoneme perception with higher levels of linguistic knowledge, and (3) a computational means of accounting for speech perception.

Revised Motor Theory

The original motor theory of speech perception was developed to account for the apparent lack of invariance among acoustic patterns across different contexts.[39] The underlying assumption of motor theory was that speech perception does not take place at the level of the acoustic signal but at the level of articulation. Listeners perceive speech because they are aware of how sounds are produced by the articulators; an intimate link exists between speech production and perception. Perception of sounds was thought to be learned through experience producing sounds and listening to others produce sounds.

Recently, motor theory has been revised in two important ways.[41] First, speech perception has been redefined as the identification of an intended gesture. A gesture is a set of movements by the articulators that result in a linguistically relevant vocal tract configuration. Each gesture has properties that are unique and distinct from other gestures. Moreover, each gesture is invariant, resulting in an underlying vocal tract configuration that corresponds to a phonetically relevant category. Second, the perception of gestures is not learned, but depends on specialized innate modules or neural structures of the brain. The biological basis is inferred from the fact that infants with limited production experience are able to perceive speech.[99] Further support comes from individuals with oral motor problems, such as adults with dysarthria; in these cases, speech is perceived even though the articulators are not volitionally controlled.

In the revised motor theory, speech input provides a listener with the phonetic intention of the talker. The intention of the talker is represented as an invariant gesture in the talker's brain. The listener is able to perceive the talker's representation via an innate perceiving module. The specialized module uses the acoustic pattern to retrieve the intended gesture, thus resulting in the perception of speech.

The primary difficulty with the revised motor theory, in our view, is the fact that there is little empirical support for or experimental demonstration of the theory. Invariant gestures cannot be identified in the acoustic signal or in static vocal tract configurations. However, the motor theory sustains prominence in the field among some researchers because of logic, parsimony, and intuitive appeal.

Fuzzy Logical Model

The fuzzy logical model was developed by Oden and Massaro as an account of feature integration in speech perception, that is, how multiple acoustic cues are integrated to arrive at a single acoustic percept.[100] The fuzzy logical model is consistent with a broader framework of auditory information processing.[101,102]

In the fuzzy logical model, three operations or processes are involved in phoneme identification, namely, feature evaluation, prototype matching, and pattern classification. Feature evaluation provides a specification of the degree to which a particular sound contains a relevant acoustic feature. Feature evaluation, as used in this sense, is unique in that *degree,* rather than mere presence of absence, of a feature is identified, with logical statements or fuzzy predicates summarizing these degrees. Prototype matching compares features to prototypes of phonemes stored in long-term memory. The prototypes are idealized representations of acoustic information stated in the form of propositions. Prototype matching thus specifies the degree to which candidate phonemes match the actual speech sound by comparing fuzzy predicates to propositions. Pattern classification is the final process involved in phoneme identification. In this process, the best match between alternate candidate phonemes and the actual speech sound is identified. Pattern classification provides the relative degree of the match, or the probability of "goodness of match." Thus the fuzzy logical model evaluates the degree of expected versus actual match between sounds and representations by means of a combination of logical rules for feature integration.

The fuzzy logical model accounts specifically for the integration of voice and place cues in stops. The model relies on syllable length (CV) units in phoneme identification and allows for dialectical and talker variation. The fuzzy logical model presents, more generally, an account of the mapping of acoustic information onto higher-level representations in long-term memory.

TRACE Model

The TRACE model of speech perception was developed by McClelland and Elman to account for the integration and parallel processing of multiple sources of information in speech perception.[103] TRACE grew out of a dynamic information-processing framework known as *interactive activation.*[104–108] Information processing through an interactive activation framework involves excitatory and inhibitory interactions among processing units. Processing units are simply hypotheses about the input being processed. Processing units are activated by the strength of the hypothesis. Constraints are imposed on processing units by connections such that units that are consistent with each other are mutually excited whereas those that are inconsistent are mutually inhibited. Moreover, when a processing unit reaches a set value of activaiton, the unit then influences (excites or inhibits) other units through connections. Therefore, each processing unit can constrain, as well as be constrained by, other processing units. During information processing, a system is constantly receiving input about processing units, updating the activation of these units, and delivering excitatory or inhibitory messages to other processing units as threshold values are reached.

TRACE is an instantiation of the interactive activation framework for speech perception. It consists of processing units or hypotheses about spoken input. Processing units are arranged on three different levels—feature, phoneme, and word—that, together, form a network. Each level includes detectors for the different and particular dimensions of sounds, and these are arranged over successive points in time, much like a stream of speech. Detectors at each of the three levels are activated as spoken input is directed into the system. Perceptual processing takes place both within and across levels of the system, with bidirectional connections among the levels. TRACE is a dyanamic model in that processing of a given portion of speech input continues as newer portions of speech are entered.

TRACE has been evaluated for both computational and psychological adequacy.[103] Thus far, TRACE has been able to account for lexical effects in phoneme perception, to replicate phonotactic constraints in English, and to describe categorical perception and trading relations among cues. TRACE has certain limitations in that it does not allow for variability (e.g., speaking rate, talker voice, or accent). In addition, it does not provide cues for word boundaries or adjust for word frequency in speech perception. TRACE further assumes that all phonemes are of equal length and that all features are equally salient. Finally, because the system is repeatedly copying information across time and levels, TRACE is encumbered by duplication and computation of processing units and connections. Nevertheless, it represents a major advance in the conception of a global approach to speech perception that can deal with a broad range of phenomena in an integrated fashion.

Future Directions

In this section, we have discussed two key primary recognition problems, the search for invariance in the speech signal and the specialization of speech processing. In the search for invariance, investigators have attempted to isolate specific acoustic cues to the perception of sounds (in particular, the perception of stop consonants). Research has identified numerous cues that signal stops, suggesting that there may not be a one-to-one mapping between acoustic signal and phonetic percept. Recent research on invariance has recognized this complex relationship between signal and percept. New approaches to invariance have concentrated on the dynamic nature of the speech signal, examining the constancy of such cues in terms of onset spectra and time-varying dimensions in perception. One area of continued study in the search for invariance is the examination of natural language contexts. Specifically, do listeners rely on dynamic cues, such as onset spectra or time-varying dimensions, in the perception of spoken fluent language? A second area of continued research focuses on language-specificity of invariant cues. Are the *invariant* dynamic cues particular to English or do these cues also signal the same contrasts in other languages? Are the invariant acoustic cues a reflection of man's general perception ability or are the cues merely a function of a specific language environment?

With regard to the second primary recognition problem, specialization of speech perception, evidence from nonspeech studies and trading relations among cues does not support an innate linguistic processor. Categorical versus continuous perception of sounds seems to be related, instead, to the specific nature of the peripheral auditory system. A fruitful line of research will be to further examine the auditory system in terms of its sensitivity, flexibility, and integrative nature in speech perception.

Speech processing problems have taken on more importance in contemporary perception research. The role of higher order linguistic and cognitive factors has been examined in the perception of speech in order to more carefully identify the levels of analysis that take place in perceptual processing. Factors such as phonological rules, prosody, and syntax have all been shown to influence the perception of a spoken message. Perception of speech thus involves an integration of bottom-up sensory information and top-down linguistic information. This integrated view is reflected in current models of speech perception, such as TRACE. Future research efforts will likely be directed at expanding and refining the data base in support of an integrated perceptual system. Research efforts will also aim at identifying the structure of the mental lexicon and how searches through the lexicon take place.[109] By understanding lexical structure, researchers will come closer to understanding functional and behavioral aspects of the perceptual system as well. This line of lexical research will also have applied consequences for improving speech recognition by machines and text-to-speech systems that generate synthetic speech by rule.

SPEECH PERCEPTION IN THE INFANT AND CHILD

Research on speech perception in infants and children over the last 15 years has been motivated primarily by findings reported in the adult speech perception literature. The fundamental issues of adult speech perception have often been treated as identical to those of infants and children. At first glance, it may appear that the study of speech perception in infants and children serves merely as a replication of perceptual research on adults. What further information about speech perception can be gained from studying young children? In our view, the study of speech perception in developing populations provides a unique window into the more complex and contemporary problems of speech perception that face researchers today. Infants and children provide a purer acoustic or sensory view of speech perception given their limited linguistic and cognitive experiences; the theories of adult speech perception must also account for these data as well. In addition, the study of infant and child speech perception provides researchers with an opportunity to answer questions associated with perceptual and cognitive development.[109a] What is the role of linguistic experience in speech perception? What is the relationship between the development of speech perception and speech production? How does the development of speech perception compare with the development of other kinds of perception and other types of complex cognitive processing?

Methodologies for Studying Perception

Although the study of developing populations offers a novel perspective on speech perception and human development, this area of research also poses unique problems. One particular problem relates to obtaining a reliable behavioral response that adequately reflects a child's perceptual capabilities. Typically, in adult research, listeners either identify or discriminate speech stimuli; infants and children are unable to respond in a comparable manner. Consequently, alternate methods of evaluating speech perception have been developed, including the heart rate paradigm, visual fixation paradigm, high-amplitude sucking procedure, and operant conditioning of head turning or pointing.

Heart Rate Paradigm

Heart rate monitoring has been used with infants 1 to 8 months of age.[110–113] In general, changes in the heart rate of infants (either accelerated or decelerated) can be elicited through presentation of any novel stimulus. The altered heart rate typically lasts 10 to 30 seconds, with the magnitude of the response gradually habituating over repeated presentations of the stimulus.

The heart rate paradigm, as used in speech perception research, begins with a baseline measure of an infant's heart rate. An auditory stimulus is presented, and a change in heart rate is observed. Presentations of the auditory stimulus are repeated over a series of trials during which the magnitude of heart rate habituates. A second novel auditory stimulus is then introduced. If a change in heart rate is noted, the experimenter infers that the infant presumably has detected a difference between the two stimuli, orienting to the novel condition. Group comparisons are typically made between changes in heart rate responses among infants presented with a second auditory stimulus versus those presented with only one auditory stimulus.

The heart rate paradigm is limited in certain ways. For example, consider two groups of infants who discriminate two sound contrasts differently as determined by different magnitudes of heart rate responding. It may seem appropriate to conclude that the sound contrast with greater dishabituation was "easier" to discriminate. However, the degree of discriminability among sound contrasts cannot be established from the heart rate procedure. As a second example, the heart rate paradigm places considerable memory demand on infants given the recovery time required between stimulus presentations and the habituation time across stimulus presentations. To decrease memory load, modifications of the heart rate paradigm have been suggested and appear to be sensitive discrimination measures.[114]

Visual Fixation Paradigm

The visual fixation paradigm uses the duration of an infant's gaze to measure speech discrimination.[115] First, a visual pattern is presented concurrently with an auditory stimulus, and the duration of an infant's gaze on the pattern is measured. The paired visual and auditory stimuli are removed for a brief period and are presented again. Additional measures of fixation time are obtained over repeated paired presentations until habituation is observed. Then a second novel auditory stimulus is presented, but is paired with the original visual pattern. A dishabituation in fixation to the same visual pattern paired with a new auditory stimulus is indicative of sound discrimination. Group comparisons are made between dishabituation responses of infants who hear a second novel auditory stimulus and those who hear and habituate to only one stimulus. The visual fixation paradigm has not been used widely, but it has been shown to be a reliable discrimination procedure.[115,116]

High-Amplitude Sucking Procedure

The most widely used procedure in the study of infant speech perception has been high-amplitude sucking.[117–121] The high-amplitude sucking procedure involves four phases: baseline, acquisition, habituation, and recovery. Initially, an infant's baseline sucking rate is measured. During acquisition, an auditory stimulus is presented contingent upon a criterion-level sucking response. Presumably, in this condition, an infant is reinforced by (1) sucking, (2) hearing the auditory stimulus, and (3) demonstrating control over presentation of the stimulus. The reinforcing value of this condition is only as durable as the novelty of the auditory stimulus; therefore sucking declines with satiation. When sucking declines and evidence of habituation can be inferred, a second novel auditory stimulus is presented, and an increase in sucking is observed. Discrimination is inferred if an infant shows recovery of the sucking response contingent upon presentation of the second novel auditory stimulus. Group comparisons are made between infants presented with two different auditory stimuli and those presented with the same auditory stimulus throughout.

The high-amplitude sucking procedure has several drawbacks. One drawback lies in the four phases of the procedure, which require approximately 15 to 20 minutes to complete. Infants often have difficulty attending for this amount of time. A second drawback is that specific levels of increased and decreased sucking must be achieved in order to demonstrate reliable shifts between each of the four phases of the procedure. A third difficulty is that there is only one opportunity to establish discrimination. An infant either recovers the sucking response rate or does not during presentation of the second novel stimulus. The basic high-amplitude sucking procedure has been varied to avoid these problems[122,123] and has been successful in establishing discrimination abilities of infants ages birth to 4 months.

Operant Conditioning of Head Turning and Pointing

The visually-reinforced head-turning paradigm is one operant conditioning procedure used with infants.[124–127] This procedure involves training an infant to orient to an auditory stimulus with a head-turning response. Reinforcement for appropriate head turning to the location of the sound is provided by lighting an animated toy located in the same proximity as the sound. The visually-reinforced head-turning paradigm has been used to evaluate detection and localization of sounds as well as discrimination in infants 5 to 18 months of age. One difficulty of the head-turning paradigm is the high attention demands required by the infant. Moreover, the procedure is only successful if the reinforcing value of the animated toy is maintained. In addition, elimination of subtle cueing of the infant by the experimenter or parent is critical.[128]

A variation of the visually-reinforced head-turning paradigm has also been developed for use with children 3 years and older.[129] This procedure involves a forced choice of two alternatives. A child is trained to point to one television in response to an auditory stimulus and a second television in response to another auditory stimulus. If the child points appropriately, the television comes on, and a brief segment of a cartoon or movie is played as reinforcement. This procedure has several advantages over other behavioral procedures used with children, such as picture identification or pressing buttons in response to sounds. First, children remain motivated and on-task during the procedure. Second, pictures are not needed and so perception of nonphonemic or isolated sounds can be evaluated. Third, there is no need for pretraining to ensure familiarity with test stimuli. Fourth, the procedure is fully automated, eliminating experimenter cueing and bias.

These four evaluation procedures have provided

basic tools for accessing speech perception abilities in developing populations. However, a word of caution is warranted in the interpretation of perceptual results from developing systems. Specifically, differences in perceptual abilities across children of different ages may be the result of "true" changes in the perceptual mechanism. Yet observed differences in perception may be side effects or consequences of other independent developmental changes, such as improvements in attention, motivation, or memory. A careful distinction must be made between developmental changes associated specifically with speech perception abilities and those attributed to more global cognitive advances.

Speech Perception in the Infant

Perceptual Cues to Simple Sound Contrasts

Virtually every perceptual distinction that has been examined in adults has also been evaluated in infants. As with adults, the bulk of these data has been collected when assessing aspects of the primary recognition problem. Several excellent comprehensive and critical reviews of the literature on infants' perception of simple sound contrasts are available;[99,109,130–132] only key findings of this line of research will be summarized. Instead, we will focus on infants' perception of more complex contrasts associated with the role of linguistic knowledge in perception.

Voicing. Of all sound contrasts, infants' discrimination of voicing has been studied most extensively. For stops, voice onset time has received primary attention. Voice onset time has been studied widely for at least three reasons: (1) it is a reliable cue to voicing in many languages of the world; (2) it is relatively easy to manipulate experimentally in synthetic speech; and (3) adult voice onset time data are available for direct comparison. The landmark study of voicing in stops was conducted by Eimas, Siqueland, Jusczyk, and Vigorito.[133] These investigators examined the bilabial voice distinction /ba/ versus /pa/ in 1- to 4-month-old infants using the high-amplitude sucking procedure. Like adults, infants displayed categorical perception, differentiating stimuli across the /b/—/p/ category, but not within either category. This finding has not only been replicated for bilabial stops, but also extended to alveolar stops.[99,134]

Voicing in fricatives has been studied to a more limited degree with regard to the /s/ versus /z/ contrast. Eilers, Wilson, and Moore demonstrated that infants 6 months of age were able to discriminate /sa/ versus /za/.[135] However, infants younger than 6 months were only able to discriminate /as/ versus /az/ but not /sa/ versus /za/.[136] These findings were interpreted as support for a developmental trend in perception, such that perception of voicing is not equivalent across contexts (i.e., initial versus final position) and that some contrasts (i.e., stops) are easier to perceive than others (i.e., fricatives). This interpretation has been criticized for underestimating infants' perceptual abilities.[137,138] Yet converging support for this position comes from the literature on the acquisition of sound production. Specifically, children do not learn to produce sounds at the same rate or in the same positions.[139,140] Moreover, children seem to acquire stops before fricatives, with stops first used in initial position and fricatives in final position.[141] These production data are consistent with claims about infant perception. Of course, whether or not perceptual and productive skills follow a parallel course of development remains to be determined.[142]

Place of Articulation. Infants, 2 months of age, were able to discriminate place of articulation in stops using two different cues, formant transition and frequency of the stop release burst.[112,143–147] Moreover, discrimination was categorical in nature. Yet which cue, formant transition or release burst, was primary for the infants? Walley, Pisoni, and Aslin addressed the question of cue primacy and trading relations in 6- to 9-month-old infants using a /b/, /d/, /g/ continuum.[148] Infants heard either full cue stimuli (5 formants plus release burst) or partial cue stimuli (2 formants minus release burst). Results indicated that either or both cues were used by infants to successfully distinguish place of articulation.[149] This demonstration of trading relations among acoustic cues supported the view that infants have a highly flexible perceptual system.

For fricatives, infants' ability to discriminate place of articulation is less clear. In some studies, infants were unable to discriminate contrasts involving /f/, and /s/, and /θ/.[135] Yet in other studies, infants not only discriminated these contrasts categorically, but did so in more than one position as well.[150–152] Methodological weaknesses and differences among these studies contribute to the difficulty in interpretation.[138]

As with stops, trading relations have been examined in fricatives. Formant transitions and spectral noise are two cues that have been manipulated. The role of formant transitions was evaluated in a study involving discrimination of the /fa/ versus /θa/ contrast.[153] Infants heard natural tokens of

/fa/ and /θa/ in one condition; in a second condition, infants heard the same tokens without frication noise (truncated stimuli). Infants only discriminated natural, but not truncated tokens; therefore formant transitions alone appeared to be an insufficient cue to fricative place distinctions. In a second study, spectral noise was manipulated in two sets of stimuli.[154] In one set, frication noise specific to /f/ versus /θ/ was appended to the vowel /a/; here, no formant transition information was available. In the second set of stimuli, a constant frication noise was appended to /a/; these stimuli contained formant transition information. Results showed that both sets of stimuli were discriminable by the infants. Spectral noise alone was a cue to fricative place distinctions, as indicated by the results obtained with the first set of stimuli. In addition, formant transitions were sufficient fricative place cues, as indicated by the results obtained with the second set of stimuli. These studies demonstrated overall that place of articulation in fricatives is discriminable by infants and that any one or combination of cues adequately signalled the distinction.

Vowels. Trehub examined infants' discrimination of natural tokens of the vowel pairs /a/ versus /i/ and /i/ versus /u/.[155] These pairs were also examined in stop contexts involving /p/ and /t/ (e.g., /pa/ versus /pi/). Infants were successful at distinguishing the vowel contrasts; moreover, no difference occurred between discrimination of vowels presented in isolation versus those presented in a consonant context. These same findings have been replicated and extended to other vowel contrasts.[125,156–159]

Perhaps the more important question was not whether infants distinguished differences among vowels, but whether infants discriminated vowels continuously. Recall that studies of adult speech perception showed that vowels are perceived continuously, whereas consonants are perceived categorically. Does the same continuous versus categorical dichotomy hold for infants as well? Swoboda, Morse, and Leavitt tested the distinction between /i/ and /I/ in 2-month-old infants and found that tokens within and between the vowel categories were discriminated equivalently.[160] Thus vowel perception for infants seems to be continuous, as in the case of adults.

Perceptual Cues to Complex Speech Contrasts

The focus on complex speech contrasts in infants has been limited to factors associated with suprasegmentals, such as stress and pitch, and normalization, such as speaker voice. This is in direct contrast to research on adults, where the focus has been on the size and structure of the linguistic unit. This difference between infant and adult research is likely associated with the prelinguistic nature of infants.

Suprasegmental Factors. There has been some debate over whether infants allocate attention to segmental or suprasegmental aspects of speech.[161–163] Do infants focus on specific sounds or the overall rhythmic pattern of speech or both?

Jusczyk and colleagues evaluated this question with regard to the particular suprasegmental, stress.[164,165] Multisyllabic units consisting of vowels plus stops and vowels plus glides were presented to 2-month-old infants. Syllables contrasted in terms of place of articulation, stress, and syllable position (e.g., /dába/ versus /dabá/, /báda/ versus /badá/). Overall, infants discriminated different places of articulation regardless of either stress pattern or syllable position. They found that stress was not distinctive; segmental information received higher priority in perception.

A second suprasegmental that has been examined is pitch.[158] Infants as young as 1 month of age were able to differentiate global pitch patterns of rising and falling intonation. However, when these pitch patterns were overlaid on segmental information, infants ignored pitch variations and focused instead on distinctive segmental properties of speech.[166]

Suprasegmental factors of stress and pitch may appear to play less of a role than segmental factors in developmental speech perception. An important question for future research is whether or not infants even rely on suprasegmental information; does suprasegmental information facilitate segmental perception in any way?

Normalization Factors. One normalization factor that has been examined in infants is variation in talker voice. In a study by Kuhl, three different talker voices were used in a vowel discrimination task with 6-month-old infants.[157,159] Results indicated that infants did not attend to the characteristics of a talker's voice, but focused on similarities among different presentations of the same vowel. Holmberg et al conducted a similar study, varying the talker's voice in infants' discrimination of fricatives, and obtained comparable results.[152] Thus infants perceived relevant phonetic differences among stimuli despite irrelevant changes in the talker's voice.[166]

Motherese. One aspect of infant speech perception that is difficult to resolve in light of the findings on stress, pitch, and talker's voice is a phenomenon known as *motherese*.[167] Researchers have demonstrated descriptively and experimentally that mothers use a particular manner of speech production when talking to their young children.[168,169] This pattern of production incorporates such features as shortened, repetitive utterances, higher pitch, exaggerated intonation, clearer, slower pronunciation, and distinct pauses between utterances. Motherese is preferred by young children; moreover, it presumably facilitates language learning. How do infants attend to features of motherese, while at the same time seemingly ignore characteristics of talker voice, stress, and pitch variation?

To address this question, Mehler, Bertoncini, Barriere, and Jassik-Gerschenfeld presented 4- to 6-week-old infants with the familiar voice of their mother and an unfamiliar female voice.[170] Intonation was varied, being either under- or overexaggerated. Infants preferred the familiar voice of their mother, but only when her productions were overinflected, suggesting that infants may focus only on certain prosodic properties of motherese.[171] Fernald and Kuhl thus examined a particular property of motherese, namely pitch contour.[172] Expanded pitch contours corresponding to motherese and nonmotherese were presented to infants. Again, infants clearly preferred the contours of motherese. Although pitch contour was identified as one property of motherese that infants attend to, it was not possible to determine precisely which aspect of pitch was preferred (e.g., level of pitch or range of pitch). Continued research is needed to further identify those acoustic properties of motherese that are most salient to infants.[173,174]

Theories of Perceptual Development

Research on infant speech perception has also been concerned with explaining the course of perceptual development. How do children learn to perceive speech? What is the role of early linguistic experience in perception? What role do genetic factors play in perceptual development? Aslin and Pisoni have outlined four cohesive frameworks to account for perceptual development (Fig. 9–3): universal theory, attunement theory, perceptual learning theory, and maturational theory.[130] Central to each theoretical framework is the interaction between innate aspects of the system and skills and capabilities that emerge with perceptual experience.

Universal Theory. This theory states that, at birth, an infant is capable of discriminating all phonetic contrasts observed in any natural language of the world. With experience, the infant learns to maintain relevant contrasts of the language; irrelevant contrasts are gradually lost. Within this framework, discrimination of speech contrasts is *maintained* through experience in the environment.

Attunement Theory. This theory states that, at birth, an infant is capable of discriminating some of the possible phonetic contrasts of natural languages. An infant's discrimination skills are incomplete and must be more finely developed. With experience, relevant contrasts are enhanced and facilitated, whereas irrelevant contrasts are lost. Here, discrimination is *sharpened* through experience.

Perceptual Learning Theory. This theory as-

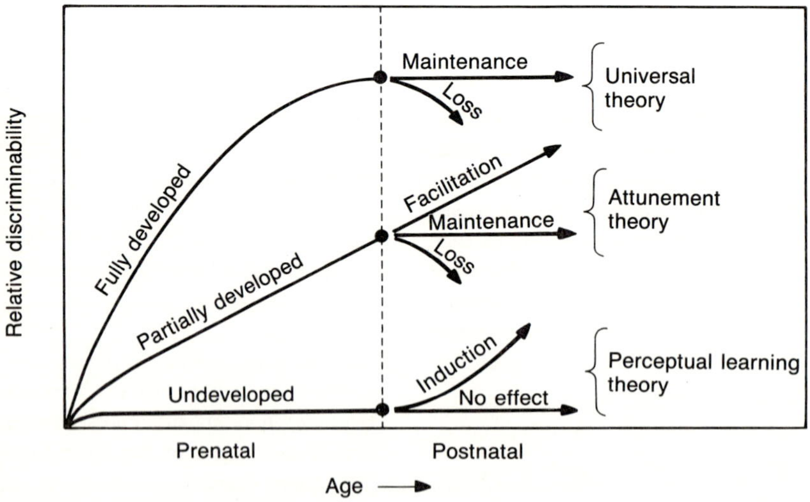

Figure 9–3 Illustration of the role of early experience in the development of speech perception. The universal theory, attunement theory, and perceptual learning theory are depicted. (From Aslin RN, Pisoni DB. Some developmental processes in speech perception. In: Yeni-Komshian G, Kavanagh JF, Ferguson CA, eds. Child phonology: perception. Vol. 2. New York: Academic Press, 1980:77.)

serts that discrimination skills are acquired solely through experience. An infant must learn to discriminate each relevant contrast of the language. Once relevant contrasts are learned, discrimination skills are strong. An infant is always able to learn new phonetic contrasts; however, discrimination skills are not as good in these cases. Discrimination of speech contrasts is *dependent* on experience.

Maturational Theory. This theory states that all phonetic contrasts of natural languages are equally discriminable by an infant at birth. The ability to discriminate particular contrasts emerges gradually over time and according to a specificed, predetermined developmental course. Within this framework, discrimination of speech is *independent* of experience.

These four frameworks make different predictions about the nature and course of perceptual development. Perhaps not one but a combination of these theories will emerge as the best characterization of developmental speech perception. Moreover, the development of speech perception may be identified as just one instance of the development of more global perceptual processes. Evidence from the literature on speech perception as well as from other perceptual systems (e.g., vision) supports this view,[109,130] further illustrating the complex interaction between genetics and experience in perceptual development.

Speech Perception in the Child

The study of speech perception in children is different from the study of infants in many ways. Although both groups display developing perceptual, cognitive, and linguistic systems, infants only provide insight into phonetic perception; whereas children also provide insight into phonemic perception.[175] *Phonetic perception* refers to the ability to distinguish between two phonetically different sounds. Phonetic perception is best associated with the sensory and perceptual coding of speech. On the other hand, *phonemic perception* refers to the ability to distinguish two phonetically different sounds that also signal meaning. This type of perception is best associated with perceptual coding and categorization of sound contrasts into functional classes in a specific language. Unlike infants, children bring general language experience to the perceptual task. In addition, unlike infants, children have experience producing relevant sounds and sound contrasts. Most importantly, by 3 years of age children have learned that certain sounds and sound sequences also carry meaning and can be used to communicate in the language.[140]

Research on phonemic perception in children, ages 2 through 6 years, has included investigations of cues to the perception of sounds as well as issues related to invariance, normalization, and phonemic constancy. Despite the breadth of this research, the majority of these studies have presented conflicting results that are difficult to interpret. Methodological weaknesses associated with certain subject, stimulus, task, and statistical variables are primarily responsible;[175–178] these variables greatly influence a child's perceptual performance. As an example, consider the type of stimuli presented. A child's performance is easily influenced by whether or not stimuli are (1) real words or nonsense syllables, (2) natural or synthetic tokens, and (3) tape recorded or presented live voice. Moreover, lack of familiarity with stimuli may bias responding. Does the child have an internal or mental representation that corresponds to the stimuli? As a second example, consider factors related to the perceptual task. Failure to perceive sound contrasts may reflect "true" limitations in a child's sensory or perceptual capabilities or an overly difficult perceptual task. Task variables that influence performance include (1) perceptual testing over a period of days, (2) number of trials for each discrimination, (3) nature of the task, either labelling or a same versus different judgment, and (4) interfering or biasing cues from the experimenter. As a final illustration, statistical treatment of data obtained from children may be inadequate, given the generally small number of responses obtained and the wide range of performance criteria used to establish perceptual mastery.

Contemporary research on the perceptual capabilities of children has focused primarily on the relationship between perception and production through examinations of trading relations among multiple acoustic cues. Recall that multiple acoustic cues arise from, and are correlated with, a number of dynamic articulatory gestures in speech production. The acoustic cues (and presumably the associated articulatory gestures) serve as perceptual cues for a listener. The purpose of multiple cue research in children has been to determine precisely what perceptual information is derived from production and, conversely, what production information is derived from perception. Specific research questions include the following: Are multiple acoustic cues equivalent for children? How are multiple cues integrated by children? What does perception of multiple cues indicate about children's productive skills?

Three recent studies have been conducted that bear upon trading relations in children. Morrongiello, Robson, Best, and Clifton examined children's perception of the fricative plus stop cluster /st/ by manipulating the cues of formant onset frequency and silence duration.[179] Mann, Sharlin, and

Dorman examined children's perception of the fricatives /s/ and /ʃ/ by manipulating frication noise and vowel context.[180] Nittrouer and Studdert-Kennedy examined children's perception of the fricatives /s/ and /ʃ/ by manipulating the spectrum of the frication noise, formant transitions, and vowel context.[181] Across these studies, several overlapping and general findings emerged.

First, children used multiple cues in perception. However, the magnitude of trading relations among cues differed significantly from that reported for adults. Second, children not only used but relied upon multiple cues in perception. Acoustic redundancies were critical to the perception of phonemic contrasts. Third, children were more sensitive to some cues than others. The value of a particular cue varied with the contrast being examined. Fourth, children assigned relative weightings to the cues. Children seemed to use primary (obligatory) cues to phonemic contrasts in the same way as adults, but their use of secondary (optional) cues varied.[182]

For perception, these findings suggest that children first attend to global aspects of speech or to the combination and integration of multiple cues in perception. With development, children shift attention to more isolated, discrete segmental cues. The ability to use isolated cues in phonemic perception improves with age and may be associated with, for example, improvements in selective attention, production of specific sounds, or additional experience listening to others produce sounds.

For production, these findings suggest that children know the acoustic effects of articulatory gestures and use this productive knowledge to perceive phonemes. A child's knowledge of production, as inferred from these studies, relates specifically to lower-level (motor) articulation of speech sounds. These data do not bear on higher-level linguistic knowledge of sounds; that is, how sounds are represented and stored in the lexicon.[183–185]

For a complete understanding of the relationship between production and perception in children, researchers need to expand their evaluations to include assessments of the perception of phonemic contrasts as well as the production of these same contrasts.[186–189] Furthermore, productive assessments need to include both auditorily and acoustically-based measures. Auditorily-based evaluations refer to relative or absolute judgments of the accuracy of a child's sound production. Acoustically-based evaluations require instrumental acoustic phonetic measurements of specific features of a child's sound production. From converging evidence employing different sources of data (perception, production, acoustic), investigators will be able to identify precisely which cues a child uses to perceive a phonemic contrast and to determine whether these same cues are also used to produce that contrast.

Future Directions

The study of infant and child speech perception over the last 15 years has advanced the general body of information on perceptual processing. Infants and children, like adults, are able to distinguish differences in voice, place, and manner of sounds given a variety of acoustic cues. Infants and children also use multiple acoustic cues in speech perception. In fact, evidence suggests that multiple redundant cues may be critical in early speech perception.

Research on infants and children has also contributed to a greater understanding of the perception of complex speech contrasts. For developing systems, it appears that segmental information plays a major role in perception; suprasegmental information may not be as critical. These results are perplexing in light of claims that infants first attend to the global rhythm of speech before attending to specific segments, and that patterns of speech which emphasize suprasegmentals (i.e., motherese) are preferred by infants. Two lines of future research may help resolve these conflicting results. First, infants' attention to segmentals may have been a consequence of inadequate methodology. That is, infants may have been unable to perceive suprasegmentals such as stress because stress may not have been implemented in the stimuli to a significant degree. Acoustic cues may not have been sufficient to signal the intention of specific suprasegmentals. Methodological improvements aimed at this potential problem may produce different perceptual results. Second, it may be that only certain suprasegmentals, or even particular aspects of one suprasegmental, are used by infants in perception. In addition, some properties of suprasegmentals may be more salient to infants than others; it will be important for future research to identify these relevant components.

Theories of perceptual development address the issue of the role of linguistic experience in speech perception. Contemporary frameworks encourage an integration of innate aspects of the system with learning and environmental experience; the two are not mutually exclusive. Moreover, the development of speech perception is not seen as an isolated ability or skill. Rather, speech perception is part of a larger perceptual and cognitive system. Evidence in support of the various theoretical frameworks comes from different sensory and perceptual systems, only one of which is speech perception.

Research on speech perception in children is different than that of infants because it focuses on phonemic rather than phonetic perception. For children, questions about the role of speech perception in relation to speech production can be asked. Current research on trading relations has suggested that young children have and use productive knowledge in the perception of sounds. Productive knowledge, as used in this sense, refers to lower-level information about the articulators and their related gestures. Productive knowledge also has been used in reference to higher-level lexical information about the structure and function of sounds in the phonological system of a child. It will be important to integrate these two types of knowledge in future research in order to fully understand the relationship between perception and production in children. One way that this might be accomplished is to obtain converging evidence from several related sources of data, perceptual, productive, and acoustic.

SPEECH PERCEPTION IN SPECIAL POPULATIONS

In this section, we turn our attention to listeners with unique language patterns and linguistic skills. We will examine the perceptual skills of children with phonological disorders and of adults acquiring a second language. These particular populations were selected for study because, for each group, researchers have claimed that difficulties in speech perception may account for concomitant deficiencies in speech production and linguistic processing. The study of special populations is of importance for understanding the nature of specific linguistic deficits and for developing appropriate training strategies to overcome these deficits. The study of special populations is of further importance in understanding the complexity of speech perception in normal populations. Given the unique nature and capabilities of special populations, researchers are forced to abandon traditional methodologies, hypotheses, and predictions about speech perception. When these basic assumptions are set aside, new insights are often gained. Here we illustrate insights that have been gained from studying perception in each of these special populations.

Children with Phonological Disorders

Children with phonological disorders can best be described as displaying numerous errors in sound production and use with no obvious or known cognitive, emotional, hearing, or motor difficulties.[190] Why then do functional speech sound disorders result?

One hypothesis is that children have disorders in sound production because of difficulties in sound perception; sound errors are the result of perceptual problems. Initial tests of this hypothesis indicated that, in general, phonologically disordered children displayed more perceptual errors than normal children; however, a wide range of variation was observed.[191–193] Some phonologically disordered children had associated perceptual difficulties, whereas other children exhibited perceptual capabilities similar to normal children. In light of these findings, the original hypothesis was refined: children with phonological disorders are likely to have difficulty perceiving those sounds produced in error in the specific context of that error.[194–199] Thus perceptual difficulties with sounds produced in error were described as "allophonic" in nature.[196]

To test the proposed allophonic nature of phonologically-based perceptual errors, it was necessary to rethink the methodology for evaluating speech perception. Locke outlined eight criteria that a clinically relevant test of perception must meet.[195,196] For example, the test must (1) examine perception of errored sounds; (2) examine perception and production of errored sounds in different contexts; (3) compare perceptual performance on errored and target sounds with a control sound; (4) provide repeated opportunities to measure perception of errored sounds; and (5) prevent nonperceptual errors associated with task difficulty from being interpreted as perceptual errors. With these criteria in mind, Locke examined available methodologies for testing speech perception (e.g., picture identification, A/X, ABX, 4IAX) and found that, although these tasks were appropriate for use with normal adults and children, they were not sensitive clinical measures of allophonic perceptual problems. Consequently, a new procedure consistent with the eight clinical criteria was developed, namely, the Speech Production-Perception Task.[196] Here, clinical research advanced the current state of knowledge by adopting a fresh perspective on the nature of children's perceptual errors and by developing an appropriate way to measure these errors that was unconstrained by traditional paradigms.

A second hypothesis regarding the origin of functional sound disorders is that difficulties in sound production are linguistically based such that a child may have errors associated with phonological rules or nontarget representations of sounds in the mental lexicon.[141,184,200] Within this perspective, a child may display a unique sound system that is structurally and functionally independent of the target sound system at a productive and/or a perceptual level. Evaluations of this hypothesis have centered primarily on what a child knows about his or her own sound system. Perceptual research has focused specifically on a child's self-perception of errored versus intended productions.

A key test of the linguistically-based hypothesis was conducted by Hoffman, Stager, and Daniloff.[201] In this study, the perception and production capabilities of children who misarticulated intended /r/ were examined and compared to children who produced /r/ correctly. All children produced sentences containing /r/ and /w/ minimal pairs (e.g., "ring" and "wing"). Sentences were tape recorded and children identified their own (and others') productions as either intended /w/ or intended /r/. Group results indicated that both normal and phonologically disordered children were able to identify correct productions of intended /w/ and intended /r/ In addition, normal children assigned misarticulated /r/ productions to the intended /w/ class. Thus normal children did not perceive distinctions between intended /r/ and intended /w/ when presented with misarticulated productions. But phonologically disordered children randomly assigned misarticulated /r/ productions to either the intended /w/ or the intended /r/ class. These results suggested that phonologically disordered children may have been perceiving distinctions in their speech that corresponded to intended /r/ versus intended /w/. Perhaps these children were somehow marking their productions in some subtle way; thus acoustic analyses were conducted. Results indicated that phonologically disordered children who perceptually identified their intended, albeit errored, productions as distinct were, in fact, marking these distinctions acoustically. Children were attending to subtle cues in their own speech at a subphonemic level. In this case, data from phonologically disordered children contributed to the general understanding of the relationship between perception and production. These data provided further motivation for studies of self-perception in normal children, supporting the integration of evidence from perception and production at phonological and acoustic levels of analysis.

Adult Second Language Learners

The study of adults acquiring a second language provides important information and a novel perspective on the role of linguistic experience in speech perception. Two key questions have been asked: (1) What is the influence of the native language on perception of target language contrasts? and (2) How does increased experience with the target language affect perception of native language contrasts?

Not surprisingly, research has shown that native speakers are better at discriminating the relevant sound contrasts of their language than nonnative speakers.[202,203] In fact, in some cases, nonnative speakers cannot even perceive these contrasts.[204] This was true, for example, in Japanese learners' perception of the English contrast /r/ versus /l/.[205] Japanese learners had great difficulty discriminating these two sounds, performing at only chance levels. Learners were unable to assign the sounds to two different phonemic categories. This inability was related, in part, to the fact that Japanese makes no phonemic distinction between /r/ and /l/. Similar findings have been reported for other second language learners, namely, English speakers acquiring Hindi.[206] Therefore the native language may prevent relevant distinctions in the target language from being perceived.

But there is evidence that speakers learning a second language are able to discriminate contrasts present in the target language but absent in the native language.[207–210] This ability seems to require increased experience with the target language. For example, Japanese learners were able to discriminate /r/ and /l/, but only following massive exposure to English.[205] Moreover, as a function of experience, learners altered their perceptual cues.[210–214] Cues that were once primary in the native language were gradually modified following significant experience with the target language.

Together, these data suggested that the native language has an initial effect on a learner's perception of relevant contrasts in the target language. With language experience, learners gradually become less sensitive to native language cues. Linguistic experience thus appears to play a critical role in speech perception.

Yet what is the pattern of perceptual development when both a native language and a target language make use of the same relevant contrast? At least four hypotheses have been advanced:

1. The nonnative speaker maintains two distinct perceptual systems corresponding to the native language and to the target language.
2. The nonnative speaker maintains one perceptual system by incorporating the new perceptual system of the target language into the existing system of the native language.
3. The nonnative speaker maintains one perceptual system by incorporating the existing perceptual system of the native language into the new system of the target language.
4. The nonnative speaker integrates both the native and target perceptual systems into a single new compromise system.[215]

Gass examined the issue of perceptual development and change in a study of voice onset time in nonnative speakers learning English.[216] The speakers spoke a variety of languages (e.g., Farsi, Thai, Italian), all of which used the voice onset time category. The only difference between a speaker's native language and the target, English, was the location of the category boundary. Results of an identification task indicated that nonnative speakers perceived stops continuously rather than categorically. Moreover, systematic areas of "disturbance" or displacement were noted in the identification functions. These areas were located specifically around the target and/or the native language boundary. Thus nonnative speakers appeared to use both the native and the target language boundaries in the perception of voice onset time, supporting a compromise perceptual system (hypothesis 4).[214,217–219] The perceptual systems of speakers acquiring a second language contributed generally to the role of linguistic experience and attenuation in perceptual development. Borrowing from this line of research, theories of perceptual development in children that explore the interaction between genetics and experience may be further refined and enhanced.

Future Directions

The study of speech in special populations offers a novel perspective on current issues, problems, and methodologies in perceptual research. Research on phonologically disordered children and adults learning a second language has contributed specifically to our understanding of the relationship between speech perception and speech production, the mechanisms of perception, and the role of linguistic experience in perception. There is much to be gained from special populations in furthering our conception of how speech is perceived and in designing models of speech perception to accommodate these findings.

SUMMARY

Speech perception is a complex multifaceted problem that has continued to perplex researchers for several decades. The study of speech perception has focused primarily on two types of problems: the primary recognition problem and the role of multiple knowledge sources in speech perception. Research on both problems has recognized the importance of the integrated and dynamic nature of perceptual processing. Perception of speech involves more than just a sensory analysis of acoustic information encoded in the signal; it also involves higher-level analyses of linguistic structure. With advanced technology, contemporary research on speech perception faces a new horizon. It will now be possible to evaluate computationally and behaviorally models and interpretations of existing data. With attention to different populations, insights will be gained about the underlying perceptual mechanisms and the time course of perceptual development. Together, these data will potentially contribute to both theoretical and applied issues, bringing us closer to understanding the nature and structure of speech perception and processing.

Acknowledgments. The preparation of this chapter was supported, in part, by National Institutes of Health Training Grant NS–07134 and National Institutes of Health Research Grant NS–12179 to Indiana University, Bloomington.

REFERENCES

1. Pisoni DB. Some current theoretical issues in speech perception. Cognition 1981; 10:249–259.
2. Pisoni DB. Speech perception. In: Estes WK, ed. Handbook of learning and cognitive processes. Vol. 6. Hillsdale, NJ: Erlbaum, 1978:167.
3. Studdert-Kennedy M. The perception of speech. In: Sebeok TA, ed. Current trends in linguistics. Vol. 12. The Hague: Mouton, 1974:2349.
4. Studdert-Kennedy M. Speech perception. In: Lass NJ, ed. Contemporary issues in experimental phonetics. New York: Academic Press, 1976:243.
5. Pisoni DB, Luce PA. Acoustic-phonetic representations in the mental lexicon. Cognition 1987; 25:21–52.
6. Liberman AM, Delattre PC, Cooper FS. The role of selected stimulus variables in the perception of the unvoiced stop consonants. Am J Psychol 1952; 52:127–137.
7. Cooper FS, Delattre PC, Liberman AM, Borst JM, Gerstman LJ. Some experiments on the perception of synthetic speech sounds. J Acoust Soc Am 1952; 24:597–606.
8. Delattre PC, Liberman AM, Cooper FS. Acoustic loci and transitional cues for consonants. J Acoust Soc Am 1955; 27:769–773.
9. Dorman M, Studdert-Kennedy M, Raphael L. Stop consonant recognition: release bursts and formant transitions as functionally equivalent context-dependent cues. Perception and Psychophysics 1977; 22:109–122.
10. Blumstein SE, Stevens KN. Acoustic invariance in speech production: evidence from measurements of the spectral characteristics of stop consonants. J Acoust Soc Am 1979; 66:1001–1017.
11. Blumstein SE, Stevens KN. Perceptual invariance and onset spectra for stop consonants in different vowel environments. J Acoust Soc Am 1980; 67:648–662.
12. Stevens KN, Blumstein SE. Invariant cues for place of articulation in stop consonants. J Acoust Soc Am 1978; 64:1358–1368.
13. Fant G. Acoustic theory of speech production. The Hague: Mouton, 1960.
14. Fant G. Speech sounds and features. Cambridge, MA: MIT Press, 1973.
15. Stevens KN. Acoustic correlates of certain consonantal features. Paper presented at the conference on speech communication and processing, Cambridge, MA, 1967.

16. Stevens KN. Airflow and turbulence noise for fricative and stop consonants: static considerations. J Acoust Soc Am 1971; 50:1180–1192.
17. Stevens KN. Further theoretical and experimental bases for quantal places of articulation for consonants. Quarterly progress report no. 108. Cambridge, MA: Research Laboratory of Electronics, MIT, 1973.
18. Stevens KN. The potential role of property detectors in the perception of consonants. In: Fant G, Tatham MAA, eds. Auditory analysis and perception of speech. New York: Academic Press, 1975:303.
19. Blumstein SE, Isaacs E, Mertus J. The role of the gross spectral shape as a perceptual cue to place of articulation in initial stop consonants. J Acoust Soc Am 1982; 72:43–50.
20. Walley AC, Carrell TD. Onset spectra and formant transitions in the adult's and child's perception of place of articulation in stop consonants. J Acoust Soc Am 1983; 73:1011–1022.
21. Blumstein SE. On acoustic invariance in speech. In: Perkell JS, Klatt DH, eds. Invariance and variability in speech processes. Hillsdale, NJ: Erlbaum, 1986:178.
22. Lahiri A, Gewirth L, Blumstein SE. A reconsideration of acoustic invariance for place of articulation in diffuse stop consonants: evidence from a cross-language study. J Acoust Soc Am 1984; 76:391–404.
23. Mack M, Blumstein SE. Further evidence of acoustic invariance in speech production: the stop-glide contrast. J Acoust Soc Am 1983; 73:1739–1750.
24. Kewley-Port D. Representation of spectral change as cues to place of articulation in stop consonants. Research on speech perception (technical report no. 3). Bloomington, IN: Speech Research Laboratory, Department of Psychology, Indiana University, 1980.
25. Kewly-Port D. Time-varying features as correlates of place of articulation in stop consonants. J Acoust Soc Am 1983; 73:322–335.
26. Kewley-Port D. Converging approaches towards establishing acoustic correlates of stop consonants. In: Perkell JS, Klatt DH, eds. Invariance and variability in speech processes. Hillsdale, NJ: Erlbaum, 1986:193.
27. Kewley-Port D, Pisoni DB, Studdert-Kennedy M. Perception for static and dynamic acoustic cues to place of articulation in initial stop consonants. J Acoust Soc Am 1983; 73:1779–1793.
28. Searle CL, Jacobson JF, Kimberley BP. Speech as patterns in the 3-space of time and frequency. In: Cole RA, ed. Perception and production of fluent speech. Hillsdale, NJ: Erlbaum, 1980:73.
29. Searle CL, Jacobson JF, Rayment SG. Stop consonant discrimination based on human audition. J Acoust Soc Am 1979; 65:799–809.
30. Kewley-Port D, Luce PA. Time-varying features of initial stop consonants in auditory running spectra: a first report. Perception and Psychophysics 1984; 35:353–360.
31. Liberman AM, Harris KS, Hoffman HA, Griffith BC. The discrimination of speech sounds within and across phoneme boundaries. J Exp Psychol 1957; 54:358–368.
32. Eimas PD. The relations between identification and discrimination along speech and nonspeech continua. Lang Speech 1963; 6:206–217.
33. Repp BH. Categorical perception: issues, methods, findings. In: Lass NJ, ed. Speech and language: advances in basic research and practice. Vol. 10. New York: Academic Press, 1984:243.
34. Fry DB, Abramson AS, Eimas PD, Liberman AM. The identification and discrimination of synthetic vowels. Lang Speech 1962; 5:171–189.
35. Pisoni DB. Auditory short-term memory and vowel perception. Memory and Cognition 1975; 3:7–18.
36. Liberman AM. The grammars of speech and language. Cognitive Psychol 1970; 1:301–323.
37. Liberman AM. Some characteristics of perception in the speech mode. In: Hamburg DA, ed. Perception and its disorders: proceedings of A.R.N.M.D. Baltimore: Williams & Wilkins, 1970:238.
38. Liberman AM. On finding that speech is special. Am Psychol 1982; 37:148–167.
39. Liberman AM, Cooper FS, Shankweiler DP, Studdert-Kennedy M. Perception of the speech code. Psychol Rev 1967; 74:431–461.
40. Studdert-Kennedy M, Shankweiler D. Hemispheric specialization for speech perception. J Acoust Soc Am 1970; 48:570–594.
41. Liberman AM, Mattingly IG. The motor theory of speech perception revised. Cognition 1985; 21:1–36.
42. Lisker L, Abramson AS. A cross language study of voicing in initial stops: acoustical measurements. Word 1964; 20:384–442.
43. Lisker L, Abramson AS. The voicing dimension: some experiments in comparative phonetics. In: Proceedings of the sixth international congress of phonetic sciences. Prague: Academia Press, 1970:563.
44. Miller JD, Wier L, Pastore R, Kelly W, Dooling R. Discrimination and labeling of noise-buzz sequences with varying noise-lead times: an example of categorical perception. J Acoust Soc Am 1976; 60:410–417.
45. Pisoni DB. Identification and discrimination of the relative onset time of two component tones: implications for voicing perception in stops. J Acoust Soc Am 1977; 61:1352–1361.
46. Fujisaki H, Kawashima T. On the modes of mechanisms of speech perception. Annual report of the engineering research institute. Vol. 28. Tokyo: Faculty of Engineering, University of Tokyo, 1969:67.
47. Fujisaki H, Kawashima T. Some experiments on speech perception and a model for the perceptual mechanism. Annual report of the engineering research institute. Vol. 29. Tokyo: Faculty of Engineering, University of Tokyo, 1970:207.
48. Fujisaki H, Kawashima T. A model of the mechanisms for speech perception: quantitative analysis of categorical effects in discrimination. Annual report of the engineering research institute. Vol. 30. Tokyo: Faculty of Engineering, University of Tokyo, 1971:59.
49. Pastore RE, Ahroon WA, Baffuto KJ, Friedman C, Puleo JS, Fink EA. Common-factor model of categorical perception. J Exp Psychol [Hum Percept] 1977; 3:686–696.
50. Pisoni DB. On the nature of categorical perception of speech sounds. Supplement to status report on speech research SR-27. New Haven, CT: Haskins Laboratories, 1971.
51. Pisoni DB. Auditory and phonetic memory codes in the discrimination of consonants and vowels. Perception and Psychophysics 1973; 13:253–260.
52. Studdert-Kennedy M. Speech perception. In: Lindblom B, MacNeilage P, Studdert-Kennedy M, eds. Biological bases of spoken language. New York: Academic Press, in press.
53. Pisoni DB. Auditory perception of complex sounds: some comparisons of speech versus nonspeech signals. In: Yost WA, Watson CS, eds. Auditory processing of complex sounds. Hillsdale, NJ: Erlbaum, 1987:247.
54. Pisoni DB, Carrell TD, Gans SJ. Perception of the duration of rapid spectrum changes in speech and nonspeech signals. Perception and Psychophysics 1983; 34:314–322.
55. Cutting JE. Plucks and bows are categorically perceived, sometimes. Perception and Psychophysics 1982; 31:462–476.
56. Cutting JE, Rosner BS. Categories and boundaries in speech and music. Perception and Psychophysics 1974; 16:564–570.
57. Lane H. The motor theory of speech perception: a critical review. Psychol Rev 1965; 72:275–309.

58. Kewley-Port D, Pisoni DB. Identification and discrimination of rise time: is it categorical or noncategorical? J Acoust Soc Am 1984; 75:1168–1176.
59. Rosen SM, Howell P. Plucks and bows are not categorically perceived. Perception and Psychophysics 1981; 30:156–168.
60. Repp BH. Phonetic trading relations and context effects: new experimental evidence for a speech mode of perception. Psychol Bull 1982; 92:81–110.
61. Hillenbrand J. Perception of sine-wave analogs of voice onset time stimuli. J Acoust Soc Am 1984; 75:231–240.
62. Parker EM, Diehl RL, Kleunder KR. Trading relations in speech and nonspeech. Perception and Psychophysics 1986; 39:129–142.
63. Repp BH. Trading relations among acoustic cues in speech perception: speech-specific but not special. Haskins Laboratories status report on speech research SR-76. New Haven, CT: Haskins Laboratories, 1983:129.
64. Mann VA, Madden J, Russell JM, Liberman AM. Integration of time-varying cues and the effects of phonetic context. Unpublished manuscript. New Haven, CT: Haskins Laboratories, 1981.
65. Massaro DW. Speech perception by ear and eye: a paradigm for psychological inquiry. Hillsdale, NJ: Erlbaum, 1987.
66. MacDonald J, McGurk H. Visual influences on speech perception processes. Perception and Psychophysics 1978; 24:253–257.
67. McGurk H, MacDonald J. Hearing lips and seeing voices. Nature 1976; 264:746–748.
68. Roberts M, Summerfield Q. Audio-visual adaptation in speech perception. Perception and Psychophysics 1981; 30:309–314.
69. Summerfield Q. Use of visual information for phonetic perception. Phonetica 1979; 36:314–331.
70. Nakatani LH, Dukes KD. Locus of segmental cues for word juncture. J Acoust Soc Am 1977; 62:714–719.
71. Nakatani LH, O'Connor-Dukes KD. Phonetic parsing cues for word perception. Unpublished manuscript. Murray Hill, NJ: Bell Laboratories, 1980.
72. Nakatani LH, O'Connor KD, Aston CH. Prosodic aspects of American English speech rhythm. Phonetica 1981; 38:84–106.
73. Nakatani LH, Schaffer JA. Hearing "words" without words: prosodic cues for word perception. J Acoust Soc Am 1978; 63:234–245.
74. Massaro DW, Cohen MM. Phonological context in speech perception. Perception and Psychophysics 1983; 34:338–348.
75. Warren RM. Perceptual restoration of missing speech sounds. Science 1970; 176:392–393.
76. Samuel AG. Phonomic restoration: insights from a new methodology. J Exp Psychol [Gen] 1981; 110:474-494. 494.
77. Samuel AG. The role of bottom-up confirmation in the phonemic restoration illusion. J Exp Psychol [Hum Percept] 1981; 7:1124–1131.
78. Foss DJ, Harwood DA, Blank MA. Deciphering decoding decisions: data and devices. In: Cole RA, ed. Perception and production of fluent speech. Hillsdale, NJ: Erlbaum, 1980:165.
79. Foss DJ, Swinney DA. On the psychological reality of the phoneme: perception, identification, and consciousness. J Verbal Learn Verbal Behav 1973; 12:246–257.
80. Morton J, Long J. Effect of word transitional probability on phoneme identification. J Verbal Learn Verbal Behav 1976; 15:43–52.
81. Foss DJ, Blank MA. Identifying the speech codes. Cognitive Psychol 1980; 12:1–31.
82. Foss DJ, Gernsbacher MA. Cracking the dual code: toward a unitary model of phoneme identification. J Verbal Learn Verbal Behav 1983; 22:609–632.
83. Cotton S, Grosjean F. The gating paradigm: a comparison of successive and individual presentation formats. Perception and Psychophysics 1984; 35:41–48.
84. Grosjean F. Spoken word recognition processes and the gating paradigm. Perception and Psychophysics 1980; 28:267–283.
85. Salasoo A, Pisoni DB. Sources of knowledge in spoken word identification. J Memory Lang 1985; 24:210–231.
86. Tyler L. The structure of the initial cohort: evidence from gating. Perception and Psychophysics 1984; 36:417–427.
87. Cole RA, Jakimik J. Understanding speech: how words are heard. In: Underwood G, ed. Strategies of information processing. New York: Academic Press, 1978:68.
88. Cole RA, Jakimik J. A model of speech perception. In: Cole RA, ed. Perception and production of fluent speech. Hillsdale, NJ: Erlbaum, 1980:133.
89. Marslen-Wilson WD, Tyler LK. The temporal structure of spoken language understanding. Cognition 1980; 8:1–71.
90. Marslen-Wilson WD, Welsh A. Processing interactions and lexical access during word-recognition in continuous speech. Cognitive Psychol 1978; 10:29–63.
91. Miller GA, Heise GA, Lichten W. The intelligibility of speech as a function of the context of the test materials. J Exp Psychol 1951; 41:329–335.
92. Miller GA, Isard S. Some perceptual consequences of linguistic rules. J Verbal Learn Verbal Behav 1963; 2:217–228.
93. Luce PA, Pisoni DB. Speech perception: new directions in research, theory, and applications. In: Winitz H, ed. Human communication and its disorders. Norwood, NJ: Ablex, 1987:1.
94. Fant G. Descriptive analysis of the acoustic aspects of speech. Logos 1962; 5:3–17.
95. Fant G. Auditory patterns of speech. In: Wathen-Dunn W, ed. Models for the perception of speech and visual form. Cambridge, MA: MIT Press, 1967:111.
96. Stevens KN. Toward a model for speech recognition. J Acoust Soc Am 1960; 32:47–55.
97. Stevens KN, Halle M. Remarks on analysis-by-synthesis and distinctive features. In: Wathen-Dunn W, ed. Models for the perception of speech and visual form. Cambridge, MA: MIT Press, 1967:88.
98. Stevens KN, House AS. Speech perception. In: Tobias J, ed. Foundations of modern auditory theory. Vol. 2. New York: Academic Press, 1972:1.
99. Eimas PD. Speech perception in early infancy. In: Cohen LB, Salapatek P, eds. Infant perception: from sensation to cognition. Vol. 2. New York: Academic Press, 1975:193.
100. Oden GC, Massaro DW. Integration of featural information in speech perception. Psychol Rev 1978; 85:172–191.
101. Massaro DW. Experimental psychology and information processing. Chicago: Rand-McNally, 1975.
102. Massaro DW, ed. Understanding language: an information processing analysis of speech perception, reading, and psycholinguistics. New York: Academic Press, 1975.
103. McClelland JL, Elman JL. The TRACE model of speech perception. Cognitive Psychology 1986; 18:1–86.
104. McClelland JL, Rumelhart DE. An interactive activation model of context effects in letter perception. Part I: an account of basic findings. Psychol Rev 1981; 88:375–407.
105. McClelland JL, Rumelhart DE, The PDP Research Group. Parallel distributed processing: explorations in the microstructure of cognition: psychological and biological models. Vol. 2. Cambridge, MA: MIT Press, 1986.
106. Rumelhart DE, McClelland JL. Interactive processing through spreading activation. In: Perfetti C, Lesgold A, eds. Interactive processes in reading. Hillsdale, NJ: Erlbaum, 1981:37.

107. Rumelhart DE, McClelland JL. An interactive activation model of context effects in letter perception. Part II: the contextual enhancement effect and some tests and extensions of the model. Psychol Rev 1982; 89:60–84.
108. Rumelhart DE, McClelland JL, The PDP Research Group. Parallel distributed processing: explorations in the microstructure of cognition: foundations. Vol. 1. Cambridge, MA: MIT Press, 1986.
109. Luce PA. Neighborhoods of words in the mental lexicon. Research on speech perception (technical report no. 6). Bloomington, IN: Speech Research Laboratory, Department of Psychology, Indiana University, 1986:573.
109a. Aslin RN, Pisoni DB, Jusczyk PW. Auditory development and speech perception in infancy. In: Mussen P, ed. Carmichael's manual of child psychology, 4th ed, Vol. 2. Haith MM, Campos JJ, eds. Infancy and the biology of development. New York: John Wiley & Sons, 1983:573.
110. Bartoshuk AK. Human neonatal cardiac responses to sound: a power function. Psychonomic Sci 1964; 1:151–152.
111. Lasky RE, Syrdal-Lasky A, Klein RE. VOT discrimination by four to six and a half month old infants from Spanish environments. J Exp Child Psychol 1975; 20:215–225.
112. Moffitt AR. Consonant cue perception by twenty- to twenty-four-week-old infants. Child Dev 1971; 42:717–731.
113. Moffitt AR. Intensity discrimination and cardiac reaction in young infants. Dev Psychol 1973; 8:357–359.
114. Leavitt LA, Brown JW, Morse PA, Graham FK. Cardiac orienting and auditory discrimination in 6-week old infants. Dev Psychol 1976; 12:514–523.
115. Boyd EF. Visual fixation and voice discrimination in 2-month-old infants. In: Horowitz FD, ed. Visual attention, auditory stimulation, and language discrimination in young infants. Monogr Soc Res Child Dev 1975; 39:5–6.
116. Colombo J, Bundy RS. A method for the measurement of infant auditory selectivity. Infant Behav Dev 1981; 4:219–233.
117. Eimas PD, Miller JL. Contextual effects in infant speech perception. Science 1980; 209:1140–1141.
118. Eimas PD, Miller JL. Discrimination of the information for manner of articulation. Infant Behav Dev 1980; 3:367–375.
119. Siqueland ER, DeLucia CA. Visual reinforcement of non-nutritive sucking in human infants. Science 1969; 165:1144–1146.
120. Trehub SE, Chang H. Speech as reinforcing stimulation for infants. Dev Psychol 1977; 13:170–171.
121. Williams L, Golenski J. Infant speech sound discrimination: the effects of contingent versus noncontingent stimulus presentation. Child Dev 1978; 49:213–217.
122. Miller CL, Eimas PD. Organization in infant speech perception. Can J Psychol 1979; 33:353–367.
123. Spring DR, Dale PS. Discrimination of linguistic stress in early infancy. J Speech Hear Res 1977; 20:224–232.
124. Eilers RE, Wilson WR, Moore JM. Discrimination of synthetic prevoiced labial stops by infants and adults (abstr). J Acoust Soc Am [Suppl] 1976; 60:S91.
125. Kuhl P. Speech perception in early infancy: perceptual constancy for vowel categories (abstr). J Acoust Soc Am [Suppl] 1976; 60:S90.
126. Suzuki T, Ogiba Y. Conditioned orientation reflex audiometry. Arch Otolaryngol 1961; 74:192–198.
127. Trehub SE, Schneider BA, Endman M. Developmental changes in infants' sensitivity to octave-band noises. J Exp Child Psychol 1980; 29:282–293.
128. Aslin RN, Pisoni DB. Effects of early linguistic experience on speech discrimination by infants: a critique of Eilers, Gavin, and Wilson (1979). Child Dev 1980; 51:107–112.
129. Kubaska CA, Aslin RN. Categorization and normalization of vowels by 3-year-old children. Perception and Psychophysics 1985; 37:355–362.
130. Aslin RN, Pisoni DB. Some developmental processes in speech perception. In: Yeni-Komshian G, Kavanagh JF, Ferguson CA, eds. Child phonology: perception. Vol. 2. New York: Academic Press, 1980:67.
131. Jusczyk PW. Auditory versus phonetic coding of speech signals during infancy. In: Mehler J, Walker ECT, Garrett MF, eds. Perspectives on mental representation. Hillsdale, NJ: Erlbaum, 1982:361.
132. Walley AC, Pisoni DB, Aslin RN. The role of early experience in the development of speech perception. In: Aslin RN, Alberts J, Peterson MJ, eds. The development of perception: psychobiological perspectives. New York: Academic Press, 1981:219.
133. Eimas PD, Siqueland ER, Jusczyk PW, Vigorito J. Speech perception in infants. Science 1971; 171:303–306.
134. Trehub SE, Rabinovitch MS. Auditory-linguistic sensitivity in early infancy. Dev Psychol 1972; 6:74–77.
135. Eilers RE, Wilson WR, Moore JM. Developmental changes in speech discrimination in infants. J Speech Hear Res 1977; 20:766–780.
136. Eilers RE. Context sensitive perception of naturally produced stop and fricative consonants by infants. J Acoust Soc Am 1977; 61:1321–1336.
137. Eimas PD, Tartter VC. On the development of speech perception: mechanisms and analogies. In: Lipsitt LP, Reese HW, eds. Advances in child development and behavior. Vol. 13. New York: Academic Press, 1979:155.
138. Jusczyk PW. Infant speech perception: a critical appraisal. In: Eimas PD, Miller JL, eds. Perspectives on the study of speech. Hillsdale, NJ: Erlbaum, 1981:113.
139. Prather ED, Hedrick DL, Kern C. Articulation development in children aged two to four years. J Speech Hear Res 1975; 40:179–191.
140. Sander E. When are speech sounds learned? J Speech Hear Disord 1972; 37:55–63.
141. Ingram D. Phonological disability in children. New York: Elsevier, 1976.
142. Straight HS. Auditory versus articulatory phonological processes and their development in children. In: Yeni-Komshian G, Kavanagh JF, Ferguson CA, eds. Child phonology: production. Vol. 1. New York: Academic Press, 1980:43.
143. Eimas PD. Auditory and linguistic processing of cues for place of articulation by infants. Perception and Psychophysics 1974; 16:513–521.
144. Miller CL, Morse PA. The "heart" of categorical speech discrimination in young infants. J Speech Hear Res 1976; 19:578–589.
145. Miller CL, Morse PA, Dorman MF. Cardiac indices of infant speech perception: orienting and burst discrimination. Q J Exp Psychol 1977; 29:533–545.
146. Morse PA. The discrimination of speech and non-speech stimuli in early infancy. J Exp Child Psychol 1972; 14:477–492.
147. Till J. Infants' discrimination of speech and nonspeech stimuli. Doctoral Dissertation. Iowa City, IA: University of Iowa, 1976.
148. Walley AC, Pisoni DB, Aslin RN. Infant discrimination of two- and five-formant voiced stop consonants differing in place of articulation. J Acoust Soc Am 1984; 75:581–589.
149. Williams L, Bush M. The discrimination by young infants of voiced stop consonants with and without release bursts. J Acoust Soc Am 1978; 63:1223–1225.
150. Abbs M, Minifie FD. Effect of acoustic cues in fricatives on perceptual confusions in preschool children. J Acoust Soc Am 1969; 44:1535–1542.
151. Eilers RE, Minifie FD. Fricative discrimination in early infancy. J Speech Hear Res 1975; 18:158–167.
152. Holmberg TL, Morgan KA, Kuhl PK. Speech perception

in early infancy: discrimation of fricative consonants (abstr). J Acoust Soc Am [Suppl] 1977; 62:S99.

153. Carden G, Levitt A, Jusczyk PW, Walley AC. Evidence for phonetic processing of cues to place of articulation: perceived manner affects perceived place. Perception and Psychophysics 1981; 29:26–36.

154. Juscyzk PW, Murray J, Murphy C, Levitt A, Carden G. Perception of place of articulation in fricatives and stops by infants. In: Haith MM, Campos JJ, eds. Carmichael's manual of child psychology. Vol. 2. Infancy and the biology of development. 4th ed. New York: John Wiley & Sons, 1983:573.

155. Trehub SE. Infants' sensitivity to vowel and tonal contrasts. Dev Psychol 1973; 9:91–96.

156. Kuhl PK. Speech perception in early infancy: perceptual constancy for the vowel categories /a/ and ŋ/ (abstr). J Acoust Soc Am [Suppl] 1977; 61:S39.

157. Kuhl PK. Speech perception in early infancy: perceptual constancy for spectrally dissimilar vowel categories. J Acoust Soc Am 1979; 66:1668–1679.

158. Kuhl PK, Miller JD. Speech perception in early infancy: discrimination of speech-sound categories (abstr). J Acoust Soc Am [Suppl] 1975; 58:S56.

159. Kuhl PK, Miller JD. Discrimination of auditory target dimensions in the presence or absence of variation in a second dimension by infants. Perception and Psychophysics 1982; 31:279–292.

160. Swoboda P, Morse PA, Leavitt LA. Continuous vowel discrimination in normal and at-risk infants. Child Dev 1976; 47:459–465.

161. Ferguson CA, Farwell CB. Words and sounds in early language acquisition. Language 1975; 51:419–439.

162. Peters AM. Language learning strategies: does the whole equal the sum of the parts? Language 1977; 53:560–573.

163. Peters AM. The units of language acquisition. Cambridge, England: Cambridge University Press, 1983.

164. Jusczyk PW, Copan HC, Thompson EJ. Perception by two-month-olds of glide contrasts in multisyllabic utterances. Perception and Psychophysics 1978; 24:515–520.

165. Jusczyk PW, Thompson EJ. Perception of a phonetic contrast in multisyllabic utterances by two-month-old infants. Perception and Psychophysics 1978; 23:105–109.

166. Carrell TD, Smith LB, Pisoni DB. Some perceptual dependencies in speeded classification of vowel color and pitch. Perception and Psychophysics 1981; 29:1–10.

167. Newport EL. Motherese: speech of mothers to young children. In: Castellan NJ, Pisoni DB, Potts GR, eds. Cognitive theory. Vol. 2. Hillsdale, NJ: Erlbaum, 1977:177.

168. Phillips JR. Formal characteristics of speech which mothers address to their young children. Doctoral Dissertation. Baltimore, MD: The Johns Hopkins University, 1970.

169. Snow CE, Ferguson CA, eds. Talking to children: language input and acquisition. Cambridge, England: Cambridge University Press, 1977.

170. Mehler J, Bertoncini J, Barriere M, Jassik-Gerschenfeld D. Infant recognition of mother's voice. Perception 1978; 7:491–497.

171. Fernald A. Four-month-olds prefer to listen to "motherese." Paper presented to the Society for Research in Child Development, Boston, MA, 1981.

172. Fernald A, Kuhl PK. Fundamental frequency as an acoustic determinant of infant preference for motherese. Paper presented to the Society for Research in Child Development, Boston, MA, 1981.

173. Hirsh-Pasek K, Kemler Nelson DG, Jusczyk PW, Cassidy KW, Druss B, Kennedy L. Clauses are perceptual units for young infants. Cognition, in press.

174. Kemler Nelson DG, Hirsh-Pasek K, Jusczyk PW, Cassidy KW. How the prosodic cues in motherese might assist language learning. Research on speech perception progress report. Eugene, OR: Speech Research Laboratory, Department of Psychology, University of Oregon, 1986:155.

175. Barton D. Phonemic perception in children. In: Yeni-Komshian G, Kavanagh JF, Ferguson CA, eds. Child phonology: perception. Vol. 2. New York: Academic Press, 1980:97.

176. Barton D. Statistical significance in phonemic perception experiments. J Child Lang 1975; 2:297–298.

177. Jusczyk PW, Shea SL, Aslin RN. Linguistic experience and infant speech perception: a re-examination of Eilers, Gavin, and Oller (1982). J Child Lang 1984; 11:453–466.

178. Strange W, Broen PA. Perception and production of approximant consonants by 3-year-olds: a first study. In: Yeni-Komshian G, Kavanagh JF, Ferguson CA, eds. Child phonology: perception. Vol. 2. New York: Academic Press, 1980:117.

179. Morrongiello BA, Robson RC, Best CT, Clifton RK. Trading relations in the perception of speech by 5-year-old children. J Exp Child Psychol 1984; 37:231–250.

180. Mann VA, Sharlin HM, Dorman M. Children's perception of sibilants: the relation between articulation and perceptual development. J Exp Child Psychol 1985; 30:252–264.

181. Nittroeur S, Studdert-Kennedy M. The role of coarticulatory effects in the perception of speech by young children. J Speech Hear Res 1987; 30:319–329.

182. Greene BG, Pisoni DB. Perception of synthetic speech by adults and children: research on processing voice output from text-to-speech systems. In: Bernstein LE, ed. The vocally impaired: clinical practice and research. Philadelphia: WB Saunders, in press.

183. Gierut JA, Elbert M, Dinnsen DA. A functional analysis of phonological knowledge and generalization learning in misarticulating children. J Speech Hear Res 1987; 30:462–479.

184. Dinnsen DA. Methods and empirical issues in analyzing functional misarticulations. In: Elbert M, Dinnsen DA, Weismer G, eds. Phonological theory and the misarticulating child (ASHA monogr no. 22). Rockville, MD: ASHA, 1984:5.

185. Gierut JA. On the assessment of productive phonological knowledge. NSSLHA J 1986; 14:83–101.

186. Baer T, Alfonso PJ. On simultaneous neuromuscular, movement, and acoustic measures of speech articulation. In: Daniloff RG, ed. Articulation assessment and treatment issues. San Diego: College-Hill Press, 1984:195.

187. Hoffman PR, Daniloff RG, Alfonso PJ, Schuckers GH. Multiple-phoneme-misarticulating children's perception and production of voice onset time. Percept Mot Skills 1984; 58:603–610.

188. Hoffman PR, Daniloff RG, Bengoa D, Schuckers GH. Misarticulating and normally articulating children's identification and discrimination of synthetic [r] and [w]. J Speech Hear Disord 1985; 50:46–53.

189. Maxwell EM, Weismer G. The contribution of phonological, acoustic, and perceptual techniques to the characterization of a misarticulating child's voice contrast for stops. Appl Psycholinguist 1982; 3:29–43.

190. Shelton R, McReynolds LV. Functional articulation disorders: preliminaries to treatment. In: Lass NJ, ed. Speech and language: advances in basic research and practice. Vol. 2. New York: Academic Press, 1979:1.

191. Kronvall E, Diehl C. The relationship of auditory discrimination to articulation defects of children with no known organic impairment. J Speech Hear Disord 1954; 19:335–338.

192. Travis L, Rasmus B. The speech sound discrimination ability of cases of functional disorders of misarticulation. Q J Speech 1931; 17:217–226.

193. Winitz H. Articulatory acquisition and behavior. New York:

Appleton-Century-Crofts, 1969.
194. Aungst L, Frick J. Auditory discrimination ability and consistency of articulation of /r/. J Speech Hear Disord 1964; 29:76–85.
195. Locke JL. The interference of speech perception on the phonologically disordered child. Part I: a rationale, some criteria, the conventional tests. J Speech Hear Disord 1980; 45:431–444.
196. Locke JL. The interference of speech perception on the phonologically disordered child. Part II: some clinically novel procedures, their use, some findings. J Speech Hear Disord 1980; 45:444–468.
197. Monnin L, Huntington D. Relationship of articulatory defects to speech-sound identification. J Speech Hear Res 1974; 17:353–366.
198. Spriestersbach D, Curtis J. Misarticulation and discrimination of speech sounds. Q J Speech 1951; 37:483–489.
199. Wolfe V, Irwin R. Sound discrimination ability of children with misarticulation of the /r/ sound. Percept Mot Skills 1973; 37:415–420.
200. Elbert M, Dinnsen DA, Weismer G, eds. Phonological theory and the misarticulating child (ASHA monogr no. 22). Rockville, MD: ASHA, 1984.
201. Hoffman PR, Stager S, Daniloff RG. Perception and production of misarticulated /r/. J Speech Hear Disord 1983; 48:210-215.
202. Marckwardt A. An experiment in aural perception. English J 1944; 33:212–214
203. Oakeshott-Taylor J. Perception and production of English sounds by German speaking subjects. Hamburger Phonetische Beitrage 1976; 17:163–199.
204. Strange W, Jenkins JJ. Role of linguistic experience in the perception of speech. In: Walk RD, Pick HL, eds. Perception and experience. New York: Plenum Press, 1978:125.
205. Miyawaki K, Strange W, Verbrugge R, Liberman A, Jenkins J, Fujimura O. An effect of linguistic experience: the discrimination of /r/ and /l/ by native speakers of Japanese and English. Perception and Psychophysics 1975; 18: 331–340.
206. Werker J, Gilbert J, Humphry I, Tees R. Developmental aspects of cross-language speech perception. Child Dev 1981; 52:349–355.
207. Flege JE. The effect of linguistic experience on Arabs' perception of the English /s/ vs. /z/ contrast. Folia Linguistica 1984; 18:117–138.
208. MacCain K, Best C, Strange W. Categorical perception of English /r/ and /l/ by Japanese bilinguals. Appl Psycholinguist 1981; 2:369–390.
209. Mochizuki M. The identification of /r/ and /l/ in natural and synthesized speech. J Phonetics 1981; 9:283–303.
210. Pisoni DB, Aslin RN, Perey AJ, Hennessy BL. Some effects of laboratory training on identification and discrimination of voicing contrasts in stop consonants. J Exp Psychol [Hum Percept] 1982; 8:297–314.
211. Elman J, Diehl R, Buchwald S. Perceptual switching in bilinguals. J Acoust Soc Am 1977; 62:971–974.
212. Garnes S. Effects of bilingualism on perception. In: Garnica O, ed. Papers in psycholinguistics and sociolinguistics. Columbus, OH: Department of Linguistics, Ohio State University, 1977:1.
213. Gottfried TL, Beddor PS. Perception of temporal versus spectral information in French vowels. Paper presented to the Acoustical Society of America, Minneapolis, MN, 1984.
214. Williams L. Phonetic variation as a function of second-language learning. In: Yeni-Komshian G, Kavanagh JF, Ferguson CA, eds. Child phonology: perception. Vol. 2. New York: Academic Press, 1980:185.
215. Flege JE. The production and perception of foreign language speech sounds. In: Winitz H, ed. Human communication and its disorders. Norwood, NI: Ablex, in press.
216. Gass S. Development of speech perception and speech production abilities in adult second language learners. Appl Psycholinguist 1984; 5:51–74.
217. Caramazza A, Yeni-Komshian G, Zurif E, Carbone E. The acquisition of a new phonological contrast: the case of stop consonants in French-English bilinguals. J Acoust Soc Am 1973; 54:421–428.
218. Flege JE. The phonological basis of foreign accent: a hypothesis. TESOL Quarterly, 1981; 15:443–455.
219. Niemi J. Noun and noun phrase stress: a phonetic study of English supplemented with an error analysis using Finnish speaker-hearers. I. Production. Lang Speech 1979; 22:221–235.

10 Auditory Linguistic Processing

Margaret L. Lemme, Ph.D.
Natalie L. Hedberg, Ph.D.

In recent years, the scope of the topic "auditory processing" has been extended from a study of the peripheral auditory mechanism to include the central processing of speech stimuli and the understanding of language. The purpose of this chapter is to view the study of central auditory linguistic processing within the framework of selected neurologic and cognitive aspects of information processing theory.

Theories of auditory processing, in the most restricted sense, deal with the analysis of the acoustic signal, whereas theories of speech perception are concerned with the analysis of acoustic patterns and their relationships to the recognition of phonemes. Other theories of linguistic processing go beyond the level of the phoneme to include the influences of all linguistic rule systems: phonology, syntax, semantics, the lexicon and pragmatics. Information-processing theories expand influences to account for how language is understood by the human. More recent discourse-processing theories take into account the situation as well. In so doing, they delineate structures and processes involved between the reception of the stimulus and the meaning response, bringing to mind the lament that "everything is related to everything else."[1]

Norman and Bobrow define process as "a set of programs that is being executed for a common purpose and for which resources are allocated as a unit."[2] Programs are activated and resources are allocated that determine the result obtained, and the results are coded and stored. The "sets of programs" carried out by the human information systems have been treated historically as isolated activities or as aspects of the mind, thus the traditional classifications of attention, perception, memory, and comprehension. To view these processes as isolated is erroneous. However, an understanding of the relationships among their functions requires consideration of the dimensions along which they vary. Four dimensions of processing are discussed here: structure and control; bottom-up and top-down; passive and active; and serial and parallel.

DIMENSIONS OF PROCESSING

Structure and Control

A comprehensive review of memory put forth by Atkinson and Shiffrin differentiated the structural, or nonvarying, features of the information-processing system from those that may vary from one task to another.[3] The structural features appear to reflect aspects, or levels of storage, that are built into the system in a fixed programmatic sense. Associated with each structural component are variable features of the system, called "control processes," that are selected by the individual and operate on the information held in the stores according to the demands of the particular situation. The variable control processes are influenced by factors such as the individual's current instructional set, the task to be performed, and the history of the individual.[3] Control processes are viewed as voluntary strategies performed by the individual in the accomplishment of a particular task. They are selected according to the aspect of processing occurring, such as coding prior to recognition, rehearsal prior to storage, and search prior to recall.

Similarly, the central nervous system is composed of fixed structures including various neuronal circuits and pools, or networks; however, its operations are known to vary and to be selective. For example, unvarying behavior would result from the "all-or-none" response of neurons—the basic functional unit of nervous system circuitry—if they were not modified by other factors. However, the qualities of variability and selectivity are provided for by synapses, influenced by excitatory and inhibitory properties, and the organization of chains of neurons. Thus neuronal circuits that transmit information are organized to facilitate or block sensory signals, to amplify or to bring them into focus, or to send them over divergent tracts.[4] Neuronal pools, located in the brain stem and cerebral cortex, which receive signals from more than one source, are engaged in the processing of information and function to determine how neuronal circuits transmit various sensory signals.

Bottom-up and Top-down

A second dichotomous representation of processing operations reflects how they are driven by the incoming data or by the concepts already known to the individual. Data driven, or bottom-up, processes are guided by the data being analyzed with increasingly finer levels of analysis being carried out between the input of the sensory stimuli and the point at which meaning is obtained. The term "bottom-up" is derived from diagrams depicting the human processing system in which the data are seen to enter the system at the bottom of the diagram and then proceed to increasingly higher levels of analysis until they reach the top, where recognition or comprehension takes place.

Conceptually driven, or top-down, processing takes into account expectations held by the individual concerning the possible nature of the incoming stimuli. These expectations derive from information stored in long-term memory as to his or her knowledge of the world in which he or she lives, and of the rules of the language he or she speaks, as well as from the context in which the stimulus is embedded. The top-down system is cued to "search" for relevant information in the available data.

Although the terms "bottom-up" and "top-down" are not used commonly in anatomic and physiologic discussions, the concept of this representation is prevalent. Auditory impulses carried by the classic auditory ascending, or afferent, system are not simply relayed to the cerebral cortex for their final integration. Rather, highly selective neurophysiologic mechanisms modify the transmission of impulses at all levels of the specific afferent pathways. Information is selected and processed for which the system is prepared. Cortical, or descending, as well as central brain stem and thalamic ascending influences have been demonstrated. Mechanisms in the midbrain control long-term, or tonic, states, including arousal and alertness. Temporary, or phasic, states, which prepare the system to receive or bias it to select certain inputs, are controlled at the thalamus.

Passive and Active

Speech perception systems have been viewed as passive or active according to whether the system operated directly or indirectly on incoming data.[5,6] In passive systems, a perceptual unit is built up by combining previously analyzed fragments. A detection mechanism responds to the unit according to the features required in the recognition of a particular pattern. Active systems contain a comparator that matches the input pattern with a pattern that is either stored or generated for purposes of mediation. Thus recognition is accomplished indirectly through a comparison process that judges the adequacy of the match. It seems probable, as will be noted in later neurologic and cognitive discussions, that processing systems are not solely passive or active; rather, both types of processing take place at various stages in the system.

Serial and Parallel

Several operations are involved between the early gross analysis of the sensory input and the determination of its meaning. These analyses might occur through successive operations—serial processing—or simultaneous operations—parallel processing. In the former strategy, the results of one level of processing are fed into a processor at the next level. For example, the analysis of a speech stimulus would begin with the extraction of the frequency, intensity, and duration of the signal. The next analyzer would synthesize this information and determine the presence or absence of certain phonemic features. Another level would group these features into bundles in order to identify phonemic characteristics, and so on until speech was understood. In contrast to the successive operations approach, parallel processing allows for multiple levels of analysis to be carried out simultaneously. An obvious problem with the serial processing strategy for speech stimuli is the factor of time required in the successive levels of processing with the speech signal being transitory in nature.

NEURAL BASIS OF AUDITORY PROCESSING

Central Auditory Nervous System

The central auditory nervous system is discussed in detail in Chapters 2 and 3. In review, the cell bodies of neurons that make up the afferent pathways are contained in five major areas—the cochlear nucleus, the superior olivary complex, the inferior colliculus, the medial geniculate body, and the auditory cortex. The functional organization of the auditory nervous system reflects serial and parallel circuits, which appear to guarantee redundancy of auditory information. Glattske suggests higher centers may make decisions, including complex sorting and discrimination, after lower nuclei strip redundancy from neural events and provide specific, well-defined sensations.[7] Although no single auditory function can be attributed to particular nuclei, a progressive increase in response specificity and central coordination from lower to higher levels is generally accepted.

The central auditory nervous system also has an efferent auditory, or descending, system, which begins with projections from the auditory cortex and exists in parallel to the ascending system. Efferent auditory system, as well as nonspecific sensory system, influences are capable of modifying afferent auditory pathway transmission.

Nonspecific Sensory System

The nonspecific sensory system distributed through the central core of the brain stem provides a diffuse, indirect route for auditory information to reach the cerebral cortex. Additionally, this system exerts modulating influences upon all specific afferent pathways and overall cerebral cortex excitability, responding especially to novel signals. The "nonspecific" sensory system, including the reticular formation, which extends from the medullary regions of the lower brain stem up through the region of the midbrain and diencephalon, provides for integrated reactions. Branches of nerve axons, or collaterals, from the lower segments of all specific afferent paths reach the sensory system,[8] and reticular formation cells respond to all modalities of sensory stimulation.[9] Collaterals of second- and third-order neurons of the specific auditory afferent pathway are given off to the reticular formation.

The reticular system is able to decrease or increase excitability of most sensory neurons, inhibiting or facilitating sensory transmission at all levels within specific afferent pathways.[8] This system then participates in regulation of activity in specific auditory afferent paths. For example, reduction or inhibition of auditory potentials recorded at the level of the cochlear nucleus during electrical stimulation of the reticular formation has been recorded.[10,11]

The discovery of the reticular formation and the diffuse thalamic projection system also advanced understanding of arousal systems. Arousal is commonly considered a neurophysiologic entity resulting from activation of the cortex by the ascending reticular activating system,[12] and it appears to respond primarily to stimulus changes.[13] Reciprocal corticoreticular influences on the control of arousal have also been demonstrated.[14] In recent years, experimental findings have suggested that the reticular formation may not be the sole site for the induction and maintenance of arousal.[15] Routtenberg, after he reviewed experimental procedures, proposed dual, mutually inhibitory subcortical arousal systems.[16] He suggested that the first arousal system, related to the reticular formation, controls the general reactivity of the organism and provides organization for response; whereas the second arousal system, related to the limbic structures, provides control of responses through incentive-related stimuli. Recognition of cortical and limbic contributions to the reticular formation made it possible to understand how internal states—thoughts and worries—might generate arousal.[17] Thus nonspecific ascending neural input can modulate, raise, or lower the overall level of excitation of extensive regions of the cortex, including auditory cortical neurons. For example, electrical stimulation of the reticular formation renders some auditory neurons more sensitive to vocalization in the monkey.[18]

Attention

Neuroscientists generally agree that attention is a selective process: a process by which an organism chooses to deal more effectively with one type of sensory stimulus at the expense of other stimuli.[19] Numerous studies of the central nervous system have attempted to localize areas of the brain that are sites of attentional activity. Neurophysiologic study of animals and regional blood flow evoked potential studies in the human, and tests of brain-damaged humans have been productive in identifying brain regions having attentional effects.

Hernández-Peón et al first remarked that "attention involves the selective awareness of certain sensory messages with the simultaneous suppression of others" (p 331).[10] Many investigators studying the effects of attention upon afferent impulses have found increased amplitude of evoked potentials in a specific modality during arousal or attention.[8,20] Inducing selective focusing of attention through conditioning, facilitation of sensory transmission has been observed at the cochlear nucleus.[21] Apparently, such facilitation of specific afferent inputs is closely coordinated with inhibition of other stimulus input. Hernández-Peón et al were the first to suggest the neural mechanisms of this process.[10] They demonstrated suppression of irrelevant auditory inputs (clicks) at the level of the cochlear nucleus while a cat attended to a meaningful visual stimulus, a mouse, or other competing stimuli. The auditory response returned to its original magnitude when competing stimuli were removed. This attenuating influence plays an important role during focusing of attention in perception. Hernández-Peón hypothesized that the reticular system was concerned with sensory information filtering and sensory integration. He suggested that the reticular formation resembles a "high command" that receives polysensory information from the external and internal environments and "filters by feedback circuits all the sensory impulses at their entrance to the central nervous system" (p 517).[8]

Thatcher and John suggest that a "possible anatomic substrate of attention is provided by examining the nature of specific-nonspecific (sensory) convergence on cortical neurons" (p 109).[17] Based on the 1967 work of Scheibel and Scheibel, these authors state that the differential organization of afferent drives in specific and nonspecific sensory systems suggests an attention-focusing mechanism that alters interactions between cortical cells and affects the routing of specific sensory control. The distribution pattern of these two sensory afferent systems results in low levels of tonic control or gradual biasing of excitability of pyramidal cells.

Human cortical evoked potential studies of auditory attention conducted by Hillyard and associates demonstrate potentials that specifically reflect selective attention and not unspecific preparatory behavior or reactive changes subsequent to attention shift.[22] These authors propose that the attentional process is a tonic influence on the incoming auditory information. Further study results suggest that the brain produces greater attentional potentials in those situations where there is the greatest demand for a selection process.[23] Knight and colleagues attempted to determine the contribution of the frontal cortex to the selective potential changes recorded during an auditory attention task in normal and brain-damaged subjects.[24] Their results indicate that the left frontal cortex may be related to global attentional processes, whereas the right may deal with more localized processes. Further, the frontal cortex may mediate the attention-related potentials, but these changes are probably not originating in the frontal cortex. Other studies show that damage to the frontal lobes yields a type of auditory neglect in man and monkey.[25,26]

Roland has attempted to localize attention sites in the human brain by measuring regional blood flow with isotopes while subjects performed various tasks.[27] When subjects were presented with visual, auditory, and somatosensory stimuli simultaneously, but asked to discriminate using only one, Roland found various cortical changes. The primary and immediate associative cortices for each modality were markedly activated in each attentional task. When subjects discriminated only auditory stimuli, blood flow increased to the auditory association cortex, midtemporal cortex, Broca's area, and the frontal eye fields. When attention was changed from one modality to another, activity changed in the superior lateral part of the prefrontal cortex regardless of the modality being switched. The results suggest that parts of the brain may be specifically related to attentional behavior and not just the sensory processing associated with any modality.

Thatcher and John, having reviewed considerable literature on brain mechanisms of attention, concluded that "a very complex, but interrelated, system involving reticular, diencephalic, limbic and cortical structures mediates attention shift and attention fixation" (p 116).[17] They have developed diagrammatic representations of anatomic components mediating attention (Figs. 10–1 and 10–2).

McGuinness and Pribram identify emotional and motivational controls on attention that operate through three neuroanatomic, neurophysiologic, and neurochemical systems.[28,29] A summary diagram of these three systems is presented in Figure 10–3. The first system controls arousal; it is based in the amygdala and is associated with phasic responses to environmental stimuli. The second system deals with activation and is defined in terms of tonic physio-

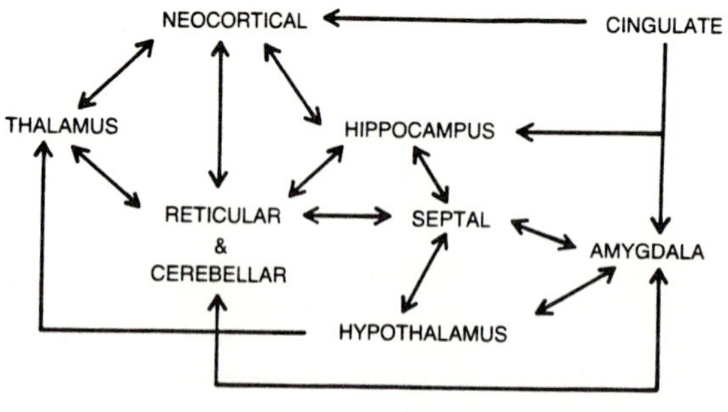

Figure 10–1 A diagrammatic representation of some of the anatomic components mediating attention. (From Thatcher RW, John ER. Functional neuroscience. Vol. I. Foundations of cognitive processes. Hillsdale, NJ: Erlbaum, 1977:115.)

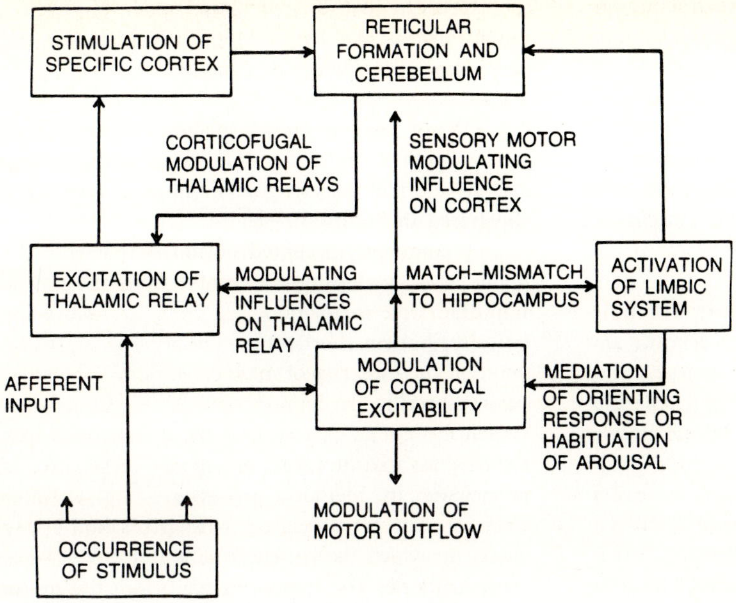

Figure 10–2 A diagrammatic representation of some of the salient features of fixation of attention mediated by anatomic systems in Figure 10–1. (From Thatcher RW, John ER. Functional neuroscience. Vol. I. Foundations of cognitive processes. Hillsdale, NJ: Erlbaum, 1977:115.)

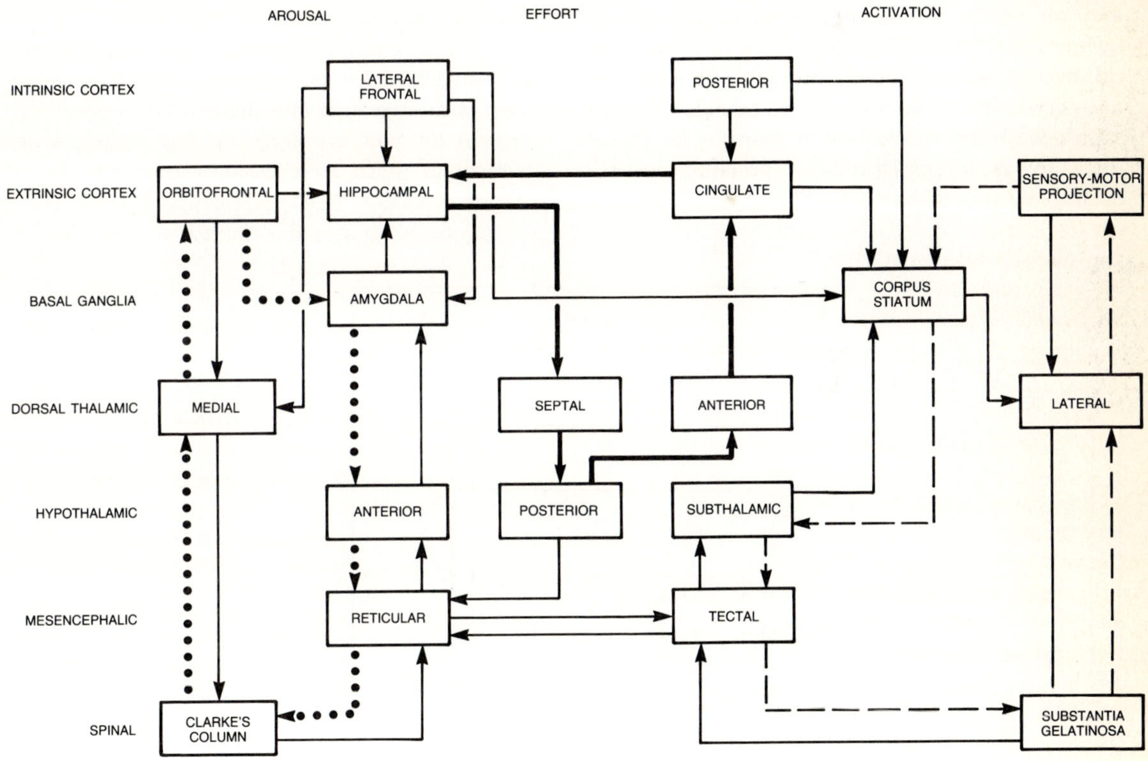

Figure10–3 A simplified diagram of the connections involved in arousal (amygdala), activation (basal ganglia), and effort (hippocampal) circuits. (From McGuinness D, Pribram KH. The neuropsychology of attention: emotional and motivational controls. In: Wittrock MC, ed. The brain and psychology. Orlando: Academic Press, 1980:130.)

logic readiness to respond; its locus is the basal ganglia of the forebrain. The third system coordinates arousal and activation processes along an effort dimension; it is centered in the hippocampus. After reviewing neurophysiologic and neurobehavioral evidence, these authors assert that emotional processes are rooted in the phasic arousal mechanisms and distinguish them from motivational processes rooted in the readiness tonic activation mechanisms. Thus "attention becomes the central process that links emotion and motivation to cognitive operations" (p 131).[28]

Brain mechanisms of attention are extremely complex, involving many transactions between different functional systems and several dynamic processes. The mechanisms of the superior brain stem and the ascending reticular activating system are considered responsible for ensuring generalized and elementary forms of attention, for example, general arousal reaction; complex forms of attention requiring selective recognition of particular stimuli and inhibition of irrelevant stimuli require contributions from higher-level brain structures, including the limbic cortex of the temporal lobe and the frontal cortex.

Memory

The nature and localization or neural location of memory are elusive, probably because memory, like language, is a complex rather than a single function. Early on, Hebb proposed that short-term memory is a dynamic process possibly attributable to reverberating neural circuits, whereas long-term memory is the result of structural change.[30] Lashley concluded in his classic essay *In Search of the Engram* that there are no special cells for special memories.[31]

Close to five decades ago, Papez designated a circuit that is of critical importance in motivation and emotion.[32] The circuit includes the neocortex, the hippocampus, the fornix, the mamillary bodies, the anterior nucleus of the thalamus, and the cingulate gyrus of the cortex. The units in that circuit also have an important role in human memory as illustrated in Figure 10–4.[33]

A commonly accepted notion is that the temporal lobes, including the limbic system, play an important role in memory function.[34–36] More specifically, human short-term memory appears to depend on the integrity of medial temporal lobe structures, especially the hippocampus.[33,37–41] In addition, evidence suggests that other cortical structures, particularly association areas, or tertiary cortical fields, participate in memory processes.[34,38,42] Amnesic memory defects associated with Korsakoff's psychosis, in which the patient retains immediate short-term memories and memories for before the lesion, frequently result from lesions in the medial diencephalon, especially the dorsal medial thalamic nuclei, or other limbic system structures.

Short-term verbal memory deficits are reported to result from left temporal lobe resections. Extension of the resection into the left cortex posteriorly, toward the posterior language area, increases these deficits as much as extension posteriorly into the

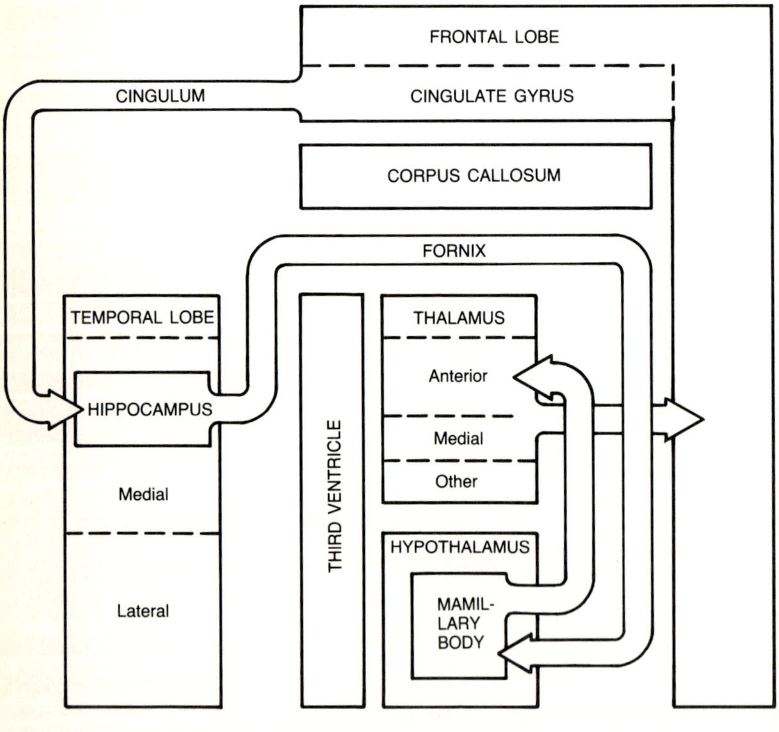

Figure10–4 Schematic diagram of the brain structures involved in memory. (From Ojemann RG. Correlations between specific human brain lesions and memory changes. Neurosciences Research Program Bulletin [Suppl] 1966; 4:6.)

hippocampus.[39] Correlating performance defects of immediate memory and regional cerebral blood flow in the left hemisphere, Hagberg concluded that memory performance involves various extratemporal regions depending upon the specific quality of memory task to be performed.[43] Correlations were demonstrated between a verbal memory task and blood flow in temporal and parietal regions; two spatial recognition tasks and blood flow in temporal and lower frontal regions; and one of two spatial memory tasks and blood flow in the temporal region.

Using electrical stimulation of human left cortex during neurosurgery, Ojemann investigated the organization of short-term verbal memory in language areas of the cortex.[38] His data suggest that cortical areas concerned with language, including generalized word memory, and those concerned with short-term verbal memory for specific, episodic material are separate, but adjacent. Further, differential roles in short-term verbal memory are suggested for cortex adjacent to the posterior and anterior language areas. Previously, Ojemann and Ward[44] and Ojemann[45] reported the effects of left ventral lateral thalamic stimulation and, in contrast to cortical data, found that language and short-term verbal memory appeared to be subserved by the same thalamic areas.

Although the hippocampus and associated structures are not the site of memory storage, consolidation or the storage process between the registration and retention phases appears dependent upon hippocampal activity.[39,46–49] The consolidation process appears to depend upon neural pathways from the neocortex, including parietal, temporal, and frontal lobes, to the hippocampal complex and then back to the neocortex, with several synaptic relays in each stage of the circuit. This circuit, the hippocampal loop in Figure 10–5, is a functional unit from cingulate gyrus through the parahippocampus to the hippocampus and then via the fornix, mammillary body, and anterior nucleus back to the cingulate gyrus. The motivational system, located in the hypothalamus (the amygdaloid complex and the orbital cortex), contributes "drives," useful in the evaluation of sensory information, to the selection unit through the septal region and the cingulate gyrus.

Recently, Squire, Cohen, and Nadel have suggested that memory consolidation best refers to a long-lived, dynamic process that is related to the medial temporal region.[49] They propose that at the time of learning, the medial temporal region establishes a relationship with memory storage sites elsewhere in the brain, primarily in the neocortex. According to Halgren, the activity of the medial temporal lobe (hippocampus, parahippocampal gy-

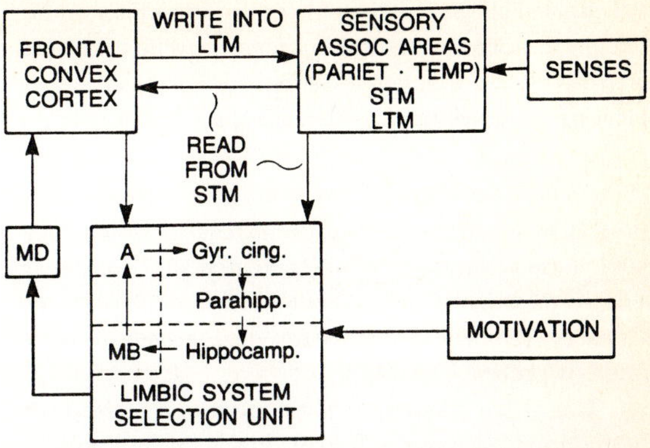

Figure 10–5 A diagrammatic scheme of anatomical structures involved in selection of information between short-term memory and long-term memory. MB = mamillary body; A = anterior thalamic nucleus; MD = mediodorsal thalamic nucleus. (From Kornhuber HH. Neural control of input into long term memory: limbic system and amnestic syndrome in man. In: Zippel HP, ed. Memory and transfer of information. New York: Plenum Press, 1973:10.)

rus, amygdaloid complex, and subicular complex) allows one to interpret current awareness, such as sensory information about emotional state and content of recent episodic memory, against a model of the external world or semantic memory elaborated in the association cortex.[50] He speculates that the medial temporal lobe structures are involved in both the initial experience of an event and in its subsequent recognition or recall. The hippocampal memory indexing theory also asserts that an interaction between the hippocampus and neocortex is involved in memory storage and retrieval.[51] According to this theory, experiential information is registered and understood primarily by multiple, specialized neocortical analyzers. The hippocampus stores the spatiotemporal pattern of these neocortical analyzers, an index of neocortical activation. Thus the hippocampus stores not a neural representation of the memory, but rather the neocortical loci, which, when reactivated in the correct sequence recreate a representation of the initial experiential event.

Although the structures in the aforementioned models may play a role in consolidation, long-term memory storage appears to be widely distributed in the cortex.[17,52,53] Many workers have concluded that memory is not localized to particular brain regions, and assumptions of nervous system activity and memory traces similar to Lashley's earlier conclusions[31] have been reported by Anderson et al.[52] Thatcher and John,[17] after reviewing extensive electrophysiologic data, suggest that

> ...the function of memory, if defined as a change in response to an event because of prior experience with that event, is broad-

ly distributed in the brain. Nonetheless, it is possible that this widespread change in response to a familiar event is initiated by changes localized in some functional system capable of influencing the activity of many brain regions (p 230).

Their own data suggest that "different anatomic regions differ quantitatively in the extent to which they participate either in the direct mediation of afferent sensory experience or the representation of past experiences, yet they all participate qualitatively in both kinds of process" (p 249).

Cognitive scientists have suggested a host of distinctions between different kinds of memories. Functionalist neuroscientists have devoted increasing energy to exploring the neurologic reality of these distinctions, searching for neural circuits and systems that correspond to subprocesses of memory. Recent data lead to the notion that the brain has distinct learning systems, one involving the hippocampus and related limbic structures and the other involving nonlimbic mechanisms.[54–56] Cohen and Squire suggest that the limbic and nonlimbic systems respectively subserve declarative and procedural memory.[57] Declarative memory denotes "data-based" memory or memory for places, events, and facts about the world; procedural memory is the repository of rules and procedures for accomplishing particular goals. Other investigators propose similar distinctions, for example, the distinction between episodic (limbic) and semantic (nonlimbic) memory processes[58] and between working (limbic) and reference (nonlimbic) memory.[59,60] This last distinction between working and reference memory is closely akin to the distinction between episodic and semantic memory proposed by Tulving in an earlier model.[61] Mishkin and associates, based on work with monkeys, propose that the brain organizes memories into two classes: recognition memory and habit memory.[62,63] Recognition memory, assumed to require higher-order level organization, is represented in higher-order areas of the cortex and involves active interaction with limbic to thalamic and cortical to neural circuits. Habit memory, based on stimulus-response association links, is assumed to be mediated by the corticostriate system.

Kesner recently presented an attribute theory concerning the neurobiologic organization of memory and attempted to integrate different theoretical positions into a single framework.[64] He suggests that there are a set of at least five interactive salient attributes, which are heterarchically organized, that characterize mnemonic information: space, time, affect, sensory perception, and response. Further, he suggests that specific neural regions subserve a single or subset of critical attributes. Kesner's comprehensive heuristic models of the structural organization memory are presented in Figures 10–6 and 10–7. He assumes that memory is organized into a

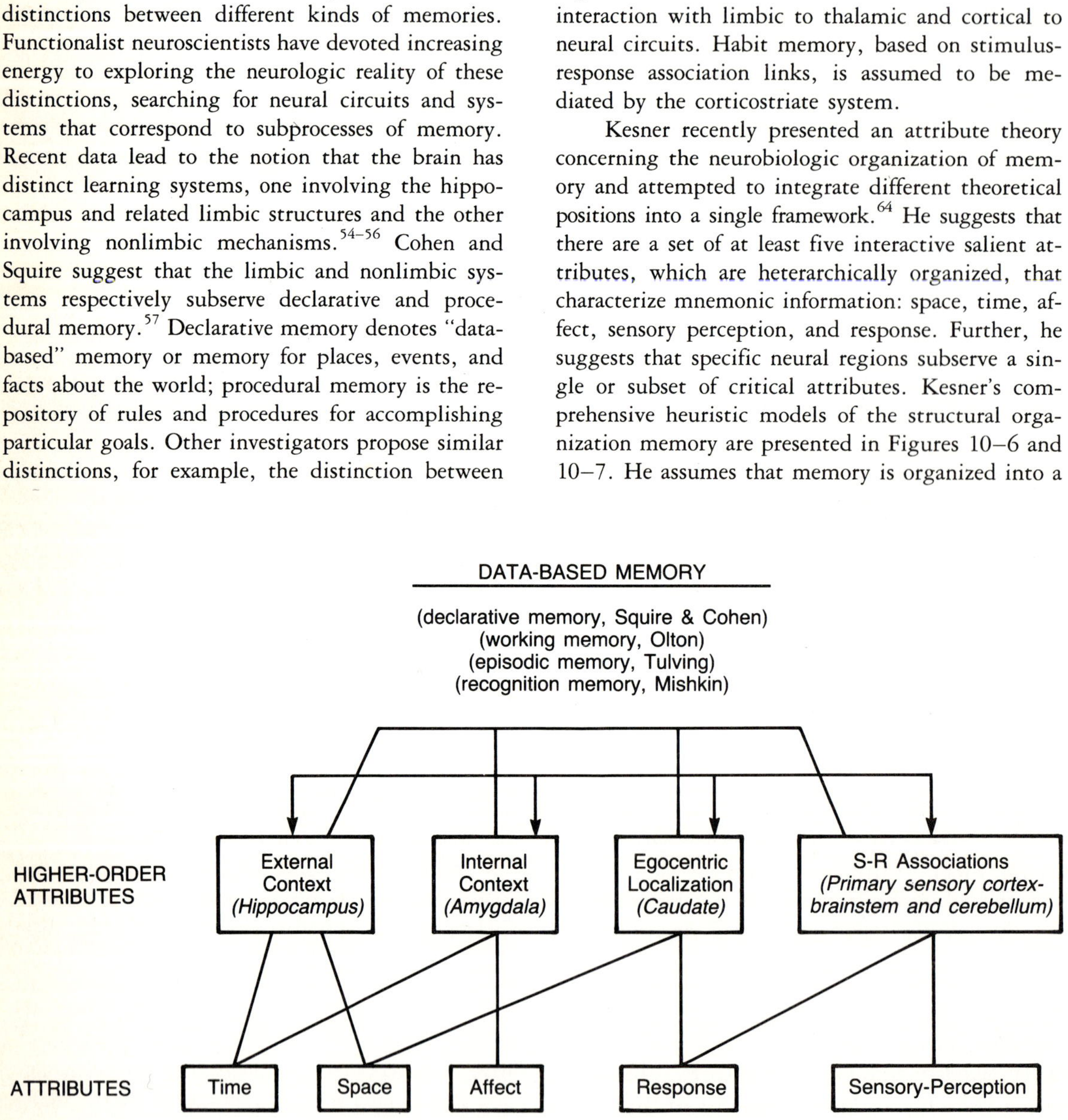

Figure 10–6 Psychological and neural organization of data-based memory. For this system the hippocampus mediates external context, the amygdala mediates the internal context, the caudate nucleus influences egocentric localization, the primary-sensory cortex and the brain stem-cerebellum circuit mediate the S-R association system. (From Kesner RP. Neurobiological views of memory. In: Martinez JL, Kesner RP, eds. Learning and memory: a biological view. Orlando: Academic Press, 1986:423, 425.)

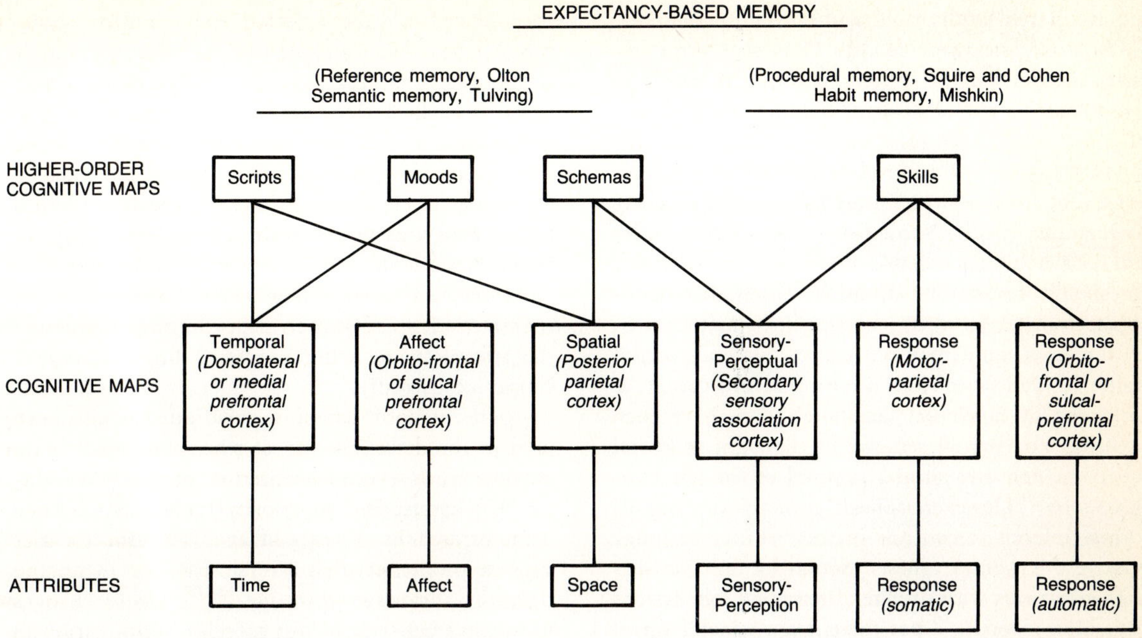

Figure 10–7 Psychological and neural organization of expectancy-based memory. For this system the posterior parietal cortex mediates the spatial cognitive map, the dorsolateral or medial-prefrontal cortex mediates the temporal cognitive map, the orbito-frontal or sulcal-prefrontal cortex mediates the affect cognitive map, the secondary sensory association cortex mediates the sensory perceptual cognitive maps, and the parietal-motor cortex influences the response cognitive map. The interaction between the dorsolateral or medial-prefrontal cortex and posterior parietal cortex serves as the neural substrate for scripts, the posterior parietal cortex and secondary sensory association cortex for schemas, the dorsolateral or medial and orbito-frontal or sulcal-prefrontal cortex for moods and the secondary sensory-association cortex and parietal-motor cortex for skills. (From Kesner RP. Neurobiological views of memory. In: Martinez JL, Kesner RP, eds. Learning and memory: a biological view. Orlando: Academic Press, 1986:424.)

data-based memory, biased toward coding incoming data with emphasis on "bottom-up processing," and expectancy-based memory, biased toward previously stored information or general knowledge of the world with emphasis on "top-down processing." Each attribute activates parallel neural regions that mediate data-based and expectancy-based information followed by subsequent interactions. The neurologic substrates are identified in the figures.

Cortical Auditory System

The primary auditory cortex for man is located within the transverse gyrus of Heschl (Brodmann's areas 41 and 42) on the superior aspect of the temporal lobe and receives auditory radiations directly from the medial geniculate body. Animal data have contributed to the understanding of auditory cortical fields as well as inter- and intrahemispheric connections in the human and are considered first.

Early cortical mapping identified two auditory areas in the temporal regions having reverse tonotopic frequency projections of each other.[65] The scheme of auditory cortical fields and tonotopic organization that is accepted today is essentially the one proposed by Woolsey,[66,67] based on cytoarchitectonic, retrograde degeneration, and evoked potential studies, and recently reexamined with essential agreement.[68,69] Celesia concluded that "the cortical auditory system of man follows closely the organization of the same system in primates" (p 411).[70]

Studies in the rhesus monkey have shown that intrahemispheric connections from the primary auditory cortex to the surrounding auditory association cortex are by short fibers.[71] Fibers from the auditory association cortex then project to the temporoparietal, parietal, and frontal regions. Some of these fields are "polysensory areas," known to receive input from visual and somatic sensory areas and to project to the cingular entorhinal cortex, providing a pathway for sensory information to reach limbic structures and the hypothalamus.[72] Study of interhemispheric connections confirms that commissural fibers connect the association areas of one hemisphere to those in the other.[73]

Findings in experimental animals have helped to indicate also the functional organization of the auditory cortex. After cortical ablation of known auditory cortex, deficits in identification of tone durations, sound localization, and change in temporal patterns of tones were found. Thus the cortex appears essential for the differentiation of sequence of stimulation or the amount of stimulation for stimulus patterns.[74] Clinical studies in human patients following unilateral removal or damage of the temporal lobe have observed similarities and differences with animal results. Similarly, unilateral cortical lesions have no appreciable effect on the absolute thresholds of pure tone stimuli[75,76] even after hemispherectomy.[77] However, hearing loss, as measured by the audiogram, may occur after bilateral cortical lesions.[78] Deficits in tonal duration identification, as measured by nonverbal (Seashore) tests, have been reported after partial removal of the right temporal lobe, but not after similar removal of the left temporal lobe.[79] However, aphasic patients were significantly inferior to controls in their ability to judge relative duration of tones.[80] Sound localization deficits in patients with unilateral temporal lobe lesions have been reported,[76] but there is not general agreement in the literature. Severe deficits in the ability to discriminate changes in the temporal order or sequence of sounds results from removal or damage to the human left auditory cortex.[81] Several studies provide evidence that the ability to perform fine temporal order judgements is located in the left hemisphere.[81–83]

Language

Lateralization of Language Function

The physiologic processes and further cortical projections of the auditory system, which are directly related to deriving meaning from aural language and part of the central language system, are less well-defined than those of the primary auditory cortex. However, cortical specialization for language function in one hemisphere of the human brain, most commonly the left, is today a well-accepted premise. Clinicopathologic studies of language function have provided much of this information.[84–87] The dichotic listening technique, discovered by Broadbent[88] and popularized as a clinical tool by Kimura,[89] has become widely used to investigate hemispheric brain asymmetry specialization of language processing capacities in normal subjects. This speech perception task has demonstrated that speech stimuli are more often perceived correctly from the right ear.[89–94] Kimura suggested that this right ear preference reflects both contralateral or left hemisphere specialization for these auditory stimuli and the "functional prepotency" of the contralateral auditory pathway.[90,91] The demonstration that the left ear was more accurate for nonspeech stimuli, that is, melody patterns,[91,95] which were thought to be processed predominantly in the right hemisphere,[79] strengthened this explanation. Additionally, studies have shown an increased electrical activity in the left cortical hemisphere subsequent to the perception of linguistically meaningful stimuli. Studies of auditory evoked responses have shown a hemispheric difference in response to identical stimuli depending upon whether the stimuli were being processed linguistically or simply acoustically.[96–98]

The dichotic listening paradigm has also been used in the determination of when functional brain asymmetry, or speech lateralization, develops. A right-ear, left-hemisphere superiority for words has been demonstrated by 3 years of age.[99] Recent theories suggest progressive left lateralization or increasing right-ear advantage with age.[100,101] Using changes in sucking behavior to test speech discrimination in infants, Eimas et al have demonstrated that some characteristics of speech perception are present as early as 4 months of age.[102] Anatomic studies indicating brain asymmetries between the left and right temporal areas in adults[103] are present also at birth,[104] and electrophysiologic studies showing evoked response asymmetries in young infants,[98] paralleling those of adults, strongly suggest that the left hemisphere is primed from birth to be the speech hemisphere.

Behavioral and electrophysiologic research findings indicate that speech perception cues are processed by a number of cortical mechanisms, some of which are bilaterally represented, and some of which are lateralized. These findings suggest some degree of redundancy in the cortical mechanisms involved in speech perception.[105] Based on their investigation of brain-damaged adults, Perceman and Kellar hypothesize that voice and place features require differential hemispheric processing.[106] They suggest voice can be processed by either hemisphere, whereas place seems to be processed by the left hemisphere. Electrophysiologic studies done by means of recordings of the brain's auditory evoked response indicate that multiple processing mechanisms, which include left hemisphere and bilateral processes, are involved in the perception of place of articulation cues, for example, formant transition.[107,108] Molfese and Erwin suggest that a number of discrete mechanisms located in both hemispheres are involved in the processing of vowels.[109]

Review of right hemisphere specialization is beyond the scope of this chapter; however, for comparison with the left hemisphere, it appears that the right hemisphere predominates for many nonlinguistic processes, notably those requiring spatial capabilities, and has some linguistic "abilities."[110] Sperry and Gazzaniga's split brain studies have demonstrated that the right hemisphere, incapable of producing speech, can comprehend many nouns, phrases, definitions, and spoken commands.[111] Thus speech comprehension may be more diversely or bilaterally represented than speech production.

Localization of Language Function

The first serious efforts in cerebral dominance, localization, and brain-language relationships began in 1861 when Broca postulated that the center for speech function or "articulated language" was in the posterior third of the left inferior frontal convolution. Later, Wernicke expressed the view that the posterior third of the left superior temporal gyrus was the center for "sensory images" of speech.

Subsequently, electrical stimulation during neurosurgery[84] and brain lesion studies[42,112] have provided more information about cortical localization of language function, although the inherent limitations of such studies are well known. Jackson in 1882 warned against the simplistic assumption that a missing function resides in an injured area. Further, a focal lesion may cause widespread disruption of brain function. Recently, approaches to brain function and localization utilizing the intact cerebral cortex have been developed, including blood flow studies[113–115] and evoked potential recordings.

Neurolinguistics, a relatively new theoretical discipline, seeks to integrate information from neuroanatomy, neurophysiology, and psycholinguistics in order to develop language organization models. Whitaker,[116,117] a neurolinguist, has developed a functional anatomic schema of the central language system comparable to clinicopathologic observations[42,112,118] and anatomic considerations,[84,85,119] as shown in Figure 10–8, which displays these left hemisphere anatomic areas subserving auditory and verbal language and the major pathways connecting them.

Although Geschwind[87,112,120] and Luria[34,42] have advanced the understanding of language processing greatly, much speculation remains as to how the central language neural structures process auditory and linguistic information. Apparently, these structures may interpret auditory patterns by deriving representational meanings based on established linguistic rules. Geschwind has discussed cortical language and connections in great detail as well as interhemispheric connections and tracts to the limbic system.[112] Luria has provided the most in-depth discussion of the status of cortical areas as "analyzers."[42]

Geschwind and Luria assign a linguistic processing role to secondary auditory cortical fields, more specifically, Wernicke's area and its interactions with the remainder of the auditory association cortex and the second and third temporal convolutions. These areas appear to have much wider projections than those of the primary auditory cortex and to work closely with adjacent areas.[42] These auditory analyzer zones are said to be responsible for analysis and synthesis of speech sound signals; significant phonemic signals of the language are differentiated from unnecessary, nonphonemic sounds, and comparisons of the differentiated phoneme signals are made to the learned language code.[42] Geschwind also suggests that the auditory association cortex, including Wernicke's area, acts to recognize and classify auditory patterns into phonemes and further speculates that they are also operational in syntactic comprehension.[121] Lesions in the secondary auditory zones, especially Wernicke's area, result in deficits in the process of isolation, differentiation, and sequencing of the pertinent phonemic system or disturbances in "phonemic hearing."[42]

Language representation, the process that completes message decoding after phonologic interpretation, appears to occur when the activities of the auditory association area and of the angular and supramarginal gyri in the inferior parietal lobe interact.[34,112,117,121] Geschwind refers to the large association area in the posterior temporoparietal or angular gyrus region, lying at the junction of the visual, auditory, and somesthetic association areas, as the "association area of association areas."[112,121] This area, suited to relate, integrate, and store multisensory information, is suggested to be responsible for mediating nonlimbic crossmodal associations[112,121] or complex simultaneous synthesis necessary for the most complex forms of information analysis.[34] The semantic aspects and logical and grammatic operations of language have been attributed to this area by Luria.[42] Lesions of the left inferior parietal area may result in a decreased understanding of grammatic structures that incorporate logical relationships communicated by inflections, prepositions, and word order while the understanding of single words and simpler grammatic structures remains unimpaired.[34,42] Luria suggests that this decreasing understanding is due to a spatial factor deficit. Integrating other views, Whitaker postulates that the cortical regions underlying the semantic and syntactic and lexical components of language are the posterior part of Wernicke's area, the auditory association area, and the supramarginal and angular gyri.[117]

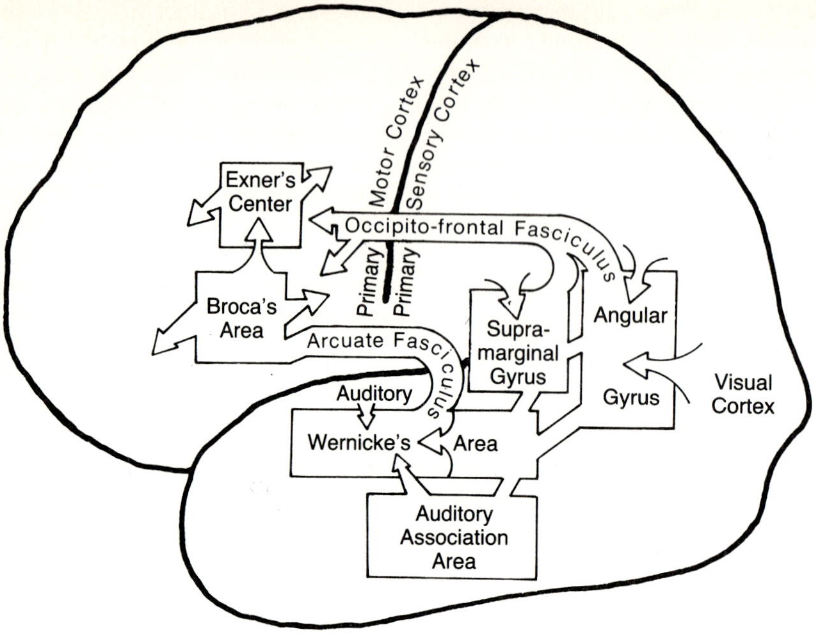

Figure 10-8 Left hemisphere anatomic areas subserving auditory-verbal language and the major pathways connecting them.

1. Auditory, Heschl's gyrus
2. Wernicke's area, middle and posterior portions of the superior temporal gyrus
3. Auditory association area, the posterior portion of the middle temporal gyrus
4. Supramarginal gyrus, at the posterior end of the Sylvian fissure
5. Angular gyrus, at the posterior end of the fissure separating the superior and inferior temporal gyri behind the supramarginal gyrus
6. Broca's area, the third frontal convolution

Cortical fields interconnect with each other as well as with subcortical and peripheral structures. (From Whitaker HA. Neurolinguistics. In: Dingwall WO, ed. A survey of linguistic science. College Park: University of Maryland, 1971:192.)

The present literature concerning brain-language theory and function emphasizes the essential role of cortical structures and cortical to cortical connections in subserving human language systems. The notion that language is subserved by a combination of cortical and subcortical structures, particularly the thalamus, remains undetermined and controversial, as reflected in a special issue of *Brain and Language* devoted to the role of the thalamus.[122] Although there are early reports in the literature of thalamic lesions in association with disorders of perception and cognition, not until Penfield and Roberts was attention focused on the thalamus in relation to language organization.[84] They proposed that the thalamus was a way station in language processing between the anterior and posterior speech zones. They suggested that the "centrencephalic system," a central coordinating and integrative mechanism in the diencephalon or higher brain stem, subserved higher integrative functions than the cortex. They viewed much of the temporal cortex as an outward projection and elaboration from the pulvinar and posterior part of the lateral nucleus of the thalamus. Speech comprehension was suggested to result during interaction between thalamic areas and posterior language areas in the cortex—posterior parts of first, second, and third temporal convolutions; supramarginal gyrus; and angular gyrus—after auditory impulses were received in both hemispheres and in higher brain stem. Penfield and Roberts concluded that information is transferred from one cortical area to another through subcortical connections and that cortical elaborations are sent back to the thalamus for coordination with other brain activities. Brown argues that the nuclei of the thalamus are not just separate control centers that influence extrinsic areas, but are rather components of more widely distributed neuroanatomic levels, since thalamic differentiation follows an evolutionary course parallel to that of the neocortex.[123,124] Thus he views the thalamus as a hierarchically organized structure that participates with its projection zones in the mediation of cognitive events specific to that structural level of which it is but one component. Whitaker suggests that the role of the thalamus in language may be to facilitate a balance between nonspecific reticular and specific cortical systems rather than to mediate linguistic decoding.[125] Synthesizing lesion and stimulation data, Mateer and Ojemann suggest that lateralization of language functions at the level of the thalamus, usually to the left, differs from language functions subserved by any cortical area.[126–128] They assert that "the left and right thalami function asymmetrically to gate access to the cortex by means of a 'specific alerting response' which is related to material-specific input'' (p 172).[126] This alerting circuit seems to represent a common thalamic mechanism for both language and memory.[126]

Abbs and Sussman have hypothesized a neurophysiologic feature detection theory of speech perception.[129] Their theory suggests that innately structured neurosensory receptive fields that operate as feature detectors decode the phonologic features of speech from the acoustic signal. Lacking sufficient evidence on the neurologic processes of speech perception, Abbs and Sussman review and use data from animal visual systems, psychophysical research, and developmental studies to support their theory.

Abbs and Sussman define feature detectors as "organizational configurations of the sensory nervous system that are highly sensitive to certain parameters of complex stimuli'' (p 24).[129] Unlike acoustic filters, which are specific to the energy within a narrow bandwidth, feature detectors respond simultaneously to multistimulus characteristics, most of which arise from spatial and temporal changes in the acoustic wave. Noting neurophysiologic evidence for feature detectors[130] and reports of lateral inhibition[131,132] in the auditory system, Abbs and Sussman postulate a complex spatial configuration of receptor cells, maximally sensitive to specific spatial and temporal physical characteristics of the auditory stimulus, as an explanation for neural decoding in speech perception. They suggest that the configurations could be located in the inner ear and be especially tuned to respond to formant patterns, specifically formant transitions that are major acoustic-speech cues for consonant identification.[133]

Wood has proposed a hypothetical organization of auditory and phonetic levels of processing within the auditory system.[96] Rejecting a strict serial model, he suggests components for a form of simultaneous, shared, or parallel processing of auditory and phonetic information, including (1) a common peripheral component for the transduction and preliminary analysis of all acoustic signals; (2) a "central" auditory component for the additional processing of nonlinguistic auditory information; and (3) a "central" phonetic component for the extraction of abstract phonetic features from the results of the preliminary auditory analysis.

Components (2) and (3) would be capable of functioning in parallel; however, both would be dependent on the output from (1). The phonetic component (3) involves mechanisms lateralized in the dominant hemisphere; however, the exact extent of lateralization and the actual subset of phonetic processes that are lateralized remain to be determined.

Cullen et al hypothesized a speech information flow model (Fig. 10–9) based on dichotic speech data from normal subjects and patients with focal cortical lesions.[134] They suggest that "speech information from two ears is functionally independent above the level of the brainstem due to the anatomical weighting given to the contralateral ear in the ascending auditory pathway and an effective ipsilateral gate mechanism, probably at the level of the medial geniculate'' (p 125). This statement extends Kimura's initial interpretation by adding the proposed thalamic ''gate'' represented in the bottom box of the model, which provides separation of ear-channel information at cortical centers while allowing intermixing of information from both ears below the medial geniculate bodies.

Nation and Aram have integrated much of the preceding information into their speech-language processing model, which attempts to delineate the interface between anatomy, physical processing, and

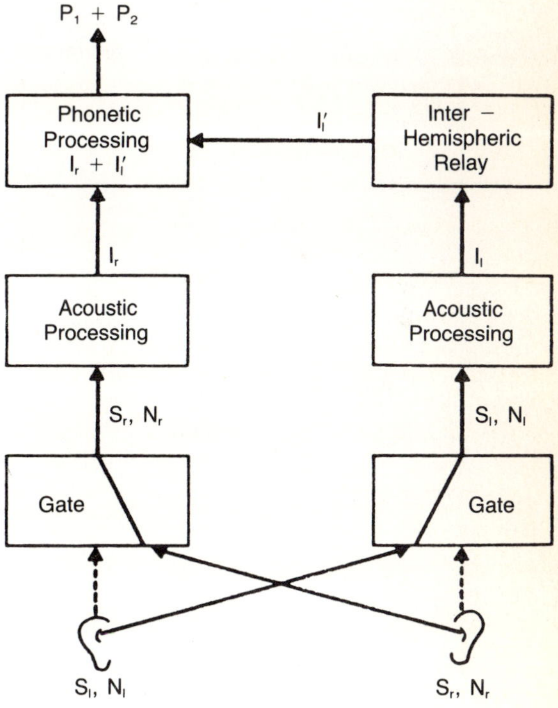

Figure 10–9 Functional flow diagram of speech information processing, based on dichotic speech data obtained with normal and cortical lesioned subjects. S = signal; N = noise; I = extracted information; P = phonemic response. (From Cullen JK Jr, Berlin CI, Hughes LF, Thompson CL, Samson DS. Speech information flow: a model. In: Sullivan MD, ed. Proceedings of a symposium on central auditory processing disorders. Lincoln: University of Nebraska Medical Center, 175:115.)

behavioral correlates.[135,136] The speech-language processing component (Fig. 10–10) of the model concerned with auditory function is composed of an auditory reception segment responsible for prelinguistic processing and a central language-thought segment responsible for linguistic decoding. Auditory sensation and perception are the suggested behavioral correlates that result from the prelinguistic processing; auditory message comprehension is the behavioral correlate of linguistic decoding.

A series of four physical processes are hypothesized with the auditory reception segment, which is made up of the bilateral structures that form the outer ear to the primary auditory cortex. These prelinguistic processes are auditory acceptance and transduction, auditory analysis and transmission, auditory reception and analysis, and auditory programming. They code and analyze the physical characteristics of the auditory signal, developing phonetic feature patterns.

Two interacting linguistic processes leading to comprehension occur within the central language segment located in the left cerebral hemisphere and composed of the anatomic areas provided in Whitaker's model.[117] These physical processes are linguistic auditory programming and language-cognitive representation.

COGNITIVE CORRELATES OF AUDITORY PROCESSING

Ebbinghaus, a German philosopher, is recognized as the first person to apply the experimental method to the study of higher mental processes. In 1885, he published the results of his studies on memory, which were patterned after the methods used in natural science, that is, isolation of a factor that can be measured and control of accompanying causal conditions.

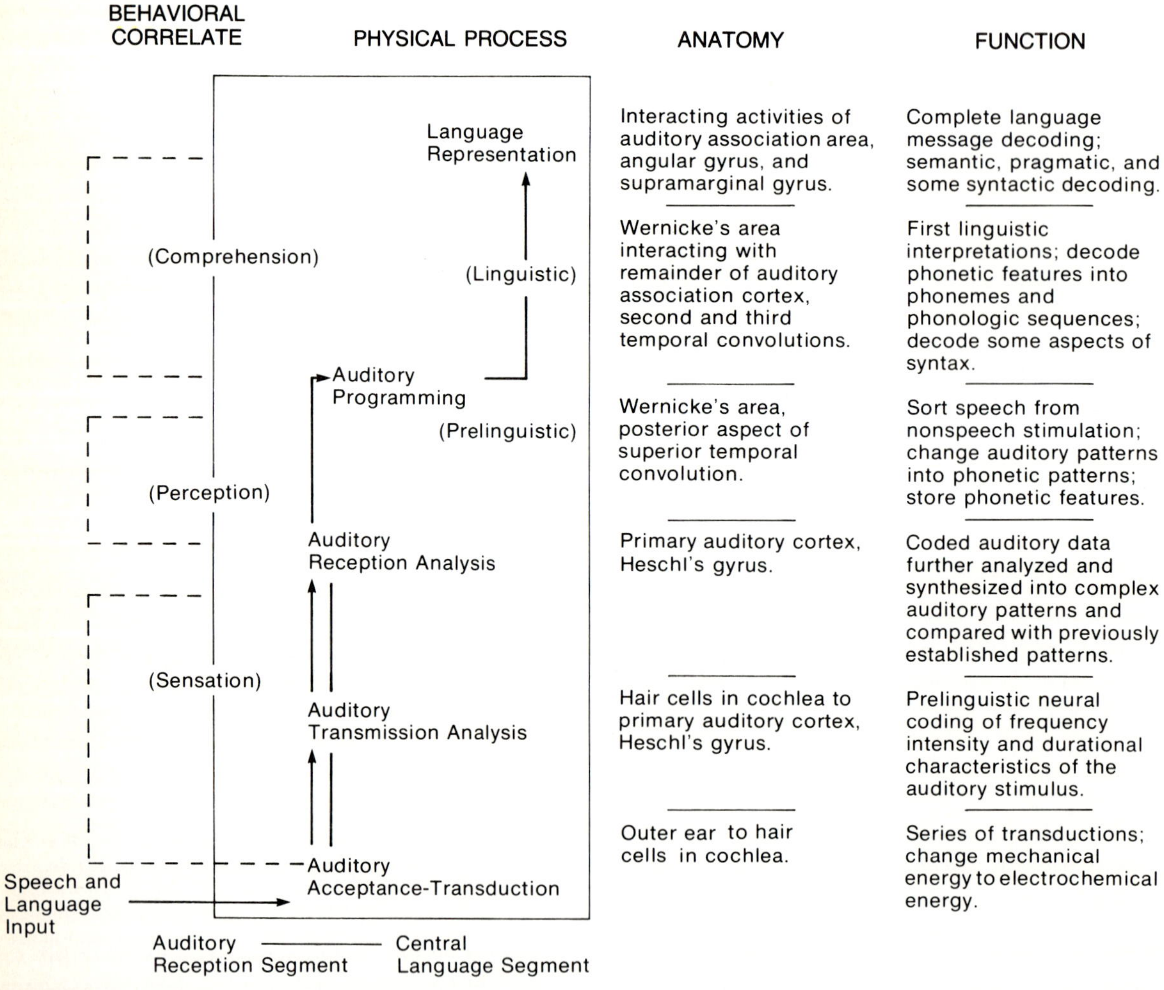

Figure 10-10 Modified speech and language processing component of the SLPM. (From Nation JE, Aram DM. Diagnosis of speech and language disorders. San Diego: College-Hill Press, 1984:28, 30, 33.)

Ebbinghaus acknowledged the dependence of memory on various factors: differences between individuals, such that one retains well whereas another retains poorly; differences within individuals, such as diurnal and age differences, differences in content of the material to be remembered, for example, melodies, forms, and colors; and differences that result from "the capriciousness of mental life . . . such as mental rigor, interest in the subject, concentration of attention, changes in the course of thought which have been brought about by sudden fancies and resolves" (p 11).[137] He also noted that "such unruly factors are of greatest importance for higher mental processes . . . the more lowly, commonplace, and constantly occurring processes are not in the least withdrawn from their influence, but we have it in our power, when it is a matter of consequence, to make this influence only slightly disturbing" (p 11).

Ebbinghaus determined to control the factors that influenced memory by selecting materials to be remembered that would not be influenced by the "unruly factors." He constructed 2,300 consonant-vowel-consonant syllables from which he randomly chose series of various lengths to be memorized. With himself as the subject, he studied variables such as the time and number of repetitions and the order of syllables that affected his learning of the material. Thus he became the first experimenter to probe the human mind beyond the initial stage of sensory perception with objective techniques that have subsequently been widely used.

After considerable experience with methodology developed by Ebbinghaus, Bartlett determined that this approach had numerous limitations.[138] He felt that it was not only impossible to eliminate the elements of meaning from stimuli, but that the attempt to do so resulted in an artificial situation in which subjective attitudes were denied as well.

Bartlett borrowed the concept of schema from Sir Henry Head's neurologic theory in order to explain the nature of memory. Schema were defined as the active organization of past experiences and reactions that were called up in response to new stimuli. Related sensory experiences, for example, visual and auditory sensations at a low level, and experiences associated with a common interest, for example, sports or art on a higher level, were grouped together. Rather than passively linked events, then, schema were composed of active integrated memories built up chronologically, with the most recent reactions dominant.

In his experimentation, Bartlett compared subjects' recall of a story they had heard with a story they constructed from an outline. When asked to remember a story, an impression or what Bartlett called "an attitude" emerged initially, followed by a construction that justified that attitude. In addition to a generalized impression, certain features were recalled either as images or in descriptive language. Thus story recall was seen as a process of reconstruction starting with a schema. This schema, which was characterized as an attitude resulting from amassed memories of past reactions, was then elaborated. In constructing a story, the same process of elaboration was observed, but in this case, schema from various events that are not usually related are combined.

By giving free rein to the factors affecting recall, which Ebbinghaus had attempted to eliminate in his experimentation, Bartlett introduced a methodology for research that takes into account the higher mental processes, concepts that are currently receiving renewed attention. As will be noted in our discussion of current information-processing models, his findings suggest that remembering is a process of reconstruction rather than reproduction.

Attention

The first attempt at a complete model of human information processing abilities was made by Broadbent in his book *Perception and Communication*, published in 1958.[88] He utilized numerous experimental tasks to study the nature of selective attention, the process of choosing which message would be attended to when competing messages were presented. His theory, which had a significant impact on the direction of subsequent research on information processing, will be the first of a group of structural models to be discussed. A second group of capacity models will conclude this section.

Structural Theories

Broadbent's model represents the human central nervous system as essentially a single communication channel that has a limited capacity for processing information. He hypothesized that input from various senses is held for seconds in a "short-term store" until certain of the sensory information is selected by a filtering mechanism. The information selected is then transmitted through a limited capacity channel for further processing. Particularly interested in competing auditory messages, he focused on the nature of the device that allows for selection of one channel of information over another and called this model "a filter theory."

In earlier studies Cherry had demonstrated that it is possible to follow or "shadow" by repeating one message of a speaker when another message by the same speaker is superimposed on the first message.[139] Popularized as "the cocktail party problem," this phenomena was further studied by Broadbent to determine the factors that made such separation possible. Broadbent's studies showed that one message could be discarded more readily when it came from a different direction, was louder or softer, and had different vocal characteristics. This evidence suggested to Broadbent that the filter is "tuned in" to the message associated with one set of physical characteristics while rejecting the second message in its entirety. Since separation of the physical characteristics from the two channels is involved, he viewed the filtering mechanism as operating on sensory data held in the short-term store. His location for the filter indicates that it operates during the early stages of perceptual analysis before the content of the messages has been determined. Only preliminary analysis of the sensory signal takes place before the decision is made as to which stimuli will receive further analysis and subsequent storage in long-term memory. The listener has, then, an efficient processor, one that utilizes its in-depth processing capacities only on selected information available to the listener.

Subsequent experimental findings showed that, under certain circumstances, some of the information in the irrelevant channel is available to the listener. For example, Moray found that subjects could hear their own names in the message that was not attended to.[140] The new evidence prompted revisions of Broadbent's theory. Treisman conducted a group of studies on the separation of competing messages that varied on three dimensions: voice characteristics, foreign languages known and unknown to the listener, and the content of the messages.[141–143] She determined that listeners have varying degrees of difficulty separating the relevant message from the irrelevant one. As with Broadbent's findings, distinct vocal characteristics made the separation easy. Separation of messages delivered in different languages varied according to the listener's knowledge of the foreign language: messages in unknown languages were separated more easily than messages in known languages. The most difficulty was encountered when both the vocal characteristics and the languages spoken were the same with the only differences being in the content of the messages.

A modification of the filter model, an attenuation model, was proposed by Treisman to account for her findings. She suggested that rather than a selective mechanism that passes all information in one incoming channel while discarding other sensory input, a more complex analysis is carried out. From the preliminary analysis of the physical properties of signals, a selective filter attenuates the strength of the multichannel input according to the dimensions deemed important. The message in the channel containing the most relevant information is analyzed fully at a subsequent stage. Simultaneously, however, the information in the attenuated channels is undergoing additional analyses as required by their contents to determine the possible relevance of this additional information. Thus all signals undergo considerable analysis before they are discarded, with selection being made at varying points along the processing continuum.

Also in response to Broadbent's model, Deutsch and Deutsch presented a theory of attention that attempted an explanation of complex discriminations. In this theory, all incoming stimuli receive extensive analysis by an alert organism, with the emerging importance of the signal determining whether a complete analysis is carried out or not. In this model, selection is made at a still later stage in processing, with considerable influence attributed to the level of arousal of the organism.

This "top-down" influence on the selection process proposed by Deutsch and Deutsch was incorporated into a comprehensive theory on memory and attention described by Norman.[144,145] His model (Fig. 10–11) illustrates the combined influences of the current sensory input and the events considered pertinent from the ongoing analysis of signals received previously. Physical signals received by the sensory system are processed automatically by stimulus-analyzing mechanisms that extract certain features from the stimuli. These features activate their representations in long-term storage. Simultaneously, the products of continuously on-going analyses relative to the changing expectations of the individual and his knowledge of perceptual, conceptual, and linguistic rule systems identify categories of events deemed currently pertinent. The pertinence input also activates stored representations so that the output from long-term storage has differing levels of excitation depending upon the level's activation from two input sources. Classes of events having the highest level of excitation are selected for further processing.

Thus a class of theories of attention that emphasize the structural aspects of information processing is available. They were dubbed "bottleneck" theories because they attempt to relate the necessity for selecting certain stimuli for further processing to the stage in processing at which the selection is made. The early theory of Broadbent places the point of selection early in the system, whereas the subsequent theory of Treisman, as well as Norman's elab-

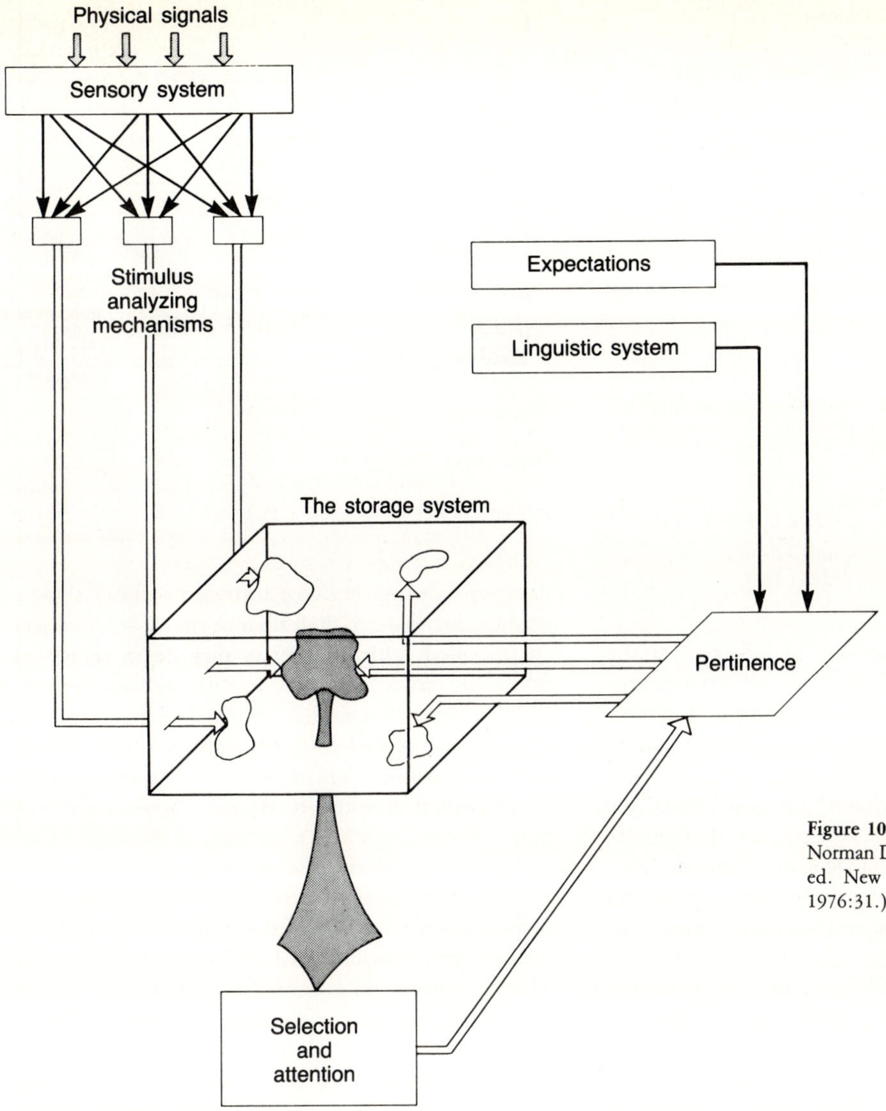

Figure 10–11 Norman's model. (From Norman DA. Memory and attention. 2nd ed. New York: John Wiley and Sons, 1976:31.)

oration of the theory of Deutsch and Deutsch, move the point of selection further along in the system. In addition to the concept of the point at which the decision is made, the second structural concept is developed in these theories: the respective roles of the data or bottom-up processes and the conceptual or top-down processes. In the later theories, conceptual processes based on individuals' expectations are seen as significant determinants in the selection process.

Capacity Theories

As a complement to these structural models, Kahneman introduced a "capacity" model of attention.[146] Although in agreement with earlier theorists on the concept of a general limitation on human's capacity to process information, Kahneman maintained, as Moray had earlier,[147] that the human has considerable control over the allocation of his or her attentional resources. This control was seen to emanate from a nonspecific input of effort that was combined with a specific sensory input. Since certain activities require no attention and others require attention only in the latter stages of processing, Kahneman theorized that concurrent activities may be carried out to the extent of the available capacity. A graphic representation of the capacity model appears in Figure 10–12.

The "possible activities" structures shown just prior to the responses output at the bottom of the model can be "activated" by the allocation of effort. The amount of effort available is closely related to

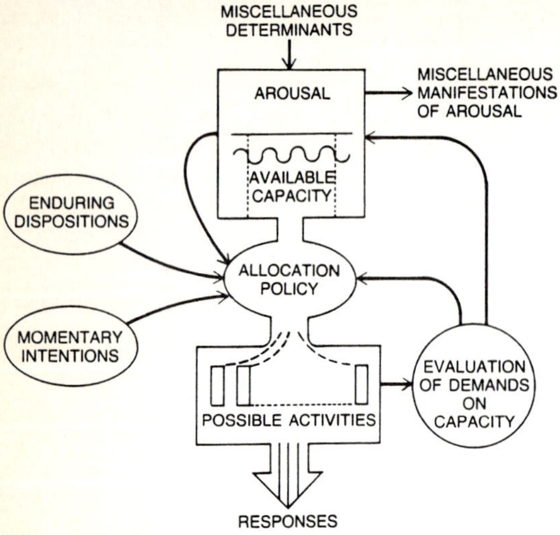

Figure 10–12 Capacity model. (From Kahneman D. Attention and effort. Englewood Cliffs, NJ: Prentice-Hall, 1973:10.)

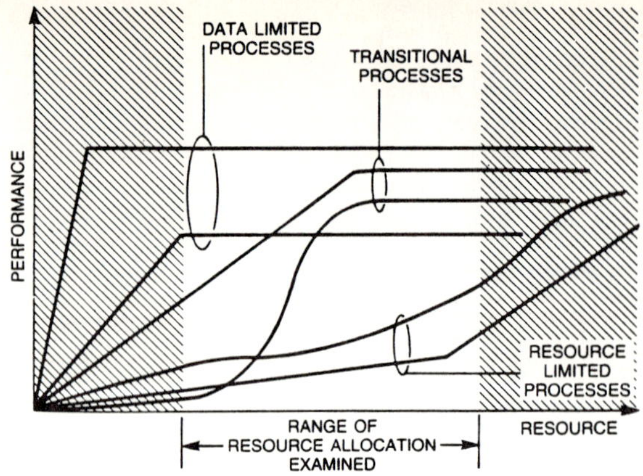

Figure 10–13 Data-limited and resource-limited processes. (From Norman DA, Bobrow DG. On data-limited and resource-limited processes. Cog Psychol 1975; 7:49.)

the level of physiologic arousal, as indicated at the top of the model. The allocation of effort is monitored by the allocation policy, a governing system that becomes a controlling force when more capacity is demanded by activities than is available. Other controls on the allocation policy, in addition to the amount of effort available and the number of demands on that effort, are momentary intentions, such as instructions and enduring dispositions, which reflect involuntary attention: for example, one's own name.

A further understanding of the nature of resource allocation is offered by Norman and Bobrow in their comparison of data-limited and resource-limited processes.[2] As noted in the earlier definition of process, the execution of a process, that is, set of programs, requires both input data and resources. Resource-limited tasks, according to Norman and Bobrow, are ones in which results can be improved by increasing the amount of resources allocated to the task, whereas data-limited tasks are those in which additional processing resources do not improve performance. Actually, most tasks are thought to be resource limited up to the point where sufficient resources have been made available to complete the task and data limited beyond that. Data limitations occur when the input signal is weak or interfered with by competing noises or where the memory capacity is insufficient to store an adequate representation of the signal. Figure 10–13 shows the relationship between performance and resource functions. The lines representing data-limited processes show a rapid increase in performance as additional resources are made available and then a plateau, indicating no further benefit from the resources. The lines representing resource-limited processes show a gradual increase in performance as more resources are allocated. Other processes may be in transition from the resource-limited to the data-limited region, as when learning is involved. These concepts may be exemplified by tasks such as those used in Treisman's studies cited earlier.[142,143] As noted, when an individual is asked to repeat a spoken message heard in one ear while a competing message is received in the other ear, he or she can do so with ease as long as physical differences in the messages can be perceived. However, if the individual is asked to perform the additional task of tapping on the desk when a target word is detected in either ear,[148] performance is high on one primary channel where he or she focuses his or her resources, but low on the secondary channel because of insufficient additional resources.[2] Thus total performance is resource limited. In another version of the first task, if the noises are the same, but the competing message is louder, thus masking the primary message, the task is data limited in that increasing the amount of resources does not improve performance.

A final theory to be discussed relative to the nature of capacity limitations on information processing is presented by Schneider and Shiffrin.[149] Their comparison of automatic and controlled modes of processing provides a further explanation of the use of information-processing capacity. An automatic process occurs when a sequence of elements, which have previously been associated with one another and stored in long-term memory, is activated by a particular input from either external and internal sources without the control of the individual and without the necessity of attentional capacity. These processes have probably developed through considerable training or experience and are difficult to suppress or change. An example of such a process is the response "I'm fine" to the frequently asked question "How are you?" A controlled process, in contrast, occurs when activation of a series of elements is accomplished under the control and with the attention of the individual. The sequential activation of the elements is temporary in that it requires the attention of the individual each time the process recurs. Since controlled processes require the individual's resources, they are limited by capacity. However, the control factor also allows for them to be established quickly and easily. Controlled processes are necessary in any situation in which automatic processes are not available. Attentional requirements allow for multiple ongoing automatic processes, but usually only a single controlled process. Little control is thought to be required during the early stage of processing when features are being abstracted and encoded. When control is required, the rate of processing by the system is the limiting factor in determining the capacity of the system.

Perception

Having considered how the human might select from the wide array of auditory sensory data available those stimuli that will receive further processing and how processing resources are allocated to that end, we now turn to the nature of the recognition process. Two major topics relative to the perception of information will be addressed. The first is the manner in which encoded stimuli are represented at the stage of recognition. The second deals with the processes through which recognition is attained.

Pattern Representation

The ability to recognize patterns is fundamental to all information-processing systems. The processing of auditory information necessitates the analysis over time of variations in the intensity, frequency, and duration of speech sounds. The results of this analysis are represented in an internal image of the physical pattern. As with the selection of input data for processing, the recognition of the image attained through the encoding process is influenced not only by the physical characteristics of the stimulus, but also by the processor's knowledge of the probabilities that any particular pattern might be encountered at any particular time. Thus the perceiver's prior experience with his or her environment and the language spoken in this environment contribute to his or her recognition of the incoming auditory signals. According to Reed, two basic theories exist as to the nature of the internal representation of patterns: template matching and feature detection.[150] On the one hand, the template matching theory suggests that each new input is compared to a standard. The degree of overlap between the pattern to be recognized and a pattern template retrieved from long-term memory is measured to determine if there is a match. On the other hand, feature detection theory holds that patterns are composed of particular features that can be combined in various ways. Pattern identification is accomplished by the detection of features in the incoming signal that are required in certain patterns. Thus the information stored in long-term memory used in the recognition of input data is an analyzable list of required elements in the feature theory as compared to an unanalyzable pattern in the template matching theory.

In 1951, the concept of distinctive features was introduced to the study of speech perception by Jakobson et al.[151] Distinctive features were viewed as the ultimate units of language. As such, the features were thought to represent the differences between phonemes. This theory proposes twelve phonemic binary contrasts such as nasal versus oral and vocalic versus nonvocalic. The choice between these polar opposites results in a finite set of distinctive features that, when grouped into simultaneous bundles, are heard as phonemes. The phonemic patterns in any language are limited in number and reflect the rules of the language for grouping features into bundles. The presence of features to be selected from the sound wave reduces the amount of information that must be processed, thus providing economy in processing. The discovery of the distinctive features and the relations among the features that create a pattern may be thought of as the first stage in forming an image of a particular pattern or the first stage in the recognition of previously learned patterns.

Reed describes two types of images that may be formed as the internal representation of a pattern.[150] The first is a concrete image, thought to be the internal representation of a pattern that was actually perceived and remembered by the individual. Once a complete pattern is learned and stored as a concrete image, differentiating that pattern from other patterns should be possible. The concrete image formed would function as a template. Using visual and tactual stimuli, studies compared recognition learning by comparing features with standards to test the efficacy of the two models. The results of three studies led to contradictory conclusions with the first study favoring the distinctive feature approach, the second study finding recognition to be equal for the two approaches, and the third study supporting the standard approach.[152–154]

The second type of image described by Reed was termed "abstract image,"[150] an evolution from the concept of schema theory described by Bartlett;[138] the abstract image theory proposes that the human abstracts redundant features from experiences and stores them as schema in order to reduce demands on information processing. The schema, then, are generalizations of experiences. An abstract image may be thought of as "an internal representation of the central tendency of a category of patterns . . . created by the subject" (p 26).[150] Also referred to as a prototype, this concept is similar to that of a template, although it consists of features that represent values derived from the calculated means of all patterns in the category. Oden and Massaro state that phoneme prototypes are described by propositions stored in long-term memory; for example, /b/ is labial and voiced, whereas /p/ is labial and not voiced.[155] Identification of the phoneme /b/ is a function of "the degree to which the sound is labial multiplied by the degree to which the sound is voiced" (p 176).[155] Prototypes have been used in experimental studies requiring both discrimination between patterns from different categories and generalization among patterns within a category.[156] A possible interpretation of the findings on the nature of the internal representation of patterns is that each theory might be appropriate for different stages in either learning or recognition.

Pattern Processing

An intriguing featural model of pattern perception entitled "pandemonium" was presented by Selfridge.[157] Pattern recognition in this model is accomplished by "demons" that search for their likenesses in input stimuli. Four successive stages of processing are carried out by different types of demons. At the first level, data or image demons register the incoming pattern prior to passing a replica to the second level, where computational demons analyze the data to determine what features are present. Cognitive demons at the next level search for their own images among the analyzed feature patterns. Upon recognition of such images, these demons "shriek" their findings to the demon at the highest level. This supreme demon must determine which of the cognitive demons is shrieking the loudest, assuming that the greatest fury is created by the demon that has found the closest resemblance; thus the decision demon is faced with the pandemonium of the shrieking demons each time it must identify a pattern. Applying this model to the perception of speech, the computational demons would analyze the acoustic representation of the auditory signal to determine the distinctive frequency, intensity, and duration present. The cognitive demons would then group these features in bundles that represent phonemic patterns. Actual recognition of the phonemes present would be decided at the final stage of processing.

Sanders classifies the pandemonium model among passive theories of perception because the input signal is directly transformed into a pattern that is recognizable as a phoneme without the mediation of a pattern generated for purposes of comparison.[6] Another passive model of perception was proposed by Fant, who described both perceptual and articulatory processes in terms of feature patterns. Fant's auditory theory suggests that separate centers exist in the brain for the acoustic and motor patterns of speech, although the two centers are closely related both physically and functionally.[158] Fant maintains that auditory processing proceeds along the course from the reception of auditory stimuli to the direct coding of the signal into distinctive auditory features to the perception of the message. He acknowledges that the motor pathway could be involved either actively, so that perceptual processing would involve mediation by the motor patterns with the resulting pathway, or passively with the simultaneous secondary activation of the pathway. However, he believes that the evidence is insufficient to conclude that articulatory recording must precede perception.

A second category of speech perception theories views pattern recognition as an active process. In these theories, decoding is accomplished through an indirect process in which a pattern is recalled or generated to match the input stimuli. Two such theories exist. The first, the motor theory of speech perception proposed by Liberman and his colleagues,[133] views speech production and perception as "two aspects of the same process." In contrast to Fant's theory, the motor theory assumes a single mechanism or center with a link between the sensory and motor areas that serve both the perception and the production of speech. Correspondence between these two processes is felt to occur not only in the central nervous system, but probably as far as the motor commands to the articulators as well.

The relationship between the perceptual and productive aspects of speech stems from the fact that the perceiver of speech is also the producer of speech. This fact enables the listener to utilize knowledge of the productive aspects of speech to segment the continuous acoustic signal into phonemic units that can be processed rapidly. The complexity of the relationship between acoustic cues and phoneme perception mandates a special mode to unlock the speech code. This special mode is thought to utilize the patterns of neural instructions for articulation as a referent for recoding of the auditory signal, as suggested by Fant as a possible alternative to this model of direct coding.

Similar in many respects to the motor theory is Stevens' and Halle's analysis by synthesis model of speech perception.[159] This model also emphasizes the close relationship between perception and production. Abstract representations of speech events consisting of segments of features are generated for comparison with the input data. Information contained in the abstract representation is derived from both the perceptual and productive processes. A diagram of the most recent analysis-by-synthesis model is presented in Figure 10–14.[160]

Auditory input receives a partial peripheral analysis, after which it is stored, whereas features that are not context specific are identified through a direct analysis of the acoustic representation. This information is transmitted to a component that controls the subsequent analysis of the data. In addition to the data from the preliminary analysis, the control component receives contextual information from the results of the previous analysis of the utterance, including its lexical, syntactic, and semantic features, from the lexicon and from the comparator, another key component in the analyzer. From this information, the control component formulates an hypothesis as to the phonetic segments and features of the utterance. The hypothesis is transmitted to a set of previously stored rules from which the relevant acoustic attributes of the hypothesized utterance are generated. These attributes are compared with the partially analyzed signal held in the temporary store. The comparator reports to the control component on the accuracy of the hypothesis it had formulated. As can be seen in the diagram, the generative rules also serve the articulatory mechanism for output production, but in contrast to the motor theory, recognition is accomplished at the acoustic rather than at the articulatory level of processing. Although it stresses the active internal generative process that produces a matching representation, this model attributes considerable importance to the direct coding of the acoustic input that takes place prior to its comparison with previously stored rules and contextual information. Models of speech perception, up until this point, have held that the preliminary analysis of speech sounds resulting in the phonetic elements of speech is accomplished in a manner different from higher levels of language processing. Phonetic structures are seen as simple, direct representations of acoustic characteristics, whereas higher levels of linguistic processing are thought to produce complex recodings of the phonetic representation. Liberman argues that this view is incorrect.[161] He proposes a model in which all levels of processing of the speech signal are carried out in a special speech mode. His model is based on Chomsky's theory of generative grammar, which posited three levels of information—phonetic, surface, and deep—related by two grammatic conversions: phonology and syntax. In this model, a third grammar is proposed that would recode the acoustic signal into a phonetic representation. The resulting abstract pattern would be obtained through application of the grammatic code in a manner similar to that in which the grammars of phonology and syntax are employed. Rather than employing a comparator, this model successively recodes the speech signal into increasingly abstract forms of representation. Liberman's model is significant in that speech perception is viewed as an integral part of the language system;

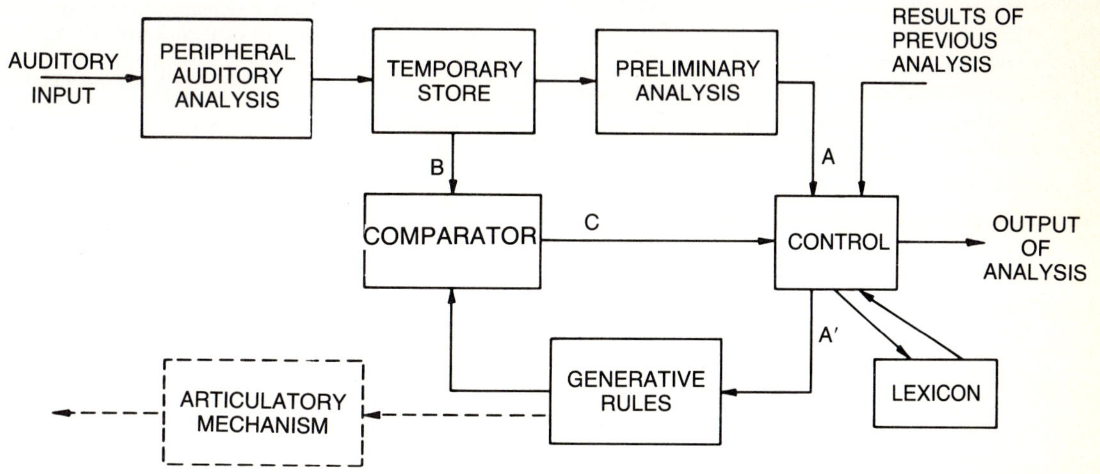

Figure 10–14 Analysis-by-synthesis model. (From Stevens KN. Segments, features and analysis by synthesis. In: Kavanagh JF, Mattingly IG, eds. Language by eye and ear. Cambridge: MIT Press, 1972:50.)

thus the study of speech provides access to further understanding of the less available higher levels of communication. Models that include the higher level processes leading to comprehension will be discussed under Comprehension.

Memory

Processing models have traditionally placed memory at a level between perception and comprehension. However, from our discussion of attention and perception, it is apparent that storage of information is an integral part of these processing stages. Recent studies of memory suggest different coding strategies rather than different storage structures, at least for short- and long-term memory. Atkinson and Shiffrin's proposed model of memory is shown in Figure 10–15.[3] Their model has three structural components: a sensory register, a short-term store, and a long-term store. The flow of information between the stores is accomplished through control processes, that is, processes that can be regulated internally. Each memory structure has associated with it a set of control processes.

At the first level of storage, sensory data entering the system are registered according to their modality. Sperling studied the limits of the sensory store by presenting arrays of random letters in multiple rows and asking subjects to report what they had seen.[162] Regardless of the number of letters presented, subjects reported only four or five items correctly. Probing further, Sperling discovered that subjects could recall all of the items in one of the rows when given a signal immediately after the presentation as to which row to report. He concluded from this finding that the visual sensory store can retain a relatively large amount of data for up to several hundred milliseconds. However, succeeding stimuli may interfere with a trace by masking it. Less is known about the nature of the sensory registers for other modalities, although structures with similar characteristics are hypothesized. A second level of storage, the short-term store, is viewed as a "working memory." Information is held in the short-term store longer than in the sensory register, that is, for 15 to 30 seconds. It may also be in a different form that it was in the sensory store; for example, visual information may be encoded in an auditory, verbal, and linguistic mode. As with the sensory

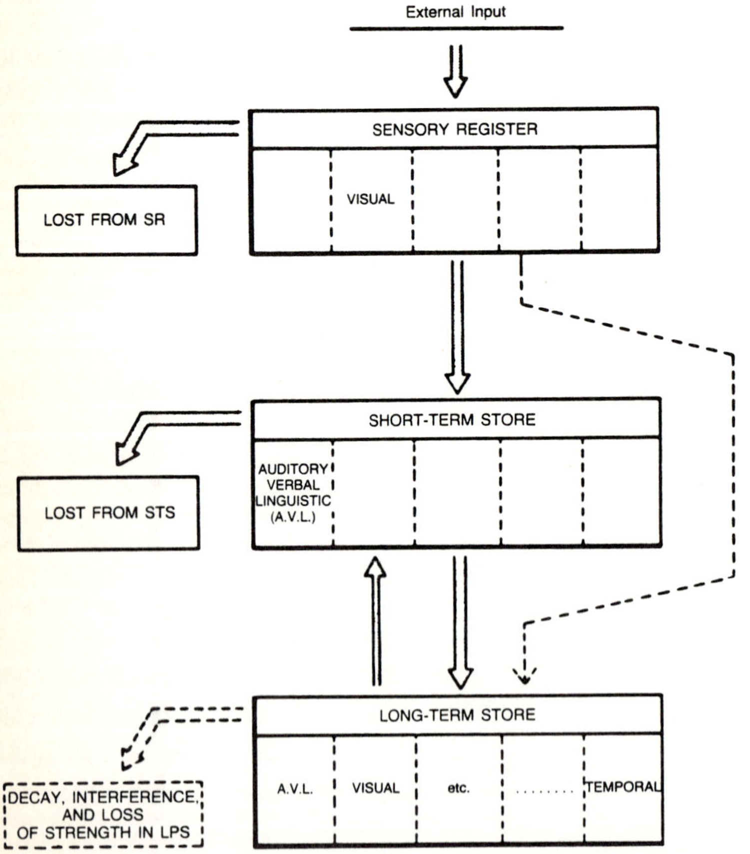

Figure 10–15 Memory components. (From Atkinson RC, Shiffrin RM. Human memory: a proposed system and its control processes. In: Spence KW, Spence JT, eds. The psychology of learning and motivation: advances in research and theory. Vol. 2. Orlando: Academic Press, 1968:93.)

register, when traces in short-term memory decay, they are assumed to be completely lost. The third and highest level of storage is the long-term store. Here information does not decay as in the two previous stores. However, other incoming information may cause traces to be modified or temporarily irretrievable. Information may be stored in the long-term store in any modality or without a specific modality, as in the case of temporal information. Many copies of traces are thought to be laid down, some of which are only partial, whereas others are complete. Interference with retrieval of memory traces is viewed in this model as structural, relating to factors that cause information to be lost or disrupted and not under the control of the individual. Additional factors, such as search mechanisms that are controlled by the individual, may also inhibit retrieval.

Control processes at the level of the sensory register relate to attention by selecting the information to be transferred to the next level. They determine which sensory register to attend to and the portion of the information in that register to transfer to the short-term store. Further strategies may be used to identify the input by matching it with information from the long-term store. Control processes associated with the short-term store regulate the transfer of information among the three stores, hence the concept "working memory." As such, the short-term store can be viewed as the center of the control system.[163] Simultaneous searches of the sensory register and long-term store result in the selection of information for transfer to the short-term store. Subsequent storage, search, and retrieval of this data occur in conjunction with the perceptual processes involved in pattern recognition. Information in the store may be rehearsed, to delay its decay, or coded. Coding refers to "a select alteration and/or addition to the information in the short-term store as the result of search of the long-term store" (p 115).[3] In addition to the short-term control processes of search, storage, retrieval, rehearsal, and coding, other processes that might occur prior to rehearsal include grouping, organizing, and chunking. The long-term store control processes are involved in storage, search, and retrieval in a manner similar to those of the short-term store, but this time they are dealing with a much larger store with more permanent memory traces and preexisting associations. Long-term memory, then, is involved in comprehension.

Atkinson and Shiffrin's model had a significant impact on information-processing theory[163] and was proposed at a time when concepts of memory were changing. Prior to this time an essentially passive role was attributed to memory: that of a structure for holding information for possible processing. The emerging view as exemplified in the Atkinson-Shiffrin model posited a more active functional role whereby storage processes were related to attention, perception, and comprehension. However, as summarized by Baddeley, subsequent research suggested certain limitations with this model. These limitations centered on the description of short-term memory and its relationship to long-term memory. Of particular interest to auditory information processing is the nature of the short- and long-term coding processes.

Acoustic and Semantic Coding

Memory research has presented conflicting evidence as to the division of memory into separate short- and long-term components.[163] Numerous studies suggest that different systems underlie each component. Short-term memory is limited in span to about seven items or "chunks," each of which may contain multiple bits of information. Recall tasks show that short-term recall is affected by the acoustic form of words, but not by the visual and semantic forms. But long-term memory has no obvious span limit; however, the amount of information in each item is limited. Long-term recall is primarily affected by the semantic form of the word. Evidence that disputes the validity of separate short- and long-term memory stores comes from recent studies of coding mechanisms.

It has been shown that both acoustic and semantic coding are present in both short- and long-term recall tasks. The differences in coding observed are not viewed as a function of the type of stimuli and/or procedures used. On the one hand, if the material to be remembered is meaningless or is presented rapidly, semantic coding is not possible. As a result, the short-term stores evidence acoustic coding, and, if the information is stored permanently, it is in an acoustic form. On the other hand, when material can be coded semantically, it appears in both stores and is remembered more readily. Current thinking enforces the view of a single memory system[164] with different types of coding possible. Acoustic and/or phonemic encoding occurs as a short-term memory process when semantic coding is not possible, such as when the rate of presentation of the information is too rapid, when the material is ambiguous, or when the listener is not paying sufficient attention to process it the first time and so "recycles" the information. When semantic encoding does occur, a permanent memory trace is laid down.

Depth and Breadth of Processing

Another aspect of encoding proposed as a determinant of retention is the elaborateness of the analysis carried out. Craik and Lockhart proposed a levels-of-processing theory of memory, which suggests that tasks allowing for only shallow processing result in less well-retained information than tasks allowing for greater depth of processing.[165] Depth of processing is associated with the elaborateness of the stimulus analysis, from the extraction of certain physical characteristics through reorganization of the features extracted; their synthesis into patterns; and the subsequent association of those patterns with meanings stored in long-term memory. A speech-processing task, for example, may require that two stimuli be identified as the same or different according to their meanings. The extraction of meaning from stimuli is thought to require more processing than the mere comparison of stimuli on nonmeaningful characteristics. It is argued that stimuli receiving sufficient processing so that they are comprehended rather than only recognized are remembered better.

Subsequent studies reported by Craik and Tulving suggest that elaboration of breadth or "spread" of the encoding operations at any processing level is an additional consideration to depth in the determination of the degree of retention.[166] Words that could be incorporated into complex sentence frames were better recalled than words for which simple sentence frames were presented. Words that did not fit either simple or complex frames were poorly retained. These findings suggest that the persistence of a representation in memory is enhanced by integration of a stimulus item into a coherent contextual framework. Degree of retention, then, is seen as more complex than the separate short- and long-term structure model would suggest. Long-term storage and retrieval appear to be related to the manner in which information is organized at the time of storage.[163]

Comprehension

As we consider increasingly higher levels of processing, long-term memory is seen to assume a more important role. In attention, knowledge of perceptual, conceptual, and linguistic rule systems is utilized in selection of certain sensory input for further processing. Additionally, associations previously stored in long-term memory allow for automatic processing of some input data, thereby reducing the attentional resources required. The perceptual process was described as a comparison of the results of stimulus analysis with patterns stored in long-term memory. Comprehension, considered in this section, is seen as totally dependent on long-term memory as perceptual information is transformed into meaningful ideas.

Representation of Knowledge

Information stored in long-term memory is accumulated through experiences and as such represents an individual's knowledge of the world. Several opinions exist as to the form of these representations. Paivio provides evidence for the existence of two independent but interrelated memory systems.[167] The first utilizes imagery in storing analogic representations that resemble the properties of events. The second system relies on verbal encoding of events according to the specific attributes of the events. Kintsch stated that two memory modes may be insufficient to account for the many types of sensory input that are stored in long-term memory.[164] He suggests that whatever the content of a memory trace, it must be coded and proposes a "multiple-coding theory."[164] Pylyshyn argues that neither images nor words can represent concepts since both need to be interpreted before they can be classified as concepts.[168] Rather, he maintains that knowledge of all kinds is stored in a propositional form, an abstracted and interpreted representation of the sensory data. An experience, then, is seen as represented by a finite set of statements or propositions that are equivalent to one's knowledge of that event and that could be asserted verbally. Whatever the representational format, it must lend itself to the kind of information that must be stored.

Three long-term storage systems are described by Tulving: procedural, semantic, and episodic memory.[169] Procedural memory, the most basic system, allows for recording connections between stimuli and responses. These action-oriented representations are then used by the individual in prescribing appropriate responses to the environment. Semantic memory, a specialized subsystem of episodic memory, represents an individual's mental model of the world. As such, it describes one individual's view of the world rather than prescribing actions upon that world. Episodic memory is, in turn, a subsystem of semantic memory. It allows for retention of information about personal experiences as they occurred in time and space. Tulving, as well as other researchers, believes that the three systems described represent the minimum number of different human memory stores.

Since retrieval of information stored in long-term memory is critical to the comprehension of auditory stimuli, the organization of semantic memory has been of considerable interest. Two major types of organizational systems have been hypothesized: network models and feature models.

Network models depict long-term memory as a vast representational system consisting of conceptual structures and relationships among concepts and words. Strategies are described that show how information extracted from sentences and nonverbal experiences can be represented meaningfully. The form in which information is stored may also be specified. In their early network model, Collins and Quillian proposed a hierarchical arrangement of supersets and subsets of relations.[170,171] The network is comprised of units or concepts that have properties that describe the units. Pointers link units to their supersets. Examples of a noun and a verb chain are "dog canine mammal animal" and "to sprint to run to go to do."[171] Comprehension is viewed as a constructive process in which incoming information is integrated into the existing structural arrangement so that a new structure is formed. This process results in a revision of the individual's representational system. Another network model presented by Rumelhart et al emphasizes the processes through which information is entered into the system, interpreted, and retrieved.[172] Processes are stored in a data base as are the data on which they operate. Both are activated as is necessary. The data base consists of nodes representing "clusters of information"[172] and relations or associations among nodes expressed by propositions. Kintsch's network model is concerned with the organization of the lexicon in long-term memory rather than the world knowledge that an individual possesses.[173,174] As such, he stresses the role of propositions which he views as "the basic building blocks of the memory model" (p 254).[173]

The human associative memory model of Anderson and Bower also uses propositions to represent information.[175] In contrast to the models of Rumelhart et al and Kintsch, in which the whole proposition is viewed as a unit of meaning or a gestalt, propositions in Anderson and Bower's model consist of associated elements that can be recalled separately.[164] Network models of long-term memory and comprehension have been extensively tested on computers. A recent computer model of speech comprehension, Hearsay-II, which emphasizes the interaction between bottom-up and top-down processing, will be presented in some detail in the next section.[176]

A second type of organizational system describes conceptual relationships in terms of features.[177,178] Concepts are represented by features on a continuum from the most important or "defining features" to the least important or "characteristic features." Abstract categories have fewer defining features, as illustrated by the example of "bird," which is the superordinate of "robin," "chicken," and "eagle" and therefore must have a feature list that can be applied to all the subordinate concept categories. Hence the defining feature list for robin would include all the features of bird and in addition at least the feature "red breast." Defining features are required in a particular concept, whereas characteristic features may only be associated with the category. A concept is defined by comparing it with a set of features stored in long-term memory. If the comparison does not readily establish a match or a clear nonmatch, then a second stage of comparison is made in which only defining features are considered. The time required for an "intermediate" match is thus greater because of the necessity of two comparison stages as opposed to the single comparison possible when the two feature sets have either an extensive overlap or no overlap.

The extent of applicability of network and feature models is viewed differently by different theorists. Klatzky suggests that the feature model is useful only for semantic memory, whereas network models may serve both semantic and episodic memories because of their broader scope.[179] But Kintsch, in cautioning against considering semantic and episodic memory as separate stores, holds that semantic memory must be derived from episodic memory.[164] This being the case, the stages of comparison in the feature model may be equated with moving from semantic to episodic memory traces in making a category decision, thus giving the more explicit feature model the greater advantage.

Models of Language Comprehension

Language comprehension, the association of meaning with information abstracted from the acoustic signal, is the end product of the auditory process. Information-processing models attempt to delineate each storage and control process between the reception of stimuli and the meaning response. Two models for understanding language will be described. The first, developed by Massaro,[180] appears in Figure 10–16.

The model has four "functional" processes (circles), each of which has a corresponding structural component (boxes) or store of information being operated on. Although both the auditory and visual systems are represented, only the auditory system will be discussed. The first functional process, feature detection, transforms sound wave patterns into acoustic features that are then held in a preperceptual auditory store. Feature detection is a passive process that operates on the acoustic signal with no input from the long-term store. Processing of fea-

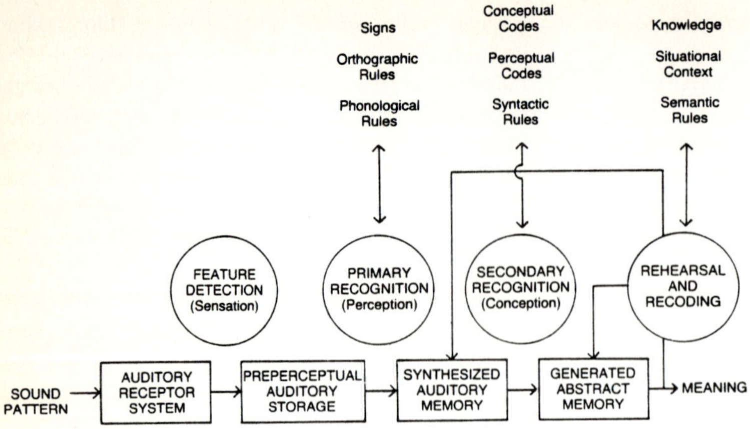

Figure 10-16 Temporal course of auditory information processing. (After Massaro DW. Understanding language. Orlando: Academic Press, 1975:6.)

tures requires varying amounts of time and may be interfered with by background noise. The first part of the auditory stimulus is held in the preperceptual auditory store until the pattern is complete and primary recognition occurs. The preperceptual image is equivalent to the sensory image referred to in earlier sections.

Primary recognition or perception, the second process, is the synthesizing of feature patterns into recognizable vowel and consonant-vowel syllables. Recognition is accomplished without reference to meaning, although phonologic rules might be employed. Massaro argues that the perceptual process does not require involvement of the motor patterns of speech.[180] The percept is held in synthesized auditory memory as a gestalt, in contrast to the pattern of separate acoustic features in preperceptual auditory storage, while the secondary recognition processes are carried out.

The lexicon, stored in long-term memory as a multidimensional representation of words, is utilized in secondary recognition or conception. Lexical representation includes both perceptual and conceptual attributes, so that when a match is obtained on the basis of the perceptual pattern, meaning is also accessed. Syntax rules may be involved at this stage, as may semantic and contextual knowledge. Conceptual units are held in generated abstract memory, so named because the events in the store are abstract meanings generated from input data and data retrieved from long-term storage. The limited capacity of this store causes forgetting to take place when new information must be processed. Additional processing or recoding of the conceptual units to obtain meanings at the phrase and sentence level utilizes whatever kind of knowledge the system has available. No changes in the nature of the information occur in this recoding. Rehearsal may also be engaged in to extend the period of retention of the information.

Unlike the previous models, which focused on a single dimension of information processing, Massaro's model incorporates the selection, perception, and comprehension processes as well as the memory stores. The speech signal is transformed into successively larger and larger chunks of information until meaning can be generated. Whereas the preperceptual stage of processing is passive and direct, the higher stages all involve utilization of certain types of information stored in long-term memory as well as the expectancies of the listener. Massaro's model for understanding language can be viewed as having a considerable top-down influence.

A second language comprehension model, Hearsay-II, has been developed as a computer speech understanding system.[176] Having recognized the many uncertainties present that can lead to errors in speech comprehension, an attempt was made to develop a system that would use knowledge of various types cooperatively so that errors would be cancelled rather than combined. To accomplish this, higher-level knowledge was felt to be particularly important. The goal of this system is to generate an hypothesis of a reasonable interpretation of an entire utterance by analyzing it from the acoustic level through the phrase level.

Speech understanding in Hearsay-II makes use of knowledge encoded in "knowledge source modules" according to specific linguistic domains, for example, acoustic-phonetic mappings, syllable recognition, syntax, and semantics.[181] The results of operations carried out by the system are recorded on a "blackboard." The blackboard is organized according to time and level of representation so that the current acoustic, phonetic, lexical, and/or phrase hypotheses for a particular temporal interval of speech may be shown. The knowledge source modules communicate with one another by modifying the hypotheses on the blackboard. Alternate hypotheses as to the interpretation of data relative to any level may be represented simultaneously.

The process that is carried out can be depicted as a "hypothesize-and-test paradigm of problem-solving."[176] When a knowledge source module detects an hypothesis to which its knowledge can be applied, it "invokes" a knowledge source procedure, that is, a modification of an hypothesis. The change activates other knowledge source modules accordingly. For example, hypothesization of the phonetic chain /t/, /e/, /l/ could invoke a lexical knowledge source that would hypothesize "tell." The lexical hypothesis could in turn evoke a syntactic knowledge source hypothesis that the following word would be from the category "us, me, her." Thus operations on hypotheses can occur as a bottom-up process, a top-down process, or along time so as to utilize contexual influences. Since multiple hypotheses may be presented, means of focusing attention so as to eliminate unlikely hypotheses are required. Two types of attentional strategies are proposed: a thresholding mechanism and priority scheduling.

Syntactic and semantic knowledge sources are thought to be particularly potent in selecting among hypotheses in a large "search" space because they can filter out the "noise" produced in the bottom-up predictions. Plausible sequences of words can be recognized and then used in filling in missing words. Without syntactic and semantic knowledge, the system is a bottom-up word recognizer. Using a 1,000-word corpus, Hearsay-II hypothesizes 80 percent of the words in an utterance correctly on the basis of word recognition. However, in addition to the correct words hypothesized, 10 to 20 incorrect words are hypothesized for each correct word. Addition of the top-down knowledge sources results in 90 percent of the utterance being correctly recognized syntactically and/or semantically.

Models of Discourse Processing

As cognitive scientists have presented increasingly integrated models of information processing and as psycholinguistic study has shifted from the successive levels of phonology, syntax, semantics, and pragmatics to the processing of entire texts, more comprehensive interdisciplinary models of discourse comprehension have evolved. Exemplifying this trend is the work of Kintsch and van Djik.[182,183] Similar to models of language comprehension that focused on linguistic levels, Kintsch and van Djik's 1978 model identified levels of textural structure such as propositions, macrostructures, and superstructures. In their more recent work,[183] Kintsch and van Djik expand their structural orientation by proposing a process or "strategical" model that describes interactive processes, both internal and external, to the language user. Understanding of words, clauses, sentences, and discourse structures result from ongoing feedback between less complex and more complex discourse segments. In addition, the model takes into account characteristics of the language user, such as interests, goals, and knowledge, as well as the situation in which the language occurs.

A central strategy of the new model is the construction of a "textbase," the representation of discourse meaning in episodic memory. The textbase consists of propositions and relations among propositions derived from the discourse. Simultaneously, a cognitive representation of persons, actions, events, and the general situation referred to in the discourse is constructed. Termed a "situation model" the cognitive representation may include related information from previous experiences and textbases, thereby making available to the comprehender all that is known about similar situations. Also entailed in the model is a control system that activates and coordinates the available strategies and knowledge to achieve understanding of the discourse.

Figure 10–17 represents the essential features of the van Dijk and Kintsch model. A central processor entailing short-term memory is shown inside the circle, and the interacting memory systems—sensory register, long-term memory, and episodic text memory—surround the central core. The sensory register briefly stores incoming perceptual data, making certain features available to the central processor as needed. Long-term memory is the repository for general knowledge derived from many experiences, as well as memories of single experiences. The episodic text memory is the memory representation being constructed for an oral or written text. It includes surface features, speech sounds, or print; propositions or units of meaning; and the macrostructure or gist of the text. A situational model accompanies the episodic text memory.

The actual processing of the text takes place in the central processor. Sentence fragments, denoted by W, are reduced to propositional units P. These are combined into complex propositions, P_k, which correspond to phrases or sentences. While a chunk of information, P_k, is being processed, a previously processed proposition, P_{k-1}, is held in a buffer. A central system at the periphery of the central processor consists of additional factors that actively in-

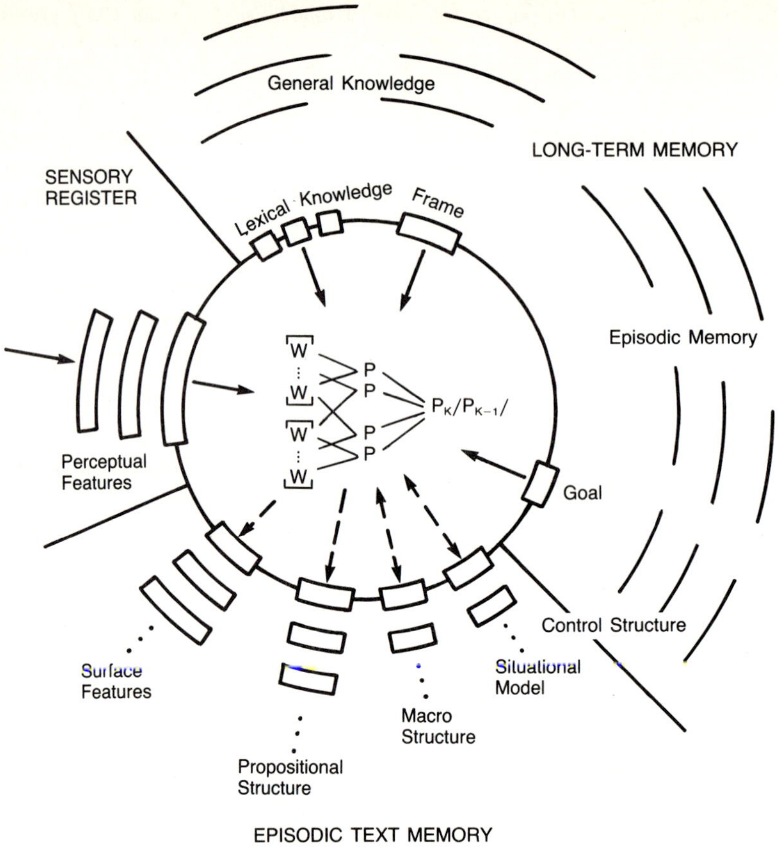

Figure 10–17 A sketch of the operation of the memory system in discourse comprehension. The circle represents working memory, containing words, and propositions; P_k is currently under construction while the previous proposition P_{k-1} is held in the limited capacity buffer. Abbreviations: W = sentence fragments; P = propositional units: P_k = complex propositions: P_{k-1} = previously proposed proposition. (From van Dijk TA, Kintsch W. Strategies of discourse comprehension. Orlando: Academic Press, 1983:347.)

fluence processing. These include goals, frames, and macrostructures related to the episode being comprehended as well as other types of knowledge that may be retrieved from memory stores and allowed to influence conscious processing. Kintsch and van Djik hypothesize that the central processor has a limited capacity and functions in an active, conscious way while the surrounding memory structures that may be accessed during processing have unlimited capacity and are beyond consciousness.

Kintsch and van Djik's model provides a theoretical framework for integrating many current cognitive and psycholinguistic theories of discourse comprehension. In effect it leads speech-language pathologists into a new era in the study of auditory and linguistic processing.

SUMMARY

Research and theoretical work have emphasized that auditory and linguistic input is never into a static system, but into one that is organized continuously by the functional state and previous experience of the individual. As such, auditory linguistic processing appears to be a function of how the acoustic signal is integrated with the existing internal states of the individual, for example, attention, knowledge, and expectations, which are in part independent of stimulus conditions. A higher level, or central, control process involving activation of appropriate mechanisms for acquisition and modification of central organization has been stressed.

Any complete theory of auditory linguistic processing needs to account at least for the capacity to organize simultaneous, successive variations in the acoustic signal into a pattern consistent with the structured verbal message as well as to account for the functional state and previous experience of the individual. Evidence has demonstrated that the central nervous system is not a passive recipient and analyzer of all auditory information, but is capable of controlling its own input and processing. Although a model that integrates neurologic, cognitive, and linguistic theories is not at present available, a shift of emphasis from invariant structures of the mind to flexible processes with the potential of variability has clinical significance. As speech-language pathologists have come to understand higher-level functioning and comprehension of language, the active involvement of the individual in constructing meaning relative to the situation contributes to central organizational patterns that prepare and directly influence the selection and processing of sensory information.

REFERENCES

1. Miller GA, Johnson-Laird PN. Language and perception. Cambridge: Harvard University Press, 1976.
2. Norman DA, Bobrow DG. On data-limited and resource-limited processes. Cognitive Psychol 1975; 7:44–64.
3. Atkinson RC, Shiffrin RM. Human memory: a proposed system and its control processes. In: Spence KW, Spence JT, eds. The psychology of learning and motivation: advances in research and theory. Vol. 2. New York: Academic Press, 1968:90.
4. Darley FL, Aronson AE, Brown JR. Motor speech disorders. Philadelphia: WB Saunders, 1975.
5. Corcoran DWF. Pattern recognition. Baltimore: Penguin Books, 1971.
6. Sanders DA. Auditory perception of speech. Englewood Cliffs, NJ: Prentice-Hall, 1977.
7. Glattske TJ. Elements of auditory physiology. In: Minifie FD, Hixon, TJ, Williams F, eds. Normal aspects of speech, hearing and language. Englewood Cliffs: Prentice-Hall, 1973:285.
8. Hernádez-Peón R. Reticular mechanisms of sensory control. In: Rosenblith WA, ed. Sensory communication. Cambridge: MIT Press, 1961:497.
9. Scheibel ME, Scheibel AB. Structural substrates for integrative patterns in the brain stem reticular core. In: Jasper HH, Proctor LD, Knighton RS, Noshay WS, Costello RT, eds. The reticular formation of the brain. Boston: Little, Brown, 1958:31.
10. Hernández-Peón R, Scherrer H, Jouvet M. Modification of electric activity in cochlear nucleus during "attention" in unanesthetized cats. Science 1956; 123:331–332.
11. Killam KF, Killam EK. Drug action on pathways involving the reticular formation. In: Jasper HH, ed. Reticular formation of the brain. Boston: Little, Brown, 1958:111.
12. Moruzzi G, Magoun HW. Brain stem reticular formation and activation of the EEG. Electroencephalogr Clin Neurophysiol 1949; 1:455–473.
13. Sharpless S, Jasper, H. Habituation of the arousal reaction. Brain 1956; 79:655–680.
14. French JD, Hernández-Peón R, Livingston RB. Projections from cortex to cephalic brain stem (reticular formation) in monkey. J Neurophysiol 1955; 18:44–55.
15. Goldstein L, Nelsen JM. Some views on the neurophysiological and neuropharmacological mechanisms of storage and retrieval of information. In: Zippel HP, ed. Memory and transfer of information. New York: Plenum Publishing, 1973:155.
16. Routtenberg A. The two-arousal hypothesis: reticular formation and limbic system. Psychol Rev 1968; 75:51–80.
17. Thatcher RW, John ER. Functional neuroscience. Vol. I. Foundations of cognitive processes. Hillsdale, NJ: Erlbaum, 1977.
18. Newman JD, Symmes D. Arousal effects on unit responsiveness to vocalizations in squirrel monkey auditory cortex. Brain Res 1974; 78:125–138.
19. Robinson DL, Petersen SE. The neurobiology of attention. In: LeDoux JE, Hirst W, eds. Mind and brain: dialogues in cognitive neuroscience. New York: Cambridge University Press, 1986:142.
20. Regan D. Evoked potentials in psychology, sensory physiology, and clinical medicine. New York: Wiley-Interscience, 1972.
21. Galambos R, Sheatz G, Vernier VG. Electrophysiological correlates of a conditioned response in cats. Science 1956; 123:376–377.
22. Hillyard SA, Hink RF, Schwent VL, Picton TW. Electrical signs of selective attention in the human brain. Science 1973; 182:177–179.
23. Schwent VI, Hillyard JA, Galambos R. Selective attention and auditory vertex potential II. Effects of signal attention and masking noise. Electroencephalogr Clin Neurophysiol 1976; 40:615–622.
24. Knight RT, Hillyard SA, Woods DL, Neville HJ. The effects of frontal cortex lesions on event-related potentials during auditory selective attention. Electroencephalogr Clin Neurophysiol 1981; 52:571–582.
25. Welch K, Stuteville P. Experimental production of unilateral neglect in monkeys. Brain 1958; 81:341–347.
26. Heilman KM, Valenstein E. Auditory neglect in man. Arch Neurol 1972; 26:32–35.
27. Roland PE. Cortical regulation of selective attention in man: a regional cerebral blood flow study. J Neurophysiol 1982; 48:1059–1078.
28. McGuinness D, Pribram KH. The neuropsychology of attention: emotional and motivational controls. In: Wittrock MC, ed. The brain and psychology. New York: Academic Press, 1980:95.
29. Pribram KH, McGuinness D. Arousal, activation, and effort in the control of attention. Psychol Rev 1975; 82:116–149.
30. Hebb DO. The organization of behavior. New York: John Wiley & Sons, 1949.
31. Lashley KS. In search of the engram. In: Beach FA, Hebb DO, Morgan CT, Nissen HW, eds. The neuropsychology of Lashley. New York: McGraw-Hill, 1960:478.
32. Papez JW. A proposed mechanism of emotion. Arch Neurol Psychiatry 1937; 38:725–743.
33. Ojemann RG. Correlations between specific human brain lesions and memory changes. Neurosci Res Program Bull [Suppl] 1966; 4:1–70.
34. Luria AR. The working brain: an introduction to neuropsychology. New York: Basic Books, 1973.
35. Milner B. Psychological defects produced by temporal lobe excision. Publ Assoc Res Nervous Ment Dis 1958; 36:244–257.
36. Penfield W. Memory mechanisms. Arch Neurol Psychiatry 1952; 67:178–198.
37. Penfield W, Mathieson G. Memory. Arch Neurol 1974; 31:145–154.
38. Ojemann RG. Organization of short-term verbal memory in language areas of human cortex: evidence from electrical stimulation. Brain Lang 1978; 5:331–340.
39. Milner B. Brain mechanisms suggested by studies of temporal lobes. In: Millikan CH, Darley FL, eds. Brain mechanisms underlying speech and language. New York: Grune & Stratton, 1967:122.
40. Drachman DA, Arbit J. Memory and the hippocampal complex, II. Arch Neurol 1966; 15:52–61.
41. Scoville WG, Milner B. Loss of recent memory after bilateral hippocampal lesions. J Neurol Neurosurg Psychiatry 1957; 20:11–21.
42. Luria AR. Higher cortical functions in man. New York: Basic Books, 1966.
43. Hagberg B. Defects of immediate memory related to the cerebral blood flow distribution. Brain Lang 1978; 5:366–377.

44. Ojemann RG, Ward A. Speech representation in ventrolateral thalamus. Brain 1971; 94:669–680.
45. Ojemann RG. Language and the thalamus: object naming and recall during and after thalamic stimulation. Brain Lang 1975; 2:101–120.
46. Kornhuber HH. Neural control of input into long term memory: limbic system and amnestic syndrome in man. In: Zippel HP, ed. Memory and transfer of information. New York: Plenum Press, 1973:1.
47. Joynt RJ. Human memory. In: Tower DB, ed. The nervous system. Vol. 2. The clinical neurosciences. New York: Raven Press, 1975:441.
48. Eccles JC. The understanding of the brain. New York: McGraw-Hill, 1977.
49. Squire LR, Cohen NJ, Nadel L. The medial temporal region and memory consolidation: a new hypothesis. In: Weingarter H, Parker ES, eds. Memory consolidation: psychobiology of cognition. Hillsdale, NJ: Erlbaum, 1984:185.
50. Halgren E. Mental phenomena induced by stimulation in limbic system. Hum Neurobiol 1982; 1:251–260.
51. Teyler TJ, DiScenna P. The hippocampal memory indexing theory. Behav Neurosci 1986; 100(2):147–154.
52. Anderson JA, Silverstein JW, Ritz SA, Jones RS. Distinctive features, categorical perception, and probability learning: some applications of a neural model. Psychol Rev 1977; 84:413–451.
53. Magoun HW. Lacunae and research approaches to them, II. In: Millikan CH, Darley FL, eds. Brain mechanisms underlying speech and language. New York: Grune & Stratton, 1967:217.
54. Moscovitch M. Multiple dissociations of functions in amnesia. In: Cernak LS, ed. Human memory and amnesia. Hillsdale, NJ: Erlbaum, 1982.
55. Brooks DN, Baddeley AD. What can amnestic patients learn? Neuropsychologia 1976; 14:111–122.
56. Cohen NJ, Squire LR. Perserved learning and retention of pattern analyzing skill in amnesia: dissociation of knowing how and knowing that. Science 1980; 210:207–209.
57. Cohen NJ, Squire LR. Retrograde amnesia and remote memory impairment. Neuropsychologia 1981; 19:337–356.
58. Kinsbourne M, Wood F. Short-term memory processes and the amnestic syndrome. In: Deutsch D, Deutsch JA, eds. Short-term memory processes. New York: Academic Press, 1975:258.
59. Olton DS. Memory functions and the hippocampus. In: Seifert W, ed. Neurobiology of the hippocampus. New York: Academic Press, 1983:335.
60. Olton DS, Becker JT, Handelmann GE. Hippocampus, space and memory. Behav Brain Sci 1979; 2:313–365.
61. Tulving E. Episodic and semantic memory. In: Tulving E, Donaldson W, eds. Organization of memory. New York: Academic Press, 1972.
62. Mishkin M. A memory system in the monkey. Philos Trans R Soc Lond 1982; 298:85–95.
63. Mishkin M, Malamut B, Bachevalier J. Memories and habits: two neural systems. In: Lynch G, McGaugh JL, Weinberger NM, eds. Neurobiology of learning and memory. New York: The Guilford Press, 1984:65.
64. Kesner RP. Neurobiological views of memory. In: Martinez JL, Kesner RP, eds. Learning and memory: a biological view. New York: Academic Press, 1986:399.
65. Woolsey CN and Walzl EM. Topical projection of nerve fibers from local regions of the cochlea to the cerebral cortex of the cat. Johns Hopkins Med J 1942; 71:315–344.
66. Woolsey CN. Organization of cortical auditory system: a review and synthesis. In: Rasmussen GL, Windle W, eds. Neural mechanisms of the auditory and vestibular systems. Springfield, IL: CC Thomas, 1960:165.
67. Woolsey CN. Organization of cortical auditory system: a review and synthesis. In: Rosenblith W, ed. Sensory communications. Cambridge: MIT Press, 1961:235.
68. Imig TJ, Ruggero MA, Kitzes LM, Javel E, Brugge JF. Organization of the auditory cortex in the owl monkey. J Acoust Soc Am 1974; 56:523.
69. Merzenich MM, Knight PL, Roth OL. Representation of cochlea within primary auditory cortex in the cat. J Neurophysiol 1975; 38:231–249.
70. Celsia GG. Organization of auditory cortical areas in man. Brain 1976; 99:403–414.
71. Pandya DN, Hallett M, Mukherjie SK. Intra- and interhemispheric connections of the neocortical auditory system in the rhesus monkey. Brain Res 1969; 14:49–65.
72. Brugge JF. Progress in neuroanatomy and neurophysiology of auditory cortex. In: Tower DB, ed in chief, Eagles EH, vol. ed. The nervous system. Human communication and its disorders. Vol. 3. New York: Raven Press, 1975:97.
73. Karol EA, Pandya DW. The distribution of the corpus callosum in the rhesus monkey. Brain 1971; 94:471.
74. Neff WD. Role of the auditory cortex in sound discrimination. In: Rasmussen G, Windle W, eds. Neural mechanisms of the auditory and vestibular systems. Springfield: CC Thomas, 1960:211.
75. Kryter KD, Ades HW. Studies on the function of the higher acoustic nervous centers in the cat. Am J Psychol 1943; 56:501–536.
76. Jerger J. Observations on auditory behavior in lesions of the central auditory pathways. Arch Otolaryngol 1960; 71:797 806.
77. Goldstein R. Hearing and speech in follow-up of left hemispherectomy. J Speech Hear Disord 1961; 26:126–129.
78. Jerger J, Weikers NJ, Sharbrough FW III, Jerger S. Bilateral lesions of the temporal lobe. Acta Otolaryngol [Suppl] 1969; 258:1–51.
79. Milner B. Laterality effects in audition. In: Mountcastle VB, ed. Interhemispheric relations and cerebral dominance. Baltimore: The Johns Hopkins University Press, 1962:177.
80. Needham EC, Black JW. The relative ability of aphasic persons to judge the duration and intensity of pure tones. J Speech Hear Res 1970; 13:725–730.
81. Efron R. Temporal perception, aphasia, and déjà vu. Brain 1963; 86:403–424.
82. Halperin Y, Nachshon I, Carmon A. Shift of ear superiority in dichotic listening to temporally patterned nonverbal stimuli. J Acoust Soc Am 1973; 53:46–50.
83. Papcum G, Krasken S, Terbeek D, Remington R, Harshman R. Is the left hemisphere specialized for speech, language and/or something else? J Acoust Soc Am 1974; 55:319–327.
84. Penfield W, Roberts L. Speech and brain mechanisms. Princeton: Princeton University Press, 1959.
85. Russell R, Espir M. Traumatic aphasia. Oxford: Oxford University Press, 1961.
86. Gazzinga M. The bisected brain. New York: Appleton-Century-Crofts, 1970.
87. Geschwind N. The organization of language and the brain. Science 1970; 170:940–944.
88. Broadbent DE. Perception and communication. London: Pergamon Press, 1958.
89. Kimura D. Cerebral dominance and the perception of verbal stimuli. Can J Psychol 1961; 15:166–171.
90. Kimura D. Some effects of temporal-lobe damage on auditory perception. Can J Psychol 1961; 15:156–165.
91. Kimura D. Functional asymmetry of the brain in dichotic listening. Cortex 1967; 3:163–178.
92. Shankweiler D, Studdert-Kennedy M. Identification of consonants and vowels presented to left and right ears. QJ Exp Psychol 1967; 19:59–63.
93. Studdert-Kennedy M, Shankweiler D. Hemispheric specialization for speech perception. J Acoust Soc Am 1970; 48:579.

94. Berlin CI, Lowe-Bell SS, Cullen JK, Thompson CL, Loovis CF. Dichotic speech perception: an interpretation of right ear advantage and temporal offset effects. J Acoust Soc Am 1973; 54:699–709.
95. Kimura D. Left-right differences in the perception of melodies. QJ Exp Psychol 1964; 16:355–358.
96. Wood CC. Auditory and phonetic levels of processing in speech perception: neurophysiological and information-processing analyses. J Exp Psychiatry 1975; 104:3–20.
97. Wood CC, Goff WR, Day RS. Auditory evoked potentials during speech perception. Science 1971; 173:1248–1251.
98. Molfese DL, Nunez G, Seibert S, Ramanaiah N. Changes in factors affecting differential hemispheric activities in infants. Ann NY Acad Sci 1976; 280:821–833.
99. Nagafuchi M. Development of dichotic and monaural hearing abilities in young children. Acta Otolaryngol 1970; 69:409–414.
100. Brown J, Jaffe J. Hypothesis on cerebral dominance. Neuropsychologia 1975; 13:107–110.
101. Porter RJ, Berlin CI. On interpreting development changes in the dichotic right-ear advantage. Brain Lang 1975; 2:186–200.
102. Eimas PD, Siqueland ER, Jusczyk R, Vigorito J. Speech perception in infants. Science 1971; 171:303–306.
103. Geschwind N, Levitsky W. Human brain: left-right asymmetries in temporal speech region. Science 1968; 161:186–187.
104. Wada J, Clarke R, Hamm A. Cerebral hemispheric asymmetry in humans. Cortical speech zones in 100 adult and 100 infant brains. Arch Neurol 1975; 32:239–246.
105. Molfese VJ, Molfese DL, Parsons C. Hemisphere processing of phonological information. In: Segalowitz SJ, ed. Language functions and brain organization. New York: Academic Press, 1983:29.
106. Perceman E, Kellar L. The effect of voice and place among aphasic, nonaphasic right-damaged and normal subjects on a metalinguistic task. Brain Lang 1981; 12:213–223.
107. Molfese DL. Left and right hemisphere involvement in speech perception: electrophysiological correlates. Perception and Psychophysics 1978; 23:237–243.
108. Molfese DL. The phoneme and the engram: electrophysiological evidence for the acoustic invariant in stop consonants. Brain Lang 1980; 9:372–376.
109. Molfese DL, Erwin RJ. Intrahemispheric differentiation of vowels: principal component analysis of auditory evoked responses to computer-synthesized vowel sounds. Brain Lang 1981; 13:333–344.
110. Searleman A. A review of right hemisphere linguistic capabilities. Pscyhol Bull 1977; 84:503–528.
111. Sperry RW, Gazzaniga MS. Language following surgical disconnection of the hemispheres. In: Millikan CH, Darley FL, eds. Brain mechanisms underlying speech and language. New York: Grune & Stratton 1967; 108–121.
112. Geschwind N. Disconnexion syndromes in animals and man, I and II. Brain 1965; 88:237–294, 585–643.
113. Ingvar DH, Schwartz MS. Blood flow patterns induced in the dominant hemisphere by speech and reading. Brain 1974; 97:273–288.
114. Lassen NA, Hoedt-Rasmussen K, Sorenssen SC, Skinhoj E, Cronquist S, Bodforss B, Ingvar DH. Regional cerebral blood flow in man determined by Krypton 85. Neurology 1963; 13:719–727.
115. Lassen NA, Ingvar DH, Skinhoj E. Brain function and blood flow. Sci Am 1978; 239:62–71.
116. Whitaker HA. A model for neurolinguistics. Occasional papers 10. Language Centre, Colchester, England: University of Essex Press, 1970.
117. Whitaker HA. Neurolinguistics. In: Dingwall WO, ed. A survey of linguistic science. College Park: University of Maryland, 1971; 136–251.
118. Green E. Psycholinguistic approaches to aphasia. Linguistics 1969; 53:30–50.
119. Magoun HW. The waking brain. Springfield: CC Thomas, 1963.
120. Geschwind N. Specializations of the human brain. Sci Am 1979; 241:180–199.
121. Geschwind N. Neurological foundations of language. In: Myklebust HR, ed. Progress in learning disabilities. New York: Grune & Stratton, 1968:182.
122. Ojernamm GA, ed. The thalamus and language. Brain Lang 1975; Vol. 2.
123. Brown J. On the neural organization of language: thalamic and cortical relationships. Brain Lang 1975; 2:18–30.
124. Brown J. Thalamic mechanisms in language. In: Gazzaniga MS, ed. Handbook of behavioral Neurobiology. Vol. 2. Neuropsychologia. New York: Plenum Press, 1979:215.
125. Whitaker HA. Neurobiology of language. In: Carterette EC, Friedman MP, eds. Handbook of perception. Vol. VII. Language and speech. New York: Academic Press 1976:121.
126. Mateer CA, Ojemann GA. Thalamic mechanisms in language and memory. In: Segalowitz SJ, ed. Language functions and brain organization. New York: Academic Press, 1983:171.
127. Ojemann RG, guest ed. The thalamus and language. Brain Lang 1975; Vol. 2.
128. Ojemann RG. Asymmetrical function of the thalamus in man. Ann NY Acad Sci 1977; 299:380–396.
129. Abbs JH, Sussman HM. Neurophysiological feature detectors and speech perception: a discussion of theoretical implications. J Speech Hear Res 1971; 14:23–36.
130. Evans EF, Whitfield IC. Classification of unit responses in the auditory cortex of the unanesthetized and unrestrained cat. J Physiol 1964; 171:476–493.
131. Carterrette EC, Friedman MP, Lovell JD. Mach bands in hearing. J Acoust Soc Am 1969; 45:986–998.
132. Katsuzi V. Neural mechanism of auditory sensation in cats. In: Rosenblith WA, ed. Sensory communications. Cambridge: MIT Press, 1961:561.
133. Liberman AM, Cooper FS, Shankweiler DP, Studert-Kennedy M. Perception of the speech code. Psychol Rev 1967; 74:431–461.
134. Cullen JK Jr, Berlin CI, Hughes LF, Thompson CL, Samson DS. Speech information flow: a model. In: Sullivan MD, ed. Proceedings of a symposium on central auditory processing disorders. Lincoln: University of Nebraska Press, 1975:108.
135. Nation JE, Aram DM. Diagnosis of speech and language disorders. St. Louis: CV Mosby, 1977.
136. Nation JE, Aram DM. Diagnosis of speech and language disorders, 2nd ed. San Diego: College Hill Press, 1984.
137. Ebbinghaus H. Memory: a contribution to experimental psychology. Ruger HA, Bussenius CA (trans). New York: Teachers College Press, 1913.
138. Bartlett FC. Remembering: a study in experimental and social psychology. Cambridge: Cambridge University Press, 1932.
139. Cherry EC. Some experiments on the recognition of speech with one and two ears. J Acoust Soc Am 1953; 25:975–979.
140. Moray N. Attention in dichotic listening: affective cues and the influence of instructions. QJ Exp Psychol 1959; 11:56–60.
141. Treisman AM. Contextual cues in selective listening. QJ Exp Psychol 1960; 12:242–248.
142. Treisman AM. Monitoring and storage of irrelevant message in selective attention. J Verbal Learn Verbal Behav, 1964; 3:449–459
143. Treisman AM. Verbal cues, language and meaning in selective attention. Am J Psychol 1964; 77:206–219.

144. Norman D. Toward a theory of memory and attention. Psychol Rev 1968; 75:522–536.
145. Norman DA. Memory and attention. 2nd ed. New York: John Wiley & Sons, 1976.
146. Kahneman D. Attention and effort. Englewood Cliffs: Prentice-Hall, 1973.
147. Moray N. Where is capacity limited? A survey and a model. Acta Psychol 1967; 27:84–92.
148. Treisman AM, Geffin G. Selective attention: perception or response? QJ Exp Psychol 1967; 19:1–17.
149. Schneider W, Shiffrin RM. Controlled and automatic human information processing, I. Detection, search and attention. Psychol Rev 1977; 84:1–66.
150. Reed SK. Psychological processes in pattern recognition. New York: Academic Press, 1973.
151. Jacobson R, Fant G, Halle M. Preliminaries to speech analysis: the distinctive features and their correlates (Tech Rep 13, MIT. Acoustics Laboratory, 1952). Cambridge: MIT Press, 1963.
152. Pick A. Improvement of musical and tactual form discrimination. J Exp Psychol 1963; 66:363–370.
153. Caldwell EC, Hall VC. Distinctive-features versus prototype learning re-examined. J Exp Psychol 1970; 83:7–12.
154. Aiken EG. Auditory discrimination learning: prototype storage and distinctive feature detection mechanisms. Perception and Psychophysics 1969; 6:95–96.
155. Oden GW, Massaro DW. Integration of featural information in speech perception. Psychol Rev 1978; 85:172–191.
156. Posner MI, Keele S. On the genesis of abstract ideas. J Exp Psychol 1968; 77:353–363.
157. Selfridge OG. Pandemonium: a paradigm for learning. Proceedings NPL symposium 1958. No. 10, Mechanization of thought processes. London: Her Majesty's Stationery Office, 1959; 513–526. As cited in Sanders DA: Auditory perception of speech, Englewood Cliffs, NJ: Prentice-Hall, 1977.
158. Fant G. Auditory patterns of speech. In: Wathen-Dunn W, ed. Models for the perception of speech and visual form. Cambridge: MIT Press, 1967:111.
159. Stevens KN, Halle M. Remarks on analysis by synthesis and distinctive features. In: Wathen-Dunn W, ed. Models for the perception of speech and visual form. Cambridge: MIT Press, 1967:88.
160. Stevens KN. Segments, features and analysis by synthesis. In: Kavanagh JF, Mattingly IG, eds. Language by ear and eye. Cambridge: MIT Press, 1972:50.
161. Liberman AM. The grammars of speech and language. Cognitive Psychol 1970; 1:301–323.
162. Sperling G. The information available in brief visual presentations. Psychol Monogr 1960; 74:498.
163. Baddeley AD. The psychology of memory. New York: Basic Books, 1976.
164. Kintsch W. Memory and cognition. New York: John Wiley & Sons, 1977.
165. Craik FIM, Lockhart RS. Levels of processing: a framework for memory research. J Verbal Learn Verbal Behav 1972; 11:671–684.
166. Craik FIM, Tulving E. Depth of processing and the retention of words in episodic memory. J Exp Psychol 1975; 104:268–294.
167. Paivio A. Imagery and verbal processes. New York: Holt, Rinehart & Winston, 1971.
168. Pylyshyn ZW. What the mind's eye tells the mind's brain: a critique of mental imagery. Psychol Bull 1973; 80:1–24.
169. Tulving E. How many memory systems are there? American Psychologist 1985; 40:385–398.
170. Collins AM, Quillian MR. Retrieval from semantic memory. J Verbal Learn Verbal Behav 1969; 8:240–247.
171. Collins AM, Quillian MR. How to make a language user. In: Tulving E, Donaldson W, eds. Organization of memory. New York: Academic Press, 1972:310.
172. Rumelhart DE, Lindsay PH, Norman DA. A process model for long-term memory. In: Tulving E, Donaldson W, eds. Organization and memory. New York: Academic Press, 1972.
173. Kintsch W. Notes on the structure of semantic memory. In: Tulving E, Donaldson W, eds. Organization of memory. New York: Academic Press, 1972:249.
174. Kintsch W. The representation of meaning in memory. Hillsdale, NJ. Erlbaum, 1974.
175. Anderson JR, Bower GH. Human associative memory. Washington: VH Winston & Sons, 1973.
176. Hayes-Roth F, Mostow DJ, Fox MS. Understanding speech in the hearsay-II system. In: Bolc L, ed. Natural communication with computers. Berlin: Springer-Verlag, 1978.
177. Rips LJ, Shoben EJ, Smith EE. Semantic distance and the verification of semantic relations. J Verbal Learn Verbal Behav 1973; 12:1–20.
178. Smith EE, Shoben EJ, Rips LL. Structure and process in semantic memory. A featural model for semantic decision. Psychol Rev 1974; 81:214–241.
179. Klatsky RL. Human memory: structures and processess. San Francisco: WH Freeman, 1975.
180. Massaro DW. Understanding language. New York: Academic Press, 1975.
181. Hayes-Roth F, Lesser VR. Focus of attention in the hearsay-II speech understanding system. Pittsburgh, Department of Computer Science, Carnegie-Mellon University, 1977.
182. Kintsch W, van Dijk TA. Toward a model of text comprehension and production. Psychol Rev 1978; 85:363–394.
183. van Dijk TA, Kintsch W. Strategies of discourse comprehension. New York: Academic Press, 1983.

11 Language Acquisition in the Child

Robin S. Chapman, Ph.D.

What is the nature of children's linguistic knowledge? This has been the central question of the past three decades of research on children's language acquisition. Throughout the work on children's words, sentences, and conversations, researchers have tried to formulate the children's rules for talking and listening. The purpose of this chapter is to provide a brief overview of issues that have arisen in these attempts to describe and explain children's linguistic knowledge and then to examine in more detail the resulting accounts of children's skill in talking and listening that carry the most immediate relevance for developmental approaches to language disorders.

A HISTORY OF SHIFTS IN RESEARCH FOCUS

Issues in research on children's language have changed as views of language have changed. Increasingly, researchers have focused on the broader context of communication. The roles of social and cognitive development in the process of language acquisition have become recognized and debated. Each broadening of vision has required old issues to be reexamined. These historical shifts have included (1) a switch away from tallying errors in language use, from the adult view, to the search for children's language rules; (2) a shift from one linguistic domain to another as an active area of inquiry—from syntax to semantics to pragmatics to their integration; (3) a shift from a search for universal aspects of language development to a search for areas of individual and cross-cultural difference; (4) shifts in the level of detail—"macro" or "micro"—brought to the developmental account; (5) changes in research goals that encompass accounting for children's linguistic performance as well as competence; (6) increased interest in older children's language development, including their developing awareness of language and the role played by literacy; and (7) renewed interest in explaining, as well as describing, the accumulating facts of language development. These seven changes in research focus are reviewed here briefly.

Adult Rules or Child Rules?

The present-day emphasis on discovering the child's knowledge differs sharply from the descriptive work of the 1940s and 1950s[1] in which adult linguistic categories were used as a basis for quantitatively summarizing the child's status. Whether the child had yet achieved some feature of the adult's system or not was the focus of the work of that period. Were sentences complete? Grammatical? The child's departures from adult forms were treated simply as mistakes. What they might mean about his or her own rules for constructing sentences, the way he or she understood a word, or the conversational conventions that he or she thought proper to follow were issues that only later assumed importance. The impetus of Chomsky's work in linguistics,[2,3] emphasizing the rule-governed nature of language, brought the modern-day emphasis on children's rules into being. With this new emphasis came a shift from prescriptive to descriptive views of language among speech clinicians.

Syntax, Semantics, or Pragmatics?

The goal of a "psychologically real" description of the children's language system has been pursued most vigorously over the past 25 years for rules of sentence construction.[4–8] In the early 1970s, children's development of word meaning began to receive attention.[9–14] Work in the late 1970s focused on children's rules of language use and the way language emerges in social contexts.[15–19] Work in the 1970s and 1980s added efforts to integrate these areas.[20–30]

Thus successive waves of research since 1960 have focused on different aspects of linguistic development: syntax, the rules for putting words together into sentences; semantics, the mapping of meaning into words; pragmatics, the reasons and rules of language use; and their integrated interaction in acquisition. Interest has shifted from a narrow concern with syntactic knowledge to a broader framework of communicative competence (see, for example, Cromer[31]). (Another aspect of linguistic development, phonology or the rules for putting sounds into words, is treated in Chapter 10.)

These systems come together in such integrated questions as the following:

1. What are the competing and listener constraints on language change?[21]
2. How do lexical, grammatical, and conversational variables affect children's sentence structure?[22,28,30]
3. How do conversational goals affect syntactic development?[23,24]
4. How do children's early sound systems constrain the words and sentences they use?[27,29]

Language Universals Versus Individual and Cultural Differences

A 1960s emphasis on universal aspects of language development gave way in the 1970s to an increased interest in language diversity. In turn, the mechanisms responsible for that diversity have been the focus of work in the 1980s. Variation in patterns of use has been a particular focus of sociolinguistic work.[32] Anthropologic linguists have shifted from studying the similarities in acquisition across languages and cultures[8,33,34] to an increased emphasis on differing patterns of acquisition.[35] Individual differences in the interactive acquisition of content, form, and use have been the object of systematic exploration by Bloom and her colleagues. Work by Nelson[36] and Ramer[37] has linked individual and dyadic differences in early acquisition differences in learning rate. Interest in identifying invariant sequences in acquisition persists, but it is balanced now by an awareness of variability in acquisition.

Cultural and linguistic sources, too, have become recognized as sources of variability.[35,38–40] Heath studied two working-class communities, black and white, that she called Trackton and Roadville.[39] She showed how they differed in the ways of talking, the value placed on talk, the role of talk in community life, and the widely differing expectations for children's verbal skills. Current accounts, drawn almost entirely from middle-class children, are biased in ways speech-language pathologists may not recognize.

The study of cross-linguistic acquisition is flowering as well.[40] Principles of acquisition such as "pay attention to the ends of words" are being tested for their universality across languages. Beliefs about what makes a language complex to learn—for example, lack of a transparent meaning for a grammatical element—can be tested through comparison of children learning languages that vary on the dimension in question.

Macrodevelopment Versus Microdevelopment

With the increased interest in individual variation has come another research trend: that of tracing the small details in development or use of a rule (e.g., Fletcher's work).[41] Thus pathologists now have not only the large outlines of developmental change in children's language—the macrodevelopment account—but also the painstakingly revealed histories of a single rule's evolution—the microdevelopment account.

For example, Bloom and her colleagues have traced differences in two- versus three-word expressions containing locative action verbs to whether the verb is new in the child's repertoire (the utterance is shorter) or old (longer).[42] In other examples, Reich,[43] Menn,[44] and Bates[45] describe the changing contextual support required for comprehension and production in the one-word period; Greenfield describes the cues required for recognition of the Peekaboo game in the first year of life.[46]

The microdevelopmental histories in each of these periods are similar in suggesting the need for active learning to generalize the rule; but some aspects of the generalization that take time and effort at an early age appear fairly automatic at older ages. At each period, microdevelopmental studies are a rich source of information for clinical application, suggesting which dimensions of generalization—time, place, speaker, lexical items, structures—will require active programming and allow progress to be identified in more detail.

The microdevelopmental accounts have become easier to construct with the advent of new technologies. Videotaping allows for analysis of context and nonverbal elements of interaction. For example, one can learn whether or not the child looks back at his or her mother after pointing to an object. Computerized event recording and analysis allows for different conditional and unconditional probabilities of an event to be compared—for example, the probability of the child talking after the mother talks or after silence.

Computers have enabled several other important changes in research on children's language. One is the creation of a computerized archive of language transcripts called "ChiLDES" (for Child Language Data Exchange System). Started by MacWhinney and Snow,[47] ChiLDES makes the contributed transcripts of many of the original child studies available to participants who themselves plan to contribute data, thereby allowing researchers to explore questions more fully before collecting their own data.

Programs to support the computerized analysis of transcribed conversation, such as Systematic Analysis of Language Transcripts (SALT),[48] allow transcripts to be analyzed quickly for a large number of quantitative characteristics (for example, mean length of utterance, number of turns, number of different words, number of questions) that, computed by hand, might take the researcher ten to 100 times longer than the computer. Such programs also support the interactive coding of transcripts. SALT transcript formats are accepted by the ChiLDES data exchange.

A third consequence of computerization has been to permit a new generation of macrodevelopmental studies that are not only longitudinal, but large-scale as well; Wells' project is such an example of the detailed exploration of semantic relations expressed by children.[49]

Competence, Learning, or Performance? A Shift to Process

The central focus of research on children's language in the past two decades—what are the child's rules?—also reveals one of the field's fundamental theoretical assumptions. Explicitly or implicitly, most researchers have sought a description of children's linguistic competence. Each performance studied—talking, complying, answering, judging, verifying, and even repeating or recalling—has been of interest primarily for what it reflects of children's underlying linguistic knowledge.

What has been assumed is that there is a single system of rules underlying these diverse performances, together with some task-specific variables affecting performance. The existence of a single competence has been asserted, rather than proposed as a hypothesis for testing. The competence to be discovered might be more or less clearly discernable through the different task windows; but researchers have assumed it to be the same competence, however blurred the image, and its description has been the critical research goal.

This view has been a legacy of the generative grammarians' attempts to characterize linguistic knowledge as a set of rules abstracted from performance demands of either speaking or listening.[2] Its result has been to distract attention from the traditional psychological pursuits of characterizing learning and performance in given tasks. These are the very pursuits that could have allowed careful modeling of the factors affecting each kind of performance and a comparison of the learning that could be inferred from each activity, thereby permitting the assumption of a single underlying system of linguistic rules to be tested.

The tasks themselves were rarely modeled as processes, although attempts to rank them in the ease or earliness with which competence is reflected has been made. For example, the generalization that "imitation precedes comprehension precedes production" has been proposed.[50] Ingram discusses the traditional meaning of the claim that comprehension precedes production.[51] That judgment tasks generally date a linguistic achievement later than production tasks has been proposed by de Villiers and de Villiers.[52]

Only in the past decade have these views been challenged; Bloom[53] proposed that the relationship between comprehension and production might differ at different developmental periods, and empirical studies showed that apparent use of a syntactic rule or word in production did not guarantee its use in comprehension.[54,55] Golinkoff and colleagues[56] have proposed that a looking paradigm,[57] in contrast to acting out methods, may yield a different answer to this question, demonstrating understanding of word order in children at early ages of use. Alternatively, understanding of word order may develop at different times for different verbs.

Some researchers are now persuaded that the fundamental assumption of a single competence requires reexamination. For example, Premack argues that the transfer of learning from one activity (e.g., talking) to the other (e.g., listening) is the surprising fact requiring explanation.[58] Description and explanation of specific performances have received attention from those interested in characterizing variation in language production[32] and predicting listener performance.[59,60] Researchers have become more cautious, too, in the conclusions about competence that can be drawn from a given performance: the continuing debate over the rules underlying early sentences is a case in point; failure of recall data to reflect meaning as indexed by judgments of acceptability is another.[61]

Interest in modeling performance processes, rather than knowledge structures, has also arisen. Process models of children's talking and listening are being constructed; MacWhinney and Bates' competition model is an example.[62,63] In principle, these models can represent separate factors bearing on production and comprehension decisions, though none have done so systematically yet. A number of adult process models for comprehension already exist; for example, Johnson-Laird's propositional model,[64] Sanford and Garrod's discourse model,[65] H. Clark's model based on speech act inference,[66] and van Dijk and Kintsch's hybrid model for comprehension of sentences and discourse.[67]

To the extent that listening depends critically on world knowledge,[68] as well as linguistic knowledge, the adult models too may fall short of accounting for performance—this is the issue of modularity or whether or not linguistic knowledge alone is the source of adult's initial interpretations of sentences, as Fodor has proposed.[69] For young children, the importance of world knowledge in their initial understanding of sentences seems great.[70]

Process models have also been constructed for adult language production—for example, Bock's interactive model[71] or Garrett's autonomous two-stage model[72]—that differ in the degree to which syntactic, semantic, and phonologic choice might interact. These models, too, treat linguistic knowledge as isolated from general world knowledge, but, in Bock's case, as interacting with it. The creation of process models for children is an important task for researchers of children's language; it is complicated by the need to model the mechanisms and outcomes of developmental change, as well as process.[73]

The Older Child's Language Development: Metalinguistics and Literacy

Most rules of interest to researchers of children's language in the past 25 years have involved no conscious awareness on the child's part. However, the development by Flavell and his colleagues[74] of a body of work on children's conscious knowledge about learning and thinking ("metamemory," "metacognition") has prompted a similar renewal of interest in children's conscious reflections on language.[75,76] Causal roles in the acquisition process have been proposed for at least two aspects of metalinguistic development: the monitoring of whether one understands the speaker as a critical aspect of learning to request clarification,[77] and the ability to judge who uses which of two forms—and which speaker is correct—in the revision of overgeneralized child rules.[78]

Older children's language development reflects both their expanded world of school, with its new social conventions and vocabulary, and their expanded world of language in print, or literacy. Written language differs from spoken langauge in discourse, syntax, and semantic structure. The processes of reading and writing differ in their demands from listening and talking. As these differences are better understood, new questions arise about the acquisition of literacy—and its effect on spoken language.[79]

Explaining Language Development

Questions seeking to elaborate the description of children's language development can be summarized as follows:

1. What are the children's rules?
2. How do the rules change?
3. How do children differ in their patterns of language acquisition?
4. How do languages and cultures differ in acquisition patterns?
5. Should rules for talking and listening be separately presented?
6. How do children come to be aware of language and its uses?

However, answers to these questions are not enough; we need explanations of the answers. Questions pursuing explanations for these facts include:

1. Where do children's rules come from?
2. Why do children's rules change?
3. Why do children differ in patterns of language acquisition?
4. Why do languages and cultures differ in acquisition patterns?
5. What role does knowledge about language play in the acquisition process?

More formally, these questions ask what generalizations can be made about rule systems and orders of acquisition; what explanations for the observed rules, changes in rules, and rates of change can be offered; what evidence exists for individual, linguistic, or cultural differences in patterns of language learning, mechanisms of acquisition, order of acquisition, or reasons for acquisition; how these arise; what course metalinguistic development takes; and what role it plays in language development. For the speech-language pathologist, a final question must be added: what are the implications of these accounts for assessment and treatment of language disorders in children?

For example, one important problem that arises in explaining children's acquisition of syntactic rules for well-formed sentences is why they should converge upon the adult solution when, according to studies of explicit adult input,[80] no feedback concerning incorrect grammatic forms is available. This is the problem of "lack of negative evidence." Some linguists have used this point to build formal constraints on adult grammars[81]—that they must be learnable through positive instances—and constraints on children's endowment for language learning[82] or ways of analyzing input. The semantic bootstrapping hypothesis for discovery of an abstract lexicalist grammar is one such proposal.[83]

Alternatively, other researchers have reevaluated the claim that no negative evidence is available, analyzing the sensitivity of mothers' repetitions[84,85] and requests for clarifications[85] to ungrammatical sentences.

A third solution lies in denying that children are learning rules couched in abstract linguistic categories. Rumelhart and McClelland describe a model of children's changing mastery of past tense production for English verbs that incorporates parallel distributed processing, rather than implicit rule learning.[86] This view holds that knowledge is stored as connections among simple processing units organized into networks ("Connectionism"); learning consists of adjusting connections between units. The behavior of such networks is lawful, but not based on rules; rather the connections capture the structure present in the input that has been provided—including both regularities and exceptions. When input concerning root forms and past tenses of English verbs is provided in groups of decreasing frequency of occurrence, the model shows the same stages of acquisition as children, including early correct production of irregular forms, then overgeneralizations, then the sorting out of exceptional patterns. Parallel distributed processing models[87,88] have become an important alternative to rule-based systems in representing adult knowledge and are likely to be increasingly applied to problems of language acquisition in children.[89]

In the foregoing example, as in explanations offered for each of the other questions, description and explanation interact; what the child is viewed as learning determines, in part, what must be explained. Explanations raise questions of their own. For example, the foregoing explanations attributed concepts, social motives, or language input to the child; these claims in their turn require empirical study.

These questions are current topics of research on children's language. The remainder of this chapter takes up selected issues in four major sections: the first dealing with the questions arising in describing and accounting for developmental changes in language use in English-speaking children; the second with comprehension development; the third with individual differences in development; and the fourth with the application of developmental information to assessment and therapy, including the problems that arise.

LEARNING TO TALK

Overview of Major Developmental Changes

Infancy

Children begin to babble repeated consonant-vowel syllables at approximately 6 to 8 months, communicate intention with conventional gestures or vocalization at 10 months, and use a first recognizable word at about 12 months. Over the next 6 months, children typically speak one word at a time, but sharply increase their frequency of talking. By 20 months, most have acquired 50-word speaking vocabularies[10] and a variety of uses for their words;[90] at least half have spoken their first true two-word sentence,[91] and the frequency of successive single word utterances is increasing.[90]

Preschool

Average sentence length increases throughout preschool years, from just above one at 20 months to four at $3^1/_2$ years and eight by 6 years.[92–96] Individual rates vary, but children tend to acquire the same structures at roughly the same mean utterance lengths, reflecting the similar sequence in which many structures are acquired despite variations in rate.[97]

As children's utterances become longer, they become more complex in structure and in sentence content and more diverse in the communicative functions served.[98] Children learn to talk about events remote in time and space from the immediate situation,[99] to use language in imaginative play;[100] to continue the other speaker's topic;[101,102] to request and give clarification;[103] to phrase requests for action in polite ways when politeness is called for;[104–106] and to vary the formality of their speech according to their speaking role,[107,108] addressee,[109] and setting.

School-Age

By the time English-speaking children are 5 years old, their speech contains examples of most of the sentence structures of the language.[100,110] Only the elaboration of sentence structures remains during the school-age years,[111,112] since the proportion of utterances in a narrative containing dependent clauses increases from approximately 16 percent in first grade to 70 percent at the end of high school.[93] Increasingly, more information is being packed into each utterance.

Semantic and pragmatic development also continues throughout the school years.[113] Not only are new words added to children's speaking vocabularies, but meanings for old words change. Developmental shifts in the word associations offered by 5 to 7 year olds[114] suggest that the children's mental "dictionary" is being reorganized from an episodic or event basis to a semantic organization reflecting similarity of word meaning.[115,116] Word definitions offered by American children shift from functional to categorical over the elementary school years, reflecting in part the greater value placed by the culture on categorical responses ("an orange is to eat" versus "an orange is a citrus fruit"). Increasing use is made of ways to create new words as children enter their teenage years.[14]

Knowing how to use words to communicate clearly to a listener can be difficult. For example, children's success as speakers in a referential communication task is limited at kindergarten age and improves slowly.[117] This is a task in which the child must describe clearly to a listener the arrangement of a set of often similar objects or nonsense figures. The listener cannot see the speaker's display. The task's difficulty depends in part, of course, on the similarity of the figures and opportunities for listener feedback; it depends critically on the speaker's considering the problem of description from the listener's point of view.

The full range of skills in using language to converse, give, and obtain new information; argue and persuade; entertain and explain; make friends and solve problems; create and tell verbal jokes, riddles, stories, and poems—these one continues to master as an adult, encountering groups, activities, and settings with new norms for use.

The foregoing sketch of children's language across time has emphasized the increasing complexity of form and content, the increasing diversity of function, the increasing separation of language comprehension from immediate context, and the increasing sensitivity of language use to context. Much work has focused on the invariant sequence in which each of these aspects develops. In Table 11–1 are summarized some of the invariant developmental sequences tentatively identified in the domains of pragmatics, semantics, and syntax. Each is discussed in turn in the following sections.

Pragmatics: Early Communicative Intents

Children's earliest communicative attempts (approximately 8 to 12 months) are usually not words at all, but actions that bring about consistent re-

TABLE 11–1 Areas in Which Approximately Invariant Sequences of Development Have Been Identified in English-Speaking Children's Production

Pragmatics
Order of emergence of communicative intents[90,118–124]
Learning to continue topic[101,102]
Learning ways to request action[104–106,125–131]
Semantics
Semantic roles of words in one- and multiword speech[49,90,97,132–139]
Semantic aspects of early negation[7,133,140–143]
Semantic aspects of Wh- questions[82,144–148]
Semantic aspects of adjacent and conjoined sentences[149,150]
Syntax
Major syntactic characteristic of Brown's (1973) five stages[97]
Mastery of 14 grammatical morphemes in obligatory contexts[97,151–156]
Syntactic aspects of sentence negation[157–159]
Syntactic aspects of yes/no questions[157,160–163]
Syntactic aspects of Wh- questions[32,144,145,147,157]
Syntactic aspects of tag questions[80,164]
Emergence of complex sentence forms[150,165–170]

sults: for example, an abbreviated reaching gesture toward an object to signal to the mother that it is wanted;[17] handing a wind-up toy to the mother to get her to activate it;[15] showing the mother an object of interest, shaking one's head, or making a pushing-away gesture with the hand to indicate refusal;[143] or acting during a pause in a familiar game to get the mother to continue it.

Vocalizations come to accompany these actions;[143,172] they become increasingly conventional and may be interpretable as words. Thus the earliest intentional vocal communication usually accompanies gestures that request or refuse objects or activities; draw the mother's attention to objects or events; or form part of a ritual game.[15,45,90,119,120] Examples of games include waving hi or bye each time mother and child come face to face and saying "peek" as one peeks in peek-a-boo; "down" as one knocks the stacked blocks down; or "ta" as blocks are given and received. The objects and activities requested or commented on are always present at this early stage; and a given vocalization ("unh!") or word ("see") is usually associated with a single pragmatic function.[90] These uses are summarized in Table 11–2 as requesting objects or activity, refusing, commenting, and playing action games (the last category is called "performative" by Greenfield and Smith).[90]

Halliday, in studying his young son Nigel's speech, found that the first intentional vocal communication began at 9 months;[121] the 9- to 12-month period included all four categories just described. Halliday, interested in capturing the social relationship associated with the child's communication, labelled the early functions a little differently from the preceding list:

Instrumental. Language serves the "I want!" function of satisfaction of material needs, for example, a generalized request for objects.

Regulatory. Language serves the "do as I tell you" function of regulating the behavior of others, for example, getting the parent to continue the game.

Interactional. Language serves the "me and you" function used in the interaction between the self and others, for example, vocalizing in response to a gift in give and take games or vocalizing in greeting.

Personal. Language serves the "here I come!" function used for the direct expression of feelings and attitudes and for the personal element in interaction, for example, vocalizing in comment on objects.

A fifth function appears at about 13 months:

Imaginative. Language serves the "let's pretend" function used to create the child's own environment. Examples of this category appear from 13 months on and include singing, noises accompanying pretend-sleeping, and lion roars; from 16 months on, Nigel supplies the final word of a rhyme.

A common example from other children is saying "vroom" as toy cars are moved about. This category, then, appears to be an extension of the early action games previously identified in which the specific functions of objects are recognized and enacted.

Midway in the second year, new communicative functions appear: asking for information through a "What's that?" question (or "Mama?" and a point) and answering specific routine questions such as "What does the cow say?" or "What's that?" in picture book reading routines.[173] Old words now serve multiple communicative intents, for example, as requests or comments. Halliday identifies a sixth function in his son's speech at 16 months, similar to the preceding "What's that?" category:[121]

Heuristic. Language serves the "tell me why" function used to investigate reality and to learn about things; "What's that?" is an early-appearing example.

Acknowledging the other speaker's comment or answer, answering yes or no questions, requesting clarification ("Hunh?"), and repeating in response to requests for clarification[103] are other speech acts observable by 2 years of age. Thus one can view the

TABLE 11–2 A Developmental Sequence of Early Communicative Intents

Stage and Age	*Intentions*	*Form*	
Intentional communication (approximately 8 to 15 mo)	Requesting objects or activity	Early:	Gesture
	Refusing	Mid:	Vocalization plus gesture
	Commenting	or	Word plus gesture
	Action games	Late:	Word only
Discourse functions (approximately 16 to 23 mo)	Requesting information		
	Answering		
	Acknowledging		
	Repeating		
Symbolic functions (approximately 24 mo on)	Symbolic play		
	Evoking absent objects and events		
	Misrepresenting reality		

latter half of the second year as a time in which children learn to use and comply with specific conversational obligations: a time of learning not only how to do things with words, but also how to carry out and respond to specific discourse acts that demand speech in return.

At approximately 2 years of age, children begin to use language to refer to events and objects outside the immediate context,[99] talking in one- or two-word sentences about events from several hours earlier; requesting or referring to objects and activities not present in or suggested by the immediate situation; and using words in symbolic play to evoke objects or relabel the objects played with,[174] for example, calling a cantaloupe slice an airplane. Children can now create an alternative to reality with their words, playfully lying ("You did it!") or denying ("no mouse; elephant!").

All of these changes may reflect children's new capacity for mentally representing the world to themselves. They have the effect, from the adult's point of view, of making the children's speech informative for the first time: the children's topics can arise from their thinking as well as from salient aspects of the immediate situation. Halliday identifies this as the seventh and last communicative function to characterize simple one-word use:

Informative. Language serves the "I've got something to tell you" function used to communicate new information about something.

It is a long time, of course, before children's language is frequently informative from the listener's point of view, nor is it known when children come to realize that they have this obligation.

These, then, are the early-appearing communicative functions; they have been summarized in Table 11–2. At least three developmental periods have been identified. The first includes gestural precursors to vocalization accomplishing the same communicative intent; the second, discourse functions; and the third, symbolic uses of language to "create" reality.

The developmental shifts in early communicative intents are believed to reflect children's cognitive growth.[15] The functions of early utterances can often be inferred from context in cases of limited utterance length or intelligibility; thus they may prove useful indices of children's pragmatic readiness for communication in the face of limited production skill.[123] How often children attempt to talk can also be clinically significant: in a study of 48 10- to 21-month-old children,[175] child utterance rates in free play with the mother increased from an average of 48 per 20 minutes at 10 to 12 months to 144 at 19 to 21 months. These figures include vocalizations as well as words.

The Older Child: Increased Diversity of Communicative Intent

A variety of ways to classify communicative intent in older children exists; Rees[176] and I[124] provide summaries. Studies include Dore's analysis of conversational acts in preschoolers playing with peers;[177] Moerk's categories of interactions likely to contribute to language learning in adult-preschooler conversations;[178] Keenan's report of the variety of communicative functions served by repetition in the conversations of her $2^1/_2$-year-old twins;[179] and Tough's study of the use of language in peer play.[100] These studies demonstrate that a wide variety of communicative intents can be identified in the speech of children by 3 years.

For example, Keenan found that repetition (with or without prosodic variation) of the other speaker's utterance served all the following functions in her $2^1/_2$-year-old twins' conversation: to comment attitudinally; to agree with; to self-inform; to query; to answer requests for information appropriately; to imitate when asked to; to make counter claims or to make claims matching the previous speaker's; to greet back; to reverse the direction of an order or request for information; and to request clarification of an utterance.[179]

Dore, using over 30 categories of conversational acts determined by utterance form, function, semantic content, and conversational role, found examples of almost every type in the peer play of 3 year olds.[177] These included requests for information in yes or no and "Wh-" question forms, requests for clarification, requests for permission, requests for action, and rhetorical questions; responses to requests, including repetitions; descriptions of objects, events, properties, locations, or times; statements of rules, evaluations, feelings, intents, beliefs, explanations, and predictions; acknowledgments of the other speaker's utterances; use of language in role playing; and organizational devices used to regulate conversation.

Tough, studying the peer play of 3 to 7 year olds, distinguished four major functions of language:[100]

Directive. Language is used to direct one's own or another's actions.

Interpretative. Language is used to report on present and past experiences and to reason.

Projective. Language is used to predict events, to express empathy for other children's feelings, and to create imaginary activities and roles.

Relational. Language is used to maintain one's own status and to interact.

Tough defined a number of specific ways in which each of these functions could be realized. She reported developmental changes in many: for example, increases from very low levels in predicting events, expressing empathy, collaborating, logical reasoning, and interpreting the past and decreases in monitoring one's own actions aloud. These categories obviously tap aspects of the children's growing social and cognitive skills.

Discourse functions in the preschool period, then, are diverse, partly because the children's increased vocabulary and complexity of sentence form allow the listener to make finer distinctions. The change across time in specific conversational functions has been studied for only a few of the many categories proposed—most notably, topic continuation and requests for action.

Topic Continuation

One of the most striking changes in the period of children's speech from 2 to 3 years is their increasing ability to continue a topic by contributing new information.[101] At an average age of 21 months with mean utterance lengths in morphemes of 1.26, the four children studied by Bloom and her colleagues continued the topic of the immediately preceding adult utterances 50 percent of the time. By 36 months, when average utterance lengths were almost 4.0, the children's topic continuation immediately following an adult utterance had increased to 75 percent of their utterances.

The way in which a topic was continued shifted markedly as well. At 21 months, the children's topic-continuing utterances were most likely to be an imitation or partial repetition of the adult (47 percent of children's topic-related utterances immediately following the adult); new information was contributed through expansion of the adult's utterances 33 percent of the time. At 3 years, topics were continued through imitation only 5 percent of the time; new information was added 51 percent of the time.

Learning to Request Action

At least six phases can be distinguished in the development of children's requests for actions (Table 11–3). The early phases will be recognized from the preceding discussion of communication intents. Up until approximately 8 or 9 months, children's cries, vocalizations,[180] and gestures[171] may result in responsive action from parents, but there is little evidence that children cry or gesture in order to achieve the effect.[15] This nonintentional stage in the development of communicative acts has been called "perlocutionary"[15] after Austin.[181]

The second phase, from approximately 9 to 13 months,[15] is marked by the use of intentional gesture and vocalization to achieve results: the illocutionary stage. Children try to get the adult to carry out actions that they themselves cannot. Bates has called these activities "proto-imperatives" and has pointed out that they share the property of being novel means to familiar ends, a characteristic of Piaget's sensorimotor stage 5.[15] (Other investigators have restricted the category of early requests to vocal communication, differentiating it from the gestural antecedents.)

A third, locutionary, phase can be identified when the child begins to use recognizable words to make requests for specific objects and actions, sometime between 12 and 18 months.[90,121]

The fourth phase, from 2 to 4 years approximately, is marked by the acquisition of a variety of syntactic forms that can be used to make requests, including need statements, imperatives, elliptical

TABLE 11–3 A Developmental Sequence for Learning to Request Action

Age	*Phase*
0–8 mo	Perlocutionary: Discovering that vocalizations and actions have predictable effects
9–13 mo	Illocutionary: Learning to request actions and objects through conventional gesture and vocalization
14 mo–2 yr	Locutionary: Learning to request specific actions and objects through words
2–4 yr	Variation in form: Learning to make explicit requests in a variety of sentence forms
4–7 yr	Variation in explicit content: Learning to make explicit and inexplicit requests matched in politeness to the imposition of the request and the listener's status and familiarity
7–14 yr	Variation in justification: Learning to make requests persuasive from the listener's point of view

mention of the desired object or action, permission requests, and formulaic questions.[125,126] These requests all have in common the explicit mention of the desired act and object, despite the variation in form.[125] The different forms are used for different addressees—formulaic questions to adults, for example,[125] and imperatives to peers.[126]

By 4 years of age, children choose politer forms for requesting favors than for defending rights in role-playing to adult dolls; politeness of form is adjusted somewhat less when speaking to peers.[106] From 4 to 7 years of age, they also begin to use the inexplicit forms of request that only hint at the desired action or object.[125,130,131] In this phase, then, children learn how to make requests politely by varying form and explicitness according to listener status, listener familiarity, and the degree of imposition of the request.

From 7 to 14 years, children's skill in making their requests persuasive to the listener increases markedly in role-playing situations.[127–129] Justifications for requests are offered with increasing frequency. Garvey showed that even young children justify some of their requests to each other and increasingly from the listener's point of view.[126]

In brief, children have learned to make requests intentionally, then conventionally, then verbally, then in a variety of forms, then politely, and, finally, persuasively. At various points along the way, cognitive growth, intelligibility, syntactic maturity, input characteristics, and social experience and skill must have played important roles in this developmental sequence.

Problems in Description

From the foregoing accounts, one can see that many different ways of describing children's communicative intents exist. Some emphasize the function of the utterance in isolation; some its function with respect to the preceding or following utterance or to the conversational structure; some its function with respect to defining and maintaining the social relationship between speaker and listener. Indeed, most utterances function at all these levels simultaneously. In addition, utterances beyond the one-word stage often express multiple functions at any one level. (For discussions of the multiple communicative levels and functions of an utterance, see Halliday,[121] Searle,[182] and myself.[124])

The choice of one or another system of classification for an interaction is complicated by the fact that most studies have required that an utterance be assigned one mutually exclusive function, although the categories used may shift level, and by the fact that the bases for distinction may often reside in semantic content or syntactic form rather than function. For example, imitation is an instance of categorization by formal similarity rather than by communicative intent.

The choice of one or another category of communicative intent depends on the level of analysis desired and the degree to which one wants to reflect specifically semantic and syntactic aspects of language acquisition in addition to pragmatic growth. The developmental changes already identified in children's speech suggest that classifications of utterances in isolation from discourse context would be informative primarily in the second year of life. The growth of conversational skill from 2 to 4 years requires that discourse context be taken into account in analyzing communicative intent; social factors clearly play a role in linguistic choices by 4 years of age.

Description in Search of a Theory

The work on pragmatic development has been primarily descriptive. Where are the theories to make the descriptions interesting?

One form of answer could be derived from linguistic and philosophical work on speech acts that outline the situational requirements for specific speech acts to be successful or felicitous.[181–184] For example, successful assertions require at least that the speaker have evidence or reasons for the truth of what he or she says, that he or she believes it, and that it is not obvious to both the speaker and the listener that the listener already knows what the speaker is saying. In following up work on specific speech acts, then, one could study not just the frequency of occurrence, but also the preconditions that the child observed as speaker, inferred as listener, and recognized as missing or unfulfilled in unsuccessful instances. That is, one could trace the change in the conventions governing the child's speech acts. These might not be the adult conventions, of course; for example, children beginning school often treat statements of intent as promises. Garvey's[126] work on requesting action and Ervin-Tripp's[125] work on interpreting action requests illustrate approaches to discovering children's conventions governing speech acts.

Philosophers and linguists have also recognized more general conventions governing cooperative conversational interchange in American English speakers. Grice sets these out as the obligations to be informative, sincere, relevant, and clear.[185] Again, one could investigate how children come to expect that both they and the other speaker should be each of these, and whether additional or different obligations are also recognized.

Much of adult conversation, of course, fails to be informative, sincere, relevant, or clear. Lakoff[186] and Brown and Levinson[187] discuss many of these departures in terms of the requirements for being polite to one another and saving both listener's and speaker's face when face-threatening speech acts are undertaken. Making the listener feel good, not imposing, and offering options are solutions discussed by Lakoff. Brown and Levinson rank solutions as a function of the weightiness of the request to be made. Weightiness is a joint function of the culturally defined imposition of the request, the power that the listener has over the speaker, and the social distance between speaker and listener. Solutions range from omitting the speech act altogether, in the case of too weighty a request; through off-record, inexplicit attempts; impersonal politeness; friendly politeness; to clear, bald, on-record requests. Tracing the developmental function relating request form to the imposition of the request, relative status, and social distance is illustrated, for example, in James'[106] and Ervin-Tripp's[125] work on requests for action.

The Spoken Narrative

Children's spoken narratives include several types:[188–190] event descriptions, personal narratives, television and movie recounts, and stories. The roots of the narratives are revealed in children's talk when they begin to mention past events at 25 months; in their brief descriptions linking events in a sequence, or cause and effect, at 3 years; in their fragments of television, movie, and story retellings at 4 years; and in their own spontaneous stories, brewed in the cauldron of sociodramatic play, at 5 years.

These early stories preserve temporal and causal order, are about goals or problems, are generally in the past tense, and contain one or more story elements: a beginning ("Once upon a time . . ."), ritualistic end (". . . and that's all."), and some episode involving stereotypic main characters.

Children's retellings of stories they have heard are influenced not only by their ideas of story elements,[191] but also by their understanding of the story, by their knowledge of the world and its usual "scripts," by the inferences they draw, and by the importance of an element's relation to the overriding goal or problem, especially its role in a causal chain.[192,193]

In children's spontaneously created stories, beginning at about 5 years, the story's problem typically concerns villainy that must be neutralized ("Monster's coming!") or a lack that must be removed (e.g., no friends). These early plots are often stereotyped. The preoccupations change with age; monsters are a typical topic of the stories of 3 to 8 year olds, and romance and science fiction typical of the stories of 8 to 14 year olds. Resolutions reflect the changing developmental problems that children are solving: learning to take initiative in preschool years, learning to feel competent in elementary school, and finding a personal identity in junior high.

Within a plot, the degree of resolution changes developmentally. At first, the villain overwhelms the victim, who makes no attempt at response ("The monster eats them up"). Later, the protagonist attempts a response to the villain, but fails, although he or she may escape or get rescued ("And he runs away, and the monster doesn't find him"). Later still, the protagonist actively nullifies the original threat or supplies what is lacking (". . . and he put the dragon to sleep"). Among the oldest storytellers, the problem is solved not only temporarily but permanently, as original circumstances are transformed so that it cannot happen again (". . . and he killed all the dragons in the kingdom").

Spontaneous story content also increases, with age, in minor detail, for example, in the increase of reports about how people feel and in the elaboration of setting information. Changes in form include increased complexity of plot structure, of sentences, of linguistic cohesion, and of story elements.

Plot complexity[194] increases developmentally from story fragments in 2 to 4 year olds to the appearance of the story dyad—problem and its resolution—to the systematic arrangement of several elements between the problem and its resolution, at about 5 to 6 years (for example, threat, chase, attack, escape). At age 7 to 8 years, children include an increasing number of these problem-response episodes in linear sequence. Later, these are each expanded; later still, embedded plots and multiple embedded plots appear between the problem and resolution of the primary plot.

Story sentences increase in length, from six words on the average at kindergarten to 12 words on the average at twelfth grade, and in the percentage containing dependent clauses (usually linked by conjunctions), from 20 percent at kindergarten to 65 percent at twelfth grade.[93]

Discourse cohesion (the degree to which linguistic choices tie one sentence to another) increases with age as well. Pronouns referring to objects or people outside the sentence average one per sentence in kindergartener's narratives, 1.5 by sixth grade. At age 7 years, about half of these instances refer appropriately to prior mentions in the story; by 9 years, about 85 percent.

Narratives present more formulation problems

than ordinary conversation; children's pauses decrease with increasing age, but repetitions, false starts, and other dysfluencies increase, particularly for longer sentences, in the period from 5 to 11 years. Individual differences in fluency seem to persist over this period.

Semantics: Word Meaning

Early Word Uses

Children's early words—for example, "hi," "doggie," "mama," "dada," "ball"—refer to people and objects or play a role in a communication game. They are restricted to contexts in which the person, object, or game is present.[10,44,45] Nelson points out that object words in children's first 50 spoken words refer primarily to things that move or that the children can act upon.[10] This observation led Nelson to propose that early word meanings had a functional core.[195] Clark, in contrast, demonstrated from diary studies that 1 to 2 year olds overgeneralized word uses on the basis of perceptual similarity.

Are early word meanings based on functional or perceptual attributes? The resolution of this conflict, reached by Clark,[9], Nelson,[196,197] and Ingram,[198] has been to agree that a wide variety of functional and perceptual characteristics may serve as a basis for understood words, but that children's word use does not always reveal what they understand the word to mean. Nor does failure to use a word necessarily mean that they do not comprehend it. Many more words are understood by children in the second year of life than are used.[199] Further, many words overextended in use are understood appropriately.[200,201]

An important consequence of the debate over the bases of word meaning and word overextension was the recognition that production data could not be used directly to infer children's semantic system or "mental dictionary." Rather, researchers have recognized that word use must reflect jointly the reasons for which children talk, what they *can* say, and what the word means from their point of view.

Pragmatic Limits

Greenfield argues that children choose to talk about what is most salient to them in the situation: what is new, changing, or most informative.[90,202,203] The choice of this last descriptor has been disputed, if it is understood to mean that information theory can explain early word choice or that children's utterances comply with the adult conversational obligation to be informative from the listener's point of view. But researchers agree that children talk about what they notice and that novelty contributes to notice.

Phonologic Limits

Schwartz and Leonard suggest that children's early production vocabularies are further limited to those words for which they can achieve reasonable phonetic approximations.[27] This restriction, of course, may reside partly in the adult's inability to recognize the children's meaning otherwise.

Conceptual and Experiential Limits

Vocabulary restriction in production arises from restrictions in children's experience, input, and conceptual representations of the world. Some content lies outside the realm of their experience. Some is not commented on in the speech addressed to them. Some lies outside the ways in which they can make sense of the experience that they do have. In the course of vocabulary development, new words are mapped onto old, familiar concepts; meaning precedes verbal comprehension, and comprehension of words precedes use.

Semantics: Changing Semantic Roles

The Holophrase Controversy

Much of the work on children's early utterances has focused on the role played by children's words: as the theoretically assigned roles have varied, so too have the presumed rules underlying the children's utterances varied. For many years, children's one-word utterances were presumed to stand for whole sentences (the holophrase position). Bloom challenged the holophrase view, pointing out that the children she studied sometimes incorporated extra phonetic material (the "empty pivot") in their utterances, but still did not produce more than one word at a time.[133]

Bloom also showed that when children begin to speak one-word utterances in succession about the same event, the utterances appeared to stand for parts of a complete comment on the event rather than a series of separate comments. Branigan has since supported this argument by showing that successive single-word utterances, though separated by pauses, have phonetic properties suggesting that they are parts of a single intended string in the sense that early elements anticipate later ones; for example, vowel length is shorter in the early words of the successive string than in the last.[204] Thus successive one-word utterances can be viewed as two-word utterances in the making; the fact that they are most frequent in the period when true two-word utterances are emerging[90] is consistent with this view.

One to Many Communicative Intents

If one-word utterances are the blocks from which children build sentences, rather than reduced versions of whole sentences, they still share the property with sentences of having communicative intent even in the earliest stage of use and the potential for multiple communicative uses by midway through the second year of life.[90,121,205]

Shifts in Semantic Roles

Greenfield and Smith, in examining the contexts of one-word use in two children, conclude that there is a developmental sequence in which semantic roles played by words emerge in the second year of life.[90] The early period of gesture-accompanied use includes commenting as objects appear and disappear, requesting, rejecting, and games. After this period, children begin to talk about action and about people and objects, particularly when they are initiators and recipients of action. These action-related roles for words are followed by comments or requests in situations of static relationships between objects, for example, possession and location begin to be encoded. Words used to modify event properties emerge latest of all, past 2 years. Mentioning absent objects and earlier nonroutine events also does not seem to occur until after 2 years.[99]

Shifts in Semantic Roles for Negation

Pea[143] traces the meanings of negation analyzed by Bloom[7,133] in six children's early gestures and one-word utterances: the earliest meanings expressed were those of rejection (gestures expressing rejection from 10 to 14 months; words from 13 to 15 months), followed by disappearance and unfulfilled expectations at 16 to 19 months, and denial of truth-value at 19 to 23 months. Researchers have speculated that these shifts in what children talk about in the second year of life reflect cognitive growth: the sensorimotor stage 5 recognition (and rejection) of the other person as agent; the sensorimotor stage 6 appreciation of object permanence, and representational thought. Correspondence of the latter with the children's talk about disappearance of objects has been demonstrated in a training study.[206]

Not all investigators agree that classification of the semantic roles of one-word utterances can be made clearly; for example, Bloom is reluctant to make these interpretations[133] because so many versions of the child's intended meaning can often be constructed. However, the roles assigned by Greenfield and Smith are similar to relations identified between words in recent accounts of multiword speech;[90] thus their account is attractive in the establishment of a continuity in the rules underlying one- and multiword utterances. This issue of how to describe the semantic basis of children's multiword utterances is taken up next.

Early Sentences: What Are the Child's Rules for Production?

How can children's rules for constructing early multiword sentences be discovered? By analysis of the sentences that they produce, has been the nearly unanimous answer of investigators. Children's early sentences include combinations unlikely to have occurred in parental speech: for example, "more hot," "more car" (meaning "drive around some more"), "no wet" (meaning "I'm not wet"), and "have-it egg" (meaning "I want egg").[207] Novel utterances such as these are one reason that children are believed to be creating utterances on the basis of their own rules, rather than simply copying stretches of adult input. Further, many of the early two- and three-word combinations that occur seem to fall into a few productive patterns. To take the previous examples, the child might combine a great many words in second position with "more," "no," and "have-it," but otherwise use single word utterances.

Shifts in Theoretical Accounts

However, the theoretical accounts of these patterns have shifted markedly over the past three decades. Early accounts, called "pivot grammars," summarized the distribution of words in sentences.[4–6] The pivot grammars gave way to grammars incorporating adult form class categories such as noun and verb.[7] Intensive attempts to fit particular adult grammars to the data, including Chomsky's[3] transformational grammar, led to their rejection in favor of categories similar to case relations[208] that captured semantic roles.[8,97,132,133]

These accounts, in turn, gave way to more restricted and idiosyncratic semantic categories,[207] often with lexical and pragmatic restrictions.[23]

With every shift but the first, the scope attributed to the children's rule has narrowed, resulting in better prediction of what children do not say, as well as what they do say. The history of these differing accounts will be reviewed here, for the issue is a critical one for clinicians.

Pivot Grammars

The distributional analyses assigned words to the same class if they occurred in the same contexts.[4–6] Rules were then written to show how words from different classes could combine. For example, a child might produce most two-word combinations by using one of a few words that occurred with high frequency, such as "no" or "more," in fixed position—the *pivot* class of words—in combination with a large number of other words that each occurred infrequently and also occurred alone—an *open* class.

There was controversy over whether or not pivot words could occur alone (it turned out that, in younger speakers, the pivot words occurred alone before they began to be used in combination) and also about whether or not some utterances involved two words both drawn from the open class, as McNeill concluded. That is, were all the rules of the pivot plus open type or not? Some children (for example, those studied by Braine[4]) had early rules exclusively of a pivot plus open type; others had rules of the open plus open type (for example, several of the children studied by Bloom[7] and Brown[97]).

The distributional analyses had the virtue of creating classes and combinatory rules on the basis of the children's utterances rather than adult categories, a virtue lacking in some of the later approaches to children's rules. However, the analyses had the defect of ignoring the speaker's meaning and communicative intent, so that an utterance such as "mommy sock," meaning "it's mommy's sock," was treated as equivalent to "Mommy sock," meaning "Mommy is putting on my sock."[209] As it turns out, children may talk about "mommy sock" in one of these senses, but not the other, and so distributional analyses ignoring meaning can fail to capture an important generalization about the limits of the child's system. Similarly, as Ervin-Tripp's data show, intent and context may need to be taken into account to describe fully the limits of some rules for some children.

A final problem with the early distributional accounts was that the link between later grammatic acquisition and the rules for two-word utterances was hard to make. Investigators wanted descriptive categories that would reveal continuities in language development from the one- to the multiword period, and descriptions imposing adult categories or couched in terms of semantic relations between words were more attractive on this count.

Syntactic Categories for Rule Writing?

Both Bloom[7] and Brown[97] analyzed children's speech samples by assigning the children's words to adult grammatical categories. Meaning had to play a role in this assignment—for example, in determining whether "Mommy" acted as subject noun or noun modifier in "Mommy sock."

Bloom found that children producing only two-word utterances might produce subject-verb, verb-object, and subject-object combinations. That they should go on later to produce subject-verb-object combinations becomes easily understandable. Indeed, Bloom argued that the underlying representation of the just cited two-word utterances should be subject-verb-object, indicating the child's awareness of the unmentioned role.[7] The shorter spoken versions were then generated by a reduction transformation that deleted one of the three elements.

Bloom's proposal of a more complex underlying structure for two-word sentences has been controversial (see discussions in Brown,[97] Bowerman,[210] and Bloom and Lahey[211]), in part because it is not clear what evidence one should bring to bear on the question. Even in its revised semantic form,[133] the proposal leaves the origins of the children's sentences difficult to link to the one-word period, a time in which Bloom has persuasively argued that there is no implicit underlying sentence representation. And it credits children with more abstract syntactic competence than evidence from comprehension tasks[212–214] would warrant.

Semantic Categories for Rules

Upon another aspect of the debate, however, Bloom[133] and Brown[97] came to agree: namely, that the syntactic accounts that they and others attempted for the early sentences were inadequate. The argument that syntactic accounts were unjustified was made most persuasively by Bowerman,[8] as she asked what it would mean to credit children with a syntactic category such as the subject of sentence. Such a category is useful in adult grammars to describe the semantically heterogeneous collection of noun phrases preceding the verb in the following sentences:

1. John broke the window.
2. The rock broke the window.
3. The window broke.

In these examples, the agent of action, the instrument of action, and the object of action can all occupy the same grammatic position of sentence subject; but the three bear different semantic relationships to the same verb. Bowerman pointed out that the category of sentence subject was justified for children's early sentences only if some narrower, semantically based category could not capture the shared attributes of words occurring in the position. Similarly, grammatical labels such as noun and verb needed to be justified by showing (1) that classes of words with similar privileges of occurrence existed and (2) that class could not be described by narrower, semantically based categories. However, data on children showed semantic restriction in the roles played by words, and so accounts were once again revised.

The descriptive language to which researchers of children's language turned, following rejection of pivot grammars and adult grammatical categories, was that of semantic relations between words in a sentence or the semantic role played by a word in an utterance.

For example, a child might use "Mommy sock" in reference to his or her mother's sock, signaling a possessive relationship, or a child might use it in asking his or her mother to put on a sock, an agent-action relationship.[209] These instances could be differentiated only if the investigator attended to the meaning of the utterance in context. With the context available to permit semantic relational interpretations, it became apparent that the majority of children's two- and three-word combinations fell into a small set of frequently occurring categories—an estimated 70 percent of children's early multiword utterance types.[97] The categories identified by Bloom, Schlesinger, and Brown are listed, with examples, in Table 11–4 (based on Bloom).[133]

The rich interpretation of children's meanings through the use of extensive context notes or video tapes constituted a major change in methodology in the early 1970s. The later shifts in the accounts of children's utterances come in part from making more use—and more precise use—of the contextual information.

Braine's Limited-Scope Formulas for First-Word Combinations

Braine reanalyzed the 16 available samples of children's early word combinations to come to the conclusions that early patterns, although semantically based, were more restricted in scope than the early applications of semantic relational categories had revealed and more variable from child to child.[207] Examples of common productive patterns that he found are listed in Table 11–5. In form, some are restricted to one particular word in combination with a varying word; others to combinations from two varying words, but semantically restricted categories. Many patterns were idiosyncratic to a child, involving, for example, movement or oral consumption.

In these positional productive patterns, the same semantic function was expressed in the same order of constituents each time; at least some of the combinations appeared novel and unlikely to be copied directly from adult speech. Braine also identified a second kind of pattern, called a "positional associative" pattern, constant-plus-variable in form, consistent in word position, but with no evidence of productivity.[207] That is, all the instances could have been copied from adult speech.

A third pattern identified by Braine, called the "groping" pattern, referred to a small set of combinations of restricted meaning but variable word order.[207] These patterns were early, temporary, and always followed by a positional productive pattern expressing the same meaning. Probably, Braine's "groping" patterns follow even earlier successive single-word utterance attempts to express the same meanings.

Important in these reanalyses has been the growing recognition that children's early speech offers little evidence for syntactic categories. Thus there is no longer justification for syntactically based approaches to intervention programming for young children's early sentences.

Pragmatic Constraints on Production Rules?

Ervin-Tripp has proposed that analyses of children's early sentences may benefit from taking even more context into account than previous work has done: not just the nonverbal, but also the conversational context of children's utterances.[23] This analysis should include, she argues, the conversational histories attached to objects or activities, the reasons for which children talk, and the prior talk to which they respond. The result of such an analysis is illustrated for one child, Elly, from 26 to 28 months in a variety of natural conversations with siblings, parents, and play group. Table 11–6 gives Ervin-Tripp's account of Elly's production rules.

TABLE 11–4 Major Semantic Categories for Two-Word Sentences*

Bloom†	*Schlesinger*	*Brown*	
Functional relations	Operations	Operators of Reference	
Existence	Introduce + X	Nomination	
This book	See boy	a	
This cleaning	There book	see + Noun	
A raisin	That blue		
Nonexistence‡	Negation + X	Nonexistence	
No pocket	No wash	Sun gone	
No fit	No wet		
	(= I am not wet)		
	No mama		
	(= I don't want to go		
	to mama)		
Recurrence		Recurrence	
More raisin		More noise	
More read			
Grammatical relations	Relations	Prevalent two-term semantic relations**	
Two-term versions of	Agent-Action	Agent-Action	Agent-Object
Agent + Action	Bambi go	Piggy squeak	Mommy pumpkin
+ Object	Mail come	Mommy fix	(= M cutting
Mommy sock	Airplane by	Car go	pumpkin)
(= M is putting			
on K's sock)			
Possessive	Agent-Object	Action-Object	Entity-Locative
Mommy sock	Eve lunch	Hit ball	Lady home
	(= have lunch)	Put light	Adam home
	Mommy sandwich		
	(= will have sandwich)		
	Betty cinna toast		
	(= will have toast)		
Attributive	Action-Object	Action-Locative	Possessor-Possession
Party hat	See sock	Put floor	My pencil
	Want more	Paper write	Adam belt
	Pick glove		
Locative	Modifier	Attribute-Entity§	Demonstrative-Entity††
Sweater chair	Pretty boat	Big drum	This
	More nut	Pretty boat	There
	Baby car		That + Noun
			Here
	Locative		
	Sat wall		
	Baby high chair		
	Dative		
	Throw Daddy		
	(= throw it to Daddy)		

* According to Schlesinger,[132] Brown,[97] and Bloom;[133] based on Bloom (p 26).[133]
† Examples from Bloom (p 22).[133]
‡ Divided into narrower categories of disappearance, cessation, and nonexistence in Bloom.[133] Rejection and denial are other negative semantic functions.
§ More + Entity utterances are treated in Brown[97] as Attribute + Entity examples.
** For English-speaking children, Brown adds Affected Person-State-Object combinations such as "I hear horn" and datives such as "give doggie."
†† Brown lists these as one of the eight prevalent two-term relations, but discusses them as a subset of nominating expressions.[97]

A Role for Communicative Function

Notice that at this stage of Elly's development, almost every rule of word combination is associated with a single communicative act. Thus pragmatically constrained rules tell us more about what Elly would say—and would not say—than would a general rule such as AGENT plus ACT plus OBJECT.

Ervin-Tripp concludes that "starting with function categories results in a massive simplification in the data for early speech, especially in natural interaction where interpersonal acts are diverse and speech is often formulaic"(p K17).[23]

A Role for Prior Discourse

Further, many of Elly's rules are *reply* rules, requiring that prior talk be taken into account in writing the grammar. Ervin-Tripp argues that the need

TABLE 11–5 Common Productive Patterns in Children's First Word Combination*

Semantic Function of Pattern	*Typical Patterns*	*Sample Utterances*
Draw attention to something	See X	See baby See pretty See train (Andrew I) Here milk There more Here balloon (Jonathan II)
Identify something	It X That X	That Scott That hole That blow (Kendall II)
Assign class membership	X is (a) Y	Mommy lady Kurt boy Kendall monkey (Kendall II)
Request	Want X	Want car Want more Want this Want read (David I)
	Have-it X	Have-it egg Have-it milk Have-it fork (Jonathan II)
Remark on specific property	Big X Little X	Big lamb Little lamb Big rock Little rock (Jonathan I)
	Hot X	Hot fire Hot tea Hot ball (Jonathan II)
	Old X	Old cookie Old cup Old stick (Jonathan II)
Plurality or iteration	Two X	Two spoon Two stick Two daddy (Jonathan II)
Recurrence	More X	More cookie More high More hot More read (Andrew I)
Alternate exemplar of a type	Other X	Other bib Other milk Other piece (Andrew I)
Disappearance	All gone X	All gone stick All gone bee All gone stone (Jonathan II)
Negation	No X	No bed No wet No fix (Andrew I)

TABLE 11–5 Common Productive Patterns in Children's First Word Combination* (Continued)

Semantic Function of Pattern	Typical Patterns	Sample Utterances
Location	X (preposition) there	Clock on there Not in there Fall down there (Andrew I)
Possession	X + Y	Daddy coffee Daddy hat Mommy tea Mommy book Daddy book (Jonathan II)
Actor-Action	X + Y	Kendall sit Kendall read Mommy read Kendall BM Mommy walk (Kendall I)

* After Braine MDS. Children's first word combinations, Monograph of the Society for Research in Child Development, No. 164, 1976.

to consider prior discourse context in writing grammars is even greater for texts taken from adult-child discourse, where adults attempt to elicit speech from the child, or from older children who increasingly choose what to say and how to say it (e.g., whether to delete elements or use pronouns) on the basis of prior utterances.

Lexical Constraints

At this time in Elly's language development, many of her production rules are limited to particular word combinations as well as particular conversational acts: "Want this?" or "Here" for offering objects, "I want OBJECT" for requesting them. In this she is similar to the children described by Braine.[207]

A Role for the Conversational Histories of Objects and Activities

Finally, examples from other children illustrate the way that different conversational histories attached to objects lead to differing reply strategies in response to topic initiations.[23] For example, "What's that?," asked about a picture in a picture book, may lead simply to naming: "cat" or "baby cat." Asked about a piece of a puzzle, the naming may be supplemented by talk about searching, manipulation, and location: "monkey," "back," "eye."

Bruner and his colleagues have provided particularly detailed accounts of earlier language development in the context of these standard dialogues around activities such as book reading and object exchange.[171,173,215]

For example, Ninio and Bruner studied picture book reading from 8 to 18 months in the free play of a child and his mother.[173] They selected this activity, because three-quarters of the mother's labelling of objects occurred in this context. They found a predictable sequence of utterances from the mother, for example, the following interaction when the child was 13 months.[173]

Mother: *Look!*
Child: (Touches picture)
Mother: *What are those?*
Child: (Vocalizes and smiles)
Mother: *Yes, they are rabbits.*
Child: (Vocalizes, smiles, and looks up at mother)
Mother: (Laughs) *Yes, rabbit.*

At least one of the first three types of mother utterance always occurred; if more than one, the order was almost invariant: "Look" preceded "what," which preceded "label."

The child's participation in the game increased over time, from at least one active response (vocalization, gesture, smile, eye contact, search for object) half the time at 8 months to all the time at 18 months.

Vocalization, absent at 8 months, was almost always a part of the child's turn by 14 months. From 14 to 18 months, these vocalizations became increasingly recognizable (up to half the time) as labels; and to the labels the mother consistently applied corrective or confirming feedback.

In a longitudinal analysis of one mother-child pair talking about pictures in a book, Snow and

Goldfield have demonstrated that the child later came to use the specific words and constructions, about a given picture, that the mother had modeled in earlier book-reading episodes.[216]

Why do Production Rules Change? The Discursive Workshop

The conversational histories of specific objects and activities in the second year of life previously discussed may not only predict later differences in what the child talks about; these repetitive, structured dialogues may be rich sources not only for the learning of lexicon, but also for the learning of conversational sequences—both the child's initial responsive role and the mother's initiating one.[25,173,217]

One important aspect for assessing the contribution of mother-child interaction in the second year of life to language acquisition, then, may be the identification of routine, gamelike aspects of the interaction over time and the associated dialogue. Both early reply strategies and early formulas for initiating a variety of conversational acts may arise from these exchanges. Competent participation in the classroom, too, may later demand the learning and use of sequences.[25]

Communicative Need and "Bursts of Syntax"

Many speculative explanations for change in young children's production rules, including the preceding discussion, turn on interaction patterns that maximize the probability that the child will comprehend a new structure. Ervin-Tripp, in contrast, has proposed an additional role for pragmatic production factors.[23] Occasions on which the child has an especially strong desire to communicate may be the first to lead to longer utterances or new syntactic complexity ("bursts of syntax") as the child attempts to get his or her point across.

Whether or not specific communicative needs are responsible for the child's first "bursts" of more complex syntactic form, clearly communicative need plays a role in the frequency with which complex constructions are sampled. Possession may be more frequently contested with peers than with adults. Receivers of goods may need to be made explicit only when multiple listeners are present. The kind of object being talked about may need to be made clear only when several similar objects are present and a particular one desired. For these reasons, the setting of a conversation can be expected to play a role in determining the constructions sampled.

TABLE 11–6 Pragmatically Constrained Production Rules for Elly's Speech* from 26 to 28 Months

Communicative Function	*Associated Production Rule*†	*Communicative Function*	*Associated Production Rule*†
Call attention	(Hey) + NAME	Assent	{OK / Kay}
Command observe	{Look / Lookit OBJ}	Refuse	{No / unh-unh}
Command	(You) + ACT (+ OBJ)		
Offer	{You like it? / Want this? / Here}	Affirm	{yeah / REPEAT}
Prohibit or mock warning	{Stop it / Don't}	Reply to rising contour	{yeah / no}
		Exchange epithet	REPEAT
Desire	I want {OBJECT / ACT (+ OBJ)}	Announce achievement	I + ACT + OBJ
		Initiate comment	That's good
Claim	(That's) {mine / my OBJECT}	Initiate identification	That OBJECT
Contrastive offer	That's NAME'S	Locate	{There he/it is / There's {NAME / OBJECT}}
Request permission	Can I + ACT?		
Solicit information	What's that?	Complete act	There

* For rules that have at least two tokens. Samples from natural conversation in the family with siblings, parents, and playgroup, including lunch and play activities.

† Categories with varying lexical content are (proper) NAME, ACT, OBJ (object of action) and (concrete) OBJECT. Examples of ACT + (OBJ) include "put it, tear this, do cape, eat my breakfast, go-peepee, see, come-here." Parentheses indicate optional elements. Braces indicate alternatives. REPEAT means that the other speaker's utterance is repeated.

After Ervin-Tripp S. From conversation to syntax. Papers Rep Child Lang Dev 1977; 13:K1–K21.

Later Semantic Sequences

Semantic Aspects of "Wh-" Questions

Children's asking and answering of "Wh-" questions show a developmental sequence reflecting in part, it is thought, the conceptual difficulty of the content queried. Questions about the semantic roles talked about in early speech—what, what-doing, where—are asked earlier than later-emerging content—why, how, when.[32,145,147,148] Similar sequences have been demonstrated in comprehension.[218–220]

The later-emerging roles for why, how, and when, concerning event modification and links between events, may be later because that content is conceptually more difficult or because the syntactic means for representing such content is more complex.[148] Pragmatic factors can also influence children's asking and answering of questions. Children who do not understand the question word or its role in the sentence are likely to supply the information that seems to be missing on the basis of the particular verb: for example, answering "When did you eat?" with "cereal."[218] Preschoolers interpret questions as requests for information or commands for action on the basis of context and expectations.[60,125]

Semantic Aspects of Conjoined Sentences

Conjoined clauses in sentences also show a predictable sequence of emergence in children's speech. Events that go together are likely to be talked about first. Additive uses of "and" are followed sequentially by talk about temporal, causal, and adversative relations.[149,150] These relations are exemplified in the following sentences.[150] "You . . . do one and I do one" (ADDITIVE); "You push that up and it turn" (TEMPORAL); "She put a Band-Aid on her shoe and it maked it feel better" (CAUSAL); "Cause I was tired. But now I'm not tired" (ADVERSATIVE). Bloom and her colleagues argue that this sequence arises through cumulative conceptual complexity: each relation includes the preceding one.

The syntactic form in which these relations are expressed may initially be successive simple sentences. When a conjunction is used, children vary in the one selected, but stick with their initial choice for a period of time before learning alternate forms for expressing the same meaning.[150]

Developmental Sequences in Syntax: Brown's Stages

The three children studied by Brown and his colleagues varied markedly in their rates of acquisition.[97] Adam and Sarah progressed from an average utterance length in morphemes of less than two at 27 months to over four at 42 months. (A morpheme is the smallest unit of meaning; "smallest," for example, consists of two morphemes.) Eve covered the same distance between 19 and 27 months. Despite this disparity among children, speech samples of similar average utterance lengths looked similar, and the change over time in speech samples was similar. For convenience in comparing the samples, Brown arbitrarily divided the average utterance length continuum into five stages and noted the major new syntactic characteristics to be found within each (Table 11–7).

Stage I (average utterance length 1.1 to 2.0) was marked by the emergence of the early word combinations previously discussed, expressing what Brown saw as a similar handful of semantic relationships. The absence of grammatic inflection in these early utterances is striking (early descriptions captured this by referring to them as telegraphic); so too is their frequently novel or creative aspect. Stage II was marked by far more frequent additions of grammatic elements obligatory in English. By the end of stage II, the locatives "in" and "on," the reg-

TABLE 11–7 Major New Syntactic Characteristics of Brown's Linguistic Stages

Linguistic Stage	*Approximate Mean Length of Utterance in Morphemes*	*New Syntactic Development*
I	1.75	Expression of semantic relations
II	2.25	Grammatical modulation of meaning
III	2.75	Differentiation of sentence types
IV	3.50	Embedded sentences
V	4.00	Conjoined sentences

ular noun plural, and the progressive "-ing" were usually being supplied by the children in 90 percent of the contexts that made clear that they were required. Stage III was characterized by the increasing differentiation of sentence type. Imperatives, declaratives, and questions more clearly differed in form as utterances lengthened and came to include auxiliary elements. Stage IV was marked by the emergence of embedded sentence constructions more elaborate than the early semiauxiliary uses of "wanna," "gonna," and "hafta"; stage V was marked by an increase in sentences containing conjoined clauses.

Fourteen Grammatical Morphemes

The development of specific structures has also been traced across Brown's stages. For example, the 14 grammatic morphemes Brown studied[97] are mastered in approximately similar order at similar stages. "Mastery" was determined by the child's use of the morpheme in at least 90 percent of the contexts in which adult grammar would require it in three successive speech samples. The usual order of mastery begins with the four cited in stage II ("-ing," "in," "on," plural) and continues through the irregular past, possessive, articles "the" and "a," "be" as a main verb in contexts in which it cannot be contracted (i.e., the uncontractible copula), and the regular past during stages III through V; it continues with the mastery of regular third person (e.g., "he play*s*"), irregular third person (e.g., "he *has* one"), auxiliary "be" in uncontractible and contractible contexts, and the contractible copula, which falls sometime after the 4.5 upper bound of stage V. Details of this sequence have been disputed,[152,153] and Brown's three children themselves often differed by one to two stages in the time of mastery of a given morpheme.

However, a more critical problem for interpretation is the fact that none of these studies has required rigorous demonstration that the morphemes studied in fact constituted separable units of meaning from the child's point of view or that their combinatory privileges were as broad as the adult system. Productivity criteria such as those discussed by Ingram[221] and Peters[222] would be useful in deciding the first problem. Bloom et al note, for example, that additions of grammatical inflections in stage II do not seem to make the utterance more complex;[223] the distribution of old and new verbs does not alter with added inflectional elements, as it does with the addition of other morphemes. This finding suggests that the grammatical inflections of stage II may not constitute separate units of meaning from the child's point of view—or that they differ in status from words.

Detailed studies of the combinatory rules suggest semantic origins. Bloom et al, reporting on the development of the verb inflections "-ing," "-s," and irregular past find that although these three inflections emerge at the same time in stage II, they are distributed selectively with different populations of verbs.[156] This distribution appears to be facilitated by the semantics of the different verbs; and the semantic differentiation upon which distribution was based appeared to reside not in verb *tense,* but in verb *aspect.* Contrasts such as state versus change of state, with or without duration and with or without completion, are aspectual contrasts in verbs. This work suggests that the activities being talked about critically affect the probability that a missing verb inflection is supplied.

The Syntax of Sentence Negation

Children's negative sentences take a variety of early stage I forms: as unusual as emphatic stress on the affirmative verb ("*Want* it!" meaning "I don't want it," an example from Lord[158]) or "no" plus a sentence,[157] or as usual as "no" or "not" plus other sentence elements. The decisive factor in the early negative morphemes and their forms appears to be the consistency with which the parents map a particular negative meaning the child is interested in expressing (e.g., rejection) with one particular form.[159] Not the frequency of the form's use, but the consistency with which it corresponds to meaning is the key. A shouted "Stop it!" may lead to "Want it!," a "No, you musn't do that" to "No, you do it."

Negative sentences in stages II and III typically include the negative morpheme within the sentence in its usual place, and more negative morphemes are used (e.g., "can't," "don't"). Uncontracted versions of auxiliary elements can be found preceding "not" in stages IV and V; the variety of contracted auxiliary elements continues to increase.

The Syntax of Questions

Yes or no questions in stage I through III are marked only by rising intonation at utterance end. Auxiliary elements, including "can," "will," dummy "do" and present tense forms of "be," begin to be preposed in stage IV; Klima and Bellugi find that provision of "do" forms lags behind.[157]

Routine or formulaic forms of "Wh-" questions are found in stage I: "What this?" "What X doing?" "Where X go?" In stage II, there is more variation in the sentence content following the interrogative word. In stage III, omitted auxiliary elements begin to be supplied, sometimes redundantly marked for tense and person with the main verb. Klima and Bellugi describe the stage as one in which the auxiliary element and the subject noun-phrase are not inverted; dummy "do" provision and inversion are also described as appearing later than other auxiliary elements.[157]

Problems in Sequence Identification for Negatives and Questions

In the case of negatives and questions, the developmental sequence of syntactic acquisition described by Klima and Bellugi[157] is based on examples from children's speech samples that fit the transformational grammar theories of the time. Relative frequency of the crucial examples in those samples was ignored, even though the rules ascribed to the child would require that they be frequent at certain stages of development. Investigators now ask if the predicted errors occur frequently in their samples, as performance becomes a concern.

For example, Maratsos and Kuczaj[162], in studying redundantly tensed questions ("Did I missed it?" "Whose is that is?") and negatives ("I didn't missed it"), show that the only frequently occurring errors were ones with redundantly tensed main verbs ("Did I caught it?"), rather than the full range of possibilities predicted by transformational accounts.[160,224] Ingram and Tyack,[147] working on "Wh-" questions, find little evidence of a stage in which the auxiliary element is supplied but not inverted ("What he can do?"). These examples point up the need for studies validating the accounts of children's language development based on examples from the child's sample.

Complex Sentences

Limber proposed a developmental sequence in which complex sentences emerge in children's speech on the basis of a longitudinal study of three children.[167] The sequence is summarized, with examples, in Table 11–8. Complex sentences differ from children's early simple sentences not only in combining content that would be expressed earlier in separate simple sentences, but also in the complexity of sentence form used to embed or conjoin content.

Earliest to appear, usually in Brown's stage II, are constructions containing the semiauxiliary or catenative elements "gonna," "wanna," "hafta," "liketa," and "trynta." From the child's point of view, these versions of complex sentences may be simple, with the catenative elements functioning as single morphemes to modify the verb. These early-appearing examples are followed by a variety of ways to elaborate the verb phrase of the sentence ("Wh-" clause embedding) and then by ways to link two separate propositions in conjoined sentences and relative clauses. In these latter constructions, the first examples lack conjoining elements or relative pronouns; these are added later. The early instances of each new construction type appear closely associated with the acquisition of specific verbs (or, in the case of relative clauses, empty head nouns such as "the place . . ." "the one . . ."). Thus early increases in frequency of use of complex constructions are likely to be associated with growth in the verb vocabulary, permitting object complementation and full propositional constructions.

As children go through the later preschool and school-age years, an increase in the proportion of utterances containing complex sentences, particularly dependent clauses, is the single most striking change

TABLE 11–8 Order of Emergence of Complex Sentence Constructions in Children's Speech Between 2 and 4 Years of Age

Structure	*Examples (from Limber[167])*
Object complementation	I wanna go. Watch me go.
Wh- clause embedding	Do it how I do it. I show you what I got.
Full propositional embedding	I think she's sick. I guess you can.
Conjoining	You play with this one, and I play with this.
Relative clauses	That's the kind I got.
Gerundive object complements	I like eating lollipops. (not found in Limber's study)

in narrative language samples.[93] These increases may reflect not only increased facility in syntax, but an increase in the organizational complexity of the narrative as well.

Factors playing a role in the development of complex sentence use must include semantic readiness to talk about relations between propositions, the syntactic means for constructing sentences, and appreciation of the pragmatic function of structural choice in marking information as new or already known. Little is known about the last question—the pragmatics of children's complex sentence use—but Bowerman offers an excellent recent review of the syntactic and semantic factors in complex sentence production and comprehension.[168]

LEARNING TO LISTEN

The development of comprehension skills must be studied experimentally to tease apart the contribution of various contributions—verbal and nonverbal—to children's understanding.[70] Further, the attribution of understanding to children is always an inference; hence many issues arising in this area of study concern just what children can or cannot understand or how children's understanding differs from the adult's. As well, the contributions of world knowledge to comprehension in everyday life make the construction of accounts based solely on linguistic knowledge problematic at all developmental levels (this is the issue of whether or not comprehension is a modular process, in the sense that only linguistic knowledge is used in the generation of possible interpretations; world knowledge, of course, could be used to choose among interpretations).

The First Year

The affective meaning of other people, objects, and events is mediated, in part, by the infants' social world. Infants' early attention to faces leads to early discrimination of basic emotional expressions, as revealed in habituation studies. Happiness is distinguished from sadness,[225] and surprise from either,[226] by 3 months. Joy is distinguished from anger or a neutral face by 4 months;[227] fear from sadness or anger by 5 months;[228] and happiness from fear, if it is seen first, by 7 months.[229]

The use of another person's emotional expression to evaluate ambiguous situations, called "social referencing,"[230] can be demonstrated in infants as young as 10 months, as they seek out and use the look on their mothers' faces as one determinant of how to respond to strangers. At 12 months, most infants use the mother's expression—fearful or happy—as a factor in deciding whether to cross an apparent drop-off (the "visual cliff") covered by plexiglass.[231] Infants use their mothers' expressions, but not strangers', as guides from 13 to 15 months.[232] Thus the mother's expressive responses to strange people, objects, and events communicate to her infant how the world is to be regarded. It is interaction, as well as the infant's initial response, that establishes the affective meaning of his or her world.[233]

The Second Year

Comprehension of words in the context of action game routines (peekaboo, pat-a-cake) can be found in children between 6 and 9 months. The order of emergence of comprehension milestones in the second year is summarized by Miller, myself, Branston, and Reichle.[234] Children show understanding (through attentive looking at the referent) of some names for people or pets in the visual field by about 10 months and of object words (for objects in front of the child) by about 13 months. In the middle of the second year, comprehension of action words outside of game contexts can be indicated through carrying out the action. Understanding of people and object words, for referents not present, can be demonstrated through children's searching behavior. For the first time, children respond as if they understand two words in the sentence, though their interpretation reveal their own expectations about how the words are related. Comprehension of "What's that?" questions emerges in the middle of the second year as well, as indicated by answers.

These milestones do not, by themselves, describe children's understanding of events—nor the impression of mothers' that children in the second year of life understand everything said to them. The use of cues in addition to linguistic ones—or in contradiction to them—in guiding children's attention and interpretation of talk is called a comprehension strategy. Comprehension strategies play a large role in children's apparent successes as listeners in the early years of life; they continue to play a role in children's responses to more complex constructions, such as conjoined sentences and relative clauses, in school-age years. Comprehension strategies that have been identified in childrens' responses to sentences are summarized in Table 11–9, based on my reviews.[70,213]

The Third and Fourth Year

Between 2 and 3 years, children come to be able to understand three words in a sentence. The

TABLE 11–9 Comprehension Strategies

Cognitive Level (approximate age)	*Development*
Sensorimotor stage 4 (8–12 mo)	Look at objects that mother looks at Act on objects that you notice Imitate ongoing action or sound if it is already within your repertoire Laugh at familiar interaction sequences
Sensorimotor stage 5 (12–18 mo)	Attend to object mentioned Give evidence of notice Do what you usually do in the situation
Sensorimotor stage 6 (18–24 mo)	Locate the objects mentioned Give evidence of notice Do what you usually do: Objects into containers. Conventional use. Act on the objects in the way mentioned Child as Agent
Early preoperations (2–4 yr)	Do what is usually done Probable location strategy for "in, on, under, beside" Probable event strategy for simple active reversible sentences Supply missing information (2 yr) Supply explanation (3 yr) Infer most probable speech act in context
Late Preoperations (4–7 yr)	
4 yr	Comprehension of word order cues to agent-object in active sentences (word order strategy) Word order strategy overgeneralized to passive Comprehension strategy for "before" and "after": order of mention of clauses
6 yr	Probable relation of events strategy for causal conjunctions
Concrete Operations (7–11 yr)	
8 yr	Understanding of contrastive conjunctions "but" and "although" as though they mean "and"

After Chapman RS. Comprehension strategies in children. In: Kavanagh JF, Strange W, eds. Speech and language in the laboratory, school and clinic. Cambridge: MIT Press, 1978:308.

tests of whether children understand word order as a clue to ACTOR and OBJECT of action in a sentence (man bit dog, dog bit man) are contradictory; some show children passing such items at 2, some at 4 years of age. One interpretation that seems consistent with all the studies so far is that understanding of word order develops verb by verb, in association with world knowledge about the ACTORS and OBJECTS usually involved in such an event. A consistent reliance on word order as a means of understanding a sentence, in the face of contradictory expectations about the world, is very late to develop.

Fast Mapping of Lexical Items

Children learn an average of eight new vocabulary words a day in the preschool period. Most of that vocabulary is learned incidentally in natural contexts. Carey has demonstrated that children can learn much about a novel word in even a single encounter with it.[235] She presented the novel word "chromium" by telling children to bring her the "chromium one, not the red one." Later testing showed that most children had learned something about the word: that it referred to color; to recognize the color referent later; or even to produce the word. This rapid initial process of learning something about the word Carey called "fast mapping," proposing that it was a different stage of lexical acquisition than the later, more extended mapping of meaning.

Dollaghan has demonstrated that even 2 year olds fast map a novel word for an object presented in the context of two familiar, and one novel, objects;[236] most show comprehension (although the name was assigned to the object only inferentially by saying, for the set of three, "where's the Koob?") and remember the location of the novel object and produce at least an approximation of its sound.

Fast mapping studies at different ages are very informative in showing us what information from a situation and a sentence context children at a given level of language skill can use; Markman's[237] and Maratsos'[238] work is illustrative.

Lexical and syntactic comprehension milestones are summarized in Table 11–10.[213] In one way, such summaries are misleading, for they truncate protracted histories of development into a single point on a chart; whereas it may be more useful to know where a child is in the process of acquiring that form. For example, comprehension of the locative prepositions "in," "on," and "under" can be shown to begin with some general appreciation of their locative nature as revealed by changing the location of

TABLE 11–10 Lexical and Syntactic Comprehension Milestones

Cognitive Level (approximate age)	*Development*
Sensorimotor stage 5 (12–18 mo)	Understanding of one word in some sentences when referents are present
Sensorimotor stage 6 (18–24 mo)	Understanding of words when referent is not present
	Understanding of action verbs out of routine context; carries out two-word commands, but often fails to understand three lexical elements
	Understanding of routine forms of questions for agent, object, locative, and action
Early preoperations (2–4 yr)	Sequence for understanding of the meaning of Wh- questions in nonroutine forms
2½ yr	What for object
	What-do for action
	Where for location (place)
3 yr	Whose for possessor
	Who for person
	Why for cause or reason
	How many for number
3 yr	Understanding of gender contrasts in third person pronouns
3½ yr	Understanding of contrasts for topological locatives ("in, on, under, beside")
	How questions for manner or instrument
Late preoperations (4–7 yr)	
4 yr	Understanding of the number of contrasts in third-person pronouns
4½ yr	Wh- questions:
	How long for duration
	How far for distance
	Understanding of noun plural "s"
5 yr	Wh- questions:
	How often for frequency
	When for time
	Understanding of tense inflections "-ing," "-ed"
5½ yr	Understanding of possessive " 's"
	Comprehension of word order cues to agent-object in passive sentences
	Comprehension of word order cues to agent-object relations in relative clauses
6 yr	Understanding of temporal conjunction "before" and "after"
	Understanding of conditional conjunctions "if" and "when" (usual rather than logical sense)
Concrete operations (7–11 yr)	
8 yr	Understanding of causal conjunctions "because" and "so"
10 yr	Contrastive conjunctions "but" and "although"

After Chapman RS, Miller JF. Analyzing language and communication in the child. In: Schiefelbush RL, ed. Nonspeech language intervention. Baltimore: University Park Press, 1980:159.

an object, but the resulting location reflects the child's action preferences for playing with toys. Later, preferred placements reflect the child's understanding of the usual locative relation of objects, especially for the preposition "under," whose comprehension is latest. Only at about 3 to 4 years of age do children consistently solve the placement or search problems for all three locatives in all conditions, including unusual locations. Thus to know what kinds of comprehension strategies the child is currently using is more useful than to know the correct performance on a single item.

A surprising characteristic of such developmental summaries, for syntax, is that children are often not credited with mastery of a form in comprehension until 1 or 2 years later than they have been credited with it in production. More stringent criteria for assessing production performance would possibly equalize estimated times of mastery. Or possibly, in both domains, acquisition is proceeding in a more piecemeal, lexically based fashion than the syntactic rules ascribed to children have recognized.

ACCOUNTING FOR SEMANTIC DEVELOPMENT

How is word meaning represented in a child's head? Theories of word meaning representation and acquisition include Clark's Semantic Feature Hypothesis[9,239] and Rosch's Prototype Theory.[11,12] Tests of the former have guided much of the research on semantic development, particularly work on semantic comprehension. What leads to reorganization of lexical knowledge? Bowerman has distinguished both "off-line" processes—something like consolidation or maturation—that may play a role and "on-line" processes that would be evident results of children's cognitive activity.[89]

Modeling the "Mental Dictionary": Semantic Features

When a child can understand a word in the absence of context, beginning at about 16 months, it becomes appropriate to ask what form his or her "mental dictionary" takes. Clark[9,239] has proposed that the "dictionary" entry for a word can be represented as a series of binary-valued semantic features—for example *+human, +adult, +male* for *man.* These features are added to the child's system as his or her understanding of the word develops. Clark initially proposed that more general features within a semantic domain, and features indicating the usual, normal value, or positive pole of a dimension, were likely to be added first to the child's system.[9] Thus the meaning of a word would change over time and would initially be broader than the adult's meaning. In particular, Clark's 1973 view predicted that words might for a time be overextended to mean their opposites as a consequence of positive pole overextension: for example, "after" understood as though it meant "before," or "less" understood as "more."

Clark's semantic feature hypothesis was an important focus for semantic research in the 1970s. It has become clear that overextension to opposite meanings seldom takes place. "Less," for example, does not mean "more,"[240–243] nor does "after" ever mean "before."[244–249] Rather, response strategies based on context or children's expectations about the world determine the systematic preferences sometimes shown in the studies—and probably children's interpretations in natural contexts as well.

Children do often link a word with the wrong dimension of meaning, rather than the opposite end of the correct continuum; this characteristic is similar to the quality of preoperational children's thinking that Piaget called "centration." The distracting dimension is typically more perceptually salient for the child in context, for example, thinking that older people are taller.[250] Clark[251,252] and myself[70] offer discussions of the role of comprehension strategies in language development. Clark, in particular, revises her account of the semantic feature hypothesis to predict dimensional mismatches rather than overextensions of positively valued features.

Prototypes

Finally, it has been recognized that word meaning in both adults and children is better represented if there can be a certain ambiguity or "fuzziness" about whether an object or event belongs to the set indicated by the word. One way to capture degrees of belongingness or typicality has been proposed by Rosch and her colleagues[11,12]; in prototype theory. Rosch argues that there are natural categories that people universally derive from experience, independently of the way words carve up the world (basic object categories), and that these and other categories possess prototypes that best exemplify the set members. "Robins," for example, are usually picked as the best examples of the category "BIRD." Membership in a set, according to prototype theory, is decided by the degree of resemblance to the prototype. Prototypes share the most features in common with other category members.

Work with 9-month-old infants has shown that they develop such conceptual categories prior to word learning and for good prototypic exemplars rather than poor ones.[253]

Developmental Changes in Dictionary Organization

Researchers have speculated that not only does the entry for a single word change over time, but also that the organization of entries changes as well. To speak of a "mental dictionary" may be an appropriate metaphor for the organization of the adult's system. It may be misleading in the case of young children. For them, words are embedded in events, and the organization of the early semantic system is thought to be episodic.[116] Bowerman details changes in children's word use over the 2- to 4-year span[13] which suggest that a reorganization of the system is gradually taking place. So too do the shifts in word associations between 5 and 7.[116] The problem of finding a way to represent mental organization of knowledge—both lexical and world knowledge—and of showing why and how knowledge changes is a current focus of work among cognitive scientists.[87,88] It is likely to be an important focus for work on children's language as well.

ACCOUNTING FOR SYNTACTIC DEVELOPMENT

Explanations of children's syntactic development depend on just what the researcher believes children have acquired, at later ages. A variety of competing accounts of older children's grammatical knowledge exist—including Schlesinger's claim that even older children's sentential rules are based on broad semantic categories, Maratsos and Chalkey's account of children's induction of syntactic categories from distributional evidence, Pinker's belief that a lexicalist grammar such as Bresnan's accounts for older children's competence, and Bates and MacWhinney's functionalist grammar. Those who ascribe highly abstract grammatical knowledge to children, knowledge for which there is no direct access or feedback, must also attribute to children innate constraints on the ways languages are learned. Thus formal issues in the learnability of grammar are of deep concern to this camp. Others, in contrast, have explored cognitive processes, language input, and interaction for sources of the mechanisms that lead to syntactic acquisition.

Among other factors that might determine rate and specific sequences in syntactic acquisition, two are frequently cited in current literature: (1) the pacing effect of cognitive development and (2) the simplified language addressed to children. These, of course, are not necessarily competing explanations; both cognitive level and input adjustments may play important roles in determining acquisition rates. So too may social experience and skill, speech motor control development, and the functioning of the auditory system. However, no study has simultaneously evaluated the contribution of each to acquisition. Here the evidence is briefly reviewed for the role of cognition and input.

The Role of Cognition

The cognition hypothesis argues that a particular conceptual achievement or level of problem solving skill is necessary to a related linguistic achievement.[254] Cognitive development is seen as the major pacer of the development of communication skills. Experience, linguistic input, perceptual salience, already acquired forms, reinforcing consequences—all play their roles only within the limits set by the child's cognitive status.

Strong Form of Cognition Hypothesis

In its strong form, the cognition hypothesis asserts that a given cognitive achievement is sufficient for the associated level of language development to emerge, except in cases of extreme linguistic deprivation or significant sensory or motor deficits.

Karmiloff-Smith's work offers a different perspective on this issue.[255,256] She argues that children learn procedures for encoding and decoding language just as they learn other problem-solving procedures; the procedures are simply additional instances of cognitive activity. In common with other cognitive activities, she goes on to argue, they profit from an inherent tendency to organization: once a procedure functions adequately and automatically, the child moves up to a metaprocedural level and considers the procedure as a unit in its own right. Thus the status and function of early-appearing forms such as determiners, pronouns, and gender markers alter predictably and spontaneously in the years after their emergence, most notably in the development of procedures that seek coherence or agreement among the differing procedures in an utterance. It is the insistence on spontaneous change in the child's system that makes Karmiloff-Smith's account a strong version of the hypothesis that cognitive development paces linguistic development: linguistic development is cognitive development, and cognitive growth occurs spontaneously as the result of cognitive activity. Given sufficient practice in encoding or decoding, interprocedural organization occurs. This view implies that a simple increase in the opportunities to interact in conversation should have therapeutic value.

Weak Form of Cognition Hypothesis

An alternative form of the cognition hypothesis, the weak form, proposes that cognitive attainments are necessary but insufficient to account for all linguistic attainment. Cromer has expressed this view:[257]

> Although the study of cognitive structures and operations and the cognitions to which they give rise are of central importance in understanding the language acquisition process, these cognitive entities by themselves are not sufficient to explain that process. Our abilities "make available," so to speak, certain meanings to be encoded, but we must also possess certain specifically linguistic capabilities in order to express these meanings in language (p 325).

Slobin argues the same point in discussing the correspondence between the 2 year old's concept of agent, actions, and location in specific situations and the similarly named linguistic relations between words.[137] Languages differ not only in the order in which words express these roles, but also in the way that the possible range of meaning is clustered in words. For example, notions of causality and change of location can be encoded together in a verb in one language—or separately in another. A child's understanding of an event cannot tell him or her how his or her meaning should be mapped into words, let alone ordered; this constitutes the specific linguistic learning that each child must carry out.

Bowerman has listed some cognitive factors believed to be necessary for language acquisition:[258]

1. The ability to use symbols to represent objects and events that may not be perceptually present.
2. The development of basic cognitive structures and operations: the ability to order spatially and temporally; the ability to classify in action; the ability to embed action patterns into each other; the establishment of concepts of basic invariance involving object permanence and conservation; the ability to apprehend relationships between objects and actions; the construction of a model of perceptual space with certain properties.
3. The ability to derive strategies for processing linguistic material from general cognitive structures and processes that are isomorphic to aspects of language structure and/or the ability to form the developmental sequences in which language-relevant cognitive knowledge is acquired on the linguistic level.
4. The ability to formulate appropriate concepts or categories to serve as the structural components upon which linguistic rules can operate.

Correlational Hypothesis

A third view of the relationship between cognitive and language measures, which also holds that they are strongly associated, might be termed the "correlational hypothesis"; common maturational or cognitive factors underlie developmental sequences in both domains, but language measures are just as likely as cognitive ones to reflect change first. Brown[97] and Bates[45] have made this more conservative proposal of relationship between the domains: Brown under the guise of attributing rate of language acquisition to a factor of general intelligence and Bates in a discussion of "local homologies" or shared features in cognitive and linguistic tasks. The correlational hypothesis is consistent with some—but not frequent—variation between language and cognitive levels in *either* direction.

Evidence for the Correlational View. Insofar as cognitive and syntactic correspondence has been studied, the evidence supports this third point of view.[259] The developmental correspondences are close, but it is not always the cognitive task that is passed first. In the second year of life, for example, the onset of communicative gestures and vocalizations appears related to successful performance on cognitive tasks assessing Piagetian sensorimotor stage 5 levels of tool use and causal reasoning. Bates, in a longitudinal study of cognition and communication in 25 9- to 13-month-old infants, found that object permanence and spatial relations items from the Uzgiris and Hunt scales[260] were poor predictors of the development of communicative gestures and language.[45] Imitation, means-ends, and play scales, particularly the last, were the best predictors of language production items. Harding and Golinkoff have reported significant correlations between causality items and the onset of intentional vocalizations in 36 children.[261] Sugarman too has reported correlations between tool use (means-ends) and requesting vocalizations in stage 5 children.[262] Nicholich, studying five children longitudinally between 13 and 22 months, reported that symbolic play and vocal imitation were both correlated with language production measures.[263]

Moore et al found a significant correlation between an experimental object permanence test and mean length of utterance in five children with Down's syndrome, even with age and IQ factored out.[264] Corrigan, in a longitudinal study of three children, reported only a rough correspondence between the onset of sensorimotor stage 6 of object permanence and the onset of single word utterances.[265] She also reported vocabulary increases and the emergence of new semantic categories of nonexistence and recurrence at an early preoperational level of object permanence. Ingram, working with data from these two production periods in Piaget's children and other diary studies, suggested a correspondence between sensorimotor stage 5 and the onset of first words.[266,267] Ingram placed sensorimotor stage 6 in correspondence to the period of rapid vocabulary acquisition, in contrast to Corrigan's findings. Miller et al found a close correspondence of all the sensorimotor measures with the development of word and sentence comprehension in 48 10- to 21-month-old infants.[234]

The relation between sensorimotor stage and production of two-word combinations has been directly evaluated by Ingram[221,267] for observations of overall sensorimotor stage; Corrigan[265] for object permanence; and Folger and Leonard[268] for means-ends and schemes. These investigators report correspondence between linguistic and cognitive stages, but little evidence that the cognitive stage is a prerequisite.

Problems in Assessing Cognition

The conceptualization and assessment of cognitive functioning have proved major problems in the course of the work on children's cognitive and linguistic development at all developmental levels. Uzgiris,[269] Corrigan,[270] and Bloom et al[271] offer useful discussions of alternative approaches at the sensorimotor (zero to 2 years) level.

Briefly, the problem resides in the fact that researchers are trying to assign cognitive stages to children. However, close examination of the theory suggests that levels or stages of development are properly assigned to mental schemas (and later mental operations), as inferred from specific task contexts, rather than to children. Variation in the context of assessment may lead to different levels of performance (a phenomenon Piaget called "horizontal decalage"). Further, the entire population of schemas (and later mental operations) that could be inferred in a given child shows a distribution of developmental levels. Thus to classify a child as sensorimotor stage 6 entails a decision about classifying the whole distribution of schemas, as inferred by measurement in particular task contexts. A variety of decision rules could be defended, with consequent variation in the child's ultimate classification.

To abandon some indication of cognitive level or stage is to abandon an important summary statement about children's thinking and problem solving, but to characterize any distribution with a single number is to omit important information about the distribution's shape. Nor is the choice of the single number clear; is it to be the highest level of performance observed? Or a reflection of average performance? If so, should a mean, median, or mode be reported? It is important, then, to be clear about how a cognitive classification for a child was derived and to provide detailed data on cognitive task performance for those who might wish to derive cognitive categories differently.

Mothers' Speech to Children Learning Language

The role of input in children's language acquisition has been investigated in stages; the first problem was simply that of characterizing mothers' (and other's) speech to children learning language.

A significant body of research demonstrates that mothers alter their speech from adult conversational patterns when talking to children learning language (see, for example, Snow and Ferguson,[217] Waterson and Snow,[272] and myself[273]). These changes are phonologic, syntactic, semantic, and pragmatic. They include exaggerated intonation contours and stress; higher fundamental frequency;[274] pauses distributed always and only at utterance boundaries;[275] shorter, syntactically simpler, more fluent, and better-formed utterances;[276] a less diverse and more concrete vocabulary;[277] higher rates of self-repetition and paraphrasing;[275] higher rates of expansion of the young child's utterances;[278] the same prevalent semantic relations found in children's speech;[138] and higher rates of questioning and lower rates of commenting than in adult-adult speech.[279] Topics are almost always about the immediate here-and-now situation and most frequently concern the child's activities.[280] In short, there is evidence for a distinctive, simplified baby talk register.

What Determines Alterations in Mothers' Speech?

Brown suggests that two motives interact to bring about the changes reported: the mother's desire to make herself understood and her desire to express affection.[281] However, only a few studies investigated the relations between the mother's input and the child's linguistic level either in comprehension or in production. Cross reports a close correspondence of indices of mother's input with comprehension measures and production measures.[280]

Rondal, in contrast, reviews literature documenting the correspondences of parental language with the child's produced language.[282,283] Rondal investigated the language-learning environments of normal children and children with Down's syndrome matched for mean length of utterance at three levels (early stage I, late stage I to stage II, and stage III).[282] Maternal speech to normal children and children with Down's syndrome did not differ except in type to token ratio for words, but many characteristics of maternal speech did vary systematically with the mean utterance length of the child. These included increases in type to token ratio for words, mean length of utterance and distribution of utterance lengths, sentence complexity, mean preverb length, number of modifiers per utterance; changes in the distribution of some semantic roles (process verbs and action or process locatives increased); decreasing nomination; decreasing requests for action; decreasing self-repetitions; expansions of child utterances, corrections, or prodding.

Retherford et al, in studying the relation between semantic roles used by mothers and children over time found that mothers' use was consistent and stable over the period; it was the children's role use that became more like the mothers' over time.[138] The basis for determining semantic roles in the mothers' speech would appear to be either the children's comprehension skills or the salient aspects of the immediate situation.

Taken together, these studies provide a picture of the ways that mothers not only use a distinctive baby talk style, but also fine tune their speech to children, though apparently some aspects are tuned to children's comprehension skills and others to their production skills. These findings make clear that measures of the effectiveness of mother input cannot be measures of the mother's language characteristics alone; rather such measures have to be based on mother language characteristics *relative* to child language characteristics.

What Aspects of Input Affect Learning?

The questions reviewed so far have been (1) Does the mother alter her speech to young children? and (2) Does she alter it as a function of the child's linguistic skills? However, the most important question in considering input is the one least often addressed in the current literature: (3) Is there evidence that these alterations make a difference in children's rate of language acquisition?

There are few longitudinal studies directly examining the relation between the rate of acquisition and the interactive measures of input effectiveness. Cross addressed the question by comparing mothers of linguistically more and less accelerated children.[284] The mothers of the accelerated children were more likely to expand and extend the semantic intentions in the children's utterances.

Golinkoff, analyzing the communicative interaction of mothers and "preverbal" infants (11 to 18 months) in their highchairs at lunchtime, found many episodes in which the interaction did not proceed smoothly. Infants initial communicative attempts (which infrequently contained words) were unsuccessful for as much as half the time. Mothers and infants negotiated such failures through extended bouts (7.3 turns on the average) of mother requests for repetition or confirmation, infant rejection of the mother's interpretation, or infant repair of communication. These negotiated episodes ended in success more than half the time, increasing from 55 to 72 percent across the 6-month span.

Other investigators report that parental expansions are much more frequent in speech to young children (1 to 2 years with average utterance lengths of less than 1.5).[97,278] A similar and parallel decline occurs in the proportion of parental utterances that children imitate.

The similarity of these findings may be more than coincidental. Folger and Chapman found that spontaneous imitations in children were much more likely to occur immediately following a parental expansion of the child's utterance.[279] One can hypothesize, then, that Cross's accelerated children continued to receive and imitate the parental expansions for a longer time period.

Is there any reason to think that the increased frequency of spontaneous imitations, as well as expansions, might help children learn to talk? This issue has been a continuing controversy in the field. There is no evidence that children's imitated utterances are syntactically more advanced than spontaneous ones,[285] and many children imitate very little at ages 2 and 3 years.[286] However, Bloom and her colleagues report that those children who do imitate do so selectively, imitating vocabulary or semantic relational combinations that are just emerging in their speech. If one places this finding in the perspective of the foregoing review, it becomes evident that the selective sensitivity to emerging forms may be the parent's as well as the child's.

DeVilliers has shown that individual children's range of grammatical use of particular verbs was strongly predicted by their own mother's variety of use, but not by her frequency of use.[287] She interpreted this to mean that children were monitoring the grammatical patterns of use of individual verbs in the input they received. Streim and myself, in a case study of fast mapping of novel verbs, found that the mother's patterns of grammatical use predicted the child's pattern of use for those four verbs in the first 14 days of her son's acquisition of them.[288] In a longitudinal analysis of one mother-child pair talking about pictures in a book, Snow and Goldfield have demonstrated that the child later came to use the specific words and constructions, about a given picture, that the mother had modeled in earlier book-reading episodes.[216]

These findings are consistent with the view of linguists such as Bresnan and Pinker who propose lexical grammars in which many of the syntactic rules, earlier thought to be neutral with respect to word choice, are instead stored in the lexicon adjacent to verb entries—that is, the view that syntax is learned verb by verb. If so, the variety of verb types modeled by mothers, and the variety of syntactic forms modeled for each verb, should predict rates of syntactic acquisition.

Mothers have been shown to repeat and request clarification of their 2-year-olds' ungrammatical utterances more often than the grammatical ones. If children are sensitive to this difference or to the feedback they receive, then interaction may provide them with more information about grammaticality than has previously been believed—including negative evidence about ungrammatical utterances. This empirical issue is a critical one for learnability theorists interested in describing formally the constraints on languages or learners.

Barnes and colleagues studied the characteristics of mother's speech at Brown's stage I as a predictor of residual gain scores 9 months later.[289] Variation in length and complexity of input was not associated with differential progress, but variation in proportion of yes or no questions with subject-auxiliary inversion was correlated with children's gains in semantic range and syntactic complexity. Frequency of directives and of utterances extending the children's subject—measures unrelated to each other—both correlated with length of utterance gains, as did the mothers' total talk.

Mothers who frequently expand their children's one- and two-word speech through the addition of new vocabulary or a familiar word in a new semantic role may have seized the perfect opportunity for teaching language. In repeating such an expanded model, the children's communicative intent and message content are preserved and expanded; the context makes it possible for children to see the meaning of the new word or role. Thus an interactive index of mothers' expansions that incorporate new roles or words is an important predictor to evaluate in a longitudinal framework.

INDIVIDUAL DIFFERENCES IN ACQUISITION

Individual differences also characterize acquisition patterns.[36,290] Among the individual differences identified or proposed in acquisition are those of Table 11–11. They include differing rates of acquisition, most often as measured by rates of change in average utterance length; differences in the interpretability of early patterns; differences in early syntactic patterns; differences in early vocabulary content and form; and differences in use to which language is put.

TABLE 11–11 Individual Differences in First Language Acquisition Identified or Proposed

- Rate of acquisition[37,97]
- Interpretability
  - Word vs. intonation babies[90,119,121]
  - Intelligibility[5]
- Syntactic differences
  - Length of initial speech units one- or multi-word (analytic vs. synthetic)[5,10,222,291]
  - Early sentences nominal vs. pronominal[223]
  - Regular vs. irregular past tense mastering first[97,156,292]
  - Differing syntactic connectives to express similar meanings in complex sentences[150]
  - Differing preferred clausal order for expressions of causation[169]
  - Greater noun phrase elaboration in precocious talkers[293]
  - Few vs. frequent presyntactic forms[37]
  - Word order errors vs. not[37]
  - Invented grammatical patterns vs. not[5]
  - All major grammatical relations expressed at syntax onset vs. predicate only[7,37]
- Semantic differences
  - Idiosyncratic position patterns or operators[5,136]
  - Referential vs. expressive early vocabulary[10]
- Pragmatic differences
  - Readiness to speak[5,119]
  - Elaborated vs. restricted codes[294]
  - Use of language for imaginative play vs. not[100]

Two Kinds of Language Learners?

Investigators have been eager to group individual difference characteristics into types. Researchers have speculated that all the first characteristics of each pair listed in Table 11–11, aside from the pragmatic ones, are associated together in a fast, noun-based, referential pattern of acquisition frequently found in girls and that the second-named characteristics are clustered together in a slower, expressive, phonologically less intelligible pattern of acquisition in boys.[37,293] As Ingram shows, these speculations appear premature;[221] added data quickly provide evidence of combinations other than the two types proposed. However, one can expect that the issue of correlation of individual differences one with another will continue to attract interest for some time. The notion that only a few underlying differences exist in learning style is theoretically appealing and conceptually simplifying; it will die hard.

What is an Individual Difference?

A problem in investigating individual differences in patterns of acquisition cross-sectionally is to rule out the possibility that one is looking at developmental differences rather than individual differences of pattern. For example, productive vocabularies include increasing proportions of verbs as children enter their third year; variation in noun to verb ratios among a group of 2 year olds, then, may reflect the differing *rate* of vocabulary development rather than noun versus verb preferences.

Short-Term or Long-Term Individual Differences?

Longitudinal studies allow one to differentiate developmental and individual differences. They often further show that individual differences apparent in one stage of development disappear or are reversed in a later stage. For example, the distinction between referential and expressive children, which is based on the question of whether the majority of the first 50 spoken words can be categorized as general nominals or not,[10] appears to correlate with few characteristics of later language development. It constitutes a dimension of individual variation, but apparently not one linked to later stages. As another example, Bloom et al showed that the early preference for pronominal or nominal syntactic constructions evidenced in their children disappeared as the children learned to produce both kinds of structures;[223] here, then, was another local divergence in paths taken to the same common end.

Because every measurable aspect of acquisition can be expected to show some variation across individuals, it is pertinent to ask whether every one of the measurable aspects of language development will one day be added to the list of individual differences in Table 11–11. In one sense, the answer is "yes." To the extent that variation can be attributed to individuals rather than to developmental change or measurement error, that dimension belongs among the list of individually varying characteristics requiring explanation.

However, inferences that there are "two kinds of people" on each of the dimensions to be listed are not warranted. For the most part, the differences listed in Table 11–11 have been studied in too few children to know much about their distribution. Do children vary along a continuum with a distribution similar to the normal curve? Or is the distribution bimodal? Where sufficient numbers of children have been examined (e.g., expressive versus referential), the answer often appears to be a normal curve. In discussing individual differences, one uses the convenient labels of the opposing ends of the continuum; but a theoretical leap to "two kinds of people" would require justification from distributional evidence of two distinct populations.

Explaining Individual Differences

The Role of Cognitive Styles or Traits

One might hypothesize that there is a persistent underlying trait of the individual that determines the path to be taken at many of these local intersections; the choice of trait would predict the way in which patterns of acquisition are correlated. Among the candidate differences in traits that have been proposed are those in cognitive style: for example, impulsivity versus reflectivity; field dependence or independence; and Gestalt or synthetic versus analytic processing. As well, social dimensions may be implicated in some of the pragmatically based differences: willingness or desire to interact; desire to please; or the skill of the child in prolonging social interaction (e.g., the value of the infant as a reinforcer). Explanations of individual differences in language acquisition on the basis of individual differences in traits of cognitive style or personality only shift the problem of explanation to a new domain, one where the consistency across tasks and persistence across time of the "trait" may be hotly contested. If supported by data, however, such condensations of the explanatory problem render the pursuit of individual differences a theoretically interesting enterprise.

Explaining Local Individual Differences by Local Mechanisms

However, most of the individual differences listed in Table 11–11 have the property of being local, in the sense that they constitute divergent paths only for a brief period in the history of the child's language development. A less ambitious attempt at explanation of individual differences, then, may pose the problem of accounting for particular local divergences one at a time. Explanations based on input, in particular, may benefit from this approach.

PROBLEMS IN CLINICAL APPLICATION

The need for assessment tools and rationally based intervention programs has led to the rapid assimilation of work on normal language development by speech-language pathologists. Problems could be expected in the process of translating evolving theory and incomplete research results into clinical practice. Those that have arisen include problems in interpretations of the existing data, overemphasis on single aspects of the language code, and failure to tie expectations to individual children's status.

Problems in Interpreting Existing Data

To construct a description of children's language development from existing data is not an easy task. Theoretical reinterpretations of the syntactic rules underlying children's early utterances continue to be made. Alternative theoretical views of semantic development are available. A theoretical view of pragmatic development has yet to be constructed. Empirically, a common reference line for ordering achievements—age, cognitive level, or linguistic stage—is needed. So, too, is information needed on the normal variability in acquisition. One must often be more precise about what is meant by "acquired" than easy textbook reading would dictate: First uses—how many? Mastery—how measured? Expectations based on speech samples must take the original sources into account because conversational purpose, speakers, and topics affect sample characteristics. The reliability of many measures needs to be established. The inherent variability in sequences of development and among individuals must be acknowledged and turned to useful account.

Shifting Bases for Early Syntax

With each reinterpretation of the underlying basis for children's early sentences has come a necessary reinterpretation of the range of sentences appropriate to model or expect in intervention. To work on teaching any NOUN plus VERB combination is one task; to work on ACTOR plus ACTION another; to work on announcing I plus ACTION following event completions still another. Thus clinicians have one of the strongest stakes in knowing the outcome of the debate on children's early sentence rules. If recent history is a guide, one cannot be complacent about the answer. Rather, it will be important to attend to what *is* learned by a child from the opportunities created and to expect microdevelopmental changes in the acquisition of sentence structure as well as macrodevelopmental change.

The Need to Know Ages or Stages of Achievement

Ages or Brown's linguistic stages have been tentatively linked with many language milestones. For example, mastery of the use of the grammatic morphemes "-ing," plural "-s," and prepositions "in" and "on" in contexts that make the form obligatory is usually associated with Brown's stage II—that is, mean utterance lengths in morphemes of 2.0 to 2.5. Production and comprehension of "why" questions is expected at $2^1/_2$ to 3 years. On the basis of the Denver Developmental Screening Test norms, one expects 50 percent of children at 20 months to be putting two words together. Knowledge of the age and stage correspondences with language milestones is critical to the identification of language delayed children and the investigation of specific linguistic deficit, but, in these examples, data bases varied radically.

Some of the established expectations are based on few observations. There is a need for sufficient data to warrant age- and stage-based expectations from representative samples of the population of interest. Although the intensive longitudinal nature of many studies permitted inferences about a sequence of acquisition in an individual, the small sample size of most of these same studies restricts the generalizability of age- and stage-related findings—and of the conclusion that the sequences identified are universal. The need for normative data is apparent to clinicians, but theoretical debate over validity of existing measurement categories has taken precedence over issues of reliability and representativeness.

The Need to Know Normal Range of Variability

Normative data are needed not just to establish the expected age or stage of an achievement, but even more critically to establish the expected range of variability in that performance as well. The significance of a child's failure to pass a language milestone at the expected age is uninterpretable without information on the usual spread of performance. How many children of the same age might be expected to fail the same item? Half? Ninety percent? If performance can be matched to other ages, what does it mean? "A year's delay" may signal marked delay in development (e.g., in failure to comprehend at least one word) or fall well within the normal range (e.g., in school-age vocabulary comprehension scores). Thus the attempts of some states to define language disorder legally in terms of number of years of delay are misconceived. A definition would be better framed in terms of percentile rank or standard deviations below the mean for the age. Without information on variability, the question of what failure signifies clinically cannot be evaluated. And as the preceding example suggests, that information must be obtained at each age to be evaluated: variability frequently increases with age, for example, in mean length of utterance measures in the preschool period.[94]

The Need to Relativize Milestone Definitions

In an informal assessment of children's language, one is tempted to search for the language milestones to be expected for the child's age without sufficient regard for how those milestones were defined in the original developmental literature. The 14 grammatic morphemes, for example, were ranked by Brown in order of mastery: presence in at least 90 percent of the verbal and nonverbal contexts in which they should have occurred for three successive free speech samples. For assessment of grammatic morphemes, the presence in a sample of a sufficient number of clear obligatory contexts is the key.

Most other work on syntactic development—for example, the development of negation, questions, complex sentences, and the auxiliary system—concerns the *first* emergence of forms in children's speech. Investigators differ in what is to count as evidence of a form's emergence: One instance? At least five different instances? Or a varying number of instances depending on the sample length? The differing problems with these decisions are discussed by Bowerman,[295] Maratsos,[296] and Bloom et al.[223] What the clinician must note for making use of the data is the number of different instances to be expected in some standard length or duration of a transcript: for example, frequency per 100 utterances or per 15-minute conversation.

The Need to Know Sample Sources

In drawing inferences about which grammatical morphemes one expects to see mastered and which forms one expects to see emerging in a speech sample, clinicians must be sure that their samples are similar to the ones of the original study in purpose, topics, and participants. Free speech samples during play, for example, yield different mean lengths of utterance and structures than description, instructional interactions, or narratives; for mothers speaking to children, speech in the latter cases is more complex. Free speech samples with an adult differ from those with a peer in structure and purpose; for example, auxiliary modal verbs are far more prevalent in samples from sociodramatic or imaginative play with peers than in conversation with adults.[297] Polite forms, in contrast, are far more frequent in speech to adults than to peers.[106,287] Samples with the mother at home may yield substantially higher values than samples with a clinician at the clinic.[298]

The complexity and amount of the child's speech varies with topic, particularly when the topic is dictated by the clinician.[299] In part, the variation occurs as a function of the child's familiarity with the implicit script associated with the topic—going to a restaurant, for example.[300] Thus the degree to which other conversational participants insist on topics unfamiliar to the child systematically affects the speech sample; this is more likely to happen with unfamiliar speakers from different cultural backgrounds.

The Need to Know Reliability of Measures

Although linguistic measures are often interpreted as reflecting children's linguistic competence, they are in fact properties of the speech sample and should be expected to vary systematically with the parameters of the interaction. Such variation is not itself evidence that the measures are unreliable. However, evidence is needed to show that currently used clinical indices of syntactic level are reliable across time when speech sample parameters are held constant.

The Need to Know Extent of Sequence Invariancy

The sequences that have been identified are not always as invariant as the textbook accounts suggest. This fact has led to unnecessary rigidity of sequencing an intervention planning. For example, the 14 grammatical morphemes studied by Brown[97] and deVilliers and deVilliers[152] do show high rank order correlations of mastery across children, but inversions of nearby ranks are common. For sequencing purposes, however, the morphemes might better be grouped into the three sets mastered early in Brown's stages (mean length of utterances of 1.1 to 2.5), late in his stages (mean length of utterances of 3.0 to 4.5), and post-stage V (mean length of utterances beyond 4.5). Similarly, "Wh-" question words can be grouped into sets emerging by 2 years, 3 years, and 4 years. Selections among these groups can then be made on the basis of which meanings the child is already marking in other ways and which meanings he or she needs to communicate in everyday settings.

Those sequences that were originally established on the basis of noting occasional error—for example, the syntactic development of yes or no questions, "Wh-" questions, and negation—should be particularly regarded as tentative until further evidence is available.

The Need to Take Individual Differences into Account

The possibility that children may differ in the ways that they learn language most easily needs further study. Deciding what to assess and what to teach is of obvious importance. The individual differences in acquisition patterns previously reviewed suggest that there are frequent local divergences in the forms children first acquire to map meaning when the forms are of equivalent linguistic complexity. The consistency with which the target meaning is encoded by a particular form in input may be the deciding factor in these local divergences.

More fundamental divergence in learning style may arise when the child follows a synthetic pattern of first learning stock phrases and only later learning to analyze these and make substitutions within patterns. Such differences in style have been especially noted in second language learners.[301] Autistic children functioning at sensorimotor stages 5 and 6 may show to an extreme degree such a pattern of associating whole sentences with the same simple meanings (e.g., prohibition) that children usually map with single words.[302]

For the clinician, the possibility of variation in synthetic versus analytic learning style[222] requires that one be able to assess the generality of *productivity*[221] of the rules attributed to the child and to provide input appropriate to the further generalization of those rules. If there exist children who learn by synthetic rather than analytic methods, for example, morpheme discovery may present a more difficult problem than syntactic acquisition for these particular learners. Alternatively, the problem of discovering morphemes that are presented by a formulaic input may account for the adoption of a synthetic learning strategy.

Overemphasis on One Aspect of Linguistic Knowledge at the Expense of Another

Just as researchers have focused on the structure of children's linguistic knowledge, so too have clinical applications focused on assessing and developing one or another aspect of the code, rather than on its expression in talking and listening in a variety of social contexts on a variety of topics. Syntax, semantics, phonology, or pragmatics: often only a single dimension of the code has received attention in any one assessment instrument or program. Further, these single dimensions have frequently been viewed only from the perspective of talking, rather than listening, and this bias has led to misplaced expectations for children's comprehension skills. Macrodevelopmental sequences identified have often been pursued at the expense of developing microdevelopmental sequences for a given step. Further, vertical progress along a particular macrodevelopmental sequence has been pursued at the expense of working across the developing communicative system on achievements likely to be concurrent. Finally, the developmentally based program has sometimes been viewed as an alternative to a program teaching functional communication skills, rather than as a means for specifying which functional skills are nearest the child's grasp and how to achieve them.

Unidimensional Applications

Early application of developmental data to intervention, like the early data itself, often focused on the language code rather than its use in communicative contexts, and on syntax development in particular. (Similarly, older articulation programs often failed to take syntactic or pragmatic characteristics of speech into account.) More recent programming has been more likely to incorporate multiple aspects of code development and use.

Assessment procedures now available for comprehension focus almost exclusively on either semantic or syntactic aspects of utterances in isolation. One's ability to teach or evaluate their interaction, or the understanding of language in conversational contexts, is in its infancy, yet these are the aspects of comprehension critical for children.

With respect to spontaneous production, only the Developmental Sentence Score procedure[303] offers a normative score, reflecting predominantly the development of the auxiliary system and grammatic speech. Other procedures are available to describe syntax (see Klee and Paul[304] for a comparison), but few exist to evaluate the semantic and pragmatic aspects of spontaneous conversation.

Overemphasis on Production

Most programs, even those focusing on multiple aspects of the language code, select target goals for production rather than comprehension. Emphasis is often placed on the child's skills as speaker, to the neglect of listening skills. Yet the classroom teacher is often more concerned about the child's comprehension than production skills; ability to follow oral instructions and to understand what is read depend on these. To take another example, no reasonable decision about whether an augmentative system is required can be made without considering production skills in relation to comprehension skills.[213]

Misplaced Expectations for Comprehension

When comprehension skills are selected as targets, it is important to base selection on direct evidence of ability to understand the given word or structure at the same developmental level in normal children. To base age and sequence expectations for comprehension, out of context, on production data may lead to expectations of mastery 2 to 6 years earlier than it actually occurs for syntactic cues to meaning.

The relationship between comprehension and production may be different for semantic cues. Information on conceptual development should suggest what word meanings children are likely to understand at each developmental level, as well as the probable limitations in how they understand them. Similarly, conceptual development can predict the interpretations that the children are likely to make of sentences in context, regardless of syntactic cues.

However, words are likely to be overextended in use at a time when children understand the same words appropriately, for example, calling all men "Daddy," but consistently picking out one's own father from other men as "Daddy." Overextended uses of the early lexicon, then, appear to reflect children's stretching of limited lexical resources for communicative purposes, rather than the actual meaning of the word.

Working on Development: One New Thing at a Time

Work on the detailed steps in a rule's acquisition and generalization (or the generalization of its expression) has been recent relative to work on macrodevelopment of children's language. Thus clinical application of the former work is just beginning. At the microdevelopmental level, behavioral principles for active teaching of generalization[305] are useful in conjunction with empirical work on children and language development.

The latter work tells us that children learn *one new thing at a time;* if the word being learned is new, then its content is already familiar to the child: it is put to familiar uses in familiar sentence structures, and it is the only word used to express that content initially. If the sentence structure is new, it expresses old meaning with old words for familiar purposes.

For intervention purposes, then, one models for the child words and structures to talk about the content he or she already wants to talk about; that is, one comments on the child's activities and topics. In this context, comprehension is likely to precede use. Out of context, comprehension of words may continue to precede their use. But one should not expect children to understand structural cues in the sentence as the only guide to meaning until much later than early use.[53,58]

Both the problem of overemphasis on production and that of misplaced comprehension expectations arise, of course, from the view that production data have given clinicians fairly direct access to a description of children's underlying communicative competence. That view, I have argued earlier, is incorrect—either in the claim that appropriate use in production is sufficient evidence of competence or else in the assumption that a competence is abstracted from what one learns to do in speaking and listening. The implication for language programming is that one works on new vocabulary, new syntactic form, new function, or revised phonology only one aspect at a time and that in every case the conceptual and experiential basis for content must already be established. That is, one uses old language to teach new concepts, and old concepts to teach new language.

Working for Concurrent Achievements Rather than Sequences

Focusing on sequential aspects of language development—changing communicative functions, lengthening sentences, stages in negation and questions, order of mastery of grammatical morphemes, emergence of "Wh-" question words and conjunctions, complex sentence development—can distract one from the many aspects of communicative skill being acquired concurrently, leading to programming of sequence from a narrow base. Given the child who has just learned to produce instances of a two-term combination—for example, ACTION plus LOCATIVE—one should be moving on to the many other two-term patterns, rather than to a three-term expansion of ACTION plus LOCATIVE, if developmental logic is to be followed.

Tying Clinical Expectations to the Individual's Status

Children referred for language disorders have often been compared to children of matched chronological age to demonstrate that a problem exists. Communicative skills, however, depend in part on children's cognitive level and information-processing skills, social development, hearing status and speech motor control skill, linguistic and social experience, development of shared knowledge about the world, and the communicative needs presented by their everyday environment. Differences in communicative skill can arise as a consequence of a difference in any of these factors, as well as through specific problems in language learning that are not yet well understood. These factors should be taken into account in interpreting the significance of a child's pattern of language use and understanding and in developing appropriate goals for therapy.

Cognitive Skills

For example, children identified as mentally retarded are significantly delayed in language development as well as other intellectual and social skills. However, determination of whether or not the child has further and specific problems in language comprehension and use can be done only if the child's performance is compared to that of other children of similar cognitive levels, rather than of similar chronological age. These comparisons depend, of course, on evidence that the sequence of cognitive development, if not rate, is similar in retarded and normal children.

Social Skills

Children's social skills reflect, in part, their general cognitive level. However, a wide variation in social skills of children at similar developmental levels can also be found, for example, in making friends or obtaining compliance.[126] Social status dimensions of relationships—relative power, relative solidarity—must be attended to because they affect culturally appropriate linguistic choices;[187] making these choices, in turn, constitute part of what is meant by social skill. When failures in pragmatic use and comprehension occur, one must ask if they are traceable to failure to learn the appropriate linguistic choices, failure to recognize the social contingency, or a differing set of pragmatic conventions.

Experience

Clinical expectations must be adjusted to the child's world. The dialect that the child is learning, his or her culture's norms of appropriate social interaction, the knowledge of the world that he or she shares with peers and adults—when these are mismatched to the expectations of clinician or teacher, the communication problems that arise can mistakenly be viewed as the child's problem, rather than as a mismatch of the expectations of the two participants.

Because adult linguistic input is continuously adjusted to the child's level of linguistic skill on many parameters, it is necessary to control the child's linguistic levels before asking if obtained input differences might have contributed to language delay; usually, equation of groups on mean length of utterance makes input appear equivalent as well.[282]

Audition and Speech Motor Control

Historically, speech-language pathologists have been sensitive to hearing and speech motor control status. Language problems may be associated with problems in the functioning of these mechanisms. It is important to differentiate when the apparent problem in language is associated with audition or speech motor control factors, rather than the previously cited ones: different remedies are dictated in the different cases.

Communicative Needs in Everyday Environments

The emphasis on generative rules of sentence construction in research work belies the frequently routine and stereotypic aspects of communicative skill. Analysis of children's communicative needs in everyday settings and the needs they encounter in the next setting to which they move can redress the balance. For example, retarded adults may need to appear communicatively more competent in the community than children of similar developmental levels and linguistic skill ordinarily appear. Simply learning to acknowledge the other speaker's topic may be a solution that takes limited cognitive and linguistic skill into account.

Analysis of everyday needs also allows one to identify the event sequences in which clients must communicate, for example, taking a bus, shopping for food or clothes, going to a restaurant, working, going to a movie, or playing soccer. Learning to anticipate the usual events in these sequences and the usual messages can facilitate communication skills for everyday settings.

Apply Developmental Principles to Meet Functional Communication Needs

The advice, as opposed to the warnings in the foregoing discussion, amounts to just this: that an individual's communication needs can often best be met by applying what is known of normal development. One wants to (1) develop clinical expectations for the client that are developmentally appropriate to his or her current status; (2) maximize his or her current communicative effectiveness; and (3) optimize his or her future communicative skill.

The use of developmental information in achieving these three goals is direct only in the case of the child delayed equally in all aspects of linguistic and cognitive development. When cognitive status is markedly higher than comprehension and production levels, one should expect that the content of the child's utterances differs from the usual pattern in reflecting his or her more advanced thought. For example, single-word utterances may be related to one another in the more complex way typical of older children's sentences—not as different aspects of the same event, but as a causal chain of events. "Paint all done. Home. TV." is an example from a 4-year-old hearing impaired child just beginning to put words together.

When comprehension and cognitive skills are similar and greater than limited production skills, one might expect differences in that child's spoken language as compared to that of a normal child at the same production level or to that of a child with deficits in comprehension as well.

Because multiple facets of language skill develop, because multiple factors play causal roles in that development, and because different groups of factors affect different strands of linguistic development, the application of a developmental logic is by no means straightforward. But knowledge of how children normally learn language—and the limitations and lacunae of that account—these are powerful tools in the hands of the thoughtful clinician attempting to identify and resolve communication problems.

Background Reading

Useful child language texts include Brown's[97] volume on first language acquisition, which lays out many of the issues in the field and the data on Adam, Eve, and Sarah; introductory texts by Dale,[306] deVilliers and deVilliers,[307] Gleason,[308] Reich,[309] and Lindfors;[310] a text on language development and language disorders by Bloom and Lahey;[211] a text on the psychology of language by Clark and Clark;[311] a discussion of selected issues in psycholinguistics by Slobin;[312] and edited volumes for the more advanced student by Wanner and Gleitman[313] and Fletcher and Garman.[314]

SUMMARY

Children acquire spoken language skills in predictable developmental sequences within the domains of sentence structure, meaning, and language use. Developmental sequences can also be identified in the acquisition of comprehension skills. Language acquisition stretches from the first year of life throughout the school years. There is general agreement about descriptions of these developmental sequences, especially in preschool children, but a variety of accounts explain them.

Explanations of developmental sequences have centered on the rules or learning attributed to children and the ease with which the rules can be learned from input. These accounts have typically focused on one domain of learning—syntax, or word meaning, for example. More complex rules, or more opaque learning situations and language input, are thought to contribute to later learning. Social and cognitive development are viewed as pacing language development in the domains of semantics and pragmatics. Identification of the rules themselves continues to be controversial.

Individual differences in language acquisition have been identified in rate of acquisition, intelligibility of speech, preferred sentence forms, referentiality of early vocabulary, and readiness to speak. Why children differ in these ways is debated; the contributions of cognitive development, social experience, language input, and intrinisic personality factors have all been cited.

The implications of work in normal language development for assessment and treatment of language disordered children are important. Normal developmental sequences provide an index for sequencing intervention goals. What children normally learn suggests what speech-language pathologists should try to teach. The roles of experience and interaction in accelerating language acquisition suggest the ways in which intervention can be effectively carried out.

Acknowledgment. The revision of this chapter was supported by NIH Core Support Grant No. 5 P30 HD03352 to the Waisman Center on Mental Retardation and Human Development. Comments by Nancy Streim on an earlier version of the chapter are gratefully acknowledged.

REFERENCES

1. McCarthy D. Language development in children. In: Carmichael L, ed. Manual of child psychology. New York: John Wiley & Sons, 1954:492.
2. Chomsky N. Syntactic structures. The Hague: Mouton, 1957.
3. Chomsky N. Aspects of the theory of syntax. Cambridge: MIT Press, 1965.
4. Braine MDS. The ontogeny of English phrase structure: the first phase. Lang 1963; 39:1–13.
5. Miller W, Ervin S. The development of grammar in child language. In: Bellugi U, Brown R, eds. The acquisition of language. Monogr Soc Res Child Dev 1964; 92:9–34.
6. Brown R, Fraser C, Bellugi U. Explorations in grammar evaluation. In: Bellugi U, Brown R, eds. The acquisition of language. Monogr Soc Res Child Dev 1964; 92:79–91.
7. Bloom L. Language development: form and function of emerging grammars. Cambridge: MIT Press, 1970.
8. Bowerman M. Early syntactic development: a cross-linguistic study with special reference to Finnish. Cambridge: Cambridge University Press, 1973.
9. Clark E. What's in a word? On the child's acquisition of semantics in his first language. In: Moore TE, ed. Cognitive development and the acquisition of language. New York: Academic Press, 1973:65.
10. Nelson K. Structure and strategy in learning to talk. Monogr Soc Res Child Dev 1973; 149.
11. Rosch E. On the internal structure of perceptual and semantic categories. In: Moore TE, ed. Cognitive development and the acquisition of language. New York: Academic Press, 1973:111.
12. Rosch E, Mervis CB, Gray W, Johnson D, Boyes-Braehm P. Basic objects in natural categories. Cognit Psychol 1976; 8:382–439.
13. Bowerman M. Systematizing semantic knowledge: changes over time in the child's organization of word meaning. Child Dev 1978; 49:977–987.
14. Clark E. Convention and innovation in acquiring the lexicon. Papers Reports Child Lang Dev 1980; 19:1–20.
15. Bates E. Language and context: the acquisition of pragmatics. New York: Academic Press, 1976.
16. Bates E, Benigni L, Bretherton I, Camaioni L, Volterra V. The emergence of symbols: cognition and communication in infancy. New York: Academic Press, 1979.
17. Lock A. Action, gesture, and symbol: the emergence of language. New York: Academic Press, 1978.
18. Ervin-Tripp S, Mitchell-Kernan C, eds. Child discourse. New York: Academic Press, 1977.
19. Ochs E, Schieffelin B, eds. Developmental pragmatics. New York: Academic Press, 1979.
20. Sinclair-DeZwart H. On pre-speech. Papers Rep Child Lang Dev 1974; 8:1–11.
21. Slobin DI. The more it changes. . . . on understanding language by watching it move through time. Papers Rep Child Lang Dev 1975; 10:1–30.
22. Bloom L. An integrative perspective on language development. Papers Rep Child Lang Dev 1976; 12:1–22.
23. Ervin-Tripp S. From conversation to syntax. Paper Rep Child Lang Dev 1977; 13:K1–K21.
24. Bates E. Functionalism and the biology of language. Papers Rep Child Lang Dev 1978; 15:K1–K26.
25. Cazden CB. Peekaboo as an instructional model: discourse development at home and at school. Papers Rep Child Lang Dev 1979; 17:1–29.
26. Clark EV. The principle of contrast; a constraint on language acquisition. In: MacWhinney B, ed. Mechanisms of language acquisition. Hillsdale, NJ: Erlbaum, 1987:1–34.
27. Schwartz R, Leonard L. Do children pick and choose? An examination of phonological selection and avoidance in early lexical acquisition. J Child Lang 1982; 9:319–336.
28. deVilliers JG. Learning how to use verbs: lexical coding and the influence of the input. J Child Lang 1985; 12:587–595.
29. Donahue M. Phonological constraints on the emergence of two-word utterances. J Child Lang 1986; 13:209–218.
30. Brown BL, Leonard LB. Lexical influences on children's early positional patterns. J Child Lang 1986; 13:219–229.
31. Cromer RF. Reconceptualizing language acquisition and cognitive development. In: Schiefelbusch R, Bricker D, eds. Early language: acquisition and intervention. Baltimore: University Park Press, 1981:51.
32. Labov W, Labov T. Learning the syntax of questions. In: Campbell RN, Smith PT, eds. Recent advances in the psychology of language. Vol. 4b. New York: Plenum Press, 1978:1–44.
33. Blount B. The pre-linguistic system of Luo children. Anthropol Ling 1970; 12:326–342.
34. Mitchell-Kernan C. Monograph No. 2, Language-Behavior Research Laboratory. Language behavior in an urban black community. Berkeley: University of California, 1971.
35. Schieffelin B. Getting it together: an ethnographic approach to the study of the development of communicative competence. In: Ochs E, Schieffelin B, eds. Developmental pragmatics. New York: Academic Press, 1979:73.
36. Nelson K. Individual differences in early semantic and syntactic development. Ann NY Acad Sci 1975; 263:132–139.
37. Ramer ALH. Syntactic styles in emerging language. J Child Lang 1976; 3:49–62.

38. Kuczaj SA, ed. Language development. Vol. II, Language, thought, and culture. Hillsdale, NJ: Erlbaum, 1982.
39. Heath SB. Ways with words. Cambridge: Cambridge University Press, 1983.
40. Slobin DI, ed. The cross-linguistic study of language acquisition. Vol. 2: Theoretical issues. Hillsdale, NJ: Erlbaum, 1986.
41. Fletcher P. The development of the verb phrase. In: Fletcher P, Garman M, eds. Language acquisition. Cambridge: Cambridge University Press, 1979:261.
42. Bloom L, Miller P, Hood L. Variation and reduction as aspects of competence in language development. In: Pick A, ed. Minnesota symposia on child psychology. Vol. 9. Minneapolis: University of Minnesota Press, 1975:169.
43. Reich P. The early acquisition of word meaning. J Child Lang 1976; 3:117–123.
44. Menn L. Pattern, control, and contrast in beginning speech: a case study in the development of word form and word function. Bloomington, IN: University Linguistics Club, 1978.
45. Bates E, Benigni L, Bretherton I, Camaioni L, Volterra V. The emergence of symbols: cognition and communication in infancy. New York: Academic Press, 1979.
46. Greenfield P. Playing peek-a-boo with a four-month-old: a study of the role of speech and non-speech sounds in the formation of a visual schema. J Psychol 1972; 82:278–298.
47. MacWhinney B, Snow C. The child language data exchange system. J Child Lang 1985; 12:271–296.
48. Miller JF, Chapman RS. Manual for SALT: a computer program for the systematic analysis of language transcripts. Madison, WI: Language Analysis Laboratory, 1985.
49. Wells G. Language development in the preschool years. Cambridge: Cambridge University Press, 1985.
50. Fraser C, Bellugi U, Brown R. Control of grammar in imitation, production, and comprehension. J Verbal Learn Verbal Behav 1963; 2:121–135.
51. Ingram D. The relationship between comprehension and production. In: Schiefelbusch RL, Lloyd LL, eds. Language perspectives—acquisition, retardation, and intervention. Baltimore: University Park Press, 1974:313.
52. deVilliers J, deVilliers P. Competence and performance in child language: are children really competent to judge? J Child Lang 1974; 1:11–12.
53. Bloom L. Talking, understanding and thinking: developmental relationship between receptive and expressive language. In: Schiefelbusch RL, Lloyd L, eds. Language perspectives—acquisition, retardation, and intervention. Baltimore: University Park Press, 1974:285.
54. Chapman RS, Miller JF. Word order in early two- and three-word utterances: does production precede comprehension? J Speech Hear Res 1975; 18:355–371.
55. Rice M. Cognition to language. Baltimore: University Park Press, 1980.
56. Golinkoff RM, Hirsh-Pasek K, Cauley KM, Gordon L. The eyes have it: lexical and syntactic comprehension in a new paradigm. J Child Lang 1987; 14:23–45.
57. Thomas DC, Campos JJ, Shucard W, Ramsay DS, Shucard J. Semantic comprehension in infancy: a signal detection analysis. Child Dev 1981; 52:798–803.
58. Chapman RS. Discussion summary: the developmental relationship between receptive and expressive language. In: Schiefelbusch RL, Lloyd L, eds. Language perspectives—acquisition, retardation and intervention. Baltimore: University Park Press, 1974:335.
59. Shatz M. The relationship between cognitive processes and the development of communication skills. In: Keasey B, ed. Nebraska symposium on motivation. Lincoln: University of Nebraska Press, 1977.
60. Shatz M. On the development of communicative understandings. An early strategy of interpreting and responding to messages. Cognit Psychol 1978; 10:271–301.
61. Johnson H, Chapman RS. Children's judgment and recall of causal connectives: a developmental study of because, so, and and. J Psycholing Res 1980; 9:243–260.
62. MacWhinney B. The competition model. In: MacWhinney B, ed. Mechanisms of language acquisition. Hillsdale, NJ: Erlbaum, 1987:249.
63. Bates E, MacWhinney B. Competition, variation, and language learning. In: MacWhinney B, ed. Mechanisms of language acquisition. Hillsdale, NJ: Erlbaum, 1987:157.
64. Johnson-Laird PN. Mental models. Cambridge: Harvard University Press, 1983.
65. Sanford AJ, Garrod SC. Understanding written language. New York: John Wiley & Sons, 1981.
66. Clark H. Inferring what is meant. In: Levelt WJM, Flores D'Arcais GB, eds. Studies in the perception of language. New York: John Wiley & Sons, 1978:295.
67. vanDijk T, Kintsch W. Strategies of discourse comprehension. New York: Academic Press, 1983.
68. Winograd T. What does it mean to understand language? In: Norman DA, ed. Perspectives on cognitive science. Hillsdale, NJ: Erlbaum, 1982.
69. Fodor J. The modularity of mind. Cambridge: MIT Press, 1983.
70. Chapman RS. Comprehension strategies in children. In: Kavanagh JF, Strange W, eds. Speech and language in the laboratory school and clinic. Cambridge: MIT Press, 1978:308.
71. Bock JK. Toward a cognitive psychology of syntax. Psychol Rev 1982; 89:1–47.
72. Garrett M. A perspective on research in language production. In: Mehler J, Walker E, Garrett M, eds. Perspectives on mental retardation. Hillsdale, NJ: Erlbaum, 1982.
73. MacWhinney B, ed. Mechanisms of language acquisition. Hillsdale, NJ: Erlbaum, 1987.
74. Flavell J. Cognitive development. Englewood Cliffs, NJ: Prentice-Hall, 1977.
75. Sinclair A, Jarvella RJ, Levelt WJM, eds. The child's conception of language. New York: Springer-Verlag, 1978.
76. Karmiloff-Smith A. From metaprocesses to conscious access: evidence from children's metalinguistic and repair data. Cognition 1986; 23:95–147.
77. Markman E. Comprehension monitoring. In: Dickson WP, ed. Children's oral communication skills. New York: Academic Press, 1981:61.
78. Slobin DI. A case study of early language awareness. In: Sinclair A, Jarvella RK, Levelt WJM. The child's conception of language. New York: Springer-Verlag, 1978:45.
79. Olson DR, Torrance N, Hildyard A, eds. Literacy, language and learning: the nature and consequences of reading and writing. Cambridge: Cambridge University Press, 1985.
80. Brown R, Hanlon C. Derivational complexity and order of acquisition in child speech. In: Hayes J, ed. Cognition and the development of language. New York: John Wiley & Sons, 1970:11.
81. Wexler K, Culicover P. Formal principles of language acquisition. Cambridge: MIT Press, 1980.
82. Pinker S. Language learnability and language development. Cambridge: Harvard University Press, 1984.
83. Pinker S. The bootstrapping problem in language acquisition. In: MacWhinney B, ed. Mechanisms of language acquisition. Hillsdale, NJ: Erlbaum, 1987:399.
84. Hirsch-Pasek K, Trieman R, Schneiderman M. Brown and Hanlon revisited: mother's sensitivity to ungrammatical forms. J Child Lang 1984; 11:81–88.
85. Demetras MJ, Post KN, Snow CE. Feedback to first language learners: the role of repetitions and clarification questions. J. Child Lang 1986; 13:275–92.
86. Rumelhart DE, McClelland JL. Learning the past tenses of English verbs: implicit rules or parallel distributed processing? In: MacWhinney B, ed. Mechanisms of language acquisition. Hillsdale, NJ: Erlbaum, 1987:195.

87. Rumelhart DE, McClelland JL. Parallel distributed processing: explorations in the microstructure of cognition. I. Cambridge: Bradford Books, 1986.
88. McClelland JL, Rumelhart DE. Parallel distributed processing explorations in the microstructure of cognition. II. Cambridge: Bradford Books, 1986.
89. Bowerman M. Commentary. In: MacWhinney B, ed. Mechanisms of language acquisition. Hillsdale, NJ: Erlbaum, 1987:444.
90. Greenfield PM, Smith JH. The structure of communication in early language development. New York: Academic Press, 1976.
91. Frankenburg WK, Dodds JB. The Denver developmental screening test. J Pediatr 1967; 71:181–191.
92. Hedrick D, Prather E, Tobin A. Sequenced inventory of communication development. Seattle: University of Washington Press, 1975.
93. Loban W. Language development: kindergarten through grade twelve, report no. 18. Urbana, IL: National Council of Teachers of English, 1976.
94. Miller JF, Chapman RS. The relation between age and mean length of utterance in morphemes. J Speech Hear Res 1981; 24:154–161.
95. Klee T, Fitzgerald MD. The relation between grammatical development and mean length of utterance in morphemes. J Child Lang 1985; 12:251–269.
96. Conant S. The relationship between age and MLU in young children: a second look at Klee and Fitzgerald's data. J Child Lang 1987; 14:169–173.
97. Brown R. A first language: the early stages. Cambridge: Harvard University Press, 1973.
98. Bloom L, Lahey M. Language development and language disorders. New York: John Wiley & Sons, 1978.
99. Sachs J. Topic selection in parent-child discourse. Discourse Processes 1979; 2:145–153.
100. Tough J. The development of meaning. New York: Halsted Press, 1977.
101. Bloom L, Rocissano L, Hood L. Adult-child discourse: developmental interaction between linguistic processing and linguistic knowledge. Cognit Psychol 1976; 8:521–552.
102. Wanska SK, Bedrosian JL. Topic and communicative intent in mother-child discourse. J Child Lang 1986; 13:523–535.
103. Gallagher T. Revision behaviors in the speech of normal children developing language. J Speech Hear Res 1979; 20:303–318.
104. Ervin-Tripp S. The comprehension and production of requests by children. Papers Rep Child Lang Dev 1974; 7:188–197.
105. Ervin-Tripp S, Gordon D. The development of requests. In: Schiefelbusch RL, ed. Language competence, assessment and intervention. London: Taylor & Francis, 1986.
106. James S. Effect of listener age and situation on the politeness of children's directives. J Psycholing Res 1978; 7:307–317.
107. Sachs J, Devin J. Young children's use of age appropriate speech styles in social interaction and role-playing. J Child Lang 1978; 5:17–24.
108. Andersen E. Young children's knowledge of role-related speech differences: a mommy is not a daddy is not a baby. Papers Rep Child Lang Dev 1977; 13:83–90.
109. Shatz M, Gelman R. The development of communication skills: modifications in the speech of young children as a function of listener. Monogr Soc Res Child Dev 1973; 152.
110. Menyuk P. Syntactic structures in the language of children. Child Dev 1963; 34:407–422.
111. Hass W, Wepman J. Dimensions of individual difference in the spoken syntax of school children. J Speech Hear Disord 1974; 17:455–469.
112. Semel E, Wiig E. Clinical evaluation of language functions. Columbus, OH: CE Merrill, 1980.
113. Palermo D, Molfese D. Language acquisition from age 5 onward. Psychol Bull 1972; 78:409–428.
114. Entwisle D. Word associations of young children. Baltimore: Johns Hopkins Press, 1966.
115. Nelson K. The syntagmatic-paradigmatic shift revisited: a review of research and theory. Psychol Bull 1977; 84:93–116.
116. Petrey S. Word associations and the developments of lexical memory. Cognition 1977; 5:57–71.
117. Asher SR. Referential communication. In: Whitehurst GJ, Zimmerman BJ, eds. The functions of language and cognition. New York: Academic Press, 1978:175.
118. Bloom L. One word at a time. The Hague: Mouton, 1973.
119. Dore J. A pragmatic description of early language development. J Psycholing Res 1974; 4:343–350.
120. Dore J. Holophrases, speech acts and language universals. J Child Lang 1975; 2:21–40.
121. Halliday MAK. Learning how to mean: explorations in the development of language. New York: Elsevier, 1975.
122. Snyder L. Pragmatics in language-disabled children: their prelinguistic and early verbal performatives and presuppositions. Boulder: University of Colorado, 1975.
123. Dale P. Is early pragmatic development measurable? J Child Lang 1980; 7:1–12.
124. Chapman RS. Exploring children's communicative intents. In: Miller JF, ed. Assessing children's language production: experimental procedures. Baltimore: University Park Press, 1981:111.
125. Ervin-Tripp S. Wait for me, roller skate! In: Ervin-Tripp S, Mitchell-Kernan C, eds. Child discourse. New York: Academic Press, 1977:165.
126. Garvey C. Requests and responses in children's speech. J Child Lang 1975; 2:41–63.
127. Clark RA, Delia JG. The development of functional persuasive skills in childhood and early adolescence. Child Dev 1976; 47:1008–1014.
128. Mitchell-Kernan C, Kernan K. Pragmatics of directive choice among children. In: Ervin-Tripp S, Mitchell-Kernan C, eds. Child discourse. New York: Academic Press, 1977:189.
129. Piché G, Rubin D, Michlin M. Age and social class in children's use of persuasive communicative appeals. Child Dev 1978; 49:773–780.
130. Wilkinson LC, Clevenger M, Dollaghan C. A sociolinguistic approach to communication in small instructional groups. Technical Report No. 505, Wisconsin Research and Development Center for Individualized Schooling, Madison, WI, June, 1979.
131. Olson D, Hildyard A. Assent and compliance in children's language comprehension: knowing and doing. In: Dickson WP, ed. Children's oral communication skills. New York: Academic Press, 1981:313.
132. Schlesinger IM. Production of utterances and language acquisition. In: Slobin D, ed. The ontogenesis of grammar. New York: Academic Press, 1971:63.
133. Bloom L. One word at a time. The Hague: Mouton, 1973.
134. Wells G. Learning to code experience through language. J Child Lang 1974; 1:243–269.
135. Howe C. The meanings of two-word utterances in the speech of young children. J Child Lang 1976; 3:29–47.
136. Braine MDS, Wells R. Case-like categories in children: the actor and some related categories. Cognit Psychol 1976; 10:100–22.
137. Slobin DI. The role of language in language acquisition. Borchers Lecture: University of Wisconsin-Madison, April 21, 1979.
138. Retherford KS, Schartz BC, Chapman RS. Semantic roles and residual grammatical categories in mother and child speech: who tunes into whom? J Child Lang 1981: 8:583–608.
139. Golinkoff RM. The case for semantic relations: evidence

from the verbal and nonverbal domains. J Child Lang 1981; 8:413–438.

140. McNeill D, McNeill NB. What does a child mean when he says "no"? In: Zale E, ed. Proceedings of the Conference on Language and Language Behavior. New York: Appleton-Century-Crofts, 1968:51.
141. Edwards D. Constraints on actions: a source of early meanings in child language. In: Markova I, ed. The social context of language. New York: John Wiley & Sons, 1978.
142. Volterra V, Antinucci F. Negation in child language: a pragmatic study. In: Ochs E, Schieffelin B, eds. Developmental pragmatics. New York: Academic Press, 1979:281.
143. Pea RD. The developmental of negation in early child language. In: Olson DR, ed. The social foundations of language and thought: essays in honor of Jerome S. Bruner. New York: WW Norton, 1980:156.
144. Smith M. The influence of age, sex and situation on the frequency form and function of questions asked by preschool children. Child Dev 1933; 4:201–213.
145. Brown R. The development of wh- questions in child speech. J Verbal Learn Verbal Behav 1968; 7:179–290
146. Ingram D. The acquisition of questions and its relation to cognitive development in normal and linguistically deviant children: a pilot study. Papers Rep Child Dev 1972; 4:13–18.
147. Tyack D, Ingram D. Children's production and comprehension of questions. J Child Lang 1977; 4:211–224.
148. Wootten J, Merkin S, Hood L, Bloom L. Wh-questions: linguistic evidence to explain the sequence of acquisition. Paper presented to the Biennial Meeting of the Society for Research in Child Development, San Francisco, March 16, 1979.
149. Clancy P, Jacobsen T, Silva M. The acquisition of conjunction: a cross-linguistic study. Papers Rep Child Lang Dev 1976; 12:71–80.
150. Bloom L, Lahey M, Hood L, Lifter K, Fiess K. Complex sentences: acquisition of syntactic connectives and the semantic relations they encode. J Child Lang 1980; 7:235–262.
151. Cazden C. The acquisition of noun and verb inflections. Child Dev 1968; 39:433–448.
152. deVilliers J, deVilliers P. A cross-sectional study of the acquisition of grammatical morphemes in child speech. J Psycholing Res 1973; 2:267–278
153. Kuczaj S. Influence of contractability on the acquisition of be: substantial, meager, or unknown? J Psycholing Res 1979; 8:1–11.
154. Block EM, Kessel FS. Determinants of the acquisition order of grammatical morphemes: a re-analysis and re-interpretation. J Child Lang 1980; 7:181–188.
155. Moerk EL. Relationships between parental input frequencies and children's language acquisition: a reanalysis of Brown's data. J Child Lang 1980; 7:105–119.
156. Bloom L, Lifter K, Hafitz J. Semantics of verbs and development of verb inflection in child language. Lang 1980; 56:386–412.
157. Klima E, Bellugi U. Syntactic regularities in the speech of children. In: Lyons J, Wales RJ, eds. Psycholinguistic papers. Edinburgh: Edinburgh University Press, 1966:183.
158. Lord C. Variations in the acquisition of negation. Papers Rep Child Lang Dev 1974; 7:78–87.
159. deVilliers P, deVilliers J. Form and function in the development of sentence negation. Papers Rep Child Lang Dev 1979; 17:57–64.
160. Hurford J. A child and the English question formation rule. J Child Lang 1975; 2:299–301.
161. Kuczaj S. Arguments against Hurford's "aux copying rule." J Child Lang 1976; 3:423–427.
162. Maratsos M, Kuczaj S. Against the transformationalist account: a simpler analysis of auxiliary overmarkings. J Child Lang 1978; 5:337–346.
163. Galligan R. Intonation with single words: purposive and grammatical use. J Child Lang 1987; 14:1–21.
164. McGrath C, Kunze L. Development of phrase structure rules involved in tag questions elicited from children. J Speech Hear Disord 1973; 16:498–512.
165. Limber J. The genesis of complex sentences. In: Moore TE, ed. Cognitive development and the acquisition of language. New York: Academic Press, 1973:169.
166. Smith MD. Relative clause formation between 29–36 months: a preliminary report. Papers Rep Child Lang Dev 1974; 8:104–110.
167. Limber J. Unraveling competence, performance, and pragmatics in the speech of young children. J Child Lang 1976; 3:309–318.
168. Bowerman M. The acquisition of complex sentences. In: Fletcher P, Garman M, eds. Language acquisition. Cambridge: Cambridge University Press, 1979:285.
169. Hood L, Bloom L. What, when, and how about why: a longitudinal study of early expressions of causality. Monogr Soc Res Child Dev 1979; 181.
170. Paul R, Chapman RS, Wanska S. The development of complex sentence use. Paper presented to the American Speech and Hearing Association Convention, Detroit, November, 1980.
171. Bruner J. On prelinguistic prerequisites of speech. In: Campbell RN, Smith PT, eds. Recent advances in the psychology of language. Vol. 4a. New York: Plenum Press, 1978.
172. Carter AL. The transformation of sensory motor morphemes into words. Papers Rep Child Lang Dev 1975; 10:31–47.
173. Ninio A, Bruner J. The achievement and antecedents of labeling. J Child Lang 1978; 5:1–16.
174. Lezine I. The transition from sensorimotor to earliest symbolic function in early development. Early Dev 1973; 51:221–228.
175. Miller JF, Chapman RS, Mackenzie H, Bedrosian J. The development of discourse skills in the second year of life. Conference of the International Association for the Study of Child Language, Vancouver, August 1981.
176. Rees N. Pragmatics of language: applications to normal and disordered language development. In: Schiefelbusch R, ed. Bases of language intervention. Baltimore: University Park Press. 1978:191.
177. Dore J. Requestive systems in nursery school conversations: analysis of talk in its social context. In: Campbell R, Smith P, eds. Recent advances in the psychology of language. New York: Plenum Press, 1978:271.
178. Moerk EL. Verbal interactions between children and their mothers during the preschool years. Devel Psychol 1975; 11:788–795.
179. Keenan EO. Making it last: repetition in children's discourse. In: Ervin-Tripp S, Mitchell-Kernan C, eds. Child discourse. New York: Academic Press, 1977:125.
180. Ricks DM. Vocal communication in pre-verbal normal and autistic children. In: O'Connor N, ed. Language, cognitive deficits, and retardation. London: Butterworths, 1975:75.
181. Austin JL. How to do things with words. Cambridge: Harvard University Press, 1962.
182. Searle J. Speech acts. Cambridge: Cambridge University Press, 1969.
183. Searle J. A classification of illocutionary acts. Lang Soc 1976; 5:1–23.
184. Cole P, ed. Syntax and semantics. Vol. 9. Pragmatics. New York: Academic Press, 1978.
185. Grice H. Logic and conversation. In: Davidson D, Harmon G, eds. The logic of conversation. Encino, CA: Dickensen Publishing Company, 1975.
186. Lakoff R. The logic of politeness; or minding your p's and q's. In: Corum C, Smith-Clark T, Weiser A, eds. Papers

from the Ninth Regional Meeting of the Chicago Linguistic Society. Chicago: Department of Linguistics, University of Chicago, 1973.
187. Brown P, Levinson S. Universals in language usage: politeness phenomena. In: Goody EN, ed. Questions and politeness: strategies in social interaction. Cambridge: Cambridge University Press, 1978:56.
188. Pitcher EG, Prelinger E. Children tell stories. New York: International Universities Press, 1963.
189. Applebee AN. The child's concept of story. Chicago: University of Chicago Press, 1978.
190. Sutton-Smith B. The folkstories of children. Philadelphia: University of Pennsylvania Press, 1981.
191. Wilenksy R. Story grammars versus story points. Behav Brain Sci 1983; 6:579–624.
192. Stein NL. The development of children's story telling skill. In: Franklin MB, Barten S, eds. Child language: a book of readings. New York: Oxford University Press, 1988.
193. Trabasso T, vanderBroek P. Causal thinking and the representation of narrative events. J Memory Lang 1985; 24:612–630.
194. Botvin GJ, Sutton-Smith B. The development of structural complexity in children's fantasy narratives. Develop Psych 1977; 13:377–388.
195. Nelson K. Concept, word, and sentence: interrelations in acquisition and development. Psychol Rev 1974; 81:267–285.
196. Nelson K, Rescorla L, Gruendel J, Benedict H. Early lexicons: what do they mean? Child Dev 1978; 49:960–968.
197. Nelson K. Features, contrasts, and the FCH: some comments on Barrett's lexical developmental hypothesis. J Child Lang 1979; 6:139–146.
198. Hoek D, Ingram D, Gibson D. Some possible causes of children's early word overextensions. J Child Lang 1986; 13:477–494.
199. Goldin-Meadow S, Seligman M, Gelman R. Language in the two-year-old. Cognition 1976; 4:189–202.
200. Huttenlocher J. The origins of language comprehension. In: Solso RL, ed. Theories of cognitive psychology. Hillsdale, NJ: Erlbaum, 1974:331.
201. Thomson J, Chapman RS. "Who is daddy?" revisited: the status of two-year-olds' over-extended words in use and comprehension. J Child Lang 1977; 4:359–375.
202. Greenfield PM. Going beyond information theory to explain early word choices: a reply to Roy Pea. J Child Lang 1980; 7:217–222.
203. Pea RD. Can information theory explain early word choice? J Child Lang 1979; 6:397–410.
204. Branigan G. Some reasons why successive single word utterances are not. J Child Lang 1979; 6:411–422.
205. Barrett MD, ed. Children's single word speech. New York: John Wiley & Sons, 1985.
206. Tomasello M, Farrar, MJ. Object permanence and relational words: a lexical training study. J Child Lang 1986; 13:495–505.
207. Braine MDS. Children's first word combinations. Monogr Soc Res Child Dev 1976:164.
208. Fillmore C. The case for case. In: Bach E, Harms RT, eds. Universals in linguistic theory. New York: Holt, Rinehart & Winston, 1968:1.
209. Bloom L. Why not pivot grammar? J Speech Hear Disord 1971; 36:40–50.
210. Bowerman M. Commentary. In: Braine MDS, ed. Children's first word combinations. Monogr Soc Res Child Dev 1976; 164.
211. Bloom L, Lahey M. Language development and language disorders. New York: John Wiley & Sons, 1978.
212. Strohner H, Nelson K. The young child's development of sentence comprehension: influence of event probability, nonverbal context, syntactic form, and strategies. Child Dev 1974; 45:567–576.
213. Chapman RS, Miller JF. Analyzing language and communication in the child. In: Schiefelbush RL, ed. Nonspeech language intervention. University Park Press, Baltimore: 1980:159.
214. Chapman RS, Kohn LL. Comprehension strategies in preschoolers: animate agents on probable events? J Speech Hear Res 1978; 21:746–761.
215. Ratner N, Bruner J. Games, social exchange and the acquisition of language. J Child Lang 1978; 5:391–402.
216. Snow CE, Goldfield BA. Turn the page please: situation-specific language acquisition. J Child Lang 1983; 10:551–570.
217. Snow C, Ferguson C. Talking to children. Cambridge: Cambridge University Press, 1977.
218. Ervin-Tripp S. Discourse agreement: how children answer questions. In: Hayes JR, ed. Cognition and the development of language. New York: John Wiley & Sons, 1970:79.
219. Stewart C. Mothers' use and children's comprehension of wh-questions. Madison: University of Wisconsin, 1976.
220. Cairns H, Hsu J. Who, why, when, how: a developmental study. J Child Lang 1978; 5:477–488.
221. Ingram D. Early patterns of grammatical development. In: Stark R, ed. Language behavior in infancy and childhood. New York: Elsevier, 1981:327.
222. Peters AM. The units of language acquisition. Cambridge: Cambridge University Press, 1984.
223. Bloom L, Lightbown P, Hood L. Structure and variation in child language. Monogr Soc Res Child Dev 1975; 160.
224. Fay D. Transformations as mental operations: a reply to Kuczaj. J Child Lang 1978; 5:143–150.
225. Keane T, Swartz K. Visual habituation to sad and happy facial expressions in three- and six-month-old infants. Paper presented at Society for Research in Child Development, Boston, 1981.
226. Young-Brown G, Rosenfeld HM, Horowitz FG. Infant discrimination of facial expression. Child Dev 1977; 48:555–562.
227. LaBarbera JD, Izard CE, Vietze P, Parisi SA. Four- and six-month-old infants' visual responses to joy, anger, and neutral expressions. Child Dev 1976; 47:535–538.
228. Schwartz GM, Izard CE, Ansul SE. The five-month-old's ability to discriminate facial expressions of emotion. Infant Behav Dev 1985; 8:65–77.
229. Nelson C, Morse P, Leavitt L. Recognition of facial expression by seven-month-old infants. Child Dev 1979; 50:1239–1242.
230. Klinnert MD, Campos J, Sorce J, Ende RN, Svejda M. The development of social referencing in infancy. In: Plutchik R, Kellerman H, eds. Emotion: theory, research and experience. 2: Emotion in early development. New York: Academic Press, 1983.
231. Sorce JF, Ende RN, Campos J, Klinnert MD. Maternal emotional signaling: its effects on the visual cliff behavior of one-year-olds. Dev Psychol 1985; 21:195–200.
232. Zarbatany L, Lamb ME. Social referencing as a function of information source: mothers versus strangers. Infant Behav Dev 1985; 8:25–33.
233. Stern D. The interpersonal world of the infant. New York: Basic Books, 1985.
234. Miller JF, Chapman RS, Branston M, Reichle J. Comprehension development in sensorimotor stages V and VI. J Speech Hear Res 1980; 9:243–260.
235. Carey S. The child as word learner. In: Halle M, Bresnan J, Miller G, eds. Linguistic theory and psychological reality. Cambridge: MIT Press, 1978:264.
236. Dollaghan C. Child meets word: "Fast mapping" in preschool children. J Speech Hear Res 1985; 28:449–454.
237. Markman E. Comprehension monitoring. In: Dickson WP, ed. Children's oral communication skills. New York: Academic Press, 1981:61.

238. Maratsos M, Gudeman R, Gerard-Ngo P, DeHart G. A study in novel word learning: the productivity of the causative. In: MacWhinney B, ed. Mechanisms of language acquisition. Hillsdale, NJ: Erlbaum, 1987:89.
239. Clark E. Knowledge, context and strategy in the acquisition of meaning. In: Dato DP, ed. Georgetown University round table on languages and linguistics. Washington: Georgetown University Press, 1975.
240. Palermo D. More about less: a study of language comprehension. J Verbal Learn Verbal Behav 1973; 12:211–221.
241. Trehub SE, Abramovitch R. Less is not more: further observations on nonlinguistic strategies. J Exp Child Psychol 1978; 25:160–167.
242. Wannemacher J, Ryan ML. "Less" is not "more." A study of children's comprehension of "less" in various task contexts. Child Dev 1978; 49:660–668.
243. Carey S. Less may never mean more. In: Campbell R, Smith PT, eds. Recent advances in the psychology of language. Vol. 4a. New York: Plenum Press, 1978:109.
244. Clark E. On the acquisition of the meaning of before and after. J Verbal Learn Verbal Behav 1971; 10:226–275.
245. Amidon A, Carey P. Why five-year-olds cannot understand before and after. J Verbal Learn Verbal Behav 1972; 11:417–423.
246. Johnson H. The meaning of before and after for preschool children. J Exp Child Psychol 1975; 19:88–99.
247. French LA, Brown AL. Comprehension of before and after in logical and arbitrary sequences. J Child Lang 1977; 4:247–256.
248. Coker PL. Syntactic and semantic factors in the acquisition of before and after. J Child Lang 1978; 5:261–277.
249. Kavanaugh RD. Observations on the role of logically constrained sentences in the comprehension of "before" and "after." J Child Lang 1979; 6:353–357.
250. Kuczaj S, Lederberg A. Height, age, and function: differing influences on children's comprehension of "younger" and "older." J Child Lang 1977; 4:395–416.
251. Clark E. Strategies and the mapping problem in first language acquisition. In: Macnamara J, ed. Language learning and thought. New York: Academic Press, 1977:147.
252. Clark E. Strategies for communicating. Child Dev 1978; 49:953–959.
253. Roberts KR, Horowitz FD. Basic level categorization in seven- and nine-month-old infants. J Child Lang 1986; 13:191–208.
254. Rice ML, Kemper S. Child language and cognition. Baltimore: University Park Press, 1984.
255. Karmiloff-Smith A. Micro- and macro-developmental changes in language acquisition and other representational systems. Cognit Sci 1979; 3:91–118.
256. Karmiloff-Smith A. A functional approach to language. Cambridge: Cambridge University Press, 1979.
257. Cromer RF. The cognitive hypothesis of language acquisition for child language deficiency. In: Morehead D, Morehead A, eds. Normal and deficient child language. Baltimore: University Park Press, 1976:283.
258. Bowerman M. Discussion summary—development of concepts underlying language. In: Schiefelbusch RL, Lloyd LL, eds. Language perspectives—acquisition, retardation, and intervention. Baltimore: University Park Press, 1974:191.
259. Beilin H. Studies in the cognitive basis of language development. New York: Academic Press, 1975.
260. Uzgiris I, Hunt J McV. Assessment in infancy. Urbana, IL: University of Illinois Press, 1975.
261. Harding C, Golinkoff R. The origins of intentional vocalizations in prelinguistic infants. Paper presented to the Society for Research in Child Development, New Orleans, March, 1977.
262. Sugarman S. A description of communicative development in the prelanguage child. In: Markova I, ed. The social context of language. London: John Wiley & Sons, 1977.
263. Nicholich L. A longitudinal study of representational play in relation to spontaneous imitation and development of multi-used utterances: final report. ERIC Document—PS007 854, 1975.
264. Moore K, Clark D, Mael M, Dawson Myers G, Ratotie P, Stoell-Gammon C. The relationship between language and object permanence development: a study of Down's infants and children. Paper presented to the Society for Research in Child Development, New Orleans, March, 1977.
265. Corrigan R. Language development as related to stage 6 object permanence development. J Child Lang 1978; 5:173–190.
266. Ingram D. Stages in the development of one word utterances. Paper presented at the Stanford Child Language Research Forum, Stanford University, April, 1974.
267. Ingram D. Sensorimotor intelligence and language development. In: Lock A, ed. Action, gesture and symbol: the emergence of language. New York: Academic Press, 1978:261.
268. Folger M, Leonard L. Language and sensorimotor development during the early period of referential speech. J Speech Hear Res 1978; 21:519–527.
269. Uzgiris I. Organization of sensorimotor intelligence. In: Lewis M, ed. Origins of intelligence: infancy and early childhood. New York: Plenum Press, 1976:123.
270. Corrigan R. Cognitive correlates of language: differential criteria yield differential results. Child Dev 1979; 50:617–631.
271. Bloom L, Lifter K, Broughton J. What children say and what they know: exploring the relations between product and process in the development of early words and early concepts. In: Stark R, ed. Language behavior in infancy and early childhood. New York: Elsevier, 1981:301.
272. Waterson N, Snow CE, eds. The development of communication: social and pragmatic factors in language acquisition. New York: John Wiley & Sons, 1978.
273. Chapman RS. Mother-child interaction in the second year of life: its role in language development. In: Schiefelbusch R, Bricker D, eds. Early language: acquisition and intervention. Baltimore: University Park Press, 1981:201.
274. Garnica OK. Some prosodic and paralinguistic features of speech to young children. In: Snow CE, Ferguson CA, eds. Talking to children. Cambridge: Cambridge University Press, 1977:63.
275. Broen PA. The verbal environment of the language-learning child. Am Speech Hear Assoc Monogr, No. 17, 1972.
276. Snow CE. Mothers' speech to children learning language. Child Dev 1972; 43:549–565.
277. Phillips JR. Syntax and vocabulary of mother's speech to young children: age and sex comparisons. Child Dev 1973; 44:192–195.
278. Seitz S, Stewart C. Expanding on expansions and related aspects of mother-child communication. Devel Psychol 1975; 11:763–769.
279. Folger J, Chapman RS. A pragmatic analysis of spontaneous imitations. J Child Lang 1978; 5:25–38.
280. Cross TG. Mother's speech adjustments: the contribution of selected child listener variables. In: Snow CE, Ferguson CA, eds. Talking to children. Cambridge: Cambridge University Press, 1977:151.
281. Brown R. Introduction. In: Snow E, Ferguson A, eds. Talking to children. Cambridge: Cambridge University Press, 1977:1.
282. Rondal J. Maternal speech to normal and Down's syndrome children matched for mean utterance length. In: Meyers CE, ed. Quality of life in severely and profoundly mentally retarded people: research foundations for improvement. Washington, DC: American Association on Mental Deficiency, 1978.
283. Rondal JA. Fathers' and mothers' speech in early language development. J Child Lang 1980; 7:353–370.

284. Cross TG. Mothers' speech and its association with rate of syntactic acquisition in young children. In: Waterson N, Snow C, eds. The development of communication. New York: John Wiley & Sons, 1978:199.
285. Ervin SM. Imitation and structural change in children's language. In: Lenneberg E, ed. New directions in the study of language. Cambridge: MIT Press, 1964:163.
286. Bloom L, Hood L, Lightbown P. Imitation in language development: if, when, and why. Cognit Psychol 1974; 6:380–420.
287. deVilliers JG. Learning how to use verbs: lexical coding and the influence of the input. J Child Lang 1985; 12:587–595.
288. Streim N, Chapman RS. A case study of acquisition of novel action verbs: possible roles of event and discourse context. Paper presented at the Boston University Conference on Language Development, October 19, 1986.
289. Barnes S, Gutfreund M, Satterly D, Wells G. Characteristics of adult speech which predict children's language development. J Child Lang 1983; 10:65–84.
290. Stark R. Language behavior in infancy and early childhood. New York: Elsevier, 1981.
291. Peters AM. Language learning strategies: does the whole equal the sum of the parts? Language 1977; 3:560–575.
292. Kuczaj S. The acquisition of regular and irregular past tense forms. J Verbal Learn Verbal Behav 1977; 16:589–600.
293. Horgan D. Nouns: love 'em or leave 'em. Ann NY Acad Sci 1980; 345:5–26.
294. Bernstein B. Elaborated and restricted codes: their social origins and some consequences. Am Anthropol 1964; 66:55–69.
295. Bowerman M. Comment on structure and variation in child language. In: Bloom L, Lightbown P, Hood L, eds. Structure and variation in child language. Monogr Soc Res Child Dev 1975; 160:80–90.
296. Maratsos M. Commentary. In: Bloom L, Lightbown P, Hood L, eds. Structure and variation in child language. Monogr Soc Res Child Dev 1975; 160:91–93.
297. Shields MM. The development of the modal auxiliary system in the verb phrase in children between three and five years. Educ Rev 1974; 26:180–200.
298. Kramer C, James J, Saxman J. A comparison of language elicited at home and in the clinic. J Speech Hear Disord 1979; 44:321–330.
299. Williams F, Naremore R. Social class differences in children's syntactic performance. J Speech Hear Res 1969; 12:778–793.
300. Nelson K, Gruendel J. At morning it's lunchtime: a scriptal view of children's dialogues. Discourse Processes 1979; 2:73–94.
301. Fillmore LW. Individual differences in second language acquisition. In: Fillmore CJ, Kempler D, Wang WSY, eds. Individual differences in language ability and language behavior. New York: Academic Press, 1979:209.
302. Kanner L. Childhood psychosis: initial studies and new insights. New York: John Wiley & Sons, 1973.
303. Lee S. Developmental sentence analysis. Evanston, IL: Northwestern University Press, 1974.
304. Klee T, Paul R. A comparison of six structural analysis procedures: a case study. In: Miller J, ed. Assessing children's language production: experimental procedures. Baltimore: University Park Press, 1981:73.
305. Stokes T, Baer D. An implicit technology of generalization. J Applied Behav Analysis 1977; 10:349–367.
306. Dale P. Language development: structure and function. New York: Holt, Rinehart & Winston, 1976.
307. deVilliers JG, deVilliers PA. Language acquisition. Cambridge: Harvard University Press, 1978.
308. Gleason JB, ed. The development of language. Columbus, OH: CE Merrill, 1985.
309. Reich P. Language development. Englewood Cliffs, NJ: Prentice-Hall, 1986.
310. Lindfors JW. Children's language and learning. Englewood Cliffs, NJ: Prentice-Hall, 1987.
311. Clark HH, Clark EV. Psychology and language: an introduction to psycholinguistics. New York: Harcourt Brace Javanovich, 1977.
312. Slobin DI. Psycholinguistics. Glenview, IL: Scott, Foresman & Co, 1979.
313. Wanner E, Gleitman LR, eds. Language acquisition: the state of the art. Cambridge: Cambridge University Press, 1982.
314. Fletcher P, Garman M. Language acquisition. Cambridge: Cambridge University Press, 1986.

Section 2

SPEECH AND LANGUAGE PATHOLOGY

Leija V. McReynolds, Ph.D.
David E. Yoder, Ph.D.

Assessment and Intervention Principles

12 Assessment Principles and Procedures

Judith Felson Duchan, Ph.D.

Evaluating children's language is something like interpreting an inkblot on a Rorschach test. To interpret the Rorschach inkblot, viewers project their own underlying ideas onto their perception of the inked shape; to do a language evaluation, clinicians project their goals and theories on their interpretation of the children's task performances. When clinicians of the present and of the past have evaluated the language of children, their preconceived frameworks have led them to decisions about what questions need answering and what aspects of the children's language need attending to. Indeed, clinicians may be drawing from several theoretical perspectives as they examine a child's language performance. Contemporary clinicians may subscribe to one theoretical perspective when administering tests, another when attempting to find out the cause for the language problem, a third when analyzing a language sample for its regularities, and yet a fourth when examining the response of the listener and the effects of the event on language performance.

This chapter will focus on how theoretic frameworks from the historical and more recent past govern our present day assessment procedures. A case will be made that past perspectives in some instances are inadequate in light of currently held views. The chapter will conclude with an appeal to speech-language pathologists to alter their approaches so that they can capture the child's competencies and communicative goals as well as communicative deficiencies and to take into consideration the situational context in which the assessment was carried out. The first half of the chapter will emphasize the historical roots and theoretical assumptions underlying approaches in current use. The second half will present the pros and cons of a structural and functional approach—an approach designed to solve some of the problems created by more traditional methods. I begin by outlining some questions which speech-language pathologists are likely to ask as they select and design their assessment procedures.

WHAT THE SPEECH-LANGUAGE PATHOLOGIST WANTS TO KNOW

There are at least four assessment questions that can be extracted from the literature and practice in speech-language pathology. A question often asked by the speech pathologist of the early 1930s was, "Does the child have a speech or language problem?" A second question also dating back to our beginnings is one of etiology: "What causes the language disorder?"[1] A third and a more recent question has emerged from borrowings from psycholinguistic theory of the 1970s: "What is the child's language like?"[2,3] Appearing most recently on the time horizon is a fourth question that derives its theoretical base from pragmatics theory of the late 1970s and early 1980s: "How well does the child succeed in communicating in different situations?"[4]

The four assessment questions are asked more or less often, depending upon the clinical setting, the severity of the child's language problem, and the theoretical orientation of the clinician. Since each question leads to a different set of assessment procedures and different reported results, it behooves us as speech-language pathologists to examine the assumptions underlying each of the four questions, the procedures tied to them, and some problems inherent in the clinical approaches emerging from them.

Does the Child Have a Language Problem?

This question of identification presupposes for most clinicians that the answer is to be found by comparing the child to a normal population. The comparison presumes that one has an idea of normal performance. It also tends to lend itself to wanting to rely on the use of formal standardized tests and usually leads to an answer based on quantitative measures. That is, children whose test scores deviate significantly from an average score are identifiable as abnormal and so diagnosed as language impaired.

The normative approach, originating from the work of evolutionist Darwin,[5] grew out of his proposed thesis that stages of ontogenetic development (development of a single organism) follow stages of phylogenetic development (evolutionary development of organisms across species).[6] In order to investigate this notion that ontogeny recapitulates phylogeny, Darwin examined stages in his own child's development in detail, spawning a movement in psychology that involved detailed studies of normal children's development.[7] Picking up on Darwin's lead, child study institutes were formed in the United States in the 1920s with the purpose of studying children in detail. The institutes located at Columbia, University of Minnesota, Berkeley, Iowa, and Yale were devoted to collecting information about children's developmental stages in a variety of areas: motor development, language development, and cognitive development.[8] Speech pathology originated as a self-declared profession in the 1930s at a time when psychologists had already discovered developmental norms for motor development, cognitive skills, and vocabulary. The earliest textbooks in the field included descriptions of developmental stages and offered a guideline from which to judge abnormality.[9]

Also in the air when the profession was first established in the 1930s was psychology's testing movement, which promoted the use of standardized observation and quantification of test results. By that time, Binet and Simon had developed the first intelligence test,[10] and Galton, Cattell, and Thorndike had refined the statistical methodology for measuring individual variation through formal test administration.[11] Van Riper's first edition of his well-worn clinical text in speech pathology contained lists of recommended tests for determining children's levels of competence in a variety of areas.[9]

Thus, from the beginning, speech-language pathologists worked from the notion that assessment of competence involved the comparison of particular individuals to an age equivalent standard and that the methodology for making normative comparisons was through the administration of standardized tests. This approach has come to be called the formal test approach.

Formal tests bring with them the supposition that in order for a test to be valid and reliable, it must be given under carefully controlled conditions, simulating as closely as possible the way the test was given to the original population upon which the test was standardized. Only when the test is given in a strictly controlled manner can comparisons be made for determining the degree of normalcy and only then is it eligible to be valid and reliable.

Careful control of context does not assure that tests are either valid or reliable. A valid test is one that measures what it is intended to measure, and careful control of context does little to help an invalid test gain validity. Face or content validity is a form of validity that involves examining the test to see if the items are related in content to what it presumes to measure. Concurrent validity has to do with whether children identified as language impaired on one measure are the same as those identified on a second measure already established as valid. Concurrent validity can exist for a test that doesn't even have language items, as long as it correlates with children's language competency and is normed on a group of children. Siegel and Broen suggest that if foot size were highly correlated with language disorders, it would be a valid measure for identifying language disordered children.[12] However, those who claim validity for their test often do so by presenting the test as a direct measure of language competence, thereby implying that normative tests are not only serving to identify which children have language problems, but also what their areas of deficit are. In so doing, testers not only try to answer the question of whether or not the child has a language problem (the "identity question"), but also aim to answer a second question about what areas the child displayed deficiency in (the area of deficit question).

To determine if a test is providing valid answers to the identity question, speech-language pathologists need to find out whether children who do poorly on it are, in fact, language disordered. The most typical way to find out if a test is valid is to look to see if the test maker provides evidence that the test correlates with other established indicators of language deviance. A major difficulty with finding a viable approach to validity testing has been raised recently in the pragmatics literature where researchers have found that children's language performances vary in important ways depending upon the accompanying social and situational contexts. Thus a child's language performance in a controlled test situation with an authority figure may differ in many respects from that same child's performance in an everyday context with a familiar family member.

This variability in performance with change in context also presents a dilemma for interpreting reliability of formal tests. The theoretic approach of pragmatics alters the value placed on reliability. Since performance is expected to vary with different contexts, reliable performance on repeated administrations of a test is no longer seen as representative of natural situations. For example, if the child's performance on a test of phonology is consistent within a test context, yet the child's phonology varies considerably with different discourse contexts, then the high test-retest reliability in the controlled testing situation is not helpful in telling one about the child's performance in more natural situations.

To determine the validity and reliability of an area of deficit test (e.g., a formal test of syntax or phonology) is even more difficult than for a general identification test. One immediate issue for an area of deficit approach to formal testing is whether it is valid to presume that knowledge or processing is divisible into separable modules. This notion of modularity in language performance is being hotly debated in the psycholinguistic literature and needs to be examined for whether it is an appropriate framework for language assessment.[13] If modularity theory goes the way of its earlier counterpart—faculty theory—the area of deficit approach will no longer be considered a valid one for assessing children's language.

A second validity issue for the area of deficit tests is whether the theoretic framework leading to the test selection is valid or not. A clinician subscribing to a processing framework would likely choose areas of deficit tests that measure processing competencies such as memory span, sequencing abilities, or auditory processing. A clinician subscribing to a linguistic framework would choose tests that measure language knowledge such as phonology, morphology, syntax, semantics. What is missing from the evaluation literature is a set of principles that help clinicians decide which tests to use for particular purposes. Said directly, clinicians must determine a framework for how to think about language before they can determine whether or not the measures are valid. Furthermore, concern about reliability must wait until clinicians are sure that the tests are testing for what they want them to.

Another problem involved in answering both identity and area of deficit questions is the powerful and often incorrect set of assumptions carried with the notion of normalcy. The most obvious assumption is that there are such things as prototypic "normal children" and that it is desirable for children to be normal. This fallacy implies a lack of consideration for the language differences in normal children from different cultural communities who speak nonstandard varieties of English. A standardization sample typically de-emphasizes the performance of the normal learners who do not speak Standard English as their first dialect.

A related problem is the tendency under a normative approach to disregard individual differences, even amoung those who speak Standard English. These differences are sometimes reflected in the scores of the standardization sample, but more than likely they are de-emphasized by the test makers. It is becoming more apparent in the literature on normal language acquisition that normally developing Standard English speakers devise idiosyncratic approaches to language learning and that our easy reliance on homogeneous developmental stages is now suspect.[14]

Even if the children tested were from the same background as the standardized sample and even if the developmental stages are usable when evaluating Standard English speakers, clinicians would still need to ask whether those stages and normal constructs are appropriate to use. Ten-year-old children who score with 2-year-old equivalencies on standardized tests are probably unlike any normal 2 year old. To extend the point to its extreme, a blind child who fails the Peabody Picture Vocabulary Test because he or she does not see the pictures cannot be compared to the sighted child who fails because of poor receptive vocabulary. Score equivalence cannot be taken to imply comparability in language competence.

The problem of using comparable scores to assume comparable competence denies the important distinction made between surface performance and the underlying structure and processes involved in producing that surface response. Although the score-equivalence fallacy is not inherent in the normative approach, it easily flows from it, as can be witnessed by examining language programs based upon normal developmental stages.

At issue here is not whether language impaired children should be identified, but rather whether the identification should be based solely on scores from formal tests and with the use of formal tests to determine areas of deficit. Also at issue, in light of research results in pragmatics and modularity theory, is whether formal tests can ever have validity and whether they should have reliability. Although the aim of the tests is to control context variability, the pragmatics literature suggests that the important thing to examine is how language varies with changes in contexts. Finally, there is a problem with the presumption that equivalent test scores come from equivalent underlying knowledge or processing. In order to solve these assessment problems, clinicians need to find a way to determine which children are in need of language intervention without relying on the age-old formal test approach. Before entertaining ideas for how to do this, a second popular assessment question will be examined, one that asks about the origin of the language disorder.

What Causes the Child's Language Problem?

A question of etiology is raised once a child has already been diagnosed as language disordered. The assumption, borrowed from the medical model, is that in order to best remedy a problem one needs to determine its cause. The medical orientation, which casts speech and language problems as symptoms of diseases, also dates back to the 1930s. Many of the first speech-language pathologists were physicians who naturally extended their medical approach to the diagnosis of speech, language, and hearing problems.[15]

There are several types of etiologies for which present day speech-language pathologists search. One is a syndrome or disease such as autism or central nervous system damage, which are seen to cause the language learning problems. Another is a psychological processing problem, such as limited memory span, which is thought to make language learning more difficult. Still another search is for a social or cultural reason for the language learning problems. These cause types vary in their therapeutic relevance, some providing a course of action, others simply offering a general explanation with no guide for medical or clinical therapies.

Clinicians have attempted to discover causes in the course of their language assessment by asking questions of the family that might lead to a hypothesis of medical etiology. Case histories are conducted wherein clinicians ask caretakers about the language impaired child's birth, disease, and emotional history in an attempt to uncover factors that may have contributed to the child's language learning problems. If the evidence seems to point to a physical or emotional problem outside their diagnostic expertise, speech-language pathologists are likely to refer the child or the family to a physician or psychologist for a diagnosis. Recently, clinicians have begun to use diagnostic checklists to arrive at an etiology.[16]

Although looking for the origin of language problems is sometimes fruitful, such endeavors can also result in further problems rather than solutions to problems. I will discuss the problems in terms of three types of causal factors: disease syndromes, psychological mechanisms, and social contexts.

Disease Syndromes

In the period of 500 to 400 B.C., Hippocrates and his followers wrote of concurrent symptoms that they attributed to malfunctioning in the organs or humors of the body. Taken from a clinical notebook of a practicing physician during the time of Hippocrates is the following passage attributing a set of symptoms to the abnormal thickening of the body's bile:

> Another disease due to thickening. It arises from bile whenever the bile flows to the liver and settles in the head. These are, then, what the patient suffers. The liver swells, and because of the swelling it enlarges toward the diaphragm, and at once pain besets the head especially at the temples. And he does not hear acutely with his ears and often does not see with his eyes.[17]

The medical methods of hypothesizing causes for symptom clusters have withstood the test of time, coming into their heyday in the area of speech pathology with the work of Myklebust.[18] Myklebust's now classic book on differential diagnosis of hearing disorders appeared in the 1950s. Differential diagnosis is a term that describes the process of determining which of several possible etiologies may be causing a particular symptom or cluster of symptoms. Myklebust identified four etiologies contributing to hearing disorders—deafness, emotional disturbance (psychic deafness), brain damage, and mental retardation (mental deficiency)—and he offered a checklist of symptoms for each etiology. His assessment procedure involved identifying the symptoms and matching the different combinations of symptoms with a particular etiology. His medically derived approach continues to be the main methodology used in today's practice of medicine and is also in frequent use in the current practice of speech-language pathology. (See, for example, the checklists of symptoms presented in American Psychiatric Association's Diagnostic and Statistical Manual, APA, 1980[19] and Emerick and Hatten's guide to diagnosis in speech-language pathology, 1979.[16])

The most common etiologies for childhood language disorders in current use are aphasia, hearing impairment, mental retardation, autism, and emotional disturbance.[16] The efforts to differentially diagnose are usually made at the time the child's language problem is first detected, usually at 2 years, when the child fails to develop first words.

A medical diagnosis made solely on the basis of the child's language delay has the potential of being based on faulty and circular reasoning. The circle starts with the child having a language problem, moves around to the point where caretakers and professionals look for an explanation, and closes when a "language disorder" is said to be the underlying etiology. This circular reasoning occurs when determining etiologies for other handicapping conditions as well: an etiology often proposed for a child with learning problems is "learning disability," and for excess activity is "hyperactivity." And so we have a child with a language problem diagnosed as "language disordered."

Most diagnoses carry with them implications that much more is wrong than just a language problem. Although etiologic explanations such as mental retardation or autism can be helpful in attaining services and establishing expectations for how a child is expected to progress, they do little to help the speech-language pathologist predict the nature of a child's language problem. That is, a child who is diagnosed as mentally retarded may have many different types of language problems. Besides not being helpful to the speech-language pathologist, some diagnostic categorizations are likely to be damaging to the language impaired child. The damage is especially likely for etiologies that have connotations of irreversibility such as the so-called "lifelong diseases" of autism or mental retardation.[20]

Along with the negative connotations of the syndrome assignation comes a change in how children so labelled are treated. Once diagnosed, children are often treated as members of that diagnostic category—their language problem is seen as an expected symptom of the "disease" and not deserving of further scrutiny. For instance, anomia in a 10-year-old Down's syndrome child went undetected because her language problem was viewed as a symptom of her retardation, and echolalia in autistic children is often treated as symptomatic rather than analyzed as a form of communication.[21]

The hypothetical syndrome problem, sometimes called the labelling problem,[22] has received considerable attention in the sociological and educational literature and has led to a nongeneric approach to handicapped children.[23] Although labels are often damaging, the impetus for them is being perpetuated because the labels bring with them an entitlement to services. The argument here is against the use of labels as comfortable explanations for language problems and against their being used as an excuse for not carrying out detailed language assessments.

Psychological Mechanisms

A second kind of explanation for why a child has a language problem is a malfunctioning psychological mechanism within the child, which affects the child's language development. Also dating back to ancient Greece, this time originating with Plato in the fourth century B.C., is the notion of divisible mind wherein one aspect of the mind controls a second part.[17] In its recent version, and one applied to a child's language problems, is the approach where clinicians test for difficulties in areas of processing in an attempt to discover a psychological mechanism deficit that may be contributing to the child's language learning problems. Bloom and Lahey[24] and Tomblin[25] have called this attempt to identify processing problems the "specific abilities approach." Processing tests have been designed to measure such things as sensitivity to the intensity and duration of the signal, pattern identification, discrimination, memory, figure-ground distinctions, and temporal sequencing. Processing assessment has tended to be conducted within one of three frameworks.

The first framework focuses on the peripheral aspects of processing such as the child's ability to detect sound (acuity), to identify isolated sounds, and to discriminate similar sounds from one another. This focus on sensation and peripheral aspects of perception was incorporated into the earliest assessment approaches, which included audiometric testing[26] and speech sound discrimination tests.[27] The attempt to measure a child's response to the sensory stimulus can be referred to as an "auditory processing" approach to assessment. This approach has had a recent resurgence from the series of studies by Tallal, which indicated that children with language disorders had difficulty identifying rapidly presented speech and nonspeech sounds.[28]

Another framework used to assess processing focuses on mental processes such as those involved in memory recognition and recall or attention.[29] The measurement of memory dates back to the studies of Ebbinghaus[30] at the turn of the century and to the digit span task that was included in the original Binet test.[10] In 1937 West, Kennedy, and Carr published a test for measuring auditory memory span for nonsense sounds,[31] and in 1939 Anderson developed a speech sound memory task, offering it as a way to determine a child's ability to process speech.[32] Today's approach to memory assessment borrows from the cognitive science literature, which adopts a computer metaphor and regards memory as a form of information processing.[33] The approach is aimed at discovering problems with the way a child is processing linguistic information. The information-processing approach, along with the auditory-processing approach have both been dubbed "bottom-up" processing approaches because the direction of processing is viewed as progressing serially from the signal to its eventual interpretation.

A third framework, the "top-down" approach to assessing processing, looks for how the higher order knowledge is used in the course of language comprehension. It was anticipated by Plato when he offered a theory of a priori concepts as a means for understanding presenting stimuli, but it was not incorporated into a speech-language pathologist's theorizing until after the Chomsky revolution of 1965. Under the top-down theory, processes such as memory, perception, and attention are viewed as active processes that work to create meaning from incoming stimuli. Avid top-down advocates expect to find contributions of higher order knowledge even at the most peripheral level of processing—hearing speech sounds. According to top-down theory, an acoustic signal conveying speech information is not simply registered, but rather is reconstructed or recoded into a sequence of speech sounds, using phonological knowledge as part of the processing procedure.

Each of the three processing frameworks leads to a different set of assessment procedures. A typical battery for assessing aspects of auditory processing skills would include measures of sound discrimination, speech sound blending, identifying auditory stimuli in noise, and of course some measure of signal detection such as pure tone or speech reception test.[34,35] Information-processing approaches include memory and attention measures,[29] and language processing focuses on the discovery of strategies used to process different areas of language knowledge such as phonology and syntax.[36]

If a language impaired child exhibits poor performance on a processing test, a bottom-up theorist is likely to presume that the language disorder is caused by the auditory processing, or memory, or attention problem.[37–39] However, a top-down theorist may regard the problem as one stemming from the child's language difficulty. For example, children who have trouble discriminating similar phonemes may do so because they do not yet have that knowledge of the language to allow them to make that distinction.[40] This language-based hypothesis is testable. Winitz, for instance, found that auditory discrimination was poorer for sounds that the children failed to distinguish in their own production, a result that calls for a higher order mental construct underlying problems in both reception and production of sounds.[41]

The need for resolving of the bottom-up, top-down debate becomes strongly felt when clinicians must decide what remedial steps need to be taken to improve the child's auditory processing or language abilities. Should a child with a hearing loss and concomitant language disorder be given auditory training to help remedy the peripheral processing problem or should he or she be given language training to help remedy the language problem? The resolution at the present time is made on the basis of the theoretical preferences of the clinician. The ones inclined toward bottom-up frameworks, especially the peripheral version of the framework, are more likely to work on improving auditory discrimination; the ones subscribing to a top-down framework are more inclined toward language intervention.

The top-down view of processing is often not a view of processing at all, but rather a view of the nature of the knowledge used for processing. For example, an apparent memory problem is seen as a problem of information storage;[42,43] a problem with sound blending is seen as difficulty with abstract phonologic representations or with the metalinguistic understandings that words are made up of sounds.[38] The assessment procedures deriving from such a view are the same used in structural analysis. That is, a language sample is analyzed to see which structures the child knows and which he or she has difficulty with. Or the child's performance on a language comprehension task is examined to see where the linguistic breakdowns occur.

To conclude, there are three distinguishable approaches to determining whether the language disordered child has processing problems: the auditory-processing approach, the information-processing approach, and the top-down language-processing approach. When a type of processing is identified as a potential cause of the child's language problem, the language clinician should ask what the nature of the relationship is. For example, a clinician would expect a child who cannot hear high-frequency sounds to have trouble with those same sounds in speech, reading, and spelling. Unless these relationships are able to be hypothesized, the clinician might be better off working directly with the language disorder rather than with the processes presumed to underlie them.

Social Contexts

The last of the approaches for answering the underlying cause questions is one that holds that the problem rests in the child's social environment. The idea that a child needs exposure to society to learn language is an early one and exquisitely expressed in the writing of Itard at the turn of the last century.[44] Itard described his attempts to teach a child found in the woods as ones where he was "civilizing" a savage wild child. The implication of Itard's description is that the child's lack of speech and savageness was attributable to his lack of exposure to civilization—a social explanation. The notion that language problems can stem from social or cultural factors permeates the literature in language pathology since its inception in the 1930s. For example, Van Riper in his 1939 edition listed lack of motivation for speech, poor speech standards, improper teaching methods, and poor economic environment as possible causes of delayed speech in children.[9] Today one hears the social contextual causes implicated when descriptors such as the following are used to describe a child or the child's family: social or cultural deprivation, troubled family, lack of environmental stimulation, disadvantaged, maternal overprotection, refrigerator mother, single parent family, poverty, neglect, and lack of semantic contingency in the language spoken to the child.

Social and cultural causal explanations are frequently applied too easily and reflect not what clinicians know to be the case for a particular child, but rather what they assume to be the case because the child and family differ from their middle-class college-educated expectations. For example, the category of "cultural deprivation" was used commonly throughout the 1960s as an explanation for a child's language problems. The idea presumed, as does the notion of normalcy, that there is a preferred culture, which is white and middle-class; this presumption prescribes a type of mother-child relationship within which language is considered to be best learned. Other cultures, the so-called culturally deprived ones, are deprived by virtue of their being different.

A corollary in the logic of this explanation is that a child whose language is different from the prestige language has language problems. Some then take it as a given that the child's language "problems" are due to his or her lack of exposure to the clinicians' culture. It is what Ryan has called "blaming the victim"[45] and what Ginsberg has called the "myth of the deprived child."[46]

Two questions should be directed to the diagnostician who designates a child culturally deprived. One is whether the child has a language learning problem or is speaking a normal child's version of the dialect of those around him. It has been repeatedly shown that a child speaking dialects different from Standard English do not do well when tested on standardized tests normed to Standard English. The question, then, is whether the child is abnormal in relation of his or her cultural context or just in terms of our culturally biased assessment tools and procedures. If the child does have a language problem when compared to age mates in his or her particular culture, what should one do about it? I suggest that calling the child culturally deprived offers nothing in the way of remedial direction. Indeed, language programs designed for a child who was labelled culturally deprived have invariably been ones that have taught the value of Standard English over nonstandard English.

The other socially oriented categorical explanations have similar faults, though perhaps not as insidious as the cultural deprivation explanation. One need only glance through case history descriptions or case history question forms to see a reflection of the cultural bias. Clinicians ask people about their marital status, their occupations, their level of education, and their family interaction and then write reports with statements that point directly or indirectly to the family as a source of the child's problems. In so doing they are blaming the victim once again.

Instead of creating prejudgements about the effect of presumed social contexts on a child's language learning, clinicians should be using some recently devised analytic techniques for examining the quality of social context in which the language impaired child operates. These techniques are discussed under the next approach to assessment, the one that evolves from asking about the nature of the child's language problem.

What is the Child's Language Like?

This question is apprehended differently depending upon the orientation of the diagnostician. Some see it as a comparison with adult language and answer it by comparing the child's language production with the adult forms. The *child to adult* comparison may involve working with a checklist of adult structures and indicating which of these the child knows or does not know.

Other clinicians may take a developmental stage approach, by which the language impaired child is compared with children of different developmental stages. This *child to child* approach takes an age-equivalent child or a stage-equivalent child as the matched comparison and uses normal children's knowledge as the model for guiding assessment and intervention.

A third and more difficult approach is to evaluate the child's language on its own terms, devising categories of description from what the child actually does rather than from what normal children do at that age or stage or from what normal adults do. This has been called structural analysis.[36] Let us take a look at the advantages and disadvantages of each of these three approaches.

Child to Adult Comparison

The adult comparison approach is one that has been used continually and challenged continually. Its prevalence comes from our adult egocentricity, which makes us believe that the way adults talk and understand language is right and that children and nonstandard English speakers are not speaking good English. In its most imperialistic form, the clinician simply matches the child's utterance to the form in which the adult would say it and considers the child's answer right or wrong depending upon the exactness of the match. Thus children are judged as normal or language impaired depending upon how well they can imitate sentences.[47,48]

A less imperialistic approach is a child to adult comparison that is obtained by recording a spontaneous language sample and analyzing it for what adult language forms it contains or does not contain. This adult checklist approach may take as its focus any of the levels of language that have been sufficiently studied in the adult language. Thus clinicians have procedures for determining which of the adult pragmatic functions are expressed in the child's language[49] and which adult syntactic structures the child expresses.[36,50,51] The most familiar and most prevalent of these checklist approaches are phonemic inventories of articulation tests that ask which of the adult phonemes the child produces or misproduces.[52,53]

Child to Normal Child Comparison

A second checklist approach is that which asks not what the child knows about preselected adult categories, but what the child knows about preselected categories found in normal children at different developmental stages. These age and stage checklists are also used for each of the linguistic levels of syntax, semantics, phonology, and pragmatics. Sometimes they are organized by stages that are demarcated according to their measured mean length of utterance developed by Brown.[54] Thus one finds Brown's five stages depicted for syntax in Lee's Developmental Sentence Scoring procedure[3] and Miller's Assigning Structural Stages procedure.[55] Sometimes the stages are determined by age equivalencies, modelled after the developmental tests, such as the Gesell, Utah, or Houston tests. Here assignments of age equivalencies are made on the basis of the tasks they can perform.[56] Most recently the stages have been based on Piaget's cognitive stages. Depending upon their task performance, children are assigned to one of the six sensorimotor stages[57] or more advanced stages of concrete or logical operations.[58]

The child-centered checklist approach has its advantage over the adult model in that the categories used in the checklist are derived from children's language rather than from adult language and may therefore be a better representation of what the disordered child knows. However, one cannot afford complacency with this method either, since the literature on stages of normal language acquisition is still in considerable flux, and also because it is not known whether the child being evaluated bears much resemblance to his or her age or stage mates. Furthermore, this approach does not ask anything about the consistencies within the child's language system, the strategies and processes being used to produce or misproduce those items on the checklist, or any structures that may be prevalent in the child's language that are not on the checklist, such as would be the case for delayed echoes in an autistic child.

In sum, the checklist approaches, whether they are adult- or child-centered, deserve the same criticism that have been levied at assessment procedures so far: they are not really geared to analyzing the child in his or her own terms.

Structural Analysis

Under the influence of the linguistics revolution, which occurred in the 1960s, a nonchecklist method has been developed for assessing children's language. It borrows from a commonly used research technique called structural analysis. The historical origin of the method has been seen as coinciding with the beginnings of modern-day linguistics in the early 1900s.[59] However, one can make a case that the method has been around since Aristotle, who proposed that language was highly regular and operated on principles of analogies. Structural analysis is also a procedure used by contemporary anthropologists to analyze the structure of myths,[60] by sociologists to analyze conversations,[61,62] by psychologists to analyze children's cognitive structures,[63] and by psycholinguists to analyze children's language acquisition.[64] The analysis is done differently in the different disciplines, but the aim is to examine data, such as a language corpus, a myth, an interaction sequence; to tease out the regularities from that data; and to hypothesize underlying designs, which could be producing the surface regularities.

Structural analysis has a long and familiar history for speech-language pathologists in some areas of their diagnosis, such as phonology, where, since the 1930s beginnings, they have listed children's "articulation" errors and then analyzed them for patterns of substitution, omission, and distortion. Recent advances in phonology have led to a more detailed procedure wherein the patterns are identified as processes according to substitution type and contextual influence, but the method has remained one of pattern discovery, in keeping with the structural approach. Once patterns are discovered, analysts may go a step further and inquire into possible reasons underlying the pattern. They may assume, for example, an underlying psychological origin such as a particular motor problem, a phonologic rule, or a high-frequency hearing loss. These hypothetical underlying causes are different from the syndrome or psychological mechanisms explanations for a disorder in that they are tied specifically to the error pattern and are not general statements, as would be the case for a diagnosis of dysarthria, mental retardation, or hearing loss.

The structural approach has advantages over the checklist approach in the same way a description has an advantage over a label for a handicapped child. That is, the structural approach commits the diagnostician to determining just what it is that makes a particular child seem unusual to other people and then leads to assessing the child in that area of "unusualness" and postulating what kinds of processes or knowledges may be leading the child to that difference. The method requires that the child's uniqueness be dealt with rather than his or her similarity to an age or stage mate or to other children in the same diagnostic category.

Structuralism has its problems as well as its advantages. Before evaluating the strengths against the weaknesses, I will elaborate on a fourth and recent approach to language assessment—one involving the social context of language. It has recently emerged in the 1980s as a guide to assessing communication between two or more participants. The approach answers a fourth assessment question about the degree to which the child's communication is successful.

How Well Does the Child Succeed in Communicating in Different Situations?

In the 1980s, the pragmatics revolution led clinicians to design assessment approaches that regard communication as a two-way interaction. The effect has been to judge a communication problem as not one emanating solely from a language disorder in the child, but as one located anywhere in the communicative context. The interaction assessment procedure is based on the view that the communicative context needs to be analyzed and that the analysis involves an assessment of how well communication functions. One may, for example, determine if the adults are responding contingently to the language impaired child's communicative efforts and if their responses are finely tuned to the child's level of communicative competence. The focus on the communicative interaction as the resource for the evaluation has created a variety of changes in the clinical procedures.

First, the focus has changed from looking at the child's "inaccuracies" or "errors" in production as isolated entities to looking at how those departures from what is expected impact upon the communicative exchange. Thus a child summarily judged unintelligible, severely language impaired, or echolalic might be seen as an adept communicator when met with a listener who understands the child's code. The same child communicating the same message might be a competent successful communicator when interacting with a familiar and sympathetic listener and an incompetent, unsuccessful communicator to a stranger who sees his or her communicative attempts as uninterpretable or bizarre.

A second focus of the interaction analysis is to identify trouble spots in the interaction and to analyze the source of difficulty and how or if the partners solved the problem. The trouble spots have been called "breakdowns," and the solutions "repairs" or "revisions."[65,66] More general terms that pertain to problems in the overall interaction have been coined, for example, "communicative distress."[67]

A third focus of the interaction assessment approach has been called "turn taking" and has taken as its metaphor a game interaction wherein partners are seen as competing for the floor and as having to devise or adhere to preestablished rules of interaction conduct.[68] Under this notion, the methods used by the child and the conversational partner are analyzed for their success and egalitarianism.

A fourth focus of interaction assessment has been to examine the situational event in which the interaction takes place. Event assessment is the most recent of the components of interaction assessment, and it stems most directly from Bruner's studies in the 1970s of ritualized routines between mothers and normally developing children. Bruner,[69] along with Nelson,[70] views ritualized interaction as crucial in a child's learning of turn taking and of the social context in which communication takes place. The analyses of event structures have begun to be incorporated into the assessment procedures of speech-language pathologists as can be seen in assessments involving analyses of children's interactions in light of dictates from their everyday "scripts."

Interaction assessment, by allowing that others must assume some of the responsibility for successful communication with a language impaired child, presents new problems for assessing communication exchange. Since evaluation implies making judgements about the quality of performances, the efforts are now being made to determine which aspects of communication dyads are desirable and which are in need of clinical intervention. These efforts can lead to the same culturally biased decisions encountered when attempting to discover social causes for a child's language problem. That is, a parent who does not respond semantically or topically to his or her child's communications is seen as a candidate for clinical intervention. The parents under scrutiny by the clinician evaluating the dyad might conclude that they have contributed to their child's language problem. The possible result is that the parent becomes indirectly and incorrectly blamed, exacerbating the communication difficulties between parent and child.

In fact, cross-cultural literature fails to show that children learn language only when the adults tailor their language complexity to the child's language level. Rather, cultures have been found in New Guinea,[71] in Guatemala,[72] and in the Piedmont mountains of West Virginia[73] where parents do not finely tune their language complexity to their child's level of competence. Instead, parents may seldom talk to their children, or if they do, they may talk in long utterances, much more complex than those used by the child. Nonetheless, the children in the cultures learn language.

The Role of Assessment Questions

I have been suggesting that the methods for assessing children's language derive from questions which the clinician is attempting to answer and from theoretical frameworks motivating the questions. The first question is whether or not the child has a language problem. Approaches to answering this question have been couched in a normative framework that carries with it tendencies to ignore cultural and individual differences and to be incorrectly satisfied with reliability and validity for measures taken under highly controlled conditions. The question is often answered by administering formal tests and obtaining standardization scores for making comparisons with normal children.

A second assessment question has been to discover a cause for a child's language difficulty. The postulated causes have been disease syndromes, psychological mechanisms, or social problems. Causes, even when found, do not always lead to therapeutic prescriptions and, in fact, may be empty in their explanatory value. Further, right or wrong, they may be detrimental in that they blame or stigmatize the child or the family or social groups with whom the child is identified. The methods used to answer the etiology question are to use syndrome checklists, which identify the disease by its often found behavioral characteristics.

A third question is one which asks what the child's language is like. It suffers from its dependency on adult and peer comparisons. When the child's language is described on its own terms, however, insights can be gained into its internal regularity, thereby offering a fruitful approach for understanding the structure and function of the child's language. The approach has traditionally been one involving structural analysis of a language sample produced by the child.

And fourth, assessments are now being developed to answer how successfully the child communicates with particular interactants, in particular events. The problem for this interaction approach is that it leads to unsubstantiated judgements by clinicians about how interactions should be conducted, creating an atmosphere where interactants are blamed for the child's communication problem. Nonetheless, the focus on the interaction and the event offers a promising potential for intervention where the target for change is not only on the child, but also on the communicative context. Since I will argue that a functional interactional version of structural analysis has in it the potential for answering all four diagnostic questions, more discussion of its features and advantages is warranted.

STRUCTURAL AND FUNCTIONAL ANALYSIS

The purpose of structural analysis is to determine the basic structures of units underlying patterns in complex events. The major effect has been to follow the direction of the structural linguists in doing analysis of children with language disorders. The linguists have led speech-language pathologists to working within analytically separable levels of phonology, syntax, and semantics and to using units of varying types with varying degrees of abstractness. The most familiar linguistic categories deriving from the research in linguistics in the 1960s have been phonemes, phonological processes, morphological inflections, phrase structures, sentence types, lexical types, and semantic relations.

In the 1970s, the examination of conceptual structures seen to underlie communication was added to linguistic analysis. Typical cognitive structures that found their way into language assessment procedures have been concepts, conceptual domains or networks, and strategies.

A more recent application of structural analysis has been in the social domain. In this case, analyses have been done to determine exchange patterns between partners, features of social control, and analyses of structures underlying social rituals. In a more functional vein, structures have been analyzed to determine what purposes they serve for speakers and listeners and the function they play in the communication endeavor.

The structures, whatever their domain, can relate to one another in various ways: some are in hierarchical relationship, some linear, and some operate in parallel fashion yet serve the same or a similar function. Furthermore, there are many types of structures: there are those that are derived by classifying similar elements; there are those that define allowable contexts for the elements to occur; and there are those that work together to serve a common purpose. These first are often called "categories," the second "contextual rules," and the third "functions." Some structures are abstract in form and seen as being used by the child in the course of communicating. These are postulated "underlying structures." They produce the patterned regularities that are found in the surface structures.

One way to do a language assessment, then, is

to operate as if one were a linguist studying a new language or an anthropologist studying a new culture. The analysis is a complex one and brings with it particular problems, which currently need to be addressed. Some of the problems are practical ones faced by clinicians who have considerable demand on their time. For example, the presumption until recently is that clinicians need to examine all aspects of a child's language in detail before a conclusion can be drawn about the nature of the child's language. Other problems are more theoretical. For example, even after having discovered regularities in the child's language performance, there is no guarantee that the structures that are the outcome of the analysis are those that best represent what the child is thinking. This concern has been one referred to in the theoretical and clinical literature as the problem of assuring "psychological reality."

Besides the problem of time expenditure and establishing psychological reality, is a third problem, which involves a theoretical criticism of the structural approach. This problem has surfaced in recent years with the emergence of the functionalist sensibility among those studying normal and abnormal language. The critics see the structural approach as not going far enough. Rather than being satisfied with representing the child's structural knowledge, researchers of functionalist persuasion would have clinicians analyze how such units work together and what purposes they serve. Although functionalists use the structural approach to find regularities in data, they do not assume those regularities are static, separate, nonmotivated units, but rather hypothesize reasons for why such structures occur. They are criticizing the *static* version of structuralism and substituting for it the *functional* version of structuralism.

To summarize, the 1970s approach to structural analysis has raised certain issues for the 1980s period. They involve (1) deciding what to analyze; (2) determining appropriate units or structures that represent the child's knowledge of language; and (3) determining the functions behind the discovered structures.

Deciding What to Analyze

Advocates of structural analytic techniques for assessing language have, until recently, either explicitly or tacitly recommended that the child's language be analyzed at all linguistic levels in order to discover the child's phonological, morphological, syntactic, and semantic systems.[12,24] I say "until recently" because the possible analyses in recent years have proliferated with the emergence of other areas of investigation such as the cognitive and social domains.

Rather than analyzing all possible areas of communication, I propose analyzing only those aspects of the child's communication system that are in question. If a child's speech production is significantly different as to render him or her difficult to understand, a phonological analysis is warranted. If the phonology is not the source for concern, then it need not be analyzed. Thus I suggest beginning the analysis by asking what it is that is most significant about the child's language and then designing a procedure to figure out the child's patterns in that area of performance.

It has been my experience that the speech-language pathologist's sense of what is important to analyze can change dramatically in the course of the analysis. That is, the clinician may begin by analyzing syntax, but realize, in the course of the analysis, that the child's semantic referencing is the greater contributor to the child's communicative difficulties. This "getting into the data" phase is an important time for selecting the structures to analyze.

Once an area is targeted for analysis, the speech-language pathologist may need to go back and collect more information from the child. This type of "deep testing" can be done over a period of time and serves as a way to track changes in the child's language as a result of clinical intervention.

These three stages of analysis—the initial period, getting into the data, and deep testing—offer different perspectives on what to analyze for. The approach being advocated is an ongoing one that is motivated by the specific communication needs of the child and the familiar interactants. It is a focused and individualized approach rather than a broad one that undertakes to analyze all areas of the child's language.

Determining Appropriate Structures

An analysis that goes beyond a behavioral description attempts to discover structures that are an abstraction away from the description. Any discussion of language assessment has this surface versus underlying structure issue lurking in it, especially if the approach being discussed is informal assessment through the use of structural analysis. But it was Chomsky's revolution in linguistics that made us focus on the fact that particular behaviors, sentences in his case, come from somewhere.[74] Chomsky said that they come from syntactic rules that operate on a base phrase structure, transforming it to its surface form. Since then linguists have postulated underlying structures for phonology, for semantics, and most recently for pragmatic levels of language. Cognitive scientists, who also are structurally inclined, have postulated underlying structural categories or systems such as prototypes, action schemes, memory networks, and story grammars.

As yet those who do structural assessment in the field of speech-language pathology have tended to stick close to the data, offering descriptions of children's language, but not explanations. While one may find idiosyncratic patterns in the child's language production and may even describe them in terms of mentalistic or underlying constructs such as rules, the rules often are not significantly different from the descriptions. For example, when a child substitutes a /t/ for a /k/, it is described as the child exhibition of a fronting process.

An example of a more abstract phonologic form is from a child in our clinic who produced all two-syllable words with a neutralized first vowel, a glottal stop for the medial consonant, and a final diminutive suffix for the final vowel. Our abstract rule was to postulate a /ĉ ʔi/ form, which the child used to produce two-syllable morphemes.[75] We regard this structure as a phonologic rule operating on an underlying adult-like form because the child had good comprehension. We postulate this rule as part of the child's abstract phonologic system and not as a motor speech disorder since the target sounds in the two-syllable words were correctly produced in other phonologic contexts. It is the two-syllable complexity that seemed to trigger this phonologic operation in the child's system.

A problem with structural analysis is that the postulated structure may not be "psychologically real" in that it is not the way the child thinks about it. One way to determine if one has represented the child's knowledge accurately is to ask whether the explanatory categories assume knowledge that is unnecessary to assume or, conversely, are sufficiently rich to explain all significant elements of the child's behavior. These mirror image errors have both been found in the literature on normal language acquisition.

The first, the problem of overrepresentation, was described by Bowerman in her argument against attributing "subjecthood" to the first noun in children's two-word utterances.[76] Bowerman noticed that children in the two-word stage seldom create sentences with inanimate subjects, such as "knife cut."[76] She was taking issue with the presumption of Bloom that children at the two-word stage had knowledge that sentences require subjects.[77] Since their use of sentence subjects was confined to animate nouns, Bowerman argued, it would be more accurate to say that the children were expressing animate nouns as semantic agents rather than to represent their first position nouns as coming from an understanding of sentence subjects.

Speech-language pathologists often make the overrepresentation mistake, ascribing adult knowledge to language impaired children. Checklist assessment techniques do it, imitation tests do it, and formal tests do it in that correct answers are seen as an indicator of adult competence. Structural analytic procedures that are sensitive to children's differences will, it is hoped, prevent so many mistakes. One test of a good analysis could be that it results in a new set of structures, rather than a list of knowledges made from a checklist of categories derived from adult or normal child models.

The underrepresentation problem is illustrated by Bloom's famous "mommy sock" example.[77] Although Bowerman found Bloom's formulation too inclusive, Bloom found the previous representations of children's language knowledge not inclusive enough. Utterances made by two-year-olds such as "mommy sock" were treated by Bloom's predecessors as pivot open constructions. Such a syntactic representation failed to show that the utterance had two possible meanings: one a request to have the mother help the child put on her sock, the other a description of the mother's sock.

Underrepresentation mistakes are just as problematic as overrepresentation mistakes. An example is the traditional assumption that austistic children absent-mindedly imitate the utterances of others. The imitation dubbed "echolalia" tended not to be analyzed for its language structure, nor for its communicative function, thereby suggesting that all the autistic children are doing when they echo is acting like a tape recorder. Recent work on autistic echolalia has shown that the imitations do indeed have communicative intent, and they often stem from the children's knowledge of language structure.[21,78] This underestimation of echolalia in autism provides an example of underrepresentation in language assessment.

A third error in determining structural units, which is perhaps worse than either the over- or underrepresentation of knowledge, is its misrepresentation. This amounts to misdiagnosis. In this case, the structural analysis of speech-language pathologists bears little resemblance to the child's underlying knowledge. This phenomenon has been felt by researchers who bring a new set of categories or a new framework to their structural analysis and discard or argue against a prior framework. Recent advances in the area of "aspectual linguistics" has made the former analysis of the role of morphologic tense seem at best shallow, at worst wrong. For example, tense markers have traditionally been considered temporal indicators of present, past, and future time. Aspect includes the linguistic indicators of activity status, such as whether an activity is ongoing, finished, repeating, or rapid. Analysts have typically seen the "-ing" form in English as a tense marker indicating present time, rather than given it its correct classification as an aspectual marker indicating ongoing activity. Thus a child who uses "-ing" to mean that an activity is continuing may or may not have a notion of tense, and one who omits "-ing" may or may not understand current time.

A second example of misrepresentation in language assessment is from phonologic process analysis. To classify a child's production of /lelo/ for "yellow" as a /l/ for /j/ substitution is a misrepresentation for the child whose pattern is one of assimilation of /j/ by the following /l/.

A fourth type of error is simply not to see what is there and to fail to represent it at all. What often is the case is that regularities in the data are missed because they are not as obvious or tangible as others. Clinicians are more likely to discover a lisp or missing copula than they are a comprehension strategy.

A key to prevention of such over-, under-, or nonrepresentation of children's knowledge is to examine the hypothesized structures to see what they predict about the child's future behavior. For example, if a rule or pattern is proposed as an underlying structure, the speech-language pathologist needs to ask what sorts of observable forms are likely to be affected by the child's structure. If the child is presumed to have a phonologic substitution process whereby the velars become alveolars, a new word containing a velar should be affected. If the finding of the analysis was that the child requests what he or she wants by reaching and saying "da," the prediction is that when tempted by a desired food, the child produces the structure of "reach + da." This predictive test is a version of what has been called the productivity test, where a structure is not judged as one the child "knows" unless the child is observed to express it at least five times and preferably in a variety of contexts.[77]

Besides testing for the psychological reality of a structure by predicting what the child will say or do in situations that require already learned knowledge, the speech-language pathologist can predict what the child will do to apply the known structure to new forms. Berko's landmark "wug" test asks children to generalize their knowledge of plurals to a newly learned word—as they are introduced to one and then a pair of fictitious animals, they are asked "Here is a wug. Here is another one. Here are two _____." Thus clinicians have a way of predicting the direction of "generalization" of a structure.

In the literature on child language learning, the most common means of refuting a proposed structural representation is to argue for or against it on the basis of scientific tests of parsimony and explanatory adequacy. Both the parsimony test and the test of explanatory adequacy are ones that tend to be called forth when a clinician needs to decide between two alternative ways of representing a child's knowledge. The clinician makes the choice on the basis of which representation accounts for the data in the simplest and most elegant way—the most parsimonious version wins—or on the basis of which representation offers the greatest insight—the most explanatory version wins. And so Bowerman's semantic relation explanation of children's first noun phrases was more parsimonious and simpler than that offered by Bloom (see previous discussion), and Bloom's semantic relation explanation of two-word utterances explained more about the double meaning of utterances such as "mommy sock" than did the pivot-open representation.

To capsulize: structural analysis in its most streamlined sense is intended to discover units in children's knowledge of their language. If structural analysts were to design boxes to fit their proposed units, as if gift wrapping them, then those who commit overrepresentation errors would pick too large a box and those who underrepresent a child's knowledge would have a box without enough compartments; the misrepresenters would try to stuff the child's knowledge into a box of the wrong size and shape, and the nonrepresenters would not even realize there was something to wrap. In order to guard against such errors, it behooves the analyst, in this case the speech-language pathologist, to examine the units for their predictability and to look out for other ways to account for the child's behavioral regularities—ways which are more parsimonious and which have greater explanatory power than the ones hypothesized.

The most recent literature on the study of children's communication offers a clear example of how changes in theories of language can provide better accounts of what children are doing as they communicate. The new shift from static structural approaches to dynamic functional approaches provides better and more parsimonious explanations of children's communicative attempts.

Discovering Underlying Functions

One side effect of the pragmatics revolution has been to view structures as tools that serve a purpose either for the initiator, the receiver, or for the text or event being created. The purposes that the structures serve have been called "functions," and the efforts to discover the functions has been called "functionalism."

Functionalism, according to Bates and MacWhinney, can be traced to the Prague school linguists who began their functionalist studies in the early 1900s.[79] In speech-language pathology, the earliest felt influences of functionalism were from "speech act" theorists, especially those studying children's language in the 1970s. The idea of speech act theory was that a speaker issues an utterance to accomplish a particular goal and that utterances can be classified by the goals they intend to accomplish. A speaker may say something with the intent of getting an object, of insulting someone, or of making an excuse. The formulations by speech act theorists doing research on children's language acquisition implied that each and every utterance had an intent underlying it, its "illocutionary force,"[49,80] and that different utterances may be serving the same intent. Further, just as children must learn about structural components of language such as phonology and syntax, they must learn how to use language to accomplish different purposes.

Speech-language pathologists borrowed from speech act theory and child language research and developed methods for analyzing intents behind children's utterances or actions.[81–83] The assessment goal for the nonspeaking children was to determine whether or not they were able to make plans or conjure up intents; for those language impaired children already communicating, the aim was to determine the different types of intents they were expressing.

Speech act analysis was an improvement over the purely structural approaches because it allowed for the discovery that utterances which were not conventional could be serving a purpose for the child and because a child regarded by others as "noncommunicative" under the structural approach could now be seen as "communicative using nonconventional means." Further, speech act analysis allowed for the discovery that linguistically different utterances, such as "Go away" and "Your mother's calling you," could be serving the same speech act intent (e.g., getting a friend to leave).

There were several difficulties with the speech act version of functionalism. One was that speech-language pathologists presumed, as did their predecessors studying normal children's language, that there was a one-to-one relationship between form and function. That is, the analysis involved examining every communicative act as an isolated unit which served to carry out a single intent. This one-to-one assumption resulted in the failure to discover what different functions a single act might be serving. For example, a child who says "Hi" when someone walks in may be accomplishing several intended goals at once: gaining attention, opening a conversation, greeting, carrying out a ritual.

A second problem with speech act functionalism was that the theory led to the separate classification of each speech act, often disregarding how acts work together within the confines of events and overall goals of the intender. The method ignored the fact that a sequence of happenings may be highly related. For example, assume the following: a child sitting in a highchair who first says "no" to an offer of food, then says "milk spill" as he or she pushes over the milk, and then says "tummy hurts." The attending adult would understand this series of speech acts as the same in kind—all with the intent of finishing eating and getting down. However, a traditional speech act analysis would miss this overall commonality and treat each act or utterance as a decontextualized event and separate from one another.

Another form of functionalism, which has become a 1980s focus of language assessment, is one that evaluates the response of the listener in light of the speaker's intent. Borrowing from the normal literature on mother-child interaction,[84] speech-language pathologists have begun to analyze how well adults respond to the child's presumed intent. This "fine tuning" version of functionalism allowed for the analysis of how often and how well adults or children were responding to the communicative efforts of the language impaired child. The literature on normal language acquisition points to the conclusion that children develop language faster (1) when they are met with frequent approval from their listeners;[85–87] (2) when the adults talk about what the child is thinking or doing;[88,89] and (3) when the adults are less directive and more inclined to give the child ample opportunity to indicate his or her own intents.[90–93] These preliminary findings for normal children have led to clinical approaches that evaluate the degree of approval and directiveness in adult responses to children's communications. If the adults are found wanting, the next step has been to remedy the "problem" by training the adults to become more finely tuned, more open to the child's initiations, and less directive.[94,95]

Besides assessing how adults fine tune each of their utterances or responses to the child's individual intents, attempts have been made in the literature on normal language acquisition to determine how adults gear their questions and demonstrations to the child's competence. The particular emphasis has been to examine the adult approaches to teaching the child routine events such as how to enact "peekaboo" or how to name pictures during book routines.[96,97] The "scaffolding" procedure for teaching the child how to carry out events involves intricate tutoring wherein the mother begins by providing considerable support by offering all the steps in the event through demonstration. Once the event is familiar to the child, the mother begins to leave slots in the scaffold for the child to fill in. The "lessons" build on one another with the mother keeping track of what the child knows and "raising the ante" when the child can supply the step with parental support.

By assessing each single act or group of acts included in a single event, fine tuning functional analysis offers clinicians a means for evaluating the degree of success the child experiences. However, this approach, like the ones before it, can be faulted for ignoring important contextual considerations. For example, the single act analysis presumes that adults best avoid directiveness. What is omitted from consideration is an attempt on the part of the analyst to determine why the adult is using the directive style. An illuminating study reported recently by Murray and Trevarthan showed that when nondirective mothers were asked to interact with their infants under conditions where the child's responses were delayed slightly, the mothers shifted to a directive style.[98] This dramatic result suggests that directive adults may be using that mode of interaction in order to gain and keep the child's attention, and so the style serves an important and useful function. Thus speech-language pathologists need to elaborate on the fine tuning functional analysis, which they now do from the child's point of view by considering the goals of the adult and how their interaction with the child accomplishes them.

A third form of the 1980s versions of functionalism takes as its point of view the object of endeavor in which the participants are engaged. Under this approach, language structures that serve the same function might be classified together. For example, one grouping can be made of structures that highlight information and another of structures that create a particular perspective for the listener. This form of functionalism goes beyond the sensibilities of particular speakers and listeners operating in specific events. Rather its endeavor is more broad in its focus, aiming to find out which linguistic devices work together to accomplish common purposes.

This sort of "linguistic functionalism" has been used to identify a variety of linguistic devices that may be brought into service to achieve the same goal,[78] in which case tne devices tend to be ones that substitute for one another and that occur locally in a text. For example, in order to emphasize or foreground information, a speaker might say it louder, place it in the beginning of the sentence, and even tell the listener it is important.

Another finding of linguistic functionalism has been to discover that linguistic devices can co-occur in a text and work together to achieve a single impression. Recent work in discourse analysis, for example, has led to the discovery of how different discourse devices are used to serve a single function. The discourse literature also offers an interesting demonstration of the static as well as the functional approaches to structuralism.

Static as well as functional analyses of discourse have been of several varieties. Some have been designed to examine discourse at the level of its overall organization, that of discourse genre; others are designed to examine more localized aspects of discourse structuring, such as those linguistic devices involved in discourse cohesion, discourse referencing, and inferencing. A review of how static and functional approaches affect the analysis of discourse genres and discourse referencing will reveal the differences between the two approaches to structural analysis.

Static studies of discourse genres have led to the finding that there are many genres of discourse and that each has a set of features that typify it. The genres most often studied are stories, lessons, conversations, and event descriptions. Methods for assessing children's understanding and production of static aspects of discourse genres have recently begun to appear in the research and clinical literature. For instance, researchers have asked children to repeat a given story and examined the relationship between the story features in the children's productions and those in the original story.[99] Other researchers have taken the features of prototypical stories as a standard and have looked to see whether the children's story formations contain the conventional features.[100]

Static analysis has also led to the discovery that exchange patterns in turn taking differ depending upon conversational rules peculiar to particular settings. For example, Mehan and others have found that a common exchange pattern occurring in classrooms is tripartite, beginning with a teacher initiation, followed by a student response, ending with a teacher evaluation.[101]

Functionalist approaches to studying discourse genre have led to the examination of how the genres differ in their communicative purposes. A functionalist perspective would lead to the conclusion that genres are organized differently so that they can best serve certain functions. Stories are organized to entertain; lessons to teach; conversations to socialize; and event descriptions to inform.

Analyses inclined to answering functionalist questions would view the exchange structure rules of classroom, which were discovered in the static analysis, as efficiency designs to achieve the goal of imparting information and managing discourse involving multiple participants. Besides seeking for the functions of classroom exchange structures, functionalists have looked for other patterns in classrooms that allow for better management such as the discourse rules, which have been found to prevent and control unwanted interruptions.[102,103]

Referencing is an area of discourse involving the organization of more localized meaning. Discourse referencing is what speakers do in order to let their listeners know what people, places, and events they are talking about. Static structural analysis has revealed that normal speakers mark new mentions of people, places, or events by using indefinite articles (e.g., a book) or by giving the necessary background information (e.g., "my friend, who lives in the Adirondacks"). Further, the structural research has shown that when speakers share information with their listeners, indicators or referents need not be as explicit as those that are not shared. A simple point of the finger to a designated object is sufficient for referencing when the object is within view of both speaker and listener, but the speaker may need to be much more specific when referring to a particular chair unknown to the listener ("a chair with blue stripes and Victorian in style").

A functionalist view of referencing has emerged from the theories of language comprehension developed in the 1980s by cognitive scientists as they study on-line processing by computers as well as adult listeners. The framework, dubbed "schema theory" by some, assumes that the listener is developing a cognitive model of what the speaker is saying and that each new piece of information serves to fill out or revise the previous model. Thus a listener who is informed at the outset of who the characters are and which ones are important forms a schema organized around those characters. When the speaker wants to add new information, it helps the listener to have it marked as new, or as significant, so that the listener knows he or she must build something new into the mental model. This keeps the listener from needlessly searching to find a previous reference when there is none. Shared referents whether they be known from previous shared experiences, or from the current context, need not be expressed as fully to the listener, since the listener already has the identifying knowledge handy in the activated model or readily retrievable from background knowledge. The "building mental models" theory of language comprehension accounts for why the language requires speakers to designate when things are being first mentioned and why shared information is less fully elaborated.[104]

Functionalist assessment approaches that focus on referencing failures have been devised. Referencing misfires are frequent, and they occur when listeners fail to understand or misunderstand what the speaker is referring to. The analysis identifying the locations of referencing failures, and then examining possible reasons for such failure, offers a potentially rich area for assessing language the functionalist way.[105]

The functionalist approach, in its speech act, fine tuning, and linguistic varieties bring with it new techniques for use in language assessment. The techniques tend to be ones that derive from static structuralism, building on an additional functional analysis either in the beginning of the analysis or at its end. The analysis may begin with a particular function in mind and then examine a sample for what structures serve that function. And so one might attempt to discover the linguistic structural categories used for requesting. Alternatively, the functional analyst may begin with a set of structures, say auxiliaries in English, and analyze what functions they serve.

An exquisite example of using structures to discover functions comes from a study by Gerhardt of children's discourse production.[106] She performed an indepth structural analysis of two types of talk of a child, Emmy, as the child progressed from 22 months to 24 months of age. Emmy often talked to herself before she went to sleep. When Gerhardt compared the language of the presleep monologues with Emmy's dialogues with her father, she found systematic differences. The monologues were descriptions of routine events and contained simple present tense, intransitive verbs, use of progressive "-ing" in sentences describing what she was currently doing. She referred to herself in the monologues as "Emmy" and "my" and frequently used temporal adverbials (now, not now) and conditional forms (maybe, when, then). But the dialogues with her father tended not to contain simple present tense or temporal adverbials and conditionals. They did contain frequent use of progressive "-ing" in concurrence with self-references of "I." Her references to herself in the dialogues tended to be as an active agent (e.g., "I'm sleeping here") as opposed to her using the patient (or object) role most often expressed in the monologues ("When Daddy come, then Daddy get Emmy").

Gerhardt summarized her findings by hypothesizing that Emmy takes two stances toward her discourse.[106] In the simple present discourse of the monologues, the stance is impersonal with Emmy assuming a decontextualized stance, outside the event. The content of the monologue discourse is to describe events as they ordinarily are done. These event descriptions are expressions of what Nelson and Gruendel have called "generalized event representations."[107] But in the dialogues Emmy was describing what Gerhardt sees as "structurally unstable events," which were not grounded in the way things ordinarily are, but instead are self-assertive challenges that are offered as a negotiation in need of outside information for resolution.

There are two bottom-line effects of functional analysis. One, it adds a step to doing structural analysis, thereby increasing the analysis time and adding to the problem of inefficiency. Second, if one can predict from the promising results of researchers such as Gerhardt, the cost of increased time is likely to be offset by the benefit of the insights gained. At this point, it certainly seems worth the try.

Problems and Advantages of Structural and Functional Assessment

The emergence of the structural analytic approach to doing language assessment in recent years has offered speech-language pathologists a means for understanding the linguistic, cognitive, and social regularities in communications of and with language impaired children. The approach has been criticized on a number of accounts. The most frequent criticisms from practising clinicians is the problem with time expenditure. The solution offered here is that clinicians abandon the attempt to analyze all areas that are analyzable and instead concentrate on those areas of analysis that seem to be most critical to the child's communication and of most concern to those who interact with that child.

A second problem, which is inherent in any structural assessment approach, is whether or not the discovered structures are psychologically real. It is the structuralist's version of the validity issue. For those doing structural analysis, the validity question has to do with whether or not the structures presumed to underly the regularities in the data analyzed are adequate representations of what the child actually uses in the course of communicating. In order to guard against incorrect representations of the child's knowledge, speech-language pathologists need to check repeatedly on the child's performance.

A problem of incompleteness raises its head for the structuralists when they become acquainted with the recent functionalist approaches to discourse analysis. The speech-language pathologist not only needs to search for structural regularities, but also must determine what purposes those structures serve. According to functionalists, without an investigation of function, the structural analysis is incomplete. The insights gained from functional analysis would suggest the criticism of the functionalists is valid, indicating that clinicians should whenever possible examine the functionality of the identified structures. The functional endeavor should not be aimed at finding a single function for a particular structure. Rather the attempt should be to find out how different structures can serve the same function; how different functions can be served by the same structure—even simultaneously; and how a variety of structures and functions work together in context.

Functionalism not only offers a useful framework for thinking about how to assess children's language, it also provides interesting insights for designing reports of assessments to fit different needs. It is to this last issue that I now turn.

THE PRAGMATICS OF REPORT WRITING

The extension of structural to functional analysis brings with it new insights into historical and current approaches to report writing. Traditionally, reports have been written as if the reader is naive about the circumstances of the report and does not know the child. The reports are written "for the record" and usually designed for whomever they may concern.[108] Because the reader is assumed to know little about the child, the report usually includes a brief introductory description of the child and a page or two about the child's family and medical, educational, and developmental history.

Traditionally, reports written "for the record" also have been intended to serve the function of answering a question about the child's level of performance in the different areas examined. Such a report works best for children who succeed on the tasks and who are found to be normal. However, it presents problems for those children who are found to be below normal. Perhaps intrinsic to the task of reporting negative results is that the report is framed to answer the question "what's wrong with this child's language?" in an attempt to justify the conclusion that the child has a problem. The question is posed in the negative, and thus leads to an answer that is cast in negative terms. The report, because of its negative function, ends up being one that documents what the child *cannot* do, focusing on deficits.

As a substitute for traditional reports, I propose that reports be tailored to their audience and with a purpose in mind. I recommend that the report writer assume a grounded perspective and write the report to a particular reader in light of that reader's background and in answer to that reader's immediate concerns. For instance, a report written to an adult familiar with the child, such as the child's parent or teacher, can be written as a direct response to the questions being asked and with the background knowledge of that person taken into account. Similarly, a report written to a physician or a psychologist would include more technical information and be designed to answer the referral question. Or if the assessment and the report is one for the speech-language pathologist's own recordkeeping, or as a log for "the clinical record," the content is more abbreviated and presumes more shared knowledge between the report writer and a future reader. Of course, all reports also reflect the perspective of the report writer in that they are a direct expression of the theoretical and historical frameworks assumed by the writer and are organized overtly or covertly to answer particular assessment questions.

I also recommend a break with tradition in what function reports are designed to serve. Rather than answering what is *wrong* with the child, reports can better serve the child when designed to tell a story about the child's communicative goals and frustrations. Oliver Sacks suggests that clinicians take as a model in their report writing the clinical reports of professionals in the 1800s such as Freud and Charcot, who wrote their results in the form of a story wherein the presenting symptoms are made sense of in light of the experiences of the client.[109] Sack's "stories" about his neurologically impaired patients offer a current model for how to organize clinical reports to convey the point of view of those experiencing the "symptoms."[110]

To gather information for "competence" rather than "deficit" reports, speech-language pathologists probably need to observe children in their everyday contexts and to analyze their performances for how successful the children might feel as they interact in those contexts. For example, the clinician might identify features of successful communicative attempts as well as when and why the child takes the interactive initiative. If the purpose of the assessment is to determine how well the context meets the child's learning needs, the report might feature the type and quality of scaffolding provided to the child and how that scaffolding fits with what the child already knows. A model for such an approach can be found in the ideas of Vygotsky and his recent followers, who attempt to determine the learning "zone" within which to offer the child to-be-learned information.[111–113]

Analysis from the child's perspective is likely to result in a report that focuses on what seems to be getting in the way of the child achieving his or her communicative attempts or of being successful. The recommendations might contain intervention suggestions for how not only to help the child learn those things that are blocks to his or her communication, but also to help those who interact with the child better tune to what the child is meaning and wanting.

Whatever perspective the assessment reports take, they will inevitably include the speech-language pathologist's framework and assessment questions. Clinicians of yore wrote reports that were medical in their orientation, focusing on answering questions of differential diagnosis.[18] Their counterparts in recent times are those clinicians working in medical settings or ones who are responding to medical referrals. Clinicians of the past as well as recent ones who are answering the normative question focus their reports on standardized test results and developmental age comparisons. Clinicians following the emerging procedures of structural analysis in the 1970s spend report space describing the child's language system or communication patterns. And those who follow the more recent focus on pragmatics and interactions may include in their report the results of an interaction analysis. Although the clinical reports are, by necessity, the result of the speech-language pathologists' Rorschachian views of the child, they can vary in the degree to which they admit another's perspective. The appeal being made here is that the report include three perspectives: that of the clinician, the child, and the audience for whom the report is intended.

SUMMARY

A speech-language pathologist who tries to assess children's language objectively and under controlled conditions is attempting the impossible. Assessments are by necessity highly complex endeavors containing as much information about the assessor and the children's social and interactive contexts as they do about the children themselves. Assessors bring to their assessment one or more theoretical frameworks, a set of tried and true assessment procedures, one or more questions to be answered, and they project these already held ideas onto their view of the child. The child becomes the assessor's inkblot to interpret, in light of the originally held frameworks, procedures, and questions.

The effort in this chapter has been to uncover some of the major ideas influencing different assessment approaches, to identify their theoretical and historical roots, and to indicate how they might work for or against the goal of obtaining a good picture of the child's communicative competence. I have favored a structural and functional analysis, which allows the speech-language pathologist to examine child's communication in an interactional and naturalistic context, and I have examined at length the possible pitfalls as well as the potential for this informal assessment approach.

Along the way, I have made a variety of recommendations for how to circumvent or solve the problems raised by different assessment approaches. I have recommended that the question about whether the child has a language problem be answered at the sociological or interactive level of analysis, by determining through observation and interviews what the child and those in the child's context take to be the problem. If formal test results are called for, I recommend administering one or two formal, well-standardized, culturally appropriate tests, rather than a group of tests in different areas of language competence. I recommended that the etiology question be de-emphasized as a guiding force in carrying out assessments and have suggested instead that it become a concern only when there appear to be medical or educational implications for discovering an original cause. I cautioned against the exclusive use of adult or child comparisons when carrying out structural and functional analysis because of the negative focus that comes with making those comparisons and because of the difficulty one may have of seeing around the a priori comparison categories. I suggested a few ways to evaluate the psychological reality of the discovered structures or functions.

In my discussion of the assessment report, I argued that the assessment results are often written "for the record" to an unknown reader about an unknown child. Although such a report might be the best form in some circumstances, it does not serve the purposes of many contexts. I made an appeal that speech-language pathologists tailor their reports to a particular audience, altering the amount of background information, the formality, and the recommendations accordingly. I have argued that the evaluation and the report be built on how the child understands the world so that they reflect a competence view of that child.

A historical perspective allows clinicians to see that assessments are not and cannot be objective views of children. They are biased views and should be evaluated accordingly. The bias expressed here was for a structural and functional approach to informal assessment, which (1) involves analyzing everyday interactions in which the child participates; (2) is done from the child's viewpoint; and (3) casts the findings in a competence frame.

REFERENCES

1. Travis L. Speech pathology. New York: D Appleton, 1931.
2. Carrow E. Test for auditory comprehension of language. Boston: Teaching Resources Corporation, 1973.
3. Lee L. Developmental sentence analysis. Evanston IL: Northwestern University Press, 1974.
4. McLean J, Snyder-McLean L. Social bases of language acquisition (Chapter 3). In: A transactional approach to early language training. Columbus, Ohio: CE Merrill, 1978.
5. Darwin C. A biographical sketch of an infant. Mind 1877; 2:285–294.
6. Kessen W. The child. New York: John Wiley and Sons, 1965.
7. Hall G. The contents of children's minds. Princeton Rev 1883; 59:249–272.
8. Senn M. Insights on the child development movement in the United States. Monogr Soc Res Child Dev 1975; 40:161.
9. Van Riper C. Speech correction: principles and methods. New York: Prentice-Hall, 1939.
10. Binet A, Simon T. The intelligence of imbeciles. English translation, 1909. Reprinted in: Significant contributions to the history of psychology. Series B. Vol IV. Washington, DC: University Publications of America, 1978.
11. Schultz D. A history of modern psychology. New York: Academic Press, 1981.
12. Siegel G, Broen P. Language assessment. In: Lloyd L, ed. Communication assessment and intervention strategies. Baltimore: University Park Press, 1976:73.
13. Fodor J. The modularity of mind. Cambridge: MIT Press, 1983.
14. Fillmore C, Kempler D, Wang W. Individual differences in language ability and language behavior. New York: Academic Press, 1979.
15. Paden E. History of the American speech and hearing association, 1925–1958. Washington, DC: American Speech and Hearing Association, 1970.
16. Emerick L, Hatten J. Diagnosis and evaluation in speech pathology. 2nd ed. Englewood Cliffs, NJ: Prentice-Hall, 1979.
17. Simon B. Mind and madness in ancient Greece: the classical roots of modern psychiatry. Cornell, NY: Cornell University Press, 1978.
18. Myklebust H. Auditory disorders in children: a manual for differential diagnosis. New York: Grune and Stratton, 1954.
19. American Psychiatric Association. Diagnostic and statistical manual of mental disorders. 3rd ed. Washington, DC: APA, 1980.
20. Duchan J. Special education for the nonhandicapped: how to interact with those who have communication problems. In: Knoblock P, ed. Special education. New York: Little, Brown, 1987: 163.
21. Prizant B, Duchan J. The functions of immediate echolalia in autistic children. J Speech Hear Disord 1981; 46:241–249.
22. Mercer J. Labeling the mentally retarded. Berkeley: University of California Press, 1973.
23. Knoblock P, ed. Special education. New York: Little, Brown, 1987.
24. Bloom L, Lahey M. Language development and language disorders. New York: John Wiley and Sons, 1978.
25. Tomblin J. Specific abilities approach: an evaluation and an alternative method. In: Perkins W, ed. Current therapy of communication disorders, 1983.
26. Fletcher H. Speech and hearing. New York: D Van Nostrand, 1929.
27. Travis L, Rasmus B. The speech sound discrimination ability of cases with functional disorders of articulation. Q J Speech Educ 1931; 17:217–226.
28. Tallal P. Rapid auditory processing in normal and disordered language development. J Speech Hear Res 1976; 19:561–571.
29. Butler K. Language processing: halfway up the down staircase. In: Wallach G, Butler K, eds. Language learning disabilities in school-age children. Baltimore: Williams and Wilkins, 1984.
30. Ebbinghaus H. On memory. Leipzig: Duncker and Humblot, 1885.
31. West R, Kennedy L, Carr A. The rehabilitation of speech. New York: Harpers, 1937.
32. Anderson V. Auditory memory span as tested by speech sounds. Am J Psychol 1939; 52:95–99.

33. Gardner H. The mind's new science: a history of the cognitive revolution. New York: Basic Books, 1985.
34. Demsey C. Selecting tests of auditory function in children. In: Lasky E, Katz J, eds. Central auditory processing disorders. Baltimore: University Park Press, 1983: 203.
35. Katz J, Illmer R. Auditory perception in children with learning disabilities. In: Katz J, ed. Handbook of clinical audiology. Baltimore: Williams and Wilkins, 1972.
36. Lund N, Duchan J. Assessing children's language in naturalistic contexts. 2nd ed. Englewood Cliffs, NJ: Prentice-Hall, 1988.
37. Eisenson J. Aphasia in children. New York: Harper and Row, 1972.
38. Duchan J, Katz J. Auditory and language processing: a synthesis. In: Lasky E, Katz J, eds. Central auditory disorders: problems of speech, language and learning. Baltimore: University Park Press, 1983.
39. Tallal P. Auditory processing disorders in children. In: Levinson P, Sloan C, eds. Auditory processing and language. New York: Grune and Stratton, 1980:81.
40. Rees N. Auditory processing factors in language disorders: the view from Procrustes' bed. J Speech Hear Disord 1976; 38:304–315.
41. Winitz H. Articulatory acquisition and behavior. New York: Appleton-Century-Crofts, 1969.
42. Kail R, Hale C, Leonard L, Nippold M. Lexical storage and retrieval in language impaired children. Appl Psycholinguist 1984; 5:37–49.
43. Masters G. Word-finding as categorization: comparisons of language learning disabled children, chronological aged peers and language age peers. Unpublished Grant Proposal to the American Speech and Hearing Foundation, 1986.
44. Itard J. The wild boy of Aveyron. 1894. Reprinted in 1962. Englewood Cliffs, NJ: Prentice-Hall.
45. Ryan W. Blaming the victim. New York: Pantheon, 1971.
46. Ginsberg H. The myth of the deprived child. Englewood Cliffs, NJ: Prentice-Hall, 1972.
47. Carrow E. A test using elicited imitation in assessing grammatical structure in children. J Speech Hear Disord 1968; 39:433–438.
48. Lee L. Northwestern syntax screening test. Evanston, IL: Northwestern University Press, 1971.
49. Halliday M. Explorations in the functions of language. London: Edward Arnold, 1973.
50. Tyack D, Gottsleben R. Language sampling analysis and training. Palo Alto, CA: Consulting Psychologists Press, 1974.
51. Miller J, Chapman R. Systematic analysis of language transcripts: users manual. Madison, WI: Language Analysis Laboratory, Waisman Center on Mental Retardation and Human Development, 1985.
52. Fisher H, Logemann J. The Fisher-Logemann test of articulation competence. Boston: Houghton Mifflin, 1971.
53. Goldman R, Fristoe M. Goldman-Fristoe test of articulation. Circle Pines, MN: American Guidance Service, 1972.
54. Brown R. A first language: the early stages. Cambridge: Harvard University Press, 1973.
55. Miller J. Assessing language production in children: experimental procedures. Baltimore: University Park Press, 1981.
56. Prutting C. Process /pr /ses/n/: the action of moving forward progressively from one point to another on the way to completion. J Speech Hear Disord 1979; 44:3–30.
57. Miller J, Chapman R, Branston M, Reichle J. Language comprehension in sensorimotor stages V and VI. J Speech Hear Res 1980; 23:284–312.
58. Ingram D. Phonological disability in children. London: Edward Arnold, 1976.
59. Saussure F. Course in general linguistics. 1st ed. 1915. Reissued New York: Philosophical Library, 1959.
60. Levi-Strauss C. Structural anthropology. New York: Basic Books, 1963.
61. Schegloff E, Sacks H. Opening up closings. Semiotica 8 1973; 289–327.
62. Schenkein J. Studies in the organization of conversational interaction. New York: Academic Press, 1978.
63. Piaget J. Structuralism. New York: Basic Books, 1970.
64. Fletcher P, Garman J, eds. Language acquisition. 2nd ed. London: Cambridge University Press, 1981.
65. Gallagher T. Revision behaviors in the speech of normal children developing language. J Speech Hear Res 1977; 20:303–18.
66. Gallagher T, Darnton B. Conversational aspects of the speech of language disordered children: revision behaviors. J Speech Hear Res 1978; 21:118–136.
67. Labov W, Fanshel D. Therapeutic discourse: psychotherapy as conversation. New York: Academic Press, 1977.
68. Sacks H, Shegloff E, Jefferson G. A simplest systematics for the organization of turn-taking for conversation. Language 1974; 50:696–735.
69. Bruner J. Early social interaction and language acquisition. In: Schaffer H, ed. Studies in mother-child interaction. New York: Academic Press, 1977:271.
70. Nelson K. Making sense, the acquisition of shared meaning. New York: Academic Press, 1985.
71. Schieffelin B. Getting it together: an ethnographic approach to the study of the development of communicative competence. In: Ochs E, Schieffelin B, eds. Developmental pragmatics. New York: Academic Press, 1979:73.
72. Pye C. Ouiche Mayan speech to children. J Child Lang 1986; 13:85–100.
73. Brice-Heath S. Ways with words: language, life and work in communities and classrooms. New York: Cambridge University Press, 1983.
74. Chomsky N. Aspects of the theory of syntax. Cambridge: MIT Press, 1965.
75. Lund N, Duchan J. Phonological analysis: a multifaceted approach. British J Dis Comm 1978; 13:119–226.
76. Bowerman M. Early syntactic development: a cross linguistic study with special reference to Finnish. New York: Cambridge University Press, 1973.
77. Bloom L. Language development: form and function in emerging grammars. Cambridge: MIT Press, 1970.
78. Schuler A. Echolalia: issues and clinical applications. J Speech Hear Disord 1979; 44:411–424.
79. Bates E, McWhinney B. A functionalist approach to the acquisition of grammar. In: Ochs E, Schieffelin B, eds. Developmental pragmatics. New York: Academic Press, 1979:167.
80. Dore J. Children's illocutionary acts. In: Freedle R, ed. Discourse relations: comprehension and production. Hillsdale, NJ: Erlbaum, 1976.
81. Beukelman D, Yorkston K. Communication interaction of adult communication augmentation system use. Top Lang Disord 1982; 2:39–54.
82. Chapman R. Exploring children's communicative intents. In: Miller J, ed. Assessing language production in children: experimental procedures. Baltimore: University Park Press, 1981:111.
83. Coggins T, Carpenter R. The communicative intention inventory: a system for observing and coding children's early intentional communication. Appl Psycholinguist 1981; 2:235–252.
84. Corsaro W. Sociolinguistic patterns in adult-child interaction. In: Ochs E, Schieffelin B, eds. Developmental pragmatics. New York: Academic Press, 1979:373.
85. Ellis R, Wells G. Enabling factors in adult-child discourse. First Lang 1980; 1:46–82.
86. Furrow D, Nelson K, Benedict H. Mothers' speech to children and syntactic development: some simple relationships.

J Child Lang 1979; 6:423–442.
87. Newport E. Motherese: the speech of mothers to young children. In: Castellan N, Pisoni D, Potts G, eds. Cognitive theory. Vol. 2. Hillsdale, NJ: Erlbaum, 1977:25.
88. Cross T. Mother's speech and its association with the rate of linguistic development in young children. In: Waterson N, Snow C, eds. The development of communication. New York: John Wiley and Sons, 1978:199.
89. Snow C. The development of conversation between mothers and babies. J Child Lang 1977; 4:1–22.
90. McDonald L, Pein D. Mother conversational behavior as a function of interactional intent. J Child Lang 1982; 9:337–358.
91. Olsen-Fulero L. Style and stability in mother conversational behavior: a study of individual differences. J Child Lang 1982; 9:543–564.
92. Kaye K, Charney R. Conversational asymmetry between mothers and children. J Child Lang 1981; 8:35–50.
93. Newport E, Gleitman L, Gleitman H. Mother, I'd rather do it myself: some effects and noneffects of maternal speech style. In: Snow C, Ferguson C, eds. Talking to children: language input and acquisitions. New York: Cambridge University Press, 1977:109.
94. Sonnenmeier R. Involving parents in the language intervention process. Masters Thesis, State University of New York, Buffalo, 1984.
95. Tiegerman E, Primavera L. Object manipulation: an interactional strategy with autistic children. J Autism Dev Disord 1981; 11:427–438.
96. Ninio A, Bruner J. The achievement and antecedents of labelling. J Child Lang 1978; 5:1–15.
97. Bruner J, Sherwood V. Early rule structure: the case of peekaboo. In: Harré R, ed. Life sentences. New York: John Wiley and Sons, 1976:55.
98. Murray L, Trevarthan C. The infant's role in mother-infant communications. J Child Lang 1986; 13:15–29.
99. Graybeal C. Memory for stories in language impaired children. Appl Psycholinguist 1981; 2:269–283.
100. Johnston J. Narratives: a new look at communication problems in older language disordered children. Lang Speech Hear Services Schools 1983; 13:144–155.
101. Mehan H. Learning lessons. Cambridge: Harvard University Press, 1979.
102. Eder D. Differences in communicative styles across ability groups. In: Wilkinson L, ed. Communicating in the classroom. New York: Academic Press, 1982.
103. Green J, Wallat C. Ethnography and language in educational settings. Norwood, NH: Ablex, 1981.
104. Johnson-Laird P. Mental models of meaning. In: Joshi A, Webber B, Sag I, eds. Elements of discourse understanding. New York: Cambridge University Press, 1981:106.
105. Liles B. Cohesion in the narratives of normal and language disordered children. J Speech Hear Res 1985; 28:123–133.
106. Gerhardt J. From discourse to semantics: the development of the verb morphology and forms of self-reference in the speech of a 2 year old. In: Nelson K, ed. Narratives in the crib, in press.
107. Nelson K, Gruendel J. Generalized event representations: basic building blocks of cognitive development. In: Brown A, Lamb M, eds. Advances in developmental psychology. Hillsdale, NJ: Erlbaum, 1981:131.
108. Pannbacker M. Diagnostic report writing. J Speech Hear Disord 1975; 40:367–379.
109. Sacks O. Tics. NY Rev Books 1987; 34:37–41.
110. Sacks O. The man who mistook his wife for a hat. New York: Summit Books, 1985.
111. Brown A, Ferrara R. Diagnosing zones of proximal development. In: Wertsch J, ed. Culture, communication, and cognition: Vygotskian perspectives. New York: Cambridge University Press, 1985:273.
112. Cazden C. Peekaboo as an instructional model: discourse development at home and at school. Papers and reports in child language development, Stanford: Stanford University, 1979; 19:1–29.
113. Vygotsky L. Thought and language. Kozulin A, ed. Revised edition. Boston: MIT Press, 1986.

13 Principles of Management and Remediation

M. N. Hegde, Ph.D.

This chapter consists of an overview of some basic principles and assumptions that govern the treatment of communicative disorders. I will be concerned mostly with a set of concepts and methods that apply across disorders of communication and individuals who exhibit them. The treatment of specific disorders is addressed in the respective chapters.

In communicative disorders, assumptions and principles of treatment have been influenced by different sources, the prominent being medicine, education, and behavioral science. Many of the pretreatment considerations relative to assessment or diagnostics have also been influenced by these disciplines.[1] The influence of the medical model is evident in the historical as well as extant philosophies of diagnostics, differential diagnostics, and treatment. An effective treatment of a disorder is thought to be contingent upon an accurate diagnosis of the disorder; treatment is thought to be most effective when the cause of a disorder is known and treatment procedures are specific to those causes.

The influence of education on treatment of communicative disorders has also been considerable mainly because of the public schools in which most speech-language pathologists provide their services. Most clinicians found that their task is to teach new skills and behaviors that the children did not possess. The clinicians have also found that it is often difficult to determine the causes of communicative disorders; therefore it is not possible to design treatment procedures based on differential etiologies. This has led to descriptive models of communicative disorders and their treatment. These models emphasize the task of describing various communicative behaviors the clients do or do not exhibit. An accurate and objective description of the communicative behaviors, or a lack thereof, provides a basis for designing intervention strategies.[2]

The applied behavioral analysis has brought behavioral science into the realm of communicative disorders. The operant model of the treatment of behavioral and developmental disorders showed that the disorders of communication are also susceptible to contingency manipulations. Because of its emphasis on the experimental method, the applied behavioral approach has been able to isolate the causes of communicative disorders that were unlike those implied in the medical model. Whereas the medical model encouraged the practitioners to look for the causes in the neurophysiologic structures and mechanisms of individuals with communicative disorders, the behavioral approach encouraged the practitioners to look for causes in the environment of those individuals. Thus the behavioral approach has led to experimental specification of the causes that typically maintain various disorders. This approach offered an alternative to the purely descriptive models. Descriptions are necessary and useful, but the clinician needs to go beyond descriptions. Clinicians seek to induce changes in the communicative behaviors of their clients and this task requires the manipulation of variables that induce those changes.[3]

Research on treatment has also been a factor in the evolution of some of the basic assumptions and practices. In recent years, the amount of treatment research has increased within the profession; and mainly because of this increase, clinicians are now able to identify some common parametric assumptions and treatment principles.

TREATMENT OF COMMUNICATIVE DISORDERS: SOME PARAMETRIC ASSUMPTIONS

It is impossible to specify a unifying philosophy of treatment that would not be controversial. In spite of an increase in the number of empirical studies on treatment, theoretic debates on the nature of the communicative behaviors and their disorders persist. Controversial theoretic positions are typically reflected in treatment philosophies. Nevertheless, it is possible to identify certain assumptions that affect various aspects of treatment of communicative disorders. These assumptions are based upon empirical observations; therefore, they may be described appropriately as parametric. Parametric assumptions to be described here are those that are based upon common clinical observations. These assumptions may or may not have been subjected to rigorous experimental tests. Regardless, they do seem to dictate certain clinical strategies and philosophic postures. It is possible to verify most of the parametric assumptions through experimental procedures.

Uniqueness and Commonalities of Individual Clients

An important parametric assumption concerns both the uniqueness and commonality of individuals who exhibit disorders of communication. However, such uniqueness and commonalities are not the special territory of communication or its disorders. It is the individuals who are unique while sharing certain common characteristics, and so the patterns of normal and disordered communication simply reflect the uniqueness and commonality of individuals who communicate with varying degrees of efficiency.[1,3]

The individual history is an important source of uniqueness of individuals. The clients who exhibit disordered communication are no exception. The individual history includes both the genetic and neurophysiologic contingencies on the one hand and the environmental contingencies on the other. The former include the genetic potentials and propensities along with the structural integrity of central and peripheral mechanisms involved in the production of speech. A normal central neural and oral-peripheral structure is necessary for the acquisition and maintenance of communicative behaviors.

What are considered normal structural patterns are not entirely homogeneous. Variations within a range are typical of normal patterns. Therefore, one needs to make a distinction between variations and deviations. All variations are not deviations. Variations are a source of uniqueness of individuals, whereas deviations may be one of the sources of clinical judgement that something is wrong and clinical intervention is warranted. Possibly subtle variations (not deviations) in neurophysiologic structures create certain unique patterns of speech and language production. It is well known that differing genetic histories are an important factor in creating unique individuals. Therefore, it is reasonable to assume that any uniqueness seen in communication and its disorders is partly a reflection of varying genetic histories of individuals as well.

The environmental contingencies that differ across individuals are another source of uniqueness of most behavioral patterns, including communication and its disorders. Varying contingencies include differing family and social interactions and the reactions of others that a speaker faces. Communication is a form of social behavior, shaped mostly by the social contingencies the individuals are exposed to. To a certain extent, both the variations and deviations in communication may be due to differing contingencies that are variable and/or deviant. Generally variable contingencies may be deviant in specific instances.

Uniqueness of individuals does not negate commonalities across individuals. This fact is also reflected in patterns of communication across individuals belonging to specific verbal communities. Similar social contingencies that prevail in particular verbal communities may create similar patterns of communication across individuals.

Both the uniqueness and commonalities of communicating individuals are significant considerations in treatment planning. Common treatment principles and unique aspects of treatment procedures stem from the basic uniqueness and commonalities of individuals who exhibit disorders of communication.

Diagnostic Categories

Whether diagnostic categories create a need for differential treatment procedures has been a controversial issue. That different disorders do create a need for different treatment procedures, and therefore the initial step in planning treatment for a client is to diagnose the disorder, is a logical extension of the medical model to communicative disorders. There is considerable emphasis on the differential diagnosis of various disorders of communication, especially those involving presumed or demonstrable organic disease. However, as noted before, the model has not necessarily worked well in the treatment of communicative disorders.

A review of treatment literature suggests that such diagnostic categories as language disorders and articulation disorders have not necessarily produced distinctly different treatment procedures.[3] Differential diagnosis of language disorders associated with "organic" versus "nonorganic" pathologies have also not produced unique treatment procedures. For example, the treatment procedures that help reduce the hypernasality of a child with a repaired cleft may not differ significantly from the procedures that help achieve the same goal in a hearing impaired client. The treatment procedures designed to teach specific language behaviors to a client with brain injury may not necessarily differ from those designed to teach the same targets to a client with no brain injury.

The main effect of successful differential diagnosis seems to be to set up different target behaviors for treatment. Diagnosis and differential diagnosis are typically a description and differential description of the behaviors of clients whose response topographies vary. For example, the description of the behaviors of a client with a voice disorder is different from the descriptions of a client with language disorders. The difference stems from the difference in the form of response being described: for example, a vocal response has a form different from the production of a grammatical feature.

Target behaviors that assume different forms do not necessarily require different treatment procedures. The procedures that are necessary to shape the correct production of a speech sound may be similar to those that are necessary to shape the production of a pronoun, a certain vocal pitch, or a fluent utterance. When we look not at the target behaviors, but at the procedures that shape them, we see more similarities than differences.

Manipulation of Relations as Against Structures

A parametric assumption inherent to most treatment procedures is that the clinicians manipulate relations but not structures. Direct manipulation of the genes that affect speech and language behaviors and disorders is obviously not possible. Some of the neurophysiologic conditions thought to create disorders of communication are also not manipulable. Brain injury, for example, is not directly manipulable. An organic condition such as a cleft palate is manipulable, but such manipulations are not the domain of speech-language pathologists. Furthermore, even after the organic manipulations are completed, some clients may need treatment for the still remaining disorder of communication. This treatment almost invariably involves the manipulation of certain relations.

In some respects, the treatment of communicative disorders is more abstract than a surgical repair of a cleft or removal of a tumor. This may be so because treatment in communicative disorders is a rearrangement of relations between the speaker and his or her environment. What is rearranged is an interactive relation between the speaker and the listening and reacting individuals. The contingencies of treatment are inherent to this abstract relation between speakers and listeners, who are often the same individuals playing different roles at different times. The speech-language clinician must manipulate those contingent events found in that relation. It is such a manipulation that alters the communicative behaviors of clients. Possibly, the listening and reacting individuals who enter into a contingent relation with the client are also changed in this process.

A contingent relation is a set of interdependent events. Like all kinds of behaviors, the communicative behaviors have their antecedents and consequences. These antecedents and consequences, for the most part and under most typical circumstances, are environmental events. It is the same as saying that people, events, and objects of the world of the speaker serve as stimuli for speech and that once speech is produced, consequences in the form of listener reactions are likely to follow. The antecedents of speech, the speech itself, and the listener responses are inexorably interrelated to form contingent relations whose essence is social communication.

The concept of the social contingency as a determinant of communicative behaviors has important consequences for the treatment of communicative disorders. The clinician selects certain communicative behaviors or characteristics as the target of clinical intervention. Then, specific antecedent conditions that set the stage for various communicative behaviors are arranged. Certain differential consequent events are then programmed for the speaker's responses, lack of responses, and inadequate or incorrect responses. While doing this, the clinician maintains a strict relation between the events that trigger the behavior, the behavior itself, and its consequences.

The neurophysiologic and genetic contingencies, though not directly manipulated by the speech-language clinician, are important in understanding the full scope of treatment. Those contingencies often serve as background variables that influence the speed or extent of learning on the part of a client. They may limit the extent of communicative behavioral improvement. In this sense, the organic and environmental contingencies interact to produce the communicative behaviors that are shaped under the influence of the treatment contingency.

Sometimes the criticism that they either ignore the influence of organic variables or assume that those variables are unimportant is levied at clinicians who focus on abstract relations. This criticism is not valid because the clinician necessarily concentrates on what he or she can and is expected to manipulate for reasons of professional training as well as legal mandate. The clinician fully realizes that contingencies not under his or her control are also important. It is fully understood that the normal or clinically shaped communicative behaviors are a product of an interaction between the organic and environmental contingencies.

Principles Versus Procedures of Treatment

Historically, treatment of various disorders of communication has been specific to the disorder. Divergent treatment procedures were used in the treatment of different disorders. There was no consistent philosophy or a conceptual approach that placed these various treatment procedures in a single perspective. Though single perspectives tend to be more or less controversial, treatment research and practice have shown that certain basic treatment principles and treatment procedures can be formulated. The distinction between treatment principles and procedures is useful in understanding the generic (common) as well as specific (unique) variables involved in the treatment of communicative disorders.

Variables that create uniqueness and commonalities across individuals give rise to treatment principles that are common and procedures that may be unique to those exhibiting disordered communication. As suggested before, the necessity for treatment procedures specific to the client stems more from the unique individual histories of clients than from the differential diagnostic categories. Clients exhibiting the same disorder may differ widely in their response to the same treatment procedure. In such cases, the clinician assumes that the unique individual histories are interacting with the treatment variables to produce the differing outcomes across individual clients.

Treatment principles are abstract statements about certain empirical relations that have been systematically investigated and found to be reliable and valid. Ideally, treatment principles are based upon experimentally verified evidence with a certain degree of demonstrated generality. Principles are broad in scope, conceptual in nature, and few in number. They are empirical rules that state that, under specified conditions, certain relations between communicative behaviors, their antecedents, and their consequences can be observed. In that sense, principles have predictive force.[3]

There have been many models of treatment in communicative disorders, but a number of them have been speculative. Many treatment models are supported only logically, not empirically. Most of the few treatment studies that were made within some of these models have been uncontrolled case studies. The behavioral approach, on the other hand, has consistently encouraged experimental treatment research. Behavioral treatment research demonstrated that a variety of response-contingent consequences can typically have predictable effects upon language, articulation, fluency, and voice behaviors and disorders.[3–15] Certain response-contingent consequences can increase the communicative behaviors upon which they are made contingent. This is the principle of reinforcement. Response-contingent presentations that increase a rate of response are known as positive reinforcers, whereas response-contingent presentations that terminate events that increase responses are known as negative reinforcers. Certain other response-contingent consequences decrease the rate of behaviors, giving rise to the principle of punishment. A response that is allowed to be made in the absence of reinforcers eventually decreases in frequency. This is the principle of extinction.

When these consequences are delivered under characteristic stimulus conditions, the stimulus conditions themselves acquire some power to either increase or decrease the rate of specified responses. The physical objects, pictures, modeling, and such other stimuli used to evoke the target responses may gain some control over them. In addition, the clinician and the physical setting in which the responses are taught may also influence the production of those behaviors. These observations have led to the formulation of the principle of stimulus control.

There are other treatment principles that have also received a certain degree of experimental support. For example, the rates of two responses can be affected differentially by arranging contrasting consequences. While increasing a desirable target response, a concomitant undesirable behavior may be decreased. This is the principle of differential reinforcement. Responses learned in one physical setting can be produced in a different setting, in relation to different stimuli, and in the presence of different audiences. This illustrates the principle of generalization. Many of these principles have been found to be applicable across both typical and disordered communicative behaviors.

Treatment principles have generality in that they are applicable across disorders and clients. Principles are general rules that work because individuals, in spite of their uniqueness, are equally susceptible to environmental manipulations of one kind or the other. In other words, the principles of positive reinforcement, punishment, discrimination, and differential reinforcement hold good regardless of the variable individual histories and diagnostic categories of their disorders.

But treatment procedures are specific technical operations derived from treatment principles. A procedure or a set of procedures is derived for a particular client. The uniqueness of the individual client typically plays a large role in the selection of treatment procedures. Therefore, treatment procedures are specific to the client, whereas principles are of general scope. And, as well, treatment procedures are operational, whereas the principles are abstract statements. A treatment procedure is stated in measurable terms so that it can be replicated by other clinicians.

Compared to the principles, treatment procedures are many, concrete, and of narrower scope. Many specific treatment procedures may be derived from a single treatment principle. For example, the principle of positive reinforcement has several specific procedures including primary reinforcers, secondary reinforcers, conditioned generalized reinforcers, high probability behaviors, and informative feedback.[16,17] Similarly, the principle of punishment has a number of procedures including response-contingent presentation of aversive stimuli, response-contingent withdrawal of reinforcement, and response-contingent imposition of work.[18,19]

Varied procedures within a limited number of principles make it possible to design treatment procedures that suit individual clients; that is, a principle allows a clinician to be flexible within certain limits. When a particular positive reinforcer (a procedure) does not work with a client, another reinforcer may be selected. When a certain stimulus, which is a known punisher, does not decrease the rate of an undesirable response in a given client, the clinician can switch to another stimulus that may be more effective. In this way, the clinician can always keep in perspective the unique response patterns of given clients and so design treatment procedures that have desirable effects on those unique patterns.

THE TREATMENT PROCESS: AN OVERVIEW

The process of treating a disorder of communication begins with the assessment of the client's communicative behaviors. The issue of assessment has been addressed by Duchan in Chapter 12. In this chapter, I will be concerned with assessment as it relates to some substantive pretreatment considerations.

Some Pretreatment Considerations

Earlier we noted that traditionally, a *diagnosis* of the disorder has been considered a precursor to treatment. However, the typical inability of the speech-language clinician to find the cause or causes of disorders of speech and language has forced a newer concept of *assessment*. Therefore, prior to the treatment, the communicative behaviors are assessed, not necessarily diagnosed.

Although assessment philosophies vary across clinicians, certain fundamental operations are a part of any assessment strategy. One of the basic aspects of assessment is the measurement of the client's target behaviors. This measurement must be reliable and, as much as possible, comprehensive. Most assessment procedures depend upon standardized tests to sample the communicative behaviors of clients seeking professional advice. However, standardized tests have several problems that make them inadequate as measurement devices.

First, standardized tests do not sample the behaviors adequately. The tests may have been "standardized" on a large sample of subjects, but the behaviors themselves are sampled inadequately. For example, a test of morphologic use may give a child one or two opportunities to produce a particular grammatical morpheme. On the basis of such limited response sampling, clinicians are expected to draw conclusions about the presence or the absence of most communicative behaviors, including the production of various grammatical, semantic, and pragmatic structures and the production of speech sounds.

Second, standardized tests give categorical answers to questions about communication patterns of given clients. A clinically more desirable and technically valid answer is quantitative, not categorical. In many cases, grammatical features or correct production of speech sounds are present at certain levels that may be inadequate, but a standardized test can give no discriminatory information about this. The behavior is either present or absent according to a test. However, when the same behavior is sampled adequately by giving multiple opportunities to produce it, the clinician may find that the behavior is present at an undesirably low level of frequency. Repeated sampling of a communicative behavior often gives a more reliable quantitative picture than do standardized tests that tend to produce yes or no answers. When behaviors are measured adequately, the rate varies from 0 to 100 percent, and the digital value of 0 or 1 is often an artifact of inadequate measurement.

Third, standardized tests give limited information about client-specific reliability. A given test may have been demonstrated to be reliable when repeatedly administered to a sample of subjects. However, there is no assurance that a given client will score similarly on a readministration of a standardized test. Therefore, the clinician cannot assume that a test known to be reliable in a sample of subjects also yields reliable results in individual clients. Reliability is data-specific. It must be demonstrated in the particular measures. The particular measure is that of the client's behavior. The only way to show that a given client's measures of communicative behaviors are reliable is to repeat the measurement. In short, the clinician must make sure that the behaviors are sampled adequately and that they are measured repeatedly.

But a thorough measurement of all aspects of a client's communication before starting the treatment is time-consuming and often impractical. The typical assessment gives the clinician enough information to select potential target behaviors that may be measured more thoroughly before initiating treatment. Such a pretreatment measurement of selected target behaviors is known as baseline measurements. Unlike standardized tests, the baselines fulfill the criteria of adequate response sampling and reliability.

Baseline Procedures

Baselines are pretreatment measures, but they are established after the initial assessment. Therefore, baselines are more appropriately considered a part of the treatment process. Baselines are measures of target behaviors in the absence of the planned intervention. Reliable baselines give a stable picture of the communicative behaviors of which the client is capable.

Baselines are needed for several reasons. First, they help establish the need for clinical services more adequately than the typical assessment results. A client who produces various elements of language at less than chance levels, or does not produce them at all, is obviously in need of clinical services. Clients whose repeatedly measured dysfluency rates or vocal pitches are too high need intervention. A child whose correct articulation of selected speech sounds is only 10 percent indicates a similar need. In essence, baselines are quantitative demonstrations of the need for treatment.

Second, baselines give a stable base against which the effects of various treatment procedures are evaluated. When the purpose is to evaluate experimentally the effects of a given treatment procedure, the clinician must establish a stable baseline of the target behaviors, which might then show a dramatic and convincing change when the treatment is introduced. The treatment may then be withdrawn to show that the behavior returned to the original baseline or approximated it. Next, the treatment may be reinstituted and continued until the client achieves a dismissal criterion. Without a stable pretreatment measure of the target behavior, it would be difficult to show that the treatment was indeed effective.

Third, baselines are needed even when the clinician simply wishes to show that the client improved under treatment. This is the question of clinician accountability: clinicians must document that their client's communicative behaviors did change while under treatment. This would be possible only when pretreatment measures of behaviors are relatively stable and a clear change in the expected direction is shown by the client's communicative behaviors. The clinician would not withdraw treatment to return the client to the baseline level even for a brief duration. In this case, the clinician would not claim effectiveness for the treatment. To claim effectiveness, the clinician must rule out such extraneous variables as history and maturation. The influence of extraneous variables is ruled out by various control measures, which include treatment withdrawal or a no-treatment control group.

Baselines are established in all of the relevant response modes. In clients with limited speech-language behaviors, the clinician might establish the baseline of imitated productions of target behaviors. Attempts may also be made to evoke target behaviors in the absence of imitation. Clients who have more advanced speech-language behaviors may be asked to imitate as well as spontaneously produce isolated target behaviors. Target behaviors may be baserated in oral reading and in conversational speech.

The discrete trial procedure is often used in establishment of the baselines of isolated target behaviors. The production of a grammatical morpheme or a speech sound at the word level may thus be baserated on discrete trials, each trial giving the client an opportunity to produce the selected response. The clinician would model the target responses when imitations are expected and avoid modeling when the responses are evoked. Whenever appropriate, the baselines of the target behaviors must be established in conversational speech.

Baselines must be repeated to establish a trend. In cases of dysfluencies and vocal characteristics, repeated samples of conversational speech and/or oral reading may be obtained. If dysfluencies or the selected vocal characteristics show a relatively consistent rate across the measures, the treatment may be instituted. In cases of language and articulation, multiple opportunities given for the production of each target behavior may be considered adequate unless the data indicate otherwise. For example, the baseline for production of the preposition "on" may be established in the context of 20 utterances, each presented on a set of modeled and evoked trials.

In the discrete trial procedure, a relevant stimulus such as a picture or an object is first presented to the client. The clinician then asks a predetermined question designed to (eventually) evoke the response from the client. Immediately, the correct response is modeled for the client to imitate it. The response is then recorded on a recording sheet. With a brief pause, to suggest that the trial is over, the clinician then initiates the next trial. The procedure would be the same for an evoked trial except that, after asking the question, the clinician would not model the correct response. Each target may be once modeled and once evoked.

Preparation of the stimulus material for baselines takes some careful planning. Pictures, objects, questions, and various conversational devices are all stimuli for speech. Depending upon the verbal skills of the client, manipulation of such concrete stimuli as pictures and objects may or may not be needed. When concrete stimuli are manipulated, the level of the client's verbal skills would determine the extent of such manipulations. Generally, clients with language and articulation disorders need more concrete stimulus manipulations than do clients with fluency and voice problems. The clients with the latter types of problems are usually able to produce conversational speech, which is probably the best response mode for establishing baselines.

Baseline data are analyzed for the percent target response rate. The number of trials on which the target behavior is produced and the total number of trials that were given help determine the percent target response rate of most isolated target behaviors. When the behaviors are baserated in conversational speech, the number of target behaviors and the total number of words or syllables spoken help determine the percentage at which those behaviors are produced by a client. This procedure can help establish baselines of such behaviors as dysfluencies or pitch breaks observed in conversational speech.

Principles of Response Selection and Specification

Most clients with disorders of communication need to learn multiple target behaviors. Whether or not the client has a disorder of articulation, language, voice, or fluency, often he or she is not able to produce a variety of behaviors and skills; and the clinician is not typically able to focus on an unlimited number of target responses, especially during the early stages of treatment. Therefore, the clinician faces the question of target behavior selection early in treatment planning.

The issue of target behavior selection is compounded by theories of speech and language behaviors. Different theories dictate different target behaviors. For example, theories of articulation and phonology have suggested somewhat different tactics of response selection in articulation training. Changing theoretic perspectives in the study of language have resulted in such divergent target responses as simple vocabulary, specific grammatical features, rules of transformational grammar, semantic notions, and pragmatic structures. In the treatment for stuttering, such varied targets as resolution of psychosexual conflicts, reduction in anxiety, increase in self-confidence, and a mastery of various skills of fluency have all been advocated. In different theoretic eras, clinicians have new targets for clients of the same diagnostic category. Different theories can be simultaneously active, in which case clinicians typically select target behaviors within the scope of the theories they subscribe to.

Evaluation of the impact of theories on the response selection process is outside the scope of this chapter. I will therefore take a more practical approach to the issue of response selection. From a practical standpoint, selected responses must be empirically valid, objectively measurable, and relevant to the individual client.

Empirical Validity of Target Behaviors

Communicative target behaviors are often selected on the basis of linguistic categories. This is especially true of target behaviors selected for treatment of language and articulation disorders. For example, in language disorders, single words, two-word phrases, and sentences may be selected as targets of clinical intervention. Different morphologic features including the production of "ing," plural /s/ in words, or the preposition "on" illustrate linguistic categories often selected as target behaviors. Such targets as the production of /s/ or /t/ in words illustrate articulatory targets based on linguistic categories of phonemic forms. Clinicians usually assume that different linguistic categories are different targets, whereas behaviors grouped under the same linguistic category are a single target.

Linguistic categories are based on the logic and theory of linguistics. The categories are also often based on the form of responses, although this is not always the case. The categories of words, phrases, and sentences are based purely on form. However, the single grammatical category of regular plural contains different forms known as the allomorphic variations. Yet verbal auxiliary ("is" and "are," for example) and copula ("is" and "are") are considered different categories even though they are the same topographically. Semantic categories and pragmatic structures are also based on theoretic grounds. Responses of various forms may be grouped as nomination (a semantic category) or request (a pragmatic structure).

Categories based purely on structure, logic, or empirically insensitive theories may or may not be valid. Linguistic theories of grammar and meaning have not been especially tuned to empirical data. They are logical theories whose terms are not always related to empirical observations. The structure of a sentence and the grammatical functions of words can be determined on logical grounds. Most linguists of the Chomskyan school have analyzed grammar and its transformations with little regard to empirical data.

But clinical operations are empirical in the sense that the clinician is in touch with communicative behaviors of individuals in everyday situations. Some of the clinical treatment research in language has shown that behaviors categorized purely on the basis of nonempirical theories and the logic of linguistics may or may not be valid. However, a clinician going strictly by linguistic theories of language may assume that the number of linguistic categories missing in a client's speech is also the number of target behaviors that must be taught. Unfortunately, that assumption can be an empirical mistake in clinical treatment. For example, the irregular plural is a single grammatical category, but it consists of as many separate target behaviors as there are irregular plural words in the English language. There is no generalization from the learning of a few irregular plural words to others not taught.[20] On the contrary, verbal auxiliary and copula are considered separate linguistically, but the clinical evidence suggests that they are the same.[21,22] Teaching one of them is sufficient to generate the correct production of both of them. Similarly, subject noun and object noun phrases are considered separate linguistic categories, but they are the same behaviors.[23] The regular plural may be a single grammatical category, but the allomorphic variations are separate targets to be taught separately.[8]

It is not known whether semantic and pragmatic categories are empirically valid behaviors that the clinician can teach according to the logical schemes presented by many theoreticians. Clinical research into whether or not they are indeed different behaviors has barely begun. However, it is clear that an empirically valid taxonomy of semantic and pragmatic behaviors will not emerge until the effects of teaching one category are experimentally evaluated on other category or categories.

Responses that are empirically related form a class, and responses within a class share similar antecedents and consequences; they can be taught by the same set of antecedents and consequences. All members of a response class need not be taught separately. When clinicians teach some of the responses belonging to a class, the other responses may be produced on the basis of generalization. Such generalized productions may be reinforced to make them last. For example, a client with a language disorder who is taught to produce six to eight phrases or sentences containing "ing" may begin to produce many new phrases and sentences in which the "ing" is appropriately used. Such generalized productions are not observed across response classes. In other words, the client who learns to produce "ing" will not begin to produce the plural /s/ without specific training. In this sense, the "ing" and the plural /s/ belong to different and discriminated response classes.

Clinicians need to know what are empirically valid response classes to determine the target behaviors for their clients. The concept of response class is clinically relevant and theoretically neutral. Any target behavior is acceptable as long as it is empirically valid. Clinicians can teach behaviors that are real, but cannot teach those that exist only in theory. If semantic and pragmatic structures are discriminated response classes with appropriate generalized responding within the classes, then they could serve as target behaviors. If phonologic processes are also empirical response classes, they too can be taught the way the phonologic theories propose. What is needed, however, is not just categorizations, but clinical and experimental evidence that shows that theoretic categories correspond to observable and measurable responses that can be taught by clinicians.

Objective Measurement of Target Behaviors

The target behaviors selected for treatment may be simply described or objectively measured. Historically, clinicians simply described what, in their judgement, was taught to their clients. Such descriptions as grammatical competence, articulatory performance, and self-confidence in speaking were considered enough in terms of target behavior specifications. But in recent years the need to measure objectively target behaviors has become apparent for scientific, legal, and professional reasons.

Subjective descriptions of target behaviors make it difficult to document the effects of treatment or the improvement shown by clients. The tradition of scientific practice requires that the treatment effects or client improvement be documented objectively. Public law 94–142 requires that the need for services provided in the public school setting and the general effectiveness of those services be documented. Various third-party payment plans also require objective determination of the need for, and the client progress under, treatment. Therefore, it is now necessary to define target behaviors such that they can be measured objectively before, during, and after treatment. And objective measurement of target behaviors requires a certain way of conceptualizing those behaviors.

First, direct measures of a behavior are more objective than indirect measures. For example, various questionnaire measures of attitudes and opinions are an indirect measure of the behaviors that they are supposed to measure. A clinician can measure a stutterer's "negative attitude" toward telephones on a questionnaire or ask the stutterer to keep a log of the number of times the incoming telephone calls were answered by him or her. The former is at best an indirect measure of the stutterer's problem with the telephone, whereas the latter is a direct measure of it.

Second, observable behaviors are more easily measured than unobservable behaviors. Therefore, the clinical targets are better described in terms of observable actions on the part of clients. Inferred entities within the mind or the brain of the client are not measurable, but, fortunately they are often inferred from some form of observable behaviors. In such cases, the observable behaviors themselves can be considered the clinical targets. For example, in the case of a client with a language disorder, the production of responses of certain classes are observable targets, whereas the inferred "linguistic competence" is not. In the case of a stuttering client, "increased confidence in speaking" is an inferred target, whereas a fluent speech rate of 98 percent is observable.

Third, target behaviors defined in operational terms are more easily measured than those that are defined in constituent terms. An operational definition describes a variable in measurable terms. Such a definition is often a description of the procedures involved in measuring the variable. For instance, a clinical target for a client with an articulation disorder may be defined as "improved articulation" or the "correct production of /s/ in 50 sentences produced during two consecutive samples of conversational speech at 90 percent accuracy." The former does not tell how to measure the target behavior, but the latter does. The example also illustrates one of the limitations of operational definitions: responses of narrow scope and specificity can be defined adequately, but broad and abstract concepts are difficult to define operationally.

Observable behaviors, defined operationally and measured directly, enhance the clinician's accountability. From the standpoint of clinical work and research, they help document the treatment effectiveness and/or client improvement.

Relevancy of Target Behaviors

Most if not all communicative behaviors have some relevancy to the client whose communication is disordered. Nonetheless, various communicative behaviors are more or less relevant to particular clients. In the process of selecting target behaviors, clinicians need to consider the relevancy of behaviors that the client will acquire.

Clinicians have selected target behaviors mostly on the basis of the normative information.[3,9] This is especially true of language and articulation disorders. The normal sequence in which children learn various aspects of speech and language is considered the standard. If there is a deviation from this standard, a disorder is usually diagnosed. The behaviors that are missing when compared to the standard are considered targets of clinical intervention. The normative approach further assumes that the target behaviors selected on the basis of norms should be taught in the same normative sequence.

The normative approach to target behavior selection is based upon the assumption that there are known normative sequences that hold good in individual clients and that the normal sequence in which the behaviors are acquired is the best sequence with which to teach those behaviors. Unfortunately, neither of these assumptions is based upon empirical evidence. The normative sequences described in the literature on speech and language development are variable across individuals—individual variations are a rule, not an exception. Normative sequences are nothing more than some broad patterns of behavioral acquisition seen in a large number of children when they are grouped under relatively large age ranges and their individual responses are averaged to mask individual differences. Consequently, those sequences are not necessarily predictive of a sequence of an individual child. Therefore, in the selection of target behaviors, normative sequences are not as helpful as they are generally thought to be.

Whether treatment should follow the normative sequence or not is a moot question when the validity and usefulness of such sequences are not assumed. Nevertheless, from a practical standpoint, clinicians can assume that such sequences do exist and then evaluate their relevance to the treatment process. It is the implicit assumption of the normative philosophy that the sequence presumably found in the normative research is the most efficient sequence to use in clinical intervention also. Unfortunately, there is no evidence that shows that the clinical intervention that follows normative sequences promotes faster learning, better generalization to the natural environment, or longer maintenance. There are a number of clinical research studies in which the sequence used was not necessarily normative.[3] No particular difficulty in teaching behaviors out of their normative sequence has been reported. In addition, Capelli[24] and De Cesari[25] have shown that normally developing children can be taught selected grammatical morphemes ahead of Brown's stages[26] and in an order that reverses Brown's rankings.

An alternative to the normative approach to target behavior selection is known as the client-specific strategy.[3,9] Within this strategy, the behaviors are selected on the basis of their relevance to the individual clients. Many of the targets thus selected may be appropriate for normative strategy as well. However, the major emphases within the client-specific strategy are the kinds of communicative demands made upon the client and the kinds of behaviors that would make the client verbally most adaptive to his or her environment. Selected behaviors, therefore, bear a special relevance to the individual client and not exclusively to the norms.

The client-specific strategy assumes that communicatively handicapped individuals cannot simply be thought of as those who are simply younger as indexed by their existing speech and language behaviors. An aphasic person's or mentally retarded adult's speech and language abilities may be comparable to those of a 10-year-old normal child, but neither the aphasic nor the retarded adult is comparable to a normal 10-year-old child. In selecting appropriate target behaviors for these two clients, clinicians need to consider the environmental demands faced by them. Behaviors that are appropriate for an aphasic person staying at home may be different from those that are appropriate for a retarded adult working in a sheltered workshop. The two sets of target behaviors may or may not be predicted by the "norms" of 10-year-old children.

The client-specific strategy further suggests that when behaviors are selected on the basis of the client's verbal environment, the client becomes verbally more adaptive and efficient. A 15-year-old child with a language handicap in a special educational program faces different demands from those in a similar child in a special jobs training program. Target behaviors selected specifically to suit a client's environment make the client a more effective communicator. Such client-relevant behaviors are also more likely to be produced by the client in his or her natural environment, and this will presumably promote better generalization and maintenance.

Stimulus Control in Treatment

The selection of target behaviors leads to a consideration of stimulus variables that constitute a part of the treatment process. Many speech-language behaviors are under the direct control of stimuli in the environment. It is common knowledge that people talk about things, events, and persons in their environment. At the same time, it must be recognized that everyday speech-language behaviors are not always under the control of physical and concrete stimuli. Two persons who engage in conversational speech are not always and necessarily reacting to sensory stimuli generated by physical environmental events. Instead, much of their conversational speech may be a response to their own speech because speech itself is stimulus for more speech. Such a control exerted by prior speech on subsequent speech is known as intraverbal control. Intraverbal control frees speech from the necessity for constant and concrete stimulus control.

In the language disordered, both the concrete stimulus control and the intraverbal control may be weak. Consequently, the quantity and quality of speech exhibited by the communicatively handicapped tend to be limited. For this and other reasons, many communicatively handicapped, especially those with language and articulation disorders, need specific and concrete stimulus manipulations during the early stages of treatment. After a significant amount of speech and language behaviors has been taught to a client, the clinician may be able to focus more upon intraverbal control, which is inherent to conversational speech. In either case, the task of the clinician is to create stimulus controls that do not exist for given clients.

Most clinicians find it necessary to use such concrete stimuli as pictures and objects especially during the early stages of treatment. This necessity is especially evident in young clients. Concrete stimuli are used to evoke single-word responses or short phrases from young children who show language, articulation, fluency, and voice problems. Subsequently, sentence productions may also be evoked with the help of concrete stimuli. With adult clients with voice and fluency problems, topic cards may be used to stimulate continuous speech. In most cases, pictures and objects are faded in later stages of treatment so that the target behaviors would come under the control of more natural stimuli, including speech from other persons and intraverbal stimuli.

Besides pictures and objects, most clinicians find it necessary to use other, even more special, stimuli to evoke the target responses in the early stages of treatment. These special stimuli include modeling, instructions, prompts, and manual guidance.[3,7,15,16]

In modeling, the clinician first asks the relevant question to evoke the target response and then immediately produces the response for the client to imitate. Imitation is a response that immediately follows a stimulus and matches its topography. Initially, the client may be reinforced even when the imitated response topography does not closely match the modeled stimulus. Eventually, more and more exact matching may be required to earn reinforcers. This process can lead to a progressive refinement of the client response topography.

Instructions on how to produce specific target responses have always been a part of clinical intervention. Many clients need instructions on how to produce given speech sounds, reduce speech rates, monitor airflow, modify vocal qualities, or use the esophageal mechanism for speech. Instructions are typically combined with modeling. This combination tells the client how to produce a target response and then shows how that response is produced. Nonetheless, the role of instructions has not been adequately researched by means of controlled experimental procedures.

Prompts are special stimuli that work like hints of everyday life. When certain target behaviors have become more likely in the presence of a modeled stimulus, the clinician may stop modeling to see if the response occurs. If it does not, the clinician may prompt that response with only a partial modeling of the correct response. For example, a child who has been taught to imitate "The girl is smil*ing*" may be shown the relevant picture, asked the question ("What is the girl doing?") and then prompted by saying "The girl is . . . ." Such prompts are often able to evoke a response when it is not readily forthcoming. In progressive steps, the extent of a prompt may be reduced and eventually eliminated.

When a client's behavior does not come under the control of a modeled stimulus, clinicians sometimes use manual guidance, which is also a form of stimulus control. The lips of a retarded person may be manually shaped into an articulatory posture to facilitate the production of a particular speech sound, or a client's hand may be physically moved by the clinician to touch a target picture or object in response to a verbal request. Such physical assistance in the execution of a response may be needed for those who would not otherwise respond to questions, requests, and modeled stimuli.

In the final stages of treatment, special stimulus manipulations must be kept to a minimum. More natural stimuli, such as events, objects, questions, requests, and other conversational devices, must control the production of target communicative behaviors. Modeling, prompts, instructions, and manual guidance must therefore be faded while the stimulus control is transferred to more natural stimuli that evoke speech in everyday life.

Management of Treatment Contingencies

As noted before, treatment consists of a strict management of the relation between certain events that are often created by the clinician. The stimulus variables of modeling, prompts, instructions, and manual guidance along with pictures and objects set the stage for the target behaviors. The clinician then evokes the imitative responses of the selected behavioral response class. However, the outcomes of these stimulus operations may be varied, though they are generally predictable. The variations of the effects of the stimulus manipulations create the need for varied response-contingent consequences to be arranged for by the clinician.

When the clinician sets the stage for the production of a target response, the client may respond appropriately, respond in the right direction but not fully correctly, or may respond totally incorrectly. An extreme but not an unusual occurrence is a client's total lack of response. As well, the client may give an irrelevant and interfering response in place of the requested appropriate response. An effective clinician knows these different response possibilities and is capable of arranging different consequences for them.

One of the early decisions the clinician must make is the acceptability of responses, especially during the initial stages of treatment. Whether imitative or evoked, responses during the early stages of treatment may not be fully accurate. A child's imitative production of modeled speech sounds, an aphasic individual's production of a three-word phrase, a stutterer's speech at reduced rate, or a voice client's imitation of a target pitch may fall short of the expected accuracy and topographic precision. Typically, most clinicians accept productions that show movement in the right direction. In gradual steps, the acceptability criterion is raised so that the desirable topographic precision of target responses is achieved eventually.

Responses that are accepted at any particular stage of treatment may be followed by those kinds of events that are known to increase the rate of responses. Such positive reinforcers as approval, verbal praise, tokens, and informative feedback may be programmed for responses that are judged correct or minimally acceptable. When responses are judged unacceptable or incorrect, the clinician may arrange a different sort of consequence known to decrease the rate of response. Such verbal statements as "No," "Wrong," or "Stop," are often used in this process. In addition, the clinician may cease all verbal interactions with the client for a short time or withdraw tangible reinforcers that the client is earning for correct responses. In some cases, incorrect or unacceptable responses may be totally ignored. It may be noted that not programming any consequence for a response is also a planned action on the part of the clinician.

Differential consequences programmed for client responses or lack thereof must be delivered immediately, forcefully, and in the most natural manner possible. For example, verbal statements of approval and disapproval must be quick, clear, and unambiguous and must be accompanied by appropriate facial expressions and emotional tone. Verbal reinforcers and punishers expressed weakly, mechanically, and in flat emotional tones may not be as effective as those that sound more natural. Clinicians often take time to decide whether a response is acceptable or not, which results in delayed action by the clinician. Such delays are not conducive to efficient learning by the client.

To begin with, clinicians select consequent events on some a priori basis. Events that are generally known to have increasing or decreasing effects on response rates are selected for potential reinforcers and punishers. However, no event is inherently and invariably a reinforcer or a punisher. Events have different effects across individuals and on the same individual across time periods. The clinician or the client judgements and feelings are unimportant in this respect. Whether a consequent event is a reinforcer, a punisher, or neutral is determined solely on the basis of its *demonstrated* effect on selected response rates. In other words, the effects of events on responses are observed and measured, not prejudged or presumed. For example, when verbal praise, selected initially to be the reinforcer, did not increase a rate of response, then that verbal praise is not a reinforcer for that particular client. The clinician then selects another potential consequence such as a token system, which may prove more effective. The same strategy is used in decreasing the rate of undesirable responses.

The management of treatment events must take into consideration the effects of different schedules (or particular methods) of arranging response consequences. Consequences are delivered initially on a continuous basis. Consequences may then be arranged on a continuous basis or on an intermittent basis. Basic and applied research has shown that the schedule of response consequence often determines whether or not and at what rate a response will be learned and once learned whether or not it will generalize and be maintained.[3,16,27] The overall strength of a target behavior is a function of the schedule on which its consequences are arranged.

In a continuous arrangement, every correct or acceptable response is positively reinforced and every incorrect response is either punished or extinguished (ignored). In the initial stages of treatment, clinicians use the continuous arrangement because it promotes relatively rapid learning of target behaviors. In the latter stages of treatment, the arrangement is more intermittent. In this arrangement, some of the responses receive consequences whereas others do not. The arrangement of response consequences can be relatively simple or complex. In a simple intermittent arrangement, every second or fifth response may receive a consequence. A more complex arrangement of response consequences requires a variable number of responses, but such variations are limited by a predetermined average. There are other complex arrangements of response consequences, but most of them have not been studied in communicative disorders.

Creating New Communicative Behaviors

More seriously affected clients often do not have a basal level of communicative behaviors whose frequency can simply be increased by contingent consequences. For example, the nonverbal or minimally verbal individuals do not present much that can be enhanced or increased. Such clients need procedures that would create new behaviors. There are treatment principles that help create nonexisting communicative behaviors in clients of all ages and diagnostic categories.

New responses are created in successive stages in which a remote, simple, and existing response is gradually changed into a final, complex, and new response. The process is known as successive approximation or shaping, but it does require an existing response that bears some relation to the final target behavior. Most nonverbal clients are able to produce some kind of a vocal response that can then be shaped into a more complex communicative behavior.

Contingencies that help create new responses are the same as those that help increase existing responses. They are made to follow responses of differing topographies at different stages of treatment.

For example, a client's infrequent and undifferentiated vocal response may be reinforced and increased in frequency initially. Then, that vocal response may be transformed into a syllable-like response by making the response consequence contingent on an appropriate topography. A syllable-like response can be refined into an acoustically less ambiguous response by making the consequence contingent on this new response. When a syllable response increases in frequency, it can be shaped into a simple word by adding another syllable to it. In this manner, a meaningful response unit can be created out of a crude and perhaps noncommunicative vocal response.

The shaping process requires a careful analysis of response topography. The terminal response, which is the new response to be created, must be broken into topographically simple, intermediate responses. An initial response the client is able to produce serves as the starting point. Selected intermediate responses are taught in a chained sequence. Consequences are programmed for the particular response in the chain at any given point in treatment. Eventually, the individually learned topographic components are "put together" in the form of the terminal, meaningful response. A single meaningful response, such as a word, can then be expanded into phrases and sentences as long as all of the words in such complex strings are also individually shaped.

Designing a Flexible Therapeutic Environment

Treatment research in the past few decades has shown that it is now possible to create reliably and increase communicative behaviors in clients who show various kinds of deficiencies.[3] However, a significant problem is to produce communicative behaviors that last in the client's natural environment and over time. It has been repeatedly found that behaviors that are reliably produced in the clinical setting when the clinician is monitoring the client productions may not be produced in the natural environment or, when produced initially, may not be maintained over time.

The difficulty in achieving permanency of target behaviors has been considered a problem of generalization.[28] Clinically taught behaviors that are produced in one setting, with the clinician as the audience, and that are related to specific stimuli may not generalize to different and nonclinical settings, audiences, or stimuli. However, a vast amount of laboratory data has shown that learned behaviors tend to generalize to new situations and stimuli without additional conditioning.[29,30] Generalization is a process that saves energy of learning as well as teaching. At its best, it can be a self-propagating process of generating more differentiated, novel, and complex response patterns.

The enormous complexity of speech and language behaviors has made it clear that it is not practical to teach every possible utterance in every possible situation. The elements of language combine into many different and highly variable response patterns. Those patterns are discriminatively produced in equally numerous and varied situations. Therefore, it appeared that what is needed for clinically established behaviors is generalization. It was thought that the establishment of behaviors in one setting and in relation to some stimulus variables should be sufficient to have those behaviors produced solely because of generalization in other settings and in relation to other stimuli. However, when it became clear that generalization of clinically established behaviors may not always be realized, clinicians began to devise strategies to promote generalization.[28] These strategies also included procedures designed to help maintain newly learned behaviors.

The strategies of generalization include such procedures as reinforcing generalized responses, bringing the behavior under the control of natural consequences, giving sufficient training with a variety of response exemplars, using stimuli that are commonly encountered by the client, and using intermittent reinforcers during training.[28] Evidently, a variety of stimulus, response, and consequent considerations are involved in programming generalization.

A critical analysis of the concept and methods of generalization shows that the approach of "programming generalization" is misleading.[3] Generalization was originally described by Pavlov in his studies on conditioning of salivary reflexes.[31] Later, the same phenomenon was observed by Skinner in his study of operant behaviors.[32,33] An operant response conditioned to a particular stimulus is likely to be emitted in the presence of similar stimuli. This laboratory phenomenon of generalization is measured during extinction. The subject is shown stimuli that are progressively different from the conditioned stimulus, and the frequency or the magnitude of the conditioned response is measured. Generalized responses are *not* reinforced (extinction). It has been repeatedly shown that generalized responses fall on a gradient. The closer the novel stimulus to the conditioned stimulus, the greater the probability of the conditioned response and vice versa. Eventually, when the stimulus is very different from the original stimulus, the response ceases to occur. In essence, when pushed to the limits, generalization terminates in extinction.

In light of the laboratory evidence on generalization, consideration of generalization as the ultimate goal of clinical interventions seems inappropriate, and the problems clinicians have had with generalization of clinically established behaviors are understandable. There is no reason to expect that behaviors will be maintained when the treatment events are terminated. If the behaviors are not reinforced, they will be extinguished. That a behavior has generalized does not mean that it will be maintained, as shown by both the basic and applied evidence.[3,30]

Many of the so-called tactics of generalization are incongruous with the basic concept and data on generalization. The incongruity is the result of setting up generalization as the goal of clinical intervention. For example, it is hard to understand why reinforcement of a generalized response is a tactic of programming generalization. If anything, it is a technique of preventing extinction of an initially generalized response. It is treatment, not generalization. Moreover, why reinforcement provided by clinicians is treatment and the same thing done by family members or friends of a client is a tactic to program generalization is not clear. It is also not clear why generalization should be implicitly redefined as behaviors reinforced by persons other than the clinician in natural environments.

Generalization is not at the heart of creating behaviors that last in natural environments. Lasting behaviors are a product of lasting contingencies. And so the same or similar contingencies that create behaviors are needed to maintain them. Therefore, the problem faced by the clinician is not the instability or tentativeness of generalization of newly learned behaviors—the phenomenon of generalization *is* unstable and tentative—the problem is one of creating flexible therapeutic environments that continually support the target behaviors, as they support any other kind of behavior. The initial therapeutic environment is the clinical setting; the therapeutic agent is the clinician. In gradual steps, the treatment setting must be changed and expanded. Treatment must be moved out of the formal clinical rooms and carried into more natural settings. The management of treatment contingencies must be shifted to significant people in the client's natural environment. In essence, the setting as well as the controlling agents must change in order for a clinically established behavior to be maintained over time and in extraclinical situations.

Designing flexible therapeutic environments needs a careful analysis of stimulus, response, and consequent considerations. Stimuli that the clients encounter in their everyday life may be more effective than arbitrarily selected stimuli that clinicians often tend to use in evoking target behaviors.[34,35] Verbal antecedents designed to evoke target responses must be common and natural, not contrived and arbitrary. As noted before, the target behaviors selected for treatment must be useful and relevant to the client. The client who learns useful responses may be expected to produce them in his or her everyday environment. Such productions may have a better chance of being reinforced by other persons, thus extending the therapeutic milieu into everyday situations.

Informal treatment sessions in which conversational speech is monitored may be held in more natural settings including the home, classroom, office, playground, and supermarket. This is done to support the production of target behaviors by the creation of new and natural discriminative stimulus control. Eventually, when significant others come to control the responses in those situations, the therapeutic control will have been further expanded.

A significant aspect of shifting the response control to the natural environment is to train significant persons in the life of a client to manage the treatment events at some level of regularity and proficiency. This is probably one of the most difficult aspects of maintenance strategies, since training others amounts to making the client's family members, teachers, colleagues, siblings, and friends clinicians. Initially, the individuals to be trained in management of treatment contingencies may be asked to observe the treatment sessions. In gradual steps, they may be trained to measure and record (chart) the production of target behaviors to make them more observant of what the client is taught and is expected to produce. Eventually, those persons must be trained in reacting appropriately and differentially to the correct, incorrect, or inadequate production of behaviors in various everyday situations.

Another important maintenance strategy is to teach the client self-monitoring skills. Self-monitoring skills are evident when a client is able to judge the accuracy of his or her own productions and in turn is able to take differential actions based upon those judgements. A stutterer who catches himself when a dysfluency is produced or imminent and uses gentle phonatory onset or reduced rate of speech in the absence of consequences is showing self-monitoring skills. A clinician teaches self-monitoring skills by imposing appropriate consequences on them. However, it must be recognized that although some research on teaching self-monitoring skills has been reported,[36,37] much experimental work needs to be done to substantiate its usefulness in maintaining clinically established behaviors.

It must be emphasized that, procedurally, many tactics of maintenance are not different from what Stokes and Baer[28] have called the tactics of generalization. The two sets of tactics are conceptually different, however. The maintenance strategy seeks to establish response-controlling mechanisms in the natural environment, whereas the generalization strategy seeks to promote generalization. Furthermore, the generalization strategy is based upon the assumption that it is programmable and when this programming is successful, responses last, but the maintenance strategy is based upon the assumption that generalization is not to be programmed and what must be programmed is the client's environment such that the process of contingency management continues beyond the clinic. Therefore, the point to be emphasized is that the major task of the clinician is to create a pervasive control mechanism that operates in the client's natural environment. Therapeutic operations should not be limited to certain physical settings, and the therapeutic agent should not be a single person: the clinician. Many tactics of generalization[28] are also appropriate as long as they are conceptualized not in terms of generalization but in terms of shifting the locus of response control.

Sequence of Treatment

There is a sequential pattern to treatment of communicative disorders. It is possible to identify some general sequences that apply across disorders and most clients. However, there is no single, invariable sequence of sufficient generality. Typically, general and broad sequences are modified to create specific sequences that suit individual clients.

Treatment must be sequenced for several reasons. The most important reasons include response topography and mode, multiple target behaviors, treatment and probe procedures, treatment and maintenance considerations, and shifts in treatment contingencies.[3] A combination of these factors results in a general sequence of treatment. However, the individual histories of clients create a need to modify that general sequence.

To begin with, target responses are trained at their simpler if not the simplest response topography. The mode of response typically used at simpler levels is imitative. An articulatory response, for example, may be initially trained at the level of syllables or simple words. The client may be asked to imitate the clinician's productions to bring the behavior under a stimulus control, which is faded in gradual steps. Simplified response topographies help establish an initial response repertoire, which is obviously limited in scope and significance. However, reduction in response topography and imitation make it possible for the client to produce a new response in the early stages of treatment. At the same time, simplified response topographies also create a need to sequence treatment so that more complex response topographies may be taught in cumulatively more complex stages. The correct imitative production of a target syllable may lead to the successive sequences of correct production of words, phrases, sentences, and conversational speech. The imitative mode may be gradually replaced by the evoked (spontaneous) mode of responses at appropriate stages.

Most clients need treatment on multiple target behaviors. Multiple phonemes are targets with most phonologically disordered clients. Clients with language disorders may need to learn a variety of vocabulary items, grammatical morphemes, syntactic structures, semantic concepts, and pragmatic behaviors. Similarly, clients of fluency and voice also need to learn multiple skills to maintain fluency or appropriate vocal quality.

In most cases, multiple targets cannot be taught all at once. The actual number of target behaviors that can be taught in a single or a set of sessions usually depends upon the client, assuming other factors such as the clinician expertise are held constant. Generally speaking, at any one time, the treatment can effectively involve only a few independent behaviors. Therefore, the clinician faces the question of what sequence should be used in which those multiple behaviors are treated. Regardless of whether one uses a normative sequence or an experimental sequence, one must use a sequence. At a more practical level, simpler behaviors may be taught before more complex behaviors are taught. Behaviors that are better imitated by the client may be taught before those that are not imitated. Behaviors may be sequenced according to baseline data. For example, behaviors that are observed more frequently on baseline trials may be taught before those that are observed less frequently.

Treatment and probe considerations create their own sequences because the clinician often has to alternate between treatment and probe. A probe procedure helps measure an initial generalization of a trained response to untrained stimuli, response contexts, and/or situations. If a response can be temporarily produced in the absence of treatment consequences, then perhaps treatment can move on to more complex response forms, a different target behavior, or different therapeutic environments. Probes help achieve economy in treatment. When a probe is successful, the treatment may be either discontinued in the clinical setting or moved to a different level in the sequence. When a probe is not successful, the treatment is continued at the same level of topography, mode, or setting.

Probes involve a presentation of stimuli not used in treatment. A child who has been taught to produce certain words in relation to certain pictorial stimuli may be shown new pictures that can evoke the same responses. If the responses are produced at some criterion level, such as 90 percent correct, treatment may be shifted to the next stage in the sequence, which may be the production of phrases. If the responses are not produced, treatment may be continued at the word level. When the responses meet certain training criterion at the phrase level, another probe may be conducted to see if the treatment can once again be shifted to the sentence level. This kind of an alternation between probes and treatment trials or sessions creates one of the most common sequences across disorders and clients.[3,9,13,38,39]

Treatment and maintenance considerations also necessitate sequences that help move from an initial establishment of target behaviors under more controlled therapeutic settings to more natural therapeutic environments. Most of the maintenance strategies described earlier are completed only after the target behaviors are established under controlled conditions to conform to a certain training and/or probe criterion. Such tactics as parent training in management of treatment contingencies and holding informal treatment sessions in everyday situations are not implemented in the first stage of treatment. They are implemented only when the client's target behaviors show some level of complexity and stability under controlled clinical situations where the treatment events are managed strictly.

Finally, necessary shifts in the treatment consequences also create certain treatment sequences because the same treatment consequences are not used from the beginning to the end. They shift across treatment phases. Initially, consequences are programmed for every occurrence of the target responses because continuous consequences promote faster learning of new responses. However, they are not very efficient in creating strong responses that can withstand some degree of extinction (lack of consequences). Since the natural environment does not always program response consequences on a continuous basis, the clinician must make sure that eventually his or her consequences approximate those in the natural environment. Therefore, in carefully sequenced stages, the frequency with which the target response productions are reinforced is reduced. The purpose of such reductions is not to create a response that will be maintained by generalization, but to have the client face clinical consequences that approximate those in the natural environment.

Treatment Modifications

Ideally, treatment programs of individual clients are written by the clinician after the first few sessions of treatment in which a planned procedure is tested out. It is better to write an entire treatment program for a client instead of weekly or daily "lesson plans." Comprehensive treatment programs help keep the final targets, the treatment sequences, and the total picture of a given intervention in proper perspective. A detailed treatment program specifies not only the initial but final target behaviors, the treatment procedures including stimulus and consequence variables, a tentative treatment sequence, probe and other measurement procedures, and maintenance and follow-up plans.

Treatment programs must be written for individual clients. They must be specific to the client and not copied from cookbooks. Nevertheless, planned treatment programs often need to be modified during various stages of implementation because the ultimate variable that determines the details of a treatment program is the client's response pattern. When the response pattern shows certain kinds of changes or does not show certain other kinds of changes, the clinician has to modify the planned intervention program.

Modifications of treatment programs result in changed procedures of treatment, not changed principles. As noted in an earlier section, a treatment principle is capable of generating a variety of treatment procedures. A procedure found ineffective with a client is either abandoned or modified. A new procedure is then selected on the basis of the relevant principle. Since ideally, treatment principles are based on laboratory evidence obtained through controlled experimental procedures, modifications of routine treatment procedures do not invalidate those principles. For example, the possibility that in a given client a verbal "No" did not decrease the number of dysfluencies in a stutterer does not negate the principle of punishment. It means only that another response consequence must be selected.

Treatment programs may have to be modified because of unique individual histories, ineffective response consequences, inadequate stimulus controls, and inappropriate response topographies.[3] Any reason to modify a procedure must be accepted since an inflexible treatment procedure is not likely to work across all clients and disorders.

It is often thought that treatment procedures are modified because of differential diagnostic categories. However, as noted before, a more valid reason to modify a treatment program is the individual client's unique history. Clients who are given the same diagnosis may react differently to particular aspects of a treatment program. Therefore, a careful measurement of the client responses throughout treatment sessions is necessary. Any time a response pattern does not show desirable change or stability, the clinician must analyze the reasons and make necessary changes.

Response consequences selected for either increasing or decreasing certain communicative behaviors may or may not be functional for given clients. It was noted earlier that the effects of any consequence are demonstrated and not just presumed or defined on an a priori basis. A clinician who selects verbal praise for a potential reinforcer in the modification of an articulation disorder may find that the correct productions do not increase in spite of several sessions of treatment. The first possibility that the clinician should consider in this case is that the verbal praise is not a functional reinforcer for the client. Perhaps a primary reinforcer, or a token system, backed up with a variety of secondary reinforcers, may be more effective. Other possibilities, to be described, must also be considered.

Inadequate stimulus controls can take various forms. Selected pictures and objects used to evoke the target behaviors may be ambiguous. They may not be effective in evoking stimuli. In addition, questions designed to evoke a target behavior, instructions given to produce that behavior, and prompts and manual guidance may all be defective. A response reliably imitated in the presence of a modeled stimulus may not be produced when modeling is discontinued. In such cases, the clinician must pay close attention to the antecedents that may not be serving their purpose. Questions may have to be changed so that they do come to evoke the response. Instructions may have to be improved and presented along with demonstrations. Stronger prompts may have to be selected. Modeling may have to be faded in gradual steps instead of an abrupt withdrawal. These and other changes may be needed to create effective stimulus control or restore lost control.

Finally, inappropriate response topographies selected for treatment may make it difficult for the client to learn the target behaviors. Many children with articulation disorders cannot respond adequately when the treatment is started at the phrase or sentence level. The most appropriate initial response topography in such cases is at the syllable or the word level. Similarly, most stutterers may not be able to modify their phonatory, respiratory, and articulatory behaviors at the sentence level during the first stage of treatment. They are better able to manage these processes at the word or phrase level. Clients with language and voice disorders also need similar topographic considerations. When desirable target responses do not increase in frequency, the clinician must make sure that a wrong response topography was not selected. Complex response topographies are typically shaped so that the client learns the various components in small, well-defined steps. When such shaping is not used, wrong response topographies often create difficulties for the client.

A clinician who carefully monitors the client response rates and defines treatment consequences only by those objectively demonstrated response rates is able to modify ineffective treatment procedures at the earliest possible time. Such a clinician is also most accountable for the treatment effects or improvement in client behaviors.

CONCLUDING REMARKS

Treatment of communicative disorders is a complex yet exciting process. Treatment is complicated by individual variations within and across diagnostic categories, unreliable diagnostic categories, speculative etiologic theories, and a lack of an inclination on the part of many clinicians to experimentally verify their procedures. In the past, treatment procedures and models in communicative disorders have often been based upon clinical experience and theoretic recommendations.

In recent years, the need to base clinical practice on scientific methods and experimental evidence has received much attention.[40–42] The need to increase the number of experimental investigations of treatment procedures is well recognized. The profession now has a set of basic principles and empirical techniques that can serve as a basis for well-controlled clinical research studies capable of producing replicated data. It is hoped that more systematic treatment-related research will help to identify strong and weak procedures and to extend the generality of effective techniques. (See Chapter 37 for a more detailed consideration of treatment-related research in communicative disorders.)

Successful treatment of communicative disorders is exciting for both the clinician and the client. A disorder of communication affects almost all aspects of a person's life, and so a successful treatment also affects almost all aspects of a treated person. Improved personal, social, and occupational life is often reported by clients who become more communicative because of treatment. In a larger sense, successful treatment of communicative disorders results in happier and productive individuals. This is what makes the endeavor of treatment of communicative disorders exciting as well as rewarding.

REFERENCES

1. Darley FL, Spriestersbach DC, eds. Diagnostic methods in speech pathology. 2nd ed. New York: Harper and Row, 1978.

2. Peterson HA, Marquardt TM. Appraisal and diagnosis of speech and language disorders. Englewood Cliffs, NJ: Prentice-Hall, 1981.
3. Hegde MN. Treatment procedures in communicative disorders. Boston: Little, Brown, 1985.
4. Costello JM. Operant conditioning and the treatment of stuttering. In: Perkins WH, ed. Strategies in stuttering therapy. Semin Speech Lang Hear 1980; 1:311.
5. Costello JM. Generalization across settings. In: Miller J, Yoder D, Schiefelbusch R, eds. Contemporary issues in language intervention. Rockville, MD: ASHA Reports No. 12, 1983:275.
6. Fitch JL. Voice and articulation. In: Lahey BB, ed. The modification of language behavior. Springfield, IL: CC Thomas, 1973:130.
7. Garcia E, DeHaven E. Use of operant techniques in the establishment and generalization of language: a review and analysis. Am J Ment Defic 1974; 79:169–178.
8. Guess D, Baer DM. Some experimental analyses of linguistic development in institutionalized retarded children. In: Lahey BB, ed. The modification of language behavior. Springfield, IL: CC Thomas, 1973:3.
9. Guess D, Sailor W, Baer DM. Children with limited language. In: Schiefelbusch RL, ed. Language intervention strategies. Baltimore: University Park Press, 1978:101.
10. Harris SL. Teaching language to nonverbal children with emphasis on problems of generalization. Psychol Bull 1975; 82:565–580.
11. Hegde MN. Treatment of fluency disorders: state of the art. In: Costello JM, ed. Speech disorders in adults: recent advances. Boston: Little, Brown, 1985:155.
12. Ingham RJ. Stuttering and behavior therapy: current status and experimental foundations. San Diego: College-Hill Press, 1984.
13. McReynolds LV, ed. Developing systematic procedures for training children's language. Rockville, MD: ASHA Monogr No. 18, 1974.
14. Schumaker JB, Sherman JA. Parents as intervention agents. In: Schiefelbusch RL, ed. Language intervention strategies. Baltimore: University Park Press, 1978:237.
15. Welch S. Teaching generative grammar to mentally retarded children: a review and analysis of a decade of behavioral research. Ment Retard 1981; 19:277–284.
16. Kazdin AE. Behavior modification in applied settings. Homewood, IL: The Dorsey Press, 1984.
17. Sundel M, Sundel SS. Behavior modification in the human services. New York: Wiley, 1975.
18. Axelrod S, Apsche J, eds. The effects of punishment on human behavior. New York: Academic Press, 1983.
19. Matson JL, DiLorenzo TM. Punishment and its alternatives. New York: Springer Publishing, 1984.
20. Hegde MN, McConn J. Language training: some data on response classes and generalization to an occupational setting. J Speech Hear Disord 1981; 46:353–358.
21. Hegde MN. An experimental-clinical analysis of grammatical and behavioral distinctions between verbal auxiliary and copula. J Speech Hear Disord 1980; 23:864–877.
22. Kearns KP, Salmon SJ. An experimental analysis of auxiliary and copula verb generalization in aphasia. J Speech Hear Disord 1984; 49:152–163.
23. McReynolds LV, Engmann DL. An experimental analysis of the relationship between subject noun and object noun phrases. In: McReynolds LV, ed. Developing systematic procedures for training children's language. Rockville, MD: ASHA Monogr No. 18, 1974:30.
24. Capelli R. An experimental analysis of morphologic acquisition. Masters Thesis, California State University, Fresno, 1985.
25. De Cesari R. Experimental training of grammatic morphemes: effects on the order of acquisition. Masters Thesis, California State University, Fresno, 1985.
26. Brown R. A first language: the early stages. Cambridge, MA: Harvard University Press, 1974.
27. Ferster CB, Skinner BF. Schedules of reinforcement. New York: Appleton-Century-Crofts, 1957.
28. Stokes TF, Baer DM. An implicit technology of generalization. J Appl Behav Anal 1977; 10:349–367.
29. Ferster CB, Culbertson S, Boren MCP. Behavior principles. 2nd ed. Englewood Cliffs, NJ: Prentice-Hall, 1975.
30. Kalish HI. From behavioral science to behavior modification. New York: McGraw-Hill, 1981.
31. Pavlov I. Lectures on conditioned reflexes. New York: International Publishers, 1928.
32. Skinner BF. The behavior of organisms. New York: Appleton-Century-Crofts, 1938.
33. Skinner BF. Science and human behavior. New York: Macmillan, 1953.
34. Faw GD, Reid DH, Schepis MM, Fitzgerald JR, Welty PA. Involving institutional staff in the development and maintenance of sign language skills with profoundly retarded persons. J Appl Behav Anal 1981; 14:411–423.
35. Welch S, Pear JJ. Generalization of naming responses to objects in the natural environment as a function of training stimulus modality with retarded children. J Appl Behav Anal 1980; 13:629–643.
36. Gajar A, Schloss PJ, Schloss CN, Thompson CK. Effects of feedback and self-monitoring on head trauma youths' conversational skills. J Appl Behav Anal 1984; 17:353–358.
37. Stevenson HC, Fantuzzo JW. Application of the "generalization map" to self-control intervention with school-aged children. J Appl Behav Anal 1984; 17:203–212.
38. Hegde MN, Noll MJ, Pecora R. A study of some factors affecting generalization of language training. J Speech Hear Disord 1979; 44:301–320.
39. McReynolds LV, Elbert MF. Generalization of correct articulation in clusters. Appl Psycholing 1981; 2:119–132.
40. Connell PJ, Thompson CK. Flexibility of single-subject experimental designs. Part III: Using flexibility to design or modify experiments. J Speech Hear Disord 1986; 51:204–214.
41. Kearns KP. Flexibility of single-subject experimental designs. Part II: Design selection and arrangement of experimental phases. J Speech Hear Disord 1981; 51:204–214.
42. McReynolds LV, Thompson CK. Flexibility of single-subject designs. Part I: Review of the basics of single-subject designs. J Speech Hear Disord 1986; 51:194–203.

14 Microcomputer Use in Assessment and Intervention with Speech and Language Disorders

Vicki Lord Larson, Ph.D.
Sylvia Steiner, Ph.D.

Bobby is an 8-year-old child with cerebral palsy. Unable to produce speech intelligible enough for most listeners to understand, Bobby is communicating with his teacher and classmates through a microcomputer linked to a printer, using a headpointer as an instrument to provide keyboard and touch screen input to the system.

Anna is a mentally retarded adolescent receiving language therapy. As part of her program, Anna goes to the computer lab in her school and uses software, allowing her to practice independently the language behaviors she is working on in therapy sessions.

Kevin is a learning disabled high school junior. He is teaching one of his friends, who does not have a learning disability, how to use the word processing program that Kevin has been using to complete some assignments for his language intervention program.

Randy is a 4-year-old with dysfluent speech. He is talking with his clinician about the Muppet microcomputer keyboard and software that has been introduced to stimulate natural conversation during the session. The objective for this intervention session is for Randy to maintain fluency, producing no more than three dysfluencies per minute in conversational speech during a structured activity with the clinician.

Mr. Franklin is a 63-year-old adult who experienced a cerebrovascular accident 4 months ago and displays moderately severe nonfluent aphasia. He owns an Apple computer, which he has employed in business-related tasks at home for several years. A speech-language pathologist sees Mr. Franklin for therapy on Monday each week and sends home therapy assignments for Mr. Franklin to do on his microcomputer on other days of the week.

Sally Taylor is a speech-language pathologist in private practice. She utilizes the microcomputer for writing reports, analyzing language samples, billing clients, generating correspondence, and as a tool during assessment and intervention sessions with clients. Recently, she has developed software that administers a single-word receptive vocabulary test to clients, and she is negotiating with a publisher interested in marketing the program. Tomorrow she will be participating in a telecommunication-based national conference without leaving her office. The conference is about the use of computer technology in delivery of service to rural clients.

The microcomputer, a device that has existed for little more than a decade, is reshaping the clinical realm of speech-language pathology. All of the types of events described in the preceding scenarios are happening now. They are not a glimpse of the future, but a glance at the existing potential of this powerful electronic assistant. Although clinical and educational disciplines have not yet exploited the full range of microcomputer operations in their professional worlds, the progress that has been made in the past few years is remarkable and exciting. The intent of this chapter is to describe microcomputer applications in speech-language pathology, examining both the potential benefits and the present limitations. Under the assumption that most clinicians have been introduced to the microcomputer and possess an understanding of basic computer terminology, some vocabulary items that may be unfamiliar to a novice in the area of computers will not be defined. Readers who lack microcomputer experience might find it helpful to consult such publications as Bear,[1] Curtis,[2] Fitch[3] and Katz[4] to develop sufficient understanding of computer terminology and fundamental ideas about microcomputer technology prior to reading this chapter. Although one of the most promising areas of microcomputer technology in the discipline of Communication Sciences and Disorders is augmentative communication systems, this chapter will address that topic to a limited degree, since another chapter in this book (Chapter 34) will address augmentative communication.[5]

Advances occur rapidly in the microcomputer world. Therefore comments about specific software and hardware characteristics become outdated quickly. For this reason, this chapter addresses ideas and principles, primarily, rather than presenting details about hardware and software. The basic tenet of the chapter is that each individual speech-language pathologist must become informed enough about microcomputers to reach appropriate decisions about whether or not to use, when to use, and how to use this flexible and influential tool.

The computer has been described frequently as a device with the potential to change the lives of individuals more than any tool developed previously. Since electronic computers were first introduced soon after World War II, the rate of change and development in computer technology has been staggering, injecting an element of "future shock"[6] into the mentality of those who are attempting to incorporate computers into their working environments and personal domains. The industrial revolution was characterized mainly by the development of mechanical machines that extended human muscle power. In contrast, the current information age is characterized by electronic devices such as the computer, which extend the mental power, the sensory capacities and the nervous systems of users.

As computers have become smaller, less expensive, and more pervasive, they have exerted an increasing influence over the daily functioning of members of modern societies. Early introduction of the general public to microcomputer technology arrived through the nonthreatening and entertaining avenue provided by computerized children's toys. Specific spheres of operation initiated the adaptation to computer technology early on, incorporated the technologic advances quickly, and changed dramatically because of the computer: industry, business, politics, and the military, for example. Within educational and clinical realms, computer applications have evolved much more slowly and have produced an impact of substantially smaller proportions.[3,7,8] As Sanders has suggested, decisions about computer applications within Communication Sciences and Disorders should be formulated carefully and gradually, rather than precipitately.[9] Fitch advised that speech-language pathologists and audiologists should examine the impact of computers in other fields such as business and industry, profiting from the experience and learning from the mistakes made in those spheres.[3]

Although the efforts of a few pioneers representing Communication Sciences and Disorders to develop computer applications can be traced back to the previous two decades, Minifie[8] was among the first to articulate a major concern about the powerful potential of computers to revolutionize the clinical process in this profession.[3] During the intervening years, evidence has accumulated that rapidly increasing numbers of speech-language pathologists and audiologists are incorporating computer technology, particularly microcomputer hardware and software, into their professional practices. Signs of growth in computerizing aspects of professional practice include the recent publication of numerous books and articles on computer applications, the expanding instances of convention presentations related to computers, the appearance of more and more computer exhibits at conventions, the changes occurring in educational curricula for future clinicians, and the burgeoning membership of the organization called Computer Users in Speech and Hearing (CUSH). In 1983, when the American Speech-Language-Hearing Association's Ad Hoc Committee on Long-Range Planning identified factors liable to exert a major influence on the profession during the next decade, one highly ranked item on their list was the developing utilization of computers and other technological advances. The American Speech-Language-Hearing Association sponsored two national leadership conferences, one in 1984 and one in 1985, to encourage incorporation of computer technology into university curricula for educating speech-language pathologists and audiologists. Those same years were marked by the first two of a series of annual conferences sponsored by the American Speech-Language-Hearing Foundation on computer technology. One of the primary objectives for these conferences has been to assist with the continuing education of professional practitioners attempting to enhance their microcomputer-related knowledge and competencies. The American Speech-Language-Hearing Association, with funding provided by a federal grant from the Department of Education, has been involved in the production of continuing education materials that individual clinicians can employ in a self-instructional mode to increase their understanding of computers (Project IMPACT). Although it is often true that mature and established practitioners within a field are more resistant to significant changes in the way they accomplish their job-related responsibilities and are less accepting of technological advances than are their younger and less experienced colleagues, it is laudable that many clinicians with 20 or more years of professional practice are adapting their professional functioning to accommodate the microcomputer. Many of the microcomputer applications developed to date are in the areas of personal productivity and administration, rather than being direct applications of the microcomputer during assessment and intervention activities with clients.

Microcomputer applications in Communication Sciences and Disorders are often at the center of professional consciousness during the current time period, the infancy of their utilization by clinicians. It is likely that in future years, when acceptance of the microcomputer as an electronic tool has become universal in this profession, it will function as a more transparent and less obtrusive device. In the not too distant future, finding a publication addressing microcomputer applications with communicatively disabled individuals may be as difficult as finding a publication now that describes applications of the pencil or the tongue depressor. The microcomputer will move from the foreground to the background and will be just one more tool, however powerful, that enriches the clinical armamentarium of speech-language pathologists. Today's challenge is to make appropriate and intelligent decisions, based on limited information and evidence, permitting evolution within Communication Sciences and Disorders in order to maximize the potential of this exciting electronic assistant, thus yielding improvement of the delivery of services to individuals with communication disabilities.

GUIDELINES FOR MICROCOMPUTER APPLICATIONS IN CLINICAL MANAGEMENT

Interpretation of comments in later segments of this chapter should be based upon an understanding of fundamental philosophical premises forming the foundation for appropriate applications of microcomputers within the clinical domain of a speech-language pathologist. Therefore this section of the chapter presents guidelines for incorporating computer technology into clinical practice.

The microcomputer is nothing more nor less than a professional tool, an electronic assistant. As is the case with each professional tool that becomes available to speech-language pathologists, individual clinicians must decide whether learning to use the new device is advantageous or not. Potential benefits of modifying a clinical operation to accommodate a new tool must be weighed against the possible drawbacks of such an action. Purchasing microcomputer hardware and software is expensive. Learning to use the hardware and software effectively is time-consuming and challenging. Only when the professional functioning of a practitioner can be enhanced through microcomputer usage should the necessary commitment of time, effort, and funds be made in order to incorporate computer technology into the clinical situation. Many speech-language pathologists have initiated attempts to employ the microcomputer clinically,[10] having decided that computer technology has substantial benefits to offer and having acknowledged that microcomputer applications are not a passing fad.[11] However, each individual clinician must formulate a judgment on this matter, basing decisions on information and evidence available.

Whether, when, and how to use the microcomputer with a given client should be considered carefully by a practitioner. Just as some clinicians respond positively to the opportunity to use a microcomputer, but others do not, some clients react favorably and others unfavorably to the introduction of a microcomputer into the clinical situation. Assessment or intervention activities that are based on computers are appropriate for some clients, but not all clients. Just as the clinician must evaluate each planned noncomputerized activity within a different referential framework for each individual client, the clinician must incorporate computer applications into the clinical plan for a client only after appraising the appropriateness of those applications for that particular client. Careful consideration of when and how to employ the microcomputer clinically produces a synthesis of computerized and noncomputerized activities in the overall clinical situation and on the individual client level.[9,12]

As microcomputer technology is incorporated into the clinical realm of speech-language pathology, it is crucial that other recent and important clinical advances not be abandoned inadvertently. Care must be taken so that emphasis on such matters as the pragmatic aspects of communication, the value of assessing and facilitating functional communication development, the need for task analysis, and the import of individualizing intervention and assessment plans are not forgotten in overly enthusiastic and ill-considered applications of computer technology.

Employment of a particular clinical procedure during assessment or intervention must be consistent with the theoretical framework of the speech-language pathologist who selects and applies it. Clinical principles that form the foundation for assessment and intervention do not change just because the microcomputer is introduced as a tool during the process. Each individual clinician must consider decisions about a specific microcomputer application by evaluating whether or not that application would violate any theoretical premises of the practitioner.

Since purchases of hardware and software involve major expenditures from tight budgets, a thorough evaluation of potential purchases prior to commitment of funds is necessary. It is crucial that hardware items that are purchased be compatible with each other and be capable of performing the tasks for which they are purchased. Software must be selected to be compatible with the particular hardware owned. Usually it is wise to decide first what types of software will be used by the clinician or the agency and then to select hardware capable of operating with the software desired. The person making a decision about software or hardware purchases must be knowledgeable about microcomputer matters and must perform a thorough assessment of needs prior to recommending expenditures. Although clinicians should make purchases following a thorough deliberation, they would be unwise to wait for ideal hardware and software to be developed. Fearing that potential purchases of microcomputer-related items might be rendered obsolete by newer technological advances, a speech-language pathologist who delays incorporation of computer technology into clinical practice runs the risk of becoming obsolete professionally.[13]

Although many practitioners are becoming computer users, with the ranks of microcomputer advocates increasing at an impressive rate, there is a remarkable lack of data supporting the efficacy of microcomputer-based intervention and assessment activities. Some available data suggest that efficiency of clinical functioning can be improved markedly by usage of the microcomputer for personal productivity tasks.[14,15] Little research has been reported in the literature on the impact of the microcomputer on client behavior or client progress. However, an article by Shriberg, Kwiatkowski, and Snyder is an outstanding example of the type of approach needed.[16] Clinicians using microcomputers are urged to disseminate data that permit others to reach clinical decisions about microcomputer utilization on the basis of factual information rather than on the basis of anecdotal reports and personal opinions of their colleagues.

There is little doubt that microcomputer applications have the potential to increase efficiency of the clinical process through their contributions to personal productivity, assessment, and intervention. However, other concerns must not be sacrificed in the effort to become more efficient. If efficiency increases, while matters related to validity, reliability, accuracy, and applicability of procedures are disregarded, the net result of microcomputer usage is a loss rather than a gain clinically. There is a continuing need to decide first what should be done and then to consider whether the use of a microcomputer will enhance accomplishment of the objective or detract from it.

Technology cannot make invalid assessment or intervention practices valid. An invalid procedure remains unacceptable when performed by a microcomputer. Data that are invalid when produced manually are still invalid when they appear in an impressive computer printout. If a clinician regards assessment of the language ability of a client to be inappropriate in the absence of contextual considerations, a microcomputer program that analyzes a spontaneous language sample devoid of situational context information yields data of limited value to that practitioner, no matter how thorough and accurate the calculations are. One of the hazards inherent in the availability of powerful software is that clinicians may use the software without understanding the limitations of programs and produce vast quantities of flawed but convincing data. Production of clinical data by the speech-language pathologist may occur without comprehension of the underlying procedures through the use of microcomputers. This possibly is dangerous since recipients of the computer information may not evaluate thoroughly the basis for the data or for the clinician's interpretations that emerge from the data.

Practitioners vary markedly in their proficiency with microcomputers, in the variety of tasks for which they use computers, and in the frequency with which they use computers. Some clinicians have never seen, touched, or read anything about a microcomputer. The professional lives of other speech-language pathologists have been modified substantially to incorporate microcomputer technology. Few clinicians have developed the skills required to write microcomputer programs. If high-quality software is to be developed in the future to meet clinical needs, it is necessary that some clinicians learn to generate microcomputer software and that others master the art of working cooperatively with experts in computer programming to produce software.[17] Some clinicians who do not use computers view the microcomputer with alarm, doubting their own abilities to learn to use it effectively and fearing that the computer may someday replace the human clinician. Those who have become proficient in the use of computers affirm that significant time and effort are required for the development of needed computer-related knowledge and competencies,[18] but they invariably feel that the struggle was worthwhile. Clinicians proficient in the use of computers realize that potential contributions of the microcomputer and the speech-language pathologist to the clinical process are complementary. Technology does not obviate the need for human interactions in clinical activities and is not capable of making the same clinical judgments that a human clinician can make. However, it is true that employers are beginning to seek for practitioners capable of using microcomputers wisely. Clinicians lacking computer proficiency are becoming less and less attractive to potential employers. Practitioners who learn to use computers, but do not evaluate carefully how they are using the technology, run the risk of becoming slaves of the microcomputer rather than its masters.

APPLICATIONS OF THE MICROCOMPUTER TO CLINICAL MANAGEMENT

Microcomputer applications for the clinical speech-language pathologist can be categorized for purposes of discussion into those related to personal productivity and those related to client assessment or intervention. This section of the chapter will discuss these categories of microcomputer applications and will illustrate contributions that can be made to the clinical process by the microcomputer in each of the categories. Personal productivity applications enhance clinical operation without being employed in the direct delivery of services to clients. Personal productivity applications such as agency administration, client recordkeeping, production of reports and other documents, management of data, and continuing education of the clinician will be addressed in later sections of this chapter. Software utilized directly in assessment or intervention may be classified as microcomputer administered or microcomputer assisted. Examples of these two varieties of clinical software will be presented in this section of the chapter. As software is employed in assessment and intervention, it may perform a variety of roles, which will also be described and illustrated in the following narrative: (1) stimulus controller, (2) response recorder, (3) data analyzer, (4) information presenter, and (5) situation generator. Assessment applications will be described for use during administration of formal and informal procedures. Intervention applications of six types will be addressed: (1) drill and practice, (2) simulation, (3) tutorial, (4) instructional games, (5) problem solving, and (6) exploration and discovery. No attempt will be made to identify exhaustively available software, since programs are being developed at such a rapid pace that attempts at creating complete directories are futile. Mention of any specific program is intended to provide an example of a type of application rather than to present an endorsement of the specific program described.

Personal Productivity

Using the microcomputer to increase personal productivity allows the speech-language pathologist to devote less time to the paper-pushing component of the job and more time to the human interaction component of the delivery of clinical services. Personal productivity includes those tasks that individuals perform to increase their efficiency in managing textual and numerical information. Microcomputer usage as a personal productivity tool assists a clinician in establishing accountability and enhancing administrative effectiveness. Personal productivity may be improved by employing the microcomputer for agency administration tasks, client recordkeeping activities, clinical research endeavors, and continuing education pursuits.

Agency Administration Tasks

Regardless of the type of setting in which a clinician is employed, certain administrative tasks must be accomplished to ensure successful operation. One such task is the development of promotional materials for public relations, to increase visibility with people who need speech-language services and with other professionals who work with communicatively disabled persons. Several software packages such as *The Print Shop,*[19] *The Newsroom,*[20] and *The Newsroom Pro*[21] can simplify and enhance the production of brochures, posters, newsletters, and pamphlets for promotion of clinical speech-language programs. *The Print Shop* is designed to generate signs, cards, and banners featuring various print styles and graphics.[19] *The Newsroom* allows the user to design, create, and print a newspaper-like publication by utilizing a built-in word processor, five different type styles, and over 600 pieces of clip art.[20] This software permits the arrangement of printed text and graphics in columns with headlines. If additional graphics are needed to enhance a particular publication, supplementary clip art collections are available. Each clip art collection provides a specific type of graphics such as business-oriented sketches or drawings related to sports and recreation. Desktop publishing software, of which *The Newsroom* is an inexpensive and relatively nonpowerful example, allows the speech-language pathologist thorough control over the layout of a publication.[20] The final product created with a desktop publishing package resembles one prepared by a commercial publisher, but can be produced at a greatly reduced cost. *The Newsroom Pro,*[21] which is a more advanced version of *The Newsroom,*[20] includes more than 2,000 pieces of clip art and sophisiticated word processing capabilities, allowing the user to create and edit an entire layout on the IBM personal computer screen. Using desktop publishing software and a modem connected to telephone lines, the speech-language pathologist can exchange newsletters with other professionals. Responsibility for production of publicity-oriented documents can be shared conveniently by a number of practitioners, each of whom owns the necessary hardware and software for the task and all of whom are attempting to achieve the same professional goal.

Scheduling is another time-consuming administrative task that can be simplified and improved by employing software such as *Pinpoint* to arrange and monitor appointments with clients or other professionals.[22] Using the database program in an integrated software package such as *AppleWorks,* the practitioner can construct a "tickler" file that provides reminders about the need for scheduling appointments with specific clients.[23] Some speech-language pathologists employ computer databases to store pertinent data on all clients seen during a specified time period, permitting easy retrieval and sorting of client data by age, disorder, assessment or intervention procedure employed, or referral source. A list of referral agencies for a given geographic area or a record of consultants who can serve as resources on certain topics might be established and maintained on a database system. Being able to access information about referral agencies or consultants efficiently is valuable when working with clients who are difficult to assess or need state-of-the-art intervention approaches.

Although the extent to which speech-language pathologists are involved in financial management varies greatly from one professional setting to another and from one individual practitioner to another, most clinicians must maintain and operate within budgets. Budgetary responsibilities may be limited to monitoring the expenditures of a designated amount of money allocated for materials in a public school or may entail accounting for the entire financial operation of a private practice. Monitoring the allocation of a set amount of money might be accomplished by using a spreadsheet found in an integrated software package such as *AppleWorks.*[23] In situations where the speech-language pathologist is responsible for billing clients directly or for third-party billing, more powerful and sophisticated business software packages such as *Businessworks* might be needed.[24] Word processing software such as *Apple writer* may be used to generate forms that are saved on a disk and employed as templates to be used during completion of forms for future individual clients.[25] Forms used frequently may be prepared in a skeletal manner, then the appropriate content can be inserted for a specific client each time the form is used, thus saving time and effort in the completion of the paperwork. Documents produced with a word processor are usually more polished in appearance than those generated by hand or on a typewriter.

Correspondence also can be prepared more easily by using a word processor. Any written communication containing repetitive words, phrases, or blocks of text is a type of form letter. The speech-language pathologist can generate various form letters through employment of a word processor, individualizing them for each client or situation. By creating slightly different sections of documents and selecting for a given document one version of each section, a process called "boilerplating," the clinician can personalize form letters and other documents. Boilerplating can be a time saver and may assist in the development of more creative and individualized documents. Correspondence that might incorporate boilerplating readily includes letters to parents or spouses regarding the client's progress, letters to referral agencies, and letters to establish meeting times with parents and other professionals. By using word processing software and *MailMerge,* the speech-language pathologist can combine names and addresses with otherwise identical form letters, so that each person receives what appears to be a personalized letter.[26]

Correspondence might also be sent through electronic mail, with messages conveyed directly from computer to computer. According to Fersko-Weiss, "The benefits of electronic mail go to the heart of the productivity issue—offering better control of time, faster dissemination of information, and more open communication flow."[27] Electronic mail systems may be expensive to implement initially and difficult for potential users to master. However, communication experts and consulting firms have determined that it takes an average of four tries to complete one phone call. To arrange a meeting among six business professionals takes approximately 100 phone calls.[28] Obviously if people who are separated by distances need to communicate frequently and rapidly with each other, electronic mail capabilities should be extremely economical. Substantial time and, therefore, money may be saved by a school district, a professional organization, or a group private practice that institutes an effective electronic mail system. To start using electronic mail, a clinician must have access to a personal computer, a modem connected to telephone lines, one of the available electronic mail software packages, and colleagues equipped with similar hardware and software. Although electronic mail is not utilized widely within Communication Sciences and Disorders, it is probably a wave of the future that could increase personal productivity by handling correspondence more effectively and efficiently than current approaches such as the telephone and traditional mail services.

Client Recordkeeping Activities

The microcomputer is a valuable asset in the personal productivity of a clinician by generating and maintaining client records. A number of software packages have been developed to assist the speech-language pathologist in writing individualized intervention plans (IEPs). The *Language Intervention Planner* includes long-term and short-term goal statements for language disordered preschool and school age children.[29] In addition, the *Language Intervention Planner* provides an option for the practitioner to develop and use a personal set of goals. This program is a therapy planner, not an IEP generator. However, its authors comment that it contains statements that could be used as goals and has the flexibility to use IEP format statements. The *IEP Writer* assists the speech-language pathologist in designing and producing IEPs.[30] This software does not contain a storehouse of goals and objectives, but provides the mechanism with which a clinician can build a bank of goals and objectives. This simplifies the process of generating IEPs with similar goals and objectives across clients or for the same client over time. *Planning Individualized Speech and Language Intervention Programs: Computer Software Adaptation* contains speech-language intervention goals and objectives in the areas of preverbal behaviors, language comprehension and production, articulation, voice, and fluency.[31] The purpose of this program is to provide clinicians with a timesaving resource for planning and implementing an IEP. The program does not allow for the addition of goals and objectives. However, space is provided after each short-term objective for further individualization of that particular item. Another software package, the *Talley Goals and Objectives Writer,* allows the speech-language pathologist to input basic student information and generate an IEP with as many as eight goals and 48 objectives per student.[32] A maximum of 25 IEPs can be stored and printed sequentially. The bank of goals and objectives is extremely flexible, permitting speech-language pathologists to devise their own or to purchase disks that contain goals and objectives based upon the various Brigance tests: *Comprehensive Inventory of Basic Skills,*[33] *Inventory of Basic Skills,*[34] *Inventory of Early Development,*[35] and *Inventory of Essential Skills.*[36] Some IEP-generating programs are quite flexible and allow the clinician to individualize goals and objectives for a client, whereas some are quite rigid and provide minimal potential for individualizing the IEP. If speech-language pathologists choose inflexible IEP-generating software, they they may be fitting clients to existing IEPs and failing to abide by the intent of the law, which is to individualize the program to fit the needs of the client.

The microcomputer can also assist the speech-language pathologist in monitoring client progress. Some software, such as *Function Pictures,* allows storage of individual client response data.[37] Other programs, such as *Progress Monitoring Program,* permit the clinician to graph performance for client behavior over a period of many sessions, showing progress toward each objective in the client's IEP.[38] By using a spreadsheet in a software package such as *AppleWorks,* the speech-language pathologist can keep numerical data from session to session.[23] Such data may be averaged by the computer for large numbers of clients or numerous clinical sessions.

By putting daily log templates on the microcomputer with a word processor, the clinician can maintain daily or weekly intervention logs for clients. This type of an approach would be excellent in those settings where the practitioner has access to the computer and appropriate software for entering client data after each client's session. Likewise, writing and updating lesson plans could be accomplished easily and rapidly with a word processor, which stores on disk the format for each lesson plan. The clinician, using a template for lesson plans, would input data pertinent for a given client into the blank framework stored on disk. Evaluation data for each client could be kept on the same disk and loaded into the report. Thus information about the lesson plan and about results of assessment and previous intervention could be accessed easily with a few keystrokes.

Word processing software can save the speech-language pathologist numerous hours in the generation of diagnostic and therapy reports. Diagnostic reports often contain a limited variety of types of information about the client, such as identification data, referral source, reasons for the referral, statement of the problem, background information about the client, assessment results and interpretations, and recommendations. The information within each of these categories tends to be expressed with repetitive phrases, sentences, and paragraphs. This type of material lends itself nicely to the idea of creating a template. The speech-language pathologist can modify the content of the template to fit each individual client. The process of producing a final diagnostic report with a traditional noncomputerized approach consumes about 15 to 20 percent of the speech-language pathologist's time and effort during assessment.[39,40] Using a template or boilerplate system can cut in half the time and effort required for writing diagnostic reports. Saving such a substantial amount of time could permit the practitioner to spend more time on creative activities and clinical decisionmaking endeavors that only a competent human clinician can perform. The concept of reducing time spent on paperwork by using templates and boilerplating with a word processor applies also to the writing of progress reports and the production of other clinical documents.

Clinical Research Activities

Because microcomputers can categorize, sort, and analyze large amounts of data accurately with remarkable speed, they are ideal tools for assisting the speech-language pathologist in conducting clinical research. For example, software designed to analyze language samples ". . . may broaden the scope and increase the reliability of research previously dependent on lengthy analysis-by-hand."[41] Statistical software allows a speech-language pathologist engaged in clinical research to analyze data quickly, releasing the clinician from the mechanical task of mathematical calculation.[42] Maintaining a database of caseload information would permit a clinical researcher to track clients from the initial assessment to termination of intervention, and after intervention has been discontinued. It has also been noted that other research-related benefits of the microcomputer are that it can be interfaced with other instrumentation to control stimulus presentation variables and can record data in real time.[13] With the use of microcomputer technology, clinical research endeavors that previously eluded the speech-language pathologist because of time limitations may now be practical.

Continuing Education

The incidence of computer networking, the connection of computers for the purpose of exchanging information, has risen sharply in the last few years.[43] By participating in national network systems, speech-language pathologists can communicate rapidly with one another and other professionals. Computer information networks such as *SpecialNet,*[44] *Compuserve,*[45] and *The Source*[46] are several of the most widely used national information network systems. *Compuserve* and *The Source* are general information services, whereas *SpecialNet* is an information network particularly for people interested in special education. The American Speech-Language-Hearing Association currently subscribes to *SpecialNet* and is investigating services that can be provided to its members through this network.

To access these information services, a user needs a microcomputer, a modem, a communications software package, and a telephone. The modem is connected to telephone lines, allowing a computer to access any other computer that can be reached by telephone. Modems operate at various speeds from 300 to 9,600 baud. The higher the baud rate, the faster information can be transmitted through the modem. Since most computer network systems charge hourly rates, a faster transmission rate usually is more economical in the long run. However, faster modems are more expensive, may not be capable of performing some tasks that slower modems can, and may incur increased hourly charges for operating at the faster baud rate.

Using computer information networks, a speech-language pathologist can share information efficiently with other professionals. Professionals across the nation can talk with each other using computer bulletin boards, reducing the need to travel many miles for a meeting that occupies a few hours. Informative inservices for professionals can be provided to all those who have access to the electronic bulletin board by a computer information network. Clinicians can exchange ideas about new methods for assessment and intervention through computer bulletin boards. Continuing education activities of clinicians can be enriched by the use of computer-assisted instructional packages devised to teach them about some specific professional content area of interest to a substantial group of individuals. For example, computer-assisted instructional materials are being developed by the American Speech-Language-Hearing Association through Project IMPACT to teach practitioners how to use microcomputers for enhancing personal productivity, clinical research endeavors, assessment practices, and intervention activities. (A. Schwartz, personal communication, January 15, 1987). In addition, *Phonological Process Tutor*[47] and *Competency Training Systems*[48] are software items that could be employed for continuing education activities by clinicians.

Assessment and Intervention

Clinical software employed during assessment and intervention may be categorized as microcomputer administered or microcomputer assisted. Microcomputer-administered programs are characterized by tasks presented by the microcomputer and responses made by the client through the use of the microcomputer. A microcomputer-assisted program performs some limited segment of a clinical activity, but does not regulate the entire activity. Existing software is marked by many more examples of microcomputer-assisted programs than microcomputer-administered programs.

One example of a microcomputer-administered assessment procedure that was developed originally for manual administration, but now is available in a software format, is *The Computerized Minnesota Child Development Inventory Report (MCDI)*.[49] This particular instrument is intended for use primarily by psychologists and early education teachers, but may be employed by speech-language pathologists working with young children. The child's mother is usually the respondent to questions about the child's development. In a computerized administration of the *MCDI*, the mother would sit at a microcomputer, receive instructions on the monitor, read questions from the monitor, and reply to the questions by keyboarding at the computer. Thus computerized administration would necessitate minimal involvement of the speech-language pathologist who could be performing other clinical procedures while the mother completed the inventory. Microcomputer-administered activities are performed by an unassisted client, or a member of the client's family, after an initial introduction to the hardware and software by the clinician. Such independent activities of the client or family member can supplement direct client-clinician procedures and can provide additional practice of emerging communication behaviors. Many of the activities that could be microcomputer-administered are repetitive tasks in which stimuli vary, but the required response type is simple and constant. For example, if a clinician decided that an adult aphasic individual needed practice at a task such as reading a paragraph and answering multiple-choice questions about its content, a program such as *Aphasia IV: Reading Comprehension* might be assigned to the client for practice between intervention sessions.[50] A child who is beginning to use the concepts of right, left, above, and below might gain additional practice by using *Juggles' Rainbow*, a program distributed now with an accompanying booklet that suggests activities for a speech-language pathologist to employ with clients.[51,52] A number of programs are accompanied now by such booklets, a visible sign of the increasing usage of microcomputers by clinicians.

The microcomputer can serve as an electronic assistant to the clinician, performing a variety of roles in assessment and intervention, even when the microcomputer is not responsible for administering any procedure entirely. Such microcomputer-assisted activities may facilitate a wide variety of aspects of the clinical process. Many stimulus presentation characteristics may be controlled by the microcomputer. Number of stimuli in an array, interstimulus interval, stimulus modality, duration of stimuli, size of stimuli, and order of stimuli in a series can be regulated by computer. Closer command over these parameters of stimulus presentation may be achieved by the clinician employing a microcomputer for stimulus control than would be possible by more traditional mechanisms. Many programs developed for use by speech-language pathologists, including *Function Pictures*, permit storage of client response data, facilitating the examination of client performance over time.[37] Such programs as *Progress Monitoring Program* allow the clinician to graph performance for almost any type of client behavior over a period of many sessions, showing progress toward an objective.[38] Thus the microcomputer can facilitate maintenance of good client records and can assist with demonstration of accountability by the clinician. One of the primary strengths of a microcomputer is that it can handle large amounts of data efficiently and accurately. Microcomputers are valuable in the storage and sorting of client data, as well as in performing calculations based on the data. Programs that analyze spontaneous language samples calculate a wide variety of measures of language behavior such as mean length of response in words or morphemes, type-token ratios, and frequency of utterance types.[53,54] Such measures, when calculated by hand, are tedious and time-consuming to achieve, but can be done quickly once a transcript is typed into the microcomputer. Microcomputer programs can deliver instructions or other information to clients or clinicians, helping with the standardization of this process. An example of software that delivers instructions is the *Computer Managed Screening Test*.[55] This screening instrument is designed with the intention that paraprofessionals should be able to administer it. The microcomputer presents on a monitor all of the instructions to the test administrator, telling the person what stimuli to present and how, as well as identifying the type of response behavior to be observed. Delivering instructions by computer may be a mechanism for standardizing procedures, reducing variability among examiners or therapists, which may be particularly important if paraprofessionals are involved in the clinical activity. Computers are capable of creating situations that simulate real-life natural communication contexts, thus contributing to the elicitation or facilitation of functional communication behaviors of a client. It may not be feasible, or at times it may be dangerous, to put the client into certain real situations in which it would be worthwhile to observe or modify the client's behavior. A clinician might wish to know how a client would function during a shopping expedition, but might prefer to simulate that experience through the use of a computer program rather than taking the client into a store immediately. Practicing some behaviors in a computer-simulated environment may be an intermediate step before introducing the client to the similar real-life situation. In other cases, the computer creates an interesting language-stimulating environment that the clinician does not intend to try to replicate realistically at some later time: for example, a visit to a haunted house, a camping expedition, flying a jet plane, or writing a newspaper story. Many computer programs contribute to assessment and intervention by performing combinations of the types of functions described previously. A given program may supply on-screen instructions and analyze client responses. Another program may simulate a situation and facilitate recordkeeping by storing and displaying data over a number of sessions.

Assessment

Some microcomputer assessment activities may be classified as formal tests, whereas others involve control of informal assessment procedures. Although examples of both formal and informal assessment applications are available, the number of formal tests programmed on the microcomputer and useful to a speech-language pathologist is relatively small.

Most formal tests available in the form of microcomputer software were developed originally for administration in a more traditional manner and for the use of professionals other than speech-language pathologists. This type of software, which may have been designed primarily for use by psychologists, early education teachers, or other professionals, may be called "CDIS-related" as contrasted with "CDIS-specific" software, which has been designed for speech-language pathologists to use with their clients. CDIS-related formal tests that are now available in computer versions include the *DTLA-2: Detroit Tests of Learning Aptitude*[56] and the *Computerized Minnesota Child Development Inventory Record.*[49]

Informal procedures employed by the speech-language pathologist during assessment also may be based on usage of the microcomputer. Informal procedures can be based upon CDIS-specific, CDIS-related, or generic software, which is software designed originally for use by a nonprofessional person. A program such as *The Factory,* which would be classified as CDIS-related, was developed initially to assist children in learning to solve problems involving analytic thinking and sequencing.[57] However, a speech-language pathologist might employ this program in a manner very different from its intended application. The program is one that presents a pattern to the user, and the user is asked to select and sequence available machines to replicate the pattern of holes and stripes on a square. It is a program that lends itself to group discussion and decisionmaking. Therefore a speech-language pathologist might use this program by introducing it to a school-age client and several friends of the client, then allowing the students to proceed through the program, talking about how to achieve the desired pattern. This activity might be selected by a clinician desiring to create a natural situation in which the client would be asking and answering functional questions or would be exhibiting turn-taking behavior. The microcomputer would administer this activity, generating the situation while the clinician could record behaviors of interest. Thus the microcomputer would create a situation in which an informal assessment procedure would be completed and would administer the entire activity after the initial introduction of the program by the clinician. A clinician wishing to have an informal procedure administered by the microcomputer would decide what behaviors are to be observed, choose software that would maximize the potential for those behaviors to occur, and employ that software to create the situation in which to observe those behaviors.

Examples of CDIS-Specific Assessment Software. Since CDIS-specific software is being developed and marketed at such a rapid rate, it would be foolish to attempt an exhaustive listing or description of available programs that might contribute to the assessment process. Therefore, the programs mentioned in this section of the chapter are included only as examples of the types of microcomputer assessment applications that are available.

Many CDIS-specific intervention programs include segments that perform probe testing that may be done to monitor progress. Although the primary purpose of such programs is not assessment, this variety of software contributes to the comprehensive assessment of clients. Some of the programs that include probe-testing sections are *Speller I,*[58] *Function Pictures,*[37] and *Microcomputer Language Assessment and Development Systems: Micro-LADS.*[59]

A variety of software packages is available for analyzing aspects of speech behavior, including the following diverse programs: *Nasometer,*[60] *Lingquest 2: Phonological Analysis,*[61] and *Computerized Assessment of Intelligibility of Dysarthric Speech.*[62]

Aspects of language behavior are assessed through the use of a number of software items such as *Systematic Analysis of Language Transcripts: SALT,*[53] *Cognitive Rehabilitation,*[63] *Computer Managed Screening Test,*[55] and *Sentence Completions: Semantics.*[64]

Although the number of CDIS-specific assessment programs is not extensive, it is expanding at an impressive rate. As more and more clinicians become capable of developing software or of collaborating in its development, the variety and quantity of CDIS-specific assessment software should increase markedly.

Intervention

Microcomputer software can assist the speech-language pathologist in accomplishing various treatment goals. Although software packages are available for both speech and language intervention, the majority of the existing software is for language rather than speech intervention.

Intervention Software for Speech Disorders. Intervention programs for use with speech disorders include a number of programs for articulation disorders, a lesser number for voice disorders, and essentially none for fluency disorders.[3] Articulation therapy programs have been developed by Fitch[65] and Weiner.[66] The articulation program developed by Fitch, a speech-language pathologist, was originally designed to be used by teachers, aides, and supervisors of Head Start programs.[65] Head Start personnel employed this program to control drill and practice routines presented on the computer screen, introducing stimuli and judging the responses of the children.[3] Weiner's *Minimal Contrast Therapy* program was developed for use with children who delete the endings of words.[66] Pictures of minimal pairs are presented on the computer screen. A clinician judges whether the child responded correctly and signals the computer, then provides feedback through the computer to the child about the accuracy of the articulation behavior. Data on the client's performance can be saved on a diskette.

The *Vocal Abuse Reduction Program (VARP)* by Johnson and Child teaches clients about (1) the physical properties of voice production and (2) how to use a wrist counter to track instances of vocal abuse.[67] Data on vocal abuse are entered into the computer, which maintains individual client records. The *Nasometer,* which measures nasal and oral energy outputs during speech, is employed during voice intervention as a biofeedback device for clients with nasality disorders.[60] A computerized version of the *Visi-Pitch,* an instrument that analyzes fundamental frequency and amplitude of the voice, provides statistical analysis of voice parameters and controls storage of client performance data as well as production of a printed record.[68] The computer-connected *Visi-Pitch* has been described as a biofeedback device that is useful during voice intervention.

Intervention Software for Language Disorders. The majority of existing CDIS-specific intervention software is associated with the area of language intervention for children and adults. Language intervention programs for children include software that might be used to teach syntactical skills. For example, *Microcomputer Language Assessment and Development System (Micro-LADS)* incorporates modules for teaching noun plurals, noun and verb agreement, verb forms, prepositions, pronouns, negatives, wh-questions, passive constructions, and deictic expressions.[59] Other programs have been designed to teach predominantly the semantic component of language. *First Words* employs animated graphics and a speech synthesizer to teach nouns to children.[69] *First Categories* teaches word categories such as animals and body parts.[70] *Exploratory Play*[71] and *Representational Play*[72] are programs that teach language skills at the single-word, two-word, and multiword utterance levels to very young children using the computer during natural play. Other programs have been designed to teach a variety of general language skills. *Computer Managed Language Treatment* was developed to teach children the concepts of colors, numbers, prepositions, and general language development skills.[73]

Language intervention software also has been designed for aphasic adults to assist them in relearning basic language skills. One example of such a program is *Word Recognition,* a program employing digitized speech, graphics, and real-time clock peripherals to assist the aphasic client in relearning common words.[74] *Cognitive Rehabilitation* assists the client in relearning a variety of language-related skills such as categorization, sequencing, association, and memory.[63] *Aphasia I*[75] teaches part-to-whole word relationships; whereas *Aphasia II*[76] teaches word association skills, and *Aphasia III*[77] teaches word categorization. The *Computerized Aphasia Treatment System (CATS)* was designed to teach reading skills to aphasic clients.[78] Other programs have been designed predominantly to teach comprehension of syntactic elements. Representative programs are *Understanding Questions,* which teaches question words of who, what, and when;[79] *Understanding Sentences,* which teaches comprehension of subject-verb-object constructions;[80] and *Understanding Stories,* which teaches the adult aphasic to comprehend short printed paragraphs.[81]

Types of Computer-Assisted Instructional Programs. Applications of the microcomputer to intervention with speech-language disorders may be classified according to the types of computer-assisted instructional activities that can be performed: drill and practice, simulation, tutorial, instructional games, problem solving, and exploration and discovery. These types of activities will be discussed briefly in relation to intervention with CDIS-specific and CDIS-related software. Software mentioned should not be assumed to be the only available programs for the purpose described, and the mention is not intended to be an endorsement.

Drill and Practice. This variety of computer-assisted instructional software is best used with those clients who need much repetition to learn a skill or concept. For example, if a clinician decides that a client needs to learn the meaning of a fixed set of nouns, an available CDIS-specific program would be *First Words.*[69] Certain types of articulation behaviors may be learned through drill and practice, using software such as *Computer Managed Articulation Treatment*[65] and *Minimal Contrast Therapy.*[66] Other language behaviors might be taught using drill and practice programs such as *Aphasia I, Aphasia II,* and *Aphasia III.*[75–77] One of the major advantages of many of these programs is that once the program's operations is illustrated by a speech-language pathologist, an aide with a client or a client alone might use the programs either in the home or in the clinician's work setting without the clinician's continual guidance. These drill and practice programs can be used to supplement the intervention program delivered directly by the speech-language pathologist.

Simulation. This type of activity allows the speech-language pathologist to place the client in situations that resemble the real world before attempting involvement in a less controlled real situation. Simulation activities work extremely well with those clients for which real-life, functional situations would be unsafe, expensive, or difficult to arrange. For example, two CDIS-related programs that might be used with an adolescent who displays a language disorder are the *Grammar Examiner*[82] and *The Whitewater Canoe Race.*[83] The *Grammar Examiner* allows the student to learn basic grammatical skills while, at the same time, experiencing what it is like to be a newspaper editor. *The Whitewater Canoe Race* simulates a camping and canoeing trip during which important decisions must be made in order to survive the trip, thus teaching problem-solving skills.

Tutorial. Tutorial programs present new information in a step-by-step process that assists the client in learning or relearning a behavior. An example of a CDIS-specific tutorial is the *Vocal Abuse Reduction Program* by Johnson and Child.[67] One CDIS-related tutorial program for use with clients is *Verbs,*[84] while another is *Analogies Tutorial.*[85]

Instructional Games. These computer-assisted instructional activities teach problem-solving strategies by means of a game format. Text or graphic adventure games are examples of this software category. Adventure games are particularly useful in language intervention with adolescents, who may expand their thinking and language skills by using the programs. While playing adventure games, adolescents may improve their map-making skills, note-taking abilities, ability to follow instructions, theory-building skills, hypothesis-testing abilities, appreciation of cause-and-effect relationships, and recognition of the importance of behavior sequences.[18] Many adventure games are available commercially. After clients become more adept linguistically and their problem-solving skills improve, software such as *Adventure Master* could be used to allow the clients to create their own adventure games.[86]

Problem-Solving Activities. Problem-solving activities permit clients to subdivide tasks into small steps and to experiment with different patterns of information. Word processors such as *Bank Street Writer,*[87] *Kidwriter,*[88] and *Keytalk*[89] permit students at various language levels to learn to organize ideas in written form. *Keytalk* employs software in conjunction with a speech synthesizer, allowing the student to write on the computer screen and produce speech output. Meyers used *Keytalk* to improve the language abilities of school-age Down syndrome children who were severely delayed in their ability to produce grammatically correct sentences.[90] The *Keytalk* program speaks the letters, words, and sentences the children type on the computer. The children were expected to learn to write more grammatically correct sentences over the course of 30 sessions: ten sessions were spent writing with paper and pencil; ten sessions were spent writing on a computer without speech output; and ten sessions were spent writing on a computer with speech output. The results of this preliminary study revealed that the children learned to speak and to write in grammatically correct multiword sentences. In addition, some children apparently learned to write grammatically correct sentences before they learned to speak them. For some children, seeing the text and hearing the synthesized speech led to improved spoken language skills.[90] An additional CDIS-related problem-solving program is *The Factory* in which the client is asked to solve a problem introduced within a game-like format.[57]

Exploration and Discovery. In this type of computer-assisted instructional activity, the computer creates an environment in which the user can pose questions, make decisions, and solve problems. One of the best examples of this type of activity is provided by Papert, who describes children learning to use the computer language called "Logo."[91] This computer language is procedure oriented, incorporating Piagetian theory and artificial intelligence concepts. Logo has been found to be successful with special children, who sometimes initially gain a degree of control over their environments through the use of this microcomputer language.[17]

Comments about Microcomputer Applications to Intervention. Whether software employed is CDIS-specific or CDIS-related, and regardless of the type of computer-assisted instructional activity, it is crucial that the speech-language pathologist should incorporate the computer only when appropriate and only as one aspect of the comprehensive intervention process. The discipline of Communication Science and Disorders has just begun to develop appropriate intervention software. Currently, the majority of the CDIS-specific programs are in the area of language disorders for children and adults and are limited to drill and practice routines. The full potential of the microcomputer as a speech and language intervention tool has not, as yet, been realized. Much clinical research is needed to demonstrate the effectiveness of the microcomputer as an intervention tool when used as part of the client-clinician intervention routines, when incorporated in home intervention programs for clients with or without the assistance of a family member, and when employed by supportive personnel such as communication aides.

LIMITATIONS OF MICROCOMPUTER APPLICATIONS TO CLINICAL MANAGEMENT

Although microcomputers have much to contribute to the clinical functioning of a speech-language pathologist, it is important that clinicians be aware of computer hardware and software limitations regarding applications possible at the current time. Limitations to be considered by practitioners as they incorporate computer technology into their professional world may be categorized as factors related to theoretical foundations of programs, to validity and reliability of programs, to flexibility of programs, to technical quality of programs, and to practicality of programs. This section of the chapter describes these limitations and their impact upon applications of the microcomputer to clinical management.

Theoretical Foundations of Programs

Some microcomputer software is accompanied by thorough and helpful documentation that explains operational characteristics of the program and provides instructions for the user. Some CDIS-specific software is sold with associated documentation that delineates explicitly the theoretical principles on which the programs are based. However, the degree to which documentation for CDIS-specific programs addresses this topic varies. When a program is distributed without concomitant explanation of underlying clinical principles, the speech-language pathologist who is deliberating about whether to purchase or use the program is forced to infer what the theoretical principles of the program are. Drawing such inferences is difficult until the program has already been purchased and used long enough for the clinician to become familiar with it. For this reason among others, it is important that clinicians consider prior to purchasing a program the distributor's policy on refunding the purchase price if the program is not satisfactory to the user. Many distributors accept a return of the software with a full refund within 30 days of purchase, but rarely is the trial period longer than 30 days. Thus clinicians must try the programs soon after receiving them to make sure within the trial period that the software is worth keeping. One of the primary criteria that must be applied in reaching a decision about whether to keep the program is that the theoretical principles for that program must be appropriate and consistent with the theoretical principles of the potential user. CDIS-related software, which is developed primarily for the use of professionals other than speech-language pathologists, is sometimes accompanied by documentation that addresses relevant theoretical issues. However, since the intended users for CDIS-related software are not speech-language pathologists, the theoretical issues addressed may or may not be the ones that would concern a clinician. CDIS-related software often is not distributed with a 30-day refund for dissatisfied users, and so careful preconsideration of whether to purchase is vital. Generic software, which is not developed for use by professionals, but is intended for the general public as consumers, rarely mentions theoretical principles in the accompanying documentation. Distributors of generic software usually are unwilling to refund the purchase price just because a buyer is not pleased with the program, but only if the program does not operate as the distributors intend it to operate. Therefore thorough familiarity with generic software must be achieved, and an evaluation of germane theoretical principles must be accomplished prior to the purchase of such programs by the potential buyer. Each individual practitioner must make a personal judgment about the appropriateness of theoretical principles that underlie a program. If a clinician rejects the notion of testing discrete aspects of language devoid of a functional context, a program such as the *DTLA-2: The Detroit Tests of Learning Aptitude* would be unacceptable theoretically to that clinician.[56] A clinician who adheres to the principle that the number of response opportunities for a client should be maximized during each session may decide that a program spending much time on the delivery of clever visual reinforcement and on switching from one graphics screen to another violates an important theoretical principle, and so the clinician might conclude that the program should not be purchased. Speech-language pathologists who feel that intervention related to semantic development should occur in functional language contexts would judge that a program teaching single words out of context is based on an inappropriate theoretical principle and so would choose not to purchase it. Because sometimes underlying theoretical principles are not delineated and sometimes inappropriate theoretical principles are incorporated into software, each clinician considering purchase must perform an evaluation personally to judge wisely what purchases are worthwhile.

Validity and Reliability of Programs

Programs classified as CDIS-specific are often field tested before they are released for purchase. However, field testing is not always as thorough as a user might wish. CDIS-related and generic software usually has not been field tested with communicatively disabled clients, the potential users of most concern to a speech-language pathologist. Whenever data from field testing are unavailable at the time when a purchase is considered, there is a danger that the program will not operate correctly, that it will be of an inappropriate difficulty level for the clients on a clinician's caseload, or that the reliability and the validity of the program have not been established adequately. Sometimes documentation does not describe thoroughly the nature and extent of the field testing that has been done, making it wise for the clinician not to purchase the program unless the distributor offers a 30-day refund policy, since the purchasing practitioner must do field testing personally before deciding whether to buy the software. Clinicians usually assume that microcomputers perform calculation routines accurately and that purchase of software to perform complex computations will improve the accuracy of the resulting data. People program computers. The microcomputer performs reliably the computations built into the program, whether the calculation routines are correct or not. Powerful but poorly programmed software may become a multiplier of errors rather than a reducer of errors. It is wise for speech-language pathologists who purchase programs to perform manual computations to check the accuracy of software and to analyze carefully any discrepancies between the manual and computer results in order to identify the source of the errors. If the error is in the software, that error must be corrected, or the clinician should probably not purchase the program. Documentation sometimes does not include an adequate explanation of the procedures employed in constructing norms for the associated software, decreasing markedly the value of any reported norms. In the rush to make software available to potential users, creators of programs seem occasionally to be taking shortcuts in establishing reliability and validity. One factor that increases the likelihood of poor program validity currently is that there are few speech-language pathologists who are capable of writing computer programs. Although more and more practitioners are developing programming skills as time passes, when programming is done by someone other than a speech-language pathologist, there is a danger that the programmer may not understand enough about the knowledge base for Communication Sciences and Disorders to make wise decisions about program content and operation. Close and effective collaboration is needed during software development between computer programmers and clinicians to ensure that program validity will be acceptable in the finished product and that high technical quality of the software will be maintained.

Flexibility of Programs

Software that is not adaptable to meet the needs of individual clients is of restricted value to a clinician. Unfortunately, many programs available currently do not include options for the clinician who wishes to customize the software for a specific client. Some of the types of valuable options that characterize certain programs, and which permit practitioners to adapt programs to fit individual clients, include the following parameters: stimulus duration, sound on and sound off, size of stimulus array, vocabulary level during the task, large print and small print, repeatability of stimuli, rate of stimulus presentation, intensity of stimuli, nature of available cues, and response mode. The more flexible a program is in presenting the clinician with options so that activities can be appropriately different for different clients, the more applicable it is liable to be to a clinician's caseload. Occasionally a unique program that fits few clients is worthy of purchase if no other mechanism exists to accomplish the same purpose. However, in general, the wider the variety of clients for whom the program is applicable, the more justifiable the purchase. Sometimes the output that is provided to the clinician by the software makes programs inflexible. For example, there are some programs that are capable of generating page after page of information about a client's language behavior, based on the analysis of a spontaneous language sample provided by a clinician. Some programs yield a massive amount of data and give the clinician no choice but to accept all of these data, not providing any possibility for the clinician to select types of analyses desired for a particular client. When software yields too much information, the ramifications may be hazardous in a variety of ways: (1) the speech-language pathologist may be overwhelmed by the printout, losing important data in a paper mountain; (2) the overall vision of the client's communication pattern may be lost in a welter of discrete numbers; (3) efficiency of operation may be reduced because the clinician needs to find the relevant information within the mass of data produced or because the clinician feels compelled to report and use all of the data available; (4) storage space may be eaten up quickly by keeping huge printouts that are not used in their entirety; or (5) the deluge of data may cause the practitioner to reject the software. One of the factors leading to a lack of flexibility in software is the limited memory capacity of many microcomputers utilized by speech-language pathologists. The more limited the computer memory, the less options are liable to be included for output or for the task presented to the client. As memory available in microcomputers increases over the years, it is likely that some of the current linear programs that permit no branching in reaction to a client's responses will disappear, to be replaced by interactive software with branching capacity that permits the program to adjust to the response of the client. Although many programmers recognize that varying the reinforcement provided to the client is desirable, some software employs a single type of reinforcement that is repeated again and again, whereas other programs vary reinforcement in inappropriate ways. Comments to the client such as "not too bad, Susan" or uninterpretable sounds that are meant to be reinforcing actually may be confusing, distracting, frightening, or insulting to clients. Flexibility of reinforcement seems not to be as crucial as the clarity of the reinforcement to the client, since working with a microcomputer often appears to be so reinforcing to the client that variety in reinforcement may not be absolutely necessary. In fact, flexibility of reinforcement is a characteristic of program design that may detract from efficiency or effectiveness of the program if the client is required to analyze each bit of feedback from the computer to decide what it means.

Technical Quality of Programs

Many of the programs used by speech-language pathologists were designed originally for microcomputers with very limited memory capacities. As a consequence, quality of graphics and clarity of text characterizing many of these programs is relatively poor. Shriberg, Kwiatkowski, and Snyder described the impact of graphics quality on the performance of children during articulation testing.[16] However, little research is available on the impact of the quality of graphics on behavior of clients in other situations. Interpreting what is being shown on the monitor screen may be a challenging task for an adult with normal eyes, superior language skills, and a lively imagination. For a child with a language disorder the task may be nearly impossible. Clients become frustrated with unclear text and graphics. Incidence of errors is likely to increase without any indication in the performance summary at the end of a program about whether the errors are linguistic errors or errors in deciphering screen displays. Not only is the clarity of text and graphics often poor, but the appearance of grammatical and spelling errors in the text displayed on the monitor screen is fairly common also. Such errors are a sign of inadequate attention to detail during the preparation of the program and lead the user to wonder what other types of errors that are less obvious may also exist in the software.

Some microcomputers are equipped with speech synthesis devices or speech digitizers that permit the microcomputer to deliver speech output to the client or to listeners with whom the client is communicating. Although it is advantageous to present auditory stimuli and audible reinforcement to clients, the quality of speech produced by many devices that create speech output is mediocre or worse. The speech often is robotic and sounds unnatural, presenting a poor speech model for clients and leading to comprehension difficulties on the part of the listeners. Such devices have improved rapidly during recent years,[92,93] and it is likely that vastly improved speech output, such as that now produced by the Apple IIgs, will be available to speech-language pathologists in the near future. Hardware that permits voice input to the computer, which would allow a client to respond to software with spoken words, is in the infancy of its development. However, as the quality of voice input devices improves so that many different speakers with a variety of speech capabilities can talk with an unlimited vocabulary into a voice input device, the contributions of the microcomputer to the clinical process will expand dramatically.

Mechanical inadequacies creep into programs when there is insufficient imposition of program standards during software development. As a consequence, some programs load easily on one microcomputer and not at all on another; some software is extremely slow during loading or in processing data. Such technical limitations are a frustration to users who are inexperienced with microcomputers and are a disappointment to more experienced computer users. Speech-language pathologists should evaluate programs, prior to purchase, for any technical limitations that might exist.

Practicality of Programs

Clinicians purchasing microcomputer hardware and software should realize that the initial period of learning to use the items effectively is liable to be of significant duration and that the task is liable to be difficult. It should be reassuring that others who have struggled to learn how to use microcomputers effectively have felt, nearly without exception, that the investment of time and money needed to become a proficient computer user is well worth it. Because this learning requires a substantial time commitment, it is advisable to consider the potential loss of client-contact time by the novice computer user to be part of the expense of purchasing a computer system. Specific software may demand a protracted learning period while the clinician masters a coding system or develops an understanding of operational characteristics of the program. This initial orientation period leads to far less frustration and loss of time in the long run than would be produced by a program that is easy to learn, but inefficient during routine usage by clients or clinicians. In general, there is a trade-off between ease of initial learning and eventual power and efficiency of the software. Clinicians should not be discouraged from attempting to master a program that is complex and difficult to learn if long-term usage of the program will increase efficiency and enhance effectiveness.

Clinicians must beware of cost and quality mismatches in purchasing both hardware and software. Higher quality does not always accompany higher costs. Clinicians will be forced to make judgments about whether it is worthwhile or not to spend hundreds or thousands of dollars for computer-related items. Such decisions must take into account flexibility in regard to the users who can benefit from the items and tasks that can be accomplished, as well as the ultimate benefits that are likely to occur in quantitative and qualitative aspects of clinical operations. The number of CDIS-specific programs is comparatively small. The market for such programs will remain somewhat limited. Consequently, the cost of CDIS-specific programs is liable to remain high. High software costs make it wise for the purchasing speech-language pathologist to do a thorough job of evaluating the software prior to purchase, so that the clinician will feel ultimately that the funds were not squandered. Because the cost of software is high, clinicians should be sure to obtain or make archival backup copies of all software and all data, protecting themselves from unnecessary replacement costs and loss of vital information. Usually software and hardware perform in a reliable and durable fashion, but it is always wise to prepare for the rare exception to such a generalization.

POTENTIAL BENEFITS OF MICROCOMPUTER APPLICATIONS IN CLINICAL MANAGEMENT

When incorporating the microcomputer into the clinical management process, it is vital that the clinician realize that this much-heralded machine has the potential to be friend or foe depending upon how wisely it is used. It is important that the microcomputer be introduced into the clinical process cautiously and judiciously. However, it is equally crucial that the possibility of misusing the new technological developments not prevent speech-language pathologists from exploring the potential values of appropriate microcomputer utilization. Possible future benefits, some of which are beginning to occur now, are addressed in the following narrative and are subdivided into four categories differentiated by the primary envisioned target of impact: (1) clinician-oriented benefits; (2) client-oriented benefits; (3) procedure-oriented benefits; and (4) data-oriented benefits.

Clinician-Oriented Benefits

There is no question that improving the efficiency of the clinical process would be of benefit to clinicians. As the efficiency of the clinical management process increases, the clinician can spend more time performing and perfecting other clinical activities that need professional attention.[3] Some software is capable of much faster analysis of data than a clinician can perform without a microcomputer. For example, some of the language analysis software packages can accomplish in a few minutes a language analysis and summary that might take an unassisted clinician many hours to complete. Even considering that the clinician would require time to learn how to use the software and time to input the coded language sample into the microcomputer, the long-range improvement in efficiency that can be obtained by using such a program is substantial. Efficiency may be improved as well by simplification of writing reports through templates and boilerplating with a word processor. Software that assists in the generation of individual intervention plans based on assessment results may decrease the time involved in program planning by 25 to 50 percent, a substantial savings of time when multiplied by the number of clients on the caseload. Krueger, delineating the steps involved in and benefits achieved from computerization of recordkeeping and production of reports in a public school, commented that time spent on paperwork dropped from 2 hours per client to 30 minutes; this drop substantially reduced the costs for this aspect of the speech-language program.[14]

In addition to increasing assessment efficiency, the microcomputer can assist in the reduction of clinician variability. Accurate microcomputer programs make fewer errors in counting, arithmetic, and tabulating than a typical clinician does, which should lead to improvement in intraexaminer reliability. Standardization of the analysis procedure and testing protocol achievable through appropriate use of microcomputers should reduce both intraexaminer and interexaminer variability. Drill and practice intervention software could be used with, or independently of, the clinician with assurance that the client would be presented stimulus items and feedback consistently. Some instructional software could be used by support personnel quite reliably, since the programs would present stimulus items consistently and store responses of the client.[3] Appropriate employment of paraprofessional aides using computerized intervention materials could free the clinician to do more creative clinical planning for the client.

Exchange of data between clinicians about a given client can be enhanced if computer technology is used wisely. In this highly mobile society, a client often changes place of residence several times, thus seeing several clinicians over a period of years. More detailed information about clinical management activities can be exchanged by successive practitioners through the use of microcomputer-generated reports. Information can be transmitted through a modem more rapidly to another clinician than would be possible through more traditional mechanisms. Electronic report transmittal and electronic mail distribution may be not only more efficient, but also more cost effective.[3] Client confidentiality and privacy of communication must be reconsidered in view of these new mechanisms of information exchange.

Recent technological advances, including microcomputers, can aid clinicians in developing and updating their knowledge of assessment and intervention devices and procedures. Microcomputer tutorials assist clinicians in learning initially about particular clinical instruments or activities, including those employing a microcomputer.[15] Thus microcomputers can be used to teach clinicians about microcomputers. A national conference about some specific clinical matter could be scheduled to allow all interested clinicians to participate through telecommunication. This type of conference would reduce the necessity for significant commitment of time and money to be spent by clinicians living in diverse areas for attending a national conference held in one specific locality. Expert systems could be developed to assist a speech-language pathologist in the development of assessment or intervention skills, enabling the clinician to learn to select and employ assessment instruments or intervention procedures more wisely.

Microcomputers possess a potential to improve storage and retrieval of clinical management information about clients. This function enables the clinician to keep permanently more data about a client than it has been reasonable to keep previously. Software such as a file management system or a database may be employed to store client information. In addition, entering client information into a microcomputer file management system would permit fast and accurate compilation of caseload information for reports that the clinician must produce. Accountability efforts of clinicians would be strengthened by the resulting available data.

Client-Oriented Benefits

Program planning for individual clients may be improved by intelligent use of the greater mass of data yielded by microcomputer activities. The accumulation of more data does not guarantee better planning of programs; however, a competent clinician can incorporate the greater quantity of information to improve quality of clinical services.

Although some programs are exceptions, most existing software is incapable of adjusting events based on client responses. As increasingly sophisticated interactive software with greater capacity for branching and real-time analysis is developed, assessment and intervention procedures can become more individualized for clients. The use of interactive video disks may allow for the presentation of simulated vignettes to be presented as lifelike, real-time events for clients to react to, without the client suffering any of the adverse consequences of the actual experience.[94]

Many clients, adults and children alike, react enthusiastically to the introduction of the microcomputer into their clinical programs. Although it is possible that their excitement is engendered simply by the interjection of change into the clinical situation, a clinical Hawthorne effect, it is often true that high levels of client interest, response, and enjoyment are sustained beyond the period of novelty. If usage of the microcomputer can encourage better cooperation, greater effort, and higher motivation on the part of clients during the assessment and intervention process, it is possible that the clinician will view behavior closer to the client's optimal level during clinical activities when the microcomputer is involved. Individualization of assessment and intervention procedures, which can be facilitated by the contributions of a microcomputer, may also lead to enhanced interest levels and motivation of clients during clinical activities.

As speech-language pathologists gain skill in using programming languages and in authoring software, more clinicians will become able to create customized software to employ in clinical activities. Under those conditions, fitting the program to the client will be possible, rather than fitting the client to existing assessment and intervention programs. If a client needs to learn more about idioms, stimuli can be selected individually based on the client's needs and presented in a variety of routines using authoring software to build the program.

Procedure-Oriented Benefits

During recent years there has been a rapid increase in the variety of input and output devices that can be used in conjunction with microcomputers. It is likely that the near future will be marked by further substantial advances in peripheral devices. For example, single switches are available for use as input devices by individuals with handicapping conditions that preclude ordinary keyboard entry of information. Single-switch devices are improving rapidly and are being employed more widely with communicatively disabled clients. Touch windows, devices that permit clients to respond to items by pointing to displays on a monitor screen, are relatively inexpensive, but not yet available to many speech-language pathologists. Other input devices for client use, such as the KoalaPad, Muppet keyboard, graphics tablet, joystick, and the mouse, have not been exploited thoroughly yet with regard to their potential for contributing to speech-language assessment and intervention procedures. Although voice input devices exist, they should improve dramatically in the next few years and should become less costly. Use of interactive videodisks in assessment and intervention protocols has vast possibilities for exploring client behavior in simulated situations, but this potential has been utilized only to a minor degree within this profession. The quality of synthesized and digitized speech is improving rapidly and will continue to do so. Technological developments in input and ouput devices have the potential to influence the clinical management process in remarkable ways.

As software for graphics and animation becomes better and as resolution of monitor screens improves, visual stimuli for speech-language activities will be enhanced. Many programs currently employ static graphics that display little or no animation and present pictures or words that are barely identifiable. Visual displays of stimuli should improve markedly in the near future as hardware developments, software production, and cost reduction permit more sophistication of graphics being employed in clinical activities. The capacity to combine high-quality animated graphics with high-quality auditory stimuli will increase the variety of clinical management tasks that can capitalize on the capabilities of a microcomputer.

Perhaps as microcomputers and telecommunication equipment become more pervasive, some clinical activities may be accomplished through these devices rather than through a face-to-face meeting of client and clinician. Although concerns must exist about issues of client privacy and about overreliance by clinicians on this medium of assessment and intervention, it might be feasible to gather through telecommunications some data for preliminary screening, for information gathering during assessment, for reassessment, for home-based intervention, for revising intervention procedures, and for follow-up purposes. The impact of telecommunication on clinical management should be especially significant in rural areas where extended distances between client and clinician tend to be the rule rather than the exception.

It is possible that microcomputer assessment and intervention procedures will lead to increased standardization of those activities, since the microcomputer can control precisely many presentation parameters, such as (1) presentation of instructions; (2) stimulus factors such as selection, organization, administration, duration, interstimulus interval, and size of array; (3) response characteristics such as type of acceptable response or enforced latency of responding; (4) use of reinforcement; and (5) stimulus repetition to check reliability of responses.

Microcomputer-controlled clinical management may reduce procedural variability that occurs because some clinicians resist adherence to the fine details in a printed administration manual. Microcomputer-controlled procedures may allow supportive personnel, or clients working independently, to use selected software during intervention. Even under such conditions, which occur while the clinician is not present, it can be assured that the stimulus items, reinforcement, and recordkeeping are being done consistently and reliably by the computer.

As technology makes it possible to simulate real-life events more realistically and less expensively, it may become easier to assist the client in bridging behaviors learned in intervention sessions to other aspects of the client's life. Software of the future and interactive videodisks will allow for teaching of communication behaviors within a meaningful context. Not only will this aid the client in learning new behaviors, but also, and perhaps more importantly, in transferring those communication behaviors to other situations. Such advances should benefit clients by promoting academic progress, enhancing personal and social interactions, and assisting in realization of vocational potential.

Data-Oriented Benefits

Microcomputers, which have the potential of serving as vast repositories of client data, may have a favorable impact upon several aspects of the development of norms related to assessment. A microcomputer, for example, is a powerful servant in the hands of a clinician who recognizes the need for development of local norms for a specific assessment instrument. In addition, collaboration among clinicians for the purpose of developing large-sample norms is facilitated by the use of microcomputers. With incorporation of the microcomputer, it should become less difficult to develop multiple sets of norms for use with clients belonging to identifiable subpopulations.

As software is evaluated more thoroughly by its developers and its users, improvements may occur in the quality, not just in the quantity, of assessment and intervention information. The quality of data being obtained in assessment and intervention research and being employed in clinical management procedures, may be enhanced by the use of the microcomputer by speech-language pathologists.

Accumulation of larger quantities of data and application of expert systems to clinical management procedures may assist speech-language pathologists to derive better clinical interpretations. Currently, physicians and psychologists are utilizing programs that supply interpretative statements to accompany results summarized by the microcomputer. In the future, such programs may be developed and utilized by speech-language pathologists to assist in the interpretation of results summarized by the microcomputer. In years to come, the microcomputer may be beneficial not only in the "objective" aspects of the clinical management process, but also in some aspects of clinical management traditionally regarded as "subjective."

Accumulation of data through the use of microcomputer records also provides ripe opportunities for clinical research. It is likely to become more feasible for selected clinicians in geographically separate parts of the country to collect data using standardized procedures under the direction of an experimenter who plans and directs the research. Thus the microcomputer may encourage more clinicians to become involved in clinical research, fostering collaboration between those who are primarily researchers and those who are primarily clinicians.

MICROCOMPUTER–RELATED RESOURCES

It is not easy for an individual to gain enough knowledge and competency to permit incorporation of microcomputers into clinical aspects of speech-language pathology. After the commitment to become a competent microcomputer user is made, usually the clinician struggles to find time for necessary learning. Part of the difficulty of the learning task is related to the amount of information to be understood and the number of skills to be mastered. However, the challenge of the task is compounded by the need to locate relevant materials, to select those that are helpful from myriad available activities and materials, to discover where one can obtain necessary hands-on experience, and to identify support mechanisms that can facilitate the learning. Frequently, advice and assistance can be obtained from professional colleagues, although valuable assistance may also come from less obvious sources such as the practitioner's students, clients, or children. The younger generation is growing up in a world that surrounds children and adolescents with computers. Often these younger people are familiar with microcomputers, comfortable using them as tools, and willing to share their expertise at little expense to the professional in need of help. Resources that may assist a speech-language pathologist to become a competent computer user are scattered rather than centralized. This section of the chapter provides some information about locating beneficial resources related to microcomputers: (1) software previews and reviews, (2) catalogues of software, (3) computer periodicals, (4) support groups and services, (5) consultants, and (6) books. Some of the resources identified in this section provide extensive and detailed information about items that belong to given categories that are described only briefly in this chapter.

Software Previews and Reviews

It is wise to preview software, trying it and evaluating it before a purchase is made. Some software that might interest speech-language pathologists may be available in local computer stores and can be examined there before a decision is reached about whether to buy it or not, although most CDIS-specific and CDIS-related software is not sold in local computer stores. The preliminary viewing of software, through the cooperation of a local computer store or an acquaintance who owns the program, may permit the potential purchaser to reach an initial decision about whether or not the software is worth examining in more depth. However, if the potential buyer wishes to field test the software with clients before making a purchase, it is wise to contact the publisher of the program to learn if it may be obtained for a preview period of several weeks' duration. Some publishers of software provide an initial trial period during which a potential purchaser may return a program without being charged for it, but other publishers do not. Reading a program evaluation written by a speech-language pathologist, or even sometimes by a nonprofessional reviewer, may provide assisstance to the individual considering whether or not to purchase a program. Software reviews and evaluations are being published frequently in the *Asha* journal and in each issue of the *Journal for Computer Users in Speech and Hearing*. In addition, many educational computing journals publish relevant software reviews. Software also is described in a number of published articles and books about microcomputers.[3,4,95,96] Criteria for evaluation of software have been suggested by Chial;[97] by Greyerbiehl, Schwartz, Clymer, Owens, and Blackstone;[98] and by Greyerbiehl, Chial, Schwartz, Owens, and Blackstone.[99]

Catalogues of Software

It is difficult to keep abreast of the rapidly developing software market, although advertisements for some programs appear in professional journals. Publicity for other programs may be mailed to a wide audience of professionals, and other programs may be demonstrated at convention exhibits. Software reviews tend to be small in number in each journal and often appear a substantial length of time after a product first becomes available to users. Therefore consideration of other sources of information about programs is worthwhile. Commonly, compilations of program descriptions are published annually for major brands of microcomputers, although not necessarily by the manufacturers of these devices. Access to such catalogues may provide the opportunity to browse through a limited amount of information about each of hundreds or thousands of software items conveniently. Silverman has produced a notebook containing brief synopses of many CDIS-specific and CDIS-related programs.[100] This information was intended for later publication as an appendix in a book.[101]

Computer Periodicals

Computer journals encompass a wide range of technicality and readability. Speech-language pathologists would likely find the *Journal of Computer Users in Speech and Hearing* to be extremely relevant, with content of interest to computer novices as well as to computer experts. Clinicians, especially those who work in public schools, might find a significant amount of beneficial material in periodicals such as *Closing the Gap* and *Computing Teacher*. Drugstores, bookstores, grocery stores, and computer stores commonly distribute periodicals such as *Personal Computing, Infoworld, A+, InCider,* and *PC Magazine,* which are publications intended for the general public. They contain articles with mass audience appeal, including occasional articles about uses of the computer by disabled individuals or by teachers. Many of these nonprofessionally oriented magazines are specific to a given brand of microcomputer, and some apply only to one model of one brand. Before buying a newsstand magazine, the practitioner would be wise to examine it to ascertain if it is pertinent to the hardware situation in which that clinician is involved. Some newsstand magazines, such as *Byte,* tend to contain articles that are much more technical in nature. Although *Byte* is usually difficult to read, being of value routinely to hardware and software developers and hackers, it has occasionally produced comprehensible issues of substantial interest to speech-language pathologists. For example, *Byte* has devoted entire issues to applications of the computer with disabled individuals (September, 1982), to information about uses of the Logo language (August, 1982), and to educational computing (February, 1987).

Support Groups and Services

Numerous support groups have emerged since the personal computer became available to the masses. There are user support groups in most geographical areas, even in small communities. These support groups may consist of members owing a similar brand of computer (e.g., an Apple users group or an IBM users group) or may include members sharing a common interest in computer applications (e.g., a microcomputer graphics users group). Most college or university campuses and some vocational schools or high schools sponsor user groups open to the general public. Being a member of one or more of these support groups affords many opportunities to anyone who joins. Such groups provide a chance to learn about new advances in hardware and software and to have these new products demonstrated before purchase is considered. If a problem about a specific piece of hardware or software arises, often a member of the user group can supply a solution. As the name implies, a support group consists of people who assist one another in solving problems and in learning about new technologic developments. The major organized support group within the profession of Communication Sciences and Disorders is CUSH, which in 1986 enrolled a roster of over 800 practitioners. This organization offers to supply a list of names of members who might be contacted for specific types of assistance with particular products or problems. Support services also are available through some hardware manufacturers, software publishers, and computer discount vendors. Some of these support services are offered without charge, even to the extent of an 800 number being available for telephone consultation, although fees are charged in other instances.

Consultants

It is beneficial to compile a list of individuals who have developed an expertise in computer technology. These individuals may assist the speech-language pathologist in a variety of ways that are dependent on the consultant's expertise areas and the needs of a specific clinician. For example, some consultants may be able to provide assistance in programming, others in illustrating how a given hardware or software item should perform or could be used with a particular type of client. CUSH has developed a list of names of practitioners who are willing to serve as consultants and who have knowledge of computer technology as it applies to Communication Sciences and Disorders. Other consultants may emerge from administrative or academic computing offices at universities, from university departments of computer science or information management, and from computer clubs at universities or high schools. In addition to obtaining lists of names for potential consultants from an organized agency, a speech-language pathologist may wish to review the publication records of professional colleagues, which may assist in the identification of specific individuals with expertise in particular areas related to computer technology. Such practitioners might be invited to provide inservice training or consultation services to an individual speech-language pathologist or to an employment agency.

Computer Books

Within the past few years, a number of documents have been published on the application of microcomputers to Communication Sciences and Disorders, with most of them addressing clinical applications to a greater or lesser degree. The December, 1985 issue of *Topics in Language Disorders,* edited by Goldman and Dahle, was devoted to the topical theme of computer technology and language disorders. Books of potential value to those interested generally in clinical applications of microcomputer technology include *Clinical Applications of Microcomputers in Communication Disorders,*[3] *Microcomputer Applications in Rehabilitation of Communication Disorders,*[102] *The Personal Computer for Speech, Language, and Hearing Professionals,*[103] *The Handbook of Microcomputer Applications in Communication Disorders,*[104] and *The Handbook of Clinical Applications for Microcomputers.*[105] Each of these books expands the general knowledge base about what to consider and how to apply the microcomputer to clinical management tasks. Those who have little prior background knowledge about microcomputers might also benefit from examining *An Introduction to Microcomputers in Speech, Language, and Hearing.*[2] Sanders, a clinician in a school district located in the state of Washington, has suggested applications of microcomputers and systems analysis for speech-language pathologists.[9] Katz has published a book about microcomputer technology and its applications with adult aphasic individuals.[4]

Prior to 1984, few publications related to microcomputer applications in Communication Sciences and Disorders had been produced. Since that time, the relevant literature has expanded rapidly, initiated with general publications about computer technology and the profession, followed later by books with a more specific focus such as a specific communication disorder or a specific work setting. The literature on computer technology and communication disorders will likely continue to expand, while the discipline struggles to incorporate microcomputer technology. The likelihood is high that when the microcomputer has been accepted by most practitioners as a valuable tool, the device will become more transparent and will assume a background status, rather than being highlighted in the titles of books and articles.

SUMMARY

A few short years ago only a small number of speech-language pathologists had ever seen or touched a microcomputer. Only a handful of visionary colleagues possessed the imagination that would permit them to predict the magnitude of the beneficial impact this desktop tool could have on the profession. Microcomputers have now become almost indispensable devices to many clinicians. It is the rare practitioner today who admits to a lack of interest in learning more about microcomputers and what they can contribute to the clinical management process. Those who have begun to implement microcomputer applications have been contagiously enthusiastic about the potential of this device to reshape the clinical world of speech-language pathology. The excitement of these computer advocates has destroyed the natural inclination of their peers to resist technological innovation and the disruptive, disquieting dissonance that accompanies fundamental modification of professional operations.

This chapter has presented a balanced perspective, discussing both the current limitations and the potential benefits of microcomputer applications in the clinical domain of speech-language pathology. Objectivity is difficult to maintain in view of the excitement spreading throughout the profession about this remarkable instrument. In the midst of their enthusiastic espousal of the microcomputer, practitioners must pause to consider guidelines and principles that should govern the integration of new techniques, procedures, materials, and instruments into the clinical management process. Therefore, this chapter has suggested guidelines and principles for incorporation of microcomputer applications into clinical realms. Although data on clinical microcomputer applications are sparse, one would be foolish to refuse to implement technological developments in a judicious and experimental fashion. However, it is necessary that practitioners evaluate each envisioned application before implementation to the extent that is possible, during implementation to provide evidence about its appropriateness, and after implementation as a basis for deciding whether it should be repeated. Microcomputers should be employed clinically when they provide the optimal means of accomplishing a clinical objective.

Speech-language pathologists should not assume that microcomputer technology is too difficult for a clinician to master. It is not. To use microcomputers effectively in the clinical situation does not require extensive understanding of what happens technically inside the computer and does not demand a knowledge of programming. The time and effort that must be expended in developing computer proficiency is more than compensated for by the long-term gains achievable in clinical operations. Computer technology should be implemented gradually, with time permitted for learning and adaptation to change. With each new aspect of computer technology that a clinician attempts to master, a period of confusion and frustration should be expected. Computers are wonderfully tolerant of the unkind words and tortured groans of their human users. The process of learning about computers, although occasionally painful and maddening, is a revitalizing experience professionally. After a person becomes proficient in the use of computers, it is difficult to imagine functioning without the assistance of the microcomputer. The microcomputer becomes a prosthetic device, rather than a crutch, permitting greater efficiency in the performance of professional responsibilities and extending the range of operations that are feasible. Although the initial expense of computerization is high, not only in dollars, but also in time and effort, cost effectiveness should be projected over a substantial time period. Probably, as more and more computer applications are developed for the clinical management situation, most computers will pay for themselves over a period of months or years.

The microcomputer is not a miracle worker. It is a limited and fallible tool with impressive potential. It may take years for speech-language pathologists to develop applications that will carry the profession beyond the stage where the computer is being used mainly for administrative tasks and repetitious drill with clients and doing old tasks in new ways, and into an era in which clinicians can perform new tasks that were impossible without the microcomputer. The metamorphosis of our clinical discipline through applications of computer technology is dawning. Clinicians are taking unsteady infant steps toward incorporation of this technological companion into their working world. Little is known and much remains to be learned about how to employ this device optimally for the improvement of clinical services. Since that must be resolved in the clinician's territory, each speech-language pathologist who applies the microcomputer clinically has the opportunity to be a pioneer and to become a contributor of ideas that will benefit future generations of communicatively disabled individuals. Clinicians must position themselves to act, rather than to react, to today's challenging era of technology.

REFERENCES

1. Bear J. Computer wimp. Berkeley: Ten Speed Press, 1983.
2. Curtis J. An introduction to microcomputers in speech, language, and hearing. San Diego: College-Hill Press, 1987.
3. Fitch J. Clinical applications of microcomputers in communication disorders. New York: Academic Press, 1986.
4. Katz RC. Aphasia treatment and microcomputers. San Diego: College-Hill Press, 1986.
5. Blackstone S. Augmentative communication. In: Lass N, McReynolds L, Northern J, Yoder D, eds. Handbook of speech-language pathology and audiology. Toronto: BC Decker, 1988:998.
6. Toffler A. Future shock. London, England: The Bodley Head, 1970.
7. Hawkridge D, Vincent T, Hales G. New information technology in the education of disabled children and adults. San Diego: College-Hill Press, 1985.
8. Minifie FD. Graduate education during a technological revolution. Proceedings of the second annual conference on graduate education. St. Louis, MO: National Council of Graduate Programs in Communication Sciences and Disorders, 1981.
9. Sanders J. Microcomputer applications for speech-language services in the schools. San Diego: College-Hill Press, 1986.
10. Hyman CS. The 1985 omnibus survey: implications for strategic planning. Asha 1986; 28(4):19–22.
11. Schwartz AH. Microcomputer applications: facts, functions, fads, and fallacies. Child Commun Disord 1984, 8(1):89–111.
12. Larson VL, Steiner S. Microcomputer applications to assess-

ment of speech and language. In: Schwartz AH, ed. The handbook of clinical applications for microcomputers. Rockville, MD: Aspen, in preparation.

13. Bull GL, Cochran PS, Lang JK, Pierce BR, Seaton W, Smaldino JJ, Mahaffey RB, Chial MR. Technology infusion: a resource guide. J Comput Users Speech Hear 1985; 1:96–116.
14. Krueger B. Computerized reporting in a public school program. Lang Speech Hear Services Schools 1985; 16:135–139.
15. Schwartz AH. Microcomputer applications: what changes hath this tool wrought? Texas Audiol Speech Pathol 1986; 12(1):4–9.
16. Shriberg LD, Kwiatkowski J, Snyder T. Articulation testing by microcomputer. J Speech Hear Disord 1986; 51:309–324.
17. Bull GL, Cochran PS. Creating tools for clinicians and teachers. J Comput Users Speech Hear 1985; 1:45–49.
18. Larson VL, Steiner S. Language intervention using microcomputers. Top Lang Disord 1985; 6(1):41–55.
19. Balsam D. The print shop [Computer program]. San Rafael, CA: Broderbund Software, 1984.
20. Springboard Software. The newsroom [Computer program]. Minneapolis, MN: Springboard, 1984.
21. Springboard Software. The newsroom pro [Computer program]. Minneapolis, MN: Springboard, 1986.
22. Skiba B. Pinpoint [Computer program]. Oakland, CA: Pinpoint Publishing, 1985.
23. Lissner R. AppleWorks [Computer program]. Cupertino, CA: Apple Computer, 1983.
24. Manzanita Software Systems. Businessworks [Computer program]. Roseville, CA: Manzanita Software Systems, 1986.
25. Lutus P. Apple writer II [Computer program]. Cupertino, CA: Apple Computer, 1984.
26. Micropro International Corp. MailMerge [Computer program]. San Rafael, CA: Micropro International, 1983.
27. Fersko-Weiss H. Electronic mail: the emerging connection. Person Comput 1985; 9(1):73.
28. Fersko-Weiss H. Electronic mail: the emerging connection. Person Comput 1985; 9(1):71–79.
29. Weiner FF, Schwartz AH. Language intervention planner [Computer program]. State College, PA: Parrot Software, 1986.
30. Weiner FF. IEP writer [Computer program]. State College, PA: Parrot Software, 1984.
31. Berryman J, Johnson R, Toman T. Planning individualized speech and language intervention programs: computer software adaptation [Computer program]. Tucson: Communication Skill Builders, 1984.
32. Talley M. Talley goals and objectives writer [Computer program]. North Billerica, MA: Curriculum Associates, 1983.
33. Brigance A. Comprehensive inventory of basic skills. North Billerica, MA: Curriculum Associates, 1983.
34. Brigance A. Inventory of basic skills. North Billerica, MA: Curriculum Associates, 1977.
35. Brigance A. Inventory of early development. North Billerica, MA: Curriculum Associates, 1978.
36. Brigance A. Inventory of essential skills. North Billerica, MA: Curriculum Associates, 1981.
37. Weiner FF, Young EC. Function pictures [Computer program]. State College, PA: Parrot Software, 1983.
38. Jennen S, Roddy D. Progress monitoring program [Computer program]. Cambridge, MN: Performance Monitoring Systems, 1986.
39. Cassidy RD, Koller DE, Schwartz AH. The uses of word processing for clinical report writing. Part I: applications, characteristics and requirements. J Child Commun Disord 1984; 8(1):7–21.
40. Schwartz AH, Koller DE, Cassidy RD. The uses of word processing for clinical report writing. Part II: program features for developing report formats. Child Commun Disord 1984; 8(1):23–35.
41. Bull GL, Cochran PS, Lang JK, Pierce BR, Seaton W, Smaldino JJ, Mahaffey RB, Chial MR. Technology infusion: a resource guide. J Comput Users Speech Hear 1985; 1:100.
42. Frankenberger W, Blakemore T. Introductory statistics software package [Computer program]. Reading, MA: Addison-Wesley, 1985.
43. Blache SE. Computer networking, information transfer, and the communication disorders specialist. J Comput Users Speech Hear 1985; 1:29–35.
44. National Association of State Directors of Special Education. SpecialNet [Computer Program]. Washington, DC: National Association of State Directors of Special Education, 1986.
45. Block H and R. Compuserve [Computer program]. Columbus, OH: H and R Block, 1984.
46. Source Telecomputing Corporation. The Source [Computer program]. McLean, VA: Source Telecomputing Corporation, 1984.
47. Weiner FF. Phonological process tutor [Computer program]. State College, PA: Parrot Software, 1985.
48. Filter MD. Competency training systems [Computer program]. Harrisonburg, VA: CTS Software, 1985.
49. Ireton H, Lun K-S. The computerized Minnesota child development inventory report [Computer program]. Minneapolis, MN: Behavior Science Systems, 1985.
50. Weiner FF, Pelletier C. Aphasia IV: reading comprehension [Computer program]. State College, PA: Parrot Software, 1984.
51. Piestrup A. Juggles' rainbow [Computer program]. Menlo Park, CA: The Learning Company, 1982.
52. Bramschreiber J, Wiegert J. Juggles' rainbow: speech-language activity booklet. Tucson: Communication Skill Builders, 1984.
53. Miller J, Chapman R. Systematic analysis of language transcripts (SALT) [Computer program]. Madison, WI: Language Analysis Laboratory, Waisman Center on Mental Retardation and Human Development, University of Wisconsin-Madison, 1983.
54. Mordecai DR, Palin MW, Palmer CB. Lingquest 1: computer-assisted language sample analysis [Computer program]. Columbus, OH: CE Merrill, 1985.
55. Fitch J. Computer managed screening test [Computer program]. Tucson: Communication Skill Builders, 1985.
56. Bryant BR. DTLA-2: Detroit tests of learning aptitude [Computer program]. Austin, TX: Pro-Ed, 1985.
57. Kosel M, Fish M. The factory [Computer program]. Pleasantville, NY: Sunburst Communications, 1984.
58. Katz RC, Nagy VT. Speller I [Computer program]. Los Angeles: VA Outpatient Clinic, Audiology and Speech Pathology Service, 1984.
59. Wilson M, Fox B. Microcomputer language assessment and development systems (Micro-LADS) [Computer program]. Burlington, VT: Laureate Learning Systems, 1983.
60. Adams L, Fletcher S, McCutcheon M. Nasometer [Computer program]. Pine Brook, NJ: Kay Elemetrics, 1986.
61. Palin MW, Mordecai DR. Lingquest 2: phonological analysis [Computer program]. Columbus, OH: CE Merrill, 1985.
62. Yorkston K, Beukelman D, Traynor C. Computerized assessment of intelligbility of dysarthric speech [Computer program]. Tigard, OR: CC Publications, 1984.
63. Smith J. Cognitive rehabilitation [Computer program]. Dimondale, MI: Hartley Courseware, 1984.
64. Volin RA, Groher ME. Sentence completions: semantics [Computer program]. Rockville, MD: Aspen, 1981.
65. Fitch J. Computer managed articulation treatment [Computer program]. Tucson: Communication Skill Builders, 1985.
66. Weiner FF. Minimal contrast therapy [Computer pro-

gram]. State College, PA: Parrot Software, 1984.
67. Johnson T, Child D. Vocal abuse reduction program (VARP) [Computer program]. San Diego: College-Hill Press, 1984.
68. Kay Elemetrics Corp. Visi-Pitch [Computer program]. Pine Brook, NJ: Kay Elemetrics, 1985.
69. Wilson M, Fox B. First words [Computer program]. Burlington, VT: Laureate Learning Systems, 1982.
70. Wilson M, Fox B. First categories [Computer program]. Burlington, VT: Laureate Learning Systems, 1983.
71. Meyers L, Fogel P. Exploratory play [Computer program]. Santa Monica, CA: Peal Software, 1985.
72. Meyers L, Fogel P. Representational play [Computer program]. Santa Monica, CA: Peal Software, 1985.
73. Fitch J. Computer managed language treatment [Computer program]. Tucson: Communication Skill Builders, 1985.
74. Mills R, Thomas R. Word recognition [Computer program]. Ann Arbor, MI: Brain-Link Software, 1983.
75. Weiner FF. Aphasia I: noun association [Computer program]. State College, PA: Parrot Software, 1983.
76. Weiner FF. Aphasia II: opposites and similarities [Computer program]. State College, PA: Parrot Software, 1983.
77. Weiner, FF. Aphasia III: categories [Computer program]. State College, PA: Parrot Software, 1983.
78. Katz RC, Nagy VT. A computerized approach for improving word recognition in chronic aphasic patients. In: Brookshire R, ed. Clinical aphasiology: conference proceedings. Minneapolis, MN: BRK Publishers, 1983:65–72.
79. Katz RC. Understanding questions [Computer program]. Los Angeles: Sunset Software, 1983.
80. Katz RC. Understanding sentences [Computer program]. Los Angeles: Sunset Software, 1983.
81. Katz RC. Understanding stories [Computer program]. Los Angeles: Sunset Software, 1983.
82. DesignWare. The grammar examiner [Computer program]. San Francisco: DesignWare, 1984.
83. Decision Development Corporation. The whitewater canoe race [Computer program]. Bloomington, IN. Agency for Instructional Television, 1985.
84. Hartley Courseware. Verbs [Computer program]. Dimondale, MI: Hartley Courseware, 1983.
85. Fleisher P. Analogies tutorial [Computer program]. Dimondale, MI: Hartley Courseware, 1983.
86. Chance C. Adventure master [Computer program]. Greenwich, CT: CBS Software, 1984.
87. Smith FE, Kusmiak G. The Bank Street writer [Computer program]. San Rafael, CA: Broderbund Software, 1982.
88. Pejsa J, Pejsa J. Kidwriter [Computer program]. Cambridge, MA: Spinnaker Software, 1984.
89. Meyers L, McNally R, Greenberg J. Keytalk [Computer program]. Santa Monica, CA: Peal Software, 1985.
90. Meyers L. Teaching language. Excep Parent 1986; 16:20–23.
91. Papert S. Mindstorms: children, computers and powerful ideas. New York: Basic Books, 1980.
92. Cohen C, Palin M. Speech syntheses and speech recognition devices. In: Grossfeld M, Grossfeld C, eds. Microcomputer applications in rehabilitation of communication disorders. Rockville, MD: Aspen, 1986:183.
93. LaRiviere C, Sherblom J. Speech synthesis and speech recognition by microcomputer. In: Northern J, ed. The personal computer for speech, language, and hearing professionals. Boston: Little, Brown, 1986: 177.
94. Salpeter J. Interactive: the truth behind the promises. Class Comput Learn 1986; Nov–Dec:26–34.
95. Rushakoff GE. Clinical applications in communication disorders. In: Schwartz AH, ed. Handbook of microcomputer applications in communication disorders. San Diego: College-Hill Press, 1984:147.
96. Schwartz AH. Microcomputer-assisted assessment of linguistic and phonological processes. Top Lang Disord 1985; 6(1):26–40.
97. Chial MR. Preliminaries to professional evaluation of software. J Comput Users Speech Hear 1986; 2:102–123.
98. Greyerbiehl DH, Schwartz AH, Clymer EW, Owens AM, Blackstone SW. User system for evaluating and reviewing software (USERS): screening and evaluation. Rockville, MD: American Speech-Language-Hearing Association, 1986.
99. Greyerbiehl DH, Chial MR, Schwartz AH, Owens AM, Blackstone SW. User system for evaluating and reviewing software (USERS): indepth review. Rockville, MD: American Speech-Language-Hearing Association, 1986.
100. Silverman F. Clinical software for speech-language pathology and audiology. Greendale, WI: CODI Publications, 1985.
101. Silverman F. An introduction to microcomputers for speech-language pathologists and audiologists. Englewood Cliffs, NJ: Prentice-Hall, 1987.
102. Grossfeld M, Grossfeld C, eds. Microcomputer applications in rehabilitation of communication disorders. Rockville, MD: Aspen, 1986.
103. Northern JL, ed. The personal computer for speech, language, and hearing professionals. Boston: Little, Brown, 1986.
104. Schwartz AH, ed. The handbook of microcomputer applications in communication disorders. San Diego: College-Hill Press, 1984.
105. Schwartz AH, ed. The handbook of clinical applications for microcomputers. Rockville, MD: Aspen, in preparation.

Articulation Disorders

15 Articulation Disorders of Unknown Etiology

Leija V. McReynolds, Ph.D.

As children begin to talk in the process of learning language, they produce errors, not only in vocabulary and syntax, but also in the speech sounds composing the words of their language. These errors may be in the form of substitutions (e.g., /t/ for /k/ in the word "cup"), distortions (e.g., unaspirated /t/ for initial /t/ in the word "top"), omissions (e.g., not producing the /p/ in the word "top"), and sometimes additions (e.g., adding a schwa between the /s/ and /t/ in the word "stop"). Other kinds of errors may occur, but they are less frequent (e.g., transpositions). The misproductions are referred to as articulation errors. Normally, children proceed through stages of sound acquisition in which these errors are gradually corrected, so that by the age of 5, 6, 7, or 8 years speech sound error productions are no longer occurring in the child's speech.

For a variety of reasons some children fail to make the appropriate corrections at a time in development when such corrections are expected. These children retain their articulation errors, continuing to misproduce sounds and showing little or no improvement over time. Such children are described as having articulation problems. The causes of these articulation errors are many—some more obvious than others. In the three chapters that follow some of the obvious causes are described and discussed. But among this group, there are a number of children who misarticulate sounds, but who exhibit no obvious etiology that could explain why they have difficulty in producing speech sounds accurately. This subgroup of children constitutes the largest single communicative disorder treated by speech-language pathologists.

FUNCTIONAL ARTICULATION DISORDER

For many years this subgroup of children was studied in an attempt to find causal variables that would explain their problem, but the studies were unable to isolate any strong variables that could account for the articulation errors. The children were not hearing impaired, had no serious perceptual deficits, had no identifiable structural defects or muscle movement insufficiency, were functioning adequately in other aspects at home, were learning appropriately in school, and were generally healthy, physically, mentally, and emotionally.[1–5] Their main problem seemed to be that they did not articulate all the speech sounds correctly. Because no single causal variable or even a cohesive group of causal variables could be identified that would explain the articulation disorder, the children were diagnosed as having a "functional articulation disorder." In essence, "functional" was used to indicate that nothing apparent could be found to account for the child's continued misarticulations.

However, it did not mean that speech pathologists did not have causal explanations for these articulation disorders. In fact, the term "functional" means different things to speech pathologists, and it is defined according to each individual's own conceptualization of the nature of articulation problems and causes thereof. For example, some speech pathologists are convinced that the children's primary problem is some form of motor deficit in that the children have difficulty in motor manipulation of the articulators to produce speech sounds accurately.[6–8]

Others define "functional" as a perceptual problem in that the children have difficulty auditorily in discriminating the acoustic aspects of speech sounds, and this difficulty is reflected in their inability to produce them.[9–11] Still others propose that the cause may lie in the child's environment; that is, perhaps the environment was inadequate in some way so that the child was unable to learn how to produce the sounds correctly.[12] Finally, for some speech pathologists, "functional" simply indicates that the cause cannot be identified, and, in any case, even if a cause could be found, it is unnecessary to seek causes; it is sufficient to describe the behavior accurately and then take steps to correct the errors in the most efficient manner possible.[12,13] However, the majority of speech pathologists appreciate the ambiguity inherent in the term "functional" and attribute the child's problem to a combination of factors, none of which singly can account for the errors, but together function to prevent the child from correcting error productions spontaneously with maturity.[1,14] Historically, exploration for etiologic variables gradually diminished as speech pathologists became more interested in trying to develop treatment programs than in discovering causes. The term "functional" was applied whenever no obvious etiologic factor or factors could be found. Thus, for most clinicians, the term continued to signify that the etiology of the articulation disorder was unknown.

From Functional to Phonologic

When linguistic theory and analysis began to be applied to the description and explanation of children's language disorders, interest in causality reawakened, albeit in a somewhat different form from the earlier interest in causality. Whereas earlier, causal factors were sought in the characteristics within the child, such as the child's visual and motor skills, perceptual skills, auditory memory, and so forth, attention shifted to more theoretic formulations concerning how language works, the components composing a language system, and how a child goes about acquiring language. In a sense, the factors considered were more abstract than the factors studied previously. The application of linguistic theory and notions to the understanding of language disorders was naturally extended to articulation disorders by way of phonologic theory, primarily phonologic theory in relation to phonologic acquisition.[15] A shift in emphasis took place in the conceptualization of what constituted an articulation disorder. The shift was from a concern with *how* speech sounds and speech sound errors are produced to *why* errors are produced in the operation of an entire linguistic system. In short, errors were viewed from a more theoretic perspective in regard to how a child learns the phonologic system of his or her community and what is important in phonologic acquisition. Much more effort was devoted to the study of the kinds of errors normal children produce as they go through the process of developing a phonologic system that would eventually match the adult phonologic system.

Thus phonologic theory, first applied to analysis of the speech of normal children in the process of acquiring phonology, was soon applied to analysis of the speech of children with articulation problems.[15–18] The extension from normal to disordered speech seemed natural and simple when it was discovered that the errors and error patterns produced by children with "functional" articulation disorders paralleled, and were similar to, those produced by normal children who were just beginning to acquire language, that is, phonology. With the discovery that articulation errors could be described within the theoretic framework of a phonologic analysis, speech pathologists took the next logical step by proposing that children's articulation disorders can also be understood better if viewed within the logic of phonologic theory.[16,18] The reasoning led to the belief that articulation errors are phonologic in nature, so that the phonology of the children is impaired rather than, for example, the motor function being involved. Consequently, the term "functional articulation disorder" has been replaced by the term "phonologic disorder" by many speech pathologists when referring to children whose articulation is disordered, but the cause for their disorder is unknown.

The term "phonologic disorder" is difficult to define because it is used differently by individual speech pathologists.[15,18–21] Ideally, it would refer to the way in which a child has organized his or her phonologic system (e.g., components of the system such as the phonetic inventory, the system of phonemic contrasts, and rules for sound production and arrangement). The term "phonologic disorder" suggests that a child's phonologic system is organized inappropriately in relation to the adult system; that is, it is "disordered." The establishment of the presence of a disordered system requires an in-depth analysis of all components in the system in order to assess the organization. Few speech pathologists conduct an in-depth phonologic analysis or have the skills to do so. Consequently, the diagnostic label of "phonologic disorder" is applied frequently to children whose articulation errors can be described in terms of error patterns derived from a surface analysis of errors rather than from an in-depth phonologic analysis, and this label is also applied to children with only a few misarticulations. The error patterns are sometimes interpreted to reflect internal (cognitive) manipulations made by the child as he or she is coping with the complexity of the ambient phonology; that is, the term "phonologic disorder" is sometimes used in an explanatory manner for a surface analysis of error patterns. Occasionally, patterns are accepted to be what they are, descriptions of errors, without attribution of deeper cognitive manipulations to the child. In-depth analyses are performed, but are rare; surface error analyses are frequent. Yet the same term is used to label the results from both kinds of analyses. Therefore, the term "phonologic disorder" appears to be used for a variety of articulation problems much as the term "functional articulation disorder" is used to refer to a variety of problems. In any case, "phonologic disorder" is used extensively to refer to the children who were formerly referred to as children with "functional articulation disorders" in the articulation literature. It is a more common term than "functional" in reference to articulation.

Although "phonologic disorders" is the prevalent term, the cause or causes of the problem remain undetermined. "Phonologic disorders" does not identify the cause for the inappropriate organization of the system; it only describes the errors in phonologic terminology. In light of the discrepancy among analyses, several models have been proposed that attempt either to explain the causes for the articulation problems or at least to explain the nature of the disorder from a linguistic and cognitive viewpoint. However, the phonologic nature of the problem is not accepted by all speech pathologists. Other conceptualizations are offered, and they can be broadly placed into two primary categories: the perceptual-motor model and the discrimination model. The three models, the perceptual-motor model, the discrimination model, and the phonologic disorders model, are briefly described in the next section.

Perceptual-Motor Skill Model

In the perceptual-motor skill model, articulation learning is viewed in the same light as the learning of other motor skills, for example, riding a bicycle. In fact, the models that are used to explain articulation learning were actually developed to explain the learning of motor skills other than articulation.[22–24] The models have been adapted to account for articulation learning.[7,8]

According to these theories, motor skill learning consists of a gradual development of a skill, starting with slow, deliberate movements that are under conscious control and ending in rapid, automatic execution of the movements, which are no longer under conscious control. These models contain a number of components that include stages of skill development, mentally analyzing and rehearsing the requirements for the movement, practice of the skilled movement, and feedback on the accuracy of the executed movement from both external and internal sources.

Two stages of learning are proposed: the acquisition stage and the automatization stage. Although the two stages are described separately, research in articulation training suggests that there is considerable overlap in that automatization begins during the acquisition stage.[25,26] However, during the skill acquisition stage, much emphasis is placed on the need for the learner to plan actively the motor movement prior to execution (to think about how the movement is to be produced) and to attend consciously to the information received after the movement has been executed. As noted, the incoming information, the feedback, is both internal and external (internally from the learner's movement and externally from the trainer's observations of the movement); therefore, during this early acquisition stage, movements are deliberate, slow, and under conscious control. But with additional practice of the movement in a variety of contexts and situations, the movements become more rapid, and conscious control is gradually relinquished. The automatization stage is reached when correct production of the movement no longer requires mental planning or conscious control. During the automatization stage the learner is given an opportunity to practice the movement in a variety of contexts and modes.

When articulation is trained as a perceptual-motor skill, the child practices producing the targeted sound many times in isolation, in syllables, in words, and in a variety of phonetic contexts; the contexts become increasingly more complex in that they change from isolated sound production to conversational speech. Initially, the child is asked to think about how the sound should be produced and after producing the sound is asked to evaluate the production for accuracy. Thus, in motor skill learning, the individual attends internally to kinesthetic and proprioceptive information from the movements and, in articulation, attends as well to the acoustic information resulting from the production of the targeted sound. External feedback is provided by the trainer who gives information on the accuracy of the specific topography (features) involved in producing the targeted sound. During the automatization stage the learner continues to practice the skill in the context of a variety of situations. Perceptual-motor skill learning entails considerable drill-like practice.

An important concept in perceptual-motor theory is the formation of a motor schema or motor plan. This schema is an ". . . internalized rule that allows the application of a particular skilled movement across a variety of contexts'' (p 134).[7] Acquisition of the rule is dependent on sufficient practice in a sufficient variety of contexts in order to allow the rule to form.

Emphasis in the perceptual-motor model on articulation learning has shifted somewhat from the motor aspect of skill learning to the cognitive and perceptual aspects during the acquisition stage. It is not sufficient that the learner simply practice the movement; it is also necessary that the learner think about the movement and plan the movement prior to execution. It is also important that the learner process the information from all sources throughout the planning, execution, and feedback phases. Attention to the feedback received from the articulatory movement and from the acoustic result of producing the movement is a pertinent component of the model. Thus, although motor practice is essential, it is not necessarily the most important component in the perceptual-motor skill learning model, at least in the early stages of acquisition.[3,7]

Discrimination Models

When articulation disorders are thought to be related to problems in discrimination, several conceptualizations have been offered. For example, in one view, the child's problem is thought to be related directly to a perceptual deficit: an inability, for whatever reason, to discriminate between speech sounds.[27] In another view, the problem is partially perceptual, but may be more closely related to the form of the word that the child has stored as a standard and to which he or she compares what is heard.[11] In this view, the possibility is considered that the child's standard is different from the adult form of a word. However, the problem could occur on one or more of several levels. In still another view, the child's discrimination is inaccurate, but the cause for the discrimination problem is in the child's inaccurate production.[9] Each of these views will be described briefly.

The first viewpoint is one that has been accepted and acted upon in the treatment of articulation problems for a number of years.[27] This approach to articulation disorders was basically derived from a servosystem concept in which a process is governed by automatic controls.[28] The system is composed of a source of energy, a motor, a regulator, and a circuit connecting the three in a continuous loop. According to Van Riper and Irwin, the regulator scans the acoustic signal produced by the mouth and compares this product with a standard that is the community language.[27] If the output from the speaker does not match the standard, modifications are made in the production until matching is accomplished. In articulation, therefore, it is necessary to learn to discriminate acoustic differences, to evaluate the adequacy of self-productions in comparison to standard productions, and then to modify the productions until they match the standard. As can be seen, discrimination is conceived as the causal variable in that production is affected by what the individual discriminates and how he or she evaluates his or her own productions.

According to this view, an articulatory defective individual fails to match the auditory feedback patterns produced by others. In other words, the child fails to discriminate the differences between his or her error productions and the productions of others, thereby preventing the necessary articulatory modifications needed to match the standard. A number of factors that might be responsible for, or contribute to, the development of defective articulation are considered. In fact, a single etiologic factor is not postulated, with the possible causes ranging from imitation of other articulatory defective speakers in the family to slow physical maturation and poor coordination. Nevertheless, poor discrimination and difficulty in recognizing self-errors are at the heart of the articulatory defective individual's articulation problems, although the origin for the inadequate discrimination may be multiply determined. The basic rationale for treatment is that the articulatory defective individual does not use the feedback (auditory, proprioceptive, and tactual) that is received to control productions automatically.

A more complex relationship between discrimination and production is visualized by Winitz.[11] He suggests that children's discrimination deficits are specific rather than general. In order to identify the problem, testing of the child's discrimination of only the sounds that are misproduced, not the sounds produced accurately, is necessary. Winitz goes even further, suggesting that if the child distorts sounds, reproductions of the distortions are necessary or else the discrimination problem will not be revealed.

However, the child's problem may not be discrimination specifically. It is possible that a child's underlying form may be different from the adult form and that the production represents the standard the child has established for him- or herself. For example, if the adult form is "cat" and the child omits the /t/ by producing [kae], perhaps for him or her there is no such word with the form of [kaet], only [kae]. The standard stored in the child's head is [kae]; that is the underlying form for the child: a CV as opposed to a CVC form.

In order to determine what the child's underlying structure may be, testing the discrimination is necessary. For example, does the child respond to [kae] and [kaet] as if they were two different words or as if they were the same word? If the child discriminates between the two by pointing appropriately to pictures of each, then the underlying form for "cat" may be said to be the same as the adult form, and so the problem lies elsewhere.

Winitz suggests four possible sources for an inaccurate production and suggests that a breakdown may occur on one or more of four levels:[11]

1. If the child does not respond correctly on a speech sound discrimination task, the child may be unable to make the discrimination.
2. If the child performs accurately on the task, the discrimination may be accurate, but the child may have formed a special phonologic rule so that the form discriminated is not the form produced.
3. The correct discrimination may be made, but motor constraints do not allow the child to produce what is heard and discriminated.
4. The child is able to make the appropriate distinctions in speech sounds, but has adopted a learning strategy that prevents him from attending to what is perceived or attaching any importance to the perception.

But whatever the source of the problem, Winitz approaches all training from a perceptual point of view.[11] The child needs to be presented with extensive perceptual training, and production is tackled only when all discrimination training has been exhausted. It is Winitz's view that with sufficient discrimination training, the child learns to produce the correct sound although the training may last as long as a year or two. However, production training can be initiated after extensive discrimination training has been provided.

Another view of the relationship between discrimination and production reverses the direction of the relationship: instead of poor discrimination causing poor articulation, poor articulation causes inaccurate speech sound discrimination.[9] Monnin has pointed out that the research on speech sound discrimination of children with functional articulation disorders has yielded equivocal results. Some studies have found that children with functional articulation problems perform more poorly on discrimination tasks than do children with normal articulation, whereas other studies have shown that they discriminate as well as normal children. However, Monnin points out that the problem is more with the kinds of discrimination tests that are administered to the children than it is with the children's ability to discriminate. Many of the tests used to explore the relationship between speech sound discrimination and articulation deficits are general speech sound tests. The tests employ many or all speech sounds in our language, sounds the children produce correctly and sounds they do not produce correctly. Monnin indicates that when articulatory defective children are tested on discrimination of sounds that they produce correctly, they perform well on the tasks. It is only when they are tested on the speech sounds that they misproduce that their performance is poor. In other words, they display selective discrimination deficits. Children with functional articulation disorders do not have a general discrimination deficit; their discrimination problem is restricted to sounds that they cannot produce correctly. It follows, Monnin suggests, that if the discrimination problem is selective, it is difficult to relate the difficulty just to an inability to process acoustic information; it would be most unusual for a child to discriminate some acoustic differences and not others. Something must be influencing the child's discrimination performance besides a general inability to discriminate. That something, according to Monnin, is articulation performance.

In attributing poor discrimination to poor articulation, Monnin[9] refers to the motor theory of speech perception that has been developed from the research at Haskins Laboratories.[29] Studies conducted at the laboratories suggest that individuals perceive what they produce, that speech is perceived by reference to production. Essentially, the ability to produce differences between speech sounds might actually come prior to the ability to perceive differences between sounds. In reference to functional articulation disorders, children cannot perceive what they cannot produce. Therefore discrimination, although faulty in these children, is best corrected not through discrimination training, but through production training, because the causal relationship is in that direction. Data supporting this view come from studies in which subjects who were learning a second language were unable to discriminate between sounds until they learned to produce them.[30] Anecdotal reports of subvocal rehearsal during discrimination tasks also suggest that discrimination is processed through production.[31] In addition, a training study by Williams and McReynolds provided evidence that when discrimination is trained, it has no effect on production, but when production is trained, both discrimination and production performance improve.[32] Finally, Monnin asks, if discrimination training is provided and correct discriminations are acquired, why is it necessary to follow the discrimination training with production training? One would expect the discrimination training to be sufficient for changing production if the problem were purely an inability to attend to acoustic differences.

Because production is the cause for the discrimination problem, training should be directed to production—not discrimination. The goal of production training is to provide the child with an internal auditory image, and this is best accomplished by teaching the child to monitor and evaluate his or her own productions.

Phonologic Disorders Model

As mentioned earlier in this chapter, linguistic theory, particularly phonologic theory, has had a strong impact on our view of articulation disorders. It started with the application of the distinctive feature theory to articulation error analysis,[33,34] moved to the derivation of phonologic rules as dictated by generative phonology,[35,36] and progressed to the application of the phonologic process analysis as exemplified in generative and natural phonology.[19,21,37–39]

Developmentally, children are assumed to produce articulation errors while attempting to produce adult forms that they are unable to articulate correctly. According to phonologists, the simplifications that result are not haphazard, they fall into patterns. In turn, these patterns are interpreted as reflecting processes that children use in their simplifications. For example, if a child consistently omits final consonants in CVC words, he or she is described as using the process of final consonant deletion because of an inability to produce CVC forms. Theoretically, normal children relinquish these simplification processes gradually as they learn to produce adult forms.

Similar error patterns can be identified in the error productions of misarticulating children. The systematic nature of their errors is interpreted as support for the conclusion that articulatory defective children are also using phonologic processes to simplify adult forms. Thus, like children developing phonology normally, their error productions are rule governed, and so their problem is a phonologic one.

Phonologic processes are not always defined in the same way by all who believe in them. Their definition depends somewhat on the particular theory referred to in the discussion of processes or on whether or not a clinician just accepts error patterns as patterns without any interpretation of what they represent. However, a commonly accepted definition is that "processes are mental substitutions which unconsciously adapt phonological intentions to phonetic capacities" (p 76).[18] Another way to state this is that children know the adult word and the adult form of the word that they want to produce, but are unable to produce it as adults do. Therefore they develop various strategies to cope with their inability to produce targeted sounds in words, and their processes reflect the strategies that they employ. Reasons for the inability to produce adult forms have not been explored empirically, but various hypotheses have been offered. On the one hand, the strategies could have developed because of perceptual limitations or because of articulatory limitations. On the other hand, perceptual and articulatory skills may be intact and accurate, but because of the way in which the child's system is organized, the correct productions are not forthcoming. The child's system is possibly unique and different from the adult system so that it does not include the forms or rules of the adult system. Regardless of the reason, the cause (or causes) for the perceptual, articulatory, or organizational problem has not been identified.

One of the most important concepts in phonologic theory and in the notion of phonologic processes is the form of the child's underlying structure, that is, the form in which the word, the lexical item, is stored in the child's mind. The assumption in al most all the phonologic process analyses by speech pathologists is that the child's underlying form is the same as the surface form produced by the adult. The word the adult produces is the word the child has stored as the underlying form with the same sounds in the same order as the adult word. This assumption has been challenged.[40,41] It is possible, say the challengers, that the child's underlying form is different from the adult form and is congruent with the form that the child produces. For example, if the child produces [kae] for [kaet], it may be that [kae] is the child's underlying form. If so, the child cannot be attributed with application of a phonologic process to simplify [kaet]; he or she may simply have no CVC forms as underlying forms, only CV forms. In order to prevent misleading interpretations, conduction of more than a surface pattern analysis of errors is necessary—testing empirically the content of the child's phonologic system is necessary in order to determine whether the child is actually applying phonologic processes, and, to do this testing, the child's underlying forms must be identified.[42]

A further criticism has been directed at the way in which present phonologic analyses are used.[43–45] These individuals suggest that there is more to phonologic analysis than just a surface pattern analysis. Further, they suggest that the term "phonologic disorders" should not be used to label all children with articulation errors because many of those children display phonetic (motor) problems rather than phonologic problems. Similar to the previous argument, in order to specify a problem as phonologic, determination of what the child intends to say is necessary. For example, if the child intends to say "dog" and produces "tog," then the error is phonetic; but if the speaker intends to produce "tog" for "dog" in the first place, then the error is phonologic because the underlying form is different from the community language. The difference between phonologic and phonetic is stated succinctly by Hewlett:

> Generative phonology models allow phonological disorders to be characterized as disorders of the phonological representation of words in the speaker's mind, and phonetic disorders to be characterized as resulting from a disorder to the mechanism of phonetic implementation of phonological representations (p 160).[44]

This issue is concerned with the need to establish the nature of the child's underlying form before labeling an articulation problem as phonologic in nature. The determination is almost never done in reaching a diagnosis of "phonologic disorder," yet implications for treatment rest on such a diagnosis.

Supporters of the phonologic disorders theory point out that articulation errors are not errors in production of single sounds; instead they reflect application of processes, each of which encompasses more than one sound. In fact, one process may affect a number of targeted sounds. For example, if a child applies the process of cluster reduction, all clusters may be affected. In this example, if the child omits the /s/ in all /s/ clusters such as /st/, /sp/, /sk/, /sm/, /sn/, and /sw/, clusters with other sounds are likely to be affected similarly. Thus the /r/ could be omitted in clusters such as /tr/, /kr/, /gr/, /dr/, /pr/, and /br/. The point is that processes operate across sounds and across classes of sounds. The general nature of process operation is considered important to treatment. The implication is that elimination of the process in one cluster should result in elimination of the process in other clusters affected by the process. Thus operation of a general process, be it cluster reduction, fronting, stopping, or others, can be halted in most of the affected sounds by treating only one or two exemplars in a sound class.

Adherents of the view that articulation disorders are phonologic disorders suggest that treatment goals should reflect the nature of the problem. Because the sound errors result from operation of phonologic processes, the goal in treatment should be the elimination of processes rather than the correct production of erroneous sounds. Instead of teaching children to articulate targeted sounds accurately, training is considered to be successful if there is any indication in the child's articulation that a process is no longer operating. Correct production of sounds is not required.

ASSESSMENT

The principal behavior submitted to an evaluation is the child's speech sound production in a number of contexts. Nevertheless, assessment consists of more than a measure of articulation. In addition to obtaining samples of speech, one must rule out a hearing problem as an etiologic or contributing factor, or the presence of an organic involvement, that could account for the misproductions. Related variables such as intelligence, language, environmental conditions, and psychological status are explored to some extent to determine whether they might have some relevance to the child's speech disorder.

However, emphasis in assessment is placed upon the examination of the child's articulation of sounds and the description of the patterns of sound errors. Assessment is a continuous activity throughout intervention, from the initial meeting between the client and the clinician to the day the client is dismissed from treatment. The functions of assessment are many when used throughout the clinical period. Initially, assessment is directed toward determining whether a child has an articulation problem. Once this decision has been reached, a more in-depth assessment is made to determine the exact nature of the articulation problem, to develop a remediation program, and to make predictions concerning the child's potential for correcting errors and the length of time it will take to remediate the disorder. During treatment, assessment is used periodically to examine the progress the child is making in treatment, that is, what has been learned; to determine what the child still needs to learn; and to plan future steps in the training program. In the final phases of treatment, assessment is designed to examine the three aforementioned aspects in order to reach a decision about dismissal from treatment if the child's errors have been corrected and if the target behaviors are used in situations outside the clinic. The various functions or purposes of assessment will be described in this section in the sequence presented, with the understanding that there is overlap in the materials and tools used to make the assessments.

Screening

The first evaluation a clinician may perform is a screening, if the clinical setting demands one. For example, in a public school setting, screening children for articulation errors is often a routine procedure, whereas in a hospital clinic it is a less likely one. Screening is conducted to identify children who produce speech sound errors in order to schedule them for further assessment. Customarily, screening consists of obtaining a short sample of spontaneous speech, but sometimes clinicians choose to administer one of the more formal screening tests.[46–48] These instruments contain items to test sounds that are frequently misarticulated. More commonly, screening consists of asking a child to count, or to name the months in a year, or to talk a few minutes about some familiar topic.

Although screening is most often conducted in school settings, a clinician may also briefly screen potential clients who have been referred to a hospital or clinical setting for an evaluation. In this case, the purpose would be to gain an indication of the material to be used when a more in-depth evaluation of a child's problem is conducted. In all cases, a screening can usually be accomplished in a matter of 2 or 3 minutes.

In-Depth Evaluation

When screening indicates that a child has a sufficient number of articulation errors to warrant a more in-depth examination, the clinician will plan to administer specific testing instruments and to present other material that will help to obtain a clear picture of the child's disorder. In this assessment, the speech-language pathologist wants to specify the form of the articulation errors, the severity and consistency of the problem, and any other factors that will help in selecting a target for training and planning a remediation program. The examination includes testing articulatory behavior in depth, but also encompasses examination of related aspects that might impinge on the child's articulation problem. The articulation assessment materials are described first.

Phonetic Inventory

A probable initial step is administration of an articulation test to obtain a more comprehensive sample of the child's production of the speech sounds of English, with emphasis on the consonants. Numerous standardized and nonstandardized tests are available, for example, Templin-Darley tests of articulation (2nd edition),[47] Goldman-Fristoe test of articulation,[49] Arizona articulation proficiency scale,[50] photo articulation test,[51] a deep test of articulation,[52] and the Fisher-Logemann test of articulation competence.[46]

The clinician first wishes to obtain spontaneous naming responses in which consonants and vowels in the names are the targets. The purpose is to evaluate the child's natural production of the sounds. To accomplish spontaneous naming, the tests contain pictures of objects thought to be familiar to the child; the child is asked to name the picture shown. Usually, just one of the consonants (or vowels) in the name is the target sound. For example, in the word "sun" the clinician listens for the child's production of the /s/. Usually each speech sound is elicited in three words in which the sound occupies a different position in the word. For example, the /s/ is elicited in the initial position as in "sun," in the medial position as in "bicycle," and in the final position as in "bus." The consonants are tested as singletons and also in clusters or blends (e.g., the /s/ in an /st/ blend in the word "stop"). Vowels are also tested, although they are less disruptive to intelligibility than consonants and so are less crucial in remediation. The articulation tests are used to obtain information on the child's phonetic inventory; that is, they are used to determine which sounds are produced correctly and which incorrectly. When the test has been completed, the clinician knows the child's complete repertoire of sounds as elicited in single words and the child's phonetic inventory as evidenced in production of single words.

The usual procedure in testing is to present a picture and to ask the child, "What is this?" The clinician attends particularly to the child's production of the targeted sound in each word. The commercially available tests include manuals with instructions for administration, scoring, and analyzing results. For some children, spontaneous naming of test pictures is a difficult undertaking. They may be shy or for other reasons speak little, or a child may not know the names of all the pictures. In such cases, a spontaneous response may not be elicited, and the clinician may have to use an imitation procedure: the clinician names the picture and then asks the child to repeat the name. There is some question as to whether imitation produces the same response as a spontaneous elicitation.[53–55] It has been suggested that imitation elicits more correct productions than a spontaneous elicitation. Even though the findings are somewhat equivocal, the clinician needs to be aware of a possible difference and to explore the possibility.

Although the articulation tests that are commercially available use different pictures and formats, the majority generally sample each consonant in three positions in words. In some versions, sentences with target words are included for older children, and the children are requested to read the sentences. Reading also possibly results in more correct responses than a spontaneously produced sample.[56] Since few clinicians rely wholly on one test or on one elicitation method to arrive at decisions regarding a child's articulation profile, the elicitation method need not be an issue. Thus a variety of elicitation methods are used, and the results from each may be compared to seek consistency across methods.

One other observation should be made about the commercially available articulation tests. The rationales on which the tests were developed differ somewhat from one test to another. For example, in the Templin-Darley test,[47] the age of acquisition is given emphasis in analyzing the data; whereas in the Arizona articulation proficiency scale,[50] a numerical index of intelligibility score is given importance in analysis. To repeat, although rationale and physical appearance differ across tests, the essential components for assessing speech sound production are similar.

Scoring

How the child's responses are scored is determined by the kind of analysis the clinician wishes to conduct. The more specific and detailed the scoring, the more information the clinician obtains about the nature of the child's articulation errors. Furthermore, the theoretic framework within which articulation disorders are viewed dictates the kind of analysis to be performed; some theories demand greater detail than others.

At the least specific level the clinician may simply indicate whether the targeted sound was produced correctly or incorrectly. For this kind of scoring it is possible to use a plus (+) for correct productions and a minus (−) for incorrect ones. Plus-minus scoring gives the clinician no information about the topography in the child's production of the targeted sound; it only identifies the sounds produced accurately and inaccurately. Correct or incorrect scoring does not help much in the selection of targeted sounds for remediation or in the development of a comprehensive intervention program; it leads, more or less, to a rather simple analysis. In all probability the scoring and analysis would not be derived from any theoretic conceptualizations; and the only information the clinician would have is a count of the sounds produced accurately and inaccurately. The plus-minus scoring is probably seldom used. Clinicians are more likely to want to specify the responses produced by the child in naming pictures.

At a more detailed level of scoring, the clinician indicates whether the child produced a variant of the targeted sound (a distortion), produced another sound in place of the targeted sound (a substitution), or did not produce the targeted sound at all (an omission). Such notation is commonly called distortion-substitution-omission (DSO) scoring and is frequently used in clinical evaluations of articulation. This scoring system might have developed from research suggesting that omission errors were more severe than substitution errors, whereas substitutions were more severe than distortions.[57] Therefore, if a clinician knew the form of error productions, remediation could be planned more efficiently. For example, distortions could be expected to respond to treatment earlier and better than substitutions. The assumption in using DSO scoring may be accurate, but remediaton data to support a hierarchy in training have not been presented.

An even better and more detailed specification of the topography of the child's articulation of targeted sounds is provided at the next level of scoring. Several analytic procedures require this kind of specificity, particularly phonologic analyses. In this scoring the clinician uses phonetic transcription to indicate the sound or sounds produced by the child. Speech pathologists commonly use the International Phonetic Alphabet (IPA) for this transcription. Several levels are possible when a child's responses are transcribed phonetically. At one level the speech-language pathologist transcribes the child's production of the targeted sound phonetically using broad transcription. Thus, if the targeted sound was /t/ and the child produced /b/ with variation as a substitution, the clinician writes /b/ on the score sheet. In this phonemic transcription, fine phonetic details of the production are not noted. However, at a more precise level of phonetic transcription, the details of productions are carefully indicated by means of diacritic markings. The use of narrow phonetic transcription allows variations in production of targeted sounds to be indicated. Thus, if a child produced aspiration on the /t/ in "stop," which normally is unaspirated, the aspiration is noted by placing an /h/ above the /t/, thusly /t^h/. Tables that illustrate diacritic marks and what they represent are available,[1,46] or speech-language pathologists can develop their own notations.

In the final level, a clinician transcribes more than just the targeted sound: the entire word with the targeted sound is transcribed. When contextual effects are explored, determination of the child's productions of the targeted sound as well as the sounds surrounding it is necessary.

The degree of specificity that is used to describe a child's production depends on the clinician's need for information in planning remediation. The need, of course, is a function of the clinician's view concerning the nature of the child's articulation problem. For instance, if a child's articulation problem is approached from a perceptual-motor aspect, fine phonetic detail may or may not be used. If the rationale for targeted sound selection is developmental so that sounds acquired early are thought to be easier to produce and learn than later appearing sounds, diacritics may not be needed. If such a rationale is used, the clinician may wish to identify only sounds produced correctly and incorrectly in order to select targeted sounds on the basis of age of acquisition.

On the other hand, if a clinician views articulation disorders as hierarchical in nature, then distortions and substitutions could be categorized separately, each requiring a different form of instruction. Furthermore, if the clinician considers treatment of inappropriate use of aspiration separately from teaching specific targeted sounds to be important, then the use of narrow transcription to determine the extent of this inappropriate use and to identify where it occurs would be important. Omissions might also be described differently by clinicians. For example, research suggests that some children mark the sound that is perceived to be absent by adults.[58] Phonemic, or even narrow phonetic transcription, is certainly essential for the speech-language pathologist who believes that articulation errors reflect a phonologic disorder. Therefore theoretic considerations determine the kind of scoring used; the finer the transcription, the more information available for planning intervention. However, fine phonetic detail may have more theoretic value than practical importance for planning intervention. That is to say, philosophical or theoretic concepts often influence the way in which a child's articulation is scored. Whether these concepts contribute realistically, or profitably, to planning remediation has not been explored, and clinicians need to define for themselves whether or not there is a need for narrow transcription.

Conversational Sample

Seldom is the administration of one articulation test considered sufficient for the initial in-depth assessment. Most speech-language pathologists believe that the structured tests of single word productions must be supplemented with data from a more natural sample of a child's everyday articulation. Therefore a sample of conversational speech is obtained frequently. To get this sample, the clinician engages the child in conversation that is directed to topics of interest to the child, for example, sports, favorite television shows, vacations, or other events in which the child has participated. If the child does not respond to such interaction, the clinician might use a more artificial method by telling the child a story and then asking for a repeat of the story or questioning the child about the story content. Sometimes pictures that can be described in more than single words are used to elicit conversational speech. Usually an attempt is made to obtain a 75- to 100-word sample. These samples are scored in the same way that the articulation test responses were scored, and the degree of specificity is dictated by the clinician's approach to articulation errors. At times, all the sounds in all the words in the sample may be transcribed if contextual or across syllable boundary influences are important in the clinician's conceptualization of articulation disorders. Conversational samples are likely to be recorded on audiotape for later transcription because conversational speech moves too rapidly for live transcription. Additional difficulties may be encountered if the child is unintelligible. To aid in transcription, the clinician provides clues concerning the topic under discussion at appropriate intervals during the conversation, and these clues orient the clinician to probable words used by the child during the conversation.

Spontaneous conversational speech is often used to obtain information on the stability of an error production in different phonetic environments, something the traditional three position single word articulation test does not do. Obtaining a sample of conversational speech is important for several reasons.

First, research suggests that articulation of a targeted sound is different in single words as opposed to free speech.[59–62] This has not always been found to be true,[21,38,63] but the possible discrepancy should be kept in mind. Moreover, if a clinician believes that context influences targeted sound production sampling, the effects of phonetic environment can be tested by administering a deep test such as the McDonald deep test of articulation.[52] In that test, each consonant is tested approximately 24 times in the arresting position and 24 times in the releasing position in different phonetic contexts (e.g., hou*s*e-cow and bed-*s*un). The deep test was developed by McDonald in order to allow clinicians to identify phonetic contexts in which the targeted sound is produced correctly. When the context is found, it can be used as an initial context for training the targeted sound. Whether context actually has a facilitating effect or not has been questioned because results from experimental studies have not supported the notion of facilitating contexts in remediation.[61,64–66]

Second, obtaining samples of conversational speech is recommended as a primary source for a phonologic process or any form of phonologic analysis. Processes operate in the context of morphologic structures or across word boundaries, not on isolated sounds. For example, final consonant deletion can be identified only if the items have a final consonant to be omitted in the context of CVC structures. However, emphasis is not placed on the need for a conversational sample in a number of phonologic process analyses. For example, a one-word delayed imitation task is used in Weiner's test,[39] and Kahn and Lewis[38] obtain a speech sample by administering the Goldman-Fristoe test of articulation.[49]

Third, the need to establish stability (consistency) of error productions constitutes the most crucial reason for obtaining conversational speech samples. Inconsistency of error productions has been established in a number of studies.[67–69] When a targeted sound is tested in each word position in only one word, the stability of that particular error cannot be substantiated, and accurate interpretation of the data for analysis purposes is at risk. A substantial number of productions of each sound are required to rule out or to reveal consistent and inconsistent errors and error patterns.

If conversational speech samples are used, it is of particular importance that the child's sample be recorded at least on audiotape. As noted, live transcription of running speech poses difficulties, and a clinician can feel more comfortable if the conversation is saved for later verification of the live transcription. Audio recordings are also useful for measuring either inter- or intraobserver reliability.

Other Assessments

Although articulatory behavior is of prime importance in the assessment of the kind of articulation problem a child exhibits, other contributing factors are checked for relevance. Some of the factors that are examined are universally evaluated, whereas others are specific to particular theoretic formulations about etiology or conceptualizations about the nature of articulation errors.

Background Information

Before conducting an in-depth evaluation of the child's articulatory performance, the speech-language pathologist obtains information from the parents about the child's problem and their concerns about him or her. Included in the case history is information on the child's general motor and mental development, performance in school, major illnesses, and general functioning at home and elsewhere. Case histories can sometimes give clues as to possible etiologic factors. The information can also be used to plan a remediation program suitable to the child's abilities and performance in other situations. The amount of information gathered in a case history interview depends largely on the severity of the articulation problem: a child with many error sounds that render speech unintelligible would need a more in-depth exploration of factors that may contribute to the articulation problem than would a child with only one or two error sounds. In either case, however, the purpose of the case history is to obtain information on the variables that contribute to the articulation problem and to obtain, from the parents and the child, some idea of the variables that concern them.

Besides interviewing the parents, and the child if appropriate, the clinician obtains information from other disciplines when others are involved with the client. Thus reports from teachers, psychologists, physicians, and other specialists are sought if they are available. If appropriate, all the specialists involved may act as a team in planning a treatment program.

Oral-Peripheral Examination

To rule out the presence of any obvious structural defects of the speech mechanism, the clinician examines various structures and functions of the articulators. Detailed instructions for conduction of an oral-peripheral examination are described by Sally Peterson-Falzone in Chapters 16 and 17. Therefore, only brief mention of the need to rule out obvious structural problems is presented in this section.

Structurally, the clinician examines dentition and occlusion of the teeth to determine whether both are within the normal range. The hard palate is examined for height and the soft palate for mobility and length. Sometimes a submucous cleft is present; although it cannot be observed directly, it should be considered. (See Chapters 16 and 17 for more details.)

Movement may be assessed by requesting the client to imitate a sequence of nonsense syllables, such as pa-ta-ka. The procedure is used to assess the client's diadochokinetic ability. Other kinds of tongue movements may be requested by asking the client to follow instructions to "touch the roof of the mouth, the right side of the mouth" and so forth.

Hearing

Audiologic testing is conducted to rule out a sensory deficit as a contributing factor. The effects of a hearing loss on articulation are explained in Chapter 29 by Osberger and Hesketh. An extensive audiometric test is usually recommended only if (1) the child does not pass an audiometric screening at 10 to 20 dB across selected frequencies or (2) in the referral, concern for the child's hearing or frequency of middle ear infections is expressed. A standard audiometric test is administered by an audiologist, whereas the speech-language pathologist is usually competent to perform a screening test.

Language, Voice, Fluency

Other communication skills are screened by the speech-language pathologist, primarily to determine whether more than articulation is deficient. Of particular interest is the child's performance on language tasks that require some knowledge of syntax, semantics, and pragmatics. Young children with severe articulation problems commonly display concomitant language problems. For this reason, the clinician may administer one of the commercially available language tests, such as the Peabody picture vocabulary test,[70] the Carrow elicited language inventory,[71] and the test for auditory comprehension of language,[72] in order to measure the child's receptive and expressive language. If problems are found, remediation can be planned to provide language training alone or in combination with articulation training.

Auditory Discrimination

Although many clinicians do not go beyond the audiometric screening for hearing loss, others who believe that there is a close relationship between discrimination and production conduct additional auditory tests in the form of speech sound discrimination tests.[11] General speech sound discrimination tests such as the Wepman auditory discrimination test[73] or the Templin speech sound discrimination test[74] may be administered, but the emphasis is generally on individualized tests designed for the child's particular speech problem.[9,11] General tests such as the Wepman and Templin tests are designed to test discrimination of pairs of speech sounds, even sounds the child produces correctly, and such tests are thought not to evaluate the child's actual discrimination problem. Therefore clinicians design tests that require the child to respond to differences between the targeted sound and the error produced by the child. For example, if the child substitutes the /w/ for the /r/, the test would require discrimination between such words as "ring" and "wing." A truly refined discrimination test would be one in which the child's productions, which have been audiotaped, are played back and the child is asked to indicate whether the production is correct or incorrect. A problem with some of these activities is that it is difficult to ascertain that the child understands the task because discrimination tests are indirect measures of a behavior that cannot be observed directly since it takes place in the child's mind. As has been noted in frequent publications, the need for discrimination testing has not been strongly supported by research.[3,32]

Stimulability

A child's ability to imitate the targeted sound is tested because it can provide the professional with valuable information for planning remediation.[75–78] Therefore testing stimulability is a routine procedure in many evaluations. In this procedure, the speech-language pathologist asks the child to imitate syllables and words containing the targeted sounds that are in error in the child's repertoire. If a child can imitate the syllables correctly, the clinician knows that providing detailed instructions on how the targeted sound is produced will not be necessary, but, instead, training can begin immediately with imitation of the targeted sound in selected contexts. Stimulability has also been interpreted as evidence that the incorrect productions are not motoric in nature because the child is able to articulate the sounds in imitation.

Analysis of Articulation

After the articulation samples are obtained, the clinician uses one or several procedures to analyze the child's performance. Selection of the analyses depends to a large extent on the theory or model of articulation disorders adhered to by a speech-language pathologist. As discussed in the previous sections, a model provides a framework within which defective articulation can be viewed. Theories, or models, are developed to conceptualize the nature of a problem and sometimes to project causal factors that might have been responsible for the defective articulation. However, they are primarily developed to help in defining what constitutes an articulation disorder. Each model uses similar articulatory data, but the data are explained in different ways. The individual's articulation is tested and analyzed with one or more of the analysis procedures to be described, but interpretation of the articulatory data differs according to the conceptualization concerning the nature of the problem. Thus, if the speech-language pathologist views the problem as a sensorimotor deficit, the data are thought to reflect a sensorimotor problem; whereas if it is viewed as a problem in the client's ability to match the auditory feedback from his or her own production with the auditory pattern produced by others, it is thought to reflect a discrimination problem. Yet the clinician who looks upon articulation errors from a phonologic disorders approach infers from the data that the child's phonologic system is inadequate. Therefore the analytic procedures are selected to conform to, and confirm, the model adopted by the speech-language pathologist. Needless to say, no one model has been thoroughly tested, although some components may have been put to an experimental evaluation. However, the analyses used assume that the articulatory behavior reflects the nature of the problem as explained in the model.

Not only does a speech-language pathologist's opinion on functional articulation disorders dictate the form of analysis to be applied to the articulatory data, but also both the model and analysis subsequently influence the treatment plan and procedures. Furthermore, the viewpoint held by the clinician determines the number of analyses to be performed on the articulatory data gathered during the assessment.

The number of analyses and the specific analyses to apply are determined mostly by the model adhered to by the speech-language pathologist, but other factors also play a part. One factor is the degree to which articulation appears to be defective; another is the speech pathologist's opinion of how extensively the disorder needs to be described before training targets can be determined. All of these considerations enter into selection of the initial targeted sound and future targets for training. The speech-language pathologist needs to decide for each client the relevance of the information inherent in the various forms of analyses. The speech-language pathologist also weighs the value of the information from each analysis in relation to her or his viewpoint concerning the nature of functional articulation disorders. The model adopted and the selection of targets are individual matters. Because no data are available to support any one viewpoint or analytic procedure, clear-cut recommendations for any specific analysis, remediation plan, and target selection are not possible. Interactive effects of individual preferences and the client's articulation sample can be illustrated with a few examples.

If a client misarticulates only a few sounds, an in-depth analysis such as is required by a distinctive feature or phonologic process analysis is obviously unnecessary. The clinician might be satisfied with a DSO analysis to determine which of the few erroneous sounds are distorted, which are substituted, and which are omitted. Taking into consideration consistency, severity, stimulability, and so forth, the clinician readily could select the first targeted sound for treatment. For example, the distorted sound might be selected for initial training. However, when a client's sample reveals a number of error sounds, individual preferences have a greater effect on selection. Depending on his or her approach, the speech-language pathologist might choose to complete more than a DSO analysis. If the clinician uses a developmental approach to remediation, he or she would eschew the use of an in-depth distinctive feature or phonologic process analysis, since the targeted sounds would be selected on the basis of training sounds that appear earlier before training sounds that appear later. For this purpose, a distinctive feature analysis is unnecessary and so is a phonologic process analysis. However, if the speech-language pathologist adhered to a phonologic disorders model, a phonologic process analysis would be mandatory for the child who makes a number of sounds in error. Training would be directed toward teaching the child to relinquish simplification processes, and, for this purpose, the articulation sample needs to be analyzed to discover the processes operating in the child's repertoire. But the same speech sample might be treated differently by the clinician whose view of articulation is based on the model proposed by Van Riper.[10] In addition to processing the sample through several analyses, the clinician would seek evidence for erroneous sounds most troublesome to the client's functioning in the environment. If the evidence was strong enough to indicate that a particular erroneous sound was bothersome to the client, the clinician might choose that sound as the target for training regardless of the results of the other analyses.

The previous examples demonstrate that individual conceptualizations, definitions, and preferences play a leading role in the choice of an analytic procedure for the development of remediation plans. Yet data to support the models, preferences, and definitions are lacking. Research has not been directed toward experimental evaluation of models, and so advocating the use of a particular approach rather than others is difficult. What is needed is a concerted effort by investigators to submit their proclamations to a serious and controlled empirical evaluation.

As is apparent from the examples presented, many factors need to be considered in the development of a remediation plan. All individual preferences aside, an attempt will be made to provide some guidelines by describing the kind of information obtained from various analytic procedures and how the information is applied in the development of remediation plans.

Basic Analysis

Examination of articulation errors for consistency, stimulability, frequency of occurrence, error type, and developmental norms is frequently the only analysis applied to articulation test results. It constitutes the traditional analysis used by most clinicians when an analysis is deemed necessary. However, parts of this analysis can also be used in conjunction with other analyses to provide supplementary information, especially for clients with more severe problems. Some of the information can serve routinely in an adjunctive capacity.

Because a number of factors are considered simultaneously in this analysis, the factors may shift in importance according to clinician preference. For example, if a clinician views stimulability as the most important factor in the selection of an initial targeted sound, stimulability would take precedence over the other factors. Conversely, another clinician might place contextual effects high on the priority list and select items (contexts) in which the erroneous sound is produced correctly for use in initial training. When normal development is considered crucial for selection, data from developmental norms would be attended to before other factors are considered.

In the basic analysis, each speech sound is commonly viewed as relatively independent of other speech sounds; thereby each erroneous sound is considered to be relatively independent of the remaining erroneous sounds. Therefore training is directed at one sound at a time. The overall remediation plan would proceed from one erroneous sound to the next in a sequential manner. When this approach is used, the effects of generalization are largely ignored, or at any rate not integrated into the plan. Relationships between phonemes are not the primary focus of the analysis.

The impact of linguistic information has caused us to reevaluate our traditional methods of analyzing and treating articulation disorders. It has been suggested that children's articulation errors should not be regarded as random errors on single phonemes, but be viewed as productions governed by rules.[16,17,41,79–81] Several analytic procedures have been introduced as a result of the influence of linguistic theory on our approaches to articulation disorders.

Place, Voice, and Manner Analysis

A place, voice, and manner analysis utilizes a classificatory system describing English consonant sounds according to three parameters. A place, voice, and manner analysis can be conducted within the framework of any of a number of phonetic charts listing the sounds according to place classifications such as bilabial, dental, alveolar, palatal, and velar and manner classifications such as plosives, fricatives, and affricates.[77,82,83] Similar to the basic analysis described before, a place, voice, and manner analysis reveals whether the child can produce a sound even though it may not be used appropriately. It also shows whether the same place or manner error occurs on more than one sound, thereby revealing a pattern of errors. Furthermore, it shows whether the child has established all the contrasts between the sounds. Turton, in discussing this analysis, draws a distinction between phonetic skills, referring to the ability to produce a sound, and phonemic skills, referring to the integration of the sounds in a linguistic system.[77] The distinction between phonetic and phonemic errors has been made by other authors as well.[43–45,78,84–86] In a place, voice, and manner analysis, the patterns of errors disclosed aid in the selection of an initial targeted sound or sounds and point to long-term goals. Examples of patterns that might be discovered are front sounds used for back sounds (errors in place), voiced sounds substituted for unvoiced sounds (errors in voicing), or plosives produced for fricatives (errors in manner).

The advantages of the place, voice, and manner examination of articulatory data are that it can be accomplished in a relatively short time and that it reveals the more obvious erroneous patterns in a child's system. A possible disadvantage is that the analysis may expose such a large array of erroneous patterns that no pattern or patterns emerge as clearly significant. Perhaps the more detailed analyses to be described are better descriptive measures. Whenever an analysis fails to reveal clear patterns, exploration of additional procedures may be useful; this problem is not unique to place, voice, and manner analysis.

Distinctive Feature Analysis

Distinctive feature analysis utilizes primarily linguistic feature systems, such as Chomsky and Halle's,[87] to isolate articulatory parameters in error in phoneme production. Distinctive feature systems are primarily theoretic and abstract constructs in which each phoneme is described in terms of the articulatory and acoustic features composing it. For example, the /t/ in the Chomsky and Halle[87] system is (+) consonantal, (+) anterior, (+) coronal and (−) vocalic, (−) high, (−) back, (−) low, (−) voice, (−) continuant, (−) nasal, and (−) strident. The features and the number of features differ across systems.[87,88] The analysis compares substituted erroneous productions to targets in order to identify particular feature(s) that account for the misarticulations. Thus the features composing the targeted sound are compared to the features composing the erroneous production. The features that do not match are the features in error. For example, if a child substitutes /t/ for /s/, two features are in error—continuancy and stridency—but the remaining features are the same for the two sounds and are therefore correct. If continuancy and stridency are found in error in other substitutions, the clinician might choose to train one (e.g., (+) continuancy) in the context of a minimal pair differing only on (+) and (−) continuancy (e.g., /s/ and /tʃ/). A distinctive feature analysis can be applied to substitutions and omissions, but not distortions. A distinctive feature analysis, although similar to a place, voice, and manner analysis, may provide more information on generality across phonemes because it is based on phonemic rather than phonetic elements. At the same time, a distinctive feature system is based on an abstract, competence model of phonology. It has been pointed out that distinctive feature theory is far removed from the phonetic aspects of sound production and therefore is not useful for analysis of articulation errors.[89,90] Specific procedures for completing a distinctive feature analysis are described completely by McReynolds and Engmann[34] and McReynolds and Huston.[91]

A disadvantage of this analysis is that it requires a large amount of time to complete. Further, as with place, voice, and manner analysis, distinctive feature analysis may not disclose any large or particular feature errors, but instead may reveal a pattern of low percentage of errors across many features. Further analyses might be desirable, although the result may not be different. In fact, other phonologic analyses have preempted distinctive feature analysis and are applied more frequently. Phonologic process analysis is the analysis most often chosen by clinicians who believe articulation errors are the products of phonologic processes. This analysis is described next.

Phonologic Process Analysis

As discussed earlier, children's misarticulations can be described as patterns that represent simplification processes similar to processes attributed to young, normally developing children. The concept of processes has been accepted by the linguistic and speech pathology community, but, as noted earlier, reservations have been expressed concerning the definition and identification of processes in children's misarticulations.[41,43,92,93]

A phonologic process analysis is conducted in order to identify the number and consistency of processes present in the child's articulation sample. A number of manuals describe the various processes that are sought in the analysis and procedures for completing an analysis.[19,21,37–39] Briefly, the procedure for analysis consists of several steps. Initially, a sample of the child's articulation is obtained, preferably a conversational sample, but single word utterances would suffice. The utterances are then phonetically transcribed by means of either a broad or narrow transcription. Errors are placed into appropriate categories that are labelled with process names. For example, each error in which a plosive is substituted for a fricative is listed in the column labelled "stopping." Omissions of final consonants in words ending in final consonants are listed under the process labelled "final consonant deletion." Thus the errors are listed and counted and categorized under process labels. Targeted processes are chosen by considering a number of factors or just one, depending on which process manual is used for the analyses; the number of processes vary across the manuals and models upon which the analyses are formed, and similarly, factors considered in the selection of targets for treatment vary across the manuals. However, regardless of the differences, the individuals writing the manuals agree that the goal is to eliminate processes. In regard to the analytic procedures, the complexity of the analysis varies, and speech-language pathologists usually choose the one that they learned to conduct during their academic program.

Phonologic Knowledge

A more in-depth analysis is used by those who believe that a phonologic process analysis is only a surface analysis and does not provide an accurate or comprehensive profile of a child's phonologic system. This kind of generative phonology approach to articulation errors requires an additional assessment and analytic procedure. In the assessment, the clinician obtains a speech sample in the customary manner. However, in addition to the phonetic inventory, system of contrasts, and phonologic process analysis, the examiner uses procedures to gain evidence of the child's underlying form.

Of prime importance is the determination of the child's degree or level of phonologic knowledge. Therefore, when an analysis reveals the presence of a process, the clinician needs to verify that a process is operating. This is accomplished with an alternation procedure, a procedure that can help to determine whether the child's stored lexical form is the same as the adult form or whether the child's production represents the form that is in his or her mind. In the alternation procedure the child is given an opportunity to produce the targeted sound in another context and in a contrasting manner. Let us say that a child does not produce the final /g/ in the word "pig," or the final /t/ in the word "cat." The child is credited with a final consonant deletion process if it is assumed that he or she knows the words have final consonants, that is, if it is assumed that the words are represented in the child's mind as "pig" and "cat" with final /g/ and /t/. To learn whether the adult forms ("pig" and "cat") are the child's underlying forms, the child is presented with an opportunity to say words such as "piggy" and "catty." If the /g/ and /t/ are produced correctly in these contexts, the child's underlying forms for the words are assumed to include final /g/ and /t/, and the final consonants are assumed to be deleted purposely by application of a neutralization rule or phonologic process. If the /g/ and /t/ continue to be omitted in the medial position words, the clinician has no evidence that the underlying form is different from the form produced by the child, that is, [pi] and [kae]. In other words, it is possible (although not proven) that there are no CVC words in the child's underlying forms—only CV forms (also not proven). If so, the child is not applying a phonologic process or neutralization rule because there is nothing to be deleted.

Not only is it necessary to test for the presence of the targeted sound in some contexts, but it is also desirable to obtain evidence that the sound is used contrastively in a minimal pair context. After all, a neutralization rule is applied for the purpose of obliterating a contrast.[40] By deleting final consonants as, for example, in producing [pi] for "pig" and [pi] for "pick," the child makes it impossible to contrast the two words because they are produced identically. Therefore, it is desirable to test whether the contrast between /g/ and /k/ is intact in the medial context. The question is, in the presence of appropriate stimuli, will the child produce "piggy" and "picky" or has the contrast been lost in all contexts?

With the added information about the child's underlying form, the clinician can gain a clearer notion about the child's level of phonologic knowledge. The child who knows about the /g/ and /t/ as final consonants is credited with a greater phonologic knowledge than the child who does not. Remediation is tailored to the child's level of phonologic knowledge; to obtain a complete picture of that knowledge, alternation procedures are used to examine all errors. Thus, for each phonologic process identified, an alternation procedure is applied to all items affected to determine whether a process can be imputed to be present. For example, if /d/, /k/, /t/ were omitted as final consonants in words, an alternation procedure would be used to examine the underlying form for each sound. In this examination, specific information would be gained about the level of the child's phonologic knowledge. For example, if the child produced the /d/ and /t/ correctly in the medial position as diminutive, but not the /k/, the child would be credited with greater phonologic knowledge of alveolar plosives than of velar plosives. Adding an alternation assessment to the other phonologic analyses would require additional time and effort on the part of the clinician.

Of all the analyses applied, the most involved and intricate are the linguistically based ones. They are appealing in regard to designing remediation procedures because they imply generalization in training. The assumption underlying the analyses is that errors are systematic. This means that each sound does not have to be taught separately. Once the system is described, sounds can be selected for training that allow a child to learn a rule or to relinquish an entire process. When the rule is learned in a few utterances, or a process eliminated in a few exemplars, the change could extend across other untrained sounds and sound classes. Each affected sound need not be treated individually.

Disadvantages of the phonologically based analyses are several. First, they require a great deal of time to conduct. Second, they require a certain degree of knowledge and experience in linguistic theory and linguistic analytic procedures. The linguistic background is absent for most speech pathologists. Third, the phonologic process and generative phonology analyses are dependent on inferential conclusions; that is, the child's underlying form is inferred, not observed. Moreover, an erroneous pattern is inferred as representing a mental manipulation by the child, but the manipulation is not observed. In reality, there is no way that the examiner can know what is in the child's mind in either instance. If the examiner's conjecture is correct, remediation could be directed to the appropriate source, but if the conjecture is incorrect, remediation planned to conform to the conjecture may be inappropriate.

Data to support the increased efficiency of training based on process or generative phonology analysis as compared to other analyses are lacking. But then no controlled comparisons have been made on the effectiveness or efficiency of any of the analyses for planning remediation, and so it is difficult to encourage or discourage use of any of the procedures. No one analysis has been supported by data as leading to the most effective intervention planning.

Within Treatment Assessment

In the beginning of the assessment section, I pointed out that evaluation is an ongoing process throughout treatment. The assessment during treatment is designed to provide information on the child's progress and to select ensuing targets for training. It also has another purpose, and that is to determine whether the target as learned in the training items has generalized to untrained contexts and situations. Specialized generalization probes are frequently developed for this purpose. The two assessments will be explained briefly.

In the assessment for progress and for new target selection, the clinician may administer the same instrument used in the initial assessment, for example, the same articulation test used originally to obtain an in-depth profile of the child's articulation status. Changes in production of the items containing the sound(s) trained are noted, and the remaining errors are identified. From the remaining errors a new target is selected.

More frequently, however, the speech-language pathologist develops specific measures known as probes. The probes are directed more at testing generalization of trained behaviors than at testing for target selection, but they may serve both purposes. However, generalization is important to test because the goal in treatment is not merely acquisition, but generalization of the behavior trained to other contexts. A few examples will illustrate the use of probes.

Suppose a clinician has chosen to train a targeted sound in the initial position of syllables and words and wishes to probe for generalization to other positions before initiating training on them. A probe may be designed to test generalization of the sound to other positions in words. Thus the clinician might present the child with ten words in which the sound is in the initial position, ten in which it is in the medial position, and ten in the final position. These 30 words are presented to the child prior to the beginning of training on the initial position. After the child reaches the training criterion on production of the sound in the initial position in the training items, the 30 words are presented again. If the child produces the sound correctly in the untrained positions, the clinician knows that the targeted sound is stable and need not be trained in the medial or final positions. If the targeted sound is produced correctly only in the initial position words, the clinician may choose to shift training to one of the other positions or to both positions.

Another example of a probe for generality might be during training for elimination of a phonologic process. In this case, the speech-language pathologist might have chosen to work on eliminating the process of cluster reduction in a few exemplars from one cluster class: the /st/ cluster as in the word "stop." In the initial assessment, the child reduced several /s/ clusters as well as /r/ clusters, such as /st/, /sp/, /sl/, and /sm/ and /tr/, /br/, and /pr/. Before training is initiated on producing /st/ in words, a probe is developed consisting of five words with the /st/ cluster, five with the /sp/ cluster, five with the /sl/ cluster, and five with the /sm/ cluster. In addition, the speech-language pathologist wishes to know whether generalization from /s/ cluster training spreads to /r/ clusters, because processes are thought to operate across sound classes. Therefore the clinician also designs five words with the /tr/ cluster, five with the /pr/ cluster, and five with the /br/ cluster for testing across sound class generalization.

Prior to training, the child's responses to these words are tested and transcribed. Only the /st/ cluster is selected as the target in training. When the child correctly produces the /st/ cluster at a stable rate in training, the 30 words containing the remaining /s/ and /r/ cluster words are presented again to determine whether or not training on the /st/ cluster has had any effect on the clusters that were not trained, that is, whether or not generalization has occurred and if the cluster reduction process has been eliminated in clusters within the /s/ and the /r/ sound classes. The child's performance on these untrained items provides the clinician with essential information concerning the generality of the cluster reduction process and whether training can be shifted to another process or continued on the process currently in treatment.

Probes developed for specific purposes in remediation can provide the clinician with valuable information on the adequacy of the training and the status of the child's articulation at selected points during treatment. They should be employed routinely to increase efficiency of training. They can give the clinician a clear indication of exactly where the child is in the treatment sequence and provide specific information for new directions in treatment. Probes are better in some ways than the standardized tests that are often used because they can be designed to obtain specific information on an individual basis. They can also be designed to test specific sounds in specific contexts to develop training steps, something the more global commercially available tests cannot do.

Final Assessment

When the probes indicate that the child has generalized to other linguistic contexts, the clinician is ready to determine whether the target behaviors will be produced in broader contexts and situations; in other words, the clinician wishes to determine whether the child is ready for dismissal either from treatment entirely or at least from treatment on that particular target. Generalization may be thought to be complete when a child produces the target behavior in normal, spontaneous conversational speech—the ultimate test. Therefore, in addition to structured probes, the clinician obtains a sample of the child's conversational speech and analyzes the speech for correct and incorrect target behavior.

TREATMENT

Treatments are as individually determined as the analytic procedures. Clinicians may plan treatment to fit their conceptualization of the nature of the articulation disorder in general, but at the same time, include procedures from other approaches if they have been shown by experience to be effective. Therefore descriptions of specific treatments in a step by step sequence is not possible, because they are too numerous to describe individually. Although each clinician would claim that his treatment is effective, and perhaps more effective than other treatments, no data have been presented to support such claims. Therefore, at this point, each clinician may be correct, but each may also be engaging in superstitious behavior regarding the efficacy of his own treatments.

Although treatments are numerous, certain principles are found in all treatments. Additionally, within each model of articulation disorders, particular phases are dictated by the model. In this section, the principles within specific approaches will be discussed first. In the final section, an attempt will be made to point out some of the similarities across treatment approaches that form general principles of intervention for articulation disorders. It should be mentioned that clinicians may use similar procedures in training, but interpret them differently to conform to their particular theoretic approach to treatment.

Discrimination Training

Discrimination training is the primary mode of treatment in Winitz's conceptualization of articulation errors that stem from perceptual deficits, inappropriate underlying forms, or inattentiveness to perceptual cues.[11] The goal is to provide the child with an accurate internal auditory model or underlying form. Although the source of the problem may vary, the appropriate treatment in each case is a series of tasks directed toward establishment of an ever more refined discrimination ability. The terminal objective is to provide the child with an ability to distinguish between the target and the child's erroneous production of the targeted sound.

During the discrimination training, the target sound is contrasted with the child's erroneous production in many phonetic environments in increasingly complex units. In essence, the recommendation is that treatment should emphasize learning correct sound patterns through experience, within contexts that serve a communicative purpose.[11] For example, in an informal training situation, minimal pairs may be presented within an actual life activity. The contrast to be learned is between the /t/ and /k/; two activities are occurring, building a table and building a cable. The clinician may request a part that goes with the table. If the child offers a part that is more appropriate to the cable activity, the clinician informs the child that the part belongs to the cable and not the table. The child is not instructed to listen and to make the discrimination; instead the child attends because of interest in the activity. The child is never requested to articulate the target, only exposed to the correct production for discrimination purposes. A number of activities can be developed by the clinician to teach a discrimination between the target and the child's erroneous sound, activities such as eating a meal or painting a picture.

After extensive discrimination training the child may spontaneously begin to produce the targeted sound, but if this does not happen, subsequent production training can be introduced. However, Winitz cautions that discrimination training should not be relinquished too early; it sometimes needs to be offered for as long as a year before introduction of articulation training.[11]

Although other options are available to clinicians, Winitz emphasizes that the best learning situation is one that involves meaningful activity and communication.[11] From an extensive exposure to contrasts, the child establishes the appropriate underlying form and may even begin to produce the targeted sound.

Although discrimination is faulty in Monnin's interpretation of the nature of articulation disorders,[9] the belief is that the child's poor articulation is responsible for the discrimination deficit. Because of this belief, it is suggested that since discrimination depends on articulation, the training should be directed at production, the source of the problem, rather than at discrimination, the product of the problem.

The goal of training is to establish an accurate internal auditory model. In order to circumvent the child's current inaccurate internal auditory model, training is started with verbal play: activities such as imitating environmental sounds and playing with other kinds of soundmaking. If the targeted sound occurs accidentally during play, production training can begin with imitation; if not, instructions and phonetic placement aid may be needed initially.

When the target sound is produced correctly, a new, internal auditory model has replaced the old, inaccurate one. At that point, extensive practice in production is provided to stabilize the new model and to establish the range of acceptable production of the targeted sound. Feedback concerning accuracy is first provided by the clinician, but the monitoring responsibility is gradually shifted to the child. In that shift, the child produces the targeted sound in a syllable, a word, or a sentence and evaluates the correctness internally. The child tells the clinician whether or not the sound was produced correctly, and the clinician only agrees or disagrees with the child's evaluation. The goal in treatment is to make the child independent by relying, not on external monitoring, but on internal monitoring of the articulation. Thus, in this approach, the child is provided only with production practice, but is gradually trained to self-evaluate his or her articulation responses. The problem may be discrimination, but the approach is articulation.

Variations of the previous two approaches have been practiced for a number of years. The specifics change from time to time and vary from clinician to clinician, but discrimination training generally precedes production practice.[10] Discrimination teaching of the target and error substitution is commonly provided at various stages of the treatment program. For example, the child may initially learn to distinguish between the targeted and erroneous sounds or other sounds presented in isolation. This phase may be followed by training on the targeted sound as produced in isolation. A period of discrimination training with the targeted and erroneous sounds embedded in syllables follows, after which the syllables are learned in production. Thus alternating periods of discrimination and production are offered as the context, in which the sound is embedded, increases in linguistic complexity.

Perceptual-Motor Training

The model from which perceptual-motor training is derived offers the clinician numerous opportunities for designing individual intervention programs. Articulation treatment has always included instructions on how sounds are produced and how the articulators should move to produce targeted sounds. The training has also included practice in producing the targeted sound in isolation, then in syllables and words, and finally in phrases, sentences, and conversational speech. The treatment usually follows a progression from imitation to spontaneous production across the levels of linguistic complexity. The goal is to provide appropriate production practice until the targeted sound is produced effortlessly in conversational speech outside the clinical environment. The treatment is directed at establishing the production of targeted sounds as a motor skill in which the articulators learn to hit the correct targets automatically.

A number of variations of the treatment can be seen by observing individual clinicians with individual clients. Some clinicians provide comprehensive step by step programs; others may incorporate a few steps while borrowing steps from other approaches to include in the treatment. Generally, however, perceptual-motor skill learning is divided into two stages, acquisition and automatization, with considerable overlap between the stages.

The acquisition stage requires mental planning, execution, and attending to feedback after the execution of the movement. Thus the child is requested to think about how the sound will be produced before production, then produces the sound, and after, attends to the proprioceptive, kinesthetic, and auditory information from the production in order to evaluate the accuracy of the response and the articulatory movements. At first, the clinician gives the child feedback on the topography of the production, but the external feedback is shifted gradually to the child's self-evaluation of the adequacy of the production. Internal feedback and self-monitoring are important components of the perceptual-motor treatment model and are the first objectives in the acquisition phase of remediation. During acquisition training, the movements are at first slow and deliberate, under conscious control of the child. After sufficient practice in production of the targeted sound in a variety of contexts, articulation becomes less deliberate and the rate increases. When the automatization stage is reached, control is no longer exerted consciously because the motor pattern has been established so well that it does not require deliberation or further effort.

Training is directed at establishing a motor schema, an internal motor rule that sets the limits and range of variation allowed in production of the targeted sound in a variety of phonetic contexts by a variety of speakers with different vocal tract configurations. Once the schema has been stabilized and production is automatic, the child is able to produce the targeted sound in any context or situation.

Phonologic Disorder

For most models of phonologic disorders, the goal is the same: elimination of phonologic processes. Means for accomplishing the elimination differ across theories and theorists. For some, a phonologic process analysis is just a way to organize the data into patterns of errors and to select targets, but the actual treatment follows a more traditional program. For example, the child may be provided with auditory stimulation for a while, followed by articulation training that includes phonetic placement instruction, feedback, and other traditional procedures.[19]

A minimal contrast approach has been described by Weiner;[94] although it includes one less traditional component, in general the treatment includes instructions for phonetic placement, presenting a model for imitation and reinforcement or for feedback on the child's accuracy in production. In the minimal contrast procedure, the child is presented with pictures of two different objects whose names differ by one element. For instance, if a child does not produce final consonants and is credited with application of a final consonant deletion process, the two pictures could be "bow" and "boat." The child asks the clinician for one of the pictures, and, if the name is produced correctly, the picture is given to the child and a star placed in a book. If the child produces "bow" but intends "boat," the clinician gives the picture of the "bow." The clinician then instructs and models the correct target by telling the child that if the child wishes to say "boat," then the /t/ has to be produced at the end of the word; otherwise the word is "bow." At the same time, the clinician describes how the /t/ should be produced and models the correct word several times.

Kahn and Lewis propose that there are three differences between a phonologic disorder remediation program and the traditional remediation program.[38] First, the child is taught to suppress or inhibit erroneous patterns, not to produce correct targeted sounds singly. Second, emphasis is placed on decreasing the frequency of occurrence of a process, and suppression does not require accurate articulation of the targeted sound. Third, selective reinforcement is given to suppression of a process aside from the actual production that indicates suppression. For example, if final consonant deletion was the process, the goal would be to teach the child to mark the final consonant in some way, not necessarily by producing the targeted sound, just by producing any sound. The rationale is that the objective is not correct sound production, but elimination of a process. Thus, selective reinforcement refers to providing positive reinforcement if a child produces something to mark the final consonant, but not to reinforce the topography of the actual production since it may be incorrect. The form of the feedback might be, "Good, you put something at the end of the word."

Even though specific aspects of treatment differ among individual speech-language pathologists, certain aspects are included in most treatments directed at elimination of phonologic processes. The commonalities include the following:

1. Most programs involve remediation of several phonemes from a class of affected sounds to suppress a process.
2. Most treatments accept misproductions as correct responses if the process is affected in treatment.
3. Although other targets are possible, many programs advocate the use of a minimal pair contrast procedure for treating suppression of processes. The contrast may be used in a communicative manner as in the procedure used by Weiner,[94] or it may be used in an imitative manner in the presence of two pictures named with a pair of minimal contrast nonsense syllables or words.[95–97]

SUMMARY

Researchers have yet to identify the etiology for a large segment of children who misproduce speech sounds. There has been a shift from the label "functional articulation disorders" to "phonologic disorders" for this group. However, neither label identifies the etiologic factors responsible for the child's articulation errors. In addition, both terms are defined in individual ways by speech-language pathologists. The labels refer more to the speech pathologist's theoretic view of the nature of articulation errors than to an explanation of errors and the cause for the errors. The tendency to label all articulation problems as phonologic is questioned by some phonologists and speech pathologists who encourage a separation of phonologic problems from phonetic ones.

Regardless of the label employed, most speech pathologists use the same assessment procedures and tools for testing children's articulation and for obtaining an adequate sample of a child's speech for analysis. When there are differences, they lie in the manner in which the speech sample is analyzed; that is, the assessment procedures are less affected by the theoretic view of the examiner than are the analytic procedures.

Treatments are individualized plans developed from the speech-language pathologist's conceptualization of the nature of articulation errors. The treatment plan is also a function of the needs of specific clients and experiences the clinician has had in the past with procedures. It is fair to state that speech pathologists often use identical procedures, although they explain the rationale for the procedures differently. For example, all of the treatments appear to rely on feedback to the child about the accuracy of the child's production. The feedback may be in different forms, but the principle of reinforcement operates across all treatments. Most of the treatments, regardless of the theory upon which they are founded, use some form of imitation, whether immediate or delayed, in the initial stages of treatment. Another similarity is the use of instructions for phonetic placement across treatments. Establishment of an internal auditory model or underlying form is an important component in practically all models. The child is treated as an active participant throughout the treatment, as, for example, in mentally planning the production prior to execution. Cognitively, the child is required to be active, either in planning the necessary movement or in self-monitoring the production. Thus the theoretical foundations may be different, but the treatments are similar. Differences are not as much in the remediation plans as the diverse analyses would lead one to believe.

REFERENCES

1. Bernthal JE, Bankson NW. Articulation disorders. Englewood Cliffs, NJ: Prentice-Hall, 1981.
2. Hanson M. Articulation. Philadelphia: WB Saunders, 1983.
3. Shelton RL, McReynolds LV. Functional articulation disorders: preliminaries to treatment. In: Lass N, ed. Speech and language: advances in basic research and practice. Vol. 2. New York: Academic Press, 1979:2.
4. Sommers RK. Articulation disorders. Englewood Cliffs, NJ: Prentice-Hall, 1983.
5. Winitz H. Articulatory acquistion and behavior. New York: Appleton-Century-Crofts, 1969.
6. McDonald ET. Articulation testing and treatment: a sensory-motor approach. Pittsburgh: Stanwix House, 1964.
7. Ruscello D. Motor learning as a model for articulation. In: Costello J, ed. Speech disorders in children. San Diego: College-Hill Press, 1984:129.
8. Shelton RL. Disorders of articulation. In: Skinner DH, Shelton RL, eds. Speech, language and hearing. Reading, MA: Addison-Wesley, 1978:173.
9. Monnin LM. Speech sound discrimination testing and training: why? why not? In: Winitz H, ed. Treating articulation disorders: for clinicians by clinicians. Baltimore: University Park Press, 1984:1.
10. Van Riper C. Speech correction principles and methods. 6th ed. New York: Prentice-Hall, 1978.
11. Winitz H. Auditory considerations in articulation training. In: Winitz H, ed. Treating articulation disorders: for clinicians by clinicians. Baltimore: University Park Press, 1984:21.
12. Mowrer DE. Behavioral application to modification of articulation. In: Wolfe D, Goulding D, eds. Articulation and learning. Springfield, IL: CC Thomas, 1973:139.
13. Garrett ER. Programmed articulation therapy. In: Wolfe WD, Goulding DJ, eds. Articulation and learning. Springfield, IL: CC Thomas, 1973:106.
14. Sommers RK, Kane AR. Nature and remediation of functional articulation disorders. In: Dickson S, ed. Communication disorders: remedial principles and practices. Glenview, IL: Scott-Foresman, 1974:104.
15. Grunwell P. Clinical phonology. Rockville, MD: Aspen Publications, 1982.
16. Edwards ML, Shriberg L. Phonology: applications in communicative disorders. San Diego: College-Hill Press, 1983.
17. Ingram D. Phonological disability in children. New York: American Elsevier, 1976.
18. Weiner F. A phonologic approach to assessment and treatment. In: Costello J, ed. Speech disorders in children. San Diego: College-Hill Press, 1984:75.
19. Hodson B. The assessment of phonological processes. Danville, IL: Interstate Press, 1986.
20. Locke JL. Phonological acquisition and change. New York: Academic Press, 1983.
21. Shriberg L, Kwiatkowski J. Natural process analysis (NPA). New York: John Wiley, 1980.
22. Fitts PM. Factors in complex skill training. In: Glaser R, ed. Training research and education. Pittsburgh: University of Pittsburgh Press, 1962:221.
23. Marteniuk RG. Information processing in motor skills. New York: Holt, Rinehart and Winston, 1976.
24. Palliard J. The patterning of skilled movements. In: Field J, ed. Handbook of physiology, neurophysiology. Vol. III, section I. Baltimore: Waverly, 1960:1679.
25. Johnson AF, Shelton RL, Ruscello DN, Arndt WB. A comparison of two articulation treatments: acquisition and acquisition-automatization. Hum Commun 1979; 4:337–348.
26. Manning W, Shirkey E. Determining articulatory automatization of newly learned sounds. In: Lass N, ed. Speech and language: advances in basic research and practice. New York: Academic Press, 1982:127.
27. Van Riper C, Irwin JV. Voice and articulation. Englewood Cliffs,NJ: Prentice-Hall, 1958.
28. Fairbanks G. Systematic research in experimental phonetics: 1. A theory of the speech mechanism as a servosystem. J Speech Hear Disord 1954; 19:133–139.
29. Liberman A, Cooper F, Shankweiler D, Studdert-Kennedy M. Perception of the speech code. Psychol Rev 1967; 74:431–461.
30. Briere E. An investigation of phonological interference. Language 1966; 42:786–796.
31. Monnin L, Huntington D. Relationship of articulatory defects to speech-sound identification. J Speech Hear Res 1974; 17:352–366.
32. Williams G, McReynolds LV. The relationship between discrimination and articulation in children with misarticulations. J Speech Hear Res 1975; 18:401–412.
33. Costello J. Onstine J. The modification of multiple articulation errors based on distinctive feature theory. J Speech Hear Disord 1976; 41:199–215.
34. McReynolds LV, Engmann DL. Distinctive feature analysis of misarticulations. Baltimore: University Park Press, 1975.
35. Compton A. Generative studies of children's phonological disorders. J Speech Hear Disord 1970; 35:315–339.
36. Compton A. Generative studies of children's phonological disorders. In: Singh S, ed. Measurements in hearing, speech, and language. Baltimore: University Park Press, 1975:55.
37. Ingram D. Procedures for the phonological analysis of children's language. Baltimore: University Park Press, 1981.
38. Kahn L, Lewis N. Kahn-Lewis phonological analysis. Circle Pines, MN: American Guidance Service, 1986.
39. Weiner F. Phonological process analysis. Baltimore: University Park Press, 1979.
40. Dinnsen DA. Methods and empirical issues in analyzing functional misarticulation. In: Elbert M, Dinnsen DA, Weismer G, eds. Phonological theory and the misarticulating child. Rockville, MD: ASHA Monogr No. 22, 1984:5.
41. Elbert M, Dinnsen D, Weismer G, eds.. Phonological theory and the misarticulating child. ASHA Monogr No. 22, 1984.

42. Elbert M, Dinnsen D, Powell T. On the prediction of phonologic generalization learning patterns. J Speech Hear Disord 1984; 49:309–318.
43. Grunwell P. Comment on the terms "phonetics" and "phonology" as applied in the investigation of speech disorders. Br J Disord Commun 1985; 29:165–170.
44. Hewlett N. Phonological versus phonetic disorders: some suggested modifications to the current use of the distinction. Br J Disord Commun 1985; 20:155–164.
45. Milroy L. Phonological analysis and speech disorders: a comment. Br J Disord Commun 1985; 20:171–179.
46. Fisher HB, Logemann JA. The Fisher-Logemann test of articulation competence. Boston: Houghton Mifflin, 1971.
47. Templin MC, Darley FL. The Templin-Darley test of articulation. 2nd ed. Iowa City: University of Iowa, Bureau of Educational Research and Service, Division of Extension and University Services, 1969.
48. Van Riper C, Erickson RL. The predictive screening test of articulation. Kalamazoo: Western Michigan University, 1969.
49. Goldman R, Fristoe R. Goldman-Fristoe test of articulation. Circle Pines, MN: American Guidance Service, 1969.
50. Fudala J. Arizona articulation proficiency scale: revised. Los Angeles: Western Psychological Services, 1970.
51. Pendergast K, Dickey S, Selmar T, Soder A. The photo articulation test. 2nd ed. Danville, IL: Interstate Press, 1969.
52. McDonald E. A deep test of articulation. Pittsburgh: Stanwix House, 1964.
53. Paynter W, Bumpas T. Imitative and spontaneous articulatory assessment of three-year-old children. J Speech Hear Disord 1977; 42:119–125.
54. Siegel G, Winitz H, Conkey H. The influence of testing instruments on articulatory responses of children. J Speech Hear Disord 1963; 28:67–76.
55. Templin MC. Spontaneous vs. imitated verbalization in testing pre-school children. J. Speech Hear Disord 1947; 12:293–300.
56. Wright V, Shelton R, Arndt W. A task for evaluation of articulation change. III. Imitative task scores compared with scores for more spontaneous tasks. J Speech Hear Res 1969; 12:875–884.
57. Weiner F, Bernthal J. The use of distinctive features in assessment of articulation. In: Singh S, ed. Diagnostic methods in speech, language, and hearing. Baltimore: University Park Press, 1978:140.
58. Weismer G, Dinnsen D, Elbert M. A study of the voicing distinction associated with omitted word-final stops. J Speech Hear Disord 1981; 46:320–328.
59. Dubois E, Bernthal J. A comparison of three methods for obtaining articulatory responses. J Speech Hear Disord 1978; 43:295–305.
60. Faircloth MA, Faircloth SR. An analysis of the articulatory behavior of a speech-defective child in connected speech and in isolated-word responses. J Speech Hear Disord 1970; 35:51–61.
61. Rigor S. An experimental analysis of articulation generalization as a function of elicitation method and sampling context during articulation training. Masters Thesis, Lawrence: University of Kansas, 1980.
62. Solomon L. Generalization of articulation in hearing-imparied children. Doctoral Dissertation. Lawrence: University of Kansas, 1981.
63. Jordan EP. Articulation test measures and listener ratings of articulation defectiveness. J Speech Hear Res 1960; 3:303–319.
64. Elbert M, McReynolds LV. Transfer of /r/ across contexts. J Speech Hear Disord 1975; 40:380–387.
65. Elbert M, McReynolds LV. An experimental analysis of misarticulating children's generalization. J Speech Hear Res 1978; 21:136–149.
66. Hoffman P. Interallophonic generalization of /r/ training. J Speech Hear Disord 1983; 48:215–221.
67. Curtis JF, Hardy JC. A phonetic study of misarticulation of /r/. J Speech Hear Res 1959; 2:244–257.
68. Gallagher R, Shriner T. Contextual variables related to inconsistent /s/ and /z/ production in the spontaneous speech of children. J Speech Hear Res 1975; 18:623–633.
69. Hoffman PR, Schuckers G, Ratusnick D. Contextual-coarticulatory inconsistency of /r/ misarticulations. J Speech Hear Res 1977; 20:631–643.
70. Dunn LM, Dunn LM. Peabody picture vocabulary test (revised). Circle Pines, MN: American Guidance Service, 1981.
71. Carrow E. Carrow elicited language inventory. Learning Concepts. Austin, TX: Author, 1974.
72. Carrow E. Test for auditory comprehension of language. Boston: Teaching Resources, 1973.
73. Wepman JM. Wepman auditory discrimination test: manual of directions. Chicago: Language Research Association, 1958.
74. Templin MC. Templin speech sound discrimination test. In: Templin MC, ed. Certain language skills in children. Minneapolis: University of Minnesota Press, 1957:61.
75. Carter ET, Buck MB. Prognostic testing for functional articulation disorders among children in the first grade. J Speech Hear Disord 1958; 23:124–133.
76. Sommers RK, Leiss R, Delp M, Gerber A, Fundrella D, Smith R, Revucky M, Ellis D, Haley V. Factors related to the effectiveness of articulation therapy for kindergarten, first and second grade children. J Speech Hear Res 1967; 10:428–437.
77. Turton LJ. Diagnostic implications of articulation testing. In: Wolfe WD, Goulding DJ, eds. Articulation and learning. Springfield, IL: CC Thomas, 1973:195.
78. Winitz H. From syllable to conversation. Baltimore: University Park Press, 1975.
79. Compton A. Generative studies of children's phonological disorders: clinical ramifications. In: Morehead DM, Morehead AE, eds. Normal and deficient child language. Baltimore: University Park Press, 1976:61.
80. Lorentz JP. An analysis of some deviant phonological rules in English. In: Morehead DM, Morehead AE, eds. Normal and deficient child language. Baltimore: University Park Press, 1976:29.
81. Oller DK. Regularities in abnormal child phonology. J Speech Hear Disord 1973; 38:36–47.
82. Calvert D. Descriptive phonetics. New York: Thieme-Stratton, 1980.
83. Ladefoged P. A course in phonetics. New York: Harcourt Brace Jovanovich, 1975.
84. Locke J. The inference of phoneme perception in the phonologically disordered child: a rationale, some criteria, the conventional tests. J Speech Hear Disord 1980; 45:431–444.
85. Moskowitz BA. The acquisition of fricatives: a study of phonetics and phonology. J Phonetics 1975; 3:141–150.
86. Pollack E, Rees N. Disorders of articulation: some clinical applications of distinctive feature theory. J Speech Hear Disord 1972; 37:451–470.
87. Chomsky N, Halle M. The sound pattern of English. New York: Harper and Row, 1968.
88. Singh S, Frank D. A distinctive feature analysis of the consonantal substitution pattern. Lang Speech 1972; 15:209–218.
89. Parker F. Distinctive features in speech pathology: phonology or phonemics. J Speech Hear Disord 1976; 41:23–39.
90. Walsh H. On certain practical inadequacies of distinctive feature systems. J Speech Hear Disord 1974; 39:32–43.
91. McReynolds LV, Huston K. A distinctive feature analysis of children's misarticulations. J Speech Hear Disord 1971; 36:156–166.
92. McReynolds LV, Elbert M. Criteria for phonological process analysis. J Speech Hear Disord 1981; 46:197–204.
93. McReynolds LV, Elbert M. Generalization of correct articulation in clusters. Appl Psycholinguist 1981; 2:119–132.
94. Weiner F. Treatment of phonological disability using the

method of meaningful minimal contrast: two case studies. J Speech Hear Disord 1981; 46:97–103.
95. Elbert M, Rockman B, Saltzman D. Contrasts: the use of minimal pairs in articulation training. Austin, TX: Exceptional Resources, 1980.
96. Elbert M, McReynolds LV. The generalization hypothesis: final consonant deletion. Lang Speech 1985; 28:281–294.
97. McReynolds LV, Bennett S. Distinctive feature generalization in articulation training. J Speech Hear Disord 1972; 37:462–470.

16 Speech Disorders Related to Craniofacial Structural Defects: Part 1

Sally J. Peterson-Falzone, Ph.D.

Orofacial structural defects affecting motor speech production occasionally occur in isolation, such as in single dental or occlusal problems or ablative defects of single structures. More often, however, they occur in complex and interrelated clusters. Cleft lip and palate affects a number of structures directly involved in speech production and is often associated with other anomalies as well. In a large number of congenital malformation syndromes, sequences, or associations,* orofacial defects are present in combination and are again accompanied by other conditions that may affect the development of communication skills. The fact that these defects tend to cluster and to have an interactive relationship with each other means that the speech pathologist's first responsibility is definitive diagnosis. Without accurate delineation of the physical problems and the speech production problems that may or may not be directly attributable to them, no therapeutic plan, whether physical or behavioral, can be realistic.

The structural problems discussed in this chapter affect articulation and resonance more frequently than other aspects of speech production. However, there are conditions in which other aspects are at risk. Laryngeal function is known to be adversely affected in a significant proportion of speakers with cleft palate, and structural anomalies of the larynx occur in some relatively rare disorders, for example, G syndrome.[1] Some craniofacial malformations affect the central nervous system, in the most severe cases producing neuromotor control problems that may affect the speech production mechanism at any level.† Finally, of course, language development is at risk in most congenital orofacial defects, although that will not be the focus of this chapter.

There are several pitfalls to be avoided in attempting to establish cause-effect relationships between orofacial defects and speech problems. The most predictable—yet the most common—is the error of assuming a one-to-one relationship between the physical findings and any perceived speech problem. Any number of physical anomalies may be present without causing a speech problem, including malocclusions and submucous clefts of the palate. And the child with physical anomalies is a child *first,*

* Most of the literature in birth defects still uses the term "syndrome" to refer to clusters of defects occurring together. However, current usage differentiates among "malformation," "association," and "syndrome." The term "malformation" refers to a defect caused by an error in morphogenesis, that is, in the earliest stages of tissue formation,[1] whereas "deformation" refers to a structural defect due to the action of unusual forces on normally developing tissue, and "disruption" refers to a defect resulting from breakdown of normal tissue. The term "syndrome" is used when multiple structural defects cannot be explained on the basis of a single initiating defect and its consequences, but rather appear to be the consequence of multiple defects in one or more tissues. "Sequence" is used if all the anomalies can be explained on basis of a single problem in morphogenesis leading to a "cascade" of subsequent defects.[1] When a pattern of anomalies recurs in another individual but has not been identified as a syndrome or a sequence, the term "association" is used. (See Cohen and Stool[2] for further details.)

† Neurogenically based speech problems are discussed in Chapters 18 and 19.

with a right to phonologic process disorders or other speech problems of presumably nonorganic origin, just like any other child.

Other pitfalls are similarly related to the tendency to oversimplify. First, the clinician may focus on only the most obvious physical problems, ending the diagnostic process prematurely. Such invisible problems as hearing loss may be overlooked. Second, the effects of previous, repaired defects must be taken into account if they were unrepaired during the speech-learning years. Examples include the compensatory articulations notorious in cleft palate and the occasional persistence of a pattern of nasal direction of the airstream after a competent velopharyngeal system has been provided through physical management. Third, the speech pathologist should never take it on faith (1) that a patient diagnosed as having a given syndrome necessarily manifests all the classic features of that syndrome; (2) that the classic features, even if present, will be of the same severity from patient to patient; or even (3) that the referral diagnosis is in fact correct.[3,4] Any one of these assumptions can easily lead to erroneous conclusions about the etiology of whatever speech or hearing problems are observed to be present. Finally, many of the physical problems discussed in this chapter can have a significant psychological effect on the individual, sometimes with a secondary effect on the desire to communicate. The speech pathologist should never forget to attempt to ascertain what is important to the patient.

WORKING DEFINITIONS

Although research has periodically pointed out the danger of assuming that a given perceptual or acoustic phenomenon is produced by, or associated with, a given set of physiologic correlates,[5,6] the speech pathologist needs a conceptual framework with which to approach speech disorders associated with structural defects. To devise such a framework, it is necessary to differentiate among commonly used—and confused—terms.

Velopharyngeal Inadequacy

In most of the older literature and even in a high percentage of more current writings, the terms velopharyngeal "inadequacy," "insufficiency," and "incompetency" are used synonymously. I have found it helpful to follow the suggestion of Trost[7] that velopharyngeal "insufficiency" be used to refer to cases in which closure is incomplete due to a lack of tissue and "incompetency" to cases in which movement is deficient. "Velopharyngeal inadequacy" is used both as an umbrella or generic term and in cases of mixed or unknown etiology.

Hypernasality

Perceptually, hypernasality refers to the resonance alteration of vowels and vocalic segments resulting from (1) abnormal coupling between the oral and nasal cavities and/or (2) increased oral impedance relative to nasal impedance of the resonated airstream. As a result of the work of Warren and associates,[8–11] we know that the size of the velopharyngeal opening is not the sole determinant of nasality and nasal emission. Neither nasality nor nasal emission is an all-or-none phenomenon. A certain amount of nasal resonance is normal in American English, and a measurable amount of nasal emission can be tolerated before speech is labelled abnormal.[8,12] Diagnostic decisions are made all the more difficult by the fact that listeners do not rate nasality with a high degree of reliability,[13] and ratings of nasality have been shown to be influenced by a number of segmental and suprasegmental features.[14–17] Although instrumental assessment of nasality has become increasingly popular,[18–28] Moll took the view that the verification of "objective measures of nasality" lies in the listener's judgment.[29,30] As pointed out by Bzoch, ". . . although several reliable methods for scaling or measuring degrees of perceived nasality have been developed, they are not necessarily valid" (p 181).[14]

Nasal Emission

The term "nasal emission" denotes loss of air through the nose during production of pressure consonants. If the airflow is sufficiently turbulent, the result sounds less like the "hissing nasal escape of air"[31] and more like a "nasal snort"[32,33] or "nasopharyngeal snort."[14,34] The "posterior nasal fricative" as described by Trost[35] in 1981 appears to be perceptually synonymous with the older term of "nasal snort." Trost described the source of frication as linguovelar contact, with the airstream shunted through an open velopharyngeal port. However, nasal deformities in patients with cleft palate frequently cause at least a partial obstruction of the airway, providing increased resistance to airflow and thus a possible source of frication.[36] By definition, posterior nasal frication cannot take place without nasal emission, although the perceptual result is dissimilar.

Nasal emission is not always audible.[36,37] In some speakers, the volume of air escaping out the nose may be so small that it is detectable only when a mirror is held beneath the nares or when aerodynamic studies are done.[10]

Nasal air loss may be inconsistent across pressure consonants for a number of reasons: (1) when the velopharyngeal port is competent, but a patent oronasal fistula is present, air loss may vary across phonemes, depending upon the size and location of the fistula;[36,38] (2) velopharyngeal closure may vary according to the content of the speech sample, for example, singleton consonants versus clusters, fricatives versus plosives, particularly in speakers with borderline closure,[36] and within speaker variation in nasal emission is likely to be greater with small as opposed to large velopharyngeal openings;[39] and (3) some speakers with competent velopharyngeal systems exhibit what has come to be labelled "phoneme-specific velopharyngeal inadequacy."[35] This topic will be discussed in a later section.

Hyponasality

Hyponasality is the resonance alteration resulting from decreased coupling of the nasal and oral tracts, that is, an inability to obtain a nasopharyngeal airway of sufficient size to allow nasal respiration and normal nasal resonance. The airway may be obstructed by inflamed or hypertrophied tissue, increased secretions, or structural deviations. Ironically, the patient with a cold typically complains of sounding "nasal." Perceptual confusions between hyper- and hyponasality are common and may stem from (1) the traditional misinterpretation of the quality associated with a cold as "nasal;" (2) confusion with cul-de-sac resonance; and (3) concurrence of hypernasality and hyponasality within a single speech sample. The latter may occur when a pharyngeal flap or prosthetic device has not completely eliminated hypernasality yet obstructs the nasopharynx to the extent that an insufficient airway is available for the normal production of nasal consonants.[40]

Cul-De-Sac Resonance

Cul-de-sac resonance is literally the quality produced by air resonating in a blind-ended cavity. Boone stated that the cul-de-sac voice is produced by deep retraction of the tongue into the oral cavity and hypopharynx.[41] This explanation would fit the definition of a cavity closed at one end, although it suggests that the airstream is blocked by the retracted tongue and does not reach the anterior oral port. Bzoch stated that

> The presence or absence of hypernasal distortion of voice can best be determined by direct clinical tests in which the abnormal effects of nasal resonance on syllabic elements is exaggerated by alternately closing and opening the nares. This changes the nasal cavity alternately into a cul-de-sac resonator and back to an open resonator. . . (p 181).[14]

By this definition, cul-de-sac resonance is the result of air flowing into the nasal cavities, but being blocked from escape by obstruction of the nasal passage. However, it is interesting to note that since many cleft palate patients exhibit aberrant tongue posture,[42,43] the two definitions may not be entirely unrelated.

INDIVIDUAL STRUCTURES

Physical deviations of each of the structures listed in this section may result in speech production problems. Tonsils and adenoids, nasal deformities, and dental deviations will be presented here, together with an overview of labial, lingual, and velopharyngeal problems. Structural problems in these last three categories will be discussed in greater detail in subsequent sections dealing with specific clinical entities such as congenital craniofacial malformations (see Chapter 17).

Tonsils and Adenoids

Although both the tonsils and adenoids are lymphoid tissue and both are parts of Waldeyer's ring, they have disparate embryologic origins and cytology.[44] The size of one is not predictive of the size of the other[44,45] (Figs. 16–1 to 16–3).

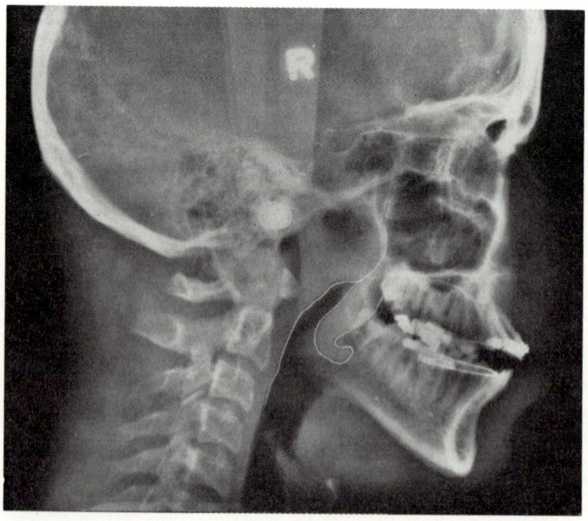

Figure 16–1 Enlarged adenoids in a male teenager. (Courtesy, Center for Craniofacial Anomalies, University of Illinois.)

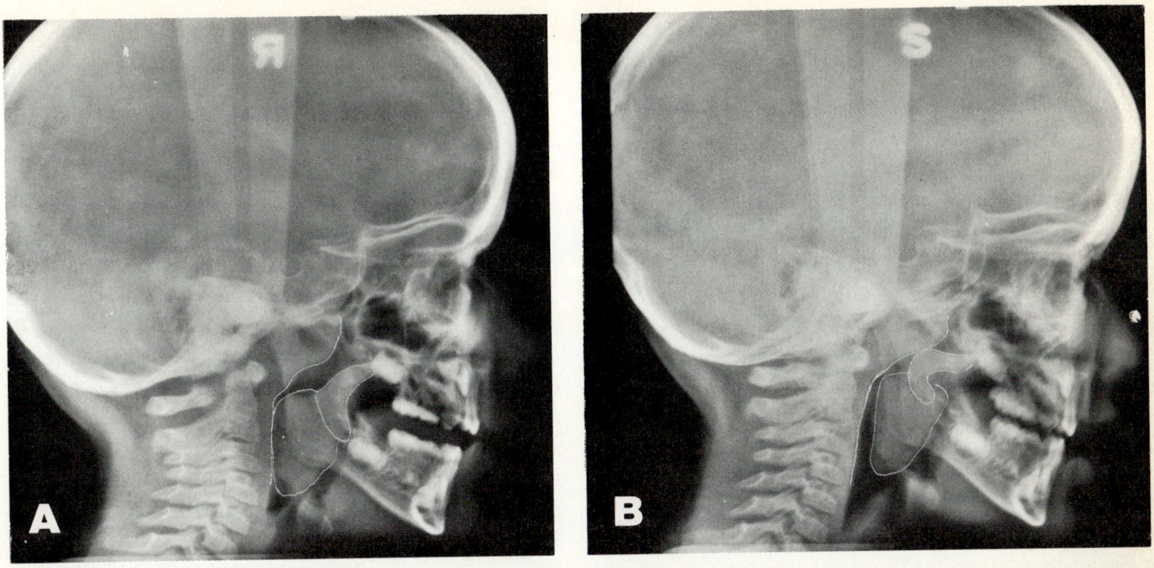

Figure 16–2 Enlarged tonsils in a 3-year old male. *A*, Note the forward positioning of the tongue. In *B* the size of the tonsil is even more clearly appreciated when the velum and tongue change position for sustained production of /s/. (Courtesy, Center for Craniofacial Anomalies, University of Illinois.)

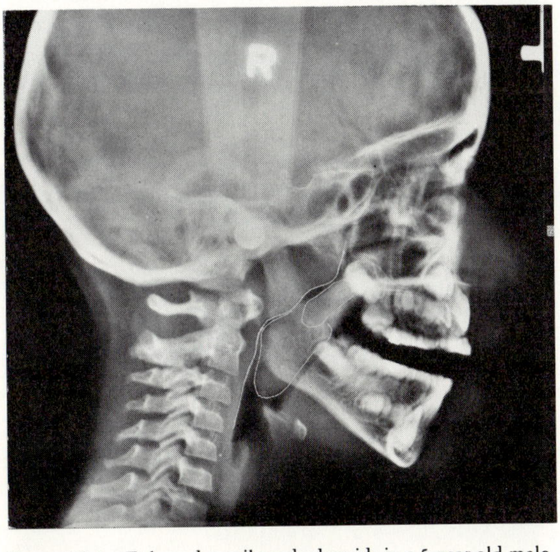

Figure 16–3 Enlarged tonsils and adenoids in a 5-year old male. Note that the length of the velum *could* be indicative of possible adenoid-dependency for "velopharyngeal" closure during speech. (Courtesy, Center for Craniofacial Anomalies, University of Illinois.)

The adenoid pad is usually visible on radiographic views of the nasopharynx by 6 weeks of age[46] and progresses in size thereafter until it reaches a "peak" size and begins to involute. Most adults do not have adenoid tissue, even if they never underwent the childhood ritual of "T and A." The literature is inconclusive about the age at which the maximum size is reached, indicating two possible peak ages. Subtelny and Koepp-Baker[46] cited ". . . as early as 9 to 10 years of age and . . . as late as 14 to 15. . . ." (p 238).[46] Linder-Aronson and Leighton[47] reported cephalometric data showing the "thickness of the soft tissue on the posterior pharyngeal wall" (p 47) in children aged 3 to 16 years to be greatest at 5 years, decreasing until age 10 with a slight increase between 10 and 11 and then decreasing again. Several authors[45,48,49] have made the mistake of citing the lymphatic growth cycle derived by Scammon, Harris, and Jackson[50] as indicative of the growth cycle of the adenoids. However, Pruzansky pointed out the error in applying this curve to tonsils and adenoids because (1) it was derived from postmortem data on a population subject to infectious diseases no longer prevalent and (2) the data did *not* include measurement of tonsils and adenoids.[44] Linder-Aronson and Leighton[47] pointed out the lack of correlation of their data to the curve of Scammon et al.[50] Pruzansky's own radiographic data on 281 normal children aged 4 to 16 years showed considerable variation in adenoid size in all age groups,[44] although Handelman and Pruzansky had earlier concluded from the same set of data that large adenoids were most frequent between the ages of 4 and 6.[51] What *is* known about the adenoid pad is that it decreases in size after the peak has been reached, undergoing natural and gradual involution until it has usually disappeared by the adult years.

In the child, adenoids play a critical role as part of both the immune system and the system for velopharyngeal closure, which is actually "velum-adenoid" closure until the tissue involutes.[44,46,52–56] In most children, the growth of the adenoids toward their peak size is offset by gradual expansion of the nasopharynx because of the natural descent of the hard palate away from the base of the skull. However, most clinicians have encountered children in whom these two factors have not remained in balance, and a hypertrophied adenoid pad has resulted in hyponasality, an habitual open-mouth posture, oronasal breathing, and so forth.

Just as the presence of too much adenoid tissue (relative to nasopharyngeal space) may be a focus of concern, absence of adenoids may lead to speech problems. Somewhat surprisingly, there have been only three reports* in the literature of cases of velopharyngeal inadequacy *apparently* consequent to natural involution of the adenoids.[57–59] By contrast, the literature is filled with (1) clinical introspection, plus a few poorly documented anecdotal reports,† on "transient hypernasality" following adenoidectomy and (2) warnings on the inadvisability of adenoidectomy in children with overt clefts, submucous clefts, or the less obvious conditions of foreshortened velum, deep pharynx, or neuromotor problems involving the velopharyngeal system.[44,46,52,56,57,60–105] The cause and duration of temporary postadenoidectomy velopharyngeal inadequacy have been poorly documented.[7,46,60,65,69,89,96,104,106] Some clinicians have attributed this phenomenon to unconscious inhibition of motion in reaction to pain or swelling,[97,107] whereas others have viewed it as a period of adjustment during which the system is adjusting to larger spatial relationships.[89] Estimates of how long this condition may last range from "days or hours"[89] to "a day or two"[108] to "within one month"[108] to "two to three weeks"[68] to "four to six weeks"[109] to "two or three months."[7]

When postadenoidectomy velopharyngeal inadequacy (VPI) does *not* resolve over time, the assumption is made that (1) the adenoid mass was masking the presence of a congenitally short palate, inadequate movement of the velopharyngeal system, disproportion of the length of the velum to the depth of the pharynx, or any combination of these‡ (see Fig. 16–3), or (2) the operative procedure resulted in inordinate scarring or other new abnormality of the structures such that velopharyngeal closure is no longer possible. Roberts[96] listed the possible causes as (1) poor development of the soft palate from disuse (owing to the hypertrophied adenoids); (2) congenitally short soft palate, congenitally deficient muscle, and nerve development; (3) (possible) creation of a larger than normal pharynx; (4) trauma to palatal and pharyngeal musculature; (5) emotional or psychological factors; and (6) neurologic disorders.§

In the past two decades, two factors have helped to reduce the risk of postadenoidectomy VPI : (1) adenoidectomy has become increasingly unpopular as a treatment for ear disease[114–117] and (2) the possible significance of the intraorally visible signs of a submucous palatal defect (discussed in Chapter 17) has been repeatedly discussed in the medical literature,[77,86,93,97,108] alerting physicians to the need for caution and for preoperative studies if an adenoidectomy is to be performed in the presence of these signs. Even when such signs are absent, other conditions predisposing towards velopharyngeal inadequacy may be present and may easily go undetected. A foreshortened velum and/or hard palate or a congenitally deep pharynx cannot be reliably diagnosed on the basis of the direct intraoral view alone, requiring at least lateral radiographic films for delineation.[60,63,70,81,84,118] Detection of muscular deficits on the nasal side of the velum, sometimes called "occult" submucous defects,[119–122] requires nasopharyngoscopy. Deficits in palatal and pharyngeal motion are best visualized on fluoroscopy[60,123–129] or nasopharyngoscopy,[77,125,130,131] but not even these studies can determine whether a lack of velar motion in the presence of a large adenoid pad is due solely to lack of room for movement or to a neuromotor deficit. As a precautionary measure, Ashley et al went so far as to recommend cinefluorography for all po-

* One probable reason for the lack of such reported cases is the extreme difficulty in accurately documenting the early status of the child, prior to the supposed adenoid involution. Even the most concerned parent is not necessarily an accurate historian or "diagnostician" in relating the condition of the child's speech.

† One reason for the poor documentation being the same as in the footnote above.

‡ Please see 1985 paper for a discussion of the multifactorial etiology of velopharyngeal inadequacy in the absence of overt cleft.[111]

§ The older literature contains frequent reference to emotional or psychological factors as causing hypernasality. Even more current articles note "psychogenic" or "psychoneurotic" disorders[112] and "emotional disturbance."[113] However, the nature of the cause-effect relationship, if any, between emotional disturbances and such speech behavior has never been delineated. In addition, the development of better diagnostic tools such as multiview videofluorography and nasopharyngoscopy has led to the discovery of previously unknown anatomic and physiologic deficits which may have been present and undetected in earlier cases presumed to have a psychogenic etiology.

tential candidates for adenoidectomy or tonsillectomy.[60] Croft et al were a little more realistic in recommending that the minimum preoperative evaluation include palpation of the hard and soft palate, observation of the uvula and palate, and at least a still radiographic study.[77]

Enlarged tonsils can obstruct the oropharynx, in extreme cases causing forward tongue carriage and an altered head-to-neck posture to protect the airway. There have been no systematic studies of the effect of tonsils on velopharyngeal activity or other aspects of speech production. The literature contains some conjecture that enlarged tonsils may aid closure in selected cases by pushing the velum upwards and backwards.[80,81,107,132] Calnan questioned whether or not tonsillectomy could ever give rise to hypernasality,[133] and Mason stated that removal of tonsils "was not linked to deterioration of velopharyngeal competency" (p 405).[54] However, others have commented on, or reported cases of, postoperative scarring of the velum and/or faucial pillars leading to restriction in velopharyngeal movement.[77,80,81,103,107,109,134–137] In fact, Beatty warned against tonsillectomy in patients with cleft palate, but not against adenoidectomy![138] Gibb and Stewart attributed their single case of post-tonsillectomy hypernasal speech to "hysterical aetiology" because of the patient's complex emotional symptomatology.[139] Richstein and Jonas drew a highly questionable conclusion of "an increase of durable open nasal speech after tonsillectomy but not after adenoidectomy" (p 29) based on a margin of one patient ($^{1}/_{7}$ after adenoidectomy, $^{2}/_{7}$ after tonsillectomy).[140]

Tonsils have been implicated as a *cause* of velopharyngeal inadequacy when their enlarged upper poles intrude between the velum and posterior pharyngeal wall.[141] Although the number of case reports is heavily outweighed by clinical introspection up to this time, such a possibility is conceivable and should not be discounted.

Guidelines for Management. Hyponasality is not amenable to speech therapy and should signal the clinician to suspect hypertrophic lymphoid tissue. The speech pathologist should record other clinical signs, such as an open-mouth posture, dark circles beneath the eyes, listlessness, and so on, and interview the family for evidence of respiratory problems at night. A careful intraoral exam should note the size of the tonsils in relationship to the apparent capacity of the oropharynx, tongue posture, integrity of the hard and soft palate (visual examination plus digital palpation), appearance of the uvula, and palatal motion on phonation. Such information should be included in the referral to an otolaryngologist. Whenever possible, it is highly recommended that the otolaryngologist and the speech pathologist examine the client together. The speech pathologist may be of assistance not only in differentiating resonance deviations,* but also in interpreting nasopharyngoscopic and radiographic data when such studies are appropriate and the tools are available.

In the case of postoperative velopharyngeal inadequacy, the speech pathologist is of course responsible for accurate delineation of the speech problem and for following the child over a period of time until it is determined that the problem has either resolved or requires further management. The topic of velopharyngeal inadequacy in the absence of overt cleft palate is discussed in Chapter 17.

Nasal Abnormalities

Nasal polyps, injected or inflamed nasal mucosa, and cartilaginous and bony deformities of the nose may result in hyponasality or cul-de-sac resonance, depending upon what conditions prevail in the remainder of the vocal tract. Nasal deformities are common in patients with cleft lip and palate, often confounding the acoustic output of speech. Ablative surgical defects of the nasomaxillary region are also encountered, the effect on resonance being dependent upon the extent and location of the defect.

Guidelines for Management. Management of such defects is, of course, not up to the speech pathologist. The clinician's responsibilities in these cases are confined to accurate delineation of the effects on speech and differentiation from the effects of whatever other physical abnormalities may be present.

Labial Abnormalities

Problems in labial articulation are most often described in reports on patients who had ablative surgery and patients who exhibit various forms of facial paresis or paralysis. A repaired cleft lip may be abnormal in length, bulk, and muscular inser-

* A review of the literature yields a disturbing number of case reports in which adenoidectomy was performed, usually not by the authors, when speech was already known to be hypernasal.[78,81,108,110,142–145] Physicians are not trained in speech disorders, but it must also be acknowledged that they are not the only professionals confused between hypernasality and hyponasality. Adenoidectomies have also been undertaken in the presence of (1) the intraorally visible stigmata associated with submucous defects[69,77,78,81,102,145] and/or (2) other "well-documented abnormalities" (the terminology of Blackfield et al).[64,81,84,110,146]

tion, yet there are few descriptions of labial articulation problems in patients with cleft lip and palate (to be discussed). Structural differences in the lips are found in several craniofacial syndromes, including orofaciodigital syndrome, type I,[1,147] Ellis-van Creveld syndrome,[1] de Lange syndrome,[1,148,149] and Van der Woude ("lip pit") syndrome,[150–153] but have not been documented to be contributory to speech production problems. Of all craniofacial syndromes, that with the most striking effect on labial articulation is Möbius syndrome[147,154–159] in which labial movement is severely reduced or totally absent due to agenesis of the nucleus of the facial nerve.

To date, no studies have documented the effects of reduced labial mobility on vowel quality or vowel intelligibility in any of these disorders.

Guidelines for Management. With few exceptions, the correction of defective production of labial consonants depends upon a change in physical structure. As we will see in the discussion of patients with cleft lip and palate, the compensatory strategies that some speakers develop in the presence of a short upper lip are often perceptually acceptable to the ear if not to the eye. The relationship of the upper lip to the lower lip must always be assessed taking into account the relationship of the maxillary to the mandibular dental arch, and the underlying maxillary and dental support for the lip. Lip incompetence may, of course, also have a neurologic origin. However, if failure to obtain appropriate placement for bilabial and labiodental consonants is indeed determined to have a structural etiology and if physical management must be postponed for some reason, the speech pathologist should assess (1) the extent to which the inappropriate productions actually interfere with intelligibility, and (2) the extent to which the patient can alter placement and maintain that alteration in contextual speech. If, for example, the distance over which the lower lip must travel to meet a short upper lip is so great that the gesture slows articulation to an artificial rate, the "correction" may be inappropriate.

Dental and Occlusal Anomalies

In reviewing the following material, the reader should bear in mind that combinations of (1) missing teeth and anomalous tooth position; (2) anterior overjet, open bite, and crossbite; and (3) molar malocclusions are common.

Missing Teeth

In general, research indicates that adjustment to edentulous spaces is highly variable. Bloomer stated that loss of teeth in childhood and excessive spacing of the central incisors (diastema) may affect sibilant production.[160] He pointed out that premature dental loss may contribute to eventual malocclusion of a serious nature or to development of habits of lingual movement which are retained after permanent teeth have erupted. Fymbo reported that edentulous spaces in the region of the upper eight anterior teeth were more prevalent in "defective" speakers than in average or superior speakers.[161] However, a high percentage of his subjects with speech defects also had either open or collapsed bite. Snow[162] and Bankson and Byrne[163] studied sibilant production in children with missing or malpositioned teeth; Bankson and Byrne reported unaffected /s/ production in some cases. Weinberg found that children who showed good articulation despite missing maxillary incisors tended to retrude the mandible and place the tongue tip below the edge of the lower incisors during /s/, whereas those with defective /s/ tended to protrude the tongue beyond the incisors and to hold the upper lip in a lower than normal position.[164]

Starr commented that the aforementioned studies pointed up the importance of the relationship between the tongue tip and the lower incisors in /s/, but that the coexistence of these phenomena does not imply a cause and effect, a point underscored by the presence of nondefective /s/ in children with missing incisors.[165]

Bloomer observed that dentures should facilitate normal articulation in the completely edentulous patient if the patient's own occlusion and articulatory habits are considered in the fabrication of the dentures.[160] Ylippo and Sovijarji found maxillary dentures in edentulous patients to be more important than mandibular dentures for /s/ and /r/, but mandibular dentures to be more critical for /t/.[166] Chierici, Parker, and Hemphill reported that the loss of natural teeth and the wearing of immediate full dentures did not alter the sensorimotor pathways that are significant to the precision of oral motor skills.[167]

The effects of edentulousness on speech and the success of denture facilitation of articulation are undoubtedly dependent in part upon such associated factors as age, hearing acuity, oral health, and adjustment to the dentures.

Verted and Malpositioned Teeth

Bloomer observed that anomalies of individual tooth position may prevent normal valving contacts of the tongue and lips, commenting that articulatory distortions caused by interference with tongue or lip activity are more frequent in open bite or severe crossbite.[160] Severe labial inclination of the maxillary incisors interferes with bilabials and may cause sibilant distortion. Anterior teeth in linguoversion may also imperil sibilants.

Ectopic eruption of teeth occurs in conditions of extreme crowding or hypoplasia of the dental arches, such as that seen in congenital hypoglossia (mandible) and Apert syndrome (maxilla). Ectopic eruption of the lateral incisor or canine is also fairly common in cleft palate. The effect on articulation has not been differentiated, to date, from the effects of other structural hazards to articulation in these conditions.

Open Bite

"Open bite" usually implies spacing between the anterior maxillary and mandibular teeth (Fig. 16–4A and B), although lateral open bite may also affect articulation. The most common associated speech problem is interdentalization of the tip-alveolar or tip-dental consonants.

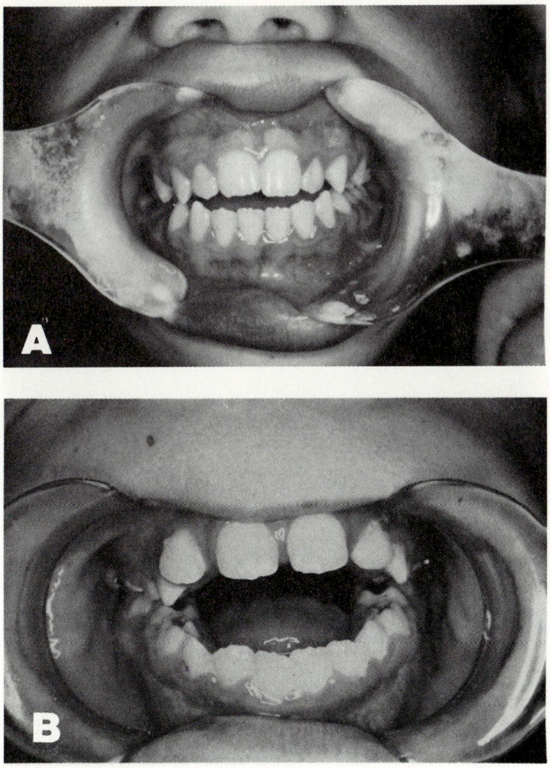

Figure 16–4 *A* and *B*, Variation in severity of anterior open bite. (Courtesy, Center for Craniofacial Anomalies, University of California—San Francisco.)

A high percentage of Fymbo's subjects[161] with speech defects had either open or collapsed bite.* Bernstein concluded from his survey of 437 children with defective speech that the only malocclusion related to the speech defects was open bite, but that the severity of the lisp was not related to the degree of the open bite.[168] However, in a study of open bite induced in normal speakers by introduction of a bite block, Warren, Allen, and King did find that the error rate increased with increased anterior incisal opening.[169]

Crossbite

"Anterior" crossbite implies that the molar relationship is normal, but that the maxillary incisors are distal to the mandibular incisors. This condition may be combined with either an open or collapsed bite. "Buccal" crossbite implies a lateral shift in the relationship of the maxilla to the mandible, with the maxillary first molar displaced medially relative to the mandibular first molar. The condition may be unilateral or bilateral.

Extreme crossbite of the buccal segments may appear in conjunction with a lateral lisp.[160] In severe cases, such as in hemifacial microsomia, the mandible may be shifted to such an extent that the tongue is placed in an unfavorable position for the production of sibilants and affricates. Anterior crossbite can also affect the production of any of the tip-alveolar consonants, since the alveolus is displaced posterior to its normal position with respect to the tongue.

Neutroclusion (Angle Class I)

Neutroclusion implies normal molar relationships, but the presence of anomalies of individual tooth position. Verted, malpositioned, or abnormally spaced teeth may affect articulation.

Distoclusion (Angle Class II, Maxillary Protrusion, Mandibular Retrusion)

In distoclusion, the mandible is in a posterior relationship to the maxilla, with the mesial groove

---

* "Collapsed" or "closed" bite means that the maxillary teeth "overclose" on the lower teeth (vertical overlap). "Overjet" refers to a horizontal overlap.

of the mandibular first permanent molar articulating posteriorly to the mesiobuccal cusp of the maxillary first permanent molar (Fig. 16–5). In Class II, Division 1 distoclusion, the maxillary incisors are in extreme labioversion (protruded). In Class II, Division 2, the maxillary central incisors are in linguoversion while the lateral incisors are tipped labially and mesially. Subdivisions designate distoclusion on only one side.

Subtelny, Mestre, and Subtelny reported that adolescents with Class II, Division 1 malocclusion showed greater mandibular retrusion and incisal opening during /s/ production than did a group with normal occlusion.[170] Defective speakers in the malocclusion group protruded the tongue tip, whereas normal speakers with malocclusion retruded the tongue tip relative to the lower incisors, thus maintaining a fairly normal position relative to the retruded mandible.

Blythe reported a correlation between Class II, Division 1 malocclusions and interdental lisp, observing that the tongue was incorrectly positioned vertically, anteroposteriorly, or both.[171] He also found a relationship between Class II, Division 2 and lateral lisp. Bloomer observed that excessive maxillary protraction may interfere with bilabials.[160] Witzel, Ross, and Munro observed errors on bilabial consonants because of an inability to close the lips in some of their patients with retrognathia.[172]

Technically, micrognathia is a form of distoclusion. However, this condition is usually associated with anomalous size or position of the tongue and will be discussed in the context of craniofacial anomalies.

Mesioclusion (Angle Class III, Maxillary Retrusion, Mandibular Protrusion)

Mesioclusion designates those conditions in which the mandibular teeth are anterior (mesial) to their normal position in relation to the maxillary teeth (Fig. 16–6). According to Bloomer, Class III malocclusions include (1) macromandibular development (prognathic or hypertrophic mandible), (2) micromaxillary development (maxillary retraction or hypoplasia), (3) marked linguoversion of the maxillary teeth so that they are distal to the mandibular anterior teeth, (4) a pseudoprognathism caused by adaptation to insufficient vertical dimension of the maxilla, with forward thrust of the mandible as it is raised to meet the occlusal plane of the maxillary teeth, and (5) mandibular abstraction created by endogenous factors or by muscular paralysis.[160] Rela-

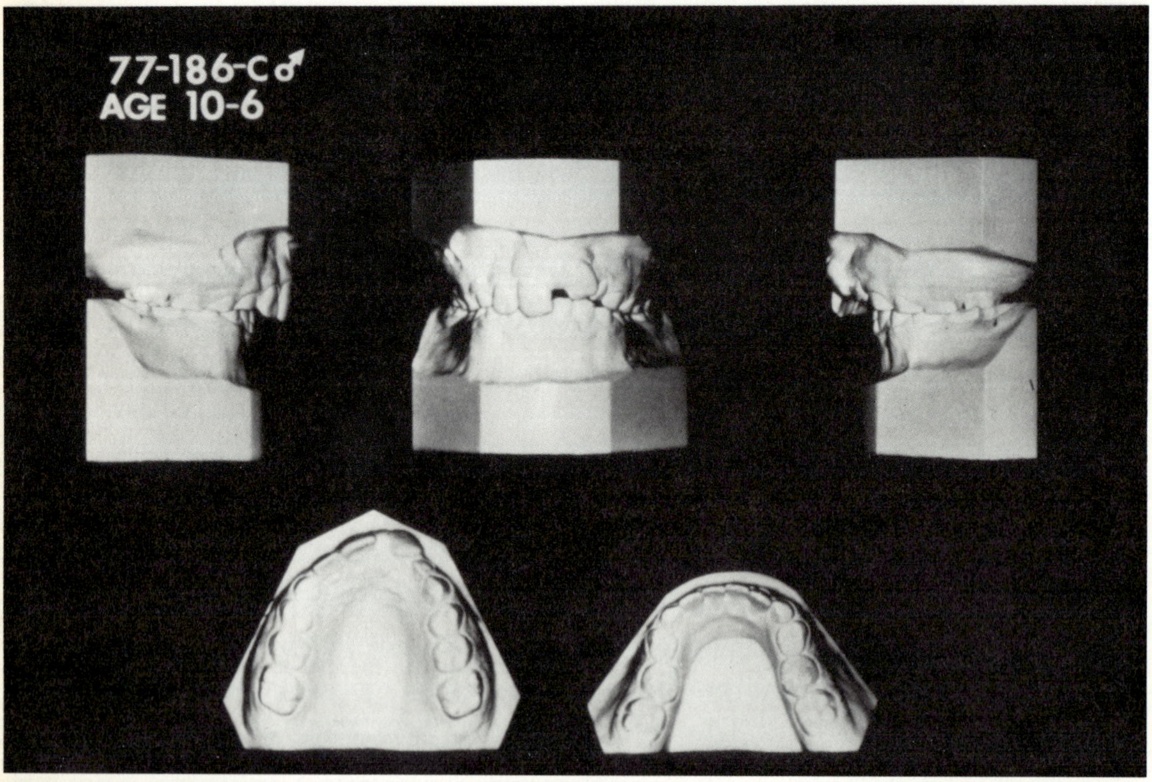

Figure 16–5 Dental models illustrating a Class II malocclusion. (Courtesy, Center for Craniofacial Anomalies, University of Illinois.)

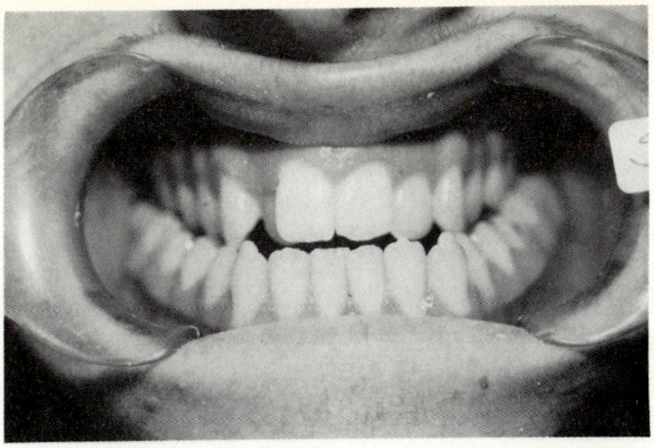

Figure 16–6 Class III malocclusion. (Courtesy, Center for Craniofacial Anomalies, University of California–San Francisco.)

tive expansion of the mandibular arch with respect to the maxillary arch brings the tongue into habitual contact with the occlusal edges of the maxillary teeth instead of the alveolar arch and the linguodental surfaces, often causing a "scalloped" appearance of the edges of the tongue. Labiodental consonants may be altered because of an inability of the lower lip to come into contact with the maxillary incisors,[172] forcing "inverted" production with contact between the lower incisors and upper lip. Tip-alveolar consonants may be produced by contact between the tongue tip and upper lip. Open bite is a frequent complication of Class III occlusions, offering yet another hazard to articulation.

Guay, Maxwell, and Beecher found a lowered and retruded tongue posture at rest in adolescents with Class III malocclusions.[173] In /s/ production, these subjects also demonstrated lingual retrusion in an apparent attempt to achieve a normal relationship of the tongue tip to the maxillary teeth, an increase in mandibular depression, and a greater than normal distance between the tongue tip and the mandibular anterior teeth. Despite these compensations, normal /s/ was found in only one of the 12 subjects. Contrasting these findings with those of Subtelny et al[170] the authors observed that Class II, Division 1 malocclusion does not restrict the operating space of the tongue. In Class III, the forward position of the anterior attachment of the tongue, with respect to the maxilla, may sabotage attempts at compensation.

A restriction in the size of the maxillary arch has been noted by several investigators to be associated with speech problems. Bruggeman concluded that there was a positive relationship between the defects of speech in children and a high palate, narrow arch width in the cuspid region, spacings in anterior dentition, and anterior open bite.[174] Fymbo also found palatal width in the cuspid region to be significant.[161] Lubit studied palatal width in both the molar and canine regions, as well as palatal height, overjet, overbite, spacing in maxillary anterior dentition, and "an occlusal feature index score."[86] He found no overall relationship to speech, but diminished palatal width and height appeared to be related to a defective /s/ production.

Guidelines for Management. The information reviewed indicates that (1) the relationship between the tongue tip and lower incisors is a critical factor in articulation; (2) individual adjustments to verted, missing or malpositioned teeth, and open bite or crossbite vary; (3) Class II malocclusions are not necessarily associated with defective articulation except perhaps in extreme cases; and (4) even Class III malocclusions may coexist with acceptable articulation, although a speech problem is more likely in these cases than in Class II. Both Bloomer[160] and Guay et al[173] observed that the correction of speech in Class III malocclusions usually requires correction or improvement of the occlusion.

Orthognathic surgery for the correction of occlusal problems generally involves one or more of the following: (1) superior repositioning of the maxilla, (2) maxillary advancement, (3) maxillary setback, (4) mandibular advancement, (5) mandibular setback, and (6) subapical osteotomies, in which the position of the teeth and alveolar bone is altered without altering the position of the maxilla or mandible itself. In cases of extreme maxillary-mandibular discrepancy, the advancement of one is often combined with the setback of the other.

There is a growing body of literature on the topic of the effect of orthognathic surgery on speech. The attempt to establish cause-effect relationships in these maneuvers has been frustrated by a number of factors, including the lack of a clear relationship between malocclusions and speech problems in the first place. For example, Witzel et al observed that almost half of their 41 patients had normal speech preoperatively despite their occlusal defects.[172] In addition, most studies have combined both types of patients (types of malocclusions) and types of operative maneuvers. Finally, studies have varied markedly in the quality and quantity of pre- and postoperative data gathered and in the amount of time between the surgery and the postoperative evaluations.

Turvey, Journot, and Epker noted a marked tendency for the preoperative speech problems associated with an open bite to self-correct following surgical correction of the malocclusion.[175] By contrast, Snidecore and Kaires found that maxillary prostheses designed to close open bites in young adults who showed sibilant distortion did not produce a significant improvement in speech.[176]

Goodstein, Cooper, and Wallace reported no significant changes in speech in five patients undergoing surgical correction of mandibular prognathism, but gave no details on the type or amount of surgical correction, and only cursory information on speech.[177] Glass, Knapp, and Bloomer reported improved /s/ production in similar patients.[178] The 41 patients of Witzel et al represented a mix of problems: one with open bite only, 12 with retrognathia only, 17 with retrognathia combined with open bite, four with prognathia only, and seven with prognathia combined with open bite.[172] These authors reported that sibilant distortions were present in all subgroups preoperatively except for the one patient with only an open bite. Postoperative improvement in articulation was not directly related to the amount of change in occlusion except in patients with retrognathia.

Garber, Speidel, and Marse reported an immediate decrease in the accuracy of articulation in patients undergoing surgical correction of maxillary protrusion, but a gradual return to preoperative levels, underscoring the importance of the time lapse between surgery and the postoperative evaluation.[179] Ruscello, Tekieli, and Van Sickels later reported similar findings in patients operated for both Class II and Class III malocclusions.[180]

Bowers, Tobey, and Shaye reported normal speech both pre- and postoperatively in five patients undergoing combinations of mandibular advancement, maxillary impaction, or mandibular setback.[181] However, they did note formant changes in vowels, which suggested to them that the speakers adjusted their articulation to accommodate to the orthognathic surgery. In an earlier review, Ewan also discussed changes in acoustic output following orthognathic surgery,[182] primarily changes in fundamental frequency and the theoretical relationship to changes in position of the hyoid bone, such as described by Wickwire, White, and Proffit.[183]

Dalston and Vig gathered both objective and subjective data on 40 patients with a variety of malocclusions prior to and following orthognathic surgery.[184] Articulation improved in one patient; two had problems with sibilants following superior repositioning of the maxilla. Although measurement by Tonar® showed improvement in denasal resonance in some patients, there was no perceptual evidence of decreased denasality. There was no change in velopharyngeal area as measured by aerodynamic studies. Dalston and Vig concluded that structural changes to the oral cavity resulting from orthognathic surgery do not typically cause perceptually significant, long-term alterations in speech. However, they noted that this conclusion does not mean that no acoustic differences occur, especially in the early preoperative period. They also noted that the lack of perceptible changes in speech does not mean that such surgery has no impact upon the motor control processes underlying speech.

Advancement of the maxilla can imperil velopharyngeal closure, since the distance between the palate and the posterior pharyngeal wall is increased. In a study of 31 patients with cleft palate and nine patients without cleft palate underoing from 3 to 20 mm of advancement, Schwarz and Gruner reported that articulation skills improved, but also that velopharyngeal closure was affected adversely in many of both groups of patients.[185] Witzel and Munro reported similar postadvancement velopharyngeal inadequacy in one youngster with a repaired cleft.[186] Mason, Turvey, and Warren described one patient with cleft palate who adapted well to a 7-mm advancement and one who showed deterioration in what was already borderline closure preoperatively.[187] One study, which included patients with Apert syndrome, Crouzon disease, cleft palate, or maxillary hypoplasia alone, reported no deterioration velopharyngeal function despite maxillary advancements averaging from 8 to 14 mm.[188,189] Similar results were reported by Dalston and Vig.[184] It must be emphasized that the likelihood of postoperative velopharyngeal inadequacy depends upon the amount of advancement and upon the status of the velopharyngeal system preoperatively.

From their review of the published studies to date on the effects of orthognathic surgery on speech, Ruscello et al concluded that 88 percent of the subjects showing preoperative errors showed a positive change in articulation, whereas 12 percent either were unchanged or showed some adverse effect.[180]

With respect to speech problems suspected in the presence of dental or occlusal problems, the speech pathologist must attempt to determine which errors are developmental or otherwise unrelated to the dentition and/or occlusion, which may be associated with the structural problem, and what changes may be made in the latter without a change in the oral environment. Planning of surgical or orthodontic intervention may have to await further tooth eruption or facial growth. Particularly in the growing child, the nearly constantly changing oral environment necessitates periodic reassessment of the structures and of the ability to make desired changes.

Lingual Abnormalities

Although lingual articulation problems have been described at some length in ablative surgery defects, cleft palate, and, to a lesser extent, craniofacial malformation syndromes, in the latter two cases actual problems of lingual structure have not always been carefully differentiated from problems of tongue carriage or posture secondary to other orofacial structural defects. For example, the literature on cleft palate in the 1940s and 1950s often implied or overtly stated that defects of lingual structure were common in this population. Discussions of this problem were generally undertaken without benefit of supportive data, and abnormalities of tongue posture and function in patients with cleft palate are now more often viewed as secondary to other factors. Abnormalities of tongue position at rest and in function have also been described in mandibulofacial dysostosis, Pierre Robin malformation sequence, Apert syndrome, Crouzon disease, and hemifacial microsomia, all of which are discussed in Chapter 17.

Abnormalities of tongue size tend to be overreported, particularly with regard to "macroglossia." Mason stated that "The size of the tongue is impossible to determine accurately in living specimens due to its adaptive nature" (p 14).[190] Although Mason suggested that macroglossia is present only if the patient cannot occlude his or her teeth without biting his or her tongue, this test may be misleading if the patient has maxillary-mandibular disproportion in the form of either a small maxilla in the presence of a normal-sized mandible or a normal maxilla in the presence of a prognathic mandible. In either case, a portion of the maxillary dentition may strike the tongue rather than occluding with the lower teeth. Similarly, suspected macroglossia must always be assessed taking into account neuromotor control of the tongue. Reports of macroglossia in Down syndrome and cretinism[1,147,160] have almost undoubtedly been influenced by this factor. True macroglossia is pathognomonic in Beckwith-Wiedemann syndrome[1] (Fig. 16–7).

Clinical reports of severe deficiency of lingual tissue in congenital "aglossia,"[191–193] more appropriately termed "hypoglossia,"[194–196] are generally replete with descriptions of the development of intelligible speech despite the marked structural defect. Hypoglossia is typically seen with concomitant reduction in the size of the mandible ("micrognathia") (Fig. 16–8). Most case descriptions of the "aglossia-adactylia" or "hypoglossia-hypodactylia" syndrome,[191,193,194,197–203] in which oral defects are accompanied by limb defects, refer to a "small mouth." If the overall size of the oral cavity is indeed reduced, an extremely small tongue may be able to manage articulatory contacts and vowel configurations sufficiently well to account for the maintenance of intelligibility.

The terms "tongue-tie" and "ankyloglossia" have been used concurrently and often indiscriminately to refer to various degrees of abnormal attachment of the tongue to the floor of the mouth.[160,204–222] The focus of concern is the lingual frenulum, which may be abnormally short and/or displaced anteriorly towards the tongue tip. However, as stated by Horton et al, "Degrees of tongue-tie vary from the very mild . . . to those in which both the frenulum and the underlying fibers of the genioglossus muscle are markedly fibrosed . . . to the rare, complete an-

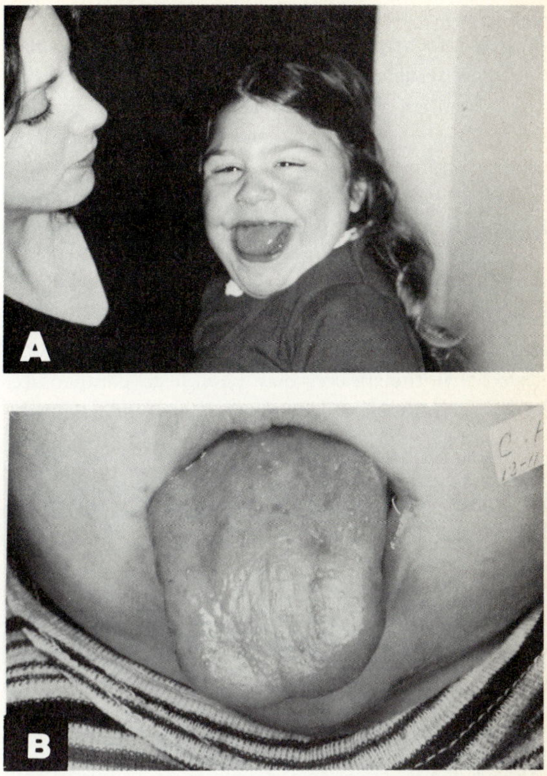

Figure 16–7 *A* and *B*, Macroglossia in a child with Beck-with-Wiedemann syndrome. (Courtesy, Center for Craniofacial Anomalies, University of California—San Francisco.)

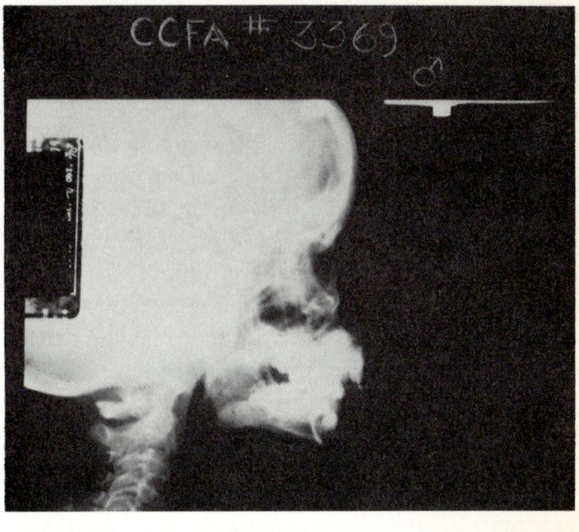

Figure 16–8 Lateral cephalometric film of a child with hypoglossia. Note that no lingual tissue can be delineated. (Courtesy, Center for Craniofacial Anomalies, University of Illinois.)

kyloglossia where the tongue is actually fused to the floor of the mouth'' (p 8).[211] Eliminating the cases of complete ankyloglossia, the clinical literature is inconsistent in the guidelines offered for deciding if the frenulum is truly abnormal and if its attachment to the tongue may be a cause of speech problems. Mason suggested evaluating the lingual frenulum by having the speaker lift the tongue tip to the maxillary alveolar ridge while biting on a tongue blade between the molars (thus creating an anterior open bite), but observed that the speaker who cannot do this may still have normal speech.[190] Mason suggested that the speaker may be able to compensate by using linguodental contacts instead of linguoalveolar contacts. Fletcher and Daly suggested that the speaker be examined for the ability to move the tongue tip to the corners of the mouth and to protrude it beyond the lower gum.[208] They noted that "notching" of the tongue tip may be seen on protrusion (due to the anchoring of the frenulum). Fletcher and Meldrum[209] and later Williams and Waldron[221] proposed a series of sublingual measurements to be made with calibrated tools. Williams and Waldron also suggested that the speaker is not a candidate for frenulectomy if the consonants /t/, /d/, /s/ and "th" are made satisfactorily. Horton et al offered the opinion of Shanks (cited as a personal communication) that "tongue-tie" probably does not *cause* articulation problems, but may *contribute* to difficulty in rate and range of articulation, particularly in the presence of other factors, for example, missing teeth.[211]

The popularity of frenulectomy or "tongue clipping" has dropped dramatically in recent decades. Clinicians have offered guidelines for deciding whether "tongue-tie" is truly present and have generally been skeptical about its role as an etiologic factor in articulation problems.

Speech pathologists are still often asked to evaluate "tongue-thrust,"[223] also called "tongue thrust swallow,"[224] "visceral swallow,"[225] "infantile swallow,"[226] "reverse swallow,"[227] "deviant swallow,"[228] "tongue thrust syndrome,"[229,230] and "orofacial muscle imbalance."[231] This concept is most popular among "myofunctional therapists" of varying credentials who propose that the pressure of the tongue against or between the teeth, primarily during swallow, contributes to malocclusion, relapse following orthodontic therapy, and articulatory disorders. Shelton pointed out that tongue-thrust is indeed observed in persons with articulatory problems, malocclusion, or both, but it is also observed in individuals with normal speech and dentition.[232]

Bloomer discussed the difficulty in defining and differentiating between normal and abnormal swallow.[233,234] Subtelny et al found malocclusion and protrusive lingual function during swallow to coexist with both normal and defective speech.[170] Fletcher et al pointed out that many children showing concurrent abnormal swallow, speech defects, and malocclusion are in a developmental stage between 6 and 9 years of age in which the structural relationships and functional patterns will later adapt maturationally without therapeutic intervention.[224] Mason later pointed out that tongue-thrust, when present, typically self-corrects at puberty, and in a still later presentation Mason pointed out that a habitual resting posture with the tongue protruding between the anterior teeth is much more likely to exacerbate or maintain an open bite than is a "tongue-thrust" swallow.[235,236] Mason and Proffit cautioned about hypertrophied tonsils and adenoids and other forms of airway obstruction *necessitating* forward carriage of the tongue.[237] In an extensive review of the literature and in their own research, they found little support for myofunctional therapy and offered guidelines for speech pathologists asked by dental specialists to provide such therapy. Mason later expanded upon these guidelines.[235] In 1975, the Joint Committee on Dentistry and Speech Pathology and Audiology reviewed over 275 papers on tongue-thrust and concluded, ". . . neither the validity of the diagnostic label tongue thrust nor the contention that myofunctional therapy produces significant consistent changes in oral form or function has been documented adequately'' (p 331).[238] The Joint Committee stressed the need for further research, as did Mason.[235] Unfortunately, scientifically rigorous studies on this topic have not emerged, in all likelihood because the variables involved are, as Bloomer pointed out,[233,234] so difficult to define and quantify.

Even if it is a valid concept, "tongue-thrust" is not a structural defect and will not be covered here in detail. Readers are referred to the excellent review by Mason.[235]

Guidelines for Management. It should be clear from the foregoing that (1) assessment of tongue size can be very difficult and must be done taking into account neuromotor control, airway adequacy, and the size of the maxilla and mandible, and (2) children born with deficient lingual tissue typically make their own articulatory adjustments. When true ankyloglossia exists, correction is the responsibility of the surgeon although a speech pathologist should assist in the assessment. Lingual abnormalities in other clinical entities are discussed in later sections.

Velopharyngeal Inadequacy

The velopharyngeal system becomes the focus of concern (1) when evidence of inadequacy persists after adenoidectomy (please see Tonsils and Adenoids), (2) when ablative surgery involves the removal of part of these structures, (3) when the initial surgical or prosthetic closure of a cleft palate does not result in adequate velopharyngeal function, and (4) when other structural or neurologic factors produce velopharyngeal inadequacy in the absence of an overt cleft.[111]

Although the velopharyngeal mechanism is appropriately viewed as an articulator responsible for the nasal and nonnasal contrast, and although the traditional focus on this mechanism is concerned with the control of resonance balance and the maintenance of appropriate air pressure and airflow relationships, it is but one in a series of valves that, together with the resonating cavities, modifies the vocal airstream. Because the velopharyngeal mechanism is an integral part of the vocal tract, its malfunction can affect more than one aspect of speech production. In other words, the consequences of an inadequately functioning velopharyngeal mechanism are not necessarily limited to hypernasality and nasal air loss.

The effects of VPI would logically be expected to be dependent in part upon the age at which the inadequacy becomes manifest and upon what other factors may be affecting speech production capabilities in the individual speaker. For example, no study or case report published to date has documented the development of the classic "compensatory articulations"[35] in speakers with noncleft VPI. Philips and Kent stated that these articulations do not develop in children who develop velopharyngeal inadequacy following adenoidectomy.[239] Since they cited no data or study addressing this point, the statement appears to reflect clinical experience.* By contrast, the child born with a cleft palate or other congenital form of velopharyngeal inadequacy may exhibit not only hypernasality and nasal air loss in speech, but also a wide variety of articulatory problems, laryngeal voice problems, and language problems that may be directly related to the inability to make certain articulatory contrasts.[36] In addition, recent studies have yielded data pointing to abnormalities in the timing and coordination of the action of laryngeal and articulatory mechanisms, including the velopharyngeal mechanism, in speakers with clefts.[239–244] The possible interrelationships of these differences to compensatory articulations and other deviant speech characteristics in such speakers will be discussed in Chapter 17.

Studies attempting to establish a quantifiable, predictable relationship between velopharyngeal function and various aspects of speech have been carried out primarily on speakers with structural defects of the mechanism (typically repaired cleft palates) and secondarily on normal speakers in whom inadequate closure was mechanically induced. In reviewing this large body of studies, it is critical that the reader keep in mind the diverse means that have been used to quantify both the independent variable (velopharyngeal closure, gap, inadequacy) and the dependent variable (speech). Investigators have typically attempted correlations between or among measures derived from the categories in Table 16–1.

Given the heterogeneity of approaches to measurement, the individual capabilities of speakers to compensate for abnormal mechanisms, and the fact that most of these studies were carried out on speakers with clefts in whom factors other than the size of the velopharyngeal port may have affected speech production, it is little wonder that Morris concluded in 1968 that the correlations between speech and velopharyngeal function in studies that had been reported up to that time averaged 0.50.[245]

A primary reason for such low correlations is the difficulty in obtaining reliable perceptual judgments of speech performance. As noted previously, listeners typically do not rate nasality with a high degree of reliability, and such ratings are influenced by a number of factors. McWilliams noted that listeners tend to perceive increased hypernasality (in speakers with clefts) when they hear seriously disordered articulation.[246] This contamination effect was illustrated by the disparate findings of two studies correlating measures of oral and nasal sound pressure levels with ratings of nasality: Weiss reported a correlation of 0.948 for speakers free of all speech problems other than hypernasality,[247] whereas a later study, in which a number of speakers exhibited articulation problems and nasal emission, reported a correlation of 0.52.[248] Note that these two studies were com-

TABLE 16–1 Approaches to Assessing Velopharyngeal Closure

Measurement of the consequences of closure or inadequacy
Perceptual studies of speech
Speech ratings (intelligibility, acceptability, nasality, etc.)
Articulation tests
Accelerometric studies
Acoustical studies
Aerodynamic studies
Photodetector studies
Visualization/measurement of the velopharyngeal port
Lateral still cephalometric radiographs
Lateral cine- or videofluorography
Multiview fluorography
Computed tomography
Ultrasound
Endoscopy (nasal and oral)

* My own clinical experience is similar.

paring one type of measurement of the consequences of velopharyngeal inadequacy (nasality ratings) with another type (oral and nasal sound pressure levels), with no direct measurement of the velopharyngeal port itself. The same is true of investigations using nasal accelerometers, which have generally reported correlations with listener ratings of nasality ranging between 0.70 and 0.90.[18–20,22,23,25–28,249,250] The fact that all of the foregoing investigators chose to validate their instrumentation against listener judgments would seem to corroborate the position of Moll noted earlier.[29,30]

Many early studies used rather simplistic methods of measuring velopharyngeal closure. Respirometers, U-tube manometers, and oral manometers provided only gross indices of the aerodynamic function of the system during blowing and sucking.[250–261] These devices have been replaced by more sophisticated aerodynamic instrumentation,[6,8–11,262–267] which not only allows estimates of velopharyngeal orifice size during speech, but also measures nasal resistance, one of the physiologic factors affecting what the listener hears. The failure to take into account nasal versus oral impedance (or resistance to airflow) may well explain in part the relatively low correlations reported between speech performance and measurements derived with the more primitive aerodynamic instrumentation. A recent study compared assessments of velopharyngeal function as yielded by listener judgments, the pressure-flow instrumentation of Warren, and Tonar II®. The authors reported a correlation of 0.80 between pressure-flow results and listener judgments, 0.76 between Tonar II® results and listener judgments, and 0.74 between the two types of instrumental assessment.

Radiologic studies of the velopharyngeal port have undergone a similar metamorphosis. Over a period of several decades, the use of lateral still cephalometric films to visualize the port, giving only a still two-dimensional view of a dynamic multidimensional system, was gradually supplanted first by lateral cinefluorography[42,43,142,254,268–285] and then by cine- and videofluorography taken in a variety of views.[123–126,128–130,286–297] The use of radiographic studies in the frontal and basal views provided a clearer indication of the participation of the lateral and posterior pharyngeal walls in velopharyngeal closure, causing Skolnick[128] to urge us to think sphincter.*

Almost simultaneously, the development of the first oral[296,297,299,300] and then nasal endoscopy[123–125,127,130,288,301–327] vastly improved the ability to visualize the velopharyngeal system during speech production, further altering the conceptions of how the system works in both normal and abnormal speakers.

Several early studies, of necessity using instrumentation less sophisticated than what is now available, attempted to establish a "cut-off" value or critical size of the velopharyngeal port that appeared to differentiate between acceptable and unacceptable speech. Subtelny and Subtelny reported that the number of plosive errors increased appreciably when the velopharyngeal opening at the midsagittal plane exceeded 5 mm as measured on lateral cephalometric laminagraphs.[328] Errors on fricatives occurred almost twice as often as errors on plosives, with subjects showing openings of 2 mm or less. In a later study, subjects with cleft palate and with velopharyngeal gaps of 0.5 to 3.0 mm on midsagittal radiographs showed a 14.3 percent loss of intelligibility as compared to subjects with complete closure, but subjects with gaps of 3.5 to 7.0 mm showed a 27.3 percent loss.[329] The authors made the point that the relationship between degree of nasality and velopharyngeal gap was not linear throughout the full range of opening. Carney and Morris, using lateral cinefluorography, found no systematic relationship between severity of nasality and measurements of velar constriction, pharyngeal constriction, oral constriction, and incisor opening.[270] Clearly, measurements of velopharyngeal opening taken from midsagittal radiographic studies (still films or cinefluorography) are only an index of that opening. Such views provide no information about what is happening on either side of the midsagittal plane or about the true area or configuration of the opening. Two studies using multiview videofluorography yielded better correlations between measurements of closure and speech ratings.[330,331]

Utilizing aerodynamic instrumentation, a number of studies have addressed this same question. Over a series of investigations, Warren and associates produced data indicating a critical port size of 0.20 cm^2.[8–11,265] Speakers with estimated orifice sizes greater than this value showed no relationship between port size and nasal emission. In 1979, Warren reported that speakers with adequate closure showed estimated orifice sizes of 0.00 to 0.09 cm^2, whereas those with borderline closure were in the range of 0.10 to 0.19 cm^2. He concluded that a speaker with a port of 0.05 cm^2 or less would rarely exhibit hypernasality or nasal emission. Data in agreement with these values had been derived in earlier studies that introduced an artificial velopharyngeal orifice of known size in normal speakers,[332,333] which indicated a critical port size of 5 mm

* Although the term "sphincter" is more descriptive than "valve" or "port," it should not be simplistically interpreted to imply a purse-string type of action taking place in a single plane of space. Frontal view fluoroscopy, in particular, reveals the tube-like nature of the velopharyngeal system, with variable muscular activity throughout the length of the tube, depending upon the task.[36,126,290,298]

in diameter or an airflow of 50 dynes per cm^2. However, data reported by McWilliams et al suggested a critical port size much smaller than 0.20 cm^2 when aerodynamic measurements were compared with listener judgments.[331] Subsequently, Warren broke his categorizations down further into 0.0–0.49 cm^2 for "adequate," 0.05–0.09 cm^2 for "adequate/borderline," 0.10–0.19 cm^2 for "borderline/inadequate," and greater than 0.20 cm^2 for "inadequate."[334] As in the 1979 study, these values for port size were derived using the PERCI®, which measures only differential pressure across the port and ignores airflow.

To date, no studies correlating speech ratings to *measured* velopharyngeal area as viewed via endoscopy ratings have appeared, probably because of the difficulties in obtaining reliable measurements using this technique.

Aerodynamic instrumentation, multiview videofluorography, and endoscopy have all provided some explanations as to why earlier correlational studies were so unsatisfactory. The instrumentation of Warren and his colleagues has allowed the study of nasal resistance, respiratory volumes, and oral port constriction, all of which may influence the perceptual judgment of speech. Endoscopy and multiview videofluoroscopy provide information on lateral defects or small central defects in velopharyngeal closure not visible on lateral radiographs, variations in amount of pharyngeal movement at different levels of the naso- and oropharynx, and differential behaviors of the port dependent upon the speech task.

With the difficulties that have been encountered in attempting to establish what constitutes "adequate" velopharyngeal closure for normal speech production, the concept of "borderline" closure warrants cautious consideration.[36] As has already been discussed, some speakers exhibit nasal air loss that is so minimal that it is inaudible or at least only inconsistently audible. Morris labelled speakers with consistent but very small gaps as the "almost-but-not-quite" group.[335] Those demonstrating inconsistency in closure, he labelled the "sometimes-but-not-always" group. The latter group reflects, at least in part, observations that have been made in the literature over several decades about the differential behaviors of the velopharyngeal mechanism dependent upon the specific content of the speech sample (fricatives versus other consonants, consonant clusters versus singletons), and the group may also include those speakers exhibiting what is now called "phoneme-specific velopharyngeal inadequacy."

In summary, the relationship between velopharyngeal port size and various measures of speech is affected by numerous variables, including but not limited to the means by which the size of the port is visualized or estimated, respiratory effort, nasal resistance, oral resistance (degree and duration of oral port constriction), speech sample, variability versus consistency of closure, and the means by which the measures of speech are derived.

Guidelines for Management. Physical management of velopharyngeal inadequacy is surgical, prosthetic, or sometimes a combination of both. This topic will be discussed in a later section on cleft palate and noncleft VPI.

The question of whether or not the behavior of the velopharyngeal system during speech production be changed through therapy is one that has incited much controversy and one to which ongoing research continues to be addressed.[36,336] Three phases of "thinking" on this topic are identifiable in the literature. In the 1940s and 1950s, and to some extent in the 1960s, a number of therapy techniques were recommended for increasing the strength, flexibility, or voluntary control of the velopharyngeal mechanism.[337–349] Among the suggested activities were blowing, whistling, sucking, swallowing, yawning, cheek inflation, playing wind instruments, and voluntary nonspeech palatal elevations. As pointed out by Shelton, Hahn, and Morris, such recommendations were based on clinical impressions and not on specific evidence that such exercises were in fact of value in increasing velopharyngeal closure.[350] In the 1960s and 1970s, skepticism arose as to the validity of the assumption the behavior of this system could be altered by either exercise techniques[34,350,351] or speech therapy.[352] This second phase of thinking began with (1) research that clearly differentiated the behavior of oropharyngeal structures in speech from that in nonspeech acts[353] and (2) a theoretical review which concluded that physical therapy approaches to altering the behavior of the speech mechanism *in speech* had no sound empirical basis.[351]

Research and clinical reports in the 1960s and 1970s addressed this question in a variety of ways. Several authors reported increased pharyngeal wall motion speakers with velopharyngeal inadequacy who had been fitted with "speech bulb" prosthetic devices, in some cases allowing a reduction in bulb size,[354–361] although one study reported no increase in pharyngeal wall motion in compensation for bulb reduction.[362] As pointed out by Cole, some authors believed that increased muscle activity resulted from resistance of the speech bulb to the movement of the palatal and pharyngeal muscles, whereas others felt that the presence of the bulb in the nasopharynx served to "stimulate" the musculature, thus producing greater activity.[363] Such reports prompted several investigators to explore the effects of "stimulation" of the velopharyngeal musculature. Lubit and Larsen devised an inflatable "palatal exerciser," which, if it had worked as described by the authors, would have in fact "exercised" the muscles that oppose palatal elevation.[364,365] Massengill, Quinn, and Pickrell reported a decrease in velopharyngeal gaps as demonstrated on cinefluorography in patients using "palatal stimulators" that were in fact palatal lifts.[366] Yules and Chase used electrical stimulation first of the palate and then of the pharyngeal walls for the purpose of obtaining "voluntary pharyngeal contractions" and then automating these into speech.[367] The initial report was optimistic, but did not allow objective evaluation of the nature and degree of change in the behavior of the mechanism, and a follow-up report indicated that only one of the seven subjects available for study 1 year later showed "a significant reduction in nasality" (p 174).[368] Peterson was unable to replicate the initially reported results of electrical stimulation using an even higher level of voltage.[369]

Shelton had earlier pointed out that one problem in trying to produce changes in behavior of the velopharyngeal mechanism through "therapeutic exercise" was the lack of a sense of palatal position.[351] In a series of studies, he and his co-workers investigated increasing the awareness of palatal position and training the voluntary movement of the velum and pharyngeal walls.[370–372] Although some subjects could be trained to produce voluntary movement of the mechanism, the movements could not be automated into speech. In addition, some subjects showed laryngeal fixation and contraction of neck musculature.[372]

Interest in increasing the sense of palatal position and in direct stimulation of velopharyngeal movement was accompanied by continuing interest in the older approaches of blowing, sucking, and swallowing exercises. Massengill et al investigated the use of each of these types of exercises, but used them in conjunction with intensive articulation therapy.[342] Although they reported positive results for only the subjects using the swallowing exercises, they did not document homogeneity of subjects across groups and gave no explanation of how a period of swallowing as an exercise accomplished what a lifetime of vegetative swallowing had not. Powers and Starr decried the use of the same types of exercises, citing a poor result on four subjects who had demonstrated "some potential for closure" (p 29).[373]

Cole reviewed the available studies on "direct muscle training."[363] He chose to interpret the results of Shelton and co-workers[371] and Tash et al[372] and others differently: "The rationale for a muscle-training program in patients with velopharyngeal inadequacy is based on the fact that the activity as well as the sense of position or of movement of oropharyngeal structures can be increased with appropriate stimulation and feedback" (p 332).[363] He recommended muscle training programs in cases where velopharyngeal closure was judged to be inconsistent or the velopharyngeal gap "relatively small." Cole pointed out that what he termed "indirect muscle training"—articulation drillwork—had been shown to be unsuccessful in producing changes in velopharyngeal closure,[353] and he recommended that "semi-direct muscle training" in the form of blowing and sucking exercises be done against resistance. He also stated that the presence of a strong gag reflex should indicate that "much of this activity could be incorporated into the speaking act through muscle training" (p 333), choosing to ignore evidence to the contrary (see previously cited studies). Cole did stress the importance of increasing sensory feedback in attempting to bring about these changes.

In the middle of the 1970s, two unrelated developments forecast the third phase of investigation into this topic. Both were directly attributable to the availability of new instrumentation. First, although earlier research using lateral cine- or videofluoroscopy had described differences between closure patterns for speech and that for blowing in both normal speakers[275] and speakers with velopharyngeal inadequacy,[330,374] research using multiview videofluoroscopy on normal subjects revealed a similarity among blowing, whistling, and speech.[126] Shprintzen, McCall, and Skolnick combined whistling and phonation in patients showing adequate function for the former, but not for the latter.[375] Positive results were reported, although the number of subjects was small.

Concurrently, the development of endoscopy provided a new means for "biofeedback" in the attempt to teach changes in velopharyngeal movement. Using an oral panendoscope linked to a video playback system, Shelton and co-workers successfully taught normal speakers to voluntarily produce closure on nonspeech tasks.[376] However, the investigators noted that the procedure induced laryngeal fixation and contraction of the neck musculature. In a much later study, Siegel-Sadewitz and Shprintzen used video feedback from nasopharyngoscopy to train one normal subject (the first author) to change from a coronal to a sagittal pattern of closure, necessitating the induction of increased mesial motion of the lateral pharyngeal walls.[377] Use of this type of instrumentation for improving closure in patients with various forms of velopharyngeal inadequacy has been reported by a number of investigators.[315,316,336,378–381] In the Japanese studies, most of the subjects achieved closure for swallowing prior to the training sessions, but did not achieve it for blowing or speech. Positive results were reported. Interestingly, the authors noted that patients who could achieve closure during blowing could be trained with comparative ease to achieve closure during speech, a finding that might have been predicted by the earlier report of Shprintzen et al.[126] Shelton et al reported increased movement toward closure in their two subjects during the training tasks, but failure of this change to be automated into speech.[380] A subsequent study on seven patients failed to produce any change in the behavior of the velopharyngeal system through endoscopic biofeedback.[379] Finally, Hoch et al recently reported positive results in eight out of nine patients in whom this approach was used, the only "failure" being one patient who exhibited arrhythmic velopharyngeal valving as a result of pseudobulbar palsy.[336] Hoch and co-workers were careful to describe both the behavior of the velopharyngeal system prior to training and the etiology of the problem. They pointed out that these factors are often *not* specified even though they have a direct influence on the feasibility of attempting "direct treatment of VPI." It should be noted that two of the eight speakers who showed positive results had exhibited phoneme-specific velopharyngeal inadequacy; Hoch and co-workers acknowledged that this problem is usually amenable to therapy even without biofeedback.

Other types of instrumentation have been utilized as forms of biofeedback in the attempt to modify the behavior of the velopharyngeal mechanism, usually by monitoring the *results* of that behavior. Moller and co-workers used a strain gauge to monitor velar elevation in one boy as they attempted to teach him to increase elevation during sustained production of /u/.[382] Radiographic studies indicated that elevation was in fact increased, but there was no reduction in either velopharyngeal gap or perceived nasality. Further analysis revealed that the results had probably been contaminated by a progressive retropositioning of the posterior pharyngeal wall during the time of the study, which the authors attributed to possible adenoid involution. Tudor and Selley reported on a palatal training appliance that consisted of (1) a palatal lift-type device that they observed caused the palate to move away (reminiscent of earlier discussions of speech bulbs as stimulators of movement) and (2) a "visual aid" monitoring device consisting of sensor electrodes connected to a light bulb.[383] They reported that the intraoral appliance itself increased "sensory perception of the soft palate . . . the patients became aware of its movement and could control them involuntarily" (p 119). The visual feedback component was added only after Tudor and Selley observed these unexpected changes in response to what they had originally planned as a palatal lift. Subsequent reports advocated the use of this instrumentation, but gave no data on results.[384,385] Kunzel described a photoelectric device he called a "velograph" that consisted of a cold light probe and a photocell inserted transnasally.[386] Registration of the light on the photocell was used to monitor the closure of the velopharyngeal port. He reported positive results in four postoperative cleft patients:

> All patients learned to actively control their velopharyngeal mechanism under feedback conditions, 2 of them also under non-feedback conditions; in these cases permanent control of newly acquired movement patterns has been established . . . Mobility of the velopharyngeal structures was increased in all patients" (p 98).[386]

Kunzel made two important points, however. First, all four patients were able to attain velopharyngeal closure "at least sometimes during speech" (p 99) prior to treatment. Second, he questioned whether the "velographic treatment" did not also involve "a certain speech-therapeutic effect" (p 98). Dalston developed a similar "photodetector" system and also discussed its potential in biofeedback, although he had no data on this application at the time.[387]

Various forms of acoustic biofeedback have also been used. Garber and Moller[388] and Burzynski and Starr [389] investigated the effects of feedback filtering. Garber and Moller reported that both normal and hypernasal speakers altered the amount of nasalization in their voices under the filtering conditions. Burzynski and Starr reported similar findings in their normal subjects, but also found that the speakers as a group were not conscious of these changes in their own speech. Burzynski and Starr concluded, "The results offer no support for the suggestion that filtering causes speakers to perceive their speech as being more nasal and therefore attempt to decrease nasalization." Tonar II®, a commercially available instrument that monitors oral versus nasal sound pressure levels, has been advocated as a biofeedback device.[19–23,390] However, it has not gained wide popularity, perhaps because of cost. To date, no clinical studies have validated the use of nasal accelerometers (energy transducers placed on the side of the nose) as biofeedback devices in speakers exhibiting velopharyngeal inadequacy.

The PERCI® is a commercially available instrument that is essentially a portable, packaged version of the airflow instrumentation first devised by Warren and his colleagues in the early 1960s.[391] Data are currently being gathered on the use of both this instrument and Dalston's photodetector[387] as biofeedback devices. "See-scape" is a simple, rather crude device for detecting (not measuring) nasal airflow; it is low in cost and easily portable, but is limited in its capabilities. For a discussion of the applications and limitations of this device, please see Glaser and Shprintzen.[392]

Finally, the recent article by Hoch and coworkers signals a renewed interest in the possibilities of modifying the behavior of the velopharyngeal system through speech therapy, specifically in attempting to eliminate compensatory articulations *prior* to surgical treatment of velopharyngeal inadequacy.[336] This approach is in direct contradiction to the results of earlier investigations of the effect of speech therapy on velopharyngeal closure.[352,393,394] Although they offered a minimum of empirical data on their results, Hoch and co-workers did provide both a detailed outline of their approach and the rationale for each step.[336] Because the focus was on the compensatory articulations occurring in speakers with cleft palate, further discussion of this article will be found in Chapter 17.

In summary, interest in the possibilities of behavioral modification of the velopharyngeal system dates back several decades. Initially, there was a more or less naive faith in (1) the ability of physical exercise of the system to increase strength and coordination and for that change to be automated into speech, and (2) the ability of speakers to learn voluntary control of the mechanism, usually through speech therapy. This faith was followed by a long period of skepticism during which various investigators nevertheless sought new approaches. That skepticism was reflected in textbooks and other sources dealing with cleft palate.[36,395] Development of various instrumental means for either visualizing the velopharyngeal port or monitoring its behavior during speech production has led to renewed enthusiasm, although it is still true, as Shelton stated in 1978, that ". . . more data are needed to determine whether and under what circumstances poor velopharyngeal closure can be corrected by behavioral methods" (p 180).[232]

OROFACIAL ABLATIVE SURGERY

Most of the information on speech defects consequent to ablative surgery has been reported in the form of individual case histories. The extreme variability in such factors as preoperative function, site and extent of lesion, preoperative health, and personal and functional adjustment to life-threatening disease and ablation typically prohibits the pooling of data. Most reports have focused on articulation and intelligibility,[396–415] with little specific reference to resonance problems.[416–423]

Ablation of the Lip

Cancer of the lip accounts for approximately 15 percent of all oral cancers.[415,424,425] Bloomer and Hawk described a patient in whom removal of nasal structures resulted in a shortened and relatively immobile upper lip.[399] There was little loss of intelligibility, although the patient was forced to substitute labiodental approximations for all bilabials. A second patient who underwent extirpation of the upper lip and the anterior two-thirds of the maxilla substituted tongue-tip adaptations for bilabials and labiodentals; /p/, /b/, /m/, /w/, /hw/, /f/, /v/ were sufficiently well imitated that her speech was reported to be moderately intelligible.

To date, no reports have been published on the effects of lower lip ablation on articulation.

Supramaxillary Excisions

According to Bloomer and Hawk, excisions in the area of the antrum, ethmoid, and nasal cavities should have a minor effect on intelligibility and resonance if the maxilla is intact and the velopharyngeal mechanism functions satisfactorily.[399] One patient illustrated in their report lost the upper lip, the anterior two-thirds of the maxilla, and all nasal structures, retaining the posterior third of the hard palate and an intact soft palate. Speech was described as impaired but intelligible due to spontaneous articulatory adaptations. Bloomer and Hawk stated, "It is difficult to state how much or in what ways vowel qualities were changed. . . . Most of the vowels seemed to be identifiable, but were obviously abnormal. Her nasal resonance was also presumed to be altered . . . but the changes that one heard are difficult to describe" (p 48).

Maxillectomy

Partial or total maxillectomy presents a severe threat to both articulation and resonance (Figs. 16–9 and 16–10). Articulation is imperiled by the removal of normal dental, alveolar, and palatal contacts, and resonance is altered if the ablation destroys the normal division between the oral and nasal cavities.[416,419,421]

Kipfmueller and Lang studied six patients with maxillectomies and with varying surgical defects.[411] Scores on pre- and postoperative and postprosthetic recordings were found to improve with increased test-retest intervals. Bloomer and Hawk subsequently reported, "Lang has commented that during a period of two years postoperatively, the prosthesis generally can be reduced in size each time the patient returns. . . . This observation leads to speculation that nature appears to be trying to obliterate the defect in its own way through tissue proliferation and aperture reduction" (p 50).[399]

A report by Majid and co-workers on six pa-

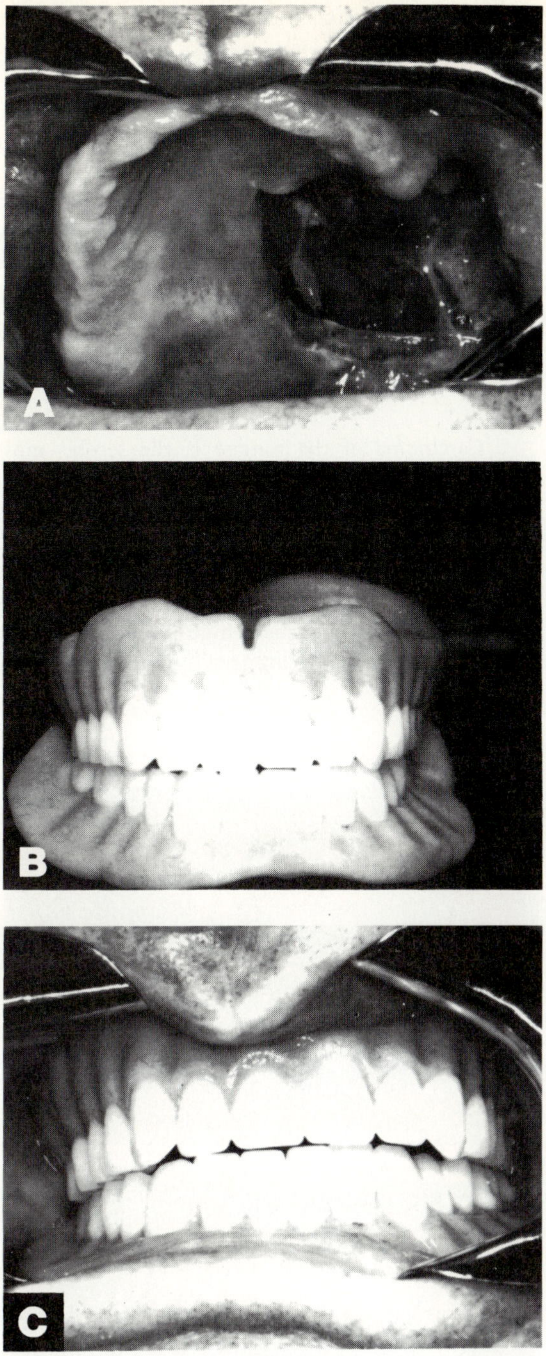

Figure 16–9 *A*, *B*, and *C*, Prosthetic rehabilitation for edentulous patient following partial maxillectomy.

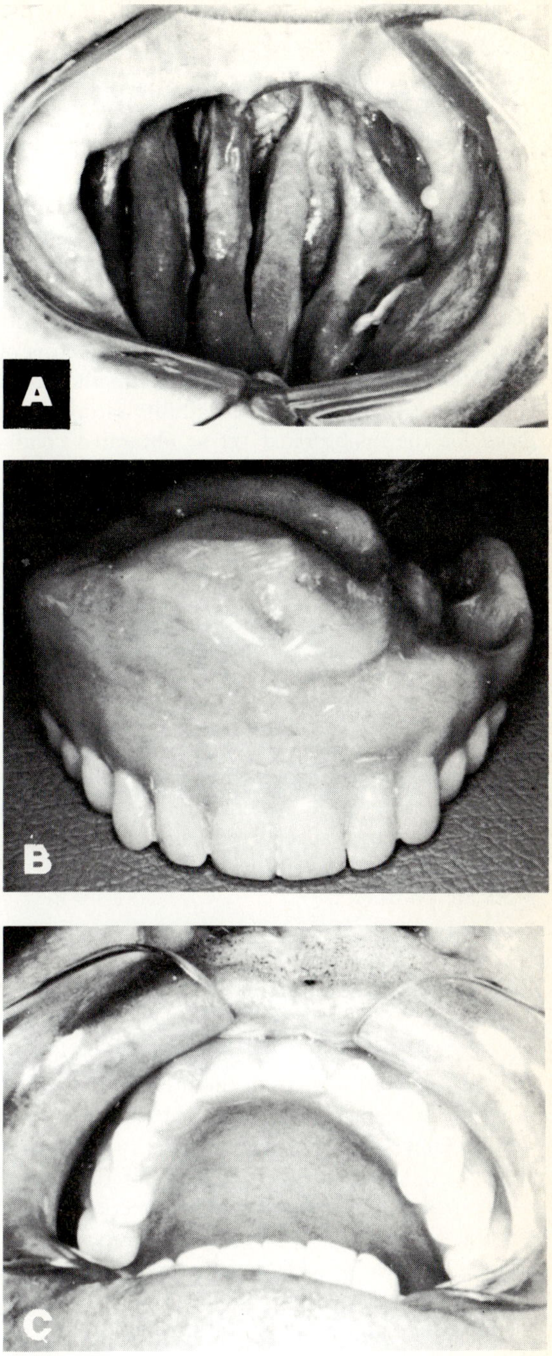

Figure 16–10 *A*, *B*, and *C*, Prosthetic rehabilitation following total maxillectomy.

tients with maxillectomies included photographic documentation of the intraoral appearance of the surgical defect as well as the intraoral appearance of each patient.[421] In view of the fact that articulation scores with prostheses in place ranged from 92 to 98 percent correct, Majid and co-workers concluded that normal intelligibility was a realistic dental treatment objective for patients with maxillectomies. However, they also noted that the articulation scores without obturation ranged from about 40 to 80 percent correct, and they urged systematic study of the specific factors responsible for these differences in individual performance. Similarly high intelligibility was reported in a study of eight patients with ablative maxillary defects whose ratings dropped from 98 percent preoperatively to only 97.25 percent postoperatively when the defects were obturated.[425]

Several reports have described different approaches to the design of prostheses for the obturation of maxillary defects.[426–444] One study of ten patients with partial maxillectomies and intact soft palates reported better speech results with a "buccal flange obturator" than with a "hollow bulb obturator."[445] The results were reported only in terms of "condition selected as best" by speech pathologists and by naive listeners; no intelligibility ratings were given for the unobturated versus obturated conditions. Moore and co-workers compared speech results obtained with rigid versus flexible obturation of a maxillary and palatal defect in one patient.[423] Both perceptual judgments and aerodynamic instrumentation reportedly indicated less hypernasality when a "semi-flexible" obturator for the velar defect was used, but Moore and co-workers did not explain how the position of the velar portion was changed or controlled by the speaker.

Although clinical reports on patients undergoing ablation of maxillary structures are difficult to evaluate because of the diversity in the surgical defects, the consensus appears to be that most patients retain excellent intelligibility once fitted with appropriate prostheses.

Ablation of the Soft Palate

To date, the only descriptions of the effects of ablation of the soft palate in the literature are those in which such ablation accompanied partial or total maxillectomy.[399,418,421,423] Hypernasality and nasal air loss would be an expected result of the loss of the normal velopharyngeal seal. Correction of the physical defect may be approached surgically, although Bloomer and Hawk expressed a preference for prosthetic treatment.[399] Bradley stated that prosthetic restoration of missing structures usually results in normal speech, and that only rarely may speech therapy be required.[446] No supportive data were offered.

Mandibulectomy

Reports describing speech after mandibulectomy (Fig. 16–11) are in fact reports on cases involving partial or total ablation of the tongue. Curtis and Cantor stated that ". . . speech distortion . . . in mandibulectomy patients results from impairment of the articulatory mechanism and/or alteration of the resonating chambers . . . reduction in tongue size and restricted mobility can prevent tongue-palate valving and result in speech distortions" (p 675).[447] Bloomer and Hawk stated that little dysfunction is found in hemimandibulectomy if bone resection does not pass the midline.[399]

Glossectomy

Carcinoma of the tongue is the second most common of oral cancers (after pharyngeal cancers), and usually involves both the tongue and the floor of the mouth.[425,448] As would be expected, the topic of partial and total glossectomy occupies by far the bulk of the literature on speech defects in ablative surgery. Several reports have highlighted the ability of some patients to develop intelligible speech with-

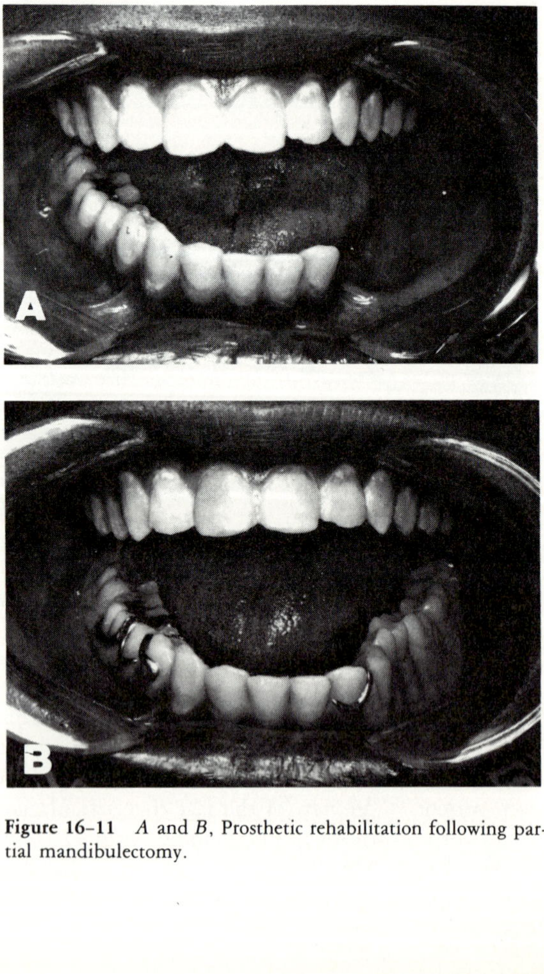

Figure 16–11 *A* and *B*, Prosthetic rehabilitation following partial mandibulectomy.

out prosthetic or surgical management of the ablative defect.[399,406,408,409] Goldstein concluded in 1940 that the tongue was *not* an indispensible articulator,[408] and Herberman that "the almost total lack* of reference to rehabilitation of glossectomy cases in the literature might imply no problems exist."[409] The repeated observation that a reserved and mobile tongue base allows usable speech[396,413] is undoubtedly related to the reports of intelligible speech in patients with congenital hypoglossia.[3,160,195,196,203] However, the assumption cannot be made that impairment in function is always proportional to the amount of tissue removed. For example, with respect to swallowing function, Logemann and Bytell found that patients with 10 percent of the tongue resected functioned almost as poorly as patients with 50 percent of the tongue removed.[412]

Most reports of glossectomies describe combined surgical ablations not only of the tongue, but also portions of the floor of the mouth, mandible, pharynx, and possibly larynx. In fact, when removal of the floor of the mouth plus or minus portions of the mandible is necessary, a portion of the tongue may be sacrificed ("tongue flap") in the surgical reconstruction of the oral floor.[419] In reviewing the literature, to keep in mind the possible effects of the combined ablative procedures of contiguous structures is more important than to dichotomize between "partial" (or "subtotal") and "total" glossectomy. For example, in an early report on a patient with a partial glossectomy, the "total lack of speech" was due to a concomitant laryngectomy (apparently with no attempt at the use of esophageal speech or an artificial larynx) rather than to the extirpation of lingual tissue.[449]

With varying degrees of thoroughness, clinical reports on patients who have undergone glossectomy typically describe the extent of the defect, speech intelligibility (or other speech parameters) postsurgically, subsequent surgical reconstruction and prosthetic treatment, and post-treatment speech capabilities. Perhaps the most interesting development of the past two decades has been the evolution in prosthetic approaches.

Many reports on partial glossectomees center on the articulatory adjustments these patients develop either independently or with training. Backus described a boy who substituted labial consonants for tongue-tip phonemes subsequent to anterolateral excision of one-third of the tongue.[398] A hemiglossectomee described by Bloomer and Hawk developed a linguoalveolar constriction between the tongue tip and the tongue blade to substitute for midline lingual grooving for production of sibilants.[399]

Skelly and co-workers described a therapy program, later elaborated by Skelly,[415] for teaching compensatory articulation to partial and total glossectomees.[448] Many of the compensatory strategies described are found in other clinical reports. After 12 months of therapy, intelligibility for the partial glossectomees increased from a pretherapy rating ranging from 6 percent to 24 percent to post-therapy values ranging from 24 percent to 46 percent. (Note how these numbers contrast to intelligibility ratings in other reports to be cited.) For the total glossectomy group, 0.0 to 8 percent intelligibility increased to 18 to 42 percent. Six total glossectomees who had an inadequate swallow made no progress from the initial 0.0 percent intelligibility. The partial glossectomees achieved their gains in shorter time and were noted to make marked use of the residual stump rather than resorting to the more varied substitutions developed by the total glossectomees. Cinefluorographic films of the patients with total glossectomies and with the highest intelligibility ratings showed consistency in (1) production of /z/ by bilabial tension obstruction of the airstream, with the lips in much closer approximation usual for this sound (a finding later reported by LaRiviere, Seilo, and Dimmick[450]); (2) production of /n/ by momentary velar contraction followed by a quick uvular relaxation, the lips concurrently almost approaching adduction; (3) production of /g/ by pharyngeal constriction, with slight bulging of the retroglossal pharyngeal wall; (4) production of /d/ by lower lip contact with the maxillary teeth or, in edentulous patients, with the maxillary alveolar ridge; and (5) /l/ and /r/ produced by combinations of pharyngeal, uvular, and buccal movements. For /l/ the uvula appeared to have some slight vibrations that possibly provided the division of the airstream usually considered critical to this phoneme. In a later report, Skelly, Donaldson, and Schinsky emphasized consistency of phoneme substitution as a critical factor in intelligibility.[451] These authors stated that, in their experience, usable gains in compensatory articulation required 6 to 8 months in cases of total glossectomy.

Duguay described several compensatory articulatory movements used by patients with glossec-

* However, this lack might also have reflected that relatively little was known about how to approach rehabilitation (prosthetic, surgical, or speech) with these patients.

tomies.[406] He observed that /l/ could be produced fairly well by retracting the lower lip and pressing it against the upper alveolar ridge. He also noted that a similar acoustic effect could be obtained by elevating the floor of the mouth (genioglossus activity) to make contact with the anterior maxillary teeth, with the tongue blade (when available) substituting for the tongue tip. A nearly identical description was given by Eskew and Shepard of an adult with congenital aglossia who approximated tip-alveolar consonants by elevating the lower lip behind the upper teeth.[452] Duguay suggested that linguovelar consonants could be approximated by pharyngeal sounds produced between the tongue base and pharyngeal wall.

LaRiviere and co-workers offered a detailed analysis of speech production in a patient with glossectomy in whom "the tongue remnant was represented by a very small (somewhat mobile) flap of tissue at a position in the median and slightly posterior to the faucial pillars" (p 202).[450] Intelligibility of initial consonants ranged from 60 to 66 percent on single word lists, final consonants 49 percent. Bilabial and labiodental consonants were highly intelligible, as would be expected, but so were /t/, /s/, /n/, /l/, and the voiced affricate. Intelligibility of vowels ranged from 90 percent for /ae/ to 9 percent for /ɝ/, with a mean of 45.8 percent. Sentence intelligibility was 88.8 percent. Confusions between /t/, /p/ and /d/, /b/ were heard perceptually, and acoustical analysis revealed that the durations of these pairs of consonants had been reversed. However, /s/ and /f/ were confused perceptually, although their durational values were not similar. On videotape, it was seen that /t/, /d/, and "th" were produced by movements normally associated with /p/, /b/, /f/, respectively. Sibilants were produced by blowing air through closed teeth, producing lateralized consonants. LaRiviere and co-workers noted that this speaker preserved manner and voicing of consonants while necessarily sacrificing the place of production.

Ablation of lingual tissue can affect the ability to attain positioning for production of vowels, as well as consonants, with consequent deleterious effects on intelligibility.[415,450,451,453–455] Skelly and co-workers noted that the value of the first formant extended over a wide frequency range in their less intelligible speakers with glossectomies, and the second formant was frequently absent.[451] As intelligibility increased, the first formant decreased in frequency range, and the second became defined more strongly. The authors concluded that, since the first formant was not a major factor in intelligibility by comparison with the second formant, compensatory vertical adjustment within the vocal tract was less important than compensatory horizontal adjustment. In a patient with a total glossectomy, La Riviere and co-workers reported that the vowels were shifted both perceptually and acoustically to more neutral vowels and that the first formant was more stable than the second.[450] Gillis and Leonard reported vowel intelligibility of 48 percent in single words in another total glossectomee.[454] In several reports describing particular prosthetic approaches to rehabilitation, the authors comment upon the effects of the prosthesis on either vowel intelligibility or resonance.[419,422,453–455]

Although resection of lingual tissue is frequently combined with partial mandibulectomy,[403,447,453,456,457] only two reports have described patients who have undergone glossectomy in combination with a *total* mandibulectomy. Shedd commented only that his patient regained communicative competence and was 70 to 80 percent intelligible, but gave no details on articulatory compensations or the treatment procedures.[458] Meyerson, Johnson, and Weitzman described a patient with a complete mandibulectomy and partial glossectomy in whom the mylohyoid, hyoglossus, genioglossus, and digastric muscles were also excised.[459] Approximately the anterior one-half of the tongue was excised. The surgical procedure was preceded by extensive radiation which produced irradiation necrosis that later complicated prosthetic care. Subsequently, multiple secondary procedures were performed to transfer skin flaps to the floor of the mouth. The initial speech evaluation showed all consonants except /h/ to be severely distorted. Even the bilabial consonants were affected due to the fact that there was no bony support for the lower lip. The vowel /i/ was also noted to be distorted, which is not surprising in view of the fact that this vowel occupies the extreme upper and anterior corner of the "vowel triangle." Intelligibility was reported to be zero at the time of the initial evaluation and 50 percent 18 months later, at which time a year of formal therapy was undertaken. Pharyngeal constrictions were taught in order to obtain a close acoustic effect of the velar stops (note that, although the anterior half of the tongue was excised, the amount of inframandibular musculature that was ablated would have affected the ability to produce these consonants). Similar to previous reports, the tip-alveolars /t/ and /d/ were approximated by contact between the lower lip and upper teeth. Meyerson and colleagues noted that adaptations were devised either by the clinician or by the patient himself for improved production of other phonemes. A slower rate was also encouraged. By the conclusion of therapy, intelligibility of contextual speech had increased to 80 percent. Acoustic analysis performed at this time showed the vowel space to be diminished in size in comparison to normal speakers, with the most limitation in the range of the second formant.

Prosthetic approaches for the glossectomee can basically be divided into attempts to provide a prosthetic tongue and attempts to lower the palatal arch in order to facilitate articulatory contacts. The latter attempts account for the term "maxillary prostheses for mandibular surgical defects."[403] Cantor and co-workers reported that such devices had a beneficial effect on velar consonant production for patients with severe restrictions in lingual mobility, but had negative effects for those with moderate restriction.[403] They interpreted this to mean that patients with some tongue mobility are able to compensate for the surgical defect and that the prosthesis interferes with, rather than assists, compensation. Wheeler and co-workers described the fabrication of "maxillary reshaping prostheses" for ten patients with ablation of the tongue ranging from 10 to 90 percent, in combination with various other resections.[457] A period of speech and swallowing therapy preceded the fitting of the prostheses. Impairment of speech intelligibility ranged from 9 to 18 percent (mean 12.5 percent).* Without the prostheses, no patient exceeded 90 percent intelligibility, whereas six of the ten exceeded this value with the prosthesis in place. Although they did not use the same terminology as Wheeler and co-workers, Lauciello and co-workers' description of the prosthetic approach used in three out of four patients included "thickening of the maxillary denture" to facilitate articulatory contacts in three patients with resections ranging from 25 to 90 percent of the lingual tissue.[419] In addition to improved articulation, the authors also noted "improved resonance" as a result of the modification of the maxillary prostheses. Knowles and co-workers made similar successive modifications to a maxillary prosthesis for a partial glossectomy patient.[456] Christensen, Hutton, Hasegawa, and Fletcher described the use of palatography (mapping of articulatory contacts sensed by electrodes imbedded in a palatal plate) for the optimal fitting of prostheses for patients with glossectomies, although they had used this instrumentation with just one patient at the time.[460] Palatograms were also suggested by McKinstry and co-workers.[455] In the approach of Aramany, Downs, Beery, and Aslan, palatal augmentation prostheses were suggested for partial glossectomees, mandibular tongue prostheses for total glossectomees.[461] No data were given on speech.

Construction of mandibular tongue prostheses has been described in a number of reports. Belsky's patients were combined laryngectomee and glossectomees, and the prostheses were fabricated for eating rather than for speech.[462] The patients were reportedly taught esophageal speech or used an electrolarynx, although no information was given as to how intelligible speech was achieved. deSouza and Martins reported that their patients with total glossectomies achieved "reasonably understandable speech" with a prosthetic tongue.[404] Moore fitted his patient first with a temporary tongue prosthesis, which reportedly produced "immediate improvement in resonance and voice quality."[422] The patient gained intelligibility quickly with practice in articulatory adjustments and substitutions. A second prosthesis was made of silicone rubber with a highly flexible tip in order to improve tongue-tip sound (no note of how the flexibility of the tip could be controlled in articulation). Gillis and Leonard designed one "rest position" tongue prosthesis for their patient, followed by six different experimental designs to improve articulation.[454] With the "typical prosthesis"† in place, it was reported that vowel intelligibility improved from 48 to 64 percent in single words, and consonant intelligibility from 82 to 90 percent. Better matches to normal vowel formants were also produced. Ballard and co-workers fitted a combination mandibular and tongue prosthesis for a patient who also had to use an electrolarynx because of a laryngectomy.[453] Intelligibility ratings (56 percent for single words, 84 percent for sentences) were given without noting whether they were derived with or without the prosthesis. One interesting observation in this article was that the patient shifted the

* Note this means that even the patient with 90 percent of the tongue extirpated had not lost more than 18 percent of his intelligibility. Compare this with the percentages of intelligibility given by Skelly et al for partial glossectomees.[448]

† Unfortunately, the article does not describe the prostheses in detail, and it is impossible to tell what the authors mean by "typical prosthesis."

anterior-to-posterior position of the mandible to achieve tip-alveolar and linguovelar consonants.

Surgical reconstruction for patients with glossectomies may attempt to reestablish function or to prepare the mandible and floor of the mouth to support a lingual prosthesis.[463-471] Those reports that do describe the recovery of function focus primarily on deglutition, with speech rarely mentioned.

Guidelines for Management. As stated by Gillis and Leonard:

> The intent of speech therapy for patients with glossectomies is the adoption of compensatory strategies, that is, new ways of producing speech sounds that approximate their typical physical characteristics, including resonances, so closely that listeners perceive them as normal. In addition, procedures for improving communicative efficiency, such as maintaining good eye contact with listeners and speaking at a lower rate, can be initiated (p 809).[454]

From the preceding reports, it is evident that many speakers may retain or regain functional intelligibility either through their own spontaneous adjustments or through a combination of these adjustments and whatever physical management (surgical and/or prosthetic) is undertaken. The studies reviewed earlier repeatedly point to the importance of the speech pathologist working with the prosthodontist during all phases of the fabrication of prosthetic devices.

As would be expected, the majority of information on therapy for patients who have undergone ablative surgery focuses on partial and total glossectomees. Depending upon the amount of extirpation, the initial phases of therapy are devoted to the functions of deglutition, which may or may not be aided by prosthetic devices.

The "compensatory physiologic phonetics" program of Skelly and her co-workers included a variety of compensatory gestures for achieving a perceptual result as similar to normally produced consonants as possible.[415,448] In addition, Skelly and her co-workers sought to improve intelligibility through manipulation of vowel duration, vocal intensity, pause length, habitual pitch, pitch range, and variety of pitch patterns.[414] Their approach recognized the need for (1) multifaceted assessment, with periodic reevaluations; (2) individualized programs based on the abilities of the patient; (3) exploration of a variety of means for increasing intelligibility rather than relying on articulation alone; (4) early success; but (5) continued therapy, despite slow gains, until such time as the patient has reached a plateau, the criterion for the plateau being no progress in 4 weeks of therapy without explanatory circumstances.[448]

The diagnostic and therapeutic principles outlined by Skelly and her co-workers in the early 1970s have generally been reflected in case reports published since that time and still appear to be highly relevant to the care of orofacial ablative patients today. With the ongoing developments in surgical care, an expanding number of options for reconstruction are available to the patient. To some extent, the same is true in prosthetic rehabilitation. Speech rehabilitation must begin with full familiarization with the patient's medical history, and should include collaboration with the surgeon and/or prosthodontist whenever possible.

Portions of this material appeared previously in Peterson-Falzone S. Velopharyngeal inadequacy in the absence of overt cleft palate. J Craniofacial Genetics and Developmental Biology, Supplement 1, 1985:97–124.

Peterson Falzone, S. Speech characteristics: Updating clinical decisions. Seminars in Speech and Language 1986; 7(3):219–296.

REFERENCES

1. Smith D. Recognizable patterns of human malformation. 3rd ed. Philadelphia: WB Saunders, 1982.
2. Cohen M, Stool S. Craniofacial anomalies and syndromes. In: Bluestone C, Stool S, eds. Pediatric otolaryngology. Vol I. Philadelphia: WB Saunders, 1983:32.
3. Peterson S. Speech pathology in craniofacial malformations other than cleft lip and palate. In: Wertz RT. ASHA Report 8: orofacial anomalies: clinical and research implications. Washington: American Speech and Hearing Association, 1973:111.
4. Shprintzen R, Siegel-Sadewitz V, Amato J, Goldberg R. Retrospective diagnoses of previously missed syndromic disorders among 1000 patients with cleft lip, cleft palate, or both. Birth Defects 1985; 21(2):85–92.
5. Carr P, Trill D. Long-term larynx-excitation spectra. J Acoust Soc Am 1964; 36:2033–2040.
6. Warren D. The determination of velopharyngeal incompetency by aerodynamic and acoustical techniques. Clin Plast Surg 1975; 2:299–304.
7. Trost J. Differential diagnosis of velopharyngeal disorders. Commun Disord Audio J Cont Educ 1981; 6(7).
8. Warren D. Nasal emission of air and velopharyngeal function. Cleft Palate J 1967; 4:148–156.
9. Warren D, Devereux J. An analog study of cleft palate speech. Cleft Palate J 1966; 3:103–114.
10. Warren D, DuBois A. A pressure-flow technique for measuring velopharyngeal orifice area during continuous speech. Cleft Palate J 1964; 1:52–71.
11. Warren D, Ryon W. Oral port constriction, nasal resistance, and respiratory aspects of cleft palate speech: an analog study. Cleft Palate J 1967; 4:38–46.
12. Lubker J, Schweiger J, Morris H. Nasal airflow characteristics during speech in prosthetically managed cleft palate speakers. J Speech Hear Res 1970; 13(2):326–328.
13. Bradford L, Brooks A, Shelton R. Clinical judgement of

hypernasality in cleft palate children. Cleft Palate J 1964; 1:329–335.
14. Bzoch K. Measurement and assessment of categorical aspects of cleft palate speech. In: Bzoch K, ed. Communicative disorders related to cleft lip and palate. Boston: Little, Brown, 1979:161.
15. Carney P, Sherman D. Severity of nasality in three selected speech tasks. J Speech Hear Res 1971; 14:396–407.
16. Counihan C, Cullinan A. Reliability and dispersion of nasality ratings. Cleft Palate J 1970; 7:261–270.
17. Moore W, Sommers R. Phonetic contexts: their effects on perceived nasality in cleft palate speakers. Cleft Palate J 1973; 10:72–83.
18. Ellis R. The Exeter anemometry system. In: Ellis R, Flack F, eds. Diagnosis and treatment of palato glossal malfunction. London: College of Speech Therapists, 1979:31.
19. Fletcher S. Contingencies for bioelectronic modification of nasality. J Speech Hear Disord 1972; 37:329–346.
20. Fletcher S. Diagnosis of speech disorders from cleft palate. New York: Grune and Stratton, 1978.
21. Fletcher S. "Nasalance" vs. listener judgements of nasality. Cleft Palate J 1976; 13:31–44.
22. Fletcher S. Perceptual skills in clinical management of nasality. Folia Phoniatr (Basel) 1973; 25:137–145.
23. Fletcher S. Theory and instrumentation for quantitative measurement of nasality. Cleft Palate J 1970; 7:601–609.
24. Fletcher S, Bishop M. Measurement of nasality with Tonar. Cleft Palate J 1970; 7:610–621.
25. Horii Y. An accelerometric approach to nasality measurement: a preliminary report. Cleft Palate J 1980; 17:254–261.
26. Horii Y. An accelerometric measure as a physical correlate of perceived hypernasality in speech. J Speech Hear Res 1983; 26:476–480.
27. Lippman R. Detecting nasalization using a low-cost miniature accelerometer. J Speech Hear Res 1981; 24:314–317.
28. Stevens K, Kalikow D, Willemain T. A miniature accelerometer for detecting glottal waveforms and nasalization. J Speech Hear Res 1975; 18:594–599.
29. Moll K. "Objective" measures of nasality. Cleft Palate J 1964; 1(3):371–374.
30. Moll K. Speech characteristics of individuals with cleft lip and palate. In: Spriestersbach D, Sherman D, eds. Cleft Palate and Communication. New York: Academic Press, 1968:61.
31. VanRiper C, Irwin J. Voice and articulation. 3rd ed. Englewood Cliffs, NJ: Prentice-Hall, 1961.
32. Backus O, Clancy J, Henry L, Kemper J. The child with the cleft palate. Ann Arbor: University of Michigan, 1943.
33. Terashima Y. Clinical and statistical study of nasality in cleft palate. Aichi-Gakuin J Dent Sci 1982; 19:168–177.
34. Morley M. Cleft palate and speech. 7th ed. Baltimore: Williams and Wilkins, 1970.
35. Trost J. Articulatory additions to the classical description of the speech of persons with cleft palate. Cleft Palate J 1981; 18(3):193–203.
36. McWilliams BJ, Morris H, Shelton R. Cleft palate speech. Toronto: BC Decker, 1984.
37. McWilliams BJ. Cleft palate. In: Shames G, Wiig E, eds. Human communication disorders. Columbus: CE Merrill, 1982:330.
38. Shelton R, Blank J. Oronasal fistulas, intraoral air pressure, and nasal air flow during speech. Cleft Palate J 1984; 21: 91–99.
39. Morris H. Evaluation of abnormal articulation patterns. In: Bzoch K, ed. Communication disorders related to cleft lip and palate. Boston: Little, Brown, 1979:192.
40. Millar R. Cleft palate and communication disorders. Ear Nose Throat J 1980; 59:54–61.
41. Boone D. The voice and voice therapy. 2nd ed. Englewood Cliffs, NJ: Prentice-Hall, 1977.
42. Brooks A, Shelton R, Youngstrom K. Compensatory tongue-palate-pharyngeal wall relationships in cleft palate. J Speech Hear Disord 1965; 30:166–173.
43. Brooks A, Shelton R, Youngstrom K. Tongue-palate contact in persons with palate defects. J Speech Hear Disord 1966; 31:14–25.
44. Pruzansky S. Roentgencephalometric studies of tonsils and adenoids in normal and pathologic states. Ann Otol Rhinol Laryngol [Suppl] 1975; 84(2):55–62.
45. Mason R, Warren D. Adenoid involution and developing hypernasality in cleft palate. J Speech Hear Disord 1980; 45(4):469–480.
46. Subtelny J, Koepp-Baker H. The significance of adenoid tissue in velopharyngeal function. Plast Reconstr Surg 1956; 17(2):235–250.
47. Linder-Aronson S, Leighton B. A longitudinal study of the development of the posterior pharyngeal wall between 3 and 16 years of age. Eur J Orthod 1983; 5:47–58.
48. Handelman C, Osborne G. Growth of the nasopharynx and adenoid development from one to eighteen years. Angle Orthod 1976; 46(3):243–259.
49. Tanner K. Ein neuer Weg in der Behandlung der Tonsillektomie-Nachblutung vorläufige Mittelung. Pract Otorhinolaryngol 1964; 26:439–442.
50. Scammon R, Harris J, Jackson C. The measurement of man. Minneapolis: University of Minnesota Press, 1930.
51. Handelman C, Pruzansky S. The size of the adenoids in normal and CPI children. Presented before the International Association of Dental Research, Washington, 1967.
52. Calnan J. Modern views on Passavant's ridge. Br J Plast Surg 1957; 10(2):89–113.
53. Fletcher S. Hypernasal voice as an indication of regional growth and developmental disturbances. Logos 1960; 3:3–12.
54. Mason R. Preventing speech disorders following adenoidectomy by preoperative examination. Clin Pediatr 1973; 12:405–414.
55. Neiman G, Simpson R. A roentgencephalometric investigation of the effect of adenoid removal upon selected measures of velopharyngeal function. Cleft Palate J 1975; 12:377–389.
56. Vrticka K. La fermeture vélo-pharyngee avant et après la tonsillectomie et l'adénotomie. Bull Audiophonol 1977; 7 (3):95–106.
57. Goode R, Ross J. Velopharyngeal insufficiency after adenoidectomy. Arch Otolaryngol 1972; 96:223–226.
58. Massengill R, Quinn G. Adenoidal atrophy, velopharyngeal incompetence and sucking exercises: a two year follow-up case report. Cleft Palate J 1974; 11:196–199.
59. Shapiro R. Velopharyngeal insufficiency starting at puberty without adenoidectomy. Int J Pediat Otorhinolaryngol 1980; 2:255–260.
60. Ashley F, Sloan R, Hahn E, Hanafee W, Miethke J. Cinefluorographic study of palatal incompetency cases during deglutition and phonation. Plast Reconstr Surg 1961; 28(4):347–364.
61. Beeden A. The bifid uvula. J Laryngol Otol 1972; 86:815–819.
62. Bergstrom L, Hemenway W. Otologic problems in submucous cleft palate. South Med J 1971; 64(10):1172–1177.
63. Berner R. Hazards of adenotonsillectomy in the child with cleft palate. J Am Med Assoc 1962; 181(6):558–559.
64. Blackfield H, Miller E, Owsley J, Lawson L. Cinefluorographic evaluation of patients with velopharyngeal dysfunction in the absence of overt cleft palate. Plast Reconstr Surg 1962; 30:441–451.
65. Calnan J. Diagnosis, prognosis, and treatment of "palatopharyngeal incompetence," with special reference to radiographic investigations. Br J Plast Surg 1956; 8:265–282.
66. Calnan J. Movements of the soft palate. Br J Plast Surg 1953; 5:286–296.

67. Calnan J. Palato-pharyngeal incompetence in speech. In: Pruzansky S, ed. Congenital anomalies of the face and associated structures. Springfield: CC Thomas, 1961:104.
68. Calnan J. Permanent nasal escape in speech after adenoidectomy. Br J Plast Surg 1971; 24:197–204.
69. Calnan J. Submucous cleft palate. Br J Plast Sug 1954; 7:264–282.
70. Calnan J. Surgery for speech. In: Calnan J, ed. Recent advances in plastic surgery. I. Edinburgh: Churchill Livingstone, 1976:39.
71. Calnan J. The investigation of nasality (nasal escape) in speech. Speech 1957; 21(2):59–74.
72. Calnan J. The mobility of the soft palate: a radiological and statistical study. Br J Plast Surg 1961; 14(1):33–38.
73. Calnan J. The surgical treatment of nasal speech disorders. Ann R Coll Surg Engl 1959; 25:119–141.
74. Chaco J, Yules R. Velopharyngeal incompetence post tonsilloadenoidectomy: an electromyographic study. Acta Otolaryngol (Stockh) 1969; 68:276–278.
75. Cotton R, Nuywayhid N. Velopharyngeal insufficiency. In: Bluestone C, Stool S, eds. Pediatric otolaryngology. Vol. II. Philadelphia: WB Saunders, 1983:1521.
76. Cotton R, Quattromani F. Lateral defects in velopharyngeal insufficiency. Arch Otolaryngol 1977; 103:90–93.
77. Croft C, Shprintzen R, Ruben R. Hypernasal speech following adenotonsillectomy. Otolaryngol Head Neck Surg 1981; 89:179–188.
78. Dey D. Nasal speech, adenoidectomy, and the Hynes' pharyngoplasty. Med J Aust 1969; 2:553–555.
79. Drettner B. The nasal airway and hearing in patients with cleft palate. Acta Otolaryngol (Stockh) 1960; 52:131–142.
80. Freud E. The otolaryngologist and the symptom of hyperrhinolalia. AMA Arch Otolaryngol 1959; 70:32–41.
81. Gibb A. Hypernasality (rhinolalia aperta) following tonsil and adenoid removal. J Laryngol Otol 1958; 72:433–451.
82. Glover D. A long range evaluation of cleft palate repair. Plast Reconstr Surg 1961; 27(1):19–30.
83. Holborow C. Conductive deafness associated with the cleft-palate deformity. Proc R Soc Med 1962; 55:305–307.
84. Jackson I, McGlynn M, Huskie C. Velopharyngeal incompetence in the absence of cleft palate: results of treatment in 20 cases. Plast Reconstr Surg 1980; 66(2):211–213.
85. Linthicum H, Body H, Keaster J. Incidence of middle ear disease in children with cleft palate. Cleft Palate Bull 1959; 9:23–25.
86. Lubit D. Before an adenoidectomy: Stop! Look! Listen! NY State J Med 1967; 67:681–685.
87. McWilliams BJ, Musgrave R. Differential diagnosis and management of hypernasal voices in children. Trans Am Acad Ophthalmol Otolaryngol 1965; 69:322–331.
88. Miller M. Hearing problems associated with cleft palate. Ann Otol Rhinol Laryngol 1959; 68:90–99.
89. Morris H. The speech pathologist looks at the tonsils and adenoids. Ann Otol Rhinol Laryngol [Suppl] 1975; 84(2):63–66.
90. Parkins F, Barbero G. The oral cavity. In: Vaughan V, McKay R, eds., Nelson's textbook of pediatrics. Philadelphia: WB Saunders, 1975:787.
91. Pickrell K, Massengill R, Quinn G, Brooks R, Robinson M. The effect of adenoidectomy on velopharyngeal competence in cleft palate patients. Br J Plast Surg 1976; 29: 134–136.
92. Pruzansky S, Richmond J. Growth of mandible in infants with micrognathia. Am J Dis Child 1954; 88:29–42.
93. Pruzansky S. Congenital palatopharyngeal incompetence: clinical, radiographic and genetic studies. J Dent Res 1968; 47:1013.
94. Pruzansky S. Contributions of roentgenographic cephalometry to the study of congenital and acquired malformations of the face. Dent Clin North Am, 1960; 4:395–417.
95. Ricketts R. The cranial base and soft structures in cleft palate speech and breathing. Plast Reconstr Surg 1954; 14 (1):47–61.
96. Roberts W. Speech defects following adenotonsillectomy. Rocky Mt Med J 1959; 56:67–69.
97. Saad E. The bifid uvula in ear, nose and throat practice. Laryngoscope 1975; 85:734–737.
98. Seeman M. Contribution à la pathogénie et la symptomatologie de la fissure sous-muqueuse du palais osseux. Arch Int Laryngol 1924; 30:388–402.
99. Severeid L. Pharyngeal disease and velopharyngeal competency and their relationship to ear disease and hearing loss. In: Graham M, ed. Cleft palate: middle ear disease and hearing loss. Springfield: CC Thomas, 1978:56.
100. Skolnik E. Otologic evaluation in cleft palate patients. Laryngoscope 1958; 68:1908–1949.
101. Thaler S, Smith H. Submucous cleft palate. Arch Otolaryngol 1968; 88:184–189.
102. Van Gelder L. Open nasal speech following adenoidectomy and tonsillectomy. J Commun Disord 1974; 7:263–267.
103. Vinicoff A. Clinical evaluation of cleft palate patients and their speech. Plast Reconstr Surg 1960; 25:496–502.
104. Wallner L, Hill B, Waldrop W, Monroe C. Voice changes following adenotonsillectomy. Laryngoscope 1968; 78(8): 1410–1418.
105. Whaley J. The otolaryngologist's role in the care of the cleft palate patient. J Can Dent Assoc 1957; 23:574–575.
106. Porterfield H, Trabue J, Terry J, Stimpert R. Hypernasality in noncleft palate patients. Plast Reconstr Surg 1966; 37(3):216–220.
107. Gibb A. Unusual complication of tonsil and adenoid removal. J Laryngol Otol 1969; 83:1159–1174.
108. Morris H, Krueger L, Bumsted R. Indications of congenital palatal incompetence before diagnosis. Ann Otol Rhinol Laryngol 1982; 91:115–118.
109. Goldstone A, Horton C. Should adenotonsillectomy be done in the cleft palate patient? Virg Med Monthly 1971; 98:133–138.
110. Greene M. Speech of children before and after removal of tonsils and adenoids. J Speech Hear Disord 1957; 22:361–370.
111. Peterson-Falzone S. Velopharyngeal inadequacy in the absence of overt cleft palate. J Craniofac Genet Dev Biol [Suppl] 1985; 1:97–124.
112. Minami R, Kaplan E, Wu G, Jobe R. Velopharyngeal incompetency without overt cleft palate. Plast Reconstr Surg 1975; 55(5):573–587.
113. Heller J, Gens G, Moe D, Lewin M. Velopharyngeal insufficiency in patients with neurological, emotional and mental disorders. J Speech Hear Disord 1974; 39(3):350–359.
114. Paradise J, Bluestone C. Toward rational indications for tonsil and adenoid surgery. Hosp Pract 1976; 11(2):79–87.
115. Paradise J. Management of middle ear effusions in infants with cleft palate. Ann Otol Rhinol Laryngol [Suppl] 1976; 25:285–288.
116. Paradise J. Primary care of infants and children with cleft palate. In: Bluestone C, Stool S, eds. Pediatric otolaryngology Vol. I. Philadelphia: WB Saunderrs, 1983:924.
117. Paradise J. Why T&A remains moot. Pediatrics 1972; 49: 648–651.
118. Calnan J. Congenital large pharynx: a new syndrome with a report of 41 personal cases. Br J Plast Surg 1971; 24:263–271.
119. Converse J, Horowitz S, Becker M. The use of tomography in the diagnosis of unusual and occult clefts of the palate. Cleft Palate J 1968; 5:311–316.
120. Croft C, Shprintzen R, Daniller A, Lewin M. The occult submucous cleft palate and the musculus uvulae. Cleft Palate J 1978; 15(2):150–154.
121. Kaplan E. The occult submucous cleft palate. Cleft Palate J 1975; 12:356–368.

122. Lewin M, Croft C, Shprintzen R. Velopharyngeal insufficiency due to hypoplasia of the musculus uvulae and occult submucous cleft palate. Plast Reconstr Surg 1980; 65(5):585–591.
123. Croft C, Shprintzen R, Rakoff S. Patterns of velopharyngeal valving in normal and cleft palate subjects: A multiview videofluorographic and nasendoscopic study. Laryngoscope 1981; 91:265–271.
124. Pigott R, Makepeace A. Some characteristics of endoscopic and radiological systems used in elaboration of the diagnosis of velopharyngeal incompetence. Br J Plast Surg 1982; 35:19–32.
125. Shprintzen R. The use of multiview videofluoroscopy and flexible fiberoptic nasopharyngoscopy as a predictor of success with pharyngeal flap surgery. In: Ellis R, Flack F, eds. Diagnosis and treatment of palato glossal malfunction. London: College of Speech Therapists, 1979:6.
126. Shprintzen R, Lencione R, McCall G, Skolnick M. A three dimensional cinefluoroscopic analysis of velopharyngeal closure during speech and nonspeech activities in normals. Cleft Palate J 1974; 11:412–428.
127. Sinclair S, Davies D, Bracka A. Comparative reliability of nasal pharyngoscopy and videofluorography in the assessment of velopharyngeal incompetence. Br J Plast Surg 1982; 35:113–117.
128. Skolnick M. Videofluoroscopic examination of the velopharyngeal portal during phonation in lateral and base projections—a new technique for studying the mechanics of closure. Cleft Palate J 1970; 7:803–816.
129. Skolnick M, McCall G, Barnes R. Sphincteric mechanism of velopharyngeal closure. Cleft Palate J 1973; 10:286–305.
130. Skolnick M, Shprintzen R, McCall G, Rakoff S. Patterns of velopharyngeal closure in subjects with repaired cleft palate and normal speech: a multi-view videofluoroscopic analysis. Cleft Palate J 1975; 12:369–376.
131. Pigott R, Bensen J, White F. Nasendoscopy in the diagnosis of velopharyngeal incompetence. Plast Reconstr Surg 1969; 43(2):141–147.
132. Leung V. Tonsils and adenoids—current thinking. J Nebraska Dent Assoc 1981; 58(2):9–12.
133. Calnan J. Investigation of children with speech defect, with particular reference to nasality. Br Med J 1958; March 29:737–740.
134. Argamaso R, Shprintzen R. Fanfare for a pharyngeal flap. Videotape presentation before the American Cleft Palate Association, Denver, 1982.
135. Crikelair G, Kastein S, Fowler E, Cosman B. Velar dysfunction in the absence of cleft palate. NY State J Med 1964; 64:263–269.
136. Mattucci K. Cleft palate patient: otologic management. NY State J Med 1979; 79:333–339.
137. Stool S, Beery Q. Diagnosis and treatment of ear disease in cleft palate children. In: Bzoch K, ed. Communicative disorders related to cleft lip and palate. 2nd ed. Boston: Little, Brown, 1979:236.
138. Beatty H. Relation between tonsil and adenoid operations and cleft palate. J Am Med Assoc 1951; 145(6):379–381.
139. Gibb A, Stewart I. Hypernasality following tonsil dissection—hysterical aetiology. J Laryngol Otol 1975; 89:779–781.
140. Richstein A, Jonas I. Offenes Naseln nach operativen Eingriffen im Oro- und Nasopharynx. Arch Otorhinolaryngol, 1981; 232:29–41.
141. Sher A, Shprintzen R. Tonsils causing hypernasal speech: a new perspective on lymphoid tissue and speech problems. Presented before the Society for Ear, Nose and Throat Advances in Children, New Orleans, 1984.
142. Abyholm F. Submucous cleft palate. Scan J Plast Reconstr Surg 1976; 10:209–212.
143. Mazaheri M, Millard R, Erickson D. Cineradiographic comparison of normal to noncleft subjects with velopharyngeal inadequacy. Cleft Palate J 1964; 1:199–209.
144. Owsley J, Chierici G, Miller E, Lawson L, Blackfield H. Cephalometric evaluation of palatal dysfunction in patients without cleft palate. Plast Reconstr Surg 1967; 39:562–568.
145. Witzel MA, Rich R, Margar-Bacal F, Cox C. Velopharyngeal insufficiency after adenoidectomy: an 8-year review. Int J Pediatr Otorhinolaryngol 1986; 11:15–20.
146. Lawson L, Chierici G, Castro A, Harvold E, Miller E, Owsley J. Effects of adenoidectomy on the speech of children with potential velopharyngeal dysfunction. J Speech Hear Disord 1972; 37(3):390–402.
147. Gorlin R, Pindborg J, Cohen M. Syndromes of the head and neck. 2nd ed. New York: McGraw-Hill, 1976.
148. de Lange C. Sur un type nouveau de génération (typus Amstelodamensis). Arch Med Enfantes 1933; 36:713–719.
149. Ptacek L, Opitz J, Smith D, Gerritsen T, Waisman H. The Cornelia de Lange syndrome. J Pediatr, 1963; 63:1000–1020.
150. Burdick A, Bixler D, Puckett C. Genetic analysis in families with Van der Woude syndrome. J Craniofac Genet Dev Biol 1985; 5:181–208.
151. Cervenka J, Gorlin R, Anderson V. The syndrome of pits of the lower lip and cleft lip and/or palate: genetic considerations. Am J Hum Genet 1967; 19:416–428.
152. Fogh-Anderson P. Fistula labii inferioris congenita. Tandlaegebladet (Dan Dent J) 1943; 47:411–417.
153. Van der Woude A. Fistula labii inferioris congenita and its association with cleft lip and palate. Am J Hum Genet 1954; 6:244–256.
154. Federman, R, Stoopack J. Moebius syndrome. J Oral Surg 1975; 33:676–678.
155. Henderson J. The congenital facial diplegia syndrome: clinical features, pathology and aetiology. Brain 1939; 62:381–403.
156. Kahane J. Pathophysiological effects of Möbius syndrome on speech and hearing. Arch Otolaryngol 1979; 105:29–34.
157. Meyerson M, Foushee D. Speech, language and hearing in Moebius syndrome: a study of 22 patients. Dev Med Child Neurol 1978; 20:357–365.
158. Rubin A. Handbook of congenital malformations. Philadelphia: WB Saunders, 1967.
159. Salinas C. Orodental findings and genetic disorders. Birth Defects 1982; 18(1):79–120.
160. Bloomer H. Speech defects associated with dental malocclusions and related abnormalities. In: Travis L, ed. Handbook of speech pathology and audiology. New York: Appleton-Century-Crofts, 1971:715.
161. Fymbo L. The relation of malocclusion of the teeth to defects of speech. Arch Speech 1936; 1:204–217.
162. Snow K. Articulation proficiency in relation to certain dental abnormalities. J Speech Hear Res 1961; 4:361–372.
163. Bankson H, Byrne M. The relationship between missing teeth and selected consonant sounds. J Speech Hear Disord 1962; 27(4):341–348.
164. Weinberg B. A cephalometric study of normal and defective /s/ articulation and variations in incisor dentition. J Speech Hear Res 1968; 11:288–300.
165. Starr C. Dental and occlusal hazards to normal speech production. In: Bzoch K, ed. Communicative disorders related to cleft palate. Boston: Little, Brown, 1979:90.
166. Ylippo A, Sovijarvi A. Sonagraphic and palatographic studies of full denture, half denture, and edentulous cases. Acta Odontol Scand 1962; 20:257–299.
167. Chierici G, Parker M, Hemphill C. Influence of immediate dentures on oral motor skill and speech. J Prosthet Dent 1978; 39(1):21–28.
168. Bernstein M. The relation of speech defects and malocclusion. Am J Orthod 1954; 40:149–150.
169. Warren D, Allen G, King H. Physiologic and perceptual

effects of induced anterior open bite. Folia Phoniatr 1984; 36:164–173.

170. Subtelny J, Mestre J, Subtelny J. Comparative study of normal and defective articulation of /s/ as related to malocclusion and deglutition. J Speech Hear Disord 1964; 29: 264–285.
171. Blythe P. The relationship between speech, tongue behavior and occlusal abnormalities. Transl J Br Soc Study Orthod 1959; 52:11–20.
172. Witzel MA, Ross RB, Munro I. Articulation before and after facial osteotomy. J Maxillofac Surg 1980; 8:195–202.
173. Guay A, Maxwell D, Beecher R. A radiographic study of tongue posture at rest and during the phonation of /s/ in Class III malocclusion. Angle Orthod 1978; 48:10–22.
174. Bruggeman C. A study of the relation of malocclusion of teeth and oral deformities to articulatory defects of speech in children. Masters Thesis, University of Iowa, Iowa City, 1934.
175. Turvey T, Journot V, Epker B. Correction of anterior open bite deformity: a study of tongue function, speech changes, and stability. J Maxillofac Surg 1976; 4:93–101.
176. Snidecor J, Kaires A. A speech corrective prosthesis for anterior "open-bite" malocclusion and its effect on two post-dental fricative sounds. J Prosthet Dent 1965; 15:779–784.
177. Goodstein D, Cooper D, Wallace L. The effect on speech of surgery for correction of mandibular prognathism. Oral Surg Oral Biol Oral Pathol 1974; 37(6):846–849.
178. Glass L, Knapp J, Bloomer H. Speech and lingual behavior before and after mandibular osteotomy. J Oral Surg 1977; 35:104–109.
179. Garber S, Speidel T, Marse G. The effects on speech of surgical premaxillary osteotomy. Am J Orthod 1981; 79(1):54–62.
180. Ruscello D, Tekieli M, Van Sickels J. Speech production before and after orthognathic surgery: a review. Oral Surg Oral Med Oral Pathol 1985; 59(1):10–14.
181. Bowers J, Tobey E, Shaye R. An acoustic-speech study of patients who received orthognathic surgery. Am J Orthod 1985; 88(5):373–379.
182. Ewan A. Aspects of speech and orthognathic surgery. In: Lass N, ed. Speech and language: advances in basic research and practice. Vol. 4. New York: Academic Press, 1980:239.
183. Wickwire N, White R, Proffit W. The effect of mandibular osteotomy on tongue position. J Oral Surg 1972; 30: 184–190.
184. Dalston R, Vig P. Effects of orthognathic surgery on speech: a prospective study. Am J Orthod 1984; 86(4):291–298.
185. Schwarz C, Gruner F. Logopedic findings following advancement of the maxilla. J Maxillofac Surg 1976; 4:40–55.
186. Witzel MA, Munro I. Velopharyngeal insufficiency after maxillary advancement. Cleft Palate J 1977; 14:176–180.
187. Mason R, Turvey T, Warren D. Speech considerations after maxillary advancement procedures. J Oral Surg 1980; 38:752–758.
188. McCarthy J, Coccaro P, Schwartz M. Velopharyngeal function following maxillary advancement. Plast Reconstr Surg 1977; 64(2):180–189.
189. Schwartz M, McCarthy J, Coccaro P, Wood-Smith D, Converse J. Velopharyngeal function following maxillary advancement. In: Converse J, McCarthy J, Wood-Smith D, eds. Symposium on diagnosis and treatment of craniofacial anomalies. St Louis: CV Mosby, 1979:277.
190. Mason R. Principles and procedures of orofacial examination. Int J Oral Myol 1980; 6(2):8–19.
191. Kelln E, Bennett C, Klingberg W. Aglossia-adactylia syndrome. Am J Dis Child 1968; 116:549–552.
192. Merson R. Speech rehabilitation in congenital aglossia. J Rehabil 1967; 33(5):32–34.
193. Tuncbilek E, Yalcin C, Atasu M. Aglossia-adactylia syndrome (special emphasis on the inheritance pattern). Clin Genet 1977; 11:421–423.
194. Nevin N, Burrows D, Allen G, Kernohan D. Aglossia-adactylia syndrome. J Med Genet 1975; 12:89–93.
195. Weinberg B, Christiansen R, Logan W, Bosma J, Wornall A. Severe hypoplasia of the tongue. J Speech Hear Disord 1969; 34(2):157–168.
196. Weinberg B, Paras N. Speech intelligibility of a seven-year-old girl with severe congenital hypoplasia of the tongue. Cleft Palate J 1969; 9:436–442.
197. Alvarez G. The aglossia-adactylia syndrome. Br J Plast Surg 1976; 29:175–178.
198. Christian J, Goldberg M, Sturman G, Ingersoll S. Orthodontic-surgical treatment of micrognathia associated with hypoglossia-hypodactylomelia syndrome. J Conn State Dent Assoc 1984; 58(3):156–159.
199. Cohen M, Pantke J, Siris E. Nosologic and genetic considerations in the aglossy-adactyly syndrome. Birth Defects 1981; 7(7):237–240.
200. Cuvelier B, Cousin J, Pauli A, Fournier A, Risbourg B, Piussan CH. L'aglossie-adactylie: deux nouvelle observations. Ann Pediatr (Paris) 1981; 28(6):433–435.
201. Deffez J, Rostand B, Allain P, Brethaux J, Grimbert N, Van Cuc E. Une forme marginale d'aglosso-adactylie. Rev Stomatol Chir Maxillofac 1981; 82(4):241–246.
202. Hall B. Aglossia-adactylia. Birth Defects 1971; 6:233.
203. Stallard M, Saad M. Aglossia-adactylia syndrome. Plast Reconstr Surg 1976; 57:92–95.
204. Browne D. Tongue tie. Br Med J 1959; 2:952.
205. Catlin F, DeHann V. Tongue-tie. Arch Otolaryngol 1971; 94:548–557.
206. DePorte J, Parkhurst E. Congenital malformations and birth injuries among children born in New York State, outside of New York City, in 1940–1942. NY State Med J 1945; 45:1097–1100.
207. Douglas B, Kresberg H. Surgical correction of ankyloglossia. NY State Dent J 1954; 20:477–479.
208. Fletcher S, Daly D. Sublingual dimensions in infants and young children. Arch Otolaryngol 1974; 99:292–296.
209. Fletcher S, Meldrum J. Lingual function and relative length of the lingual frenulum. J Speech Hear Res 1968; 11:382–390.
210. Greene J. Anomalies of the speech mechanism and associated voice and speech disorders. NY State J Med 1945; 45(6):605–608.
211. Horton C, Crawford H, Adamson J, Ashbell T. Tongue-tie. Cleft Palate J 1969; 6:8–23.
212. Mathewson R, Siegel M, McCanna D. Ankyloglossia: a review of the literature and a case report. J Dent Child 1966; 33:238–243.
213. McEnery E, Gaines F. Tongue-tie in infants and children. J Pediatr 1941; 18:252–255.
214. Rogers J, Douglas B. Surgical correction of ankyglossia. United States Armed Forces Med 1952; 31(5):695–697.
215. Spencer W, Cade S. Diseases of the tongue. London: HK Lewis and Company, 1931.
216. Spitzer R. Partial ankyloglossia—report of a case. Oral Surg Oral Med Oral Pathol 1960; 13:787–790.
217. Tuerk M, Lubit E. Ankyloglossia. Plast Reconstr Surg 1959; 24:271–276.
218. Wallace A. Tongue tie. Lancet 1963; 2:377–378.
219. Wallace A. The tongue-tie controversy. Nurs Times 1964; 60:527–528.
220. Whitman C, Rankow R. Diagnosis and management of ankyloglossia. Am J Orthod 1961; 47:423–428.
221. Williams W, Waldron C. Assessment of lingual function when ankyloglossia (tongue-tie) is suspected. J Am Dent Assoc 1985; 110:353–356.
222. Young E, Sacks M. Examining for tongue tie. Clin Pediatr 1979; 18(5):298.

223. Hanson M. Some suggestions for more effective therapy for tongue thrust. J Speech Hear Disord 1967; 32:75–79.
224. Fletcher S, Casteel R, Bradley D. Tongue-thrust swallow, speech articulation and age. J Speech Hear Disord 1961; 26:201–208.
225. Ward M, Malone H, Jann G, Jann H. Articulation variations associated with visceral swallowing and malocclusion. J Speech Hear Disord 1961; 26:334–341.
226. Leighton B. Early development of the deciduous dentition. Dent Practit 1960; 10:100–111.
227. Barrett R. On approach to deviate swallowing. Am J Orthod 1961; 47:726–736.
228. Garliner D. The deviant swallow: a functional approach. J Mass Dent Soc 1964; 13:26–30.
229. Jann G, Ward M, Jann H. Longitudinal study of articulation, deglutition, and malocclusion. J Speech Hear Disord 1964; 29:425–435.
230. Palmer J. Tongue thrusting: a clinical hypothesis. J Speech Hear Disord 1962; 27:323–333.
231. Garliner D. Myofunctional therapy in dental practice. Brooklyn: Bartel Dental Book Company, 1971.
232. Shelton R. Disorders of articulation. In: Skinner P, Shelton R, eds. Speech, language and hearing: normal processes and disorders. Reading, MA: Addison-Wesley Publishing, 1978: 173.
233. Bloomer H. Oral manifestations of dysdiadochokinesis, with oral astereognosia. In: Bosma J, ed. Symposium on oral sensation and perception. Springfield: CC Thomas, 1967: 336.
234. Bloomer H. Speech defects in relation to orthodontics. Am J Orthod 1963; 49(12):920–929.
235. Mason R. Tongue thrust. Oral motor behavior: impact on oral conditions and dental treatment. Proceedings of the Workshop. United States Department of Health, Education, and Welfare, Public Health Service, National Institutes of Health, 1979.
236. Mason R. Update on dental research in relation to speech pathology. Presented before the Illinois Speech-Language-Hearing Association, Chicago, 1987.
237. Mason R, Proffit W. The tongue thrust controversy: background and recommendations. J Speech Hear Disord 1974; 39(2):115–132.
238. Joint Committee on Dentistry and Speech Pathology-Audiology. Position statement on tongue thrust. Asha 1975; 17:331–340.
239. Philips BJ, Kent R. Acoustic-phonetic descriptions of speech production in speakers with cleft palate and other velopharyngeal disorders. In: Lass N, ed. Speech and language: advances in basic research and practice. Vol. 11. New York: Academic Press, 1984:113.
240. Forner L. Speech segment durations produced by five and six year old speakers with and without cleft palates. Cleft Palate J 1983; 20:185–198.
241. Jones D, Folkins J. Effect of speaking rate on judgments of disordered speech in children with cleft palate. Cleft Palate J 1985; 22(4):246–252.
242. Karnell M, Folkins J, Morris H. Relationships between the perception of nasalization and speech movements in speakers with cleft palate. J Speech Hear Res 1985; 28:63–72.
243. Leder S, Lerman J. Some acoustic evidence for vocal abuse in adult speakers with repaired cleft palate. Laryngoscope 1985; 95:837–840.
244. Warren D, Dalston R, Trier W, Holder M. A pressure-flow technique for quantifying temporal patterns of palatal pharyngeal closure. Cleft Palate J 1985; 22:11–19.
245. Morris H. Etiological bases for speech problems. In: Spriestersbach D, Sherman D, eds. Cleft Palate and Communication. New York: Academic Press, 1968.
246. McWilliams BJ. Some factors in the intelligibility of cleft-palate speech. J Speech Hear Disord 1954; 19(4):524–527.
247. Weiss C. Oral and nasal sound levels as related to judged severity on nasality. Doctoral Dissertation, Purdue University, 1954.
248. Shelton R, Knox A, Arndt W, Elbert M. The relationship between nasality score values and oral and nasal sound pressure level. J Speech Hear Res 1967; 10:549–557.
249. Edgerton M, Sadove M, Compton M, Bull G, Blomain E, McDonald W, Bralley R. Nasal vibration analysis: a noninvasive objective technique to evaluate the speech of patients with palatal pharyngeal disorders. Plast Reconstr Surg 1981; 68:153–157.
250. Horii Y, Lang J. Distributional analyses of an index of nasal coupling (HONC) in simulated hypernasal speech. Cleft Palate J 1981; 18:279–285.
251. Barnes I, Morris H. Interrelationships among oral breath pressure ratios and articulation skills for individuals with cleft palate. J Speech Hear Res 1967; 10:506–514.
252. Brandt S, Morris H. The linearity of the relationship between articulation errors and velopharyngeal incompetence. Cleft Palate J 1965; 2:176–183.
253. Morris H. The oral manometer as a diagnostic tool in clinical speech pathology. J Speech Hear Disord 1966; 31:362–369.
254. Pitzner J, Morris H. Articulation skills and adequacy of breath pressure ratios of children with cleft palate. J Speech Hear Disord 1965; 30(1):26–40.
255. Shelton R, Brooks A, Youngstrom K. Articulation and patterns of palatopharyngeal closure. J Speech Hear Disord 1964; 29(4):390–408.
256. Shelton R, Brooks A, Youngstrom K. Clinical assessment of palatopharyngeal closure. J Speech Hear Disord 1965; 30 (1):37–43.
257. Spriestersbach D, Powers G. Articulation skills, velopharyngeal closure, and oral breath pressure of children with cleft palates. J Speech Hear Res 1959; 2:318–325.
258. Spriestersbach D, Moll K, Morris H. Subject classification and articulation of speakers with cleft palates. J Speech Hear Res 1961; 4(4):362–372.
259. VanDemark D. A comparison of the results of pressure articulation testing in various contexts for subjects with cleft palates. J Speech Hear Res 1970; 13:741–754.
260. VanDemark D. A factor analysis of the speech of children with cleft palate. Cleft Palate J 1966; 3:159–170.
261. VanDemark D. Misarticulations and listener judgements of the speech of individuals with cleft palates. Cleft Palate J 1964; 1:232–245.
262. Lubker J. Aerodynamic and ultrasonic assessment techniques in speech-dentofacial research. In: Fricke IE, ed. ASHA Reports #5: speech and the dentofacial complex: the state of the art. Washington: American Speech and Hearing Association, 1970:207.
263. Machida J. Air flow rate and articulatory movements during speech. Cleft Palate J 1967; 4:240–248.
264. Warren D. Velopharyngeal orifice size and upper pharyngeal pressure-flow patterns in cleft palate speech: a preliminary study. Plast Reconstr Surg 1964; 34:15–26.
265. Warren D. Velopharyngeal orifice size and upper pharyngeal pressure-flow patterns in normal speech. Plast Reconstr Surg 1964; 33:148–162.
266. Warren D, Duany L, Fischer N. Nasal pathway resistance in normal and cleft lip and palate subjects. Cleft Palate J. 1969; 6:134–140.
267. Warren D, Mackler S. Duration of oral port constriction in normal and cleft palate speech. J Speech Hear Res 1968; 11:291–301.
268. Bjork L. Velopharyngeal function in connected speech. Acta Radiol [Suppl] (Stockholm) 1961.
269. Dalson R, Warren D. Comparison of Tonar II, pressure-flow and listener judgments in the assessment of velopharyngeal function. Cleft Palate J 1986; 23:108–115.

270. Carney P, Morris H. Structural correlates of nasality. Cleft Palate J 1971; 8:307–321.
271. Fritzell B. The velopharyngeal muscles in speech: an electromyographic and cineradiographic study. Acta Otolaryngol [Suppl] (Stockholm) 1969.
272. Hoopes J, Dellon A, Fabrikant J, Edgerton M, Soliman A. Cineradiographic definition of the functional anatomy and pathophysiology of the velopharynx. Cleft Palate J 1970; 7:443–453.
273. Lubker J. An electromyographic-cinefluorographic investigation of velar function during normal speech production. Cleft Palate J 1968; 5:1–18.
274. Lubker J, Moll K. Simultaneous oral-nasal air flow measurements and cinefluorographic observations during speech production. Cleft Palate J 1965; 2:257–272.
275. Moll K. A cinefluorographic study of velopharyngeal function in normals during various activities. Cleft Palate J 1965; 2:112–122.
276. Moll K. Cinefluorographic techniques in speech research. J Speech Hear Res 1960; 3:227–241.
277. Moll K. Velopharyngeal closure on vowels. J Speech Hear Res 1962; 5:30–37.
278. Powers G. Cinefluorographic investigation of articulatory movements of selected individuals with cleft palates. J Speech Hear Res 1962; 5(1):59–69.
279. Shaw R, Folkins J, Kuehn D. Comparison of methods for measuring velar position from lateral-view cineradiography. Cleft Palate J 1980; 17(4):326–329.
280. Subtelny J, McCormack R, Subtelny J, Worth J, Cramer L, Runyon J, Rosenblum R. Synchronous recording of speech associated with physiological and pressure-flow dynamics: instrumentation and procedures. Cleft Palate J 1968; 5:93–116.
281. Subtelny J. Physio-acoustic considerations in radiographic study of speech. Cleft Palate J 1964; 1:402–410.
282. Wada T, Yasumoto M, Ideoka N, Fujiki Y, Yoshinaga R. An approach for the cinefluorographic study of articulatory movements. Cleft Palate J 1970; 7:506–522.
283. Warren D, Hofmann F. A cineradiographic study of velopharyngeal closure. Plast Reconstr Surg 1961; 28(6):656–669.
284. Williams W, Eisenbach C. Assessing VP function: the lateral still techniqiue vs. cinefluorography. Cleft Palate J 1981; 18(1):45–50.
285. Williams W. Radiological measures of abnormal speech physiology. In: Bzoch K, ed. Communicative disorders related to cleft lip and palate. Boston: Little, Brown, 1979:249.
286. Griffith B, Monroe C, Hill B, Waldrop W, White H. Motion of the lateral pharyngeal walls during velopharyngeal closure. Plast Reconstr Surg 1968; 41(4):338–342.
287. LaRossa D, Brown A, Cohen M, Spackman T. Videoradiography of the velopharyngeal portal using the Towne's view. J Maxillofac Surg 1980; 8:203–205.
288. Pigott R. An assessment of some surgical techniques used in the management of palatal incompetence. In: Ellis R, Flack F, eds., Diagnosis and treatment of palato glossal malfunction. London: College of Speech Therapists, 1979:67.
289. Shprintzen R, Lavorato A, Rakoff S, Skolnick M. Incongruous movements of the velum and lateral pharyngeal walls. Cleft Palate J 1977; 14:148–157.
290. Shprintzen R, McCall G, Skolnick M, Lencione R. Selective movement of the lateral aspects of the pharyngeal walls during velopharyngeal closure for speech, blowing and whistling in normals. Cleft Palate J 1975; 12(1):51–58.
291. Skolnick M. Video velopharyngography in patients with nasal speech, with emphasis on lateral pharyngeal motion in velopharygeal closure. Radiology 1969; 93:747–755.
292. Skolnick M. Velopharyngeal function in cleft palate. Clin Plast Surg 1975; 2(2):285–297.
293. Skolnick M, McCall G. Velopharyngeal competence and incompetence following pharyngeal flap surgery: a videofluoroscopic study in multiple projections. Cleft Palate J 1972; 9:1–12.
294. Stringer D, Witzel MA. Waters projection for the evaluation of lateral pharyngeal wall movement in speech disorders. Am J Roentgenol 1985; 145:409–410.
295. Zwitman D, Gyepes M, Sample F. The submentovertical projection in the radiographic analysis of velopharyngeal dynamics. J Speech Hear Disord 1973; 38(4):473–477.
296. Zwitman D, Gyepes M, Ward P. Assessment of velar and lateral wall movement by oral telescope and radiographic examination in patients with velopharyngeal inadequacy and in normal subjects. J Speech Hear Disord 1976; 41:381–389.
297. Zwitman D, Sonderman J, Ward P. Variations in velopharyngeal closure assessed by endoscopy. J Speech Hear Disord 1974; 39(3):366–372.
298. McWilliams BJ. Unresolved issues in velopharyngeal valving. Cleft Palate J 1985; 22(1):29–33.
299. Taub S. The Taub oral panendoscope: a new technique. Cleft Palate J 1966; 3:328–346.
300. Willis C, Stutz M. The clinical use of the Taub oral panendoscope in the observation of velopharyngeal function. J Speech Hear Disord 1972; 37:495–502.
301. Albery E, Bennett J, Pigott R, Simmons R. The results of 100 operations for velopharyngeal incompetence—selected on the findings of endoscopic and radiological examination. Br J Plast Surg 1982; 35:118–126.
302. Bell Berti F, Baer T, Harris K, Niimi S. Coarticulatory effects of vowel quality on velar function. Phonetica 1979; 26:187–193.
303. David D, White J, Sprod R, Bagnall A. Nasendoscopy: significant refinements of a direct-viewing technique of the velopharyngeal sphincter (with comment by Makepeace and Pigott). Plast Reconstr Surg 1982; 70:423–428.
304. Dellon A, Hall C, Chretien P. Fiberoptic endoscopy in the head and neck region. Plast Reconstr Surg 1975; 55(4):466–471.
305. Fujimura O. Model studies of tongue gestures and the derivation of vocal tract area functions. In: Sawashima M, Cooper F, eds. Dynamic aspects of speech production. Tokyo: University of Tokyo Press, 1977:225.
306. Gilbert S, Pigott R. The feasibility of nasal pharyngoscopy using the 70° Storz-Hopkins nasopharyngoscope. Br J Plast Surg 1982; 35:14–18.
307. Goto T. Tightness in velopharyngeal closure and its regulatory mechanism. J Osaka Univ Dent School 1977; 22(1):87–106.
308. Harris K. Physiological measures of speech movements: EMG and fiberoptic studies. In: Fricke JE, ed. ASHA Report #5: speech and the dentofacial complex. Washington: American Speech and Hearing Association, 1970:271.
309. Heiner H, Schumann D, Erler U. Endoskopie und Elektromyographie zur Beuteilung der velopharyngealen Funktion beim Spalttrager. Stomatol DDR 1981; 31:819–827.
310. Honjo I, Mitoma T, Ushiro K, Kawano M. Evaluation of velopharyngeal closure by CT scan and endoscopy. Plast Reconstr Surg 1984; 74(5):620–627.
311. Huskie C, McGrouther D. The applications of nasendoscopy to the diagnosis of speech problems. In: Ellis R, Flack F, eds. Diagnosis and treatment of palato glossal malfunction. London: College of Speech Therapists, 1979:22.
312. Ibuki K, Karnell M, Morris H. Reliability of the nasopharyngeal fiberscope (NPF) for assessing velopharyngeal function. Cleft Palate J 1983; 20(2):97–104.
313. Karnell M, Ibuki K, Morris H, VanDemark K. Reliability of the nasopharyngeal fiberscope (NPF) for assessing velopharyngeal function: analysis by judgment. Cleft Palate J 1983; 20(3):199–208.
314. Matsuya T, Miyazaki T, Yamaoka M. Fibroscopic examinations of velopharyngeal closure in normal individuals. Cleft Palate J 1974; 11:286–291.

315. Matsuya T, Yamaoka M, Miyazaki T. A fiberoptic study of velopharyngeal closure in patients with operated cleft palates. Plast Reconstr Surg 1979; 63(4):497–500.
316. Miyazaki T, Matsuya T, Yamaoka M. Fiberscopic methods for assessment of the velopharyngeal closure during various activities. Cleft Palate J 1975; 12:107–114.
317. Niimi S, Bell-Berti F, Harris K. Dynamic aspects of velopharyngeal closure. Folia Phoniatr (Basel) 1982; 34:246–257.
318. Osberg P, Witzel M. The physiologic basis for hypernasality during connected speech in cleft palate patients: a nasendoscopic study. Plast Reconstr Surg 1981; 67(1): 1–5.
319. Pigott R. The development of endoscopy of the palatopharyngeal isthmus. Proc R Soc Lond, 1977; 195:269–275.
320. Pigott R. The nasendoscopic appearance of the normal palato-pharyngeal valve. Plast Reconstr Surg 1969; 43(1):19–24.
321. Pigott R, Makepeace A. Technique of recording nasopharyngoscopy. B J Plast Surg 1975; 28(1):26–33.
322. Sawashima M, Ushijima T. The use of fiberscope in speech research. In: Hirschberg J, Szepe G, Vass-Kovacs E, eds. Papers in interdisciplinary speech research. Budapest: Akademiai Kiado, 1971:229.
323. Sawashima M. Current instrumentation and techniques for observing speech organs. Technocrat 1976; 9:19–26.
324. Sawashima M. Fiberoptic observation of the larynx and other speech organs. In: Sawashima M, Cooper F, eds. Dynamic aspects of speech production. Tokyo: University of Tokyo Press, 1977:31.
325. Sommerlad B, Hackett M, Watson J. A simplified method of recording nasal pharyngoscopy. Br J Plast Surg 1975; 28: 34–36.
326. Sugai T, Ibuki K, Matusuya T, Miyazaki T, Wada T, Iwasaki H. Video-fiberscopic examination for velopharyngeal movement: a new field by field analysis using video tape recording procedures. J Jpn Cleft Palate Assoc 1983; 8(2): 217–227.
327. Ushijima T, Sawahima M. Fiberscopic observation of velar movements during speech. Ann Bull Res Inst Logoped Phoniatr 1972; 6:25–38.
328. Subtelny J, Subtelny J. Intelligibility and associated physiological factors of cleft palate speakers. J Speech Hear Res 1959; 2:353–360.
329. Subtelny J, Koepp-Baker H, Subtelny J. Palatal function and cleft palate speech. J Speech Hear Disord 1961; 26(3): 213–224.
330. McWilliams BJ, Ratings of velopharyngeal closure during blowing and speech. Cleft Palate J 1965; 2:46–55.
331. McWilliams BJ, Glaser E, Philips B, Lawrence C, Lavorato A, Beery Q, Skolnick M. A comparative study of four methods of evaluating velopharyngeal adequacy. Plast Reconstr Surg 1981; 68(1):1–9.
332. Honjow I, Isshiki N, Morimoto M. Aerodynamic patterns of cleft palate speech. Plast Reconstr Surg 1968; 42:465–471.
333. Isshiki N, Honjow I, Morimoto M. Effects of velopharyngeal incompetence upon speech. Cleft Palate J 1968; 5:297–310.
334. Warren D. The velopharyngeal sphincter: a control factor in the speech regulating system. Presented before the American Speech-Language-Hearing Association, Detroit, 1986.
335. Morris H. Cleft palate. In: Weston A, ed. Communicative disorders. Springfield: CC Thomas, 1972:128.
336. Hoch L, Golding-Kushner K, Siegel-Sadewitz V, Shprintzen R. Speech therapy. Semin Speech Lang 1986; 7(3):313–326.
337. Berry M, Eisenson J. Speech disorders: principles and practices of therapy. New York: Appleton-Century-Crofts, 1956.
338. Buck M, Harrington R. Organized speech therapy for cleft palate rehabilitation. J Speech Hear Disord 1949; 14:43–52.
339. Eckelmann D, Baldridge P. Speech training for the child with a cleft palate. J Speech Disord 1945; 10:137–147.
340. Kantner C. The rationale of blowing exercises for patients with repaired cleft palates. J Speech Disord 1947; 12:281–286.
341. Luchsinger R, Arnold G. Voice, speech and language: clinical communicology. Belmont, CA: Wadsworth Publishing, 1965.
342. Massengill R, Quinn G, Pickrell K, Levinson C. Therapeutic exercise and velopharyngeal gap. Cleft Palate J 1968; 5:44–47.
343. Morley M. Cleft palate and speech. 1st ed. Baltimore: Williams and Wilkins, 1945.
344. Moser H. Diagnostic and clinical procedures in rhinolalia. J Speech Disord 1942; 7(1):1–4.
345. VanRiper C. Speech correction: principles and methods. New York: Prentice-Hall, 1947.
346. VanRiper C. Speech correction: principles and methods. 4th ed. Englewood Cliffs, NJ: Prentice-Hall, 1963.
347. Wells C. Improving the speech of the cleft palate child. J Speech Disord 1945; 10:162–168.
348. Wells C. Practical techniques in speech training for cleft palate cases. J Speech Hear Disord 1948; 13:71–73.
349. West R, Ansberry M, Carr A. The rehabilitation of speech. New York: Harper, 1957.
350. Shelton R, Hahn E, Morris H. Diagnosis and therapy. In: Spriestersbach D, Sherman D, eds. Cleft palate and communication. New York: Academic Press, 1968:225.
351. Shelton R. Therapeutic exercise and speech pathology. Asha 1963; 5(12):855–859.
352. Shelton R, Chisum L, Youngstrom K, Arndt W, Elbert M. Effect of articulation therapy on palatopharyngeal closure, movement of the pharyngeal wall, and tongue posture. Cleft Palate J 1969; 6:440–448.
353. Hixon T, Hardy J. Restricted motility of the speech articulators in cerebral palsy. J Speech Hear Disord 1964; 29(3):294–306.
354. Blakeley R. The complementary use of speech prostheses and pharyngeal flaps in palatal insufficiency. Cleft Palate J 1964; 1:194–198.
355. Blakeley B. The rationale for a temporary speech prosthesis in palatal insufficiency. Br J Disord Commun 1969; 4:134–139.
356. Cole R. Cleft lip and palate: problems and progress. Chicago Med School Q 1966; Fall:129–136.
357. Fletcher S, Haskins R, Bosma J. A movable bulb appliance to assist in palato-pharyngeal closure. J Speech Hear Disord 1960; 25:249–258.
358. Harkins C, Harkins W, Harkins J. Principles of cleft palate prosthesis. New York: Columbia Unviersity Press, 1960.
359. Rosen M, Bzoch K. The prosthetic speech applicance in rehabilitation of patients with cleft palate. J Am Dent Assoc 1958; 57:103–120.
360. Warren D. A physiologic approach to cleft palate prosthesis. J Prosthet Dent 1965; 15(4):770–778.
361. Weiss C. Success of an obturator reduction program. Cleft Palate J 1971; 8:291–297.
362. Shelton R, Lindquist A, Arndt W, Elbert M, Youngstrom K. Effect of speech bulb reduction on movement of the posterior wall of the pharynx and posture of the tongue. Cleft Palate J 1971; 8:10–17.
363. Cole R. Direct muscle training for the improvement of velopharyngeal activity. In: Bzoch K, ed. Communicative disorders related to cleft lip and palate. Boston: Little, Brown, 1979:328.
364. Lubit E, Larsen R. A speech aid for velopharyngeal incompetency. J Speech Hear Disord 1971; 36(1):61–70.
365. Lubit E, Larsen R. The Lubit palatal exerciser: a preliminary report. Cleft Palate J 1969; 6:120–139.

366. Massengill R, Quinn G, Pickrell K. The use of a palatal stimulator to decrease velopharyngeal gap. Ann Otol Rhinol Laryngol 1971; 80:135–137.
367. Yules R, Chase R. Pharyngeal flap surgery: a review of the literature. Cleft Palate J 1969; 6:303–308.
368. Weber J, Jobe R, Chase R. Evaluation of muscle stimulation in the rehabilitation of patients with hypernasal speech. Plast Reconstr Surg 1970; 46:173–174.
369. Peterson S. Electrical stimulation of the soft palate. Cleft Palate J 1974; 11:72–86.
370. Shelton R, Harris K, Sholes G, Dooley P. Study of nonspeech voluntary palate movements by scaling and electromyographic techniques. In: Bosma J, ed. Second symposium on oral sensation and perception. Springfield: CC Thomas, 1970:432.
371. Shelton R, Knox A, Elbert M, Johnson T. Palate awareness and nonspeech voluntary palate movement. In: Bosma J, ed. Second symposium on oral sensation and perception. Springfield: CC Thomas, 1970:416.
372. Tash E, Shelton R, Knox A, Michel J. Training voluntary pharyngeal wall movements in children with normal and inadequate velopharyngeal closure. Cleft Palate J 1971; 8: 277–290.
373. Powers G, Starr C. The effects of muscle exercises on velopharyngeal gap and nasality. Cleft Palate J 1974; 11:28–35.
374. Peterson S. Velopharyngeal closure: some important differences. J Speech Hear Disord, 1973; 39:89–97.
375. Shprintzen R, McCall G, Skolnick M. A new therapeutic technique for the treatment of velopharyngeal incompetence. J Speech Hear Disord 1975; 40(1):69–83.
376. Shelton R, Paesani A, McClelland K, Bradfield S. Panendoscopic feedback in the study of voluntary velopharyngeal movements. J Speech Hear Disord 1975; 40:232–244.
377. Siegel-Sadewitz V, Shprintzen R. Nasopharyngoscopy of the normal velopharyngeal sphincter: an experiment of biofeedback. Cleft Palate J 1982; 19(3):194–200.
378. Nishio J, Yamaoka M, Matsuya T, Miyazaki T. How to exercise the velopharyngeal movement by the velopharyngeal fiberscope. Jpn J Oral Surg 1974; 20:450–457.
379. Shelton R, Ruscello D. Palatal and articulation training in patients with velopharyngeal closure problems. Presented before the American Clelft Palate Association, San Diego, 1979.
380. Shelton R, Beaumont K, Trier W, Furr M. Videoendoscopic feedback in training velopharyngeal closure. Cleft Palate J 1978; 15(1):6–12.
381. Yamaoka M, Matsuya T, Miyazaki T, Nishio J, Ibuki N. Visual training for velopharyngeal closure in cleft palate patients: a fiberscopic procedure. J Maxillofac Surg 1983; 11 (4):191–193.
382. Moller K, Path M, Werth L, Christiansen R. The modification of velar movement. J Speech Hear Disord 1973; 38:323–334.
383. Tudor C, Selley W. A palatal training appliance and a visual aid for use in the treatment of hypernasal speech. Br J Disord Commun 1974; 9:117–122.
384. Curle H. Therapeutic methods for the incompetent soft palate. In: Ellis R, Flack F, eds. Diagnosis and treatment of palato glossal malfunction. London: College of Speech Therapists, 1979:62.
385. Flack F. Experiments with a simple monitor for soft palate movement. In: Ellis R, Flack F. Diagnosis and treatment of palato glossal malfunction. London: College of Speech Therapists, 1979:45.
386. Kunzel H. First applications of a biofeedback device for the therapy of velopharyngeal incompetence. Folia Phoniatr (Basel) 1982; 34:92–100.
387. Dalston R. Photodetector assessment of velopharyngeal activity. Cleft Palate J 1982; 19:1–8.
388. Garber S, Moller K. The effects of feedback filtering on nasalization in normal and hypernasal speakers. J Speech Hear Res 1979; 22:321–333.
389. Burzynski C, Starr C. Effects of feedback filtering on nasalization and self-perception of nasality. J Speech Hear Res 1985; 28(4):585–588.
390. Daly D, Johnson H. Instrumental modification of hypernasal voice quality in retarded children: case reports. J Speech Hear Disord 1974; 39:500–507.
391. Warren D. PERCI: a method for rating palatal efficiency. Cleft Palate J 1979; 16:279–285.
392. Glaser E, Shprintzen R. See-scape: instrument and manual (review). Cleft Palate J 1979; 16:213–214.
393. Chisum L, Shelton R, Arndt W, Elbert M. The relationship between remedial speech instruction activities and articulation change. Cleft Palate J 1969; 6:57–64.
394. Shelton R. Modification of oral-facial function during speech. In: Fricke JE, ed. ASHA Report No. 5: speech and dentofacial complex: the state of the art. Washington: American Speech and Hearing Association, 1970:146.
395. Peterson-Falzone S. Articulation disorders in orofacial anomalies. In: Lass N, McReynolds L, Northern J, Yoder D, eds. Speech, language, and hearing, Vol. 2. Philadelphia: WB Saunders, 1982:611.
396. Amerman J, Laminack C. Evaluation and rehabilitation of glossectomy speech behavior. J Commun Disord 1974; 7:365–374.
397. Luchsinger R, Arnold G. Voice, speech and language: clinical communicology. Belmont, CA: Wadsworth Publishing, 1965.
398. Backus O. Speech rehabilitation following excision of the tip of the tongue. Am J Disabl Child 1940; 60:368–370.
399. Bloomer H, Hawk A. Speech considerations: speech disorders associated with ablative surgery of the face, mouth and pharynx—ablative approaches to learning. In Wertz RT, ed. ASHA Report No. 8: orofacial anomalies: clinical and research implications. Washington: American Speech and Hearing Association, 1973:42.
400. Brodnitz F. Speech after glossectomy. In: Current problems in phoniatrics and logopedics. Basel: Karger, 1960:42.
401. Brodnitz F. Vocal rehabilitation. Rochester: American Academy of Otolaryngology, 1965.
402. Cantor R, Curtis T. Prosthetic management of edentulous mandibulectomy patients. Part I. Anatomic, physiologic and psychologic considerations. J Prosthet Dent 1971; 25:446–457.
403. Cantor R, Curtis T, Shipp T, Beumer J, Vogel B. Maxillary speech prostheses for mandibular surgical defects. J Prosthet Dent 1969; 22(2):253–260.
404. deSouza I, Martins O. Swallowing and speech after radical total glossectomy with tongue prosthesis. Oral Surg 1975; 39(3):356–360.
405. Donaldson R, Skelly M. Paletta F. Total glossectomy for cancer. Am J Surg 1968; 116:585–590.
406. Duguay M. Speech after glossectomy. NY State J Med 1964; 64:1836–1838.
407. Fleming S, Weaver A, Rourke D. A correlational study of speech intelligibility of glossectomy patients. Presented before the American Speech-Language-Hearing Association, San Francisco, 1978.
408. Goldstein J. Speech without a tongue. J Speech Hear Disord 1940; 5:65–69.
409. Herberman M. Rehabilitation of patients following glossectomy. Arch Otolaryngol 1958; 67:182–183.
410. Kalfuss A. Analysis of the speech of the glossectomee. Doctoral dissertation, Wayne State University, Detroit, 1968.
411. Kipfmueller L, Lang B. Treating velopharyngeal inadquacies with a palatal lift prosthesis. J Prosthet Dent 1972; 27:467–477.
412. Logemann J, Bytell D. Articulation patterns of five groups

of head and neck surgical patients. Presented before the American Speech-Language-Hearing Association, San Francisco, 1978.

413. Massengill R, Maxwell S, Pickrell K. An analysis of articulation following partial and total glossectomy. J Speech Hear Disord 1970; 35:170–173.

414. Skelly M, Donaldson R, Fust R, Townsend D. Changes in phonatory aspects of glossectomee intelligibility through vocal parameter manipulation. J Speech Hear Disord 1972; 37(3):379–389.

415. Skelly M. Glossectomee speech rehabilitation. Springfield: CC Thomas, 1973.

416. Arndt W, Shelton R, Bradford L. Articulation, voice, and obturation in persons with acquired and congenital palate defects. Cleft Palate J 1965; 2:377–383.

417. Davidson T, Drane J, Matalon V. Emotional aspects of new prostheses for previously treated maxillofacial patients. J Prosthet Dent 1975; 34(1):55–58.

418. Fletcher S, Sooudi I, Frost S. Quantitative and graphic analysis of prosthetic treatment for "nasalance" in speech. J Prosthet Dent 1974; 32(3):284–291.

419. Lauciello R, Vergo T, Schaaf N, Zimmerman R. J Prosthet Dent 1980; 43(2):204–211.

420. Logemann J, Wheeler R. A maxillary reshaping prosthesis for head and neck surgical patients. Presented before the American Speech-Language-Hearing Association, Houston, 1976.

421. Majid A, Weinberg B, Chalian V. Speech intelligibility following prosthetic obturation of surgically acquired maxillary defects. J Prosthet Dent 1974; 32(1):87–96.

422. Moore D. Glossectomy rehabilitation by mandibular tongue prosthesis. J Prosthet Dent 1972; 28(4):429–433.

423. Moore D, Pishney J, Welch T. Comparison of rigid and flexible obturation for surgical cleft of the soft palate. J Prosthet Dent 1985; 54(4):548–552.

424. United States Department of Health and Human Services. Progress against cancer of the mouth. 1985.

425. Plank D, Weinberg B, Chalian V. Evaluation of speech following prosthetic obturation of surgically aquired maxillar defects. J Prosthet Dent, 1981; 45(6):626–638.

426. Ackerman A. The prosthetic management of oral and facial defects following cancer surgery. J Prosthet Dent 1955; 5:413–432.

427. Adisman I. Removable partial dentures for jaw defects of the maxilla and mandible. Dent Clin North Am 1962; 6: 848–870.

428. Aramany M, Drane J. Effect of nasal extension sections on the voice quality of acquired cleft palate patients. J Prosthet Dent 1972; 27:197–202.

429. Baden E. Prosthetic therapy of congenital and acquired clefts of the palate. J Hist Med Allied Sci 1955; 10:290–301.

430. Boucher L, Heupel E. Prosthetic restoration of the maxilla and associated structures. J Prosthet Dent 1966; 16:154–168.

431. Chalian V, Barnett M. A new technique for constructing a one-piece hollow bulb obturator after partial maxillectomy. J Prosthet Dent 1972; 28:448–453.

432. Drane J, Guerra L. Prosthetics and reconstruction. J Am Med Assoc 1972; 219:351–353.

433. Gutman D, Malberg E, Neder A. Management of surgical defects of the maxilla. J Oral Surg 1964; 22:244–248.

434. Hammond J. Dental care of edentulous patients after resection of maxilla. Br Dent J 1966; 12:591–594.

435. King G. Maxillofacial prosthetic rehabilitation. J Oral Surg 1971; 29:805–811.

436. Migliani D, Drane J. Maxillofacial prosthesis and its role as a healing art. J Prosthet Dent 1959; 9:159–168.

437. Nadeau J. Special prosthesis. J Prosthet Dent 1968; 20:62–76.

438. Nidiffer T, Shipmon T. The hollow bulb obturator for acquired palatal openings. J Prosthet Dent 1957; 7:125–134.

439. Payne A, Welton W. An inflatable obturator for use following maxillectomy. J Prosthet Dent 1965; 15:759–763.

440. Pettit L, Williams B, Ryan R. Prosthesis after maxillectomy. J Prosthet Dent 1960; 10:983–986.

441. Rahn A, Boucher L. Maxillofacial prosthetics. Philadelphia: WB Saunders, 1970.

442. Robinson J. Prosthetic treatment after surgical removal of the maxilla and the floor of the orbit. J Prosthet Dent 1963; 13:178–184.

443. Sala H, Spear J. Resection of the upper jaw and its immediate restoration. Oral Surg Oral Med Oral Pathol 1960; 13:1033–1037.

444. Zarb B. The maxillary resection and its prosthetic replacement. J Prosthet Dent 1967; 18:268–281.

445. Oral K, Aramany M, McWilliams BJ. Speech intelligibility with the buccal flange obturator. J Prosthet Dent 1979; 41(3):323–327.

446. Bradley D. Congenital and acquired palatopharyngeal insufficiency. In: Bzoch K, ed. Communicative disorders related to cleft lip and palate. Boston: Little, Brown, 1979:77.

447. Curtis T, Cantor R. The forgotten patient in maxillofacial prosthetics. J Prosthet Dent 1974; 31(6):662–680.

448. Skelly M, Spector D, Donaldson R, Brodeur A, Paletta F. Compensatory physiologic phonetics for the glossectomee. J Speech Hear Disord 1971; 36(1):101–114.

449. Lehman W, Hulicka I, Mehringer E. Prosthetic treatment following complete glossectomy. J Prosthet Dent 1966; 16(2):344–350.

450. LaRiviere C, Seilo M, Dimmick K. Report on the speech intellibility of a glossectomee: perceptual and acoustic observations. Folia Phoniatr (Basel) 1975; 27:201–214.

451. Skelly M, Donaldson R, Schinsky L. Substitution consistency as a factor in glossectomee intelligibility. J Missouri Speech Hear Assoc 1972; 5:21–23.

452. Eskew H, Shepard E. Congenital aglossia. Am J Orthod 1949; 35:116–119.

453. Ballard J, Kerner E, Tyson J, Ashford J, Rees R. Adenocarcinoma of the tongue complicated by a hemimandibulectomy: soft tissue support for a tongue prosthesis in an edentulous glossectomy patients. J Prosthet Dent 1986; 56(4):470–473.

454. Gillis R, Leonard R. Prosthetic treatment for speech and swallowing in patients with total glossectomy. J Prosthet Dent 1983; 50(6):808–814.

455. McKinstry R, Aramany M, Beery Q, Sansome F. Speech considerations in prosthodontic rehabilitation of the glossectomy patient. J Prosthet Dent 1985; 53(3):384–387.

456. Knowles J, Chalian V, Shanks J. A functional speech impression used to fabricate a maxillary speech prosthesis for a partial glossectomy patient. J Prosthet Dent 1984; 51(2):232–237.

457. Wheeler R, Logemann J, Rosen M. Maxillary reshaping prostheses: effectiveness in improving speech and swallowing of postsurgical oral cancer patients. J Prosthet Dent 1980; 43(3):313–319.

458. Shedd D. Rehabilitation problems of head and neck cancer patients. J Surg Oncol 1976; 8:11–21

459. Meyerson M, Johnson B, Weitzman R. Rehabilitation of a patient with complete mandibulectomy and partial glossectomy. Am J Otolaryngol 1980; 1(3):256–261.

460. Christensen J, Hutton J, Hasegawa A, Fletcher S. Evaluation of the effects of palatal augmentation on partial glossectomy speech. J Prosthet Dent 1983; 50(4):539–543.

461. Aramany M, Downs J, Beery Q, Aslan Y. Prosthodontic rehabilitation for glossectomy patients. J Prosthet Dent 1982; 48:78–82.

462. Belsky M. Prosthetic reconstruction of mandibular tongue prostheses. J Prosthet Dent 1978; 39(6):650–653.

463. Chamber R, Jaques D, Mahoney W. Tongue flaps for intraoral reconstruction. Am J Surg 1969; 18:783–786.
464. Corso P, Gerald F. Immediate and secondary reconstruction of the floor of the mouth and rehabilitation of the tongue by a new method. Am J Surg 1963; 104:727–731.
465. DeSanto L. Lingual flap reconstruction after resection for cancer. Trans Am Acad Ophthalmol Otolaryngol 1974; 78:135–139.
466. Helpser J, Fister H. Use of skin grafts in the mouth in the management of oral cancer. Am J Surg 1967; 114:596–600.
467. Myers E. Reconstruction of the oral cavity. Otolaryngol Clin North Am 1972; 5:421–422.
468. Papioannou A, Farr H. Reconstruction of the floor of the mouth by a pedicle tongue flap. Surg Gynecol Obstet 1966; 122:807–810.
469. Sessions D, Dedo D, Ogura H. Tongue flap reconstruction in cancer of the oral cavity. Arch Otolaryngol 1975; 101: 166–169.
470. Som M, Nussbaum M. Marginal resection of the mandible with reconstruction by tongue flap for carcinoma of the floor of the mouth. Am J Surg 1971; 121:679–683.
471. Washio H. Use of a pterygoid muscle sling to provide glossomimic function after total glossectomy. Plast Reconstr Surg 1973; 51:497–500.
472. Schoenborn K. Ueber eine neve Nethche ves Verhandl de Deutsch. Arch Klin Chir 1876; 10:527–531.

17 Speech Disorders Related to Craniofacial Structural Defects: Part 2

Sally J. Peterson-Falzone, Ph.D.

CLEFT PALATE AND NONCLEFT VELOPHARYNGEAL INADEQUACY

Because cleft palate and noncleft velopharyngeal inadequacy present many similar hazards to speech production and because there is a significant overlap in approaches to treatment, they will be treated together.

Clefts of the lip and palate constitute the third most common birth defect.* Combining all types, these defects occur approximately one in every 750 to 1,000 live births in Caucasians. The incidence is approximately doubled in the Mongolian races (which include American and Canadian Indians as well as most Asian groups) and halved in blacks. Incidence is influenced not only by racial background, but also by sex, type of cleft, and method of ascertainment. Unfortunately, a large majority of studies on the incidence of cleft have relied upon information recorded on birth certificates, and all congenital malformations are notoriously underreported on birth records. For example, Green, Nelson, Gaylor, and Holson found that only 65 percent of all clefts were noted on birth records (53 percent cleft lip, 31 percent cleft palate, 59 percent cleft lip and palate), and the *accuracy* of reporting (of cleft type) was only 48 percent.[2] Studies on the incidence and genetics of clefting have further been limited by the failure to record even easily visible submucous defects,[2,3] and by the failure to record other physical defects that could signal the presence of a malformation syndrome, association, or sequence, thus altering the epidemiologic and genetic picture.[4,5]

In most racial groups, clefts of the lip and palate combined occur approximately twice as often as clefts of either the lip alone or the palate alone.[†,6–12] Unilateral clefts occur twice as often on the left as on the right, the reason for this discrepancy being unknown.[6,8,10,13,14] Bilateral clefts of the lip, with or without accompanying cleft of the palate, occur about half as often as unilateral clefts.[6,8,14,15] The majority of studies have shown a higher occurrence of cleft lip with or without cleft palate in males and of isolated cleft palate in females.[6–8,10–12,16,17] However, in some studies of Asian populations the male to female ratio for cleft lip alone has been found to be virtually 1:1.[18–22] It appears that sexual differences in incidence gradually disappear as the severity of the defect diminishes. For example, clefts of the soft palate only occur with about equal frequency in males and females, the predominance of females becoming apparent only as the cleft extends into the hard palate.[23] Similarly, the frequency of submucous

* This chapter will not deal with the topic of lateral facial clefts, which are etiologically and structurally different from clefts of the lip and palate.[1]

† The terms "cleft palate alone" and "isolated cleft palate" can be a source of confusion. In most of the literature, they are used to mean a cleft confined to the secondary palate, with no involvement of the lip, alveolus, or anterior hard palate. However, in discussions of dysmorphology and syndromology, either of these terms may be used to refer to a cleft (even one of lip *and* palate) occurring without any associated defects.

clefts, which constitute one form of isolated cleft palate if no associated cleft of the lip is present, has appeared to be nearly equal in males and females in some studies.[24,25]

Just as the incidence of cleft is generally recognized to have been underestimated by early studies that relied on birth records, the frequency with which clefts occur in combination with other birth defects is also known to have been seriously underestimated in the majority of the literature up to the current decade. For example, MacMahon and McKeown reported a frequency of associated malformations in 9.1 percent of cases of cleft lip, 14.9 percent of those of cleft palate, and 21.0 percent of those of cleft lip and palate as recorded on hospital records.[11] Greene et al used birth certificate data to report a frequency of associated defects in 7 percent of infants with cleft lip, 24 percent of those with cleft palate, and 14 percent of those with cleft lip and palate.[13] Meskin and Pruzansky reported similar numbers: 5.6 percent of cleft lip cases, 17.8 percent of cleft palate, and 10.3 percent of cleft lip and palate.[26] However, in one early study in which the individuals were actually *examined* for associated defects, the frequency was found to be 16 percent in cleft lip with or without cleft palate and 51 percent in isolated cleft palate.[27] (The majority of studies have agreed on a higher occurrence of such defects in cleft palate alone rather than cleft lip with or without cleft palate,[8,15,27–36] the figures of MacMahon and McKeown being an exception.) Beder et al reported that the more extensive clefts had the greatest number of associated anomalies,[15] and Greene et al found more associated malformations in bilateral than in unilateral clefts.[13] Recent studies have shown just how seriously underreported associated defects have been. Rollnick and Pruzansky reported that 44 percent of 2,512 cases of all types of clefts had associated malformations,[37] and Jones found an incidence of $^{17}/_{30}$ (56.6 percent) among children with isolated cleft palate.[4] In a study of 1,000 cases of cleft, Shprintzen et al reported that at least one minor or one major associated anomaly was found in 44.6 percent of those with cleft lip, 50.3 percent of those with cleft lip and palate, and 56.2 percent of those with clefts of the secondary palate alone (including submucous clefts).[5] Associated anomalies occurred in a total 63.4 percent of their sample. These included an identified syndrome, sequence, or association in 31 percent and "provisionally unique pattern syndromes"* in another 22 percent. In about 11 percent of the cases, minor findings occurred that either were not part of an anomaly pattern or were familial characteristics. Discounting these, Shprintzen et al concluded that only 47 percent of their sample had "clefts in isolation."[†5]

The importance of a fully accurate diagnosis is not just the indication of how often a child with a cleft may be expected to have other problems requiring attention (in fact, most "minor" malformations do not require treatment), but rather it is the impact upon the understanding of the etiology of clefts. When clefts occur as part of a known genetic syndrome, the risks of recurrence are dramatically altered. Similarly, when clefting occurs as a secondary defect consequent to other intrauterine growth disturbances, as it does in the Pierre Robin malformation sequence, the risk of recurrence is actually less than would be the case in truly "isolated cleft palate."

TYPES OF OVERT CLEFTS

The median section of the upper lip and the anterior wedge-shaped section of the alveolar ridge and hard palate back to the incisive foramen evolve from the embryonic "primary palate." Clefts of the primary palate vary from a unilateral or bilateral notch (incomplete cleft) of the lip to a complete unilateral or bilateral cleft (Figs. 17–1 and 17–2) extending back to the incisive foramen.‡ If the cleft is bilateral and complete, the infant presents with a "floating premaxilla" unattached to anything but the columella. True median or midline clefts of the lip and alveolus are rare[40] and should not be confused with the more "common" paramedian clefts. Midline clefts may occur in conjunction with either severe hypotelorism (close spacing of the eyes) or hypertelorism (wide spacing of the eyes). The combination of midline clefts and severe hypotelorism signals the presence of midline defects of the central nervous system, and is not compatible with life.[41]

The remainder of the hard palate and the soft palate are derived from the embryonic "secondary palate." Clefts of the secondary palate range from a bifid uvula and/or submucous deficiency in the bulk of the musculus uvulae[42–45] to either submucous (Figs. 17–3 and 17–4) or overt clefts extending as far forward as the incisive foramen (Fig. 17–5). Combinations of overt and submucous defects of the secondary palate are seen, the submucous defect con-

* A term used to denote a pattern of anomalies not yet described in other individuals, e.g., "provisionally unique" until it is reported in other cases.

† See previous note about the use of the term "isolated cleft."

‡ Submucous clefts of the lip and alveolus have also been reported.[38,39]

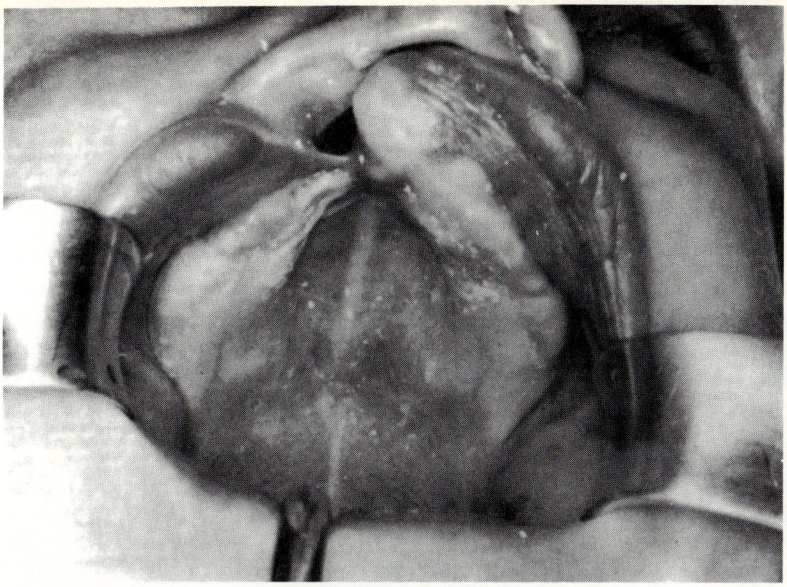

Figure 17–1 Incomplete unilateral cleft of the primary palate.

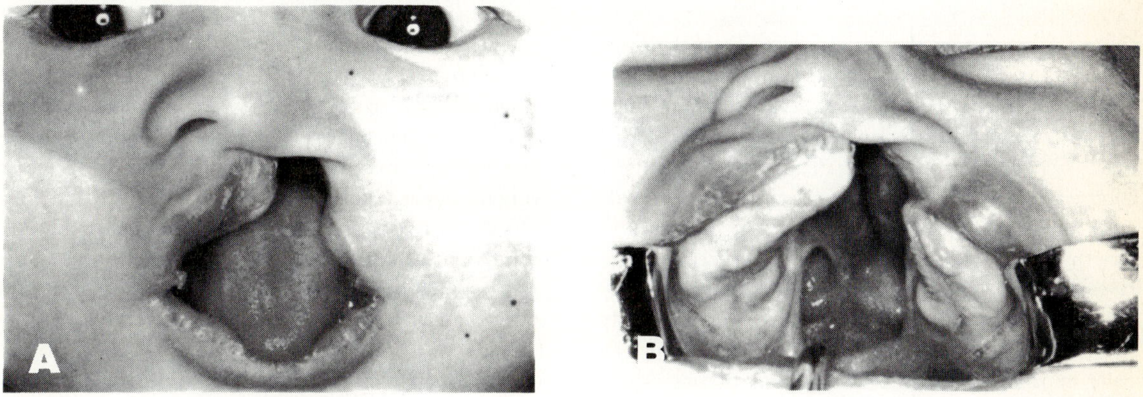

Figure 17–2 *A*, Unilateral complete cleft of the lip and palate. *B*, Note partial fusion of the right lateral palatine process to the vomer bone.

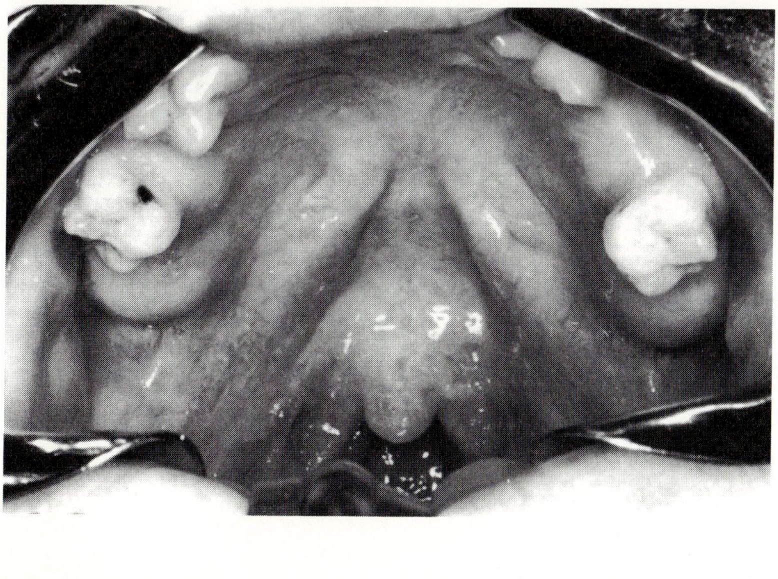

Figure 17–3 Submucous defect of the hard palate with muscular diastasis of the soft palate and an apparently intact uvula, at least as viewed intraorally.

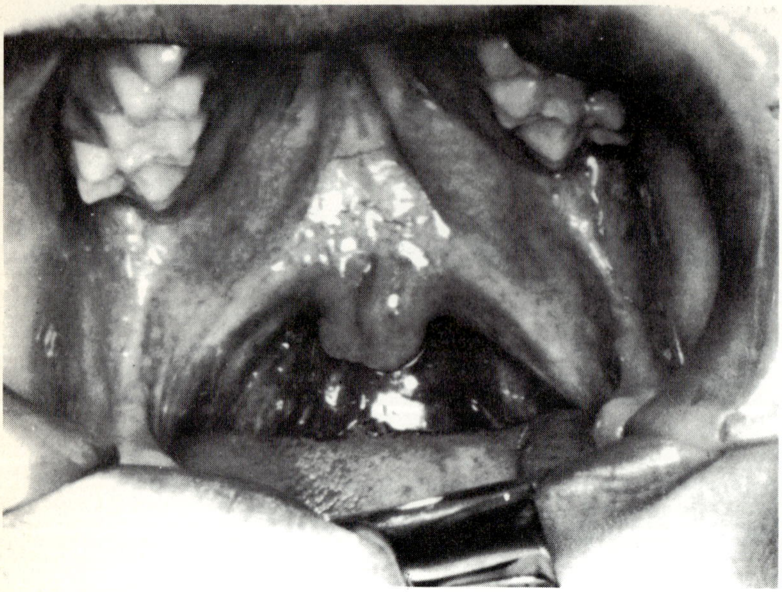

Figure 17–4 Full triad of the intraorally-visible signs of submucous cleft: Submucous defect of the hard palate, muscular diastasis of the soft palate, bifid uvula.

tinuing forward from the anterior margins of the overt defect[46–50] (Fig. 17–6). Mitts, Garrett, and Hurwitz reported one rather unusual case in which there was an overt cleft of the posterior 7 mm of the hard palate and anterior 4 mm of the soft palate, with a submucous cleft of the remainder of the soft palate.[51] Clefts of the secondary palate vary not only in length but in width as well, with the extreme case resembling a horseshoe. Technically, a cleft of the secondary palate is termed "bilateral" when only partial fusion or total lack of fusion of each of the palatine shelves with the vomer bone occurs.

The term "cleft lip and palate" implies combined clefting of both the primary and secondary palate, "unilateral" meaning the cleft of the primary palate is present on only one side, "bilateral" that it is present on both the right and left sides (Figs. 17–7 to 17–9). The adjective "complete" is used when there is no continuity of tissue across the line of the cleft. Thus, in a "complete unilateral cleft lip and palate," there is a cleft through the lip, alveolar ridge, and anterior portion of the hard palate *back* to the incisive foramen, combined with a cleft through the uvula, soft palate, and hard palate *up* to the incisive foramen. Some bilateral clefts are complete on one side of the primary palate and incomplete on the other.

Clefts vary along the five dimensions of unilateral to bilateral, complete to incomplete, anterior to posterior extent, width, and submucous versus overt, with combinations possible as noted previously. Several systems have been developed for the

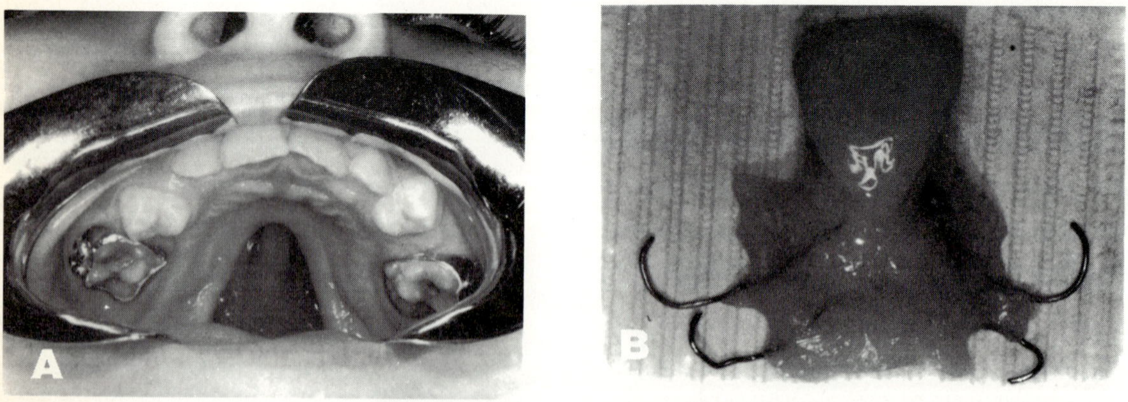

Figure 17–5 *A*, Isolated cleft of the soft palate, and *B*, the prosthetic device for obturation.

categorization of clefts.[38,52–59] However, because clinics and individual professionals differ in the systems used, if any, and because significant variation can occur *within* a given category, it is more efficient to describe the cleft fully than to simply label it.

SUBMUCOUS CLEFTS

It has already been noted that submucous clefts constitute one type of cleft of the secondary palate and are considered by most investigators to be mi-

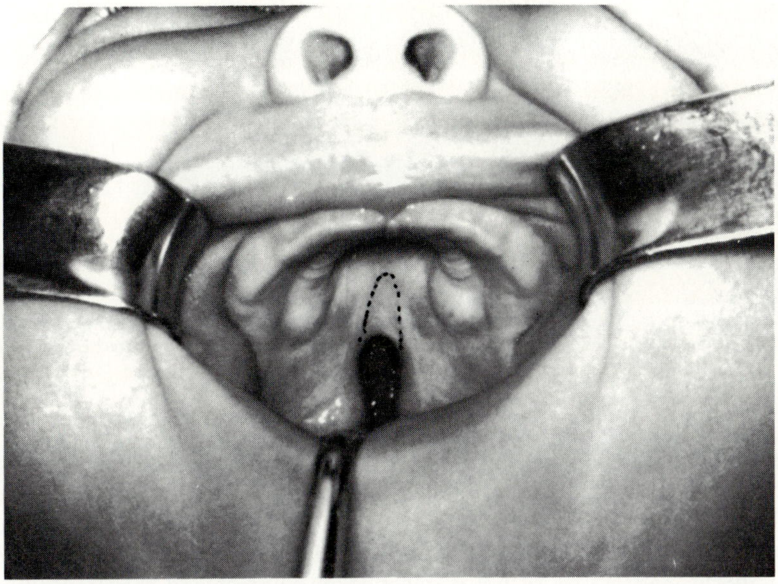

Figure 17–6 Cleft of the soft palate combined with a submucous defect of the hard palate.

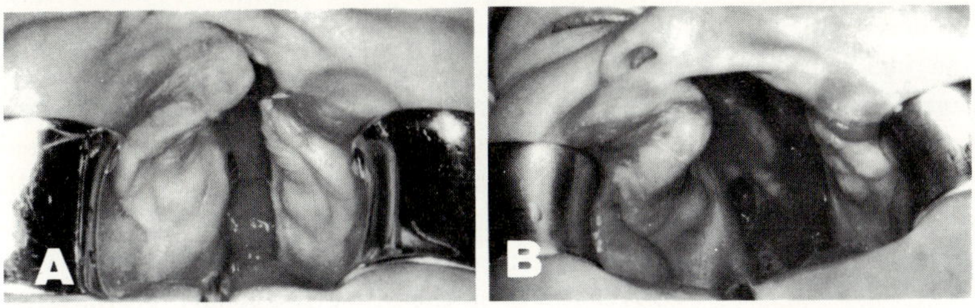

Figure 17–7 *A* and *B*, Within-type variability of cleft. These two infants both present with complete unilateral cleft lip and palate, but note difference in the width of the clefts.

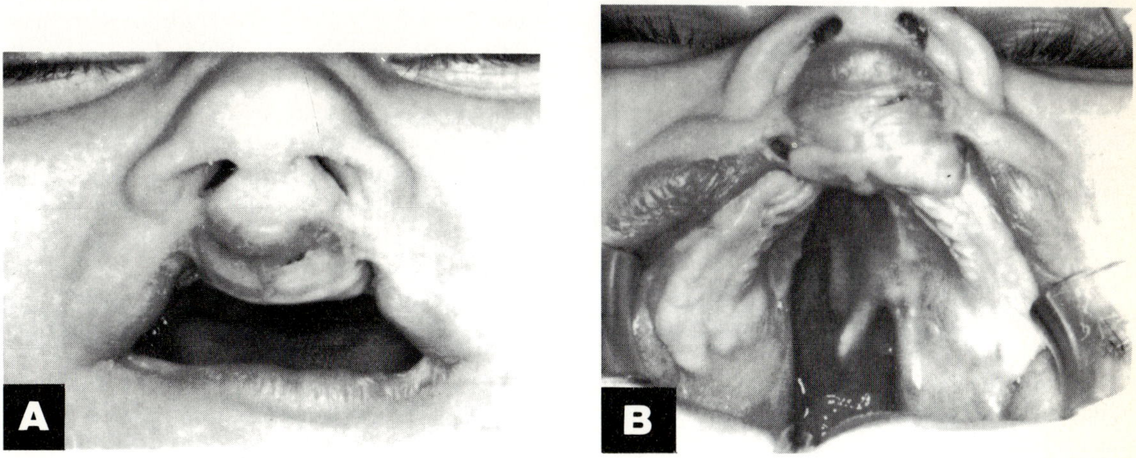

Figure 17–8 *A*, Frontal and *B*, intraoral views of bilateral incomplete cleft of the lip and palate.

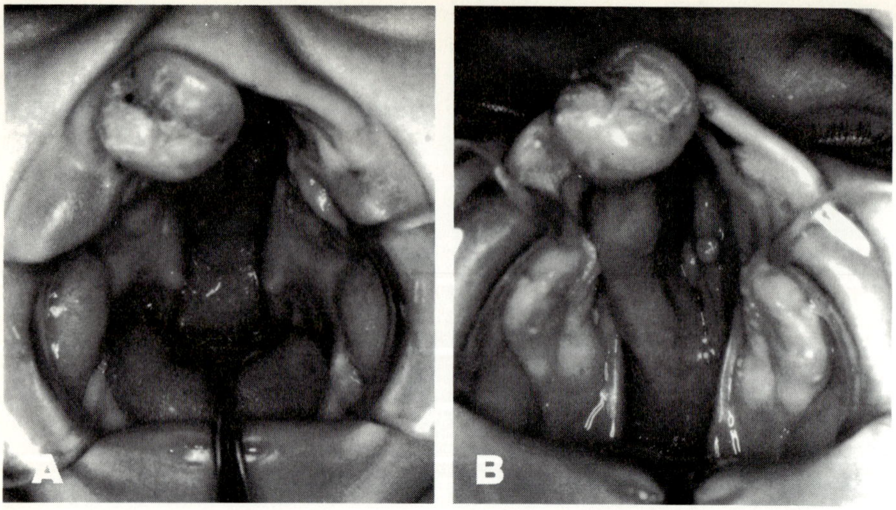

Figure 17-9 *A* and *B*, Intraoral views of infant with complete bilateral cleft lip and palate. Note that premaxilla is not attached to either palatine process.

croforms of cleft palate.[60–62] Combinations of submucous clefts with overt clefts of either the primary or secondary palate are relatively common.[63] Shprintzen et al noted that 42 of their 364 cases of "cleft lip and palate" had overt clefts of the lip and alveolus with submucous clefts of the palate and that such cases would have been categorized as "cleft lip only" in epidemiologic studies that ignored all but overt defects.[5] In fact, they found an incidence of associated anomalies in their submucous clefts of the secondary palate ($^{192}/_{250}$ = 76.8 percent) that was similar to the incidence in their overt clefts of the secondary palate ($^{224}/_{330}$ = 67.8 percent),a finding that attests to the commonality of these two types of defects.

Four problems regarding submucous defects have arisen which have both clinical and empirical impact:

1. Without knowing how many submucous clefts are present in any given population, it is impossible to accurately estimate the frequency of "genes" for clefting in that population. Counting only "overt" clefts is not sufficient.

2. Many people have submucous clefts without showing any evidence of velopharyngeal inadequacy.[24,64–82] Thus, the only way to estimate the frequency of submucous defects in a given population is to conduct random examinations of a large *nonclinical* sample, such as a school population or visitors to a shopping mall. Two surveys of school children have been published. Bagatin and Barkovic found submucous defects in five of 9,720 (0.05 percent) children examined (four of the five were asymptomatic), but did not specify the criteria used to determine the presence of these defects.[64] Weatherley-White and co-workers found nine submucous clefts in 10,836 children (0.08 percent), but insisted that all three intraorally visible stigmata of a bifid uvula, muscular deshiscence of the soft palate, and bony notch of the hard palate be present for such a designation to be made and specifically excluded those with "only a bifid uvula and a bony notch."[81,82] Shprintzen and coworkers found 82 cases of bifid uvula in "approximately 2,500 peroral examinations" (32 percent) of children in a pediatric practice.[76] These studies point up the next problem.

3. Investigators have not consistently agreed on what findings must be present to signify a submucous cleft. Prior to the advent of nasopharyngoscopy, investigators typically described varying combinations of the three intraorally visible stigmata, sometimes adding data from lateral radiographic studies or intraoperative examinations.[24,25,47,68–70,72,74,78,81–96] Although most investigators consider each of the three intraorally visible stigmata to constitute an anatomical abnormality of the secondary palate, Shapiro, Meskin, Cervenka, and Pruzansky considered bifid uvula "to fall in the borderland between malformation and normal development"(p 82).[97] It is known that the concordance among the three stigmata is variable. For example, submucous defects of the hard or soft palate may be present when the uvula appears to be intact.[76,91] What is *not* known is the concordance between one or more of the easily seen stigmata and the "occult" muscular deficiencies. The reason is explained in number 4.

4. Less than a fraction of 1 percent of all individuals reported in the literature as presenting with one or more of the intraorally visible stigmata of submucous defects or with evidence of velopharyngeal inadequacy in the absence of these stigmata have

been subjected to nasopharyngoscopic examination. Shprintzen and co-workers used nasopharyngoscopy to examine 25 of the 82 subjects with bifid uvula in the study cited previously and reported that 23 showed "some or all of the landmarks of submucous cleft palate."[76] However, these landmarks included at least three subject to possible questions of interpretation with regard to their validity as markers for submucous clefts: "flatness" of the nasal surface of the velum, absence of the salpingopharyngeal fold, and hypoplasia of the eustachian tube orifice. The fact that abnormal muscle insertions and deficient muscular bulk can be present when the velum and uvula appear normal on the peroral examination [42,43,45,69] constitutes one more reason why one cannot know the true incidence of submucous defects.

OCCULT MUSCULAR DEFICIENCIES

Several surgeons writing about submucous clefts have described abnormal orientation and insertion of the velar musculature, primarily the levator palatini.[24,69,85,98,99] However, Kaplan described such muscular abnormalities in 26 patients who showed none of the three classic intraorally visible stigmata.[69] This condition was definitively diagnosed only on the operating table, and Kaplan labeled it "occult submucous cleft palate." Converse et al, in an earlier report on the use of tomography to detect such defects, used the same term.[100] Trier described similar findings both in patients with visible stigmata and in patients whose palates seemed normal on intraoral inspection.[99] Somewhat earlier, Pigott et al described a deficiency in the bulk of the musculus uvulae as seen via nasopharyngoscopy in four patients with repaired clefts.[44] Although a midline deficiency in muscular bulk was hardly a surprising finding in repaired clefts, the hypernasal speech in these four patients was directly attibutable to a type of postoperative velopharyngeal insufficiency that would not have been detected on oral examination or lateral radiographic studies. Subsequently, extensive nasopharyngoscopic studies showed a similar muscular deficiency in hypernasal speakers whose palatal morphology appeared normal on intraoral inspection.[42,43] Shprintzen[45] reported that either an absence of the musculus uvulae on the nasal surface of the velum or diastasis of muscle tissue on the nasal surface was found in 20 hypernasal speakers with normal intraoral findings.*

The majority of investigators writing on this topic have viewed this muscular deficiency as a lack of bulk of the musculus uvulae, which they felt contributed substantially to the bulk of the velum and the "velar" eminence on palatal elevation.[42-45] This view was substantiated by anatomic studies showing the musculus uvulae to be a paired muscle, with each bundle originating from the tendinous palatal aponeurosis posterior to the hard palate (*anterior* to the insertion of the levator palatini), converging with its counterpart is an area overlying the levator sling and coursing over the dorsum of the soft palate to divide again into two separate bundles that terminate at the uvula proper.[102] However, Trier disagreed.[99] Noting that none of the authors using nasopharyngoscopy had validated their "hypothetical absence of a uvular muscle" (p 215) via surgical exploration of the velar muscles, Trier placed greater faith in the anatomic descriptions of Fara and Dvorak[103] and of Kriens,[104,105] in the state-of-the-art reviews of Dickson, Grant, Sicher, DuBrul, and Poltau[106] and Maue-Dickson,[107,108] and in his own intraoperative findings and those of Kaplan[69] in stating that the crucial muscular deficiency in both classic and occult submucous clefts was in the levator and not the musculus uvulae.

PALATOPHARYNGEAL DISPROPORTION

Disproportion between the size of the palate and the size of the nasopharynx (Fig. 17–10) has been described as a cause of velopharyngeal insuffiency by a number of authors.[24,69,70,86,98,109-123] In many cases reported by these authors, a foreshortened palate and/or overly large pharynx coexisted with other anatomic abnormalities, such as a submucous cleft. Kaplan reported that 75 percent of his 240 cases of velopharyngeal inadequacy had a short soft palate, but that all of these were subsequently shown to have either classic or occult submucous clefts.[69]

Crikelair et al pointed to foreshortening of the hard palate, with consequent anterior displacement of the points of insertion of the velar musculature, as a cause of velopharyngeal insufficiency.[115] However, foreshortening of the hard palate has most often been described in conjunction with either classic submucous clefts[70,124] or occult submucous clefts.[70]

Palatopharyngeal disproportion, with or without the presence of either a classic or occult submucous cleft, may remain undetected so long as an adenoid pad is present in the nasopharynx. However, unless surgery to remove the adenoids is careless or overly aggressive, thus causing a structural change in an otherwise normal nasopharynx, postad-

* Chaco and Yules used electromyography to diagnose midline muscular deficiencies (which they then labeled "submucous clefts") in six of nine patients who had developed hypernasal speech following adenotonsillectomy.[101]

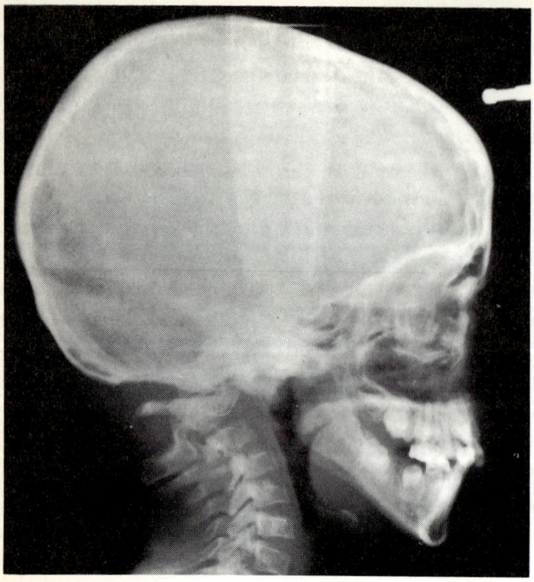

Figure 17–10 Lateral cephalometric rest film of patient with congenital palatopharyngeal disproportion due to abnormal pharyngeal depth consequent to anomalies of the cervical spine. Note posterior displacement of C-2 and lack of fusion of the odontoid process.

enoidectomy palatopharyngeal disproportion should in fact be viewed as a *congenital* condition, the presence of which is simply unmasked by—not caused by—the adenoidectomy. This point is well illustrated by the three case reports of such a disproportion apparently unveiled as the result of normal adenoid involution.[125–127]

ABNORMALITIES OF THE FAUCIAL PILLARS

Congenital anomalies of the faucial pillars have been described in the literature since the 1800s.[128] Fridenburg described a patient with a "supernumerary anterior faucial pillar" that ran from the lateral margin of the soft palate to the dorsum of the tongue on each side, "entirely free of the oral or pharyngeal wall."[129] The anterior pillars themselves were also separated from the lateral pharyngeal walls. Speech was described as nasal. Oldfield and MacNaughtan described one case of congenital absence of an anterior pillar and one in which the posterior pillars formed a thin diaphragm extending from the posterior pharyngeal wall to the posterior border of the soft palate, with an elliptical hiatus in the middle.[130] Speech was affected in both cases. Longacre described an infant similar to the second case, in whom the soft palate was continuous with the base of the tongue; the opening into the oropharynx was described as being a partial cleft of the velum.[131] Infants with similar findings were also described by Kouyoumdjian and McDonald;[132] Hub and Jirasec,[133] Seghers,[134] and Chandra, Yadava, and Sharma.[135] Several of these authors labeled the condition "persistent buccopharyngeal membrane," the latter being an embryonic structure that normally disintegrates. Hoffman used this label in describing a patient with a severe speech problem in whom a membrane stretched between the anterior pillars and from the soft palate to the base of the tongue, with a small central opening.[136] Crikelair et al described two patients with "cleft palate speech" in whom the velum was anchored inferiorly by abnormalities of the pillars, secondary to massive lymphangioma of the floor of the mouth in the first case and to posttonsillectomy scarring in the second.[115] Warren, Bevin, and Winslow described two patients with posterior pillar webbing behind the uvula and a third patient with webbing with palatopharyngeal displacement, all with limitation in velar motion and hypernasal speech.[137]

NEUROMOTOR DEFICITS AFFECTING THE VELOPHARYNGEAL SYSTEM

There is limited information on any effect of apraxia on velopharyngeal function. To date, only one study of apraxia has focused on velar motion.[138] The single patient in this study showed marked variation in velar movement and abnormal movement patterns, including lack of coordination (inappropriate timing) of velar movements with those of other articulators, but the report does not mention hypernasality or nasal emission. Noll speculated that the apparent paradox may have been due to the subtlety of the abnormalities of velar motion, being so minor as to have no perceived effect on speech.[139] Logically, apraxia could indeed affect velopharyngeal function since this system is in fact an "articulator" (responsible for the nasal/nonnasal contrast), the programming for which could be affected just as the programming for the rest of the articulatory system is affected.

Extensive information is available on velopharyngeal incompetency in various types of dysarthria, a large portion of it found in textbooks on neurologic disorders of speech. Clinical case reports in the literature have described two phenomena:

1. Neuromuscular problems *apparently* affecting primarily the velopharyngeal system* or this system

* Some investigators (i.e., Netsell[140]) have seriously questioned the existence of neuromotor deficits affecting the velopharyngeal system exclusively.

together with "other muscle complexes of the oral-facial-pharyngeal-laryngeal complex."[141] Paresis or paralysis of the velum alone or together with the pharyngeal musculature has been described by Ardan and Kemp;[142] Ashley et al;[143] Blackfield et al;[144] Calnan;[68,84,145,146] Cohn, Garver, Metz, McWilliams, Skolnick and Garrett;[147] Crikelair et al;[115] Hoopes, Dellon, Fabrikant, and Soliman;[148] Jackson et al;[117] Jafek, Balkany, Wong, and Bryant;[149] Kelly;[70] Keogh;[150] Lawshe, Hardy, Schweiger, and Van Allen;[151] Mazaheri et al;[152] Minami et al;[153] Owsley et al;[154] Pitt and Ingram;[155,156] Pollack, Shprintzen, and Zimmerman-Manchester;[157] Shprintzen et al;[158] Sturim and Jacob;[159] Stueber and Wilhelmsen;[120] and Worster-Drought.[160] The impairment in velopharyngeal motion may be bilateral or unilateral, as often seen in cases of hemifacial microsomia.[161,162] Also of interest are a number of reports of "palatal myoclonus" or "nystagmus" in a majority of which, unfortunately, speech is only vaguely mentioned. (Please see my 1985 paper for a complete list of references.[110])

2. Abnormalities of velopharyngeal muscular motion occurring as part of a generalized neurologic deficit.[115,117,141,144,146,153–155,163–186]

Two problems become apparent in reviewing information on neuromotor deficits affecting the velopharyngeal system. First, authors are not consistent in how they label some neurologic disorders. Second, the information is sometimes presented in relation to the type of dysarthria, sometimes in relation to the level or site of neurologic damage, and sometimes in relation to the disease process itself. Please see my 1985 paper for a table listing reports organized by these three categories.[110]

TWO SPECIAL TYPES OF VELOPHARYNGEAL INADEQUACY

In recent years, two particularly intriguing types of velopharyngeal inadequacy (VPI) have been described in the literature. Although one type usually occurs *without* structural or neurologic deficits and the physical findings in the other have been highly variable, they are worth a brief mention.

Phoneme-Specific VPI

In an article describing postadenoidectomy VPI in 1972, Lawson and co-authors wrote, "For some patients, the nasal emission appeared only on specific phonemes or combinations"(p 394).[187] In 1975, I described "nasal emission as a component of the misarticulation of sibilants and affricates" both in children who had been treated for cleft palate or for other forms of structural velopharyngeal inadequacy and in children for whom no history of such inadequacy could be documented. In all cases, all pressure consonants except /s/ and /z/, all four sibilants, or the sibilants and affricates together were free of nasal distortion.† Aberrant lingual position for these phonemes could be identified on lateral radiographic studies. (Fig. 17–11). Trost, in describing "posterior nasal frication," commented upon "a notable occurrence in noncleft velopharyngeal disorders, including the neurogenic problems of the dysarthrias and phoneme-specific velopharyngeal inadequacy" (p 197).[188] She used this term, which has now become the preferred label, "to define the occurrence of nasal air emission and audible posterior frication on certain pressure consonants only." Riski offered a later case description and suggestions for therapy, but reverted to the older term "functional velopharyngeal incompetence" (p 197).[188] In 24 cases I recently reviewed, age at ascertainment ranged from 3.1 to 12.4 with a mean age of 6.6.[190] Eight different patterns of occurrence of the phoneme-specific behavior were identified in these subjects; no apparent relationship existed between the number of phonemes so affected and the number of other articulatory/phonologic problems present in the same child. The nasal emission or nasal frication

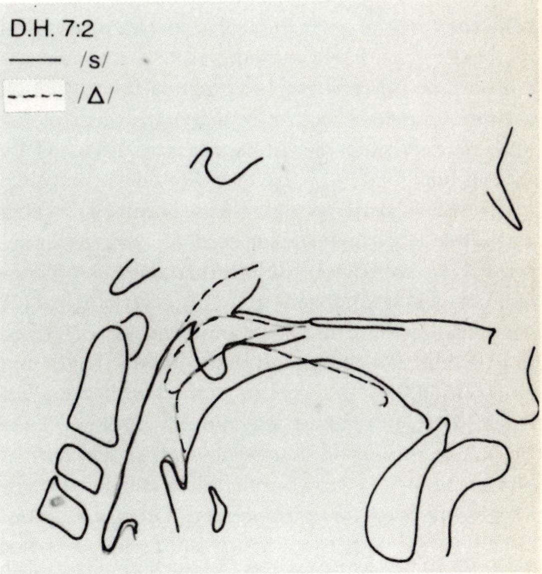

Figure 17–11 Tongue and velar position, indicated by --- line, in a child producing a posterior nasal fricative which he habitually substitutes for /s/. The solid line illustrates tongue and velar position after he was taught appropriate /s/ production.

† The perceptual consequence of phoneme-specific inadequacy was limited to the label "nasal emission" in the 1975 article, but may also be heard as "posterior nasal frication."[188]

was heard as a coarticulation in some speakers, with correct or incorrect (i.e., interdentalized) oral placement, whereas in others it *replaced* the normal oral gesture. When nasopharyngoscopy was performed, velopharyngeal gaps were evident only on those phonemes that were "vulnerable" in each speaker.

To date, it is not known why phoneme-specific inadequacy develops. Why is the speaker unaware or unconcerned that he or she is emitting these consonants nasally, whereas all others are appropriately produced orally? It is tempting to speculate that the nasal emission or posterior nasal frication is somehow sufficiently similar, in the ears of the developing child, to the frication heard in normal sibilants so that it may be adopted as a reasonable approximation to the adult model. We do not know what type of breakdown occurs in learning, or when. What *is* known is that, unlike other forms of velopharyngeal inadequacy, correction of phoneme-specific VPI is solely the task of the speech pathologist. Physical management of the system (prosthetic or surgical) is doomed to failure.

"Stress" VPI

In 1970, Weber and Chase described an oboe player who developed "continuous nasal snorting" after the first 10 minutes of playing, causing problems only during playing and not during speech.[191] No structural abnormality of the velopharyngeal mechanism could be detected on oral exam, oral endoscopy, or cineradiographic examination, although the ratio of palatal length to pharyngeal depth ($^{30}/_{31}$ mm) on cephalometric films was not discussed by the authors and *may* have indicated a marginal mechanism, based on Subtelny's norms.[192] Weber and Chase labeled this phenomenon "stress velopharyngeal incompetence." (Note that there is no connotation or implication here of psychological or emotional factors.) A similar problem was described in a bassoon and saxophone player by Massengill and Quinn in 1974.[126] In this case, the liability was attributed to progressive adenoid involution. However, such involution is normal, and, if this normal process results in velopharyngeal inadequacy, some underlying mechanism is present. Of two cases reported by Dibbell, Ewanowski, and Carter, one had a submucous cleft, whereas the other showed "herniation" of the soft palate into the nasopharynx under the stress imposed by the high intraoral pressures required for playing a wind instrument: with continuous playing the soft palate was literally blown into the nasopharynx.[193] Argamaso and Shprintzen described velopharyngeal inadequacy in a trumpet player who had undergone a tonsillectomy that resulted in scarred musculature.[194] In the single case that I saw, a clarinet player developed nasal leakage after approximately 30 minutes of playing. This leakage first occurred only after she enrolled as a music major in college and began playing 6 to 8 hours a day. Nasopharyngoscopy revealed a slight V-shaped defect on the nasal surface of the velum, resulting in a small inconsistent central velopharyngeal gap.

Reviewing the few cases of "stress" velopharyngeal inadequacy in musicians reported to date, it is clear that some actually did have at least some minor structural findings. Others may have had either a structural defect, which was undetected, or some predisposing minor muscular weakness that became symptomatic only under sustained use of extremely high intraoral pressures. (Please see Dibbell et al for a table of required pressures in wind instrument playing.[193])

SPEECH PROBLEMS

The literature on speech production in patients with clefts is extensive. Unfortunately, a large number of studies have suffered from problems in research design, including heterogeneity of subjects and poor control of independent variables. Approaches to answering the same questions have varied dramatically from study to study. Although such problems account for some of the conflicting results reported over the years, the most pervasive limitation until recent years was the attempt to correlate speech findings to the size of the velopharyngeal gap with inadequate means for viewing the port. Despite such limitations, a sufficient body of data has emerged to allow some cautious generalizations.

Nasal Air Loss and Resonance Deviations

Speakers with both cleft palate and noncleft velopharyngeal inadequacy exhibit varying degrees of (1) nasal air loss on pressure consonants with consequent weakening of those consonants, (2) possible posterior nasal frication, and (3) hypernasal resonance. The lack of a one-to-one correlation between the occurrence of audible nasal emission and hypernasality was discussed in the previous chapter. Varying degrees of hyponasality or cul-de-sac resonance may be heard after surgical or prosthetic treatment, and even prior to treatment as a result of the nasal deformities common in cleft lip and palate. In evaluating any of these deviations, it is critical that the speech pathologist keep in mind that incomplete closure of the velopharyngeal port is not the *only* independent variable. Please see Chapter 7 for a review of those physiologic factors affecting nasal air loss and resonance deviations.

Compensatory Articulations

The literature in cleft palate is replete with references to the substitution of glottal and pharyngeal articulatory gestures for oral consonants (e.g., Bzoch;[195] McWilliams et al;[196] Morley;[197] Morris;[198] and Wells[199]).* The general concept has been that a child learning speech with an open cleft or inadequate velopharyngeal closure tends to develop and retain "backed" articulations in an attempt to make effective use of the airstream before it escapes through the nose. Infants with clefts demonstrate more glottal articulations than infants without clefts.[200,201] Most compensatory articulations represent a sacrifice of the *place* feature for retention of the *manner* feature,[188] although the child with severely disordered articulation may substitute glottal stops for continuants and even for liquids and glides, as well as for stops.[202] Trost, together with most investigators, viewed compensatory articulations as the result of the child's effort to approximate a perceptual or acoustic target.[188,203] But Warren hypothesized that these articulations serve to preserve respiratory homeostasis: by stopping or at least diminishing the loss of air before it reaches an open velopharyngeal port, the speaker is responding only to the physiologic need to maintain a constant subglottic pressure head.[204] However, neither of these views explains why many speakers with unrepaired clefts or marked postsurgical VPI do not develop compensatory articulations.

Compensatory articulations are notorious for their persistence even after an adequate velopharyngeal system has been provided through surgical or prosthetic care.[188,196,203,205] Thus the speech pathologist cannot assume that their presence is indicative of a current physical problem. They are typically observed to be more deleterious to speech intelligibility than nasal air loss or hypernasal resonance.

Glottal Stops. Transcribed as /ʔ/, glottal stops are normal replacements for /t/ and /d/ in some dialects in the United States (for example, /wʌʔnt/ for "wouldn't"). Speakers with past or present velopharyngeal inadequacy may substitute this gesture for both voiced and voiceless stops, or, in more severe cases, for other classes of consonants. The glottal stop is sometimes produced simultaneously, or "coarticulated," with the normal oral gesture, in which case it is transcribed as a superscript, for example, /p̉/.[188,195]

Pharyngeal Fricative. The pharyngeal fricative is the other classic compensatory articulation mentioned in the literature on cleft palate and has been documented in toddlers.[200,201,206] This gesture is produced by the turbulent flow of air through a constriction between the tongue dorsum and the posterior pharyngeal wall,[188,197,203] and it is usually heard as a replacement for sibilants and affricates. Weinberg and Horii delineated the acoustic features of the pharyngeal /s/ as produced by speakers with clefts.[207] As with glottal stops, this gesture may occur simultaneously with normal articulatory placement. The voiced pharyngeal fricative is transcribed as /ʕ/ and the unvoiced as /ʕ̵/.[188]

Pharyngeal Affricate. Trost-Cardamone also described the pharyngeal affricate, a gesture that appears to consist of the combination of a glottal stop and a pharyngeal fricative, /ʔʕ/ or /ʔʕ̵/.[208]

Pharyngeal Stop. In 1971, Honjow and Isshiki described the radiographic and spectrographic appearance of what they termed "pharyngeal stop" substitutions for /k/ and /g/.[209] Previous investigators had described compensatory tongue, palate, and pharyngeal wall contacts in speakers with clefts.[210,211] Trost reported identical radiographic findings to those of Honjow and Isshiki, namely contact between the tongue dorsum and the posterior pharyngeal wall, and suggested that the pharyngeal stop be described as /ʕ̍/ when voiced and /ʕ̵̍/ when unvoiced.[188]

Velar Fricatives. Velar fricatives, transcribed as /γ/ when voiced and /χ/ when unvoiced, are phonemic in some languages, but Trost discussed them as compensatory articulations.[188,203] This gesture is produced by airflow through a constriction between the tongue dorsum and the velum, and it is typically heard as a substitution for oral fricatives or velar stops.[188,203,206,212] It was Trost's impression that this gesture occurs more often in neurogenic velopharyngeal incompetency than in speakers with clefts.

Palatal Fricatives. There are also some references to palatal fricatives as compensatory articulations.[196] Palatal fricatives, like velar fricatives, are normal phonemes in some languages, including some dialects of Spanish. The task of determining the occurrence of these particular "compensatory" articulations in any linguistically mixed population is thus complex.

Mid-dorsum Palatal Stops. The palatal stop

* The literature to date lacks a single empirical study on the occurrence of compensatory articulations in the various noncleft forms of velopharyngeal inadequacy. The article by Trost briefly mentions the occurrence of certain compensatory gestures in neurogenically based velopharyngeal inadequacy.[188]

appears to represent a place compromise between /t, k/ or /d, g/.[188] Perceptually, the phoneme boundaries between the tip-alveolar and the velar stops are lost. The voiceless mid-dorsum stop /k̟/sounds equally like /t/ or /k/, and the voiced cognate /ɟ/ sounds equally like /d/ or /g/. When the speaker substitutes this gesture for the tip-alveolar stops, this compensatory articulation fits the general pattern of "backing." When substituted for /k/ or /g/, it does not.

In radiographic studies of speakers with clefts, Brooks and co-workers[210,211] and Lawrence and Philips[213] described abnormal contacts or constrictions between the tongue and various points on the palate and the pharyngeal wall. The majority of these abnormal gestures were posterior to normal placement. However, since there were no data on the perceptual or acoustic effects on these gestures, one cannot know how closely they were related to the pharyngeal, velar, and midpalatal articulations that Trost later described.[188,203]

Posterior Nasal Fricatives. Trost described the posterior nasal fricative /Δ/ as a compensatory articulation substituted for sibilants or occurring simultaneously with oral production of fricatives, affricates, and stops.[188,203] In the latter case, it is one variant of the perceptual result of nasal air loss accompanying either normal or deviant articulatory placement and is not strictly speaking a compensatory gesture. Trost found posterior nasal fricatives to be the most frequently occurring form of phoneme-specific velopharyngeal inadequacy.

Ingressive Airflow. McWilliams and Philips described the use of ingressive airflow as an apparent compensatory gesture in some speakers with cleft palate.[214] In my own clinical experience, I have observed the occurrence of this gesture on sibilants and even on stop-plosives in children who could not build sufficient intraoral air pressure to produce the normal frication or plosive spike. The audible impression was of a short "sucking" sound.

One final point must be made about "compensatory" articulations: except for the glottal stop and pharyngeal fricative, speech pathologists have no data about the occurrence of these patterns in speakers without velopharyngeal inadequacy. Thus the term "compensatory" may be presumptive.

Other Articulation Problems

Prior to the 1980s, the majority of studies of articulation in children with cleft palate reported the phonemes most often affected without describing the nature of the problems beyond the classic categorizations of omissions, distortions, and substitutions. For example, many studies reported that speakers with clefts have more problems with fricatives than with plosives.[202,212,215–221] The single most vulnerable phoneme has been repeatedly reported to be /s/.[217,221–225]

Early studies of the prevalence of omissions, distortions, and substitutions yielded results varying at least in part as a function of the subjects' age. Distortions were more frequent than omissions or substitutions in adults[217] and also in two groups aged 8 to 18 years[225] and 5 to 14 years,[226] but omissions were more frequent in a study of children aged 3 to 8 years.[218] Philips and Harrison reported a decline in omissions with increasing age from 36 to 71 months,[227] a trend similar to that seen in children with normal oral structures.[228]

As pointed out by McWilliams et al, phonemes may be transcribed as "omitted" when the speaker has actually substituted glottal stops.[196] Furthermore, consonant deletions may signify a phonologic process such as cluster reduction or final consonant deletion.

Few studies described specific types of distortions in speakers with clefts. Bzoch[202,212] and Van-Demark,[226] among others, recorded percentages of "nasal distortions" in their subjects, but this label does not describe articulatory placement or other features relevant to production.

Until recent years, descriptions of substitutions were limited to compensatory articulations, primarily the glottal stop.[195,202,212,229,230] Recently, phonologic analyses of three children with repaired clefts and reportedly adequate velopharyngeal closure were reported in two different studies.[206,231] The 5-year-old-child studied by Hodson et al fit the pattern of earlier studies on children in this age group: the majority of the child's errors fell into some category of deletions (omissions), and replacement phonemes were glottal stops or nasal consonants. Of the two children described by Lynch et al, ages 2 years 8 months and 2 years 5 months, one tended to substitute stops for fricatives, whereas the other more frequently substituted fricatives for stops.[206] For the latter child, however, the majority of substitutions again consisted of nasal consonants and glottal stops.

The other traditional way in which errors have been analyzed has been by place, manner, and voicing. These categories are not easily segregated to determine what factor most affects accuracy of articulation.[232] For example, the place designation of "tip-alveolar" includes fricatives and affricates as well as the simpler plosives /t/ and /d/. Also, in analyzing voicing errors, one must take into account that devoicing of word-final obstruents is a natural consequence of the aerodynamics of the vocal tract. When the tract is obstructed, oral air pressure posterior to the obstruction rises until it equals subglottic pressure. Air no longer flows across the vocal folds, and phonation stops.[233] Velar stops are more vulnerable to devoicing than bilabial stops because distance is less from the place of obstruction to the vocal folds. This model, in fact, would predict *fewer* devoicing errors in speakers with velopharyngeal inadequacy since the speakers cannot equalize the pressure above and below the folds with normal articulatory placement of obstruents.

Analyzing the place of articulation in speakers with cleft palate can mean identifying both the normal place of articulation or error consonants and the place of production of substituted consonants. With regard to the former, Moll concluded that place was not as likely as manner to identify vulnerable consonants.[232] When he combined the results of several previous studies,[212,217,218,222,230] it was evident that fricatives were far more vulnerable to error than plosives, glides, or nasals, regardless of the place of articulation. Moll concluded that data on place contributed little except to suggest that labials were less vulnerable than linguals. In a study using distinctive feature analysis, a subgroup of subjects identified only as "cleft palate" reportedly showed peak performance on labiality and poorest performance on the front/back distinction.[234]

With regard to manner of articulation, fricatives, particularly the sibilant fricatives, have consistently been found to be most often in error, followed by plosives.[216,220,223,225,227,232] Glides, liquids, and nasals are far less vulnerable.[220,225,227,230] These differences have generally been consistent across age groups.

As would be expected, errors classified according to place and manner of articulation are inextricably related to errors that may be caused primarily by specific oral structural differences. This topic will be discussed.

Although most studies have consistently reported fewer errors on voiced than on voiceless consonsants,[212,217–219,221,235] this difference may vary with the particular consonant and specific age group under study. Spriestersbach et al found that, although voiced plosives and affricates were indeed produced correctly more often than their voiceless cognates, the reverse was true for fricatives.[219] They suggested that age might be a factor in this apparent paradox, since the voiceless fricatives are learned earlier than the voiced fricatives, whereas the reverse is true for plosives. The consistency of the voiceless and voiced differential in studies of adolescents[221,235] and adults[217] supported this theory, as did the results of Philips and Harrison,[227] who found no difference in voiced and voiceless performance in children aged 36 to 71 months.

As noted before, a diminished ability to make normal voicing contrasts would be predicted in the speaker with inadequate velopharyngeal closure. Leder and Lerman reported spectrographic evidence of inappropriate voicing of voiceless stop consonants in adults with clefts and severe hypernasality.[236] Although they interpreted these findings as evidence of vocal abuse, it appears more reasonable that the inappropriate voicing reflected the aerodynamics of the speech mechanism, as previously discussed. That is, in a speaker with an inadequate velopharyngeal mechanism, the air pressure in the vocal tract above and below the vocal folds does not equalize when the tract is obstructed (as for an obstruent consonant), allowing the folds to continue vibrating.

It is important to note that in the studies on voicing errors, as in most studies on sound production errors, it is not known to what extent either residual velopharyngeal inadequacy or the persistence of patterns learned in the presence of such inadequacy may have affected results.

Investigators have also attempted to study the effect of phonetic context and word position on articulatory errors. They have largely dichotomized data on the influence of phonetic context into singleton versus cluster productions, rather than addressing specific phonetic content of the cluster or the elements of coarticulation. Speakers with clefts have demonstrated better production on singletons than on the same consonants in clusters.[198,218,219,224] Two-element blends appear to differentiate speakers with clefts from those without clefts,[202,212,217,221,230,235] and consonants are more likely to be defective in three-element than in two-element blends.[224,237] McDermott specifically studied /s/ and found no differences in production based on its place within a cluster.[224] Spriestersbach et al[218] and McWilliams et al[196] pointed out that poorer articulation of consonants in clusters is in contrast to the observation that embedding a consonant in a cluster may facilitate production in children with nonorganically based speech problems. The assumption is that the impaired oral structures prevent the child with a cleft from making the rapid adjustments that would facilitate better production in a cluster (please see the section Timing).

Studies on effects of word position on accuracy of articulation have yielded variable results. Bzoch's preschoolers made more errors on consonants in the medial position than in the initial or final positions.[202,212] However, children of the same age studied by Philips and Harrison showed decreasing accuracy, going from the initial to the medial to the final position.[227] The same results were reported by Singh et al in school-age cleft children, but were also found in children described as articulation disordered, language disordered, mentally retarded, and hearing impaired.[234] Starr studied different types of errors and found omissions more often in the final position than in the other two positions in children aged 6 to 11 years.[230] Substitutions, indistinct productions, and "indistinct productions resulting from nasal emission" occurred equally in all three positions. Byrne et al found no consistent differences from initial to medial to final position across phonemes, although small differences occurred between phonemes.[222] Counihan's young adults also showed no relationship between word position and articulation.[221,235] Finally, McDermott reported greater accuracy of /s/ articulation in the "syllable-releasing" than in the "syllable-arresting" position.[224]

The child with a cleft has every right to the same presumably developmental errors as every other child. There is some evidence that children with clefts may show more errors even on consonants independent of normal velopharyngeal closure and normal dentition,[202,212,238] and certainly there is no reason to withold therapy for these errors simply because structural anomalies are present.

In children with clefts and other forms of velopharyngeal inadequacy, one wants to know the extent to which problems in sound production reflect (1) the inability to produce a given phoneme correctly because of past or present structural problems, (2) the inability to produce a given phoneme correctly because of maturational or other factors, and (3) the failure to use certain sounds consistently despite a demonstrated ability to produce them under some conditions. McWilliams et al would apply the term "phonetic misarticulation" to the first two cases and "phonologic misarticulation" to the third.[196] Using this dichotomy, a child with a cleft would be exhibiting phonetic misarticulation in using pharyngeal fricatives for sibilant fricatives regardless of the word position or the elements of phonetic context. Another child using glottal stops for, say, tip-alveolar plosives in the prevocalic position despite appropriate use of these plosives in other positions would be exhibiting a phonologic misarticulation.

McWilliams et al pointed out that the description of articulation by distinctive feature or phonologic process analysis, although providing more information, does not identify etiology.[196] Such analyses only identify patterns. For example, speech pathologists do not know why a child may replace velar stops with tip-alveolar stops until they examine both the pattern of these replacements and the child's physical ability to raise the tongue dorsum. In children with clefts, the etiology of phonetic misarticulations may be either structural or developmental. Even the presumably phonologically-based errors may have a physical etiology, for example, cluster reduction suspected to reflect problems in making rapid articulatory adjustment.

Those few studies that used distinctive feature analysis to describe speech in children with clefts have not revealed a wealth of new information.[206,231,234] Their results largely reflected those of much earlier studies. Trost-Cardamone reported that phonologic process analysis did not yield more thorough or useful data for her subject with cleft lip and palate than did traditional segment analysis.[239] However, the combined number of subjects with clefts examined in these studies is 23, and the results for the majority—the 18 included in the study of Singh et al[234]—were not presented in detail. Thus, to date, speech pathologists have little information derived from the use of these forms of analysis. As pointed out by Shriberg and Kwiatkowski, child phonologists disagree about what constitutes a proper phonologic analysis,[240] and the several published procedures for describing phonologic processes differ markedly in underlying theory and method. It appears that this still evolving field has the potential for more significant contributions to the study of speech in cleft palate speakers than has yet been realized.

Timing

In the past two decades, investigators have reported data related to timing and coordination of the action of the laryngeal and articulatory mechanisms, including the velopharyngeal system, in speakers with clefts. Aerodynamic data provided by Warren and Mackler suggested that pressure consonant duration changes significantly as a function of velopharyngeal inadequacy,[241] as did spectrographic data on plosives reported by Rolnick and Hoops.[242] A cinefluorographic study of timing interactions among the velum, tongue, and larynx showed more variable temporal correspondence of velopharyngeal closure and linguopalatal constriction in relation to voice-onset time in poor speakers with clefts than in good speakers.[243,244] The poor speakers also showed more variability in the onset time of tongue movement, time of linguopalatal constriction, time of constriction release, and offset time of tongue movement. Unfortunately, speakers were classified as "good" or "poor" based solely on their production of the Japanese /k/. Fletcher reported that polysyllabic diadochokinesis, presumably reflecting coordination of the tongue, jaw, and velopharyngeal and laryngeal activity, accounted for 60 percent of the variance in his subjects.[223]

Three relatively recent studies have utilized spectrographic data,[245] aerodynamic data,[246] and a combination of radiographic and spectrographic data.[247] In her study of 5 and 6 year olds with and without clefts, Forner found that speech segment durations were significantly longer in children with clefts, that the stop gaps of the plosives and fricatives were the most deviant single acoustic finding, and that the subjects with moderate or severe hypernasality had significantly increased vocal onset times; Forner hypothesized that these increased times might have been due to an increased time requirement for the buildup of sufficient pressure for the release of a plosive or affricate.[245] Alternative or additional theories included that an increase in voice onset times may be a form of perceptual compensation for damped sound energy and that the backing of articulatory gestures may alter the aerodynamic interaction of labial, lingual, velar, and laryngeal valving.[245] Previous investigators had also conjectured that compensatory articulations may alter normal temporal characteristics of speech.[210,211,241] A cause-effect dilemma occurs in such observations: Do compensatory articulations cause the temporal disruptions? Or do the demands of attempting to coordinate laryngeal, velopharyngeal, lingual, and labial activity in the presence of velopharyngeal inadequacy cause compensatory articulations?

Warren et al[246] reexamined timing characteristics in normal speakers and in three groups of speakers with clefts who were categorized into adequate closure (velopharyngeal orifice areas 0.00 to 0.09 cm^2 as estimated by aerodynamic studies), borderline (0.10 to 0.19 cm^2) and inadequate (greater than 0.19 cm^2).* The speech sample was limited to the word "hamper," requiring subjects to make the transition from a nasal to an oral consonant. Comparisons were made among the four groups on eight aerodynamic variables reflecting timing of velopharyngeal closure. The borderline and inadequate groups both showed increased duration of the overall airflow curve compared with both the adequate group and the normal speakers. The inadequate group showed an air pressure curve duration longer than the normal speakers, but shorter than the adequate group; that is, they could not maintain the pressure over a similar length of time. Only two of eight variables differentiated the inadequate and borderline groups, which was interpreted as reflecting simply different degrees of inadequacy. Nasality was rated in all speakers, and the investigators reported that only in the borderline group did pressure-flow timing differences consistently coincide with subjective ratings of speech, that is, the greater the disturbances in timing in this group, the greater the rating of nasality. However, it should be pointed out that only in this group would there be the "room" to demonstrate correlation. The adequate and normal speakers presumably all received low ratings of nasality, whereas the inadequate group all received high ratings. The results of this study revealed different adjustments in timing in the three groups of cleft speakers, apparently reflecting differing strategies in dealing with the effects of velopharyngeal opening.

* Note differences in categories from those subsequently reported by the same investigator.

Karnell et al used spectrographic measures of time of voice onset and of voice offset and cinefluorographic records of movement of the tongue tip, tongue dorsum, jaw, velar knee, velar tip, and posterior pharyngeal wall to examine temporal relationships in four speakers with repaired clefts.[247] Whereas the expected velopharyngeal opening movements were coordinated with prevocalic constriction release in CVC and CVN (nasal consonant) syllables in the two subjects who exhibited nasalized CVC utterances, two subjects who had been judged as less nasal did not show such opening. The investigators speculated that the absence of these movements could reflect an abnormally tight mechanical linkage between the tongue and velum via the palatopharyngeal muscles in speakers with repaired clefts or an attempt to avoid nasal emission at the initial and terminal portions of the syllable when oral pressure would build up. It was thus suggested that

> it may be counterproductive to assume that decreased nasalization may be achieved best by attempting to adjust the timing of articulatory and vocal events so that movement patterns more closely approximate those patterns found in non-cleft speakers. The most successful patients may be those who can best reorganize their motor system to accommodate their unique structure (p 71).[247]

That timing differences exist seems clear. However, investigators are just learning how particular deviations, and their magnitude, may affect one's perception of nasality and other speech deviations in these speakers. The data of both Warren et al[246] and Karnell et al[247] appear to constitute a reason for reconsidering the usual goal of "normalization" in speech therapy. If indeed, one had therapeutic techniques for teaching better coordination of laryngeal, velopharyngeal, lingual, and labial activity, one might disrupt favorable adaptations already learned.

Suprasegmental Features

Some data on vocal pitch, intensity, and speaking rate in speakers with clefts are available. Studies of pitch have addressed two questions: Do speakers with clefts habitually use higher or lower pitch level? And is there a consistent relationship between pitch and perceived nasality? This information was sought primarily for the purpose of determining if speakers with clefts either already used or should be taught to use higher or lower pitch levels in order to minimize hypernasality. Unfortunately, several studies used "functionally nasal" speakers as well as cleft and normal speakers; experimental procedures varied drastically; and none of the studies could address the ultimate question of whether a particular pitch level causes speech to be perceived as more or less hypernasal, or, conversely, whether or not hypernasal speakers choose to use certain pitch levels to mask hypernasality. Results have varied from no consistent relationship between nasality and pitch[248] to lower fundamental frequencies for females with clefts and no differences for males[249,250] to a positive relationship between nasality and higher pitch[251] to a negative relationship between nasality and higher pitch.[252] Tarlow and Saxman found no significant differences in fundamental frequencies between cleft and noncleft children aged 7 to 9 years, but they did report differences in some inflectional measures.[253] Thus it appears that the answer to the two primary questions stated earlier is negative.

Clinical descriptions of speakers with clefts often describe the use of reduced loudness levels.[195,196,198,254–256] This vocal behavior has been thought to be, at least in part, an attempt to mask hypernasality. However, vowel amplitude is known to decrease as oronasal coupling increases.[257–259.] This energy loss may account for the use of increased respiratory volumes and vocal effort levels in some speakers with clefts,[260] a cycle that can end in vocal abuse and aberrant laryngeal vocal quality, to be discussed. Attempts to relate intensity level to severity of perceived nasality have produced nearly as confusing results as those attempts to relate pitch and nasality. Weiss reported a negative correlation between intensity level and nasality ratings, with severely hypernasal speakers using lower levels than mildly hypernasal speakers.[261] However, Hess found higher intensity levels to produce lower nasality ratings.[252] Williamson reported a similar inverse relationship in "functionally nasal" speakers.[262] Counihan and Cullinan found this same effect for males, with cleft palate but not females.[263] These investigators found a contaminating effect in playback levels, and Rampp and Counihan concluded that such judgments were confounded by the interaction among intensity, vowel, and sex of speaker.[250] In addition, results are undeniably affected by the particular intensity levels used and the method of rating nasality. Thus another question remains unanswered: do speakers with velopharyngeal inadequacy elect to use a lower loudness level in order to mask the effect of the inadequacy, or is the "soft voice syndrome"[196] dictated by the physiologic constraints of inadequate closure?

Traditional studies of rate investigated the number of syllables or words per minute. Lass and Noll[264] and Tarlow and Saxman[253] reported slower speaking rates in speakers with clefts. McDermott reported that speakers with clefts used more breath units and that this difference increased with speech therapy.[224] As noted earlier Forner's 5 and 6 year olds with clefts demonstrated significantly longer durations for both syllables and total sentences than did their peers without clefts.[245]

Two recent studies investigated the effects of increased rate on listeners' perception of the speech of adults with clefts. D'Antonio found that an increased rate did not increase the perception of nasality.[265] Jones and Folkins reported similar findings in speakers whose velopharyngeal closure as judged from midsagittal radiographic studies varied from complete (two subjects) to a small extent of velopharyngeal contact (three subjects) to a small velopharyngeal gap in one subject.[266] Only one of the subjects was free of any nasal emission, nasality, or articulatory problems. Ratings of the severity of speech disorder did not increase with an increased rate. Jones and Folkins noted the apparent disparity between these results, as well as those of D'Antonio, and those of earlier studies indicating that speakers with clefts used a slower rate. They hypothesized that the higher rate in both their study and that of D'Antonio was not sufficiently high to tax the speech production mechanisms of their subjects. They also noted that maintaining velopharyngeal closure may actually become easier when articulatory positions are held for a shorter period of time and pointed out that "the temporospatial factors involved in control of the velopharyngeal mechanism, and its interaction with other articulatory systems, are still not clear" (p 252). (Please see the section on timing.)

Findings with regard to pitch level are generally negative and uninformative. It does appear that reduced intensity is a common clinical finding, but the cause-effect relationship is not clear. Findings of slower rate in cleft speakers probably reflect production level problems as discussed in the preceding section on timing.

Laryngeal Disorders

As noted previously, increased oronasal coupling leads to dissipation of the accoustic energy of the speech signal. Curtis hypothesized that speakers with velopharyngeal inadequacy would have to expend more effort to attain a given intensity,[267] and studies by Warren et al demonstrated increased respiratory volumes in speakers with clefts.[260] In an ultrasound study of the vocal folds in normal speakers producing normal and nasalized vowels, Hamlet found that the reduced open quotient of the vibratory cycle characteristic of nonnasalized vowels produced with loud phonation was also seen in nasalized vowels.[268] She interpreted her data to mean that a stronger adductory force was being used in both cases and hypothesized that such force in nasal speakers could lead to vocal abuse with consequent damage to the folds and abnormal laryngeal vocal quality.

These hypotheses lead to the expectation that speakers with clefts would exhibit a higher incidence of voice disorders than is found in speakers without clefts. However, the available incidence figures show wide variation. In normal speakers, the incidence of voice disorders in nine studies reviewed by Marks, Barker, and Tardy ranged from 0.5 to 7.1 percent.[269] In studies reviewed by McWilliams et al,[196] the figures ranged from 16 to 23 percent in children[270,271] and 2.7 to 7.2 percent in adults.[272,273] The incidence in speakers with cleft palate was 0.6 percent in a retrospective study of hospital records,[274] 10 percent in a group of 76 patients examined by Brooks and Shelton,[275] 15.8 percent in a questionnaire survey by Greenberg,[276] and 34 percent in 102 patients with clefts and other structural forms of velopharyngeal inadequacy examined by Marks et al.[269] The latter investigators found no relationship between velopharyngeal closure on /s/ as shown on lateral still radiographs and laryngeal voice ratings. Twenty-four of the 35 subjects exhibiting abnormal laryngeal vocal quality were laryngoscoped: 18 showed abnormalities of the cords, with five showing vocal nodules.

Leder and Lerman interpreted their findings of inappropriate voicing of voiceless consonants to be evidence of vocal abuse in patients with clefts.[236] Such an interpretation is not necessarily inaccurate, but as pointed out previously it ignores the more fundamental explanation based on the aerodynamics of the vocal tract in the absence of complete velopharyngeal closure.*

Obviously, there are wide methodological variations affecting the results of such investigations in speakers with or without clefts, including the method of ascertainment and the standards by which abnormal laryngeal vocal quality was judged.

Of more importance than the relative incidence of voice disorders, however, are the practical implications for management. From the preceding discussion, it is clear that the child with breathy or aspirate phonation in the presence of inadequate velopharyngeal closure should *not* be urged to use an increased loudness level since this may lead to vocal abuse. In fact, McWilliams, Bluestone, and Musgrave,[277] McWilliams,[255] and McWilliams et al[196] warned about the possibility of speech therapy causing vocal hyperfunction with resultant hoarseness in children with borderline inadequacy when that therapy is undertaken for the purpose of improving closure. In 86 percent of the children with clefts and hoarseness who McWilliams et al successfully laryngoscoped, bilateral vocal nodules were the most common finding.[277] In a follow-up study in which 27 of the orginal 43 children were examined $4^1/_4$ years later, 70 percent had retained their vocal abnormalities.[278] Eight who had normal cords at the time of the follow-up study nevertheless persisted in hoarseness. Physical management of the velopharyngeal mechanism in seven children was found generally to improve the condition of the vocal cords, but completely eliminated vocal symptoms (both physical and perceptual) in only one. However, the investigators noted that "removal of the nodules without attention to the valving mechanism proved to be ineffective" (p 1751). They felt that age played a role in the remission of nodules, since the average age of those who showed remission was 15 years 8 months, whereas the average age for those who did not was 12 years 1 month.

McWilliams et al noted two other categories of laryngeal disorders: "Soft-voice-syndrome," already discussed, and "strangled voice."[196] In the latter, they described phonation as associated with extreme tension in the abdominal, diaphragmatic, thoracic, laryngeal, and supraglottal muscles. They attributed this to an attempt to mask hypernasality. This quality thus seems to represent an extreme of the presumed compensation discussed earlier. McWilliams et al readily admitted the lack of empirical data proving that either of these two laryngeal behaviors is more prevalent in speakers with clefts than in those without clefts. Their remarks were based on clinical experience rather than on controlled studies.

At least one study has indicated a higher incidence of perceived laryngeal voice disorders in speakers with clefts and other forms of velopharyngeal inadequacy,[269] but other incidence figures are equivocal. The clinician should be aware of the possible role that velopharyngeal inadequacy may play in producing abnormalities of laryngeal quality and of the potential for causing or exacerbating laryngeal hyperfunction in attempting to improve borderline closure through therapy.

* Note how studies on timing, laryngeal function, and rate of speech interrelate.[236,245–247,265,266]

ETIOLOGICAL BASES OF SPEECH PROBLEMS

Although recognizing the principal role of velopharyngeal inadequacy in producing the speech associated with cleft palate, investigators have also pursued relationships between speech and other structural problems, specifically of the lips, teeth, and tongue. Attempts to establish such relationships have generally been futile.

Labial

Both research evidence[219] and clinical opinions[196,198,279] consistently reflect the view that the repaired cleft lip has little significance in articulation. McWilliams et al noted that the repaired lip in bilateral clefts may be short and tight, resulting in labiodental production of bilabials.[196] The same result may be seen when the maxillary dentition is positioned far anteriorly to the mandibular dentition, as in a severe overjet or Class II malocclusion, but this is not due to the cleft lip *per se.* When the lip, particularly the bilateral cleft lip, is repaired without establishment of the integrity and normal insertions of the orbicularis, rounded phonemes such as /w/ may be visually distorted. However, there are no reports in the literature of perceptual distortion of such phonemes.

Maxillary/mandibular discrepancy together with inappropriate bony and dental support for the upper lip may lead to disturbances in the production of labiodental consonants that are not attributable to a structural problem of the lip itself.

Dental

Given both the extreme variability in individual ability to adapt to structural deviations and the number of other factors that can affect speech in individuals with clefts, it is not surprising that Morris deemed it unreasonable to expect evidence of a relationship between dentition and speech for this population in general.[198] However, the clinician faced with the patient exhibiting both speech problems and dental and/or occlusal anomalies wants to know to what extent the former is caused by the latter and whether speech may be expected to improve in the presence of such anomalies (Figs. 17–12 and 17–13).

Bzoch,[212] Counihan,[221] and Starr[230] concluded that relationships between articulation and dentition in children with clefts could not be delineated until articulation skills were well advanced. Maxillary arch width appeared significant in 6- to 11-year old subjects[230] and 13- to 24-year old subjects,[221] but not in preschoolers.[212] Foster and Greene reported a relationship between maxillary arch collapse and "lateral defects in articulation," but none between articulation and lateral open bite or defects in the

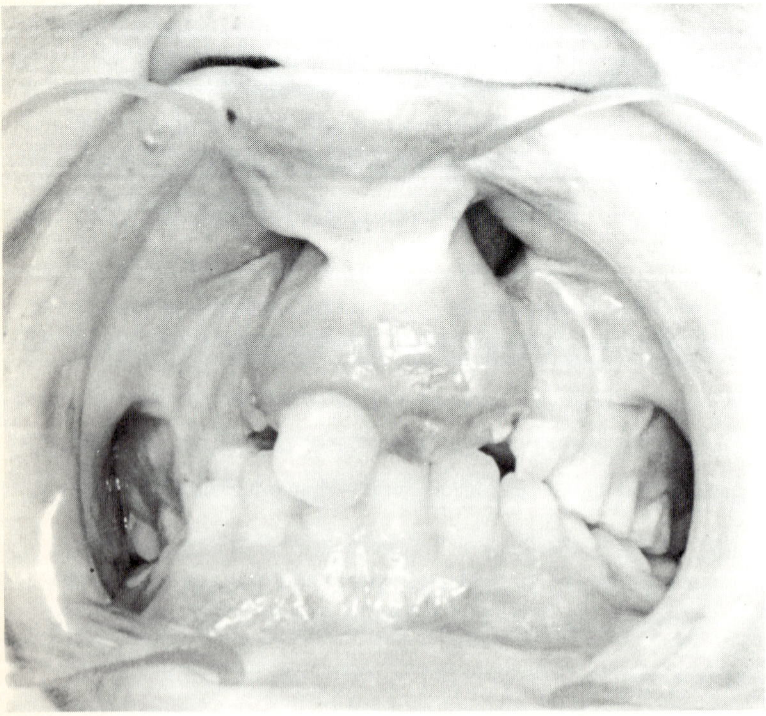

Figure 17–12 Dental and occlusal hazards to speech in bilateral cleft lip and palate. Note collapsed right lateral segment, producing a crossbite, and residual defects through the alveolus.

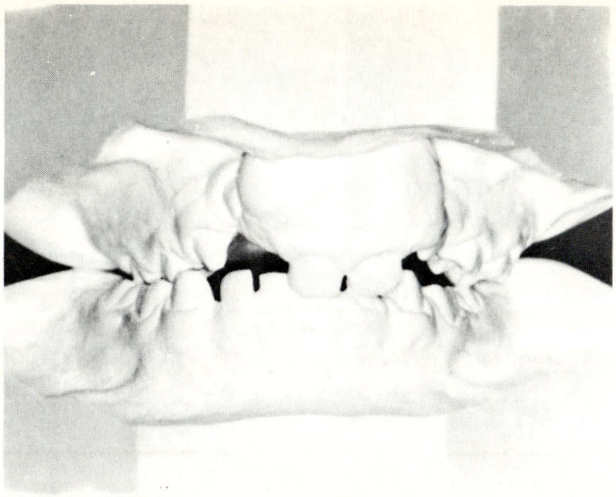

Figure 17–13 Articulated dental casts demonstrating malocclusion in bilateral cleft lip and palate.

alveolus in the area of the cleft.[280] McDermott related /s/ articulation to anteroposterior relationships of the dental arches, continuity of the cutting edges of the anterior teeth, and vertical relationships between the maxillary and mandibular teeth in children with clefts aged 8 to 18 years.[224] He found that /s/ varied with the number and severity of dental problems, the only single significant factor being anteroposterior dental arch relationships. However, Subtelny and Subtelny found no such relationship in adults with clefts.[281] Similarly inconclusive observations were made by Bishara, VanDemark, and Henderson in 1975 when they studied the relationship of articulation to a number of orofacial features, including malocclusions.[282] These investigators reported that subjects with good or poor articulation did not differ systematically in their facial and dental relationships.

The findings of Bruggeman,[283] Fymbo,[284] and Lubit[285] all implicated a narrow palatal arch as possible causal factor in articulation problems in normal children. This has particular relevance to the cleft palate population, since restriction of the maxillary arch postoperatively is a relatively common clinical finding.

As noted previously, anterior positioning of the mandibular dentition with respect to the maxillary dentition, as in a Class III malocclusion or anterior crossbite, may result in "inversion" of the labiodental fricatives and tip-labial production of normally tip-alveolar consonants.

Although the data from speakers both with and without clefts (reviewed earlier) are nebulous, it appears that the clinician questioning a relationship between dental abnormalities and speech problems in a given speaker might direct attention to (1) restrictions in maxillary arch width, (2) Class III malocclusion, (3) missing maxillary incisors, and (4) the relationship between the tongue tip and the lower incisors, although none of these is guaranteed to be responsible for problems with anterior consonants. The majority of authors, whether speaking from data or from clinical observation, emphasize that speech problems are more likely to result when dental and/or occlusal anomalies are present in number rather than in isolation and during the speech-learning years as opposed to later years. McWilliams et al emphasized the role of dentition and occlusion in establishing the size of the oral cavity and the fluctuating status of the oral environment as children go through the change from deciduous to permanent dentition as well as through the surgical management of the dental arches often required in clefts.[196]

Lingual

Several early authors discussed abnormal tongue posture and mobility in speakers with clefts, basing their remarks on clinical observations rather than on physiologic data.[286–289] Some postulated that the tongue itself was structurally abnormal or poorly innervated, whereas others felt that aberrant lingual function was secondary to velopharyngeal inadequacy.

Concern over innervation of tongue musculature motivated a study of coordination and flexibility in speech and nonspeech movements by Mathews and Byrne.[290] The results showed a significant difference between children without clefts and children with cleft lip and/or palate on two of three speech tasks. However, Morris pointed out that all of the subjects with clefts in this study were in fact in speech therapy and that they may have slowed the rate of production in order to produce the best speech of which they were capable.[198] Morris concluded that the available information failed to document problems in tongue coordination and flexibility in patients with clefts.

Several studies focused on tongue carriage, abnormal lingual contacts in speech, or both. Buck reported some small differences in tongue carriage measurements between normal children and children with cleft palate aged 7 to 19, but felt that these were explained by significant differences in the size of the oral cavity.[291,292] In a later study, Buck reported that (1) the total tongue area above the incisal line was markedly greater in subjects with cleft palate than in normal subjects, (2) the vertical tongue-palate distance was significantly smaller in patients with unrepaired clefts, and (3) the horizontal position of the high point of the tongue was more posterior in the unrepaired than in the normal and repaired groups.[293] Koepp-Baker discussed the possible effect of reduced oral cavity size (due to narrow or shallow palatal vaults) on tongue carriage.[279] The clinical descriptions by Starr[294] and the study of Guay et al[295] indicated that at least extreme reduction in vault size may affect speech, although the effect may be more directly linked to the spatial relationship between the tongue tip and the anterior teeth. However, Morris concluded that "Not even for cases where the intraoral cavity is restricted in size and where the tongue is habitually positioned unusually high or unusually posteriorly . . . is evidence available to demonstrate that such malpositioning interferes with normal articulation" (p 133).[198]

Despite the fact that Morris was unimpressed with the data in 1968, several studies have demonstrated posterior tongue carriage and/or abnormal lingual contacts at least in some speakers with clefts. Shohara, using palatography, showed a shift from more posterior articulatory contacts to more anterior contacts in a patient with cleft palate as a consequence of obturation.[296] Powers reported that two speakers with cleft palate and with poor articulation showed posterior tongue carriage, whereas two speakers with good articulation did not.[297] No consistent differences were found in tongue height. One of the subjects with poor articulation also showed a large velopharyngeal gap on midsagittal radiographic studies and exhibited what Powers termed "compensatory tongue movements." Powers felt that the retracted and elevated tongue dorsum described by McDonald and Koepp-Baker[288] might be seen clinically in patients with cleft palate and with certain kinds of structural and speech inadequacies, but was not typical of subjects with cleft palate as a group.

Brooks et al described "compensatory" tongue, palate, and posterior pharyngeal wall contacts in patients with surgically and prosthetically repaired palates and unrepaired palatal insufficiency.[210] Those who showed tongue and pharyngeal wall contact during speech were inferior in articulation and in velopharyngeal closure to those who did not. Four subjects appeared to use lingual assist to elevate the velum. In a later study, subjects who showed tongue and velum or tongue, velum, and pharyngeal wall contacts were again reported to show poorer articulation, but not greater velopharyngeal gaps.[211]

Massengill and Spoerl found no significant differences between cleft palate subjects with and those without velopharyngeal closure on measures between the tongue and various points along the cervical spine and midpharyngeal cavity, although the subjects with velopharyngeal gaps demonstrated larger variances.[298]

As noted previously, Honjow and Isshiki described tongue and pharyngeal wall contact in the production of pharyngeal stops.[209] Lawrence and Philips described deviant lingual articulatory contacts in three groups of subjects with clefts designated as having adequate, borderline, or inadequate velopharyngeal closure.[213] Seventy-five of the deviant contacts were posteriorly displaced but 25 consisted of anterior displacements on /k/ and /g/.* Subjects showing linguovelar contacts also demonstrated poorer articulation and velopharyngeal closure. Those for whom physical management had provided velopharyngeal adequacy before the age of mastery of consonants showed fewer deviant contacts.

Trost provided radiographic examples of the deviant contacts associated with the pharyngeal fricative, pharyngeal stop, and mid-dorsum palatal stop.[188] In light of the findings of Lawrence and Phillips,[213] it is pertinent to note that Dorf and Curtin documented a statistically significant difference in the occurrence of the compensatory patterns described by Trost in children whose clefts had been repaired before the age of 12 months as opposed to children operated after this age.[299]

The only study that has contradicted clinical observation or radiographic evidence of a tendency towards posterior tongue carriage in speakers with clefts was that of Dickson, in which he used a mixture of cleft palate and functionally nasal speakers.[251] The most nasal of his subjects showed a lower and more anterior tongue carriage—but also greater velopharyngeal gaps—than the remaining subjects. Several studies have shown a correlation between tongue height and velar height,[300–303] but the interrelationships between tongue and velar musculature have not received much attention in studies of deviant lingual posture in speakers with clefts.

The interpretation of abnormal tongue posture and/or deviant lingual contacts has taken several forms. Most investigators have felt that these findings were in some way linked to current or past velopharyngeal inadequacy. The data could support either or both of the theories that (1) the posterior carriage is assumed in the unconscious effort to assist in velopharyngeal closure either by lingual assist in velar elevation or by the use of the tongue dorsum to obstruct the velopharyngeal port or (2) the posterior carriage either facilitates or results from the habitual use of the generally posteriorly displaced compensatory articulations.

One must recognize that the data interrelating velopharyngeal inadequacy, abnormal tongue carriage, and deviant lingual contacts are incomplete. For example, we do not have complete radiographic

---

* See earlier discussion of the substitution of "mid-dorsum palatal stops" for /t/, /d/ and /k/, /g/ as described by Trost.[188,203]

studies of tongue movement on large samples of subjects with and without compensatory articulations or on subgroups with varying degrees of velopharyngeal inadequacy. Furthermore, we have no data on the possible occurrence of posterior tongue carriage in subjects *without* clefts or other forms of velopharyngeal inadequacy.

There does seem to be sufficient indication that some speakers with clefts tend towards posterior or retracted tongue carriage and deviant lingual contacts in speech. Most investigators have interpreted these findings as being related to present or past inadequate function of the velopharyngeal system. Although the data interrelating velopharyngeal problems and tongue posture and/or articulatory contacts are incomplete, few if any investigators now view the tongue in cleft palate as being inherently defective in structure or innervation.

Velopharyngeal

The velopharyngeal system has already been discussed in detail. Although this system is certainly viewed as the primary culprit in the speech problems common to speakers with clefts, the number and interrelationships of other structural anomalies present in these speakers complicates the process of making cause-effect conclusions. An additional complication is encountered when speakers retain long-established patterns such as compensatory articulations or nasal direction of the airstream after physical management has supposedly provided an adequate mechanism. Definitive diagnosis of the status of the velopharyngeal mechanism must usually be relegated to medical facilities where such procedures as radiographic, aerodynamic, and endoscopic studies can be done. However, diagnosis begins with the perceptual evaluation of speech, and the responsibility for deciding whether further evaluations are necessary falls to the speech pathologist. As noted earlier, some portable but rather expensive instrumentation is available for measuring the aerodynamic or acoustic consequences of velopharyngeal opening.[223,304–311] However, each type of instrumentation is subject to mechanical or electrical sources of error; the data provided must be interpreted taking into account *all* factors that might affect the output of the instrument, that is, oral resistance, or speech sample; and data derived from instrumentation cannot be used as a substitute for the clinician's own judgment. Augmentative use of such instrumentation may help to clarify a perceptually confusing situation, for example, in phoneme-specific velopharyngeal inadequacy or when nasal air loss is so minimal as to be only inconsistently audible.

Oronasal Fistulas

Patients with clefts, particularly complete unilateral or bilateral clefts of the lip and palate,[312] may have postoperative fistulas either in the alveolus in the line of the cleft or in the hard or soft palate (Fig. 17–14). In the alveolus, it is quite common for surgeons not to attempt bony union of the segments in the initial palate surgery. Fistulas in the palate itself occur as a result of postoperative breakdown, inability to mobilize enough tissue to obtain complete closure, or the surgeon's use of primary veloplasty.[313,314] In the latter procedure, only the soft palate is closed (together with the lip if the lip is involved) in the initial palatal surgery, leaving the hard palate open for a period of years in the attempt to allow better midfacial growth.

With the exception of the results of primary veloplasty,[315] few quantitative data exist that pertain to the effects of fistulas on speech. Information on the effects of labionasal fistulas is limited to sporadic case descriptions. Some speakers have been reported to show a visible inflation of the upper lip on bilabi-

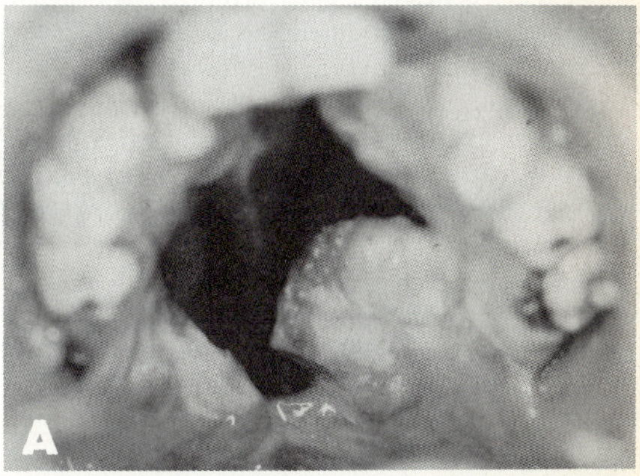

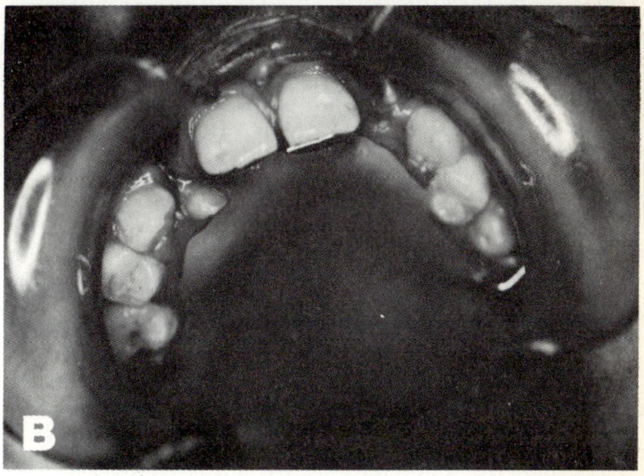

Figure 17–14 *A*, Large palatal fistula due to postoperative breakdown following palatal repair, obturated in *B* (Courtesy, Center for Craniofacial Anomalies, University of California–San Francisco.)

al plosives (the "Bing Crosby syndrome") and occasional leakage of saliva through the defect. One of the subjects of Shelton and Blank had a large maxillary defect that reportedly distorted fricatives and affricates. She showed low intraoral air pressure and the presence of nasal airflow during production of /p/ and /f/ in CV syllables.[316]

The only quantitative data on the effects of palatal fistulas were provided by Shelton and Blank.[316] Their remaining six patients had either one or two fistulas at various sites in the hard palate. Unfortunately, fistula size was described only subjectively. Also, not all subjects produced the same pressure consonants in the CV syllables. The data showed the expected drop in intraoral pressure with the fistulas open, with generally greater effects on /p/ and /f/ than on /k/. All subjects had articulation errors, but these were not described in detail. Two were noted to show errors in place of articulation, with one showing posterior placement.

Witzel, Salyer, and Ross reviewed the results of primary veloplasty on both facial growth and speech.[317] (The reader should be aware that the residual hard palate cleft is sometimes obturated and sometimes unobturated until definitive hard palate repair and that this difference is not well documented in studies of speech results.) With few exceptions, all the information regarding effects on speech was subjective. A number of investigators reported that sizeable percentages of patients undergoing the "Schweckendiek procedures" required secondary pharyngoplasties.[381–321] Schweckendiek's commentary on speech consisted only of an estimate that no more than 5 to 10 percent of his patients required pharyngoplasty.[314] Perko simply reported that the residual hard palate defect did not affect speech "to a relevant degree."[322]

Only one data-based report has been positive. Hotz, Gnoinski, Nussbaumer, and Kistler compared speech results between two groups of children who had had early palatal closure and delayed hard palate closure.[323] They found fewer glottal stops and pharyngeal substitutions and less hypernasality in the latter group, both before and after hard palate closure. However, the soft palate in the second group was repaired earlier than the complete palatal repair in the first group, thereby invalidating the results of the study. When Bardach et al reexamined 43 of Schweckendiek's patients in Marburg, more than 80 percent exhibited evidence of velopharyngeal inadequacy, glottal or pharyngeal articulations, or both.[315]

Two studies carried out on patients before hard palate closure reported extensive articulation problems as well as nasal air loss and hypernasality.[324,325]

The studies on primary veloplasty point to serious effects on speech production both before and after closure of the anterior palatal defect. However, the amount of objective data is slim. Both the objective and subjective reports represent a mixture with regard to use of obturation before hard palate closure, timing of both the early velar closure and the later palatal closure, and size of the residual defect. Speech pathologists also know little about the effects of the size of unintentional postoperative fistulas. The only available information about the differential effects of location[316] confirms the clinical expectation that anterior consonants are more affected by fistulas than are velar consonants when the velopharyngeal port is functioning adequately.

Oral Sensory Function

The possible role of oral sensory function in the acquisition and maintenance of articulatory skills was the focus of a surge of studies in the 1960s and 1970s. With respect to cleft lip and palate, attempts were made to determine (1) if patients with clefts showed poorer oral sensory discrimination than speakers without clefts and (2) if patients with cleft palate and with decreased sensory function were more apt to exhibit articulation errors, or vice versa. The question of oral sensory function in speakers with congenital oral anomalies is particularly intriguing in view of evidence that sensory nerve fibers serve a trophic function,[326,327] which might lead one to expect sensory deficits in congenital structural defects.

In speakers without structural defects, the research generally showed (1) more difficulty with oral form recognition in articulatory defective speakers than in normal speakers,[328–330] in children as well as in adults,[331] and (2) varying results on the ability of oral form discrimination to differentiate between degrees of articulation proficiency.[328,329,332] Ringel felt that some articulatory disorders of unknown etiology might eventually be found to result from disorders of sensory function, and some disorders attributable to motor factors might be found to involve sensory function.[333]

Both Ringel[334] and Shelton[335] felt that the type of feedback important during speech acquisition could be different from that controlling stabilized speech activities, and both raised the question of the implications of the research in oral sensory function for therapy. Ringel et al[331] questioned whether training in oral form discrimination might be used to facilitate improvement in articulation. Shelton felt that the nonspecific nature of traditional recommendations for the use of tactile and kinesthetic feedback, coupled with the failure to test clinical methods experimentally, cast doubt on past therapeutic use of oral sensation.

Interestingly, a few of the studies of the effects of experimental oral sensory deprivation, usually in the form of nerve block anesthesia, produced results that bore a similarity to articulation characteristics reported in speakers with cleft palate: production of intended fricatives as stops;[336] retracted placement for /t/, /d/, /k/, /g/, upper lip inactivity for /p/ and /b/; and delabialization of /w/;[336a] and general loss of precision of articulation.[336a,337,338] Prosek and House[339] followed a suggestion by Perkell[340] that intraoral air pressure is sensed in the oral cavity and monitored by myotactic feedback. Despite the fact that their sensory-deprived subjects showed articulatory distortions identical to those reported in other studies that used the same nerve blocks, Prosek and House concluded that their results did not support intraoral air pressure as an important parameter in controlling articulation. However, they did not state how feedback from intraoral air pressure could be distinguished from that for articulatory contacts.

The two earliest studies comparing oral form discrimination between speakers with and without cleft palate reported conflicting results: Hochberg and Kabcenell found poorer performance for the cleft subjects,[341] whereas Mason did not.[342] Neither study included articulation assessment. Catalanotto and Moss reported essentially normal performance on tasks of oral and manual stereognosis in patients with clefts.[343] Andrews found decreased oral form discrimination among children and adults with cleft palate, but only in subjects who also showed poor articulation; subjects with mild to moderate articulation errors performed normally.[344] Pressel and Hochberg reported inferior mean performance on oral form discrimination among 60 children with repaired clefts.[345] However, no measure of speech was included, and the significance of the difference between subjects with clefts and controls was accounted for by only 3.5 percent of the variance between groups. LaPointe and Williams found no significant difference between subjects with cleft palate and controls on form identification, two-point discrimination, weight and thickness discrimination, and pattern recognition.[346] Acknowledging that varying instrumentation and methodology might account for the discrepancy between their results and those of Hochberg and Kabcenell[341] and Andrews,[344] LaPointe and Williams nevertheless concluded that the consistent findings of no significant difference in scores across the seven components of their test supported the view of no real differences between the two groups.

The contradictory evidence on presence or absence of problems in oral sensory function among patients with clefts might have been due to differences in methodology or to heterogeneity in ages of subjects and severity of clefts. Failure to document severity of cleft ("type" of cleft is not synonymous with "severity") was universal in all of these studies. In addition, only Andrews included information on speech.[344] The coexistence of reduced orosensory ability and articulation errors in subjects without clefts should signal for caution in interpreting results in subjects with clefts. Andrews' findings support the view that the differentiating factor may be the presence or absence of articulation errors, rather than the cleft, although the lack of information on severity of the cleft is frustrating, since it is reasonable to assume that patients with more severe clefts could be those with more severe articulation problems.

The data derived in the studies cited did not allow the establishment of a cause-effect pattern among the factors of severity of cleft (and/or inadequacy of repair), orosensory deficit, and articulation problems. That this area of research essentially proved unfruitful is attested to by the fact that no new studies have appeared in recent years.

Hearing Loss

Children with clefts have long been known to be subject to middle ear disease and to conductive hearing loss. In her review of 1979, Heller pointed out that historical reports linking cleft palate to hearing problems date back to the 1870s.[347] A review of the large body of literature that has accumulated on this topic reveals the changes in findings that would be expected as technologic advances were made in the diagnosis of middle ear disease, the assessment of auditory function, and the medical treatment of both ear disease and clefts. In addition, however, one finds conflicting results and conclusions attributable, especially in the earlier research, to poor study design and marked inconsistency in such factors as the criteria set for hearing loss. Such problems were not, of course, exclusive to studies related to cleft palate.

The majority of reports in the 1940s, 1950s, and 1960s pointed to high frequency of occurrence of conductive hearing loss and/or middle ear diseases.[348–376] As pointed out by Heller,[347] extreme variability in the criteria for and means of determining hearing loss led to the reported incidence of loss ranging from 0.0 percent in one study, which nevertheless reported a 50 percent incidence of pathology of the middle ear[377] to 90 percent.[372]*

Part of the variability was due to differences in the age groups of subjects. Earlier investigators lacked

* Goetzinger et al also stated that over 50 percent of the audiograms in their subjects "revealed conductive components."[377]

the means currently available for assessing auditory function in young children. In addition, the incidence of both hearing loss and middle ear pathology has been shown to vary with age. Spriestersbach et al reported significantly worse thresholds for children aged 33 to 71 months than for children in three older age groups.[375] Heller, Hochberg, and Milano found improved hearing sensitivity with increasing age in both normal and cleft palate children, which was most evident above the age of 6.[378] Webster and Eldis reported an incidence of 94 percent of hearing loss of 10 dB or more at the age of 4 years, which decreased to an incidence of 43 percent at 20 years.[379] However, Shimo reported a higher incidence of middle ear pathology in 5 to 16 year olds with clefts than in 1 to 4 year olds.[380] Skolnik also reported a gradual increase in middle ear pathology with age, rising from 27 percent between the ages of 1 and 4 years to 69 percent between the ages of 3 and 8 years.[373] He felt the incidence increased up to school age and then leveled off. The ears of the children in these studies were *not* examined under a microscope, and Heller pointed out that a routine otologic examination does not always reveal a pathologic condition.[347] Her point is illustrated by the fact that one study utilizing microscopic examination showed a 100 percent incidence of mucoid material present in the middle ears of 40 children with cleft palate under the age of 2 years.[381] Graham reported that hearing stabilized by about 8 years of age.[354]

Although Goetzinger et al considered middle ear disease to have run its course in patients with cleft palate by adolescence, several studies have yielded contradictory data.[377] Incidence of middle ear pathology was reported to be 78 percent in patients aged 10 years to 40 years in one study[348] and 40 percent in a subject group aged 14 to 29 in another study.[382] An incidence of around 50 percent for middle ear disease and/or conductive hearing loss in adults with clefts was also reported by Bennett,[383] Caldarelli,[384] Smith,[374] and Swigart,[385] although criteria for determining the presence of diseases or hearing loss varied from study to study.

In addition to the factor of age, investigators attempted to determine the influence of the type of cleft and the type and age of physical management of the cleft on the incidence of ear disease and hearing loss. Unfortunately, the majority of these studies occurred before the advent of tympanometric testing and brain stem evoked response audiometry, and again they suffered from inconsistency in criteria and methods. Skolnik reported a decreasing incidence of middle ear pathology, going from children with overt cleft of the palate only to submucous clefts to complete unilateral clefts.[373] He also reported that there was no apparent relationship between the width of cleft and the incidence of ear disease. However, both Masters et al[364] and Paulsen[371] concluded that ear disease was more likely the wider the cleft. Masters et al also concluded that patients with clefts of the palate only were more likely to have ear disease than those with clefts of the lip and palate.[364] Heller et al[378] and Caldarelli [384] later reported similar findings. However, Drettner[352] and Pannbacker[370] found a higher incidence in patients with clefts of both the lip and palate. Bennett reported that patients with bilateral clefts were more vulnerable than patients in other cleft categories.[383] In her review in 1979, Heller stated that "the evidence of a relationship between hearing loss and type of cleft is inconclusive" (p 108).[347] No data have emerged in the interim to contradict this conclusion.

A number of early studies looked at ear disease in relation to both the type of palatoplasty and the age at which it was performed.[358,364,375,386,387] Results were conflicting,primarily due to poor study design. Koch et al concluded that surgical repair of the palate neither caused nor improved ear disease.[381] However, Bluestone did report that only infants whose clefts had been repaired showed function of the eustachian tube.[388] Some investigators attempted to establish a relationship between ear disease and whether or not the palatoplasty had in fact provided velopharyngeal closure,[375,384,386,389] without the benefit of currently available methods for assessing the latter. Reported results were again conflicting. Heller concluded in 1979 that no firm conclusions could be drawn about any of these three variables based on the data in these studies.[347] However, Morgan, Dellon, and Hoopes later reported less frequent and milder hearing loss in children undergoing palatal repair that included levator retrodisplacement as opposed to repair without such displacement.[390]

Studies of the effects of obturators and pharyngeal flaps initially focused on whether or not they might cause additional problems with the function of the eustachian tube and thus a higher incidence of hearing loss. Several early investigators warned about deleterious effects of obturators, based either on results of audiometric studies or on clinical intuition that such devices blocked the pharyngeal orifice of the eustachian tube.[361,364,371,375] However, Graham, Schweiger, and Olin reported that the incidence of ear problems was not increased in patients treated prosthetically,[391] and a later assessment of their patients after several years of wearing obturators confirmed the original conclusion.[392] Swigart found no significant differences among groups of patients treated prosthetically, surgically, or by a combination of surgery and obturation.[385]

Other investigators attempted to determine if

pharyngeal flaps had either a positive or negative effect on auditory function. Graham and Lierle reported no effect of flaps.[355] Aschan found the incidence of hearing loss to be reduced from 40 percent to 33 percent following flaps.[348] Bennett's findings were similar to those of Graham and Lierle: those patients who had tubal dysfunction preoperatively continued to show dysfunction postoperatively.[383] Yules reported that the incidence of air bone gaps 15 dB or greater decreased from 58 percent preoperatively to 46 percent postoperatively.[389] LeWorthy and Schliesser studied hearing acuity before and after pharyngeal flap in patients aged 3 to 17 years.[393] They reported that 13 percent had a hearing loss both pre- and postoperatively, 26 percent had a loss preoperatively that disappeared postoperatively, and hearing deteriorated postoperatively in two patients.

In reviewing studies of the effects of any type of physical management, remember that the increasing age of the patient from the pre-management to the post-management state may contaminate results.

The majority of studies on hearing in cleft palate that emerged after the mid-1960s were influenced by three technological advances, namely the development of instrumentation and techniques for tympanometric testing, brain stem evoked response audiometry, and microscopic examination of the ears of infants—all of which made assessment possible at much younger ages than had previously been possible.

Microscopic examinations of the ears of children with clefts became routine in the late 1960s and dramatically changed the incidence figures on ear problems. Middle ear pathology was found to be virtually universal in infants with clefts.[381,389,394–397] Although abnormalities in eustachian tube function had long been known to be the primary culprit in ear disease in clefts,[354,356,357,371] the discovery of the early onset of otitis media (conceivably prior to birth) spurred a series of studies of the anatomy and physiology of this structure in children, adults, and animal models.[382,398–407] Early insertion of ventilating tubes became popular.[394,406,408–419]

Bluestone, Paradise, Beery, and Wittel studied eustachian tube function in 22 infants undergoing two types of palatoplasty and reported improved tubal function in all following surgery, echoing Bluestone's earlier report in 1971.[420] Doyle, Reilly, Jardini, and Rovnak also reported improved passive function of the eustachian tube following palatoplasty.[421] Too-Chung conducted tympanometric testing on infants prior to and following palatal surgery performed at varying age levels and found an incidence of middle ear problems (based on tympanometry only) in children repaired at or before 4 months, which was no greater than that in normal children.[422]

Studies in the 1970s and 1980s continued to demonstrate a high incidence of ear disease and conductive hearing loss in patients with cleft palate.[362,385,396,423–426] When auditory testing at extremely high frequencies became possible, Ahonen and McDermott found a statistically significant difference between the hearing of normal and cleft palate subjects *only* about 9,000 Hz.[427]

Most reports agreed on a rare incidence of sensorineural loss in patients with clefts,[347,369,428,429] although Bennett reported that 31 percent of his adults with clefts had either sensorineural or mixed hearing loss.[383] Bluestone[430] conjectured that this finding might be explained by the work of Paparella, Oda, Hiraida, and Brady who found sensorineural loss in some patients with otitis media and ascribed this loss to associated pathologic changes in the inner ear, presumably mediated via the round window.[431]

The development of tympanometric testing contributed greatly to the ability to delineate middle ear function, sometimes revealing pathology not revealed by either routine audiometric testing or otologic examination. A series of studies in the 1970s reflected the initial excitement about the application of this technique in detection of middle ear pathology associated with clefting.[381,432–436]

A sizeable body of data has been accumulated, indicating that patients with submucous clefts as well as most other types of velopharyngeal inadequacy experience the same incidence and type of ear disease as patients with overt clefts.[66,75,93,374,380,423,429,437–441] Bergstrom and Hemenway reported that 39 percent of their patients with submucous clefts had middle ear disease.[437] Thirty-four percent had conductive hearing loss, and interestingly 25 percent had either sensorineural or mixed losses. In a later report by Bergstrom, the incidence figures were 38 percent conductive loss, 16 percent sensorineural, and 10 percent mixed.[423] Caldarelli reported a 67 percent incidence of serous otitis media in patients with the visible stigmata of a submucous cleft and 74 percent in patients with velopharyngeal inadequacy in the absence of such stigmata.[438] His results were similar to Calnan's earlier reported incidence of 79 pecent.[24] In a study initiated out of concern for how often a bifid uvula signals the presence of an occult submucous cleft, the authors determined that children with bifid uvula might be at only a slightly increased risk for otitis media, but that the magnitude of the increase, if any, was small.[442]

The topic of the influence of hearing impairment on speech, language, and cognitive development in normal children has generated a large series of studies.[443–452] Although authors have frequently voiced concern about this influence in children with cleft palate,[348,381,453] only a few studies specifically addressed the question. Galkowski, Gassowski, and Grossmann reported a "smaller" speech development in children with cleft palates and an "accompanying serious defect of hearing" than in other children with clefts without an accompanying hearing loss.[454] However, two later studies reported essentially negative results. Freeland and Evans concluded that treatment of middle ear effusions produced "no advantage for speech and language."[455] Hubbard, Paradise, McWilliams, Elster, and Taylor found that mean verbal performance, full-scale IQs, and scores on psychosocial indices were normal both in one group of children with cleft palate who had undergone myringotomy with placement of ventilating tubes at 3 months and another group for whom that procedure had not been performed until the age of nearly 31 months as well as in two subjects for whom it was not done at all.[456] However, consonant articulation was significantly better in the first group.

In summary, patients with clefts are known to be particularly vulnerable to middle ear disease, which has its beginnings with effusion present virtually at birth. The primary etiology is malfunction of the eustachian tube. Patients with submucous clefts and other forms of velopharyngeal inadequacy are similarly vulnerable. Incidence figures on both the middle ear disease and the consequent conductive hearing loss have been strongly influenced by changing methods of investigation and criteria for the presence of a loss. Both hearing acuity and the health of the ear appear to improve with age, although approximately 50 percent of adults with clefts continue to exhibit a hearing loss, evidence of middle ear pathology, or both. The relationship between ear problems and the type or severity of cleft is unclear, and it is not likely to be further delineated since infants with clefts are now treated much earlier than was previously the case. Studies of the effects of specific strategies of physical management of the cleft on the incidence of ear problems have been contaminated by a number of interrelated factors. Again, current otologic management makes the accrual of future data on this topic unlikely unless patients are arbitrarily assigned to a no-treatment group.

For further review of the topic of hearing loss in cleft palate, please see Graham,[457] Heller,[347] Hudson,[458] Jardini,[428] Litton, Severeid, and Tharp,[459] and Swigart.[429]

PHYSICAL MANAGEMENT

The physical management of clefts consists of either prosthetic or surgical closure of the cleft and, similarly, either prosthetic or surgical approaches to residual velopharyngeal inadequacy following palatal closure. Combinations of prosthetic and surgical procedures are fairly common. Other categories of physical management, not discussed here, include cosmetic revisions of the lip and nose, orthodontia, and prosthetic replacement of missing teeth.

An extremely large body of literature has accumulated on the efficacy of innumerable surgical approaches for closure of the lip and palate and amelioration of velopharyngeal inadequacy. Unfortunately, in only a small percentage of those studies on palatal closure or various surgical procedures for velopharyngeal inadequacy was a speech pathologist one of the investigators. Conclusions about speech results have largely been drawn by the surgeons themselves and have typically consisited of broad judgmental categories rarely supported by quantitative data. To a certain extent, the same is true for studies of speech results in prosthetically treated patients. In addition, only in the last 20 or so years have multiview videofluoroscopy, endoscopy, and aerodynamic studies been available for the assessment of surgical or prosthetic results. Finally, the majority of the published studies were characterized by the failure or the inability to control for a number of independent variables (type and severity of cleft, surgical technique).

Space does not permit an exhaustive review of all the investigations of various types of physical management. Rather, some fundamental information will be offered here, together with information from some recent studies. For a comprehensive review of this topic, the reader is referred to McWilliams et al.[196]

Surgical Care

The reader must be aware that philosophies on the timing and type of surgical care for the child with a cleft vary widely, making it difficult to make generalizations. The following, therefore, is a cautious summary.

Lip Closure

In the child with a cleft lip who is otherwise healthy, surgical closure often occurs between the second and third month (Fig. 17–15). The "rule of 10s" (10 lbs of weight, 10 g of hemoglobin, 10 weeks of age)[460] is popular with some surgeons, but not with others. In the case of a bilateral cleft of the lip, some surgeons prefer to close one side at a time, whereas others prefer to close both simultaneously. In this as in other surgical questions, the size of the cleft and the availability of tissue in the individual baby may affect the timing of the procedure.

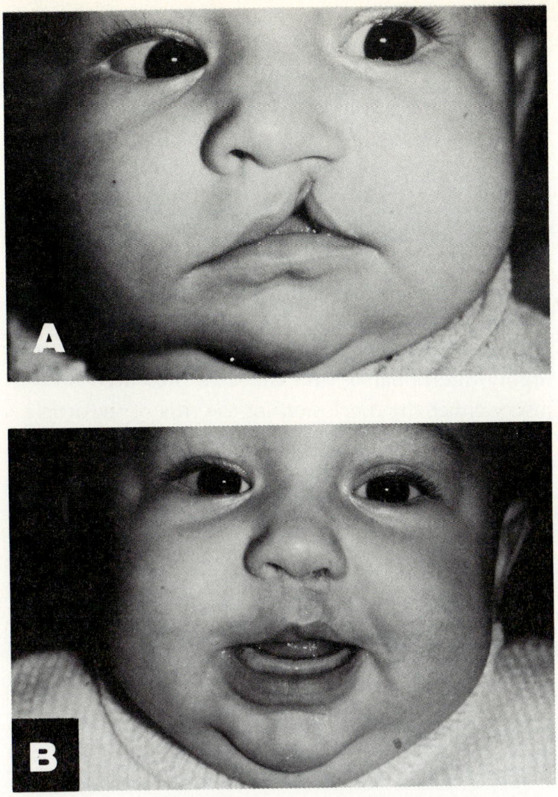

Figure 17–15 Incomplete cleft lip, *A*, prior to and *B*, following repair. (Courtesy, Dr. William Hoffman and the Center for Craniofacial Anomalies, University of California–San Francisco.)

Closure of the Alveolar Cleft

Primary bone grafting of the alveolar cleft is a point of long and vehement controversy, with some surgeons advocating it,[461,462] whereas others, typically orthodontists, see no need for it and fear for deleterious effects on growth and later interference with orthodontic therapy.[463,464] This procedure is more popular in Europe than in the United States. However, one set of English investigators who had earlier advocated primary bone grafting later published negative long-term results.[465] Secondary bone grafting at a later age to provide bone so that teeth may erupt and the lip will have bony support is much less controversial.[466–468]

Palatal Closure

There are several basic surgical approaches to closing the palatal cleft (Fig. 17–16), with variations of each which are typically given yet another name. Combinations of approaches are also used. The most popular approach is the "V-Y pushback," also variously known as the Oxford technique, the Wardill-Kilner, and the Veau-Wardill-Kilner,[68,196,469] and has generated variations based on the number of unipedicled mucoperiosteal flaps raised.[470,471] The Von Langenbeck procedure raises bipedicle flaps and has also generated variations.[312] The vomer flap mobilizes the base of the vomer bone to close the cleft.[472–475] In a primary pharyngeal flap, closure of the palate is combined with incorporation of a pharyngeal flap.[476–483] This procedure became less popular when it was pointed out that a relatively low percentage of patients undergoing palatal closure later require flaps and as other techniques for obtaining a longer and more mobile palate were developed.[484]

Levator reconstruction, also called intravelar veloplasty, is not actually a procedure for closing the palatal cleft, but is often used in conjunction with a pushback or Von Langenbeck in an attempt to restore the normal muscular action of the velum.[485–490] Similarly, the island flap is used in conjunction with a V-Y procedure, with a flap of palatal mucoperiosteum repositioned and the levator muscles dissected from their abnormal attachment on the posterior border of the hard palate.[491–501] Any of the aforementioned procedures may be used for the closure of submucous defects as well.[83,502]

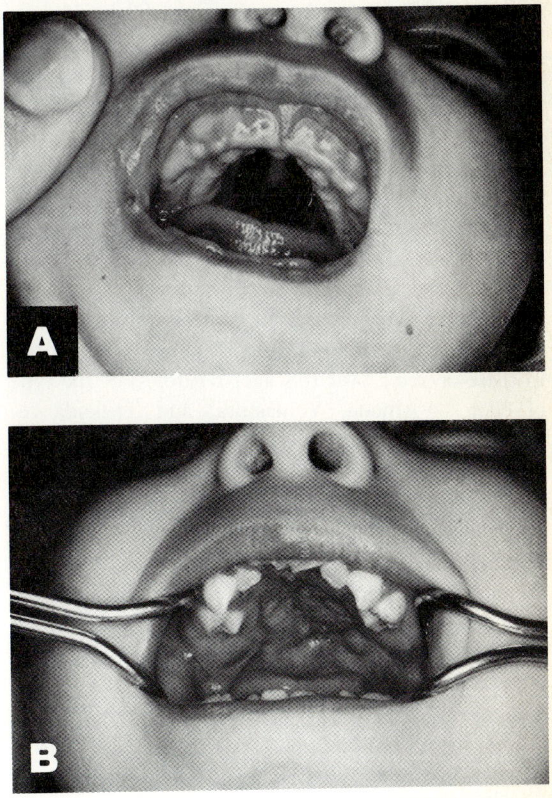

Figure 17–16 Palatal cleft, *A*, prior to and *B*, following repair. (Courtesy, Center for Craniofacial Anomalies, University of California–San Francisco.)

As noted earlier, "primary veloplasty" refers to closure of the velum with the hard palate left open for closure some years later.[313,314,322,503,504] A large amount of literature is accumulating on this subject, which basically indicate that the desired beneficial effect on midfacial growth may be achieved,[315,505] although one study found no significant differences in occlusion or facial profile at the age of 4½ years between children whose hard palates had been closed at the age of 11 months versus children whose palates were still unrepaired at the time of assessment.[506] Evidence indicates that the effects on speech are devastating,[315,317,319,321,507] although more objective data are needed.

Age of Palatal Closure

Philosophies on the age at which surgical closure of the palate should be performed vary dramatically, although most standard surgical texts today still recommend "18 to 24 months." Such recommendations obviously ignore the fact that speech development begins long before this time period in the normally developing child. Knowledge that earlier surgery generally produces better speech results dates back at least to Veau, who in 1933 (as cited by Morley,[508]) reported "normal speech" in 75 percent of children operated on prior to 12 months, 60 percent in those operated on between 2 and 4 years, and 28 percent in those operated on over the age of 9 years. Other studies have produced similar results.[359,509–513] In attempting to balance speech results against effects of surgery on maxillary growth, Koberg and Koblin settled on the age of 2 to 3 years as being optimum for palatal closure.[514] Dorf and Curtin found a statistically significant difference in the occurrence of compensatory articulations in children operated at 12 months or younger as opposed to those operated over this age, regardless of the type of cleft.[299] Ainoda, Yamashita, and Tsukada reported "abnormal articulation" in 48 percent of children operated on between the ages of 12 and 22 months (mean = 15.2 months), but no comparable group was operated on earlier or later.[515] Randall, LaRossa, Fakharaee, and Cohen reported significantly better speech results and a lower incidence of later need for pharyngoplasties in a series of children operated on between 3 and 7 months as opposed to a comparable group operated on between 12 and 18 months.[516]

It should be noted that what is considered "early" by most European investigators is not considered early by others. This discrepancy is best illustrated in a recent article by Blijdorp and Muller in which they compared speech results in children operated around the age of 3 years to those in children operated around age 6.[517] More "compensations" (unspecified) were found in the first group. Oddly, "nasal escape" was judged with a mirror held beneath the nose while the speaker produced "ee" and "oo." Despite the authors' conclusions, the soft palate was reported to be longer and more mobile in the first group, although no difference occurred between the groups in incidence of poor palatal function (approximately 50 percent in both groups if no pharyngoplasty had been performed). The ages at which surgery was performed in this study were too late to make a difference in speech,[299] the methods of assessment were highly questionable, and the data presented do not justify either the conclusions or the title of the article.

Desai reported that none of 100 children whose palates were closed prior to the age of 16 weeks demonstrated nasal escape, but offered neither details on how this judgment was made nor any other information about speech.[518]

The controversy over timing of closure is based on the concern that early closure, although benefiting speech, may be deleterious to midfacial growth. Extensive reviews on this topic have been offered by Berkowtiz,[519] Egyedi,[520] Kaplan,[521] McWilliams et al,[196] and Ross and Johnston.[23] Egyedi concluded that the optimum time for closure would be between the ages of 12 and 18 months, although the majority of the studies he reviewed were European.[520] Kaplan concluded from his review of the available data that the age of palatal closure might soon move below 3 months.[521] However, to date no data are available on speech development that would support such early surgery. As of this writing, the best data indicate that, in the normally developing child, 12 months may indeed be a critical cut-off time for surgery considering speech results *only*.[299]

Comparative Speech Results Across Surgical Procedures

Data comparing speech results across surgical approaches are usually contaminated by such factors as age both at the time of surgery and at the time of assessment, severity of cleft, specific variations of surgical procedures used, and methods of assessment.

McWilliams et al[196] reviewed 13 studies on the results of the V-Y procedure and found that the reported percentages of success ranged from 21 to 95 percent, with the majority reporting an average of over 70 percent.[312,318,486,509,512,522–530] Aaronson, Fox, and Cronin reported "readily intelligible speech" in 78 percent, normal articulation in 66 percent, and normal resonance in 78 percent of 92 patients repaired with the Cronin version of the pushback procedure.[531]

In the reports on the success of the Von Langenbeck procedure reviewed by McWilliams et al,[196] success rates ranged from 51 percent to 73 percent, with a mean of 60 percent, the most frequently reported rates being between 50 and 60 percent.[318,525–527,529] McWilliams et al concluded that the preponderance of the evidence indicated a lower success rate for his procedure than for the pushback.[196] Kaplan, Labandter, Ben-Bassat, Dresner, and Nachmani reported "normal speech" in 68 percent of patients undergoing the Von Langenbeck procedure.[532] Witzel, Clarke, Lindsay and Thomson found no significant differences in velopharyngeal closure or conversational speech between two matched groups whose palates were closed by a pushback or a Von Langenbeck procedure.[533] McWilliams et al pointed out that such results reflect the differences in results obtained in the hands of different surgeons.[196] Similarly, Palmer, Hamlen, Ross, and Lindsay reported comparable results for these two procedures.[534] The Von Langenbeck and a four-flap version of a pushback were two of the four operative procedures used in a series of 249 patients reviewed by O'Riain and Hamond.[535] Unfortunately, the information offered on speech in this study is uninterpretable. Holtmann, Wray, and Weeks reviewed the results of the V-Y pushback, the Von Langenbeck, and the latter procedure used in conjunction with a pharyngeal flap.[536] However, all of these essentially amounted to primary veloplasty, since the anterior palatal defect was not closed, thereby making it difficult to interpret their statement that no differences in speech were found among the three groups. Interpretation is also prohibited by the fact that no assessment data on speech were offered. This study typifies virtually all of the problems in such research listed previously. Dreyer and Trier compared speech results among three groups repaired with the Von Langenbeck procedure with no palatal lengthening, "palate lengthening procedures" consisting of a V-Y or island procedure," and Von Langenbeck with the addition of levator reconstruction.[537] They found no differences between the first two groups: the incidence of excellent speech was approximately 30 percent in each group, acceptable speech approximately 35 percent in each group, and poor speech 38 percent. In the third group, excellent speech was achieved in 50 percent and acceptable speech in 41 percent. VanDemark and Hardin reported that more children whose clefts were closed by the Von Langenbeck procedure required pharyngeal flaps than children who had undergone the Wardill pushback.[538]

Lewin et al reported that the Millard island flap procedure produced "acceptable speech" in 71 percent of patients with overt cleft palate and 60 percent in patients with velopharyngeal insufficiency.[502] They concluded that this procedure offered no advantage over the pushback procedure. Luce et al reported that the incidence of severe or moderately severe hypernasality in the island flap was "distressingly high," being 40 percent in their 96 patients.[495]

Marks and Wynn reported an incidence of 81.5 percent of "near-normal or normal resonance" in 413 patients undergoing Wynn's bilateral osteotomy" (vomer flap or bone flap).[539] Unfortunately, subjective judgment of resonance was the only assessment result offered.

As noted previously, speech results in primary veloplasty have generally been poor. Schweckendiek reported that 57 percent of his patients had "normal" speech, as judged by intelligibility, even before closure of the hard palate.[314] Nevertheless, Schweckendiek stated that only 5 to 10 percent needed pharyngoplasty. Cosman and Falk reported that only 34 percent of their patients had acceptable speech.[319] In the 43 patients reviewed by Bardach et al, only 16 percent had velopharyngeal adequacy, and the incidence of compensatory articulations was high.[315] The conclusions of Hotz et al about the beneficial effects of delayed hard palate closure were invalid, as discussed previously.[323] Witzel et al pointed out that, of the six studies of primary veloplasty in which speech pathologists were authors, five (all except that by Hotz et al) demonstrated that this procedure results in severe speech problems both before and after hard palate closure.[317]

Morris reviewed the available studies up to 1971 and concluded that palatal cloure is generally successful about 75 percent of the time, notwithstanding all the ways in which that success is measured.[484] Shprintzen reported an 86 percent success rate with closure of the anterior hard palate at 12 months (technique unspecified) and closure of the soft palate with a lengthening procedure at 18 months.[540]

Exactly what constitutes a pushback, Von Langenbeck, or other procedure varies from surgeon to surgeon and study to study, with success rates varying accordingly. Studies to date indicate a higher percentage of successful results of palatal closure when the procedure incorporates palatal lengthening or repositioning of the levator. Success rates with the island flap have not been favorable, and insufficient data exist to judge the effect of the bone or vomer flap. However, data gathered to date indicate unfavorable results on speech when primary veloplasty is used.

Pharyngeal Flaps

Technically, the term "pharyngoplasty" is applied to any surgical procedure on the pharyngeal musculature. However, the term "pharyngeal flap" is commonly reserved for a procedure that produces an attachment of musculature between the velum and the posterior pharyngeal wall (Fig. 17–17). This is a generic term, encompassing many brand names. Passavant first described a posterior pharyngeal flap in 1865, but this flap was apparently the creation of adhesions between the velum and pharyngeal wall.[541] Schoenborn described an inferiorly based flap in 1876,[542] but the procedure did not become popular until Rosenthal revitalized it in 1924;[543] it was introduced in the United States by Padgett in 1930.[469,541] In this procedure, a three-sided pocket-shaped flap of tissue is raised from the posterior pharyngeal wall, leaving an attachment inferiorly. In the superiorly based flap described by Sanvernero-Rosselli in 1935, the "pocket" is inverted, leaving the flap attached to the wall superiorly.[544] These are the two main types of flaps. Kapetansky described a "transverse" flap in which two pedicles are raised from the pharyngeal wall and transposed into the soft palate.[545] Another bipedicled flap was described by McCoy and Zahorsky in 1972.[176] Hogan popularized the "lateral port control" flap in which the flap is constructed so as to leave lateral ports the size of catheters of a certain gauge, which are then left in place for a period of time as the tissue heals.[546–548] He based this approach on Warren's aerodynamic data that indicated that a velopharyngeal port of 0.20 cm^2 or over results in hypernasality.

It is quite common for a pharyngeal flap to be combined with either a pushback[549–554] or levator retropositioning.[555] A pharyngeal flap alone or in combination with another procedure may be used as the primary means of repair in submucous clefts or

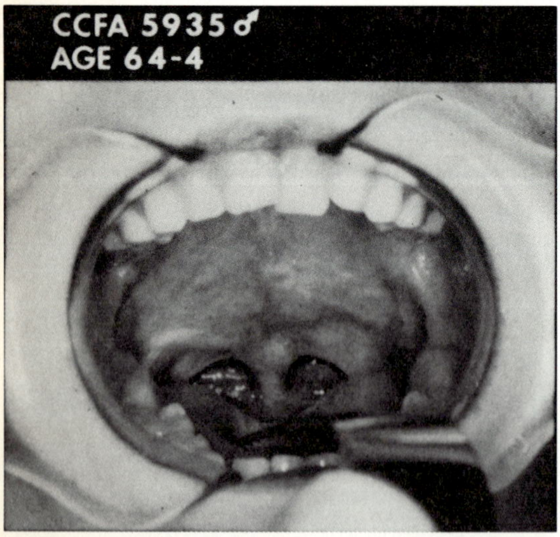

Figure 17–17 Downward migration of pharyngeal flap base on the posterior pharyngeal wall. (Courtesy, Center for Craniofacial Anomalies, University of Illinois.)

various forms of noncleft velopharyngeal inadequacy.[83,549,550,553,556–559]

At one time, it was thought that the transposed musculature incorporated into the flap retained its mobility. Subtelny, Oya, Subtelny, Curtin, and McCormack reported an association between successful speech results and "mobility of the flap and/or adjacent structures."[560] Skoog felt that inferiorly based flaps retained mobility better than superiorly based flaps, although he felt the speech results were comparable.[561,562] Fara and Vele reported that inferiorly based flaps retained their electromyographic (EMG) activity, whereas superiorly based ones did not.[563] McCoy and Zahorsky devised their bipedicled or "chevron" flap in the effort to avoid the denervation they found in superiorly based flaps; however, the evidence of preserved innervation in their flaps was based on evaluations made less than 6 months postoperatively.[176] Owsley, Creech, and Dedo also found a lack of EMG activity in superiorly based flaps and concluded that, if the velum-flap mechanism moves, the movement is due to the action of the velum itself.[564]

Whitaker, Randall, Graham, Hamilton, and Winchester conducted a randomized study on inferiorly and superiorly based flaps and found no significant difference in speech results.[565] This finding reflected the earlier opinion published by Skoog,[561,562] but conflicted with the results of another study that reported a 48 percent success rate with high-attached flaps, but only 19 percent in low-attached flaps.[559] A later study compared the relative technical advantages and disadvantages of each and expressed a preference for inferiorly based flaps in some situations, particularly in patients in whom the nasopharynx is difficult to access.[566]

Moll, Huffman, Lierle, and Smith reported that wide pharyngeal flaps (as judged on the intraoral view) were more likely to provide good speech results than narrow flaps and that less successful results were obtained on patients operated over the age of 15 years.[567] Lierle, Huffman, and Smith pointed out in 1967 that successful speech results from pharyngeal flaps were dependent upon the suitability of the size of the flap to the width of the velopharyngeal area and the movement of the lateral pharyngeal walls toward the flap.[568] Morris and Spriestersbach found that patients with successful pharyngeal flaps showed either mesial movement of the lateral walls or superoposterior movement of the palatal flap structure, with the mesial movement proving to be the better predictor of success.[569] The critical role of mesial motion of the lateral walls was borne out in extensive studies using multiview videofluoroscopy[549,570–572] and nasopharyngoscopy.[549,553,554,573,574]

Studies on pharyngeal flap, as well as studies

on other kinds of pharyngoplasty and on prosthetics, have typically been characterized by the design problems discussed previously. Assessment of speech results is gross at best and often not done by a speech pathologist. With few exceptions, the operated patients represent a variety of etiologies of velopharyngeal inadequacy, although some authors have taken care to report their results by patient type. An additional problem is that most studies have counted patients with postoperative denasality as "successes" in terms of speech. Finally, the time between surgery and postoperative assessment varies widely in these studies as it does in studies of other forms of physical management, with few investigators offering long-term results.

Yules and Chase[575] and Yules et al[541] offered extensive reviews on the information available on pharyngeal flap, as well as other types of procedures for velopharyngeal inadequacy. In the 24 studies they reviewed, the reported failure rate (generally by surgeons) ranged from 0.0 to 29 percent. Studies published since that time have claimed success rates (usually including denasal patients) ranging from 74 to 97 percent.[120,546,549,551,554,556,558,565,570,576–578] The criteria for success used in these studies varied greatly, with most authors hedging to a degree by mentioning "slight hypernasality, slight residual nasal air loss" among those they counted as successes.

The advent of multiview videofluoroscopy and nasopharyngoscopy made it possible for surgeons to attempt to gauge their procedure to the size of the velopharyngeal port and the amount and level of motion of both the velum and the pharyngeal walls. Shprintzen et al reported on "tailor-made flaps" in which three different methods of attaching the flap to the velum resulted in flaps of narrow, moderate, or wide lateral dimensions.[554] The success rate in 60 patients examined with multiview videofluoroscopy and nasopharyngoscopy preoperatively and subsequently receiving the appropriate-sized flap was 97 percent (although 18 percent were hyponasal) as opposed to an 80 percent success rate in patients for whom the surgical procedure had not been preceded by such examination. Similar approaches to suiting the particular procedure to the size and behavior of the velopharyngeal port were described by Albery et al[549] and Pigott.[553,573] Skolnick and McCall demonstrated the different behaviors of the lateral pharyngeal walls, which, together with the appropriateness of the size of the pharyngeal flap, determine whether or not closure is achieved postoperatively.[572] The 1980 report by Argamaso et al similarly illustrated that flaps can fail because they are too narrow for the amount of pharyngeal wall motion present, because they are skewed to one side, or because they are not placed at the level of maximum mesial motion of the lateral pharyngeal walls, usually being too low.[570] The latter finding is the main reason why most surgeons have expressed a preference for the superiorly based as opposed to inferiorly based flap.

Several studies looked at changes in pharyngeal wall behavior after attachment of a pharyngeal flap. Shprintzen, McCall, and Skolnick, using nasopharyngoscopy and multiview videofluoroscopy, found that only 16 of 100 patients showed a change in pharyngeal wall motion 6 or more months postoperatively.[579] An equal number showed increased or decreased motion. Lewis and Pashayan reported change in five of 20 patients, with an increase in two, but a decrease in three, which they attributed to the flap impeding mesial excursion of the walls.[580] Zwitman, using oral endoscopy, reported a decrease in lateral pharyngeal wall motion in 13 of 14 patients.[581,582]

The importance of the timing of assessment of surgical results is underscored by those studies reporting changes over time. Bzoch noted in 1964 that 29 of 40 cases who were at first hyponasal improved over a period of 1 to 3 years.[583] Of the 140 cases reported by Brondsted et al, 39 percent were hyponasal 6 weeks postoperatively, but by 5 years only 6 percent showed evidence of obstruction, and, in a number of these, allergies were a factor.[556] VanDemark and Hardin also reported a tendency for hyponasality to disappear with time.[538] Dalston and Stuteville found a similar trend in primary pharyngeal flaps.[477] Neiman, Peterson, and Pruzansky reported on one case of a "failed flap" in which pharyngeal activity appeared for the first time 5 years postoperatively and evidence of persistent velopharyngeal inadequacy disappeared.[584]

Early reports on the success rate in pharyngeal flaps either lacked speech results or offered information on speech that was impossible to interpret.[476,479,481,482] Stark and Frileck claimed "excellent speech" results in three of 31 cases, and "good" in 26 more.[480] One report claimed better speech results in primary than in secondary flaps, but the speech data in the article are difficult to interpret.[478] Dalston and Stuteville reported that 62 percent of their 50 patients had no discernible degree of nasality, whereas 32 percent manifested a degree of nasality "inaudible to all but a trained observer."[477] The overall success rate was thus considered to be 94 percent. However, 22 percent of the subjects were still moderately hyponasal after 5 years.

The problem of hyponasality and other signs of airway obstruction in patients with pharyngeal flap is currently receiving more attention in the literature than was previously the case. Albery et al reported "an unacceptably high proportion of hyponasality" across 100 patients treated for velopharyngeal inadequacy by a variety of procedures, with a 63 percent occurrence after a Honig pharyngoplasty and 30 percent after a superiorly based flap.[549] Smith, Cohen, Skef, and Dorf reported a 35 percent occurrence of obstruction, as judged by aerodynamic studies after attachment of superiorly based pharyngeal flaps in 31 patients, and a 60 percent occurrence of hyponasality.[585] Flap revision, whether to open the ports when evidence of obstruction persists or reconstruct the flap when evidence of velopharyngeal inadequacy persists, is not an easy task.[564,577,586,587]

Success rates with pharyngeal flaps have tended to fall in the 80- to 90-percent range in recent years, especially when hyponasal patients are counted as successes. However, most of these results are based on subjective perceptual judgments alone, and there is evidence that the failure rate is higher when state-of-the-art instrumentation is used either to observe the port directly[570] or to assess aerodynamic results.[585]

Other Types of Pharyngoplasty

Other types of pharyngoplasty were initially of two main types, both intended to bring the pharyngeal wall forward in order to accomplish velopharyngeal closure. These included (1) transplants of cartilage, fat, or muscular tissue and (2) injection or implantation of various types of synthetic materials. More recently, the "sphincter pharyngoplasty" has gained popularity.

Gersuny in 1900 injected vaseline into the pharyngeal wall as a subcutaneous prosthesis, with one fatality and several cases of blindness.[588] Eckstein injected paraffin, not only with no reported complications, but also with no reported speech results.[588] Hollweg and Perthes reported the first attempts with autogeneous cartilage.[589] Von Gaza inserted fat grafts.[590] Lando inserted cadaveric cartilage.[591] Cartilage pharyngolasty was reported in later studies.[592–595] Although the authors were optimistic, graphs of speech results in one of these reports indicated that none of the subjects reached a normal level of nasal resonance,[593] and another report states that midsagittal velopharyngeal gaps on lateral radiographic studies averaging 5.00 mm persisted in eight of 31 subjects.[595] Calnan expressed more enthusiasm for cartilage pharyngoplasty than the use of synthetics, but did not offer speech results.[68]

In 1965, Lewy, Cole, and Wepman reported on the injection of Teflon® in a patient with velopharyngeal insufficiency.[596] This report inspired a series of studies in which reported success rates clustered around 50 to 60 percent for "normal" resonance or total elimination of evidence of velopharyngeal inadequacy, higher if those with "improved" resonance were counted.[159,597–602] There was some variation in the form of Teflon® used, but the most common was the injectable form. Reinjection was used in some studies when the first treatment failed. Bluestone et al reported that hypernasality was eliminated in 16 of 27 patients after the first injection and five more after a second injection, with a persistent problem in the remaining six (22 percent).[598] Furlow et al reported success in 18 of 35 on the first injection, and eight more after a second injection, giving them an overall success rate of 74 percent.[601] Kuehn and VanDemark reported a continuous change in competency for speech in 69 patients, with significant improvement occurring 3 or more months postoperatively.[603] They pointed out that the best results were likely to be achieved in patients with a midsagittal velopharyngeal gap of 2 mm or less, with mild-to-moderate hypernasality and with a good palatal mobility. The requisite of good palatal mobility and a velopharyngeal gap not exceeding a specific size was included in most of the aforementioned studies, although the designation of "1 cm or less" by Furlow et al[599] was far in excess of what most authors thought could be treated by this approach. Enthusiasm for injectable Teflon® in the treatment of velopharyngeal inadequacy was partially based on the fact that the procedure could be carried out in many patients under a topical anesthetic, allowing the investigator to judge the immediate effect on speech as the substance was injected. Also, obturation of the defect could be observed via endoscopy as the subject spoke. However, this enthusiasm came to a necessary end in 1978, at least in the United States, when the Food and Drug Administration withdrew approval of the use of Teflon® in the velopharyngeal system after a fatality.

Use of various forms of silicone was reported in the literature from the mid-1960s to the mid-1970s.[541,604–606] None of the reports contained data on speech other than "improved" in a certain percentage, and the use of this material never became popular.

In the late 1970s and early 1980s, implantation of Proplast® on the posterior pharyngeal wall to treat VPI was reported at some professional meetings, but no reports have been published.

A few inventive techniques of muscle transplantation have appeared in the literature but have generally failed to gain support. Hynes transferred the salpingopharyngeal muscles from their lateral insertions to a medial location on the posterior pharyngeal wall in an attempt to create a bulge on the wall.[607,608] Neither report contained speech results. Harding reported in 1979 that the procedure had fallen into disrepute,[609] and Calnan in 1976 decried his own results with this procedure.[68] Kiehn, DesPrez, Tucker, and Moore tried transplanting the temporalis or masseter muscle in order to suspend the nonfunctioning soft palate.[610] No interpretable speech results were given in their report, and the procedure never gained popularity. The same was true for the "bilateral pharyngoplasty" of Sullivan in which lateral superior constrictor flaps were raised from both sides of the pharynx to the superior surface of the soft palate.[611] Gold and Song advocated transplantation of the tendon of the palmaris longus to the velopharynx;[612] again, no speech results were given, and no further reports appeared.

By contrast, the "sphincter pharyngoplasty" described by Orticochea in 1968 continues to attract attention.[613] In this procedure, the posterior faucial pillars containing the palatopharyngeus muscles are freed from their inferior attachments and lifted posteriorly to be inserted into a pocket created by raising a flap on the posterior pharyngeal wall. (The posterior flap serves the purpose of housing the insertions of the lateral flaps and is not extended into the velum itself.) When the lateral defects where the flaps were taken have healed, the procedure in theory leaves one small central sphincter that closes during speech. In 1983, Orticochea reported an 89 percent success rate on 236 cases.[614] However, he made this judgment based on the range of motion of the sphincteric mechanism on intraoral examination. Stradoudakis and Bambace reported evidence of persistent velopharyngeal inadequacy in five of 16 cases operated on by means of this procedure and hyponasality in three when seen from 6 months to 4 years postoperatively.[615] Jackson varied this procedure by substituting a superiorly based midline flap for the inferiorly based flap of Orticochea.[616–618] In one report, severe nasal escape persisted in two of 26 patients, moderate in six, and mild in eight, meaning that some degree of velopharyngeal inadequacy persisted in 62 percent of the speakers 12 months postoperatively.[616] The figures of Jackson and Silverton indicated persistence of some evidence of velopharyngeal inadequacy in 36 of 74 cases, or 49 percent.[618] However, these judgments were made by a panel of speech pathologists listening to taped samples, and no indication was given of how long postoperatively the judgments were made. With regard to the latter point, the observation of Lendrum and Dhar that the central sphincter in this surgery can remain incompetent for up to 3 years postoperatively is particularly pertinent.[619] Lendrum and Dhar reported elimination of nasal escape in 20 of 53 patients and improvement in an additional five (for a total of 58 percent).

Meyer, Failat, and Kelly offered a modification of the Orticochea method, which involved the creation of bilateral z-flaps; no speech results were given.[620] Two reports argued for moving the site of insertion of the palatopharyngeal flaps upward from what Orticochea had described.[621,622] Riski et al reported "successful resolution of nasality" in 43 of 55 patients (78 percent), including in 16 of 26 patients in whom the ultimate height of flap insertion was still below the level at which velopharyngeal closure was attempted (evaluated radiographically) prior to surgery.[621]

Augmentation of the anatomy of the velopharyngeal system by building out the pharyngeal wall by the use of muscle transplants have not met with notable success according to the published reports. Success rates with the use of both cartilage and synthetic implants were mostly in the 60 to 70 percent range, and these procedures have similarly fallen into disuse, in one case (Teflon®) by law. Reported success rates with the most popular type of pharyngoplasty—the Orticochea or "sphincter" pharyngoplasty—have not been as high as in most studies on pharyngeal flaps.

Prosthetic Management

Prosthetic management of cleft palate and noncleft velopharyngeal inadequacy takes the following forms.

1. Placement of feeding obturators for infants with clefts, advocated by some authors but deemed unnecessary by most.[196,623–626]
2. Placement of "articulation development" prostheses in children, generally first fitted under the age of 12 months, when such development would be otherwise threatened due to delay in surgical closure of the palate.[627]
3. Fabrication of prostheses that obturate both the unoperated cleft and the velopharyngeal area when surgical repair is not a viable option.[625,628–640]
4. Fabrication of "speech bulbs" (Fig. 17–18) either for postoperative cleft patients for whom palatal surgery has not provided an adequate mechanism or for patients with noncleft velopharyngeal inadequacy, in both cases as an alternative to pharyngeal flap or pharyngoplasty.[628,629,631,633,640–643] In both unoperated and operated clefts, prosthetics may be used as an adjunct to surgery.[583,632,644,645]
5. Fabrication of "palatal lifts" (Fig. 17–19) in patients for whom palatal length is adequate, but movement is deficient.[151,166,183,646–656]
6. Palatal plates[625,628,640,657] or temporary material[658] for the obturation of palatal fistulae.

In the fitting of either a speech bulb or a pal-

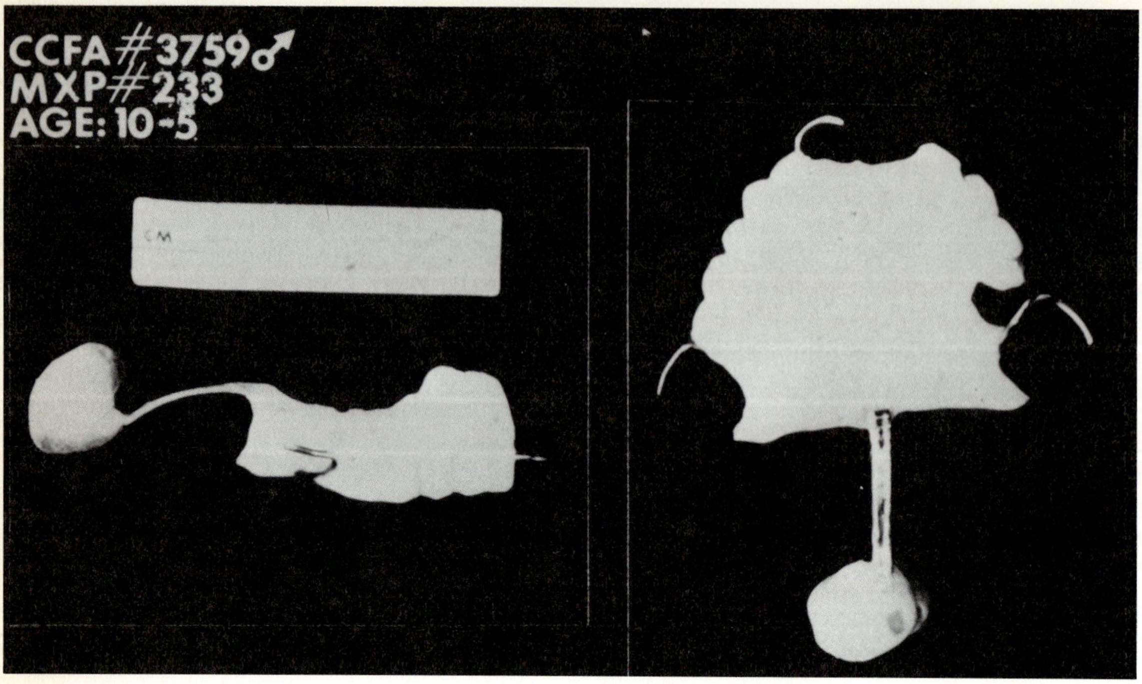

Figure 17–18 Prosthetic speech bulb. (Courtesy, Center for Craniofacial Anomalies, University of California–San Francisco.)

atal lift, it is of course critical that one fits the device taking into account the same factors that must be taken into account in the creation of a midline pharyngeal flap, namely level, amount, and symmetry of pharyngeal wall motion. Radiographic studies served as the primary means of making these determinations[659–661] until the advent of oral and nasal endoscopy.[662–664] In judging the efficiency of obturation, aerodynamic studies are also useful[665–670] as are acoustic studies.[671]

Several authors, particularly in earlier literature, talked about prosthetic devices, usually bulbs but occasionally lifts, as serving as "muscle stimulators" or "velopharyngeal activity stimulators."[636,657,672–675] Blakeley advocated the use of a temporary speech prosthesis* to force appropriate oral pressure during speech training.[676] He reported that the use of such a device could stimulate activity prior to surgery, occasionally to such an extent that closure would be achieved and the surgery would not be required.[678,679] Weiss also reported obturator reduction programs.[645,680,681] However, Shelton and co-authors[682] failed to produce increased pharyngeal wall motion with a similar program and observed a breakdown in articulatory skills and velopharyngeal closure[661] after minimal amounts of reduction.

Bzoch[583] and Blakeley[678] described the relative advantages and disadvantages of prosthetic devices as opposed to pharyngeal flaps, the obvious advantage being the ability to modify the device at will. Byrne et al reported no differences in articulatory skills between children treated prosthetically and those treated surgically.[222] Marsh and Wray reported a higher failure of compliance rate in children treated prosthetically than surgically, illustrating the fact that both clinicians and parents must be somewhat aggresive if a prosthetic program is to be successful.[558]

Shelton and Lloyd[683] and Subtelny, Sakuda, and Subtelny[684] reviewed the factors influencing the effect of a prosthetic device on speech. Although instrumentation approaches to the fitting and assess-

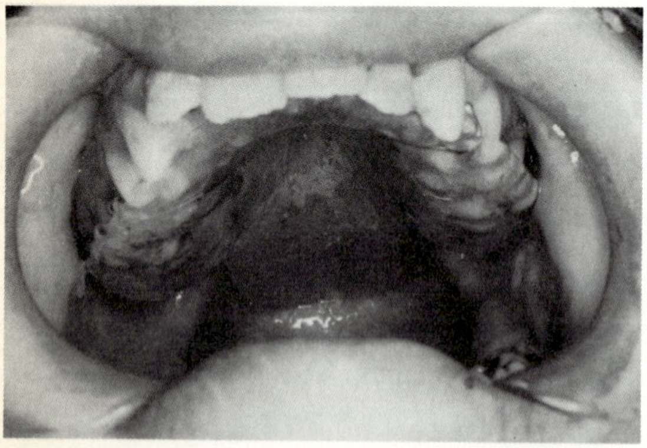

Figure 17–19 Palatal lift in place. (Courtesy, Center for Craniofacial Anomalies, University of California–San Francisco.)

* Curtis and Chierici described the temporary fitting of a prosthesis in order to determine whether surgery would in fact affect speech or not.[677]

ment of prostheses have changed dramatically in the intervening decades, their conclusions would not be changed noticeably.

Those few studies that have reported speech results in prosthetic treatment have cited numbers comparable to those on pharyngeal flap. For instance, Gallagher reported 74 percent normal nasal resonance and 13 percent more "improved" resonance in a series of 80 postoperative patients with clefts.[641] Success rates with palatal lifts reflect the difficulty in treating neurogenic patients and in obtaining accurate assessment of the behavior of the velopharyngeal system in the presence of the other speech problems occurring in these patients.

The goals of prosthetic treatment of the velopharyngeal system are the same as those of surgical management. Many of the same variables that affect the results of surgical treatment also affect prosthetic results, that is, the amount of mesial motion of the lateral pharyngeal walls. Prosthetic treatment often requires more aggression on the part of parents and clinicians, but has the advantage of "instant" change in the status of the system and the opportunity for as many adjustments as are needed to obtain an optimal result.

SPEECH THERAPY

Speech therapy in cleft palate is concerned with (1) early stimulation of both language and appropriate sound production, beginning in infancy and incorporating parent training;[685–687] (2) remediation of language problems when they are detected;[196] (3) remediation of vocal abuse, when present, and counseling for subsequent prevention;[196] (4) exploration of behavioral means for improving use of the velopharyngeal system when inconsistent closure or a minimal velopharyngeal inadequacy is diagnosed;[196,205,688] (5) training for correct articulatory placement to prevent or replace inappropriate compensatory articulations;[195,196,199,205,689,690] and (6) when moderate or severe velopharyngeal inadequacy must be endured with no prospect of remediation by physical management, exploration of ways to minimize the effect of that inadequacy. Speech therapy for hyponasality is not appropriate. Therapy for speakers with noncleft velopharyngeal inadequacy, excluding those with neurogenic disorders in whom other aspects of speech production are likely to be involved, will most likely focus on numbers 4 and 6, since there is as yet no documentation of the occurrence of compensatory articulations in the absence of clefting.

Therapy for language disorders and voice problems is discussed in other chapters. With particular regard to the child with a cleft, the speech pathologist must bear in mind the possible role of hearing loss in causing or exacerbating a language problem and the role of either past or persistent velopharyngeal inadequacy in habitual vocal abuse.

Hahn was one of the first to point out the importance of early intervention with infants with cleft palate, beginning with parent counseling about the cleft, the possible effects on speech and hearing, and ways in which the parents can assist in the establishment of correct speech production patterns.[685,686] Information should not, of course, be given before the parents are ready for it. In the early weeks, some parents do not focus on speech at all, but are preoccupied with possible feeding problems, the impact of the child upon the family, and their own grief over the "loss" of a perfect child. If no questions are forthcoming by the second or third month, however, the speech pathologist should begin counseling. That counseling may include a wide variety of information (in addition to reassurance), but should begin to teach the parents about the importance of language stimulation and the emphasis they should place on "front sounds" (labial and tongue-tip) as they play with their baby. Teaching the child to produce a Bronx cheer is not a bad idea. Later the speech pathologist can begin regular visits with the child and parents, demonstrating the stimulation of appropriately *placed* speech sounds even if the child of necessity produces them with nasal emission because the cleft has not yet been repaired. Once palatal surgery has been accomplished, the parents should be taught ways in which to stimulate and reinforce oral direction of the airstream. In this instance, blowing tasks are used not as exercise for the velopharyngeal system, but as a means of teaching the child the feeling of an orally emitted airstream. As development progresses, the speech pathologist accompanies these activities with stimulation and reinforcement of oral direction of the airstream in the production of fricatives and plosives.

As of this writing, instructional videotapes on therapy for infants and toddlers with clefts are appearing with regularity. One set of such tapes is currently available through Children's Hospital in Vancouver, British Columbia.

Possible behavioral means for improving the amount or consistency of velopharyngeal closure were discussed in Chapter 16.

The teaching of correct articulatory placement is, of course, much easier if it is done during early speech development. Trost-Cardamone has found that a didactic approach can be successful even with very young children, using diagrams to teach them about the parts of the speech mechanism and how they are used to produce consonant sounds.[208] If compensatory articulations or inappropriate direction of the airstream have already been established, the very young child may respond to various blowing games, again not as physical exercise for the velopharyngeal system. Biofeedback even in simple forms such as a See-scape is extremely useful in therapy.

Several reports on the use of palatography in remediation of articulation in speakers with clefts have appeared in the literature, primarily from investigators in Japan.[691–693] Such devices are beyond the reach of most clinicians, but have demonstrated what another form of biofeedback can accomplish in eliminating inappropriate articulatory placement.

As noted earlier, Hoch et al offered information not only on improvement of velopharyngeal function through nasopharyngoscopic feedback, but on techniques for eliminating glottal and pharyngeal compensatory articulations.[205] In the experience of those authors, elimination of compensatory articulations can and should be accomplished prior to the physical management of an inadequately functioning velopharyngeal system, which is contrary to the experience and recommendations of most other authors writing on therapy, for example, Shelton et al[682] and Wells.[199] Whether prior to or following such management, the therapeutic regimen of Hoch et al included a series of criteria for phoneme selection, a list of techniques ("facilitators") for teaching the new articulation, and criteria for correct responses.[205] The criteria for phoneme selection included stimulability, anterior place of production, visibility, maturational appropriateness, and voicelessness. Facilitators included whispering the phoneme; using aspirate /h/ as a bridge between the consonant and the vowel; a series of steps for proceeding from the simple to the complex; use of visual, tactile, and auditory cues; and use of coarticulation of a nasal consonant to facilitate production of a target phoneme produced in the same place. They recommended a criterion of 70 to 100 correct responses per session, at least in children older that 4 years of age.

Some of the suggestions of Hoch et al[205] are found in earlier recommendations for therapy programs.[197,199]

Although Hoch et al recommended the use of nasopharyngoscopic feedback in the elimination of phoneme-specific velopharyngeal inadequacy, the clinician may use other approaches.[205] Depending upon the maturity of the child, an explanation of how an appropriate /s/ is produced and how it is different from what he or she is producing, together with training in discriminating his or her own productions, may be all that is required. For other children, it may be necessary first to force oral direction of the airstream by closing the nares (typically, the child at first emits no air at all, blocking the oral route by elevating the tongue against the palate). Once oral production with the nares closed is established, the clinician can use the approach of "successive approximations," partially blocking the nose or just touching the nose. Some clinicians approach this problem by having the child "prolong a 't'," working towards oral production of "tssss." Another approach is to intentionally teach the child the temporary use of a frontal lisp if his or her production of "th" is appropriately oral. One can then use another form of progressive approximations going from the "th" (or "sh") to the target phoneme(s). The crucial point is to break the child's habit of automatically elevating the tongue and forcing the air through the nose. Biofeedback is very helpful and can be provided in a variety of ways, including the use of earphones with the microphone placed directly beneath the child's nose.* It is not unusual to encounter complete discouragement in a phoneme-specific child the moment he or she is asked to produce the /s/ orally, that is, "I can't." Some clinicians have found it useful to avoid the use of the phoneme label altogether, describing the correct means of production and inventing a new name for the phoneme. Once oral direction of the airstream on the problem phoneme(s) is accomplished, whether or not the new oral consonant is perfectly produced, it is critical both to give appropriate reinforcement and to obtain a large number of productions (as indicated by Hoch et al[205]) before the therapy session is ended. In fact, it is also critical *not* to end the first therapy session before oral production is obtained. The child must leave the session knowing he or she can produce the target phoneme orally.

Hodson et al advocated the use of phonologic therapy in children with clefts.[231] Certainly this therapy is appropriate so long as the structural hazards to articulation present in any given child are taken into account. Given the probability that a number of phonemes are affected in a child with cleft palate for whom speech sound acquisition has not progressed normally, teaching a set of features or a class of sounds should be more efficient than teaching a single phoneme at a time.

Albery and Enderby reported that intensive speech therapy as opposed to weekly therapy not only

* Earphones of the type used on commercial airplanes are especially useful. They are simple listening tubes with no electronic components, and the dual plug fits nicely beneath the nares of a small child. When a pressure consonant is produced appropriately, no air emission is heard through the tube. When the consonant is produced with nasal emission or nasal frication, the sound of the rush of air in the child's ears is louder than the speech signal itself.

produced significantly greater improvements in speech, but also improvements that were maintained over a longer period of time.[694] The results of VanDemark and Hardin on an intensive therapy program were less favorable.[690] However, 23 percent of their subjects were known to have marginal velopharyngeal adequacy, and possibly traditional articulation therapy would not have worked as well for them as, for example, the approach outlined by Hoch et al.[205] Results of an earlier study by VanDemark did in fact show greater progress in therapy for children with adequate as opposed to marginal velopharyngeal closure.[695]

When significant velopharyngeal inadequancy is present and there is no prospect for either surgical or prosthetic treatment, the patient and the speech pathologist may choose to explore ways to minimize the problem. Use of various forms of biofeedback in the attempt to alter the behavior of the system is an obvious first choice, although the clinician must be alert for signs of inappropriate muscular tension at the laryngeal or supralaryngeal level brought about by the effort to make changes that are perhaps physically impossible. In addition, patient and clinician may explore perceptual changes induced by altering the rate, effort level, and mouth opening. Elimination of compensatory articulations, when present, may alter the severity of perceived hypernasality even if no change has been effected in the size of the velopharyngeal defect.

Because clefts and other craniofacial anomalies are relatively infrequent in the average school or clinic caseload, speech pathologists often approach these speakers with timidity. The clinician must first learn to discriminate both the resonance deviations and the compensatory articulations described previously before he or she can teach the patient. Replacement of compensatory articulations with appropriately produced phonemes *is* possible. Many older children and adults are completely unaware of what they are doing in speech production and how that differs from normal speech production. Learning a new speech behavior is typically easier for them by first learning what constitutes that behavior—not by aiming blindly for an acoustic target provided by the clinician.

EXAMPLES OF OTHER CRANIOFACIAL DEFECTS

It is not within the scope of this chapter to cover all craniofacial syndromes, sequences, or associations and the communicative deficits that may accompany them. Rather, a few clinical entities will be discussed in order to illustrate the complexity of problems and the necessity for accurate diagnosis.

The majority of craniofacial malformation syndromes, sequences or associations vary greatly in expressivity. This variability means that (1) all but the most astute diagnosticians may miss the minimally affected case, (2) those features affecting communicative function are not affected to the same degree from case to case, and so (3) the clinician must approach each patient individually *without* an a priori assumption of what the physical and behavioral findings will be.

Assessment and treatment of speech problems in craniofacial malformations is complicated by the relatively high incidence of such associated problems as hearing loss and mental retardation. Conversely, undiagnosed or inaccurately delineated primary handicaps in communicative function can lead to an erroneous assumption of mental retardation or untreatable hearing loss and thus "secondary" or institutional retardation. For a concrete example: a tour of any large school for the deaf turns up at least one patient with mandibulofacial dysostosis—a syndrome in which the hearing loss is typically conductive and intellectual function is normal if the loss is recognized and treated early.

Two factors contribute to the confusion in attempting to understand craniofacial defects and the communicative problems they may produce. First, because of the variability in expression of these disorders, the diagnosis is based more on a pattern of anomalies than on the presence or absence of "obligatory" or "pathognomonic" features. Second, as with cleft lip and palate, speech pathologists are becoming increasingly aware of how often a given syndrome, sequence, or association may occur together with findings of yet another clinical entity, thus changing the etiology and possibly the management requirements.

Apert Syndrome

There is a large group of syndromes, known under the general rubric of "premature craniofacial synostosis," in which one or more of the sutures of the skull and face fuse prematurely.[696,697] Growth of the craniofacial complex is restricted in the area of the fused sutures, and there is a compensatory overdevelopment of the unaffected parts of the skull.[698] Apert syndrome, or acrocephalosyndactyly type I, was first described by Troquart in 1886, with several other case descriptions before the report by Apert.[696,699,700] It is estimated to occur in one in 100,000 to one in 160,000 births.[697]

In this syndrome, premature closure of several of the cranial sutures, most often those in the coronal complex alone or together with the sagittal

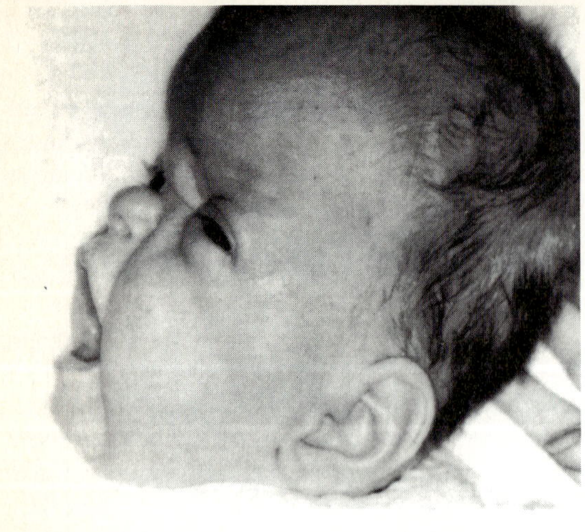

Figure 17-20 Infant with Apert syndrome. Note frontal bossing, midface hypoplasia, acrocephaly, and brachycephaly.

suture, results in a skull that is vertically long, but shortened in the anteroposterior dimension (Fig. 17–20).[41,696,697,701–703] The synostosis and resultant failure of growth affects the skull base as well.[704] There is a commonly held theory that the synostosis in the cranial base is in fact responsible for the secondary deformation of the face and synostosis of other cranial sutures,[705–707] although there is some disagreement on this point.[708,709] Central nervous system abnormalities in this syndrome have been documented primarily in the rhinencephalon[709] and include the absence of olfactory bulbs and tracts. Mental retardation is commonly reported,[710,711] but normal intelligence has been observed.[712] Although early craniectomy is recommended to prevent brain damage,[713–715] there have been no studies comparing intelligence in patients who had such surgery as opposed to patients who did not.

Hypoplasia of the middle third of the face, including the maxilla, contributes in part to exophthalmus and relative prognathism.[701,716,717] The primary cause of the exophthalmus is the flattening of the orbit. The mandible is actually shorter than the normal mandible,[718] but appears prognathic in relation to the extremely hypoplastic maxilla. The cranial and facial deformities in children with Apert syndrome become worse with time. These patients also have syndactyly of the hands and feet, as well as other skeletal abnormalities,[701,703] which again tend to become worse with time because of progressive synostosis.[719–721] Synostosis is also found in the cervical spine.[721,722]

The maxillary hypoplasia leads to a compressed, V-shaped arch with ectopic eruption of dentition (Fig. 17–21). It is not unusual for the maxillary arch to fit within the mandibular arch, resulting in a severe Class III malocclusion. The palatal vault is further crowded by lateral swellings of soft tissue caused by an accumulation of acid mucopolysaccharides (Fig. 17–22).[723] These swellings are present in infancy and increase as the child matures to a point where they are separated only by a narrow median groove.[724,725] This configuration often leads to a misdiagnosis of cleft palate, although true clefts are estimated to occur in approximately 30 percent of these cases.[717] The hard palate is significantly decreased in length,[726] whereas the soft palate is abnormally long and thick.[725,726] The nasopharynx is decreased both in height and depth.[726–729] The combination of a long, thick soft palate and a shallow nasopharynx contributes to airway problems that can lead to mouthbreathing, denasality, forward carriage of the tongue to protect the airway, and even sleep apnea.[730–732] As would be expected,

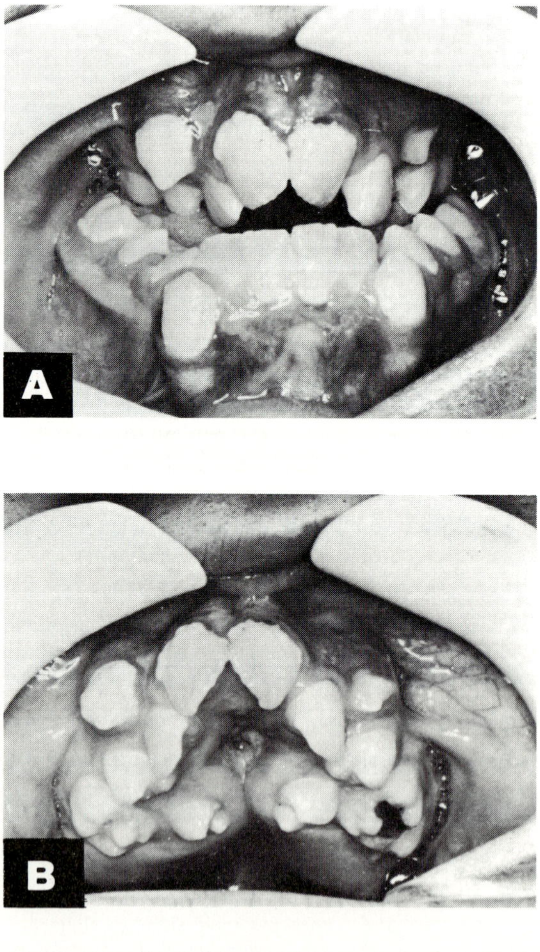

Figure 17-21 *A* and *B*, Malocclusion, ectopic eruption of teeth and anomalous configuration of the palatal vault in Apert syndrome.

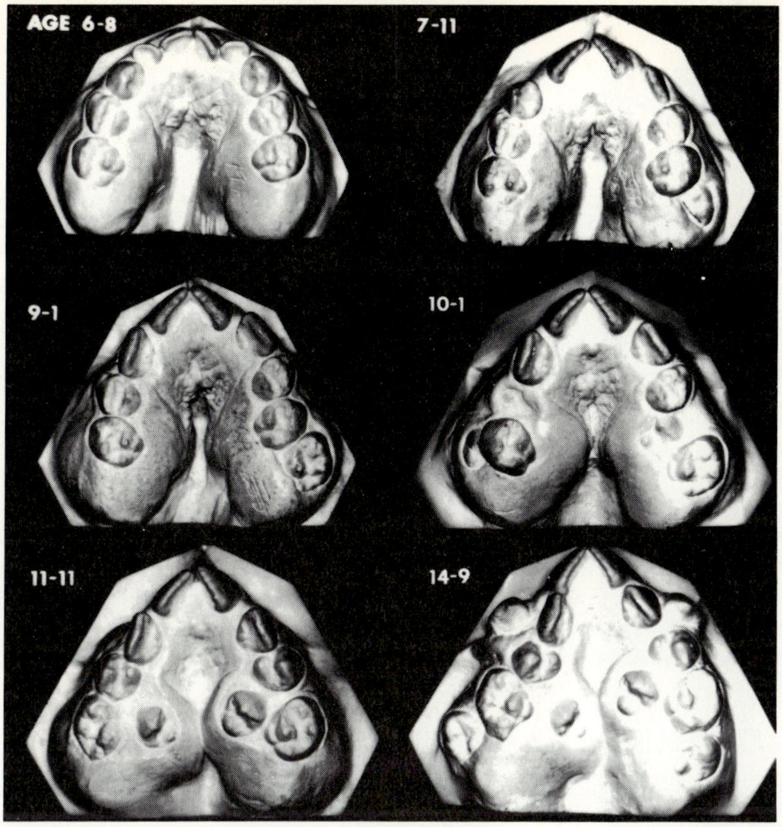

Figure 17–22 Increasing severity of palatal vault deformity in Apert syndrome. Note ectopic eruption of teeth and progressive accumulations of soft tissue (acid mucopolysaccharide deposits) along the lateral palatine shelves.

palatal elevation on phonation is typically minimal, since there is simply no room for superoposterior movement.

Although craniofacial surgery (Fig. 17–23) involving advancement of the midface in early childhood has been advocated for a number of reasons, including improvement of the airway,[715,733–735] such advancement does not necessarily relieve the airway obstruction,[736] pointing to the possibility of other etiologies for the obstruction, such as posterior atresia of the nasal airway.

Otologic findings in this syndrome include minor external ear malformation[737] and frequent conductive hearing loss that may be due to malformations of the stapes and oval window[731,738–743] or the prevalent otitis media that has been attributed to the crowding of the nasopharynx.[697,744,745] Gould and Caldarelli reported that serous otitis media in this syndrome develops in infancy and persists into adulthood.[739]

Hazards to speech production in this syndrome are myriad: possible mental retardation, crowding of the palatal vault obliterating normal points of tongue and palate contact, cleft palate, Class III malocclusion (Fig. 17–24), nasopharyngeal obstruction, and hearing loss. Most clinical reports have described articulation problems due to the malocclusion[711,728,729,745a] that may improve after midface advancement has brought the jaws into a normal relationship.[728,729,746,747] However, midface advancement may also change denasality into velopharyngeal inadequacy if the velopharyngeal system cannot accomodate to the enlarged dimensions of the nasopharynx.[748] The crowding of the oral and pharyngeal cavities is reflected in the crowding of the vowel triangle: the articulators cannot reach the normal configurations for the vowels, altering the formants towards neutralized ("schwa") vowels.[749]

Crouzon Disease

Crouzon disease (Fig. 17–25), also known as craniofacial dysostosis, is another syndrome involving premature cranial synostosis and was first described in 1912. Although Cohen stated in 1979 that no estimate of incidence had ever been given,[697] Walker gave an incidence of one in 600,000 live births, without citing a source for this figure.[750]

In this syndrome, the coronal, sagittal, lamboidal, and metopic sutures may be involved.[696] The cranial deformity depends upon the order and rate of progression of the sutural synostosis,[697] with the ultimate skull shape often very hard to distinguish

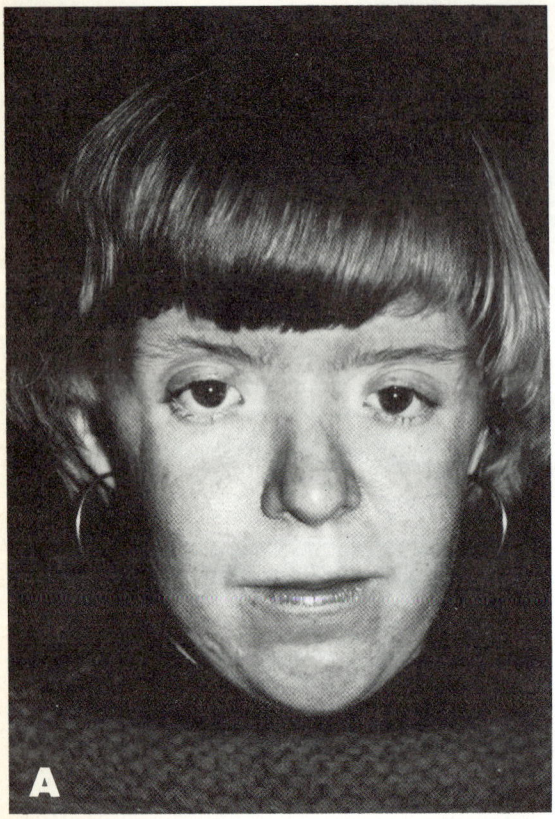

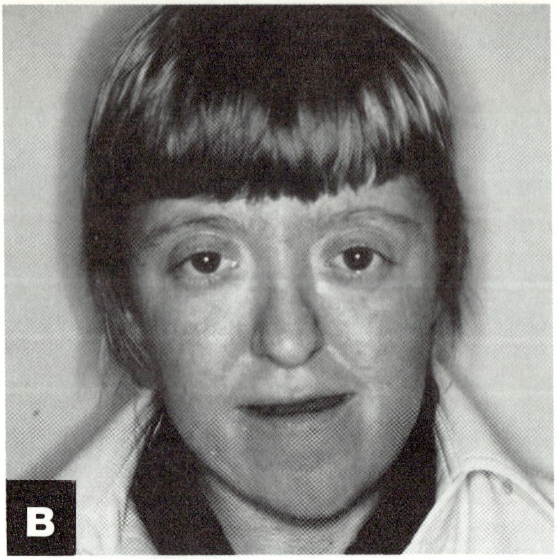

Figure 17–23 Female with Apert syndrome, *A*, prior to and, *B*, following craniofacial surgery (midface advancement). Note retruded midface and proptotic eyes in the first picture. (Courtesy, Dr. Douglas Ousterhout and the Center for Craniofacial Anomalies, University of California–San Francisco.)

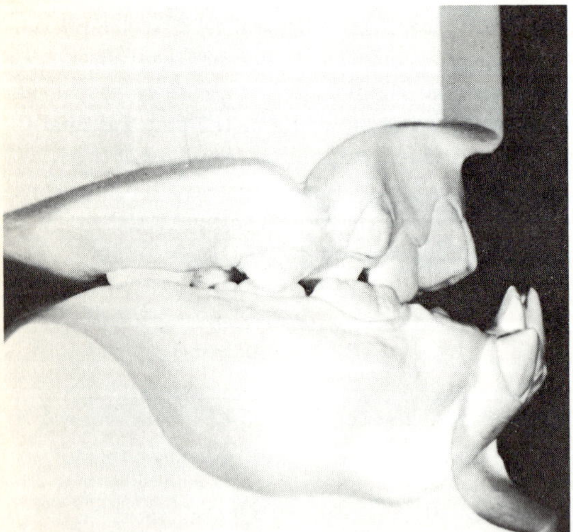

Figure 17–24 Articulated dental casts of Apert patient demonstrating severe maxillary/mandibular disproportion with resultant Class III malocculsion presenting hazard to speech.

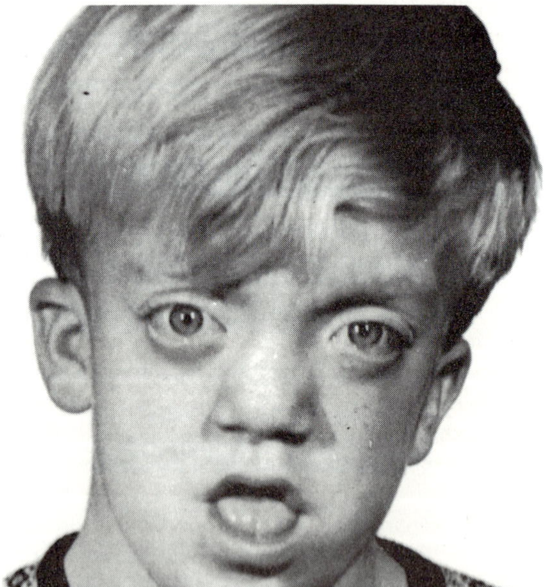

Figure 17–25 Patient with Crouzon disease (craniofacial dysostosis). Note exophthalmos, midface hypoplasia, and obligatory mouth-breathing with forward carriage of the tongue.

from that seen in Apert syndrome.[751] Typically, the skull is foreshortened in the anteroposterior dimension[41,697] and wider in the lateral dimensions.[41] As in Apert syndrome, the synostosis also appears in the skull base,[704,752–755] and shallow orbits cause ocular proptosis. Hypertelorism has also been described.[41,708]

Crouzon disease is more variable in expression than Apert syndrome,[696] but shares many of the same features. Maxillary hypoplasia leads to a V-shaped dental arch.[696] Descriptions of a high-arched palate[696,756] are probably attributable to this V-shape and to the accumulation of soft tissue along the lateral palatine shelves that is seen, but that is less consistent and less severe than in Apert syndrome.[725] Cleft palate has been reported, but is not a frequent finding.[757] Again, the mandible often appears prognathic, with a Class III malocclusion, but is actually abnormally short in body length.[718]

Although mental retardation has been reported in Crouzon disease,[697,710,711,716] it is not as frequent a finding as in Apert syndrome. Again, early craniectomy has been advocated,[713–715,758] but no one has related the presence or absence of mental retardation to early surgical intervention.

Patients with Crouzon disease exhibit the same reduced dimensions of the nasopharynx as those with Apert syndrome,[697,726–729,731,759] together with vulnerability to airway obstruction and sleep apnea.[697,730–732,736,756,759] Moore, Moore, and Brown described bony obstruction of the nasal passages in one patient.[760] Tracheal stenosis has been reported.[761] The patients also show frequent hearing impairment of the same type and etiology as seen in Apert syndrome.[731,741,742,756] Farkas reported the same tendency towards low-set ears as seen in Apert syndrome.[737]

The hazards to speech production are virtually the same as in Apert syndrome with the exception that the variability of expression is greater in Crouzon disease and so more patients exhibit minimal or no speech problems. As in Apert syndrome, midfacial advancement (Fig. 17–26) can change preoperative denasality into postoperative velopharyngeal inadequacy, but can also improve articulation problems that were due to the Class III malocclusion.[728,729,746–748]

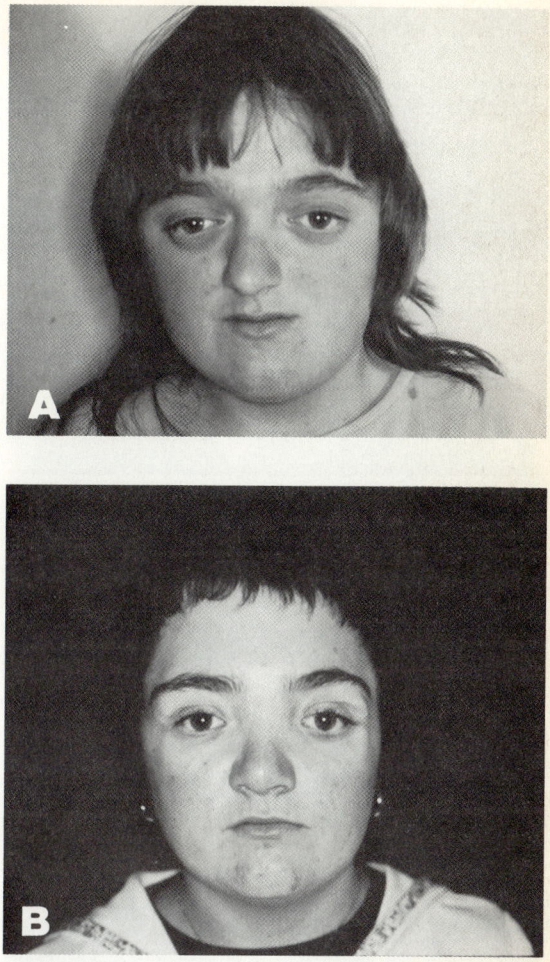

Figure 17–26 Female with Crouzon disease, *A*, prior to and, *B*, following craniofacial surgery. Note similarity of facial features to those of the Apert female in Figure 17–23. (Courtesy, Dr. Douglas Ousterhout and the Center for Craniofacial Anomalies, University of California–San Francisco.)

Fetal Alcohol Syndrome

Alcohol is now recognized as the most common teratogen to which the human fetus is likely to be exposed.[41] According to one Swedish study, one in 300 infants is born with fetal alcohol effects, with half of these having the fetal alcohol syndrome that was first described by Lemoine in 1968.[762] Olegard et al estimated that 10 to 20 percent of mental deficiency with an IQ in the range of 50 to 80 is a result of alcohol, and that one in six cases of cerebral palsy stems from the same cause.[762] Incidence in the United States has been estimated to be greater than one in 1,000 live births.[763]

The features of this syndrome include pre- and postnatal growth deficiency, mental retardation with an average IQ of 63, fine motor dysfunction and poor eye-hand coordination, irritability in infancy and hyperactivity in childhood, mild to moderate microcephaly, short palpebral fissures, maxillary hypoplasia, short nose with a smooth philtrum and thin and smooth upper lip, joint anomalies, and cardiac defects (Fig. 17–27).[41,764,765] Associated abnormalities include, among other findings, hydrocephalus, cleft lip with or without cleft palate, micrognathia, prominent lateral palatine ridges, and dysplastic dental

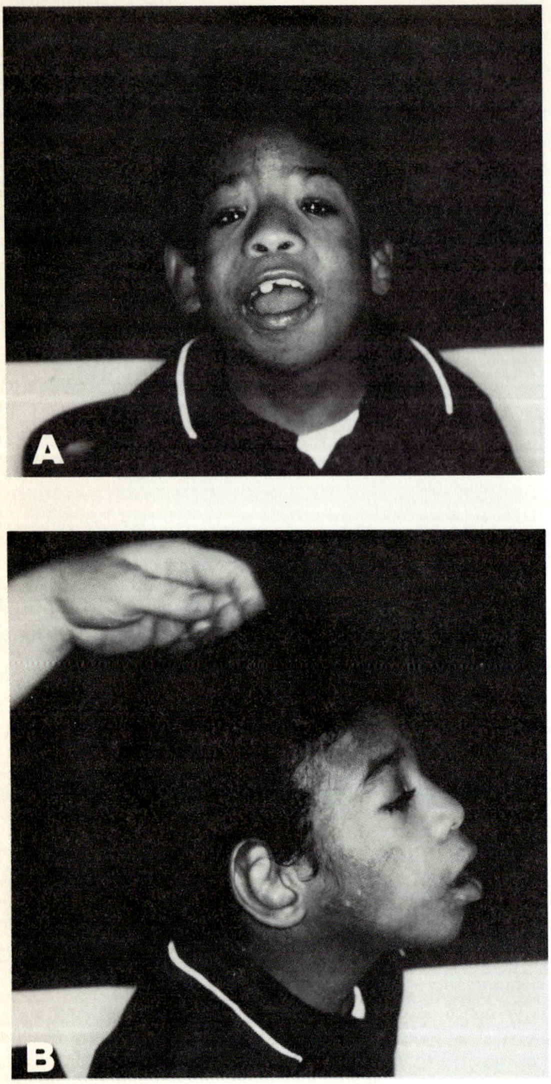

Figure 17–27 *A* and *B* Male with fetal alcohol syndrome. Note microcephaly, short palpebral fissures, smooth philtrum and upper lip. (Courtesy, Center for Craniofacial Anomalies, University of California–San Francisco.)

enamel. Riekman concluded that the midface was not truly flat in this syndrome, but was an "optical illusion" caused by the short palpebral fissures, broad nasal base, and absence of a normal philtrum.[766] Relative prognathia may appear in later childhood.[764,767] Shprintzen reported "deficient palatal growth" in this syndrome.[768] One cephalometric study concluded that the craniofacial abnormalities as seen radiographically were secondary to abnormal growth and development of the central nervous system.[769]

Although well over 50 studies of fetal alcohol syndrome have been published to date, few have dealt with communication deficits. One study reported speech or language defects in 84 percent of 63 subjects.[770] Language abilities were reported to be positively correlated with IQ scores. Another report mentioned fluency and rate problems, articulation and voice quality disorders and language delays, but did not state whether or not these observations were based on personal experience with the syndrome.[771] Siegel-Sadewitz and Shprintzen reported "frequent" problems with articulation, cognition, and resonance in addition to conductive hearing loss.[772] Sparks concluded from her review that whether the language development in this syndrome is consistent with overall developmental delay or has another characteristic pattern is unknown.[773] Hanson et al noted that these children do not show catch-up growth or performance during infancy or early childhood.[763] As stated by Sparks, prognosis is poor for improvement in cognition even when the child receives good care and intellectual stimulation.[773]

Hemifacial Microsomia

"Hemifacial microsomia" is one term for a large family of disorders in which structures on one side of the face do not grow normally (Fig. 17–28). Current alternative umbrella terms covering the same association of anomalies are "facio-auriculo-vertebral spectrum"[41] and "facio-auriculo-vertebral complex."[162] Older literature used the terms unilateral facial dysplasia, lateral facial dysplasia,[774] microtia syndrome, hemicraniofacial microsomia,[775] craniofacial microsomia,[776] first branchial arch syndrome,[777] first and second branchial arch syndrome,[778,779] and otomandibular dysostosis.[780]

Hemifacial microsomia is a classic example of the confusion that can accrue to the delineation of clinical entities. The severity of expression is highly variable, and dysmorphologists do not agree on an obligatory set of features. The most commonly cited clinical findings include variable combinations of mandibular hypoplasia; maxillary hypoplasia; and ear deformities including microtia, preauricular tags or pits, and malformations of the external auditory meatus and middle ear. Some dysmorphologists feel minimal diagnostic criteria should include deformity of both the ear and the mandible.[713] Others view microtia occurring alone as a microform of hemifacial microsomia.[781–783]

Goldenhar described the occurrence of eye malformations, specifically epibulbar dermoids or lipodermoids, in conjunction with malformations of the ear.[784] Gorlin, Jue, Jacobsen, and Goldschmidt noted a high frequency of vertebral malformations occurring together with the anomalies described by Goldenhar and used the term "oculoauriculovertebral dysplasia."[785] Most of the literature uses this term

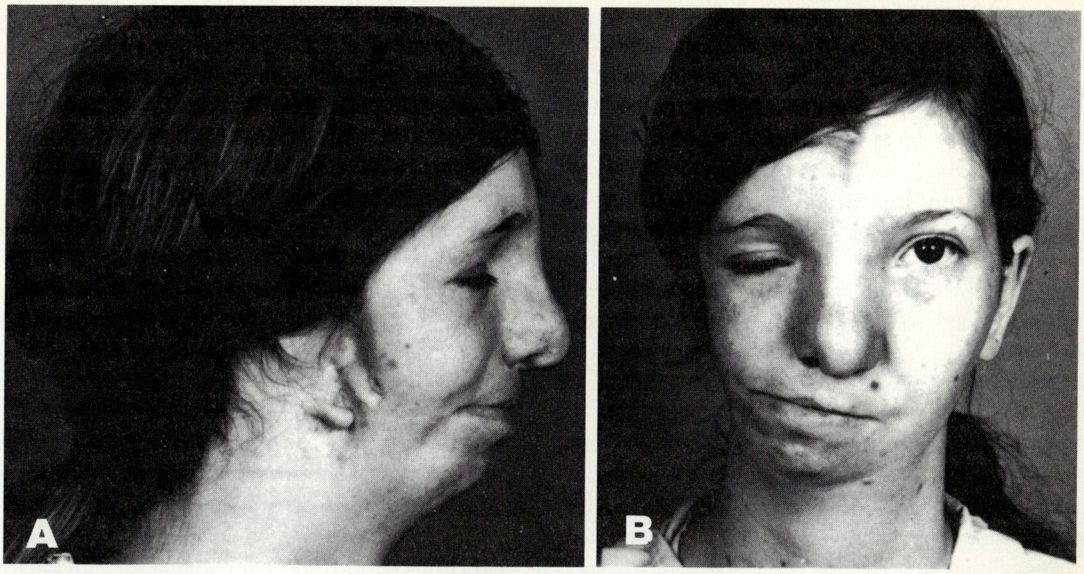

Figure 17–28 *A*, Lateral and *B*, frontal views of young adult with hemifacial microsomia.

and "Goldenhar syndrome" interchangeably.[786–796] Several papers have pointed out overlapping features between hemifacial microsomia and Goldenhar syndrome,[797,798] although Heffez and Doku insisted that epibulbar dermoids, auricular appendices, pretragal fistulae, and vertebral anomalies were absent in hemifacial microsomia.[799] Smith stated, "the occurrence of various combinations and gradations of [these] anomalies...has suggested that hemifacial microsomia and the Goldenhar syndrome may simply represent gradations in severity of a similar error in morphogenesis."[41] Taking all variations into account, Smith gave an estimate of occurrence of between one in 3,000 and one in 5,000, with a slight (3:2) male predominance.

A further point of confusion is the fact that, although "hemifacial" denotes involvement of only half the face, hemifacial microsomia often occurs in a bilateral but asymmetric form.[41,800,801] Smith stated that the anomalies were unilateral in about 70 percent of the cases.[41] He catalogued the anomalies as "variable combinations" of hypoplasia of the malar, maxillary, and/or mandibular region; lateral cleft-like extension of the mouth (macrostomia); hypoplasia of facial musculature; microtia; preauricular tags and/or pits; middle ear anomalies with variable "deafness"; diminished to absent parotid secretion; anomalies in function or structure of the tongue; malfunction of the soft palate; and vertebral anomalies that are most commonly cervical, but may also be thoracic or lumbar. "Occasional" anomalies included various eye abnormalities, including microphthalmia, inner ear defects with "deafness," cleft lip and palate, and cardiac defects, in addition to other scattered findings. A number of authors have tried to develop systems for either grouping or segregating the clinical findings into a classification system with little resultant agreement or clarification.[717,783,802,803]

The anomalies of hemifacial microsomia do *not* constitute a syndrome. Rather, the features can occur in conjunction with a number of malformation syndromes. These include, to date, Klippel-Feil syndrome,[797,804] Klinefelter syndrome,[805] cri du chat syndrome,[806] Saethre-Chotzen syndrome,[807] and Seckel syndrome.[807]

A number of authors have described the wide variety of malformations of the external ear and canal.[782,808–814] Caldarelli and Valvassori concluded that the severity of the external ear malformation parallels the severity of mandibular deformity, but not necessarily in terms of the specific grade of severity.[809] These authors also reported that ossicular malformations and malformations of the external auditory meatus paralleled *either* the severity of the microtia or the severity of the mandibular deformity. Figueroa and Pruzansky reported that more severely affected mandibles were likely to be associated with more severely affected external ears, but that there were exceptions.[811] In their patient series, the frequency of severely affected mandibles increased as hemifacial microsomia became associated with other findings.

Malformation of the temporal bone has been described in several reports.[809,810,815] Chandra-Sekhar reported sensorineural hearing loss and malformation of the cochlea.[775] One report described an anomalous internal auditory meatus in Goldenhar syndrome,[816] and another a progressive hearing loss.[817]

Notwithstanding the confusion about which features should be considered typical and which "associated," several investigators have reported the frequency of cervical spine anomalies. Grabb reported malformation of vertebrae and/or ribs in 11 percent of his sample of "first and second branchial arch syndrome."[779] Ross estimated an incidence of cervical vertebral anomalies of between 20 and 30 percent,[774] and Figueroa and Friede found an incidence of slightly over 29 percent.[797] The point of interest in these particular anomalies is their possible role in producing craniofacial defects in the embryo.[722]

Concurrence of hemifacial microsomia with clefts of the lip and/or palate has been noted repeatedly,[162,579,789,804,818,819] and one recent report described tracheoesophageal anomalies.[820] Cardiac malformations have been frequently reported.[821–824] There are also reports of upper airway obstruction, sleep apnea, and resultant cor pulmonale.[804,825,826] An association between urogenital anomalies and ear malformations is always suspected because of the timing of morphogenesis in the embryo,[827,828] and the syndrome of "branchio-oto-renal dysplasia" must be considered in differential diagnosis.[829–834]

Neuromuscular involvement of one side of the face (or both in the bilateral form) has long been noted in hemifacial microsomia. Asymmetric function of facial muscles could theoretically stem from (1) primary hypoplasia of the muscle itself, (2) abnormality of the bony structures to which the muscles attach, (3) deficiency in innervation, and/or (4) secondary overdevelopment of the musculature on the nonaffected or lesser affected side. Since the facial nerve courses through the middle ear cavity, it is vulnerable to deformation or malformation in hemifacial microsomia.[809,810,815] Converse et al noted cranial nerve anomalies, the most common being the facial nerve.[776] Although Grabb and others mentioned underdevelopment of facial and oral muscles, including the tongue, no one has systematically investigated tongue function.[779] Extensive EMG studies of facial muscle function in hemifacial microsomia have recently been reported.[835–837]

Three studies have investigated symmetry of velopharyngeal motion and its relation to velopharyngeal inadequacy in speech in hemifacial microsomia. I reported asymmetrical palatal elevation in 37 of 51 patients (72.5 percent).[838] In two of the 37, elevation was stronger on the affected, rather than the supposedly unaffected, side of the face. Only three of the 37 showed velopharyngeal inadequacy as judged by the presence of audible nasal emission and hypernasality. Of 18 patients studied by Luce et al, 14 showed either partial or total unilateral palatal paralysis, but only six showed evidence of velopharyngeal inadequacy.[161] Shprintzen et al investigated 22 patients, six of whom had cleft palates.[162] Of the remaining 16, ten showed unilateral gaps in closure as viewed via nasopharyngoscopy, and all ten were reported to show either mild or moderate hypernasality. Of the entire group of 22 subjects, all but one showed asymmetrical lateral pharyngeal wall motion during speech. Shprintzen et al reported that there was no clear relationship between the severity of the malformation complex and the presence of velopharyngeal inadequacy or the severity of hypernasal resonance. Although they stated that "examination of the subjects failed to reveal any cranial-nerve abnormalities," (p 137) both their own findings and previous descriptions of abnormalities in the course of the facial nerve leave this open to question.

Because of the extreme variability in expression in hemifacial microsomia, patients may present with a clinical picture ranging from virtually no speech production problems to severe problems. The possible hazards to speech include hearing loss, aberrant tongue posture and asymmetric function, cleft palate, velopharyngeal inadequacy due to asymmetric palatal and pharyngeal wall motion, malocclusion, and secondary retardation in intellectual development if the hearing loss is bilateral and if amplification is not provided early. (Smith cited an IQ below 85 in 13 percent, a finding that may reflect associated syndromes or malformation, or untreated hearing loss, or both.[41]) The most obvious and critical need for these children is early audiologic testing and otologic evaluation, including roentenographic evaluation of the temporal bone, regardless of how mild the external ear findings might be.[839]

Mandibulofacial Dysostosis

Mandibulofacial dysostosis is known by a number of names, the most common being Treacher Collins syndrome. According to Smith, the first case was reported by Thomson in 1846.[41] A later case description was given by Berry,[840] and the syndrome was eventually associated with the ophthalmologist (Treacher Collins) who described two cases in 1900. As of 1982, more than 250 cases had been reported, but no incidence figures were available.[41]

Mandibulofacial dysostosis is another syndrome in which there is wide variation in expressivity, and it is not unusual for the affected parent of a more severely affected child (the syndrome is an autosomal dominant, with a 50 percent recurrence risk) to have gone through life undiagnosed. A number of authors have catalogued the features, with most listings including antimongoloid slant of the palpebral fissures, hypoplasia of the malar bones, lower lid defects (colobomata and partial to total absence of lower eyelashes), bilateral malformations of the auricle and middle ear, and hypoplasia of the maxilla and mandible (Fig. 17–29).[41,717,794,841–844] When present, the mandibular hypoplasia results in curvature of the lower border of the mandible ("antegonial notching") with consequent malocclusion including an open bite that may become worse in time.[727,845] Gorlin et al reported an incidence of 30 percent of cleft palate (Fig. 17–30).[717] Submucous clefts and noncleft velopharyngeal inadequacy were reported by Fara et al,[86] Shprintzen,[768] Walker,[846] and Weatherley-White et al.[81] Pruzansky and I reported an incidence of 32 percent of cleft palate and 32 percent of noncleft velopharyngeal inadequacy in a series of 25 patients.[847] Pharyngeal hypoplasia, with extreme narrowing of the pharyngeal airway,[847,848] causes difficulties in trying to treat cleft or velopharyngeal inadequacy when it occurs and may be related to frequent reports of sleep apnea and other signs of upper airway obstruction.[736,843,849,850] Crysdale described one child (Fig. 17–31) with mandibulofacial dysostosis who required an emergency tracheotomy after cleft palate repair (the open cleft apparently having provided a necessary airway) and another who required tracheotomy after a pharyngeal flap.[731] Several reports have noted frequent neonatal death.[780,843,850–853] In light of such reports, it is of interest that one postmortem examination on a 7-month-old child with mandibulofacial dysostosis revealed laryngeal dimensions largely comparable to those of a newborn.[854]

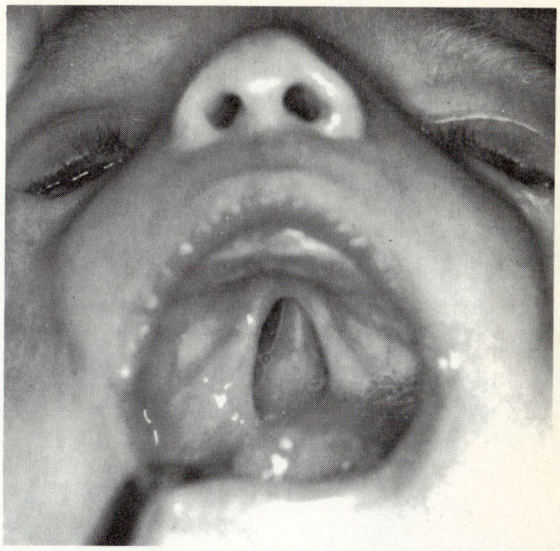

Figure 17-30 Cleft palate in infant with mandibulofacial dysostosis.

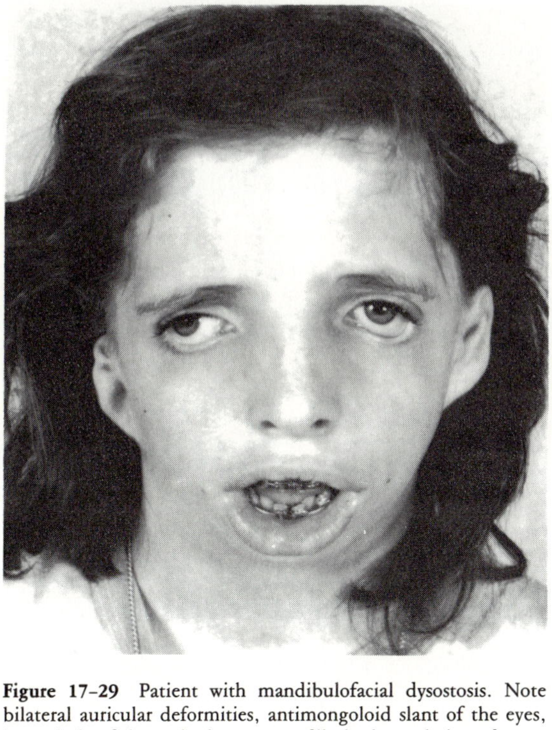

Figure 17-29 Patient with mandibulofacial dysostosis. Note bilateral auricular deformities, antimongoloid slant of the eyes, hypoplasia of the malar bones, mandibular hypoplasia and open bite.

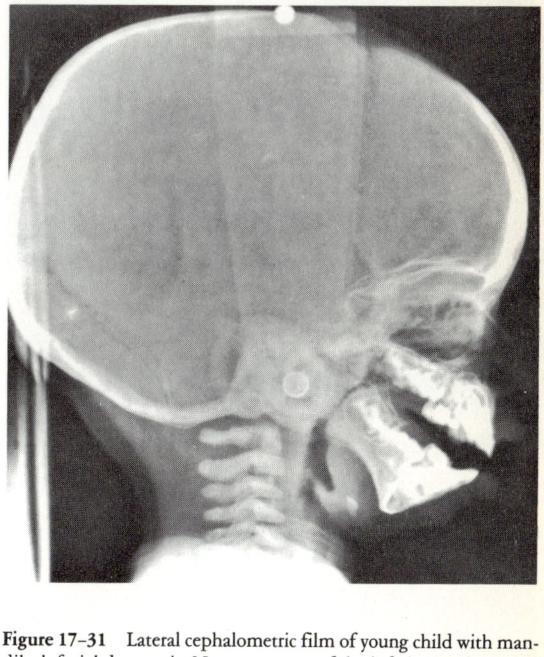

Figure 17-31 Lateral cephalometric film of young child with mandibulofacial dysostosis. Note curvature of the inferior border of the mandible and crowding of the nasopharyngeal airway.

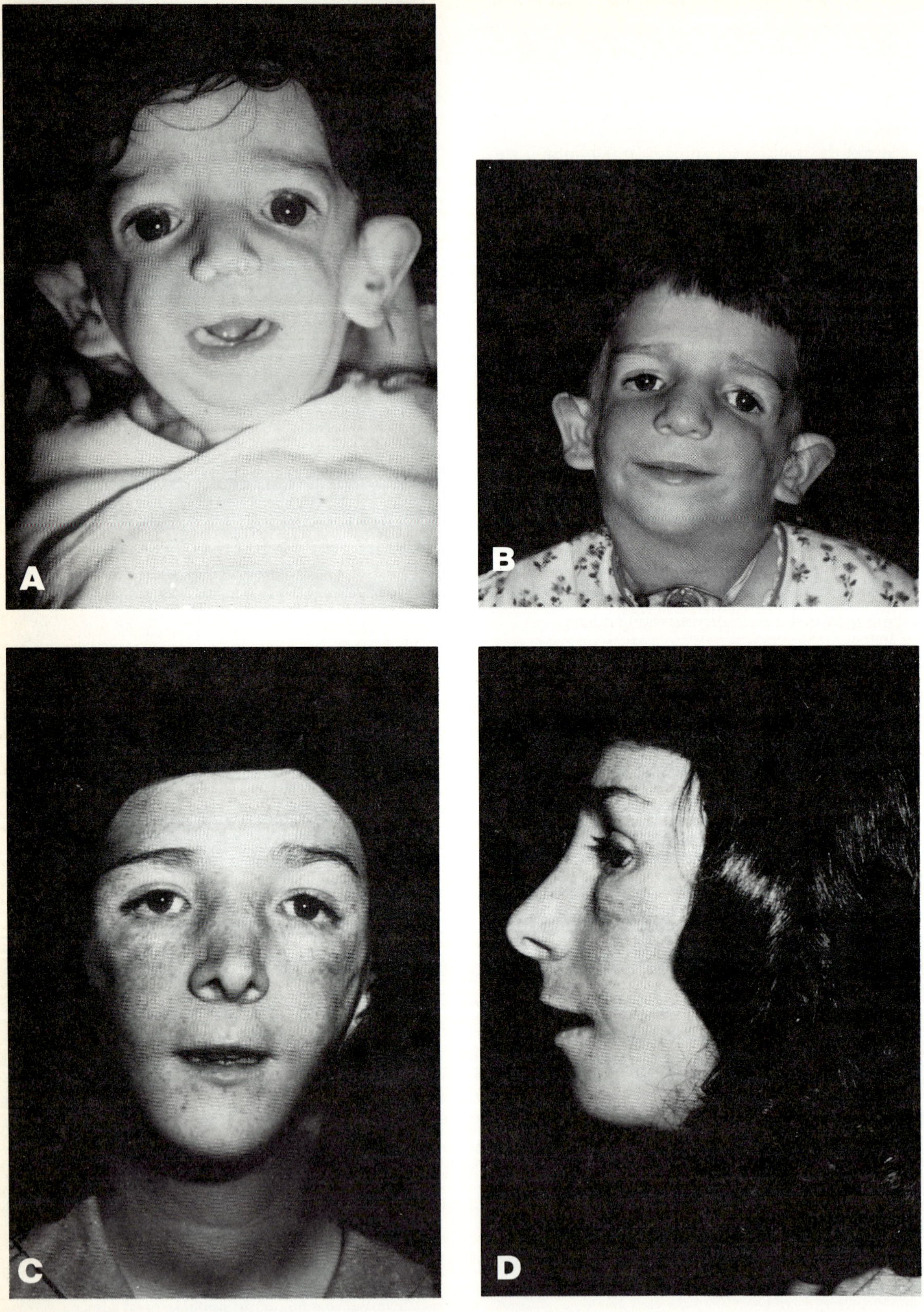

Figure 17–32 Female with mandibulofacial dysostosis at the ages of *A*, 5 months, *B*, 4 years, 5 months, and *C* and *D*, following craniofacial surgery as a teenager. (Courtesy, Dr. Douglas Ousterhout and the Center for Craniofacial Anomalies, University of California–San Francisco.)

The malformations of the external and middle ear in mandibulofacial dysostosis vary in severity as they do in hemifacial microsomia, even though they are two entirely separate disorders.[737,814,855,856] As in hemifacial microsomia, the hearing loss is typically reported to be a maximum conductive loss, with normal structure and function of the inner ear.[741,855*]

Abnormally acute cranial base angulation has been reported in mandibulofacial dysostosis in both postmortem and radiographic studies,[842,858,859] and it may play a role in the crowding of the naso- and oropharyngeal airway. One recent longitudinal study of 24 cases revealed this finding in 50 percent, with seven of the cases decreasing from normal angulation in infancy or early childhood to abnormal angulation at the time the last set of records were taken.[859a]

When present in even a moderate degree of severity, mandibulofacial dysostosis (Fig. 17–32) is a syndrome that seems specifically designed to sabotage speech production. Hazards to the development of normal communication skills include hearing loss, cleft palate or noncleft velopharyngeal inadequacy, malocclusion, and secondary mental retardation when the loss is unrecognized and so is not treated early. In addition, the crowding of the oral cavity and pharyngeal space leads to damping and abnormal frequency location of the vowel formants.[860] Even when blatant VPI is present, the effect of this crowding on the vowel formants overrides what would otherwise be clearly hypernasal resonance.

Pierre Robin Sequence

Pierre Robin, a French physician, described the role of glossoptosis[861] and mandibular "hypotrophy"[862] in producing respiratory distress in infants. In 1930, Eley and Farber described four cases in the United States with micrognathy, glossoptosis, cleft palate, and respiratory distress (Fig. 17–33).[863] For many years, the term "Pierre Robin syndrome" and then "Pierre Robin anomalad" was applied to the concurrence of micrognathy, glossoptosis, and cleft of the secondary palate, although Robin had not originally described cleft as part of the picture. Many authors still include cleft palate as a pathognomonic feature,[417,697,864–869] whereas others do not.[870–878] Dennison considered cleft palate to be a common, but not a constant feature.[871] Fletcher et al concluded from the studies they reviewed that cleft palate was present in over 50 percent of the cases.[872] Oka et al estimated that clefts occurred in approximately 70 percent of the cases in Japan.[874]

Estimates of the incidence of the Robin sequence are obviously influenced by what criteria are used for diagnosis. Rubin cited an incidence of one in 30,000.[879] Bush and Williams cited one in 8,500, but this figure was based on admissions to a cleft palate unit in a large hospital, thereby introducing ascertainment bias.[864] However, a recent report yielded a frequency of four cases in 10,000 consecutive births.[880] In the latter study, diagnostic criteria were not given. Shprintzen reported an incidence of one in 2,000 live births in a large metropolitan hospital if the three classic criteria were used for ascertainment, one in 1,250 if the requirement of a U-shaped cleft palate was dropped.[881]

The replacement of the term "syndrome" with "sequence" stemmed from the realization that the features are not the result of multiple errors in morphogenesis, but rather the result of a sequence of events. Most of the authors writing on this subject have considered sequence to be (1) failure in normal growth of the mandible in utero, which itself could be caused by a number of different factors,[697,865,865a,866] leading to (2) inability of the tongue to drop down from between the palatal shelves, leading to (3) cleft palate.[41,882–884] However, other theories have been advanced, including primary hypotonia of the tongue,[885–887] and primary growth deficiency of the maxilla as well as the mandible.[888–890] A primary neuromuscular problem could be compatible with a theory based either on the mandible (failure of the mandible to lift off the ster-

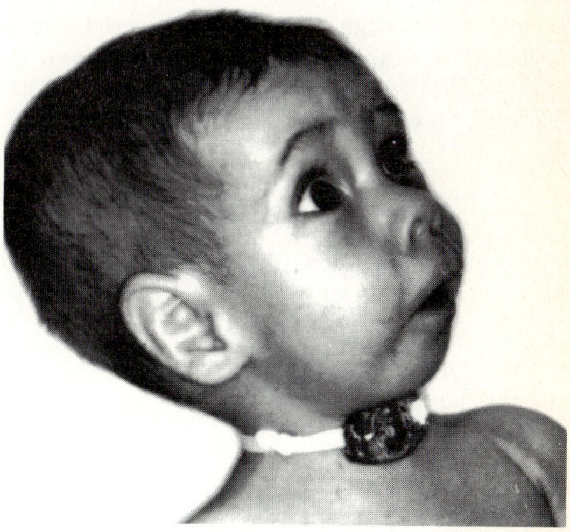

Figure 17–33 Infant with Pierre Robin malformation sequence. Note micrognathia and tracheostomy.

* A sensorineural loss in one patient described by Lynn and Pirkey in 1965 was ascribed to drug toxicity in utero.[857]

num in utero with the resultant restriction of growth) or the tongue.[697,865,865a,866,891]

The Robin sequence can occur in isolation, as part of numerous syndromes, or associated with other nonsyndromic congenital anomalies.[697,865–866,891–897] Cohen listed 18 different clinical entities in which the Robin sequence appears as one feature.[697,865–866] Williams et al reported that 25 percent of their 55 cases had abnormalities other than retrognathia and cleft palate and noted a particularly high incidence (5 in 55) of peripheral limb defects, which they did not specify.[896] Wood and Sandlin reported hand abnormalities in three of eight cases, but this incidence was subject to ascertainment bias since the report emanated from an orthopaedic department.[897] In a series of 60 cases reported by Siegel-Sadewitz and Shprintzen, 32 percent had Stickler syndrome,* 14 percent had the velo-cardio-facial syndrome, 9 percent had the fetal alcohol syndrome, and 9 percent had provisionally unique syndromes.[894,895] In only 19 percent did the sequence appear in isolation. Such findings underscore not only the etiologic heterogeneity of this sequence as discussed by earlier investigators,[697,865–866,875–878] but also the necessity for *not* expecting the same development and consequences of treatment in each case.

By far the bulk of the literature on this topic has been devoted to the neonatal problems, primarily the causes and management of airway obstruction and its sequelae.[417,868,870–872,875,878] Fletcher et al concluded that the condition was incompatible with life in 25 to 50 percent of affected infants, based on the reports they reviewed.[872] Williams et al reported 14 deaths in the first 3 months of life in the 55 cases they reviewed.[896] Cardiac problems, presumably secondary to respiratory stress, were frequently reported,[904–906] although the association between clefting in general and cardiac problems has long been established.[907–915]

Early reports such as those by Robin himself[861,862] and Dennison[871] focused on the micrognathia and glossoptosis as the cause of the airway obstruction. Champion blamed the tongue intruding into the cleft and blocking the airway, and advocated cleft palate closure in the first 48 hours of life as a preventative measure.[885] However, Hoffman, Kahn, and Seitchik felt the respiratory problems and consequent anesthetic risk constituted a good reason for delaying palate repair until late in the second year of life.[916] Routledge agreed with Champion on the cause of obstruction, but preferred the tongue-adhesion procedure of Douglas[917–918] to keep the tongue out of the cleft and out of the airway.[887] Fletcher et al conducted pharyngeal and esophageal manometric studies in a 4 month old and concluded that the "glossoptosis" was not a primary but, in fact, a secondary result of negative pressure in the pharynx, which became progressively more severe with repeated attempts to swallow and breathe, the negative pressure sucking the tongue back against the pharyngeal wall.[872] Ogborn and Pemberton recently cited the theory of Fletcher et al to explain the development of airway obstruction in five infants after the neonatal period.[920] Because most investigators implicated the tongue position as causing the respiratory difficulties, a number of variations of the Douglas tongue-lip adhesion[917–919] or "glossopexy" were developed.[867,921–924] Others advocated prosthetic palatal plates to keep the tongue out of the cleft,[869,886,925] use of nasopharyngeal tubes,[926] gastrostomy to prevent aspiration,[927] or simply an aggressive program of prone positioning.[873,893] Para-

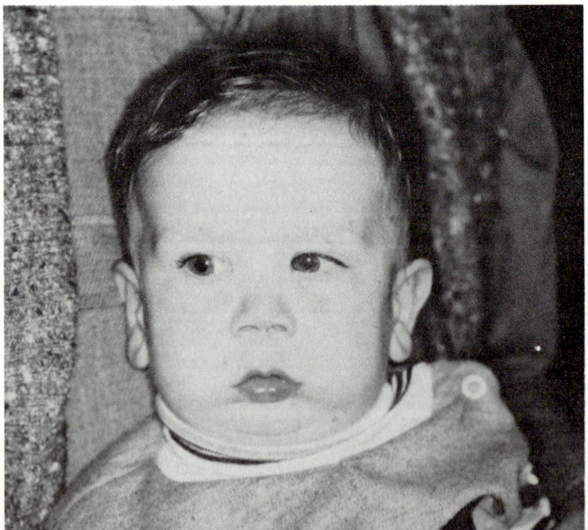

Figure 17–34 Infant with Stickler syndrome. Note flat facies, depressed nasal bridge, epicanthal folds, and micrognathia. (Courtesy, Center for Craniofacial Anomalies, University of California–San Francisco.)

* Stickler syndrome (Fig. 17–34), or hereditary progressive arthro-ophthalmopathy, was first described in 1965,[898] with further case descriptions by Stickler and Pugh in 1967;[899] Spranger in 1968;[900] Herrmann, France, Spranger, Opitz and Wiffler in 1975;[901] and Hall in 1974.[902] This is an autosomal dominant syndrome characterized by multiple ocular findings including myopia, which appears by age 10, and possible retinal detachment with eventual blindness if the condition is not recognized early, together with abnormalities of the bones and joints.[41] Several authors have commented on its frequent association with the Robin sequence[768,894,901] The report of "limb defects" in five cases and ocular findings in two cases of Williams et al may have signalled undiagnosed Stickler syndrome.[896] The same is true of the report of Smith and Stowe in which 13 of 39 cases of Robin sequence had ocular findings.[903] Stickler should be ruled out in any case of dominant cleft palate, hereditary myopia, or Pierre Robin sequence.[41,901]

dise suggested that tracheotomy should be tried only if positioning failed.[417]

Pruzansky and Richmond documented "catch-up" growth of the mandible in the first few months of life, which they believed provided a natural resolution to "the symptoms attending the glossoptosis."[928] They also reported continued mandibular growth in early childhood that reduced the retrognathic profile. However, as pointed out by Siegel-Sadewitz and Shprintzen, expectations of mandibular growth are not the same in the Robin sequence that appears as part of a syndrome as they are in the isolated Robin.[894,895] Mallory and Paradise described a $3^1/_2$-month-old infant who could tolerate closure of the tracheotomy and ascribed this tolerance, not to catch-up growth of the mandible, but to increasing control of the tongue musculature.[929]

Recent nasopharyngoscopic and videofluorographic findings reported by Siegel-Sadewitz and Shprintzen[894] provided a possible explanation why previous authors[873,893] had expressed dissatisfaction with the results of procedures designed to anchor the tongue-tip forward, namely the fact that the site of upper airway obstruction is often *below* the level of the tongue base. The narrowed lower pharyngeal airways demonstrated by these investigators may have reflected the mechanism described earlier by Fletcher et al.[872] The findings of Siegel-Sadewitz and Shprintzen may also help to explain persistent respiratory distress and death in later childhood.[892]

The palatal anomalies in the Robin sequence have been a topic of considerable discussion. The majority of sources describe a "U-shaped" cleft, and Hanson and Smith considered this unusual shape to be indicative of the role of an intruding tongue in producing the cleft.[882] However, V-shaped clefts have also been described.[889,890,930] In fact, Poradowska et al reported the presence of submucous clefts as well.[930]

Children with the Robin sequence are known to be vulnerable to conductive hearing loss,[930a] the incidence possibly reflecting the influence of cleft palate. In addition to the probability of otitis media, however, the possible role of congenital malformations of the middle ear and ossicles should be considered.[904,931]

Hazards to speech production in the Robin sequence include possible developmental sequelae to early respiratory distress and other neonatal problems, hearing loss, cleft palate and possible post-repair velopharyngeal inadequacy, possible malocclusion in early childhood until "catch-up" growth of the mandible takes place (if it does), and possible difficulties in laryngeal voice production in cases in which a tracheotomy is performed and especially if weaning the child from this is difficult. Pharyngeal flap may be contraindicated as a secondary procedure even in later childhood due to airway problems and certainly carries a possible danger of exacerbating problems in early childhood if performed as a primary procedure.[932] Obviously the hazards to communication development become more complex when the sequence occurs as part of a syndrome. Levinson, Massengill, Pickrell, and Bryson described deficits in lingual and labial movements, primarily in nonspeech tasks, in five children who had undergone the Douglas tongue-tip adhesion; however, the amount of data was small.[933] Bloomer also mentioned possible problems in tongue-tip articulation following this procedure.[934] Apart from these brief notes, there are no other reports in the literature of communication deficits that might be specific to the Robin sequence itself and not consequent either to cleft palate or concurrence with a syndrome.

Van der Woude Syndrome

Demarquay described congenital fistulas of the lower lip in 1845.[933a] Fogh-Andersen described three cases of congenital paramedian fistulae of the lower lip and stated that there was a genetic connection with cleft lip and palate (Fig. 17–35).[935] However, the "lip pit syndrome" was later given the name of Van der Woude, who called attention to about 14 reports in the literature with familial occurrence, 80 percent of which were in association with facial-oral clefts of various types.[936] Seventy-five percent of the cases she reviewed showed dominant inheritance. She added three new pedigrees, and she attributed the disorder to a "a single gene of variable expressivity," with expression varying from the "full triad of cleft lip, cleft palate, and fistulae of the lower lip to no detectable departure from normal."*

Since that time, the association of lower lip pits and clefting has been described in nearly 100 reports (see review by Burdick et al[937]). Cervenka et al estimated penetrance at 80 percent and frequency at one in 75,000 to one in 100,000 in Caucasians.[938] Glass, Stewart, and Miles reported submucous clefts as well as overt clefts in affected kindreds.[939] In 67 cases described by Shprintzen, Goldberg, and Sidoti in 1980, there was variable expression of clefting and lower lip pits, but the penetrance was 97 percent.[940] Rintala, Lahti, and Gylling described 22

* The term "penetrance" is used in genetics to denote the frequency with which any expression at all of a gene is manifested. For example, if a trait known to be dominantly inherited is present in generations I and III in a family, but not in II, it is known that the gene was still present in generation II, but simply did not "penetrate." "Expression" or "expressivity" refers to the severity of the trait when it is in fact manifested.

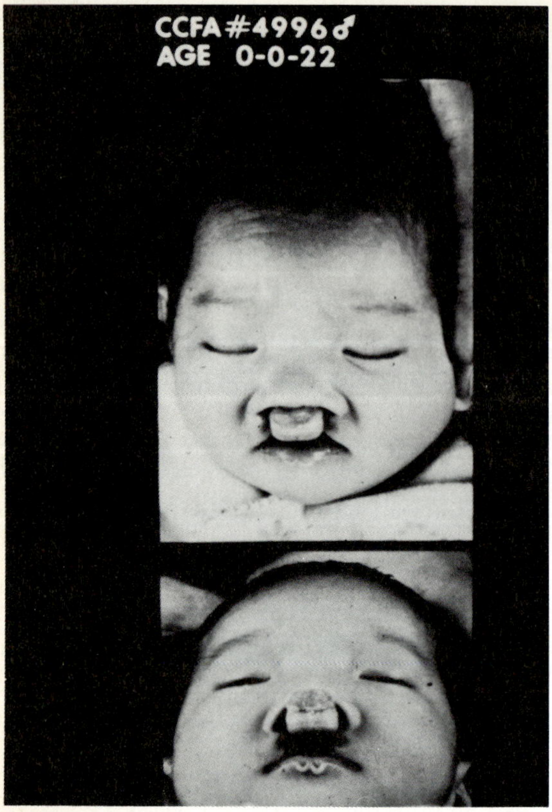

Figure 17–35 Infant with Van der Woude syndrome, the expression in this case including bilateral cleft lip and palate together with paramedian lip pits. (Courtesy, Center for Craniofacial Anomalies, University of Illinois.)

cases, in one of which there was only one lip "sinus," which was contralateral to the cleft.[941] Two studies described the variabililty in appearance of the lip pits, microforms of which could account for missed cases.[942,943] In their 1983 report, these authors also described hypodontia in these patients; Schneider had earlier reported the association of lip pits and absent second molars.[944] Pauli and Hall described three cases with associated congenital heart disease.[945] In 258 members of an affected family reported by Janku, Robinow, Kelly, Bralley, Baynes, and Edgerton, lip pits were the only manifestation in 64 percent, and overall penetrance was 96.7 percent.[946] Burdick et al concluded from their review that both cleft palate alone and cleft lip and palate together with lower lip pits segregated in an autosomal dominant mode with penetrance estimated to be between 89 and 99 percent.[937]

Patients with Van der Woude syndrome are not known to exhibit problems in speech production other than what may be encountered in any speaker with a cleft. However, the topic is raised here because, as pointed out by Glass et al, speech pathologists can play an important role in identifying these patients.[939] Identification of this disorder changes the recurrence risk for clefting from what would normally be only a few percentage points higher than in the general population to 50 percent.

Velo-cardio-facial Syndrome

In 1955, Sedlackova described a series of patients with velopharyngeal inadequacy, unusual facies, and reduced facial expression together with manifestations of ectodermal dysplasia.[947] Other descriptions of palatal problems, including submucous clefts and/or reduced motion of the velopharyngeal system, associated with reduced facial expression and minor morphologic differences in the face appeared in subsequent reports by Calnan,[110] Fara et al,[86] Kaplan,[69] Kruk and Tronczynska,[948] Pitt and Ingram,[155] Saad,[949] and Sedlackova et al.[119] A 1978 report described the "velo-cardio-facial syndrome" that bore a facial resemblance to the "Sedlackova syndrome,"[948] but lacked the features of ectodermal dysplasia and added a variety of cardiac findings.[950] In a later report on 39 cases, overt or submucous cleft palate was observed to be present in 100 percent of the cases, as were learning disabilities.[951] Cardiac malformations were present in 85 percent.[952] In a later report, Arvystas and Shprintzen listed the frequent features as being overt or submucous clefts, cardiac anomalies, characteristic facies (prominent nose with a broad nasal root, narrow alar base, narrow palpebral fissures, flattened malar eminences, vertical maxillary excess, retrognathia), learning disabilities and/or mental retardation, pharyngeal hypotonia, slender hands and digits, abundant scalp hair, and anomalous ears (Fig. 17–36).[953] Arvystas and Shprintzen also reported obtuse angulation of the cranial base with retrodisplacement of the mandibular complex, which they postulated could explain the occurrence of the Robin sequence in this syndrome, an alternative explanation being the neurogenic factors and lack of mandibular exercise in utero.

Golding-Kushner, Weller, and Shprintzen offered detailed information on the language and psychological profiles in 26 children with this syndrome.[954] The children tended to score within the normal range on tests of intellectual and language development prior to age 6, except for immature language usage. However, problems in motor coordination and poor development of numerical concepts were consistently evident, and, together with bland affect, proved to be better predictors of later academic problems than did preschool IQ tests. These children did not appear to progress beyond a relatively concrete level of cognitive development.

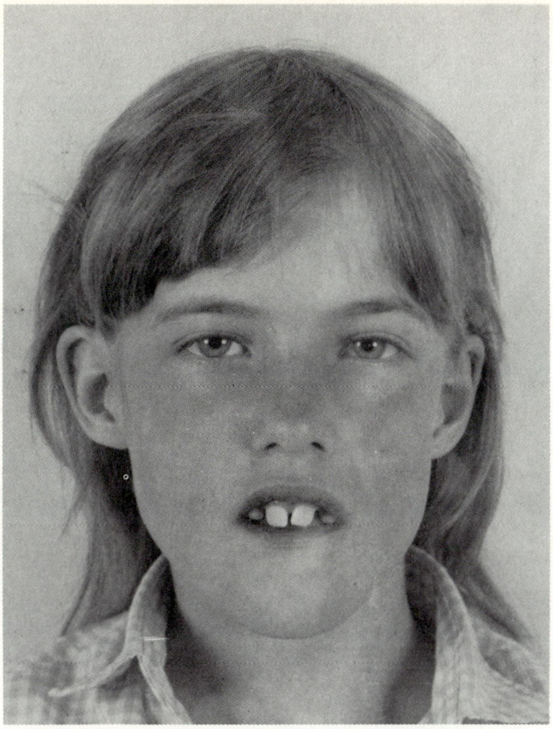

Figure 17–36 Female with velo-cardio-facial syndrome. Note prominent nose with broad nasal root, narrow alar bas, narrow palpebral fissures, vertical maxillary excess, retrognathia and reduced facial expression. (Courtesy, Center for Craniofacial Anomalies, University of Illinois.)

Shprintzen et al reported frequent episodes of serous otitis media in the velo-cardio-facial syndrome,[951] and Siegel-Sadewitz and Shprintzen noted conductive hearing loss as well as problems in articulation, resonance, and cognition as being frequent in this population.[772] The hazards to communication development obviously go beyond what could be expected simply on the basis of an inadequately functioning velopharyngeal system and associated hearing loss.

Guidelines for Management

By this point it is clear that intelligent management of craniofacial syndromes, sequences, or associations is dependent upon accurate diagnosis. Although he was not speaking of speech production problems, Dennison's statement about the Pierre Robin "syndrome" is relevant: "In its recognition lies half the treatment" (p 336).[871]

Responsibilities of the speech pathologist in dealing with these patients is fourfold: (1) obtaining appropriate information on the features, genetics, physical management, and possible communicative deficits present in the disorder; (2) early intervention, including assistance in obtaining audiologic and otologic assessment in those fortunate cases where the diagnosis is made in infancy; (3) assistance in obtaining accurate, complete diagnosis and genetic counseling if this has not already been accomplished; and (4) coordination of speech and language therapy with the complex and multiple physical management procedures that may be required. The wisdom of learning the genetics of a disorder is not the ability of the speech pathologist to offer genetic counseling, but rather increased awareness of the risk of recurrence and thus of the need for such counseling by a qualified geneticist. Of the disorders discussed in this section, six (Apert syndrome, Crouzon disease, mandibulofacial dysostosis, Stickler syndrome, Van der Woude syndrome, and the velo-cardio-facial syndrome) are dominantly inherited. Similarly, the speech pathologist should be aware of the dramatic surgical advances made in the management of craniofacial anomalies since most families and even a large number of physicians are not.[735]

The most difficult task may be the on-going process of tailoring the goals and techniques of speech and language therapy to the needs and capabilities of the individual patient. Virtually all craniofacial anomalies vary in severity, and the severity of expression is not necessarily related clearly to the severity of communication deficits. Furthermore, given the psychosocial impact of these anomalies, it is quite possible that improvement of speech is not the patient's own first priority.

Portions of this material appeared previously in Peterson-Falzone S. Velopharyngeal inadequacy in the absence of overt cleft palate. J Craniofac Genet Devel Biol 1985; [Supplement] 1:97–124.

Peterson-Falone S. Speech characteristics: updating clinical decisions. Sem Speech Lang 1986; 7(3):269–296.

REFERENCES

1. Tessier P. Anatomical classification of facial, cranio-facial and latero-facial clefts. J Maxillofac Surg 1976; 4(2):69–92.
2. Green H, Nelson C, Gaylor D, Holson J. Accuracy of birth certificate data for detecting facial cleft defects in Arkansas children. Cleft Palate J 1979; 16(2):167–170.
3. Abyholm F. Cleft lip and palate in Norway. I. Registration, incidence and early mortality of infants with CLP. Scand J Plast Reconstr Surg 1978; 12:39–44.
4. Jones M. Etiology of facial clefts: prospective evaluation of 428 patients. Cleft Palate J (in press).
5. Shprintzen R, Siegel-Sadewitz V, Amato J, Goldberg R. Anomalies associated with cleft lip, cleft palate, or both. Am J Med Genet 1985; 20:585–595.
6. Fogh-Andersen P. Inheritance of harelip and cleft palate. Copenhagen: Arnold Busck, 1942.
7. Fraser F, Baxter H. The familial distribution of congenital clefts of the lip and palate. Am J Surg 1954; 87(5):656–659.

8. Fraser G, Calnan J. Cleft lip and palate: seasonal incidence, birth weight, birth rank, sex, site, associated malformations and parental age. A statistical survey. Arch Dis Child 1961; 36:420–423.
9. Greene J. Anomalies of the speech mechanism and associated voice and speech disorders. NY State J Med 1945; 45(6):605–608.
10. Hixon E. A study of the incidence of cleft lip and cleft palate in Ontario. Can J Public Health 1951; 42:508–511.
11. MacMahon B, McKeown T. The incidence of harelip and cleft palate related to birth rank and maternal age. Am J Hum Genet 1953; 5(2):176–183.
12. Mazaheri M. Statistical analysis of patients with congenital cleft lip and/or plate at the Lancaster Cleft Palate Clinic. Plast Reconstr Surg 1958; 21:193–203.
13. Greene J, Vermillion J, Hay S, Gibbens S, Kerschbaum S. Epidemiologic study of cleft lip and cleft palate in four states. J Am Dent Assoc 1964; 68:387–404.
14. Phair G. Wisconsin cleft palate program. J Speech Disord 1947; 12:410–414.
15. Beder O, Coe H, Braafladt R, Houle J. Factors associated with congenital cleft lip and cleft palate in the Pacific Northwest. Oral Surg Oral Med Oral Pathol 1956; 9(12):1267–1273.
16. Oka S. Epidemiology and genetics of clefting: with implications for etiology. In: Cooper H, Harding R, Krogman W, Mazaheri M, eds. Cleft palate and cleft lip: a team approach to clinical management and rehabilitation of the patient. Philadelphia: WB Saunders, 1979:108.
17. Tanaka K, Fujino H, Tashiro H, Sanui Y. Recurrent risk of cleft lip and palate among relatives of patients, with special considerations of sex and racial differences. Jpn J Hum Genet 1967; 12(3):141–149.
18. Fujino H, Tanaka K, Sanui Y. Genetic study of cleft-lips and cleft-palates based upon 2828 Japanese cases. Kyushu J Med Sci 1963; 14:317–331.
19. Fujino H, Tashiro Y, Sanui Y, Tanaka K. Empirical genetic risk among offspring of cleft lip and cleft palate patients. Jpn J Hum Genet 1967; 12:62–68.
20. Kobayashi Y. A genetic study of harelip and cleft palate. Jpn J Hum Genet 1958; 3:73–107.
21. Koguchi H. Population data on cleft lip and cleft palate in the Japanese. In: Melnick M, Bixler D, Shields E, eds. Progress in clinical and biological research. Vol. 46. Etiology of cleft lip and palate. New York: Alan R Liss, 1980:297.
22. Kurozumi S, Okazaki H, Kosaka N, Kido N, Tanaka T, Nakagawa Y, Fujiwara K, Yasuhara K, Ohsaki K, Konishi S, Ohkura K. A genetic study of harelip and cleft palate. Jpn J Hum Genet 1963; 8(2):120–127.
23. Ross RB, Johnston MC. Cleft lip and palate. Huntington, NY: Robert E Kreiger, 1979.
24. Calnan J. Submucous cleft palate. Br J Plast Surg 1954; 7:264–282.
25. Gylling U, Soivio A. Submucous cleft palates. Acta Chir Scand 1965; 129:282–287.
26. Meskin L, Pruzansky S. A malformation profile of facial cleft patients and their siblings. Cleft Palate J 1969; 6(3):309–315.
27. Spriestersbach D, Spriestersbach B, Moll K. Incidence of clefts of the lip and palate in families with children with clefts and families with children without clefts. Plast Reconstr Surg 1962; 29(4):392–401.
28. Chi S. Cleft lip and cleft palate in New South Wales. Aust Dent J 1974; 19:111–117.
29. Conway H, Wagner K. Congenital anomalies of the head and neck: as reported on birth certificates in New York City, 1952 to 1962 (inclusive). Plast Reconstr Surg 1965; 36(1):71–79.
30. Conway H, Wagner K. Incidence of clefts in New York City. Cleft Palate J 1966; 3:284–290.
31. Curtis E. Genetic and envrionmental factors in the etiology of cleft lip and cleft palate. J Can Dent Assoc 1957; 23:576–580.
32. Czeizel A, Tusnadi G. An epidemiologic study of cleft lip with or without cleft palate and posterior cleft palate in Hungary. Hum Hered 1971; 21:17–38.
33. Gilmore S, Hofman S. Clefts in Wisconsin: incidence and related factors. Cleft Palate J 1966; 3:186–199.
34. Ingalls T, Taube I, Klingberg M. Cleft lip and palate: epidemiologic considerations. Plast Reconstr Surg 1964; 34(1):1–10.
35. Knox G, Braithwaite F. Cleft lips and palates in Northumberland and Durham. Arch Dis Child 1963; 38(197):66–70.
36. Wilson M. A ten-year survey of cleft lip and cleft palate in the south west region. Br J Plast Surg 1972; 25:224–228.
37. Rollnick B, Pruzansky S. Genetic services at a center for craniofacial anomalies. Cleft Palate J 1981; 18:304–313.
38. Berlin A. Classification of cleft lip and palate and related craniofacial disorders. In: Bzoch K, ed. Communicative disorders related to cleft lip and palate. Boston: Little, Brown, 1979:20.
39. Pruzansky S. Description, classification analysis of unoperated clefts of the lip and palate. Am J Orthod 1953; 39(8):590–611.
40. Patten B. Embryology of the palate and the maxillofacial region. In: Grabb W, Rosenstein S, Bzoch K, eds. Cleft lip and palate: surgical, dental and speech aspects. Boston: Little, Brown, 1971:21.
41. Smith D. Recognizable patterns of human malformation. 3rd ed. Philadelphia: WB Saunders, 1982.
42. Croft C, Shprintzen R, Daniller A, Lewin M. The occult submucous cleft palate and the musculus uvulae. Cleft Palate J 1978; 15(2):150–154.
43. Lewin M, Croft C, Shprintzen R. Velopharyngeal insufficiency due to hypoplasia of the musculus uvulae and occult submucous cleft palate. Plast Reconstr Surg 1980; 65(5):585–591.
44. Pigott R, Bensen J, White F. Nasendoscopy in the diagnosis of velophrayngeal incompetence. Plast Reconstr Surg 1969; 43(2):141–147.
45. Shprintzen R. Velopharyngeal insufficiency in the absence of overt or submucous cleft palate: the mystery solved. In: Ellis R, Flack F, eds. Diagnosis and treatment of palato glossal malfunction. London: College of Speech Therapists, 1979:37.
46. Crikelair G, Cosman B. On submucous cleft palate (letter). Plast Reconstr Surg 1977; 59:424–425.
47. Crikelair G, Striker P, and Cosman B. The surgical treatment of submucous cleft palate. Plast Reconstr Surg 1970; 45(1):58–65.
48. Demarquay J. Tissue fibrineux remplaçant au voile du palais et à la voute palatine les muscles palatine. Bull Soc Anat Paris 1846; 21(1):11–12.
49. Roux J. Memoire sur la staphylorraphie, ou suture du voile du palais. Paris: JS Chaude, 1825.
50. Veau V. Division palatine. Paris: Masson, 1931.
51. Mitts T, Garrett W, Hurwitz D. Cleft of the hard palate with soft palate integrity. Cleft Palate J 1981; 18(3):204–206.
52. Elsahy H. The modified striped Y: a systematic classification for cleft lip and palate. Cleft Palate J 1973; 10:247–250.
53. Harkins C, Berlin A, Harding R, Longacre J, Snodgrasse R. A classification of cleft lip and cleft palate. Plast Reconstr Surg 1962; 29(1):31–39.
54. Kernahan D, Stark R. A new classification for cleft lip and cleft palate. Plast Reconstr Surg 1955; 22:435–441.
55. Kernahan D. The striped Y: a symbolic classification for

cleft lip and palate. Plast Reconstr Surg 1971; 47:469–470.

56. Kernahan D. Letter to the editor. Plast Reconstr Surg 1973; 51:578.
57. McCabe B. A coding procedure for classification of cleft lip and cleft palate. Cleft Palate J 1966; 3:383–391.
58. Millard D. Cleft craft. Vol. I. The unilateral deformity. Boston: Little, Brown, 1977.
59. Whitaker L, Pashayan H, Reichmann J. A proposed new classification of craniofacial anomalies. Cleft Palate J 1981; 3:161–176.
60. Meskin L, Gorlin R, Isaacson R. Abnormal morphology of the soft palate: I. The prevalence of cleft uvula. Cleft Palate J 1964; 1(3):342–346.
61. Meskin L, Gorlin R, Isaacson R. Abnormal morphology of the soft palate: II. The genetics of cleft uvula. Cleft Palate J 1965; 2(1):40–45.
62. Meskin L, Gorlin R, Isaacson R. Cleft uvula—a microform of cleft palate. Acta Chir Plast (Prague) 1966; 8(2):91–95.
63. Kono D, Young L, Holtmann B. The association of submucous cleft palate and clefting of the primary palate. Cleft Palate J 1981; 18(3):207–209.
64. Bagatin M, Barkovic M. Submukozni rascjep nepca. Chir Maxillofac Plast 1982; 12(1):7–10.
65. Bagatin M. Submucous cleft palate. J Maxillofac Surg 1985; 13:37–38.
66. Beeden A. The bifid uvula. J Laryngol Otol 1972; 86:815–819.
67. Blakeley R. Variations in the soft palate of school children. Presented before the American Speech and Hearing Association, Chicago, 1965.
68. Calnan J. Surgery for speech. In: Calnan J, ed. Recent advances in plastic surgery. I. Edinburgh: Churchill Livingstone, 1976:39.
69. Kaplan E. The occult submucous cleft palate. Cleft Palate J 1975; 12:356–368.
70. Kelly AB. Congenital insufficiency of the palate. J Laryngol Rhinol Otol 1910; 25:281–358.
71. Kinnebrew M, McTigue D. Submucous cleft palate: review and two clinical reports. Pediatr Dent 1984; 6(4):252–258.
72. Lowry R, Courtemanche A, MacDonald C. Submucous cleft palate and the general practitioner. Can Med Assoc J 1973; 109:995–996.
73. Massengill R, Pickrell K, Robinson J. Results of pushback operations in treatment of submucous cleft palate. Plast Reconstr Surg 1973; 51:432–435.
74. Porterfield H, Mohler L, Sandel A. Submucous cleft palate. Plast Reconstr Surg 1976; 58(1):60–65.
75. Saad E. The bifid uvula in ear, nose and throat practice. Laryngoscope 1975; 85:734–737.
76. Shprintzen R, Schwartz R, Daniller A, Hoch L. Morphologic significance of bifid uvula. Pediatrics 1985; 75(3):553–561.
77. Starr C, Meskin L, Shapiro B, Weist K. Nasality and cleft uvula. Cleft Palate J 1971; 8:189–195.
78. Stewart J, Ott J, LaGace R. Submucous cleft palate. Birth Defects 1971; 7(7):64–66.
79. Tolarova M, Havlova Z, Ruzickova J. Distribution of signs considered to be microforms of lip and/or palate clefts in a normal population of 3 to 6 year old individuals. Acta Chir Plast (Prague) 1967; 9:184–194.
80. Tolarova M, Havlova Z, Ruzickova J. The distribution of characters considered to be microforms of cleft lip and/or palate in a population of normal 18–21-year-old subjects. Acta Chir Plast (Prague) 1967; 9:1–14.
81. Weatherley-White R, Sakura C, Brenner L, Stewart J, Ott J. Submucous cleft palate. Plast Reconstr Surg 1972; 49(3):297–304.
82. Weatherley-White R. Submucous cleft palate. In: Calnan J, ed. Recent advances in plastic surgery. Edinburgh: Churchill Livingstone, 1976:58.
83. Abyholm F. Submucous cleft palate. Scand J Plast Reconstr Surg 1976; 10:209–212.
84. Calnan J. The investigation of nasality (nasal escape) in speech. Speech 1957; 21(2):59–74.
85. Fara M, Weatherley-White R. Submucous cleft palate. In: Converse J, ed. Reconstructive plastic surgery. Vol. 4. Cleft lip and palate, craniofacial deformities. Philadelphia: WB Saunders, 1977:2104.
86. Fara M, Hrivnakova J, Sedlackova E. Submucous cleft palates. Acta Chir Plast (Prague) 1971; 13(4):221–234.
87. Massengill R, Fetterolf J. A cleft palate condition not easily detected during routine examination. Folia Phoniatr (Basel) 1968; 20:7–12.
88. Means J. Clefts of the hard and soft palate. South Med Record 1894; 24:24.
89. Passavant G. Über die Beseitigung der naselnden Sprache bei angeborenen Spalten des harten und weichen Gaumens. Arch Klin Chir 1865; 6:333–349.
90. Passavant G. Zweiter Artikel über die Operation der angeborenen Spalten des harten Gaumens und der damit complizirten Hasenscharten. Arch Heilk 1862; 3:305–338.
91. Pruzansky S, Peterson-Falzone S, Laffer J, Parris P. Hypernasality in the absence of overt cleft: commentary on nomenclature, diagnosis, classification research design. Presented before the 3rd International Congress on Cleft Palate and Related Craniofacial Anomalies, Toronto, 1977.
92. Rees T, Wood-Smith D, Swinyard C, Converse J. Electromyographic evaluation of submucous cleft palate: a possible aid to operative planning. Plast Reconstr Surg 1967; 40(6):592–594.
93. Thaler S, Smith H. Submucous cleft palate. Arch Otolaryngol 1968; 88:184–189.
94. Trelat U. Imperfect intonation and its cause. Lancet 1870; 1:553.
95. Trelat U. Malformation de la voute et la voile du palais. Circonstances exceptionelles. Bull Soc Chir (Paris) 1868; 8:450.
96. Trelat U. Vice de conformation voile du palais—etiologie rapport entre la brièveté de la voute palatine et la cacophonie spécial. Dental Cosmos 1870; 12:329.
97. Shapiro B, Meskin L, Cervenka J, Pruzansky S. Cleft uvula: a microform of facial clefts and its genetic basis. Birth Defects 1971; 7(7):80–82.
98. Dorrance G. Congenital insufficiency of the palate. Arch Surg 1930; 21:185–248.
99. Trier W. Velopharyngeal incompetency in the absence of overt cleft palate: anatomic and surgical considerations. Cleft Palate J 1983; 3:209–2 17.
100. Converse J, Horowitz S, Becker M. The use of tomography in the diagnosis of unusual and occult clefts of the palate. Cleft Palate J 1968; 5:311–316.
101. Chaco J, Yules R. Velopharyngeal incompetence post tonsilloadenoidectomy: an electromyographic study. Acta Otolaryngol (Stockh) 1969; 68:276–278.
102. Azzam N, Kuehn D. The morphology of musculus uvulae. Cleft Palate J 1977; 14:78–87.
103. Fara M, Dvorak J. Abnormal anatomy of the muscles of palatopharyngeal closure in cleft palates. Plast Reconstr Surg 1970; 46:488–497.
104. Kriens O. An anatomical approach to veloplasty. Plast Reconstr Surg 1969; 43:29–41.
105. Kriens O. Anatomy of the velopharyngeal area in cleft palate. Clin Plast Surg 1975; 2:261–283.
106. Dickson D, Grant J, Sicher H, DuBrul E, Poltau J. Status or research in cleft palate anatomy and physiology. Part I. Cleft Palate J 1974; 11(3):471–492.
107. Maue-Dickson W. Cleft lip and palate research: an updated state of the art. Section II. Anatomy and physiology. Cleft Palate J 1977; 14:270–287.

108. Maue-Dickson W. The craniofacial complex in cleft lip and palate: an updated review of anatomy and function. Cleft Palate J 1979; 16:291–317.
109. Birrell J. Palatal disproportion in children. J Laryngol 1966; 80:706–717.
110. Calnan J. Congenital large pharynx: a new syndrome with a report of 41 personal cases. Br J Plast Surg 1971; 24:263–271.
111. Calnan J. Diagnosis, prognosis, and treatment of "palatopharyngeal incompetence," with special reference to radiographic investigations. Br J Plast Surg 1956; 8:265–282.
112. Calnan J. The mobility of the soft palate: a radiological and statistical study. Br J Plast Surg 1961; 14(1):33–38.
113. Cotton R, Nuywayhid N. Velopharyngeal insufficiency. In: Bluestone C, Stool S, eds. Pediatric otolaryngology. Vol. II. Philadelphia: WB Saunders, 1983:1521.
114. Cotton R, Quattromani F. Lateral defects in velopharyngeal insufficiency. Arch Otolaryngol 1977; 103:90–93.
115. Crikelair G, Kastein S, Fowler E, Cosman B. Velar dysfunction in the absence of cleft palate. NY State J Med 1964; 64:263–269.
116. Dorrance G, Shirazy E. The operative story of cleft palate. Philadelphia: WB Saunders, 1933.
117. Jackson I, McGlynn M, Huskie C. Velopharyngeal incompetence in the absence of cleft palate: results of treatment in 20 cases. Plast Reconstr Surg 1980; 66(2):211–213.
118. Porterfield H, Trabue J, Terry J, Stimpert R. Hypernasality in noncleft palate patients. Plast Reconstr Surg 1966; 37(3):216–220.
119. Sedlackova E, Lastova M, Sram R. Contribution to knowledge of soft palate innervation. Folia Phoniatr 2973; 25:434–441.
120. Stueber K, Wilhelmsen R. Use of the pharyngeal flap in the treatment of congenital palatopharyngeal incompetence. Plast Reconstr Surg 1984; 73(2):219–222.
121. Szabo S, Rehak G, Hirschberg J. Phoniatrische und kieferorthopädische Untersuchungen in Fallen mit kongenital verkurztem Gaumensegel. Proc XVIth Int Congr Logoped Phoniatr 1974; 478–482.
122. Winters H. Congenital short palate. Lochem, 1975.
123. Winters H. Some historical remarks on congenital short palate. Br J Plast Surg 1966; 19(4):308–312.
124. Ricketts R. The cranial base and soft structures in cleft palate speech and breathing. Plast Reconstr Surg 1954; 14(1):47–61.
125. Goode R, Ross J. Velopharyngeal insufficiency after adenoidectomy. Arch Otolaryngol 1972; 96:223–226.
126. Massengill R, Quinn G. Adenoidal atrophy, velopharyngeal incompetence and sucking exercises: a two year follow-up case report. Cleft Palate J 1974; 11:196–199.
127. Shapiro R. Velopharyngeal insufficiency starting at puberty without adenoidectomy. Int J Pediatr Otorhinolaryngol 1980; 2:255–260.
128. Newcomb J. Anatomical defects in the faucial pillars. Laryngoscope 1897; 2:220–224.
129. Fridenburg P. Congenital detachment of faucial pillars and isolation of palato-glossus muscle. Laryngoscope 1908; 18:567–571.
130. Oldfield M, MacNaughtan I. Congenital abnormalities of the pillars of the fauces and the action of the posterior pillars and nasopharyngeal valve during speech. J Laryngol Otol 1946; 61:594–600.
131. Longacre J. Congenital atresia of the oropharynx. Plast Reconstr Surg 1951; 8:341–348.
132. Kouyoumdjian A, McDonald J. Association of congenital adrenal neuroblastoma with multiple anomalies including an unusual oropharyngeal cavity (imperforant buccopharyngeal membrane?). Cancer 1951; 14:784–788.
133. Hub M, Jirasec J. Perzistence stredni casti membrane buccopharyngicae. Cas Lek Cesk 1961; 99:1297–1299.
134. Seghers M. Une malformation rare: l'imperforation oropharyngienne. Acta Paediatr Belg 1966; 10:130–137.
135. Chandra R, Yadava V, Sharma R. Persistent buccopharyngeal membrane. Plast Reconstr Surg 1974; 54:678–679.
136. Hoffman R. Persistent pharyngeal membrane. Arch Otolaryngol 1979; 105:286–287.
137. Warren D, Bevin A, Winslow R. Posterior pillar webbing and palatopharyngeus displacement. Possible causes of congenital palatal incompetency. Cleft Palate J 1978; 15:68–72.
138. Itoh M, Sasanuma S, Ushijima T. Velar movements during speech in a patient with apraxia of speech. Annu Bull Res Inst Logoped Phoniatr 1977; 11:67–75.
139. Noll JD. Remediation of impaired resonance among patients with neuropathologies of speech. In: Lass N, McReynolds L, Northern J, Yoder D, eds. Speech, language, and hearing. Philadelphia: WB Saunders, 1982:556.
140. Netsell R. The velopharynx in perspective. Presented before the Symposium of Treatment of the Velopharynx for Individuals with Dysarthria. Omaha: Boys Town Institute, 1983.
141. Johns D, Salyer K. Surgical and prosthetic management of neurogenic speech disorders. In: Johns D, ed. Clinical management of neurogenic communicative disorders. Boston: Little, Brown, 1978:311.
142. Ardran G, Kemp F. Radiology in the study of neurological diseases affecting the pharynx and larynx. Proc R Soc Med 1975; 18:641–644.
143. Ashley F, Sloan R, Hahn E, Hanafee W, Miethke J. Cinefluorographic study of palatal incompetency cases during deglutition and phonation. Plast Reconstr Surg 1961; 28(4):347–364.
144. Blackfield H, Miller E, Owsley J, Lawson L. Cinefluorographic evaluation of patients with velopharyngeal dysfunction in the absence of overt cleft palate. Plast Reconstr Surg 1962; 30:441–451.
145. Calnan J. Palato-pharyngeal incompetence in speech. In: Pruzansky S, ed. Congenital anomalies of the face and associated structures. Springfield: CC Thomas, 1961:104.
146. Calnan J. The surgical treatment of nasal speech disorders. Ann R Coll Surg Eng 1959; 25:119–141.
147. Cohn E, Garver K, Metz H, McWilliams B, Skolnick M, Garrett W. Velopharyngeal incompetence in a patient with multifocal eosinophilic granulumoa (Hand-Schuller-Christian disease). J Speech Hear Disord 1982; 47:320–323.
148. Hoopes J, Dellon A, Fabrikant J, Soliman A. Idiopathic hypernasality: cineradiographic evaluation and etiologic considerations. J Speech Hear Disord 1973; 35:44–50.
149. Jafek B, Balkany T, Wong M, Bryant K. Surgical management of the hypodynamic palate. Arch Otolaryngol 1979; 105:347–350.
150. Keogh C. Paralysis of the pharynx. J Laryngol Otol 1956; 70:344–351.
151. Lawshe B, Hardy J, Schweiger J, Van Allen M. Management of a patient with velopharyngeal incompetency of undetermined origin: a clinical report. J Speech Hear Disord 1971; 36(4):547–555.
152. Mazaheri M, Millard R, Erickson D. Cineradiographic comparison of normal to noncleft subjects with velopharyngeal inadequacy. Cleft Palate J 1964; 1:199–209.
153. Minami R, Kaplan E, Wu G, Jobe R. Velopharyngeal incompetency without overt cleft palate. Plast Reconstr Surg 1975; 55(5):573–587.
154. Owsley J, Chierici G, Miller E, Lawson L, Blackfield H. Cephalometric evaluation of palatal dysfunction in patients without cleft palate. Plast Reconstr Surg 1967; 39:562–568.
155. Pitt M, Ingram T. The radiology of speech disorders in childhood. Part 1. Disorders and their study. Radiogra-

phy 1975; 41(483):53–59.
156. Pitt M, Ingram T. The radiology of speech disorders in childhood. Part 2. Radiology in the diagnosis of speech disorders. Radiography 1975; 41(484):90–104.
157. Pollack M, Shprintzen R, Zimmerman-Manchester K. Velopharyngeal insufficiency: the neurological perspective. A report of 32 cases. Dev Med Child Neurol 1979; 21:194–201.
158. Shprintzen R, Lavorato A, Rakoff S, Skolnick M. Incongruous movements of the velum and lateral pharyngeal walls. Cleft Palate J 1977; 14:148–157.
159. Sturim H, Jacob C. Teflon pharyngoplasty. Plast Reconstr Surg 1972; 49:180–185.
160. Worster-Drought C. Congenital suprabulbar paresis. J Laryngol Otol 1956; 70:453–456.
161. Luce E, McGibbon B, Hoopes J. Velopharyngel insufficiency in hemifacial microsomia. Plast Reconstr Surg 1977; 60(4):602–606.
162. Shprintzen R, Croft C, Berkman M, Rakoff S. Velopharyngeal insufficiency in the facio-auriculo-vertebral malformation complex. Cleft Palate J 1980; 17:132–137.
163. Darley F, Aronson A, Brown J. Clusters of deviant speech dimensions in the dysarthrias. J Speech Hear Res 1969; 12:462–496.
164. Darley F, Aronson A, Brown J. Differential diagnostic patterns of dysarthria. J Speech Hear Res 1969; 12:246–269.
165. Darley F, Aronson A, Brown J. Motor speech disorders. Philadelphia: WB Saunders, 1975.
166. Hardy J, Netsell R, Schweiger H, Morris H. Management of velopharyngeal dysfunction in cerebral palsy. J Speech Hear Disord 1969; 34(2):125–137.
167. Hardy J, Rembolt R, Spriestersbach D, Jayapathy B. Surgical management of palatal paresis and speech problems in cerebral palsy: a preliminary report. J Speech Hear Disord 1961; 26:320–325.
168. Hegarty I. Case study of velar and facial paralysis. J Speech Hear Disord 1960; 25:409–411.
169. Heller J, Gens G, Moe D, Lewin M. Velopharyngeal insufficiency in patients with neurological, emotional and mental disorders. J Speech Hear Disord 1974; 39(3):350–359.
170. Hirose H, Kiritani S, Sawashima M. Patterns of dysarthric movement in patients with amyotrophic lateral sclerosis and pseudobulbar palsy. Folia Phoniatr 1982; 34:106–112.
171. Honjow I, Isshiki N, Kitajima K. Congenital and acquired hypernasalities Folia Phoniatr 1969; 21:266–276.
172. Hoopes J, Dellon A, Fabrikant J, Soliman A. Cineradiographic assessment of combined Island flap pushback and pharyngeal flap in the surgical management of submucous cleft palate. Br J Plast Surg 1970; 23:39–44.
173. Hoopes J, Dellon A, Fabrikant J, Edgerton M, Soliman A. Cineradiographic definition of the functional anatomy and pathophysiology of the velopharynx. Cleft Palate J 1970; 7:443–453.
174. Kent R, Netsell R. Articulatory abnormalities in athetoid cerebral palsy. J Speech Hear Disord 1978; 43(3):353–373.
175. Leach W. Generalized muscular diseases presenting as pharyngeal dysphagia. J Laryngol Otol 1962; 76:237–240.
176. McCoy F, Zahorsky C. A new approach to the elusive dynamic pharyngeal flap. Plast Reconstr Surg 1972; 49(2):160–164.
177. McWilliams BJ, Musgrave R. Differential diagnosis and management of hypernasal voices in children. Trans Am Acad Ophthalmol Otolaryngol 1965; 69:322–331.
178. Mullendore J, Stoudt R. Speech patterns of muscular dystrophic individuals. J Speech Hear Disord 1961; 26:252–257.
179. Netsell R. Evaluation of velopharyngeal function in dysarthria. J Speech Hear Disord 1969; 34(2):113–122.
180. Pollack M, Shprintzen R. Velopharyngeal insufficiency in neurofibromatosis. Int J Pediatr Otorhinolaryngol 1981; 3:257–262.
181. Randall P, Bakes F, Kennedy C. Cleft palate-type speech in the absence of cleft palate. Plast Reconstr Surg 1960; 25(2):484–495.
182. Rosenbek J, LaPointe L. The dysarthrias: description, diagnosis and treatment. In: Johns D, ed. Clinical management of neurogenic communication disorders. Boston: Little, Brown, 1978:251.
183. Schweiger J, Netsell R, Sommerfeld R. Prosthetic management and speech improvement in individuals with dysarthria of the palate. J Am Dent Assoc 1970; 80:1348–1353.
184. Weinberg B, Bosma J, Shanks J, DeMyer W. Myotonic dystrophy initially manifested by speech disability. J Speech Hear Disord 1968; 33:51–59.
185. Wolski W. Hypernasality as the presenting symptom of myasthenia gravis. J Speech Hear Disord 1967; 32(1):36–38.
186. Worster-Drought C. Speech disorders in children. Dev Med Child Neurol 1968; 10:427–440.
187. Lawson L, Chierici G, Castro A, Harvold E, Miller E, Owsley J. Effects of adenoidectomy on the speech of children with potential velopharyngeal dysfunction. J Speech Hear Disord 1972; 37(3):390–402.
188. Trost J. Articulatory additions to the classical description of the speech of persons with cleft palate. Cleft Palate J 1981; 18(3):193–203.
189. Riski J. Functional velopharyngeal incompetence: diagnosis and management. In: Winitz H, ed. Treating articulation disorders. Baltimore: University Park Press, 1984:223.
190. Peterson-Falzone S. Analysis of phoneme-specific velopharyngeal inadequacy in 24 children. Presented before the American Society of Plastic and Reconstructive Surgery, Los Angeles, 1986.
191. Weber J, Chase R. Stress velopharyngeal incompetence in an oboe player. Cleft Palate J 1970; 1:858–861.
192. Subtelny J. A cephalometric study of the growth of the soft palate. Plast Reconstr Surg 1957; 19:49–62.
193. Dibbell D, Ewanowski S, Carter S. Successful correction of velopharyngeal stress incompetence in musicians playing wind instruments. Plast Reconstr Surg 1979; 64(5):662–664.
194. Argamaso R, Shprintzen R. Fanfare for a pharyngeal flap. Videotape presentation before the American Cleft Palate Association, Denver, 1982.
195. Bzoch K. Measurement and assessment of categorical aspects of cleft palate speech. In: Bzoch K, ed. Communicative disorders related to cleft lip and palate. Boston: Little, Brown, 1979:161.
196. McWilliams BJ, Morris H, Shelton R. Cleft palate speech. Toronto: BC Decker, 1984.
197. Morley M. Cleft palate and speech. 7th ed. Baltimore: Williams and Wilkins, 1970.
198. Morris H. Etiological bases for speech problems. In: Spriestersbach D, Sherman D, eds. Cleft palate and communication. New York: Academic Press, 1968:119.
199. Wells C. Cleft palate and its associated speech disorders. New York: McGraw-Hill, 1971.
200. O'Gara M, Logemann J. Longitudinal phonetic analyses of the speech development of cleft palate babies. Presented before the American Speech-Language-Hearing Association, Detroit, 1986.
201. Olson D. A descriptive study of the speech development of a group of infants with unoperated cleft palate. Doctoral Dissertation. Northwestern University, Evanston; 1965.

202. Bzoch K. Articulation proficiency and error patterns of pre-school cleft palate and normal children. Cleft Palate J 1965; 2:340–350.
203. Trost J. Differential diagnosis of velopharyngeal disorders. Commun Disord Audio J Cont Educ 1981; 6.
204. Warren D. Compensatory speech behaviors in cleft palate: a regulation/control phenomenon? Cleft Palate J 1986; 23(4):251–260.
205. Hoch L, Golding-Kushner K, Siegel-Sadewitz V, Shprintzen R. Speech therapy. Semin Speech Lang 1986; 7(3):313–326.
206. Lynch J, Fox D, Brookshire B. Phonological proficiency of two cleft palate toddlers with school-age follow-up. J Speech Hear Disord 1983; 48:274–285.
207. Weinberg B, Horii Y. Acoustic features of pharyngeal /s/ fricatives produced by speakers with cleft palate. Cleft Palate J 1975; 12:12–16.
208. Trost-Cardamone J. From diagnosis to treatment: speech remediation for persons with cleft palates and related velopharyngeal disorders. Short course presented before the California Speech-Language-Hearing Association, Anaheim, 1985.
209. Honjow I, Isshiki N. Pharyngeal stop in cleft palate speech. Folia Phoniatr (Basel) 1971; 23:347–354.
210. Brooks A, Shelton R, Youngstrom K. Compensatory tongue-palate-pharyngeal wall relationships in cleft palate. J Speech Hear Disord 1965; 30:166–173.
211. Brooks A, Shelton R, Youngstrom K. Tongue-palate contact in persons with palate defects. J Speech Hear Disord 1966; 31:14–25.
212. Bzoch K. An investigation of the speech of pre-school cleft palate children. Doctoral Dissertation, Northwestern University, Evanston, 1956.
213. Lawrence C, Philips B. A telefluoroscopic study of lingual contacts made by persons with palatal defects. Cleft Palate J 1975; 12:85–94.
214. McWilliams BJ, Philips BJ. Velopharyngeal incompetence. Audio seminars in speech pathology. Philadelphia: WB Saunders, 1979.
215. Brandt S, Morris H. The linearity of the relationship between articulation errors and velopharyngeal incompetence. Cleft Palate J 1965; 2:176–183.
216. Hess D. Effects of certain variables on speech of cleft palate persons. Cleft Palate J 1971; 8:387–398.
217. McWilliam BJ. Articulation problems of a group of cleft palate adults. J Speech Hear Res 1958; 1(1):68–74.
218. Spriestersbach D, Darley F, Rouse V. Articulation of a group of children with cleft lips and palates. J Speech Hear Disord 1956; 21(4):436–445.
219. Spriestersbach D, Moll K, Morris H. Subject classification and articulation of speakers with cleft palates. J Speech Hear Res 1961; 4(4):362–372.
220. VanDemark D. Consistency of articulation of subjects with cleft palate. Cleft Palate J 1969; 6:254–262.
221. Counihan C. A clinical study of the speech efficacy and structural adequacy of operated adolescent cleft palate persons. Doctoral dissertation, Northwestern University, Evanston, 1956.
222. Byrne M, Shelton R, Diedrich W. Articulatory skill, physical management, and classification of children with cleft palates. J Speech Hear Disord 1961; 26(4):326–333.
223. Fletcher S. Diagnosis of speech disorders from cleft palate. New York: Grune and Stratton, 1978.
224. McDermott R. A study of /s/ sound production by individuals with cleft palates. Doctoral dissertation, University of Iowa, Iowa City, 1962.
225. VanDemark D, Morris H, VandeHaar C. Patterns of articulation abilities in speakers with cleft palate. Cleft Palate J 1979; 16:230–239.
226. VanDemark D. A factor analysis of the speech of children with cleft palate. Cleft Palate J 1966; 3:159–170.
227. Philips BJ, Harrison R. Articulation patterns of preschool cleft palate children. Cleft Palate J 1969; 6:245–253.
228. Milisen R. A rationale for articulation disorders. J Speech Hear Disord [Monogr Suppl] 1954; 4:5–17.
229. Sherman D, Spriestersbach D, Noll JD. Glottal stops in the speech of children with cleft palates. J Speech Hear Disord 1959; 24:37–42.
230. Starr C. A study of some of the characteristics of the speech and speech mechanisms of a group of cleft palate children. Doctoral Dissertation, Northwestern University, Evanston, Illinois. 1956.
231. Hodson B, Chin L, Redmond B, Simpson R. Phonological evaluation and remediation of speech deviations of a child with a repaired cleft palate: a case study. J Speech Hear Disord 1983; 48:93–98.
232. Moll K. Speech characteristics of individuals with cleft lip and palate. In: Spriestersbach D, Sherman D, eds. Cleft palate and communication. New York: Academic Press, 1968:61–118.
233. Locke J. Epigenetic paths to phonological disorders. In: Children's Phonology Disorders: Pathways and Patterns. Conference Proceedings. Washington: American Speech-Language-Hearing Association, 1985:1–8.
234. Singh S, Hayden N, Toombs M. The role of distinctive features in articulation errors. J Speech Hear Disord 1981; 46(46):1745–183.
235. Counihan C. Articulation skills of adolescents and adults with cleft palates. J Speech Hear Disord 1965; 25(2):181–187.
236. Leder S, Lerman J. Some acoustic evidence for vocal abuse in adult speakers with repaired cleft palate. Laryngoscope 1985; 95:837–840.
237. Morris H, Spriestersbach D, Darley F. An articulation test for assessing competency of velopharyngeal closure. J Speech Hear Res 1961; 4(1):48–55.
238. Pitzner J, Morris H. Articulation ills and adequacy of breath pressure ratios of children with cleft palate. J Speech Hear Disord 1965; 30(1):26–40.
239. Trost-Cardamone J. Phonological process analysis: its role in diagnosis of the child with cleft palate. Presented before the American Cleft Palate Association, Miami, 1985.
240. Shriberg L, Kwiatkowski J. Phonological disorders I: a diagnostic classification stem. J Speech Hear Disord 1982; 47:226–241.
241. Warren D, Mackler S. Duration of oral port constriction in normal and cleft palate speech. J Speech Hear Res 1968; 11:291–301.
242. Rolnick M, Hoops H. Plosive phoneme duration as a function palato-pharyngeal adequacy. Cleft Palate J 1971; 8:65–76.
243. Wada T. Cinefluorographic analysis of articulatory movements. J Osaka Univ Dent Soc 1968; 13:105–122.
244. Wada T, Yasumoto M, Ideoka N, Fujiki Y, Yoshinaga R. An approach for the cinefluorographic study of articulatory movements. Cleft Palate J 1970; 7:506–522.
245. Forner L. Speech segment durations produced by five and six year old speakers with and without cleft palates. Cleft Palate J 1983; 20:185–198.
246. Warren D, Dalston R, Trier W, Holder M. A pressure-flow technique for quantifying temporal patterns of palatal pharyngeal closure. Cleft Palate J 1985; 22:11–19.
247. Karnell M, Folkins J, Morris H. Relationships between the perception of nasalization and speech movements in speakers with cleft palate. J Speech Hear Res 1985; 28:63–72.
248. Sherman D, Goodwin F. Pitch level and nasality. J Speech Hear Disord 1954; 19:423–428.
249. Flint R. Fundamental vocal frequency and severe nasality in cleft palate speakers. Masters thesis, University of Oklahoma, 1964.
250. Rampp D, Counihan D. Vocal pitch-intensity relation-

ships in cleft palate speakers. Cleft Palate J 1970; 7:846–857.
251. Dickson D. A radiographic study of nasality. Cleft Palate J 1969; 6:160–165.
252. Hess D. Pitch, intensity, and cleft palate voice quality. J Speech Hear Res 1959; 2:113–125.
253. Tarlow A, Saxman J. A comparative study of the speaking fundamental frequency characteristics in children with cleft palate. Cleft Palate J 1970; 7:696–705.
254. Bzoch K. Etiological factors related to cleft palate speech. In: Bzoch K, ed. Communicative disorders related to cleft lip and palate. Boston: Little, Brown, 1979:67.
255. McWilliams BJ. Communication problems associated with cleft palate. In: VanHattum R, ed. Communication disorders: an introduction. New York: Macmillan, 1980:379.
256. McWilliams BJ. Cleft palate. In: Shames G, Wiig E, eds. Human communication disorders. Columbus: CE Merrill, 1982:330.
257. Bernthal J, Beukelman D. The effect of changes in velopharyngeal orifice area on vowel intensity. Cleft Palate J 1977; 14:63–77.
258. Fant G. Acoustic theory of speech production. The Hague: Mouton, 1960.
259. House A, Stevens K. Analog studies of the nasalization of vowels. J Speech Hear Disord 1956; 21(2):218–232.
260. Warren D, Wood M, Bradley D. Respiratory volumes in normal and cleft palate speech. Cleft Palate J 1969; 6:449–460.
261. Weiss C. Oral and nasal sound levels as related to judged severity on nasality. Doctoral Dissertation, Purdue University, 1954.
262. Williamson A. Diagnosis and treatment of eighty-four cases of nasality. Q J Speech 1944; 36:471–479.
263. Counihan C, Cullinan A. Some relationship between vocal intensity and rated nasality. Cleft Palate J 1972; 9:101–108.
264. Lass N, Noll J. A comparative study of rate characteristics in cleft palate and noncleft palate speakers. Cleft Palate J 1970; 7:275–283.
265. D'Antonio L. An investigation of speech timing in individuals with cleft palate. Doctoral dissertation, University of California at San Francisco, 1982.
266. Jones D, Folkins J. Effect of speaking rate on judgments of disordered speech in children with cleft palate. Cleft Palate J 1985; 22(4):246–252.
267. Curtis J. Acoustics of speech production and nasalization. In: Spriestersbach D, Sherman D, eds. Cleft palate and communication. New York: Academic Press, 1968:27.
268. Hamlet S. Vocal compensation: an ultrasonic study of vocal vibration in normal and nasal vowels. Cleft Palate J 1973; 10:267–285.
269. Marks C, Barker K, Tardy M. Prevalence of perceived acoustic deviations related to laryngeal function among subjects with palatal anomalies. Cleft Palate J 1971; 8(2):201–211.
270. Senturia B, Wilson F. Otorhinolaryngologic findings in children with voice deviations. Preliminary report. Ann Otol Rhinol Laryngol 1968; 77:1027–1040.
271. Silverman E, Zimmer C. Incidence of chronic hoarseness of school-age children. J Speech Hear Disord 1975; 40:211–215.
272. Brindle B, Morris H. Prevalence of voice quality deviations in the normal adult population. J Commun Disord 1979; 12:439–445.
273. Laguaite J. Adult voice screening. J Speech Hear Disord 1972; 37:147–151.
274. Takagi Y, McGlone R, Millard R. Speech disorders of individuals according to the type of cleft. Cleft Palate J 1970; 7:271–274.
275. Brooks A, Shelton R. Voice disorders other than nasality in cleft palate children. Cleft Palate Bull 1963: 13:63–64.
276. Greenberg R. The incidence of hoarseness among children enrolled in speech therapy. J Pennsylv Speech Lang Hear Assoc 1982; 15:20.
277. McWilliams BJ, Bluestone C, Musgrave R. Diagnostic implications of vocal cord nodules in children with cleft palate. Laryngoscope 1969; 79:2072–2080.
278. McWilliams BJ, Lavorato A, Bluestone C. Vocal cord abnormalities in children with velopharyngeal valving problems. Laryngoscope 1973; 83(11):1745–1753.
279. Koepp-Baker H. The treatment of orofacial clefts: surgical, orthopedic, and prosthetic. In: Travis L, ed. Handbook of speech pathology and audiology. New York: Appleton-Century-Crofts, 1971:783.
280. Foster T, Greene M. Lateral speech defects and dental irregularities in cleft palate. Br J Plast Surg 1960; 12:367–377.
281. Subtelny J, Subtelny J. Intelligibility and associated physiological factors of cleft palate speakers. J Speech Hear Res 1959; 2:353–360.
282. Bishara S, VanDemark D, Henderson W. Relation between speech production and oro-facial structures in individuals with isolated clefts of the palate. Cleft Palate J 1975; 12:452–460.
283. Bruggeman C. A study of the relation of malocclusion of teeth and oral deformities to articulatory defects of speech in children. Masters thesis, University of Iowa, Iowa City, 1934.
284. Fymbo L. The relation of malocclusion of the teeth to defects of speech. Arch Speech 1936; 1:204–217.
285. Lubit D. Before an adenoidectomy: Stop! Look! Listen! NY State J Med 1967; 67:681–685.
286. Berry M. Lingual anomalies associated with palatal clefts. J Speech Hear Disord 1949; 14:359–362.
287. Brown S, Oliver D. A qualitative study of the organic speech mechanism abnormalities associated with cleft palate. J Speech Hear Disorder 1940; 5:265–270.
288. McDonald E, Koepp-Baker H. Cleft palate speech: an integration of research and clinical observations. J Speech Hear Disord 1951; 16:9–20.
289. Morley M. Cleft palate and speech. 1st ed. Baltimore: Williams and Wilkins, 1945.
290. Matthews J, Byrne M. An experimental study of tongue flexibility in children with cleft palates. J Speech Hear Disord 1953; 18:43–47.
291. Buck M. An x-ray study of cleft palate oropharyngeal structures and their function during vowel formation. Cleft Palate Bull 1952; 2:5.
292. Buck M. Facial skeletal measurements and tongue carriage in subjects with repaired cleft palates. J Speech Hear Disord 1953; 18:121–132.
293. Buck M. Velopharyngeal movement and tongue carriage during speech in adults with unrepaired incomplete cleft palate. Cleft Palate Bull 1960; 10:8–10.
294. Starr C. Dental and occlusal hazards to normal speech production. In: Bzoch K, ed. Communicative disorders related to cleft palate. Boston: Little, Brown, 1979:90.
295. Guay A, Maxwell D, Beecher R. A radiographic study of tongue posture at rest and during the phonation of /s/ in Class III malocclusion. Angle Orthod 1978; 48:10–22.
296. Shohara H. Speech rehabilitation in a case of postoperative cleft palate and malocclusion. J Speech Hear Disord 1942; 7:381–388.
297. Powers G. Cinefluorographic investigation of articulatory movements of selected individuals with cleft palates. J Speech Hear Res 1962; 5(1):59–69.
298. Massengill R, Spoerl A. Lingual positions of cleft palate patients with and without velopharyngeal closure. Folia Phoniatr (Basel) 1970; 22:185–190.
299. Dorf D, Curtin J. Early cleft palate repair and speech

outcome. Plast Reconstr Surg 1982; 68:153–157.
300. Bzoch K. Variations in velopharyngeal valving: the factor of vowel changes. Cleft Palate J 1968; 5:211–218.
301. Hardy J, Arkebauer H. Development of a test for velopharyngeal competence during speech. Cleft Palate J 1966; 3:6–21.
302. Lubker J. An electromyographic-cinefluorographic investigation of velar function during normal speech production. Cleft Palate J 1968; 5:1–18.
303. Moll K. Velopharyngeal closure on vowels. J Speech Hear Res 1962; 5:30–37.
304. Edgerton M, Sadove M, Compton M, Bull G, Blomain E, McDonald W, Bralley R. Nasal vibration analysis: a noninvasive objective technique to evaluate the speech of patients with palatal pharyngeal disorders. Plast Reconstr Surg 1981; 68:153–157.
305. Horii Y. An accelerometric approach to nasality measurement: a preliminary report. Cleft Palate J 1980; 17:254–261.
306. Horii Y. An accelerometric measure as a physical correlate of perceived hypernasality in speech. J Speech Hear Res 1983; 26:476–480.
307. Horii Y, Lang J. Distributional analyses of an index of nasal coupling (HONC) in similated hypernasal speech. Cleft Palate J 1981; 18:279–285.
308. Lippmann R. Detecting nasalization using a low-cost miniature accelerometer. J Speech Hear Res 1981; 24:314–317.
309. Stevens K, Kalikow D, Willemain T. A miniature accelerometer for detecting glottal waveforms and nasalization. J Speech Hear Res 1975; 18:594–599.
310. Tronczynska J. Electrorhinopneumography as an objective measure as an assessment of velopharyngeal insufficiency in cleft palate patients. Folia Phoniatr 1972; 24:371–380.
311. Warren D. PERCI: a method for rating palatal efficiency. Cleft Palate J 1979; 16:279–285.
312. Lindsay W. Von Langenbeck palatorrhaphy. In: Grabb W, Rosenstein S, Bzoch K, eds. Cleft lip and palate: surgical, dental and speech aspects. Boston: Little, Brown, 1971:393.
313. Schweckendiek W. Primary veloplasty. In: Schuchardt K, ed. Treatment of patients with cleft lip, alveolus and palate. Stuttgart: Thieme, 1966:850.
314. Schweckendiek W. Primary veloplasty: long-term results without maxillary deformity. Cleft Palate J 1978; 15:268–274.
315. Bardach J, Morris H, Olin W. Late results of primary veloplasty: the Marburg project. Plast Reconstr Surg 1984; 73:207–215.
316. Shelton R, Blank J. Oronasal fistulas, intraoral air pressure, and nasal air flow during speech. Cleft Palate J 1984; 21:91–99.
317. Witzel MA, Salyer K, Ross R. Delayed hard palate closure: the philosophy revisited. Cleft Palate J 1984; 21:263–265.
318. Blocksma R, Leuz C, Mellerstig K. A conservative program for managing cleft palates without the use of mucoperiosteal flaps. Plast Reconstr Surg 1975; 55:160–169.
319. Cosman B, Falk A. Delayed hard palate repair and speech deficiences: a cautionary report. Cleft Palate J 1980; 17:27–33.
320. Fara M, Brousilova M. Experiences with early closure of velum and later closure of hard palate. Plast Reconstr Surg 1969; 44:134–141.
320a. Jackson I, McLennan G, Scheker L. Primary veloplasty or primary palatal plasty: some preliminary findings. Plast Reconstr Surg 1983; 72:153–157.
321. Schroder F. Operation der Spalte in harten Gaumen in Auschluss an Velumplastik nach Schweckendiek. Acta Chir Plast (Prague) 1966; 8:268–274.
322. Perko M. Two-stage closure of cleft palate. J Maxillofac Surg 1979; 7:76–80.
323. Hotz M, Gnoinski W, Nussbaumer H, Kistler E. Early maxillary orthopedics in CLP cases: guidelines for surgery. Cleft Palate J 1978; 15:405–411.
324. Henningsson G, Karling J. Early or late surgery of the hard palate? A comparison of speech at four years of age. Plast Reconstr Surg (in press).
325. Kuo J, Noordhoff S, Wong F, Witzel MA. Articulation skills in patients with cleft palate before delayed hard palate closure. Presented before the American Cleft Palate Association, Indianapolis, 1983.
326. Sidman R, Singer M. Stimulation of forelimb regeneration in the newt, Triturus viridescens, by sensory nerve supply isolated from the central nervous system. Am J Physiol 1951; 165:257–260.
327. Singer M. The nervous system and regeneration of the forelimb of adult Triturus. II. The role of the sensory supply. J Exp Zool 1943; 92:197–315.
328. Moser H, LaGourgue J, Class L. Studies of oral stereognosis in normal, blind and deaf subjects. In: Bosma J, ed. Symposium on oral sensation and perception. Springfield: CC Thomas, 1967:244.
329. Ringel R, Burk K, Scott C. Tactile perception: form discrimination in the mouth. In: Bosma J, ed. Second symposium on oral sensation and perception. Springfield: CC Thomas, 1970:410.
330. Weinberg B, Lyons M, Liss G. Studies of oral, manual and visual form identification skills in children and adults. In: Bosma J, ed. Second symposium on oral sensation and perception. Springfield: CC Thomas, 1970:340.
331. Ringel R, House A, Burk K, Dolinsky J, Scott C. Some relations between oral sensory discrimination and articulatory aspects of speech production. J Speech Hear Res 1970; 13:3–11.
332. Arndt W, Elbert M, Shelton R. Standardization of a test of oral stereognosis. In: Bosma J, ed. Second symposium on oral sensation and perception. Springfield: CC Thomas, 1970:379.
333. Ringel R. Studies of speech related oro-sensory monitoring systems. Presented before the American Speech and Hearing Association, Chicago, 1967.
334. Ringel R. Oral sensation and perception: a selective review. In: Fricke JE, ed. ASHA report #5: speech and the dentofacial complex: the state of the art. Washington: American Speech and Hearing Association, 1970:188.
335. Shelton R. Oral sensory function in speech production and remediation. In: Bzoch K, ed. Communicative disorders related to cleft lip and palate. Boston: Little, Brown, 1979:120.
336. Gammon S, Smith P, Daniloff R, Kim C. Articulation and stress/juncture production under oral anesthetization and masking. J Speech Hear Res 1971; 14:271–278.
336a. Scott C, Ringel R. Articulation without oral sensory control. J Speech Hear Res 1971; 14:804–818.
337. Putnam A, Ringel R. A cineradiographic study of articulation of two talkers with temporarily induced oral sensory deprivation. J Speech Hear Res 1976; 19:247–266.
338. Ringel R, Steer M. Some effects of tactile and auditory alterations on speech output. J Speech Hear Res 1963; 6:369–378.
339. Prosek R, House A. Intraoral air pressure as a feedback cue in consonant production. J Speech Hear Res 1975; 18:133–1147.
340. Perkell J. Physiology of speech production: results and implications of a quantitative cineradiographic study. Cambridge: MIT Press, 1969.
341. Hochberg I, Kabcenell J. Oral stereognosis in normal and cleft palate individuals. Cleft Palate J 1967; 4:47–57.
342. Mason R. Studies of oral perception involving subjects with alterations in anatomy and physiology. In: Bosma J, ed. Symposium on oral sensation and perception. Springfield: CC Thomas, 1967:294.

343. Catalanotto F, Moss J. Manual and oral stereognosis in children with cleft palate, gonadal dysgenesis, pseudohypoparathyroidism, oral facial digital syndrome and Kallman's syndrome. Arch Oral Biol 1973; 18:1227–1232.
344. Andrews J. Oral form discrimination in individuals with normal and cleft palates. Cleft Palate J 1973; 10:92–98.
345. Pressel G, Hochberg I. Oral form discrimination of children with cleft palate. Cleft Palate J 1974; 11:66–71.
346. LaPointe L, Williams W. Oral sensory-perceptual profiles of cleft palate individuals. Proceedings of the XVIth International Congress of Logopedics and Phoniatrics. Basel: Karger, 1976.
347. Heller J. Hearing loss in patients with cleft palate. In: Bzoch K, ed. Communicative disorders related to cleft lip and palate. 2nd ed. Boston: Little, Brown, 1979:100.
348. Aschan G. Hearing and nasal function correlated to postoperative speech in cleft palate patients with velopharyngoplasty. Acta Otolaryngol 1966; 61:371–379.
349. Bennett M, Ward R, Tait C. Otologic-audiologic study of cleft palate children. Laryngoscope 1968; 78:1011–1019.
350. Berry M, Eisenson J. Speech disorders: principles and practices of therapy. New York: Appleton-Century-Crofts, 1956.
351. Chapman J, Birch D. An orthodontic and otolaryngologic review of thirty-four cleft-lip and cleft-palate patients. Br J Surg 1965; 52(9):646–650.
352. Drettner B. The nasal airway and hearing in patients with cleft palate. Acta Otolaryngol (Stockh) 1960; 52:131–142.
353. Gaines F. Frequency and effect of hearing losses in cleft palate cases. J Speech Disord 1940; 5(2):141–149.
354. Graham M. A longitudinal study of ear disease and hearing loss in patients with cleft lips and palate. Ann Otol Rhinol Laryngol 1964; 73:34–47.
355. Graham M, Lierle D. Posterior pharyngeal flap palatoplasty and its relationship to ear disease and hearing loss. Laryngoscope 1962; 72:1750–1755.
356. Halfond J, Ballenger J. An audiologic and otorhinologic study of cleft-lip and cleft-palate cases. AMA Arch Otolaryngol 1956; 64:335–340.
357. Holborow C. Conductive deafness associated with the cleft-palate deformity. Proc R Soc Med 1962; 55:305–307.
358. Holmes E, Reed G. Hearing and deafness in cleft-palate patients. AMA Arch Otolaryngol 1955; 62:620–624.
359. Lindsay W, LeMesurier A, Farmer A. A study of the speech results of a large series of cleft palate patients. Plast Reconstr Surg 1962; 29(3):273–288.
360. Linthicum H, Body H, Keaster J. Incidence of middle ear disease in children with cleft palate. Cleft Palate Bull 1959; 9:23–25.
361. Loeb W. Speech, hearing and the cleft palate. Arch Otolaryngol 1964; 79:4–14.
362. Lowry L, Billings B, Leonard J. Otolaryngic findings in a cleft palate population. Cleft Palate J 1974; 11:62–65.
363. MacCollum D, Richardson S, Swanson L. Habilitation of the cleft palate patient. N Engl J Med 1956; 254:299–307.
364. Masters F, Bingham H, Robinson D. The prevention and treatment of hearing loss in the cleft palate child. Plast Reconstr Surg 1960; 25(5):503–509.
365. McWilliams BJ, Musgrave R. EENT considerations in the management of children with cleft palate. EENT Digest 1969; 31:61–67.
366. Means B, Irvin J. An analysis of certain measures of intelligence and hearing in a sample of the Wisconsin cleft palate population. Cleft Palate Bull 1954; 4(2):4.
367. Miller M. Hearing losses in cleft palate cases. Part I. Nature of the study. Laryngoscope 1956; 66:1492–1496.
368. Miller M. Hearing problems associated with cleft palate. Ann Otol Rhinol Laryngol 1959; 68:90–99.
369. Nober E. Hearing problems associated with cleft palate. In: Lencione R, ed. Cleft palate habilitation: proceedings of the fifth annual symposium on cleft palate habilitation. Syracuse, NY: Syracuse University, 1967:37.
370. Pannbacker M. Hearing loss and cleft palate. Cleft Palate J 1969; 6(1):50–56.
371. Paulsen J. Studies on the hearing and the tubal function in a series of children with cleft palates. Acta Otolaryngol (Stockh) [Suppl] 1964; 188:36–44.
372. Sataloff J, Fraser M. Hearing loss in children with cleft palates. AMA Arch Otolaryngol 1952; 55:61–64.
373. Skolnik E. Otologic evaluation in cleft palate patients. Laryngoscope 1958; 68:1908–1949.
374. Smith J. Cleft palate: auditory and otologic findings. Tex Med 1968; 64:69–71.
375. Spriestersbach D, Lierle D, Moll K, Prather W. Hearing loss children with cleft palates. Plast Reconstr Surg 1962; 30(3):336–347.
376. Whaley J. The otolaryngologist's role in the care of the cleft palate patient. J Can Dent Assoc 1957; 23:574–575.
377. Goetzinger C, Embrey J, Brooks R, Proud G. Auditory assessment of cleft palate adults. Acta Otolaryngol (Stockh) 1960; 52:551–557.
378. Heller J, Hochberg I, Milano G. Audiologic and otologic evaluation of cleft palate children. Cleft Palate J 1970; 774–783.
379. Webster J, Eldis F. Ear disease in relation to age in the cleft palate child and adolescent. Clin Otolaryngol 1978; 3:455–461.
380. Shimo G. Middle ear problems associated with cleft palate. Can J Otolaryngol 1972; 1:9–20.
381. Koch H, Neveling R, Hartung W. Studies concerning the problem of ear diseases in cleft palate children Cleft Palate J 1970; 7:187–193.
382. Cole R, Cole J, Intraprasong S. Eustachian tube function cleft lip and palate patients. Arch Otolaryngol 1974; 99:337–341.
383. Bennett M. Symposium on ear diseases. III. The older cleft palate patient. Laryngoscope 1972; 82:1217–1225.
384. Caldarelli D. Incidence and type of otologic disease in the older cleft-palate patient. Cleft Palate J 1975; 12:311–314.
385. Swigart E. Hearing sensitivity of adults with cleft lip and/or palate. Cleft Palate J 1979; 16:72–80.
386. Glover D. A long range evaluation of cleft palate repair. Plast Reconstr Surg 1961; 27(1):19–30.
387. Miller A, Wynn S. Better hearing results in cleft palate repaired by the bone flap technique. Cleft Palate J 1970; 7:455–458.
388. Bluestone C. Eustachian tube obstruction in the infant with cleft palate. Ann Otol Rhinol Laryngol [Suppl] 1971; 2(80):1–30.
389. Yules R. Hearing in cleft palate patients. Arch Otolaryngol 1970; 91:319–323.
390. Morgan R, Dellon A, Hoopes J. Effects of levator retrodisplacement on conductive hearing loss in the cleft palate patient. Ann Plast Surg 1983; 10(3):306–308.
391. Graham M, Schweiger J, Olin W. Hearing loss and ear disease in cleft palate patients with obturators. Plast Reconstr Surg 1962; 30(3):348–358.
392. Anthony P, Anthony L. Hearing loss in prosthetically treated adults with cleft palate. Arch Otolaryngol 1976; 102:151–153.
393. LeWorthy G, Schliesser H. Hearing acuity before and after pharyngeal flap procedure. Plast Reconstr Surg 1975; 56(1):49–51.
394. Paradise J, Bluestone C. Early treatment of the universal otitis media of infants with cleft palate. Pediatrics 1974; 53(1):48–54.
395. Paradise J, Bluestone C, Felder H. The universality of otitis media in 50 infants with cleft palate. Pediatrics 1969; 44(1):35–42.
396. Soudijn E, Huffstadt A. Cleft palates and middle ear ef-

fusions in babies. Cleft Palate J 1975; 12:229–233.
397. Stool S, Randall P. Unexpected ear disease in infants with cleft palate. Cleft Palate J 1967; 4:99–103.
398. Bluestone C, Wittel R, Paradise J. Roentgenographic evaluation of Eustachian tube function in infants with cleft and normal palates. Cleft Palate J 1972; 9:93–100.
399. Casselbrant M, Doyle W, Cantekin E, Ingraham A. Eustachian tube function the rhesus monkey model of cleft palate. Cleft Palate J 1985; 22(3):185–191.
400. Doyle W, Cantekin E, Bluestone C. Eustachian tube function cleft palate children. Ann Otol Rhinol Laryngol [Suppl] 1980;89(68):34–40.
401. Doyle W, Cantekin E, Bluestone C, Phillips D, Kimes K, Siegel J. Nonhuman primate model of cleft palate and its implications for middle ear pathology. Ann Otol Rhinol Laryngol [Suppl] 1980; 89(68):41–45.
402. Doyle W, Kitajiri M, Sando I. The anatomy of the auditory tube and paratubal musculature in a one month old cleft palate infant. Cleft Palate J 1983; 20(3):218–226.
403. Falk B, Magnuson B. Eustachian tube closing failure: occurrence in patients with cleft palate and middle ear disease. Arch Otolaryngol 1984; 110(1):10–14.
404. Gopalakrishna A, Goleria K, Raje A. Middle ear function in cleft palate. Br J Plast Surg 1984; 37:558–565.
405. Shprintzen R, Croft C. Abnormalities of the Eustachian tube orifice in individuals with cleft palate. Int J Pediatr Otorhinolaryngol 1981; 3:15–23.
406. Stool S, Beery Q. Diagnosis and treatment of ear disease in cleft palate children. In: Bzoch K, ed. Communicative disorders related to cleft lip and palate. 2nd ed. Boston: Little, Brown, 1979:236.
407. Webster J. Middle ear function in the cleft palate patient. J Laryngol Otol 1980; 94(1):31–37.
408. Bluestone C, Felder H. The role of the otolaryngologist in secondary surgical management of the cleft palate patient. Trans Am Acad Ophthalmol Otolaryngol 1969; 73:715–719.
409. Bluestone C, Klein J. Otitis media with effusion, atelectasis, and eustachian tube dysfunction. In: Bluestone C, Stool S, eds. Pediatric otolaryngology. Vol. I. Philadelphia: WB Saunders, 1983:356.
410. Bluestone C, Beery Q, Cantekin E, Pardise J. Eustachian tube ventilatory function in relation to cleft palate. Ann Otol Rhinol Laryngol 1975; 84:333–338.
411. Donaldson J. The role of the artificial Eustachian tube in cleft palate patients. Cleft Palate J 1966; 3(1):61–66.
412. Frable M, Brandon G, Theogaraj S. Velar closure and ear tubings as a primary procedure in the repair of cleft palates. Laryngoscope 1985; 95:1044–1046.
413. Mattucci K. Cleft palate patient: otologic management. NY State J Med 1979; 79:333–339.
414. Meyerhoff W, Shea D, Foster C. Otitis media, cleft palate and middle ear ventilation. Otolaryngol Head Neck Surg 1981; 89:288–293.
415. Paradise J. Management of middle ear effusions in infants with cleft palate. Ann Otol Rhinol Laryngol [Suppl] 1976; 25:285–288.
416. Paradise J. Middle ear problems associated with cleft palate. Cleft Palate J 1975; 12:17–22.
417. Paradise J. Primary care of infants and children with cleft palate. In: Bluestone C, Stool S, eds. Pediatric otolaryngology. Vol. I. Philadelphia: WB Saunders, 1983:924.
418. Paradise J, Bluestone C. Diagnosis and management of ear disease in cleft palate infants. Trans Am Acad Ophthalmol Otolaryngol 1969; 73:709–714.
419. Potsic W, Cohen M, Randall P, Winchester R. A retrospective study of hearing impairment in three groups of cleft palate patients. Cleft Palate J 1979; 16:56–58.
420. Bluestone C, Paradise J, Beery Q, Wittel R. Certain effects of cleft palate repair on Eustachian tube function. Cleft Palate J 1972; 9:183–193.
421. Doyle W, Reilly J, Jardini L, Rovnak S. Effect of palatoplasty on the function of the Eustachian tube in children with cleft palate. Cleft Palate J 1986; 23(1):63–68.
422. Too-Chung M. The assessment of middle ear function and hearing by tympanometry in children before and after early cleft palate repair. Br J Plast Surg 1983; 36:295–299.
423. Bergstrom L. Congenital and acquired deafness in clefting and craniofacial syndromes. Cleft Palate J 1978; 15(3):254–261.
424. Harrison R, Philips BJ. Observations on hearing levels of preschool cleft-palate children. J Speech Hear Disord 1971; 36:252–256.
425. Moller P. Hearing, middle ear pressure and otopathology in a cleft palate population. Acta Otolaryngol (Stockh) 1981; 92:521–528.
426. Riberti C, Baldo D, Tirone L, Collini M. Hearing impairment in children with cleft lip and palate: a clinical and statistical study. Pediatr Med Chir 1984; 6:131–136.
427. Ahonen E, McDermott J. Extended high-frequency hearing loss in children with cleft palate. Audiology 1984; 23:467–476.
428. Jardini L. Hearing problems in cleft palate patients. Semin Speech Lang 1986; 7(3):241–254.
429. Swigart E. Hearing and audiology. In: Cooper H, Harding R, Krogman W, Mazaheri M, Millard R, eds. Cleft palate and cleft lip: a team approach to clinical management and rehabilitation of the patient. Philadelphia: WB Saunders, 1979:484.
430. Bluestone C. Prevalence and pathogenesis of ear disease and hearing loss. In: Graham M, ed. Cleft palate: middle ear disease and hearing loss. Springfield: CC Thomas, 1978:27.
431. Paparella M, Oda M, Hiraida F, Brady D. Pathology of sensorineural hearing loss in otitis media. Ann Otol Rhinol Laryngol 1972; 81:632–647.
432. Arora M, Sharma V, Gudi S, Balakrishnan C. Acoustic impedance measurements and their importance in cleft palate patients. J Laryngol Otol 1979; 93:443–445.
433. Bess F, Lewis H, Cieliczka D. Acoustic impedance measurements in cleft-palate children. J Speech Hear Disord 1975; 40(1):13–24.
434. Bess F, Schwartz D, Redfield N. Audiometric, impedance, and otoscopic findings in children with cleft palate. Arch Otolaryngol 1976; 102:465–469.
435. Billings G, Lowry L. Tympanometry, impedance, and aural reflex testing in a cleft palate population. Cleft Palate J 1974; 11(1):21–27.
436. Paradise J, Smith C, Bluestone C. Tympanometric detection of middle ear effusion in infants and young children. Pediatrics 1976; 58:198–210.
437. Bergstrom L, Hemenway W. Otologic problems in submucous cleft palate. South Med J 1971; 64(10):1172–1177.
438. Caldarelli D. Incidence and type of otopathology associated with congenital palatopharyngeal incompetence. Laryngoscope 1978; 88(12):1–15.
439. Heller J, Gens G, Croft C, Moe D. Conductive hearing loss in patients with velopharyngeal insufficiency. Cleft Palate J 1978; 15(3):246–253.
440. Jaffe B, DeBlanc G. Cleft Palate, cleft lip, and cleft uvula in the Navaho Indians: incidence and otorhinolaryngologic problems. Cleft Palate J 1970; 7:300–305.
441. Taylor G. The bifid uvula. Laryngoscope 1972; 82:771–778.
442. Schwartz R, Hayden G, Rodriguez W, Shprintzen R, Cassidy J. The bifid uvula: is it a marker for an otitis prone child? Laryngoscope 1985; 95:1100–1102.
443. Bluestone C, Klein J, Paradise J, Eichenwald H, Bess F, Downs M, Green M, Berko-Gleason J, Ventry I, Gray S, McWilliams G, Gates G. Workshop on effects of otitis

media on the child. Pediatrics 1983; 71(4):639–652.
444. Brookhouse P, Hixson P, Matkin N. Early childhood language delay: the otolaryngologist's perspective. Laryngoscope 1979; 89:1898–1913.
445. Cook R, Teel R. Negative middle ear pressure and language development. Clinical Pediatr (Phila) 1979; 18(5):296–297.
446. Dobie R, Berlin C. Influence of otitis media on hearing and development. Ann Otol Rhinol Laryngol [Suppl] 1979; 88(60):48–52.
447. Holm V, Kunze L. Effect of chronic otitis media on language and speech development. Pediatrics 1969; 43(5):833–839.
448. Horowitz F, Leake F. Effects of otitis media on cognitive development. Ann Otol Rhinol Laryngol [Suppl] 1980; 89(68):264–268.
449. Menyuk P. Effect of persistent otitis media on language development. Ann Otol Rhinol Laryngol [Suppl] 1980; 89(68):257–263.
450. Naremore R. Influences of hearing impairment on early language development. Ann Otol Rhinol Laryngol [Suppl] 1979; 88(60):54–63.
451. Rapin I. Conductive hearing loss: effects on children's language and scholastic skills. A review of the literature. Ann Otol Rhinol Laryngol [Suppl] 1979; 88(60):3–12.
452. Zinkus P, Gottlieb M, Schapiro M. Developmental and psychoeducational sequelae of chronic otitis media. Am J Dis Child 1978; 132:1100–1104.
453. McWilliams BJ. The role of otolaryngological problems in speech disorders associated with cleft palate. Trans Am Acad Ophthalmol Otol 1969; 7:720–723.
454. Galkowski T, Gassowski P, Grossman J. Influence of hearing disorders on development of speech in children with cleft lip/palate. Folia Phoniatr (Basel) 1970; 22:72–78.
455. Freeland A, Evans D. Middle ear disease in the cleft palate infant: its effect on speech and language development. Br J Plast Surg 1981; 34:142–143.
456. Hubbard T, Paradise J, McWilliams B, Elster B, Taylor F. Consequences of unremitting middle-ear disease in early life: otologic, audiologic, and developmental findings in children with cleft palate. N Engl J Med 1985; 312(34):1529–1534.
457. Graham M. Cleft palate: middle ear disease and hearing loss. Springfield: CC Thomas, 1978.
458. Hudson W. Otologic and related problems in cleft palate children. In: Georgiade N, ed. Symposium on management of cleft lip and palate and associated deformities. St Louis: CV Mosby, 1974:195.
459. Litton W, Severeid L, Tharp R. Cleft palate and otitis media. In: Glorig A, Gerwin K, eds. Otitis media: proceedings of the national conference. Callier hearing and speech center, Dallas. Springfield: CC Thomas, 1972:86.
460. Wilhelmsen H, Musgrave R. Complications of cleft lip surgery. Cleft Palate J 1966; 3:223–231.
461. Brauer R, Cronin T. Maxillary orthopedics and anterior palate repair with bone grafting. Cleft Palate J 1964; 1:31–42.
462. Rosenstein S, Monroe C, Kernahan D, Jacobson B, Griffith B, Bauer B. The case for early bone grafting in cleft lip and cleft palate. Plast Reconstr Surg 1982; 70(3):297–305.
463. Berkowitz S. Cleft lip and palate research: an updated state of the art. Section III. Orofacial growth and dentistry. Cleft Palate J 1977; 14(4):288–301.
464. Pruzansky S. Pre-surgical orthopedics and bone grafting for infants with cleft lip and palate: a dissent. Cleft Palate J 1964; 1(2):164–187.
465. Robertson N, Jolleys A. An 11-year follow-up on the effects of early bone grafting in infants born with complete clefts of the lip and palate. Br J Plast Surg 1983; 36:438–443.
466. Abyholm F, Bergland O, Semb G. Secondary bone grafting of alveolar clefts. Scand J Plast Reconstr Surg 1981; 15(2):127–140.
467. Enemark H, Krantz-Simonsen E, Schramm J. Secondary bonegrafting in unilateral cleft lip palate patients: indications and treatment procedures. Oral Surg 1985; 14:2–10.
468. Turvey T, Vig K, Moriarty J, Hoke J. Delayed bone grafting in the cleft maxilla and palate: a retrospective multidisciplinary analysis. Am J Orthod 1984; 86(3):244–256.
469. Grabb W. General aspects of cleft palate surgery. In: Grabb W, Rosenstein S, Bzoch K, eds. Cleft lip and palate: surgical, dental and speech aspects. Boston: Little, Brown, 1971:373.
470. Cronin T, Brauer R, Alexander J, Taylor W. Pushback repair using nasal mucosal flaps: results. Cleft Palate J 1964; 1:269–274.
471. Cronin T. Pushback palatorrhaphy with nasal mucosal flaps. In: Grabb W, Rosenstein S, Bzoch K, eds. Cleft lip and palate: surgical, dental and speech aspects. Boston: Little, Brown, 1971:432.
472. Butow K-W, Steinhauser E. Follow-up investigation of palatal closure by means of a one-layer cranially-based vomer-flap. Int J Oral Surg 1984; 13:396–400.
473. Kobus K. Extended vomer flaps in cleft palate repair: a preliminary report. Plast Reconstr Surg 1984; 73(6):895–901.
474. Wynn S. Bone-flap technique in cleft palate surgery. In: Georgiade N, ed. Symposium on cleft lip and palate and associated deformities. St Louis: CV Mosby, 1974:153.
475. Wynn S. Long-term results after cleft palate closure by bilateral osteotomy technique. Plast Reconstr Surg 1976; 58(1):71–79.
476. Bingham H, Suthunyarat P, Richards S, Graham M. Should the pharyngeal flap be used primarily with palatoplasty? Cleft Palate J 1972; 9:319–325.
477. Dalston R, Stuteville O. A clincial investigation of the efficacy of primary nasopalatal pharyngoplasty. Cleft Palate J 1975; 12:177–192.
478. Fara M, Sedlackova E, Klaskova O, Hrivnakova J, Chmelova A, Supacek I. Primary pharyngofixation in cleft palate repair. Plast Reconstr Surg 1970; 45(5):449–458.
479. Stark R, DeHaan C. The addition of a pharyngeal flap to primary palatoplasty. Plast Reconstr Surg 1960; 26:378–387.
480. Stark R, Frileck S. Primary pharyngeal flap and palatorrhaphy. In: Grabb W, Rosenstein R, Bzoch K, eds. Cleft lip and palate: surgical, dental and speech aspects. Boston: Little, Brown, 1971:404.
481. Stark R, DeHaan C, Frileck S, Burgess P. Primary pharyngeal flap. Cleft Palate J 1969; 6:381–383.
482. Stark R. Primary pharyngeal flap. In: Lencione R, ed. Cleft palate habilitation. Proceedings of the Fifth Annual Symposium on Cleft Palate Habilitation. Syracuse, NY: Syracuse University, 1967:25.
483. Stellmach R. Prevention of velopharyngeal insufficiency following palatoplasty by velopharynx adhesion. Fortschr Kiefer Gesichtschir 1985; 30:145–147.
484. Morris H. Velopharyngeal competence and primary cleft palate surgery, 1960–1971: a critical review. Cleft Palate J 1973; 10(1):62–71.
485. Braithwaite F, Maurice D. The importance of the levator palati muscle in cleft palate closure. Br J Plast Surg 1968; 21:60–62.
486. Braithwaite F. Cleft palate repair. In: Gibson T, ed. Modern trends in plastic surgery. London: Butterworth,

1964:38.
487. Edgerton M, Dellon A. Surgical retrodisplacement of the levator veli palatini muscle Plast Reconstr Surg 1971; 47:154–167.
488. Honjo I, Harada H, Okazaki N. Significance of levator muscle sling formation in cleft palate surgery: evaluation by electrical stimulation. Plast Reconstr Surg 1980; 65(4):443–446.
489. Kaplan E. Soft palate repair by levator muscle reconstruction and a buccal mucosal flap. Plast Reconstr Surg 1975; 56(2):129–136.
490. Trier W, Dreyer T. Primary von Langenbeck palatoplasty with levator reconstruction: rationale and technique. Cleft Palate J 1984; 21(4):254–262.
491. Batstone J, Millard D. Pushback palatorrhaphy with island flap to the nasal surface. In: Grabb W, Rosenstein S, Bzoch K, eds. Cleft lip and palate: surgical, dental and speech aspects. Boston: Little, Brown, 1971:441.
492. Edgerton M. The island flap pushback and the suspensory pharyngeal flap in surgical treatment of the cleft palate patient. Plast Reconstr Surg 1965; 36:591–630.
493. Georgiade N, Mladick R, Thorne R, Massengill R. Preliminary evaluation of the island flap in cleft palate repair. Cleft Palate J 1969; 6:488–494.
494. Greminger R. Island soft palatoplasty for early reconstruction of the posterior muscular ring. Plast Reconstr Surg 1981; 68(6):871–877.
495. Luce E, McClinton M, Hoopes J. Long-term results of the island flap palatal pushback. Plast Reconstr Surg 1976; 58(3):332–339.
496. McNeill K. Experiences with island flap in palate surgery. Arch Otolaryngol 1967; 85:75–77.
497. Millard D. A new use of the island flap in wide palatal clefts. Plast Reconstr Surg 1966; 30:330–335.
498. Millard D, Batstone J, Heycock M, Bensen J. Ten years with the palatal island flap. Plast Reconstr Surg 1970; 46(6):540–547.
499. Millard D. The island flap in cleft palate surgery. Surg Gynecol Obstet 1963; 116:297–300.
500. Noordhoff M. The island flap in secondary cleft palate surgery. Plast Reconstr Surg 1970; 46(5):463–467.
501. Rintala A, Rantala S. Secondary palatal repair by the island flap technique. Scand J Plast Reconstr Surg 1978; 12:257–260.
502. Lewin M, Heller J, Kojak D. Speech results after Millard island flap repair in cleft palate and other velopharyngeal insufficiencies. Cleft Palate J 1975; 12:263–269.
503. Herfert O. Two-stage operation for cleft palate. Br J Plast Surg 1963; 16:37–45.
504. Slaughter W, Pruzansky S. The rationale for velar closure as a primary procedure in the repair of cleft palate defects. Plast Reconstr Surg 1954; 13(5):341–357.
505. Friede H, Lilja J, Johanson B. Cleft lip and palate treatment with delayed closure of the hard palate. Scand J Plast Reconstr Surg 1980; 14:49–53.
506. Robertson N, Jolleys A. The timing of hard palate repair. Scand J Plast Reconstr Surg 1974; 8:49–51.
507. Poupard B, Coornaert H, Debaere P, Treanton A. Cleft lip and palate: can the hard palate be left open? A study of sixty-two cases with a follow-up of six years or more. Ann Chir Plast Esthet 1983; 28:325–336.
508. Morley M. Cleft palate and speech. 6th ed. Baltimore: Williams and Wilkins, 1966.
509. Battle R. Speech results of palate repair when performed before two years of age. Trans Fourth Int Congr Plast Reconstr Surg 1967; 425–428.
510. Holdsworth W. Cleft lip and palate. 3rd ed. New York: Grune and Stratton, 1963.
511. Jolleys A. A review of the results of operations on cleft palates with reference to maxillary growth and speech function. Br J Plast Surg 1954; 7:229–241.
512. McWilliams BJ. Cleft palate management in England. Speech Pathol Ther 1960; 3(1):3–7.
513. Peet E. The Oxford technique of cleft palate repair. Plast Reconstr Surg 1961; 28(3):282–294.
514. Koberg W, Koblin I. Speech development and maxillary growth in relation to technique and timing of palatoplasty. J Maxillofac Surg 1973; 1(1):44–50.
515. Ainoda N, Yamashita K, Tsukada S. Articulation at age 4 in children with early repair of cleft palate. Ann Plast Surg 1985; 15(5):415–422.
516. Randall P, LaRossa D, Fakhraee S, Cohen M. Cleft palate closure at 3 to 7 months of age: a preliminary report. Plast Reconstr Surg 1983; 71(5):624–627.
517. Blijdorp P, Muller H. The influence of the age at which the palate is closed on speech in the adult cleft patient. J Maxillofac Surg 1984; 12:239–246.
518. Desai S. Early cleft palate repair completed before the age of 16 weeks: observations on a personal series of 100 children. Br J Plast Surg 1983; 36:300–304.
519. Berkowitz S. Timing cleft palate closure—age should not be the sole determinant. J Craniofac Genet Dev Biol [Suppl] 1985; 1:69–83.
520. Egyedi P. Timing of palatal closure. J Maxillofac Surg 1985; 13:177–182.
521. Kaplan E. Cleft palate repair at three months? Ann Plast Surg 1981; 7(3):179–190.
522. Cacnan J. V-Y pushback palatorrhaphy. In: Grabb W, Roesenstein S, Bzoch K, eds. Cleft lip and palate: surgical, dental, and speech aspects. Boston: Little, Brown, 1971:422.
523. Evans D, Renfrew C. The timing of primary cleft palate repair. Scand J Plast Reconstr Surg 1974; 8:152–155.
524. Greene M. Speech analysis of 263 cleft palate cases. J Speech Hear Disord 1960; 25(1):43–48.
525. Krause C, Tharp R, Morris H. A comparative study of results of the Von Langenbeck and the V-Y pushback palatoplasties. Cleft Palate J 1976; 13:11–119.
526. Krause C, VanDemark D, Tharp S. Palatoplasty: a comparative study. Trans Am Acad Ophthalmol Otolaryngol 1975; 80:551–559.
527. McEvitt W. The incidence of persistent rhinolalia following cleft palate repair. Plast Reconstr Surg 1971; 47(3):258–261.
528. Morris H. Velopharyngeal competence and the Demjen W/V-Y technique. In: Morris H, ed. The Bratislava project: some cleft palate surgical results. Iowa City: University of Iowa Press, 1978:49.
529. Musgrave R, McWilliams BJ, Matthews J. A review of the results of two different surgical procedures for the repair of clefts of the soft palate only. Cleft Palate J 1975; 12:281–290.
530. Trauner R, Trauner M. Result of cleft lip and palate operations. Trans Fourth Int Congr Plast Reconstr Surg 1967; 429–434.
531. Aaronson S, Fox C, Cronin T. The Cronin push-back palate repair with nasal mucosal flaps: a speech evaluation. Plast Reconstr Surg 1985; 75(6):805–809.
532. Kaplan I, Labandter H, Ben-Bassat M, Dresner J, Nachmani A. Long-term follow-up of clefts of the secondary palate repaired by Von Langenbeck's method. Br J Plast Surg 1978; 31:353–354.
533. Witzel MA, Clarke J, Lindsay W, Thomson H. Comparison of results of pushback or Von Langenbeck repair of isolated cleft of the hard and soft palate. Plast Reconstr Surg 1979; 64(3):347–352.
534. Palmer C, Hamlen M, Ross RB, Lindsay W. Cleft palate repair: comparison of the results of two surgical techniques. Can J Surg 1969; 12:32–39.
535. O'Riain S, Hammond B. Speech results in cleft palate surgery: a survey of 249 patients. Br J Plast Surg 1972; 25:380–387.

536. Holtmann B, Wray R, Weeks P. A comparison of three techniques of palatorrhaphy: early speech results. Ann Plast Surg 1984; 12(6):514–518.
537. Dreyer T, Trier W. A comparison of palatoplasty techniques. Cleft Palate J 1984; 21(4):251–253.
538. VanDemark D, Hardin M. Longitudinal evaluation of articulation and velopharyngeal competence of patients with pharyngeal flaps. Cleft Palate J 1985; 22(3):163–172.
539. Marks S, Wynn S. Speech results after bilateral osteotomy surgery for cleft palate: a review of 413 patients. Plast Reconstr Surg 1985; 86(2):230–238.
540. Shprintzen R. Factors related to the development of normal speech following palate repair. Presented before the 4th International Congress on Cleft Palate and Related Craniofacial Anomalies, Acapulco, 1981.
541. Yules R, Chase R, Blocksma R, Lang B. Secondary techniques for correction of palatopharyngeal incompetence. In: Grabb W, Rosenstein R, Bzoch K, eds. Cleft lip and palate: surgical, dental and speech aspects. Boston: Little, Brown, 1971:451.
542. Schoenborn K. Ueber eine neve Nethche ves Verhandl de Deutsch. Arch Klin Chir 1876; 10:527–531.
543. Rosenthal W. Vur Farge der Gaumenplastik. Zentralbl Chir 1924; 51:1621–1624.
544. Sanvenero-Rosselli G. Division palatina e sua aura chirurgico alu. Congress Int Stomatol 1935; 36:391–395.
545. Kapetansky D. Transverse pharyngeal flaps: a dynamic repair for velopharyngeal insufficiency. Cleft Palate J 1975; 12:44–50.
546. Hogan VM. A biased approach to the treatment of velopharyngeal incompetence. Clin Plast Surg 1975; 2(2):319–325.
547. Hogan VM. A clarification of the surgical goals in cleft palate speech and the introduction of the lateral port control (L.P.C.) pharyngeal flap. Cleft Palate J 1973; 10:331–345.
548. Hogan VM, Schwartz M. Velopharyngeal incompetence. In: Converse J, ed. Plastic and reconstructive surgery: cleft palate and craniofacial anomalies. Philadelphia: WB Saunders, 1977:2268.
549. Albery E, Bennett J, Pigott R, Simmons R. The results of 100 operations for velopharyngeal incompetence—selected on the findings of endoscopic and radiological examination. Br J Plast Surg 1982; 35:118–126.
550. Buchholz R, Chase R, Jobe R, Smith HJ. The use of the combined palatal pushback and pharyngeal flap operations: a progress report. Plast Reconstr Surg 1967; 39(6):554–461.
551. Dixon V, Bzoch K, Habal J. Evaluation of speech after correction of rhinophonia with pushback palatoplasty combined with pharyngeal flap. Plast Reconstr Surg 1979; 64(1):77–83.
552. Moore F. A new operation to cure nasopharyngeal incompetency. Br J Surg 1960; 47:424–428.
553. Pigott R. The results of nasopharyngoscopic assessment of pharyngoplasty. Scand J Plast Reconstr Surg 1974; 8:148–152.
554. Shprintzen R, Lewin M, Croft C, Daniller A, Argamaso R, Ship A, Strauch B. A comprehensive study of pharyngeal flap surgery: tailor made flaps. Cleft Palate J 1979; 16:46–55.
555. Fisher J, Edgerton M. Combined use of levator retrodisplacement and pharyngeal flap for congenital palate insufficiency. Cleft Palate J 1975; 12:270–273.
556. Brondsted K, Liisberg W, Orsted B, Prytz S, Fogh-Andersen P. Surgical and speech results following palatopharyngoplasty operations in Denmark 1959–1977. Cleft Palate J 1984; 21(3):170–179
557. Hamlen M. Speech changes after pharyngeal flap surgery. Plast Reconstr Surg 1970;46(5):439–444.
558. Marsh J, Wray R. Speech prosthesis versus pharyngeal flap: a randomized evaluation of the management of velopharyngeal incompetency. Plast Reconstr Surg 1980; 65(5):592–594.
559. Owsley J, Lawson L, Miller E, Harvold E, Chierici G, Blackfield H. Speech results from the high attached pharyngeal flap operation. Cleft Palate J 1970; 7:306–317.
560. Subtelny J, Oya N, Subtelny J, Curtin J, McCormack R. Pre- and post-operative analysis of velar and pharyngeal flap mobility. Cleft Palate J 1970; 7:748–762.
561. Skoog T. The pharyngeal flap operation in cleft palate. Br J Plast Surg 1965; 18:265–282.
562. Skoog T. The pharyngeal flap operation for cleft palate patients. J Am Med Wom Assoc 1966; 21(12):1022–1027.
563. Fara M, Vele F. The histology and electromyography of primary pharyngeal flaps. Cleft Palate J 1972; 9:64–72.
564. Owsley J, Creech B, Dedo H. Poor speech following the pharyngeal flap operation: etiology and treatment. Cleft Palate J 1972; 9:312–318.
565. Whitaker L, Randall P, Graham W, Hamilton R, Winchester R. A prospective and randomized series comparing superiorly and inferiorly based posterior pharyngeal flaps. Cleft Palate J 1972; 9:304–311.
566. Randall P, Whitaker L, Noone R, Jones W. The case for the inferiorly based posterior pharyngeal flap. Cleft Palate J 1978; 15(3):262–265.
567. Moll K, Huffman W, Lierle D, Smith J. Factors related to the success of pharyngeal flap procedures. Plast Reconstr Surg 1963; 32(6):581–588.
568. Lierle D, Huffman W, Smith J. Correction of palatal insufficiency. Minn Med 1967; 50:945–947.
569. Morris H, Spriestersbach D. The pharyngeal flap as a speech mechanism. Plast Reconstr Surg 1967; 39:66–70.
570. Argamaso R, Shprintzen R, Strauch B, Lewin M, Daniller A, Ship A, Croft C. The role of lateral pharyngeal wall movement in pharyngeal flap surgery. Plast Reconstr Surg 1980; 66(2):214–219.
571. Kelsey C, Ewanowski S, Crummy A, Bless D. Lateral pharyngeal-wall motion a predictor of surgical success in velopharyngeal insufficiency. N Engl J Med 1972; 287(2):64–68.
572. Skolnick M, McCall G. Velopharyngeal competence and incompetence following pharyngeal flap surgery: a videofluoroscopic study in multiple projections. Cleft Palate J 1972; 9:1–12.
573. Pigott R. An assessment of some surgical techniques used in the management of palatal incompetence. In: Ellis R, Flack F, eds. Diagnosis and treatment of palato glossal malfunction. London: College of Speech Therapists, 1979:67.
574. Shprintzen R. The use of multiview videofluoroscopy and flexible fiberoptic nasopharyngoscopy as a predictor of success with pharyngeal flap surgery. In: Ellis R, Flack F, eds. Diagnosis and treatment of palato glossal malfunction. London: College of Speech Therapists, 1979:6.
575. Yules R, Chase R. A training method for reduction of hypernasality in speech. Plast Reconstr Surg 1969; 33(2):180–185.
576. Engstrom K, Fritzell B, Johanson B. A study of speech improvement following palatopharyngeal flap surgery. Cleft Palate J 1970; 7:419–431.
577. Owsley J, Lawson L, Chierici G. The re-do pharyneal flap. Plast Reconstr Surg 1976; 57(2):180–185.
578. Schulz R, Heller J, Gens G, Lewin M. Pharyngeal flap surgery and voice quality—factors related to success and failure. Cleft Palate J 1973; 10:166–175.
579. Shprintzen R, McCall G, Skolnick M. The effect of pharyngeal flap surgery on the movements of the lateral pharyngeal walls. Plast Reconstr Surg 1980; 66(4):570–573.
580. Lewis M, Pashayan H. The effects of pharyngeal flap sur-

gery on lateral pharyneal wall motion: a videoradiographic evaluation. Cleft Palate J 1980; 17(4):301–304.

581. Zwitman D. Oral endoscopic comparison of velopharyngeal closure before and after pharyngeal flap surgery. Cleft Palate J 1982; 19(1):40–46.
582. Zwitman D. Velopharyngeal physiology after pharyngeal flap surgery as assessed by oral endoscopy. Cleft Palate J 1982; 19(1):36–39.
583. Bzoch K. Clinical studies of the efficacy of speech appliances compared to pharyngeal flap surgery. Cleft Palate J 1964; 1:275–286.
584. Neiman G, Peterson S, Pruzansky S. Delayed pharyngeal flap success: report of a case. Cleft Palate J 1975; 12:244–246.
585. Smith B, Cohen M, Skef Z, Dorf D. Aerodynamic assessment of the results of pharyngeal flap surgery: a preliminary investigation. Plast Reconstr Surg 1985; 76(3):402–408.
586. Cosman B, Falk A. Pharyngeal flap augmentation. Plast Reconstr Surg 1975; 55(2):149–155.
587. Hoffman S. Correction of lateral port stenosis following a pharyngeal flap operation. Cleft Palate J 1985; 22(1):51–55.
588. Eckstein H. Demonstration of paraffin prosthesis in defects of the face and palate. Dermatologica 1904; 11:772–778.
589. Hollweg E, Perthes G. Treatment of cleft palates. Franz Pietzcher, 1912.
590. Von Gaza W. Über freie Fettgewebstranplantins in der retropharyngealen Raum bei Gaumenspalte. Arch Klin Chir 1926; 142:590–599.
591. Lando R. Transplant of cadaveric cartilage into the posterior pharyngeal wall in treatment of cleft palate. Stomatologiia (Mosk) 1950; 4:38–39.
592. Hagerty R, Hill M. Cartilage pharyngoplasty in cleft palate patients. Surg Gynecol Obstet 1961; 112:350–356.
593. Hagerty R, Hess D, Mylin W. Velar motility, velopharyngeal closure, and speech proficiency in cartilage pharyngoplasty: the effect of age at surgery. Cleft Palate J 1968; 5:317–326.
594. Hagerty R, Mylin W, Monat R. Augmentation pharyngoplasty. In: Georgiade N, ed. Symposium on management of cleft lip and palate and associated deformities. St Louis: CV Mosby, 1974:192.
595. Hess D, Hagerty R, Mylin W. Velar motility, velopharyngeal closure, and speech proficiency in cartilage pharyngoplasty: an eight year study. Cleft Palate J 1968; 5:153–162.
596. Lewy R, Cole R, Wepman J. Teflon injection in the correction of velopharyngeal insufficiency. Ann Otol Rhinol Laryngol 1965; 74:874–879.
597. Bluestone C, Musgrave R, McWilliams B, Crozier P. Teflon injection pharyngoplasty. Cleft Palate J 1968; 5:19–22.
598. Bluestone C, Musgrave R, McWilliams B. Teflon injection pharyngoplasty—status 1968. Laryngoscope 1968; 78:558–564.
599. Furlow L, Williams W, Eisenbach D, Bzoch K. A long term study on treating velopharyngeal insufficiency by Teflon injection. Cleft Palate J 1982; 19(1):47–61.
600. Smith J, McCabe B. Teflon injection in the nasopharynx to improve velopharyngeal closure. Ann Otol 1977; 86:559–563.
601. Ward P, Goldman R, Stoudt R. Teflon injection to improve velopharyngeal insufficiency. J Speech Hear Disord 1966; 31(3):267–273.
602. Ward P, Stoudt R, Goldman R. Improvement of velopharyngeal insufficiency by Teflon injection. Trans Am Acad Ophthalmol Otolaryngol 1967; 71:923–933.
603. Kuehn D, VanDemark D. Assessment of velopharyngeal competency following Teflon pharyngoplasty. Cleft Palate J 1978; 15(2):145–149.
604. Blocksma R. Correction of velopharyngeal insufficiency by silastic pharyngeal implant. Plast Reconstr Surg 1963; 31(3):268–274.
605. Blocksma R. Silicone implants for velopharyngeal incompetence: a progress report. Cleft Palate J 1964; 1:72–81.
606. Brauer R. Retropharyngeal implantation of silicone gel pillows for velopharyngeal incompetence. Plast Reconstr Surg 1973; 51:254–262.
607. Hynes W. Observations on pharyngoplasty. Br J Plast Surg 1967; 20:244–256.
608. Hynes W. Pharyngoplasty by muscle transplantation. Br J Plast Surg 1950; 3:128–135.
609. Harding R. Surgery. In: Cooper H, Harding R, Krogman W, Mazaheri M, Millard R, eds. Cleft palate and cleft lip: a team approach to clinical management and rehabilitation of the patient. Philadelphia: WB Saunders, 1979:162.
610. Kiehn C, DesPrez J, Tucker A, Malone M. Experiences with muscle transplants to incomplete soft palates. Plast Reconstr Surg 1965; 35(2):123–130.
611. Sullivan D. Bilateral pharyngoplasty as an aid to velopharyngeal closure. Plast Reconstr Surg 1961; 27:31–39.
612. Gold A, Song I. A tendon transplant pharyngoplasty. Cleft Palate J 1980; 17(4):283–290.
613. Orticochea M. Construction of a dynamic muscle sphincter in cleft palates. Plast Reconstr Surg 1968; 41:323–327.
614. Orticochea M. A review of 236 cleft palate patients treated with dynamic muscle sphincter. Plast Reconstr Surg 1983; 71(2):180–188.
615. Stradoudakis A, Bambace C. Sphincter pharyngoplasty for correction of velopharyngeal incompetence. Ann Plast Surg 1984; 12(3):243–248.
616. Huskie C, Jackson I. The sphincter pharyngoplasty—a new approach to the speech problems of velopharyngeal incompetence. Br J Disord Commun 1977; 12(1):31–35.
617. Jackson I. Sphincter pharyngoplasty. Clin Plast Surg 1985; 12(4):711–718.
618. Jackson I, Silverton F. The sphincter pharyngoplasty as a secondary procedure in cleft palates. Plast Reconstr Surg 1977; 59(4):518–524.
619. Lendrum J, Dhar B. The Orticochea dynamic pharyngoplasty. Br J Plast Surg 1984; 37:160–168.
620. Meyer R, Failat A, Kelly T. Bilateral Z-flap pharyngoplasty in the treatment of rhinolalia. Head Neck Surg 1981; 3:366–370.
621. Riski J, Serafin D, Riefkohl R, Georgiade G, Georgiade N. A rationale for modifying the site of insertion of the Orticochea pharyngoplasty. Plast Reconstr Surg 1984; 73(6):882–894.
622. Roberts T, Brown B. Evaluation of a modified sphincter pharyngoplasty in the treatment of speech problems due to palatal insufficiency. Ann Plast Surg 1983; 10(3):209–213.
623. Jones J, Meade P, Edwards A. Treating cleft lip and palate infants. Dent Assist 1985; 4(5):20–25.
624. Markowitz J, Gerry R, Fleishner R. Immediate obturation of neonatal cleft palates. Mt Sinai J Med (NY) 1979; 46(2):123–129.
625. Moore D. The continuing role of the prosthodontist in the treatment of patients with cleft lip and palate. J Prosthet Dent 1976; 36:186–193.
626. Razek M. Prosthetic feeding aids for infants with cleft lip and palate. J Prosthet Dent 1980; 44(5):556–561.
627. Dorf D, Reisberg D, Gold H. Early prosthetic management of cleft palate. Articulation development prosthesis: a preliminary report. J Prosthet Dent 1985; 53(2):222–226.

628. Adisman I. Cleft palate prosthetics. In: Grabb W, Rosenstein S, Bzoch K, eds. Cleft lip and palate: surgical, dental and speech aspects. Boston: Little, Brown, 1971:617.
629. Aram A, Subtelny J. Velopharyngeal function and cleft palate prostheses. J Prosthet Dent 1959; 9(1):149–158.
630. Arndt W, Shelton R, Bradford L. Articulation, voice, and obturation in persons with acquired and congenital palate defects. Cleft Palate J 1965; 2:377–383.
631. Birnbach S. Physiologic recording of the soft palate for fabrication of obturatory speech prostheses. J Prosthet Dent 1978; 39(5):539–545.
632. Coursin D. Treatment of the patient with cleft palate. Am J Dis Child 1950; 80:442–453.
633. Harkins C, Koepp-Baker H. Twenty-five years of cleft palate prosthesis. J Speech Hear Disord 1948; 13:23–30.
634. Harkins C, Harkins W, Harkins J. Principles of cleft palate prosthesis. New York: Columbia University Press, 1960.
635. Hotz M, Gnoinski W. Effects of early maxillary orthopaedics in coordination with delayed surgery for cleft lip and palate. J Maxillofac Surg 1979; 7:201–210.
636. Mazaheri M. Prosthodontic care. In: Cooper H, Harding R, Krogman W, Mazaheri M, Millard R, eds. Cleft palate and cleft lip: a team approach to clinical management and rehabilitation of the patient. Philadelphia: WB Saunders, 1979:268.
637. Mazaheri M. Prosthodontics in cleft palate rehabilitation. In: Lencione R, ed. Cleft palate habilitation: proceedings of the fifth annual symposium on cleft palate habilitation. Syracuse University, 1967:73.
638. Mazaheri M. Speech aid prosthesis in cleft palate rehabilitation. J Am Med Wom Assoc 1971; 21(11):926–934.
639. Posnick W. Prosthetic management of palatopharyngeal incompetency for the pediatric patient. J Dent Child 1977; 44:117–121.
640. Rosen M, Bzoch K. The prosthetic speech appliance in rehabilitation of patients with cleft palate. J Am Dent Assoc 1958; 57:103–120.
641. Gallagher B. Prosthesis in velopharyngeal insufficiency: effect on nasal resonance. J Commun Disord 1982; 15:469–473.
642. Olin W. Cleft lip and palate rehabilitation. Am J Orthod 1966; 52:126–144.
643. Olin W. Cleft lip and palate rehabilitation. Springfield: CC Thomas, 1960.
644. McKinstry R, Aramany M. Prosthodontic considerations in the management of surgically compromised cleft palate patients. J Prosthet Dent 1985; 53(6):827–831.
645. Weiss C. The significance of Passavant's pad in post-obturator patients. Folia Phoniatr (Basel) 1972; 24:51–56.
646. Enderby P, Hathorn I, Servant S. The use of intra-oral appliances in the management of acquired velopharyngeal disorders. Br Dent J 1984; 157(5):157–159.
647. Gonzalez J, Aronson A. Palatal lift prosthesis for treatment of anatomic and neurologic palatopharyngeal insufficiency. Cleft Palate J 1970; 7(1):91–104.
648. Gibbons P, Bloomer H. The palatal lift, a supportive type speech aid. J Prosthet Dent 1958; 8:362–369.
649. Holley L, Hamby G, Taylor P. Palatal lift for velopharyngeal incompetence: report of a case. J Dent Child 1973; 40:467–470.
650. Kerman P, Singer L, Davidoff A. Palatal lift and speech therapy for velopharyngeal incompetence. Arch Phys Med Rehabil 1973; 54:271–276.
651. Kipfmueller L, Lang B. Treating velopharyngeal inadequacies with a palatal lift prosthesis. J Prosthet Dent 1972; 27:467–477.
651a. Lang B, Kipfmueller L. Treating velopharyngeal inadequacy with the palatal lift concept. J Prosthet Dent 1969; 43:467–477.
652. LaVelle W, Hardy J. Palatal lift prostheses for treatment of palatopharyngeal incompetence. J Prosthet Dent 1979; 42(3):308–315.
653. Marshall R, Jones J. Effects of a palatal lift prosthesis upon the speech intelligibility of a dysarthric patient. J Prosthet Dent 1971; 25(3):327–333.
654. Millard R. Cleft palate and communication disorders. Ear Nose Throat J 1980; 59:54–61.
655. Netsell R. Dysarthria in adults: physiologic approach to rehabilitation. Arch Phys Med Rehabil 1979; 60(11):502–508.
656. Wedin S. Rehabilitation of speech in cases of palatophayngeal paresis with the aid of an obturator prosthesis. Br J Commun Disord 1972; 7:117–130.
657. Thompson R, Ferguson J, Barton M. The role of removable orthodontic appliances in the investigation and management of patients with hypernasal speech. Br J Orthod 1985; 12:70–77.
658. Reisberg D, Gold H, Dorf D. A technique for obturating palatal fistulas. Cleft Palate J 1985; 22(4):286–289.
659. Falter J, Shelton R. Bulb fitting and placement in prosthetic treatment of cleft palate. Cleft Palate J 1964; 1:441–447.
660. Mazaheri J, Millard R. Changes in nasal resonance related to differences in location and dimension of speech bulbs. Cleft Palate J 1965; 2:167–175.
661. Shelton R, Lindquist A, Knox A, Wright V, Arndt W, Elbert M, Youngstrom K. The relationship between pharyngeal wall movements and exchangeable speech appliance sections. Cleft Palate J 1971; 8:145–158.
662. Beery Q, Aramany M, Katzenberg B. Oral endoscopy in prosthodontic management of the soft palate defect. J Prosthet Dent 1985; 54(2):241–244.
663. Beery Q, Rood S, Schramm V. Pharyngeal wall motion prosthetically managed cleft palate adults. Cleft Palate J 1983; 20(1):7–17.
664. Walter J. The design of prostheses used in the treatment of velopharyngeal insufficiency. Br Dent J 1981; 151:338–342.
665. Lubker J, Schweiger J. Nasal airflow as an index of success of prosthetic management of cleft palate. J Dent Res 1969; 48(3):368–375.
666. Lubker J, Schweiger J, Morris H. Nasal airflow characteristics during speech in prothetically managed cleft palate speakers. J Speech Hear Res 1970; 13(2):326–328.
667. Reisberg D, Smith B. Aerodynamic assessment of prosthetic speech speech aids. J Prosthet Dent 1985; 54(5):686–690.
668. Schneiderman C, Mann M. Air flow and intelligibility of speech of normal speakers and speakers with a prosthodontically repaired cleft palate. J Prosthet Dent 1978; 39(2):193–199.
669. Warren D. A physiologic approach to cleft palate prosthesis. J Prosthet Dent 1965; 15(4):770–778.
670. Watson R, Gray B. Assessing effective obturation. J Prosthet Dent 1985; 54(1):88–93.
671. Fletcher S, Sooudi I. Joint prosthetics and speech treatment of hypernasality: report of a case. J Am Dent Assoc 1973; 87:1418–1425.
672. Dalston R. Prostodontic management of the cleft-palate patient: a speechpathologist's view. J Prosthet Dent 1977; 2:190–195.
673. Massengill R, Quinn G, Pickrell K. The use of a palatal stimulator to decrease velopharyngeal gap. Ann Otol Rhinol Laryngol 1971; 80:135–137.
674. Mazaheri M, Mazaheri E. Prosthodontic aspects of palatal elevation and palatopharyngeal stimulation. J Prosthet Dent 1976; 32(3):319–326.
675. Millard R. Training for optimal use of the prosthetic speech appliance. In: Bzoch K, ed. Communicative disorders re-

lated to cleft lip and palate. Boston: Little, Brown, 1979:341.
676. Blakeley R. Temporary speech prosthesis as an aid in speech training. Cleft Palate Bull 1960;10(3):63–65.
677. Curtis T, Chierici G. Prosthetics as a diagnostic aid in pharyngeal flap surgery. Cleft Palate J 1964; 1:95–98.
678. Blakeley R. The complementary use of speech prostheses and pharyngeal flaps in palatal insufficiency. Cleft Palate J 1964; 1:194–198.
679. Blakeley R. The rationale for a temporary speech prosthesis in palatal insufficiency. Br J Disord Commun 1969; 4:134–139.
680. Weiss C. Success of an obturator reduction program. Cleft Palate J 1971; 8:291–297.
681. Wong L, Weiss C. A clinical assessment of obturator-wearing cleft palate patients. J Prosthet Dent 1972; 27(6):632–639.
682. Shelton R, Lindquist A, Chisum L, Arndt W, Youngstrom K, Stick S. Effect of prosthetic speech bulb reduction on articulation. Cleft Palate J 1968; 5:195–204.
683. Shelton R, Lloyd R. Prosthetic facilitation of palatopharyngeal closure. J Speech Hear Disord 1963; 28(1): 58–66.
684. Subtelny J, Sakuda M, Subtelny J. Prosthetic treatment for palatopharyngeal incompetence: research and clinical implications. Cleft Palate J 1966; 4:130–158.
685. Hahn E. Directed home training program for infants with cleft lip and palate. In: Bzoch K, ed. Communicative disorders related to cleft lip and palate. Boston: Little, Brown, 1979:311.
686. Hahn E. Speech therapy for the pre-school cleft palate child. J Speech Hear Disord 1958; 23(5):605–609.
687. Philips BJ. Stimulating syntactic and phonological development in cleft palate infants. In: Bzoch K, ed. Communicative disorders related to cleft lip and palate. Boston: Little, Brown, 1979:304.
688. Shelton R, Hahn E, Morris H. Diagnosis and therapy. In: Spriestersbach D, Sherman D, eds. Cleft palate and communication. New York: Academic Press, 1968:225.
689. McWilliams BJ. Speech therapy for cleft-palate patients. Speech Pathol Ther 1959; 2(1):3–7.
690. VanDemark D, Hardin M. Effectiveness of intensive articulation therapy for children with cleft palate. Cleft Palate J 1986; 23(3):215–224.
691. Michi K-I, Suzuki N, Yamashita Y, Imai S. Visual training and correction of articulation disorders by use of dynamic palatography: serial observation in a case of cleft palate. J Speech Hear Disord 1986; 51:226–238.
692. Okazaki K, Abe M, Suzuki N, Kato M. Speech therapy of the palatalized articulation by use of a dynamic palatograph. J Jpn Cleft Palate Assoc 1980; 5:154–161.
693. Okazaki K, Onizuka T, Abe M, Sawashima M. Palatalized articulation as a type of cleft palate speech: observation by dynamic palatograph and cineradiograph. Jpn J Logoped Phoniatr 1980; 22:109–120.
694. Albery L, Enderby P. Intensive speech therapy for cleft palate children. Br J Disord Commun 1984; 19:115–124.
695. VanDemark D. Some results of speech therapy for children with cleft palate. Cleft Palate J 1974; 11:41–49.
696. Cohen M. An etiologic and nosologic overview of craniosynostosis syndromes. Birth Defects 1975; 11(2):137–189.
697. Cohen M. Craniosynostosis and syndromes with craniosynostosis: incidence, genetics, penetrance, variability and new syndrome updating. Birth Defects 1979; 15(5B):13–63.
698. Buchanan R. Acrocephalosyndactyly, or Apert's syndrome. Br J Plast Surg 1968; 21(4):406–418.
699. Apert E. De l'acrocéphalosyndactylie. Bull Mem Soc Med Hop Paris 1906; 23:1310–1313.
700. Buckley R, Yakovlev P. Dysostosis of skull, face and extremities (acrocephalosyndactyly). Am J Dis Child 1948; 75: 688–694.
701. Blank C. Apert's syndrome (a type of acrocephalosyndactyly)—observations on a British series of thirty-nine cases. Ann Hum Genet 1960; 24:151–163.
702. Ferriman D. Acrocephaly and acrocephlosyndactyly. Oxford: Oxford University Press, 1941.
703. Park E, Powers G. Acrocephaly and scaphocephaly with symmetrically distributed malformations of the extremities. Am J Dis Child 1920; 20(4):235–315.
704. Matras H, Watzek G, Perneczky A. Cephalometric observations in premature craniosynostosis. J Maxillofac Surg 1977; 5:298–303.
705. Ousterhout D, Melsen B. Cranial base deformity in Apert's syndrome. Plast Reconstr Surg 1982; 69(2):254–263.
706. Stewart R, Kawamoto H. Acrocephalosyndactyly (Apert's syndrome): a cause for reconsideration of its pathogenesis. In: Converse J, McCarthy J, Wood-Smith D, eds. Symposium on diagnosis and treatment of craniofacial anomalies. St Louis: CV Mosby, 1979:258.
707. Stewart R, Dixon G, Cohen A. The pathogenesis of premature craniosynostosis in acrocephalosyndactyly (Apert's syndrome). Plast Reconstr Surg 1977; 59(5):699–707.
708. Ebel Kl-D. Craniostenosis. Pediatr Radiol 1974; 2:1–14.
709. Maksem J, Roessmann U. Apert's syndrome with central nervous system anomalies. Acta Neuropathol (Berl) 1979; 48:59–61.
710. deCastro P, Pascual Castrojiejo I. Evolucion mental de 108 casos con craneosinostosis. An Esp Pediatr 1981; 15(5):443–448.
711. Elfenbein J, Waziri M, Morris H. Verbal communication skills of six children with craniofacial anomalies. Cleft Palate J 1981; 18(1):589–64.
712. Musallam S, Poley J, Riley H. Apert's syndrome (acrocephalosyndactyly): a description and a report on seven cases. Clin Pediatr 1975; 14(11):1054–1062.
713. Bergsma D, ed. Birth defects: atlas and compendium. 2nd ed. Baltimore: Williams and Wilkins, 1979.
714. Giuffre R, Vagnozzi R, Savino S. Infantile craniosynostosis: clinical, radiological, and surgical considerations based on 100 surgically treated cases. Acta Neurochir (Wien) 1978; 44:49–67.
715. Rougerie J, Tessier P. Craniosynostosis and craniofacial dysmorphia: a study of 335 cases with reference to neurosurgery and craniofacial surgery. Zeistschr Kinechir 1981; 34(2):179–183.
716. Bertelsen T. The premature synostosis of the cranial sutures. Acta Ophthalmol (Copenh) 1958; Suppl 51.
717. Gorlin R, Pindborg J, Cohen M. Syndromes of the head and neck. 2nd ed. New York: McGraw-Hill, 1976.
718. Costaras-Volarich M, Pruzansky S. Is the mandible intrinsically different in Apert and Crouzon syndromes? Am J Orthod 1984; 85(6):475–487.
719. Beligere H, Harris V, Pruzansky S. Progressive bony dysplasia in Apert syndrome. Radiology, 1981; 139:593–597.
720. Palacios E, Schimke R. Craniosynostosis-syndactylism. Am J Roentgenol Radium Ther Nucl Med 1969; 106(1):144–155.
721. Schauerte E, St-Aubin P. Progressive synostosis in Apert's syndrome (Acrocephalosyndactyly). Am J Roentgenol Radium Ther Nucl Med 1966; 97(1):67–73.
722. Sherk H, Whitaker L, Pasquariello P. Facial malformations and spinal anomalies: a predictable relationship. Spine 1982; 7(6):526–531.
723. Solomon L, Medenica M, Pruzansky S, Kreiborg S. Apert syndrome and palatal mucopolysaccharides. Teratology 1973; 8(3):287–292.
724. Miani C, Pagnacco A. Observations on a case of acrocephalosyndactyly with special reference to the oro-facial picture. Minerva Stomatol 1966; 17:541–548.
725. Peterson S, Pruzansky S. Palatal anomalies in the syn-

dromes of Apert and Crouzon. Cleft Palate J 1974; 11(4):394–403.

726. Peterson-Falzone S, Pruzansky S, Laffer J, Parris, P. Nasopharyngeal dysmorphology in the syndromes of Apert and Crouzon. Cleft Palate J 1981; 18:237–250.
727. Goldberg J, Enlow D, Whitaker L, Zins J, Kurihara S. Some anatomical characteristics in several craniofacial syndromes. J Oral Surg 1981; 39:489–498.
728. McCarthy J, Coccaro P, Schwartz M. Velopharyngeal function following maxillary advancement. Plast Reconstr Surg 1977; 64(2):180–189.
729. Schwartz M, McCarthy J, Coccaro P, Wood-Smith D, Converse J. Velopharyngeal function following maxillary advancement. In: Converse J, McCarthy J, Wood-Smith D, eds. Symposium on diagnosis and treatment of craniofacial anomalies. St Louis: CV Mosby, 1979:277.
730. Crysdale W. Malformations and syndromes. In: Bluestone C, Stool S, eds. Pediatric otolaryngology. Vol. I. Philadelphia: WB Saunders, 1983:55.
731. Crysdale W. Otorhinolaryngologic problems in patients with craniofacial anomalies. Symp Congenit Disord Otolaryngol Otolaryngol Clin North Am 1981; 14(1):145–155.
732. Lauritzen C, Lilja J, Jarlstedt J. Airway obstruction and sleep apnea in children with craniofacial anomalies. Plast Reconstr Surg 1986; 77(1):1–5.
733. Tessier P. Les cranio-facio-stenoses (C.F.S.) maladies de Crouzon et d'Apert. Ann Laringol Otol Rinol Faringol 1979; 77(1–2):19–30.
734. Tessier P. Osteotomies totales de la face. Syndrome de Crouzon. Syndrome d'Apert. Oxycephalies. Scaphocephalies. Turricephalies. Ann Chir Plast 1967; 12:273–286.
735. Tessier P. The definitive plastic surgical treatment of the severe facial deformities of craniofacial dysostosis: Crouzon's and Apert's diseases. Plast Reconstr Surg 1971; 48(5):419–442.
736. Schafer M. Upper airway obstruction sleep disorders in children with craniofacial anomalies. Clin Plast Surg 1982; 9(4):555–567.
737. Farkas L. Ear morphology in Treacher Collins', Apert's and Crouzon's syndromes. Arch Otorhinolaryngol 1978; 220:153–157.
738. Bergstrom L. Causes of severe hearing loss in early childhood. Pediatr Ann 1980; 9(1):23–27.
739. Gould H, Caldarelli D. Hearing and otopathology in Apert syndrome. Arch Otolaryngol 1982; 108(6):347–349.
740. Lindsay J, Black F, Donnelly W. Acrocephalosyndactyly (Apert's syndrome): temporal bone findings. Ann Otol Rhinol Laryngol 1975; 84:174–178.
741. Selder A. Hearing disorders in children with otocraniofacial syndrome. In: Wertz RT, ed. ASHA report #8: orofacial anomalies: clinical and research implications. Washington: American Speech and Hearing Association, 1973:95.
742. Terrahe K. The ear in Crouzon's and Apert's craniofacial abnormalities. Z Laryngol Rhinol Otol Ihre Grenzgeb 1971; 50(11):784–802.
743. Warkany J, Lemire R, Cohen M. Mental retardation and congenital malformations. Chicago: Chicago Year Book Medical Publishers, 1981.
744. Bergstrom L, Neblett L, Hemenway W. Otologic manifestations of acrocephalosyndactyly. Arch Otolaryngol 1972; 96:117–123.
745. Pellant A. Hearing disorders caused by dysplasia of the skull bones. Cesk Otolaryngol 1972; 21(4):158–162.
745a. Peterson S. Speech pathology in craniofacial malformations other than cleft lip and palate. In: Wertz RT, ed. ASHA report #8: orofacial anomalies: clinical and research implications. Washington: American Speech and Hearing Association, 1973.
746. Glass L, Knapp J, Bloomer H. Speech and lingual behavior before and after mandibular osteotomy. J Oral Surg 1977; 35:104–109.
747. Witzel MA, Ross RB, Munro I. Articulation before and after facial osteotomy. J Maxillofac Surg 1980; 8:195–202.
748. Witzel MA, Munro I. Velopharyngeal insufficiency after maxillary advancement. Cleft Palate J 1977; 14:176–180.
749. Peterson-Falzone S, Landahl K. Effect of aberrant supralaryngeal vocal tracts on transfer function. In: Lass N, ed. Speech and language: advances in basic research and practice. Vol. 6. New York: Academic Press, 1981:265.
750. Walker J. Crouzon's disease. Br Dent Assis 1981; 40:30–31.
751. Kreiborg S, Pruzansky S. Craniofacial growth in premature craniofacial synostosis. Scand J Plast Reconstr Surg 1981; 15:171–186.
752. Kreiborg S. Craniofacial growth in plagiocephaly and Crouzon syndrome. Scand J Plast Reconstr Surg 1981; 15:187–197.
753. Burdi A, Kusnetz A, Venes J, Gebarski S. The natural history and pathogenesis of the cranial coronal ring articulations: implications in understanding the pathogenesis of the Crouzon craniostenotic defects. Cleft Palate J 1986; 23(1):28–39.
754. Rosen H, Whitaker L. Cranial base dynamics in craniofacial dysostosis. J Maxillofac Surg 1984; 12:56–62.
755. Silla I. I rapporti della faccia e della base cranica nella disostosi cranio-facciale. Dent Cadmos 1966; 34:1029–1054.
756. Baldwin J. Dysostosis craniofacialis of Crouzon: a summary of recent literature and case reports with emphasis on involvement of the ear. Laryngoscope 1968; 78:1660–1667.
757. Selle G, Jacobs H. Cleft palate in two syndromes. Cleft Palate J 1977; 14(3):230–233.
758. Nathan V. Craniofacial dysostosis: Crouzon's disease. West Indian Med J 1983; 32(4):237–240.
759. Chandra-Sekhar H. Airway problems in craniofacial dysostosis. In: Converse J, McCarthy J, Wood-Smith D, eds. Symposium on diagnosis and treatment of craniofacial anomalies. St. Louis: CV Mosby, 1979:274.
760. Moore S, Moore A, Brown J. Crouzon's deformity with hyperostosis frontalis interna. Plast Reconstr Surg 1953; 2:1–9.
761. Schmid H. Synchondrosis of the laryngotracheal skeleton and tracheostenosis in the Apert-Crouzon syndrome. Zentralbl Allg Pathol 1971;114(3):326–337.
762. Olegard R, Sabel K, Aronsson M. Effects on the child of alcohol abuse during pregnancy. Acta Paediatr Scand [Suppl] 1979; 275:112–121.
763. Hanson J, Streissguth A, Smith D. The effects of maternal alcohol consumption during pregnancy on fetal growth and morphogenesis. J Pediatr 1978; 92:457–460.
764. Barnett R, Shusterman S. Fetal alcohol syndrome: review of literature and report of cases. J Am Dent Assoc 1985; 111:591–593.
765. Jones K, Smith D, Ulleland C, Streissguth P. Patterns of malformation in offspring of chronic alcoholic mothers. Lancet 1973; 1:1227–1231.
766. Riekman, G. Oral findings of fetal alcohol syndrome patients. J Can Dent Assoc 1984; 11:841–842.
767. Tollaro I, Pagni L, Casini Raggi G. Maxillofacial anomalies in a case of fetal alcohol syndrome. G Stomatol Orthognatod 1983; 2(4):19–26.
768. Shprintzen R. Palatal and pharyngeal anomalies in craniofacial syndromes. Birth Defects 1982; 18(1):53–78.
769. Frias J, King G, Williams C. Cephalometric assessment of selected malformation syndromes. Birth Defects 1982; 18(1):139–150.
770. Iosub S, Fuchs M, Bingol N, Gromisch D. Fetal alcohol syndrome revisited. Pediatrics 1981; 68:475–479.
771. Sanger D, Stick S, Sanger W, Dawson K. Specific syn-

dromes and associated communication disorders: a review. J Commun Disord 1984; 17:385–405.
772. Siegel-Sadewitz V, Shprintzen R. The relationship of communication disorders to syndrome identification. J Speech Hear Disord 1982; 47:338–354.
773. Sparks S. Birth defects and speech-language disorders. San Diego: College-Hill Press, 1984.
774. Ross RB. Lateral facial dysplasia (first and second branchial arch syndrome, hemifacial microsomia). Birth Defects 1975; 11(7):51–59.
775. Chandra-Sekhau H. Audiology and temporal bone disease in craniofacial anomalies. In: Converse J, McCarthy J, Wood-Smith D, eds. Symposium on diagnosis and treatment of craniofacial anomalies. St. Louis: CV Mosby, 1979.
776. Converse J, McCarthy J, Coccaro P, Wood-Smith D. Clinical aspects of craniofacial microsomia. In: Converse J, McCarthy J, Wood-Smith D, eds. Symposium on diagnosis and treatment of craniofacial anomalies. St. Louis: CV Mosby, 1979:461.
777. Stark R, Saunders D. The first branchial syndrome: the oral-mandibular-auricular syndrome. Plast Reconstr Surg 1962; 29(3):229–239.
778. Converse J, Coccaro P, Becker M, Wood-Smith D. On hemifacial microsomia. Plast Reconstr Surg 1973; 51(3):268–279.
779. Grabb W. The first and second branchial arch syndrome. Plast Reconstr Surg 1965; 36(5):485–508.
780. Francois J. Hereditary in ophthalmology. St Louis: CV Mosby, 1961.
781. Bennun R, Mulliken J, Kaban L, Murray J. Microtia: a microform of hemifacial microsomia. Plast Reconstr Surg 1985; 76(6):859–863.
782. Kaye C, Rollnick B, Pruzansky P. Malformations of the auricle: isolated and in syndromes. IV. Cumulative pedigree data. Birth Defects 1979; 15:163–169.
783. Rollnick B, Kaye C. Hemifacial microsomia and the branchio-oto-renal syndrome. J Craniofac Genet Dev Biol 1985; Suppl 1:287–295.
784. Goldenhar M. Associations malformatives de l'oeil et de l'oreille. J Genetique Humane 1952; 1:243–283.
785. Gorlin R, Jue K, Jacobsen U, Goldschmidt E. Oculoauriculovertebral dysplasia. J Pediatr 1963; 63:991–999.
786. Feingold M, Baum J. Goldenhar's syndrome. Am J Dis Child 1978; 132:131–138.
787. Hussain A, Dutta N. Oculo auriculo vertebral dysplasia. Indian J Ophthalmol 1979; 2:65–66.
788. Kallor A, Hendricks W. Oculoauriculovertebral dysplasia (Goldenhar's syndrome). Cutis 1979; 24(1):41–42.
789. Kruk J. Simultaneous external ear deformities and cleft palate and lip. Czas Stomatol (Warsaw) 1978; 31(12):1141–1146.
790. Maser E. Oculoauriculovertebral dysplasia. J Pedodont 1979; 3(3):Spring:253–258.
791. Mellor D, Richardson J, Douglas D. Goldenhar's syndrome. Arch Dis Childh 1973; 48:537–541.
792. Rao V, Rao S, Lamba P. Goldenhar's syndrome. Indian J Ophthalmol 1982; 30:147–149.
793. Scott A, Jamsky R. Oculoauroculovertebral dysplasia. J Pedodont 1982; 7(1):75–79.
794. Sugar H, Berman M. Relationship between the mandibulofacial dysostosis syndrome of Franceschetti and the oculo-auriculo-vertebral dysplasia syndrome of Goldenhar. Am J Ophthalmol 1968; 66(3):510–514.
795. Sugar H. The oculo auriculo vertebral dysplasia syndrome of Goldenhar. Am J Ophthalmol 1966; 62:678–682.
796. Thomas P. Goldenhar syndrome and hemifacial microsomia: observations on three patients. Eur J Pediatr 1980; 133:287–292.
797. Figueroa A, Friede H. Craniovertebral malformations in hemifacial microsomia. J Craniofac Genet Dev Biol [Suppl] 1985; 1:167–178.
798. Pashayan H, Pinsky L, Fraser F. Hemifacial microsomia: oculo-auriculo-vertebral dysplasia: a patient with overlapping features. J Med Genet 1970; 7:185–188.
799. Heffez L, Doku H. The Goldenhar syndrome: diagnosis and early surgical management. Oral Surg 1984; 58(1):2–9.
800. Converse J, McCarthy J, Coccaro P, Wood-Smith D. Bilateral craniofacial microsomia. In: converse J, McCarthy J, Wood-Smith D, eds. Symposium on diagnosis and treatment of craniofacial anomalies. St. Louis: CV Mosby, 1979:506.
801. Farkas L, Ross RB, James J. Anthropometry of the fact in lateral facial dysplasia: the bilateral form. Cleft Palate J 1977; 14(1):41–51.
802. Lauritzen C, Munro I, Ross RB. Classification and treatment of hemifacial microsomia. Scand J Plast Reconstr Surg 1985; 19:33–39.
803. Tenconi R, Hall G. Hemifacial microsomia: phenotypic classification, clinical implications, and genetic aspects. In: Harvold E, Vargervik K, Chierici G, eds. Treatment of hemifacial microsomia. New York: Alan R Liss, 1983:39–50.
804. Puckett C, Pickens J, Reinisch J. Sleep apnea in mandibular hypoplasia. Plast Reconstr Surg 1982; 70(2):213–216.
805. Poonawalla H, Kaye C, Rosenthal I, Pruzansky S. Hemifacial microsomia in a patient with Klinefelter syndrome. Cleft Palate J 1980; 17(3):194–196.
806. Laderkarl S. Combinations of Goldenhar's syndrome with the cri-du-chat syndrome. Acta Ophthalmol (Lopenh) 1968; 46:605–610.
807. Smith D. Recognizable patterns of human malformation. 2nd ed. Philadelphia: WB Saunders, 1976.
808. Bellucci R. Ear-related developmental anomalies of branchial clefts and arches I and II. In: Converse J, McCarthy J, Wood-Smith D, eds. Symposium on diagnosis and treatment of craniofacial anomalies. St. Louis: CV Mosby, 1979:512.
809. Caldarelli D, Valvassori G. A radiographic analysis of first and second branchial arch anomalies. In: Converse J, McCarthy J, Wood-Smith D, eds. Symposium on diagnosis and treatment of craniofacial anomalies. St. Louis: CV Mosby, 1979:476.
810. Caldarelli D, Hutchinson J, Pruzansky S, Valvassori G. A comparison of microtia and temporal bone anomalies in hemifacial microsomia and mandibulofacial dysostosis. Cleft Palate J 1980; 17(3):103-110.
811. Figueroa A, Pruzansky S. The external ear, mandible and other components of hemifacial microsomia. J Maxillofac Surg 1982; 4(10):200–211.
812. Phelps P, Lloyd G, Poswillo D. The ear deformities in craniofacial microsomia and oculo-auriculo-vertebral dysplasia. J Laryngol Otol 1983; 97:995–1005.
813. Rapin I, Ruben R. Patterns of anomalies in children with malformed ears. Laryngoscope 1976; 86:1469–1502.
814. Sando I, Suehiro S, Wood R. Congenital anomalies of the external and middle ear. In: Bluestone C, Stool S, eds. Pediatric otolaryngology. Vol. 1. Philadelphia: WB Saunders, 1983:309.
815. Sedee G. Facial nerve and dysplasia of the temporal bone. J Otol Rhinol Laryngol 1973; 35:222–228.
816. Yanagihara N, Yanagihara H, Kabasawa I. Goldenhar's syndrome associated with anomaloud internal auditory meatus. J Laryngol Otol 1979; 93:1217–1222.
817. Parving A. Progressive hearing loss in Goldenhar's syndrome. Scand Audiol 1978; 7:101–103.
818. Belenchia P, McCardle P. Goldenhar's syndrome: a case study. J Commun Disord 1985; 18:383–392.
819. Cohen M. Variability versus "incidental findings" in the first and second branchial arch syndrome: unilateral variants with anophthalmia. Birth Defects 1971; 7(7):103–108.

820. Mendelberg A, Ariel I, Mogle P, Arad I. Tracheo-oesophageal anomalies in the Goldenhar anomalad. J Med Genet 1985; 22(2):149–150.
821. Friedman S, Saraclar M. The high frequency of congenital heart disease in oculo-auriculo-vertebral dysplasia (Goldenhar's syndrome) (letter). J Pediatr 1974; 85(6):874.
822. Abe K, Ishikawa N, Murakami Y. Goldenhar's syndrome associated with cardiac malformations. Helv Paediatr Acta 1975; 30:57–60.
823. Greenwood R, Rosenthal A, Sommer A, Wolff G, Craenen J. Cardiovascular malformations in oculoauriculovertebral dysplasia (Goldenhar syndrome). J Pediatr 1974; 85(6):816–818.
824. Morand P, Chantepie A, Moraine C. Microsomies hemifaciales et malformations cardiac. Arch Mal Coeur 1978; 71(10):1154–1159.
825. James D. Obstructive sleep apnoea syndrome (letter). Br Med J 1982; 285:736.
826. Mealer W, Fisher J. Cor pulmonale and facio-auriculovertebral sequence. Cleft Palate J 1984; 21(2):100–103.
827. Longenecker C, Ryan R, Vincent R. Malformations of the ear as a clue to urogenital anomalies. Plast Reconstr Surg 1965; 35(3):303–309.
828. Melnick M. Hereditary hearing loss and ear dysplasia-renal adysplasia syndromes: syndrome delineation and possible pathogenesis. Birth Defects 1980; 16(7):59–72.
829. Carmi R, Binshtock M, Abeliovich D, Bar-Ziv J. The branchio-oto-renal (BOR) syndrome: report of bilateral renal agenesis in three sibs. Am J Med Genet 1983; 14:625–627.
830. Fraser F, Ling D, Clogg D, Norgrady B. Genetic aspects of BOR syndrome—branchial fistulae, ear pits, hearing loss, loss, and renal anomalies. Am J Med Genet 1978; 2:241–252.
831. Fraser F, Sproule J, Halal F. Frequency of the branchio-oto-renal syndrome in children with profound hearing loss. Am J Med Genet 1980; 7:341–349.
832. Melnick M, Bixler D, Silk K, Yune H, Nance W. Autosomal dominant branchio-oto-renal dysplasia. Birth Defects 1975; 11(5):121–128.
833. Melnick M, Bixler D, Nance W, Silk K, Yune H. Familial branchio-oto-renal dysplasia: a new addition to the branchial arch syndromes. Clin Genet 1967; 9:25–34.
834. Melnick M, Hodes M, Nance W, Yune H, Sweeney A. Branchio-oto-renal dysplasia and branchio-oto-dysplasia: two distinct autosomal dominant disorders. Clin Genet 1978; 13:425–442.
835. Miller A, Vargervik K. Electromyography as a technique to study neuromuscular characteristics in hemifacial microsomia and other congenital anomalies. In: Harvold E, Vargervik K, Chierici G, eds. Treatment of hemifacial microsomia. New York: Alan R Liss, 1983:89.
836. Vargervik K, Miller A. Assessment of facial and masticatory muscles in hemifacial microsomia. In: Harvold E, Vargervik K, Chierici G, eds. Treatment of hemifacial microsomia. New York: Alan R Liss, 1983:113.
837. Vargervik K, Miller A. Neuromuscular patterns in hemifacial microsomia. Am J Orthod 1984; 86(1):33–42.
838. Peterson-Falzone S. Structural and functional anomalies in hemifacial microsomia: panel on the first and second branchial arch syndrome. Presented before the American Cleft Palate Association, San Francisco, 1976.
839. Caldarelli D, Hutchinson J, Gould H. Hemifacial microsomia: priorities and sequence of comprehensive otologic management. Cleft Palate J 1980; 17(3):111–115.
840. Berry B. Note on a congenital defect (coloboma?) of the lower lid. R Lond Ophthalmol Hosp Rep 1889; 12:255–257.
841. Axellson A, Brolin I, Engstrom H, Liden G. Dysostosis mandibulo-facialis. J Laryngol Otol 1963; 77(7):575–592.
842. Behrents R, McNamara J, Avery J. Prenatal mandibulofacial dysostosis (Treacher Collins syndrome). Cleft Palate J 1977; 14:13–34.
843. Franceschetti A, Klein D. The mandibulofacial dysostosis, a new hereditary syndrome. Acta Ophthalmol (Copenh) 1949; 27:141–224.
844. Rogers B. Mandibulofactial dysostosis: Treacher Collins syndrome. In: Converse J, McCarthy J, Wood-Smith D, eds. Symposium on diagnosis and treatment of craniofacial anomalies. St Louis: CV Mosby, 1979:423.
845. Roberts F, Pruzansky S, Aduss H. An x-radiocephalometric study of mandibulofacial dysostosis in man. Arch Oral Biol 1975; 20:265–281.
846. Walker F. Apparent autosomal recessive inheritance of the Treacher-Collins syndrome. Birth Defects 1974; 10(8):135–139.
847. Peterson-Falzone S, Pruzansky S. Cleft palate and congenital palatopharyngeal incompetency in mandibulofacial dysostosis: frequency and problems in treatment. Cleft Palate J 1976; 13(4):354–360.
848. Shprintzen R, Croft C, Berkman M, Rakoff S. Pharyngeal hypoplasia in Treacher Collins syndrome. Arch Otolaryngol 1979; 105:127–131.
849. Johnston C, Taussig L, Koopmann C, Smith P, Bjelland J. Obstructive sleep apnea in Treacher-Collins syndrome. Cleft Palate J 1981; 18(1):39–44.
850. Sando I, Hemenway W, Morgan W. Histopathology of the temporal bones in mandibulofacial dysostosis. Trans Am Acad Ophthalmol Otolaryngol 1968; 72:913–924.
851. Book J, Fraccaro M. Genetical investigations in a North-Swedith population with mandibulo-facial dysostosis. Acta Genet Stat Med 1955; 5:327–333.
852. Fagen L, Elmore J, Nadler H. Mandibulo-facial dysostosis. Am J Dis Child 1967; 113:405–410.
853. Rogers B. Berry-Treacher Collins syndrome: a review of 200 cases. Br J Plast Surg 1964; 17:109–137.
854. Herring S, Rowlatt U, Pruzansky S. Anatomical abnormalities in mandibulofacial dysostosis. Am J Med Genet 1979; 3:225–259.
855. Holborow C. Deafness and the Treacher Collins syndrome. J Laryngol Otol 1961; 75(11):978–984.
856. Hutchinson J, Caldarelli D, Valvassori G, Pruzansky S, Parris P. The otologic manifestations of mandibulofacial dysostosis. Trans Am Acad Ophthalmol Otolaryngol 1977; 84:520–528.
857. Lynn G, Pirkey W. Oto-audiological findings in Treacher Collins' syndrome. J Speech Hear Disord 1965; 30(2):188–191.
858. Dahl E, Kreiborg S, Bjork A. A morphologic description of a dry skull with mandibulofacial dysostosis. Scand J Dent Res 1975; 83:257–266.
859. Garner L. Cephalometric analysis of Berry-Treacher-Collins syndrome. Oral Surg Oral Med Oral Pathol 1967; 23(2):320–327.
859a. Peterson-Falzone S. Longitudinal changes in cranial base angulation in mandibulofacial dysostosis. Presented before the Society for Ear, Nose and Throat Advances in Children, Dallas, December, 1985.
860. Forner L, Peterson-Falzone S, Kretschmer L. Acoustic characteristics of speech in mandibulofacial dysostosis. Presented before the American Speech-Language-Hearing Association, San Francisco, 1984.
861. Robin P. Backward lowering of the root of the tongue causing respiratory disturbances. Bull Acad Natl Med (Paris) 1923; 89:37–41.
862. Robin P. Glossoptosis due to atresia and hypotrophy of mandible. Am J Dis Child 1934; 48:541–547.
863. Eley R, Farber S. Hypoplasia of the mandible (micrognathy) as a cause of cyanotic attacks in the newly-born infant: report of four cases. Am J Dis Child 1930; 39:1167–1175.
864. Bush P, Williams A. Incidence of the Robin anomalad

(Pierre Robin syndrome). Br J Plast Surg 1983; 36:434–437.
865. Cohen M. Dysmorphic growth and development and the study of craniofacial syndromes. J Craniofac Genet Dev Biol [Suppl] 1985; 1:43–55.
865a. Cohen M. Syndromology's message for craniofacial biology. J Maxillofac Surg 1979; 7:89–109.
866. Cohen M. The Robin anomalad—its nonspecificity and associated syndromes. J Oral Surg 1976; 34:587–593.
867. Goldberg M, Eckblom R. The treatment of the Pierre Robin syndrome. Pediatrics 1962; 30:450–458.
868. Grignon J, Flageul G. Pitfalls in the diagnosis and primary treatment of the Pierre Robin syndrome. Glosso-palato-mandibular distress in the hypotrophic infant. Rev Stomatol Chir Maxillofac 1984; 85(3):224–227.
869. Poole A, Greene I, Greenstein R. Feeding problems in Robin anomalad: a report of 4 cases. Birth Defects 1982; 18(1):151–159.
870. Cozzi F, Pierro A. Glossoptosis-apnea syndrome in infancy. Pediatrics 1985; 75(5):836–843.
871. Dennison W. The Pierre Robin syndrome. Pediatrics 1965; 36(3):336–341.
872. Fletcher M, Blum S, Blanchard C. Pierre Robin syndrome: pathophysiology of obstructive episodes. Laryngoscope 1969; 79(4):547–560.
873. Lewis M, Pashayan H. Management of infants with Robin anomaly. Clin Pediatr 1980; 19(8):519–528.
874. Oka H, Saisho H, Hamanaka T, Moriguchi T, Tani T. Some experiences with the Pierre Robin syndrome with particular emphasis on the associated cleft palate. Bull Jpn Plast Surg Assoc 1983; 3(3):337–342.
875. Randall P. The Robin anomalad: micrognathia and glossoptosis with airway obstruction. In: Converse J, ed. Reconstructive plastic surgery: cleft lip and palate, craniofacial deformities. Philadelphia: WB Saunders, 1977:2235.
876. Randall P, Hamilton R. The Pierre Robin syndrome. In: Grabb W, Rosenstein S, Bzoch K, eds. Cleft lip and palate: surgical, dental and speech aspects. Boston: Little, Brown, 1971:559.
877. Randall P, Krogman W, Jahina S. Pierre Robin and the syndrome that bears his name. Cleft Palate J 1965; 2:237–246.
878. Randall P. The Pierre Robin syndrome. In: Georgiade N, ed. Symposium on management of cleft lip and palate and associated deformities. St Louis: CV Mosby, 1974:217–221.
879. Rubin A. Handbook of congenital malformations. Philadelphia: WB Saunders, 1967.
880. Van Regemorter N, Dodion J, Druart C, Hayez F, Vamos E, Flament-Durand J, Perlmutter-Cremer N, Rodesch F. Congenital malformations in 10,000 consecutive births in a university hospital: need for genetic counseling and prenatal diagnosis. J Pediatr 1984; 104(3):386–390.
881. Shprintzen R. Syndromic cleft lip and palate. ACPA Workshop on Heterogeneity of Cleft Lip and Palate, San Antonio, 1987.
882. Hanson J, Smith D. U-shaped palatal defect in the Robin anomalad: developmental and clinical relevance. J Pediatr 1975; 87:30–33.
883. Latham R. The pathogenesis of cleft palate associated with the Pierre Robin syndrome. Br J Plast Surg 1966; 19(3):205–214.
884. Poswillo D. Mechanisms and pathogenesis of malformation. Br Med Bull 1976; 32(1):59–64.
885. Champion R. Treatment of cleft palate associated with micrognathia. Br J Plast Surg 1954; 7:283–290.
886. Hotz M, Gnoinski W. Clefts of the secondary palate associated with the "Pierre Robin syndrome." Swed Dent J [Suppl] 1982; 15:89–98.
887. Routledge R. The Pierre-Robin syndrome: a surgical emergency in the neonatal period. Br J Plast Surg 1960; 13:204–218.
888. Edwards J, Newall D. The Pierre Robin syndrome reassessed in the light of recent research. Br J Plast Surg 1985; 38:339–342.
889. Ranta R, Laatikainen T, Laitinen S. Cephalometric comparisons of the cranial base and face in children with the Pierre Robin anomalad and isolated cleft palate. Proc Finn Dent Soc 1985; 81:82–90.
890. Rintala A, Ranta R, Stegars T. On the pathogenesis of cleft palate in the Pierre Robin syndrome. Scand J Plast Reconstr Surg 1984; 18:237–240.
891. Carey J, Fineman R, Ziter F. The Robin sequence as a consequence of malformation, dysplasia, and neuromuscular syndromes. Pediatrics 1982; 101(5):858–864.
892. Haberland C, Daniels A, Dawson G. Pierre Robin syndrome. Acta Neuropathol (Berl) 1974; 30:91–107.
893. Pashayan H, Lewis M. Clinical experience with the Robin sequence. Cleft Palate J 1984; 21(4):270–276.
894. Siegel-Sadewitz V, Shprintzen R. Pierre Robin: a new look at an old disorder. Videotape presented before the American Cleft Palate Association, New York 1986.
895. Siegel-Sadewitz V, Shprintzen R. The Robin sequence: an analysis of its heterogeneity. Presented at the annual meeting of the Society for Ear, Nose and Throat Advances in Children. Philadelphia, 1986.
896. Williams A, Williams M, Walker C, Bush P. The Robin anomalad (Pierre Robin syndrome)—a follow-up study. Arch Dis Child 1981; 56:663–668.
897. Wood V, Sandlin C. The hand in Pierre Robin syndrome. J Hand Surg 1983; 8(3):273–276.
898. Stickler G, Belau P, Farrell F, Jones J, Pugh D, Steinberg A, Ward L. Hereditary progressive artho-ophthalmopathy. Mayo Clin Proc 1965; 40(6):433–455.
899. Stickler G, Pugh D. Hereditary progressive arthro-ophthalmopathy, II. Additional observations on vertebral abnormalities, a hearing defect, and a report of a similar case. Mayo Clin Proc 1967; 42:495–500.
900. Spranger J. Arthro-ophthalmopathia hereditaria. Ann Radiol (Paris) 1968; 11:359–364.
901. Herrmann J, France T, Spranger J, Opitz J, Wiffler C. The Stickler syndrome (hereditary arthoophthalmopathy). Birth Defects 1975; 11(2):76–103.
902. Hall J. Stickler syndrome. In: Bergsma D, ed. Clinical cytogenetics and genetics. Birth defects 1974; 10(8):157–171.
903. Smith JL, Stowe F. The Pierre Robin syndrome (glossoptosis, micrognathia, cleft palate): a review of 39 cases with emphasis on associated ocular lesions. Pediatrics 1961; 27:128–133.
904. Bergstrom L, Hemenway W, Sando I. Pathological changes in congenital deafness. Laryngoscope 1972; 82(10):1777–1792.
905. Cogswell J, Easton D. Cor pulmonale in the Pierre Robin syndrome. Arch Dis Child 1974; 49(11):905–908.
906. Jeresaty R, Huszar R, Basu S. Pierre Robin syndrome: cause of respiratory obstruction, cor pulmonale, and pulmonary edema. Am J Dis Child 1969; 117:710–716.
907. Boesen I, Melchior J, Terslev G, Vendel S. Extracardiac congenital malformations in children with congenital heart disease. Acta Paediatr Scand [Suppl] 1963; 146:28–33.
908. Calli L. Cleft lip/palate with tetralogy of Fallot. Birth Defects 1971; 7(7):261.
909. Caramelli Z, Reginato L. The role of the association between congenital heart disease and cleft lip and palate in surgical mortality. Br J Plast Surg 1959; 12:76–77.
910. Geis N, Seto B, Bartoshesky L, Lewis M, Pashayan H. The prevalence of congenital heart disease among the population of a metropolitan cleft lip and palate clinic. Cleft Palate J 1981; 18(1):19–83.
911. Kitamura H, Kraus B. Visceral variations and defects associated with cleft lip and palate in human fetuses: a macroscopic description. Cleft Palate J 1964; 1:99–115.
912. Mackeprang M, Hay S. Observations on congenital heart

disease in a mortality study of children with cleft lip and palate. J Chronic Dis 1971; 24:34–43.

913. Poswillo D. Otomandibular deformity: pathogenesis as a guide to reconstruction. J Maxillofac Surg 1974; 2(2):343–349.

914. Shah C, Pruzansky S, Harris W. Cardiac malformations with facial clefts. Am J Dis Child 1970; 119:238–244.

915. Wallgren E, Landtman B, Rapola J. Extracardiac malformations associated with congenital heart disease. Eur J Cardiol 1978; 7:15–24.

916. Hoffman S, Kahn S, Seitchick M. Late problems in the management of the Pierre Robin syndrome. Plast Reconstr Surg 1965; 35(5):504–510.

917. Douglas B. A further report on the treatment of micrognathia with obstruction a plastic procedure. Plast Reconstr Surg 1950; 5(2):113–122.

918. Douglas B. The treatment of micrognathia associated with obstruction a plastic operation. J Am Med Wom Assoc 1966; 21(12):1027–1033.

919. Douglas B. The treatment of micrognathia associated with obstruction by a plastic procedure. Plast Reconstr Surg 1946; 1(3):300–308.

920. Ogborn M, Pemberton P. Late development of airway obstruction in the Robin anomalad (Pierre Robin syndrome) in the newborn. Aust Paediatr J 1985; 21:199–200.

921. Chassagne J, Monin P, Maxant P, LeFevre J, Mougenot A, Flot F, Stricker M. Management of Pierre Robin syndrome. Rev Stomatol Chir Maxillofac 1985; 86(3):195–202.

922. Hadley R, Johnson J. Utilization of the Kirschner wire in Pierre Robin syndrome. Plast Reconstr Surg 1963; 31:487–495.

923. Parsons R, Smith D. A modified tongue-lip adhesion for Pierre Robin anomalad. Cleft Palate J 1980; 17(2):144–147.

924. Smith JD. Treatment of airway obstruction in Pierre Robin syndrome. Arch Otolaryngol 1981; 107:419–421.

925. Kelly J, Sorenson H, Turner E. Prosthodontic treatment for Pierre Robin syndrome. J Prosthet Dent 1978; 39(5):554–560.

926. Heaf D, Helms P, Dinwiddie R, Matthew D. Nasopharyngeal airways in Pierre Robin syndrome. J Pediatr 1982; 100(5):698–703.

927. Crow M, Holder T, McCoy F, Chandler R. The use of temporary gastrostomy to prevent aspiration in Pierre Robin syndrome. Plast Reconstr Surg 1965; 35(5):494–503.

928. Pruzansky S, Richmond J. Growth of mandible in infants with micrognathia. Am J Dis Child 1954; 88:29–42.

929. Mallory S, Paradise J. Glossoptosis revisited: on the development and resolution of airway obstruction the Pierre Robin syndrome. Pediatrics 1979; 64(6):946–948.

930. Poradowska W, Reszke S, Lenkiewicz T. Pierre Robin syndrome. Pediatr Pol 1981; 56(6):607–611.

930a. Gould H, Caldarelli D, Parris P, Toney L. Audiologic and otologic findings in Pierre Robin anomalad. Presented before the American Cleft Palate Association, San Diego, 1979.

931. Igarashi M, Filippone M, Alford B. Temporal bone findings in Pierre Robin syndrome. Laryngoscope 1976; 86(11):1679–1687.

932. Jackson P, Whitaker L, Randall P. Airway hazards associated with pharyngeal flaps in patients who have the Pierre Robin syndrome. Plast Reconstr Surg 1976; 58(2):184–186.

933. Levinson C, Massengill R, Pickrell K, Bryson M. Lingual and labial movements of Pierre Robin syndrome patients treated by Beverly Douglas procedure. Cleft Palate J 1969; 6:45–49.

933a. DeMarquey J. Quelques considérations sur le bec-de-lièvre. Gazette Med (Paris) 1845; 13:52–53.

934. Bloomer H. Speech defects associated with dental malocclusions and related abnormalities. In: Travis L, ed. Handbook of speech pathology and audiology. New York: Appleton-Century-Crofts, 1971:715.

935. Fogh-Andersen P. Fistula labii inferioris congenita. Tandlaegebladet (Dan Dent J) 1943; 47:411–417.

936. Van der Woude A. Fistula labii inferioris congenita and its association with cleft lip and palate. Am J Hum Genet 1954; 6:244–256.

937. Burdick A, Bixler D, Puckett C. Genetic analysis in families with van der Woude syndrome. J Craniofac Genet Dev Biol 1985; 5:181–208.

938. Cervenka J, Gorlin R, Anderson V. The syndrome of pits of the lower lip and cleft lip and/or palate: genetic considerations. Am J Hum Genet 1967; 19:416–428.

939. Glass L, Stewart R, Miles J. The speech-language pathologist's role in understanding the genetics of Van der Woude syndrome. J Speech Hear Disord 1979; 44(4):472–478.

940. Shprintzen R, Goldberg R, Sidoti E. The penetrance and variable expression of the Van de Woude syndrome: implications for genetic counseling. Cleft Palate J 1980; 17(1):52–57.

941. Rintala A, Lahti A, Gylling U. Congenital sinuses of the lower lip in connection with cleft lip and palate. Cleft Palate J 1970; 7(1):336–345.

942. Ranta R, Rintala A. Correlations between microforms of the Van Der Woude syndrome and cleft palate. Cleft Palate J 1983; 20(2):158–162.

943. Rintala A, Ranta R. Lower lip sinuses: I. Epidemiology, microforms and transverse sulci. Br J Plast Surg 1981; 24:26–30.

944. Schneider E. Lip pits and congenital absence of second premolars. Varied expression of the lip pit syndrome. J Med Genet 1973; 10:346–349.

945. Pauli L, Hall J. Lip pits, cleft lip and/or palate, and congenital heart disease. Am J Dis Child 1980; 134:293–295.

946. Janku P, Robinow M, Kelly T, Bralley R, Baynes A, Edgerton M. The van der Woude syndrome in a large kindred: variability, penetrance, genetic risks. Am J Med Genet 1980; 5:117–123.

947. Sedlackova E. Insufficiency of the palatopharyngeal passage disorder. Casopis Lekaru Ceskych (Prague) 1955; 94:1304–1307.

948. Kruk J, Tronczynska J. Velopharyngeal insufficiency in children with Sedlackova's syndrome. Acta Chir Plast (Prague) 1978; 20(1):13–17.

949. Saad E. The underdeveloped palate in ear, nose and throat practice. Laryngoscope 1980; 90:1371–1377.

950. Shprintzen R, Goldberg R, Lewin M, Sidoti E, Berkman M, Argamaso R, Young D. A new syndrome involving cleft palate, cardiac anomalies, typical facies, and learning disabilities: velo-cardio-facial syndrome. Cleft Palate J 1978; 15:56–62.

951. Shprintzen R, Goldberg R, Young D, Wolford L. The velo-cardio-facial syndrome: a clinical and genetic analysis. Pediatrics 1981; 67(2):167–172.

952. Young D, Shprintzen R, Goldberg R. Cardiac malformations in the velo-cardio-facial syndrome. Am J Cardiol 1980; 46:643–648.

953. Arvystas M, Shprintzen R. Craniofacial morphology in the velo-cardio-facial syndrome. J Craniofac Genet Dev Biol 1984; 4:39–45.

954. Golding-Kushner K, Weller G, Shprintzen R. Velo-cardio-facial syndrome: language and psychological profiles. J Craniofac Genet Dev Biol 1985; 5:259–266.

18 Articulation Disorders in the Child with Neurogenic Pathology

Cynthia K. Thompson, Ph.D.

This chapter will discuss two types of articulation disorders associated with neuropathologic conditions occurring in children. These include developmental dysarthria and developmental apraxia of speech. The discussion begins with definitions of the disorders and a brief historical review. Basic neurologic correlates of speech production, neuropathology, and etiologies associated with each are addressed. Subsequent sections focus on behavioral pathology and methods for assessment and treatment.

DEFINITIONS

Both developmental dysarthria and developmental apraxia of speech are relatively new terms in the communication disorders literature, although the disorders have existed for a very long time. Historically, the terms "dysarthria" and "apraxia of speech" have referred to acquired neuromotor speech deficits seen in adults and have only recently come into use by speech-language pathologists to describe speech disorders of children. Developmental dysarthria is a term used to describe speech disorders associated with disturbances in muscular control of the speech mechanism, often associated with speech disorders seen in cerebral palsy;[1] whereas developmental apraxia of speech has been associated with deficits in articulatory or motor programming.[2] Developmental apraxia of speech is a controversial term and some professionals have questioned its use.[3,4] Others use the term and treat children accordingly. Therefore it is important for practicing clinicians to understand what is meant by developmental apraxia of speech and issues pertaining to use of the term.

In order to best understand the meaning of developmental dysarthria and apraxia of speech, it is necessary to provide a definition of each word comprising the diagnostic categories.

Developmental

"Developmental" disorders refer to those occurring sometime during the course of maturation. "Developmental" neurogenic speech disorders result from an insult or lesion to the brain occurring prior to or during the course of speech development, whereas "acquired" disorders are those resulting from a lesion to the adult brain after speech development has been completed. Therefore developmental and acquired speech disorders are not directly comparable. Lesions to the developing brain disrupt systems as they develop, whereas lesions to the adult brain disrupt systems that are fully developed anatomically and physiologically.

Dysarthria

The second term to be defined, "dysarthria," composed of the prefix "dys" meaning faulty and the root "arthria" meaning articulation is, as pointed out, a term used to describe speech disorders caused from "disturbances in muscular control of the speech mechanism resulting from impairment of any of the basic motor processes involved in the execution of speech."[5] There may be paralysis, weakness or decreased muscle strength, alterations in speed of movement, range of motion, coordination, or altered muscle tone because damage to the peripheral or central nervous sytem has disrupted neurologic connections to and from the muscles involved in production of speech. The term is used when both isolated and coexisting components or subsystems of speech production including respiration, phonation, resonance, and articulation are involved because disruption of one or several of these components may result in abnormal speech production. Therefore perhaps the term "the dysarthrias" is more accurate than "dysarthria" because specific characteristics of the disorder vary, depending upon which subsystem(s) is involved.

It may appear unusual to consider respiration, phonation, resonance, and articulation within a discussion of articulation disorders, but as pointed out by Brain,[6] who defines dysarthria as a disorder of articulation, articulation is most accurately defined in a broad sense because "movement of the lips, tongue, palate, vocal cords and muscles of respiration {constitute} the motor function whereby sounds ... are converted into words" (p 122).[6] The term "dysarthria," then, is more than "imperfect articulation of speech," the medical dictionary definition.[7] A comprehensive definition of dysarthria is common in both the adult and child literature.[1,8]

One other important aspect of a definition of dysarthria is that it is restricted to speech disorders manifest secondary to neurologic impairment. Therefore disorders of respiration, phonation, resonance, and/or articulation caused from psychological or structural defects are not considered dysarthria.

Apraxia of Speech

Apraxia of speech is a motor speech disorder quite different from dysarthria. Apraxia, made up of the prefix "a," meaning loss of, and the root "praxia," referring to movement, occurs in the absence of weakness, paralysis, and incoordination of the speech musculature. The disorder has been defined as one of motor programming of "the volitional production of individual speech sounds and their combination into sequences to form words."[5] More recently, Wertz, LaPointe, and Rosenbek modified this definition as follows:

> Apraxia of speech is a neurogenic phonologic disorder resulting from sensorimotor impairment of the capacity to select, program, and/or execute in coordinated and normally timed sequences, the positioning of the speech musculature for the volitional production of speech sounds. The loss or impairment of phonologic rules of the native language is not adequate to explain the observed pattern of deviant speech, nor is the disturbance attributable to weakened or misdirected actions of specific muscle groups. Prosodic alteration, that is, changes in speech, stress, intonation, and/or rhythm, may be associated with the articulatory disruption either as a primary part of the condition or in compensation for it (p 4).[9]

In adults, the disorder is most often associated with infarction of the left or language dominant hemisphere of the brain. Some writers have also suggested a similar lesion in children presenting with the disorder, indicating that "developmental apraxia of speech is an articulation disorder subsequent to brain damage . . . characterized by impaired ability to accomplish the volitional production of speech sounds and sound sequences" (p 13).[10] However, research has shown that children with developmental apraxia of speech do not present with identifiable neurologic lesions.[3]

HISTORY

Developmental Dysarthria

As pointed out, the term "developmental dysarthria" originated from the adult literature or what is termed "acquired dysarthria." Descriptions of dysarthria, or neurogenic speech disturbances in adults, have been noted as early as 3500 B.C.,[11] although not until the 19th century did writers such as Jackson[12] note a distinction between neurogenic speech disturbances and language or symbolic disorders. In 1950, an article by Peacher appears to have marked a "turning point in attention to dysarthria" (p 99).[11] In this and other articles appearing around that time, the disorder was reviewed, and classification systems were posed.[13–16]

The most comprehensive and influential research guiding contemporary thinking about dysarthria was reported in a series of two articles in 1969.[17,18] In these articles, Darley and his colleagues at the Mayo Clinic attempted to describe deviant speech characteristics associated with specific neuropathologies. At least 30 subjects from each of seven diagnostic groups including bulbar palsy, pseudobulbar palsy, cerebellar disease, Parkinson's disease, dystonia, and chorea were selected and their speech analyzed. Judges rated speech samples from each subject on 38 dimensions of speech and voice, using a seven-point scale of severity.

Analysis of the results by means of a correlational matrix revealed clusters of deviant speech dimensions associated with each of the neuropathologies studied, suggesting that disruption of different neurologic mechanisms resulted in different speech disorders or dysarthrias. The authors were therefore led to label each of the dysarthrias identified based upon their neurologic underpinnings. In Chapter 19, Kearns and Simmons present a detailed description of the Mayo Clinic research and list the types of dysarthria and speech behaviors associated with each.

The types of dysarthria seen in children with neurologic disorders have not been studied as extensively. However, a review of the history of children with cerebral palsy suggests a gradual recognition that these children make up a heterogeneous population with regard to neuromotor symptomatology. Therefore it follows that heterogeneity in speech behavior also exists in these children as it does in adults.

What is known today as cerebral palsy was first described by Little in the *Lancet* in the 19th century,[19,20] and it was labelled Little's disease. Little's description indicated that children with the disease had neuromotor involvement of the upper and/or lower extremities and that some had involvement of the speech musculature. Later writers noted variability in the type of motor problems seen. For example, hypertonic muscles were seen in some children, whereas flaccidity and/or tremors were present in others. By the late 1800s and early 1900s, there was some agreement that several types of cerebral palsy existed, and, not long after that, classification systems began to appear in the literature.[21,22] For example, Minear summarized the results of a survey of the American Academy of Cerebral Palsy, indicating that at least eight different types of cerebral palsy were being observed at the time.[21] These included (1) spasticity, (2) athetosis, (3) rigidity, (4) ataxia, (5) tremor, (6) atonia, (7) mixed, and (8) unclassifiable cerebral palsy.

Recognizing the variety of neurologic problems associated with cerebral palsy, Crothers and Paine streamlined classifications into three subtypes including spasticity, involuntary motion disorders (dyskinesia, extrapyramidal cerebral palsy), and mixed.[23] They further differentiated spastic patients based on the topographic distribution of neuromotor signs (e.g., hemiplegia, paraplegia). These classifications of cerebral palsy continue to be used at the present time,[1] and they remain problematic since patients within each classification are heterogeneous.

Given this heterogeneity, it is not surprising that speech disorders or dysarthrias seen secondary to cerebral palsy may also vary. Depending upon the type of cerebral palsy and the motor systems involved, however, clinicians can predict with some reliability whether or not the speech musculature is involved. For example, in spastic quadriplegia involving the upper and lower extremities of the body, speech is more likely to be involved than in spastic diplegia involving only the lower extremities because of the topographic arrangement of cortical motor control. (This topographic arrangement will be explained further in Neurologic Correlates section in this chapter.) However, the pattern of speech disruption is much more difficult to predict based upon this information. Further, not all children with neuromotor problems carry a diagnosis of cerebral palsy; that is, dysarthria may be present in children with a variety of neurologic disorders. Unfortunately, many developmental disorders resulting in dysarthria have not been studied extensively. Perhaps research with children similar to that conducted by Darley et al.[17,18] with adults may lead to a better understanding of the relationship between neurologic impairment and speech disorders in children.

Developmental Apraxia of Speech

The term "apraxia of speech" did not appear in the literature until the late 1960s and early 1970s. The disorder was described long before that time, however, with several different terms being used to label it including aphemia,[24] cortical dysarthria,[25] apraxic dysarthria,[26] verbal aphasia,[27] phonetic disintegration,[28,29] and apraxia of verbal expression.[30] In fact, as pointed out by Darley,

> when we review the behavior that Broca[31] described which has since gone by the name of motor aphasia, many of us believe that it should be called a name other than aphasia, because it is in a different, a non-linguistic dimension. The gropings of the motor aphasic patient for correct positioning of his articulators, his clumsiness in finding the right pattern of movement to produce a polysyllabic word, his near misses phonemically and his retrials are predominant. This is coupled with no reduction in auditory comprehension—a specific modality bound deficit better labelled an apraxia, to be exact, an oral verbal apraxia (p 46).[31]

Articles appearing around the 1970s were the first in which articulatory programming or motor speech disorders occurring secondary to neurologic infarction were set apart from aphasia.[29,33–38] Although this separation was not accepted without critisism from Martin[39] and others, the term "apraxia of speech" began to appear in texts,[5,40,41] and in 1984 a text devoted solely to the disorder and its treatment was published.[9]

Interestingly, the major persons responsible for coining and popularizing the term "apraxia of speech" in adults were also instrumental in introducing the concept in the developmental literature in this country,[2,42] although the phenomenon had previously been observed and described in the British literature.[43–45] Rosenbek and Wertz presented a review of 50 cases of developmental apraxia of speech, describing the motor speech behaviors of these children and suggesting that the currently in vogue term "childhood expressive aphasia"[46] was inappropriate for these children.[2] A similar thesis was advanced in a later article by Yoss and Darley.[42]

Since the early 1970s, researchers have taken a closer look at what was termed "developmental apraxia of speech" by Rosenbek and Wertz,[2] Yoss and Darley,[42] and others. Some writers have attempted to more clearly define the disorder,[47] whereas others have questioned the use of the term. For example, Guyette and Diedrich, in a comprehensive, scholarly review of the disorder, suggested that developmental apraxia of speech is a "label in search of a population" (p 39).[3] That is, they found wide variability across children labelled with the disorder and questioned the difference between children with developmental apraxia of speech and those with functional articulation disorders. Further, they questioned the usefulness of the label for treatment. Guyette and Diedrich's comments will be discussed further in later sections on Developmental Apraxia of Speech.

NEUROLOGIC CORRELATES

I have already established that developmental dysarthria and developmental apraxia of speech are derived from disorders observed in adults and that these adult disorders are caused from damage to the central and/or peripheral nervous system. In order to understand the underlying neuropathology of these speech disorders when seen in children, one must understand the basic motor processes involved in speech production and then understand how speech is disrupted when certain of these processes are impaired in the adult brain. In this section, a basic overview of neuromotor mechanisms related to speech production will be presented along with a discussion of speech disorders and other problems resulting from damage to various aspects of the system. Speech disorders resulting from acquired brain damage are listed in Table 18–1 along with the primary site of lesion for each.

Neuromotor control of speech production is best explained within a general discussion of the motor system of the human body. The neuromotor system is composed of several interconnected components, each of which contributes a particular function. It is the dynamics or integrated workings of these as well as sensory components that result in coordinated motor activity. For this discussion, the motor system will be divided into four components including (1) cortical motor programming, (2) descending motor pathways (upper motoneurons), (3) control circuits, and (4) final common pathways (lower motoneurons). Motor behavior is programmed at the cortical level; information is transmitted to the brain stem or spinal cord via the direct and indirect pathways and modified en route by control circuits; and, finally, information reaches the muscles via final common pathways arising from brain stem and spinal cord nuclei. Each of these components will be discussed briefly. For more complete information and understanding, the reader should consult a textbook on neuroanatomy and neurophysiology.[48–52]

Cortical Motor Programming

In order to perform any skilled, volitional movement, one must somehow preplan or program the movement such that the sequence of movements necessary for its execution are carried out. Although the neurologic mechanisms involved in motor programming are not totally clear, researchers have suggested that the primary area of the brain responsible for this activity is the premotor cortex.[5] Another important area is located in the posterior aspect of the brain where perceptual information is processed and concepts about a particular motor behavior are formulated.

The motor cortex, premotor cortex, and posterior aspects of the left hemisphere of the brain are shown from a lateral view in Figure 18–1. Broca's area, associated with programming speech production, is also shown. Damage to areas of the brain involved in motor programming results in an inability to program sequences of voluntary motor activity. Because the motor area is spared in such a

TABLE 18–1 Acquired Neurogenic Speech Disorders and Primary Site of Lesion

Speech Disorder	*Site of Lesion*
Apraxia of speech	Premotor Cortex
Dysarthria	
Spastic	Motor cortex
	Direct and indirect motor pathways
Hyperkinetic	Basal ganglia
Hypokinetic	Basal ganglia
Ataxic	Cerebellum
Flaccid	Final common pathway

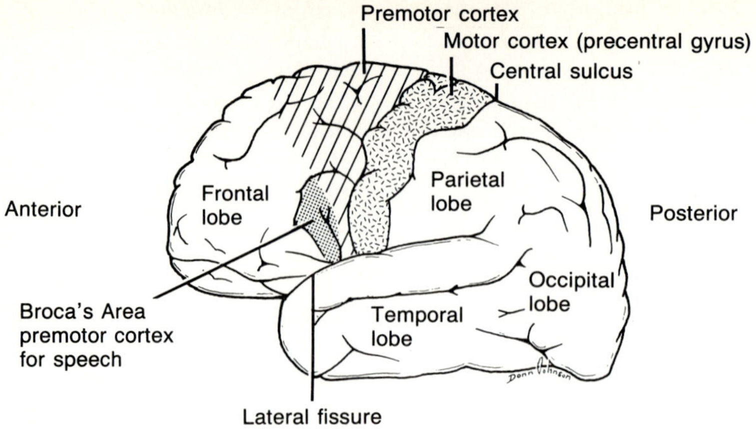

Figure 18–1 Lateral view of the cerebral cortex. The motor cortex, premotor cortex, and posterior aspect of the left hemisphere are shown.

lesion, no muscle weakness or paralysis is present, and so involuntary or automatic motor movements may be performed. The disorder resulting from such a lesion in adults is called "apraxia" and when programming areas for speech are involved, apraxia of speech may occur.

Descending Motor Pathways (Upper Motoneurons)

Descending motor pathways include direct and indirect bundles of fibers (tracts) that make connections with nuclei in the brain stem and spinal cord. These tracts are considered upper motoneurons, whereas tracts arising from brain stem and spinal cord nuclei that ultimately connect with the muscles are considered lower motoneurons. The direct motor pathways, also referred to as pyramidal tracts, include two major bundles of nerve fibers: the corticospinal tract and the corticobulbar tract. These tracts are responsible for carrying out voluntary activity of the body and head, respectively, given "commands" to do so from the premotor cortex. They originate in the motor cortex and are primarily excitatory in function.

The topographic arrangement of cell bodies in the motor cortex giving rise to corticospinal and corticobulbar fibers is an important aspect of the direct motor system. Specifically, these cell bodies are arranged such that fibers arising from certain areas of the cortex course to specific muscle groups. A schematic representation of this topographic arrangement is shown in Figure 18–2. As can be seen, corticobulbar fibers arise from the areas of the brain involved in motor activity of the neck, face, and mouth; therefore it is the corticobulbar system that is most important for speech production.

The corticospinal and corticobulbar tracts are considered to be direct because from their origin in the motor cortex they course without interruption (synapse) to either the spinal cord in the case of the corticospinal tract or to the brain stem (bulb) in the case of the corticobulbar tract. Before synapsing in the spinal cord, most corticospinal fibers cross over or decussate to the opposite (contralateral) side. Some corticobulbar fibers also cross over to the contralateral side; however, others remain uncrossed (ipsilateral). This crossing of fibers influences the side of the body or head on which clinical signs are seen when a lesion occurs.

Lesions of the direct motor pathways result in disrupted conduction of neural information to the motor nuclei of the brain stem and spinal cord. This blockage causes weakness or paralysis of muscles innervated by the portion of the tract involved. In addition, a reduction in muscle tone or hypotonia results because of a loss of input to the muscle fibers. Reflexes are often reduced, and some abnormal reflexes (e.g., Babinski's reflex) are manifested because of a reduction in the suppressive functions of the pathways. Lesions occurring above the level of decussation result in clinical signs on the opposite side of the head or body. Of course, when portions of the pathways that do not decussate are involved, clinical signs are on the same side of the body as the lesion.

In addition to the direct pathways coursing from the cortex to the spinal cord and brain stem nuclei, there is another set of pathways that are also involved in motor activity. These pathways are considered indirect because before reaching the lower motoneurons, they synapse or make connections with subcortical nuclei. There are three major indirect motor pathways including the rubrospinal tract, the reticulospinal tract, and the vestibulospinal tract, which are considered the extrapyramidal tract because they do not course with the pyramidal tract.

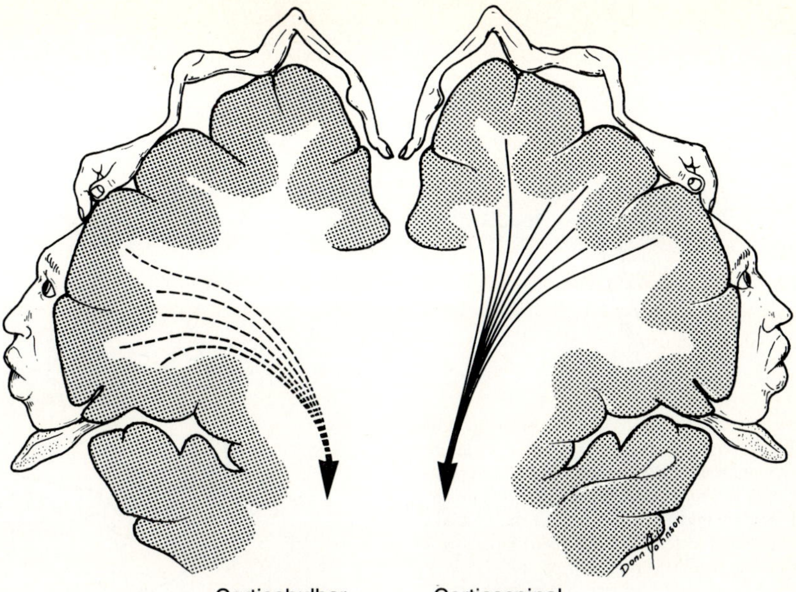

Figure 18–2 Schematic representation of topographic arrangement of the motor cortex of the brain (frontal section), indicating the origin and parts of the head and body innervated by the corticobulbar and corticospinal tracts.

The indirect pathways function mainly to maintain posture, tone, and associated movement, primarily by inhibiting pyramidal tract activity. Therefore normal motor behavior is dependent on both the direct and indirect pathways. Disruption of the direct motor pathways results in decreased muscle tone, leaving the indirect pathways unchecked. This causes overexcitation of muscles, a condition known as increased tone or spasticity. Muscles in which spasticity is seen depends upon the level of brain damage, following the same topographic schema as the direct activation pathways.

Lesions of the motor pathways of the cerebral hemispheres are common and are called "upper motoneuron lesions." Direct and indirect motor pathways are rarely damaged in isolation; therefore clinical findings are usually a combination of effects from a disruption of both. A unilateral lesion results in weakness, slowed motor activity, spasticity, and abnormal reflexes on the side opposite to the lesion. Whereas a bilateral lesion results in these signs in muscles on both sides of the body. Upper motoneuron lesions involving muscles of speech production in an adult result in dysarthria often labelled "spastic dysarthria."

Control Circuits: Basal Ganglia and Cerebellum

Two major groups of nuclei and their connections, the basal ganglia and the cerebellum, serve to integrate and coordinate direct and indirect pathway activity such that efficient and smooth motor behavior is accomplished. These groups of nuclei are considered control circuits because they modify information transmitted by way of the direct and indirect descending pathways that, in turn, influence lower motoneurons.

The basal ganglia are important for the modification of posture for movements initiated in the cerebral cortex and for controlling movements associated with those initiated in the cortex. The basal ganglia consist of subcortical nucleus centers including the caudate nucleus, the putamen, and the globus pallidus. The substantia nigra and subthalamic nucleus are closely related to the basal ganglia and are also considered to be part of the system. Like the indirect activation pathways, the basal ganglia and its connections are considered part of the extrapyramidal tract because they are concerned with motor activity, but are not part of the pyramidal tract. Pathways of the basal ganglia are simply a series of loops that interconnect the various nucleus centers with each other and with the cortex, as shown in Figure 18–3.

In general, excess discharge in the basal ganglia produces slowing, whereas a lack of discharge produces hyperactivity. Disruption of the basal ganglia, then, results in abnormal movements and changes in muscle tone. Specifically, a reduction in mobility (hypokinesia) results in increased tone known as rigidity, or involuntary movements (hyperkinesia) may be manifested. Hypokinetic movements are slow, stiff,

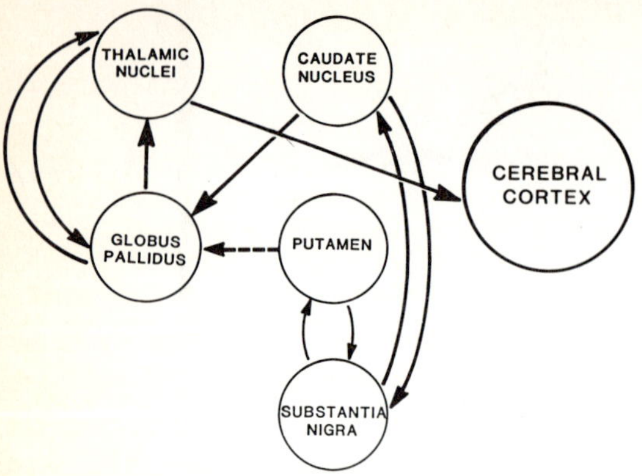

Figure 18–3 Schematic representation of the basal ganglia (caudate nucleus, putamen, and globus pallidus), other nuclei involved (thalamic nuclei, substantia nigra), and connections: caudate nucleus and putamen to globus pallidus to thalamus to cortex to caudate nucleus and putamen; caudate nucleus and putamen to substantia nigra to caudate nucleus and putamen; globus pallidus to thalamus to globus pallidus.

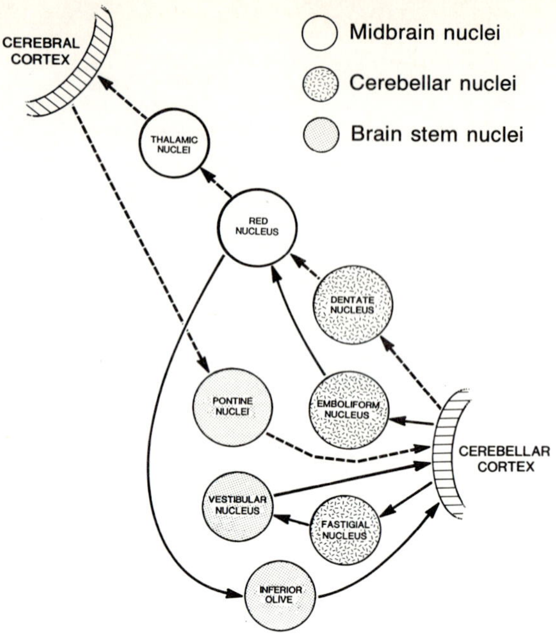

Figure 18–4 Schematic representation of interconnections of the cerebellar cortex, cerebellar nuclei (dentate, emboliform and fastigium), brain stem nuclei (vestibular, pontine, and inferior oliva), midbrain nuclei (red nucleus, thalamus), and cortex. Three cerebellar pathways are shown: the cerebellodentatorubrothalamocorticopontocerebellar loop; the cerebellorubroolivocerebellar loop; the cerebellovestibulocerebellar loop.

and initiated or stopped with great difficulty, and abnormal postures are often seen. Hypokinetic movements are seen in muscles at rest (resting tremor) and during movement. With a lesion in the basal ganglia, one may see these abnormal movements in the speech musculature as well as in other muscles of the body. Either hypokinetic or hyperkinetic dysarthria may result.

The cerebellum, the second major control circuit, is concerned with the regulation and coordination of muscle activity, especially skilled movements. This function is carried out in conjunction with the basal ganglia and depends upon input from sensory systems (visual, auditory, proprioceptive, somatic, vestibular) and from sensory and motor aspects of the cerebral cortex. In turn, the cerebellum sends outputs to brain stem neurons and to the motor cortex. Nerve fibers enter and leave the cerebellum by means of three loops, as shown in Figure 18–4.

As can be seen, pathways of the cerebellum are highly connected with other structures and pathways involved in motor activity. These connections are designed to modulate activities of other centers in controlling activities including equilibrium, posture and gait, and voluntary movements. Lesions of the cerebellum may result in impaired balance, an inability to stand or sit without swaying or falling (truncal ataxia), unsteady walking or staggering gait (gait ataxia), irregular movements of the limbs (limb ataxia), loss of muscle coordination (dyssynergia), loss of ability to measure range of motion (dysmetria), tremor with voluntary activity (intention tremor), and abnormal head and eye movements (nystagmus). When speech is disrupted secondary to a lesion of the cerebellum, ataxic dysarthria results.

Final Common Pathways

The final common pathways, also known as the lower motoneuron system, is the peripheral mechanism by which all motor activity is mediated. Motor information from the direct and indirect pathways, the basal ganglia, and cerebellum all influence information transmitted to muscles via the final common pathways.

The final common pathways important for speech production arise from motor nuclei in the brain stem and are called "cranial nerves." There are twelve pairs of cranial nerves; those involved in motor aspects of speech production include (1) the fifth, the trigeminal nerve; (2) the seventh, the facial nerve; (3) the ninth, the glossopharyngeal nerve; (4) the tenth, the vagus nerve; (5) the eleventh, the accessory nerve; and (6) the twelfth, the hypoglossal nerve. Table 18–2 lists each of these nerves along with muscles innervated by each. Some of these and other cranial nerves also serve sensory functions that are important in speech production.

Some cranial nerves are bilaterally represented, innervating muscles on the opposite (contralateral) side and on the same (ipsilateral) side of the head and neck (the ninth, tenth, and eleventh nerves); some are primarily contralateral with just a few ip-

TABLE 18–2 Muscles Innervated by Cranial Nerves Involved in Speech Production and Their Primary Function

Cranial Nerve	*Muscle Innervated*	*Primary Function*
Trigeminal (the fifth)	Muscles of mastication	Chewing
	Anterior belly of digastricus	Moves hyoid bone upward and forward
	Mylohyoideus	Moves hyoid bone in initial phase of swallowing
		Depresses lower jaw
	Tensor tympani	Moves tympanic membrane
	Tensor veli palatini	Moves soft palate
Facial (the seventh)	Muscles of facial expression	
	Buccinator	Moves cheeks
		Pulls mouth angle laterally and posteriorly
		Tenses cheek
		Narrows mouth opening
		Presses lips and cheeks against teeth
	Levator anguli oris	Elevates corner of mouth
		Elevates lower lip
	Mentalis	Chin muscle
		Protrudes lower lip
		Expression of doubt
	Orbicularis oris	Adducts lip
		Narrows lip against teeth
	Platysma	Protrudes lip
		Elevates lower lip
		Pulls corner of mouth downward & outward
		Pouting
	Depressor labii inferioris	Moves lip downward and laterally
	Levator labii superioris	Moves lip upward and laterally
	Risorius	Retracts corner of mouth
	Depressor anguli oris	Pulls mouth angle down
	Zygomaticus minor	Pulls corner of mouth upward and laterally
		Smiling
	Posterior belly of digastricus	Moves hyoid bone upward and backward
	Stylohyoideus	Elevates, retracts, and tilts hyoid bone
Glossopharyngeal (the ninth)	Stylopharyngeus	Elevates pharynx during swallowing and speech
Vagus (the tenth)	Muscles of the palate	
	Palatoglossus	Draws tongue up and back
	Levator veli palatini	Major mass of soft palate
		Lifts soft palate up and back
		Elevates and widens pharyngeal opening of eustacian tube during swallow
	Palatopharyngeus	Depresses soft palate
		Raises and lowers larynx in first stage of swallow
	Tensor veli palatini	Lifts soft palate for velopharyngeal closure
	Uvulae	Elevates uvula
	Muscles of the pharynx	
	Cricopharyngeus	Valving of pharyngoesophageal junction
	Contrictor pharyngis inferior	Sphincter action of pharynx during swallow
	Constrictor pharyngis medius	Sphincter action of pharynx during swallow
	Constrictor pharyngis superior	Sphincter action of pharynx during swallow
	Palatopharyngeus	Depresses soft palate
		Raises and lowers larynx during first stage of swallow
	Salpingopharyngeus	Opens eustacian tube
		Elevates pharynx in first stage of swallow
	Stylopharyngeus	Sphincter action of pharynx in area of soft palate
		Elevates larynx and pharynx
	Intrinsic muscles of the larynx	
	Cricoarytenoideus posterior	Inspiration
	Arytenoideus transversus	Widens glottis
		Adducts vocal folds

TABLE 18–2 Continued

Cranial Nerve	*Muscle Innervated*	*Primary Function*
	Arytenoideus obliquus	Adducts vocal folds
	Aryepiglotticus	Adducts aryepiglottic folds
	Cricoarytenoideus lateralis	Adducts and abducts vocal folds
	Thyroarytenoideus	Shortens vocal folds
	Cricothyroideus	Lengthens vocal folds
	Vocalis	Vibrates vocal folds
	Ventricularis	Ventricular fold movement
	Thyroepiglotticus	Depresses epiglottis
Accessory (the eleventh)	Muscles of the palate	
	Palatoglossus	Draws tongue up and back
	Levator veli palatini	Major mass of soft palate
		Lifts soft palate up and back
		Elevates and widens pharyngeal opening of the eustacian tube during swallow
	Palatopharyngeus	Depresses soft palate
		Raises and lowers larynx in first stage of swallow
	Tensor veli palatine	Lifts soft palate for velopharyngeal closure
	Uvulae	Elevates uvula
	Intrinsic muscles of the larynx	
	Cricoarytenoideus posterior	Inspiration
	Arytenoideus transversus	Adducts vocal fold
	Arytenoideus obliquus	Adducts vocal folds
	Aryepiglotticus	Adducts aryepiglottic folds
	Cricoarytenoideus lateralis	Adducts and abducts vocal folds
	Thyroarytenoideus	Shortens vocal folds
	Cricothyroideus	Lengthens vocal folds
	Vocalis	Vibrates vocal folds
	Ventricularis	Ventricular fold movement
	Thyroepiglotticus	Depresses epiglottis
Hypoglossal (the twelfth)	Intrinsic muscles of the tongue	
	Longitudinal inferior linguae	Shortens tongue from front to back
	Longitudinalis superior linguae	Shortens tongue to make it thicker and wider
	Traversus linguae	Narrows and protrudes tongue
	Verticalis linguae	Flattens and broadens tongue
	Muscles connecting the tongue to the hyoid and mandible	
	Genioglossus	Protrudes tongue, moves tip, and depresses medially for food
	Hyoglossus	Moves tongue downward and backward
	Palatoglossus	Elevates tongue posteriorly
	Styloglossus	Retracts and elevates tongue

silateral fibers (the fifth and twelfth nerves); and some are mixed, with some fibers being only contralateral and others being both contralateral and ipsilateral (the seventh nerve). The portion of the seventh cranial nerve that innervates the upper half of the face is contralateral and ipsilateral, whereas the portion of the seventh nerve that innervates the lower half of the face is completely crossed.

The arrangement of cranial nerve innervation of muscles is important when upper motoneuron damage occurs. That is, with a unilateral upper motoneuron lesion, muscles innervated by the ninth, tenth, and eleventh nerves remain unaffected because they are bilaterally innervated. Mild and probably transient contralateral loss of functioning of muscles innervated by the fifth and twelfth nerves may occur, and the lower facial muscles (the seventh nerve) is affected, while the upper facial musculature is preserved. Lower motoneuron lesions involving nerve fibers of the final common pathways result in weakness on the same side of the lesion. Such lesions are called lower motoneuron lesions and result in flaccid dysarthria.

Sensory and Motor Integration

Motor activity is highly dependent upon sensory input from the nervous system. That is, motor activity occurs in response to sensations arising from stimuli external or internal to the body, including tactile, proprioceptive, auditory, visual, and other. This sensory input is processed at several levels of the nervous system. For example, simple reflexes such as the knee jerk are controlled at the level of the spinal cord by tactile stimuli, whereas more complex motor behavior is controlled at the cortical level. At this level, the nervous system processes input from sensory receptors throughout the body, modifying them as needed in response to environmental conditions.

The specific neuromechanisms involved in processing and integrating sensory information will not be described here. However, it is important to note that disruption in sensory processing often occurs along with disruption of motor systems, adding to the complex motor problems seen secondary to brain damage. Without normal sensory input, motor behavior is abnormal.

DEVELOPMENTAL DYSARTHRIA

Etiology and Behavioral Pathology

There are many conditions that interfere with neurologic development that may occur before birth (prenatal), during or immediately following birth (perinatal), or later during early childhood (postnatal). Any of these conditions may result in dysarthria depending upon which brain mechanisms are involved.

Prenatal problems include genetic factors such as blood incompatibilities of mother and child, metabolic disturbances, and others. One prenatal factor that has been widely studied is Rh incompatibility when the mother's blood is Rh negative and the child's is Rh positive. This problem is now easily detected prior to birth and can be managed through medical intervention. Other genetic problems can also be detected prior to birth through amniocentesis, wherein amniotic fluid is extracted from the mother and analyzed for genetic makeup. Some disorders can be managed medically and others cannot.

Other problems causing brain damage result from abnormal conditions occurring during pregnancy. These include problems that disrupt oxygen supply to the fetus such as compression of the umbilical cord and bleeding of the placenta. Maternal infections, exposure to roentgenograms, chemicals, and other problems occurring during early pregnancy may also cause damage to the neurologic system of the fetus.

Perinatal factors include problems occurring during or soon after birth. For example, head trauma may occur in difficult deliveries either from the use of forceps during delivery or from cranial pressure exerted by contact between the baby's head and the mother's pelvis. Premature and rapid deliveries may also be problematic in that they do not allow for gradual adjustment of the fetal circulatory system to extrauterine conditions. Respiratory problems that occur during and following birth may also result in brain damage.

Many other problems may occur well after birth. These include infections such as encephalitis and meningitis,[53] brain abscesses, tumors, stroke, and other encephalopathies resulting in disorders such as Reye's syndrome.[54] Head injuries among children are also common. It has been estimated that the annual brain-injury rate per 100,000 children is 185 and that major causes of pediatric brain injury are falls, recreational activities, and motor vehicle accidents.[55]

Any of the aforementioned conditions and others may result in developmental dysarthria, depending upon the site and extent of brain damage. The neurologic basis for developmental dysarthria found in children is similar to that described for acquired adult disorders. That is, dysarthria results when, during the course of development, damage to the motor cortex, direct and indirect motor pathways, basal ganglia, and/or cerebellum occurs. Brain injury in any of these areas disrupts information communicated via the final common pathway to and from the muscles involved in speech production. I should point out that brain damage affecting the motor system occurring prenatally and perinatally is often labelled cerebral palsy. When damage occurs postnatally, it may or may not be labelled cerebral palsy. For example, some head-injured children evidence motor disorders similar to those seen in cerebral palsy, but may not be labelled as such. Criteria used for labelling neurologically impaired children as having cerebral palsy are unclear and vary, depending upon the age of the child, severity of motor impairment, and cause of brain damage.

There are two major types of dysarthria that are commonly discussed with regard to developmental neuromotor disorders. These include spastic dysarthria and dyskinetic dysarthria. Spastic dysarthria results from infarction of the upper motoneuron system (motor cortex and/or direct and indirect motor pathways), whereas dyskinetic dysarthria results from primary involvement of the basal ganglia and connections. Mixed dysarthrias among neurologically impaired children also occur when aspects of both the upper motoneuron system and the basal ganglia are involved.[56] Other types of dysarthria (e.g., ataxic dysarthria resulting from cerebellar infarction and flaccid dysarthria resulting from lower motoneuron involvement) appear to be less common in children than in adults.[1]

Abnormal Movement Patterns

A unique aspect of neuromotor disorders in children relates to the fact that the neurologic system is damaged prior to completion of its development. In this regard, developmental disorders are different from acquired disorders. In addition to weakness and changes in muscle tone that result from malfunctioning of the neuromotor system, abnormal movement patterns—not seen in adults—may be present. These abnormal patterns result because of alterations in neurologic development. In a normal child, some components of the motor system develop before others and therefore dominate motor behavior until other systems are completely developed. For example, excitatory motor components develop before inhibitory ones. When the normal motor system has completely developed, some of the early motor patterns disappear, some remain but are no longer dominant, and some continue as in infancy throughout life.

When the neurologic system is damaged during the course of development, early patterns of behavior that normally disappear, do not; whereas other early dominant movement patterns that normally become nondominant, remain dominant or become exaggerated. In addition, children often develop compensatory motor patterns in an attempt to overcome movement problems. These exaggerated, retained, and/or compensatory behaviors result largely because normal inhibitory mechanisms do not develop. Therefore excitatory muscle activity remains unchecked as the brain matures following a lesion. For example, the Moro embrace reflex may persist, and tonic neck reflexes and other postural reactions may become overly dominant and exaggerated.*

Several writers, including Ingram,[61] Sheppard,[62] Alexander,[63] and McDonald and Chance,[64] have described specific infantile oral reflexes that involve aspects of speech production including labial, lingual, velar, pharyngeal, mandibular, laryngeal, respiratory, and others. Table 18–3, taken from McDonald and Chance,[64] provides a list of some of these reflexes involving structures used in articulation of speech. Abnormal and compensatory oral motor behaviors seen in neurologically impaired children are listed in Table 18–4, which is taken from Alexander.[63] Researchers have suggested that these and other infantile reflexive behaviors may be critical to the development of speech production in neurologically impaired children. That is, Mysak,[65–68] Sheppard,[62,69] and others have suggested that abnormal oral motor reflex patterns may interfere with speech production. However, this assertion has been questioned. For example, Hixon and Hardy indicated that nonspeech and speech movement patterns are controlled by different neurologic mechanisms and are therefore unrelated.[70]

Love, Hagerman, and Taimi studied the relationship between infantile oral reflexes and speech performance in 60 children and young adults diagnosed with spastic, athetoid, and mixed spastic and athetoid cerebral palsy.[71] Nine reflexes were tested including rooting, lip, mouth opening, biting, chewing, sucking, cephalic, auriculocephalic, and nasocephalic. In addition, speech proficiency was measured by means of the Irwin Integrated Articulation Test for Cerebral Palsied Children,[72] yielding a percent correct articulation score for each subject.

Results of the study indicated that only 25 percent (15 of 60) of the subjects presented with infantile oral reflexes, and the mean number of abnormal reflexes displayed by each subject was 2.2. (This finding contrasted with data reported by Sheppard, who found that 43 of 52 dysarthric subjects [84 percent] displayed abnormal reflex patterns.)[62] When Love et al examined speech performance of the 15 subjects displaying these abnormal oral reflexes, eight of the children demonstrated no speech, and all but one of the remaining seven evidenced some articulatory impairment.[71] However, a clear pattern between the number of abnormal reflexes present and the level of articulatory proficiency was not found.

While examination of the data reported by Love et al indicates that there may be some relationship between the presence of abnormal reflexes and abnormal speech production,[71] there were a number of children with dysarthria (N = 11) in the study who did not evidence abnormal oral reflexes, and one subject who evidenced abnormal reflexes and no dysarthria. These data, coupled with the findings reported by Sheppard,[62] indicate that the presence of abnormal reflexes and dysarthria varies greatly across neurologically impaired children. Furthermore, keep in mind that correlative data do not suggest a cause and effect relationship. That is, even if all children with developmental dysarthria had abnormal oral reflexes, this would not mean that the abnormal oral reflexes cause or even influence the occurrence of dysarthria in these children. The point here is that

* These reflexes and postural reactions are common among children with cerebral palsy. The Moro embrace or startle reflex occurs when the head and shoulders are raised off of a table and the head is suddenly dropped back. It also occurs in response to loud noise, resulting in the arms and head extending backward. The tonic neck reflexes involve movement of the head and extremities. In the symmetrical tonic neck reflex, when the head is moved backward, the arms extend and the legs flex; when the head is moved forward and down, the arms flex and the legs extend. In the asymmetrical tonic neck reflex, when the head is turned to one side, the arm on that side is extended, and the opposite arm is flexed. There are other abnormal movement patterns seen in neurologically impaired children. These have been well described in several sources.[57–60]

TABLE 18–3 Infantile Oral Reflexes Observed in Neurologically Impaired Children

Reflex	*Stimulus*	*Response*
Cephalic reactions	Stroking the lobe of the ear or the nostril	Turns head away from stimulus
Facial response	Sharp tapping around mouth	Rounding and protrusion of lips as in pouting
Rooting reflex	Repeated light stroking of the cheek or around the mouth	Movement of the head as if trying to get a nipple into the mouth
Mouth opening	Sight of an object such as a nipple, finger, or tongue depressor, which is usually associated with mouth opening	Lowering of the mandible and separation of lips
Lip reflex	Tapping around the angle formed at the corner of the mouth	Involuntary movements of the lips—lip closure and pouting
Biting reflex	Object placed between teeth (or gums)	Strong, sustained elevation of the mandible
Sucking reflex	Gentle pushing and pulling on a nipple or finger placed in mouth	Alternating protruding and retracting movement of the tongue, often with elevation of the tip
Chewing reflex	Tapping with teeth or gums with a tongue blade	Alternating elevations and depressions of the mandible
Laughing	Light stroking or tickling, particularly of the sides of the thorax	Involuntary twitching of the body, opening of the mouth, disruption of breathing rhythm, often accompanied by sound production on both inhalation and exhalation
Swallowing (Oral)	Presence of food or liquid in oral cavity	Waveline motion of tongue to propel food into oropharynx
Swallowing	Contact of food or fluid with mucosa of faucial pillars and pharyngeal wall	Contraction of faucial pillars and walls of pharynx, elevation and closing of larynx, and momentary suspension of respiration

From McDonald ET, Chance B. Cerebral palsy. Englewood Cliffs, NJ: Prentice-Hall, 1964:123.

neurologically impaired children with developmental dysarthria have complex motor problems that may be complicated by abnormal reflexes and postural reactions. The extent to which these behaviors are considered in management of children with dysarthria will be discussed in sections addressing assessment and treatment of developmental dysarthria in this chapter.

Spastic Disorders

Children with developmental spastic dysarthria may have a wide range of speech problems resulting from damage to the neuromotor system. In general, hyperreflexia and hypertonia of muscle groups involved in speech production is seen. One should keep in mind that variability across children with spastic dysarthria is common. Because of subtle variations in patterns of brain injury, speech pathology may be different in different children. In addition to variability across children, variability may also be seen across muscle groups within the same child. For example, involvement of respiratory and laryngeal muscle groups may be present in the absence of motor impairment of the oral mechanism.

Many children with spastic dysarthria also evidence spastic involvement of the upper and lower extremities and are classified as such. These classifications include spastic hemiplegia, spastic paraplegia, spastic diplegia, and spastic quadriplegia. All of these motor disorders result from impairment of portions of the upper motoneuron system. It is important to understand the extent of neurologic involvement found in children carrying these classifications because they provide information on the distribution of brain damage. Because of the close proximity of corticobulbar and corticospinal tracts at the cortical level and during their course to the brain stem and spinal cord, damage to one system often occurs concomitant with the other. Therefore classifications may

TABLE 18–4 Abnormal and Compensatory Oral Motor Behaviors of Infants and Young Children with Cerebral Palsy

Behavior	*Description*
Cheek-lip retraction	Abnormal pulling back of cheeks; lips appear thin and form a tight line across mouth; often seen with head and neck hyperextension and tongue retraction
Exaggerated jaw closure	Abnormal jaw closure on objects such as feeding utensils
Exaggerated tongue protrusion	Forward-backward suckling movement with exaggerated forward motion; tongue appears thick
Jaw thrusting	Strong depression of lower jaw; jaw may be stuck in open position; position occurs with head-neck hyperextension
Jaw thrusting with protrusion	Compensatory strong depression of lower jaw occurring in an attempt to close jaw
Jaw thrusting with retraction	Strong depression and retraction of lower jaw seen concomitant with head and neck hyperextension and tongue retraction
Lip pursing	Lips pursed and protruded with tension extended to the cheeks; corners of lips retracted slightly
Tongue retraction	Posterior movement of tongue into oropharyngeal area occurring with head and neck hyperextension; back of tongue appears humped; the tongue is thick
Tongue retraction with anterior elevation	Tongue assumes posterior position in oral cavity with tongue tip elevated and pushing against hard palate and alveolar ridge; compensatory for tongue instability
Tongue thrusting	Strong forward pushing of the tongue; tongue appears thick
Tonic biting	Strong jaw closure in response to tactile stimulation on biting surface of teeth or gums; jaw is stuck in closed position; increased head, neck, trunk extension occurs in attempt to overcome abnormal pattern

After Alexander R. Oral-motor treatment for infants and young children with cerebral palsy. Semin Speech Lang 1987; 8:87.

be helpful in predicting the extent to which muscles involved in speech production are affected.

Spastic Hemiplegia

In spastic hemiplegia, the upper and lower extremities of one side of the body are involved, resulting from unilateral infarction of the corticospinal system. The corticobulbar system may or may not be involved. When it is involved, hemiparesis and spasticity may be seen in the lower half of the face and oral musculature on the side contralateral to the lesion, resulting in dysarthria. However, because of the bilateral neurologic control of many of the muscles involved in speech production, dysfunction of the speech musculature often resolves in these children. As pointed out by Kamalashile in a study of 110 children with cerebral palsy, only two of the children with hemiplegia evidenced dysarthria.[73]

Spastic Paraplegia

Spastic paraplegic children present with involvement of both lower extremities while the upper extremities remain unaffected. In addition, the muscles of the torso walls may be involved. When torso muscle functioning is impaired, respiration may be impaired, and, in some cases, a mild dysarthria may result. For example, in the Kamalashile study, dysarthria was seen in two paraplegic children.[73] In most cases, however, respiratory impairment does not affect speech production, and dysarthria is not present. Only when other aspects of the speech musculature are affected, is a significant dysarthria manifested.

Spastic Diplegia

The extent of neuromotor involvement in spastic diplegia exceeds that of hemiplegia and paraplegia, with the muscles of both the upper and lower extremities and the torso being involved. The spastic involvement in diplegia also often extends to the neck musculature; however, involvement of the arms and neck area are less severe than that of the legs. In children with spastic diplegia, speech production may or may not be impaired. Some children may evidence rather mild speech problems such as dysprosody resulting from involvement of the respiratory system coupled with impairment of the extrinsic laryngeal musculature. But other children may evidence severe dysarthria resulting from involvement of the oral, laryngeal, and respiratory musculature.[1] As pointed out by Hardy,[1] oral and laryngeal motor involvement may not be extensive in these cases. However, with a marked reduction in respiratory support, mild dysfunction of oral and laryngeal mechanisms may result in significant dysarthria. Kamalashile reported that nine of the diplegic children studied had speech problems.[73]

Spastic Quadriplegia

Spastic quadriplegia is the most severe of the spastic motor classifications. In these children, involvement is apparent in both the upper and lower extremities in equal degrees of severity. In addition, motor involvement extends to the oral and laryngeal musculature. Therefore, in spastic quadriplegic children, developmental dysarthria is often seen, and it is often severe. Speech production problems were reported in 63 of the spastic quadriplegic children studied by Kamalashile.[73]

Dyskinetic Disorders

In children with dyskinetic dysarthria, as in spastic dysarthria, variability exists with regard to the various dimensions of speech production that may be disrupted. Movement of the lips, tongue, mandible, soft palate, laryngeal mechanism, and the respiratory mechanism may be impaired secondary to involvement of the thoracic wall and orofacial musculature. In children with dyskinetic dysarthria, all four extremities are often involved; therefore they may be labelled quadriplegic, with the upper extremities being more seriously involved than the lower extremities. In general, movement patterns in impaired muscle groups are lacking in coordination, and involuntary motion is seen. The involuntary movements associated with dyskinesia may vary in frequency and type. For example, athetoid movements, chorea, and other abnormal movement patterns may be seen. Athetoid movements are usually described as slow and writhing, whereas chorea is characterized by rapid, flailing, and jerking movements of the extremities.

Speech Pathology

Review of the literature focused on identification of speech pathology associated with the developmental dysarthrias is limited. Although several studies have compared performance of dyskinetic and spastic children on certain speech and nonspeech tasks, many paramenters of speech production have not been studied extensively. Further, research methodologies employed in many studies have been problematic. For example, some studies have not controlled for important variables such as hearing ability and intelligence, and children presenting with wide ranges of severity have been included for study in a single group. Therefore these sources of uncontrolled variability in subjects studied make it difficult to draw conclusions about specific speech patterns occurring in children with dysarthria. In addition to these limitations, it is interesting to note that most of the studies that focused on speech production problems associated with developmental dysarthria were published in the mid to late 1960s. By the 1970s, literature discussing dysarthria in children focused primarily on prespeech, oral motor behaviors, feeding, and positioning with little discussion of speech production behavior. This focus has perhaps been influenced by factors such as (1) changes in legislation, for example, passage of the Handicapped Children's Early Education Act (1968) and The Education of All Handicapped Children's Act (PL 94–142) that together influenced the delivery of speech-language pathology services to younger and more severely impaired children; (2) popularity of neurodevelopmental theories and approaches to treatment;[74–79] and (3) discussion and development of early feeding programs for neurologically impaired children.[80]

Hardy appears to be the first to refocus on speech production problems in these children, specifically in children with cerebral palsy.[1] The following discussion is presented from a point of view perhaps similar to that of Hardy's. That is, speech pathologists need to understand, carefully assess, and treat speech problems seen in children with dysarthria, without overlooking the importance of their concomitant impairments. Therefore the following discussion will focus primarily on speech production problems seen in children with developmental dysarthria. Specifically, each of the subsystems involved in speech production (respiration, phonation, resonance, and articulation) will be discussed. Where possible, literature will be cited comparing the performance of spastic and dyskinetic dysarthric children.

Respiration

Respiratory functioning may be impaired in speakers with both spastic and dyskinetic dysarthria. Specifically, when the torso musculature is involved in spastic paraplegia, diplegia, and quadriplegia and in dyskinetic disorders, respiration may be abnormal. Most often, however, malfunctioning of the respiratory system alone does not result in significant speech production problems. It is when other subsystems of speech production are impaired along with respiration that the impaired respiratory component becomes important. Hardy presents perhaps the most comprehensive discussion of respiratory function problems seen in developmental dysarthria.[1] In that discussion, Hardy pointed out that children with spastic and dyskinetic dysarthria have similar problems with their expiratory and inspiratory abilities and that a similar progression of difficulty is seen with increased severity of neurologic involvement. In mildly and moderately involved children, expiratory functioning is relatively more impaired than inspiratory functioning; whereas severely involved children evidence severe restriction of both inspiration and expiration.

A breathing pattern often seen in children with cerebral palsy and with dysarthria is "reversed breathing."[81] This breathing pattern occurs when inhalation movements of the thoracic musculature and exhalation movements of the abdominal musculature occur simultaneously. This breathing pattern, according to Westlake and Rutherford,[82] results in reduced air volume of the rib cage and concomitant reduction in the quantity of air inhaled. Children with dysarthria may also evidence reduced lung volume or vital capacity[81,83] in the absence of a "reversed breathing" pattern. Problems with expiration and inspiration coupled with decreased vital capacity may result in reduced efficiency in generating expiratory air pressure to drive the vocal tract.

Studies of respiration in children with dysarthria have shown that breathing patterns are often disrupted in children with spastic, athetoid, and ataxic cerebral palsy. However, athetoid children appear to evidence more severe involvement than others. Athetoid children with dyskinetic dysarthria present with "varying gradations of a pattern of irregular, shallow, and noisy breathing" (p 358),[84] resulting in disruption in volume, rate, and rhythm of speech.[85] In a study in which the breathing patterns of 58 children with athetoid cerebral palsy were studied, Palmer reported that every subject had at least one breathing abnormality.[86] In contrast, children with spastic dysarthria presented with relatively better respiratory control, although these children evidenced reductions in chest movement and greater abdominal breathing movement than did normal children.

There are several speech problems that may result from these and other impairments in respiratory functioning in children with dysarthria. Some abnormal breathing patterns and speech production problems that may result from respiratory dysfunction are listed in Tables 18–5 and 18–6, respectively.

Phonation

A variety of phonation problems may be seen in children with dysarthria, some of which result from impairments in respiratory functioning. Phonation problems also commonly result from abnormal body postures and reactions. For example, when hyperextension of the head occurs in the symmetrical tonic neck reflex, breathy vocal quality may result. As explained by Davis, head "hyperextension

TABLE 18–5 Abnormal Breathing Patterns Seen in Children with Dysarthria

Rapid breathing[64]
Shallow breathing[86]
Noisy breathing[84]
Involuntary movement of respiratory musculature[64]
Irregular cycline[84]
"Reversed breathing"[81]

TABLE 18–6 Speech Production Problems Seen in Children with Developmental Dysarthria that may Result from Respiratory Dysfunction

Short phrasing[1]
Frequent inspiration[1]
Reduced syllabic repetitions[102]
Decreased rate of speech[89]
Uncontrolled prolonged exhalation[64]

biochemically facilitates vocal fold abduction'' (p 103).[81] Other phonation problems result from involvement of the vagus (tenth cranial) nerve. In this case, strained vocal quality may be seen because of hypertonicity and spasticity of the intrinsic laryngeal musculature. This problem is common in spastic dysarthria.

Reactions to decreased lung volume and other compensatory learned behaviors may also contribute to hypertension of the vocal folds. For example, children with low vital capacity may use increased body tension to push expiratory air for speech production. This causes an increase in general tension in the laryngeal mechanism, and the child with dysarthria sounds as if she or he is using "residual air phonation."[81]

There are three general dimensions of phonation that may be disrupted in dysarthric speakers. These include (1) pitch, which is determined by the longitudinal tension of the vocal folds, (2) loudness, which is determined by the amount of medial compression of the folds, and (3) periodicity, which is determined by patterns of vocal fold vibration. In children with dysarthria, any of these dimensions may be impaired. Pitch may be high or low, and reduced pitch range may be evident. Loudness is often reduced, and breathiness and aperiodicity may occur.

Few studies are reported in the literature that have attempted to describe phonation problems in developmental dysarthria. Early studies by Rutherford[87] and Leith and Steer[88] indicated, based on listener judgments, that pitch, loudness, and rate are often affected in dysarthria. Examining aspects of phonation in 48 children with athetoid cerebral palsy and 74 with spastic cerebral palsy, Rutherford reported a greater degree of impairment in the children with athetoid as compared to those with spastic cerebral palsy.[87] Specifically, she found decreases in pitch range, increases in loudness, and breathiness to be greater in the athetoid children. Further, athetoid speech was slower, and abnormal rhythm was often noted. Laryngeal dysfunction noted in the athetoid children in the Rutherford study included dilator spasm, constrictor spasm, and phonation out of phase with articulation. Structural and functional abnormalities of the vocal folds are less often noted in children with spastic dysarthria, although phonation problems are common.

In the more recent literature, only one study focused in this area was found in which fundamental frequency was examined in 50 children.[89] Results indicated that the mean fundamental frequency in dysarthric speakers is similar to that in normal children and that children with spastic and dyskinetic dysarthria perform similarly. Unfortunately, the standard deviation for each group was not reported; therefore the data are of little use in terms of understanding differences among children with dysarthria.

Further study is needed in this area such that phonatory problems in developmental dysarthria can be better understood. Manifestations of phonation problems that have been reported, but that have not been well studied in children with dysarthria are listed in Table 18–7. In addition, possible reasons for each phonatory characteristic are listed.

Resonance

Children with dysarthria may also evidence resonatory and other articulatory problems because of insufficient velopharyngeal functioning. In one study, the authors estimated that approximately 30 percent of children with dysarthria secondary to cerebral palsy had velopharyngeal closure problems.[90] In another study, 34 of 54 children presented with nasality (rhinophonia).[56] These problems may result from malfunction in timing, range of motion, changes in muscle tone, reduced movement (unilateral or bilateral paresis), and/or random reflexive behaviors of the soft palate and/or posterolateral pharyngeal walls. For example, Pruszewicz et al reported that ten of 54 children with dyskinetic dysarthria had disordered velar functioning resulting in hypernasality; four presented with distinct velar asymmetry, and six presented with reduced bilateral movement.[56] Physiologic problems causing perceived hypernasality were undetermined in another 22 children in the study.

Examples of patterns of velopharyngeal dysfunction among speakers with cerebral palsy are presented by Netsell.[91] Specifically, he reported five abnormal velopharyngeal movement patterns seen in these children, using simultaneous recording of in-

TABLE 18–7 Phonation Problems Seen in Children with Developmental Dysarthria and Possible Laryngeal Abnormalities

Phonatory Problem	*Laryngeal Abnormality*
Decreased sustained phonation[56]	Decreased medial compression of vocal folds
Breathy vocal quality[1,87]	Decreased medial compression of vocal folds
"Strained" vocal quality[81]	Hypertension, spasticity of laryngeal musculature
Decreased loudness[1]	Decreased medial compression of vocal folds
Bursts of loudness[81]	Aperiodicity resulting from involuntary activity of laryngeal musculature
Increased loudness[87]	Constrictor spasm; hypertension of laryngeal musculature
Monoloudness; decreased loudness range[1]	Decreased medial compression of vocal folds and immobility of vocal folds
Sudden changes in pitch[81]	Changes in longitudinal tension resulting from involuntary activity of laryngeal mechanism
Monopitch; decreased pitch range[1]	Decreased longitudinal tension and immobility of vocal folds
Slow rate[87]	Out of phase phonation and articulation
Abnormal rhythm[87]	Out of phase phonation and articulation
"Residual air phonation"[81]	Hypertension of vocal folds

traoral air pressure, the rate of nasal air flow, and the speech signal. These patterns included gradual opening, gradual closing, anticipatory closing, retentive opening, and premature opening. In children with gradual opening patterns, early segments of connected speech were produced normally, with the onset of nasal airflow occurring in later segments. In gradual closing, the opposite was observed. That is, the velopharynx gradually opened as connected speech progressed. In anticipatory opening, nasal airflow was seen as speech was initiated and subsided thereafter, and, in children with retentive opening patterns, slow closure of the velopharyngeal port occurred during the formation of individual consonants. Finally, in premature opening, the velopharyngeal seal was broken at inappropriate times during consonant production, thereby disrupting the acoustic form of the consonant. Other patterns of velopharyngeal functioning may also be observed in children with dysarthria. For example, Kent and Netsell reported intermittent velopharyngeal closure resulting from instability of velar elevation in athetoid children.[92]

Disruptions in velopharyngeal functioning result in abnormal intraoral breath pressure needed for production of all speech sounds except nasals. Therefore hypernasality and/or nasal emission may be detected during speech production. Other speech problems such as slow rate of speech may also be manifested secondary to velopharyngeal incompetence, occurring in compensation for slow palatopharyngeal movement.

Articulation

Articulation errors seen in children with dysarthria have been reported by several investigators including Byrne,[93] Clarke and Hoops,[89] Irwin,[94] and Rutherford.[87] These data have indicated that children with dysarthria have complex articulation problems secondary to weakness, decreased range of motion, alterations in timing, changes in muscle tone, abnormal oral movement patterns such as extensor jaw thrust and tongue thrust, and other neuromotor problems of the lips, jaw, and tongue.

In general, studies have shown that dyskinetic dysarthric speakers present with more severe articulation problems than do spastics.[93–97] That is, spastic dysarthric speech is generally more intelligible and less articulatorily impaired than athetoid dysarthric speech.[93,95,98] This finding is perhaps due to the many aberrations in tongue, mandibular, and lip control seen in children with extrapyramidal damage. As pointed out by Palmer, athetoid children evidence difficulty in elevation of the tip of the tongue, gross clumsy tongue movement, bizarre lip closing and facial grimacing, resulting in speech sound production errors.[86]

Studies describing articulatory errors seen in children with dysarthria have pointed out a number of error patterns, some of which remain consistent as these children mature.[95] Specifically, in terms of manner of articulation, children with dysarthria evidence great difficulty with production of fricatives, affricates, and liquids in both initial and final word positions, and stops, nasals, and glides are somewhat easier at least in the initial word position. As pointed out by Byrne, in a study of 61 children with developmental dysarthria with cerebral palsy aged 2 to 7 years, 75 percent of the total group studied produced /w/, /b/, /j/, /m/, and /d/ correctly, and at least 60 percent of the children produced /n/, /h/, /g/, /k/, and /t/ correctly in the initial word position.[93] However, these sounds were produced correctly in the final position in less than 50 percent of responses as were fricatives and affricates in both initial and final positions. In a similar study with older dysarthric speakers, Platt et al indicated that these individuals continue to evidence problems with fricatives and affricates, although productions in the initial position become more accurate with age.[95]

With regard to place of articulation, most errors are noted in production of postdental fricatives (/ð/, /θ/), alveolar fricatives and affricates (/s/, /z/, and /ʤ/), palatal liquids (/r/), and labiodental fricatives (/f/, /v/), but bilabial and velar articulations are more often produced accurately. These patterns, again, are consistent in older children and adults with developmental dysarthria although final word productions of postdental fricatives remain particularly difficult. Figure 18–5 presents data reported by Byrne[93] for children and by Platt et al[95] for adults with developmental dysarthria aged 17 to 55 years.

Phonemic errors made by children with developmental dysarthria have also been studied and classified.[93,96,99] The most comprehensive phonemic analysis reported in the literature was completed by Platt et al on their data with adults with congenital dysarthria.[99] Using a confusion matrix paradigm, they studied articulation errors made in initial and final word positions in 50 subjects. Findings indicated that most errors consist of within-manner (place and voicing errors) as compared to between-manner errors. Specifically, in the initial word position, within-manner fricative, stop, and affricate errors were noted. Fricative errors were most frequent, consisting of devoicing and place errors. Stop errors were largely of place, voicing, and devoicing, and affricate errors were characterized by devoicing. Similar error patterns were noted in the final position. Within-manner fricative errors were most prevalent, with both devoicing and place errors occurring frequently. All affricate within-manner errors were devoicing, nasal errors were place errors, and within-manner stop errors consisted of both place and devoicing.

Between-manner errors were observed less frequently in the Platt et al study.[99] In the initial position, these errors consisted of liquid-to-glide substitutions (/w/ for /l/), affricate-to-stop substitutions (/t/ for /tʃ/), and fricative-to-stop errors (/b/ for /v/). In the final position, between-manner errors consisted primarily of affricate-to-stop and affricate-to-fricative changes.

Vowel productions have also been studied in children with dysarthria,[93–95,100,101] indicating that vowels requiring neutral tongue positions such as /ʌ/ and /a/ are produced more accurately than others. This finding is not surprising given reductions in range of motion of the tongue and other oral structures found in these children. That is, limitations in movement result in an inability to achieve full vocal tract shapes for formation of some vowels, particularly those in the extreme positions of the vowel diagram. These limitations have been demonstrated in cineradiographic studies reported by Kent and Netsell.[92]

Diadochokinetic rate has also been studied in children with dysarthria in both speech and nonspeech conditions.[70,97,102] Results of these and other studies have indicated that these children evidence difficulties with both activities. However, mixed findings have been reported with regard to the correlation between these activities and speech production ability. That is, alternate motion rates using speech stimuli have correlated highly with speech intelligibility in several studies;[70,97,102] whereas conflicting results have been reported with regard to correlations between nonspeech alternate motion rates and speech intelligibility. In a study of 50 children with developmental dysarthria, Hixon and Hardy indicated that of five nonspeech activities including (1) opening and closing of the lips and teeth together, (2) retracting and rounding the lips, (3) raising the tongue to the alveolar ridge and lowering it, (4) lateralizing the tongue from one corner of the mouth to the other, and (5) opening and closing the jaw, only one (lateralizing the tongue) correlated with speech production ability.[70] In a similar study of 15 adults with developmental dysarthria aged 16 to 51 years, Schliesser found three nonspeech activities to be strongly related to severity of dysarthria.[102] These included opening and closing the jaw, retracting the tongue to the alveolar ridge, and retracting and rounding the lips. Tongue lateralization did not correlate with speech production in the Schliesser study. These conflicting findings may indicate differences between younger and older individuals with dysarthria and/or reflect the great heterogeneity seen in developmental dysarthria. Whatever the source(s) of variability in these studies, one can say that most children with developmental dysarthria evidence difficulty in performance of both speech and nonspeech diadochokinetic tasks and that these problems may or may not relate to the severity of dysarthria.

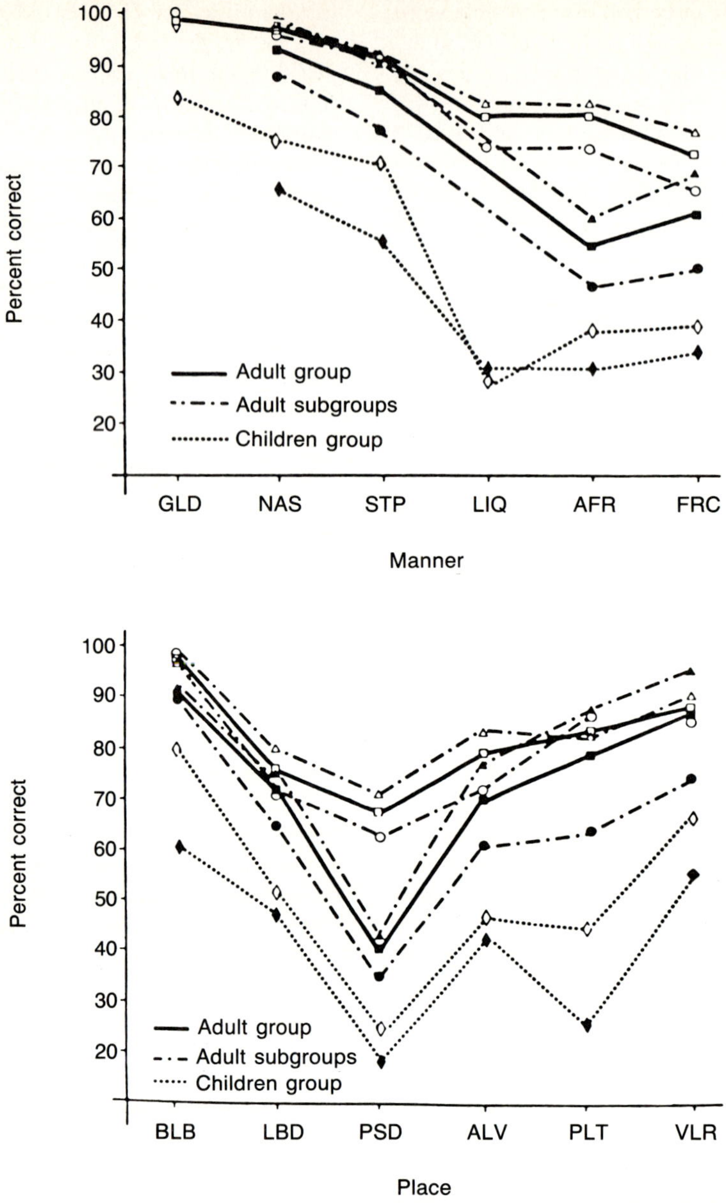

Figure 18–5 Profile of articulatory accuracy (percent subjects correct per phoneme) for manner and place features of English consonants in adults with dysarthria and cerebral palsy.[95] The children's data and profiles were computed from percent correct phoneme values reported by Byrne.[93] Abbreviations: GLD = glide; NAS = nasal; STP = stop; LIQ = liquid; AFR = affricate; FRC = fricative; BLB = bilabial; LBD = labiodental; PSD = postdental; ALV = alveolar; PLT = palatal; VLR = velar; open symbols refer to initial consonants, solid symbols refer to final consonants; o = athetoid adults, △ = spastic adults; □ = adult group; ◇ = children's group. (From Platt JF, Andrews G, Young M, Quinn PT. Dysarthria of adult cerebral palsy: I. Intelligibility and articulatory impairment. J Speech Hear Res 1980; 23:35.)

Assessment

Assessment of dysarthria in children should include an oral motor examination, evaluation of all subsystems of speech production including respiration, phonation, resonance, and articulation, evaluation of prosody, and assessment of intelligibility. During the course of the evaluation, identification of compensatory strategies for potential enhancement of speech production is also necessary. The major purposes of the evaluation are to (1) identify physiologic deficits of the speech-producing musculature, (2) identify the involved speech production subsystems and complete an articulatory profile, (3) estimate the severity of dysarthria based on intelligibility testing, and (4) establish the modifiability of speech through stimulability testing and identification of compensatory strategies that may improve speech. There are no standardized test batteries designed for use with children to obtain all of this information. Therefore it is necessary to employ a variety of activities and test protocols. Many of the tools used to assess these behaviors in neurologically impaired children with dysarthria are the same as those used with other speech impaired children. However, some techniques are different, and they vary depending upon the age of the child being tested.

In testing children, some assessment tools may be borrowed from the adult literature. One test designed for use with adults, the Frenchay Dysarthria Assessment,[103] may be easily adapted for use with children. This assessment tool addresses the first three components of a dysarthria evaluation. It attempts to determine physiologic deficits, identify subsystems involved, and estimate intelligibility. However, the test does not provide an articulatory profile nor does it address compensatory strategies.

The test is divided into eight major sections: reflex, respiration, lips, jaw, palate, laryngeal, tongue, and intelligibility. Each section consists of a series of subtests presented for systematic observation of aspects of the various systems tested. For example, subtests for tongue functioning include observation at rest, upon protrusion, elevation, lateralization, during an alternating motion task, and of speech. Each subtest is scored on an eight-point equal interval rating scale ranging from no function to normal function. Enderby provides profiles for adult dysarthrias including upper motoneuron (spastic), lower motoneuron (flaccid), mixed upper and lower motoneuron, cerebellar (ataxia), and extrapyramidal (hypokinetic and hyperkinetic).[103] Although these profiles may not be useful for children, the test design provides a systematic approach to observation that is appropriate for analysis of dysarthria in children. A standardized instrument similar to this one is needed for evaluation of developmental dysarthria.

The following sections present other methods for analysis of physiologic deficits, subsystem involvement, intelligibility, and compensatory strategies for children with dysarthria.

Testing Physiologic Deficits

Oral Motor Examination. The oral motor examination includes evaluation of the peripheral speech structures at rest and during nonspeech activities, as is common in an oral peripheral examination.[104] At rest, the lips, face, mandible, tongue, and palatopharyngeal musculature are observed and judgements about general symmetry, size, and configuration are made. In addition, any other signs of neuromotor impairment such as fasciculations and involuntary movements are noted. Signs of lip and facial weakness include parting of the lips at rest and asymmetry of the angles of the mouth. In addition, there may be flattening of the nasolabial fold on one or both sides. Mandibular weakness may be suspected when the mandible hangs lower than normal in a resting position. The size of the tongue in relation to the oral cavity should also be checked, with a shrunken appearance of one or both sides indicating unilateral or bilateral involvement, respectively. Abnormal patterns may also be noted at rest such as anterior or posterior tongue elevation. As well, observation of the palatopharyngeal mechanism should be accomplished with the child's tongue relaxed on the floor of the mouth and with the mouth open wide. With bilateral involvement, both sides of the soft palate rest near the posterior aspect of the tongue; whereas with unilateral damage, only the weak side appears lower than normal. However, keep in mind that many normal children present with asymmetry of the soft palate; therefore neurologic impairment cannot be inferred from this observation alone.

Other observations that may be made when the oral structures are at rest include any pocketing of food in the anterior or lateral sulci, indicating abnormal oral motor functioning. In addition, the child's ability to control oral secretions should be noted. Finally, structural relationships of the lips, jaw, tongue, and palate should be checked (e.g., tongue size, palatal arch, and maxillary arch). Children with dyskinetic dysarthria often present with a high palatal arch and narrow maxillary arch that, coupled with restricted mobility of the tongue, influences articulatory precision.

In assessment of nonspeech movement of the articulators, strength, range of motion, coordination, and accuracy of movement are assessed. Symmetry of structures is also assessed, and the presence of abnormal oral reflexive or compensatory behaviors as listed by Alexander[63] are noted (see Table 18–4). Common nonspeech movements of the lips and facial musculature include tasks such as spreading of the lips and puffing out the cheeks. During these activities, the examiner evaluates symmetry of the corners of the mouth and lip strength, respectively. When one or both sides of the lip do not elevate during lip spreading and/or when the lip closure seal is broken by exertion of pressure on the child's puffed out cheeks, muscle weakness is indicated. Lip-pursing may be noted during these activities.

To assess mandibular control, range of motion is tested as the child opens and closes the mouth and moves the mandible from side to side without resistance. Movement with imposed resistance is checked to determine the strength of muscles that open and close the mandible. The examiner tests the muscles involved in opening the jaw or depressing the mandible by attempting to close the child's mouth when the child is given instructions to open the mouth as widely as possible and to try to prevent the examiner from forcing it closed. Muscles involved in closing the mouth are evaluated as the child attempts to overcome resistance when closing the mouth. This time, the examiner exerts force to keep the jaw open as the child attempts to close it. For example, the examiner may place a tongue blade on the lower teeth and instruct the child to close her or his mouth against the examiner's resistance. Jaw thrusting may be noted.

The tongue is also checked for strength and range of motion, the latter by testing tongue protrusion, elevation, and lateralization. Upon tongue protrusion, weakness may be observed on one or both sides, and, with a unilateral weakness, the tongue deviates toward the side of weakness. Exaggerated tongue protrusion and/or tongue thrust may be observed. In tongue elevation to the upper lip and alveolar ridge and in lateralization from side to side, weakness is noted when the child is unable to move the tongue in desired directions and when slowness or irregularity of movement is noted. Tongue strength is tested by exerting pressure against it upon protrusion with a tongue blade or by observing the child's ability to place the tongue in her or his cheek and resist the examiner's attempts to force the tongue inward.

Movement of the soft palate during production of "ah" provides a basis for evaluation of palatopharyngeal movement. In unilateral involvement, no movement of the involved side is noted, and the uvula deviates toward the unimpaired side.

Diadochokinesis. Activities performed in assessment of rapid alternating motion of the lips, jaw, and tongue include (1) productions of /u/ and /i/ and repetition of /pʌ/ for observation of the lips; (2) repetition of /tʌ/ for observation of tongue tip articulation; (3) repeated productions of /kʌ/ for evaluation of posterior tongue activity; (4) repetitions of /pʌtʌkʌ/ for evaluation of sequential motion; and (5) counting and contextual speech sampling for evaluation of articulatory ability in connected speech production.

Syllables per second of /pʌ/, /tʌ/, /kʌ/ and /pʌtʌkʌ/ repetitions are calculated as well as duration of sustained repetitions. These data and observations of coordination and rhythm are used to evaluate neuromuscular involvement. Slowness (decreased number of syllables per second) and short duration of syllabic repetition often indicate neuromuscular weakness of the lips, tongue, and/or mandible. However, they may also be seen secondary to respiratory insufficiency, velopharyngeal incompetence, and/or laryngeal involvement. Observable incoordination of the articulators and abnormal rhythm (e.g., pauses between syllables or words, variable rate) also indicate neuromuscular involvement.

Other Related Behaviors. In addition to examination of the structure and function of the speech articulation mechanism, other oral motor behaviors may also be examined. For example, some test protocols examine oral reflexes such as the gag reflex even though there may be no relationship between movement noted during these reflexive activities and speech production.[1] Other protocols examine gross motor development, feeding (during which many abnormal oral patterns such as tonic biting may be noted), and other nonspeech behaviors. Most tests of this nature are not standardized; therefore scoring may be unreliable, and the validity of findings may be questionable. Nevertheless, these protocols are often used, particularly with infants and young children.

The Preschool Oral Motor Examination is one nonstandardized protocol designed to assess aspects of the peripheral speech mechanism, oral reflexes, oral postural control, control of oral secretions, eating, voluntary nonverbal behaviors, and vocal behaviors.[69] The protocol provides a guide to elicitation and observation of a variety of behaviors within each category. For example, guidelines for elicitation of several oral reflexes are given including the gag, cough, swallow, rooting, lip, mouth opening, biting, lateral tongue, and Babkin reflex. Specific scoring criteria are not provided with the protocol, although it is suggested that by using this systematic approach to observation, developmental levels of each oral behavior, the presence of pathologic motor patterns, and symptoms of subsystem involvement can be obtained. The severity of involvement is also estimated based on the number of involved subsystems, deficient subskills, and incorrect responses observed.

Another similar protocol designed for use with neurologically impaired children is the Pre-Speech Assessment Scale.[105] Rating scales are used to assess gross motor development and prespeech behaviors in children functioning below the 2-year level. Among the prespeech behaviors examined are feeding, respiration, phonation, and sound play. Gross motor observations include head and neck control, response to sensory stimulation, and overall postural tone and movement patterns. These and other behaviors are then rated on two scales, one providing a rating of normal developmental level and the other providing a rating of abnormal movement patterns. The derived rating scale profile is then analyzed based on normative data for normal and developmentally delayed children. Therefore the scale determines a general developmental level for children tested along with a profile of abnormal behavior.

Another assessment protocol designed for use with neurologically impaired infants and young children was developed by Mysak.[68,106] This protocol labelled "Evaluation of Basic and Early Skilled Speech Movements" is an outgrowth of a previous assessment tool, the Neuorphysiological Speech Index, described in 1980.[106] Mysak's approach to assessment is based on a neuroevolutional view of speech whereby early reflexive behaviors, body postures, and movement patterns form the basis for speech development. Therefore this evaluation tool purports to assess speech readiness through testing of basic and skilled speech, hand, listening, and oral movements. Speech postures and hand movements tested largely consist of gross motor skills, whereas listening and oral movements addressed are primarily reflexive activities. Based on observed behavior, the examiner rates each as present, absent, or immature. A discussion of this assessment protocol is provided by Mysak.[68] All targeted behaviors are listed, and general developmental norms are provided for some of them. However, guidelines for interpretation of findings are not provided.

Testing Subsystems of Speech Production

An important aspect of assessment of dysarthria in children is focused on identification of disordered speech production subsystems (respiration, phonation, resonance, articulation) that contribute to abnormal speech patterns. This is accomplished through perceptual analysis of a series of selected speech activities. Instrumental evaluation methods are also available and have been described elsewhere.[107,108] One should keep in mind that it is difficult, if not impossible, when using perceptual analysis to separately assess certain subsystems of speech production, such as respiration and phonation. Therefore many of the speech tasks used in a subsystem analysis involve more than one subsystem. Further, one should recognize that perceptual analyses are subjective, and error is common. Thus reliability may not be high from examiner to examiner. That is, one clinician may judge a given child's voice to be excessively loud, whereas another may estimate it to be within normal limits. In order to decrease error, clinicians need extensive training in listening. Finally, one should note that it is the dynamic interworkings of respiration, phonation, resonance and articulation that result in speech production. Therefore as abnormal subsystems are identified, their contribution to the overall pattern of speech exhibited by the child must be estimated.

Respiration and Phonation. Common activities used to evaluate respiration and phonation include (1) inspiration and expiration of a deep breath, (2) prolongation of a neutral vowel, (3) consonant-vowel (CV) productions using voiced and/or voiceless cognates with a neutral vowel, (4) counting from one to ten, and (5) production of contextual speech during reading or conversation.[1,5] Loudness and pitch variation tasks for evaluating respiration and phonation, respectively, have also been suggested. Loudness tasks include (1) prolongation of /a/ with abrupt loudness change from loud to soft keeping pitch constant and (2) prolongation of /a/ with gradual increase and decrease in loudness. Tasks concerned with pitch include (1) prolongation of /a/ with abrupt pitch change keeping loudness constant and (2) prolongation of /a/ with rapid fluctuations in pitch from high to low.[11] The first four activities are timed to yield a mean length of inspiration, expiration, and vowel prolongation, and mean number of syllables produced per second are calculated for voiced CV repetitions, voiceless CV repetitions, counting, and contextual speech. In addition, for counting and contextual speech, the mean length of utterance per inhalation is calculated.

Inspiration and expiration activities indicate general control of the respiratory mechanism. Shallow inspiration, short exhalation, and/or interruptions during inhalation and exhalation indicate respiratory problems. The duration of vowel phonation reflects the general capability of the child's respiratory system to drive the vocal tract and the ability of the laryngeal mechanism to modify the airstream. The child who evidences difficulty in prolonging vowels also evidences decreased CV repetitions; however voiced CV productions may be longer than voiceless CV productions. Loudness variation tasks indicate strength and coordination of respiration. Children with difficulty in this area are unable to perform these tasks.

The length of utterances per inhalation provide information on respiratory support for connected speech production. The child who requires frequent inhalation and produces few syllables of speech per inhalation is either not taking in enough air to support connected speech production or not appropriately valving the airstream and so allowing expiration of more air than is necessary during production of speech. Other observations to be made about respiratory functioning during connected speech include the general respiratory effort exerted, signs of "residual air phonation" such as strained vocal quality occurring at the end of phrases, and rapid interphrase rate.

Aspects of phonation are also observed as the child performs the aforementioned speech activities.

For example, laryngeal pathology may be suspected when there is a marked difference between duration of voiced CV repetitions and voiceless CV repetitions. As pointed out earlier, a pattern often seen in children with dysarthria is better production of voiced than voiceless syllables, perhaps reflecting abduction and adduction problems of the larynx. Pitch, loudness, and vocal quality are also evaluated. Laryngeal coordination is evaluated as the child performs pitch variation tasks. Habitual pitch and pitch range is noted as well as the presence of pitch breaks or any unusual pitch patterns. A lower than normal pitch may be indicative of weakness of the vocal folds (causing a decrease in longitudinal tension). Loudness and loudness range are also observed, providing an indication of adduction ability of the vocal folds. A breathy voice and/or inhalation stridor indicates hypoadduction, whereas a loud voice (sometimes noted in dyskinetic dysarthria) is indicative of hyperadduction. Vocal quality should also be observed. A hoarse, harsh, strained or strangled vocal quality may result from spasticity and hypertonicity of the vocal folds; whereas an inconsistent, fluctuating vocal pattern with sudden uncontrolled variation, phonation breaks, and vocal tremor may suggest dyskinesia.

Velopharyngeal Function. Speech tasks commonly used to evaluate velopharyngeal competence include (1) prolongation of a voiceless continuant (/s/); (2) production of CV voiced and/or voiceless stops (/p/, /b/) and nasals (/m/) with neutral vowels and with vowels requiring more extreme tongue positions (/i/, /u/); (3) counting one to ten; and (4) contextual speech production. The examiner listens for nasal resonance (hypernasality) and nasal emission in each task. Nasal airflow or nasal resonance should not be apparent in /s/, /p/, or /b/ productions nor during nonnasal consonant productions in counting from one to ten. Hardy suggests using a mirror held below the nares during counting, explaining that

> fogging of the mirror should be detectable in association with the /n/ in "one"; the fogging may continue to expand as a result of retentive opening of the port as the individual produces the /t/ in "two." However, no detectable nasal emission of air should be associated with the consonant productions thereafter until the word "seven" is produced. . . . Anticipatory port opening may be observable for the /s/ in "seven," and with retentive opening after that nasal and the anticipatory port opening associated with the following /n/s in the words "nine" and "ten," there may be consistent fogging throughout the remainder of the act (p 129).[1]

Listening for abnormal nasal resonance during conversation or reading provides a means for evaluating the extent to which velopharyngeal involvement influences speech intelligibility.

Articulation

There are several commercially available articulation tests that may be used with children with dysarthria. For many children, a single-word articulation test is appropriate; however analysis of speech in a sentence articulation task should also be undertaken for children with sentence production ability.

One test that can be recommended for testing both single words and sentences is the Screening Deep Test of Articulation.[109] Because it is designed to sample a variety of phonetic contexts in which a particular sound is produced, it is particularly useful for children with dysarthria. These children present with restrictions in motor function; therefore production of some sound combinations may be possible, whereas others may not be. Administration of the test provides a profile of misarticulated sounds and phonetic contexts in which the misarticulations occur. Other sound inventories such as the Fisher-Logemann Test of Articulation Competence,[110] The Templin-Darley Tests of Articulation,[111] and others may also be employed.

Regardless of the test instrument chosen, consonant errors should be analyzed with regard to place of articulation (bilabial, labiodental), manner of articulation (stop, fricative) and voicing, error type (substitution, omission, distortion), and word position of errors. A place-manner-voicing analysis provides a method for identification of patterns such as substitution of linguovelar by linguoalveolar sounds (place errors), substitution of fricatives by stops (manner errors), and substitution of voiceless by voiced sounds (voicing errors). In addition, an analysis of vowel production errors should be undertaken with regard to place (front, central, back), height (high, mid, low), tension, and lip rounding. These analyses are well described in other sources focused primarily on articulation.[112]

Sound productions should also be analyzed phonetically by means of narrow phonetic transcription. Because sound distortion is common in dysarthria, resulting from weakness and incoordination of the articulators, this analysis may be particularly useful for children with dysarthria. For example, children with dysarthria may produce bilabials as fricatives instead of as stops because of incomplete lip contact. Table 18–8 provides a narrow transcription system that may be useful in analysis of dysarthric speech.

Phonologic process analysis may also be useful in assessment of dysarthria. This analysis has been discussed by several writers.[113–117] Using phonologic process analysis, one may identify modifications or simplifications of adult phonology. Common errors seen in children with dysarthria that may be considered phonologic process errors include cluster re-

TABLE 18–8 Narrow Phonetic Transcription System: Consonant Allophones

For the Phoneme	*Allophonic Symbol*	*Modifier*	*Description of Modification of Production Indicated by This Symbol*
p, b, m	p̪, b̪, m̪	̪	Labiodental articulation instead of bilabial
p, b	Φ, β	x	Fricative instead of stop (incomplete contact of lips)
θ, ð	ɹ̣ɹ	⊢	Tip-alveolar articulation instead of tip-dental, but still fricative (sound more like /s/ and /z/)
θ, ð	t̪, d̪	•	Stop production instead of fricative, but still tip-dental articulation
	J̣J		Affricate production instead of fricative (articulators touch completely before frication begins)
t, d, n, l	t̪, d̪, n̪, l̪	̪	Tip-dental articulation instead of tip-alveolar
t, d, n, l	ţ, ɡ, ɲ, λ	ɹ	Tip-lowered instead of raised ("tongue-tied")
t, d, n	ţ, ɖ, ɳ	ι	Retroflex articulation (tongue tip turns back to touch palate)
t, d	ɹ̣ɹ	x	Fricative instead of stop (incomplete contact of tongue tip to alveolar ridge)
l	L		Back-velar articulation instead of tip-alveolar (and no lifting of the tongue tip)
s, z	θ ð		Tip-dental articulation instead of blade-alveolar ("frontal" or "dental" lisp)
s, z	ɹ̣ɹ		Tip-alveolar articulation instead of blade-alveolar
s, z	ɬ̣ɬ	⁀	Lateral emission of fricative ("lateral lisp")
s, z		T	Tongue blade lowered, producing reduced constriction (a "thick" or "mushy" production)
s, z	ts, dz		Affricate production instead of fricative (articulators touch completely before frication begins)
ʃ, ʒ, ʃ, d, ʒ		⁀	Lateral emission of fricative ("lateral lisp")
	ç, ɹ	⊢	Front-palatal articulation instead of blade-prepalatal (retracted articulation)
t ʃ d ʒ	ţ ç, ḍ ɹ	⊢	Blade and front-palatal articulation instead of tip and blade-prepalatal (retracted articulation)
r	ɟ	ɹ	No lifting of the tongue tip for /r/, (but still a central-palatal articulation)
r			Labiodental articulation accompanying /r/
r	я		Back-velar articulation of /r/ and no lifting the tongue tip
k, g	c, ɟ	⊣	Front-palatal articulation instead of back-velar (an advanced tongue position)
k, g	χ, j	x	Fricative instead of stop (incomplete contact of back of tongue to velum)
Any stop or fricative	h̃ (following the phonemic symbol)	~	Nasal emmission with the consonant
Any stop consonant	ʔ		Glottal stop instead of articulation in oral cavity
Any fricative consonant	ħç		Pharyngeal fricative (articulated by the tongue against the pharyngeal wall instead of articulation in oral cavity)
Any consonant having lip rounding	•	m	Unrounded
Any consonant not having lip rounding		ɯ	Rounded
Any voiced consonant		O	Voiceless instead of voiced
Any voiceless consonant		v	Voiced instead of voiceless

From Fisher HB, Logemann JA. The Fisher-Logemann test of articulation competence. Boston: Houghton Mifflin, 1971.

duction (deletion of one sound in a cluster), final consonant deletion (omission of final word consonants), and stopping (substitution of stops for fricatives).

Speech Intelligibility

Speech intelligibility is commonly estimated in assessments of speech production in children and is particularly important in assessment of dysarthria. Intelligibility measures are useful for estimating severity of speech deficits;[97] they provide a method for evaluating the extent to which neurophysiologic impairments and abnormal subsystems of speech production influence speech. And they provide a functional dependent variable or outcome measure for use in evaluating the effects of treatment for some children.

Intelligibility in developmental dysarthria has received little attention, as have other aspects of speech production in this population. However, methods used to estimate intelligibility in adult dysarthric speakers may be used with children. The Assessment of Intelligibility of Dysarthric Speech provides a set of word and sentence stimuli that when read or produced imitatively are analyzed to yield a percent single-word intelligibility score, a score for rate of intelligible and unintelligible speech, and a communication efficiency ratio.[118] Although normative data have not been gathered for children, this test could easily by adapted for assessment of developmental dysarthria.

Another more informal method for evaluating single-word intelligibility was advanced by Yorkston and Beukelman.[119] From a set of 50 cards on which individual words are printed, the examiner randomly selects ten and presents them to the child to read. Without knowledge of words selected, the examiner simply writes down what word she or he thinks that the child said. Intelligibility is calculated by comparing these words with their targets. For children with developmental dysarthria who cannot read, single-word intelligibility may be measured by means of pictures instead of written words in a manner similar to this.

Compensatory Strategies and Stimulability Testing

A final aspect of assessment is focused on evaluation of the modifiability of abnormal speech production. This activity, sometimes referred to as diagnostic therapy,[11] provides a basis for making prognostic statements and for planning treatment. Although the direction of this portion of the evaluation is guided by the presenting behaviors of an individual child, a few guidelines can be offered.

One major adjustment that often improves speech production is posture. The best posture for efficient speech production for most people is when the spine is straight and the head is held at midline. Therefore attempts should be made to position children in this posture. Because children with dysarthria often evidence complex abnormal postural reactions (e.g., tonic neck reflexes), special chairs are often needed. For example, a child with strong extensor tone in the neck, shoulders, and hips, tongue thrust and jaw thrust may benefit from a chair designed to support the hips such that hip extension is inhibited. This posture may then also decrease general body tension; the child may be able to align the head with the body; and tongue and jaw thrust may be decreased. The speech pathologist should consult with a physical therapist or occupational therapist to determine optimal posturing for speech production for individual children.

Other compensatory techniques directed toward specific subsystems should be evaluated for their effect on other subsystems and on overall intelligibility of speech. First, alterations in breath support may be made. For example, instructions to inhale more deeply before speaking may improve overall speech production by providing a greater amount of air volume for driving the system. Forced laryngeal adduction may also compensate for respiratory[120] weakness and facilitate loudness variation.[11] Next, alterations in vocal intensity might be tested. For children presenting with hypertonic muscle tone and strain strangled vocal quality, instructions to speak with reduced intensity may improve vocal quality. Conversely, for children with generalized muscular weakness and breathy vocal quality, but who appear to speak with minimal effort, instructions to speak more loudly may improve vocal quality. Finally, attempts to modify articulatory precision should be made. For example, slowing the speech rate may facilitate better articulation.

Attempts should also be made to modify articulatory placement for production of errored phonemes, both in isolation and in CV segments. Given simple placement instructions, some articulatory contacts may be relatively easy for a child to accomplish. Others find this more difficult because of motoric constraints of articulatory structures. Attempts to approximate these more difficult postures should be made so that an acoustically acceptable signal is produced. For example, a child who has difficulty with the tongue tip elevation necessary for production of /t/, may be able to produce an acoustically acceptable /t/ by coupling the blade of the tongue and the alveolar ridge.

Other Assessment Considerations

Children with dysarthria, like children with other types of speech disorders, often present with a variety of additional problems. These include auditory processing, intelligence, language development, and other neuropsychologic factors;[121] visual perception; and somatosensory impairments.[1] These factors will not be discussed here; however it is necessary that they be considered in both assessment and treatment of these children.

Treatment

Treatment for developmental dysarthria has been approached from several directions based upon the age of the child being treated, behavioral deficits with which the child presents, severity of deficit, and the clinician's theoretical framework for the development of speech in neurologically impaired children. These treatments have developed largely as an outgrowth of theories of neuromotor speech development and the clinical experience of authorities in the field. Among them are three major orientations to treatment, including (1) neurodevelopmental treatments focused on motor development and prespeech behavior,[63,68,76,77,79,106,122] (2) treatments focused directly on disrupted subsystems of speech production,[1] and (3) treatments focused on provision of nonspeech, alternative and augmentative communication systems.[123]

In this section, each of these treatment approaches will be described. Before doing so, however, it is necessary to point out that experimental data indicating the effects of these treatments are lacking. As pointed out by Jaffe, "treatment for dysarthria is not researched in the most recent literature" (p 163).[124] Data are unavailable to indicate the extent to which these treatments improve communicative functioning; data on subject variables important for successful application of a particular treatment have not been reported; and many of these treatments have not been well described and are difficult to apply. Therefore central to this discussion is the need for applied, clinical research documenting the effects of these and other treatments for developmental dysarthria.

Neurodevelopmental Approaches

Several writers have advanced methods focused on neurodevelopmental treatment such as oral motor treatment,[63] feeding treatment,[80] and neurospeech therapy.[106] These methods, developed largely for intervention with infants and young, preverbal children with cerebral palsy, emphasize positioning, handling, and sensory stimulation in an attempt to inhibit development of abnormal postures and reactions. Treatments of this type have derived from neurodevelopmental theory advanced by Bobath and Bobath, who suggest that special posturing and handling inhibits abnormal movement patterns and allows facilitation of more normal movement patterns prerequisite for speech development.[125]

A review of these treatments[63,68,80,105,106,122,126,127] indicates a common philosophy upon which they are based. This philosophy can be summarized as follows:

1. The overall goal of treatment is to facilitate normal motor development as much as possible because the development of coordinated oral motor behavior is directly influenced by movement patterns of the body.
2. Abnormal movement patterns reduce opportunity for normal movement and sensory feedback and so are inhibited through special posturing and handling techniques.
3. Normal movement patterns are facilitated by means of visual, auditory, tactile, and other stimulation methods.
4. Facilitation of normal oral motor reflexive and volitional movements provides a basis for speech production.
5. Training techniques are implemented throughout the day and are emphasized during activities of daily living such as feeding.
6. Early intervention is essential.
7. Family involvement is encouraged.

One major treatment of this nature was developed by Mysak.[68,106,126] This treatment, labelled "neurospeech therapy," is "designed to stimulate early skilled speech movements" (p 55).[68] Specifically, patterns of behavior identified from assessment of "speech movement readiness," discussed earlier, provide the basis for treatment. Two major components of Mysak's approach include stimulation of basic movements and stimulation of skilled movements.

The first tasks required in neurospeech therapy involve stimulation of (1) basic listening movements, (2) speech postures, (3) hand movements, and (4) speech movements deemed necessary for speech production. These basic movements consist largely of reflexive behaviors and body postures. Listening movements include protective reflexes (such as the Moro embrace reflex), listening reflexes (quieting in response to sound), and tuning reflexes (changes in respiration, heart rate in response to sound). One stimulates these reflexes using a variety of auditory stimuli (e.g., loud, soothing, familiar, unfamiliar sounds) in an attempt to increase selective responding to different auditory signals.

Speech postures include back postures (e.g., head and body alignment), elbow postures (e.g., arm support in prone), sitting patterns, and standing patterns. These postures are accomplished to facilitate early reflexive vocalization, improve visual and auditory perceptual input, and establish appropriate positioning for speech production. Hand movements include protective and vegetative reflexes such as arm support reactions and hand-to-mouth movements, and basic speech movements include protective reflexes (e.g., glottic closing and opening, cough reflex), emotional reflexes (e.g., cry, smile, laugh), vegetative reflexes (associated breathing and feeding), and reflexive vocalization (e.g., vocalizations during movement and feeding).

Once these reflexive behaviors and postures have been established, neurospeech treatment centers on skilled movements: (1) listening movements, (2) imitative vocalization, (3) speech movements, and (4) expressive communication. During this portion of the program, treatment is focused on activities such as vocal imitation. Attempts to facilitate speech production are made, and communication is addressed by focusing on gestural communication, spoken language, and compensatory strategies.

Mysak provides a discussion of methodologies for elicitation and training of these basic and skilled behaviors using "neurofacilitation" techniques.[106] For example, "movement-to-posture sequences" for facilitating basic body postures are presented. Methods recommended for facilitation of speech include (1) "conditioning movements" such as "stretching, shaking, and tapping upper and lower lips" (p 294);[106] (2) "stimulating-feedback maneuvers" such as holding the child's lips together and instructing her or him to blow open the contact for stimulation of bilabials; (3) "movement facilitation maneuvers" such as "resisted movement maneuvers" that simply require the child to move aspects of the speech mechanism while the clinician applies resistive pressure, and "reflex-movement maneuvers" such as facilitation of velopharyngeal closure through elicitation of the gag reflex as the child produces /a/; and (4) "movement exercises" such as production of CV sequences.

There are several other neuromotor treatment approaches reported in the literature that are similar to Mysak's.[63,105,122,127] Morris emphasizes the interaction of sensory, physical, and communicative environments.[122] The focus of treatment is to facilitate normal development sequences as much as possible. Body postures and reactions and oral motor behaviors are studied, and methods for modifying abnormal patterns are implemented. Morris involves parents in determining appropriate postures and handling methods, indicating that there are several postures for children that are dependent upon the situation. Also emphasized are the use of visual, auditory, tactile, and other stimulation methods to "increase the child's awareness and discrimination of the sensory stimulus and expand the sensorimotor options for responding to the input" (p 80).[122]

Morris is one of many advocates of feeding treatment. Underlying this intervention is the notion that oral motor control for feeding is a precurser of oral motor control for speech production. Once postural adjustments have been made, intervention is focused on reduction of abnormal oral motor behaviors during feeding, such as active suckle movements of the tongue, and facilitation of normal movement patterns, such as lip closure around a spoon.[80] Alexander also discusses feeding as a major focus of oral motor training.[63]

As can be recognized from this discussion, neurodevelopmental treatments are comprehensive, encompassing a wide range of activities. Although this treatment may be helpful for some children, specialized training is necessary before implementing certain aspects of it. For example, positioning and handling motorically involved children requires skills not in the repertoire of most speech-language pathologists. Further, several aspects of this treatment are controversial with regard to their effect on speech production. The notion previously discussed regarding the relationship between reflexive activity and volitional speech behavior has been questioned, and data are unavailable to indicate that the accomplishment of some aspects of treatment is possible, such as training selective responding to auditory stimuli or modifying abnormal respiratory patterns. Advocates of neurodevelopmental approaches to treatment have not published data to support these or any other aspects of this treatment. These data are badly needed.

A Subsystems Approach

A perhaps more traditional approach to intervention for developmental dysarthria involves modification of disrupted subsystems of speech production identified during assessment. Treatment is focused on respiration, phonation, resonance, and articulation with the overall goal of treatment being facilitation of the best speech possible given the neuromotor limitations of a particular child. This approach to treatment is most appropriate for preschool and school-age children. Younger children and infants probably do not present with the ability to participate in treatment of this nature. Like neurodevelopmental treatment, positioning is emphasized. As pointed out earlier, professionals trained in positioning neurologically impaired individuals assist in determining the best posture(s) for speech production. These may vary with the subsystem being targeted in treatment. Suggestions for posturing children and adults have been described in several sources.[1,11,81,106,122]

A subsystems approach to treatment has been recommended for both acquired and developmental dysarthria.[1,11] In the following discussion, suggestions taken from the adult and child literature will be presented. Many of these intervention methods were borrowed from those used with other speech impaired populations (e.g., methods for managing resonance are like those used with individuals with cleft palate and methods for managing phonation are like those used with children with voice disorders). Suggestions for both speech and nonspeech training will be discussed where appropriate for each subsystem. One should keep in mind that these are only suggestions and that data supporting their use are unavailable. In fact, not one study focusing on evaluation of the effects of any of these methods with children with dysarthria has been published to my knowledge.

Respiration. The major goals of intervention concentrated on respiration include (1) modification of inspiration to provide sufficient air intake for speech production, (2) modification of expiratory patterns to facilitate controlled exhalation, (3) modification of inspiration and expiration relationships, and (4) production of speech within respiratory limits. Once an appropriate posture for respiration has been established (neck elongation, head and shoulder alignment, and stability of the vertebral column[81]), inspiration training may begin. This training consists of tasks designed to gradually increase air intake. The child's mean duration of inhalation is measured, and a target duration is set. The child is instructed to breathe deeply, and air intake is monitored using a variety of methods. The clinician may place her or his hand on the child's torso or may place the child's hand there to provide tactile feedback. A light-weight object (such as a feather) attached to a string may be suspended in front of the child's mouth, which, upon inhalation, moves toward the child's mouth. Or an instrument such as a spirometer may be used to provide visual feedback. When air intake has been modified in these nonspeech activities, inspiration is monitored during speech production. This requires carry-over of the newly acquired inhalation behavior to breathing and speaking tasks with a gradual increase in the length of spoken utterances. Finally, treatment is focused on interphrase breathing. The optimum length of phrase produced per breath is identified, and the child is trained to inhale at these intervals.

Some caution is warranted with regard to inhalation training. This training is inappropriate for children for whom increased effort results in increased dysfunction. Further, as pointed out by Davis,[81] deep inspiration prior to speech production is an atypical speech-breathing pattern; for some children, it may disrupt coordination of inspiration, expiration, and phonation. For these children, concentration on controlled exhalation may be more appropriate.

Exhalation training also often begins with nonspeech tasks, with the major goal of such training being facilitation of controlled exhalation. Blowing is one such task that has been suggested. Blowing exercises are implemented to increase the pressure and/or duration of expired air in an attempt to improve the strength and coordination of respiratory muscles. However, whether or not blowing exercises improve respiratory support for speech production is an empirical question, and, as pointed out by Hardy,[1] there may be no relationship between these activities.

A variety of devices are available for measuring air pressure and duration during blowing. One simple device suggested by Hixon, Hawley, and Wilson can be made using a water glass, a straw, and a paper clip.[128] A water manometer or an oscilloscope with an air pressure transducer may also be used. As pointed out by Rosenbek and LaPointe, subglottic air pressure for normal speech production ranges from 5 to 10 cm of water, and less than 5-seconds duration is necessary for production of normal breath groups.[11] Therefore one may design treatment to approximate these levels.

As soon as possible, controlled exhalation training should involve speech production. A logical beginning point is sustained vowel phonation with the goal being to increase the duration of phonation. Consonant productions are then incorporated as are strings of consonants and CV productions. During these activities, pitch and loudness should be kept constant, and consonants and vowels chosen for practice should be in the sound repertoire of the child. A Visipitch (Kay Elemetrics Corporation) may be useful for providing visual feedback regarding pitch and loudness variation during this training.

Modification of inspiratory and expiratory relationships involves a combination of inspiration training activities and expiration training activities. Maximum inspiration is facilitated followed by controlled expiration. This training may begin with monitoring of breathing during nonspeech tasks (e.g., deep inhalation followed by blowing at desired pressure and duration levels). Training may then move to speech tasks (e.g., deep inhalation followed by controlled vowel prolongation and deep inhalation followed by consonant repetitions, CV repetitions, and so on).

The final aspect of respiration training is focused on connected speech production and training the child to talk within the physiologic limits of her or his mechanism. As discussed, the child is trained to recognize the length of utterance per breath that can be accomplished and to inhale at appropriate times during speech production. At the same time, the child is trained to control exhalation during connected speech. One may begin this training using word repetition and advance to incorporate production of short phrases, short sentences, and paragraphs.

Phonation. Intervention focused on improved phonation is applied in accordance with the type of laryngeal pathology seen in a particular child. As discussed in the assessment section, there are three major aspects of phonation that may be disordered, which include loudness, quality, and pitch. In children with dysarthria, any of these may be impaired. The voice may be too soft (breathy) or too loud, vocal quality may be abnormal, or pitch may be too high or too low. Treatment methods used to improve laryngeal problems secondary to neurologic involvement (dysarthria) are similar to those used to improve laryngeal problems secondary to other problems. A few of the more common treatment methods will be discussed here, keeping in mind that no data exist to support their use. For other methods, a textbook on voice disorders may be consulted.[129]

Common problems seen in children with dysarthria concern the loudness dimension of phonation. Specifically, laryngeal weakness and hypo-adduction result in breathy phonation, whereas hypertonicity and hyper-adduction result in overly loud phonation. Breathy phonation may be modified by means of exercises used to increase speaking effort. These include various "pushing" exercises as originally advocated by Froeschels, Kastein, and Weiss.[130] This method simply requires simultaneous pushing with the arms and phonating. This method may not be used with some children with dysarthria, however, because in addition to weakness of the larynx, they may also evidence upper extremity weakness that precludes pushing activity. Children may also be instructed to tighten the muscles of the abdomen and oral mechanism prior to and during speech production in the hope that this effort will generalize to the laryngeal mechanism. Voiced bilabial plosives and labiodental fricatives are good speech sounds for use in practicing this activity because of the visible articulatory contact inherent in their production.

Methods to decrease loudness or adduction involve maneuvers that decrease effort and muscle tension. General muscular relaxation techniques may in some cases be helpful; however, most neurologically impaired children are probably unable to undergo procedures necessary to accomplish this (e.g., progressive muscular relaxation,[131] the chewing method.[132]) A technique that may be useful for more children is laryngeal massage, done either manually or with vibration. Aronson presents instruction in manual laryngeal massage.[129] Once relaxation has been induced, vowels, CV sequences, words, and phrases are practiced. The effects of the yawn-sigh[133] and other easy-onset techniques may also be evaluated. For some children, reduced laryngeal tension and concomitant reduced loudness may result from use of these techniques. Similar techniques may be used for altering vocal quality (e.g., strained or strangled vocal quality seen in spasticity).

When pitch is targeted for treatment, attempts to raise pitch, lower it, or increase its variability are often therapeutic goals. This may be done by means of visual feedback such as is possible with the Visipitch or a variation of this instrument. Using this type of biofeedback, the targeted pitch or pitch pattern is displayed along with the child's production. In this manner, immediate feedback is provided.

Closely related to pitch and loudness training and perhaps more important with regard to intelligibility is stress and intonation. Children presenting with monopitch and/or monoloudness also evidence reduced stress patterns or flat intonation contour in speech production. Therefore treatment focuses on improving stress patterns. This training may begin as soon as the child is able to prolong vowels. During vowel prolongation, intonation variation is introduced. The clinician simply models a down, up, down pattern while phonating /a/ and the child imitates. Visual feedback using a Visipitch, voice light, or other instrument is helpful during this training.

As soon as the child has learned to produce a few consonants, these are incorporated into intonation training. First meaningless CV or CVC syllables are produced using the down, up, down intonation pattern (e.g., ↓ ba, ↑ ba, ↓ ba). Next, meaningful stimuli are used in which speech sounds in the child's repertoire are embedded. When this level is achieved, contrastive stress drill may be implemented.[11] This drill involves a dialogue between the clinician and child: the clinician asks questions to which the child responds by placing stress on one of the words in a target phrase or sentence. This is illustrated as follows for the target sentence "Tom hit Bob":

Clinician: Who *hit Bob?*
Child: Tom *hit Bob.*
Clinician: *Did Tom hit* Jack.
Child: *No. Tom hit* Bob.

Resonance. Intervention focused on resonance in developmental dysarthria is approached in a manner similar to that in children with cleft palate, although some unique considerations are involved in managing dysarthria. One major treatment strategy is prosthetic or surgical management. In children presenting with significant hypernasality and nasal emission, a palatal lift prosthesis or pharyngeal flap surgery may be recommended to improve articulation and speech intelligibility. Deciding whether or not this type of management is appropriate requires some special considerations. These include

1. Prosthetic or surgical management is contraindicated when other subsystems of speech physiology are severely involved such that speech production remains unintelligible even with decreased hypernasality.
2. In cases of disproportionately severe hypernasality relative to other speech subsystems, prosthetic or surgical management may be recommended to improve physiologic support for development of speech.
3. Some children may be unable to tolerate a palatal lift, for example, if a hyperactive gag reflex is present.
4. Palatal lifts may be difficult to manage for some children with dysarthria because motor involvement of the upper extremities precludes independent insertion and removal.

A prosthodontist is consulted to fit palatal lifts when they are recommended. In general, prostheses are fitted at a young age, and numerous adjustments are required as speech develops.

When prosthetic or surgical intervention is recommended and when mild to moderate cases of hypernasality are present, which preclude the use of the management strategies just described, speech therapy procedures may be applied to improve resonatory functioning. Nonspeech procedures include the use of whistling and blowing exercise aimed at facilitation of oral airflow and elimination of nasal airflow,[134] elicitation of the gag reflex with simultaneous production of /a/,[106] and palatal massage[135–137] aimed at improving velopharyngeal closure. Speech tasks for improving resonance in dysarthria have not been specifically described. A logical progression of activities might begin with nonnasal vowel training, followed by nonnasal CV training, CVC, word, phrase training, and so on. During these tasks, instructions to overarticulate (open mouth wider, exaggerate oral contacts) may be given to improve oral airflow.

As with treatment focused on respiration and phonation, incorporation of visual feedback techniques is recommended during resonance activities. A variety of these are presented by Rosenbek and LaPointe[11] and range from simple devices such as a mirror or feather placed under the child's nose to an oscilloscope equipped with airflow and air-pressure transducers.

Articulation. Treatment to improve articulation in developmental dysarthria may include (1) training of nonspeech behavior in an attempt to increase strength, range of motion, and/or tone of the lips, tongue, and mandibular musculature and (2) speech training to improve speech sound production. The same considerations discussed concerning nonspeech activities for improving other subsystems are salient for the former. That is, data have not been published that support these activities, and so their validity is questionable. Further, it has been reasoned that because oral exercises involve individual muscle groups, this practice may not improve speech production involving the integration of several muscle groups. Finally, it has been suggested that many oral exercises require movements not needed in speech production (e.g., tongue lateralization) and so are probably unnecessary. It would not be difficult to experimentally evaluate the effects of oral exercise on speech production. Methods for doing this are suggested in the summary section in this chapter.

Two types of oral exercises have been discussed: isotonic and isometric.[11] Isotonic exercises simply involve repetitive movement of the articulators without resistance, and isometric exercises involve movement of specific structures with imposed resistance. Exercises involving the lips (lip rounding [pursing], spreading, opening, and closing), the tongue (protrusion, retraction, elevation), and the jaw (protrusion, opening, and closing) can be performed both isotonically and isometrically. Of course, when this type of activity is included in treatment, only those structures that appear weak need to be treated, and often only one or two movements per structure may be necessary (e.g., tongue elevation, but not protrusion and retraction).

In the accomplishment of this treatment, visual and tactile stimulation may be required to facilitate desired movement patterns. For example, with a mirror placed in front of the child, the clinician may manually manipulate the lips into a pursed position. Once the movements have been approximated, treatment is focused on increasing the number of repetitions of a particular movement and on increasing the duration of sustained movement (e.g., tongue protrusion) with imposed resistance. It may be possible to incorporate instrumentation into this training. As pointed out by Rosenbek and LaPointe,[11] Netsell[138] reported a biofeedback technique using EMG feedback in which muscle potentials were converted to audible tones. With electrodes attached to a patient's upper lip, for example, muscle activity could be monitored and modified with instructions to keep the tone within a specified frequency range.

Speech training proceeds much like articulation training in other populations with regard to target selection and training activities. Target selection is guided by results of diagnostic testing. Sound errors and patterns are identified through place, manner, and voicing analysis and/or phonologic process analysis; the types of errors that a child makes are noted (e.g., distortion, substitution, omission), as are the word position(s) in which they occur. And using narrow phonetic transcription, the clinician identifies the nature of the articulatory distortions. Results of stimulability testing are analyzed, indicating error patterns that are easily modified and those that are not. From these data, targets for treatment are chosen. General guidelines for target selection include (1) erroneous sounds that are stimulable are chosen for treatment instead of those that are not, (2) sounds that are produced correctly in one position but not in another are chosen as opposed to those that are never produced correctly in any word position, (3) distorted sounds are usually chosen for remediation before substituted or omitted sounds, (4) visible sounds are frequently chosen instead of ones that are not (e.g., bilabials instead of linguovelar), and (5) early developing sounds are chosen before later developing ones. In addition, targets from a particular place, manner, or voicing category or phonologic process may be selected.

While this list of suggestions for choosing articulatory targets for training is not exhaustive, nor is it intended to be, some additional considerations in treatment for developmental dysarthria are necessary. These pertain largely to the presenting neurophysiologic limitations of children with dysarthria. That is, it may be impossible for certain articulations to be accomplished by a particular child due to restrictions in movement and/or abnormal movement patterns. For example, a child who cannot accomplish linguovelar coupling is likely unable to produce /g/ or /k/. Therefore /g/ and /k/ would be inappropriate targets for treatment. This is not to say that this child should never be trained to produce these sounds. However, postponing treatment that focuses on them may be indicated, with treatment instead that focuses on sounds that are within the neurophysiologic limits of the child's system.

Another, perhaps unique, aspect of target selection with children with dysarthria pertains to training compensatory articulations. In many cases of developmental dysarthria, when normal articulatory coupling cannot be accomplished, compensatory placements may be trained to yield an acceptable acoustic product. The example provided earlier with regard to production of /t/ with more anterior placement of the tongue than is normal is salient here. Although training of this nature should be attempted only when attempts to train normal articulations have failed, these compensatory patterns often become targets with children with developmental dysarthria.

Strategies used in articulation treatment for children with developmental dysarthria are also similar to those used with other speech impaired children, with a few exceptions. Two major phases in training are targeted including establishing production of target sounds and facilitating production of target sounds in linguistic contexts. These training phases have been described in depth in several sources[112] and in Chapter 15 and so will only be described here briefly.

Whether training individual sounds, compensatory behaviors, sound patterns, or processes, the first phase of treatment is often focused on establishing production of target behaviors in isolation. This production may be accomplished by means of phonetic placement, shaping, and/or "watch me, listen to me, and do what I do" (p 137) therapy.[11] These procedures utilize a variety of stimuli such as tactile positioning of the child's articulators, visual models of articulatory placement (e.g., pictures, drawings, and/or the clinician's model), and auditory cues (e.g., spoken models, articulatory placement instructions). Feedback is also important in this phase of treatment using a mirror and/or tape recorder.

As soon as target behaviors are produced successfully in isolation, sound production training is done in syllable and word contexts, with treatment moving to meaningful contexts and incorporating production in utterances of increasing length as soon as possible. Procedures similar to those used to train sound production in isolation are used. In addition, contrast drill may be useful. This drill simply requires production of contrasts such as voiced versus voiceless segments in words (pat versus bat; pit versus bit; pie versus buy).

During this phase of training, attention should be given to generalization to untrained sounds, word positions, and linguistic contexts. Treatment probes designed to assess such generalization may be helpful in guiding treatment and in understanding speech acquisition in children with dysarthria. The process of generalization has not been studied in this population. Data are unavailable that indicate whether or not training in the initial position, for example, facilitates transfer to the final and medial position in words. Clinicians also do not know whether generalization occurs across sounds similar in place, manner, voicing, or a particular process. And, as well, the extent to which generalization from phrases to sentences to conversational speech occurs is unknown as is the extent to which trained responses are used in nontraining situations or the natural environment. In children with functional articulation disorders, articulation generalization is variable;[139,140] therefore it is likely to be in children with dysarthria as well.

Another focus of treatment that is related to articulation is the rate of speech production. As mentioned earlier about assessment of compensatory strategies, articulation is often improved when children are given instructions to reduce their rate of speech. When such is the case, rate reduction treatment might be incorporated into articulation training using devices such as a metronome, a flashing light, or a pacing board with the goal of treatment to facilitate production of one word per beat of the metronome, flash of the light, or touch of the pacing board. Many other techniques may be designed and utilized depending upon the motor ability of the child being treated. It is important to point out here that rate reduction often produces changes in pitch and loudness variation. Therefore the clinician must decide which abnormal prosodic variable is the least disruptive to speech intelligibility: rate or intonation.

Intelligibility. The final consideration in a subsystems approach to treatment for developmental dysarthria is concerned with speech intelligibility. Speech intelligibility reflects the interworkings of all subsystems of speech production and therefore provides an index for evaluating the effects of training one or several aspects of speech production. Because improved speech intelligibility is the ultimate goal of treatment, it is suggested that periodic assessment of intelligibility be undertaken to evaluate treatment effectiveness and to modify treatment when appropriate.

Nonspeech Alternative or Augmentative Communication

Another major treatment approach for dysarthria pertains to provisions of an alternative or augmentative communication system or device. These devices are often used with children with dysarthria and range from simple to complex, depending upon the presenting behaviors and abilities of the child.[123,141,142] For example, simple picture communication boards may be used with some children,[143] whereas, with others, computer based systems may be provided.[123,141] Selection of a nonspeech communication system is based on the child's physical ability, level of cognitive functioning, visual processing ability, and other considerations such as the communicative environment in which the system will be used. Based on these data, a system is prescribed with appropriate symbols,[144,145] vocabulary size, access mechanism, and output ability. Blackstone (Chapter 34), Cook and Coleman,[141] Shane and Bashir,[146] Vanderheiden and Harris-Vanderheiden,[143] and others have discussed matching nonspeech communication systems to children.

As with other treatments for dysarthria, little data have been published indicating the benefits of providing nonspeech communication systems to nonspeaking children. Although several authors have presented case studies suggesting the usefulness of these systems,[147,148] the need for controlled experimental research in this area is apparent. Culp presents a review of outcome research, indicating that there is a high percentage of communication board rejection and a low percentage of communication board use among nonspeaking individuals and suggests specific directions for research in this area.[149] Research evaluating the usefulness of specific alternative or augmentative communication systems and treatment methods for facilitating optimum use of these systems is badly needed.

DEVELOPMENTAL APRAXIA OF SPEECH

Etiology and Behavioral Pathology

The etiology of developmental apraxia of speech is unknown. As pointed out earlier, apraxia of speech in adults results from brain damage. The left or language dominant hemisphere is involved, and both anterior lesions in and around Broca's area[5] and posterior lesions[150] have been reported. However, research investigating localization in children has indicated an absence of such clear lesions. For example, using a battery of neurodiagnostic tests including computerized tomography (CT scan), electroencephalography (EEG), and clinical examination, Horowitz found no consistent neurologic problems or specific sites of lesion in a study of children with developmental apraxia of speech.[151] Other studies investigating neuropathology in these children have resulted in similar findings. Aram reported normal CT scans in four of six children with dyspraxia,[152] and Rosenbek and Wertz reported that 22 of 36 children with dyspraxia were essentially free of neuropathology "except for the presence of a generalized apraxia" (p 25).[2]

Other research in developmental apraxia of speech has indicated that "soft" neurologic signs or neurobehavioral findings such as fine and gross motor problems and muscle weakness are often seen in these children. Such problems were reported in 36 of 60 children studied by Ferry, Hall, and Hicks,[153] 14 of 36 children studied by Rosenbek and Wertz,[2] and in six of seven children studied by Aram.[152] Specifically, behaviors including orofacial dyspraxia, motor retardation, hand tremor, hyporeflexia, hyperreflexia, gait, and coordination problems were found. However, it is important to note that in several of these and other studies reporting positive neurologic "soft" signs, mentally retarded subjects, who often present with motor dysfunction, were included in the subject pool. In addition, reliability data were not reported, which, as pointed out by Myklebust, Bosher, Olson, and Cole,[154] may be low when measuring these behaviors in children. Finally, "soft" signs such as clumsiness are common among nonspeech impaired children,[155] and some children with "functional" articulation disorders present with these problems.[156] It appears, then, that because abnormal brain functioning in children with developmental apraxia of speech has not been clearly or consistently demonstrated, the disorder is probably not caused from brain damage as in adults.

There are some data indicating familial tendencies for developmental apraxia of speech. For example, Aram,[152] Ferry et al,[153] and Morley[157] have noted a family history of speech disorders in several children with dyspraxia. These reports suggest a possible genetic basis for the disorder. Developmental apraxia of speech has also been associated with learning disability.[2,42] Perhaps as these disorders become better understood a clear etiology will be revealed.

The literature describing behaviors seen in children with developmental apraxia of speech is confused. As pointed out by Guyette and Diedrich, most reports are not based on data, and findings from the few that are based on data are contradictory and inconclusive.[3] Further, there is little agreement regarding subject selection criteria in studies of developmental apraxia of speech because there is no agreed upon definition of the disorder. Therefore researchers have studied children varying in age, intelligence quotient (IQ), language ability, and other variables. For example, Yoss and Darley[42] studied children ranging in age from 5 to 10 years old as did Williams, Ingham, and Rosenthal.[4] However, subjects studied by Rosenbek and Wertz ranged from 2 to 14 years,[2] and Ferry et al studied subjects up to 30 years old.[153] IQs in children studied have also varied. Ferry et al studied subjects with IQs ranging from 40 to 120,[153] whereas Yoss and Darley[42] and Williams et al[4] studied subjects with IQs of 90 or above. Finally, with regard to language functioning, "no effort was made to exclude children with language delay or mental retardation" (p 24) by Rosenbek and Wertz.[2] But children studied by Yoss and Darley[42] and Williams et al[4] presented with a language age no more than 6 months below chronological age with no known organic disability.

The lack of homogenity across studies of children with developmental apraxia reflects the lack of agreement in the literature about symptoms characterizing the disorder. Clearly, as pointed out by Guyette and Diedrich, researchers select subjects based upon opinion about salient characteristics that define the disorder.[3] If a researcher or group of researchers believe that developmental apraxia of speech concurs with language delay, then language delayed children are included in the group of children studied. Similarly, if researchers believe that developmental apraxia of speech occurs concomitant with poor oral motor control, then only children with oral motor problems are studied. That results of such investigations, describing the important characteristics of the disorder, are tautologic is not surprising. That is, chosen subject selection variables are found to be prevalent in children studied; therefore these variables become characteristic of the disorder.

Table 18–9 lists some symptoms of developmental apraxia of speech that have been reported. As can be seen by examination of these findings, numerous speech and nonspeech problems have been noted. Even though it may appear from this list that a clear diagnostic profile of developmental apraxia is available, this is not the case. The first problem, as pointed out by Guyette and Diedrich,[3] is that many of these characteristics were derived from clinical observation and were not studied empirically. This problem is true for behavioral characteristics reported by Rosenbek and Wertz, whose data were obtained largely from retrospective analysis of medical and speech histories of children diagnosed with apraxia of speech.[2] Therefore data collection and analytic procedures were not standardized. Observations made by Chappell,[158] Edwards,[44] Morley,[157] and others are also questionable since these authors presented no data to substantiate them.

A second problem with this listing of charac-

TABLE 18–9 Speech and Nonspeech Symptoms Reported in the Literature as Characteristic (or Not Characteristic) of Developmental Apraxia of Speech

Presenting Symptoms	*Characteristic*	*Not Characteristic*
Speech Symptoms		
Inconsistent errors	Rosenbek and Wertz[2] Edwards[44] Morley[157]	Yoss and Darley[42]
Inability to imitate speech sounds	Chappell[158] Edwards[44] Macaluso-Haynes[159] Rosenbek, Hansen, Baughman, and Lemme[10]	
Vowel distortion	Rosenbek and Wertz[2]	Morley[157] Yoss and Darley[42]
Omission errors	Yoss and Darley[42] Williams, Ingham, and Rosenthal[4] Rosenbek and Wertz[2] Smartt, LaLance, Gray, and Hibbett[160]	
Distortion errors	Yoss and Darley[42] Rosenbek and Wertz[2]	Williams et al[4] Smartt et al[160]
Addition errors	Yoss and Darley[42] Williams et al[4] Rosenbek and Wertz[2]	Smartt et al[160]
One feature errors	Williams et al[4] Yoss and Darley[42]	
Two to three feature errors	Yoss and Darley[42] Williams et al[4]	
Prolongations	Yoss and Darley[42] Rosenbek and Wertz[2]	
Repetition errors	Yoss and Darley[42] Rosenbek and Wertz[2]	
Consonant cluster errors	Rosenbek and Wertz[2]	Yoss and Darley[42]
Fricative errors	Rosenbek and Wertz[2]	
Affricate errors	Rosenbek and Wertz[2]	
Methathetic errors	Edwards[44] Morley[157] Rosenbek and Wertz[2]	
Sequencing errors	Chappell[158] Edwards[44] Morley[157] Rosenbek and Wertz[2]	
Articulatory groping	Rosenbek and Wertz[2]	Yoss and Darley[42]
Voicing errors	Yoss and Darley[42]	
Increased errors with increased length and complexity	Rosenbek and Wertz[2] Edwards[44]	
Prosodic disturbance	Rosenbek and Wertz[2] Edwards[44] Yoss and Darley[42]	
Non-speech Symptoms		
Oral apraxia	Chappell[158] Rosenbek and Wertz[2] Yoss and Darley[42] Aram[152] Ferry, Hall and Hicks[153]	Court and Harris[161]
Diadochokinetic difficulty	Aram[152]	Yoss and Darley[42]
Language deficits	Green[43] Rosenbek and Wertz[2] Edwards[44] Aram[152] Ekelman and Aram[162]	Williams et al[4] Yoss and Darley[42] Chappell[158]

teristics is that reports in the literature disagree. As noted in Table 18–9, disagreement about error consistency, vowel errors, distortions, additions, cluster reduction, and articulatory groping have been reported. Further, disagreement about the presence of oral apraxia, language deficits, and other nonspeech variables exists. This lack of agreement is highlighted in one of the few studies based on data on developmental apraxia of speech. That is, Williams, Ingham, and Rosenthal,[4] in an attempt to replicate findings published by Yoss and Darley,[42] reported agreement on only two of six variables found by Yoss and Darley to discriminate children with developmental apraxia of speech from others.

Another problem with the characteristics of developmental apraxia of speech is that children with functional articulation disorders also present with many of them (e.g., feature errors, fricative errors, affricate errors, consonant cluster errors, and increased difficulty with increased length and complexity of utterance). Because studies have not always made comparisons between children with functional articulation disorders and developmental apraxia of speech, the characteristics listed are probably unhelpful when diagnosing speech impaired children. That is, the presence of one or several of these characteristics in the speech of a particular child does not indicate that that child has developmental apraxia of speech.

Behaviors symptomatic of developmental apraxia are unclear. As pointed out by Jaffe, apraxia is defined as a symptom cluster; however, "not all symptoms must be present; no one characteristic or symptom must be present; and the typically reported symptoms are not exclusive to developmental apraxia of speech" (p 170).[124] This observation coupled with the lack of empirical support for many symptoms of developmental apraxia of speech makes it difficult to understand the disorder—if it exists.

In the most recent literature, researchers have approached the disorder from a linguistic perspective, analyzing errors using a phonologic process approach.[47] In general, this research has indicated that phonologic process errors as well as other linguistic problems can be found in the speech of children diagnosed with developmental apraxia of speech. Although such research may provide new symptoms and perhaps lead to new linguistically based treatments for developmental apraxia of speech, the same problems already discussed remain salient when this approach is taken. That is, it is difficult, if not impossible, to define behaviors characteristic of a particular population without a clear definition of the population being defined.

Assessment

Because the behaviors or symptoms of developmental apraxia of speech are unclear, a discussion of assessment of this disorder is difficult. Only one assessment tool, the Screening Test for Developmental Apraxia of Speech (STDAS),[163] has appeared in the literature for use with children of this nature. This test, as the name implies, is intended to be used for screening children for apraxia of speech. Development of the test was based on the assumption that a cluster of symptoms are available that define the disorder. Children are tested for the presence of these symptoms in each of the following subtests: I, expressive language discrepancy; II, vowels and diphthongs; III, oral-motor movement; IV, verbal sequencing; V, articulation; VI, motorically complex words; VII, transpositions; and VIII, prosody.

There are several problems with this assessment tool; therefore it may not be useful for its intended purpose. Guyette and Diedrich explain why.[164] Specifically, they reviewed each of the "agreed upon"[163] symptoms of the disorder and indicated that there is little agreement that these symptoms are diagnostically characteristic of developmental apraxia of speech. For example, Blakeley suggested that vowel and diphthong errors are indicative of the disorder.[163] However, Guyette and Diedrich pointed out that "the only experimental evidence relating to the vowel and diphthong issue is presented by Yoss and Darley. These investigators found that vowel errors did not help discriminate between children labeled as apraxic and children with functional articulation disorders" (p 203).[164]

Guyette and Diedrich also presented a critique of test construction, administration, scoring, and interpretation of the STDAS, pointing out problems in each area.[164] For example, test-retest reliability data for either examiners or children tested are not presented, and no attempts to validate the test were made. Further, test interpretation is questionable because no scoring guidelines are presented for making referrals for further testing. As well, even if there were a well-defined, valid score indicating a need for further testing, there are not other tests available to administer; and because children with developmental apraxia of speech do not necessarily have clear neurologic lesions or even neurologic "soft" signs, referral for neurologic examination may also not be useful. As suggested by Guyette and Diedrich, a clear definition of a disorder and a complete test battery to test for the disorder should precede the development of any screening tool.[164]

Clearly, no specific assessment tools exist for developmental apraxia of speech that will lead to such a diagnosis at the present time. Therefore assessment of these children should proceed as with other speech impaired children. Haynes suggests that tools to assess the following should be included within a diagnostic battery: (1) tests of articulatory proficiency, (2) tests of diadochokinesis, (3) tests of volitional movements of the oral musculature, (4) tests of orosensory perception and oral awareness, and (5) tests of language ability.[165]

Treatment

Treatment of developmental apraxia of speech is reportedly a difficult process. Therapy has been described as requiring "an inordinate amount of . . . time [resulting in] minimal improvement" (p 24).[166] In fact, some clinicians base their diagnosis of the disorder on this observation, at least in part.[161]

Several writers have suggested methodologies for treatment of developmental apraxia of speech. Unfortunately, few of these suggestions are based on data. Many have been taken from the treatment literature dealing with acquired apraxia in adults, and some are derived from clinical reports and case studies with children. Therefore the effects of most treatments for developmental apraxia are essentially unknown. That is, methods advanced for adults may not be useful for children because the two disorders may be unrelated,[3] and further the effects of many treatments for adult apraxia have not been empirically tested even with adults. Problems with clinical reports and case studies in developmental apraxia of speech are many. First, many treatment strategies have not been well described and so are difficult to replicate. Second, a variety of treatment methods have often been simultaneously applied, making it difficult to determine which aspect(s) of treatment were most useful. Third, behaviors treated have not been measured objectively. And fourth, experimental control for maturation or other threats to internal validity have not been demonstrated. Therefore any changes or improvements noted during the course of treatment cannot be attributed to the treatment given. With these limitations in mind, a few treatment strategies found in the existing literature for developmental apraxia of speech will be summarized.

Oral Motor and Oral Sensory Training

Oral exercises of the lips and tongue have been discussed by several writers. Specifically, Yoss and Darley suggested that imitation training and mirror work be used to facilitate increased range of motion and accurate placement of the articulators and to decrease "irrelevant, searching, extraneous movements" (p 30).[166] Haynes, Johns, and May also suggested that oral movement exercises emphasizing both isolated movements and movement sequences may be helpful.[167] In a case study report of an adult with developmental apraxia, Haynes et al noted improvement in movement of the articulators and a concomitant improvement in speech articulation by training oral movement patterns.[167] Training incorporated the use of food placed on a tongue depressor, food placed in specific areas of the oral cavity, and mouthwash placed on the tongue tip and in the buccal area. The patient was simply required to move the tongue to remove food from the mouth or from the tongue depressor held at various angles and distances outside of the mouth and to move the tongue to areas of the mouth swabbed with mouthwash.

Similarly, oral sensory programs to improve sensorimotor patterning and feedback have been advocated. For example, Edwards discussed the use of proprioceptive neuromuscular facilitation, involving the use of tactile stimulation to facilitate orosensitivity and awareness with children with developmental apraxia.[44] Haynes et al also reported using oral awareness training as a part of treatment of developmental apraxia of speech, suggesting that therapy sessions begin with such training.[167] Specifically, they suggested using (1) various textures of sandpaper to stimulate oral sites including the lips, tongue tip, and tongue blade; (2) swabbing sites within and around the oral cavity with sour food, including lemon and grapefruit juice; (3) olfactory stimulation using noxious odors, including ammonia and rubbing alcohol; and (4) stimulating various areas on the lips and tongue, requiring the patient to identify the stimulated area by pointing to a diagram of the mouth. Experimental data are needed to establish the usefulness of such treatment.

Training Articulatory Postures

There is some controversy in the literature with regard to treatment emphasizing articulatory placement. For example, Rosenbek et al suggested that training "the elusive sound in isolation" (p 15) is inappropriate for the child with apraxia, indicating that such training may be particularly difficult for children with apraxia because of limitations in the ability to imitate.[10] Jaffe has expressed a similar opinion.[124] However, Logue advocates motor speech training, beginning with articulatory placement training.[168] Specifically, Logue advanced a training program, called "Monitoring Articulatory Postures," designed to train children to program articulatory movements.[168] The program is divided into three phases. Phase I, articulatory posture training, focuses on training articulatory placement for vowel and consonant production. Phase II, speech shadow imitation, focuses on speech sound production, initially using visual stimuli followed by auditory stimuli; and phase III, competitive articulatory posturing, emphasizes training in rapidly changing articulatory postures. For example, the clinician instructs the child to place the articulators in a position to produce a specific sound and to then produce a sound requiring a competing articulatory placement. Logue suggests that this training facilitates improvement in speech production of children with developmental apraxia; however, no data have been reported to substantiate this claim.

Speech Training Paired with Rhythm, Hand, and/or Body Movement

Several treatment approaches for developmental apraxia of speech have been suggested utilizing nonspeech behaviors such as syllabic tapping, pacing boards,[124] arm swinging and body movement,[42] and gesture.[124,169] These techniques are used to accentuate speech sequencing and changes in placement of the articulators. For example, Haynes explains that "movements of the extremities, such as foot tapping or finger tapping . . . increases the accuracy of patient's responses" (p 263),[165] and Jaffe suggests that manual signs "can help the child's speech by the association of a meaningful gross motor movement with units of speech" (p 175).[124]

Two reports in the literature are salient here. One method was reported by Klick, called an "adapted cuing technique" (ACT).[169] This treatment strategy pairs manual signs with speech training. Manual signs or cues used reflect the shape of the oral cavity, articulatory placement, and movement patterns and the manner in which sounds are produced. For example, "in cuing place of production . . . the hand is held near the side of the face, moving as the tongue does, to the front, middle, or back of the oral tract" (p 256), and manner of stop consonant production is marked by "quick, forward movements away from the speaker" (p 257).[169] Changes in hand configurations are made as speech sound changes are made, thereby guiding articulatory motion. Klick presented a case study utilizing this treatment approach with a child with dyspraxia, reporting positive results.[169] However, no data were presented.

The second report is one by Helfrick-Miller, who investigated the effects of melodic intonation therapy paired with signed English with two children with developmental dyspraxia.[170] Melodic intonation therapy was originally designed for use with aphasic patients to improve production of propositional language through the use of intoned language sequences paired with hand tapping.[171] It has since been used with adult patients with apraxia.[172] The melodic intonation therapy adaptation used by Helfrick-Miller incorporated manual signs instead of hand tapping and consisted of three levels of training; at each level, length of phrases used for training were lengthened, phonemic complexity was increased, and reliance on the clinician and on intonation and signing were decreased.

At level I, phrases were two to three words in length, consisting of particle plus word sequences with few grammatic morphemes. At level II, four to five word phrases were used, alveolars, glottals, and sibilants were used, and plurals and possessives were embedded in noun phrase and verb phrase constructions; at level III, more complex phonologic, morphologic, and syntactic constructions were used in the training stimuli. Imitation training at each level was utilized with delayed imitation introduced at level II and normal prosody introduced at level III.

The effects of melodic intonation therapy for the two children with developmental apraxia of speech were evaluated by measuring articulation errors and sequencing error rate at four intervals: pretreatment, midtreatment, posttreatment, and 6 months following treatment. Results, as shown in Figure 18–6, indicate that both children evidenced a gradual decrease in articulation errors and in sequencing errors throughout the course of training. However, interpretation of these data is difficult because experimental control was not demonstrated. That is, factors other than treatment may have influenced speech production. Further, it is impossible to determine which aspect of treatment, for example, signing, intoning, delayed imitation, increased complexity of stimuli, influenced changes in responding. Further investigation in this area is needed using controlled experimental methods.

Training Sound Sequences

Several writers have suggested that training children to produce sequences of sounds is the most appropriate tactic for improving speech production in developmental apraxia. Writers advocating this approach believe that the inability to sequence sounds is one of the salient characteristics of the disorder and therefore advance that treatment be focused at this level, using meaningful stimuli when possible.[10,42,165] In general, this training begins with production of visible consonants in CV, VC, CVC sequences, moving to words and phrases when appropriate. Because children with apraxia may have difficulty producing complex syllable shapes such as consonant clusters, introduction of the intrusive schwa has been recommended[2] to train sound ordering. Use of word lists requiring front-to-back and back-to-front placement have also been recommended[167] (e.g., "back" versus "cab").

One experimental study, investigating the effects of a sound-referenced rebus approach for facilitating production of consonant clusters and ambisyllabic consonant productions, has been reported in the literature. Young and myself,[173] using a multiple baseline design across behaviors,[174,175] trained two adults with developmental articulation problems to produce initial word fricative plus liquid and fricative plus stop clusters and ambisyllabic or abutting consonants in bisyllabic words. Both subjects had been diagnosed as having developmental apraxia, but were not labelled as such by the investigators because of the controversy and lack of meaning inherent in the diagnosis. Both subjects presented with low normal IQ and had histories of learning problems. Speech development was delayed and intelli-

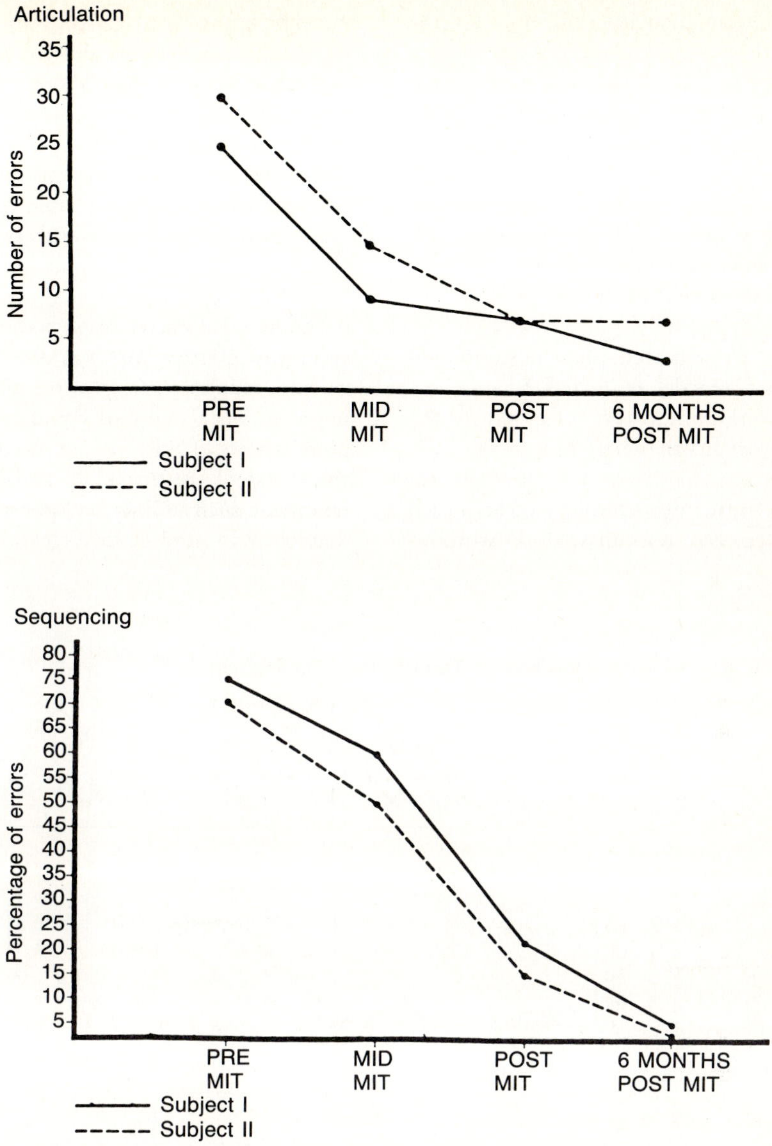

Figure 18–6 Number of articulation errors and percent sequencing errors prior to (PRE MIT), during (MID MIT), upon completion (POST MIT), and 6 months following (6 MONTHS POST MIT) melodic intonation therapy treatment for subjects I and II (children with developmental apraxia of speech). (From Helfrick-Miller KR. The use of melodic intonation therapy with developmentally apractic children: a clinical perspective. J Penn Speech Lang Hear Assoc 1983; XVI: 13.)

gibility was poor characterized by omission of sounds and syllables especially in words requiring complex sound sequences.

A total of 35 target words were selected for study; 15 words were trained, 15 were utilized to assess generalization to untrained words, and five with initial affricate were tested throughout the study, but never trained. Following baseline testing, Subject 1 was first trained to produce words with ambisyllabic consonants, followed by training on initial word fricative plus liquid clusters, and finally, initial word stop plus liquid clusters were trained. To control for order effects, Subject 2 was trained first on initial word stop plus liquid clusters, followed by training on initial word fricative plus liquid clusters, and, finally, ambisyllabic consonants were trained.

Target words were trained using a rebus-cued training technique with backward chaining. Colored pictures of target nouns with corresponding rebuses were utilized as visual stimuli (e.g., for the target noun "magnet," a picture of a magnet and a picture of a net were used; for the target noun "train," a picture of a train and a picture of rain were used). Each set of target words was trained to an 80-percent criterion level in four steps:

1. The target picture and rebus were presented

together. The clinician modeled the rebus for the subject to repeat, then modeled the entire target word using equal stress on each syllable for ambisyllabic words and pausing between consonants comprising the consonant cluster for cluster words. The subject repeated.

2. The target picture and rebus were presented as in step 1; words with ambisyllabic consonants were modeled with normal stress, and cluster words were modeled without separation of the consonants. The subject repeated.

3. The rebus was removed, and the subject repeated the clinician's model as in step 2.

4. Target word stimuli were presented for the subject to name without the clinician's model.

Following each treatment session in which each target word was presented ten times, all 35 stimulus items were presented for the subject to name, as in the baseline. Responses to these probes served as the dependent variable throughout the study.

Results of the study are presented in Figures 18–7 and 18–8 for Subjects 1 and 2, respectively. As can be seen, treatment was effective in facilitating production of ambisyllabic consonants and initial consonant clusters in both subjects, and generalization to untrained words was noted, although Subject 2 showed a stronger generalization effect than did Subject 1. Generalization both within cluster types and across cluster types was observed for Subject 2, whose production of fricative plus liquid clusters improved when stop plus liquid clusters were trained. More studies of this type are needed to demonstrate the effects of treatment. In addition, the effects of treatment such as this on spontaneous speech production is in need of investigation.

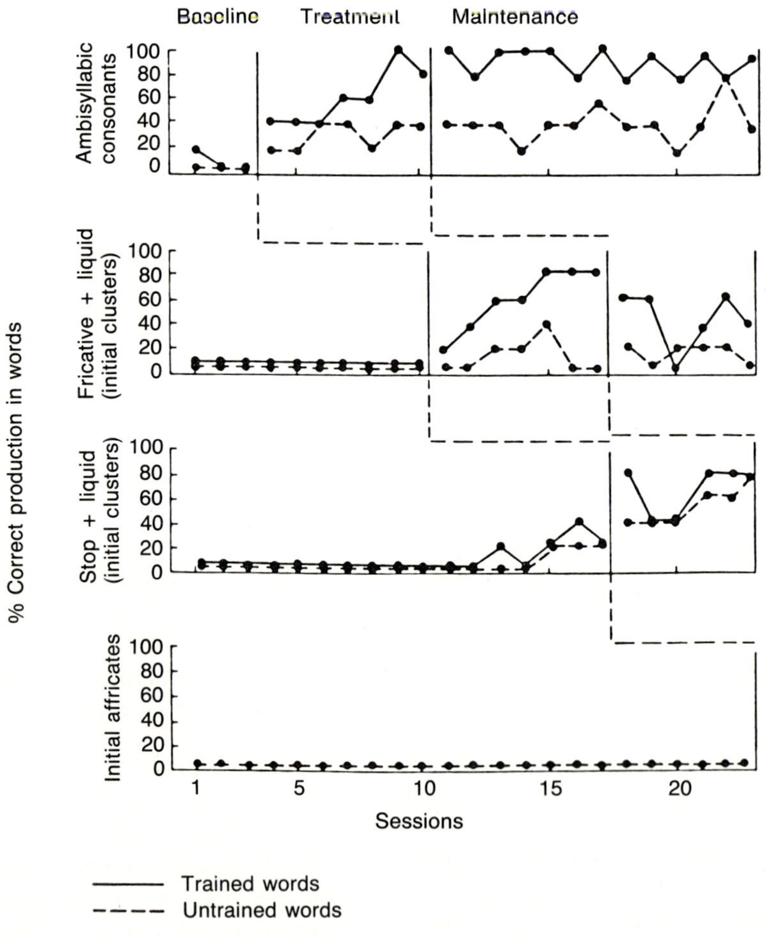

Figure 18–7 Multiple baseline across behaviors indicating effects of a sound-referenced rebus approach to training ambisyllabic consonants, fricative + liquid clusters, stop + liquid clusters and initial fricatives during baseline, experimental, and maintenance phases of the study for Subject 1. (From Young EC, Thompson CK. An experimental analysis of treatment effects on consonant and ambisyllabic consonants in two adults with developmental phonological problems. J Commun Disord 1987; 20:144. Reprinted by permission of the publisher, Elsevier Science.)

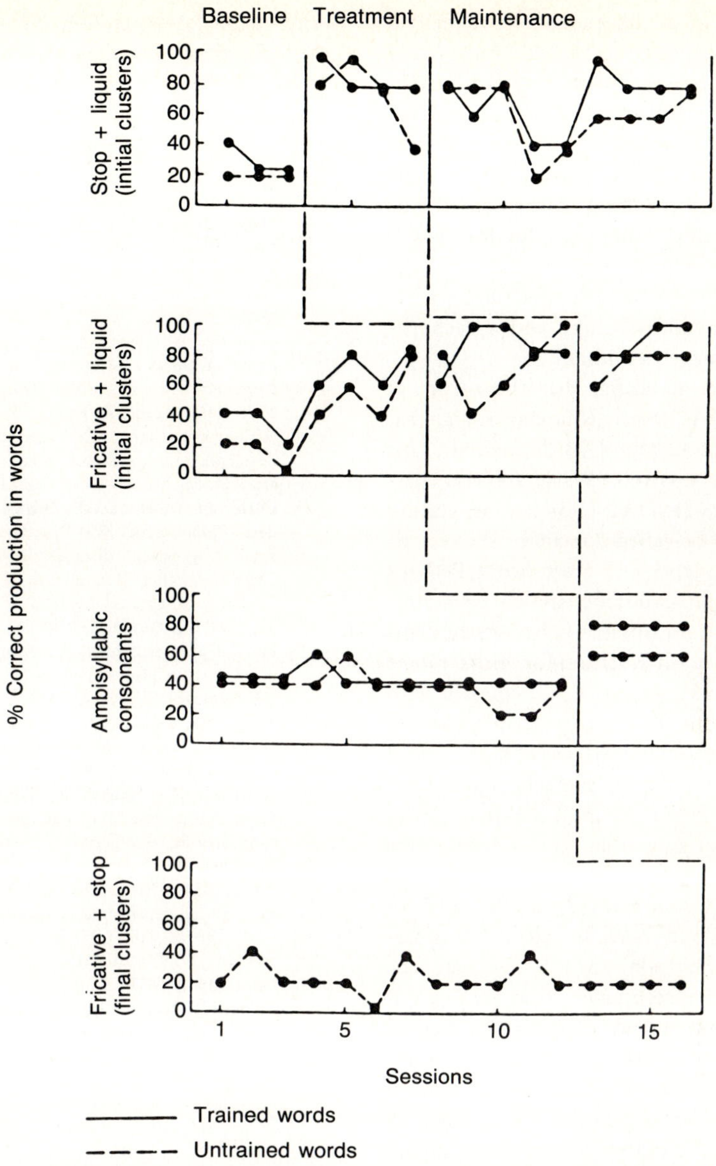

Figure 18–8 Multiple baseline across behaviors indicating effects of a sound-referenced rebus approach to training ambisyllabic consonants, fricative + liquid clusters, stop + liquid clusters and initial fricatives during baseline, experimental, and maintenance phases of the study for Subject 2. (From Young EC, Thompson CK. An experimental analysis of treatment effects on consonant clusters and ambisyllabic consonants in two adults with developmental phonological problems. J Commun Disord 1987; 20:144. Reprinted by permission of the publisher, Elsevier Science.)

Other Treatments

Many other suggestions for treatment for developmental apraxia of speech have been made in the literature such as rate control training, use of carrier phrases, stress and intonation variation, linguistic approaches, and others. Many of these are reviewed by Jaffe[124] and Haynes,[165] and, like most treatments reviewed here, they have not been empirically tested. Certainly, there is a need for treatment research investigating the effects of these and other treatments for developmental apraxia of speech.

SUMMARY

This chapter has reviewed two disorders, developmental dysarthria and developmental apraxia of speech, and has highlighted significant needs for research in both areas. In terms of the nature of these disorders, questions remain with regard to developmental dysarthria. Speech-language pathologists know little about neurologic disease processes or disorders, other than cerebral palsy, that result in dysarthria. Further speech-language pathologists know little about the types of dysarthria seen in children or if different types of dysarthria can be identified reliably. Further research in this area is needed. For example, children presenting with a variety of disorders, such as Reye's syndrome, need to be studied using neuroradiologic techniques to document the site and extent of brain damage, and, at the same time, well-controlled behavioral testing should be accomplished to establish speech production deficit patterns. With data such as these, speech-language pathologists may begin to better understand the relationship between neuropathology and speech pathology in brain damaged children.

This chapter has indicated that the nature of developmental apraxia of speech is unknown and that controversy and chaos surround its discussion. This controversy must be resolved. What are the characteristics of these children that clinicians are calling apraxic? Should they be called apraxic or should clinicians abandon the label and start over? Perhaps clinicians should begin studying speech characteristics of children with measurable behaviors in common (e.g., children with fine and/or gross motor deficits, children with learning deficits, children with visual perceptual difficulty) rather than studying children based on an undefined variable or set of variables. It appears that researchers have been studying an heterogeneous group of children; therefore it is not surprising that the findings are inconclusive.

This chapter has also pointed out the need for better assessment tools for both disorders. For dysarthria, standardized tests designed to evaluate the various subsystems of speech production are needed. Conversely, for developmental apraxia of speech, perhaps clinicians need to use already existing standardized tests to determine what differences exist (if any) between children being diagnosed as apraxic and other speech impaired children. It seems a fruitless exercise to spend time developing new tests to test for an undefined disorder.

Finally, and perhaps most importantly, this chapter has pointed out that a paucity of treatment research exists on evaluating the effects of treatment for either developmental dysarthria or developmental apraxia of speech. I have suggested that single-subject experimental research designs be used to demonstrate the effects of treatment suggestions summarized in this chapter. The advantages of using these designs in clinical research and guidelines for using them have been discussed in several sources including Connell and Thompson,[176] Kearns,[177] McReynolds and Kearns,[174] McReynolds and Thompson,[175] in Chapter 37. Clinicians and researchers working with children with developmental dysarthria or developmental apraxia of speech are encouraged to consult these sources and to begin gathering scientific data to document the effects of treatment for these disorders.

REFERENCES

1. Hardy JC. Cerebral palsy. Englewood Cliffs, NJ: Prentice-Hall, 1983.
2. Rosenbek, JC, Wertz RT. A review of 50 cases of developmental apraxia of speech. Lang Speech Hear Serv in Schools 1972; 3:23–33.
3. Guyette TW, Diedrich WM. A critical review of developmental apraxia of speech. In: Lass N, ed. Speech and language: advances in basic research and practice. Vol. 5. New York: Academic Press, 1981:1.
4. Williams R, Ingham R, Rosenthal J. A further analysis for developmental apraxia of speech in children with defective articulation. Speech Hear Disord 1981; 24:496–505.
5. Darley FL, Aronson AE, Brown JR. Motor speech disorders. Philadelphia: WB Saunders, 1975.
6. Brain WR. Speech disorders: aphasia, apraxia and agnosia. 2nd ed. London: Butterworth, 1964.
7. Dorland's illustrated medical dictionary. 26th ed. Philadelphia: WB Saunders, 1981.
8. McNeil MR, Rosenbek JC, Aronson AE. The dysarthrias: physiology, acoustics, perception, management. San Diego, CA: College-Hill Press, 1984.
9. Wertz RT, LaPointe LL, Rosenbek JC. Apraxia of speech in adults. The disorder and its management. Orlando, FL: Grune & Stratton, 1984.
10. Rosenbek JC, Hansen R, Baughman CH, Lemme M. Treatment of developmental apraxia of speech: a case study. Lang Speech Hear Serv in Schools 1974; 5:13–22.
11. Rosenbek JC, LaPointe LL. The dysarthrias: description, diagnosis, and treatment. In: Johns DL, ed. Clinical management of neurogenic communicative disorders. Boston: Little, Brown, 1985:97.
12. Jackson JH. On affections of speech from disease of the brain. Brain 1878; 1:304.
13. Canter GJ. Neuromotor pathologies of speech. Am J Phys Med 1967; 46:659–666.
14. Grewel F. Classifications of dysarthrias. Acta Psychiatr Scand Neurol 1957; 32:325–337.
15. Froeschels E. A contribution to the pathology and therapy of dysarthria due to certain cerebral lesions. J Speech Hear Disord 1943; 8:301–321.
16. Morley DE. The rehabilitation of adults with dysarthric speech. J Speech Hear Disord 1955; 20:58–64.
17. Darley FL, Aronson AE, Brown JR. Differential diagnostic patterns of dysarthria. J Speech Hear Res 1969; 12:246–269.
18. Darley FL, Aronson AE, Brown JR. Clusters of deviant speech dimensions in the dysarthrias. J Speech Hear Res 1969; 12:462–478.
19. Little WJ. Course of lectures on deformation of the human frame, lecture no. 8. Lancet 1843; 1:318.
20. Little WJ. On the influence of abnormal parturition, difficult labor, premature birth, and asphysia neonatorum, on the mental and physical condition of the child, especially in relation to deformities. Lancet 1861; 2:378–380.
21. Minear WL. A classification of cerebral palsy. Pediatrics 1956; 18:841–852.
22. Phelps WM. Classification of athetosis with special reference to the motor classification. Am J Phys Med 1956; 35:24–31.
23. Crothers B, Paine RS. The natural history of cerebral palsy. Cambridge, MA: Harvard University Press, 1959.
24. Critchely MacD. Aphasiological nomenclature and definitions. Cortex 1967; 3:3–25.

25. Bay E. Aphasia and nonverbal disorders of language. Brain 1962; 85:412–426.
26. Nathan PW. Facial apraxia and apraxic dysarthria. Brain 1947; 70:449–478.
27. Head H. Aphasia and kindred disorders of speech. London: Cambridge University Press, 1926.
28. Alajouanine T, Ombredane A, Durand M. Le syndrome de desintegration phonetique dans l'aphasie. Paris: Masson, 1939.
29. Shankweiler D, Harris K. An experimental approach to the problem of articulation in aphasia. Cortex 1966; 8:265–283.
30. Denny–Brown D. Physiological aspects of disturbances of speech. Aust J Exp Biol Med Sci 1965; 43:455–474.
31. Broca P. Remarques sur la de la facueté du langage articulé suives d'une observation d'aphemie. Bulletin de la Societé d'Anthropologie 1861; 2:235–257.
32. Darley FL. Lacune and research. Approaches to them, IV. In: Millikan CH, Darley F, eds. Brain mechanisms underlying speech and language. New York: Grune & Stratton, 1967:236.
33. Aten JL, Johns DL, Darley FL. Auditory perception of sequenced words in apraxia of speech. J Speech Hear Res 1971; 14:131–143.
34. Deal JL, Darley FL. The influence of linguistic and situational variables on phonemic accuracy in apraxia of speech. J Speech Hear Res 1972; 15:639–653.
35. Johns DL, Darley FL. Phonemic variability in apraxia of speech. J Speech Hear Res 1970; 13:556–583.
36. LaPointe LL, Johns DL. Some phonemic characteristics in apraxia of speech. J Commun Disord 1975; 8:259–269.
37. Rosenbek J, Wertz RT, Darley FL. Oral sensation perception in apraxia of speech and aphasia. J Speech Hear Res 1983; 16:22–36.
38. Trost JE, Canter GJ. Apraxia of speech in patients with Broca's aphasia: a study of phonemic production accuracy and error patterns. Brain Lang 1974; 1:63–79.
39. Martin AD. Some objections to the term apraxia of speech. J Speech Hear Disord 1974; 39:53–64.
40. Johns DL, ed. Clinical management of neurogenic communicative disorders. Boston: Little, Brown, 1978.
41. Johns DL, ed. Clinical management of neurogenic communicative disorders. 2nd ed. Boston: Little, Brown, 1985.
42. Yoss KA, Darley FL. Developmental apraxia of speech in children with defective articulation. J Speech Hear Res 1974; 17:399–416.
43. Green MCL. Speech and backward at three. Br J Disord Commun 1967; 2:134–145.
44. Edwards M. Developmental verbal dyspraxia. Br J Disord Commun 1973; 8:64–70.
45. Morley ME. The development and disorders of speech in childhood. 2nd ed. London: Livingstone, 1965.
46. Wilson LF. Characteristics of aphasia in children. In: Rappaport SR, ed. Childhood aphasia and brain damage. Vol. 1. Narberth, PA: Livingstone, 1964:7.
47. Crary MA, Landess J, Towne R. Phonological error patterns in developmental verbal dyspraxia. J Clin Neuropsychol 1984; 6:157–170.
48. Carpenter MB. Human neuroanatomy. Baltimore: Williams & Wilkins, 1976.
49. Chusid JG. Correlative neuroanatomy and functional neurology. Los Altos, CA: Lange Medical Publications, 1985.
50. Daube JR, Sandok BA. Medical neurosciences. An approach to anatomy, pathology, and physiology by systems and levels. Boston: Little, Brown, 1978.
51. Gazzaniga MS, Steen D, Volpe BT. Functional neuroscience. New York: Harper & Row, 1979.
52. Gilman S, Winans SS. Manter and Gantz's essentials of clinical neuroanatomy and neurophysiology. Philadelphia: FA Davis, 1982.
53. Yost GC, Kaplan AM, Bustamante R, Ellison C, Hargrave A III, Randall DL. Bacterial meningitis in Arizona American Indian children. Am J Dis Child 1986; 140:943–946.
54. Holtzhauer FJ, Campbell RJ, Hall LJ, Halpin TJ. Reye's syndrome: an epidemiologic analysis of mild disease. Am J Dis Child 1986; 140:1231–1236.
55. Kraus JF, Fife D, Cox P, Ramstein K, Conroy C. Incidence, severity and external causes of pediatric brain injury. Am J Dis Child 1986; 140:687–693.
56. Pruszewicz A, Obrebowski A, Zgorzalewicz B. Selected problems in the hearing, voice, and speech disturbances in the extra-pyramidal form of cerebral palsy. Folia Phoniatr 1977; 29:302–310.
57. Bobath K. The motor deficit in patients with cerebral palsy. England: Spastics International Medical Publications, 1976.
58. Florentino MR. Normal and abnormal development. Springfield, IL: CC Thomas, 1972.
59. Mitchell RG. The Moro reflex. Cereb Palsy Bull 1960; 2:135–141.
60. Parr C, Routh DK, Byrd MT, McMillan J. A developmental study of the asymmetric tonic neck reflex. Dev Med Child Neurol 1974; 16:329–335.
61. Ingram TTS. Clinical significance of the infantile feeding reflexes. Dev Med Child Neurol 1962; 4:159–169.
62. Sheppard J. Cranio-oropharyngeal motor patterns in dysarthria associated with cerebral palsy. J Speech Hear Res 1964; 7:373–380.
63. Alexander R. Oral-motor treatment for infants and young children with cerebral palsy. Semin Speech Lang 1987; 8:87–100.
64. McDonald ET, Chance B. Cerebral palsy. Englewood Cliffs, NJ: Prentice-Hall, 1964.
65. Mysak E. Significance of neurophysiological orientation to cerebral palsy habilitation. J Speech Hear Disord 1959; 24:221–231.
66. Mysak E. Dysarthria and orthopharyngeal reflexology: a review. J Speech Hear Disord 1963; 28:252–260.
67. Mysak E. Neuroevolutionary approach to cerebral palsy and speech. New York: Teachers College Press, 1968.
68. Mysak ED. Assessment of speech movement readiness in cerebral palsy. Semin Speech Lang 1987; 8:41–56.
69. Sheppard JJ. Assessment of oral motor behaviors in cerebral palsy. Semin Speech Lang 1987; 8:57–70.
70. Hixon TJ, Hardy JC. Restricted motility of the speech articulators in cerebral palsy. J Speech Hear Res 1964; 29:293–306.
71. Love RJ, Hagerman EL, Taimi EG. Speech performance, dysphagia and oral reflexes in cerebral palsy. J Speech Hear Res 1980; 45:59–75.
72. Irwin OC. Communication variables of cerebral palsied and mentally retarded children. Springfield, IL: CC Thomas, 1972.
73. Kamalashile J. Speech problems in cerebral palsy children. Lang Speech 1975; 18:158–165.
74. Bobath K. The motor deficit in patients with cerebral palsy. London: William Heinemann Medical Books, 1966.
75. Bobath K. The normal postural reflex mechanism and its deviation in children with cerebral palsy. Physiotherapy 1971; 57:515–525.
76. Bobath B. The very early treatment of cerebral palsy. Dev Med Child Neurol 1967; 9:373–391.
77. Bobath B. Abnormal postural reflex activity caused by brain lesions. London: William Heinemann Medical Books, 1971.
78. Bobath B. Motor development: its effect on general development and application to the treatment of cerebral palsy. Physiotherapy 1971; 57:526–532.
79. Bobath K, Bobath B. Cerebral palsy. Part 1: diagnosis and assessment of cerebral palsy. Part 2: the neurodevelopmental approach to treatment. In: Pearson PH, Williams CE, eds. Physical therapy services in the developmental disabilities. Springfield, IL: CC Thomas, 1972.
80. Morris SE. Program guidelines for children with feeding

problems. Edison, NJ: Childcraft Education, 1977.
81. Davis LF. Respiration and phonation in cerebral palsy: a developmental model. Semin Speech Lang 1987; 8:101–106.
82. Westlake H, Rutherford D. Speech therapy for the cerebral palsied. Chicago: National Easter Seal Society for Crippled Children and Adults, 1961.
83. Hardy JC. Intraoral breath pressure in cerebral palsy. J Speech Hear Disord 1961; 26:309–319.
84. Berry MF, Eisenson J. Speech disorders: principles and practices of therapy. New York: Appleton-Century-Crofts, 1956.
85. Blumberg ML. Respiration and speech in the cerebral palsied child. Am J Dis Child 1955; 89:48–53.
86. Palmer MF. Speech therapy in cerebral palsy. J Pediatr 1952; 40:514–524.
87. Rutherford B. A comprehensive study of loudness, pitch, rate, rhythm, and quality of children handicapped by cerebral palsy. J Speech Hear Disord 1944; 9:263–271.
88. Leith W, Steer M. Comparison of judged speech characteristics of athetoids and spastics. Cereb Palsy Rev 1958; 19:15–19.
89. Clark WM, Hoops HR. Predictive measures of speech proficiency in cerebral palsied speakers. J Commun Disord 1980; 13:385–394.
90. Dawes VA. Palatal dysfunction in cerebral palsy. Unpublished paper presented at American Speech and Hearing Association Convention, New York, 1958.
91. Netsell R. Evaluation of velopharyngeal function in dysarthria. J Speech Hear Res 1969; 34:113–122(a).
92. Kent RD, Netsell R. Articulatory abnormalities in athetoid cerebral palsy. J Speech Hear Res 1978; 43:353–373.
93. Byrne MC. Speech and language development of athetoid and spastic children. J Speech Hear Res 1959; 24:231–240.
94. Irwin OC. Correct status of vowels and consonants in the speech of children with cerebral palsy as measured by an integrated test. Cereb Palsy J 1968; 29:9–12.
95. Platt JF, Andrews G, Young M, Quin PT. Dysarthria of adult cerebral palsy. I. Intelligibility and articulatory impairment. J Speech Hear Res 1980; 23:28–38.
96. Farmer A. Voice onset time production in cerebral palsied speakers. Folia Phoniatr 1980; 32:267–273.
97. Platt LJ, Andrews G, Young M, Neilson PD. The measurement of speech impairment of adults with cerebral palsy. Folia Phoniatr 1978; 30:50–58.
98. Clement M, Twitchell T. Dysarthria in cerebral palsy. J Speech Hear Disord 1959; 24:118–122.
99. Platt LJ, Andrews G, Howie PM. Dysarthria of adult cerebral palsy. II. Phonemic analysis of articulation errors. J Speech Hear Res 1980; 23:41–55.
100. Irwin OC. Phonetic equipment of spastic and athetoid children. J Speech Hear Disord 1955; 20:54–57.
101. Kent RD, Netsell R, Bauer LL. Cineradiographic assessment of articulatory mobility in the dysarthrias. J Speech Hear Res 1975; 40:467–480.
102. Schliesser HF. Alternate motion rates of the speech articulators in adults with cerebral palsy. Folia Phoniatr 1982; 34:258–264.
103. Enderby PM. Frenchay dysarthria assessment. San Diego: College Hill Press, 1983.
104. Dworkin J, Culatta R. D-COME: Dworkin Culatta oral mechanism examination. Nicholasville, KY: Edgewood Press, 1980.
105. Morris SE. The pre-speech assessment scale. Clifton, NJ: JA Preston, 1982.
106. Mysak ED. Neurospeech therapy for the cerebral palsied. A neuroevolutional approach. 3rd ed. New York: Teachers College Press, 1980.
107. Ludlow CL, Bassich CJ. The results of acoustic and perceptual assessment of two types of dysarthria. In: Berry WR; ed. Clinical dysarthria. San Diego: College Hill Press, 1983.
108. Netsell R. Physiologic studies of dysarthria and their relevance to treatment. In: Rosenbek JC, ed. Current views of dysarthria: nature, assessment, and treatment. Seminars in speech and language. New York: Thieme-Stratton, 1984.
109. McDonald FI. Screening deep test of articulation. Pittsburg: Stemwix House, 1964.
110. Fisher HB, Logemann JA. The Fisher-Logemann test of articulation competence. Boston: Houghton Mifflin, 1971.
111. Templin M, Darley F. The Templin-Darley tests of articulation. Iowa City, IA: Bureau of Educational Research and Service, University of Iowa, 1969.
112. Bernthal JE, Bankson NW. Articulation disorders. Englewood Cliffs, NJ: Prentice-Hall, 1981.
113. Compton A. Generative studies of children's phonological disorders: a strategy of therapy. In: Singh S, ed. Measurements in hearing, speech, and language. Baltimore: University Park Press, 1975.
114. Ingram D. Phonological disability in children. New York: American Elsevier, 1976.
115. Weiner F. Phonological process analysis. Baltimore: University Park Press, 1978.
116. Hodson B. The assessment of phonological processes. Danville, IL: Interstate Press, 1980.
117. Shriberg L, Kwiatkowski J. Natural process analysis. New York: John Wiley & Sons, 1980.
118. Yorkston KM, Beukelman DR. Assessment of intelligibility of dysarthric speech. Tigard, OR: CC Publications, 1984.
119. Yorkston KM, Beukelman DR. A clinician-judged technique for quantifying dysarthric speech based on single word intelligibility. J Commun Disord 1980; 13:15–31.
120. Nober EH. Assessment of auditory processing in cerebral palsy. Semin Speech Lang 1987; 8:19–39.
121. Wilson BC, Davidovicz HM. Neuropsychological assessment of the child with cerebral palsy. Semin Speech Lang 1987; 8:1–18.
122. Morris SE. Therapy for the child with cerebral palsy: interacting frameworks. Semin Speech Lang 1987; 8:71–85.
123. Ferrier LJ, Shane HC. Computer-based communication aids for the nonspeaking child with cerebral palsy. Semin Speech Lang 1987; 8:107–122.
124. Jaffe MB. Neurological impairment of speech production: assessment and treatment. In: Costello J, ed. Speech disorders in children. San Diego: College Hill Press, 1984:157.
125. Bobath K, Bobath B. The facilitation of normal postural reactions and movements in the treatment of cerebral palsy. Physiotherapy 1964; 50:246–262.
126. Mysak ED. Treatment of deviant phonological systems: cerebral palsy. In: Perkins WH, ed. Current therapy of communication disorders. New York: Thieme-Stratton, 1983.
127. Davis L. Pre-speech. In: Connor FD, Williamson GG, Siepp JM, eds. Program guide for infants and toddlers with neuromotor and other developmental disabilities. New York: Teachers College Press, 1978.
128. Hixon TJ, Hawley JL, Wilson KJ. An around-the-house device for the clinical determination of respiratory driving pressure: a note on making simple even simpler. J Speech Hear Disord 1982; 47:413–415.
129. Aronson AE. Clinical voice disorders. An interdisciplinary approach. 2nd ed. New York: Thieme-Stratton, 1985.
130. Froeschels E, Kastein S, Weiss DA. A method of therapy for paralytic conditions for the mechanisms of phonation, respiration, and glutination. J Speech Hear Disord 1955; 20:365–370.
131. Jacobson E. You must relax. 5th ed. New York: McGraw-Hill, 1976.
132. Froeschels E. Chewing method as therapy. Arch Otolaryngol 1952; 61:427–434.
133. Boone DR. The voice and voice therapy. Englewood Cliffs, NJ: Prentice-Hall, 1977.
134. Shprintzen RJ, McCall GN, Skolnick MD. A new therapeutic technique for the treatment of velopharyngeal incompetence. J Speech Hear Disord 1975; 40:69–83.

135. Cole RM. Direct muscle training for the improvement of velopharyngeal function. In: Grabb WC, Rosenstein SW, Bzoch KR, eds. Cleft lip and palate. Boston: Little, Brown, 1971.
136. Lubit EC, Larsen RE. The Lubit palatal exercise: a preliminary report. Cleft Palate J 1969; 6:120–133.
137. Yules RB, Chase RA. A training method for reduction of hypernasality in speech. Plast Reconstr Surg 1969; 43:180–185.
138. Netsell R. Instrumentation in the rehabilitation of dysarthria. Presented at the Veterans Administration Workshop on motor speech disorders, Madison, WI, 1975.
139. Bankson N, Byrne M. The effect of a timed correct sound production task on carryover. J Speech Hear Res 1972; 15:160–168.
140. Powell J, McReynolds L. A procedure for testing position generalization from articulation training. J Speech Hear Disord 1969; 12:625–645.
141. Cook AM, Coleman CL. Selecting augmentative communication systems by matching client skills and needs to system characteristics. Semin Speech Lang 1987; 8:153–167.
142. McDonald ET, Schultz AR. Communication boards for cerebral palsied children. J Speech Hear Disord 1973; 38:73–88.
143. Vanderheiden GC, Harris-Vanderheiden D. Communication techniques and aids for the nonvocal severely handicapped. In: Lloyd L, ed. Communication assessment and intervention strategies. Baltimore: University Park Press, 1976:607.
144. Clark CR, Woodcock RW. Graphic systems of communication. In: Lloyd L, ed. Communication assessment and intervention strategies. Baltimore: University Park Press, 1976:549.
145. Carlson F. PicSyms categorical dictionary. Lawrence, KS: Baggeboda Press, 1984.
146. Shane HC, Bashir AS. Election criteria for the adoption of an augmentative communication system: preliminary consideration. J Speech Hear Disord 1980; 45:408–414.
147. Buzolich MJ. Children in transition: implementing augmentative communication systems with severely speech-handicapped children. Semin Speech Lang 1987; 8:199–213.
148. Glennen SL, Calculator SN. Training functional communication board use: a pragmatic approach. Augmentative and Alternative Commun 1985; 1:134–142.
149. Culp PM. Outcome measurement: the impact of communication augmentation. Semin Speech Lang 1987; 8:169–181.
150. Mohr JP, Pessen MS, Finklestein S, Funkenstein HH, Duncan GW, Davis KR. Broca aphasia: pathologic and clinical. Neurology 1978; 28:311–324.
151. Horowitz SJ. Neurological findings in developmental verbal apraxia. In: Aram D, ed. Assessment and treatment of developmental apraxia. New York: Thieme-Stratton, 1984.
152. Aram M. Developmental apraxia of speech. Paper presented at the annual convention of the American Speech and Hearing Association, Atlanta, 1979.
153. Ferry PC, Hall SM, Hicks JL. Dilapidated speech: developmental verbal apraxia. Dev Med Child Neurol 1975; 17:749–756.
154. Myklebust HR, Bosher B, Olson DA, Cole CH. Minimal brain damage in children (final report). Washington, DC: Department of Health, Education, and Welfare, Neurological and Sensory Disease, National Institutes of Health, 1969.
155. Gubbay SS, Ellis E, Walton JN, Court SDM. Clumsy children: a study of apraxia and agnosic defects in 21 children. Brain 1965; 88:295–312.
156. Dickson S. Differences between children who spontaneously outgrow and children who retain functional articulation errors. J Speech Hear Res 1962; 5:263–271.
157. Morley ME. The development and disorders of speech in childhood. 3rd ed. London: Livingstone, 1972.
158. Chappell GE. Childhood verbal apraxia and its treatment. J Speech Hear Disord 1973; 38:362–368.
159. Macaluso-Haynes S. Developmental apraxia of speech: symptoms and treatment. In: Johns DF, ed. Clinical management of neurogenic communicative disorders. Boston: Little, Brown, 1978:243.
160. Smartt J, LaLance L, Gray J, Hibbett P. Developmental apraxia of speech: a Tennessee Speech and Hearing Association subcommittee report. J Tenn Speech Hear Assoc 1976; 20:21–39.
161. Court D, Harris M. Speech disorders in children-Part II. Br Med J 1965; ii:409–411.
162. Ekelman BL, Aram DM. Syntactic findings in developmental verbal apraxia. J Commun Disord 1983; 16:237–250.
163. Blakely RW. Screening test for developmental apraxia of speech. Tigard, OR: CC Publications, 1980.
164. Guyette TW, Diedrich WM. A review of the screening test for developmental apraxia of speech. Lang Speech Hear Serv in Schools 1983; 14:202–209.
165. Haynes S. Developmental apraxia of speech: symptoms and treatment. In: Johns DF, ed. Clinical management of neurogenic communicative disorders. Boston: Little, Brown, 1985:259.
166. Yoss KS, Darley FL. Therapy in developmental apraxia of speech. Lang Speech Hear Serv in Schools, 1974; V:23–31.
167. Haynes SM, Johns DF, May EB. Assessment and therapeutic management of an adult patient with developmental apraxia of speech and orosensory perceptual deficits. Texas Audio Speech Path 1978; 3:6–15.
168. Logue RD. Disorders of motor-speech planning in children: evaluation and treatment. In: Communicative disorders: an audio journal for continuing education, 3. New York: Grune & Stratton, 1978.
169. Klick SL. Adapted cuing technique for use in treatment of dyspraxia. Lang Speech Hear Serv in Schools 1985; 16:256–259.
170. Helfrick-Miller KR. The use of melodic intonation therapy with developmentally apractic children: a clinical perspective. J Pennsylvania Speech-Language-Hearing Association 1983; XVI:11–15.
171. Albert M, Sparks R, Helm N. Melodic intonation therapy for aphasia. Arch Neurol 1973; 29:130–131.
172. Sparks RW, Holland AL. Method: melodic intonation therapy for aphasia. J Speech Hear Disord 1976; 41:287–297.
173. Young EC, Thompson CK. An experimental analysis of treatment effects on consonant clusters and ambisyllabic consonants in two adults with developmental phonological problems. J Commun Disord 1987; 20:137–149.
174. McReynolds L, Kearns K. Single-subject experimental designs in communicative disorders. Baltimore: University Park Press, 1983.
175. McReynolds LV, Thompson CK. Flexibility of single-subject experimental designs. Part I. Review of the basics of single-subject designs. J Speech Hear Disord 1986; 51:194–203.
176. Connell PJ, Thompson CK. Flexibility of single-subject experimental designs. Part III. Using flexibility to design or modify experiments. J Speech Hear Disord 1986; 51:214–225.
177. Kearns KP. Flexibility of single-subject experimental designs. Part II. Design selection and arrangement of experimental phases. J Speech Hear Disord 1986; 51:204–213.

19 Motor Speech Disorders: The Dysarthrias and Apraxia of Speech

Kevin P. Kearns, Ph.D.
Nina N. Simmons, M.S.

The term "motor speech disorders" refers to speech disturbances associated with lesions of the motor system, the dysarthrias, and apraxia of speech. The purpose of this chapter is to discuss current trends in the literature on motor speech disorders and to provide an introduction to the assessment and treatment of these disorders. This review will be restricted to acquired disorders of adults. Motor speech disorders associated with developmental problems, such as those evident in cerebral palsy and developmental apraxia of speech, are considered elsewhere in this volume (see Chapter 18).

The dysarthrias and apraxia of speech encompass the entire spectrum of speech problems seen by speech-language pathologists, and, as such, they represent a microcosm of speech-language pathology. Virtually all of the motor systems involved in speech production, including respiration, phonation, articulation, and palatopharyngeal valving, may be impaired in dysarthric individuals. Furthermore, disturbances of articulation and prosody (i.e., intonation, stress, and rhythm) are prevalent in apraxia of speech. Clinical management of motor speech disorders is further complicated by the fact that the dysarthrias and apraxia of speech frequently co-occur with one another and with aphasic language problems.[1,2]

Given the pervasiveness and inherent complexity of the dysarthrias and apraxia of speech, it is clear that advanced study and training may be needed for clinicians involved in the clinical management of these disorders. The range of clinical skills required to assess and treat the dysarthrias and apraxia include an understanding of normal and disordered anatomy and physiology,[3,4] knowledge of medical terminology and procedures, an understanding of disease processes,[5] and skills in behavioral assessment and programming.[6] Moreover, physiologic and acoustic measures of speech production are becoming commonplace in clinical research in this area,[7–10] and instrumental measurement and biofeedback are being used to develop and evaluate treatment procedures.[11–13] Consequently, it is becoming increasingly necessary that clinicians who assess and treat motor speech problems familiarize themselves with physiologic and acoustic measures of speech production. Scholarly and comprehensive summaries of the dysarthrias and apraxia of speech are now available to the interested clinician.[1,3,14–21] Our summary owes much to these sources.

NATURE

The Dysarthrias

Current views of the dysarthrias have their origin in the seminal work of Darley[22] and his colleagues at the Mayo Clinic and the early physiologic efforts of Hardy.[23] Their studies of the perceptual characteristics of the speech of groups of neurologically impaired patients with dysarthria[22,24,25] were summarized in the text *Motor Speech Disorders.*[15] Darley defined the dysarthrias as a group of speech impairments resulting from muscular weakness, slowness, or incoordination that occur as a result of central or peripheral nervous system involvement.[26] As previously noted, all of the motor systems involved in speech production can be impaired in individuals with dysarthria. Motoric involvement in dysarthria can be restricted to a single system, such as laryngeal valving. More typically, however, multiple motor speech systems are simultaneously impaired in individuals with dysarthria. For example, following multiple cerebrovascular accidents (CVAs), a patient may exhibit pseudobulbar palsy and spastic dysarthria. The deviant perceptual characteristics of such a patient would likely involve some or all of the following: imprecise consonant articulation, monopitch, reduced stress, harsh voice quality, monoloudness, reduced pitch level, reduced rate of speech, and mild hypernasality (Table 19–1).

Imprecise consonant articulation is the common denominator shared by the various dysarthrias. However, the results of the Mayo Clinic study demonstrated that six types of dysarthria can be distinguished on the basis of perceptual characteristics.[22,24] The six types include flaccid, spastic, ataxic, hypokinetic, hyperkinetic, and mixed (see Table 19–1). It is important to emphasize, therefore, that "it is proper to speak of the dysarthrias (plural) rather than of dysarthria (singular), and that the dysarthrias are clinically differentiable."[15] The types of dysarthria can be identified by the trained clinician because of the unique clusters of deviant perceptual dimensions that characterize them (see Appendix 1). Thus the "trained ear" was viewed by the Mayo group as an important instrument for aiding in the differential diagnosis of disease processes. Recent acoustic studies have demonstrated that perceptual analysis techniques validly differentiate types of dysarthric speakers.[27,28]

The perceptual classification system is based on the neuromuscular status of the muscles whose dysfunction causes the dysarthria. For example, lesions or diseases that result in upper motoneuron involvement classically result in spasticity to the involved muscles. Thus, when motor speech systems are impaired as a result of upper motoneuron damage, the resultant dysarthria is labelled "spastic" dysarthria. This approach is based to a large degree on the fact that Darley and his colleagues felt strongly that the deviant perceptual characteristics of the speech of individuals with dysarthria reflects the underlying pathophysiology of the impaired nervous system. Consistent with the earlier suggestions of Grewel,[29] the dysarthrias are viewed as having value for lesion localization within the nervous system.

Although the Mayo Clinic taxonomy has become the standard for both clinical and research endeavors, several words of caution are necessary about perceptually based analyses. First, deviant perceptual characteristics of dysarthric speech may be relatively difficult to identify as compared to normal perceptual characteristics, even for experienced clinicians.[30] Specialized training and experience are required for differential diagnosis of motor speech disorders through perceptual analyses.[9] In addition, perceptual (and acoustic) analyses may not be sufficient to infer the underlying pathophysiology.[31] Motor systems for speech production may be differentially affected in the dysarthrias, and these differences may not be apparent from an auditory analysis of taped speech samples. Perceptual ratings of dysarthric speech are increasingly being supplemented with acoustic[13,32,33] and physiologic measures.[8,34] These and related findings led Darley to the conclusion that the simultaneous use of perceptual, acoustic, and physiologic measurements may increase the reliability of dysarthria assessment procedures.[35] Despite the inherent shortcomings of this approach, perceptual analysis continues to be the primary clinical tool available for evaluating and treating individuals with dysarthria. Perceptual analyses have also been widely used to evaluate apraxia of speech, our next topic of discussion.

Apraxia of Speech

Apraxia of speech remains one of the most controversial topics in the speech-language pathology literature. Darley discussed the historical bases for the controversy in his paper entitled *Apraxia of speech: 107 years of terminological confusion.* In this presentation, he highlighted differences between apraxia, dysarthria, and aphasia, and he called for adoption of the term "apraxia of speech." His rationale for the distinction between these disorders was largely clinically motivated. Darley stated, "If we apply unclear or overlapping labels and let our language do our thinking for us, we may end up misunderstanding the disorder of apraxia of speech and mistreating the patient who is handicapped by it."[36] Johns and LaPointe's extensive literature review led them to the same conclusion.[37] Considerable research has been conducted in the 3 decades since Darley's historic paper, and contemporary reviews trace the evolution of progress in this area.[1,38–41] In the most comprehensive treatise available, Wertz et al provide the following definition:

> . . . apraxia of speech (is) a neurogenic phonologic disorder resulting from sensorimotor impairment of the

TABLE 19–1 Perceptual Characteristics of the Dysarthrias

Type	*Rank Order of Characteristics*	*Explanation*	*Predominant clusters*
Flaccid dysarthria	Hypernasal Imprecise consonants Breathy (continuous) Monopitch Nasal emission Audible inspiration Harsh Phrases short Monoloudness	Lower motoneuron	Resonatory incompetence Phonatory incompetence Phonatory prosodic insufficiency
Spastic dysarthria	Imprecise consonants Monopitch Reduced stress Harsh Monoloudness Pitch level Rate Hypernasal Strained or strangled Phrases short	Upper motoneuron	Prosodic insufficiency Phonatory stenosis Prosodic excess
Ataxic dysarthria	Imprecise consonants Excess and equal stress Irregular disintegrating articulation Vowels distorted Harsh Phonemes prolonged Intervals prolonged Monopitch Monoloudness Rate	Cerebellar	Articulatory inaccuracy Prosodic excess Phonatory prosodic insufficiency
Hypokinetic dysarthria	Monopitch Reduced stress Monoloudness Imprecise consonants Inappropriate silences Short rushes Harsh Breathy (continuous) Pitch level Variable rate	Extrapyramidal	Prosodic insufficiency
Hyperkinetic dysarthria Predominantly quick	Imprecise consonants Distorted vowels Harsh Irregular disintegrating articulation Strained or strangled Monopitch Monoloudness Inappropriate silences Short phrases Prolonged intervals	Extrapyramidal	Prosodic excess Prosodic insufficiency Articulatory and resonatory incompetence Phonatory stenosis
Predominantly slow	Imprecise consonants Prolonged intervals Variable rate Monopitch Harsh Inappropriate silences Distorted vowels Excess loudness variation Prolonged phonemes Monoloudness	Extrapyramidal	Articulatory inaccuracy Prosodic excess Phonatory stenosis Prosodic insufficiency

TABLE 19–1 (Continued)

Type	*Rank Order of Characteristics*	*Explanation*	*Predominant clusters*
Mixed dysarthria (e.g., Spastic-flaccid)	Imprecise consonants Hypernasal Harsh Rate Monopitch Short phrases Distorted vowels Pitch level Monoloudness Excess and equal stress	Upper and lower motoneurons	Prosodic insufficiency Prosodic excess Articulatory and resonatory incompetence Phonatory stenosis

After Darley FL, Aronson AE, Brown JR. Motor speech disorders. Philadelphia: WB Saunders, 1975.

capacity to select, program, and/or execute incoordinated and normally timed sequences, the positioning of speech musculature for the volitional production of speech sounds . . . Prosodic alteration, that is, change in speech stress, intonation and/or rhythm, may be associated with the articulatory disruption either as a primary part or in compensation for it (p 4).[21]

Wertz et al also stress that the motor speech impairment in apraxia is not a result of aphasic language deficits.[21] Stimilarly, apraxia of speech is not a consequence of the muscular weakness, slowness, or incoordination seen in the dysarthrias.

Canter stressed the importance of underlying neuropsychologic mechanisms when trying to understand neurogenic communication disorders.[42] That is, the ability to identify the behaviors that characterize dysarthria and apraxia is not enough; the clinician must also understand the nature of the disorders. Although the underlying mechanisms that result in dysarthric impairments are relatively easy to comprehend and observe, explanations for apraxia of speech have, by comparison, been comparatively obtuse. In the dysarthrias, the relationship between abnormalities in muscular speed, range, strength, and coordination can frequently be observed and, therefore, logically attributed to damage to the central or peripheral nervous system. Moreover, other nonspeech motor system impairments frequently cooccur with dysarthria, thus confirming our observation that the pattern of dysarthric speech is directly related to muscular involvement. By contrast, motor speech deficits in apraxia are usually explained by analogy to hypothetical processes, a motor programmer, that cannot be directly observed or analyzed.[40,41] The problems inherent in specifying the nature of apraxia of speech has been a proverbial double-edged sword. On the one hand, the definition by analogy problem has contributed to the controversy that continues to surround the topic of apraxia of speech. On the other hand, the definitional problems associated with this disorder stimulated considerable research that has influenced current notions of apraxia of speech.[43]

A Motor Programming Deficit

Much of the controversy surrounding apraxia of speech has centered on whether or not this disorder is a unique phenomenon that is distinct from other neurogenic communicative disorders, particularly aphasia. As noted earlier, Darley argued that apraxia resulted from inhibition or impairment of the programming of motor speech movements.[26] While programming notions are being reevaluated,[44] an understanding of the historical roots of the motor programming model is prerequisite to understanding the apraxia of speech literature. Darley felt that the articulatory and prosodic impairments that were observed in patients with apraxia should be treated directly and that language treatment was inappropriate for treating apraxic symptoms. Although apraxia of speech and aphasia may coexist, they were viewed as distinct disorders that required entirely different treatment approaches. Early support for this view was derived from studies that revealed phonemic variability in apraxic speakers. The issue of variability is inextricably linked to the motor programming position. Researchers reasoned that if the capacity to program timing, positioning, sequencing, and coordination of motor movements for speech is impaired, then inconsistent and variable articulatory impairment should result. Indeed, early perceptual analyses of individuals with apraxia revealed the presence of variable and inconsistent articulatory performances according to traditional error classifications of substitution, omissions, and distortions.[45–48] Relatedly, results that distinguished subjects with apraxia from those with dysarthria lend further support to the notion that apraxia of speech was indeed a distinct clinical entity.[46] The broad transcription techniques used in this early research demonstrated that substitution errors predominated for the subjects with apraxia, whereas distortion errors were common to those with dysarthria.

Additional support for the motor programming position was also provided by reports of "pure" cases of apraxia in the absence of aphasic language disturbances.[49] Finally, this position was also upheld by the findings that apraxic deficits could not be attributed to auditory perceptual[50,51] or oral sensory impairments.[52]

In contrast to the motor programming viewpoint, there appeared to be growing sentiment for the position that apraxia of speech was not a distinct clinical entity. This linguistic viewpoint attributed the articulatory deficits of apraxic speakers to aphasic language impairments.[53,54] Support for this position was obtained from several sources. First, unlike traditional articulatory assessments, linguistic analyses, including distinctive feature, markedness, and phonologic process analyses, revealed a considerable degree of lawfulness in the speech of patients with apraxia.[55–60] That is, investigators systematically accounted for much of the seemingly random variability apparent in the speech of subjects with apraxia by using linguistic analysis procedures. Since the observed lawfulness was consistent with linguistic hypotheses about the organization of language, these findings were interpreted as supporting the notion that apraxic errors resulted from a breakdown in linguistic processing (i.e., aphasia).[61]

The linguistic view of articulatory breakdown in apraxia was given further impetus by studies that failed to distinguish between aphasic patients with (presumed) coexisting apraxia and aphasic patients without coexisting apraxia.[55,62] A final line of research that supported the notion that apraxia is a linguistic rather than a motor programming deficit involved studies that demonstrated the influence of linguistic variables on articulatory performance in individuals with apraxia.[63,64]

The linguistic view of apraxia is based, in part, on tautologic reasoning.[9,41,65] That is, this position assumes speech production and errors are lawful (rule governed) because verbal output is controlled by phonologic, linguistic rules. The finding that lawfulness (less variability) exists in the speech of patients with apraxia is subsequently used to substantiate the hypothesis that apraxic errors are governed by linguistic rules. As Kent and Rosenbek indicate,[9] there is a danger of confusing one's method of analysis with the results of the analysis. The fact that most linguistic studies cited as refuting the existence of apraxia of speech as a motor speech phenomenon have used subjects that are both aphasic and apraxic is also problematic for the linguistic position.[41] It is not surprising that linguistic factors interacted with articulatory impairments[63,66] in this population of linguistically impaired subjects. Albeit so-called pure apraxic patients are rare and not readily available for study. However, the fact that these patients have been reported[49,51,67] is also problematic for the linguistic view of apraxia.

Ultimately, working hypotheses about the nature of any disorder should be based on data and scientific principles rather than logic or opinion. Therefore recent trends in the literature on apraxia of speech are briefly reviewed next.

Research in this area has gradually taken on an instrumental flavor as the perceptual and descriptive linguistic studies of the past have given way to acoustic and physiologic studies.[21,39–41,68] Acoustic analyses using spectrographic techniques have examined voice onset time in patients with aphasia and apraxia. Acoustic analyses of voice onset times provide a sensitive measure of the timing and coordination of voicing and other articulatory dimensions. In normal individuals, voice onset time ranges for voiced and voiceless cognates (e.g., /b/ and /p/) do not overlap. However, considerable overlap and variability have been found for the patients with apraxia.[9,62,70,71] These results highlight motoric timing and coordination problems that are consistent with the motor programming position. Recent acoustic studies have also demonstrated that apraxic speakers have slow, inaccurate, and variable movements during consonant and vowel production, overall reduced speaking rates, initiation difficulties, prolongations, and prosodic disturbances that are consistent with deficient motor programming abilities.[9,72,73]

Physiologic studies of apraxic speech production have supported and expanded acoustic observations of apraxic speech. Fiberoptic observations of a "pure" apraxic patient documented variability of velar movements and phonetic production errors that were not evident in normal subjects.[67] In a subsequent study of the same patient, an x-ray microbeam system was used to simultaneously track and time movements of several articulators.[70] Results demonstrated highly variable movement patterns and incoordinated timing between velar, labial, and lingual movements for the patient with apraxia as compared to a normal subject. Results of simultaneous physiologic measurements, including electromyography (EMG), muscular movement, and voicing measures, also document pervasive motoric timing and coordination deficits in adults with apraxia.[7]

Cumulatively, results of recent acoustic and physiologic studies indicate that individuals with apraxia have difficulty programming the timing, coordination, and articulatory adjustments necessary for normal speech production. These findings are generally consistent with the motor programming explanation of the disorder espoused by Darley[26] over 20 years ago. However, the concept of apraxia as a motor programming disorder has not remained static and our notions about the appropriateness of the terminology used to describe these deficits are being reevaluated.[44] Recent data have influenced speech-language pathologists' concept of the disorder, and these changes have begun to influence patient management. For example, studies that highlight timing and coordination problems in apraxia have also demonstrated the frailty of perceptual analysis techniques that rely on broad phonetic transcription. That is, studies of voice onset time, phoneme and segment durations, and articulatory movement patterns demonstrate that apraxic timing and dyscoordination deficits result in phonetic distortions that are perceived as substitutions.[7,9,62,69,70] Thus early studies that used broad phonetic transcription probably classified many distortions as substitution errors. As Rosenbek et al point out,[40] in the absence of instrumental measurement, future research and clinical endeavors should utilize narrow phonetic transcription to classify apraxic errors.

The concept of apraxia has also evolved from the notion that it is an articulatory disorder to the current notion that apraxia is a movement disorder that results from deficient motor programming.[21,40] The current view is eloquently summarized by Rosenbek et al:

> If we begin to think of apraxia of speech as a movement disorder rather than as an articulation or even a speech disorder, and if we think of even perceived substitutions . . . as resulting from distortions of the temporal sequence of component movements, then our attitudes about apraxic errors and our treatment approaches are altered . . . In treatment, speech targets are replaced by movement targets. In this revised view, the speech sounds one selects (for treatment) are merely facilitators of movement on par with other facilitators such as rate, rhythm, and stress (p 58).[40]

Further consideration will be given to this view of apraxia of speech and its influence on clinical practice in our discussion of treatment for this disorder. In the section that follows, we turn our attention to assessment issues.

ASSESSMENT

A Philosophy of Clinical Process and Assessment

Traditional teaching in speech-language pathology separates the clinical process into discrete phases including assessment, treatment, generalization, and follow-up. In this approach, clinical assessment is conceived of as a brief period of evaluation that occurs at the initiation of, and periodically throughout, clinical contact. This view of the clinical process fosters the notion that patient care activities are relatively independent and sequential. As one phase of the process (e.g., assessment) is concluded, the following phase (e.g., treatment) begins.

Kearns discussed the pitfalls of the sequential, discrete phase view of the clinical process and suggested an alternative model.[75] In this alternative schema, the clinical process consists of a number of overlapping and interdependent activities that cannot be divided artificially into discrete phases. This approach can be conceptualized as a closed loop system whereby assessment, treatment, generalization, and maintenance activities occur simultaneously rather than sequentially. Each clinical activity is integrally related to all others. In this model, assessment is an ongoing activity that serves as the basis for treatment decisions. From the outset, ongoing evaluation procedures are used to establish goals and criteria for generalization and maintenance of improvements on treated behaviors. Assessment and intervention activities are continuously fine tuned according to the change in a client's performance on the ongoing evaluation probes of treatment, generalization, and maintenance situations. This integrated model of the clinical process necessitates the development of a comprehensive assessment and treatment plan, and it requires consideration of *all* aspects of patient management prior to beginning treatment. This approach encourages advanced planning for and continuous assessment of components of intervention, such as generalization and maintenance, that may otherwise not be considered until the final "phases" of clinical intervention.

Although the two views of patient care outlined previously are superficially similar, they lead to very different approaches to patient management. For example, by separating assessment, treatment, and generalization activities, the discrete phase model reinforces a test-*then*-treat approach to assessment. Because assessment is only conducted periodically, the administered tests tend to be global measures of performance. Measurement of performance on actual treatment tasks is seldom conducted. Thus an overall measure of intelligibility may be administered to evaluate a patient with dysarthria who is experiencing a decreased conversational loudness level, but loudness (intensity level) may not actually be evaluated. The results of this type of assessment document whether or not overall improvement occurs, but insufficient information is available to determine *why* progress occurred. Continuing our previous example, a dysarthric individual's increase in overall intelligibility may have resulted from therapy or extraneous factors such as general improvement in neurologic or health status.

Purpose

Although we have argued that the clinical assessment of motor speech disorders should be an ongoing activity, the purpose of assessment tends to vary throughout the clinical process. McNeil and Kennedy listed ten reasons for assessing dysarthria. Their list is equally applicable to the assessment of apraxia of speech:

> (1) to detect or confirm a suspected problem; (2) to establish a differential diagnosis . . .; (3) to classify within a specified disorder; (4) to determine site of lesion or disease process; (5) to specify degree of severity of involvement; (6) to establish a prognosis; (7) to establish candidacy for treatment; (8) to specify more precisely the treatment focus; (9) to establish criteria for treatment termination; (10) to measure any change in the patient that accompanies treatment, lack of treatment, or exacerbation of the original etiological factor (p 337).[6]

More often than not, several of these purposes are of equal interest at a given point in the assessment process. For example, a clinician may initially be interested in determining if a communication problem exists, establishing the nature and severity of identified problems, assisting with differential diagnosis, and obtaining information for intervention purposes. The nature of the information needed and the focus of the assessment tend to vary throughout the clinical process. Thus assessment procedures administered in conjunction with therapy may be very different from the procedures used to establish the nature and severity of a disorder. Individualized treatment probes are needed to obtain information about the effectiveness of specific treatment techniques and the need for modification of treatment.

There are no standard motor speech assessment batteries, and it is unlikely that one will be available in the near future. Consequently, the accurate assessment of motor speech impairments largely rests on the clinician's knowledge of these disorders, and so the characteristics of the motor speech disorders are reviewed in the sections that follow.

Characteristics of Motor Speech Disorders

Few standardized procedures currently exist for assessing the dysarthrias and apraxia of speech. Attempts are underway to develop objective clinical assessments in this area,[76,77] and the instrumental assessments based on acoustic and physiologic studies show promise for clinical application.[10,79] At the present time, however, clinicians rely primarily on analysis and interpretation of performance on nonstandard tasks to assess motor speech disorders. Ultimately, assessment of motor speech disorders is based on a knowledge of the behavioral and perceptual characteristics associated with the dysarthrias, apraxia of speech, and related disorders. Factors that distinguish these disorders are reviewed in the following sections. Our discussion closely follows the levels of analysis suggested by Canter.[42] He suggested that information concerning site of lesion, underlying neuropsychological mechanisms, speech characteristics, and related impairments can be used to distinguish the dysarthrias, apraxia, and aphasia from one another.

Site of Lesion

As previously noted, clinicians involved in the management of motor speech disorders must be familiar with medical terminology, pathophysiology, and the various medical conditions that can result in the dysarthrias and apraxia of speech. As Wertz and his colleagues indicate,[2,21] this information is essential during the assessment process because the medical and biographical histories can help to confirm or dispute a diagnosis. This information can be supplied, in part, from the history supplied by the patient, but it is often obtained from reviewing the patient's hospital medical records. Of most concern to our present discussion, information such as medical history and etiology can be useful if one understands the neuropathologic conditions that underlie the dysarthrias and apraxia of speech. For example, as a general rule, chronic, debilitating dysarthria is usually the result of bilateral subcortical damage to the nervous system. The speech musculature is bilaterally innervated, and most individuals readily compensate for unilateral damage. By contrast, the volitional programming deficits associated with apraxia of speech most frequently result from unilateral cortical damage to the left hemisphere.[40] The most frequent site of damage in apraxia, Broca's area, is considered the major cortical region associated with programming or planning motoric activities, including speech production. Consequently, damage to this cortical region often results in apraxia of speech, a motor programming deficit.

There are notable exceptions to these generalities. For example, multiple CVAs (strokes) that damage the cerebral cortex can cause lasting dysarthric symptoms. Similarly, unilateral damage to the nervous system can, occasionally, result in surprisingly severe and persistent dysarthria. Kertesz's observation that apraxia can occur in patients with subcortical damage[78] is also contrary to the general rule. However, these exceptions do not diminish the fact that knowledge of a patient's site of lesion and related information about underlying neuropathology can contribute to the assessment of motor speech disorders. Knowledge of pathophysiology can also prove valuable when the clinician is faced with the task of differentiating types of dysarthria and/or planning dysarthria treatment.[3,4,79]

Given the controversy surrounding apraxia of speech and its occasional confusion with aphasia, a brief description of the expected site of lesion for aphasic articulatory errors (phonemic or literal paraphasias) is in order. Lesions associated with aphasic phonologic errors are frequently localized to the posterior (temporoparietal) areas of the left hemisphere of the cerebral cortex (Wernicke's area) and/or the deep fibers that connect the anterior (Broca's area) and posterior (Wernicke's area) language zones. These lesions are in contrast to the more anterior (Broca's area) left hemisphere lesions associated with apraxia and to the subcortical damage frequently seen in the dysarthrias.

Underlying Mechanisms

In addition to site of lesion, knowledge of the neuropsychological mechanisms that characterize the motor speech disorders can be of great value in distinguishing apraxia, the dysarthrias, and aphasia. Earlier in our discussion, we distinguished the deficient motor programming deficits underlying apraxia of speech and the muscular execution problems of the dysarthrias. Relatedly, Darley defined aphasia as an acquired language disturbance, resulting from brain damage, that affects all language modalities (i.e., verbal formulation, auditory comprehension, reading, and writing).[26] Motor speech deficits must be differentiated from linguistic impairments in aphasia. Underlying mechanisms that distinguish the disorders are briefly contrasted in Table 19–2. Speech and related characteristics that may be of value in distinguishing apraxia, the dysarthrias, and aphasia are considered next.

Speech and Related Characteristics

Apraxia of Speech. After an extensive review of the apraxia literature, Wertz et al summarized the following clinical characteristics of apraxia of speech:

1. Effortful, trial and error, groping articulatory movements and attempts at self correction.
2. Dysprosody unrelieved by extended periods of normal rhythm, stress, and intonation.
3. Articulatory inconsistency on repeated productions of the same utterance.
4. Obvious difficulty initiating utterances.[21]

This succinct list can serve as a guidepost for signaling the presence of apraxia of speech, particularly when combined with other hallmarks of the disorder. Specifically, apraxia is viewed as a problem of *volitional* motor programming, and performance differences may be apparent on tasks that vary in the degree of volition required to complete them.[15,20,21] For example, automatic speech tasks—those that require little or no volition such as counting—may be performed with relatively little difficulty as compared with more volitional tasks such as repetition or confrontation naming. Relatedly, patients with apraxia often produce "islands of error free speech." That is, they may produce a fluent phrase or sentence in the context of effortful speech.

Performance variability can also be observed when motoric or linguistic elements of task difficulty are systematically altered. For example, an increase in articulatory errors, effortful groping, and prosodic disturbance may be evident as the length of a verbal stimulus item increases on a repetition task. Similarly, phonemes that require exceptionally fine motor control for their production (affricates, fricatives, and blends) result in error productions more frequently than other speech sounds. Moreover, all else being equal, polysyllabic words are more difficult to produce than monosyllabic words on a given speech task.

Another distinguishing characteristic of the patient with apraxia is the type of articulatory error produced. Although these patients produce both substitution and distortion errors, their speech is replete with errors that are perceived as substitutions.

The Dysarthrias. The speech characteristics associated with the dysarthrias are markedly different from the characteristics associated with apraxia. As previously noted, the pattern of deficits in dysarthria varies according to the site of lesion and the specific type of dysarthria (see Table 19–1). However, several general aspects of the dysarthrias help to distinguish them from other neurogenic communicative disorders. A common denominator of the dysarthrias is the presence of imprecise consonant articulation and distortions. Unlike apraxic speakers, dysarthric speakers rarely exhibit frank substitution errors.

A second distinguishing characteristic of the dysarthrias is the relative consistency of patient performance. The muscular weakness that underlies the dysarthrias is everpresent. Therefore, repeated trials on a given speech task usually result in similar performances across repeated trials. All else being equal, the performance of patients with dysarthria is also relatively consistent over time. By contrast, patients with apraxia and aphasia exhibit considerable variability in their performance over time and across repeated attempts at the same speech task.

Impairment of multiple motor systems involved in speech production is another defining feature of the dysarthrias. Dysarthric speakers often have simultaneous impairment of articulation, respiration, phonation, and/or laryngeal valving. Multiple systems involvement of this nature is not evident in apraxia of speech nor aphasia. With the possible exception of ataxic dysarthria,[73] the characteristics of dysarthric speech can be readily distinguished from apraxic articulatory and prosodic disturbances.

Phonemic Paraphasias. Phonemic or literal paraphasias can be viewed as phoneme substitutions produced by fluent aphasic speakers. These errors are produced in the context of fluent, melodic speech. By contrast, the speech of patients with apraxia is often nonfluent and characterized by initiation difficulties and effortful groping for articulatory targets. The robotic dysprosody that occurs in apraxia is also markedly different from the near normal melodic line apparent in patients with aphasia who produce phonemic paraphasias. Another factor that helps to differentiate phonemic paraphasias from apraxia of speech is the relationship of articulatory errors to their intended targets. Whereas phonemic paraphasias frequently appear to be only remotely related to intended targets (e.g., /z/ for /k/), apraxic errors are frequently only one or two features from intended targets (e.g., /t/ for /d/).

Associated Problems

Problems that frequently co-occur with the dysarthrias, apraxia, and phonemic paraphasias can provide confirmatory information on an initial diagnosis. In addition, the presence of associated problems must also be considered during treatment planning.

Disorders that coexist with the dysarthrias relate to the fact that the neurologic damage that caused the speech problem also impairs other nonspeech functions. In fact, the perceptual characteristics of the speech of individuals with dysarthria may closely parallel more generalized motoric involvement. Thus an individual with myasthenia gravis who exhibits the perceptual characteristics of flaccid dysarthria (see Table 19–1) may also exhibit flaccidity of the arms and legs. This finding is not surprising since the disease process impairs communication between the nerves and their muscles regardless of whether the muscles are used for walking or for speech production. Other associated problems that result from muscular weakness, slowness, or incoordination, such as swallowing disorders (dysphagia), may also accompany dysarthria.

Occasionally the absence of an associated disorder can also be revealing. For example, assessment often reveals that many individuals with dysarthria have normal cognitive and language skills. This finding is not surprising given the site of lesion (i.e., bilateral subcortical) typically found in the dysarthric population. But apraxia of speech usually results from cortical damage to the dominant (left) hemisphere for language, and so, predictably, apraxia most often co-occurs with Broca's aphasia.

Apraxia of Speech. Patients with Broca's aphasia and apraxia of speech generally have relatively functional auditory comprehension skills. Consequently, a common finding among patients with apraxia is that they are aware of their speech impairments. Their ability to monitor their speech is frequently accompanied by a high level of frustration.

In addition to the accompanying language deficits, the site of lesion (unilateral cortical) that most frequently results in apraxia of speech also results in weakness or paralysis to the opposite side of the body. This weakness often includes the facial muscles on the right side of the body.

Perhaps one of the most reliable associated signs in apraxia of speech is the presence of an oral, nonverbal apraxia. Although apraxia of speech can be found without an accompanying nonverbal apraxia, these two impairments are frequently found together. Obvious signs of apraxia for oral nonspeech movements (e.g., puckering lips) are not found in purely dysarthric or fluent aphasic individuals.

Phonemic Paraphasias. In marked contrast to the patient with apraxia, patients that produce phonemic paraphasias often have a fluent, Wernicke's aphasia without any concomitant motor impairments. In addition, auditory comprehension skills are markedly impaired, and error awareness is diminished. Finally, the site of lesion that results in fluent paraphasic speech (posterior and unilateral cortical area) also frequently causes visual field defects that can affect performance on assessment tasks.

To briefly summarize, Canter has observed that the dysarthrias, apraxia of speech, and aphasic articulatory errors can be distinguished on the basis of the site of lesion, the neuropsychologic mechanisms that underlie the disorders, speech-related characteristics, and associated impairments that occur with each problem (Table 19–2).[42] Approaching the assessment process with a knowledge of factors associated with each level of analysis may enhance the clinician's ability to evaluate motor speech disorders. In the section that follows, we consider examples of assessment tasks that may help to further structure the assessment process.

The assessment techniques described here should be viewed as a representative sample of available procedures rather than a comprehensive list of diagnostic possibilities. Our goal is to describe the areas that are usually evaluated during an assessment of motor speech abilities as an introductory framework for our later discussion of treatment procedures.

Our discussion is geared toward assessment procedures that assist with differential diagnosis and treatment planning. As noted earlier, assessment procedures that evaluate patient's performances on specific treatment tasks, assess treatment progress, and narrow the focus of therapy must be tailor made for individual patients and treatment tasks. Guidelines for developing measurement procedures that accomplish these goals are described elsewhere.[6,19,21,77,80]

Expecting the Unexpected

Identification of the patient with moderately severe apraxia or dysarthria who does not have significant language or cognitive involvement is relatively easy. The knowledgeable clinician analyzes relevant medical and behavioral information and examines the data for patterns of impairment that fit the previously described characteristics of these disorders. Unfortunately, the clinical picture is often complicated by the coexistence of related disorders and atypical patterns that do not fit neatly into the classic descriptions of the motor speech disorders. For example, apraxia of speech usually co-occurs with aphasia, and the presence of a moderately severe language deficit can mask the symptoms of apraxia. In addition, it is now recognized that there may be subtypes of apraxia[81] whose speech and related characteristics can differ considerably from one another.[40] The symptom picture can also be confounded in the dysarthrias. Patients with dysarthria can sometimes exhibit coexisting language and cognitive deficits. There is also a wide range of variability in the perceptual characteristics of even the more common types of dysarthria. Here too, unusual and perplexing combinations of symptoms challenge even the highly skilled clinician. As Netsell has pointed out,[85] the classic types of dysarthria identified by Darley et al[22,24] were never intended to cover all of the possibilities.

It should be clear from the previous discussion that evaluation of the motor speech disorders requires looking beyond the obvious symptoms and explaining what appear to be incongruous clinical findings. This usually involves testing nonspeech areas, including language and cognition, in order to isolate the nature of the communication deficit. The assistance of other health care providers may also prove valuable.

TABLE 19–2 Differences in Sites of Lesion, Underlying Mechanisms, Speech Characteristics, and Associated Problems for the Dysarthrias, Apraxia of Speech, and Phonemic Paraphasias

	Dysarthrias	*Apraxia of Speech*	*Phonemic (Literal) Paraphasia*
Frequent sites of lesion	Bilateral, subcortical	Unilateral, anterior cortical (Broca's area)	Unilateral, posterior cortical temporal (Wernicke's area) and/or parietal
Underlying mechanisms	Disturbed execution of speech movements due to impairment of upper and lower motoneuron systems	Impairment of volitional motor speech programming	A phonologic selection/retrieval deficit associated with aphasic language disturbance
Speech-related characteristics	Errors of articulatory distortion predominate; phonation, resonance, respiration, and prosody disturbed	Perceived errors of phoneme substitution predominate; prosody disturbed; initiation of speech particularly difficult	Errors of phoneme substitution predominate; unrelated substitutions; normally fluent prosodic speech pattern
Related impairments	Impairment of nonspeech musculature (paralysis, weakness); drooling and dysphagia possible	Right hemiplegia; right central facial weakness; impairment of language (Broca's aphasia); error awareness; frustration	Little or no motor impairment; impairment of language (Wernicke's or conduction aphasia); visual field defects

After Canter GJ. Dysarthria, apraxia of speech and literal paraphasia: three distinct varieties of articulatory behavior in the adult with brain damage. Paper presented to the American Speech and Hearing Association, Detroit, MI, 1973.

Assessment Techniques

The procedures used to assess the dysarthrias and apraxia of speech overlap considerably. The clinician often begins an initial assessment session attempting to determine whether or not the patient exhibits signs of dysarthria or apraxia and then selects appropriate additional tasks once this question is answered satisfactorily. Assessment proceeds into diagnostic therapy as the clinician gathers information to establish the need for therapy and focus the direction of treatment.

Test batteries for assessing motor speech disorders generally include (1) a test of language function; (2) articulation testing; (3) an oral peripheral mechanism examination; (4) the Motor Speech Evaluation,[21] and (5) disorder specific evaluation procedures.[15,76,77,83] Normally not all of the components of such a battery would be necessary or desirable; the patient's pattern of deficits dictate the direction of the evaluation. The selective use of components of a motor speech test battery to assess the dysarthrias and apraxia of speech are considered next.

The Dysarthrias

Although many patients with dysarthria would not be expected to have coexisting language problems, some individuals (e.g., stroke victims) may also be aphasic. Whenever a language impairment is suspected, one of the standardized aphasia batteries can be administered (see Chapter 25). In cases of uncertainty, a screening test of language function, such as the Shortened Version of the Token Test,[84] can be administered to rule out language impairment. The presence of a significant language deficit must, of course, be considered in treatment planning.

Sometimes it is apparent that the patient has dysarthria, and the primary question relates to the differential diagnosis. For the purposes of differentiating among the types of dysarthria, an analysis of the perceptual characteristics in combination with a measure of overall intelligibility may suffice. At a minimum, a tape recorded sample of a reading sample from a standard reading passage is sufficient for conducting a perceptual analysis.[15] Whenever possible a spontaneous speech sample should also be obtained. Occasionally, in the case of severely involved patients, the clinician may have to obtain the sample through sentence repetition. Once an adequate sample is available, a seven-point equal-appearing intervals scale of severity can be used to rate perceptual dimensions listed in Appendix 1. Rating a group of characteristics, for example, all those pertaining to voice, separately may enhance the ability to complete the complex task. Clinicians may have to listen to the taped samples several times, often once for each group of perceptual characteristics, before they complete a perceptual analysis. The final stage of the perceptual analysis involves comparing the ratings with the list of characteristics that typify each type of dysarthria (see Table 19–1) and, whenever possible, affixing a diagnostic label.

Until recently, the assessment of speech intelligibility has been a subjective process that was conducted according to the whims of each individual clinician. However, Yorkston and Beukelman's *Assessment of Intelligibility for Dysarthric Speech*[77] now provides an objective means of assessing intelligibility. In addition to providing a means for quantifying single word intelligibility and sentence intelligibility, this battery also serves as a means of analyzing the speaking rate of individuals with dysarthria.

More often than not, a clinician is primarily concerned with gathering information for treatment planning. Unfortunately, a perceptual analysis of dysarthric speech alone or in combination with intelligibility measures, may not be adequate for focusing treatment. The additional information obtained from a standard articulation test, particularly one that examines the influence of phonetic context, is helpful, but also insufficient. The information needed for intervention comes from an evaluation of the functional systems (structures that generate or valve the air stream)[4] that contribute to the dysarthria. For the purpose of treatment planning, knowing only the degree of impairment present for each motor speech system is insufficient. The evaluation must attempt to evaluate the integrity of the functional systems and to relate this information to the dysarthric symptoms. This general approach to the clinical management of the dysarthrias, the physiologic approach, has been pioneered by Netsell and his colleagues.[3,4,19,23,65,79,82,85,86] The physiologic approach encourages clinicians to gather information about the status of the impaired functional systems and to hypothesize about the relative contribution of the impairments to each deviant perceptual characteristic. In essence, the clinician's task is to determine *why* speech sounds aberrant so that treatment tasks can be developed that directly attack the source of the problem. The heart of this approach is the systematic assessment of each functional component alone and in combination. Ideally, this component analysis approach reveals a hierarchy of impairments that contribute to the overall pattern of deficient speech.

Both speech and nonspeech tasks are used to evaluate the integrity of the functional components of the motor speech system. Many appropriate tasks are routinely administered during a comprehensive oral peripheral mechanism examination. Still others have been compiled as the Motor Speech Evaluation.[21] Comprehensive discussions of the evaluation of the functional systems are available.[3,19,85]

The functional components of the motor speech examination include the respiratory, laryngeal, velopharyngeal, posterior tongue, anterior tongue, jaws, and lips. The primary goals of assessment are to determine how severely each component is affected and to evaluate the functional impact of that impairment. Netsell suggests using a seven-point severity rating scale to estimate the severity of involvement of each component.[82] For example, a rating of "1" might indicate the presence of mild intermittent hypernasality during the assessment of velopharyngeal valving, and a rating of "7" could indicate severe persistent hypernasality. Evaluation of the functional impact of velopharyngeal valving problems might include testing production of test phrases with the nares open versus occluded. It might also include having a temporary palatal prosthesis made for the patient so that one could evaluate speech with and without the speech appliance.

As previously noted, it is important to attempt to evaluate each functional component alone and in combination whenever possible. This type of evaluation is sometimes easier said than done. For example, to separately assess respiratory and laryngeal functions is difficult. Speech tasks that measure a patient's ability to speak loudly as an indication of respiratory function, can also be influenced by laryngeal valving problems. Clinicians and researchers alike are becoming more adept at separating functional components. For example, a bite block can be used to stabilize jaw movement and thereby permit independent testing of lower lip and tongue mobility.[87]

Although considerable clinical acumen is needed to evaluate systematically the influence of each component on speech production, the principle of testing each variable alone and in combination with other components is a critical factor in dysarthria assessment. For example, we once evaluated a patient with Wilson's disease[15] who exhibited a mixed type of dysarthria. A primary characteristic of this patient's dysarthria was a marked degree of inconsistent hypernasality. An analysis of the functional components contributing to the patient's overall speech pattern revealed that she had poor lingual control. She routinely kept her tongue tip down and elevated the dorsum of her tongue during speech. An interesting result of our component analysis was that the hypernasality was primarily due to lingual posturing rather than to deficient velopharyngeal valving. Without systematic testing of each functional component alone and in combination for this patient, the reason for her hypernasality would not have been apparent, and any attempted intervention for this problem would have been misdirected. Failure to tease out the underlying reason for an impairment can lead to misdiagnosis and mismanagement.

Apraxia of Speech

Wertz et al provide comprehensive coverage of the appraisal of patients with apraxia of speech.[21] Their battery includes tests of language; functional communication; speech production; oral, nonverbal movements; and intelligence. This comprehensive protocol provides ample information for diagnosing apraxia of speech and ruling out nonapraxic impairments that might influence the patient's performance during assessment or treatment. Our concern here is primarily with speech and nonspeech tests that provide information directly relevant to assessing the apraxic symptomatology. However, our discussion begins with a brief consideration of language testing since apraxia usually coexists with aphasic language impairments.

Language Testing. Although clinical and neuroanatomic relationships are not easily defined,[88] apraxia of speech frequently occurs in patients with Broca's aphasia. Therefore, language tests that provide information about this aphasic syndrome clearly serve a useful clinical function in the assessment of apraxia. Two standardized aphasia tests, the Boston Diagnostic Aphasia Examination (BDAE)[89] and the Western Aphasia Battery (WAB),[90] provide a means of diagnosing the classical types of aphasia, including Broca's aphasia. Although classification of patients with aphasia on the BDAE is based on subjective criteria, it is a comprehensive test of language function, and typical BDAE profiles of patients with aphasia and apraxia are available in the published literature.[21] In addition, the BDAE's profile of speech characteristics includes ratings of parameters, such as melodic line and articulatory agility, that are relevant to the assessment of apraxia. Prosodic disturbances are a cardinal feature of apraxia, and melodic line refers to changes in one element of prosody (intonation). Relatedly, lack of articulatory agility is also a hallmark of apraxia of speech. Overall, the BDAE profile of speech characteristics heightens clinicians' awareness of key aspects of motor speech performance prior to planning intervention goals.

In contrast to the subjective BDAE rating scales, the WAB uses a numerical taxonomy to classify patients with aphasia. The WAB's objective profiling of patient performance takes the guesswork out of classifying patients. Ultimately, however, the clinician, not the aphasia test, decides whether or not a patient fits the clinical profile of a patient with Broca's aphasia and apraxia of speech. Data from the BDAE, WAB, or any other language test merely provides information that contributes to the decisionmaking process.

In addition to the BDAE and the WAB, other equally useful standardized aphasia tests are available for examining the language abilities of patients with aphasia and apraxia. For example, Wertz et al provide patterns of performance on the Porch Index of Communicative Ability (PICA)[91] that are suggestive of apraxia. Inordinately low PICA verbal scores in conjunction with significantly better gestural and graphic performance should alert the clinician to consider the diagnosis of apraxia of speech. Relatedly, Wertz, Rosenbek and Collins also demonstrated that the PICA verbal subtests alone assist the diagnosis.[92] They accurately identified over 70 percent of a sample of subjects with apraxia using performance on PICA verbal tasks as the basis for their categorization. The use of other verbal and nonverbal tasks to assess patients with apraxia is considered next.

The Motor Speech Evaluation. Tests of speech production and oral, nonverbal movements commonly serve as the core of any apraxia assessment battery. The Motor Speech Evaluation consists of a compilation of such tasks that have been found to be particularly sensitive to detecting the problems of patients with motor speech problems. Although these tasks have not been standardized, research and clinical practice have demonstrated the face validity of the motor speech battery. Wertz et al discuss the Motor Speech Evaluation at length and describe its usefulness for assessing apraxia of speech.[92] Our overview is presented to demonstrate the range of tasks that are typically used to assess motor speech disorders.

The areas tested with the Motor Speech Evaluation are outlined in Table 19–3. Three types of tasks—nonspeech, speech, and oral, nonverbal—are included in the battery. Nonspeech tests included in the motor speech protocol include vowel prolongation, diadochokinetic tasks (repetition of monosyllables, e.g., /pa-pa-pa/ and repetition of combined monosyllables, e.g., /pa-ta-ka/). The speech tasks include repetition of polysyllabic words, multiple repetitions of the same word, repetition of words of increasing length, repetition of words having the same initial and final phoneme, sentence repetition, counting forwards and backwards, picture description, and oral reading. Patients are also probed to determine the consistency of their productions by having them repeat sentences that they produced volitionally during the examination. Finally, tasks designed to detect oral, nonverbal apraxia such as "lick your lips" are also included in the Motor Speech Evaluation.

In analyzing the results of motor speech testing, the clinician uses his or her knowledge of the characteristics of apraxia and determines whether or not the observed pattern of performance is consistent with that information. Once the diagnosis is confirmed through this process, he or she must proceed to the task of establishing the focus of therapy by systematically evaluating the collected data to determine where the patient begins to break down and what factors (e.g., stimulus length) contribute to that breakdown.

The Apraxia Battery for Adults (ABA) is a commercially available test that consists of non-

TABLE 19–3 Motor Speech Evaluation

Nonspeech Tasks
Vowel production: /a/, /i/, /u/
Diadochokinetic tasks:
Repeating monosyllables /p/, /t/, /k/
Repeating combined monosyllables: /p-t-k/
Speech Tasks
Multisyllabic words: "snowman," "gingerbread," "impossibility"
Words of increasing length: "please," "pleasing," "pleasingly"
Words with the same initial and final phoneme: "coke," "dad," "gag,"
Repeating sentences: 'Please put the groceries in the refrigerator"
Describing a picture:
Repeat "error" sentences made in spontaneous picture description
Counting: 1 to 20 forward and backward
Days of the week: forward and backward
Oral, Nonverbal Apraxia
Tongue movements: "Stick out your tongue," "Lick your lips"
Lip movements: "Smile," "Show how you would kiss a baby"
Miscellaneous: "Cough," "Make your teeth chatter," "Clear your throat"

After Wertz RT. Neuropathologies of speech and language: an introduction to patient management. In: Johns DF, ed. Clinical management of neurogenic communication disorders. Boston: Little, Brown, 1985:1.

speech, speech, and oral, nonverbal assessment tasks.[83] Standardization data are not available for the ABA. There are six subtests in this battery, including diadochokinetic rate, increasing word length, limb apraxia and oral apraxia, latency and utterance time for polysyllabic words, repeated trials test, and an inventory of articulation characteristics of apraxia. Like all nonstandardized test batteries, the ABA should be viewed as an organized compilation of tasks that may assist the experienced clinician with the task of differential diagnosis.

Articulation Testing. Since apraxia of speech is manifested primarily in prosodic and articulatory disturbances, it is not surprising that articulation tests are routinely included in apraxia assessment batteries. The usefulness of articulation testing in this population may vary for individual patients. Individuals with dyspraxia are highly variable on repeated trials of speech tasks, and this variability is often evident on articulation tests. This variability can be counteracted somewhat by ensuring that a large sample of behavior is obtained. Administration of a "deep" test of articulation accomplishes this goal while also providing information on the influence of the phonetic environment on articulation.[93] Similarly, assessments of articulatory or phonologic performance that attempt to capture patterns of production may also provide information that will assist with treatment planning.[57] Articulation tests, and all speech tests for that matter, are obviously of limited value for patients with severe apraxia who have a restricted phonemic repertoire.

Prosody. Prosody involves the perceptual attributes of rhythm stress and intonation. Recent acoustic studies have demonstrated that disturbances of prosody are an integral component of apraxic impairments.[9] Although information on the clinical assessment of prosody is sparse, Rosenbek and LaPointe provide clinical guidance that is equally valuable for assessing apraxia and the dysarthrias.[19] They note that changes in loudness, pitch, articulation time, and pause time contribute to the perception of prosodic aspects of speech. Clinical decisions involved in the assessment of prosody include ''whether (1) the patient's overall loudness, pitch, and pattern of loudness and pitch changes are appropriate to the context; (2) the pattern of stressed and unstressed syllables is normal; and (3) the pattern of rate change, duration of sounds, and location and length of pauses are right for the context'' (p 117).[19] Rosenbek and LaPointe use a "contrastive stress" drill to assess aspects in their patients. This drill involves having the clinician ask a series of questions that require the patient to alter the prosodic elements of their answers in each successive attempt. This drill provides a controlled sample of connected speech that permits analysis of pitch, loudness, articulation, and pause time.

Objective analysis of the prosodic aspects of speech production is also available to many clinicians. Appropriate clinical instrumentation that is reliable, relatively inexpensive, and easy to use is now available. The Visi-Pitch (KAY Elemetrics), for example, extracts fundamental frequency (perceived as pitch) and intensity (loudness) information and graphically displays it in real time on a display screen. This type of instrumentation can be used to measure and observe prosodic aspects of speech production, and it can also prove useful for measuring performance changes resulting from treatment. The treatment of motor speech disorders is reviewed in the remainder of this chapter.

TREATMENT

Apraxia of Speech

Historic Perspective on Treatment

Traditionally the emphasis has been on differentiating the language approaches of aphasia from the motor speech and articulation approaches of apraxia of speech. In the frenzy to separate apraxia therapy, clinicians have had a tendency to forget that the motor speech mechanism is largely driven by the language system. Rosenbek, Kent, and LaPointe feel that apraxia requires speech-language therapy that emphasizes the relationship between movement and meaning.[40] In other words, therapy must be directed at improving movement and articulatory transitions within the context of the language system.

Acoustic and physiologic studies of apraxic speakers have also shaped current thinking about apraxia therapy. Understanding that apraxic speech is not simply a series of "articulation substitutions," but rather a symptom of a motor system unable to make rapid transitions and to implement dynamic motor subprograms for speech helps one understand why pure articulation therapy is usually insufficient.

Not only has the concept of apraxia of speech as an articulation disorder been replaced by the concept of apraxia as a movement disorder,[40] but also the definition clearly takes into account the disruption of prosody as a primary feature. It has even been suggested that prosodic abnormalities might cause the listener to "perceive" articulatory substitutions.[94] For example, shortening the vowel in the word "pod" could result in the listener hearing the word "pot." Thus a treatment philosophy for apraxia must reflect the dynamic nature of the speech process that is disrupted.

Prognosis

Much of what speech-language pathologists know about apraxia of speech is embedded in research on aphasia since the two frequently occur together. Thus prognostic variables associated with aphasia tend also to be associated with apraxia of speech. These include severity of the disorder, time post onset of impairment, age of the patient, associated disorders, and etiology. Wertz studied patients with coexisting apraxia and aphasia and found that a change in one did not appear to be significantly related to a change in the other.[5] He also reported that of the treated patients with apraxia studied, 74 percent improved. Others support the contention that patients with apraxia improve with time and treatment. Rosenbek suggests that the diagnosis of apraxia of speech itself is associated with a positive prognosis, but cautions that severe apraxia should not be confused with severe aphasia.[95] Rosenbek, Kent, and LaPointe point out the existence of patients who begin and remain speechless;[40] the ability to predict recovering patients with apraxia from those resistant to improvement remains poor. Frequently the best indication of potential for change is the patient's response to treatment. An extensive review of the literature on prognosis is available in Wertz, LaPointe, and Rosenbek.[21]

Treatment Rationale

Traditional treatment methodology in apraxia of speech frequently involves "facilitation" of accurate responding and repeated "practice" of the response. One might assume that repetition and practice helps to reprogram the speech-motor system. Thus the clinician and patient work to reestablish "subprograms" for speech production by practicing increasingly difficult tasks. This assumption is consistent with the current knowledge of apraxia of speech. For example, in an effort to explain substitution versus distortion behavior, Rosenbek, Kent, and LaPointe suggest the possibility that failure in the implementation of an action results in a loss of information about succeeding actions.[40] On a broader scale, we all experience such "loss of information" when in the course of a relatively automatic and overlearned task (preprogrammed), we are interrupted or lose our place; the result is frequently a momentary confusion relative to the next step. Perhaps the patient with apraxia experiences this repeatedly within the speech-motor system. Treatment aimed at reestablishing the programs might diminish the frequency of such interruptions and thereby reestablish fluent speech.

Probably, most of the methodology in apraxia of speech treatment also involves establishing compensatory mechanisms to overcome a faulty motor system or somehow reorganize the act of speaking.[95]

Treatment Principles

Shewan proposed that the treatment of apraxia of speech involves systematic drill organized in a hierarchy that maximizes the patient's ability to respond.[96] Similarly, Duffy proposed eight principles to be incorporated in treatment of apraxia of speech as follows:

1. Insure a high level of success.
2. Use intensive and extensive drill.
3. Concentrate on articulation and prosody.
4. Introduce meaningful and useful material as soon as possible.
5. Systematically manipulate variables that affect response accuracy.
6. Encourage self-monitoring and self-correction.
7. Employ both auditory and visual stimulation.
8. Recognize the limits of therapy and shift into compensatory strategies or alternative systems when other approaches fail to move in the direction of functional speech.[97]

To this list might be added the suggestion that patients with apraxia need to understand their disorder and to learn how to avoid undermining their own progress. These patients are usually frustrated by their noncompliant speech system. They need to learn how to approach the task of speaking productively. In other words, counseling and education are necessary to successful management. Rosenbek uses the term "prophylaxis" to describe prevention of maladaptive attitudes and behaviors and urges that counseling is the key ingredient.[17]

Treatment Hierarchies

Many approaches to apraxia treatment rely on a progression through a series of graded difficulty levels. This hierarchy of treatment tasks is usually based on what research tells clinicians is more or less difficult for individuals with apraxia and on what clinicians know about the individual patient. For example, Rosenbek et al designed the widely used "eight-step continuum" to move patients from limited, clinician-assisted speech to volitional, purposeful speech production.[98] Deal and Florance successfully used a modification of this hierarchical approach with patients with apraxia.[99]

Task continuums that allow the patient with apraxia to successfully practice nonspeech or speech productions of varying levels of difficulty are used widely. Where a patient begins and what variables influence difficulty must be evaluated individually. A number of variables might be considered.

Stimuli. Although nonspeech stimuli might be appropriate in severe cases, usually tasks requiring some level of speech production are chosen. The phonetic features of target sounds, frequency of occurrence of words or sounds, position of target sounds or words within an utterance, utterance length and complexity, phonetic distances, and stress characteristics should be considered in the choice of stimuli. Although stimuli are obviously chosen to suit the movement needs of the patient, linguistic influences cannot be overlooked.

Mode of Presentation. Stimuli can be presented through one or more of the following modes: auditory input, watching the face of the clinician, reading, looking in the mirror, tactile-kinesthetic input, or gestures. In addition, the degree of reliance on clinician input must be taken into account when determining difficulty. For example, imitation or simultaneous production of a word is usually easier than producing the word in response to a question. The amount of time that elapses between the presentation of the stimulus and the patient's response, and what the patient is doing during delayed responses (e.g., silent rehearsal), can also be a powerful influence on response accuracy.

Response Requirements. Patients can be asked to provide speech, nonspeech, gestural, graphic, or a combination of responses. Melody or rhythm can be superimposed on vocalization, or prosodic elements can be altered.

Facilitators

In order to meet the criteria of "successful practice" of responses, the clinician is met with the task of discovering what variations in stimulus or response help wheedle an accurate response from a faulty mechanism. Varying stimulus and response characteristics to help the patient reach a target response is the foundation of facilitation. The literature is replete with suggestions for what helps or hinders response accuracy in apraxia of speech.[21] Armed with this knowledge, the clinician must then determine exactly which variables are the most powerful and efficient facilitators for the individual patient.

Specific Approaches

Melodic Intonation Therapy. Melodic intonation therapy uses melody to increase the verbal expression of nonfluent patients with aphasia.[100–102] Criteria for selection of candidates implies that certain individuals with verbal apraxia might be appropriate candidates. The program follows a highly structured hierarchy that moves the patient from intoning an utterance in unison with the clinician through graded levels until ultimately the patient is using utterances purposefully to answer questions. The program incorporates a number of characteristics that appear to facilitate the production of speech in apraxia. Melody and slow intoning might facilitate production by increasing the time allowed to make articulatory transitions. Other elements that might contribute to success for patients with apraxia are the controlled attention to stress, prosody, and linguistic content of utterances; accompaniment of pacing gestures; hierarchical organization of tasks; repetition; emphasis on successful production; multimodality stimulation; and use of controlled delays between stimulus and patient response. Modifications in the program have been proposed by Dunham and Newhoff[103] and Marshall and Holtzapple.[104]

Duffy and Gawle raise an interesting issue in their study of apraxic speech.[94] They found that the apraxic speakers studied tended to have shortened vowel durations, which resulted in the listener perceiving a sound substitution where none existed. Duffy and Gawle speculate that treatment approaches such as melodic intonation therapy and contrastive stress drills[19] might in fact help "normalize" these abnormal durational elements and so inadvertently improve our perception of surrounding consonants.

PROMPT System. Square, Chumpelik, Morningstar, and Adams report successful application of the PROMPT system of therapy to three patients with apraxia.[105] This approach is described as an articulatory prosodic treatment with dynamic tactile and kinesthetic cues delivered during speech production. The cues or prompts provide input on multiple factors relative to speech production such as place and manner of sound production, voicing, and durational elements.

Gestural Reorganization. Many apraxic speakers seem to benefit from "talking with their hands." That is, gesture paired with the act of speaking has been observed to facilitate speech production with patients with apraxia. Skelly et al reported that training in American Indian sign language (Amerind) resulted in improved oral communication for the patient with oral, verbal apraxia.[106] Rosenbek, Collins, and Wertz proposed that systematic pairing of speech and limb gestures may facilitate the reorganization of verbal communication.[107] Gestural facilitation approaches include using meaningful signs such as Amerind or using timing gestures such as tapping in rhythm with speech.[17,108]

Visual Cueing. Reading as an approach to facilitating oral production has been discussed by Rosenbek[17] and Wertz, LaPointe, and Rosenbek.[21] In addition, visual cues to sound productions and positions can be presented in drawings or by observing the clinician. Berman and Peelle suggest having patients use writing to cue themselves to the first letter of problem words.[109] Possibly combining such a technique with phonetic placement and visual imagery ("picture in your mind how you make the sound for this letter") assists the patient with apraxia in producing words. Such a technique has potential as an aid in carry-over training also, since the patient functions with self-generated cues rather than clinician-generated cues.

Articulation Therapy. Traditional methods of teaching speech sound production can be adapted to the patient with apraxia. During the early stages of treatment, some patients need repeated practice on individual sounds, syllables, or words before moving into phrases, sentences, or connected speech. Imitation, phonetic placement, successive approximation, and phonetic derivation[17] might be used to assist patients in moving from nonspeech positioning to speech sound production. Rosenbek recommends moving quickly from establishing sounds in isolation to production of sounds in syllables and words.[95] He also suggests helping the patient practice moving back and forth between target sounds by drilling with contrast words such as "bat" versus "back."

Contrastive Stress Drill. This approach, described by Rosenbek,[17,19] involves production of a phrase or sentence with variations in stress. For example, the meaning of the sentence "Jay writes books" changes somewhat depending on which word in the sentence receives primary stress. Clinicians can develop programs that help patients practice altering stress patterns while also practicing articulation. Attention is thus directed at the durational and prosodic elements of the disorder.

Relaxation. EMG feedback on activity of the frontal muscle (forehead) has been used as a means of helping patients monitor muscle tension; decreasing the muscle activity tends to result in relaxation. McNeil, Prescott, and Lemme used this approach to teach relaxation to patients with apraxia of speech and aphasia.[110] Similarly Rubow and Rosenbek used this approach to improve fluency in one patient with apraxia.[111]

Other approaches include using automatic responses as a means of eliciting speech attempts; using an intrusive schwa to assist in difficult articulatory transitions; using starter or carrier phrases, integral stimulation, and fading of clinician cues; using key words to help approximate similar words; prolonging phonemes; using silent rehearsal; using rhythmic speech activities; pacing speech with a metronome; and using cued speech.[97]

Treatment of apraxia of speech is a dynamic process. Approaches and focus of treatment change with individual characteristics of the patient and over time with individual patients. Patients with mild apraxia require different treatment than patients with severe apraxia. The techniques discussed have only been introduced and are most often used in combinations rather than in isolation.

Alternatives to Speech

Unfortunately, there are patients with apraxia for whom speech is an unattainable goal. These patients are recognizable when repeated, vigorous, and intelligently devised treatment fails. Providing such patients with options for augmenting the speech system is important. Writing, gesturing, or using communication boards or electronic systems might be feasible alternatives. Lyon suggests drawing as an expressive mode for speechless patients.[112] The degree of coexisting aphasia, motivation of the patient, and a range of other variables influence the choice of system.

Carry-over of Gains

Drill and graded tasks must ultimately lead toward functional speech production in a variety of settings and tasks. Generalization training strategies[113] must be applied to aid the patient in moving from clinician-assisted speech to functional independence. Generalization is accomplished partially through gradually fading clinician cues during treatment and working in more difficult and varied speech activities. Rosenbek recommends using homework as a means of reinforcing transfer of training.[95] Others find that teaching family members how to work with patients and how to facilitate, not just speech, but communication as a whole enhances communication outside the clinic.[114] Self-cueing strategies can shift responsibility to the patient. Work on self-monitoring and repair strategies can assist the patients in dealing with novel conversational situations.

The Dysarthrias

The Historic Perspective

Early approaches to treatment of dysarthria followed a "do whatever works" mentality as little data existed to support specific treatment methodologies for specific patients. Later, based on the seminal work of Darley, Aronson, and Brown,[15] clinicians learned to more clearly identify and classify types of dysarthria. However, in spite of an attempt by Darley et al to relate the perceived speech characteristics to an underlying pathophysiology of the disorder, resulting treatment approaches tended to embrace perceptual symptoms as the focus of therapy. In other words, clinicians analyzed the speech characteristics and treated the deviant dimensions. Thus imprecise consonant production resulted in articulation treatment; decreased loudness resulted in work on voice intensity. Recently, researchers have shown that perceived symptoms or a neurologic diagnosis per se does not always predict exactly what physiologic variables are contributing to a given patient's speech symptoms.[34,85,115] Netsell[82,86] and Netsell and Rosenbek[85] warn that in order to treat patients with dysarthria efficiently, evaluation must also focus on how the perceived speech characteristics specifically relate to the integrity of each functional component of the speech system. In other words, clinicians must not only identify what a speaker sounds like and relate this to the disorder, but they also must clearly understand *why* a speaker sounds the way he or she does. This "physiologic" approach[82] requires that one look beyond symptoms and the disorder to the underlying movement and control abnormalities: in other words, not only identifying that a patient has consonant imprecision, but also recognizing that this imprecision is due to decreased range and force of anterior tongue movement.

The physiologic approach suggests a need to consider focusing treatment based on knowledge obtained from several levels of analysis. For example, a patient is assessed as evidencing "imprecise consonant production" (a perceptual characteristic), which is described as impaired "articulation" (a functional system); the problem is attributed to diminished force (physiologic correlate) of anterior tongue movement (functional component). This evaluation process requires a multilevel analysis because one level cannot be automatically assumed from knowledge of another level. Continuing our example, the evaluation might have revealed that imprecise consonant production, though a characteristic of poor articulation, was, in fact, due to inadequate intraoral air pressure caused by poor respiration secondary to abdominal weakness. As this example demonstrates, a multilevel evaluation is necessary to insure appropriate treatment. In the aforementioned example, articulation treatment aimed at improving the perceived symptom might not only be inefficient, but ineffective as well.

Finally, treatment requires consideration of the dysarthric speaker as part of a communication context. This "pragmatic approach" to dysarthria evaluation and management allows clinicians to take into account environmental and social influences on communication adequacy. The fact that people do not communicate in isolation is obvious. However, clinicians often fail to consider that many things in addition to the motor speech mechanism can influence how well one "uses" speech. For example, increased processing requirements on a dysarthric speaker might result in a division of attention and energy between language processing and motor-speech production, possibly resulting in a lessened ability to consciously control the compensations needed for speech. Many nonspeech variables must be considered such as the physical demands on the speaker (walking and talking simultaneously, maintaining posture), linguistic and cognitive demands (imitation, easy versus difficult formulation, discourse characteristics), and environmental demands (speaking distance, noise).

Thus management requires consideration of many levels of analysis:

1. A perceptual analysis to arrive at a picture of relative involvement of various speech characteristics and an estimate of severity and bizarreness.
2. A functional systems approach to determine the relative involvement of respiration, phonation, resonance, articulation, and prosody.
3. A functional components evaluation,[79] which looks at the integrity and interaction of nine structures required for production of speech: diaphragm, abdomen, rib cage, larynx, velopharynx, posterior tongue, anterior tongue, lips, and jaw.
4. A knowledge of coexisting cognitive and language deficits and how these might influence learning.
5. A knowledge of contextual influences such as language context, environment, speaker roles, stress, and physical context.

When combined with appropriate treatment

principles, the information obtained from a multilevel evaluation leads directly to the establishment of appropriate treatment goals. Treatment principles and goals are considered in the following sections.

Treatment Principles

Darley et al suggest that the following principles apply to dysarthria treatment:

1. Compensation—patients must learn to make maximum use of what they have.
2. Purposeful activity—patients must learn to impose conscious control and effort on speaking rather than rely on their prior ability to speak automatically.
3. Monitoring—patients must learn to be self-critical, recognize "good" speech production, and adjust production on-line.
4. An early start—therapy should begin immediately after the time of onset in order to obviate entrenchment of bad habits or, in cases of progressive disease, to teach compensations to conserve speech for as long as possible.
5. Motivation—treatment should provide sufficient information to help the patient understand the disorder and the rationale of treatment, graded activities that insure success, feedback about results, and emotional support in order to maintain patient motivation.[15]

Treatment Goals

Rosenbek and LaPointe suggest that treatment consists of improving what patients have *and* improving what patients do with what they have.[19] Thus, one might consider the goals of treatment to include reestablishing motor control and/or developing compensatory strategies for using residual motor ability. Rosenbek and LaPointe add that the overall goal of treatment is rarely normal speech, rather it is usually to establish compensated intelligibility.[19] Similarly, Beukelman notes that disability is often diminished in dysarthria by moving *away* from normal production as when speakers improve intelligibility by adopting a slower than normal speech rate.[116]

In addition to the goal of maximum intelligibility, Beukelman adds the goals of maximum efficiency, the most socially acceptable and natural communication approach possible, and communication that most adequately satisfies the patient.[116]

Goals might not only reflect the expected level of intelligibility, efficiency, and naturalness, but also the expected "functional independence." That is, is the patient able to use the optimum speech production in all situations with all people; does he or she need external cues? Thus treatment gains must be judged not only against the clinician's assessment of progress within the clinic, but also against the clinician's, patient's, and others' assessment of intelligibility, efficiency, and social acceptibility across a variety of settings and contexts.

Prognosis

Single case studies cited throughout this chapter point out the efficacy of various techniques for improving the communication of various patients with dysarthria. Fortunately, the field of motor speech has not fallen into the trap of large group efficacy studies. There has been a recognition that large group studies of "treatment" are inappropriate because of the variety of disorders and approaches. Studies demonstrate that individual patients who fail to respond to one type of treatment, may respond well to an alternative intervention approach.[4,117] Netsell summarized the state of the art in motor speech treatment by stating that treatment of dysarthria has shown significantly positive outcomes, and even the most severely impaired dysarthric speaker can respond favorably to appropriate intervention.[82]

While the overall prognosis for functional improvement of impaired communication is favorable for dysarthric speakers, establishment of a precise prognosis for an individual with dysarthria remains an inexact science. Additional data are needed to establish the efficacy of specific treatments for individual patients with dysarthria. Clinicians must, therefore, carefully weigh a myriad of factors in order to arrive at an accurate prognostic statement for a given patient.

There are a number of factors that influence the outcome in the treatment of dysarthria and thus also influence one's choice of treatment methods.[82,85] These include the following:

1. Neurologic status and history: including the location, extent, and cause of the neurologic insult and whether the disorder is progressive or stable. An understanding of the pathophysiology of disease is obviously helpful for predicting the patient's potential response to treatment and type of treatment.
2. Age.
3. Automatic adjustments to the disorder: including knowledge of adaptive versus maladaptive responses to the speech breakdown.
4. Treatment: implementing the most appropriate

and efficient approach for each patient insures a better outcome. In addition, the availability of treatment, the experience of the clinician, the time available for treatment, and the tools and equipment available to the clinician influence the outcome.

5. Personality and intelligence: more optimistic and purposeful clients tend to respond best to treatment.
6. Support systems: the availability of someone to reinforce carry-over of skills tends to enhance treatment outcome.
7. Sensory, cognitive, and language abilities: including coexisting problems such as aphasia or memory disorders, influence patient's response to treatment.
8. Severity.
9. Motivation: the clinician must take into account what the dysarthric speaker wants to achieve and set goals based on the patient's needs. Motivation must be considered not only in light of whether or not a person wants and needs to communicate, but also in light of the amount of opportunity that he or she has to communicate.

Approaches to Treatment

The clinician can choose from several general treatment approaches in developing a plan for intervention. Netsell and Rosenbek define behavioral, prosthetic, and instrumental approaches to managing dysarthric speech.[85] We add the pragmatic approach to their list of treatment options. These general approaches are briefly introduced below as a prelude to our discussion of specific treatment techniques.

Behavioral treatment refers to what has traditionally been delivered to individuals with dysarthria as speech therapy. It involves a variety of activities including education and counseling, training recognition of problem behaviors, teaching alternative responses, providing feedback and reinforcement, and practicing responses until they are well established. Behavioral approaches need not be protracted; for example, teaching a patient to use a different sitting position might be a fast and efficient means of altering speech. Yet any approach that requires an individual to "learn a new way of doing something" might require extended practice in many conditions. Developing a hierarchy of what is easier and more difficult for a given patient is usually necessary. Working up the continuum from easier to more difficult tasks insures adequate practice of accurate responding rather than repeated failure.

Prosthetic treatment includes any alterations to the physical properties related to speech production such as surgery, medication, palatal lift prostheses, or splints.

Instrumental approaches include the use of technology that provides information on physiologic or acoustic parameters. Acoustic information derived from commercially available instruments includes voice intensity, voice onset time, pitch, and pause time. Instrumentation can provide physiologic information such as force or range of movement, oral or nasal air pressure, and muscle activity or tension.

Instrumental approaches often fall under the rubric of biofeedback. This is the process of providing an individual with *moment to moment* feedback on the state of some physiologic variable, for example, the rate of airflow during expiration or lip muscle tone.[118,119] The process usually involves transducing a physiologic variable into an auditory or visual signal, which allows the patient to monitor and hopefully modify the behavior. The benefit of biofeedback is that feedback can be provided instantaneously and continuously in an efficient fashion. Rubow provides an overview of the use of biofeedback with individuals with dysarthria.[120]

Pragmatic approaches teach the patient with dysarthria how to use residual speech to be an effective communicator. Pragmatic treatment does not focus so much on the dysarthric impairment per se, but on the patient as a communicator in various contexts. One example of a pragmatic approach is teaching the patient and family how to maximize the communication environment by altering noise and speaking distance.[121]

It is worth noting that the general treatment approaches outlined herein are not mutually exclusive. Clinicians often, for example, utilize a combination of behavioral, instrumental, and pragmatic methods with a given patient at any point in therapy. Moreover, the clinician may elect to focus intervention on a variety of approaches at different stages of the treatment process.

Focusing Treatment

A number of factors can influence the choice of what to treat and in what order. The following principles will assist in appropriately focusing treatment.

First, treatment targets should present a reasonable probability of success and make a difference in the speech production.[6] For example, based on knowledge of what is required for normal speech production, one might assume that a patient with spastic dysarthria who evidences a unilateral left facial weakness would be unlikely to find marked benefit in speech production from work directed toward increasing left-sided facial motor activity.

Second, identification and mobilization of existing compensations or adaptations is both efficient and useful in achieving early positive results. Consequently, appropriate compensations should be explored as an early focus of treatment.

Another important factor that influences the treatment focus is the relative degree of impairment that is evident for the functional components. Targeting treatment on a specific functional component that is most impaired and/or most influences the intelligibility of speech can often result in immediate functional change. For example, the individual with severe hypernasality and nasal emission and distortion of anterior tongue sounds would most likely achieve more functional improvement with the elimination of velopharyngeal incompetence. Importantly, Netsell and Rosenbek caution that components are interdependent, and a malfunction in one area can diminish function in another area.[85] An example of this concept of peripheral dependencies might be seen in the unintelligible patient who exhibits articulatory imprecision, short phrasing, low volume, breathy voice, and hypernasality. An evaluation of the components reveals major velopharyngeal incompetency and poor respiratory control; in such a case, the "articulation and prosodic" problems could be partially dependent on the failure of respiration and velopharyngeal function.

In some cases, it may prove more efficient to work on tasks that affect all functional systems at once. Rosenbek states that enhancing the coordinated activity of all components often has a more significant effect on intelligibility than does the manipulation of separate components.[39] For example, altering the rate of speech often improves articulation, resonance, and voice possibly because it takes the system out of the "overdrive" mode and gives the muscles more time to carry out and coordinate the work of speaking.

As noted previously, attention to prosthetic and postural adjustments early in the course of treatment often eliminates immediately certain problems, thereby allowing focus on other aspects of the disorder. For example, fitting a palatal lift prosthesis might eliminate velopharyngeal incompetence and so free the clinician to focus treatment on altering laryngeal and respiratory control problems.

Additionally, clinicians must make decisions on whether to work on "speech" tasks (phonation, articulation) or nonspeech tasks (muscle strengthening, coordination exercises). Rosenbek suggests that nonspeech drills might be most appropriate if speech is impossible, improved physiology would benefit speech production, nonspeech treatment techniques are available, and the nonspeech or "physiology" can, in fact, be modified.[39]

The time and tools available also determine the focus of treatment to some degree. The patient whose funding allows only six sessions might be treated differently than the patient who has the time, funding, and motivation to work from the underlying physiology on up.

Treatment should be adjusted to suit what the clinician knows about a person's disease. Goals and tactics used for a patient with mixed dysarthria resulting from a single onset CVA might differ from those for a patient with a similar speech pattern but resulting from a progressive disease. What has gone before also influences one's thinking in designing treatment; a patient who has had considerable behavioral treatment to improve dysarthria in the past, but has "lost ground" in spite of a stable disease process might need more work on the carry-over environment rather than a repeat of direct training methods.

The choice of a general treatment approach also depends, in part, on severity. Netsell and Rosenbek suggest that behavioral methods might be sufficient for motivated patients with milder dysarthria.[85] However, a combination of behavioral, prosthetic, and instrumental managements might be necessary for patients with more severely involved dysarthria.

As Beukelman warns,[116] clinicians should intervene as little as possible in order to avoid teaching strategies that will have to be "removed" later in the course of therapy. For example, teaching patients to pause after each word early after the onset might result in disrupted prosody even after physiology has improved.

In the final analysis, choices of treatment focus should depend on what the patient wants and needs.

Treatment Methods

Following the precedent of Rosenbek and his colleagues,[19,39,85] our discussion of treatment methods is organized according to the following functional components: respiratory, laryngeal, velopharyngeal, orofacial, and combined. The reader must remember that dividing the speech-motor system into functional components does not imply that each component works in isolation. A malfunction in one component can seriously hinder perceived characteristics associated with another. Thus treatment *must* be based on an accurate evaluation of *why* perceived speech impairments occur. Furthermore, the need to measure and adjust task difficulty according to patient ability applies to all training approaches.

The Respiratory System. The goal of respiratory management is to improve the respiratory support and control of respiration for speech, that is, to be able to initiate on and off control, inhale and exhale the proper amount of air, and sustain a smooth flow of air appropriately. A thorough knowledge of normal and disordered respiration is needed in order to approach management. Moreover, an understanding of the neuropathology and underlying pathophysiology assists in treatment focus. For example, many patients with ataxia demonstrate respiratory irregularity and must learn to coordinate breathing for speech.[122] Alternately hypotonia in patients with flaccid dysarthria would generally respond more favorably to activities that increase tone and strength.

Positioning changes provide one of the most immediate approaches available for modifying the respiratory support for speech production. An upright sitting position is not always the best position for maximizing respiratory control and normal posture may not be the most advantageous position for speech respiration. Therefore, various positions should be tried, and their influence on speech noted to determine the posture that best suits a given client. In addition to aiding in postural evaluations, a trained physical therapist might assist in improving the strength and tone of respiratory muscles.

Another approach to respiratory management is to train controlled expiration. Whereas Murry suggests beginning with unvoiced exhalation,[122] others begin by sustaining speech sounds, either voiced or unvoiced, and use loudness level and loudness change as a monitor. This approach can be accomplished with simple or sophisticated instrumentation, or by teaching the patient to self-monitor loudness level, and length of sustained exhalation or speech sound. The patient can learn to recognize what postural or behavioral adjustments are needed to maintain respiratory control. This activity can be broadened to include combinations of sounds and variations of loudness. A similar approach uses biofeedback to provide information on the control of air pressures. Instruments that provide the biofeedback can vary from readily available and simple devices measuring the acoustic parameters of loudness, such as the volume meter on a tape recorder or "voice lite," to more sophisticated aerodynamic systems.

Acoustic Feedback. Berry and Goshorn provided a patient with immediate visual feedback on loudness level via a graphic signal on an oscilloscope. By using the continuous feedback from his productions and comparing it to a visual model, the patient was able to successfully alter his speech pattern.[123]

Rubow and Swift trained a patient with Parkinson's disease to use a wearable device that provided feedback on voice intensity relative to a target intensity level.[12] The patient was able to use the device both within and outside the clinic to achieve generalized loudness improvement.

Hardware and software systems that provide feedback on acoustic parameters such as voice intensity are now available commercially.

Physiologic Feedback. Aerodynamic biofeedback measuring subglottal air pressure generated by the respiratory system has also proven successful as a means of improving respiratory control and breath support.[4] The easiest of such systems is a simple water manometer such as that described by Netsell and Hixon.[124] They suggest that the ability to exert 5 cm of water pressure for 5 seconds demonstrates sufficient pressure for speech production. In hospital settings, the respiratory therapy department may be able to provide a simple spirometer to assist work on sustaining and controlling airflow.

A more sophisticated aerodynamic system, consisting of oscillographic visual feedback of air pressures exerted through a pressure transducer, can also be used for providing on-line feedback to patients with dysarthria.

Many patients require a combination of approaches, for example, defining the optimum postural adjustment for speech, using biofeedback to increase respiratory support, and using behavioral methods to carry over altered patterns to connected speech activities. The astute clinician also monitors treatment effects, be they positive or negative, on other speech systems. Furthermore, knowledge of the influence of speech changes on motor activities other than speech is equally important. For example, postural adjustments that improve speech respiratory support at the cost of the physical therapist's goal of establishing sitting balance and normalization of tone may not be desirable. Coordinated and prioritized goal setting is necessary to meet all of the patient's rehabilitation goals.

When respiratory support has been maximized, compensatory strategies for using residual abilities may be needed. For example, the patient may need to learn to alter phrase length to accommodate an inability to sustain exhalation throughout a sentence. This approach requires a clear understanding of physiologic as well as linguistic constraints. An unwitting clinician may turn a patient with diminished loudness into a patient with unintelligible speech because of choppy and inappropriate application of breath groupings. Patients must learn *how* to shorten phrases and recharge the respiratory system without compromising prosody and intelligibility.

When sufficient loudness cannot be generated

for communication purposes, a wearable voice amplifier is an alternative. Relatedly, when the respiratory support for speech cannot be improved physiologically, a respiratory prothesis[19] might be considered as a brace for weakened respiratory structures.

The Larynx. Treatment of the laryngeal component includes procedures to reduce laryngeal tone and hyperadduction of the vocal folds. Postural adjustments or relaxation activities might assist in reducing the consequent harsh or strained or strangled voice quality. Conversely, approaches to increasing laryngeal tone and overcoming hypoadduction might include pushing exercises, practicing glottal attacks, or increasing tone and laryngeal closure by speaking while exerting downward force with the arms against a surface, such as the arms of a chair.[19] Postural adjustments such as turning the head to assist a weakened vocal fold in approximating closure or digital manipulation of the larynx have also been suggested in cases of unilateral cord weakness.

In addition, one may use a hierarchy of speech tasks similar to that described under "The Respiratory System" in order to gain increasing laryngeal control over progressively longer or more difficult utterances, beginning with single sounds.

Instrumental approaches that measure airflow and subglottal air pressure may be appropriate for training laryngeal and respiratory control. Also, Netsell and Rosenbek suggest the potential application of videofiberoptic feedback as a means of improving laryngeal control of patients with dysarthria.[85]

Finally, individuals that have a unilateral vocal cord weakness may benefit from a Teflon injection to help position the margin of the weakened cord toward the midline.

The Velopharynx. Hypernasality is the most frequent dysarthric speech problem associated with the velopharynx. Resonance problems in dysarthria relate to marked weakness of the palate resulting in continuous hypernasality and nasal emission, incoordination of palatal closure and speech sound production, slowed velar movement, and hyperfatiguability of the palate.

Activities designed to increase strength and movement of the soft palate have been used to treat velopharyngeal problems. However, they have rarely been studied to determine their efficacy. Palatal retraining techniques include massaging the palate and assisting elevation with a finger or wrapped tongue depressor.

Traditional tactics, such as using a mirror held below the nares to provide the patient with feedback on nasal airflow, have been employed to treat the velopharyngeal problems in patients with dysarthria. Numerous other approaches that provide more sophisticated feedback have the potential for altering velopharyngeal closure. These include the Scapescope[125] or aerodynamic measures of intraoral air pressure, oral airflow, and nasal airflow.[126,127]

In cases of severe velopharyngeal incompetence, prosthetic management such as a palatal lift prosthesis or surgical placement of a pharyngeal flap might be indicated. Comprehensive reviews of this subject are available.[128]

The Orofacial System. Intelligible speech production requires adequate strength and movement of the lips, tongue, and jaw. Thus attention can be directed at graded exercises geared towards progressive muscle retraining. Rosenbek and LaPointe describe isotonic and isometric exercises designed to increase the strength of the lips, tongue, and jaw.[19] Although such nonspeech activities should not be overlooked, it is most efficient to begin incorporating speech activities along with or instead of nonspeech activities as soon as possible. The speech focus relative to orofacial components is similar to traditional behavioral articulation training. However, the goal is intelligible production rather than normal production. Movement of the lips, tongue, and jaw are progressively differentiated in an effort to move towards recognizable speech sounds. This progressive differentiation relies partly on a clear knowledge of the physiologic substrates of the articulation errors and partly on the application of traditional methodology such as imitation and integral stimulation (watch, listen, and do), phonetic placement, immediate feedback of results, and training in the ability to self-monitor. An individually designed task continuum is used to move the patient from shorter, easier speech units to longer, more difficult utterances.

Orofacial prostheses have not been used frequently in dysarthria; however, clinicians should be alert to potential applications. Netsell suggests the use of a bite block prosthesis to assist in stabilizing the jaw during speech.[87] Other possible approaches include using slings to maintain jaw closure, and palatal prostheses to lower the palate and assist the tongue to reach its contact point.

Instrumentation has proven useful for both increasing and decreasing motor activity of the orofacial system. For example, several studies have reported the successful use of EMG biofeedback to facilitate return of motor control after cranial nerve anastomosis.[129–131] Others have used biofeedback to decrease excess movement or muscle activity. For example, hypertonicity of lip muscles and abnormal lip retraction was decreased in a patient with Parkinson's disease through training with biofeedback.[132] Similarly, Rubow, Rosenbek, Collins, and Celesia reduced facial spasms using EMG feedback with coincident improvement in speech intelligibility.[119]

Treatment of Combined Systems. Many dysarthric speakers require treatment approaches that effect the interaction of functional components. Often such combined approaches focus on altering the overall physiologic support for speech. In addition these approaches may target prosodic features of speech such as variations in pitch, timing, loudness, and proportions of silence to articulation time, that create intonation, stress, and rhythm of speech.

Physiologic Support. Modifying posture and increasing the overall effort for speech either through conscious efforts to exaggerate speech production or by exerting a force against an external object, such as the arms of a chair, can modify the physiologic support for speech and increase tone. Conversely, progressive relaxation exercises or postural changes may decrease excess muscle tone.

In an effort to improve naturalness and intelligibility, patients can systematically practice altering intonation patterns, pause time, and loudness variation. However, the variables that influence the perception of speech prosody are complex and interrelated. For example disruptions in timing of articulatory movements, speech rate, loudness, pause time, and pitch variation can alter intelligibility and quality of speech. These variables are often difficult for patients to monitor perceptually. Consequently, clinicians may attempt to alter prosody by providing graphic representations of these parameters. Berry and Goshorn used visual feedback from an oscilloscope to teach a patient with severe dysarthria to monitor loudness, speech rate, and improve intelligibility.[123] Similarly, Caligiuri and Murry demonstrated the effectiveness of feedback training upon articulatory precision, speaking rate, and prosody.[133] Treatment also resulted in an overall decrease in the severity of the patient's impairment.

Clinicians frequently attempt to alter the rate of speech in order to increase intelligibility of dysarthric speech. For example, using acoustic biofeedback procedures, Yorkston and Beukelman employed rate modification with a patient with ataxia.[77] Use of delayed auditory feedback has also been suggested as a means of modifying the rate of speech. Hanson and Metter, for example, reported a marked reduction in speech rate using delayed auditory feedback for two patients with hypokinetic dysarthria secondary to Parkinson's disease.[134] Although neither patient generalized the gains to speaking situations in which the delayed auditory feedback device was not used, both continued to use the device to improve intelligibility outside the clinic. The possibility of using a wearable delayed auditory feedback device can be investigated as a possible treatment option.

Behavioral methods of rate modification have also proven useful as a treatment option. Thus, pacing or tapping gestures paired with speech production have been suggested as a means of reorganizing the speaking process.[19] The patient simply accompanies each word or syllable with a gestural motion such as finger tapping. For appropriate candidates, the result is an alteration in rate, timing, and consequently intelligibility of speech. Helm used such a gestural system with tactile feedback from a "pacing board" to modify prosody and intelligibility.[135] Beukelman suggests avoiding an overcompensated rate as a result of such treatment approaches by helping patients learn to reduce rate, while maintaining appropriate phrase groupings.[116] There appears to be a "critical point" for each patient where maximum intelligibility is reached with the least disturbance of rate and prosody.

Contrastive stress drills have also been described as a means of correcting prosodic and stress abnormalities.[19] This approach can be successfully combined with rate control and articulation work to produce a more natural quality while maintaining an acceptable level of intelligibility.

Pragmatic Treatment

The literature on dysarthria focuses on the alteration of articulatory and prosodic elements of speech, whereas it largely ignores the modification of context and linguistic content as a means of improving the listener's understanding of what the dysarthric speaker is saying. In addition, it has been suggested that clinicians sometimes might overestimate the intelligibility of dysarthric speakers because of familiarity with the patient and so assume that gains observed within the treatment setting will result in improvements in other situations and with unfamiliar listeners.[136,137] Moreover, the recent emphasis on physiologic and acoustic parameters could result in an inadvertent failure to incorporate more functional and contextual variables along with speech training. Suggestions for maintaining a functional treatment perspective are reviewed in the following discussion.

Environmental Manipulation. Alterations in the "communication environment" of the dysarthric speaker can enhance communication. This principle is especially useful when significant residual speech problems exist after treatment or when the dysarthric condition is a result of a progressive degenerative disease. Berry and Sanders suggest that clinicians teach patients and families principles such as (1) avoid communicating in dark or noisy places; (2) reduce the distance between the speaker with dysarthria and the listener rather than forcing the dysarthric speaker to increase his or her volume; (3) attend to position and orientation of speakers: a full face view maximizes intelligibility; and (4) learn to utilize situational, nonverbal, and gestural cues.[121]

Utterance Length. Research results suggest that mildly impaired dysarthric speakers tend to be more intelligible when complete sentences are used, whereas severely impaired speakers tend to be more intelligible when short words and phrases are used.[137] Thus patients can be taught to use the utterance structure and length that most improves function.

Repair Strategies. Clinicians who have worked with patients with dysarthria are undoubtedly familiar with the frequent observation that when a patient with dysarthria is not understood and is asked "what," *many* patients simply repeat the utterance without any modification; many patients do not seem to spontaneously adopt effective repair strategies for communication failures. Interestingly, Ansel, McNeil, Hunker, and Bless concluded that the intelligibility-impaired dysarthric speakers studied did not respond to their own communication failures with consistently effective modifications to improve intelligibility.[138] They suggested that either the dysarthric speakers did not know or could not use effective repair strategies. One might conclude that treatment could logically include training in the most effective repair strategies.

Self-Monitoring. Ansel et al also suggested that their dysarthric speakers seemed unaware of their own lack of intelligibility.[138] In other words, they failed to monitor the need to make adjustments that would assist their listeners. Perhaps attention to training in self-monitoring would help patients carry over treatment gains. This would necessarily include not only relearning what to look, listen, or feel for within the speech motor system, but also learning how to monitor input from the listener relative to the adequacy of message transmission.

Topic and Attention Getting. People are easier to understand when one knows the topic and context. Dysarthric speakers can be taught to control context and alert others to topic shifts by utilizing alerting carrier phrases such as "Now I want to talk about . . . (pause) the children."[121] Similarly, alerting the listener that they must attend carefully can be accomplished by teaching the dysarthric speaker to use techniques such as stating the listener's name or touching the listener.

Many other approaches relative to controlling the contextual, social, linguistic, emotional, physical, and cognitive constraints of communication are available to the creative clinician.

Communication Augmentation

When speech communication fails, an alternative or adjunctive system is frequently in order. This alternative can range from the simple alphabet board or universal gesture system to highly sophisticated microcomputers that talk for the patient. Patients require training and practice to become confident and comfortable with such systems; it is an injustice to the patient to assume that a simple introduction to an alternative system suffices. Excellent reviews are available that address this extensive area.[139]

Carry-Over and Maintenance of Treatment Gains

Treatment cannot stop when the patient achieves improved speech production with the therapist. How the patient performs with speech tasks, speakers, and settings beyond the treatment situation determines if the therapy has been successful. The goal must be to teach carry-over of patterns. To achieve this goal often requires a carefully designed continuum of activities that successively approximate more natural settings and slowly fade the constraints of the original training context. Carry-over training must take into account all variables that influence production, including speech-motor demands of the situation (rate, loudness, utterance length and difficulty, utterance similarity to trained responses), emotional influences (stress, embarrassment, nonsupportive responses of listeners), linguistic variables (utterance length, complexity, formulation demands), and cognitive variables (attentional demands).

Maintenance of gains after treatment is rarely a topic addressed in the literature. However, clinical experience often suggests that patients with dysarthria who have obtained intensive behavioral treatment frequently lose ground over a period of months or years after treatment is terminated. Years and years of normal automatic speech is poor training for the dysarthric speaker who must adopt new ways of talking. When the external forces that reinforce the "new way of talking" are removed, there could be a tendency to revert to that overlearned and habitual manner of talking that an entire life has reinforced. This is a primary reason for insuring adequate attention to the carry-over environment and, if necessary, for setting up a mechanism for maintenance reinforcement of compensated speech.

Progressive Diseases

Because of the progressive nature of degenerative diseases such as multiple sclerosis, Parkinson's disease, amyotropic lateral sclerosis, Huntington's chorea, patients with such diagnoses are often overlooked as appropriate candidates for referral to speech-language pathologists. In fact, the speech-language pathologist can play an important role in maximizing the communicative effectiveness of individuals in spite of the progression of disease. Teaching compensatory strategies can help the patient preserve and maximize residual skills. Training and counseling can help prevent the acquisition of maladaptive strategies. Family members can be taught how to facilitate communication, and counseling can assist with adjustment. Frequently external aids such as delayed auditory feedback, augmentative communication devices, and voice amplifiers can be introduced. Early intervention is needed to insure that patients are taught how to use such alternative systems while they still have the capacity and stamina to practice and become proficient; frequently frustration and failure results when patients are not taught these systems until they have lost a functional means of communicating.

SUMMARY

The purpose of this chapter was to survey the literature on the dysarthrias and on apraxia of speech and to summarize the available information on their assessment and treatment. Following a brief historical overview, the dysarthrias and apraxia were distinguished on the basis of site of lesion, underlying neuropsychological mechanisms, speech characteristics, and related impairments. In addition, these motor speech disorders were briefly contrasted with aphasic language impairments. Throughout our discussion, the need for ongoing clinical assessment was stressed. Although examples of specific assessment procedures were described, emphasis was on information of possible value for differential diagnosis and treatment planning. For example, assessment procedures for the dysarthrias were discussed from a physiologic approach, thereby challenging clinicians to go beyond traditional perceptual analyses and to hypothesize *why* a specific pattern of deficits exists; thus, clinicians are better prepared for treatment planning.

Recent physiologic and acoustic studies have helped reshape our thinking about the nature of motor speech disorders, and this, in turn, has begun to alter our approaches to clinical management. For example, the current view of apraxia of speech as a movement disorder has directed intervention efforts toward selection of treatment tasks and behaviors (e.g., articulatory, stress, rhythm) that facilitate movement. Likewise, the aforementioned physiologic approach to the dysarthrias encourages clinicians to select treatment goals that attempt to improve physiologic impairments presumed to cause the more obvious speech impairment. Broadly speaking, recent approaches require that clinicians avoid treating the symptoms of motor speech disorders and rather attempt to treat basic processes or conditions that underlie the dysarthrias and apraxia of speech. Once treatment targets are selected, special emphasis should be placed on pragmatic treatment approaches that incorporate generalization prompting strategies.

Although the proliferation of studies of motor speech disorders has affected our clinical thinking and intervention, it should be cautioned that many of the treatment procedures described herein are based on only limited data. As in other areas of speech-language pathology, the clinical management of apraxia and the dysarthrias in an evolving, but as yet underdeveloped, clinical science. Clinicians therefore, should critically and continuously evaluate suggested procedures and attempt to determine which approaches are best suited to their individual patients.

Acknowledgments. The authors gratefully acknowledge the assistance of Dr. J. Rosenbek.

The writing of this manuscript was supported, in part, by Veterans Administration Rehabilitation Research and Development funds.

APPENDIX 1

Dimensions Used in The Mayo Clinic Dysarthria Study*

Dimension	*Description*
Pitch level	Pitch of voice sounds consistently too low or too high for individual's age and sex.
Pitch breaks	Pitch of voice shows sudden and uncontrolled variation (falsetto breaks).
Monopitch	Voice is characterized by a monopitch or monotone. Voice lacks normal inflectional changes. It tends to stay at one pitch level.
Voice tremor	Voice shows shakiness or tremulousness.
Monoloudness	Voice shows monotony of loudness. It lacks normal variations in loudness.
Excess loudness variation	Voice shows sudden, uncontrolled alterations in loudness: sometimes loud, becoming too loud, sometimes too weak.
Loudness decay	There is a progressive diminution in loudness.
Loudness level (overall)	Voice is insufficiently or excessively loud.

APPENDIX 1

Dimensions Used in The Mayo Clinic Dysarthria Study*

Dimension	*Description*
Harsh voice	Voice is harsh, rough, and raspy.
Hoarse (wet) voice	There is a wet "liquid sounding" hoarseness.
Breathy voice (continuous)	Voice is continuously breathy, weak, and thin.
Breathy voice (transient)	Breathiness is transient, periodic, and intermittent.
Strained or strangled voice	Voice (phonation) sounds strained (an apparently effortful squeezing of voice through glottis).
Voice stoppages	There are sudden stoppages of the voiced airstream (as if some obstacle along the vocal tract momentarily impedes airflow).
Hypernasality	Voice sounds excessively nasal. Excessive amount of air is resonated by nasal cavities.
Hyponasality	Voice is denasal.
Nasal emission	There is nasal emission of the airstream.
Forced inspiration and expiration	Speech is interrupted by sudden, forced inspiration and expiration sighs.
Audible inspiration	There is audible breathy inspiration.
Grunt at the end of expiration	There is a grunt at the end of expiration.
Rate	Rate of actual speech is abnormally slow or rapid.
Short phrases	Phrases are short (possibly because inspirations occur more often than normal). Speaker may sound as if he or she has run out of air. He or she may produce a gasp at the end of a phrase.
Rate increase in segments	Rate increases progressively within given segments of connected speech.
Increase of rate overall	Rate increases progressively from beginning to end of a sample.
Reduced stress	Speech shows reduction of proper stress or emphasis pattern.
Variable rate	Rate alternates from slow to fast.
Prolonged intervals	Interword or intersyllable intervals are prolonged.
Inappropriate silence	There are inappropriate silent intervals.
Short rushes of speech	There are short rushes of speech separated by pauses.
Excess and equal stress	There is excess stress on usually unstressed parts of speech, for example, monosyllabic words and unstressed syllables of polysyllabic words.
Imprecise consonants	Consonant sounds lack precision. They show slurring, inadequate sharpness, distortions, and lack of crispness. There is clumsiness in going from one consonant to another.
Prolonged phonemes	Phonemes are prolonged.
Repeated phonemes	Phonemes are repeated.
Irregular articulatory breakdown	There is intermittent, nonsystematic breakdown in accuracy of articulation.
Distorted vowels	Vowel sounds are distorted throughout their total duration.
Intelligibility (overall)	This is a rating of overall intelligibility or understandability of speech.
Bizarreness (overall)	This is a rating of degree to which overall speech calls attention to itself because of its unusual, peculiar, or bizarre characteristics.

* After Darley FL, Aronson AE, Brown JR. Motor speech disorders. Philadelphia: WB Saunders, 1975.

REFERENCES

1. Wertz RT, Rosenbek JC, Deal JL. A review of 228 cases of apraxia of speech: classification, etiology, and localization. Paper presented to the American Speech and Hearing Association, New York, 1970.
2. Wertz RT. Neuropathologies of speech and language: an introduction to patient management. In: Johns DF, ed. Clinical management of neurogenic communication disorders. Boston, MA: Little, Brown, 1985:1.
3. Netsell R. A neurobiologic view of speech production and the dysarthrias. San Diego, CA: College-Hill Press, 1986.
4. Netsell R, Daniel B. Dysarthria in adults: physiological approach to rehabilitation. Arch Phys Med Rehabil 1979; 60:502–508.
5. Wertz RT. Response to treatment in patients with apraxia of speech. In: Rosenbek JC, McNeil MR, Aronson AE, eds. Apraxia of speech: physiology, acoustics, linguistics, management. San Diego, CA: College-Hill Press, 1984:257.
6. McNeil MR, Kennedy JG. Measuring the effects of treatment for dysarthria: knowing when to change or terminate. In: Rosenbek JC, ed. Seminars in speech and language. Vol. 5, No. 4. Current views of dysarthria. New York: Thieme-Stratton, 1984.
7. Fromm D, Abbs JH, McNeil MR, Rosenbek JC. Simultaneous perceptual physiological method of studying apraxia of speech. In: Brookshire RH, ed. Clinical aphasiology conference proceedings. Minneapolis, MN: BRK Publishers, 1982:189.
8. Hunker CJ, Abbs JH. Physiological analysis of parkinsonian tremors in the orofacial system. In: McNeil MR, Rosenbek JC, Aronson AE, eds. The dysarthrias: physiology, acoustics, perception, management. San Diego, CA: College-Hill Press, 1984:69.
9. Kent R, Rosenbek JC. Acoustic patterns of apraxia of speech. J Speech Hear Res 1983; 26:231–249.
10. Weismer G. Acoustic descriptions of dysarthric speech: perceptual correlates and physiological inferences. In: Rosenbek JC, ed. Seminars in speech and language. Vol. 5, No. 4. Current views in dysarthria. New York: Thieme-Stratton, 1984:293.
11. Rubow R. A clinical guide to the technology of treatment in dysarthria. In: Rosenbek JC, ed. Seminars in speech and

language. Vol. 5, No. 4. Current views of dysarthria. New York: Thieme-Stratton, 1984:315.

12. Rubow R, Swift. Microcomputer based wearable biofeedback device to improve treatment carryover in Parkinsonian dysarthria. J Speech Hear Disord 1985; 50:178.
13. Simmons NN. Acoustic analysis of ataxic dysarthria: an approach to monitoring treatment. In: Berry WR, ed. Clinical dysarthria. San Diego, CA: College-Hill Press, 1983:283.
14. Berry WR, ed. Clinical dysarthria. San Diego, CA: College-Hill Press, 1983.
15. Darley FL, Aronson AE, Brown JR. Motor speech disorders. Philadelphia: WB Saunders, 1975.
16. McNeil MR, Rosenbek JC, Aronson AE, eds. The dysarthrias: physiology, acoustics, perception, management. San Diego, CA: College-Hill Press, 1984.
17. Rosenbek JC. Treating apraxia of speech. In: Johns DF, ed. Clinical management of neurogenic communication disorders. 2nd ed. Boston, MA: Little, Brown, 1985:267.
18. Rosenbek JC, ed. Seminars in speech and language. Vol. 5, No. 4. Current views of dysarthria. New York: Thieme-Stratton, 1984.
19. Rosenbek JC, LaPointe LL. The dysarthrias: description, diagnosis, and treatment. In: Johns DF, ed. Clinical management of neurogenic communication disorders. Boston, MA: Little, Brown, 1985:97.
20. Rosenbek JC, McNeil MR, Aronson AE, eds. Apraxia of speech: physiology, acoustics, linguistics, management. San Diego, CA: College-Hill Press, 1984.
21. Wertz RT, LaPointe LL, Rosenbek JC. Apraxia of speech in adults: the disorder and its management. New York: Grune & Stratton, 1984.
22. Darley FL, Aronson AE, Brown JR. Clusters of deviant speech dimensions in the dysarthrias. J Speech Hear Res 1969; 12:462–496.
23. Hardy JC. Suggestions for physiological research in dysarthria. Cortex 1967; 3:128–156.
24. Darley FL, Aronson AE, Brown JR. Differential diagnostic patterns of dysarthria. J Speech Hear Res 1969; 12:246–269.
25. Darley FL, Brown JR, Goldstein JR. Dysarthria in multiple sclerosis. J Speech Hear Res 1972; 15:229–245.
26. Darley FL. Aphasia input and output disturbances in speech and language processing. Presented in dual session on aphasia, Chicago, IL: ASHA 1969.
27. Ludlow CL, Bassich CJ. The results of acoustic and perceptual assessment of two types of dysarthria. In: Berry WR, ed. Clinical dysarthria. San Diego, CA: College-Hill Press, 1983.
28. Ludlow CL, Bassich CJ. Relationships between perceptual ratings and acoustic measures of hypokinetic speech. In: McNeil MR, Rosenbek JC, Aronson AE, eds. The dysarthrias: physiology, acoustics, perception, management. San Diego, CA: College-Hill Press, 1984:163.
29. Grewel F. Classification of dysarthrias. Acta Psychiatr Neurol Scand 1957; 32:325–337.
30. Kearns KP, Simmons NN. Interobserver reliability and perceptual ratings: more than meets the ear. J Speech Hear Res (in press).
31. Abbs JM, Hunker CJ, Barlow SM. Differential speech motor subsystem impairments with suprabulbar lesions: neurophysiological framework and supporting data. In: Berry WR, ed. Clinical dysarthria. San Diego, CA: College-Hill Press, 1983:165.
32. Murry T. The production of stress in three types of dysarthric speech. In: Berry WR, ed. Clinical dysarthria. San Diego, CA: College-Hill Press, 1983:69.
33. Yorkston KM, Beukelman DR, Minifie FD, Sapir S. Assessment of stress patterning. In: McNeil MR, Rosenbek JC, Aronson AE, eds. The dysarthrias: physiology, acoustics, perception, management. San Diego, CA: College-Hill Press, 1984:131.
34. Netsell R, Daniel B, Celesia G. Acceleration and weakness in Parkinsonian dysarthria. J Speech Hear Disord 1975; 40:326–330.
35. Darley FL. Perceptual analysis of the dysarthrias. In: Rosenbek JC, ed. Seminars in speech and language. Vol. 1, No. 4. Current views of dysarthria. New York: Thieme-Stratton, 1984:267.
36. Darley FL. Apraxia of speech: 107 years of terminological confusion. Presented to the American Speech and Hearing Association. Chicago, 1969.
37. Johns DF, LaPointe LL. Neurogenic disorders of output processing: apraxia of speech. In: Whitaker H, Whitaker HA, eds. Studies in neurolinguistics. Vol. 7. New York: Academic Press, 1976.
38. Buckingham HW. Explanations for the concept of apraxia of speech. In: Sarno MT, ed. Acquired aphasia. New York: Academic Press, 1981.
39. Rosenbek JC. Treating the dysarthric talker. In: Rosenbek JC, ed. Seminars in speech and language. Vol. 5, No. 4. Current views of dysarthria. New York: Thieme-Stratton, 1984:359.
40. Rosenbek JC, Kent RD, LaPointe LL. Apraxia of speech: an overview and some perspectives. In: Rosenbek JC, McNeil MR, Aronson AE, eds. Apraxia of speech: physiology, acoustics, linguistics, management. San Diego, CA: College-Hill Press, 1984:1.
41. Roy EA, Square PA. Common considerations in the study of limb, verbal and oral apraxia. In: Roy EA, ed. Neuropsychological study of apraxia and related disorders. North Holland: Elsevier, 1985.
42. Canter GJ. Dysarthria, apraxia of speech and literal paraphasia: three distinct varieties of articulatory behavior in the adult with brain damage. Paper presented to the American Speech and Hearing Association, Detroit, 1973.
43. Kearns KP. Apraxia of speech: avoiding clinical and research myopia. Paper presented to the American Speech/Language Hearing Association, Toronto, Canada, 1982.
44. Abbs JH, Rosenbek JC. Some motor control perspectives on apraxia of speech and dysarthria. In: Costello J, ed. Speech disorders in adults. San Diego: College-Hill Press, 1985:21.
45. Deal JL, Darley FL. The influence of linguistic and situational variables on phonemic accuracy in apraxia of speech. J Speech Hear Res 1972; 15:639–653.
46. Johns DF, Darley FL. Phonemic variability of apraxia of speech. J Speech Hear Disord 1970; 13:556–583.
47. LaPointe LL, Horner J. Repeated trials of words by patients with neurogenic phonological sequencing impairment (AOS): stimulus mode and response condition revisited. In: Brookshire RH, ed. Clinical Aphasiology Conference Proceedings, Minneapolis, MN: BRK Publishers, 1976.
48. Shankweiler D, Harris KS. An experimental approach to the problem of articulation in aphasia. Cortex 1966; 2:277–297.
49. Lecours, Lhermitte. The 'pure form' of the phonetic disintegration syndrome (pure anarthria); anatomo-clinical report of a historical case. Brain Lang 1976; 3:88–112.
50. Aten JL, Johns DF, Darley FL. Auditory perception of sequenced words in apraxia of speech. J Speech Hear Res 1971; 14:131–143.
51. Square PA, Darley FL, Sommers RI. Speech perception among patients demonstrating apraxia of speech, aphasia, and with disorders. In: Brookshire RH, ed. Clinical Aphasiology Conference Proceedings. Minneapolis, MN: BRK Publishers, 1982:83.
52. Rosenbek JC, Wertz RT, Darley FL. Oral sensation and perception in apraxia of speech and aphasia. J Speech Hear Res 1973; 16:22–36.
53. Buckingham HW. Explanation of apraxia of speech. Brain Lang 1979; 8:202–226.
54. Martin AD. Some objections to the term apraxia of speech. J Speech Hear Disord 1974; 39:53–63.

55. Blumstein SE. A phonological investigation of aphasic speech. The Hague: Mouton, 1973.
56. Bowman E, Hodson B, Simpson R. Oral apraxia and aphasic misarticulations. In: Brookshire RH, ed. Clinical Aphasiology Conference Proceedings. Minneapolis, MN: BRK Publishers, 1980.
57. Kearns KP. The application of phonological process analyses to adult neuropathologies. In: Brookshire RH, ed. Clinical Aphasiology Conference Proceedings. Minneapolis, MN: BRK Publishers, 1980.
58. Martin AP, Rigrodsky S. An investigation of phonological impairment in aphasia. Part 2: distinctive feature analysis of phonemic communication errors in aphasia. Cortex 1974; 10:329–346.
59. Marquardt TP, Reinhart JB, Petersen HA. Markedness analysis of phonemic substitution errors in apraxia of speech. J Commun Disord 1979; 12:481–494.
60. Trost JE, Canter GJ. Apraxia of speech in patients with Broca's aphasia: a study of phoneme production, accuracy and error patterns. Brain Lang 1974; 1:63–79.
61. Blumstein SE. Phonological aspects of aphasia. In: Sarno MT, ed. Acquired aphasia. New York: Academic Press, 1981.
62. Blumstein SE, Cooper WE, Goodglass H, Statlender S, Gottlieb J. Production deficits in aphasia: a voice-onset time analysis. Brain Lang 1980; 9:153–170.
63. Dunlop J, Marquardt T. Linguistic and articulation aspects of single word production in apraxia of speech. Cortex 1977; 13:17–39.
64. Martin AP, Wasserman NH, Gilden L, Gerstman L, West JA. A process model of repetition in aphasia: an investigation of phonological and morphological interaction in aphasic error performance. Brain Lang 1975; 2:434–450.
65. Rosenbek JC. Advances in the evaluation and treatment of speech apraxia. In: Rose FC, ed. Advances in neurology. Vol. 42. Progress in aphasiology. New York: Raven Press, 1984:327.
66. Hardison D, Marquardt T, Petersen H. Effects of selected linguistic variables on apraxia of speech. J Speech Hear Res 1977; 20:334–343.
67. Itoh M, Sasanuma S. Velar movements during speech in a patient with apraxia of speech. Brain Lang 1979; 7:227–239.
68. Itoh M, Sasanuma S. Articulatory movements in apraxia of speech. In: Rosenbek JC, McNeil MR, Aronson AE, eds. Apraxia of speech: physiology, acoustics, linguistics, management. San Diego, CA: College-Hill Press, 1984:135.
69. Blumstein SE, Cooper WE, Zurif EB, et al. The perception and production of voice-onset time in aphasia. Neuropsychologia 1977; 15:371–382.
70. Itoh M, Sasanuma S, Tatsumi IF, et al. Voice onset time characteristics in apraxia of speech. Brain Lang 1982; 17:193–210.
71. Sands ES, Freeman FJ, Harris KS. Progressive changes on articulatory patterns in verbal apraxia: a longitudinal study. Brain Lang 1978; 6:97–105.
72. Collins MJ, Rosenbek JC, Wertz RT. Spectrographic analysis of vowel and word duration in apraxia of speech. J Speech Hear Res 1983; 26:224–230.
73. Kent R, Rosenbek JC. Prosodic disturbances and neurologic lesion. Brain Lang 1982; 15:259–291.
74. Itoh M, Sasanuma S, Hirose H, Yoshioka H, Ushyima T. Abnormal articulatory dynamics in a patient with apraxia of speech: X-ray microbeam observation. Brain Lang 1980; 11:66–75.
75. Kearns KP. Methodologies for studying generalization. Presented to the Kansas University Spring Symposium, Generalization strategies in treatment of communicative disorders. Overland Park, KS, 1987.
76. Enderby P. The standardized assessment of dysarthria is possible. In: Berry WR, ed. Clinical dysarthria. San Diego, CA: College-Hill Press, 1983:109.
77. Yorkston KM, Beukelman DR. Assessment of intelligibility of dysarthric speech. San Diego: College-Hill Press, 1981.
78. Kertesz A. Subcortical lesions and verbal apraxia. In: Rosenbek JC, McNeil MR, Aronson AE, eds. Apraxia of speech: physiology, acoustics, linguistics, management. San Diego, CA: College-Hill Press, 1984:73.
79. Netsell R. A neurobiologic view of the dysarthrias. In: McNeil MR, Rosenbek JC, Aronson AE, eds. The dysarthrias: physiology, acoustics, perception, management. San Diego, CA: College-Hill Press, 1984:1.
80. McReynolds LV, Kearns KP. Single subject experimental designs in communicative disorders. Austin, TX: Pro-Ed, 1983.
81. Deutsch SE. Prediction of site of lesion from speech apraxic error patterns. In: Rosenbek JC, McNeil MR, Aronson AE, eds. Apraxia of speech: physiology, acoustics, linguistics, management. San Diego, CA: College-Hill Press, 1984:133.
82. Netsell R. Physiological studies of dysarthria and their relevance to treatment. In: Rosenbek JC, ed. Seminars in speech and language. Vol. 5, No. 4. Current views of dysarthria. New York: Thieme-Stratton, 1984:279.
83. Dabul B. Apraxia of speech: battery for adults. Tigard, ME: CC Publications, 1979.
84. De Renzi E, Faglioni P. Normative data and screening power of the shortened version of the Token test. Cortex 1978; 14:41–49.
85. Netsell R, Rosenbek J. Treating the dysarthrias. In: Darby J, ed. Speech and language evaluation in neurology: adult disorders. Orlando, FL: Grune & Stratton, 1985.
86. Netsell R. Speech motor control: theoretical issues with clinical impact. In: Berry WR, ed. Clinical dysarthria. San Diego, CA: College-Hill Press, 1983:1.
87. Netsell R. Construction and use of a bite block for evaluating and treating speech disorders. J Speech Hear Disord 1985; 50:103–106.
88. Marquardt TP, Sussman M. The elusive lesion—apraxia link in Broca's aphasia. Ln: Rosenbek JC, McNeil MR, Aronson AE, eds. Apraxia of speech: physiology, acoustics, linguistics, management. San Diego: College-Hill Press, 1984.
89. Goodglass H, Kaplan E. The Boston diagnostic aphasia examination. Boston: Lea & Febiger, 1983.
90. Kertesz A. Western aphasia battery. New York: Grune & Stratton, 1982.
91. Porch BE. Porch index of communicative ability. 3rd ed. Palo Alto, CA: Consulting Psychologists Press, 1981.
92. Wertz RT, Rosenbek JC, Collins MJ. Identification of apraxia of speech from PICA verbal tests on selected oral-verbal apraxia tests. In: Brookshire RH, ed. Clinical aphasiology, collected conference proceedings, 1978. Minneapolis, MN: BRK Publishers.
93. McDonald ET. A deep test of articulation. Pittsburgh: Stanwix House, 1964.
94. Duffy JR, Gawle CA. Apraxic speaker's vowel duration in consonant-vowel-consonant syllables. In: Rosenbek JC, McNeil MR, Aronson AE, eds. Apraxia of speech: physiology, acoustics, linguistics, management. San Diego, CA: College-Hill Press, 1984:167.
95. Rosenbek J. Treatment of apraxia of speech in adults. In: Perkins W, ed. Current therapy of communication disorders: dysarthria and apraxia. New York: Thieme-Stratton, 1983:49.
96. Shewan CM. Phonological processing in Broca's aphasics. Brain Lang 1980; 10:71–88.
97. Duffy J. Assessment and treatment of apraxia of speech. Presented at the Ochsner clinic foundation annual meeting, New Orleans, 1987.
98. Rosenbek JC, Lemme ML, Ahern MG, Harris EH, Wertz RT. A treatment for apraxia of speech in adults. J Speech Hear Disord 1973; 38:462.
99. Deal JL, Florance CL. Modification of the eight-step con-

tinuum for treatment of apraxia of speech in adults. J Speech Hear Disord 1978; 43:89–95.
100. Sparks RW, Deck JW. Melodic intonation therapy. In: Chapey R, ed. Language intervention strategies in adult aphasia. 2nd ed. Baltimore, MD: Williams & Wilkins, 1986:320.
101. Sparks R, Holland A. Method: melodic intonation therapy. J Speech Hear Disord 1976; 41:287–297.
102. Sparks R, Helm N, Albert M. Aphasia rehabilitation resulting from melodic intonation therapy. Cortex 1974; 10:303–316.
103. Dunham M, Newhoff M. Melodic intonation therapy: rewriting the song. In: Brookshire RH, ed. Clinical Aphasiology Conference Proceedings. Minneapolis, MN: BRK Publishers, 1979:283.
104. Marshall N, Holtzapple P. Melodic intonation therapy, variations on a theme. In: Brookshire RH, ed. Clinical Aphasiology Conference Proceedings. Minneapolis, MN: BRK Publishers, 1976:115.
105. Square P, Chumpelik D, Morningstar D, Adams S. Efficacy of the PROMPT system of therapy for the treatment of acquired apraxia of speech. In: Brookshire RH, ed. Clinical Aphasiology Conference Proceedings. Minneapolis, MN: BRK Publishers, 1986:221.
106. Skelly M, Schinsky L, Smith R. Fust R. American Indian sign (Amerind) as a facilitator of verbalization for the oral verbal apraxic. J Speech Hear Disord 1974; 39:445.
107. Rosenbek JC, Collins MJ, Wertz RT. Intersystemic reorganization for apraxia of speech. In: Brookshire RH, ed. Clinical Aphasiology Conference Proceedings, Minneapolis, MN: BRK Publisher, 1976.
108. Simmons N. Finger counting as an intersystemic reorganizer in apraxia of speech. In: Brookshire RH, ed. Clinical Aphasiology Conference Proceedings. Minneapolis, MN: BRK Publishers, 1978:174.
109. Berman M, Peelle L. Self-generated cues: a method of aiding aphasic and apraxic patients. J Speech Hear Disord 1967; 32:372.
110. McNeil M, Prescott I, Lemme M. An application of EMG biofeedback to aphasia/apraxia treatment. In: Brookshire RH, ed. Clinical Aphasiology Conference Proceedings. Minneapolis, MN: BRK Publishers, 1976.
111. Rubow R, Rosenbek JC. Stress management in the treatment of apraxia of speech. Proceedings of the Biofeedback Society of America (abstract), 1984.
112. Lyon J. Drawing: its communicative effectiveness for the expressively restricted aphasic adult. Workshop presented in conjunction with the American Speech, Language and Hearing Association Convention, Detroit, MI, 1986.
113. Stokes T, Baer D. An implicit technology of generalization. J Appl Behav Anal 1977; 10:349–367.
114. Florance C, Rabidoux P, McCauslin L. An environmental manipulation approach to treating apraxia of speech. In: Brookshire RH, ed. Clinical Aphasiology Conference Proceedings. Minneapolis, MN: BRK Publishers, 1980:285.
115. Barlow S, Abbs J. Orofacial fine motor control impairments in congenital spasticity: evidence against hypertonus-related performance deficits. Neurol, 1984; 34:145–150.
116. Beukelman D. Management of dysarthric speakers. Workshop presented in conjunction with the American Speech and Hearing Association Convention, Detroit, MI, 1986.
117. Seif M, Netsell R. Restoration of speech production thirteen years post trauma. Paper presented at the Clinical Dysarthria Conference, Tuscon, AZ, 1984.
118. Davis SM, Drichta CE. Biofeedback theory and application in allied health. Biofeedback Self Regul 1980; 5:159–174.
119. Rubow R, Rosenbek J, Collins M, Celesia G. Reduction in hemifacial spasm and dysarthria following EMG biofeedback. J Speech Hear Disord 1984; 49:26–33.
120. Rubow R. Role of feedback, reinforcement, and compliance on training and transfer in biofeedback-based rehabilitation of motor speech disorders. In: McNeil MR, Rosenbek JC, Aronson AE, eds. The dysarthrias: physiology, acoustics, perception, management. San Diego, CA: College-Hill Press, 1984:207.
121. Berry W, Sanders S. Environmental education: the universal management approach for adults with dysarthria. In: Berry W, ed. Clinical dysarthria. San Diego, CA: College-Hill Press, 1983:203.
122. Murry T. Treatment of ataxic dysarthria. In: Perkins W, ed. Current therapy of communication disorders: dysarthria and apraxia. New York: Thieme-Stratton, 1983:79.
123. Berry WR, Goshorn EL. Immediate visual feedback in the treatment of ataxic dysarthria: a case study. In: Berry WR, ed. Clinical dysarthria. San Diego, CA: College-Hill Press, 1983:253.
124. Netsell R, Hixon T. Noninvasive method for clinically estimating subglottal air pressure. J Speech Hear Disord 1978; 43:326–330.
125. Shprintzen RJ, McCall GN, Skolnick ML. A new therapeutic technique for the treatment of velopharyngeal incompetency. J Speech Hear Disord 1975; 40:69.
126. Collins JJ, Rubow RT, Rosenbek JC, Gracco V. An instrumental approach to reduction of nasal emission in dysarthria. Paper presented to the American Speech and Hearing Association, Los Angeles, CA, 1981.
127. Fletcher S. Time-by-count measurement of diadochokinetic syllable rate. J Speech Hear Res 1972; 26:297–304.
128. Johns D. Surgical and prosthetic management of neurogenic velopharyngeal incompetency in dysarthria. In: Johns D, ed. Clinical management of neurogenic communicative disorders. Boston, MA: Little, Brown, 1985.
129. Balliet R, Shinn JB, Bach-y-Rita P. Facial paralysis rehabilitation: retraining selective muscle control. Int Rehabil Med, 1982; 4:67–74.
130. Booker HE, Rubow R, Coleman P. Simplified feedback in neuromuscular retraining: an automated approach using electromyographic signals. Arch Phys Med Rehabil 1969; 50:621–625.
131. Daniel B, Guitar B. EMG biofeedback and recovery of facial and speech gestures following neural anastomosis. J Speech Hear Disord. 1978; 43:9–20.
132. Netsell R, Cleeland C. Modification of lip hypertonia in dysarthria using EMG feedback. J Speech Hear Disord 1979; 38:131–141.
133. Caligiuri MP, Murry T. The use of visual feedback to enhance prosodic control in dysarthria. In: Berry WR, ed. Clinical dysarthria. San Diego, CA: College-Hill Press, 1983:267.
134. Hanson WR, Metter EJ. DAF as instrumental treatment for dysarthria in progressive supranuclear palsy. J Speech Hear Disord 1983; 34:123–127.
135. Helm N. Assessing candidacy for melodic intonation therapy. Paper presented to the American Speech & Hearing Association, Houston, TX, 1976.
136. Beukelman D, Yorkston K. The influence of passage familiarity of intelligibility estimates of dysarthric speech. J Commun Disord 1980; 13:33–41.
137. Yorkston KM, Beukelman DA. Comparison techniques for measuring the intelligibility of dysarthric speech. J Commun Disord 1978; 11:499–512.
138. Ansel BM, McNeil MR, Hunker EJ, Bless DM. The frequency of verbal and acoustic adjustment used by cerebral palsied-dysarthric adults when faced with communicative failure. In: Berry WR, ed. Clinical dysarthria. San Diego, CA: College–Hill Press, 1983.
139. Beukelman DR, Yorkston KM, Dowden PA. Communication augmentation: a casebook of clinical management. San Diego, CA: College-Hill Press, 1984.

Fluency Disorders

20 Dysfluency in the Child

Meryl J. Wall, Ph.D.

Since "dysfluency" infers a difficulty with the smooth and easy flow of speech production, several communicatively disordered groups may be considered dysfluent. Dysarthric and apraxic individuals may be dysfluent, as may speakers with severe or profound hearing loss. However, the most frequent interpretation of dysfluency is that of stuttering, with cluttering a close second. Some use "disfluency" to refer to stuttering and cluttering, whereas "nonfluency" is usually used to describe disruptions observed in the developing speech and language of the young child or the natural interruptions of mature speech. Sorting out the terminology is difficult because of inconsistent use within the speech-language pathology profession. However, "dysfluency" is the term associated frequently with disordered fluency as in stuttering and cluttering, with "disfluency" used synonymously by some professionals.

What to call a fluency disorder in young children, and how to spell it, is only part of a more global problem of definition, a problem that appears to lessen as the child matures. Clinicians seem more at ease in defining and therefore in diagnosing a fluency disorder in an elementary school-age and high school-age child than in a preschooler. The reason for this discrepancy is that many regard a confounding variable to be present in the preschooler; that of normal nonfluency. How to distinguish between early nonfluency and stuttering, or what some call incipient (beginning) stuttering, has therefore become a major issue in the differential diagnosis of stuttering in the young child. However, the distinction between the two conditions, nonfluency and stuttering, is by no means a consistently difficult one to make.

For an historical perspective on this issue, one needs to reexamine Johnson's theory of the onset of stuttering,[1,2] since Johnson was the first to emphasize a possible relationship between early nonfluency and stuttering. He believed that at the time of the onset of stuttering, children's nonfluencies were within normal limits, and that the direct cause of stuttering was the stressful effect of parental reaction to the nonfluencies. The implication was that the parents were perfectionists who demanded unusually high standards of their children in speech production and perhaps in other ways as well. As a result, they created stuttering from essentially normal speech. This was referred to as the diagnosogenic theory. Later, in a refinement of the theory, Johnson stressed the disruption of relationships between the child and those in the environment subsequent to the diagnosis of stuttering. However, it was Johnson's earlier, well-received concept—that children who stutter had been, in fact, normally nonfluent, were misdiagnosed as stutterers by their parents, and as a result became self-conscious and tense about speech and developed into stutterers—that had such impact. His theory has probably contributed to the apprehension some clinicians feel when required to evaluate and/or treat a young stutterer; they apparently fear making the condition worse.

Although there is no absolute or discrete categorization between early nonfluency and stuttering, nonfluency is likely to consist of word and phrase repetitions, revisions of utterances, and interjections, whereas early stuttering is likely to consist of sound and/or syllable repetitions (part-word repetitions) and sound prolongations. Normally nonfluent children may also experience part-word repetitions or even prolongations, but the same characteristics in the young stutterer are excessive in number. No firm data exist on early clutterers. However, reports on older clutterers suggest that one looks for the youngster who speaks indistinctly, at a fast rate, with some language disorganization, and possibly simple sound and/or syllable repetitions and prolongations.[3–5] The section at the end of this chapter on Cluttering, further addresses cluttering and its symptoms.

Therefore, the clinician's task is to differentiate the dysfluent child from the nonfluent child. Some children fall into an indeterminate area between the two categories, which is to be expected since the two entities are not entirely dichotomous. However, fears of misdiagnosing the nonfluent child as dysfluent, and vice versa, are largely unwarranted since there are reasonable guidelines for evaluation, which will be discussed later in this chapter.[6–12] (See Assessment of Dysfluency, The Physiologic Factor.) Two conditions appear to operate to create clinical caution in dealing with preschool dysfluent children. One is the fear of exacerbating the condition or even of causing stuttering. (For a review of Johnson's influence on theory and therapy in this area, see Bloodstein.)[13] The other condition concerns reports that a high percentage of young stutterers develop into fluent speakers without professional help. It should be noted that the recovery studies on stutterers give widely disparate results on spontaneous remission. Van Riper reports that such recovery rates range from 40 to 94 percent.[10,11] The numbers do not inspire confidence and may reflect the difficulties and differences in methodology of such studies. Differences in definition of stuttering, for example, and difficulties of parental or personal recall of the condition render the studies difficult to assess and to compare.

Although most stuttering originates in the preschool years, some cases begin later, with new cases diminishing at about 13 years of age. New cases are rare after puberty, and the medical and psychosocial history should be evaluated carefully. Little has been reported about the child who acquires dysfluent symptoms after the preschool and early elementary school years. Personal observation is that these children may have a rapid escalation of symptoms, thus militating against deferring therapy. Some such children have a history of rapid and indistinct speech, suggesting the presence of cluttering before the symptoms of stuttering occurred, a position espoused by Weiss.[5]

Early stuttering usually has a gradual onset. Parents may notice mild repetitions of sounds, as in "m-m-mommy," repetitions of syllables, as in "mo-mo-mommy," or, less frequently, prolongations, as in "mmmmmommy." The repetitions and prolongations are likely to be effortless, though occasional children have extremely forceful symptoms from the onset of the dysfluencies. The usual pattern reported is that the symptoms come and go, perhaps appearing for 2 to 3 weeks and then subsiding, only to return. This pattern may continue for weeks or months before the periodicity subsides and the dysfluency is consistent, or nearly so. Increasing tension, extended repetitions and prolongations, and hard blocks may ensue and occur more frequently. Associated symptoms may develop, such as body movements, grimacing, and eventually avoidances of situations and speech. Not all stutterers follow this pattern through to its conclusion, and it is unknown why some stutterers who start out with modest symptoms maintain a relatively simple level of stuttering, whereas others may develop severe symptomatology or even recover. Bluemel referred to the easy, effortless repetitions that come and go in many young stutterers as "primary stammering."[14] He referred to the more forceful and consistent stuttering, which was accompanied by an awareness of the condition, as "secondary stuttering." Van Riper elaborated upon Bluemel's developmental stages by adding a "transitional" stage, in which the beginnings of forceful repetitions and prolongations were manifested. These were among the earlier efforts to define and describe childhood stuttering.

Van Riper has since made a concerted effort to trace the development of dysfluency, attempting to order the complexities of stuttering and the heterogeneity of stutterers.[10,11] Analyzing data from 44 case histories, which met his criteria for completeness of information, he sorted the subjects' histories into four tracks of development. The largest number of cases fell into track I, where the onset of stuttering was at $2^1/_2$ to 4 years of age following a period of fluent speech. Briefly, the initial symptoms were usually effortless syllabic repetitions that were intermittent. The repetitions became increasingly frequent and irregularly timed; prolongations developed, as did tension, fear, and avoidance. Advanced physiologic symptoms of tremor and struggle developed in some track I stutterers. Track II children were different in that their dysfluent symptoms were present from the onset of connected speech, and many children showed manifestations of "retarded speech development." The children tended to repeat "long strings of syllables or words" at a rapid rate; a few complete blockings and struggle reactions occurred, though later than for the track I subjects. Van Riper noted that track II children developed symptoms that are closely allied to both stuttering and cluttering, and, unlike the track I children, these youngsters showed little or no awareness of dysfluency at onset, but developed awareness over time. Relatively few children belonged to track III, a group whose onset was late, 5 to 9 years, and may have followed a traumatic experience. Such children exhibited severe blocking, including laryngeal blocks, from the start and progressed to associated or secondary characteristics of struggle, body movements, fears, frustration, and avoidances. Those who did not remit spontaneously became chronic stutterers. Track IV stutterers are unusual, having had a period of fluency before the onset of a rather stereotyped pattern of stuttering, to which there is no concerned reaction. They appear to be aware of the stuttering, but remain relatively detached from it, demonstrating little or no avoidance or fear of the condition. Based upon the previous categorization, one would expect most stutterers to belong to tracks I and II. One would also expect childhood stutterers, with the exception of those perhaps in track IV, to undergo changes in symptoms with maturation.

Bloodstein, also working from case material, described the development of stuttering as occurring in four phases.[15] The progression is from phase 1, in which whole word repetitions occur periodically, primarily at clause and phrase onsets, with little observable reaction from the child, through to phase 4. In phase 4, the most advanced phase, the stutterer uses word substitution and circumlocution to cope with severe blocking. In this phase, the stutterer's reactions to the condition may be severe to the point of impairing relationships with others.

Stuttering, then, is primarily a disorder of early childhood. It may begin after a period of fluency or at the time connected speech emerges. The initial symptoms are usually, though not always, easy sound or syllable repetitions and perhaps prolongations. A variety of manifestations of physical tension may ensue: hard blocks, eye closure, facial grimacing, body movements. Fears and avoidances may well occur as the child matures. Wingate describes the repetitions and prolongations as the "elemental units" of stuttering,[16] and the overlaid associated or secondary symptoms are imposed upon these units.

MODELS OF DYSFLUENCY

Many models have been proposed in an attempt to explain the onset of stuttering; most lack supportive data. However, the heterogeneity of stuttering and stutterers forces the recognition that there must be more than one explanation for the occurrence of stuttering; there may be a mosaic of factors that shift in importance from stutterer to stutterer. Genetics, for instance, may be paramount in one case, whereas language delay and environmental stress may be components of the mosaic in another beginning stutterer. Speech-language pathologists do not actually "know" why one child becomes a stutterer and another does not. At best, they make educated guesses. The following is an attempt to summarize theorists' answers to the parental question, "why does my child stutter?"

Myers and Wall, in order to organize information on this topic, suggested a model of three overlapping factors that may influence the onset of stuttering.[17] The model, composed of physiologic, psychosocial, and psycholinguistic factors, might also serve to give direction for evaluation and therapy for the young stutterer. Information subsumed under the physiologic factor would include, for example, genetic influences on stuttering and physiologic differences between stutterers and nonstutterers. The psychosocial factor would include influences of environment and of the interaction between the child and the environment. Under the psycholinguistic factor might be the potential effects of language and speech delay on fluency or the effect of a rapid rate of parental speech production. The component parts of each factor are not considered to be discrete entities, but to interact with each other. A child with a language and speech delay who becomes dysfluent, for example, may elicit reactions from the environment and, in turn, reduce his or her speech output or become tense about speaking and increasingly dysfluent. In this case, the psycholinguistic factor interacts with the psychosocial factor.

The Physiologic Factor and Etiology

The most powerful documented physiologic influence on the etiology of stuttering is that of genetics. One method of determining a genetic influence on a disorder is to carry out a concordance study. In such studies, identical twins and fraternal twins are compared for the frequency of occurrence of certain characteristics. If a characteristic occurs with significantly greater frequency in each member of monozygotic twin pairs, who share identical genetic information, than in each member of dizygotic twin pairs, who are, genetically speaking, like any two siblings, then the genetic make-up of the subjects is considered to be responsible for the particular characteristic. The concordance rate, or frequency with which a characteristic occurs in monozygotic twins versus dizygotic twins has been found to be high for stuttering in twin pairs, indicating genetic involvement in many, but not all, stutterers.[18,19] In addition to the concordance studies, genetic research by Andrews and Harris,[20] Kidd,[21] and Kidd, Kidd, and Records[22] supports a familial basis to stuttering. The precise nature of the genetic transmission is still to be determined. Howie noted that environmental factors are instrumental in causing at least some cases of stuttering since she found a higher percentage of stutterers in the dizygotic twin pairs than would be expected between siblings.[19] The plausible explanation for this finding appears to be that environmental factors were responsible for the onset of the stuttering, though the nature of environmental influences was not clear.

Physiologic studies have been carried out with the intent of discovering whether or not stutterers differ from nonstutterers in their basic physiologic make-up or "constitution" and, on a more focal level, whether or not stutterers' speech production mechanisms function differently from nonstutterers'. Research on the physiology of stuttered speech and of the fluent speech of stutterers has produced some interesting findings, primarily with adult stutterers who are more amenable to physiologic studies than young children. Some examples of the findings of research on the speech production of adult stutterers are as follows. Most studies cite stutterers as having longer voice onset times than nonstutterers.[11,15,23–26] Also, adult stutterers have demonstrated slower manual, vocal, and articulatory reaction times than nonstutterers.[23,25] There are suggestions of other physiologic differences between the two groups, for example, hemispheric dominance for language and speech, but most other areas studied have been studied too little to offer firm results or have been studied through a variety of methods, thus rendering comparisons difficult.

The importance of the positive findings in speech physiology research on adult stutterers for the childhood population is as follows. If the differences in voice onset time or other physiologic aberrations were present at or near the time of the onset of stuttering, the findings would support a theory of the onset of stuttering that states that mistimings and incoordinations of the speech production system underly stuttering from its inception. That is, these molecular mistimings, if present at the onset of stuttering, would support a physiologic theory of stuttering.

Attempts have been made to test the integrity of the speech production mechanism of young stutterers by applying voice onset time and reaction time paradigms. Agnello, Wingate, and Wendell found that 5- and 7-year-old stutterers exhibited longer voice onset times and voice termination time than adult controls.[27] This finding suggests that the voice onset mistimings of adult stutterers are present close to the time of the onset of stuttering.

Reaction time studies have also yielded differences between young stutterers and nonstutterers. According to Luper and Cross, finger reaction time is longer in childhood stutterers aged 5 and 9 years than in similarly aged nonstutterers.[28] Cross and Luper, examining voice reaction time in the 5 and 9 year olds, again found significant differences between stutterers and nonstutterers at both age levels with the stutterers having the slower reaction times.[29] Adult stutterers and controls included in the Cross and Luper study demonstrated similar findings. Adams conducted a small-N study of voice onset time of preschool stutterers, finding longer times in the experimental group than in the control groups.[30] In addition, using measures of initial consonant duration and vowel duration, he found significant differences between the two groups, with the stutterers having the longer durations for consonants and vowels.

Other voice reaction and voice initiation time studies (for example, Cullinan and Springer,[31] Murphy and Baumgartner,[32] Reich and Till[33]) have yielded inconsistent results, whereas Zebrowski, Conture, and Cudahy detected subtle asynchronies in the temporal characteristics of speech in young (3 to 7 years) stutterers.[34] Using the technique of spectrographic analysis, they examined plosive production and noted a difference between the stutterers and matched controls in the timing of aspiration and duration of the stop gap, which reflects closing of the articulators.

This brief section has summarized work considered pertinent to the physiologic etiology of stuttering. Genetic support for a physiologic basis of stuttering is strong, but not for all cases of stuttering. It appears that, although a definitive statement about physiologic mistimings and their relevance to speech production of young stutterers cannot be made, a body of research is accumulating that lends support to the concept of poorer motor speech control in this group than in nonstutterers. However, given the variability of physiologic performance in young children and the difficulties of getting large-N, well-controlled studies, speech-language pathologists await further confirmatory evidence of a speech motor problem in early stuttering.

The Psychosocial Factor and Etiology

This theory infers that the stutterer has certain personality characteristics and/or a certain way of relating to the environment that induces stuttering. For this reason, psychiatrists and psychoanalysts have hypothesized a variety of causal factors. For example, they have described the stutterer as having an oral fixation,[35–37] an anal fixation,[38,39] a conflict between the id and the superego,[40] inadequate interpersonal relationships and generally poor adjustment to life situations,[41,42] and "unspeakable feelings."[43] This quick summary cannot reflect the depth of thought and interest that the early psychoanalysts brought to the study of stuttering. However, the fact remains that these highly specific inferences were not verifiable. Attempts by psychologists, using accepted standardized procedures to evaluate the personality make-up and relationships of stutterers to the environment, were unsuccessful in establishing a particular personality type or the presence of neurosis in stutterers. Yet stutterers do exhibit some difficulties of social adjustment that, according to Andrews et al,[23] are more likely a *consequence* of stuttering than a cause. However, the fact that psychosocial (or at least nonphysiologic) causes exist for some stutterers was, as previously stated, in evidence in Howie's twin study, though Howie was unable to specify the nature of the psychosocial influences.[19]

Moving more specifically to theories pertaining to the early childhood population, Johnson's diagnosogenic theory and interactional hypothesis must be reconsidered since these theories seemed plausible and have had considerable impact on speech-language pathology over the years.[1,2] These were psychosocial theories of stuttering. Johnson maintained that stuttering was caused by the parents' misperceptions of their child's speech; a misevaluation of stuttering for normal nonfluency. The parents required of the child a level of performance that the child could not attain, and subsequent reactions on the part of child and parents resulted in further deterioration of speech. Starkweather later referred to similar dissonances between the young child and the environment as a "demands and capacities" model of the onset of stuttering.[44] He noted that the child might have a level of speech development, for example, which does not meet the demands of the environment. The ensuing effort to resolve the dissonance between the child's capacity and the environmental demands may lead to dysfluent speech. In support of Johnson's theory, Johnson and his associates amassed a large body of data on parents' recollections of young stutterers' early stutterings and compared them with the recollected early nonfluencies of nonstuttering controls. The object was to establish that the two groups exhibited the same nonfluencies at the onset of stuttering, thereby inferring that changes in the stuttering group occurred as a result of psychosocial factors. The nonfluencies examined were syllable, word, and phrase repetition; sound prolongation; silent interval (pause); interjection; and complete block. In reporting results, Johnson stressed that some of each category of nonfluency occurred in each group of children, with the exception of complete block, of which there were few and which occurred only in the children who stuttered. He stressed the overlap of symptoms, the fact that neither group could be distinguished solely on the basis of nonfluencies exhibited. But subsequently, McDearmon found that some significant differences did indeed exist in the frequency of occurrence of certain types of nonfluency between the stutterers and nonstutterers.[45] The stutterers used sound and syllable repetitions and prolongations more frequently than the nonstutterers, whereas the nonstutterers used word and phrase repetitions more frequently than the stutterers. Johnson's original interpretation of his data, however, (that at the time of the diagnosis of stuttering the child's speech was normally nonfluent) contributed to a psychosocial theory of the onset of stuttering because the implication was that parental reaction caused the nonfluencies to become dysfluencies. Interestingly, because of the later analysis of Johnson's work, his data, in the long run, served to help distinguish young stutterers from nonstutterers.

The diagnosogenic theory of the onset of stuttering lost some of its appeal with the advent of genetic research, which suggests a strong inherited component in stuttering. In addition, most contemporary theorists and clinicians reject the notion that parents may be the sole "cause" of stuttering in a youngster. This rejection does not negate the fact that environment is assumed by many to play a role in the onset, maintenance, and development of stuttering.

Some learning theorists believe that environmental conditions affect the course of stuttering development, whereas others offer learning theory as an explanation for the onset of stuttering. On the one hand, Brutten and Shoemaker suggest that classical conditioning is the basis of the onset of early dysfluencies, and the child's efforts to deal with speech disruptions result in the development of coping behaviors such as speaking on inhalation, eye closure, or body movement.[46] The coping behaviors (secondary or associated behaviors) are reinforced by instrumental or operant conditioning and result in the development of more complex symptomatology. On the other hand, Shames and Sherrick propose operant conditioning as the reason for the onset of stuttering.[47] They suggest that the normal nonfluencies of childhood are reinforced by an environmental event, usually parental attention, and a complex schedule of punishment and negative reinforcement serves to exacerbate the child's disruptions to create secondary stuttering.

Although the research on the effects of operant conditioning on established stuttering is voluminous, it has not clarified the role of operant conditioning in the onset of stuttering. Rather, operant conditioning has become a clinical tool frequently used in the treatment of stuttering (see, for example, Starkweather[48]). Some theorists would argue that, although neither classical nor operant conditioning can be firmly associated with the onset of stuttering, the development and maintenance of stuttering may be rationally explained by operant conditioning.

The Psycholinguistic Factor and Etiology

The relationship between language acquisition and fluency is an interesting though sparsely studied phenomenon. During the language learning years, the nature of nonfluency differs from the nonfluency of developed language. For example, some of the early nonfluencies, such as phrase repetition, subside as the child matures, whereas natural pauses associated with the syntax of a sentence increase.[49,50] In studying the relationship of nonfluency to the acquisition of semantic and syntactic structures, Colburn and Mysak noted, in a small-N study, that nonfluencies increased on new semantic and syntactic structures and subsided when the structure had been practiced and learned.[51] Such relationships are interesting to clinical researchers of dysfluency since some have hypothesized that dysfluency is an outgrowth of normal nonfluency.[2,52] However, there are others who view early stuttering and nonfluency as relatively dichotomous events.[6,7,16] Therefore, the developmental characteristics of nonfluency have intrigued students of stuttering,[53–58] but like so many controversial areas surrounding this complex topic, a specific relationship between developmental nonfluency and stuttering has not been established.

Observation and research on language and speech acquisition in young stutterers have revealed that some, probably at least one-third, experience a delay in these areas. Positive findings from structured language tests or subtests were reported by Kline and Starkweather,[59] Murray and Reed,[60] Westby,[61] and Williams and Marks,[62] though not for all subjects. Fewer researchers, for example Haynes and Hood,[63] reported negative findings. Muma used a transformational analysis on 4 year olds' spontaneous speech and found that the fluent group used significantly more double-based transformations (resulting in complex sentences) than the "highly disfluent" group.[64] In a similar vein, Wall examined the spontaneous speech of four preschool stutterers and four matched nonstutterers.[65] She found that the stutterers used more sentence complexity than the nonstutterers. The aforementioned data point to differences in language development and language use between some stutterers and nonstutterers. Andrews et al, in their extensive review, estimate that stutterers' language is delayed an average of 6 months.[23]

Focusing on the school-age stutterer, Williams and Silverman found the incidence of speech disorders in 115 stutterers to be 23.5 percent as opposed to 8.7 percent for nonstutterers.[66] Blood and Seider surveyed more than 1,000 stutterers from schools in 31 states and found that 10 percent of the stutterers had language problems; 7 percent exhibited language, learning, and articulatory disorders; and 91 percent of the group received both stuttering and articulation therapy.[67] Clearly, then, language and speech difficulties, with or without a learning disorder, may accompany childhood stuttering. The co-occurrence of disorders is the case particularly with the preschool stutterers and to some extent with the school-age population also. Whether there is a causal relationship between the stuttering and language and learning disorders or not is unknown, but the numbers arouse suspicion—at least for a subgroup of stutterers.

Another interesting and rather curious phenomenon regarding early stuttering and language is that the stutterings occur in predictable places in the utterance. Bloodstein and Gantwerk noted that young stutterers stutter more on pronouns and conjunctions than on other parts of speech.[68] They pointed out that pronouns and conjunctions usually occur at the onset of children's utterances, as in "I want . . .," "And then . . .," "My daddy . . ." Bloodstein pursued this line of thought in examining the utterances of six preschool stutterers and found that most of the stutters occurred on the initial words of clauses or phrases.[69] Bloodstein and Grossman confirmed these findings,[70] while Wall, Starkweather, and Cairns[71] and Wall, Starkweather, and Harris[72] found significantly more stuttering at the onset of clauses than at nononset positions in preschool stutterers. They also noted that words beginning with vowels (most likely "I" and "and") were stuttered more frequently than words beginning with consonants, perhaps because of their position at the head of a clause. They hypothesized that both psycholinguistic and physiologic events were plausible explanations for speech breakdown at these particular points in an utterance for the following reasons. Psycholinguists have suggested that sentence planning takes place at clause boundaries, reflecting increased cognitive activity. Physiologically, respiration for speech occurs primarily at clause boundary positions as, of course, does the onset of voicing. Therefore, one has a complex array of linguistic and speech motor variables occurring simultaneously. This may explain why the clause onset position has been found to be the primary site of normal nonfluencies and is the location of most stuttering—particularly in the early stages of the condition.

Wall and Myers proposed a theory of the onset of stuttering, which includes a genetic factor and which could be manifested in a slight incoordination of the speech musculature.[12] Working in concert with the linguistic stress of a language and speech delay or, in some cases, with the linguistic stress of normal speech and language acquisition, the physiologic incoordinations could account for the breakdown of speech in many young stutterers. And, since the clause boundary position is the most vulnerable point in an utterance, the word at the onset of the clause is the one most likely to be stuttered.

Finally, the area of pragmatics may illuminate the reasons for speech breakdown in stutterers in specific conversational contexts. Does a child stutter more when giving directions to another than when responding to instructions? Is a child more likely to stutter when confronted by a critical verbal reaction from an adult? Although there are few hard data in this area, such research has begun to appear. Guitar, Kopfs, Kilburg, and Conway analyzed conversational interaction between a preschool stutterer and her mother.[73] They found a high correlation between verbal "nonacceptingness" in the mother and the presence of secondary stuttering in the child. Meyers and Freeman examined the interrupting behaviors of mothers of young stutterers with their own and others' children, since parents of stutterers are frequently admonished not to interrupt their children's speech.[74] Meyers and Freeman found that mothers of stutterers in fact interrupted their children's speech less than the mothers of nonstutterers. However, both groups of parents interrupted stuttered speech significantly more often than they interrupted fluent speech. Further in the psycholinguistic mode, Meyers and Freeman examined various aspects of speech rate in mothers of the young stutterers and nonstutterers. An important finding here was that mothers of stutterers talk significantly faster to all children than do mothers of nonstutterers. Meyers and Freeman acknowledge that this finding does not imply a causal relationship between rapid-talking mothers and the onset of stuttering. However, it is clearly a finding that deserves closer scrutiny. It may have relevance to the onset of stuttering in some children and to the management of stuttering in the childhood population.

The psycholinguistic factor offers interesting possibilities for the etiology of stuttering in some children. Speech-language pathologists know that one subgroup of stutterers is language and speech delayed and that a further subgroup exhibits a more broadly based language deficit that includes a learning disability. There is documentation that early stuttering is an integral part of the structure of the child's sentences and suggestions that pragmatic variables may influence stuttering in ways that can be clearly documented. As well, parental speech rate has come under scrutiny with, to date, positive findings.

ASSESSMENT OF DYSFLUENCY

This section will begin with some general statements about the assessment of childhood stuttering, then proceed to areas of enquiry according to physiologic, psychosocial, and psycholinguistic factors; a discussion of specific tests available; and a discussion of the testing procedures recommended in some of the commercially available programs for children who stutter.

Like assessments for other disorders, the assessment of childhood stuttering requires the gathering of data from a broad base of information. Not for the purpose of learning the "cause" of the stuttering (since no one cause is known), but rather to piece information together; to evaluate the role of genetics, for example; and to evaluate conditions that may exacerbate and maintain the stuttering. To this end, a comprehensive case history is taken, one that delineates many aspects of childhood development: birth and developmental, medical, social, genetic, and educational history, together with an account of parental perception of the onset of stuttering and its subsequent developmental pattern, for instance, whether the periods of dysfluency are lessening or becoming more severe and more frequent. Specific examples of such information will be included in the discussion of the physiologic, psychosocial, and psycholinguistic factors. And since stuttering frequently varies from situation to situation, it behooves the clinician to be sensitive to this issue in taking the case history and in collecting speech samples. The parent whose child is fluent in the professional office, but who states that the child's speech deteriorates at home, should be taken seriously. An audiotaped sample of the child's spontaneous speech at the evaluation session may be used for an analysis of dysfluencies and later compared to a sample taped at home. Language and fluency analyses may be derived from the same tapes. A videotaped analysis of the child's spontaneous speech is desirable in order to evaluate the visual aspects of stuttering. Videotaping parent-child interaction and, ideally, the child's interaction with peers allows the clinician to evaluate the child's pragmatic use of language and possible effects of situational influences on stuttering.

At the end of the diagnostic evaluation, the clinician has both qualitative and quantitative data on the child's stuttering. Qualitative data refers to descriptions of the child's symptoms, such as sound and syllable repetition, hard block, and secondary or associated characteristics. The quantitative characteristics comprise a measure such as the percent of stuttered words or the percent of stuttered syllables or the rate of speech (stuttered words or syllables per minute). A compilation of all data gathered from the adult informants (usually the parents), from the child, and from the clinician's observations, testing, and fluency analyses should serve to differentiate the stutterer from the nonstutterer. In addition, the evaluation should reveal underlying difficulties, such as a speech motor problem or language and speech delay.

The Physiologic Factor

Under the physiologic factor, assessment enquiries become highly specific to the family history of stuttering, cluttering, rapid speakers, language, and speech and learning disorders. Attention is directed to the child for examination of the physiology of speech production. Beginning with the subglottal component, one is interested in the way the child uses respiration for speech. Some of the commonly noted respiratory anomalies of childhood stuttering are speaking on inhalation, forcing speech out on expiratory reserve volume, and gasping for breath—perhaps in an effort to get speech started. Such anomalies may be present in preschool as well as school-age stutterers. Body tension around the thorax and clavicular area may be a by-product of effortful speech production. Moving to the glottal level of production, the subtle aberrations of voice onset time, voice initiation time, and the like can be detected only with the use of instrumentation. Also, because there is still a need for ongoing research in these areas, such techniques have not become a routine part of diagnostic procedure. However, the clinician may note less precise phonatory aberrations such as prevoicing, apparently used to get speech started; strained initiation of phonation; the use of glottal fry; or delayed phonation when phonation is inhibited by hyperadduction of the vocal folds. Young stutterers may use a pitch glide wherein the pitch changes in an upward direction in an apparent effort to escape from a block. With regard to the supraglottal area, the clinician evaluates, as far as observation permits, articulator tension and performs an oral peripheral examination. In addition, coordinated, rhythmic speech attempts may be checked through diadochokinetic tasks. Included under the physiologic factor is a description of the end result of the physical aberrations, the actual blocks. These constitute the qualitative descriptions of stuttering suggested earlier in this section.

Assuming that qualitative and quantitative data have been gathered, what is the significance of these data? Clinicians generally agree that the child who exhibits part-word repetitions is more likely to be diagnosed as a stutterer than a child who exhibits word and phrase repetitions or one who uses frequent fillers. However, the child who is diagnosed as a stutterer may well also exhibit some word and phrase repetitions, and the child who is considered normally nonfluent may have occasional part-word repetitions. The quantitative data do not precisely agree, but there are some commonalities to be addressed. In reviewing this literature, Adams,[6,7] Curlee,[9] McDearmon,[45] Ryan,[75] and Van Riper[10,11] agree upon part-word repetition as a diagnostic clue for early stuttering. The frequency of repetitions per unit is considered to be an additional clue in the diagnosis of stuttering. That is, "mo-mo-mo-mommy" is more likely to be considered stuttering than "mo-mommy." Curlee suggests that two repetitions per word, plus obvious vocal tension, are clues for stuttering, whereas Van Riper designates three repetitions per word as critical to the perception of stuttering. Other signs of early stuttering are prolongation of sounds,[10,11,45,75] cessation of voice,[6] and dysfluencies lasting 2 seconds or longer.[9–11] Curlee recommends that two instances of dysfluency per 100 words be a diagnostic criterion; Adams suggests 10 instances of any type of fluency disruption, and Ryan recommends three dysfluencies per minute as the criterion level for diagnosing stuttering.

At first glance, several diverse points of view seem to appear here. However, as previously stated, some commonalities emerge; children are likely to be diagnosed as stutterers if they exhibit sound and syllable repetitions that contain a minimum of two or three repetitions per unit ("mo-mo-mommy" or "mo-mo-mo-mommy"). Children are also likely to be considered stutterers if they prolong sounds and if their dysfluencies last for 2 seconds or longer. The presence of tension or struggle is considered to be a diagnostic clue, as is disruption of phonation. Additionally, "child awareness" is cited by Curlee[9] and Van Riper[10,11] as a danger sign. However, one should keep in mind that not all children are overt in demonstrating concern; some are, in fact, quite subtle about it. The quantitative indices of stuttering are still not firmly determined, but they, along with the descriptive clues of differential diagnosis and a complete case history, help us to distinguish, in most cases, stutterer from nonstutterer.

The Psychosocial Factor

Since the influence of psychosocial factors on the etiology of stuttering remains unclear, enquiry into this area during the evaluation might be regarded as having uncertain relevance. Nevertheless, it is usually a well-researched area in the diagnostic evaluation because of its relevance to the development and maintenance of stuttering even if it is not considered by the clinician vital to the etiology of the stuttering. However, those who follow Johnsonian thinking focus on investigating parental relationships with the child, particularly the demanding and perfectionist requirements of the client for general behavior and for speech. Myers and Freeman have pointed out that clinicians pursue certain lines of exploration and parent counseling even without data to confirm that parents of stutterers behave in certain ways.[74] Clinicians make certain assumptions about the way children respond to modeled speech, for instance. Similarly, clinicians may assume certain emotional differences between the parents of stutterers and nonstutterers, yet there is no firm evidence that such parents differ emotionally or have different types of personalities.

Wall and Myers suggested the following psychosocial lines of exploration for the young stutterer: try to determine if the child is aware of the dysfluency.[12] The preschool child may be verbal and demonstrative about the difficulties experienced with speech or may give subtle signs, such as brief eye aversion at the moment of a block, or no reaction at all. A range of reactions is possible with the school-age child. Some discuss their reactions to stuttering in a mature fashion; others deny the existence of pronounced symptoms. Explore parental reactions to stuttering as well as to other aspects of the child's use of speech and language. Explore how they refer to the problem (by use of the word "stuttering?") and how they deal with the child's moment of stuttering. Furthermore, seek information on the child's overall adjustment to self, to speech, and to the reactions of others. Information gleaned from these personal and interpersonal characteristics depend in part upon the age and maturity of the child. Young children, for example, appear to have little awareness of specific situational problems with their speech, though they may be aware of a general difficulty with talking from time to time. Parental reports of conditions that usually exacerbate stuttering in preschoolers refer to excitement, fatigue, and perhaps illness. More specific situational influences, such as speaking to authority figures, speaking on the telephone, speaking in front of a group, emerge as the child matures. The school-age child may well develop reactions to speaking situations in the school setting.

In evaluating the psychosocial aspects of childhood stuttering, then, the clinician deals with the child's inter- and intrapersonal behavior, which includes reactions to speech together with environmental circumstances that might serve to maintain or exacerbate the symptoms of stuttering. The clinician should bear in mind that no data exist to support a concept of disordered personalities in the parents of stutterers or in the stutterers themselves. Therefore it seems wise to keep an open mind in evaluation of such clients and to probe appropriately if indicated, but not to assume certain personality findings, either in children or in parents.

The Psycholinguistic Factor

Examining the psycholinguistic aspects of both child and parent use of language and speech is advisable. For the child, standardized language and speech tests may be used and/or less formal measures such as mean length of utterance and a language analysis of the spontaneous speech sample. Also important is a description of the pragmatic variables that interfere with communication or that appear to influence the fluency of the child. An example of an interaction of psychosocial and psycholinguistic factors is to be found here. If, for instance, the child reacts to the dysfluencies and limits language output or begins to circumlocute or to substitute one word for another, he or she alters the language and speech use in the broadest sense, in a pragmatic sense.

The clinician usually explores the complexity and sophistication of the language used by the parents with the client on the assumption that the youngster may have difficulty in processing overly complex language, thereby resulting in linguistic pressures. Also, since parents usually act as the child's primary models for language and speech, the child may try to match the parents' language complexity, creating a "linguistic overload" in this attempt and so resulting in speech breakdown. Such thinking is still hypothetical; nevertheless, it is considered by many to offer a reasonable course of enquiry at the diagnostic session. Observation and measurement of parental speech rate is a verifiably legitimate diagnostic procedure (see Meyers and Freeman's findings[74]), as is evaluation of parent pragmatics. Poor communicative style on the part of the parents may result in unnecessary interruptions during the child's talking, for example, as found by Myers and Freeman.

The preceding discussion on assessment summarizes Wall and Myers proposal that childhood stutterers be evaluated according to the three factors of physiologic, psychosocial, and psycholinguistic aspects of stuttering.[12] This profile should act as a guide to the differential diagnosis of stuttering as well as a guide to the planning of therapy. In addition, the profile guide may be updated as necessary when therapy and circumstances create a shift in the profile pattern.

Formal Tests

Instruments for testing adults and children have been commercially produced, some as part of therapy packages. Riley focused on assessment only in his *Stuttering Severity Instrument for Children and Adults*.[76] For nonreaders, the test provides a picture description task. For readers, it provides a verbal task as well as a reading task. The scoresheet allows for a count of blocks for each test section, estimated length of the longest blocks, and an inclusion of physical concomitants based on a severity scale of 0 to 5. A total overall score is converted to a percentile and then to a severity rating of stuttering of very mild, mild, moderate, severe, and very severe.

Other assessment procedures may be culled from commercial packages. Ryan and Van Kirk describe their "fluency interview," in which the client performs various speaking tasks such as imitation, reading, and conversation.[77] If the child exhibits three or more stuttered words per minute (SW/M), therapy is instituted. Stocker presents a set of pretherapy probes to the child who stutters.[78] The probes consist of questions, 50 in all, about common objects, and they reflect five levels of demand or communicative responsibility. For example, a level I probe would require a one-word response, such as a response to an either/or question. On level V, however, the child is required to make up a story. Working from the corpus of utterances and the stutterings resulting from the probes, Stocker rates the stuttering from mild to severe, depending on the total number of stutters.

Cooper and Cooper use a chronicity prediction checklist for children from 3 to 8 years of age as part of a therapy package for children and adults.[79] The checklist includes historical, attitudinal, and behavioral indicators of chronicity, a teacher assessment inventory, and a parent assessment inventory. Shames and Florance use a total of 17 measures to determine changes in speech, self-concept, perceptions of others, self-reinforcing tendencies, and coping styles.[80] Specific measures include speaking rate, stuttering frequency, syllable rate, and continuity of phonation. The child evaluation includes a videotape for parent-child interaction analysis. Shine administers a stuttering interview in which he determines the rate of stuttering according to SW/M.[81] He also makes an informal assessment of physiologic speaking processes (phonation, respiration, articulation, resonance) throughout the diagnostic session.

Many, but not all, of the foregoing assessment procedures were devised by behaviorally oriented clinicians and reflect a strong interest in quantifying information to provide base rates of stuttering. In some instances, quantitative measures appear to be the only source of evaluation. Others incorporate evaluation of the psychosocial factor.[79,80] Stocker's evaluation, although part of a behavioral program, has a strong psycholinguistic bent. The clinician needs to evaluate available assessment procedures, using those that are rational in light of current theoretical knowledge and clinical practice.

MANAGEMENT OF DYSFLUENCY

Management decisions begin when the diagnostic evaluation of the dysfluent child is complete. The evaluation has indicated if the child is normally nonfluent, if the child is a stutterer in the initial or more advanced stages of the condition, or, as is sometimes the case, if the child appears to be borderline between normal nonfluency and stuttering. If the child's fluency is within normal limits, parent counseling is indicated in order to attune the parents to the range of normal speech, language, and fluency behaviors expected of young children. If the child appears to be borderline between normal nonfluency and stuttering, parent counseling is indicated and possibly intervention with the child. Therapy might be instituted for the borderline dysfluent child in the presence of, for example, a language and speech delay, a genetic history of stuttering, frequent fluency disruptors in the environment, or marked parental anxiety about speech. If intervention is deemed unnecessary for the borderline dysfluent child, follow-up appointments are instituted in order to monitor the dysfluency. For the borderline dysfluent child and the dysfluent child, parent counseling following evaluation would include information sharing on speech, language, and fluency development in children; management of parental speech rate and language complexity if indicated; management of situations that are likely to exacerbate the dysfluency; and management of the parents' reactions to the child's stuttering.

For the school-age child, the diagnosis of stuttering is usually a more clear-cut issue, though cases of mild dysfluency may cause a dilemma for the clinician. In my experience, in cases of mild dysfluency in school-age children, the clinician may wonder if therapy is indicated, perhaps assuming that the child might still "grow out of it." Since mild dysfluencies may escalate quickly, therapy, or at least monitoring of the dysfluency, is advisable.

THERAPY FOR THE DYSFLUENT PRESCHOOL CHILD

Several therapy options are available for the dysfluent preschooler: direct therapy, for example, which is working on the child's speech in a one-to-one or small group situation. Or working indirectly on the child's speech by working with the parents and not the child, or by working with the child in such a way that the child remains unaware that speech is the focus of the interaction. The clinician may choose to work with the parents and also with the child, as opposed to working with one (parent(s)) or the other (child). In addition, the clinician may choose a behavioral approach, a language-based approach, or both in working with the child.

Proponents of direct therapy with preschool stutterers are Ryan and Van Kirk, who tell the youngster that he or she is there to work on speech, before presenting fluency shaping tasks;[77] Stocker, who incorporates direct techniques into a language-based and behavioral approach;[78] Gregory and Hill;[82] Shine;[81] and Wall and Myers,[12] who direct the child's attention to easier ways of speech production at propitious moments in the therapy session. Therapy tends to become more direct when there is considerable physiologic involvement. Respiratory abnormalities, for example, may receive direct attention if other, less direct methods, do not achieve the desired results. Wall and Myers put such direct approaches within the context of therapy that attends to the physiologic, psychosocial, and psycholinguistic aspects of the child's stuttering. They advocate attempting to alleviate the child's dysfluency by using fluency enhancement strategies, to be discussed later, prior to or in addition to using direct techniques.

Johnson described indirect methods of treating the preschool stutterer through parent counseling.[83] Bloodstein argues that Johnson also treated the child, but that this point is not clear in Johnson's writings.[13] In addition to areas of counseling already mentioned before, Johnson proposed that parents be helped to accept their child's speech and nonspeech efforts and be less demanding of the child and less anxious about the child's speech performance. Although this advice may still be useful in individual cases, clinicians have modified their use of Johnson's counseling procedures because clinicians no longer necessarily assume that the parents have been demanding of the child or unusually anxious about speech generally. The parents may have reacted justifiably to their child's dysfluency. In addition, clinicians no longer assume that the parents have created the condition of stuttering through their misdiagnosis of the condition. Hence counseling procedures, whether used as the sole treatment method or in conjunction with child therapy, are less likely to assume parental guilt or create parental guilt.

Van Riper used indirect therapy with both parents and child. His counseling included the suggestion that parents reinforce fluency by encouraging speech on fluent days, but not on dysfluent days. He helped the parents to be good listeners for their child and to deal with their reactions to stuttering. For the child, he used a process of systematic desensitization to demonstrate that stuttering does not necessarily result from an intense or threatening situation. That is, through play, he reinforced fluency throughout increasingly stressful situations: situations wherein the increments of stress were carefully graded hierarchically.

Most clinicians incorporate both parents and child into therapy for the preschool dysfluent child.[8,12,81,84] Fewer focus primarily or solely on the parents[83,85] or primarily or solely on the child.[77,78] Wall and Myers proposed that therapy for the preschool dysfluent child be based upon the diagnostic profile of psychosocial, psycholinguistic, and physiologic factors, making use of direct or indirect techniques as needed. Their therapy is included in the following section.

The Psychosocial Factor

This factor involves work with the parents and the child to reduce conditions in the child's life that may exacerbate or maintain stuttering. In addition to information covered previously in counseling on how to deal with fluency disruptors and the like, parents are helped to find alternatives to possibly negative or punitive reactions to the dysfluencies. During observation of therapy, their attention is drawn to the acceptance of the dysfluencies by the clinician—for example, no gaze aversion and maintenance of eye contact. Parental counseling keeps abreast of therapy with the child, so that what is asked of the parents makes sense in light of what is happening in therapy sessions. Parent reactions are monitored, and they are increasingly involved in the therapy process. The parents may be helped to find for themselves appropriate responses to their child's dysfluency; these may be verbal or nonverbal responses that they are encouraged to use judiciously, thus reducing the tension surrounding stuttering moments. Information is also shared with the parents on general knowledge of stuttering and child raising practices, as indicated: for example, the need for most children to have a fairly well-regulated environment and an adequate amount of sleep. Parental counseling may be necessary with regard to the child's overall adjustment and behavior. If such problems are of a chronic or consistent nature, appropriate referral for more intensive counseling is made.

The child's negative reactions to stuttering should be reduced upon discovering that the dysfluencies are lessening. For this reason, it is highly desirable to facilitate fluency as soon as possible. This facilitation is usually done by eliciting a slightly slower rate of speech using "easy" or nonforced speech production on shorter-than-usual utterances, and building upon that production (see the next section The Psycholinguistic Factor). Due praise for successful use of easy speech and, of course, for other nonspeech tasks reinforces fluency and increases a sense of self-esteem. Although specific situational fears usually do not require attention in the preschooler, the client benefits from practicing his or her easy speech in circumstances that might provoke stuttering, such as situations that are exciting, or rushed, or argumentative. This aspect of therapy is phased in when the child has achieved easy speech in less demanding situations. With regard to reactions to dysfluency, occasionally a preschool child is quite verbal and specific about reactions, but more often the clinician is dealing with more subtle indications and reactions or no discernible reactions at all.

The psychosocial factor in therapy, then, may involve the parents and the child. It may also involve others important in the child's life, such as relatives, siblings, and preschool teachers. At this early stage, it is less likely to involve peers, whose reactions are important to therapy with the school-age stutterer. The parent counseling is probably best handled by regular weekly meetings in the first part of therapy, with contacts becoming less frequent as the parents achieve satisfactory levels of coping with their child's dysfluency and learning to reinforce fluency.

The Psycholinguistic Factor

This factor may also involve both parents and children. Parents are taught to modify their speech and language use, if necessary, in order to provide better models for their dysfluent child and to allow the child to perceive and manage the incoming message more calmly and efficiently. This may mean heightening the parents' attention to their own speech rate, to the length and complexity of the utterances used with their young child, and to their pragmatic use of language. Any specific counseling or therapy on language and speech use is designed to meet individual needs of the parents.

Because of the potential relationships between language and dysfluency described earlier in this chapter and because clinicians have found that stutterers are, on the whole, more fluent using shorter utterances than longer utterances, therapeutic techniques have evolved which capitalize on this knowledge. Such techniques encourage fluency from the child on short utterances, then proceeding to longer and syntactically more complex utterances. This therapy also uses language structure to elicit fluent utterances through questions. Asking "WH" questions, for example, frequently elicits complex responses on which the child in the early stages of therapy is dysfluent. However, asking questions requiring a yes or no response or an either/or response[78] elicits a brief, probably fluent response. Thus, using knowledge of semantic and syntactic structures and being sensitive to pragmatic variables, one may facilitate the child's fluency. Several therapies approach the treatment of the young and older childhood stutterer with this language-based approach,[77,78,81,82] though not always for the same reasons.

Wall and Myers suggest a language-based therapy for the young stutterer with a low-structured, natural setting in which the child is encouraged to play and talk along with the clinician.[12] "WH" questions are kept to a minimum or avoided. Parallel play is used if the child is unable to participate on an interactive level. The clinician uses a slow to normal rate of speech and, within the context of the play situation, elicits one- and two-word utterances from the client in an unhurried manner, keeping the atmosphere of the session calm and low key. The short utterances in this situation are usually fluent. When the child has become proficient at this level, utterance length is increased to two- and three-word utterances, three and four words, and so on. It will be noted that the therapy so far is indirect. That is, fluency is elicited and reinforced through play without mention to the child that speech is involved. This situation can change, of course, if the child is a severe stutterer and in need of more direct intervention (see the next section The Physiologic Factor). However, milder preschool stutterers may do well with the indirect fluency facilitation, as described before. A slightly more direct approach is when the clinician offers occasional reinforcement of "easy speech"—"I like the way you said that; it was nice and easy," or "I like your easy talking." Lengthening the utterances of the child usually also increases the complexity of the sentence, and care is taken to lengthen utterances in the first instance without altering sentence complexity; increases in complexity are then introduced. Examples of increases in complexity may be the conjoining of clauses and the introduction of different types of clauses, but only within the limits of the child's language capacities. With the advent of conjoined clauses, simple story telling is encouraged, leading to conversational speech. More complex questions may now be asked of the child, requiring complex responses. Pragmatic aspects of communication such as turn taking, maintaining eye contact, assuming different roles are instituted, with easy speech encouraged throughout these activities. Thus generalization, carryover, or transfer of easy, fluent speech production is addressed.

For the child with a language delay, Wall and Myers recommend limiting fluency enhancement procedures to vocabulary and semantic-syntactic structures that the child already possesses at the time of entering therapy. As fluency increases, new lexical items and appropriate structures may be introduced gradually, maintaining a balance between the acquisition of new language and fluency. For the child who has an articulatory disorder, when should it be treated? Prior to treating the fluency disorder? After the fluency disorder? There is, of course, no firm answer to these questions. Wall and Myers suggest, therefore, that the clinician be guided by the severity of the problem as well as by reactions of the child. In the case of an intelligibility problem, clarifying the speech production in order to relieve the child of the communicative effort of being understood seems essential. In itself, this increase in intelligibility might facilitate fluency. Any work on articulation needs to be carried out in small, incremental steps, with an emphasis on ease of production. Another reason for instituting gentle articulation therapy is if the child is upset about the speech production difficulty. However, relatively minor problems may be dealt with later in therapy prior to discharge.

Observation of language-based, fluency facilitation sessions allows the parents, with appropriate counseling and guidance, to facilitate fluency at home, sometimes in casual conversation, at other times in play sessions with their child. As stated previously, the young mild stutterer may require fluency facilitation only. The client with more severe symptoms may require help in modifying the blocks, as described next in the Physiologic Factor.

The Physiologic Factor

Some, perhaps all, of the aberrant physiology associated with stuttering subsides with the slower rate of speech and the encouragement of easy speech production. For the young child, modification of blocks is also possible, though technicalities of techniques, such as Van Riper's "pull-out," are not introduced. Rather, attention is drawn to the physical effort and strain of the speech production by referring to "hard" speech. The clinician may comment that some of the child's speech was "hard" at that moment and demonstrates "easy" speech,[86] or the clinician has the child say it over the easy way. Other descriptive words, such as "bumpy" and "smooth," may assist the child in beginning to monitor the contrast between effortful speech and smooth, relaxed production. Casual, polite attention to tense speech production and equally casual, polite suggestions for remediation usually are not threatening to the child. If the child is threatened, the clinician proceeds at a slower pace.

This type of physiologic modification of the block is particularly important if the child is considered to have a motor component to the stuttering.[8,87–89] The child, having learned the difference between hard and easy speech and what must be done to achieve the latter as opposed to the former, may then simply be cued by the clinician when he or she tightens for speech.

When stuttering is severe in the preschooler, with marked physiologic involvement, it may be necessary to address directly the respiratory and phonatory aspects of the child's speech production. Breathing anomalies in the young child, such as forcing the air out to the limits of expiratory reserve and gasping for breath, may be handled by the slower speech rate and by the simple process of teaching the child to pause periodically during speech production, that is, teach the child how to phrase the sentence string. Phrasing allows time at appropriate points in the utterance to take a breath and to organize linguistically and physiologically for the next part of the sentence. In some instances, the child may be taught to generate easy onsets by feeling a little breath emerge from the mouth prior to vowel production. This easy-onset vowel may then be shaped into actual words (particularly "I" and "and," which are frequently stuttered by young children) and incorporated into short phrases. Nelson describes some simple exhalation games for the young stutterer that she shapes to easy onsets of vowels, leading to connected speech.[87]

Stuttering blocks in young children, then, may be modified in some cases through language-based fluency facilitation techniques, by using a slightly slower speech rate, and by paying some attention to hard and easy speech production. Further assistance, when indicated, may take the form of teaching phrasing for speech to help regulate the breathing pattern and, more specifically, easy onset of phonation may be taught.

THERAPY FOR THE DYSFLUENT SCHOOL-AGE CHILD

Circumstances of therapy for the school-age child as compared with the preschool child clearly differ. The preschool child is brought to therapy apparently to play and talk with a benign adult and, for the most part, this works out very well. The school-age child, however, usually more aware of the communicative disorder, is more likely to show resistance. Yet if therapy takes place in the school, the clinician is able to observe the client in a variety of situations and so to assist in transfer or generalization activities in constructive ways. Since "school-age" refers to a wide span of ages and maturity, the clinician needs to adapt therapy strategies to accomodate the client's needs with regard to language use and activities. The principles underlying therapy for the dysfluent preschooler, for example, often may be applied to the school-age child with appropriate adjustments. However, particularly for the moderate and severe school-age stutterer, techniques that help him or her to modify the stuttering block (Van Riper's loose contacts, pull-outs, cancellations) are likely to be used in addition to fluency facilitating techniques. The following are considerations for therapy specifically for the school-age child.

The Psychosocial Factor

The clinician may have to deal with reactions to stuttering ranging from embarrassment and guilt to denial of the problem; other children may show appropriate discomfort and be willing and ready to participate in a constructive therapy program. Although some clients seem to benefit from discussion of the stuttering, at least on some days, others seem to abhor the topic and may wish to communicate as little as possible. For the latter group, involvement in activity in which talking is not a focal point sometimes leads to freer communication. Increasing the child's skill with easier speech production is certainly one way to help reduce negative reactions to speech and elicit more verbal interaction. Some situations, such as being teased by peers and having to deliver oral reports in school, are specific to the school-age child and deserve special mention. The clinician may assist the child in understanding and managing such situations through role playing, in which the child and clinician play each role in turn and alternate strategies for management are acted out. In addition, judicious intervention by the clinician with a sympathetic teacher might help to ease a difficult situation.

That parents of school-age children understand the principles of therapy and be updated on goals and progress appropriately is important. Stuttering is a difficult condition to understand and to treat, and parental cooperation and participation is more likely forthcoming if parents are well informed. In addition, parental understanding of stuttering should help to reduce anxiety and any negative reactions to the condition. The parents of school-age children may need counseling on whether or not to discuss the stuttering with their child, how to do so, and how to handle moments of severe stuttering. They may need help in managing speaking situations at home so that the client has adequate time to speak—for instance, at the dinner table when they may institute turn taking for family conversations. As therapy progresses parents may participate in therapy, thus helping in the transfer process and fostering communication about stuttering.

Since stutterers and their parents have not been found to be emotionally disturbed, speech-language pathologists are equipped to counsel parents of stutterers. Again, appropriate referral should be made if there are indications of chronic behavioral difficulties on the part of the client or substantial family maladjustment. If parents remain inaccessible to the school clinician despite all efforts to involve them, the clinician might consider treating the child with the view to increasing the child's skills in managing speech in a variety of different, and sometimes difficult, situations.

The Psycholinguistic Factor

The clinician should be alert to the possibility of residual language and speech problems in the school-age child and incorporate those areas into therapy planning as necessary. However, the prevalence of such disorders is reduced in this older population. As with the preschooler, using the smaller language units and working towards larger units is a rational way to begin therapy in order to elicit fluent or near fluent speech. Easy speech, or for this older child, work on loose contacts,[84,90] as discussed under the Physiologic Factor next, may be incorporated into the increasingly long and complex structures. For the younger school-age child, play is still a useful method of eliciting the desired-length utterance, though the clinician is more direct in instructing the client to maintain easy speech or loose contacts during his or her responses. Question and answer sessions about topics of interest to the child, word games, and card games serve as vehicles to facilitate fluency. Question and answer sessions are graded so that the clinician is at first eliciting short responses, then eliciting longer and longer responses, including complex responses to "WH" questions. Spontaneous conversation, particularly with the older school-age child, becomes a valuable tool for the practice of loose contact speech and, ultimately, any stuttering modification strategies the client has learned in therapy. As fluency improves, more subtle linguistic phenomena, such as poor vocal variation, may require attention.

If the client habitually uses word substitution and/or circumlocution, creating discomfort for him- or herself and possibly for others who may not follow his or her line of thought, assistance can be given by having the client move ahead on feared words, using loose contacts, and using other available modification strategies. Through a gradual process of desensitization of the feared words and incorporation of these "physiologic" strategies, the client's style of conversation should become more appropriate.

The Physiologic Factor

Slowing down the speech rate allows the school-age child to experience a more coordinated speech attempt, one in which smooth coarticulatory movements are more likely to occur, leading to a reduction in stuttering. A further step to alleviating the physiologic aspects of stuttering is to teach the child to use loose contacts. Loose contacts means reducing the tension in the articulators so that the lips and tongue make light contact with any opposing surface during speech. Analogies may be made, such as speaking like a rag doll or speaking as though weary. The older and more mature the child, the more direct and explicit is the explanation, to the point of explaining to an interested client the difference between muscle contraction and relaxation and the difficulties that arise during speech production with muscle overshoot. For severe stutterers, the clinician may begin this work with exaggerated loose contacts and then shape the speech to be closer and closer to normal production, all the while incorporating the technique into increasing length of utterances and more complex utterances, as described previously.

Slower speech rate and loose contacts may suffice as stuttering modification strategies for some school-age stutterers; others may need help, again provided by Van Riper some years ago in the form of pull-outs and cancellations. With regard to pull-outs, the client is advised, upon finding him- or herself in a block, to reduce the tension, stop pushing, and allow the word to emerge easily and naturally. The important issues are that the client reduces contraction of the articulatory muscles and moves on to coarticulate with the rest of the word and sentence. The child may be helped by likening a pull-out to loose contacts that are used after the block has started. Cancellation refers to Van Riper's method of having the stutterer pause after the stuttered word, consider the nature of the interference to the emerging word (Lips tightly compressed? Vocal folds tightly together?) and repeat the word using easier stuttering. Since children often react negatively to what they feel is "stuttering again," a modified form of cancellation would be to repeat the word using looser or easier speech. A child's ability to use cancellation suggests considerable skill in monitoring speech and in taking responsibility for therapy. In addition, cancellation permits the client to reinforce an easier or a fluent production.

As with the aforementioned strategies, strategies for handling breathing anomalies, such as shallow, strained exhalation, or phonation difficulties, such as hard onsets of words, should be instituted if indicated by the physiologic profile of the child and if the preceding strategies have not resulted in improvement in respiration and phonation. Associated symptoms, such as poor eye contact or devices designed to postpone speech production, such as fillers "er er er er" or "um um um," may have subsided with the psycholinguistic and physiologic work already carried out. More habituated associated symptoms may require specific behavioral approaches, such as negative practice, wherein the response is duplicated by the client voluntarily, or massed practice, wherein the response is voluntarily duplicated many times in an attempt to extinguish the response. It is important to note that psychosocial, psycholinguistic, and physiologic factors of therapy may proceed concurrently; they have been separated here for ease of presentation.

Transfer Procedures

When the child, regardless of age, has mastered steps of increased fluency and methods to reduce the severity of the blocks, the clinician moves to see that these new-found skills are used in situations other than the one-to-one or small group situation. This transfer of skills is done by, as stated previously, involving parents (and siblings and friends) in the therapy session; teaching parents to work with their children appropriately, according to client age and willingness (parents who are unable to participate constructively in this activity and who show no promise of improvement are discouraged from working with the child); helping the client to participate in a variety of activities in which he or she can try out his new skills, such as telephoning, oral reading in school, or whatever activity is appropriate to the child; and grading these activities carefully from least to most difficult. Maintaining or stabilizing the child's gains may take place over months or years with clinical visits becoming less often as time proceeds.

In conclusion, some therapies for childhood stutterers are comprehensive in that they attempt to deal with many aspects of the child's life that might possibly affect the child's stuttering, reactions, responses to therapy, and the like, as well as deal with the symptoms of stuttering,[79,80,82,84,86,91] while some therapies have a highly specific focus, for example, a behavioral focus.[77,92,93] Some of the more specific therapies have been organized into "programs," which give precise instructions to the clinician about the goals of therapy and steps to attain those goals. Clinicians need to become enlightened critics and educated consumers of therapies in order to apply the best of available information to their young clients, since well-controlled studies of the effectiveness of therapies for childhood stutterers are still lacking.

CLUTTERING

Cluttering is a fluency disorder that is characterized minimally by rapid speech rate, disordered articulation, and a lack of awareness of the problem on the part of the speaker. Because of the presence of sound, syllable, or word repetitions, and even sound prolongations, the condition is sometimes confused with stuttering. However, in some cases, the two conditions—cluttering and stuttering—likely coexist. The most prominent feature of cluttering as opposed to stuttering in individuals as young as school-age (there is a dearth of information on preschool clutterers) is a lack of awareness of the condition exhibited by the clutterer. The stutterer is usually highly aware and is discomfited by the stuttering, whereas the clutterer thinks his or her (usually his) speech is satisfactory and sees no reason for intervention. Although thousands of research articles have been published on stuttering, this is not so for cluttering. Most writings consist of observational reports. Weiss has postulated a central language imbalance, which includes reading and writing difficulties as well as a short attention span, as the basis of the clutterer's expressive difficulties.[5] A similar position was taken by Arnold.[94]

Daly, in his excellent review of cluttering, cites the following areas of possible communicative impairment in the clutterer: tachylalia (excessive rate); respiratory, phonatory, and articulatory symptoms; problems of rhythm and monotony; disorganized thought processes; language difficulties; and reading and writing difficulties.[3] Myers specifies the core features of cluttering as fast rate, disynchrony (between thought, language, and speech), and an inefficient feedback system.[4] She divides the possible symptoms of cluttering among four categories of behavioral characteristics—fluency, prosodics, linguistics, and articulation. There is agreement in the literature, then, that cluttering may involve various language and speech production processes together with a poor system of self-monitoring, though not all clutterers exhibit all symptoms.

When evaluating the clutterer, Daly suggests, in addition to the acquisition of a comprehensive case history, the administration of language tests including tests of auditory comprehension, auditory memory, and auditory processing; articulatory assessment; and speech rate measure. Few specific suggestions are offered in the literature on therapy for the clutterer, though the use of a tape recorder to increase speech monitoring skills is frequently mentioned, as is slowing down the rate of speech and improving articulatory skills. In addition to these aspects of therapy, Myers suggests the following: implementation of strategies to improve language formulation; phrasing, which should facilitate coordination of inhalation with articulatory functions; using new strategies on increasingly long and complex utterances; reading poetry to practice phrasing and prosodic variations and to acquire more speech rhythm and syllabic stress; and paying attention to the pragmatics of communication.

The precise relationship between cluttering and stuttering is unknown, but they do appear to occur simultaneously in some individuals, and to some extent the therapy strategies for the two conditions overlap. Although information on cluttering in children is lacking, clinicians should be aware of the possibility of this syndrome of symptoms existing in the school-age, and even preschool, populations. The school-age clutterer may be notable not only because of the speech symptoms, but because of language and learning difficulties also. Data on the preschool clutterer are simply lacking. Cluttering in children deserves attention in future research.

SUMMARY

This chapter attempts to define childhood dysfluency, to present it within an historical context, and to address current issues related to childhood dysfluency—particularly genetic, physiologic, and psycholinguistic issues. The differentiation of nonfluency and dysfluency in early childhood has presented difficulties of diagnosis, but the difficulties have lessened with increased information from clinical research. More data are needed to compare characteristics of stuttering with cluttering, particularly in the preschool population. The tendency to treat stutterers at a young age appears to be a worthwhile trend because early stuttering frequently is less complex than advanced stuttering, the speech pattern is less habituated, and the children are accessible and responsive to a therapeutic environment. However, as yet we have no clinical research results to confirm that early therapy produces better long-term gains than therapy carried out in older children. Assessment and management strategies are presented here within the framework of psychosocial, physiologic, and psycholinguistic factors; a broad-based approach to stuttering opposed to a more focused approach, such as learning theory or psychoanalytic theory.

Consideration of the 3 factors allows the clinician to touch all known theoretical and pragmatic bases in the evaluation and to design therapy procedures based upon the diagnostic profile of the client. Management strategies from a variety of sources are incorporated into the discussion on therapy for childhood stutterers. Mention is made of structured, programmed therapies that are now available for children who stutter. I would like to suggest to those clinicians interested in the programs that they become enlightened consumers; examine the programs in light of their knowledge of historical and current issues of the field, and in light of the needs of their particular clients.

REFERENCES

1. Johnson W. A study of the onset and development of stuttering. In: Johnson W, Leutenegger RR, eds. Stuttering in children and adults. Minneapolis: University of Minnesota Press, 1955:37.
2. Johnson W, and Associates. The onset of stuttering. Minneapolis: University of Minnesota Press, 1959.
3. Daly DA. The clutterer. In: St. Louis K, ed. The atypical stutterer: principles and practices of remediation. New York: Academic Press, 1985:155.
4. Myers FL. Acoustic and perceptual characteristics of cluttering. Presented at the 22nd Annual Convention of the New York State Speech-Language-Hearing Association, Ellenville, 1982.
5. Weiss DA. Cluttering. Englewood Cliffs: Prentice-Hall, 1964.
6. Adams MR. A clinical strategy for differentiating the normally nonfluent child and the incipient stutterer. J Fluency Disord 1977; 2:141–148.
7. Adams MR. Fluency, nonfluency and stuttering in children. J Fluency Disord 1982; 7:171–185.
8. Adams MR. The young stutterer: diagnosis, treatment and assessment of progress. In: Perkins WH, ed. Stuttering disorders. New York: Thieme-Stratton 1984:41.
9. Curlee RF. A case selection strategy for young disfluent children. Semin Speech Lang Hear 1980; 1:277–288.
10. Van Riper C. The nature of stuttering. Englewood Cliffs: Prentice-Hall, 1971.
11. Van Riper C. The nature of stuttering. 2nd ed. Englewood Cliffs: Prentice-Hall, 1982.
12. Wall MJ, Myers FL. Clinical management of childhood stuttering. Austin: PRO-ED, 1984.
13. Bloodstein O. Semantics and beliefs (postscript). In: Shames GH, Rubin M, eds. Stuttering then and now. Columbus: Charles E Merrill, 1986:130.
14. Bluemel C. Primary and secondary stammering. Q J Speech 1932; 18:187–200.
15. Bloodstein O. A handbook on stuttering. 3rd ed. Chicago: National Easter Seal Society, 1981.
16. Wingate ME. Stuttering: theory and treatment. New York: Irvington, 1976.
17. Myers FL, Wall MJ. Issues to consider in the differential diagnosis of normal childhood nonfluencies and stuttering. J Fluency Disord 1981; 6:189–196.
18. Nelson SE, Hunter N, Walter M. Stuttering in twin types. J Speech Disord 1945; 10:335–343.
19. Howie PM. Concordance for stuttering in monozygotic and dizygotic twin pairs. J Speech Hear Res 1981; 24:317–321.
20. Andrews G, Harris M. The syndrome of stuttering. Clinics in developmental medicine, no. 17. London: Heinemann, 1964.
21. Kidd KK. Genetic models of stuttering. J Fluency Disord 1980; 5:187–202.
22. Kidd KK, Kidd JR, Records MA. The possible causes of the sex ratio in stuttering and its implications. J Fluency Disord 1978; 3:13–23.
23. Andrews G, Craig A, Feyer AM, Hoddinott S, Howie P, Neilson M. Stuttering: a review of research findings circa 1982. J Speech Hear Disord 1983; 48:226–246.
24. Freeman FJ. Phonation in stuttering: a review of current research. J Fluency Disord 1979; 4:78–89.
25. Starkweather CW. Stuttering and laryngeal behavior: a review. Asha Monogr 1982:21.
26. St. Louis KO. Linguistic and motor aspects of stuttering. In: Lass N, ed. Speech and language: advances in basic research and practice, vol. 1. New York: Academic Press, 1979:89.
27. Agnello J, Wingate ME, Wendell MV. Voice onset and voice termination times of children and adult stutterers. Presented at the ASHA Convention, Las Vegas, 1974.
28. Luper HL, Cross DE. Finger reaction time of stuttering and non-stuttering children and adults. Presented at the ASHA Convention, San Francisco, 1978.
29. Cross D, Luper H. Voice reaction time of stuttering and non-stuttering children and adults. J Fluency Disord 1979; 4:59–77.
30. Adams MR. Voice onsets and segment durations of normals and beginning stutterers. Presented at the ASHA Convention, Detroit, 1986.
31. Cullinan WL, Springer MT. Voice initiation and termination times in stuttering and nonstuttering children. J Speech Hear Res 1980; 23:344–360.
32. Murphy M, Baumgartner JM. Voice initiation and termination time in stuttering and nonstuttering children. J Fluency Disord 1981; 6:257–264.
33. Reich A, Till J. Reaction-time experiments with stuttering and nonstuttering children. Presented at the ASHA Convention, Los Angeles, 1981.
34. Zebrowski PM, Conture EG, Cudahy EA. Acoustic analysis of young stutterers' fluency: preliminary observation. Presented at the ASHA Convention, Cincinnati, 1983.
35. Coriat IH. The oral-erotic components of stammering. Int J Psychoanal 1927; 8:56–69.
36. Coriat IH. The nature and analytic treatment of stuttering. Proc Am Speech Corr Assoc 1931; 1:151–156.
37. Coriat IH. The psychoanalytic concept of stammering. Nervous Child 1943; 2:167–171.
38. Fenichel O. The psychoanalytic theory of neurosis. New York: Norton Press, 1945.
39. Heilpern E. A case of stuttering. Psychoanal Q 1941; 1:95–115.
40. Glauber IP. The psychoanalysis of stuttering. In: Eisenson J, ed. Stuttering: a symposium. New York: Harper & Row, 1958:71.
41. Barbara DA. Stuttering: a psychodynamic approach to its understanding and treatment. New York: Julian Press, 1954.
42. Barbara DA. New direction in stuttering: theory and practice. Springfield: CC Thomas, 1965.
43. Travis LE. The unspeakable feelings of people, with special reference to stuttering. In: Travis LE, ed. Handbook of speech pathology. Englewood Cliffs: Prentice-Hall, 1977:1009.
44. Starkweather CW. Stuttering in children: an overview. In: Luper H, ed. Intervention with the young stutterer. Special issue of J Childhood Commun Disord 1982; 6(1):5–14.
45. McDearmon J. Primary stuttering at the onset of stuttering: a re-examination of data. J Speech Hear Res 1968; 11:631–637.
46. Brutten EJ, Shoemaker DJ. The modification of stuttering. Englewood Cliffs: Prentice-Hall, 1967.
47. Shames GH, Sherrick CE Jr. A discussion of nonfluency and

stuttering as operant behavior. J Speech Hear Disord 1963; 28:3–18.
48. Starkweather CW. A multiprocess behavioral approach to stuttering therapy. In: Perkins WH, ed. Stuttering disorders. New York: Thieme-Stratton, 1984:129.
49. DeJoy DA, Gregory HH. The relationship of children's disfluencies to the syntax, length and vocabulary of their sentences. Asha Abstract 1973; 15:472.
50. Starkweather CW. Speech fluency and its development in nonvocal children. In: Lass N, ed. Speech and language: advances in basic research and practice, vol. 4. New York: Academic Press, 1980:143.
51. Colburn N, Mysak E. Developmental disfluency and emerging grammar. II. Co-occurrence of disfluency with specified semantic-syntactic structures. J Speech Hear Res 1982; 25:421–427.
52. Bloodstein O. Stuttering and normal nonfluency—a continuity hypothesis. Br J Disord Commun 1970; 5:30–39.
53. Bjerkan B. Word fragmentations and repetitions in the spontaneous speech of 2–6 year old children. J Fluency Disord 1980; 5:137–148.
54. Silverman EM. Generality of disfluency data collected from preschoolers. J Speech Hear Res 1972; 15:84–92.
55. Silverman EM. Clustering: a characteristic of preschoolers' disfluency. J Speech Hear Res 1973; 16:578–583.
56. Silverman EM. The influence of preschoolers' speech usage on their disfluency frequency. J Speech Hear Res 1973; 16:474–481.
57. Silverman EM. Word position and grammatical function in relation to preschoolers' speech disfluency. Percept Mot Skills 1974; 39:267–272.
58. Silverman EM. Effect of selected word attributes on preschoolers' speech disfluency: initial phoneme and length. J Speech Hear Res 1975; 18:430–434.
59. Kline ML, Starkweather CW. Receptive and expressive language performance in young stutterers. Asha Abstract 1979; 21:797.
60. Murray H, Reed C. Language abilities of preschool stuttering children. J Fluency Disord 1977; 2:171–176.
61. Westby C. Language performance of stuttering and nonstuttering children. J Commun Disord 1979; 12:133–145.
62. Williams A, Marks C. A comparative analysis of the I.T.P.A. and P.P.V.T. performance of young stutterers. J Speech Hear Res 1972; 15:323–329.
63. Haynes WO, Hood SB. Disfluency changes in children as a function of the systematic modification of linguistic complexity. J Commun Disord 1978; 11:79–93.
64. Muma JR. Syntax of preschool fluent and disfluent speech: a transformational analysis. J Speech Hear Res 1971; 14:428–441.
65. Wall MJ. A comparison of syntax in young stutterers and non-stutterers. J Fluency Disord 1980; 5:321–326.
66. Williams D, Silverman F. Note concerning articulation of school-age stutterers. Percept Mot Skills 1968; 27:713–714.
67. Blood GW, Seider R. The concomitant problems of young stutterers. J Speech Hear Res 1981; 46:31–33.
68. Bloodstein O, Gantwerk BG. Grammatical function in relation to stuttering in young children. J Speech Hear Res 1967; 10:787–789.
69. Bloodstein O. The rules of early stuttering. J Speech Hear Disord 1974; 39:379–394.
70. Bloodstein O, Grossman M. Early stutterings: some aspects of their form and distribution. J Speech Hear Res 1981; 24:298–302.
71. Wall MJ, Starkweather CW, Cairns HS. Syntactic influences on stuttering in young child stutterers. J Fluency Disord 1981; 6:283–298.
72. Wall MJ, Starkweather CW, Harris KS. The influence of voicing adjustments on the location of stuttering in the spontaneous speech of young child stutterers. J Fluency Disord 1981; 6:299–310.
73. Guitar BE, Kopfs H, Kilburg GD, Conway P. Parent verbal interactions and speech rate: a case study in stuttering. Presented at the ASHA Convention, Los Angeles, 1981.
74. Meyers SC, Freeman FJ. Mother and child speech rates as a variable in stuttering and disfluency. J Speech Hear Res 1985; 28:436–444.
75. Ryan BP. Stuttering therapy in a framework of operant conditioning and programmed learning. In: Gregory HH, ed. Controversies about stuttering therapy. Baltimore: University Park Press, 1979:129.
76. Riley G. Stuttering severity instrument for children and adults. Tigard, OR: CC Publications, 1980.
77. Ryan B, Van Kirk B. The establishment, transfer and maintenance of fluent speech in 50 stutterers using delayed auditory feedback and operant procedures. J Speech Hear Disord 1974; 39:3–10.
78. Stocker B. The Stocker probe technique: for diagnosis and treatment of stuttering in young children. Tulsa: Modern Education, 1980.
79. Cooper EB, Cooper CS. Cooper personalized fluency control therapy—revised. Allen: DLM Teaching Resources, 1985.
80. Shames GM, Florance SL. Stutter-free speech: a goal for therapy. Columbus: Charles E Merrill, 1980.
81. Shine RE. Direct management of the beginning stutterer. Semin Speech Lang Hear 1980; 1:339–350.
82. Gregory HH, Hill D. Stuttering therapy for children. Semin Speech Lang Hear 1980; 1:351–364.
83. Johnson W. Speech handicapped school children. New York: Harper & Row, 1967.
84. Van Riper C. The treatment of stuttering. Englewood Cliffs: Prentice-Hall, 1973.
85. Johnson L. Facilitating parental involvement in the therapy of the disfluent child. Semin Speech Lang Hear 1980; 1:301–309.
86. Williams D. Stuttering therapy for children. In: Travis LE, ed. Handbook of speech pathology and audiology. Englewood Cliffs: Prentice-Hall, 1971:1073.
87. Nelson LA. Language formulation related to disfluency and stuttering. Stuttering therapy: prevention and intervention with children. Memphis: Speech Foundation of America, 1985.
88. Riley GD, Riley J. A component model for diagnosing and treating children who stutter. J Fluency Disord 1979; 4:279–293.
89. Riley GD, Riley J. Motoric and linguistic variables among children who stutter: a factor analysis. J Speech Hear Disord 1980; 45:504–514.
90. Luper HL, Mulder RL. Stuttering: therapy for children. Englewood Cliffs: Prentice-Hall, 1964.
91. Conture EG. Stuttering. Englewood Cliffs: Prentice-Hall, 1982.
92. Costello JM. Treatment of the young chronic stutterer: managing fluency. In: Curlee RF, Perkins WH, eds. Nature and treatment of stuttering: new directions. San Diego: College-Hill Press, 1984:375.
93. Mowrer DE. A program to establish fluent speech. Columbus: Charles E Merrill, 1979.
94. Arnold GE. An attempt to explain the causes of cluttering with LLMM theory. Folia Phoniatr 1970; 22:247–260.

21 Stuttering in the Adult

Thomas W. Guyette, Ph.D.
John M. Baumgartner, Ph.D.

HISTORY

In the 19th century, behavior therapies were available to the stutterer. These therapies often involved intensive drill, breathing exercises, vocalization training, and vowel prolongation. Behavioral treatment declined in popularity once it became associated with the commercial stuttering schools. The major disappointment with this approach was in the lack of transfer and maintenance of the newly acquired fluency. Many of the stuttering therapists of this era disassociated themselves from behavioral therapy[1,2] because of this problem.

Orton[3] and Travis[4] proposed one of the earliest formal theories of stuttering. These scholars proposed a theory of stuttering that was based on the idea that persons who stuttered lacked adequate cerebral dominance. This lack resulted in dysfluency because both hemispheres would function "independently" and the neurologic signals sent to the speech musculature would be poorly synchronized. This model of stuttering suggested that if dominance could be established then the dysfluency would disappear. Travis' work laid the foundation for three other University of Iowa graduates (i.e., Bryngelson, Johnson, and Van Riper) whose work would dominate thinking about stuttering for the first half of the 20th century.

Bryngelson, like Travis, pursued the cerebral dominance theory of stuttering.[1,2] As a result, the establishment of dominance was considered an important part of treatment during this time of history. His approach to treatment also involved teaching the stutterer to have an "objective attitude" toward his or her stuttering. He reasoned that if the powerful negative emotional feelings associated with speaking were reduced, then the motor system would be less likely to breakdown when speaking. He also developed a technique called "voluntary stuttering," which the patient used to gain control over the stuttering moment.

Johnson's approach to stuttering moved away from physiologic explanations and viewed stuttering as a learned response resulting from negative listener reactions.[5] The stutterer, he believed, was taught to attempt to avoid what was in reality normal dysfluency. Stuttering was explained as an avoidance reaction. Johnson believed that fear of being dysfluent was the main cause of the problem. Psychotherapy and training in general semantics were recommended to help the stutterer resolve the negative feelings toward speech.

Van Riper's approach to stuttering has always been more oriented to manipulating the symptoms of stuttering than was either of his colleagues.[2,6] Therapy started with identifying and analyzing the stuttering behavior, systematically desensitizing feelings toward this behavior, and finally learning techniques to modify and reduce the stuttering. Van Riper recommended the use of concepts from both psychotherapy and behavior therapy with the goal of helping the patient stutter more fluently.

In the 1960s, behavior therapists began to exert a stronger influence on the treatment of stuttering. As Ingham points out, the influence of the behavior therapists increased consistently throughout the 1960s and 1970s until behavior therapy dominated the treatment literature.[7] During this period, learning concepts did indeed dominate the literature, but this is not to say there was agreement in the literature. Debate on both a theoretical and applied (treatment) level was lively and included interpretations of stuttering as an operant behavior, avoidance behavior, the result of approach and avoidance conflict, and a combination of two-factor learning principles. All of these were based in learning theory, yet all led to different treatment procedures. For an excellent review of these classic theoretical positions see Shames and Rubin.[8]

Although current treatments for stuttering are still predominantly behavioral, models of the etiology of stuttering are increasingly focused on a physiologic explanation of the disorder. If this trend continues, then it may well lead to more physiologically based treatment programs in the near future. It remains to be seen whether or not this change of focus would solve the problems of transfer and maintenance. We also want to point out that learning theory models and specific physiologic variables are not mutually exclusive, and a synthesis of learning theory and physiology may form the basis for new, more comprehensive theoretical formulations.

DEFINITION

One problem in defining stuttering is separating normal dysfluency from stuttering. There are at least two dimensions to this: type of dysfluency and frequency of dysfluency. According to Johnson's classification, there are eight types of dysfluency: interjections ("uh," "well"), part-word repetitions ("ba–ba–ba–baby," "ca–ca–ca–cat"), word repetitions ("I–I–I am tired"), phrase repetitions ("I am—I am—I am tired"), revisions ("I was—I am tired"), incomplete phrases ("I wish—he should have called"), broken words ("I was t—ired"), and prolonged sounds ("ssssssaw").[9] Of these eight types of dysfluency, certain types are more likely to be perceived as stuttering. For example, part-word repetitions are more likely to be perceived as dysfluency than are revisions, prolongations, or hesitations.[10,11] Prolongations and broken words also appear to have more saliency as types of stuttering dysfluency than interjections, whole-word repetitions, and revisions,[12] which tend to be perceived as more normal types of dysfluency. Bjerkan suggests that dysfluencies that fragment the word (e.g., part-word repetitions, prolongations, broken words) are likely to be perceived as stuttering, whereas those that do not (e.g., word repetitions, revisions, incomplete phrases) are perceived as normal dysfluency.[13] However, even the "normal" dysfluencies are perceived as stuttering if their frequency, severity, or duration is increased sufficiently.[14,15] Bloodstein defines stuttering as "whatever is perceived as stuttering by a reliable observer who has relatively good agreement with others"(p 9).[1] Although this definition may be accurate, it offers little help to the clinician investigating the characteristics that are used to identify the disorder.

Another approach is to define stuttering in terms of the behaviors normally associated with stuttering. The definition of the International Classification of Diseases is more descriptive of behavior, defining stuttering as a disorder "in the rhythm of speech, in which the individual knows precisely what he wishes to say, but at the time is unable to say it because of an involuntary repetitive prolongation or cessation of a sound"(p 202).[16] This definition is helpful in that it describes some of the characteristics of stuttering; however, it may not readily differentiate the stutterer from the nonstutterer unless, as Perkins argues, the word "involuntary" distinguishes normal from abnormal dysfluency.[17] For several points of view on this controversy, see Martin and Haroldson,[18] Perkins, [19,20] and Wingate.[21]

EPIDEMIOLOGY

The prevalence of stuttering in the adult population is unknown.[22] Estimates for school-age children range between 0.7 and 1.0 percent. Since the prevalence is highest in children under 12 years (1.0 percent) and decreases in older school-age children to 0.8 percent,[23] the trend would suggest that the prevalence is somewhere below 0.8 percent in the adult population. The incidence is between 4.0 to 5.0 percent.[1,22,23] The onset of stuttering is typically in early childhood usually between 3 and 5 years, with a gradually decreasing frequency after 5 years of age.[24] The ratio of male to female stutterers is approximately 3:1 in children,[24] and this ratio increases with age.[22] Specific estimates of sex ratio in the adult stuttering population were not found in the literature.

CHARACTERISTICS OF STUTTERERS

There is an extensive literature comparing attributes of the stutterer with the nonstutterer. Only a sample of the literature selected for its clinical relevance is presented here, and most of the publications cited are in themselves reviews. A more complete review of these and other characteristics can be found in Andrews et al,[22] Bloodstein,[1] or Curlee and Perkins.[25] In this literature, positive findings describe stutterers as a group and should be interpreted with caution. An individual stutterer may or may not exhibit any of these characteristics.

Hemispheric Dominance

In normal adults, the right hemisphere acts as a "holistic-gestalt, time independent processor and the left hemisphere as an analytic-segmental, time dependent processor."[26] It has been suggested that stutterers differ from nonstutterers in the hemisphere used to process language and speech. Evidence for differences in the hemisphere processing of language have been inferred from dichotic listening tasks. Rosenfield and Jerger in a review of these studies conclude that the evidence supporting this claim is inconsistent.[27] However, Moore reviewed similar data, controlling for the nature of the stimuli used in the testing, and found that meaningful linguistic stimuli tended to evoke right hemisphere processing in stutterers.[26] The results of lateral dominance testing using the Wada test have been inconclusive.[26,28,29]

Motor Speech Behavior

A number of studies have looked at parameters of the speech production system. Differences in the laryngeal behavior between stutterers and nonstutterers have been reported. Adams reviewd the literature on laryngeal reaction times in stutterers and nonstutterers and concluded that the voice onset times, voice initiation times, and speech initiation times were more likely to be slower in stutterers than in normal subjects.[30] Freeman, reviewing electromyographic (EMG) research, concluded that not only does muscle activity increase during stuttered speech, but more importantly the abductor and adductor laryngeal muscles appear to cocontract as well.[31] This cocontraction also occurs during silent periods prior to otherwise fluent utterances. Observation of the vocal folds by means of fiberoptics indicates that the glottis is usually inappropriately open or closed during a dysfluency.[32] These studies implicate the larynx in the moment of stuttering, but a specific causal relationship between laryngeal behavior and stuttering has not been established.

The movement and velocity of the lips and jaw have also been studied in both perceptually fluent and dysfluent utterances.[33–35] Zimmerman's work suggests that the fluent utterances of stutterers contain lower velocities of movement and smaller displacements than do those of nonstutterers. The time between movement onsets for different phonemes is also longer in fluent utterances. Stuttered speech was found to be preceded and followed by aberrant movement patterns. Thus both the stuttering moments and fluent speech differed between stutterers and nonstutterers.

Delayed Speech and Language

Stutterers are more likely than nonstutterers to have a history of either delayed speech or delayed language development.[1,22,36–38] Whether these differences continue into adulthood or not is unclear.

Intelligence

Stuttering appears to be negatively related to intelligence such that the prevalence for stuttering goes up as level of intelligence goes down,[23,36] resulting in a prevalence as high as 3 percent in the mentally retarded.[1,22]

Familial Tendency

Stuttering tends to run in successive generations of the same family. Generally, the risk is considered to be three times that of the nonstuttering population for first-degree relatives.[22] Kidd has argued that an inherited genetic susceptibility can explain these data.[39] Certainly, if stuttering is found to have a genetic etiology, then this finding will not only alter theoretical models that view stuttering as a learned behavior, but also alter the kind of information and counseling provided to the adult stutterer.

Personality

Stutterers and nonstutterers do not differ on measures of neurotic behavior.[22,23,40] However, stutterers do have more social adjustment problems,[1] which appear to result from the speech disorder. We will come back to this topic when discussing assessment of adults who stutter.

CURRENT MODELS

It is a well-known fact and has already been discussed elsewhere in this volume (Chapter 20) that stuttering usually begins in childhood. Stuttering or stuttering-like speech can also begin in adulthood and, in these cases, it is referred to as acquired stuttering. A review of formal theories on childhood onset stuttering and their current status is beyond the realm of this chapter, but for the interested reader we want to again recommend the text edited by Shames and Rubin.[8] In this unique work, articles representing each of the major theories are reprinted and then critiqued (by the original authors whenever possible) in view of what has been learned in the last 25 years. Original and then revised theoretical positions of Wingate, Perkins, Travis, Johnson (revised by Bloodstein), Brutten, Sheehan, Flanagan, Goldiamond and Azrin, and Shames and Sherrick are included in this volume. Other chapters in this volume are devoted to the then and now of management. For the serious student of theory, this work makes fascinating and enlightening reading. What becomes clear is that people who develop stuttering as children are a heterogeneous population and that no single theory adequately explains either the disorder or the population. What has evolved in the recent literature is the construction of models rather than full-blown theories. These models provide a general framework from which to view what is clearly a multidimensional disorder. Meyers and Wall,[41] Wall in Chapter 20, and Riley and Riley[42] have described general models for looking at the onset of stuttering in children. Less general components such as genetics, motor programming and timing principles, laryngeal dynamics, and articulatory dynamics have been discussed in other recent publications (see chapters in Curlee and Perkins' 1984 book for a detailed presentation of these models[25]). A thorough review of the previously mentioned theories and models leads to the conclusion that stuttering which begins in childhood is a breakdown in motor control that affects respiratory, laryngeal, and/or supralaryngeal structures. Control over the speech production system can be disrupted by any of a number of factors including genetic, anatomic, physiologic, emotional, linguistic, and/or cognitive. When a clinician sees an adult whose problem began in childhood, the picture is further complicated by whatever adjustments or maladjustments have occurred over time, and this is true regardless of what model or theory best explains the original onset.

Models for explaining the onset of stuttering or stuttering-like speech in adulthood (acquired stuttering) are less well developed than those that pertain to childhood onset. Acquired stuttering can be neurogenic, psychogenic, or idiopathic. The formulation of models to explain acquired stuttering is hampered by small sample size in particular. In addition, the specific speech, language, and other characteristics of these patients are frequently not described in detail. No type or site of neurologic lesion is either necessary or sufficient to produce stuttering in adults. The same can be said for psychiatric conditions and stuttering. Models for acquired stuttering will improve as the number of patients studied and reported on in the literature increases.

ASSESSMENT

As with other disorders, assessment of stuttering in adults should be conducted with several goals in mind. At a very general level, the assessment should lead to a decision as to whether the stuttering problem in the adult is idiopathic and of childhood onset, idiopathic of adult onset, neurogenic of adult onset, or psychogenic of adult onset. More specific categories may be established in given patients. Although this chapter deals primarily with adults whose stuttering began in childhood, the clinician who sees adults should be aware of the distinct possibility that patients with adult onset fluency problems also present for evaluation and treatment. Detailed discussion of differential diagnostic, etiologic, and treatment aspects of adult onset stuttering problems are available in helpful reviews and case reports.[43–46]

Achieving the goal of determining onset and possible etiology and moving from there to treatment decisions depends on the collection of information relevant to more specific goals. It is toward this end that we believe an adequate assessment of stuttering in an adult should include the acquisition of information on at least the type and frequency of dysfluencies, associated physical struggle behavior, aspects of nonstuttered speech including rate; the attitude regarding speech, stuttering itself, and the perceived influence of stuttering on day-to-day function; and the onset of the problem and concomitant or related problems. In addition, variability of the problem with respect to frequency and/or type of dysfluency, amount of struggle, and attitude, as well as the patient's prior experience with treatment, should be evaluated. Severity of the stuttered speech itself is usually measured as a function of type and frequency of dysfluencies plus duration and type of struggle behavior (e.g., Riley[47]). Frequency, duration, and struggle, plus the other variables we have mentioned, collectively form a picture of the overall extent and type of communicative disorder. This overall picture is necessary for specific differential diagnostic and therapeutic decisions.

We think that all of these variables should be measured or considered in some way and to some extent in order to provide competent clinical services to adults who stutter. However, the specific procedures utilized as well as the scheduling and time devoted to each area vary as a function of the question being asked (differential diagnosis versus evaluation and treatment) and the environment in which the clinician works (university clinic, private practice, medical practice, rehabilitation facility, acute care, inpatient, outpatient). The following procedural section is not meant to be detailed in all respects. Rather, specific procedures are described or recommended in some instances, whereas in others more general possibilities are raised.

Speech Measures

As has been previously described, the type of dysfluencies should be described, and those that qualify as "stuttered" (see earlier comments about controversies over the issue of definition) should be expressed either as percent syllables or words stuttered (see Costello and Ingham for a discussion of percent words versus percent syllables[48]). This percentage should be calculated for at least the following tasks: general conversation, discussion of patient history, reading (at an appropriate level for the patient), and monologue. Repeated readings in order to check for the well-known adaptation effect may be helpful in terms of differential diagnosis, identification of common loci of dysfluencies, and in identifying changes the patient makes on his or her own in order to attempt to deal with the task. The clinician should not just label the type of dysfluencies, but should also describe the nature of the breakdown in coordination between the respiratory, phonatory, and articulatory systems. During these tasks, the type of struggle behavior (if any) and its variability should be described. Duration of dysfluent moments should be either estimated or actually timed. It is impractical to do this for every dysfluent moment, and usually it is most useful to address only the longest moments (or "blocks"). Frequency of stuttering, duration, and type of struggle are components of a commonly used commercially available severity instrument.[42,47] Rate of speech should also be calculated during conversation and reading. Rate can be quantified in either words per minute (WPM) or syllables per minute (SPM), and, increasingly, SPM is the preferred measure. Measures of rate that include time spent stuttering are indicative of how many different words or syllables the patient communicates per unit of time rather than the actual speed of speech movements. Clearly, the time the patient spends repeating, prolonging, or struggling with a given syllable reduces the overall number of syllables produced per unit of time. Measures of speech rate that do not include the time spent stuttering should also be made (see the section Measures of Nonstuttered Speech).

The degree to which the patient can describe the type of dysfluent behavior and identify instances of occurrences should also be evaluated.[49,50] These specific behaviors can be further categorized on the basis of those that are reported to be involuntary and those that the patient describes as voluntary (even though not readily controllable). Behaviors may also be thought of as representing core stuttering, escape or physical struggle, and avoidance. Early specification of these types of behavior is helpful to both the clinician and the patient in terms of management decisions. Discussion of these issues should be a part of the history and description of the current problem, and the clinician can expect that some adults describe readily and accurately the specific types of behavior and how they have changed (or not changed) over time, whereas others are unable to do so. Specification of behaviors that make up the problem may be supplemented by the use of written checklists if the clinician desires (as an example, see Brutten for a description of checklists[49]).

Attitude

The measures already mentioned have to do with relatively (although not always) observable and quantifiable types of behavior. A less obvious and quantifiable (from a validity and reliability standpoint) but just as important an area is the measurement of attitude. The patient's attitudes and feelings about his or her speech, the effects of his or her problem on day-to-day life (vocational, social), and previous treatment are all important in the formulation of an overall impression of severity, selection of treatment approach, and likely outcome. Pretreatment attitude has been shown to be related to short- and long-term treatment outcome,[51] and posttreatment attitude may be related to long-term outcome,[52] but clinicians are far from understanding either the extent to which this is true or the dynamics. As will be discussed later, some treatment approaches focus on attitude at an early stage and continue to emphasize it, whereas others deal with attitude at later stages. The patient's attitude about the extent to which he or she is "handicapped" in vocational and social activities helps fill out the overall impression of how the patient perceives him- or herself and his or her disorder. Attitude regarding perceived handicap may play a role in medicolegal issues as well (issues of vocational rehabilitation, disability). Patient attitude about expectations and/or past experiences with therapy help give the clinician needed information on the type and amount of counseling that needs to be accomplished as an early part of treatment. When working with adults whose stuttering began in childhood, considerable adjustment or readjustment of expectations regarding treatment outcome may be needed. In patients with acquired stuttering, inquiry into attitude and extent of perceived handicap is equally as important, particularly if the clinician suspects a major psychogenic component to the problem.

If one looks through the literature on evaluation and treatment of stuttering, the topic of attitude is nearly always mentioned. Agreement on how well it can be measured is another story. A combination of interview, cautious probing and reprobing, plus paper and pencil measures should be adequate at least in the initial stages of patient evaluation and management. The clinician should be aware of two issues. The first is the extent to which stutterers as a group show adjustment problems in addition to or separate from their stuttering problem. Comprehensive reviews of this topic suggest strongly that, as a group, stutterers do show higher social anxiety, reduced self-esteem, and increased general anxiety in comparison to nonstutterers (see Bloodstein,[1] and Cox[53] for excellent reviews). However, these are grouped data; the specific assessment procedures varied, and the findings may or may not apply to a particular patient. The clinician should be sensitive to signs of significant maladjustment or other emotional disorders and ready to make appropriate referrals. The other and more specific issue is the assessment of attitude toward and/or anxiety about speech and speech situations. Interview approaches to this are well described elsewhere.[6,49,50]

There are also paper and pencil measures that can be used including Stutterers Self Ratings of Reactions to Speech Situations,[50] the Iowa Scale of Attitude Toward Stuttering,[50] and the Perceptions of Stuttering Inventory.[54] However, these forms do not yield quantifiable scores that can be used readily. Brutten describes the Speech Situations Checklist (SSC), which attempts to measure separately perceived emotional reactions and speech disruption in 51 different speech situations.[49] The SSC has not truly been standardized, but it has been used to the extent that means and standard deviations for various populations are available.[49] Hanson, Gronhovd, and Rice performed a discriminant analysis of the SSC and identified 21 (of the 51 total) items that separate stutterers with high speech anxiety from normals.[55] These authors did not include the speech disruption section of the SSC, and the usefulness of their study remains to be more fully demonstrated, but studies such as this one are certainly a step in the right direction. A paper and pencil attitude scale that has received considerable attention in recent years is the S-24 scale,[56] which is a modified version of the Erickson S-scale.[57] The S-24 scale has been used on enough patients to develop means and standard deviations for both stutterers and nonstutterers. It would be helpful if scores on attitude scales like the SSC or S-24 gave clinicians specific information on what to include in treatment and what kind of short- and/or long-term outcome to expect, but such is not the case. These scales are helpful in a general way, but they lack specificity. Further research is needed in order to better develop and standardize attitude scales and to determine their usefulness.

Measures of Nonstuttered Speech

It is no longer thought that the problem of stuttering consists solely of dysfluent interruptions in what is otherwise normally fluent speech. This nonstuttered speech has been shown to differ from that of nonstutterers both before and after treatment. Adams and Runyan reviewed studies on physiologic and aerodynamic components of nonstuttered speech and other studies on listener reactions to nonstuttered speech.[58] The majority of both groups of studies reported significant differences. We recommend that one at least measures rate during nonstuttered speech. Other dimensions of nonstuttered speech that one might look at include aerodynamic variables, duration of voicing, fundamental frequency or variations in fundamental frequency, voice initiation time, voice onset time, and articulatory transitions to name a few. Such an instrumented approach is probably not practical for most clinicians. Another way to look at nonstuttered speech, and one that is more practical than instrumented approaches for most clinicians, is the use of rating scales that pertain to the "quality" of stutterer's nonstuttered speech. For example, Martin, Haroldson, and Triden have addressed this issue and demonstrated considerable reliability in the use of their scale.[59] This topic (speech quality and "normalcy") will be discussed further in the following section on treatment. As more information is obtained, clinicians will be better able to specify how the overall speech pattern of adults who stutter differs from normal. This comparison to normal raises another thorny issue, and that is the question of what is normal fluency? The answer is that not all of (or perhaps even many of) the specific components of fluent speech are known yet. As has been shown in reviews of this issue,[60,61] clinicians still tend to describe fluency as the absence of stuttering.

TREATMENT

Many treatments are available for stuttering. Some focus on changing the form of the stuttering behavior, some attempt to increase the frequency of fluent utterances, and others concentrate on the attitude of the person who stutters. The diverse nature of these treatments makes classification difficult. Treatments for dysfluency will be discussed in terms of whether the major focus is on modifying the stuttering or shaping the fluent speech.[62]

Stuttering Modification

The approaches that fall into the stuttering modification category (e.g., Brutten, re type II behaviors,[49] Sheehan,[63] Van Riper[2]) attempt to teach the patient first to stutter and struggle less severely by the use of techniques to reduce the patient's fear of stuttering and then to teach the patient to exercise more "control" over stuttering behavior. In this treatment, goals related to modification of attitudes and feelings are equally as important as the goals related to reduction of the struggle behavior and more important initially than goals of reduced frequency of stuttering.

There are many variations on the stuttering modification approach, but the most widely known and the model for others is Van Riper's.[2] The first step in this treatment is to heighten the stutterer's awareness of the form of his or her dysfluencies. The patient is also taught to analyze blocks, describe secondary behaviors, and identify areas of tension. The patient is asked to analyze feelings and to confront fears associated with the block; he or she is asked to confront fears of specific speaking environments, persons, words, and phonemes. As the patient becomes aware of specific stuttering behavior and associated feelings, he or she is led by the clinician toward the realization that he or she is responsible for much of this behavior. The clinician emphasizes that stuttering is something the patient does, not something that is done to him or her. Identification is often taught by means of a hierarchy that begins with reading and proceeds through conversation with the clinician and then into more difficult transfer situations. However, identification activities can occur throughout the treatment program and not just at the beginning.

Modification of negative communication attitudes is also a goal of this kind of therapy. The clinician attempts to help the patient reduce fears associated with stuttering. Elimination or reduction of these fears is important because it is hypothesized that the patient is unable to gain control at the moment of stuttering if strong emotions are present.

As progress toward desensitization and fear reduction occurs, the patient is taught methods to bring the loss of physical control that forms the block under "control" or possibly to eliminate it entirely. These methods attempt to reduce the amount of struggle and tension in the dysfluent speech and to increase the patient's ability to produce a smooth transition out of a dysfluency. Typical examples of these modification procedures include Van Riper's use of variation, cancellation, "pull-out," and preparatory set.[2] In the variation stage, the patient is asked to change something about the dysfluency. He or she still stutters, but the stuttering is different in some way. For example, if the patient taps his or her leg as a "starter," then he or she could be asked to tap his or her chest instead. Introduction of purposeful variation into the involuntary struggle is the first step in gaining control. Cancellation is a form of self-confrontation in which the patient stops immediately after stuttering and reviews in his or her mind the previous dysfluency, hoping to gain some insight into the physical mechanics of the block. After analyzing the dysfluency, the patient repeats the stuttered word, hopefully with more control. The pull-out is difficult because the stutterer must gain control during the dysfluency. Using this technique, the patient attempts to gain control during the actual stuttering moment and to finish the block voluntarily. In the final stage, the patient is taught various preparatory sets when speaking, which can be used to eliminate stuttering prior to its occurrence. In this approach, fluent speech may not be a goal of therapy. In fact "successful treatment" does not necessarily imply speech free of dysfluencies; a successful treatment involves confrontation and elimination of fears and negative communication attitudes along with acquisition of ways to modify and control the form of dysfluency. The successful patient learns to "stutter more fluently."

Fluency Shaping Therapy

Fluency shaping therapies usually involve teaching the patient a technique that eliminates overt dysfluencies, establishing this manner of speaking in conversation, then gradually fading the technique and shaping the patient's speech so that it sounds more normal. This stage is followed by a transfer stage in which the fluent speech is used in situations outside of the clinical setting. The third phase is teaching the patient how to maintain over time the newly learned speech control. Generally, the fluency shaping approaches do not deal with the patient's attitude as a goal separate from speech control. Changes in attitude are thought to occur secondary to improved speech control achieved by the use of the control technique(s).

Fluency Establishment

Fluency establishment procedures result in a reduction in dysfluency when used by the stutterer. In most fluency shaping treatments, the patient is shown or instructed in a technique with an immediate goal of zero percent syllables stuttered. In some treatment programs, the technique is used immediately in conversation and monologue,[64] whereas in others, the patient practices the technique in simple utterances (e.g., words and short phrases); as the patient progresses, the length and complexity of utterances are measured until the patient is using the technique in conversation. As the patient progresses through a program, speech measures usually include (1) percent syllables stuttered and (2) SPM. Once the fluent speech is firmly established, measures of speech quality are taken and used to help the patient develop the most natural but still stutter-free speech possible.[65] As previously discussed, speech quality is most practically measured by means of a scaling procedure.

In the following section, the fluency establishment techniques have been organized into categories based on their ability to manipulate rate, prosody, duration, speech breathing, articulatory effort, or a combination of these techniques. The techniques are listed individually with the understanding that, in most therapy programs, individual techniques are used in combination with other techniques to form a treatment "package." Many techniques can fall into more than one category, and the selection of one category over another is usually arbitrary.

Rate, Prosody, and Duration. ***Delayed Auditory Feedback (DAF).*** Persons speaking with an auditory feedback delay usually produce speech characterized by prolonged syllables, reduced rate, occasional blurring of the distinction between consonants, and a high rate of fluency. Typically, programs start the patient using maximum auditory delay times (between 200 and 250 msec), which are reduced as the patient progresses through the program.[66] The intent is to reduce the delay time while increasing the "quality" of the patient's speech. Fluency is maintained and eventually the device is removed.

Prolonged Speech. Prolonged speech is similar to "DAF speech" in that it is characterized by elongated syllables, reduced rate, and continuous vocalization. The difference is that prolonged speech does not have to be induced by delayed auditory feedback. Usually prolonged speech is learned through clinician modeling and instruction. For example, Ingham and Andrews used clinician modeling of the target behavior to replace delayed auditory feedback.[67] Prolonged speech is the most widely used of the fluency establishment techniques[7] and is used frequently in combination with other techniques.[64,68]

Rhythmic Speech. Syllable timed speech is characterized by even stress across syllables and enunciation of each syllable after a specific time interval.[69] This technique does not necessarily involve prolongation of sounds, rate reduction, or continuous vocalization. Usually syllable timed speech is achieved either through instruction and modeling by the clinician or through the use of timing aids such as the metronome. In some treatments, the metronome is used to establish syllable timed speech and then is faded as the patient acquires skill. However, in some cases, the metronome is used as a speech aid and is worn continuously.

Rate Reduction or Slowed Speech. This refers primarily to techniques that attempt to establish fluent speech through the use of slowed rate. Typically, these programs start at greatly reduced rates (30 SPM for example) and gradually increase rate while maintaining fluency. Usually rate reduction programs are used in combination with delayed auditory feedback or prolonged speech programs because rate reduction achieved solely through increased pausing is not an effective fluency establishment technique.[70]

Speech Breathing. ***Airflow.*** Airflow techniques involve modification of speech breathing patterns. For example, Schwartz recommends that the patient begins passive expiration just prior to initiating speech for each breath.[71] Coupled with the airflow, the patient is instructed to prolong the first syllable of each breath unit. This approach overlaps with prolonged speech and easy onset in the manner in which vocalization is modified.

The regulated-breathing method is a habit reversal procedure that involves among other things adjustments in speech breathing.[72,73] These alterations in speech breathing are used because they are "incompatible" with stuttering and include relaxed deep breathing, beginning speaking immediately after taking a deep breath, emphasizing the initial part of the utterance, and short phrase durations.

Blending or Continuous Phonation. This technique involves teaching blending of one sound into another with no stoppage of the airflow within phrase units.[64,66] This procedure is often included as a part of a program package and is rarely used alone.

Breathy Voice. This technique involves teaching the patient to speak with a breathy voice and usually is used along with other techniques in fluency shaping programs.[64]

Articulatory Effort. ***Soft Contact.*** Using this technique, the patient learns to speak with less articulatory effort. For example, consonant sounds have less pressure and are released with less aspiration. Contacts between the articulators have a reduced duration and reduced muscular effort. Any indications of tension in the articulation process are discouraged. Loudness tends to be reduced slightly. Often this approach is taught by means of a combination of modeling by the clinician and negative practice on the part of the patient. Soft contact is used with many of the prolonged speech programs.[24,64]

Easy Onset. Although soft contact refers to effort involved in oral cavity articulation, easy onset usually refers to a reduction in effort during the onset of phonation. Easy onset is also a component of several treatment programs.[64,68] It is similar in many respects to breathy voice techniques although some specific differences do exist.

Combining Establishment Techniques. Most treatment "programs" for stuttering incorporate more than a single fluency establishment technique. For example, Perkins describes using rate control, phrasing, easy voice onset, soft contact, breathy voice, and blended words in his program.[64] He uses delayed auditory feedback initially to establish rate and the prolonged speech features. The Prince Henry Program offered by Andrews and his colleagues uses "smooth motion speech," which is a combination of gentle onset of phonation, continuous airflow, continuous movement of the articulators with increased vowel and consonant durations, soft articulatory contact, and rate control.[24] This program uses instruction and clinician modeling to teach the new speech pattern. Another treatment package is the Precision Fluency Shaping Program, which involves teaching a speech pattern altered by prolongation of syllables, smooth transitions, gentle onset of phonation, and altered breathing.[68] A voice onset monitor is used in this program to provide feedback to the patient.

Many program packages are available to the fluency clinician, and the interested reader is referred to Ingham, which is the most comprehensive review of fluency shaping and other available behavior therapy programs.[7]

Transfer

Transfer occurs when a patient exhibits newly learned behavior in situations other than those in which the behavior was originally learned. Research on treatment effects indicates that skills learned in the clinic do not necessarily transfer to other communication situations without specific training, and so a specific transfer stage of therapy is needed.[74] The purpose of the transfer phase is to teach the patient to use the skills gained in establishment in the more difficult situations of the real world.

In the transfer stage the patient is often given specific assignments that involve using speech control techniques in new situations. These speaking situations are usually hierarchically arranged based on the difficulty of the situation as perceived by the patient. The results of an instrument such as the SSC[49] or the S-24[56] plus interview results can be used to develop this hierarchy. The patient begins transfer by entering into the least difficult speaking situations while attempting to maintain the level of fluency achieved in the establishment phase. Patients often tape record conversations during these encounters and later analyze the recordings for the use of the fluency establishment techniques, frequency of stuttering, naturalness of speech, and conversational technique. Progress may be slowed by anxiety or fear of a specific speaking situation. In these cases, techniques to reduce anxiety and/or autonomic arousal (e.g., systematic desensitization) can be implemented. Practice in the real situation itself can be viewed as in-vivo desensitization. Self-reinforcement[75] and self-responsibility[76] are concepts introduced in the transfer phase, and specific transfer activities may be preceded by a discussion of and training in these skills.

A variety of procedures have been suggested as methods to facilitate transfer. For example, Stokes and Baer use the following nine categories to describe generalization techniques: train and hope, sequential modification, use natural maintaining contingencies, train sufficient exemplars, train loosely, use indiscriminable contingencies, program common stimuli, mediate generalization, and train to generalize.[77] Ingham reviews these nine categories with respect to stuttering treatment and concludes that although many of these techniques have promise, few have been demonstrated to be effective.[78] For further discussion of this topic, see Boberg and Kully[75] and Ingham.[79]

Maintenance

Maintenance refers to the continuation of speech and attitudinal changes over time while contact with the clinician is reduced. Data on the long-term effects of treatment programs indicate that maintenance of fluent speech is a major problem for all stuttering treatments.[80] A relatively recent development in stuttering therapy is the use of specific procedures to teach the patient the skills needed to maintain the recently acquired fluency. One general maintenance technique involves teaching the patient to become his or her own therapist. For example, the patient learns the ability to evaluate his or her own speech[81] or to self-administer reinforcement contingent on compliance with the program procedures. Hanna and Owen suggest a self-control phase that involves teaching the client to self-monitor, self-reinforce, and use self-help groups.[82] Part of maintenance involves the patient setting up regular sessions for the practice of fluency establishment techniques. Self-evaluation is critical if these practice sessions are to be carried out independently and effectively. In publications that specifically address maintenance procedures, reduction in contacts with the clinician is usually contingent on the maintenance of high levels of fluency.[83] Ingham suggests that clinicians need to consider at least three factors when designing a maintenance program: (1) the type of behavior needed to sustain fluency, (2) environmental contingencies that can be linked into that fluency maintaining behavior, and (3) the use of self-management principles whenever possible.[78]

Other topics related to maintenance involve counseling the patient about the possibility of relapse and preparing him or her for changes in his or her social life that result from the increased fluency. The patient is also introduced to the idea that attendance at booster sessions and support groups may be necessary to maintain the fluency. For further discussion of this topic, see Boberg,[80] Florance and Shames,[76] and Ingham.[7,78]

Combined Approach

The stuttering modification approach differs from the fluency shaping approach on several major points.[62] For example, in the modification approach, acceptable stuttering can be a terminal goal of therapy, whereas in the shaping approach, any dysfluency is usually considered a negative outcome. Another major difference is that the fluency shaping therapies usually do not target the patient's attitudes and feelings, whereas this target is a major part of the modification approach. Also, the shaping programs have more "structure" than the modification programs. Finally, as Cheasman points out,[69] the stuttering modification approach does not usually insist upon the distinction between establishment and transfer as do the fluency shaping programs.

Since Guitar[51] and Guitar and Bass[52] reported that the stutterers' "attitude" may be a predictor of long-term outcome in behavioral therapy, (see Ingham[84] for a critique of Guitar and Bass' study[52]) more of a focus on attitude has occurred in the treatment literature. Their article suggests that patients can be fluent and still maintain negative attitudes toward communication. They further argue that these attitudes are predictive of relapse. Guitar and Peters suggest that stuttering modification and fluency shaping approaches are not incompatible and that stutterers who respond well to fluency establishment techniques and who also have negative attitudes may benefit most from treatment that focuses on both attitude and behavior.[62] The therapist should not be afraid to combine stuttering modification with fluency shaping if the patient would appear to benefit from the components of each approach. Cheasman also reports on the benefits of combining these two types of therapies.[69]

Other Stuttering Treatments

Contingency Stimulation

In the operant approach, the patient is not required to modify the manner in which he speaks in a specific way. Instead, this approach uses positive and/or negative stimulation, which is contingent on the presence or absence of a specified level of fluency.[85] These programs use a hierarchy of difficulty based on gradually increasing the length and complexity of the utterance in which the target behavior is exhibited. At each program step, the target behavior is reinforced until it is produced consistently.

Treatments using punishment have also been reported.[86,87] Punishment in these programs has usually involved either forced periods of silence on the part of the speaker or the listener "timing out" the speaker each time the criterion level of stuttering is exceeded. These programs, like those using reinforcement, typically have gradually increased the length and complexity of the utterance in order to organize the establishment phase of therapy. Some clinicians report using a combination of reinforcement and punishment. (e.g., Ingham and Packman;[74] see Ingham for a detailed review of contingent-response programs[7]).

Auditory Masking

Masking of auditory feedback results in a reduction in dysfluency for many stutterers. In this approach, a device that generates a level of noise loud enough to mask perception of speech is worn by the patient. In many patients, this level of noise facilitates fluent speech. Once fluency is established, use of the device may be faded, or the device is worn permanently as a speech aid. Probably the most publicized use of auditory masking involves the "Edinburgh Masker."[88]

Biofeedback

Clinicians have attempted to teach stutterers to reduce muscular effort using instrumental techniques. For example, electrodes that sense muscle activity are placed on the appropriate sites, and either visual or auditory feedback on the level of muscle activity is provided immediately to the patient. Guitar has reported on the use of biofeedback with stutterers.[89]

Reciprocal Inhibition

The reduction of fear and anxiety associated with speaking often results in improvements in fluency. The desensitization of patient anxiety can be accomplished through the use of reciprocal inhibition therapy. Reciprocal inhibition therapy is composed of two main parts.[90] First, a relaxation response is developed. Muscle relaxation achieved through progressive relaxation exercises is the response used most frequently. This procedure is used until the patient can induce the relaxation response consistently and quickly. Second, the patient and therapist put together a hierarchy of anxiety producing situations. The patient is then asked to imagine the least anxiety producing situation of the hierarchy while in a relaxed state. When the patient can do this for a specified time, the next situation on the hierarchy is introduced. This procedure continues until the patient is able to imagine all the situations on the hierarchy without feelings of anxiety. The best description of reciprocal inhibition or systematic desensitization therapy as an approach to stuttering is by Brutten.[49]

Hypnosis

Hypnosis can have a positive impact on the reduction of fear and anxiety in the stutterer. The power of suggestion itself may give the stutterer the confidence he or she needs to reduce dysfluency. Limited research on the effect of hypnosis treatments is available,[91] and long-term treatment effects are unknown.

Drug Treatments

Many different drugs have been used to decrease the severity of stuttering.[1] In particular, the drug haloperidol has been shown to have some effect in reducing the severity of the stuttering,[92] but not the overall frequency.[7] Because of the significant side effects of this drug, many patients are reported to "drop out" of treatment.[1]

Efficacy of Treatment

Almost any of the treatments for stuttering have been able to demonstrate fairly dramatic short-term treatment effects. The nemesis of stuttering therapy has been long-term maintenance of treatment gains. In a review of available treatment literature, Martin estimated that about one-third of the patients achieved and maintained satisfactory fluency, one-third responded to treatment positively, but experienced significant regression, and one-third either did not respond to treatment or dropped out.[93] After reviewing several 5-year follow-up studies, Silverman suggests that the rate of relapse is probably between 40 and 90 percent.[94] Although these estimates are probably an accurate summary of the combined data, they may or may not reflect the success of a particular program. Also, the definition of a "success" varies depending on the perspective of the program. For example, some program evaluations include attitude data, whereas others do not. The treatment evaluation data for individual programs will be discussed next with the full understanding that in many instances comparison is inappropriate.

The data on the long-term effectiveness of the stuttering modification approach are mainly provided by Van Riper.[95] The long-term outcome data on stuttering modification approaches suggest that 50 percent of the patients maintain a high level of fluency and are essentially free of avoidance and fear over a five-year follow-up period.[95] Unfortunately, these data are based primarily on patient self-report and informal observation and are dated in comparison to evaluations of effectiveness of other treatment approaches.

The most effective of the fluency shaping treatments for stuttering involve some form of prolonged speech.[22,96] Andrews et al report that the average stutterer enters his or her intensive prolonged speech program with 14 percent of his or her syllables stuttered and by the end of treatment exhibits 0.0 percent of syllables stuttered during overt recording of speech.[22] Covert samples are slightly higher immediately after treatment, but the size of the difference between covert and overt recordings decreases such that statistical differences do not persist past the sixth month. Approximately 18 to 24 months posttreatment, the stutterer exhibits an average of 1 to 2 percent of syllables stuttered. Five-year follow-up data were not found. After treatment, the patients regard themselves as stutterers who can control their fluency, not as normal speakers. Even with a maintenance program, some experience significant relapse and require additional treatment. The quality of their speech is close to normal, but can be detected as different from normal speech.

Syllable timed speech is less frequently used as a fluency establishment technique than it was 10 years ago. Cheasman suggests that the change from syllable timed speech to prolonged speech was based primarily on the higher maintenance of fluency found using prolonged speech.[69] Also, patients' dissatisfaction with the sound of their speech when using this technique probably was associated with poor transfer and maintenance. Most studies report improvements in speech following programs using a metronome.[97,98] However, Silverman reports that the effects decreased over time and were absent by the third year.[99] Other studies report maintenance of gains over time, but either their follow-up interval is too short or the follow-up period is so broad that it is difficult to interpret the data.[7]

Controlled and clinically reliable supporting research for auditory masking devices is lacking. Current data suggest only that the device may work in reducing dysfluency for some subjects.[100] Criteria describing which subjects might benefit from the use of masking devices have yet to be identified. We would agree with Ingham[7] that auditory masking may have limited clinical value.

The data on the effect of airflow programs is also unimpressive. Ladouceur et al examined effectiveness of the Regulated-Breathing Method and report pretreatment data of 11.5 percent syllables stuttered along with immediate posttreatment data of 5.6 percent.[101] Two months after treatment, the mean had increased to 8.4 percent, and the treatment gains were primarily lost. These results are less optimistic than the data provided by Azrin and colleagues.[72,73] Andrews and Tanner [102] evaluated an airflow therapy similar to Schwartz's[71] and found that stutterers demonstrated a 90 percent reduction in stuttering frequency during treatment, but that within a year all six subjects relapsed. By month 12, there was no longer a statistical significance between the pre- and posttreatment data.

Data on the effectiveness of biofeedback therapy are positive but limited. Guitar investigated subjects' ability to reduce EMG feedback from different electrode placements on different stutterers.[89] Results for the one subject who received the full treatment program indicated stuttering had completely disappeared up to 1 year after therapy. Studies by Lanyon have also reported marked improvement related to the use of EMG feedback.[103,104] Problems in research design and the small number of subjects involved suggest the need for more research.

Reciprocal inhibition therapy is usually one part of a larger treatment program based on the two-factor theory of stuttering.[105,106] The findings related to the effectiveness of this treatment are generally positive. However, this treatment is reported to reduce stuttering, not eliminate it, and long-term follow-up data are lacking.[7]

Studies investigating the effect of reinforcement as the primary treatment variable have indicated that reinforcement alone does reduce stuttering, but usually does not completely eliminate it.[107,108] Treatments using the combination of reinforcement and punishment have not yielded better results than those obtained from administering either condition separately.[7] Follow-up data are also lacking.

SUMMARY

There continues to be many unresolved issues in both the etiology and management of stuttering. Currently, intensive research is focused on the physiology of stuttering, and hopefully the issue of brain and neuromuscular function will yield fruitful developments in the near future. The trend in recent years has been to use instrumented approaches to look at basic physiologic parameters of stutterers and stuttering. Continued work in this area may lead to a formation or reformulation of theory.

Continued investigation into the nonstuttered speech of stutterers both in terms of etiology (theory) and evaluation of treatment is another area that deserves attention.

Although something is known about the effectiveness of treatment packages such as prolonged speech, little is known about the contribution of the individual components to the overall success of the program.[109] Currently, treatment programs often incorporate many different components. Continued clinical research is needed in order to further delineate those components that are truly necessary and those that are not. Cost effectiveness and scheduling issues are related to these clinical questions. For example, specifically, if or in what way intensive programs are better than nonintensive programs is unknown. According to Andrews et al,[22] the primary variable may be the total number of hours in therapy. The importance of the scheduling of these hours is not clear.

The measurement of attitude, the need to treat it, and the way to treat it are still unresolved questions. There are authors who suggest that because attitude and dysfluency vary independently, the clinician should consider working directly on negative feelings and attitudes.[62] Others do not appear to be convinced that the data indicate a need to address attitudes separately from fluency.[22,84,110] Resolution of this issue would certainly benefit clinicians and may also contribute to the formulation of a comprehensive theory.

The discussion of attitude leads to the topic of outcome measures in general. Currently, there is a trend toward the incorporation of more than just stuttering counts and speech rate data as outcome measures. Bloodstein suggests the need to include data on the attitude of the patient toward communication and self-concept.[1] Bloodstein,[1] Ingham and Costello,[111] and Onslow and Ingham[65] argue for the need to incorporate speech quality data. As the measurement of "speech quality" develops, it will be interesting to see what parameters of quality (natural, normal) are deemed to be appropriate for scaling. In addition, the relationship between ratings of quality and variables, such as relapse and attitude, may well prove enlightening.

As has always been true, maintenance of fluent speech is still an issue. There remains a paucity of data demonstrating effective treatment procedures for maintaining fluent speech over long-term (5 years) periods. Research that develops maintenance technology and/or identifies characteristics of those stutterers who do maintain treatment gains should continue to be a high priority.

Finally, we want to mention again the fact that acquired stuttering in both neurogenic and psychogenic types is a real clinical entity, and clinicians who treat adults would do well to familiarize themselves with the literature. Unfortunately, the literature on psychogenic acquired stuttering in particular is limited. Further attention to these patients and publication of differential diagnostic and treatment information are needed.

REFERENCES

1. Bloodstein D. A handbook on stuttering. Chicago: National Easter Seal Society, 1981.
2. Van Riper C. The treatment of stuttering. Englewood Cliffs, NJ: Prentice-Hall, 1973.
3. Orton ST. A physiological theory of reading disability and stuttering in children. New Engl J Med 1928; 199:1045–1052.
4. Travis LE. Speech pathology. New York: Appleton-Century, 1931.
5. Johnson W. The Indians have no word for it. I. Stuttering in children. Q J Speech 1944; 30:330–337.
6. Van Riper C. The Nature of stuttering. Englewood Cliffs, NJ: Prentice-Hall, 1982.
7. Ingham RJ. Stuttering and behavior therapy: current status and experimental foundations. San Diego: College-Hill Press, 1984.
8. Shames GH, Rubin H. Stuttering: then and now. Columbus: Charles E Merrill, 1986.
9. Johnson W. Measurements of oral reading and speaking rate and disfluency of adult male and female stutterers and nonstutterers. J Speech Hear Disord Monogr [Suppl] 1961; 1-20.
10. Boehmler RM. Listener responses to non-fluencies. J Speech Hear Res 1958; 1:132–141.
11. Huffman ES, Perkins WH. Dysfluency characteristics identified by listeners on "stuttering" and "stutterer." J Commun Disord 1974; 7:89–96.
12. Young MA. Identification of stuttering and stutterers. In: Curlee RF, Perkins WH, eds. Nature and treatment of stuttering: new directions. San Diego: College-Hill Press, 1984.
13. Bjerkan B. Word fragmentations and repetitions in the spontaneous speech of 2–6 year old children. J Fluency Disord 1980; 5:137–148.
14. Hegde MN, Hartman DE. Factors affecting judgements of fluency. I. Interjections. J Fluency Disord 1979; 4:1–11.
15. Hegde MN, Hartman DE. Factors affecting judgements of fluency. II. Word repetitions. J Fluency Disord 1979; 4:13–22.
16. World Health Organization. Manual of the international statistical classification of diseases, injuries and causes of death. Vol. 1. Geneva: World Health Organization, 1977.
17. Perkins WH. The problem of definition: commentary on stuttering. J Speech Hear Disord 1983; 48:246–249.
18. Martin RR, Haroldson S. Stuttering as involuntary loss of speech control: barking up a new tree. J Speech Hear Disord 1986; 51:187–190.
19. Perkins WH. Stuttering as a categorical event: barking up the wrong tree: reply to Wingate. J Speech Hear Disord 1984; 49:430–434.
20. Perkins WH. More bite for a bark: epilogue to Martin and Haroldson's letter. J Speech Hear Disord 1986; 51:190–191.
21. Wingate ME. Definition is the problem. J Speech Hear Disord 1984; 49:430–431.
22. Andrews G, Craig A, Feyer A, Hoddinott S, Howie P, Nielson M. Stuttering: a review of research findings and theories circa 1982. J Speech Hear Disord 1983; 48:226–245.
23. Andrews G, Harris M. The syndrome of stuttering. Clin Dev Med 1964; 17.
24. Andrews G. The epidemiology of stuttering. In: Curlee RJ, Perkins WH, ed. Nature and treatment of stuttering: new directions. San Diego: College-Hill Press, 1984:1.
25. Curlee RF, Perkins WH. Nature and treatment of stuttering. San Diego: College-Hill Press, 1984.
26. Moore WH. Central nervous system characteristics of stutterers. In: Curlee RF, Perkins WH, eds. Nature and treatment of stuttering: new directions. San Diego: College-Hill Press, 1984:49.
27. Rosenfield D, Jerger J. Stuttering and auditory function. In: Curlee RF, Perkins WH, eds. Nature and treatment of stuttering: new directions. San Diego: College-Hill Press, 1984.
28. Jones RK. Observations on stammering after localized cerebral injury. J Neurol Neurosurg Psychiatry 1966; 29:192–195.
29. Andrew G, Quinn P, Sorby W. Stuttering: an investigation into cerebral dominance for speech. J Neurol Neurosurg Psychiatry 1972; 25:414–448.
30. Adams MR. Laryngeal onset and reaction time of stutterers. In: Curlee RJ, Perkins WH, eds. Nature and treatment of stuttering: new directions. San Diego: College-Hill Press, 1984:89.
31. Freeman FF. Laryngeal muscle activity of stutterers. In: Curlee RF, Perkins WH, eds. Nature and treatment of stuttering: new directions. San Diego: College-Hill Press, 1984:104.
32. Conture EG. Observing laryngeal movements of stuttering. In: Curlee RF, Perkins WH, eds. Nature and treatment of

stuttering: new directions. San Diego: College:Hill Press, 1984:116.

33. Zimmerman G. Articulatory behavior associated with stuttering: a cinefluorographic analysis. J Speech Hear Res 1980; 23(1):95–107.
34. Zimmerman G. Articulatory dynamics of fluent utterances of stutterers and nonstutterers. J Speech Hear Res 1980; 23(1):108–121.
35. Zimmerman G. Articulatory dynamics of stutterers. In: Curlee RF, Perkins WH, eds. Nature and treatment of stuttering: new directions. San Diego: College-Hill Press, 1984:131.
36. Wingate ME. Speaking unassisted comments on a paper by Andrews et al. J Speech Hear Disord 1983; 48(3):255–263.
37. Westby CE. Language performance of stuttering and nonstuttering children. J Commun Disord 1979; 12:133–145.
38. Wall NJ. A comparison of syntax in young stutterers and nonstutterers. J Fluency Disord 1980; 5:345–352.
39. Kidd KK. Stuttering as a genetic disorder. In: Curlee RF, Perkins WH, eds. Nature and treatment of stuttering: new directions. San Diego: College-Hill Press, 1984:149.
40. Prins D. Personality, stuttering severity, and age. J of Speech Hear Res 1972; 15:148–154.
41. Meyers FL, Wall MJ. Toward an integrated approach to early childhood stuttering. J Fluency Disord 1982; 1:47–54.
42. Riley GD, Riley J. Motoric and linguistic variables among children who stutter: a factor analysis. J Speech Hear Disord 1980; 45:504–515.
43. Baumgartner JM, Duffy JR. Adult onset stuttering: psychogenic and/or neurogenic. Paper presented at American Speech, Language and Hearing Association Convention, Detroit, 1986.
44. Deal JL. Sudden onset of stuttering: a case report. J Speech Hear Disord 1982; 47:301–304.
45. Helm-Estabrooks N. Diagnosis and management of neurogenic stuttering in adults. In: St. Louis KO, ed. The atypical stutterer: principles and practices of rehabilitation. San Diego: Academic Press, 1986:193.
46. Rosenbek JC. Stuttering secondary to central nervous system damage. In: Curlee RF, Perkins WH, eds. Nature and treatment of stuttering: new directions. San Diego: College-Hill, 1984.
47. Riley GD. A stuttering severity instrument for children and adults. J Speech Hear Disord 1972; 37:314–322.
48. Costello JM, Ingham RJ. Assessment strategies for stuttering. In: Curlee RF, Perkins WH, eds. Nature and treatment of stuttering: new directions. San Diego: College-Hill, 1984:303.
49. Brutten GJ. Stuttering: topography, assessment and behavior change. In: Eisenson J, ed. Stuttering: a second symposium. New York: Harper & Row, 1975:199.
50. Williams DE. Differential diagnosis of disorders of fluency. In: Darley FL, Spriestarsbach DC, eds. Diagnostic methods in speech pathology. New York: Harper & Row, 1978:409.
51. Guitar B. Pretreatment factors associated with the outcome of stuttering therapy. J Speech Hear Res 1976; 19:590–600.
52. Guitar B, Bass C. Stuttering therapy: the relationships between attitude change and long term outcome. J Speech Hear Disord 1978; 43:392–400.
53. Cox MD. The psychologically maladjusted stutterer. In: St. Louis KO, ed. The atypical stutterer: principles and practices of rehabilitation. San Diego: Academic Press, 1986:93.
54. Woolf G. The assessment of stuttering as struggle, avoidance, and expectancy. Br J Disord Commun 1967; 2:158–171.
55. Hanson BR, Gronhovd KD, Rice PL. A shortened version of the SIU-SSC for identification of speech-related anxiety. J Fluency Disord 1981; 6:351–360.
56. Andrews G, Cutler J. Stuttering therapy: the relation between changes in symptom level and attitudes. J Speech Hear Disord 1974; 39:312–319.
57. Erickson RL. Assessing communication attitudes among stutterers. J Speech Hear Res 1969; 12:711–724.
58. Adams MR, Runyan CM. Stuttering and fluency: exclusive events or points on a continuum. J Fluency Disord 1981; 6:197–218.
59. Martin RR, Haroldson SK, Triden KA. Stuttering and speech naturalness. J Speech Hear Disord 1984; 49:53–58.
60. Adams MR. Fluency, nonfluency and stuttering in children. J Fluency Disord 1982; 7:171–185.
61. Hegde MN. Fluency and fluency disorders: their definition, measurement and modification. J Fluency Disord 1978; 3:51–71.
62. Guitar B, Peters T. Stuttering: an integration of contemporary therapies. Memphis: Speech Foundation of America, 1980.
63. Sheehan JG. Stuttering: research and therapy. New York: Harper & Row, 1970.
64. Perkins WH. Techniques for establishing fluency. In: Perkins WH, ed. Stuttering disorders. New York: Thieme-Stratton, 1984:173.
65. Onslow M, Ingham R. Speech quality measurement and the management of stuttering. J Speech Hear Disord 1987; 52(1):2–17.
66. Shames GH, Florence C. Stutter-free speech: a goal of therapy. Columbus: Charles E Merrill, 1980.
67. Ingham RJ, Andrews G. Details of a token economy stuttering therapy program for adults. Aust Hum Commun Disord 1973; 1:13–20.
68. Webster RL. The precision fluency shaping program: speech reconstruction for stutterers. Roanoke, VA: Hollins Communication Research Institute, 1974.
69. Cheasman C. Therapy for adults: an evaluation of current techniques for establishing fluency. In: Dalton P, ed. Approaches to the treatment of stuttering. London: Croom Helm, 1983:76.
70. Perkins WH, Bell J, Johnson L, Stocks J. Phoneme rate and the effective planning time hypothesis of stuttering. J Speech Hear Res 1979; 22:747–755.
71. Schwartz MF. Stuttering solved. New York: McGraw-Hill, 1976.
72. Azrin N, Nunn R. A rapid method of eliminating stuttering by a regulated breathing approach. Behav Res Ther 1974; 12:279–286.
73. Azrin N, Nunn R, Frantz S. Comparison of regulated-breathing versus abbreviated desensitization on reported stuttering episodes. J Speech Hear Disord 1979; 44:331–339.
74. Ingham RJ, Packman A. Treatment and generalization effects in an experimental treatment for a stutterer using contingency management and speech rate control. J Speech Hear Disord 1977; 42:394–407.
75. Boberg E, Kully D. Techniques for transforming fluency. In: Perkins WH, ed. Stuttering disorders. New York Thieme-Stratton, 1984:183.
76. Florance CL, Shames H. Stuttering treatments: issues in transfer and maintenance. In: Perkins WH, ed. Stuttering disorders. New York: Thieme-Stratton, 1984:189.
77. Stokes TF, Baer DM. An implicit technology of generalization. J Appl Behav Analysis 1977; 10:349–367.
78. Ingham RJ. Techniques for maintaining fluency. In: Perkins WH, ed. Stuttering disorders. New York: Thieme-Stratton, 1984:209.
79. Ingham RJ. Evaluation and maintenance in stuttering treatment: a search for ecstacy with nothing but agony. In: Boberg E, ed. Maintenance of fluency. New York: Elsevier, 1981.
80. Boberg E. Maintenance of fluency: proceedings of the Banff conference, 1979. New York: Elsevier, 1981.
81. Ingham RJ. The effects of self-evaluation training on main-

tenance and generalization during stuttering treatment. J Speech Hear Disord 1982; 47:271–280.
82. Hanna R, Owen N. Facilitating transfer and maintenance of fluency in stuttering therapy. J Speech Hear Disord 1977; 42:65–76.
83. Ingham RJ. Modification and maintenance and generalization during stuttering treatment. J Speech Hear Disord 1980; 23:733–745.
84. Ingham RJ. Comment on "stuttering therapy: the relation between attitude change and long-term outcome." Speech Hear Disord 1979; 44:397–400.
85. Mowrer D. An instructional program to increase fluent speech of stutterers. J Fluency Disord 1975; 1:25–35.
86. Costello JM. The establishment of fluency with time-out procedures: three case studies. J Speech Hear Disord 1975; 40:216–231.
87. Egolf D, Shames G, Seltzer H. The effects of time-out on the fluency of stutterers in group therapy. J Commun Disord 1971; 4:111–118.
88. Dewar A, Dewar A, Barnes H. Automatic triggering of auditory feedback masking on concomitant movements of stammering. Br J Disord Commun 1976; 11:95–102.
89. Guitar B. Reduction of stuttering frequency using analog electromyographic feedback. J Speech Hear Res 1975; 18:672–685.
90. Wolpe J. Psychotherapy by reciprocal inhibition. Palo Alto, CA: Stanford University Press, 1958.
91. Lockhart M, Robertson A. Hypnosis and speech therapy as a combined therapeutic approach to the problem of stammering: a study of thirty patients. Br J Disord Commun 1977; 12:97–108.
92. Prins D, Mandelkorn T, Cerf A. Principal and differential effects of haloperiodol and placebo treatments upon speech disfluencies in stutterers. J Speech Hear Res, 1980; 23:614–629.
93. Martin RR. Introduction and perspective: review of published studies. In: Boberg E, ed. Maintenance of fluency: proceedings of the Banff conference. New York: Elsevier, North Holland, 1981.
94. Silverman F. Relapse following stuttering therapy. In: Lass N, ed. Speech and language: advances in basic research and practice. New York: Academic Press, 1981.
95. Van Riper C. Experiments in stuttering therapy. In: Eisenson J, ed. Stuttering a symposium. New York: Harper & Row, 1958.
96. Andrews G, Guitar B, Howie P. Meta-analysis of the effects of stuttering treatment. Speech Hear Disord 1980; 45:287–307.
97. Brady J. Metronome conditioned speech retraining for stuttering. Behav Ther 1971; 2:129–150.
98. Silverman F, Trotter D. Impact of pacing speech with a miniature electronic metronome upon the manner in which a stutterer is perceived. Behav Ther 1973; 4:414–419.
99. Silverman F. Long term impact of a miniature metronomic on stuttering: an interium report. Percept Mot Skills 1976; 42:1322.
100. Ingham RJ, Southwood H, Horsburgh G. Some effects of the "Edinburgh masker" on stuttering during oral reading and spontaneous speech. J Fluency Disord 1981; 6:135–154.
101. Ladouceur R, Cote C, Lablond G, Bouchard L. Evaluation of regulated-breathing method and awareness training in the treatment of stuttering. J Speech Hear Disord 1982; 47:422–426.
102. Andrews G, Tanner S. Stuttering treatment: an attempt to replicate the regulated breathing method. J Speech Hear Disord 1982; 47:138–140.
103. Lanyon R. Effect of biofeedback based relaxation on stuttering during reading and spontaneous speech. J Consult Clin Psychol 1977; 45:860–866.
104. Lanyon R. Behavioral approaches to stuttering. In: Hersen M, Eisler R, Miller PM, eds. Progress in behavior modification. Vol. 6. New York: Academic Press, 1978:47.
105. Adams MR. The use of reciprocal inhibition procedures in the treatment of stuttering. J Commun Disord 1972; 5:59–66.
106. Brutten GJ. Stuttering: reflections on a two factor approach to behavior modifications. In: Gray BB, England RS, eds. Stuttering and the conditioning therapies. Monterey: Monterey Institute for Speech and Hearing, 1969:81.
107. Peters A. The effect of positive reinforcement on fluency: two case studies. Lang Speech Hear Serv Schools 1977; 8:15–22.
108. Rickard H, Mundy M. Direct manipulation on stuttering behavior: an experimental-clinical approach. In: Ullman LP, Kramer L, eds. Case studies in behavior modification. New York: Holt, Rinehart & Winston, 1965.
109. Hegde MN. Treatment of fluency disorders: state of the art. In: Costello J, ed. Speech disorders in adults: recent advances. San Diego: College-Hill Press, 1985:155.
110. Ryan B. Programmed therapy for stuttering children and adults. Springfield, IL: Charles Thomas, 1974.
111. Ingham RJ, Costello JM. Stuttering treatment outcome evaluation. In: Costello JM, ed. Speech disorders in adults. San Diego: College-Hill Press, 1985:189.

Language Disorders

22 Language Delay in the Child

Anne van Kleeck, Ph.D.
Alice Richardson, Ph.D.

The incredible diversity of individuals that constitute the population of children with delayed language development, although perhaps overwhelming, is not terribly surprising given both the complexity of language itself and the complexity of the other systems with which language development interacts. Children are growing, changing human beings who adapt to the communication demands of their individual environments in a variety of ways. The time of onset, the extent of the delay in language, and the aspects of language that are delayed affect these adaptations. Delayed language development may be the first symptom that anything is wrong with the child, and the clinician's job is to explore the reasons for that symptom and the implications for the child's development in language and in other areas. The characteristics manifested by four of the 3-year-olds with whom we are currently working illustrate the diversity among children with delayed language development:

Joey has normal intelligence, but a mild to moderate hearing loss, which was first aided at 18 months of age. His speech is rapid and difficult to understand, despite normal development of all the speech sounds. From age $2^1/_2$ to 3 years, the most striking characteristics of Joey's language were his echolalia and his limited ability to combine words into sentences. During this period, his behavior was marked by frequent temper tantrums, pronounced disobedience, and refusal to acknowledge or interact with his younger sibling. From age 3 to $3^1/_2$, echolalia decreased, but the majority of Joey's utterances were jargon supplemented by a few stereotypic sentences that appeared to have been learned as unanalyzed wholes. His compliance had improved, but his symbolic play skills were poor, and he did not interact with other children. At age $3^1/_2$, Joey's pattern of learning language through unanalyzed wholes persists, and his marked comprehension problems stand out because he typically fails to respond to questions and directives that he does not understand. Joey speaks in three- to four-word sentences, plays symbolically with toys, interacts with other children, and has begun to express his feelings verbally rather than acting them out behaviorally. His language comprehension and expression remain a year below age level.

Jennifer is also $3^1/_2$, but uses crying, gestures, and a few single words to communicate. Her language comprehension and expression are at approximately the 12-month level. Her range of performance on nonverbal cognitive tasks varies from the 14- to the 30-month levels, depending on the nature of the task. She has poor eye contact and a fleeting attention span. Her mother reports that she does not do anything at home unless it is her idea. Resistance to modelling and direction has been characteristic of her behavior during therapy sessions as well.

At age 3 years, Bobby has normal intelligence and hearing and good language comprehension, but has a year delay in expressive language development. He communicates with gestures and by positioning himself near an adult to signal that he wants the adult to start guessing what he wants. He then responds with a yes or no to the adult's questions. He rarely initiates conversation verbally, but is a willing responder. His spontaneous utterances are one to two words long and show marked phonologic difficulty. For example, he uses few bilabials, nasals, or fricatives in his speech. Oral motor control of the lips and tongue is good for imitative tasks.

Jonathan will be 3 in 2 months. He communicates by gesturing, using a few single words, and jabbering extensively in unintelligible jargon with an occasional string that sounds like a well-formed adult sentence. Although Jonathan would not cooperate for intelligence tests, he has had difficulty learning perceptual-motor problem solving tasks such as sorting and stringing beads. He has a history of chronic otitis media, but hearing sensitivity is within normal limits. His comprehension of what is said to him is extremely poor, and he follows only two to three simple commands.

How does one begin to construct a framework for assessing and providing remediation to language delayed children when the heterogeneity of the population is so great? Although the theories that the field of child language disorders borrows from offer a variety of answers on assessment and intervention, none of the theories addresses all of the critical questions successfully. The clinician is left with the task of picking and choosing among available theoretic perspectives or developing her or his own perspective. Most often clinicians borrow valuable components from several different theoretic orientations to create their own "eclectic" view. This borrowing is a necessary enterprise, both because no current theory addresses adequately all of the questions critical to assessment and intervention planning for the heterogeneous population of children with language delay and because each clinician must make explicit her or his own beliefs and assumptions about language learning and language delay. The potential problem with an eclectic theoretic frame is that elements of the theory may be inconsistent, incompatible, and eventually self-defeating.[1] For example, the clinician who believes that language develops from meaningful interactions with supportive and responsive others, but who trains language through drill and practice rewarded by tangible reinforcers, may realize the incompatibility of this theory and practice when the child fails to use the trained language interactively in her or his natural environment.

In providing this review of some of the major theories of language development and models of language disorders, we suggest that the perspectives we will discuss may be used as a series of lenses that the clinician may hold up in succession or in combinations to find those that give the clearest picture of the unique language delayed child under consideration. Although all of these perspectives have something to offer the clinician who is planning for assessment or intervention, different sets of lenses provide the best fit of theory with practice for different children. Although delayed language development may be the primary symptom noticed by those who refer the child for testing and intervention, the job of the interventionist is to identify each child's particular constellation of strengths and deficits so that the most appropriate treatment for each particular child may be planned. The theories and models to be discussed address many of the variables clinicians must consider in adapting to the needs of individual children. Integrating these variables into a coherent framework for addressing the individual needs and differences of each language delayed child is the clinician's task for the future. The purpose of this chapter is to provide a preliminary framework for understanding how to plan for each child's individual needs, to discuss how current theories of language acquisition and disorders contribute valuable insights at various stages in the planning process, and to provide specific examples of the contributions our theoretic bases make to assessment and intervention planning. In addition, because of the dangers inherent in borrowing from a variety of theoretic perspectives, we will offer suggestions for testing the compatibility of components of a treatment plan for any particular child.

In this chapter, we will first present a brief overview of the assessment and intervention planning process. Next we will discuss the major theories and models that have influenced the field of language intervention, and we will consider the implications and contributions of each for conducting a language assessment, for selecting what we work on (the goals of intervention), and for choosing how to facilitate those goals (the procedures for intervention). Once we have done this, we will consider how many simultaneously held beliefs might interact to influence our selection of goals and procedures and how they might be integrated into a theoretically compatible perspective for dealing with language delayed children's individual differences.

ASSESSING AND PLANNING FOR INDIVIDUAL NEEDS

To continue the analogy of lenses for viewing the language delayed child, conceptualize the process of planning as one of viewing the child with successive levels of magnification. Five such levels are critical to language assessment and intervention (see Table 22–1). The levels are comparable to allowing our lens to zoom in more and more directly on the child's specific strengths and weaknesses, and then zoom back out as we consider how the specific difficulties we have identified affect each other and the functioning of the whole child. At the first level, an intersystem analysis level, the goal is to see the whole child and to develop an overview of the child's functioning in each domain of his or her life. These domains include the child's linguistic system, cognitive system, social system, and physical system. To achieve this overview, one must be clear about what one is looking for within each of these systems. An example of one way these systems might be viewed is presented in Table 22–2. At the intersystem analysis level, our questions ask which systems are intact and which require further evaluation.

At the second level of magnification, an intrasystem analysis level, one examines in great detail each of the impaired subsystems. This process must occur for every impaired subsystem, and language

TABLE 22–1 Levels in the Process of Assessment and Intervention Planning

	Level	Purpose	Assessment and Intervention Questions
Zoom In	Intersystem analysis	To obtain an overview of the whole child and the child's life situation To identify the systems to be assessed	Which systems are intact? Which systems require further evaluation?
	Intrasystem analysis	To identify specific areas of impairment	Which areas require intervention?
	Developmental	To compare the child to normal developmental sequence data For each impaired area, to identify the child's stage within a developmental sequence To identify the child's expected next step in each area of impairment	Is the child following a normal developmental sequence within each area of impairment? What is the next step the child might be expected to take in each impaired area?
Zoom Out	Intrasystem interaction	To examine each impaired area in relation to the larger system it is a part of	What impact does the impaired area have on the rest of the system? What effect might the rest of the system have on remediation of the impaired area?
	Intersystem interaction	To examine each impaired area in relation to the other systems that make up the whole child	How does the impaired area affect the child's overall development? How should the child be taught? What should the contexts for intervention be?

clinicians work with several other professionals in examining systems other than the linguistic system. An example of the areas that might be explored when examining the form and content subsystems at an intrasystem level is provided in Table 22–3. Questions at this level focus on the areas that may require intervention.

The third level of examination, the developmental level, maintains an intrasystem focus, but adds the dimension of developmental sequence. It involves comparing the child with whatever developmental information is available in order to specify the order or sequence of development for the areas

TABLE 22–2 Systems to Consider in Intersystem Analysis

Linguistic System	*Cognitive System*
Form Phonology Grammar Content Use Communicative intent Discourse	Level of functioning Concept formation Reasoning and problem solving Learning style Information processing Achievement
Social System	***Physical System***
Self-help skills Nonverbal communication Play Interaction skills Emotional/behavioral factors Environmental factors	Gross motor skills Fine motor skills Hearing Vision Sensory integration Neurologic integrity

of primary impairment. This level is pivotal for planning because the focus begins to shift from assessment for diagnostic purposes to assessment for intervention planning. For example, the questions asked at this level are, where is the child in the normal developmental sequence for this skill or area and what is the next logical step?

Once a fine-grained picture of the child has been obtained in each area, the process of magnification reverses. One must reconsider each of the areas requiring intervention within the system it is a part of. We call this fourth level an intrasystem interaction level because we are still concerned with the impaired subsystem, but we now consider it in relation to the larger system of which it is a part. For example, if limited verb vocabulary has been identified as delayed and requiring intervention, how does the child's learning of verb vocabulary interact with other aspects of the child's linguistic system, that is, with other lexical development? With syntactic development at the clause, phrase, and morphologic levels? With the child's ability to sustain conversation? This fourth level, where the interaction among areas is explored, somewhat alleviates the anguish sometimes experienced at the intrasystem analysis level when the clinician tries to neatly segment complex behaviors into component areas. For example, deciding whether a child's difficulty with understanding questions is more of a lexical (wh- words), grammatic (S-V inversion), or discourse phenomenon may be difficult. This difficulty arises because all of these aspects (as well as others such as cog-

TABLE 22–3 Intrasystem Analysis of Form and Content

Form	*Content*
Phonology	Semantic roles and relations
Phonetic inventory by word position	Word knowledge and use
Percentage correct use of phonetic inventory	Vocabulary
Phonologic processes	Lexical diversity by part of speech
Word shapes	Word retrieval
Favorite/avoided sounds	Synonyms
Effects of phonetic context	Antonyms
Intelligibility	Definitions
Prosody	Multiple meanings
	Idiomatic expressions
Grammar	Question comprehension
Mean length of utterance	Wh- questions
Word level	Perceptual-language complexity[2]
14 grammatical morphemes	Language concepts
Prefixes and suffixes	
Phrase level	
Noun phrase elaboration	
Verb phrase elaboration	
Clause level	
Sentence patterns	
Sentence transformation	
Complex sentences	
Conjunctions	

nitive complexity) are involved.[2] At the intrasystem analysis level each of these aspects is examined separately. At the intrasystem interaction level each is examined in relationship to the others. Kirchner and Skarakis-Doyle argue that "communication should be considered as a dynamic system comprised of inseparable parts which directly influence each other and the system as a whole."[3] Examining intrasystem interaction allows the clinician to reexplore each aspect of the system as it relates to other aspects and to the whole.

The fifth and final level involves exploring interactions at an intersystem level. How can the area requiring intervention affect or be affected by the other domains of functioning? For the verb vocabulary need mentioned before, the clinician must first ask how the child's cognitive skills (e.g., cognitive stage, knowledge of the world, attention, memory, etc.), social skills (e.g., peer interaction, parent-child interaction, self-concept, etc.), and physical abilities (e.g., hearing, oral motor control, gross motor skills, etc.) affect the teaching of verb vocabulary; and second, she or he must ask how the child's verb vocabulary development has affected or will affect functioning in these other areas. Questions at this intersystem interaction level involve how the identified problems affect overall development, what strengths might be used for compensation or instruction purposes, what the contexts for intervention should be, and how the child should be taught.

With this five-stage model of the assessment and intervention process in mind, we will next examine the major theories of language acquisition and models of language disorders that have influenced the field of child language intervention. After a brief summary of each theory or model, we will consider the perspective it provides for viewing the language delayed child and the levels of the planning process at which it has the most to offer. Then we will reverse our perspective and examine how a language delay affects other aspects of development, and the implications of these findings for assessment and intervention planning. An overview of the topics to be covered is provided in Table 22–4.

THEORIES OF LANGUAGE ACQUISITION

Theories of language acquisition differ in the degree to which they consider that either innate (i.e., biologic) factors or the environment play a key role in learning language. Chomskyan linguistic theory lies at one extreme, touting that syntax is an innate

TABLE 22–4 Theories, Models, and Roles of Language in Development that Interact to Determine Language Assessment and Intervention

Theories of Language Disorders	*Models of Language Disorders*	*Role of Language in Development*
Nativism	Medical	Developing and maintaining social relationships
Cognitive bases	Processing	Developing self-concept
Social bases	Descriptive	Academic success
Operant learning		

skill, the development of which is merely "triggered" by environmental input. Learning theory is at the opposite extreme, positing great importance to environmental antecedents and consequences in the development process.[4]

These extreme theories have been dubbed by George Miller as either "impossible" (learning theory) or "miraculous" (nativism).[5] It is not surprising that they have spurred the development of more moderate theories on the role of nature and nurture in language development. We shall refer to these theories, which allow for an interaction between the child and the environment in guiding development, as the cognitive and social theories. Recently, Katherine Nelson's work on event knowledge has attempted to marry the cognitive and social theories into one theoretic framework, and her work will be discussed as a bridge between the two.[6] Table 22–5 depicts this continuum of theories. Although learning theory has few advocates in the 1980s as a theory of language development, it continues to have great impact upon some language intervention. The other theories are all alive and well in various incarnations.

In the following, we will briefly explain these theories (summarized in Table 22–5) and the critical questions related to intervention with language delayed children that they address. Since the majority were not developed specifically to deal with language intervention or language delay, we will also identify the elements language interventionists have found beneficial to borrow from each theory in their efforts to adapt to individual children's needs.

Operant Learning Theory

In Skinner's account of operant learning, language, like all behavior, is explained using the doctrines of behaviorism.[4] That is, the input from and reaction of the environment explain learning. The sequence of events in any learning situation includes an original stimulus (discriminative stimulus), a response to that stimulus, and then an outcome (reinforcing stimulus). Favorable outcomes (positive reinforcers) increase the likelihood that future occurrences of the discriminative stimulus result in the same response, and unfavorable outcomes decrease that likelihood. The operant learning lens for viewing language delayed children focuses on determining (1) what is reinforcing and punishing for a particular child and (2) how the child responds to a situation structured entirely by the adult. For example, in observing parent-child interaction the clinician would want to determine the natural contingencies that the parent uses to reinforce (either positively or negatively) the child's communicative attempts.

Operant learning theory does not suggest which domains of behavior should be assessed or which skills within a domain to explore. As such it is not helpful in diagnosis or in goal selection. Any behavior that is overtly observable and hence measurable may be targeted. The techniques of operant learning can be applied to absolutely any skill area (e.g., syntax, vocabulary, answering questions) or any "problem" area interfering with learning language (e.g., lack of eye contact, failure to attend) that can be operationally defined by discrete, observable behavior. Operant learning theory also does not suggest developmental sequences to follow in the determination of the skills that have been mastered and the next steps to implement.

The power of operant learning theory lies in its contribution toward procedures for intervention. It suggests breaking complex behaviors into small manageable steps that allow the child to achieve and maintain success; it provides a technology for increasing the frequency of the desired behavior and for decreasing undesirable behaviors. An example of this technology in intervention contexts is when a "token economy" is set up: the child receives intrinsically unrewarding but concrete reinforcers (such as plastic chips, blocks, or check marks on a paper) that are periodically exchanged for back-up reinforcers that are rewarding for the individual child (such as stickers, little toys, getting to play a favorite game). The child earns token reinforcers for correct responses on a predetermined schedule (every time, every *n*th time, randomly) and either does not receive a reinforcer or is forced to forfeit a reinforcer when her

TABLE 22–5 Theories of Language Acquisition

Strong role for biology ←——————————→ *Strong role for environment*

Nativism	Cognitive theories	Event knowledge	Social theories	Operant learning theory
	Piagetian theory Component skills model Information processing theory		Transactional learning theory Social learning theory	

or his response is not the desired one. Many additional techniques for increasing or decreasing the strength of a behavior are specified in operant conditioning technology.[7] A criterion for success is explicitly established, and so, for example, a child may be required to produce nine out of ten correct target responses before the clinician considers the goal to have been met. Although operant learning techniques can be effective in altering specified behaviors in trained contexts, their failure to achieve generalization to untrained contexts is becoming more widely recognized, and many interventionists are turning to more naturalistic procedures for this reason.[8]

Another contribution operant learning theory has made to procedures for language intervention is its tools for measuring treatment effectiveness and for comparing the effects of different treatments. Single-subject research designs have been employed extensively in the behavioral literature and offer clinicians a way to look at each child individually as they examine the effects of treatment.[9] Such tools are critical for dealing with heterogeneous populations such as children with language delay. Although single-subject designs such as multiple baseline and alternating treatments are most useful in the examination of behaviors that can be brought easily under stimulus control (as opposed to behaviors that are learned, cumulative, and interact in complex ways with the child's entire system), they have been extremely useful to our field so far and point us in the direction of developing similar tools for measuring learning of more complex behaviors in individual language delayed children.[10]

Nativism

Chomsky's well-known view of language development, which developed in response to the learning theory view, is that children are born with a special capacity to derive the structural rules of grammar. This innate linguistic knowledge (sometimes called the language acquisition device) consists in part of the basic grammatic categories and relationships that are universal to all languages. The language acquisition device relies only remotely on environmental experience and is not related to other learning processes, such as cognition.

The nativist perspective offers little to the identification of delay across the variety of domains that interact with language, but it does provide a detailed view of the linguistic system itself. Specifically, it provides tools for the intrasystem analysis of the syntax of the language. Language assessment has been influenced by nativism more because of the syntactic focus of the theory than because of how the theory explains development. As McLean notes, "it got us beyond the phoneme as a clinical preoccupation and also allowed us to quantify deficits in language through application of syntactic measures."[11] The influence of Chomskyan theory on goals selected for intervention has been especially strong. A large percentage of the language intervention studies reported in the literature in the past 10 years have focused on the training of syntax. In addition to its emphasis on syntax, Bruner states that nativist theory has "turned attention to the problem of rule learning, even if it concentrated only on syntactic rules."[12] Duchan discusses this step in the assessment process as attempting to determine underlying rules that are generating surface behaviors.[13] Ingram has reported a more detailed procedure for assessing productivity specifically in early syntactic development (i.e., assuring that forms are generated by an underlying grammar and are not just rote).[14] In intervention, we have applied nativist theory by focusing on syntax and teaching in such a way as to foster the child's induction of syntactic rules.

Although providing us with goals, Chomskyan theory leaves us empty-handed regarding procedures. Lacking the ability to rewire faulty language acquisition devices, the language specialist, espousing a pure form of the innate hypothesis, would find little other direction for how to teach or facilitate language development since the theory downplays the role of the environment in language learning. This theory also fails to account for the interactions that occur among components of the linguistic system. Dissatisfied with the examination of syntax in isolation from the rest of the linguistic system, some recent research and intervention efforts have begun to explore more fully the interaction between syntax and semantics, pragmatics and phonology.[14,15] For example, phonologic interventions have begun to emphasize early work on those phonemes that also carry grammatic information, such as /s/ and final clusters.[16]

Cognitive Theories

Numerous theories developed subsequent to Chomsky's notions on an innate language acquisition device have considered language learning not as an entirely unique process, but as part of learning in general. Piaget's theory has had by far the strongest impact on cognitive explanations of language development. However, models of cognition that consider component skills and information processing are also relevant to discussions of language and communication development. Furthermore, Katherine

Nelson's recent formulation of "event knowledge" contains a strong cognitive component, as well as acknowledging the role of social interaction in language development. It provides a bridge between the cognitive theories to be discussed in this section and the social theories to be discussed next. Because Nelson emphasizes cognitive aspects of event knowledge, we will discuss the theory she developed with her colleagues in this section.

Piagetian Theory

Although Piaget himself said little about language development, his work in cognitive development had a great impact on many language development theorists in the 1970s. This view proposes that children learn first about the world (cognition) and then learn to convey their ideas through language. The ideas about the world they develop prior to learning language are conveyed through the early semantic relations discussed originally by Bloom and Brown.[17,18] Furthermore, to develop "true" (displacable) language at all, children first need to develop the ability to think symbolically: a hallmark of Piaget's sensorimotor stage of development, occurring at about 18 months of age.

The universals needed to develop language are cognitive and not specifically linguistic. The system is semantically driven, in that children learn ideas and then learn to convey those ideas linguistically. Syntax is merely the vehicle for transmitting these meanings. Schlesinger recently put forth a weaker version of this theory by postulating that children continue to develop concepts by using language throughout the course of development (i.e., cognition does not always necessarily "come first").[19] Rice and Kemper discuss numerous possible relationships between language and cognition.[20]

At an intersystem analysis level, this approach has led interventionists to explore the cognitive abilities of language delayed children within a Piagetian frame.[21] The focus created by this approach is also exemplified in Lois Bloom's pioneering work, which moved the field of child language from its exclusive focus on syntax to also considering cognitive and semantic aspects of early language.[17,22] The clinical area that has been an outgrowth of this approach to language development is the assessment and subsequent facilitation of early semantic relations, such as agent-action, possessor-object possessed, and attribute-object.[23,24,25]

Piagetian theory also offers strong support for language intervention at the developmental level. The notions of sequential stages of development within domains and of the ordinal sequencing of skills are distinctively Piagetian. Such stage and ordinal scale information helps interventionists identify where in a normal developmental sequence the language delayed child falls behind and what the developmentally most appropriate next steps might be.

At the intersystem interaction level, researchers have explored the cognitive precursors to language skills—both prelinguistically and throughout early language development. Prelinguistically, this exploration has involved a focus on Piaget's sensorimotor domains of imitation skills, knowledge of means-end relationships, and the related areas of object permanence (knowing that objects continue to exist when out of sight) and symbolic function (being able to "hold in mind" nonpresent objects and events). During intervention, the clinician may attempt to facilitate the development of cognitive precursors not yet acquired by the child prior to attempting to focus on language goals per se. Owens provides an excellent summary of research to date on the relationship of the various sensorimotor cognitive domains to early linguistic achievements.[26] After language development has begun, the clinician may assess (and later teach) cognitive concepts, such as time and space, believed to underlie and hence be prerequisite to the child's production of the linguistic forms encoding these concepts.

Piagetian theory does not directly advocate specific procedures for teaching concepts to children. As Duckworth explains, from this theoretic perspective you "document a child's unaided development; you don't intervene."[27] In fact, Piagetian theory views the child as "self-pedagogic" if the right environmental stimulation is provided. The adult's role is limited to providing the right opportunities for learning to take place spontaneously. The title of Duckworth's 1979 article sums up this stance—"Either we're too early and they can't learn it or we're too late and they know it already: the dilemma of 'applying Piaget.'" Duckworth states that this dilemma is false, yet she seems to agree with it when she concludes that "left to their own rhythm and given the opportunity, children develop the basic frameworks as naturally as walking."[27] Unfortunately, this natural development is not so for many language delayed children.

The Component Skills Model

It is a fact of human development that many complex behaviors consist of the coordination of simpler behaviors. First the infant learns separately to look at interesting objects and to grasp them. Later, these skills are combined into the beginnings of eye-hand coordination. A failure to develop this skill might be attributed to either a visual problem, a motoric problem, or a general delay in the cognitive mechanism responsible for coordinating them. Similarly, breaking far more complex behaviors such as language into a set of component skills has an intuitive appeal, especially for those in the business of trying to facilitate the development of those complex behaviors.

The component skills model was originally applied to areas of communicative competence such as referential skills and the more general area of role-taking.[5,28,29] For example, in their review of the development of referential skills, Glucksberg et al concluded that "acquisition of the language itself may be a necessary condition but it is clearly insufficient. To language competence must be added component skills and processes . . . including knowledge of other persons, the ability to predict the potential effectiveness of messages, and the ability to provide alternative encodings when appropriate and necessary."[5]

More recently, a version of the component skills model has been applied specifically to language acquisition by Fischer and Corrigan.[30] These authors state that "language involves many different sets of skills, including vocalization (articulation, motor control, intonation, etc.), hearing, concepts to be talked about, social interactions, and much more. A skill analysis of language development in general would require an analysis of the many sets of skills in each of these domains and a determination of how the skills in each domain are combined with each other and with skills in other domains."

Although clearly endorsing the notion of component skills, these authors also integrate the idea that general processing limits "account for the overall course of development." In this respect, they have incorporated information processing theory (to be discussed in the next section) into their skill theory approach to language acquisition.

The component skills perspective does not focus on any particular domain of communication or behavior, since any complex task can be subdivided into simpler tasks. However, it does offer the clinician a powerful tool at the intrasystem analysis level: task analysis. The component skills perspective strongly emphasizes the need to understand the demands imposed by the tasks and the measurement instruments used to assess a child's language. This assessment is done by determining the particular skills the tasks require of a child. If it is possible to derive a model of subskills needed to perform a particular task (and the possibility has been questioned), then one would attempt to assess the various subcomponents individually when a child failed on the overall task.[31]

Another suggestion from the component skills orientation takes into account that task analyses may not always be feasible. Hence, an error in performance cannot be unambiguously interpreted as a specific subskill deficit. Furthermore, even an adequate performance cannot be taken as proof that the subskills are all intact, since as Fischer and Corrigan explain, "children may use very different strategies to produce superficially identical behaviors . . . [and] different strategies will involve different skills."[30] Because of this, we must obtain a "coherent pattern of performances" before meaningful interpretations can be made.[32] Thus the component skills model suggests that our assessment should provide collaborative evidence from several kinds of tasks before one draws conclusions about specific deficit areas.

The component skills model offers little in the way of developmental data to compare a language delayed child to, except within the specific content areas that have been empirically tested from this perspective, such as referential communication skills. The component skills model does emphasize the interaction among domains and among aspects of the domain under study; thus it encourages the clinician to look across the domain boundaries for component skills.

Procedures used in intervention from the component skills orientation might best be understood by example. Let us consider a school-age child's performance on word problems in math. Such a task requires the integration of a number of skills in both the linguistic and cognitive domains. To mention just a few of these, linguistically the child needs to know vocabulary related to math (number words, specialized math vocabulary) and must be able to understand complex, often unusual syntactic constructions. Cognitively, in order to understand number concepts and operations, the child must have a grasp of classification, seriation, conservation, spatial and temporal concepts, causality, and transitivity. In addition, word problems in math require abstract thinking and general organizational abilities. For a child having difficulty with these kinds of math problems, it may be fruitful to understand her or his errors by (1) attempting to determine which component skill areas the child is deficient in, (2) working on that area in "isolation," and (3) once the subskill has been mastered in an easier context, reintegrate it back into the overall task.

Although the word problem in math seems a viable enough application of this model, the reader should be aware of the assumptions the approach makes. According to Sharz, the model assumes that (1) a model of subskills needed to perform a particular task can be derived, (2) these skills can be "acquired and utilized independently of one another," and (3) errors or deficits in performance can be attributed to a deficit in one or more presumably isolable and measurable component skills.[31] Shatz questions the validity of these assumptions in building her case for an information-processing approach to communication.

Information-Processing Theory

The information-processing approach to cognitive development focuses on children's strategies for attending to, interpreting, and remembering their experiences. Human resources for carrying out this mental work are limited. Developmentally, "children are more subject to failure only because they have fewer means (i.e., well-learned techniques) for distributing their limited resources efficiently."[31] The general application of information-processing theory to work with language delayed children has led to an assessment and intervention focus on memory and attention. Recently, interest has also developed in assessing children's information-processing style and in exploring the implications of individual processing style differences for intervention.[33,34,35]

Specifically related to communication, Shatz critiqued the component skills approach to communication by suggesting that finding particular lacking skills is exceedingly hard. Moreover, it does not explain why children are likely to be variable in their display of a particular skill; that is, "skills found lacking in one experimental situation are often displayed in another."[31] Because of this variability, Shatz believes performance to be more a matter of information processing, that is, the amount of and type of mental work required to carry out the cognitive operations involved in successful communication.

At an intersystem analysis level, information-processing theory alerts one to the need to consider memory, attention, and (recently) processing style as one examines individual children's cognitive systems. A variety of tools have been developed for intrasystem analysis of the processing subsystems.[36,37]

Little is offered to interventionists in the way of sequences for the normal development of processing abilities. The developmental literature in this area has shifted more toward examination of the strategies children use to assist them with difficult processing tasks. This parallels a shift in intervention practices away from direct drill on memory (which seems to have little long-term effect on memory) and toward the identification and training of compensatory strategies.[38]

At the intrasystem interaction level, information-processing theory focuses on careful observation of how a child approaches tasks, rather than focusing entirely on accuracy of performance. From observing how processing factors interact with task performance, the clinician can determine both the variables that influence a child's memory and attention and how the child may be compensating for processing problems. For example, an eight-year-old we work with who has memory and auditory processing problems managed to recall a series of four digits by counting how many digits were in the string and how many he had said so far. Such strategy information suggests compensatory techniques that may be used in particular problem situations. This child was failing the sentence dictation portion of his spelling tests, not because he did not know how to spell the words, but because he could not remember the sentences long enough to write them down. He was taught to reauditorize each sentence, counting how many of the total number of words he remembered. He then asked for repetitions of the sentence until he was sure he remembered the correct number of words. Only at that point was he ready to start writing the sentence. Another important source of compensatory techniques emerges as the clinician examines the relationship between the child's processing weaknesses and processing strengths. For example, children with strong visual memory skills and weak auditory memory skills often can be taught to use visual techniques to assist memory.

At an intersystem interaction level, information-processing theory alerts the clinician to be extremely careful during assessment about assuming that an error represents a deficient skill and not a processing limitation. Before coming to such a conclusion, one would need to probe for the skill in question with tasks, materials, and contexts that were clearly familiar to the child.

From a little different processing perspective, Kaufman and Kaufman have explored the implications of differences in children's information-processing styles for how they are taught.[34] Utilizing the constructs of simultaneous (i.e., holistic or Gestalt) versus sequential (or analytic) processing styles, they compared matched groups of learning disabled students who had reading comprehension problems on reading tests before and after treatment. The group that received intervention designed to match their processing style made greater gains than the group receiving intervention with conventional published materials. A growing awareness of processing and learning style differences among normal and delayed children learning language suggests the need to explore further the implications of these processing differences for language intervention.[39,40]

The information-processing approach also provides some concrete ideas for what the contexts for language intervention should be that share much in common with the application of Katherine Nelson's event knowledge theory, to be discussed next. Specifically, information processing supports the use of familiar contexts for facilitating language intervention. Using activities familiar to a child in a sense frees up cognitive space. Hence the nonlinguistic components of the event can be dealt with more automatically, allowing the child to place more focus on the linguistic and communicative dimensions of the event. Thus, as Constable concludes, the familiar activities act as an "organizational prosthetic; resources that ordinarily are required to organize information could be used by children to organize communicative acts and display their emerging linguistic skills."[41] Indeed, Lucariello, Kyratzis, and Engel document that in the language accompanying mother-child interaction in familiar, routine events, children's linguistic skills appear to be far in advance of the language produced when mothers and their children talked about novel toys in a spontaneous free-play setting similar to most language sampling.[42]

Although information-processing theory advocates using familiar events because it frees up mental energy, so to speak, Katherine Nelson and her colleagues discuss specifically how this freeing up occurs.

Event Knowledge

Nelson and their colleagues view children's knowledge of routine everyday experiences as the initial content of their mental representations and hence as the foundation for "thinking, talking, and acting."[6] The event representations are cognitive entities, formed by cognitive processes. This account of the cognitive aspects of language development goes beyond the information-processing view to discuss why familiar events free up mental energy. They do so by creating a scaffolding "cognitive context" for the interaction. The event knowledge encoded in children's event representations includes understanding of the invariant temporal sequence of subevents making up the overall event and the roles of the participants and props in that event. For the young child, daily activities of eating, dressing, and bathing constitute such routine events. Grocery shopping, eating in a restaurant, feeding pets, and doing laundry are some further examples.

The data Nelson and her colleagues have collected demonstrates vividly that the talk embedded in familiar events is more advanced than talk accompanying traditional toy-oriented, "free-play" data collection procedures.[42] In their study, one of the toy-oriented "nonevent" contexts (meaning "nonroutine" event) involved a model castle and associated figures that were unfamiliar to the children, and the other nonevent context consisted of the following toys: a hand puppet, a tea set, a shape register, a stack-toy dog, and a pull-toy train (no child had precisely the same toys in his or her own collection). The children's language in the nonevent contexts contained virtually no reference to future and past, whereas the routine event context contained 15 percent future talk and 13 percent past talk. Questions were answered far better in the routine event context and greater semantic complexity and diversity in the children's language occurred. In the nonevent contexts, the adults used directives and attention focusing devices more frequently.

The authors conclude that "when mother and child both possess and share event knowledge for the interactive context, the child's competence in using language is greatly enhanced."[42] And it appears that the mother is the catalyst for this fuller expression of the child's linguistic potential: "The semantic topics were introduced to the conversation largely by the mother . . . (and) these mothers never failed to pick up on a topic introduced by the child. The factors of mother as catalyst and the allocation of processing capacity to linguistic behavior on the part of the child may combine to make these conversations possible in the Event Context."[42]

Using an event knowledge lens for viewing the language delayed child focuses, at the intersystem analysis level, on examination of both the cognitive and social domains of the child's development. Specifically, it encourages us to look for the kinds of event knowledge the child brings to the assessment or intervention experience. At the developmental level, it forces us to reanalyze much of the existing normative data used for planning purposes, because, if a familiar and routine context is tapped, some skills seem to develop considerably earlier than was previously supposed.

The event knowledge perspective offers its greatest contributions at an intersystem interaction level. It helps explain and directs the search for relationships between the cognitive and social domains. In the planning for language intervention, it stresses the importance of using or building familiar contexts within which to train language. The event knowledge perspective also provides a simple but somewhat revolutionary suggestion for language assessment—namely, that our language samples involving parent-child interaction include not just talk accompanying play with our clinic toys but also having parents engage their children in a familiar routine event.

Event knowledge acknowledges the importance of mental resource allocation and as such incorporates information-processing theory. However, routine events also take place in interactive social contexts, and, as such, the mother's role as the catalyst to the child's successful communication is recognized. From this perspective, Nelson and her colleagues duly acknowledge their allegiance to a Vygotskian social approach to language development in addition to the cognitive perspective they discuss. Bruner and others, however, have been far more explicit about how social interaction with routine events facilitates language development. We will discuss his work under Vygotskian theory, although it shares much in common with event knowledge theory discussed here.

Social Theories

In this section, we will discuss Vygotskian theory and social learning theory as explanations for language development. Both theories view social interaction as the basis for language acquisition. Vygotskian theory requires an active, directly participatory role of the adult; it requires that the adult be a "consenting partner, willing to negotiate with the child."[12] In social learning theory, the adult's role is somewhat less active—to provide language models for the developing child.

Vygotskian Theory

Recently, interest in work conducted by Russian psychologist L.S. Vygotsky in the 1920s and 1930s has been rather vigorously revived. Vygotsky's ideas on the social basis of learning, or transactional learning, provides the theoretic underpinnings of much recent thinking on the nature of language development.

The notion of transactional learning suggests that all individual psychological functioning, including language, is acquired through social interaction with a more experienced, competent member of the culture. According to Vygotsky, "Any function in the child's cultural development appears twice, or on two planes. First it appears on the social plane, and then on the psychological plane: first it appears between people as an interpsychological category, and then within the child as an intrapsychological category."[43] This process of moving from other-regulation to self-regulation allows for the eventual independent problem solving by the child.

The notion of a "zone of proximal development" is the crux of Vygotsky's transactional learning: "It is the distance between the actual developmental level as determined by independent problem solving and the level of potential development as determined through problem solving under adult guidance or in collaboration with more capable peers."[43] Herein lies the contribution of this theory to examining a child's development at both an intrasystem analysis level and a developmental level. Determination of a child's proximal zone requires exploration of how modifiable the child's behavior is with support from an adult. In effect, it is an effort to assess at what rate and how the child learns best. Brown and Ferrera discuss research on diagnosing the proximal zone in tasks found on traditional IQ tests such as letter series completion tasks.[44] Feuerstein outlines an extensive program for both assessment and intervention that relies on the proximal zone notion.[45] Olswang, Bain, Rosendahl, Oblak, and Smith have applied the proximal zone notion to assessing two language disordered children in the single-word stage of development.[46] From the combination of both a static (traditional, unassisted performance) and dynamic (aided, zone of proximal development) assessment, these researchers were able to predict the children's onset and rate of correct performance. Olswang et al believe such information is helpful in determining who should receive language therapy.

Although Vygotskian theory focuses on the social domain and its relationship to cognitive development at an intersystem interaction level, it offers no real guidance regarding what to teach. For interventionists, the strength of the theory lies in the procedures it delineates for teaching. In the language development literature, Bruner has used the term "scaffolding" to refer to the process of transactional learning.[12,47] Adults scaffold the child's language learning of a task by (1) providing simpler talk, sometimes called "motherese," and by (2) capitalizing on familiar, routine, highly constrained events, which Bruner calls formats. The format contains a sequential structure, clearly marked roles, and scripts for the accompanying communication. Bruner and his colleagues have focused much research on game formats such as peekaboo, build-and-bash, and object exchange.[48,49] Others have studied book reading formats.[50]

The process by which skills are transmitted in the kinds of routine events discussed previously offers a more viable framework for teaching than any other theories discussed so far. The transactional learning approach is more viable because it clearly specifies the role of the adult in facilitating learning from an interactional framework compatible with current pragmatic approaches to language intervention. In addition, other theories recommend a consistent response to the child regardless of his or her stage of learning. The clinician would model the correct response following social learning theory or reinforce following operant learning theory if the new behavior were just being introduced or if it were being stabilized and generalized. In contrast, transactional learning suggests a sequence of stages in the learning process. Both the adult's role and the expected level of participation from the child vary at each of these stages. Likewise, responses to errors vary.

In our own application of transactional learning to the clinical enterprise (combined with the event structure notion of Bruner and Nelson), we have formulated four stages in acquiring new behavior. This process of passing on a skill or of moving from other-regulation to independent action or self-regulation is presented in skeletal form in Table 22–6.

As shown in Table 22–6, stage 1 involves setting up a positive relationship and enticing the child into attending to the task. At this point, the adult familiarizes the child with the nature of the overall task rather than expecting specific responses. The overall task, like Bruner's formats or Nelson's event structures, is constructed to allow multiple opportunities for the child to produce one or more targeted areas of behavior. The clinician chooses a routine daily activity or begins establishing a clinical routine activity into which she or he can embed the language goals for the child in a pragmatically meaningful manner.

In stage 2, we assume the child has gained enough familiarity with the event structure of the activity that "cognitive space" (i.e., mental energy) is freed up to allow the child to begin to participate more actively. The adult's goal is at first to increase the child's willingness to participate, to take the risk of trying the new behavior, and to build the child's confidence. "In effect, the child is permitted to do as much as he can spontaneously do; whatever he cannot do is filled in or 'held up' by the mother's scaffolding activity."[51] In practice, this would mean that the adult would respond to the child's less-than-mastery-level response by providing that response for her or him.

In stage 3, the child is so familiar with the event structure of the activity that she or he often initiates segments of the activity and can successfully reverse roles with the adult in the activity (e.g., the child may begin asking the adult, "What's that?" during the book "reading" routine). The adult begins to abdicate to the child some of the responsibility for structuring the task. In addition, they begin to mutually negotiate who will take what roles in the completion of component segments of the activity. The child continues to practice the target behaviors embedded in the activity until they become stabilized and more automatic. At this point, the adult might begin to introduce variations of the original activity. A book reading routine might be applied to looking at a different book or a wall poster. A grocery shopping routine might be extended to other types of shopping.

Stage 4 involves moving from doing an activity to thinking and talking about the activity. The adult verbally models the planning of the activity before doing the activity, and the child begins to internalize the adult's thinking "out loud" and can begin to verbally plan as well. In addition, the target behaviors embedded in the activity itself are in a sense decontextualized from the concrete activity in that they are now produced without the immediate perceptual support of the ongoing activity. The adult also helps the child identify errors himself so that the child can begin to self-monitor while carrying out the activity. In this process, what began as a completely adult regulated activity in stage 1 becomes child regulated by stage 4.

Social Learning Theory

Social learning theory as explained by Bandura incorporates some aspects of operant learning theory (such as stimulus, response, and reinforcement), but it also differs in some important ways.[52] First of all, in social learning theory, learning can and most often does take place through observation rather than overt production of behavior. Furthermore, the child's attention to this modeled event is essential if learning

TABLE 22–6 Stages of Transactional Learning

Stage	*Adult's Role*	*Child's Role*
1	Entice; introduce event structure	Take risk of becoming involved; attend; learn to anticipate some aspects of event structure
2	Scaffold success	Learn target responses; become familiar with event structure
3	Vary task; abdicate control of task	Stabilize response; initiate control and interchange roles in event structure
4	Verbally model planning; help child identify errors to develop self-monitoring; help child generalize to new contexts	Verbally plan activity; decontextualize language; self-monitor; generalize behavior to new contents

is to occur. In addition to external reinforcement, reinforcement can be vicarious, as when a child observes another person being rewarded for a behavior, or it can be provided by the child himself (self-reinforcement).

According to this theory, language behavior is learned via a process of "abstract modeling" wherein the child abstracts the common attributes of many modeled utterances in order to "formulate rules for generating behavior with similar structural characteristics."[52]

As a lens for viewing the language delayed child at an intersystem analysis level, social learning theory focuses on the social domain, especially on examination of the opportunities the child has to learn from adult and peer models and the appropriateness of those models for the child's language level. Like operant learning theory, social learning theory really provides no direction in intrasystem analysis of the child's system or in determination of the developmental level. Thus, it has not been helpful in specifying goals of intervention, since any behavior that can be observed is an appropriate target. The impact of both these theories has been on how to teach—not on what to teach. Fey discusses the specific influence of social learning theory on language intervention. He outlines five steps the clinician would take to "motivate the child to attend closely to the target linguistic behavior:"[24]

> (1) selecting a model with whom the child closely identifies, such as a parent or a peer; (2) having the model produce numerous examples of the target behavior (e.g., subject-verb-object constructions to describe pictures with varying content); (3) reinforcing the model for correct productions; (4) after the presentation of several uninterrupted models, encouraging the child to "talk just like the model"; and (5) reinforcing the child for correct productions of the target.

MODELS OF LANGUAGE DISORDERS

In this section, we will consider major models that have been used as frameworks for considering children's language delays. As with theories of language acquisition, the framework or frameworks through which one chooses to view language delay has a direct impact upon how one would assess a child and subsequently intervene to facilitate language growth. We will explore three general models. The first two—medical and processing models—were developed primarily to explain why children have language delays. The third general model, which we refer to as a descriptive model, was developed to a large extent in reaction to the inability to derive goals for intervention from explanations for language delays. As such, this framework espouses the importance of describing a child's actual communicative skills.

Medical Model

The medical model or categorical orientation focuses on assigning language delayed children to a particular category based on patterns of both linguistic and nonlinguistic behavior that they exhibit. It is exemplified in the pioneering work of Myklebust, who discussed language delay in children by differentiating among the global categories of peripheral deafness, aphasia, psychic deafness (emotional disturbance), and mental deficiency.[53] Historically, this approach to language delay was the earliest in the field, but it is by no means considered archaic today. Three recent textbooks on child language disorders, for example, are organized into chapters by similar categories.[54,55,56]

A variation on this model attempts to determine the causes underlying various categorical labels. For example, McCormick and Schiefelbusch consider language and communication problems associated with (1) motor disorders (cerebral palsy, spina bifida), (2) sensory deficits (hearing and visual impairment), (3) central nervous system dysfunction (learning disabilities, aphasia), (4) severe emotional and social dysfunction (autism), and (5) cognitive disorders (mental retardation).[57]

Rapin and Allen discuss the process of nosology, which refers to the process of delineating a pathologic condition.[58] The various aspects of this process are often not considered separately in the application of the medical model in our field. The steps they discuss include (1) diagnosis—isolating clusters of symptoms in order to recognize a particular condition; (2) determining pathogenesis—discovering what causes specific symptoms by understanding the underlying anatomic, physiologic, and metabolic pathologies (i.e., due to tumor, infection, allergic reaction, genetic defect); (3) determining the cause or etiology of the various pathogeneses (i.e., due to tumor or infection); and (4) providing efficacious therapy.

Given these nosologic distinctions, one can see that Myklebust focused on diagnosis, while McCormick and Schiefelbusch highlighted pathogenesis. An etiologic approach would in turn involve determining the cause of the motor, sensory, central nervous system, emotional and social, or cognitive disorders McCormick and Schiefelbusch listed. The myriad etiologies of these diagnostic and pathogenic categories is discussed in this volume in chapters focusing on special populations.

The multifaceted nature of determining the diagnosis, pathogenesis, and etiology of language delay often requires input from numerous other professionals such as neurologists, psychologists, psychiatrists, ophthalmologists, and audiologists. For the speech-language pathologist presented with a child with delayed language development, the major goal of assessment from the medical model orientation is diagnosis—to determine which category or categories best characterize a particular child. The task of assigning a child to a category is by no means straightforward. Several problems in determining a classification include the following:

1. Behavioral characteristics of categories sometimes overlap, and identical behaviors can have different causes. Hence, a hearing impaired child can appear to be mentally retarded; an autistic child can appear deaf.
2. Children rarely fit neatly into one category.
3. Identifying the medical condition does not insure it is the singular or even the most important cause of the problem.
4. Each of the categories may be the result of a wide variety of causes. Furthermore, different causes may indicate different treatments. And so, for example, mental retardation may be due to environmental deprivation, malnutrition, a seizure disorder, or a large number of congenital syndromes, to name just a few. Management for the seizure disorder would include medication, whereas management for environmental deprivation may involve drastically different measures, such as parent training or removal of the child from the problematic environment.

In spite of these kinds of problems inherent in attempting to categorize a child, it is often important to do so for one or more of the following reasons:

1. Some of the problems are treatable, as we shall discuss.
2. To obtain funding or adequate educational placement, categorization of the child may sometimes be required.
3. Having a diagnostic label can sometimes help parents move through the grieving process that is a natural part of coming to accept their handicapped child.
4. Knowing the category may alert the clinician to look for special language characteristics sometimes found in that category, such as echolalia in autistic children, special syntactic problems of deaf children, and "cocktail" speech in hydrocephalic children. Although the category, if known, can alert the clinician to these special characteristics, it is perhaps more often the case that these characteristics are part of the data used to determine the child's category.
5. Knowing the cause can give the clinician some general guidelines for how best to obtain information about the child's actual communication abilities during assessment. The same guidelines provide general procedures for presenting information during intervention. They will be discussed further on.

The medical model is a helpful lens for viewing the child's symptoms, especially the physical symptoms. But one of the major difficulties with the medical model is that once the domains of impairment have been diagnosed at an intersystem analytic level and the child's category has been determined, recommendations may be made without exploration of the child's individual needs at the other levels of our assessment and planning process model. For example, the medical model orientation frequently results in recommendations for physical interventions such as surgery (e.g., repair of cleft lip and/or palate, myringotomy), prosthesis (e.g., fitting with a hearing aid, providing a wheelchair for locomotion), or biochemical therapy (e.g., medication, a special diet). Another common practice is the prescription of a particular type of therapy (e.g., speech therapy, physical therapy) or special school (e.g., school for the blind, residential school for the retarded). It is then incumbent upon each of the other professionals who becomes involved with the child to investigate the child's individual needs in sufficient depth and breadth to assure that those needs are being met. Unfortunately, without organized collaboration among both the family and the variety of professionals involved, there is no guarantee that the whole child is being served appropriately.

Another problem sometimes encountered is that a particular intervention may be applied indiscriminately to all children with a language delay regardless of its relevance to an individual child's needs or to her or his language delay. For example, Seiben reviews both biochemical and physical therapies that have been used with learning disabled children.[59] One physical therapy he discusses is patterning, which has been used to treat mental retardation, cerebral palsy, epilepsy, autism, and hyperactivity. This approach, also known as the Doman-Delacato treatment, attempts to treat neurologically handicapped children by "moving the abnormal brain through a normally sequenced developmental pattern by sensory stimulation and the imposition of passive movement on the patient."[59] The intensive program, involving hours and hours a day, is supposed to induce the brain to reorganize neural patterns and hence correct the presumed damage. The efficacy of the procedure has been refuted in a joint statement issued by the American Academies of Pediatrics, Neurology, Orthopedics, Cerebral Palsy, Physical Medicine, and Rehabilitation and by the National Association of Retarded Children.

Although diagnosis and prescription at the intersystem analytic level are the most familiar applications of the medical model, the medical model can also offer useful concepts and guidance at the intrasystem analytic and intrasystem interactions levels. The notion of determining pathogenesis is an important part of intrasystem analysis. Interventionists must search for the stumbling blocks that are preventing normal development in each impaired area. For example, the almost three-year-old named Jonathan that we described in the introduction to this chapter has long strings of unintelligible jargon with occasional strings that sound like intelligible sentences. At an intersystem analytic level, we identified his history of recurrent middle ear problems as the most likely etiology for his language delay; but this history was not helpful in explaining the reasons for his jargon. It was only at an intrasystem analytic level when we examined the effects of our speech rate and prosody on his imitation ability that we discovered the problems he has segmenting the speech stream. This segmentation difficulty could also explain why he occasionally is able to use a well-formed sentence in appropriate situations (i.e., he has not segmented the sentence, but uses it as an unanalyzed whole) although he uses only eight to ten words generatively. Thus the pathogenesis of his jargon appears to be his segmentation problem, although the etiology of his language delay is probably his middle ear problems.

At the intrasystem interaction level, the medical model lens suggests guidelines and techniques for how best to accommodate to the common problems experienced by children with various categories of impairment. These guidelines are useful both for assessment of children and for planning how to teach them. Some examples of guidelines for blind, visually impaired, hearing impaired, austic, and learning disabled children are found in Tables 22–7 to 22–11.

Processing Models

Processing models attempt to identify the mental processes causing or contributing to language delay in children. In general, the various models that fall under this rubric have been generated to explain language delay in developmental aphasia or dysphasia, when no other obvious cause exists such as hearing impairment, mental retardation, or emotional disturbance.

Because developmental aphasia has no obvious cause, researchers have turned their attention to specifying central nervous system damage or to considering what kinds of mental processing deficits might account for difficulty in language learning.[60,61] As such, processing models have primarily arisen to explain the developmental aphasia category of the medical model, although there is no reason to assume that children classified in the other medical categories do not sometimes have processing deficits as well. To date, two types of processing models have emerged in the literature, (1) those postulating deficits specific to auditory-linguistic processing and (2) those suggesting that deficits are, in general, cognitive processes that might influence other learning in addition to language learning.

Auditory Processing Models

The notion of auditory processing deficits has a rather long history in the study of language delay in children, although the terminology has varied. In 1929, Worster-Drought and Allen discussed the "auditory imperception" of a child with congenital word deafness.[62] The same general notion has subsequently been referred to as "auding" by Hardy,[63] "auditory perceptual dysfunction" by Myklebust,[64] "central auditory dysfunction" by Keith,[65] and "defects of auditory perception" by Tallal and Piercy.[66] The auditory processing models (or the specific abilities approach, as it has been labelled by Bloom and Lahey) share much in common with the component skills approach to language acquisition discussed earlier.[23] Advocates of this approach attempt to break into component skills the auditory processes deemed necessary for learning language such as attention, sequencing, discrimination, and memory.

In extending the specific abilities approach to language assessment and intervention, Bloom and Lahey call to question numerous unsupported or faulty assumptions underlying such an approach, noting:

> (1) that the abilities for language are distinct from each other in the learning and use of language; (2) that each ability is a necessary prerequisite for the development and use of language, and weak abilities therefore interfere with the learning or use of language; and (3) that weak abilities can be strengthened by training, and that strengthening specific abilities through remediation training will transfer somehow to general improvement in knowledge and use of language.[23]

Tomblin adds a fourth assumption to this list, namely, that these processes occur prior to percep-

TABLE 22–7 Tips for Assessing Blind Children

Orient the child to the test room before beginning your evaluation so that the child becomes familiar with her or his surroundings. This may mean that you have to act as a sighted guide for the child so that the child can explore her or his physical environment. For ease and safety of movement, the child should grasp the guide's upper arm just above the elbow (a younger child with an adult may hold the adult's wrist) so that the thumb is on the outside and the fingers are on the inside of the guide's arm. Both the visually handicapped child and the guide hold their upper arms close to their own bodies. This should automatically position the child one-half step behind the guide. For negotiating narrow passageways, the guide can either press her or his arm close to her or his body or place her or his arm behind her or his body so that the blind child knows she or he must stand directly behind her or him. Verbal cues are also important: the guide should inform the child of any obstacles, including ascending and descending walking surfaces.
You may need some sort of a boundary on the table so that the child can distinguish test items from nontest items. With younger children you might use a tray for test objects to keep them from rolling away. In general, limit the number of objects used in a particular instance to avoid confusing the child.
Make sure you test the child's inventory of basic concepts because there are times when a child's expressive skills outstrips his or her knowledge. For example, a child may talk about gasoline wars—which she or he has heard about on the T.V. or radio—but know almost nothing about cars.
Talk in a normal voice to the child.
Provide verbal boundaries to your conversations that might normally be supplied by nonverbal cues. For example, if you are making some subtle change in an activity, verbally alert the child by saying such things as "Now we are going to. . . ."
Feel comfortable using words such as "see" and "look." These words are as much a part of the vocabulary of the child with a visual handicap as they are of anyone else's. Pragmatically, these verbs signal that there is something specific that the child needs to notice or attend to.
When you have to move somewhere, irrespective of whether or not you are acting as a sighted guide, let the child know where you are going. If you must leave the room, leave the child in contact with some piece of furniture so that she or he does not become disoriented.
When approaching a blind child, unless she or he knows you extremely well, always state your name. Voices are not always easy to identify.
You may want to keep track of the amount of time within which a particular test is normally expected to be completed vs. the amount of time that it takes for the visually impaired child to complete the test.
If you are going to substitute tactile information for pictorial information, it is better to simulate the texture of the intended object instead of presenting a miniature model of the object. For example, the child may have real world experience with an object such as an airplane (at its normal size), but not with a miniature model of an airplane.
Some of these tips may also be adapted to students with poor vision (but not legally blind) because the boundary that separates the two groups may often be fuzzy.

tion and cognition.[67] Tomblin discusses how recent cognitive research indicates that, on the contrary, our knowledge base interacts with incoming stimuli before resources are allocated for such processes as attention and memory.

Although the literature reviewed by both Bloom and Lahey and Tomblin offers convincing evidence that these assumptions are not true, complete elimination of the possible explanatory and subsequent intervention value of the auditory processing model may be premature.[23,67] Most of Bloom and Lahey's argument rests on measuring specific abilities by the Illinois Test of Psycholinguistic Abilities, a test spawned by this approach.[68] It is by now widely accepted, as Bloom and Lahey also pointed out, that this test taps children's ability to consciously focus on properties of language. Thus it is a measure of metalinguistic abilities rather than auditory processing abilities.[69] Keith clarifies the issue somewhat by distinguishing between these tests of auditory language function and tests of auditory neuroanatomic level function.[70] The latter are exemplified by tests of central auditory function, which should utilize nonlinguistic signals or at least require no linguistic manipulation of the signal. Such tests yield information on the integrity or maturity of the auditory neurologic system. Tallal and her colleagues have been able to convincingly isolate the *duration* aspect of an acoustic signal and provide solid evidence that some language delayed children do have difficulty processing brief acoustic events.[66] Clinically feasible methods for measuring at least some aspects of auditory processing, based on work such as Tallal's, are becoming available and may be helpful assessment tools. Such tests might allow us to delineate subgroups of children in all populations of language delay who do have difficulty processing information auditorily as well as the specific nature of the processing problems displayed.

The auditory processing lens reminds us to pay attention to how the child processes auditory information and not just whether or not she or he hears it. To understand the child's learning strengths and weaknesses, one must examine how the child learns through the auditory modality. To know whether the child benefits from supplemental cues from other modalities, longer processing time, or a louder signal and to know how the child is affected by competing messages and degraded signals are critical for intervention planning. Although tests are available to explore auditory language functioning (e.g., the Goldman-Fristoe-Woodcock Auditory Skills Battery) and auditory neuromaturational level functioning, the attentive clinician finds that closely ob-

TABLE 22–8 Tips for Assessing Visually Impaired Children

There is a misconception that as much bright light as possible benefits the visually impaired child. However, there are children who are overly sensitive to light (photophobia)—in such instances you may need to block out some of the light and glare from the environment with sun visors and other shields. Generally speaking, one should make sure that the light is even.
Use materials that are not shiny; glare can create perceptual problems.
Visually presented materials, in general, should be of high contrast—dark figures on a white, low glare ground. Few visually impaired children have color vision losses—which you would need to be aware of prior to doing an evaluation—and so color contrasts also may be helpful. Purple ditto materials are bad; occasionally a yellow transparency might be placed over such materials in order to darken the figures that the child views.
Keep the testing field uncluttered; try to present just one test item at a time. Be aware of whether or not the child experiences any loss of vision in any of the visual fields (right, left, upper, lower). If so, avoid presenting materials in the area where there is a visual field loss.
Visually impaired children may require extra time to complete test items. A general rule of thumb is to allow the child 1.5 times the amount of time you would the normal child.
You need to know whether the child uses low vision aids—devices for magnification such as a monocular (a little telescope)—in the classroom. With such an aid, the child may be able to read normal print size.
Try not to stand with your back to any window. Glare and light create a silhouette that may fatigue the visually impaired child.
Dim light does not harm the eyes. As a result of some eye conditions (cataracts, albinism), a child may require dim lighting in order to feel more comfortable.
Make sure that doors and cupboards (and any other obstacles) are all the way open or all the way shut.
You may have to provide many more verbal cues than you are used to because the child cannot read facial expressions, head nods, or arm movements, which are usually employed by individuals to modulate their conversations.
Behavior: A totally blind child or a child with severe visual impairment may exhibit certain mannerisms (fingers in the eyes or eye poking, rocking, extra movements).

TABLE 22–9 Tips for Assessing Hearing Impaired Children

Check the child's ability to understand oral language both with and without visual cues.
Check the child's hearing aid to make sure it is functioning properly before you begin the assessment.
Speak as naturally as possible. You may need to speak at a slower than normal rate, with slightly lower than normal pitch, or at a slightly louder than normal volume, but shouting or exaggerating your mouth movements makes you more difficult to understand.
Background noise makes it difficult for the hearing impaired person to understand you. So make sure your evaluation is done in a quiet place. However, part of your assessment may be to determine how well the individual communicates in noisy vs. quiet situations.
Distance is important. The best distance for communicating with a hearing impaired person is between 3 and 6 feet. This distance makes your voice louder. It also makes your voice sound clearer if there is any background noise.
Arrange the environment so that the hearing impaired person is in the best possible position to see and hear. Good lighting on the speaker's face is important. If possible, the hearing impaired person should sit away from sources of background noise and with his or her hearing aid toward the speaker.
For maximum comprehension, speak in short sentences and pause slightly between them. Also, rephrase misunderstood messages rather than just repeating them—expanding on ideas in the sentence may be useful.
Be a patient and accepting listener. Don't think the person is ignoring you if she or he fails to respond appropriately to your communication efforts. Avoid saying "never mind" or "it's not important" when the hearing impaired person does not understand what you have said. Your communication efforts are very precious to the person, and the communication breakdown that can occur because of the hearing loss can be a source of sadness and frustration for the hearing impaired person.
Do not be afraid to consult with the audiologist, and other appropriate people, in order to gain a clearer picture of the child's communicative abilities. Remember, part of being a good professional is knowing when to ask others questions.

TABLE 22–10 Tips for Assessing Autistic Children

Most of these children do not respond to a typical standardized test. Therefore, the clinician must be prepared to use nontraditional assessment procedures in order to assess the child's level of communicative functioning. This means that the assessment may take more than 1 day and may involve observing the child in a variety of contexts (e.g., eating meals) in which communication could be built into the daily routine.
Informants (such as classroom teachers and caregivers) who spend a significant amount of time with the child may be necessary in gaining a complete diagnostic picture of the child's current level of functioning. You may wish to do assessment procedures with teachers and/or caregivers who are familiar with the child.
Assessment and intervention need to go hand in hand. That is, you may not be able to assess the child's level of functioning without trying some intervention procedures.

serving the child's performance during assessment and treatment tasks is also helpful.[36,70] Thus, at the intersystem interaction level, the clinician should watch how well the child performs language tasks in quiet versus noise and what effects alterations in loudness, prosody, or rate of speech have on performance. Many of the learning disabled college students we see who have residual language problems still have difficulty learning the lyrics of songs, following conversations in noisy situations, and understanding lectures by nonnative speakers. To the attentive clinician, these kinds of difficulties serve as red flags that further exploration of auditory processing abilities is needed.

Rather than making improvement of auditory processes specific goals for language intervention, the clinician needs to delineate such deficits and take them into account in devising procedures for intervention. Johnston mentions that auditory attentional deficits might be dealt with by either capitalizing on the child's already established focus or creating attention grabbing events that have "unusual perceptual salience, novelty, or significance for the child."[71] From the opposite viewpoint, information lost because of some type of perceptual deficit might in a sense be scaffolded or compensated for by using familiar activities. After many successes in the familiar context, the child's knowledge base might become adequate to fill in missing perceptual information, even in less familiar contexts. Johnston also notes that the clinician might compensate for presumed auditory processing problems by using visual techniques such as written language, pictured sentences, and signed English.[71] Williford offers several suggestions for classroom teachers, including seating the child near the front of the classroom and away from noise sources (such as windows, doors, and air conditioners), facing the child when speaking, arranging for parents to preview content material with the child prior to its presentation in class, and assessing the effects of assistive listening devices.[72] These intervention procedures are all similar to those one would consider using with hearing impaired children.

Cognitive Processing Models

By definition, developmentally aphasic children exhibit normal cognitive abilities on nonverbal intelligence tests such as the Leiter International Performance Scale and the Columbia Mental Maturity Scale.[73,74] Numerous researchers have nonetheless attempted to demonstrate that these children may have cognitive deficits in domains important to language development, but not tapped by such tests.

Some of these explanations are extensions of the auditory processing approach to include other modalities. For example, some researchers have suggested that difficulty with sequential processing and memory may be a more general deficit that extends beyond the auditory modality and includes the visual modality as well. Johnston notes that research testing this possibility contains contradictory findings and is at present inconclusive.[71]

Another extension of the auditory processing model proposed by Rosenthal was labelled the "efferent adjustment deficit." It postulates a variable "critical band" in processing sensory stimuli. Johnston explains this notion as follows:[75]

TABLE 22–11 Tips for Assessing Learning Disabled Children

Be particularly sensitive to keeping the test environment uncluttered and free from distractions. In fact, you may wish to observe differences in performance in quiet vs. noisy environments (including visual and auditory noise).
Talk to the child at a slow rate of speed and allow a substantial amount of time for responses. Tests that place time constraints on the child may adversely affect performance.
If possible, obtain information on the child's classroom performance and interaction with peers prior to conducting your evaluation.
Be sensitive to both the perspective of the caregivers and the child in regard to the nature of the child's difficulty.

> In lay terms, the ear and mind process only portions of the available acoustic signal—enough to enable identification. When the signal is brief, the "band" of frequencies to which we attend widens or shifts to maximize the information available. Rosenthal speculates that if this efferent adjustment were slow, a brief signal would be gone or unrecognizable. . . . Similar problems might arise with rapidly changing signals of any physical sort, since the locus of difficulty would reside not in particular sensory mechanisms, but in those central executive functions that tune them.[71]

Other cognitive processing explanations of language delay have no analog in the auditory modality. Several researchers have used Piaget's notion of symbolic function to suggest that the general ability to symbolize, of which language is only a part, may be impaired in these children. And numerous studies have demonstrated representational deficits in language disordered children. Moreover, such deficits have been documented across a number of tasks or activities that are believed to make particularly high representational demands. These include symbolic play,[76] anticipatory imagery,[77] and haptic recognition.[78]

Another possible cognitive processing deficit suggested by Cromer—one in hierarchical structuring—stems from linguistic theory rather than Piagetian theory and was developed in reaction to the notion of sequencing deficits in language delayed children.[79] Cromer argued that language structure does not consist of mere associative links between adjacent elements, but that meaning is derived from the whole structure. This is most apparent when some kind of interruption occurs in the surface features of a sentence as in the case of relative clauses. The written language samples of the language disordered children Cromer studied in fact did not contain relative clause structures. He interpreted this omission to mean that these children were not able to hierarchically organize language structure. A logical extension of Cromer's notion would be to suspect that children with language problems have difficulty with any learning requiring the ability to hierarchically organize information.

Recently, Kamhi and his colleagues tested the possibility that hypothesis testing deficits might underlie difficulty in learning language.[79,80] These authors argue that such a deficit is plausible, given the widely accepted view that language learning involves formulating and testing hypotheses about both conceptual domains and linguistic rules. Contrary to expectations, in the two empirical studies designed to test this notion, the hypothesis testing abilities of the language impaired children were generally intact. It is important to note, however, that a careful analysis of individual data indicated that as many as 10 to 20 percent of the language impaired children did seem to demonstrate hypothesis testing problems, a fact obscured in the grouped data. This may well be true of all of the processing models discussed in this section—that each may have explanatory value for some children's language delay. Rapin and Allen suggest that "Since the processes that underlie language are so complex and so numerous, language must be vulnerable to many different deficits."[58]

The various potential cognitive processing problems we have described are still too incompletely understood for us to specify all of their ramifications for planning intervention with language delayed children. However, they do alert us to the fact that traditional tests of intelligence may not tap many of the particular cognitive functions thought to be related to language development. Assessment of most of the cognitive processes just discussed, with perhaps the exception of symbolic function, is at present an imprecise and speculative venture. Yet, because of the possible benefits of such information for determining the most efficacious language intervention procedures for any given child, such speculation may be worthwhile. Thus, at the intrasystem analysis level, clinicians need to supplement standardized tests with procedures drawn from the experimental literature. For example, the assessment of symbolic function is greatly assisted by the existence of experimental procedures for haptic recognition[78] and anticipatory imagery[77] that can be borrowed for informal clinical evaluation. Furthermore, symbolic play can be evaluated by an observational measure,[81] or by more formal procedures set forth in Nicholich,[82] or by the symbolic play test,[83] a formalized test that provides a language-free assessment of play.

If deficient cognitive processing abilities are found, the clinician must turn clinical scientist and carefully examine, at an intersystem interaction level, the possible relationships between those processes and a particular child's delayed language development. The implications of this examination process relate both to determinations of pathogenesis and to planning the goals and procedures of intervention. The clinician must address several groups of questions and consider the impact of her or his answers on treatment:

Question 1. Is the cognitive processing deficit the particular stumbling block preventing normal language development? If so, can it be treated directly? If it can, would improving the processing deficit resolve all of the symptoms of the child's language delay? When viewing hierarchical structuring, sequencing, memory, or hypothesis testing with these questions in mind, the treatment implications become clearer. The field of speech-language pathology does have experience with attempting to train some specific cognitive processing abilities such as memory. Unfortunately, such efforts have not led to resolution of the child's language problems.[23]

Question 2. Is the language delay causing the cognitive processing deficit; that is, could limited experience using language for cognitive processing purposes account for the child's poor performance on the processing tasks? If so, would improving the child's language skills resolve the cognitive processing problem? These questions have been asked less frequently; in fact, group research studies try to control for this possibility by matching children studied by language age. Nevertheless, careful clinicians may want to test these questions for themselves.

Question 3. Is some other factor or combination of factors causing the language delay and the cognitive processing problem? Can the factor(s) be treated directly? For example, a general symbolic deficit or representational problem might underlie both the language delay and the performance on tests of symbolic play, anticipatory imagery, or haptic recognition. No obvious way currently exists to treat an abstract problem such as a symbolic deficit, other than to teach the specific symbolic skills the child needs to learn for life success.

Question 4. What language skills might the cognitive processing most affect? As an example, hierarchical structuring may be taxed during language tasks such as learning kinship terms and geographical relationships, outlining, the rules of grammar, and diagramming sentences. A child with hierarchical structuring problems may need particular help in these areas.

Question 5. What life skills might the cognitive processing deficit interfere with and should the interventionist address these? An example that seems relevant to consider here is symbolic play. Although there is no reason to suspect that working on symbolic play improves language ability (i.e., although these two skills are correlated developmentally, this in no way implies that one is a causal factor in the development of the other), the clinician may wish to work on symbolic play for social reasons. For example, she or he may believe that the ability to play is essential to peer relations. The clinician might in such a case be indirectly facilitating language development, since, as stated by McCune-Nicholich and Carroll, "by becoming somewhat isolated from the mainstream of players, the child loses valuable opportunities for developing language and social skills through play."[84]

Descriptive Models

Descriptive models are simply aimed at describing the actual observable language and related behaviors of a language delayed child. Our allegiance to this approach is evident throughout this chapter, although we have suggested going beyond describing observable behavior as well. The pioneers of the most extensive version of this approach, Bloom and Lahey, spelled out the rationale for and details of this orientation in their classic 1978 text. Descriptions can be derived from reported or observational data. Three major types of observational data include standardized tests, informal elicitations, and spontaneous language samples. Different data sources, Bloom and Lahey convincingly argue, are useful for answering different kinds of questions. Descriptions can focus on any component of language. Bloom and Lahey considered form, content, and use. More traditional categories include syntax, morphology, phonology, semantics, and pragmatics.[85]

Since this model has received such extensive attention elsewhere, we will not go into detail here regarding (1) the multitude of tests available for assessing the various components of language, (2) the types of informal tasks one can use to elicit language behaviors, or (3) the numerous analytic procedures for coding spontaneous language samples. The reader is referred especially to books by Bloom and Lahey,[23] Lund and Duchan,[85] Crystal,[86] and Miller.[87]

Describing various components of a child's linguistic system via language sample analysis is essential for establishing intervention goals for that child and is relatively useless for discovering how to teach those goals. Although the value of this approach cannot be overemphasized, certain limitations, which should be acknowledged, include the following:

1. Huge gaps still exist in normative data essential for comparison with the language delayed child's behavior, especially for children beyond the preschool level.
2. Child language researchers currently have little understanding of what range of time is normal for the development of various linguistic behaviors.
3. When normative data on normal children are available, assessment procedures have not always been developed for analyzing language delayed children's language.
4. There is an ever present threat that the language sample a speech-language pathologist analyzes is not representative of a particular child's typical language ability.

THE ROLE OF LANGUAGE IN DEVELOPMENT

In the section on theories of language acquisition, we discussed various ways in which social factors, cognition, and innate endowments might affect language development. In this section, we wish to consider the opposite side of the coin—how language affects other domains of development. Specifically, we will consider the role of language in developing and maintaining social relationships, developing self-concept, and achieving academic success. These are areas in which language delayed children might experience problems secondary to their language problems. At times, work in these areas constitutes goals of therapy. At other times, such problems might be avoided altogether by direct work on facilitating language development.

The issue of how language affects other aspects of development is often alluded to in the literature that discusses the various functions of language. Indeed, a look at some of the major taxonomies of language functions reveals that the three categories listed previously are often addressed in these lists. Halliday, for example, considers the following functions of language:[88] (1) instrumental: to get things done; (2) regulatory: to regulate the behavior of others; (3) interactional: interaction between self and others; (4) imaginative: to create reality; (5) personal: expression of identity, of self; (6) heuristic: to explore the environment and to learn; and (7) representational: to express propositions (convey information).

The first three functions listed obviously relate to the role of language in developing and maintaining social relationships. We suggest that the imaginative function would be included here as well, because of its importance in the development of peer relationships. Halliday's personal function corresponds to our "development of self-concept" category, and he argues that language plays an essential role in the development of personality. The heuristic function, or using language to learn, is one of the ways in which language impacts upon academic success.

Unlike Halliday and many others, we have chosen not to list functions of language in this section, but rather to focus on the role of language in other domains of development. The reason for this is that most people tend to think of communicative functions only when they think of the functions of language. As Halliday notes,

> We tend to underestimate both the total extent and the functional diversity of the part played by language in the life of the child. His interaction with others, which begins at birth, is gradually given form by language, through the process whereby at a very early age language already begins to mediate in every aspect of his experience. It is not only as the child comes to act on and to learn about his environment that language comes in; it is there from the start in his achievement of intimacy and in the expression of his individuality.[88]

Furthermore, focusing on the role of language in other domains of development provides, we believe, a better conceptual framework for guiding assessment and intervention by emphasizing the rationale for doing so than does a list of language functions. It somehow seems less urgent and compelling if we say a child completely lacks the "personal" function of language than if we say a child is experiencing severe self-esteem problems due to her or his language delay.

Development and Maintenance of Social Relationships

From birth, communicative ability influences and shapes social relationships. In this section, we consider the impact of a language delay on parent-child and peer interaction. We have chosen these particular social relationships because the former has been extensively studied with language delayed children and because the latter has been studied with normal children, but is all too rarely considered in our work with language delayed children.

Parent-Child Interaction

A body of literature now exists that documents the impact of impaired communicative ability upon parent-child, particularly mother-child, interaction from birth onward. Elicitors of parental responses in infancy include the communicative behaviors of crying, smiling and laughter, looking, and nondistressed vocalizations. A growing body of literature documents that numerous populations of infants who are at high risk for later communication disorders (e.g., Down's syndrome, developmentally disabled, brain damaged, malnourished, blind, and high risk) exhibit communicative behaviors in infancy that are more difficult to detect than in normal infants.[89] For example, cries may be of lower intensity, sustained for shorter periods of time, less differentiated, and arrhythmical, making them less apparent to parents.

The probable effect of a less "readable" infant on the parent-infant interaction has been discussed by Dunst,[89] Goldberg,[90] and Harter.[91] According to Goldberg, the chain of events is as follows: "When the infant is unpredictable and difficult to read, decisions [on the parents' part] require a longer time, are difficult to make, and are less likely to be appropriate"[90] The interaction leaves both parties feeling ineffective—the infant because she or he cannot predictably influence the environment and the parent because he or she cannot figure out an appropriate response. Eventually these feelings of helplessness and inefficacy make both parties less likely to initiate or respond to communicative bids. The decreased motivation to communicate leads to less opportunity for the infant to practice communicative skills and hence leads to a further lowering of skill level and of self-concept as a communicator.

As children with communicative impairments mature, parent-child interaction continues to be characterized by withdrawal. That is, significantly less overall interaction occurs between parents and their language delayed children than between parents and their normally developing children. The interaction that does take place between parents and their language delayed children is often characterized as controlling and intrusive, containing (1) attempts to elicit rather than respond to behavior, (2) a preponderance of parent initiated interactions, and (3) a large amount of parental directiveness. These patterns of interaction have been documented in numerous studies of children with language delay, mental retardation, and hearing impairment and their mothers. It seems that mothers attempt to compensate for their child's passivity by attempting to get the child to respond more and by initiating more themselves.

The high frequency of directives in maternal speech to these children may have a different explanation. Parents are highly motivated to socialize their babies successfully, that is, to get them to act in socially acceptable ways. As well, babies learn a lot by simply observing socially appropriate behavior. But much behavior seems to be taught by overt direction—the child hears a lot of "Do this" and "Don't do that." Indeed, many research studies have documented the directive nature of early adult-child interaction. Most infants become increasingly self-regulatory, and mothers of normally developing children correspondingly decrease the amount of directiveness in the language that they address to their children. However, self-regulation is mediated primarily through language. Children who may not adequately develop the ability to self-regulate because they have language deficits, may be more regulated by their parents in a compensatory fashion.

The previous discussion clearly indicates that the basic interaction patterns of the extremely important mother-child relationship can fall into a negative cycle early on with communicatively impaired children, thereby leading to a decreased desire to communicate on the part of both participants. Without intervention, this cycle develops into a continued low frequency of interaction for the children who most desperately need practice and success with communication. When interaction does occur, parents may be controlling and intrusive, unknowingly reinforcing the communicative passivity they are working so hard to draw the children out of.

The parent-child interaction lens is evidently a critical one for viewing the language impaired child, and clinicians need to address the parent-child interaction in their intervention efforts. It is the foundation, the crucial platform, on which the success of all other intervention goals depends. The earlier we can intervene, the less entrenched a negative interaction pattern will be, and the easier it will be to successfully teach alternate interaction patterns.

Assessing parent-child interaction at an intrasystem level can be accomplished by coding both parent and child behaviors in a spontaneous language sample or by an observational checklist such as the "Home Observation for Measurement of the Environment"* by Caldwell and Bradley.[92]

In coding a spontaneous language sample, the clinician might first of all indicate the range and frequency of communicative intentions used by the parent. This indication would highlight an excessive use of directives and questions, both considered controlling interaction devices. In addition, on a discourse level, the clinician could code the parent's type and frequency of responsiveness to any communicative attempts on the child's part, either verbal or nonverbal. This encoding would reveal how often and in what ways the adult follows the child's lead, consequently providing the child with a sense of the power of communication to affect the environment.

Once the pattern of parent-child interaction is determined, the clinician must examine that interaction in relation to the child's language development and life needs. When the interaction is facilatory for language growth and the parents' own personal needs have been assessed, the parents' role in the overall intervention program should be considered. Many parents can play an active and important role in building their child's language skills. This role may range from carrying out home assignments to implementing a full program with direction from the interventionist. Assuming a maximally supportive environment, to in effect train the parents to be the language facilitators is often most efficacious, especially for very young children. Certainly they spend much more time with their children than the therapist and have many more opportunities to facilitate language in natural contexts.

When assessment indicates a less than ideal parent-child interaction and the parent is a viable candidate for becoming involved in intervention (see "Why Parent Programs Fail" by Nygard and Adair[93]), improving the parent-child interaction becomes a most appropriate goal for intervention. This goal is especially appropriate for infants and preschoolers who

---

* The HOME manual is available from the Center for Child Development and Education, University of Arkansas, Little Rock, Arkansas 72204.

spend a great deal of time interacting with one or both parents.

If parents' behaviors are targeted, an essential first step involves a careful and convincing explanation that their current interaction patterns are a completely natural adaptation to interacting with a communicatively handicapped child. Although a natural adaptation, clinicians need to explain that it may not be the best for facilitating language development. Because these children are already experiencing difficulty learning language, clinicians want to provide the maximal environmental support possible. The point that must be made manifestly clear is that the parents are not to blame for the child's language problems (except in the rare instances when this may indeed be the case). We often explain to parents that we have to work long and hard in training clinicians to repress the same natural reaction of "taking over" for the child who has difficulty communicating.

Some structured parent training programs, such as the Hanen program, "It Takes Two to Talk," focus on the parent-child interaction.[94] This particular program trains parents to systematically (1) observe the child's attempts to communicate, (2) follow the child's lead, (3) respond so that the child learns, (4) keep the conversation going, and (5) prompt for better turns. Although the Hanen program was designed for the parents of prelinguistic and very-early-language-level children, the same principles can guide intervention in the parent-child relationship regardless of the child's level of communicative ability.

Peer Interactions

From another point on the age continuum, the social problems of older children with language disorders and learning disabilities provide further evidence of the detrimental effect a language delay can have on development. In a review of the communication skills and peer relations of learning disabled adolescents, Donahue and Bryan describe the kinds of social interaction difficulties older language impaired children may encounter.[95] Included are problems with making and keeping friends, interacting cooperatively with others in the classroom, fitting into cliques, and learning the slang that is currently popular. These problems may persist into adulthood; Blalock found that 50 percent of the adults she studied with residual language and learning disabilities had few friends, made inappropriate social comments, or showed inappropriate use of personal space.[96]

There are several reasons why children with delayed language development may have peer interaction problems. First, some children with language delays also have problems in social perception. They have difficulty perceiving and interpreting the nonverbal cues of social communication, such as facial expression, intonation, social space, and gesture.[97] Second, language delayed children sometimes also have motor problems that may interfere with their mastery of social activities such as sports and learning dance steps. A third and major reason language delayed children may have peer interaction problems relates specifically to the language impairment. Gottman and Parker identified several conversational processes that are highly related to children hitting it off with each other in the first steps of friendship building.[98] In order of importance, these processes are communication clarity and connectedness (especially the provision of clarification following a request), the successful exchange of information, exploration of interpersonal similarities and differences, the establishment of joint play activities, the amicable resolution of conflicts, and disclosure of private thoughts and information. Language delayed children may have considerable difficulty with many of these communicative exchange processes. In addition, numerous other communication problems of language delayed children can influence their peer relationships: they frequently have difficulty understanding verbal humor; they have trouble learning ritual insults; they take teasing very literally; they are slow to master slang; their problems understanding rapid speech and following topic shifts may make it hard to keep up with conversations; they may have problems learning the rules of games, especially word games; they may not know the rules for when and how to initiate and terminate conversations; or they may be excluded because they "sound different." And fourth, language delayed children may develop poor peer interaction skills because they have more limited opportunities to learn them. Children who are socially and linguistically less mature than their age mates may become social isolates, thereby further decreasing their opportunities to learn appropriate peer interaction skills. Educational settings can contribute to this problem as well. Children who are served in special education classrooms may have little opportunity to learn appropriate peer interaction skills from normal peers.

Awareness of the probabilities of peer interaction problems among children with delayed language development alerts clinicians to the need to assess peer interaction as a subsystem of the social domain. Clinicians have several techniques available for such an assessment at an intrasystem level. These include observing the frequency and type of social interaction the child engages in within the classroom, on the playground, and in small group situations; interviewing parents and teachers about the child's activities, including friendships, groups the child participates in, and special interests; and sociograms of the relationship dynamics in groups. At an intersystem interactions level, the clinician can pay particular attention to the role language plays in each of these situations. If the child is found to be at risk for peer interaction problems, several methods of intervention are available. First, the child's environment can be structured so that more opportunities arise for successful social interaction. These opportunities may include having the parent arrange small playgroups, finding a few potential friends and arranging for more frequent contact with them, mainstreaming the child to increase opportunities to learn social behavior from normal peers, and having the teacher arrange peer tutoring opportunities. Helping the child develop special interests in which she or he can excel is useful for boosting the child's self-concept and can also afford opportunities to interact with peers who have similar interests. Teachers can be encouraged to reinforce cooperative group performance on tasks, rather than rewarding individual competition.[95] For children who do not interact successfully with normal peers, opportunities can be arranged for the child to interact with younger normal children, who may be more comparable in language age and social maturity to the language delayed child.

A second approach to intervention for language delayed children with peer interaction problems involves direct teaching of social interaction skills. The techniques used for direct teaching include using films for modelling prosocial behavior,[24] applying programs for social training (such as magic circle[99] or personal effectiveness training[100]), and training specific social communication skills.[97] Researchers at the University of Kansas are developing a strategies training approach for use with learning disabled adolescents.[101] Students are taught specific strategies for resisting peer pressure, giving positive and negative feedback, negotiating, and personal problem solving.

Development of Self-Concept

Two aspects of self-concept were distinguished by William James—the social self and the private self. The social self consists of the many social roles we play, which expand and change throughout development. The toddler soon adds to the roles of child, daughter, and sibling those of playmate, pupil, and so forth. The private self is one's inner essence—those thoughts, feelings, intentions, and memories of a unique set of experiences that are hidden from the purview of others. Although anthropologists such as Rosaldo have recently suggested that this dichotomy may be culturally shaped and not a universal characteristic of human beings everywhere,[102] it is a helpful framework for considering the self-concept of the language delayed child. On the one hand, one needs to consider how well a child has absorbed the role attributes and relationships that are required in various social contexts. This consideration requires a social view of the child in myriad social contexts. On the other hand, one should be attuned to the inner emotional world of the child.

The self-esteem of language and learning disabled children often becomes a glaring clinical problem by the time the children reach adolescence.[97] We would hope that a conscious consideration of the role of language in the development of self-concept would alert clinicians to pay attention to this dimension of the child's development from the earliest stages of intervention and to intervene when problems are evidenced.

In order to consider the impact of a language delay upon a child's developing self-concept, consideration of the process of development is helpful. In the following, we will consider two possible avenues of development of self-concept—the "looking glass self" and learning social roles—and how a language delay might interfere in both of these processes.

The Looking Glass Self

Mead stresses the impact of the child's experiences with others on her or his developing self-concept.[103] He discusses the "looking glass self" wherein children's developing understanding of their own identity represents a reflection of how others see and respond to them. Mead distinguished between the "I"—the personality—and the "me"—which is built on attitudes of others. We tend to agree with the anthropologist Rosaldo, who recently suggested that undoubtedly both aspects are socially created, not just the "public" self.[102] Indeed, in the following discussion, we consider how others' opinions might shape the innermost emotional landscape of the language delayed child.

We might extend Mead's "looking glass" metaphor and consider factors that might cause others to give the language delayed child a poor reflection of himself, an image eventually internalized to form the child's own poor "self-image." First of all, from Mead's perspective the development of the self-concept is inextricably bound to social interaction. As such, the issues discussed earlier in the section on the development of social relationships point out potential problems in the development of self-concept as well. The parent who cannot "read" the infant and who eventually feels helpless because of this inability probably initially reflects any number of negative emotions back onto the child, such as frustration and anger. Later, the parent protects himself from these less than satisfactory interactions by simply avoiding them altogether. Meanwhile, the child is internalizing these negative feelings in the initial formation of his self-concept. The lack of interaction that ensues may also have a disintegrative effect on the emotional health of the child (e.g., Bowlby and Spitz both have studied the extremely deleterious effects of extreme social deprivation on all aspects of infant development[104,105]).

In addition to the day to day frustrations of interacting with a child who is difficult to interact with, the parents' emotional "reflections" may stem from the broader impact of dealing with the extreme disappointment of having a handicapped child at all. An emotionally healthy adjustment to such a disappointment often requires months, or even years, of moving through the grieving process, with its stages of denial, anger, guilt, and depression that may precede acceptance of the handicap. These emotions are undoubtedly also "reflected" back onto the child. In addition, siblings may naturally become jealous of the special attention given to the handicapped child, leading to yet another source of negative reflections on the "looking glass" that serves as the basis of the child's self-concept.

Negative reflections are not restricted to family members alone. The "different" child is also exposed to the reflections of a society at large in which attitudes toward handicaps may be manifested in ridicule, scorn, revulsion, pity, overprotection, and so forth. One mother we worked with relayed a heartrending story of the appalled reaction of a woman in a neighboring car at a red light to the behavior of her autistic son. The mother felt so humiliated by the other woman's reaction that she followed her for blocks to give her a card she carried for just such occasions. It said, "Please excuse my child's unusual behavior. He is autistic. For more information on autism, call ________" (here she provided the phone number of the state society for autistic citizens).

The notion of the "looking glass self" reminds the clinician doing the initial inter- and intrasystem analyses to look closely at the child's emotional self-concept, at the reflections of self she or he is receiving from significant others, and at the needs of those others as well. We must sensitize ourselves to the many ways in which the child might allow us glimpses of the state of her or his own inner emotional world that has developed as a result of many of these experiences. Children sometimes provide such glimpses by fleeting comments they make. More often, we are able to discern their feelings by reading the sometimes subtle and sometimes poignantly direct symbols manifested in their play, drawings, and fantasy stories.

Interviewing the parents and siblings and examining parent-child and sibling-child interactions aid the clinician in identifying the child's mirrors in the immediate environment. In addition, the clinician might specifically assess the parents' feelings and attitudes about having a handicapped child as well as their resources for coping with these problems. Too often clinicians react to parents' expressions of guilt, anger, fear, denial, or depression without understanding the functions these feelings serve in helping the parents cope with having a handicapped child. Moses has provided helpful explanations of the functions of these feelings and suggestions for how clinicians might deal with them productively rather than reactively.[106]

At the developmental level, Greenspan's work provides a framework for discerning the normal emotional concerns of children at different developmental stages.[107] This framework provides a backdrop to use in determining whether a language delayed child is having emotional problems above and beyond the normal unconscious struggles toward growth.

When self-concept problems are suspected or identified through analysis of the "looking glass self," clinical intervention aimed at either preventing or remediating the language delayed child's poor self-concept might include a number of approaches. These include (1) improving the parent-child interaction, (2) connecting the parents with resources (such as counseling, support groups, and financial assistance) for coping with the added stress of having a handicapped child, (3) helping parents through the grieving process, and (4) being alert to signals from the handicapped child regarding her or his inner emotional world. In addition, involving siblings in the intervention process can serve to abate the natural and potentially destructive rivalries that often attend having a handicapped sibling.

Learning Social Roles

Much of our identity is defined by the various social roles we play. During development, a child learns the norms or prescriptions for behavior associated with various roles. Language is related to this process in several ways. First, at the most global level, a child's mastery of the language of her or his community is a prerequisite to full participation in that society. Second, language is the principal avenue for conveying attitudes and social beliefs to the child. Third, knowing the language of cultural subgroups is essential to a sense of belonging to those groups.[108]

Language delayed children are clearly at a disadvantage in learning the variety of social roles that provide access to social groups and to society in general. Because these children have less skill with language, they are deprived of the most important channel for learning about social roles. This undoubtedly leads to an experiential deficit, since the language delayed child does not learn the many roles that the normal child can pick up incidentally by observing others converse in various roles. In addition, normal children often practice roles such as mother, father, doctor, or teacher by role playing them in their dramatic play. We have already mentioned that some language delayed children appear to have deficits in their ability to engage in such symbolic play. Here again, the language delayed child, because of a lack of skill, would be deprived of practice in learning social roles.

For older children, being a member of the childhood culture in part requires the rather advanced linguistic skills involved in playground chants, jump rope rhymes, handclap songs, punning, ritualized insults, and secret languages. These types of language play are transmitted by children to children. Bernstein notes that such play with language makes the child "sensitive to roles and status and also to the customary relationships connecting and legitimizing the social positions within his peer group."[109] Regarding secret languages specifically, Sherzer notes that "a common function of play languages is concealment and a corresponding delineation of social groups and subgroups."[110] Not surprisingly, these various forms of language play are beyond the capacity of many language disordered children. They are unable to use such language skills to reinforce group solidarity and achieve access to important aspects of the childhood culture.

The preceding discussion offers some guidelines for the assessment of a child's knowledge of social roles at an intrasystem analysis level. One may want to observe the child interacting in a variety of social roles—as a daughter or son, student, playmate, sibling, and so forth—in an attempt to determine the child's role attribute knowledge. If the child engages in role play during dramatic play, one is provided with yet another window into such competencies. For the older child, one would need to assess the ability to engage in language play.

At an interaction level, the notion of social roles suggests that the interventionist consider potential language goals for their usefulness in the various social roles the child must function in. In addition, children may need to be taught to recognize the different social roles of others and to adjust their language accordingly. As was discussed when we addressed peer interaction, particular types of language required for some roles might need to be taught directly. Many language delayed children must be taught to understand and enjoy jokes, slang, and the rituals of their peer groups. Social role learning also raises the issue of who is the best agent to teach different social roles. Peers may be the best agents for teaching play group roles; parents may be best for son or daughter roles; teachers may be best for student roles. Often clinicians want to engage others in the child's intervention to increase carryover effects. However, many times clinicians ask others to play a clinician role. The social role learning perspective suggests that these others may be more naturally equipped to teach the language related to roles they already engage in with the child. The most successful clinician may be the one who can convey critical information about how the child learns and what language the child needs to learn for particular roles and may also be the one who can guide others to assist in the teaching.

Academic Success

In the preschool years, children's dual task of both learning language and deriving meaning in social contexts is bolstered by the fact that the language they hear is usually embedded in concrete, daily life experiences. The nonlinguistic context and numerous nonverbal devices provide cues to meaning. As the child enters school, there are increasing demands to derive meaning from the linguistic code alone in both reading and following classroom discussions. In our culture, language is the primary medium of formal education. It is not surprising then that language delayed children are at risk for academic failure.

Language plays a crucial role in nearly all the academic tasks children encounter. Many kinds of language skills interact to influence classroom success, including (1) literacy knowledge, (2) metalinguistic skills, (3) comprehension monitoring,[111] (4) classroom pragmatic and discourse skills,[112–114] (5) the role of language in concept formation,[115,116] (6) the role of language in reasoning,[2,45] (7) using language to plan,[45,117] (8) strategies for learning and study skills,[38] and (9) language necessary for specific academic content areas.[97] Entire books have been written about many of these areas. We shall briefly discuss only the first two areas listed and refer readers to the references listed after each of the other areas for comprehensive coverage of the issues involved.

Literacy Knowledge

In recent years, anthropologists who have become interested in literacy as a cultural phenomenon have documented the vast knowledge about literacy that children acquire before they ever learn to actually decode print. Van Kleeck and Schuele summarize the domains of literacy knowledge possessed by preschoolers that are indicated in this research.[117] Some of these areas of knowledge include (1) the nature of print (i.e., that it corresponds to oral language and hence meaningful ideas), (2) the multiple functions of print (for entertainment, communicating, self-expression, acquiring information, carrying out daily affairs, practicing religion), (3) many conventions of print (e.g., front to back of book, left to right on line of print, top to bottom on page), and (4) how to take meaning from books (i.e., answer questions about their content in a school-like fashion).

Researchers in this area all suggest that these kinds of knowledge facilitate a smooth transition into learning how to actually read. Van Kleeck and Schuele posit that, in addition to focusing on oral language skills, intervention with preschool language delayed children should be aimed toward developing such literacy knowledge.[117] In a second article, these authors offer numerous concrete suggestions for both assessment and intervention aimed at these skill areas.[118]

Metalinguistic Skills

Metalinguistic refers to language awareness. These skills are manifested when a child is able to consciously focus on the linguistic code as an object in its own right. This ability underlies numerous skills,[119] not the least of which numerous researchers believe is learning to decode print in early reading acquisition. In addition, learning secret languages and many other forms of language play discussed earlier require a conscious focus on the linguistic code. Many classroom language arts skills—such as defining words, forming synonyms and antonyms, and rhyming—are clearly metalinguistic in nature.

Many language delayed children experience difficulty with various metalinguistic skills.[120] Here again, as with literacy knowledge, intervention can begin in the preschool years. Van Kleeck and Schuele discuss the normal development of numerous early emerging metalinguistic skills believed to be important to early reading and provide assessment and intervention suggestions in a subsequent article.[118,119]

SUMMARY

In this chapter, we have reviewed the theories and models upon which much current language intervention practice is based. We have suggested that the variety of available theoretic perspectives provide a set of lenses through which the clinician might view individual children who present with the symptom of language delay. There are two final considerations we must address before leaving the clinician to use these lenses to explore language delayed children's individual differences.

The first consideration involves the problem of fragmentation. There is a danger in the artificiality of viewing the child as a series of separate systems. Damico has discussed the strong reliance on fragmentation in language assessment and the fallacy of breaking "the elements of language apart and trying to test them with little or no attention to the way those elements interact in the larger context of communication."[121] Neither language nor children function this way; both are complex, synergistic systems in which the whole is significantly different from the sum of the parts. Unfortunately, as Schacter et al have pointed out, interventionists have tended to take either a fragmented view and attempted to "fix" one part of the system or a whole child view and attempted to provide general stimulation.[122] Neither approach is successful in meeting all of the individual needs of language delayed children.

We would suggest that the nature of the problem lies not so much in the initial fragmentation, but in the failure to put the parts back together again. The complexity of language and its social, cognitive, and physical bases requires the careful scrutiny of its parts if the clinician hopes to examine the child's strengths and weaknesses in sufficient depth to understand them. What speech-language pathology has spent less time doing is examining the inter- and intrasystem interactions in order to understand the reciprocal relationships among the specific language problems, the contexts in which they occur, the other systems involved, and the whole child. We hope that more careful attention to levels four and five in our intervention planning model will remedy many of our former oversights.

The final consideration is the potential theoretic incompatibility that can arise from clinicians viewing children through lenses of different and possibly conflicting theoretic perspectives. One type of problem that may arise is a mismatch between assumptions about language and actual intervention practices. For example, Rice has discussed the mismatch between the premises of most language intervention (that the problem resides within the child, that the focus of treatment should be on discrete skills, that language skills can be hierarchically organized) and the premises of the communication competence model, which takes into account the complex interactions among language, cultural expectations, and the context of communication.[1] Another type of problem springs from the clinician's lack of awareness of and commitment to her or his own theoretic assumptions. In order to adapt to the individual needs of language delayed children, the clinician may switch assumptions with each child. As Johnston quips, "If this is Elmer, I must provide reinforcing consequent events."[71]

The necessity to draw from numerous theoretic perspectives in assessing and planning for the language delayed child should be obvious by this point. None of the theoretic orientations we have reviewed is comprehensive enough to yield an adequately broad view of the whole child. Few models account for the heterogeneity we find among children with delayed language. And no one perspective addresses all of the levels that need to be considered in intervention planning, even within the primary domain it focuses on. So how can the interventionist integrate many simultaneously held beliefs into one theoretically consistent perspective for dealing with children's individual differences? We agree with Johnston that the solution lies in taking theory seriously and in making explicit one's basic beliefs.[71] The clinician who is sensitive to individual differences expects children to differ in the etiology and pathogenesis of the language difficulties, in the effects of context and the environment, in the interactions that occur within and among systems, in the goals selected for intervention, and in the optimal intervention agents and procedures. However, despite viewing the child through many different lenses, it is unlikely that the clinician can switch basic beliefs on the following questions without considerable soulsearching:

1. What is the nature of language?
2. What is language intervention?
3. What makes children's language behavior change?

The clinician must make explicit her or his answers to these questions and then must test the assessment and intervention practices selected to be sure that they are compatible with these basic assumptions.

Acknowledgment. We wish to thank Dana Kovarsky for his help in compiling the information in Tables 22–7 to 22–11.

REFERENCES

1. Rice M. Mismatched premises of the communicative competence model in language intervention. In: Schiefelbusch RL, ed. Language competence: assessment and intervention. San Diego: College-Hill Press, 1986:261.
2. Blank M, Rose SA, Berlin L. The language of learning: the preschool years. New York: Grune and Stratton, 1978.
3. Kirchner DM, Skarakis-Doyle E. Developmental language disorders: a theoretical perspective. In: Gallagher T, Prutting C, eds. Pragmatic assessment and intervention issues in language. San Diego: College-Hill Press, 1983: 215.
4. Skinner BF. Verbal behavior. New York: Appleton-Century-Crofts, 1957.
5. Glucksberg S, Krauss R, Higgins ET. The development of referential communication skills. In: Horowitz F, ed. Review of child development research. Vol. 4. Chicago: Chicago University Press, 1975:305.
6. Nelson K. Event knowledge: structure and function in development. Hillsdale, NJ: Erlbaum, 1986.
7. Reese E. The analysis of human operant behavior. Dubuque, IA: WC Brown, 1966.
8. Warren SF, Kaiser AP. Incidental language teaching: a critical review. J Speech Hear Disord 1986; 51:291–299.
9. Barlow DH, Hersen M. Single case experimental designs. New York: Pergamon Press, 1984.
10. McReynolds LV, Kearns K. Single-subject experimental designs in communicative disorders. Austin, TX: Pro-Ed, 1983.
11. McLean J. Historical perspectives on the content of child language programs. In: Miller J, Yoder D, Schiefelbusch R, eds. Contemporary issues in language intervention. Rockville, MD: The American Speech-Language-Hearing Association, 1983:115.
12. Bruner J. Child's talk: learning to use language. New York: Norton, 1983.
13. Duchan JF. The elephant is soft and mushy: problems in assessing children's language. In: Lass N, McReynolds L, Northern J, Yoder D, eds. Speech, language, and hearing. Vol. II. Pathologies of speech and language. Philadelphia: WB Saunders, 1982:741.
14. Ingram D. The psychological reality of grammatical rules in children's language. Paper presented at the University of Washington, 1979.
15. Panagos JM, ed. Children's phonological disorders in language contexts. Semin Speech Lang Hear 1982; 3:101.
16. Hodson BW, Paden EP. Targeting intelligible speech. San Diego: College-Hill Press, 1983.
17. Bloom L. Language development: form and function in emerging grammars. Cambridge: MIT Press, 1970.
18. Brown R. A first language. Cambridge: Harvard University Press, 1973.
19. Schlesinger IM. Steps to language: toward a theory of native language acquisition. Hillsdale, NJ: Erlbaum, 1982.
20. Rice M, Kemper S. Child language and cognition. Baltimore: University Park Press, 1984.
21. Dunst CJ. Infant learning: a cognitive-linguistic intervention strategy. New York: Teaching Resources, 1981.
22. Bloom L. One word at a time: the use of single word utterances before syntax. The Hague: Mouton, 1973.
23. Bloom L, Lahey M. Language development and language disorders. New York: John Wiley and Sons, 1978.
24. Fey M. Language intervention with young children. San Diego: College-Hill Press, 1986.
25. McDonald J. Environmental language inventory. Columbus, OH: CE Merrill, 1978.
26. Owens R. Language development: an introduction. Columbus, OH: CE Merrill, 1984:100.
27. Duckworth E. Either we're too early and they can't learn it or we're too late and they know it already: the dilemma

of "applying Piaget." Harvard Educ Rev 1979; 49:297–312.

28. Rosenberg S, Cohen BD. Referential processes of speakers and listeners. Psychol Rev 1966; 73:208–231.
29. Flavell F, Botkin P, Fry C, Wright J, Jarvis P. The development of role-taking and communication skills in children. New York: John Wiley and Sons, 1968.
30. Fischer K, Corrigan R. A skill approach to language development. In: Stark R, ed. Language behavior in infancy and early childhood. New York: Elsevier North-Holland, 1981:245.
31. Shatz M. The relationship between cognitive processes and the development of communication skills. In: Keasey CB, ed. Nebraska symposium on motivation. Vol. 25. Lincoln, NB: University of Nebraska Press, 1977:1.
32. Cole M, Gay J, Glick J, Sharp D. The cultural context of learning and thinking. New York: Basic Books, 1971.
33. Das JP, Kirby JR, Jarman RF. Simultaneous and successive cognitive processes. New York: Academic Press, 1979.
34. Kaufman AS, Kaufman NL. Kaufman assessment battery for children; interpretive manual. Circle Pines, MN: American Guidance Service, 1983.
35. Orzbut JE, Orzbut A, Bryden MP, Bartels SB. Information processing and speech lateralization in learning disabled children. Brain Lang 1985; 25:87–101.
36. Goldman R, Fristoe M, Woodcock R. GFW auditory skills battery. Circle Pines, MN: American Guidance Service, 1974.
37. Kaufmann AS, Kaufman NL. Kaufman assessment battery for children. Circle Pines, MN: American Guidance Service, 1983.
38. Deshler DD, Warner MM, Shumaker JB, Alley GR. Learning strategies intervention model. In: McKinney J, Feagans L, eds. Current topics in learning disabilities. Vol. I. Norwood, NJ: Ablex, 1983:245.
39. Peters A. Language learning strategies: does the whole equal the sum of the parts? Language 1977; 53:560–573.
40. Prizant B. Language acquisition and communicative behavior in autism: toward an understanding of the "whole" of it. J Speech Hear Disord 1983; 48:296–307.
41. Constable CM. The application of scripts in the organization of language intervention contexts. In: Nelson K, ed. Event knowledge: structure and function in development. Hillsdale, NJ: Erlbaum, 1986:205.
42. Lucariello J, Kyratzis A, Engel S. Event representations, context, and language. In: Nelson K, ed. Event knowledge. Hillsdale, NJ: Erlbaum, 1986:137.
43. Vygotsky LS. Mind in society: the development of higher psychological processes. Cambridge: Harvard University Press, 1978.
44. Brown AL, Ferrera RA. Diagnosing zones of proximal development. In: Wertch J, ed. Culture, communication, and cognition: Vygotskian perspectives. Cambridge: Cambridge University Press, 1985:273.
45. Feuerstein R. Instrumental enrichment: an intervention program for cognitive modifiability. Baltimore: University Park Press, 1980.
46. Olswang L, Bain B, Rosendahl P, Oblak S, Smith A. Language learning: moving performance from a context-dependent to -independent state. Child Lang Teach Ther 1986; 2:180–210.
47. Bruner JS. On cognitive growth. In: Bruner JS, Oliver RR, Greenfield PM, eds. Studies in cognitive growth. New York: John Wiley and Sons, 1966:1.
48. Nineo A, Bruner JS. The achievements and antecedents of labelling. J Child Lang 1978; 5:1–16.
49. Ratner N, Bruner JS. Games, social exchange, and the acquisition of language. J Child Lang 1978; 5:391–402.
50. Snow CE, Goldfield BA. Turn the page please: situation specific language acquisition. J Child Lang 1983; 10:551–569.
51. Bruner J. Vygotsky: a historical and conceptual perspective. In: Wertsch J, ed. Culture, communication, and cognition: Vygotskian perspectives. Cambridge: Cambridge University Press, 1985:21.
52. Bandura A. Social learning theory. Englewood Cliffs, NJ: Prentice-Hall, 1977.
53. Myklebust H. Auditory disorders in children. New York: Grune and Stratton, 1954.
54. Bernstein D, Tigerman E. Language and communication disorders in children. Columbus, OH: CE Merrill, 1985.
55. Carrow-Woolfolk E, Lynch J. An introduction to language disorders in children. New York: Grune and Stratton, 1982.
56. Reed V. An introduction to children with language disorders. New York: Macmillan, 1986.
57. McCormick L, Schiefelbusch R. Early language intervention. Columbus, OH: CE Merrill, 1984.
58. Rapin I, Allen D. Developmental language disorders: nosological considerations. In: Kirk U, ed. Neuropsychology of language, reading, and spelling. New York: Academic Press, 1983:155.
59. Seiben RL. Medical treatment of learning problems—a critique. In: Canine D, Elkind D, Hendrickson D, Meichenbaum D, Seiben RL, Smith F, eds. Interdisciplinary voices in learning disabilities and remedial education. Austin, TX: Pro-Ed, 1983:157.
60. Rudel R, Denckla M. Relation of forward and backward digit repetition to neurological impairment in children with learning disabilities. Neuropsychologia 1974; 12:109–118.
61. Johnston R, Stark R, Melitts E, Tallal P. Neurological status of language impaired and normal children. Ann Neurol 1981; 10:159–163.
62. Worster-Drought C, Allen I. Congenital auditory imperception: report of a case with congenital word deafness. J Neurol Psychopathol 1929; 9:193–203.
63. Hardy W. On language disorders in young children: a reorganization of thinking. J Speech Hear Disord 1965; 30:3–16.
64. Myklebust H. Childhood aphasia: an evolving concept. In: Travis L, ed. Handbook of speech pathology and audiology. New York: Appleton-Century-Crofts, 1971:1181.
65. Keith RW, ed. Central auditory dysfunction. New York: Grune and Stratton, 1977.
66. Tallal P, Piercy M. Defects of auditory perception in children with developmental aphasia. In: Wyke M, ed. Developmental dysphasia. New York: Academic Press, 1978:63.
67. Tomblin JB. Specific abilities approach: an evaluation and an alternative method. In: Perkins WH, ed. Language handicaps in children. New York: Thieme-Stratton, 1984:27.
68. Kirk S, McCarthy J, Kirk W. The Illinois test of psycholinguistic abilities. Urbana, IL: University of Illinois Press, 1968.
69. van Kleeck A. Assessment and intervention: does "meta" matter? In: Wallach G, Butler K, eds. Language learning disabilities in school-age children. Baltimore: Williams and Wilkins, 1984:179.
70. Keith RW, ed. Central auditory and language disorders in children. San Diego: College-Hill Press, 1981.
71. Johnston J. The language disordered child. In: Lass N, McReynolds L, Northern J, Yoder D, eds. Speech, language, and hearing. Vol. II. Pathologies of speech and language. Philadelphia: WB Saunders, 1982:780.
72. Williford JA, Burleigh J. Handbook of central auditory processing disorders in children. New York: Grune and Stratton, 1985.
73. Arthur B. The Arthur adaptation of the Leiter international performance scale. Washington, DC: Psychological Service Center Press, 1952.
74. Burgemeister B, Blum L, Long I. Columbia mental maturity scale. 3rd ed. New York: Harcourt, Brace, Jovanovich, 1972.
75. Rosenthal W. The role of perception in child language dis-

orders: a theory based on faulty signal detection strategies. Paper presented at the American Speech and Hearing Association, 1974.
76. Brown J, Redmond A, Bass L, Liebergott J, Swope S. Symbolic play in normal and language impaired children. Paper presented at the American Speech and Hearing Association, Washington, DC, 1975.
77. Savich P. Anticipating imagery ability in normal and language-disabled children. J Speech Hear Res 1984; 27:494–501.
78. Kamhi A, Catts H, Koenig L, Lewis B. Hypothesis-testing and nonlinguistic symbolic abilities in language-impaired children. J Speech Hear Disord 1984; 49:169–176.
79. Cromer R. The basis of childhood aphasia: a linguistic approach. In: Wyke M, ed. Developmental dysphasia. New York: Academic Press, 1978:85.
80. Kamhi A, Catts H, Lee R, Gholson B. The ability of language-disordered children to use and modify hypotheses in discrimination learning. Appl Psycholinguist 1985; 6:435–452.
81. Westby C. Assessment of cognitive and language abilities through play. Lang Speech Hear Services Schools 1980; 11:154–168.
82. Nicholich L. Beyond sensorimotor intelligence: assessment of symbolic maturity through analysis of pretend play. Merrill-Palmer Q 1977; 23:89–101.
83. Lowe M, Costello A. Symbolic play test. Berkshire, UK: NFER-Nelson, 1976.
84. McCune-Nicholich L, Carroll S. Development of symbolic play: implications for the language specialist. Top Lang Disord 1981; 2:1–16.
85. Lund N, Duchan J. Assessing children's language in naturalistic contexts. Englewood Cliffs, NJ: Prentice-Hall, 1983.
86. Crystal D. Profiling linguistic disability. London: Edward Arnold, 1982.
87. Miller J. Assessing language production in children: experimental procedures. Baltimore: University Park Press, 1981.
88. Halliday M. Relevant models of language. Educ Rev 1969; 22:26–37.
89. Dunst C. Communicative competence and deficits: effects on early social interactions. In: McDonald E, Gallagher D, eds. Facilitating social-emotional development in the young multiply handicapped child. Philadelphia: Home of the Merciful Savior Press, 1985.
90. Goldberg S. Social competence in infancy: a model of parent-infant interaction. Merrill-Palmer Q 1977; 23:163–177.
91. Harter S. Effectance motivation reconsidered: towards a developmental model. Hum Dev 1978; 21:34–64.
92. Caldwell B, Bradley R. Home observation for measurement of the environment. Little Rock, AK: Center for Child Development and Education, 1966.
93. Nygard NK, Adair M. Why parent programs don't work. Paper presented at the American Speech-Language-Hearing Association, Atlanta, 1979.
94. Manolson A. It takes two to talk: a Hanen early language parent guide book. Toronto: Hanen Early Language Resource Center, 1983.
95. Donahue M, Bryan T. Communication skills and peer relations of learning disabled adolescents. Top Lang Disord 1984; 4:10–21.
96. Blalock J. Persistent problems and concerns of young adults with learning disabilities. In: Cruickshank W, Silver A, eds. Bridges to tomorrow: the best of ACLD. Vol. 2. Syracuse: Syracuse University Press, 1981:35.
97. Wiig E, Semel E. Language assessment and intervention for the learning disabled. 2nd ed. Columbus, OH: CE Merrill, 1984.
98. Parker J. Becoming friends: conversational skills for friendship formation in young children. In: Gottman J, Parker JG, eds. Conversations of friends: speculations on affective development. New York: Cambridge University Press, 1986: 103.
99. Gerber ER. The magic circle program: how to involve teachers? Element School Guid Counsel 1973; 8:86–91.
100. Liberman RP, King LW, DeRisi WJ, McCann M. Personal effectiveness. Champaign, IL: Research Press, 1975.
101. Hazel J, Schumaker J, Sherman J, Sheldon J. Application of a group training program in social skills and problem solving skills to learning disabled and non-learning disabled youth. Learn Disabil Q 1982; 5:398–408.
102. Rosaldo M. Toward an anthropology of self and feeling. In: Shweder R, Levine R, eds. Culture theory: essays on mind, self, and emotion. Cambridge: Cambridge University Press, 1984:137.
103. Mead GH. Mind, self and society. Chicago: University of Chicago Press, 1934.
104. Bowlby J. Maternal care and mental health. New York: Columbia University Press, 1952.
105. Spitz R. Infantile depression and the general adaptation syndrome In: Hoch P, Zubin J, eds. Depression. New York: Grune and Stratton, 1954.
106. Moses K. Counseling: a critical part of our practice. American Speech-Language-Hearing Association teleconference, 1986.
107. Greenspan S. The clinical interview of the child. New York: McGraw-Hill, 1981:15.
108. Bram J. Language and society. New York: Random House, 1963.
109. Bernstein B. Review of "the lore and language of school children" by I and P Opie. Br J Sociol 1969; 11:178–181.
110. Sherzer J. Play languages: implications for (socio) linguistics. In: Kirshenblatt-Kimblett B, ed. Speech play. Philadelphia: University of Pennsylvania Press, 1976.
111. Dolloghan C. Comprehension and monitoring in normal and language-impaired children. Top Lang Disord 1987; 7:45–60.
112. Ripich D, Spinelli F, eds. School discourse problems. San Diego: College-Hill Press, 1985.
113. Simon C, ed. Communication skills and classroom success: assessment of language-learning disabled students. San Diego: College-Hill Press, 1985.
114. Simon C, ed. Communication skills and classroom success: therapy methodologies for language-learning disabled students. San Diego: College-Hill Press, 1985.
115. Johnston J, ed. Cognition and language in the preschool years. Top Lang Disord 1981:2.
116. Werner H, Kaplan B. Symbol formation. New York: John Wiley and Sons, 1963.
117. van Kleeck A, Schuele M. Precursors to literacy: normal development. Top Lang Disord 1987; 7:13–21.
118. Schuele M, van Kleeck A. Precursors to literacy: assessment and intervention. Top Lang Disord 1987; 7:32–44.
119. van Kleeck A. Metalinguistic skills: cutting across spoken and written language and problem-solving abilities. In: Wallach G, Butler K, eds. Language learning disabilities in school-age children. Baltimore: Williams and Wilkins, 1984:128.
120. Kamhi A. Metalinguistic abilities in language-impaired children. Top Lang Disord 1987; 7:1–12.
121. Damico J. The lack of efficacy in language therapy. Unpublished manuscript, Louisiana State University, 1986.
122. Schachter F, Kirshner K, Klips B, Friedricks M, Sanders K. Everyday preschool interpersonal speech usage: methodological, developmental, and sociolinguistic studies. Monogr Soc Res Child Dev 1974; 39:1–88.

23 Specific Language Disorders in the Child

Judith R. Johnston, Ph.D.

The fact that most children learn to talk easily, rapidly, and within a predictable age range is a touchstone of contemporary psycholinguistics. This chapter concerns one group of children who do not. Variously labelled as developmentally aphasic, dysphasic, language impaired, language disabled, or language disordered, these children acquire language more slowly, at a later age, and with less success than do their peers.

A typical definition of this population opened the Proceedings of the Institute on Childhood Aphasia, which met at Stanford in the Fall of 1960:

> Impairment of language function (expressive and receptive) resulting from maldevelopment or injury to the central nervous system, prenatally, paranatally, or postnatally (not later . . . than the normal time for the development of speech . . .). The language deficiency may or may not be associated with other cerebral or neurological pathology or dysfunction.
>
> Excluded are language problems associated primarily with:
>
> (1) mental deficiency
> (2) hearing impairment
> (3) central nervous system damage affecting the peripheral speech mechanism
> (4) emotional disturbance
> (5) delayed maturation in language development resulting from social and emotional factors or physical factors not primarily due to central nervous system involvement. (p 1).[1]

Children of this sort had been studied as early as 1835,[2] but the Stanford conference represented a modern surge of interest in the identification and treatment of children who had difficulty learning language and did not fit the more common etiological or pedagogical categories.

The significance of the Stanford meeting lies not in the answers it provided, but in the questions that were asked. These questions presaged two decades of investigation and thus set the stage for this review. The purpose of this chapter is to summarize the research with language disordered children in three areas pertinent to population description: language acquisition patterns, perceptual function, and intellectual development.* In each topic area, the Institute on Childhood Aphasia shall serve as a point of reference.

What has been learned about developmental language disorders since 1960? Do views of the language disordered child and hence of language intervention need revision? What questions remain unanswered?

Before pursuing this task, two methodological notes are in order. The first concerns the problem of population. The opening statement of the Institute on Childhood Aphasia will be used as a working definition of language disordered children. Although many of the studies reviewed here provide only a portion of the necessary descriptive information, none of the reports concerns children who clearly violate this working definition, and all of them concern children who meet at least the minimal criteria of significant language delay, normal-range performance intelligence quotient (IQ), and adequate peripheral hearing. The key feature of the working definition is, of course, the developmental gap between language and other aspects of growth. Similar gaps may exist for some children with subnormal performance IQ,[3] but such children have not yet been systematically studied and will not be discussed further in this chapter. Finally, recent longitudinal studies suggest that language disordered children comprise a notable portion of the school-

* The burgeoning literature on language disorders makes it impossible to review material pertinent to emotional and social health or central nervous system disorders. The reader is referred to the earlier edition of this book for a survey of those areas.

age population currently known as learning disabled.[4-6] Some of the research with such children is undoubtedly pertinent to this review. However, since studies of learning disabilities do not typically report measures of oral language nor identify subjects by type of disability, that literature will not be systematically covered.

The second note concerns terminology. As mentioned earlier, a wide range of terms has been applied to those children who do not learn to talk normally and who generally fit the working definition. Since differences in labels usually reflect theoretical emphasis rather than differences in population, this chapter will speak of children with language disorders,[7,8] regardless of the particular term that individual authors may have used.

LANGUAGE ACQUISITION PATTERNS

Language disordered children, by definition, do not speak like their peers. The goal of linguistic research with this population has been not to discover differences but to characterize them. Participants at the Institute on Childhood Aphasia voiced the opinions that prevailed in 1960:

> Linguistically, the child shows a marked amount of retardation in both the comprehension, evaluation, and production of language, and a disproportion and unevenness in the anticipated comprehension-production ratio . . . Developmentally, the child does not show expected increments or the "ordered" pattern by which most children increase their linguistic abilities (p 82).[1]

A virtual revolution in theoretical linguistics and numerous studies of normal language development have made it possible to examine this portrait in detail. This section considers research in syntax, grammatical morphology, relational semantics, lexical semantics, and pragmatics, emphasizing studies that have analyzed spontaneous conversational speech.† What is now known about the language of language disordered children?

Syntax

Sentence Patterns

The first linguistically based studies of disordered language development were reported by Adams and Pace,[8a] Leonard,[9] and Menyuk.[10] These investigators compared the spontaneous speech of 3- to 5-year-old language disordered children with that of age-matched peers. The language disordered children were found to use fewer complex sentences, elaborated verb phrases, pronouns, adjectives, and auxiliaries.‡ However, Leonard notes that although they used them less frequently, his language disordered children did use advanced structures that were appropriate for their age. Menyuk disagrees, claiming that "at no age level did the grammatical production of a child with deviant speech match or closely match . . . a child with normal speech."[10]

Morehead and Ingram approached this question directly by setting aside the traditional age-matched paradigm.[11] They gathered spontaneous speech samples from 15 language disordered children and 15 younger normal children, matched at five levels of language development, indexed by mean length of utterance. Linguistic analyses revealed that at each level, the same sentence patterns were being used by children in the two groups, at approximately the same frequencies of occurrence. Both Johnston and Kamhi[12] and Meline and Sanders[13] likewise report that groups of language disordered and normal children matched for mean length of utterance produced sentence patterns of equivalent developmental complexity, though the language disordered children did make more grammatical errors.

These data indicate that language disordered children's knowledge of major syntactic categories and sentence-level combinatorial rules resembles that of younger, normal children. Furthermore, since this resemblance has been noted throughout a range of developmental levels, language disordered children may be acquiring sentence patterns in much the normal order.

Discourse Patterns

Since children normally learn most English sentence patterns by the age of 6,[14] it was long believed that syntactic knowledge was an achievement of early childhood. It is now clear that this belief reflected a bias towards "sentence-level" and "function-blind" syntactic analyses. Once children learn to combine words into grammatical sentences, they must learn to combine sentences into larger dis-

† Data pertinent to phonological development are reviewed elsewhere in this volume.

‡ Space constraints make it impossible to report specific means, standard deviations, and significance values for each of the studies that are reviewed. However, the group differences and/or experimental effects that are mentioned do meet accepted levels of reliability. Nevertheless, since much of the research with language disordered children consists of small sample studies, the reader should generalize with caution.

course units and to select the sentence patterns that best serve their communicative task of the moment. This learning continues throughout the school years. To study this growth, researchers have looked at one particularly appealing and universal human form, the story.

Oral narratives are typically organized in a predictable fashion, regardless of specific content. Units such as initiating events, attempts, and consequences are ordered within episodes, and the episodes themselves are ordered to convey temporal and causal connections.[15,16] The principles for constructing and combining narrative units are conventional, abstract, and fundamentally communicative.[17] A speaker may have full knowledge of circumstances and plot, yet be unable to relate the story in a coherent, comprehensible manner. For example, normal 6 year olds are inclined to switch settings without informing the listener, ignore psychological motives and reactions, and forget to resolve the problems they originally introduced.[16,18,19] They may also have difficulty using familiar linguistic tools such as pronominalization or conjoining to convey the discourse structure.[20,21] Given the striking parallels between syntax as traditionally defined and the structure inherent in narratives, it is not surprising that there is now a considerable literature on the acquisition of "story grammar."

Language disordered children, from 6 to 13 years of age, have participated in at least nine studies of narrative ability. Some experimenters have asked children to view a movie and then tell the story to a naive listener. Others have asked children to relate a television plot, retell a story they have just heard, or make one up. Despite differences in methodology, a consistent picture of narrative abilities emerges from this work. As might be expected, the stories of language disordered children tend to be shorter than those of age-matched peers.[21a§,22§,23] They contain the same number of episodes, but are less elaborated. The language disordered children provide less information about the physical setting and the characters and pay little attention to psychological aspects such as motives, plans, and emotional responses. The resultant narratives, like those of younger normal children, focus on the action sequence: initiating events, deeds, and consequences.[21,21a,24–26]

Narratives require specific linguistic skills as well as skill in organizing content. The speaker must convey the connections among events and the hierarchical relationships among episodes. For language disordered children, this complexity apparently leads to general difficulties in sentence formulation[27] and misleading use of conjunctives.[21] The speaker must also use language to construct a well-bonded "text," that is, to tie the elements of one sentence to those of another in ways that clarify reference and simplify linguistic processing. In comparison to their normal age peers, language disordered children are less expert in using such "cohesion devices."[21a,22,23,25,28,29] For example, they frequently fail to use anaphoric pronouns when the text invites them and use them ambiguously when they do.

There is little doubt that story telling challenges the communicative skills of school-age language disordered children. However, the source and extent of their deficits is not yet clear. Organizational weaknesses could reflect the children's poor understanding of story content[21a,29] and/or ignorance of the principles of story telling. Studies of language disordered children have typically ignored this distinction.[30] Linguistic problems with cohesion and reference could reflect special difficulties with text or the "normal" course of acquisition for speakers who were late in mastering sentence-level syntax. Only one study of disordered narrative has included a language-level control group to explore such issues.[27] It looked exclusively at sentence breakdowns, but suggests that language impaired children may know more about narrative structure than their syntax peers and less about expressing it than their age peers.

Grammatical Morphology

Studies of grammatical morphology focus on noun and verb inflections, prepositions, articles, auxiliaries, and other minor syntactic categories, which, as Brown observes,[31] serve to express secondary modulations of basic sentence meaning. Most studies of grammatical morphology have looked at the acquisition of specific forms. Johnston and Schery analyzed conversational samples from 287 language disordered children, noting those grammatical morphemes that appeared at each stage of language development and the consistency with which each was used.[32] Their data yielded two major findings. First, taking consistent (90 percent) use as the criterion for acquisition, language disordered children seemed to acquire grammatical morphemes in much the same order as normal children. Second, although many grammatical morphemes appeared at the earliest stages of language development, they were not used consistently until later than is normal. Data from other investigators corroborate these findings.[9,12,33–36]

These studies of grammatical morphology indicate that language disordered children learn to use

§ This sign indicates that the subjects in study cited may not fit the operational criteria of language disorder used in this chapter.

minor syntactic categories in normal sequence, but over a protracted span of stages. Since developmental stages were indexed by mean length of utterance, there may be some atypical relationship between their proficiency with major sentence patterns and their proficiency with grammatical morphemes—a topic that will be explored further in the section on language deviance.

Semantics

Relational Semantics

The study of meaning can be arbitrarily divided into two subfields: relational semantics, the study of the meanings expressed through word combination, and lexical semantics, the study of the meanings of individual words. Researchers interested in language disordered children have drawn upon the work of Brown,[31] Chafe,[37] Fillmore,[38] and Schlesinger[39] to study relational meaning. Using data from adult or child speech, these writers schematized the relational meanings that may be expressed through sentences. To illustrate briefly, the sentence "The boy caught the fish" tells us that an ACTION occurred, that a boy was the AGENT of that action, and that a fish was the OBJECT acted upon. Stated differently, this sentence expresses two types of relational meaning: AGENT-ACTION, and ACTION-OBJECT. Categories of this sort capture general aspects of the speaker's intention and have been used to characterize the first phases of normal language growth. For example, Bowerman notes that her children's earliest subject noun phrases expressed AGENT-ACTION relations.[40] And Slobin observes that children learning a variety of languages express the same set of basic relational meanings in their first word combinations.[41] Do language disordered children, acquiring language at later than normal ages, show these same patterns?

Leonard, Bolders, and Miller analyzed the speech of normal and language disordered children, age-matched at 3;6 and 5;0, according to the type and number of meaning relations that were encoded in each sentence.[42] Comparisons were restricted to those meaning types that were used by at least half of the children in a given group. The resultant analyses revealed that the children were expressing a single set of relational meanings, regardless of age or group. Differences between groups consisted solely in frequencies of use. When portions of the data were reanalyzed to control for language level, however, even these differences in frequency disappeared. Freedman and Carpenter[43] and Lee[44a] report similar lack of differences. But Leonard, Steckol, and Schwartz using groups matched for mean length of utterance, again detected significant differences in the frequency with which certain meaning relations occur.[45] Normal children were more likely to talk about psychological experiences, that is, EXPERIENCER + VERB, whereas language disordered children expressed more of those relations that normally appear before EXPERIENCER, that is, AGENT + VERB, OBJECT + VERB.

A study by Johnston, Kamhi, and McDonald shed some light on these discrepancies.[46] Language disordered 5 year olds were compared to two control groups, one matched for mental age, the other for mean length of utterance. Samples of spontaneous conversation were collected, and each finite verb was classified according to its meaning type: causal action on objects, locational state, self-movement, modality, and so forth. In contrast to the earlier studies, this analysis differentiated among more types of relational meaning, for example, agent of causal action on objects versus agent of self-movement. It also ignored surface syntax; relational meanings that were implicit in the verb were coded regardless of whether they were fully expressed. Research with normal children had suggested that this approach would be more likely to capture developmental trends.[31,40,47] Distinct profiles of meaning were found for each of the three groups, revolving in particular around the use of modality, aspect, and knowledge-state predicates. The language disordered children expressed modality and aspectual notions less often than either peer group, but resembled the younger, mean length of utterance–matched normals in the frequency with which they spoke about knowledge states. It seems that language disordered children, once past the initial phases of learning, may not express the relational meanings that would be expected for either their mental age or grammatical level.

Lexical Semantics

Developmental studies of the lexicon look beyond broad features of meaning such as +AGENT or +EXPERIENCER to observe the order in which specific words are acquired and the evolving ways in which they are used. Studies with language disordered children have thus far focused on early action and object words, attributive adjectives, and *Wh*-question words.

Leonard and his colleagues observed normal and language disordered children as they learned new labels for objects and events.[48,48a] All of the children were at the one-word level and had vocabularies of 25 to 75 items. Each child heard 16 new words used five times during an unstructured play session. The words that were presented were unlikely to be heard outside of the experiment. Comprehension and production of the new vocabulary items were measured over the course of ten sessions. By both criteria, the language disordered children learned as many of the new words as did the normal children. They were also more likely to produce the action terms. This latter fact is especially interesting given arguments that verb meanings are more difficult to acquire.[49] In related studies of the same subjects, Chapman, Leonard, Rowan, and Weiss[50] and Leonard, Camarata, Schwartz, Chapman, and Messick[51] analyzed aspects of their spontaneous speech. Children in the language disordered group used the same proportion of homonyms as the normal children, and they "overextended" their vocabulary no more than was normal for their language level. However, there was some indication that the disordered children had more words mapped "in competition" to the same referent.

These early vocabulary studies suggest that many aspects of lexical development in language disordered children are appropriate to their language level. Investigations of attributive adjectives and questions seem to corroborate this view. Illerbrun[52] and Peach[53] assessed the comprehension of terms such as *tall, short, happy,* and *red* by language disordered and normal children matched for mean length of utterance and receptive syntax, respectively. No major group differences were found. Ingram[54] and Lee and Ashmore[55§] observed the *Wh-* questions (for example, "*Wh*ere is . . ." or "*Wh*o gave . . .") asked by language disordered children and noted their success on the various sorts. Again, the disordered children seemed to be learning *Wh-* question words in the normal order and during the normal phase of syntax acquisition.

Conclusion

Given the range of potential topics, the semantic research with language disordered children has scarcely begun. Researchers have as yet paid little attention to the evolution of meaning or the progressive structuring of lexical fields, though recent work suggests that such studies will be revealing.[56§–58] The most striking fact about the research to date is that, apart from the Leonard et al finding on verbs,[48a] there is no indication of relative linguistic strength. Indeed, where group differences have been found, they suggest deficits in comparison to normal children at equivalent levels of language development.

Research with young normal children suggests that some aspects of semantic development reflect conceptual growth.[59–63] The observed deficits in relational semantics could thus be symptomatic of unrecognized intellectual deficiencies in language disordered children. This possibility will be explored further in the section on intellectual development. However, other explanations deserve equal consideration. It might be that language disordered children, even more than is normal, find it difficult to infer meanings that have no observable physical correlates. The "late" arrival of knowledge-state predicates could be explained in this way as easily as by appeal to conceptual difficulty. It might also be that language disordered children, because of poor memory access or habits acquired during a prolonged preverbal period, fail to integrate language symbols into the reasoning process. Infrequent expression of modality notions such as POSSIBILITY or epistemic NECESSITY could be a consequence of such failure.[12]

Even the "negative" lexical findings raise similar questions. Barring evidence of conceptual delay, a language disordered child of 6 years might be expected to know more advanced expressions than a normal child of 3 years, rather than to perform at merely comparable levels. After all, standardized test scores have long indicated vocabulary "peaks."[9,64] The lexical data suggest that theorists have either overestimated the conceptual resources of language disordered children or underestimated the role of nonconceptual factors, such as frequency of use, perceptual access, or syntactic correlates, in lexical acquisition. Different sectors of the lexicon may also be differentially sensitive to these factors. Relational terms, for example, may reflect conceptual resources, and nonrelational terms may reflect language experience. Since standardized vocabulary measures such as the Peabody Picture Vocabulary Test are frequently biased towards nonrelational terms, the reported "peaks" may misrepresent the total lexicon. Additional research is needed to explore these alternatives.

Pragmatics

The past decade has brought an energetic proliferation of research on pragmatics, that is, the *use* of language in context. Included in this area of study are topics such as communicative function, conversational skill, stylistic variation, and syntactic form as it is conditioned by context of use. Language disordered children have been noted to use fewer than normal questions[54] and more than normal "back channel" responses such as "uh-huh"[65]—formal facts that might indicate pragmatic weakness. However, other writers have noted that they are responsive, even "chatty," conversationalists[66] and that they are effective in nonverbal communication[67,68]—facts that suggest pragmatic strength. How may these observations be reconciled? It is possible to be an effective user of language despite restrictions in grammatical knowledge?

Communicative Function

Comparative studies of language disordered and autistic children indicate that language use strongly differentiates between the two groups.[69,70] Even when matched for mean length of utterance and IQ, language disordered children are more likely to comment spontaneously on events and report past experiences and are less likely to perseverate on inappropriate conversational topics. Are similar strengths seen in comparisons with normal peers?

From the earliest phases of language growth, normal children use language for a wide variety of social purposes. They gather information, gain attention, influence action, seek permission, describe, explain—in short, use words to accomplish all the goals of human interaction.[47,71,72] The first look at speech functions in language disordered children suggested restrictions in language use. Snyder used structured games to elicit comments and requests for action from normal and language disordered children at the early one-word level.[73] Her disordered children were less likely to use language for both of these functions. However, a replication study that controlled for knowledge of the specific words required by the experimental tasks found no group differences.[74] Subjects in this study were at slightly higher cognitive and language levels than Snyder's, but it seems likely that lexical control accounted for the different results.

Broader surveys of communicative function have similarly revealed no deficits. Leonard, Camarata, Rowan, and Chapman categorized the spontaneous speech acts of children at the one-word level into 16 functional types, including regulate attention, describe, announce intention, answer question, name, and request action.[48] Both the language disordered and normal speakers engaged in a variety of speech acts, at equivalent proportional frequencies. Only two categories differentiated the groups. The disordered children were more likely to be answering questions and less likely to be naming. Since the examiner tended to ask children for any object label that was not offered spontaneously, many of the question responses were in fact naming acts. The reported group difference may thus be one of reticence rather than function. Leonard et al also report similar findings from an earlier study of children with mean lengths of utterance of 3 or more.[48] A final experiment looked at the ability of language disordered listeners to infer functional intent.[75] Utterances in the form of questions were presented to children with mean lengths of utterance of around 2.5. From trial to trial, a given question functioned either as a request for information or as a request for action. The intended function was signaled by prior discourse context. The disordered children interpreted the questions in a manner that was appropriate to their language level. They showed a bias toward action, but clearly could use context to differentiate between the two functional types.

Studies of communicative function thus far indicate that language disordered children use words to pursue an appropriate range of social purposes. Scattered reports of infrequent question asking may have paid too much attention to surface syntax and insufficient attention to function.[11,54,76]

Conversational Topic

Conversations are verbal interactions in which people talk together, about something. The introduction and subsequent management of a conversational topic requires complex skills that develop well into the school years. Children must learn, for example, to consider the listener's attentional focus and prior knowledge, presupposing only that information that is available. The foundations of this learning are most probably nonlinguistic in nature. The human mind is preset to attend to novelty. This bias leads toddlers to use their single words to label the *changing* elements in a stream of events, rather than to label the background "topic."[77,78] Eventually children extend this bias to discourse, topicalizing those elements that have been established in joint attention through language or current experience and commenting on them. Success in this effort requires knowledge of the presuppositional features of language forms and accurate estimates of the listener's knowledge state.[79]

Research on topic-related phenomena with language disordered children is piecemeal but provocative. In her investigation of early communication schemes, Snyder assessed the degree to which children verbalized the new aspect of an event, for example, saying "boat" when a boat followed a long series of blocks in an object movement game.[73] Her normal toddlers verbally coded new, as opposed to old, elements some 94 percent of the time; the disordered children coded new elements only 69 percent of the time. As was true for speech functions, however, this difference disappeared when lexical resources were controlled.[74] Similar findings are reported by Skarakis and Greenfield for children with more advanced language.[80] These experimenters asked children with mean lengths of utterance from 2.8 to 6.0 to label a set of pictured events. Each of the pictures was presented in two different discourse contexts, establishing either the AGENT or the OBJECT as "old" information. Language disordered children focused their descriptions on whatever was contextually "new" just as often as the normal children, though they made more use of pronominalization to do so.

Additional reports concern specificity of reference and pertinence. In blind communication tasks, school-age language disordered children proved as effective as their age peers in describing objects so that a listener could find them.[81] Conversational responsivity and topic maintenance may also be areas of strength. Leonard reports that language disordered preschoolers at the one-word level actually responded more often, and with a wider range of response types, to the directives, statements, and questions of their adult partners.[82] Similarly, Reichle, Busch, and Doyle found that disordered preschoolers maintained their partner's topic to the degree expected for their language level.[83] Unlike Leonard's subjects, disproportionate amounts of these children's responsivity consisted of imitative utterances, a fact that may have reflected their severe phonological deficits. The only theme that runs counter to this picture of responsive and effective communication is found in scattered reports that language disordered preschoolers have difficulty answering their partner's questions.[75,76,84]

The fact that research to date has revealed no marked deficiencies in topic-related discourse skills is surprising. Given reports of attentional problems in this population,[85–87] their apparent sensitivity to listener and context might not have been expected. It seems worth noting that all of these studies used highly structured elicitation tasks and/or adult partners, thus minimizing the child's attentional effort. More demanding conversational environments may reveal more difficulties with topic management.

Conversational Repair

The challenges of conversation make breakdowns inevitable. Speakers miscalculate their partners' attention or knowledge; listeners are distracted or have difficulty following a line of thought. The health of a conversation frequently depends on the participants' ability to *repair* such breakdowns, to seek clarification, and to reformulate the problematic utterances. Normal preschoolers are already responsive to requests for repair.[88–90] They answer from 70 to 100 percent of such queries, usually trying to revise their original utterances. The nature of these revisions changes with age from phonetic alteration to syntactic and semantic paraphrase. Preschoolers also request repairs, asking for repetitions, confirmations, and elaborations.[90] However, the frequency of such requests is low.

Unlike many of the pragmatic skills reviewed thus far, conversational repair requires considerable linguistic expertise. Speakers must be able to express an idea in more than one way; listeners must be able to monitor the likelihood of their first readings. How do language disordered children fare in such tasks?

Gallagher and Darnton recorded hour-long conversations with language disordered children at stages I through III.[91] An adult experimenter periodically pretended not to understand the child's speech in order to see what modifications the child might make. The language disordered children did revise their utterances, generally showing the same progression of revision types as normal children at comparable language levels. However, the stage III children used fewer paraphrases and more phonetic revisions than their normal peers. The stage I children were also more likely to reduce their already brief utterances. Using much the same methodology, Brinton, Fujiki, and Channell observed repair sequences in school-age language disordered and normal children matched for age.[91a] The disordered children were more likely to make syntactic revisions and less likely to provide additional information. Meline and Meline measured the degree to which such revisions actually improved the communicative effectiveness of a message.[92] Language disordered children, ages 7 to 11 years, essentially equalled their age peers in the degree of improvement, though they were somewhat less likely to revise. Both groups performed better than a younger group of normal children matched to the disordered children by utterance length.

The three studies that look at children's own requests for repair offer contradictory findings. In one experiment, language disordered and normal children matched at two levels of mean length of utterance, 2.5 and 5.4, were asked to assist an adult in a role-playing activity.[93] Nonsense words were embedded in the instructions. Children in each group requested clarification about 50 percent of the time, but different groups preferred different types of queries. Older children, disordered and not, were likely to ask for specific clarification, for example, "The what?" Younger disordered children were likely to make nonverbal requests, while their normal peers used all query types with equal frequency. In a similar vein, Leonard's disordered children at the one-word level actually made more requests for clarification in free conversation than did the controls matched for mean length of utterance.[82] But Brinton and Fujiki report that their language disordered kindergarteners made fewer requests for clarification than their age peers.[76] The fact that this study analyzed peer rather than adult-child interactions and compared age mates rather than language mates may account for the difference in results.

Like the work on speech functions and topic management, these investigations of conversational repair reveal the communicative strengths of language disordered children. At least in the initial years of language learning, they seem to monitor their own understanding, to inform the speaker when they fail to understand, and to make honest, often effective, attempts to clarify their own intents. But here for the first time, one also sees clear deficiencies. Language disordered children appear to be limited by their inadequate command of linguistic tools. In comparison to both their mean length of utterance and age peers, their revisions are less mature in form and content. In particular, they seem unable to formulate alternative expressions for the same intent[94] and may also have difficulty diagnosing the root of the breakdown.

Speech Style Variation

Think for a moment about the variety of situations in which speech is used. We yell encouragement to our favorite team, whisper questions about obscure movie plots, discuss vacation plans with our families, make formal presentations to school boards—the list is endless. Not surprisingly, competent speakers vary their speech style from situation to situation. Factors such as the absence of referents, the status and knowledge of the listener, and the nature of the task determine our choice among styles that are more or less formal and elaborated.[95]

In her recent developmental review of style switching, Shatz concludes that children's ability to adjust their speech according to the age of the listener is "one of the best documented facts in the communication literature."[79] Beginning as early as 2 years of age, children talk more, use fewer directives, and are more informative with listeners of older age or higher status. By age 5, they can also mimic the speech styles associated with such social roles as "teacher" or "doctor." These achievements indicate considerable knowledge about social relationships and an impressive command of linguistic resources. Do language disordered children do as well?

Fey and his colleagues designed two experiments to address this question.[96,97] The second one nicely illustrates the findings in both.[97] Five-year-old language disordered children were videotaped as they interacted with an adult, an age peer, and a toddler. The researchers then measured ten parameters of speech style, including percentage of imperatives, percentage of internal state questions, and mean length of utterance. These procedures were repeated for control groups of age-matched and mean length of utterance-matched normal children. Without exception, the language disordered children adjusted *functional* and *semantic* aspects of their speech from listener to listener, in the same manner as their age peers. They asked the toddlers more questions about their feelings or perceptions, for example, and were more apt to direct the toddler's activities. The only variables that did not show listener-related adjustments were the *structural* measures, mean length of utterance, and preverbal utterance complexity. Trends for the younger control group children were unclear, but they seemed to show less variation in speech style than either of the older groups. Results from studies that focused on stylistic variation in the requests made by older language disordered children are in harmony with Fey's findings. Both Messick and Newhoff[98] and Prinz[99,100] conclude that it was primarily syntactic deficiencies that limited their subjects' ability to make "polite" requests.

This research on stylistic variation suggests the same mixture of pragmatic strengths and weaknesses that was evident in the literature on repairs. Language disordered children can use social and communicative schemes to adjust their speech in an age-appropriate manner, but only when this variation requires minimal grammatical knowledge.[101,102]

Not all researchers would agree with this characterization. Donahue,[§] for one, argues that her data on request strategies "clearly implicate deficits in the understanding of social relationship" (p 229) by learning disabled children.[103] Her subjects did adjust their speech styles, but in an abnormal direction, showing greater degrees of politeness with friends than strangers. Disagreement of a different sort is evident in the Liles data on narratives.[21,23] Here, cohesion patterns did vary with the listener's degree of prior knowledge, but episode elaboration did not. It seems that grammatical skills are not the only point of potential pragmatic vulnerability. Together, these studies challenge researchers to tease apart the cognitive, social, and linguistic aspects of stylistic variation in disordered groups.

Conclusion

Researchers and clinicians in speech-language pathology have tended to treat pragmatics as the

[§] This sign indicates that the subjects in study cited may not fit the operational criteria of lar ·.·age disorder used in this chapter.

fourth aspect of language competence, complementing the trio of syntax, semantics, and phonology. It would be better to view it as a distinct perspective that illuminates all aspects of language knowledge. This posture is explicit in the literature on functional grammar. Writers like Bates and MacWhinney[104] and Givon[105] argue that all language forms exist for a purpose and that these purposes are the key to understanding both grammatical structure and patterns of acquisition. The importance of studying language *use* is powerfully illustrated by the literature on language disordered children. Despite their evident interactional strengths, these children are communicatively handicapped exactly because they lack command of language form. Without sufficient grammatical resources, they have difficulty constructing cohesive texts, repairing conversational breakdowns, and varying their speech to fit the social situation.

Pragmatically oriented studies are inherently complex since they admit, if not examine, the role of situational variables on language performance. Some of the discrepancies in current findings are undoubtedly due to differences in partner and task. Others, for example those concerning the "assertiveness" of language disordered children, seem to reflect differences in comparison groups. (See Fey and Leonard for a review.[106]) Researchers may need to reexamine their predominant use of mean length of utterance-matched controls.[107] This strategy may be appropriate only when specific language forms are at stake. In other cases, language comprehension[108,109§] or social cognition may be the more pertinent control variables.

Researchers have not begun to exhaust the topics implied by the pragmatic perspective on language. Do the speech style limitations of language disordered children persist into adolescence or do they vanish once the requisite forms are learned? Are these children delayed in learning to provide feedback signals like "uh-huh" to the speaker when there is no breakdown? If so, why? Can speech-language pathologists manipulate functional contexts to help children master language form? Answers to questions such as these will illuminate the nature of language disorder and the interplay of form and function for all speakers.

Summary

Linguistically based research with language disordered children has investigated their knowledge of syntax, grammatical morphology, relational semantics, lexical semantics, and pragmatics. Further work is needed in each of these areas, but there are now sufficient data for an interim, global conclusion. At the sentence level, language disordered children seem to acquire major grammatical categories and rules of combination in the same order as do normal children, although more slowly and at a later age. Their learning of grammatical morphology also follows the normal patterns, though this course of development is markedly protracted. Text level grammars are clearly delayed, but whether they emerge along normal lines remains to be seen. Semantic studies suggest some failure to use language for reasoning purposes, but they also indicate that language disordered children follow normal acquisition patterns for certain lexical domains and can express stage-appropriate relational meanings. And finally, language disordered children appear to be purposeful and responsive conversationalists, limited only by their relatively poor mastery of grammatical form.

Thus stated, there is scant support in the linguistic research for the long-standing clinical distinction between language *delay* and language *deviance.*[110–113] "Blockages" in development[114] and deviation from the ordered patterns of normal acquisition seem not to occur. However, the clinical wisdom may be closer to the facts than this summary would indicate.

The Question of Language Deviance

The studies reviewed above focused on one linguistic domain at a time. It now appears that the realities of disordered language can be captured only across domains. For example, consider the relationship between major sentence patterns and inflectional morphology. The normal child generally masters the progressive "-ing" and the plural "-s" while using simple sentences. If language disordered children have difficulty mastering grammatical morphemes, their sentences might be relatively more complex before these noun and verb inflections are acquired. Case studies by Bax and Stevenson,[115] Kerschensteiner and Huber,[116] Trantham and Pedersen,[117] and Weiner[118] had suggested that such was true. Moreover, research studies using control groups matched for mean length of utterance had often reported morphological deficiencies, thus implying a developmental gap between syntax and morphology.[32,34,36] Alternately, if language disordered children have difficulty mapping related propositions onto a single sentence, they might use abnormally high proportions of inflectional morphology just prior to

§ This sign indicates that the subjects in study cited may not fit the operational criteria of language disorder used in this chapter.

the advent of complex sentences.[119] In either case, the developmental associations between primary sentence form and use of inflections would be atypical.

Consider also the relationship between lexical and syntactic competence. The fact that normal children master relational meanings for the prepositions *behind* and *in front of* at about the same time that they master modal inversion in Wh- questions may well be a developmental accident. No obvious connection exists between these two achievements other than the fact that the normal 3 year old is busy learning both forms. As argued earlier, if the acquisition of relational terms is linked to conceptual growth, older language disordered children with normal intelligence should use vocabulary items that are developmentally in advance of syntactic patterns. Lee had noted such discrepancies in a language disordered 4 year old.[120] And again, research studies using vocabulary-matched control groups had reported syntactic deficiencies, thus implying a developmental gap between syntax and the lexicon.[9,64]

Given such hints in the literature, it is surprising that the debate over language *deviance* continued for as long as it did. Johnston and Kamhi finally tackled the issue in a multidomain study of language disordered 5 year olds.[12] Samples of spontaneous language were assessed for evidence of syntactic, morphological, semantic, and pragmatic knowledge. These data were then compared to data from younger normal children matched to the disordered group at a mean length of utterance from 4.2 to 5.5. Language profiles for the two groups of speakers were dissimilar. Many of the sentence patterns produced by the disordered children were developmentally equivalent to those of the normal children. The disordered group also used ellipsis, pronominalization, and imperatives at normal rates. However, they differed from the control group in their poor mastery of grammatical functors and low level of propositional embedding.

Apparently, language disordered children acquire some aspects of linguistic ability more rapidly than others. Thus, even when forms in each domain develop along normal lines, some of the children's utterances are unlike those of any normal speaker. The course of such asynchronies invites further study. Data from Liles and Watt suggest that propositional embedding may be in advance of morphology at an earlier period of learning.[110] In any case, the Johnston and Kamhi findings seem to provide one resolution to the delay versus deviance controversy.[12]

Coming Attractions

Linguistic research on language disordered children has thus far emphasized the oral language patterns used by relatively young children. However, there are recent signs of broadening interests. This section takes a brief look at research on three of these new topics: the language learning process, literacy, and the longitudinal course of language disorders.

The Language Learning Process

There is now strong evidence that language disordered children learn language slowly and have particular difficulty with certain form classes. However, the evidence reveals little about the mechanisms that conspire to bring this about. Depending upon one's view of the mind, these mechanisms involve either general cognitive processes such as attention and memory or processes specific to language.[121] If the former, studies with nonverbal tasks can shed light on language learning disability. Subsequent sections of this chapter will review such work in detail. If the mind is "modular," however, greater insight may come from microdevelopmental studies of language learning itself.

These and related concerns have motivated three recent studies of language disordered children. In the first, Johnston, Blatchley, and Streit presented artificial miniature languages to 8 year olds, integrating them into competitive board games.[122] Each child had to learn two languages merely by listening to the experimenter use them while playing, a situation analogous to natural language learning. On alternate trials, the child either produced or comprehended an ACTION (AGENT, OBJECT) utterance, using the grammer of the language specific to that game. As the game progressed, changes in verbal performance revealed the evolution of the child's grammatical knowledge. Among other findings, the slow language learners seemed to use a different strategy than the fast learners. Instead of paying attention to several aspects of the grammar at once, the slow learners mastered one pattern before moving on to the next. Four of the 15 children in this experiment were language disordered; they all fell within the group of six slow learners who employed this attentional strategy.

The second study focused on an aspect of lexical acquisition known as "fast mapping." Normal preschoolers form approximate representations of the form and meaning of a new word after only one or two exposures. Would disordered children evidence any of this rapid learning? Dollaghan embedded an unfamiliar object within a brief hiding game and referred to it, once, as a "koob."[123,124] At the end of the game, she asked children to choose the "koob" from an object array, to name it and other objects in a second array, and to recall where it had been hidden. Language disordered 4 year olds, like their age peers, could identify the "koob" on command and could recall where it had been hidden. However, they could not use the word to name the object. Dollaghan suggests that this failure implicates some specific difficulty with accessing phonological representations in memory.

The final study concerned learning "style." Current evidence suggests that normal language learning can proceed in two directions.[125] Large units corresponding to adult phrases or clauses can be acquired whole and subsequently broken down into their constituent parts. Alternatively, small units corresponding to adult words can be acquired and subsequently combined into larger schemes. Some children seem to prefer one of these starting points, whereas others make equal use of both. Weiss looked for signs of language learning style in a small group of language disordered toddlers, noting such indices as the presence of jargon and the use of formulaic phrases.[126] Different children did seem to prefer one or the other of these styles, but these preferences were not linked to patterns of play. This finding may indicate that language learning styles are solutions born out of the special demands of the language learning task.

Each of these studies suggests important ramifications for intervention practice. Clinicians will want to follow subsequent efforts to confirm or elaborate them. Equally important, this research reminds one that however it may incorporate general cognitive mechanisms, language learning proceeds in a unique problem space. This fact may prove crucial to our understanding of language disorder.

Written Language, Literacy, and Metalinguistics

There is widespread evidence that children who are slow to acquire oral language are likely to have difficulty learning written language as well. Sample-based estimates range from 40 to 100 percent, depending upon the rigor of the original assessment and the cut-off criteria employed. Longitudinal studies have documented the poor performance of language disordered children in elementary school reading programs,[4–6,127–130] and the one study of their written language suggests a wide variety of grammatical and expressive deficiencies.[131] In fact, problems with literacy are evident even before formal schooling begins. Gillam and Johnston report that language disordered preschoolers are less able to interpret environmental print such as words from food product labels, than their age peers.[132]

These problems with written language most probably result from some unknown interaction between poor knowledge of oral language and general cognitive processing deficiencies. One pertinent aspect of oral language knowledge may be evidenced in "metalinguistic" behaviors. Throughout the preschool and elementary school years, children not only become competent speakers and listeners, but they also show an increased ability to reflect on the language "object." By self-correction, word play, and explicit judgements of grammaticality, they demonstrate their growing conscious control of language knowledge. Van Kleek, among others, has argued that this ability to think about language structure is a vital prerequisite to literacy.[133,134] If so, metalinguistic thought may be a major stumbling block for language disordered children. In all of the studies conducted thus far, such children have been less able to notice and correct grammatical errors, or to segment language units, than their age or language peers.[64,135–140] If further research confirms the causal role of metalinguistic skill in the acquisition of written language, clinicians may have a new line of attack on the problem of literacy.

The Longitudinal Course of Language Disorders

The recent spurt of metalinguistic studies is just one facet of a growing interest in the oral language problems of school-age children and their connection to reading disabilities. Longitudinal studies indicate that large percentages of children with early language disorder go on to have difficulty with school achievement. Speech-language pathologists have also suspected that large percentages of poor achievers have oral language deficits. Efforts to establish this fact have been hampered by varying criteria for school achievement and by poor language assessment tools.[141] Two recent attempts may be harbingers of coming success. Gibbs and Cooper tested all of the learning disabled students from 8 to 12 years of age in one school district, some 242 children.[142] They report that 91 percent of them evidenced some oral language deficit. Similarly, Lieberman, Moore, and Hutchinson administered oral language measures to language disordered and learning disabled school-age children.[143] The language disordered children had more difficulty in the area of syntax, but virtually all of the children in both groups performed below the twentieth percentile on at least three subtests.

Implicit in these findings is the strong likelihood that many of the preschoolers identified as *language disordered* are later identified as *learning disabled.*[144, 145] This fact might indicate only the illogic of institutions or the vulnerability of symptomatic labels. In a recent study, however, Scarborough and Dobrich suggest a more interesting possibility—"illusory recovery from language delay."[146] As part of an ongoing longitudinal study of child literacy, these researchers took repeated measures of oral language ability from age 2 onward. For many of the measures, normal children evidenced a plateau that began about 42 months and lasted a year and a half. The four language disordered children in the sample followed much the same pattern at a 1-year lag. The disordered children thus entered their plateau period before growth curves for the normal children again accelerated. For a brief period then, around age $4^1/_2$, the disordered children performed as well as the normal children. But this recovery was indeed illusory. The normal children's scores soon improved, but the disordered group's scores remained at the plateau. Perhaps children are identified as language disordered at one age and learning disabled at another because there is in fact an interim age at which measurement tools can no longer see their problems. Bishop and Edmundson's longitudinal study of language disordered and normal preschoolers lends support to this interpretation.[147] After reviewing test scores taken at 4, $4^1/_2$, and 5 years of age, these researchers conclude that 44 percent of their disordered children had "good outcomes," that is, were no longer performing below normal levels. However, a careful look at their data reveals that much of this "improvement" can be attributed to test ceiling and plateau effects in the normal group.

Implications for Assessment and Intervention

Each of the studies reviewed thus far have implications for clinical practice, some of which have been mentioned in passing. However, a few major implications deserve special attention. The first ones stem from the notion of developmental asynchronies in language development. Besides providing a more accurate picture of disordered language, cross-domain studies provide new ways of talking about differences *within* the population of language disordered children. For example, de Ajuriaguerra and his colleagues[§] have identified two groups of such children.[148] One group prefers simple sentences, is consistent in language level from day to day, provides concrete but intelligible narratives, and evidences a narrow comprehension-production gap. The second group uses more complex sentences, is inconsistent in language level, provides imaginative but largely incoherent narrative, and evidences a wide comprehension-production gap.

Judging from this description, de Ajuriaguerra's second group should show greater developmental disparity between their control of sentence patterns and their mastery of grammatical morphology. Other clinical researchers have described somewhat different constellations of phonological, semantic, syntactic, and pragmatic deficit.[7,149,150] The importance of all such categorizations is that they are based on linguistic profiles, estimates of relative proficiency across several domains of language knowledge.

Once one accepts the possibility that language disordered children acquire different aspects of language knowledge at different rates, two modifications of assessment and intervention practice seem inescapable.

First, descriptions of a child's linguistic level by means of a single index such as mean length of utterance are no longer justifiable. Global "stage" values make sense only when there are predictable relationships between mastery of sentence patterns, grammatical morphology, lexicon, and communicative functions. Researchers may eventually develop a comprehensive picture of disordered language that will again allow clinicians to employ global indices. However, Bishop and Edmundson's work suggests that linguistic profiles will continue to have the greater utility.[147] They found that by characterizing performance in a number of language domains, they could predict severity of impairment and future levels of communicative success. With this in mind, clinicians will probably want to assess a child's expertise in each area of language instead of relying on single test scores or stage designations.

Second, educators need to reconsider the use of normal acquisition data in intervention programming. Despite continuing debate on this issue,[151,152] many clinicians have developed program outlines that mirror the facts of normal language learning.[153,154] The rationale for this strategy rests on the orderliness that pervades the evolution of early language patterns. Such predictability suggests that each linguistic achievement depends upon certain prerequisite learning. By using normal data as a basis for programming, the clinician attempts to insure that such prerequisites have been met. The crucial point here is that normal language *facts* are important only insofar as they indicate the set of structural and functional dependencies that shape language learning. The past decade of research on children's language has made it clear that some of these dependencies are linguistic in nature, and some are not. Children's current world knowledge, conceptual understanding, organizational abilities, and social needs

§ This sign indicates that the subjects in study cited may not fit the operational criteria of language disorder used in this chapter.

influence their language achievements just as surely as does their current linguistic knowledge. For any two language patterns, Form B may normally be learned after Form A for linguistic reasons, for example, because B incorporates A, or for nonlinguistic reasons, for example, because B requires an understanding of perspective and A does not. In the latter case, learning A may in no way prepare the child for learning B and in fact may be unnecessary.

The research on developmental asynchronies supports this multifactored view of language growth and suggests that interventionists may, when evidence warrants it, program "abnormal" patterns of language acquisition. If the typical language disordered child is indeed still mastering the plural "-s" while acquiring catenative verbs like "gonna," no direct dependency would seem to exist between these two patterns, despite the fact that the plural "-s" is normally learned prior to "gonna." In such cases, the therapist may comfortably violate normal guidelines, setting higher-level phrase structure and lexical goals simultaneously with lower-level morphological goals. Adherence to the normal course of acquisition would deprive the child of appropriate learning opportunities.

A second set of implications rises out of the work in pragmatics. As researchers moved away from studies of grammar to focus on communicative functions, it became fashionable to question the wisdom of targetting syntactic forms for assessment or intervention. Sentiment favored those "who opt for overthrowing our previous conceptions that language is what we are assessing, and propose that we move toward a new conceptualization which examines communication and context, and, if called for, the language within it" (p 178).[155] Recalcitrant goals such as the copula, the auxiliary, or pronoun case were gratefully abandoned in favor of "pragmatic" goals such as turn taking or topic maintenance.

If the functional grammarians are right, however, this substitution will prove to have been misguided. Language forms exist because they have work to do, somewhere. When children reach the point at which a form is needed, its absence will get in the way of communication. Recall, for example, the research on narrative. The language disordered children were less effective as story tellers exactly because they lacked control of pronominalization and conjoining schemes. Nouns may seem as effective as pronouns for establishing reference, and the substitution of *him* for *he* a minor irritant—until our communicative goal is to create a text. Nothing works as well as a case-marked pronoun for binding sentences together, clarifying relationships between participants and directing the listener's attention from new to old information. Whenever linguistic forms appear to be "syntactic doilies," pretty but unnecessary, one needs to look further for their legitimizing contexts of use. The point is not that turn taking and topic maintenance are inappropriate targets for intervention, but that the mastery of grammatical schemes is equally important. The challenge is to present these schemes in contexts that make them both learnable and useful.

PERCEPTUAL FUNCTIONS

Normal language acquisition certainly requires the effective functioning of a variety of perceptual mechanisms, both those that are bound to specific senses and those that span the senses. Participants at the Stanford Institute frequently suggested that specific perceptual dysfunctions, particularly auditory ones, were an important, if not prime, source of language learning difficulty:

> Early in life, the normally developing child learns how to use an auditory self-monitoring system, a kind of servo-mechanism, which becomes the control center of his capacity to hear, to listen, and to reproduce meaningful utterances. Some children cannot naturally do this: among this group are (the) aphasoid . . . It seems clear that one of the deficits of a highly distractible child who is not learning language is a fundamental inability to pay consistent attention to the succession of stimuli which makes the learning of verbal-auditory meanings possible (p 40).[1]

Researchers have spent considerable effort attempting to support such clinical impressions with experimental facts. What is known about perceptual dysfunctions in language disordered children? Are these dysfunctions specifically auditory? Do they remain viable explanations for the syndrome?

Studies of Auditory Perception

To answer these questions, consider first the research on auditory perception. Studies by Reichstein[156] and Rosenthal[157] indicated that language disordered children show greater auditory threshold variation than their age peers and do not show a normal decrease in threshold with increase in duration for brief low-frequency sounds. Holloway,[158] McReynolds,[159] and Wilson, Doehring, and Hirsh[160] reported that language disordered children have relative difficulty recognizing complex speech and nonspeech acoustic stimuli, particularly at short duration or low frequency. These studies of signal detection and identification are probably best interpreted in the light of a further body of research, which explores auditory temporal resolution.

Experiments by Efron,[161] and Hirsh and Sherrick[162] established the background for studies of auditory temporal resolution with language disordered children. When normal and brain-injured adults were asked to judge which of two brief auditory stimuli occurred first, normal subjects required an interstimulus interval (ISI) of 20 to 60 msec to reach 75-percent accuracy, whereas brain-damaged subjects required significantly longer ISIs. In 1965, Lowe and Campbell used this paradigm to study language disordered and normal children, ages 7 to 14.[163] The ISI at which language disordered children could decide whether one or two events had *occurred* did not differ from normal. But the ISI necessary for accurate judgments of *order* was significantly longer, 357 msec versus 36 msec.

Subsequent investigations substantiated and broadened these findings. Rosenthal confirmed the general deficit in auditory temporal resolution and also reported that his language disordered children required longer ISIs for acoustic events that differed in rise time and duration as opposed to frequency; whereas for normal children, this pattern was reversed.[157] Using two complex tones that varied in fundamental frequency, Tallal and Piercy also found that language disordered children required abnormal ISIs for judgments of temporal order.[164,165] These subjects, mean age 8;6, performed more poorly than 4½-year-old normals at ISIs under 305 msec. With longer ISIs, however, they performed as well as their age peers. These findings were substantially replicated with a second population[166,167] and are mirrored by findings with fixed ISIs.[168]

The fact that language disordered children have abnormal difficulty judging the order of two brief acoustic events raises three important questions. First, which signal property creates this difficulty: duration or order? Second, what is the relationship between this aspect of auditory perception and the language disorder? Third, is this perceptual deficit truly auditory? The next sections review research pertinent to these questions.

Duration Versus Order

Signal duration has been of importance in several studies of auditory perception,[157,158,169] but it is considered most directly in the work of Tallal and Piercy.[165,170–172] Seven to 9 year olds were presented with two 75-msec tones separated by varying intervals and were asked to judge either the order of the tones or their similarity. Normal children had no difficulty with these tasks, but language disordered children performed poorly whenever the ISI was 150 msec or less. Since this finding was true for judgments of similarity as well as for judgments of order, Tallal and Piercy argued for a basic "failure of discrimination of auditory quality" to which the errors in order judgment were secondary. Pursuing this notion, they varied the length of the stimuli as well as the ISI and found that, for the language disordered children, accuracy of response was directly related to total duration of the stimulus pattern. With shorter ISIs and/or shorter tones, identification of the sequences proved difficult.

Noting the rapidity of normal speech signals, Tallal and Piercy next studied their subjects' perception of pairs of synthesized vowels or stop consonants, again requiring judgments of order and similarity across varying ISIs. Each speech sound lasted 250 msec, including, for the stops, a transition segment of 30 msec. There was no difference between groups for the vowel pairs, but the language disordered children had significantly greater difficulty with consonant pairs, generally requiring ISIs in excess of 428 msec. Tallal's replication study again confirmed this pattern,[166] as did Frumkin and Rapin's findings for a group of language disordered children with persistent phonological deficits.[173] Their second group without phonological manifestations did not, but age and task differences make it difficult to interpret this fact. In general, results from the speech sound studies seem to implicate some problem in processing the brief transition segments that distinguished the stop consonant from the vowel stimuli.

Recognizing that these transitions were marked by frequency change and brevity, Tallal and Piercy synthesized stimuli that could tease these parameters apart. They presented pairs of pseudodiphthongs that had brief, steady-state initial segments with no glide, and pairs of stop consonants that had transition segments of twice-normal duration. Total stimulus length was again held at 250 msec. In contrast to earlier findings, the language disordered children now judged the consonant items normally and found the vowel items virtually impossible. Tallal and Piercy conclude that duration, not change, is the critical parameter, and that language disordered children show "an impaired rate of processing auditory information." However, findings from Tallal and Stark[174] suggest that this statement may not yet capture the problem.[175] Disordered children in the replication sample were successful in recognizing brief vowel segments. But here, unlike the first study, the vowels were not immediately followed by other stimuli.[173,174] Brief, *rapidly sequenced* signals seem to be the point of vulnerability.

The experiments by Tallal and her colleagues provide good evidence of difficulties in processing certain brief acoustic events for at least two groups of language disordered children. If typical, such a deficit could help to explain the more general observations of poor sound detection and identification, which were reviewed earlier. This work also suggests that order judgments per se, even for auditory stimuli, may not be impaired. When stimulus duration was long enough, language disordered children were well able to judge order.

Relationships to Language

The fact that language disordered children have difficulty processing brief, rapidly sequenced acoustic events may or may not help to explain their problems in language learning. Debate on this issue has raged for 15 years and has generally brought more heat than light. Some writers have taken Tallal's work as an occasion to criticize the larger literature on "central auditory processing."[175–177] They rightly note that this literature frequently ignores the role of knowledge or higher cognitive functions in perception and memory. Nowhere is this more evident than when complex linguistic stimuli are used as a measure of the auditory mechanism. (See Rees for a review.[173]) In contrast to this larger literature, the claims of Tallal and her colleagues have been modest. "Such rapid changes are highly characteristic of the speech signal . . . difficulty in processing these events in the auditory speech stream could conceivably be detrimental to the acquisition of language" (p 121).[166] Lubert agrees with this opinion,[178] but Rees asks "just what kind of and how severe a language deficit should this kind of difficulty cause?" (p 109)[179]

No one can answer this question. Data from both Tallal projects have been used to document general relationships between performance on the rapid auditory processing tasks and various measures of language. Language disordered children who have difficulty identifying stop consonants also have difficulty producing them. Timing of the movements that signal the voicing contrast seems particulary problematic.[180,181] Such children also are unsuccessful in recognizing syllables in words when those syllables consist of a stop consonant and a vowel.[182] And finally, when Tallal, Stark, and Mellits examined all of their demographic, psychological, "soft" neurological, motor, and perceptual variables to see which ones would predict receptive language level, they found that four measures of rapid auditory processing were the most effective.[183] In concert, these four measures had a correlation coefficient of 0.85 with receptive language scores.

Unfortunately, establishing general relationships of this sort does not yet make the case for causality. Correlational data alone can never reveal the direction of causal influences. More specifically, however, virtually all of the perceptual tasks that contribute to these correlations involved speech-like stimuli. Given the role of knowledge schemes in perceptual activity, one could predict that children who knew more about speech and language would be more successful in perceiving the speech-like events.[184] It is not surprising that language disordered children performed less well than their age peers and performed similarly on the "perceptual" and "language" tasks. As Leonard notes, their difficulty with the perceptual tasks could be as much a *product* of the general language learning limitation as an explanation.[175] This argument applies less convincingly to nonverbal auditory abilities, but there is scant evidence of linkage between performance on nonverbal tasks and language behavior.[185]

The explanatory power of the research represented by Tallal and her colleagues depends ultimately on the degree to which it taps basic perceptual mechanisms as opposed to higher level cognition. If difficulty in processing rapidly sequenced nonverbal stimuli does indicate the dysfunction of some basic mechanism, then it seems reasonable to imagine that such dysfunction could, in some fashion, impede language learning. Ironically, it is a body of nonauditory findings that may ultimately justify this claim.

Visual Perception

A small body of research growing out of the early work on auditory temporal resolution has examined the modality specificity of this function. Hirsh and Sherrick's study had shown that normal adults required ISIs of 20 msec regardless of stimulus modality, implicating some central perceptual process as the key factor in judgments of order.[162] Yet clinical reports of language disordered children, bolstered by results from standardized and nonstandardized test batteries,[186–188] had suggested deficits that were uniquely auditory.

Two studies by Furth attempted to resolve this issue.[189,190] Age-matched deaf, normal, and language disordered children were asked to learn associations between sequences of auditory or visual stimuli and specific response buttons, one for each possible sequence. In the first study, 10 year olds were tested on two-item temporal sequences of unfamiliar geometric forms. There were no significant differences between the groups. In a second study, however, 6-year-old deaf and language disordered children did have more difficulty than normals in learning three-unit temporal sequences, both auditory and visual. Likewise, Poppen, Stark, Eisenson,

Forrest, and Wertheim found that their language disordered 9 year olds were less succcessful than normals in pressing visual panels in the order in which they had just been lit.[191]

These studies, though intriguing, seem biased towards higher-level mental processes. In comparison to studies of auditory temporal resolution, the tasks here involve longer durations, more units, and much slower rates, for example, 1-second events with an ISI of 1 second[190] versus 75-msec events with ISIs of up to 357 msec.[163]

More convincing data have been generated in the Tallal replication project.[167] These researchers presented exact visual analogues for each of their nonverbal auditory processing tasks. Children in the language disordered group had difficulty judging order for brief, rapidly sequenced *visual* events (e.g., lights and nonsense figures), requiring abnormally long ISIs to solve these problems. This was particularly true for the younger children in the sample, ages 5 and 6. Moreover, when a discriminant function analysis of 160 variables was performed to discover which ones could identify children in the language disordered group, five of the six best predictors involved the perception of brief events presented either simultaneously or in succession. Only one of them was auditory! Poor tactile and visual perception also proved crucial to characterizing the disordered group.[192] Similar nonauditory deficits had not been found in the Tallal and Piercy study,[165] but this seems to have been due to the somewhat older age of their subjects. It is clearly premature to draw conclusions about the modality specificity of the perceptual problems associated with language disorder. However, corroboration of findings from the second Tallal project would prove valuable in the interpretation of all of the work on "temporal resolution." Free of the specter of "speech perception," the visual and tactile rapid processing tasks do indeed seem to tap into basic perceptual mechanisms. And if they do, why not the nonverbal auditory tasks as well?

Efferent Perceptual Deficits: A Unifying Hypothesis

The perceptual studies reviewed thus far have largely proposed dysfunctions that are conceived as discrete entities: poor auditory signal detection, poor processing of rapidly sequenced auditory (or visual) events, and so forth. One writer has challenged this approach, suggesting instead that a single deficiency may be responsible for all of the perceptual findings. Rosenthal begins his explanation with theories of auditory function, which hypothesize a variable "critical band."[193] In lay terms, the ear and mind process only portions of the available acoustic signal, enough to enable identification. When the signal is brief, the band of frequencies to which one attends widens or shifts to maximize the information available. Rosenthal speculates that if this efferent adjustment were slow, a brief signal could fade from sensory memory before it was recognized. Similar problems might arise with rapidly changing signals of any physical sort since the locus of difficulty would reside not in particular sensory mechanisms, but in those central *executive* functions that tune them.

Contemporary models of the mind, particularly those identified with the cognitive sciences, have broadened the notion of attention to include the entire range of functions that serve to arouse, to allocate mental resources, to select among activities, and to coordinate them. Some of these functions appear to be automatic, others are under the more or less conscious control of intellect.[194] Little is known about the development of attentional processes during the early years, but behavioral changes seem to result from structural maturation, increased knowledge, and increased procedural efficiency, in some unknown interaction. (See Brown, Bransford, Ferrara, and Campione[195] and Kail and Bisanz[196] for reviews.)

There have been no direct studies of dysfunction in the tuning mechanisms that Rosenthal hypothesizes to underly perceptual deficits. However, such mechanisms clearly lie within the scope of attentional processes as outlined previously. A brief look at the research on attention in language disordered children may thus provide some indication of the plausibility of Rosenthal's proposal.

Otto, Honck, Finger, and Hart[§] made electroencephalographic recordings during a visual matching task and characterized the waveforms that occurred during the alert, interpretation, and response intervals.[197] Records from their language disordered subjects evidenced somewhat less negative variation during the alert interval, indicating abnormal expectancy states. They also evidenced prolonged and larger shifts during the interpretation interval, suggesting some difficulty in identifying the stimuli. Edwards cites similar findings,[198] and Mason and Mellor[§] report other abnormalities in late cortical evoked responses.[199] Behavioral evidence from Mackworth, Grandstaff, and Pribram seems to mirror these EEG findings.[87] Language disordered and normal children were filmed while they observed a periodically changing array of geometric forms. The

[§] This sign indicates that the subjects in study cited may not fit the operational criteria of language disorder used in this chapter.

language disordered children either were slow to notice a change in one of the forms or stared at a new figure for prolonged periods.

Some of the most interesting recent findings on attention are found in the work of Ceci.[85,86] In one experiment, language disordered and normal children were conditioned to expect a loud noise whenever they heard a specific target word. Skin conductance response was used to confirm the efficacy of the conditioning. The children were then given a listening task in which they had to repeat all of the words presented to one ear while ignoring those presented to the other ear. When the conditioned word was presented to the *un*attended ear, the two groups of children evidenced comparable autonomic reactions.

In a second experiment, Ceci contrasted this automatic sort of attention with more conscious processes. Four- and 10-year-old normal children, and 10-year-old language disordered children were trained extensively in a naming task. After a verbal cue, "Here's a picture of a __________ you know," the children were to name a slide as quickly as possible. The cues were either neutral ("something"), facilitating (e.g., "animal" for a picture of a horse), or misleading ("animal" for a picture of an orange). Patterns of reaction time across various conditions indicated whether a child made *active* use of information in the cues. Only the 10-year-old normal children did so. The language disordered children showed the same pattern of *automatic* level facilitation as their age peers, indicating that their language knowledge was comparable. But they, like the 4 year olds, either could not determine the reliability of cue information or had no ability to consciously "expect" a given type of input. Martinius[§] reported a similar failure to establish an attentional set.[200] In the context of such findings, it seems worth noting that all of the perceptual tasks reviewed earlier had a similar potential for "set," or expectation.

Rosenthal's hypothesis is consonant with most of the perceptual studies reviewed earlier. It predicts the relative difficulty of brief or low-frequency stimuli and the increased demands of the auditory world where rapid change is the rule. These studies of attentional processes add further support. Language disordered children do seem to have difficulty with the alerting and control functions basic to intellect. Work on impulsivity[201,202] and capacity limitations[203] is as yet preliminary, but suggests additional facets of disorder.

§ This sign indicates that the subjects in study cited may not fit the operational criteria of language disorder used in this chapter.

Conclusions

Investigations of perceptual processes in language disordered children are as yet inconclusive. The major lines of research have explored the stimulus properties of duration and modality. It seems likely that language disordered children do have difficulty discriminating and identifying brief, rapidly sequenced events, both auditory and visual, linguistic and nonlinguistic. These problems may be viewed as local or as symptoms of a general dysfunction in controlled processing. Whatever the case, their relationship to delays in language acquisition has yet to be defined. The fact that hyperactive boys *without* language disorders or academic problems nevertheless perform poorly on rapid auditory processing tasks[204] reminds one that this relationship cannot be simple. Despite earlier hopes,[119] researchers are unlikely to explain developmental language disorders by a simple appeal to perceptual deficit.

Implications for Intervention

Regardless of how one views them, as correlates or as contributing causes, the likelihood of perceptual and attentional deficits in language disordered children suggests specific intervention strategies.

The first of these concerns the role of attention. The essential task of the language learner is to discover the relational mapping between linguistic forms and their meanings. In the early stages, such discovery depends upon the child's ability to determine the probable meaning of an utterance in context.[61] Shared attentional focus between the child and the speaker insures that these first estimates of meaning are at least good approximations. However, if the child fails to notice significant changes in the stream of events or ignores the speaker's line of regard, his or her estimates of meaning are likely to be inaccurate and his or her language learning thus slowed.

Given this characterization, the most effective intervention strategies are those that promote shared attention, either by attracting or by following the child's attentional focus. This general principle suggests at least two specific techniques. First, the therapist may create event contexts that have unusual perceptual salience, novelty, or significance for the child, events likely to capture attention and hence to be adequate keys to language. One clue to the nature of such attention-grabbing events can be found in Leonard's study, which demonstrated that children learn language faster when shown three-dimensional, real-time events than when shown pictures.[205] Second, the therapist may model language forms that express those topics and ideas to which the child is already attending. Schwartz et al's vertical discourse structuring is a good example of one such technique.[206] Child-oriented approaches demand a certain flexibility and ingenuity, but obviously increase the likelihood that the prerequisite of shared attention will be met.

The consequences of auditory dysfunction are less easily addressed. As was emphasized earlier, the specific relationships between perceptual deficiencies and language learning are unknown. Nevertheless, one can imagine that if a child cannot reliably assess the shape of an acoustic event, he or she will have difficulty recognizing its recurrence in the speech stream. Such pattern recognition is fundamental to language acquisition, particularly at the earliest stages when a child's prior language knowledge plays a small role in perceptual search and cannot yet supplant an accurate and thorough reading of the acoustic signal.

To mitigate the presumed effects of auditory dysfunction, some therapists have attempted to slow the speed of the speech signal[64,207] or use exaggerated pauses between major sections of an utterance.[208] With refinement, both techniques appear promising. Other therapists have turned to visualization techniques such as written language,[209] pictured sentences,[210] and more recently, signed English.[211] The work of Tallal and Rosenthal provides some insight into the role of such visual techniques. By using written, pictured, or signed versions of a language simultaneously with its spoken form, one gives the language disordered child a relatively static, spatial correlate for the rapidly changing temporal event. Such correlates may guide perception, aid in segmentation, and enable pattern discovery even when the acoustic signal goes partially unrecognized. Thus viewed, visualization techniques are not so much visual as they are slower, spatial, and static.**

INTELLECTUAL DEVELOPMENT

By traditional definition, language disordered children exhibit normal-range nonverbal intelligence, typically operationalized via performance scales such as the Leiter, Columbia, Ravens, or Wechsler. Despite this fact, participants at the Institute on Childhood Aphasia alluded to a wide range of possible conceptual or cognitive deficits:

> . . . intellectual inefficiency over and above any "measurable" intellectual deficit. . . (p 20).
>
> . . . lack of tracking . . . being unable to process an indefinite variety of incoming information, employing all the attributes of the sensorium, and to relate this to previous and presently pertinent experience (p 42).
>
> . . . predict that the aphasic . . . does not have these prerequisite organizations (symbolic and cognitive) for language function. . . (p 73).[1]

Until recently, notions such as intellectual efficiency, tracking, or symbolic organization provided little competition for psychometry. It was as though the fact of normal nonverbal intelligence had obviated further inquiry. The rapid acceleration of studies in early normal development now seems to have reversed that trend. With normative guidelines, effective methodology, and theoretical constructs of considerable power, the task of studying *disordered* cognition seems more possible. Do language disordered children function normally in all intellectual areas except language? If not, what is the nature of their conceptual or reasoning deficiencies?

Conceptual Development

The research literature provides good evidence that language acquisition depends in part upon nonverbal concepts and knowledge of the world.[62] Ideas motivate the quest for expressive means and constitute meanings. This perspective on language invites one to question the adequacy of conceptual growth in language disordered children. Certain aspects of their language deficiency may reflect conceptual lags.

Initial evidence on this issue came from Piagetian studies of *operative,* or logical, thought at two developmental extremes. Snyder observed 30 children at the one-word stage, half of whom had been diagnosed as language disordered.[73] Each child was given the Uzgiris and Hunt intelligence scales,[212] as well as a series of tasks designed to elicit comments on novel events or requests for assistance. Performance in these communication situations correlated highly with achievement on the means-ends subscale. Language disordered children used simpler communicative means and were less competent in tool use. Their delay in language acquisition was apparently accompanied by an analogous lag in nonverbal cognition.

In a longitudinal study of 17 school-age language disordered children, de Ajuriaguerra and his colleagues§ also found developmental delays on operative tasks.[148,213] Nine of the children showed clear reasoning deficiencies, four were erratic, and four

** This claim applies only to signed English as it is typically used in a remediation setting, not to signed systems in general.

§ This sign indicates that the subjects in study cited may not fit the operational criteria of language disorder used in this chapter.

showed operative strengths. Of these latter four, however, the two children who had reached the age at which hypothetical and deductive reasoning would be expected had not yet achieved this level of thought. (But see also Inhelder.[214]) Similar evidence of intellectual deficiency was provided by Johnston and Ramstad.[215,216] A battery of Piagetian tasks was administered to seven preadolescent language disordered children. The tasks included problems from the domains of space, number, and class and required both logical and image-based reasoning. Average performance was about 3 years below age expectations. Like Snyder's toddlers, the school-age language disordered children in these studies evidenced conceptual as well as linguistic deficits.

Recent work with preschool and kindergarten children completes the developmental continuum. Kamhi compared the conceptual development of language disordered and normal 5 year olds.[217] Children were asked to group similar objects, judge quantity across perceptual transformations, replicate spatial arrays of objects, recognize objects by touch, predict the appearance of a tilted transparent jar of water, and imagine the superimposition of geometric forms. In all cases, the language disordered children performed less well than their mental age peers. Few of the group differences were statistically significant, but the consistency of the results across tasks is convincing. Moreover, reports of classification and perspective-taking abilities in language disordered 4 year olds[218,219] confirm this picture of delay.

The tasks used in these studies were presented in ways that minimized the need for verbal skills. Yet across conceptual domains and ages, language disordered children performed much less well than would be expected for their mental ages. A second generation of studies has attempted to identify the bases for these conceptual delays and relate them to language disorder. Analysis of performance IQ scales has failed to reveal any specific strengths or weaknesses,[220] but analysis of nonstandardized cognitive tasks has suggested problems in three areas: symbolic function, heirarchical planning, and hypothesis testing. Researchers argue that disability in these areas might impede both verbal and nonverbal cognitive growth. The following sections summarize their efforts to document such impairments.

Symbolic Function

Toward the end of the second year, normal children manifest their first symbolic acts—speech, communicative gestures, deferred imitation, and pretend play—thus reaching a crucial milestone in intellectual growth. With the advent of symbols, children can move beyond perceived reality to discover the abstract relations and problem solving strategies that characterize mature thought.[221] Often referred to as the symbolic function, the mental events that underlie symbol use are not well understood. Children must certainly be able to differentiate a part of an event, evoke it at will, and use it to hold in mind, or represent, the meaning of the whole. Processes of this sort are common to language and other symbolic forms despite the unique conventionality and complexity of the verbal system. Could it be that language disorders are but one facet of a broader symbolic deficit[222] and that conceptual deficits in this population reflect a limited ability to create, store, and manipulate symbols in the service of thought? Researchers to date have explored this question by looking primarily at two types of nonverbal symbols: symbolic play and mental imagery. They argue that difficulties with these forms in conjunction with language disorder would support the symbolic deficit hypothesis.

Symbolic Play

At least six different studies have compared the symbolic play activities of language disordered and normal children, varying in age from 3 to $6^1/_2$.[223–228] Samples of free play, responses to play prompts, and/or performances on a standardized test were analyzed to see how often the children engaged in pretend play and to determine the complexity of their play. Without exception, the language disordered children differed from their chronological or mental age peers, pretending less often and using fewer advanced play schemes, that is, those that involve symbolic substitutions of one object for another or combinations of schemes around a theme. Since higher levels of play may require social cooperation via language and are more easily recognized when accompanied by verbal labels, there is some confounding of symbolic play abilities and language abilities in this body of work. However, scoring of the Symbolic Play Test[229] is based solely on nonverbal aspects of individual play. The three studies that use this test as well as nonstandardized measures report similar findings with both methods of assessment.

Visual Imagery

Studies of visual imagery are by nature more inferential. It is impossible to observe imagery as one observes play; instead, experimenters must present conceptual puzzles that seem to invite the use of visual imagery and then observe a child's degree of success. For example, in one such Piagetian task, children are asked to imagine how a three-dimensional display would appear from a different point of view. This type of thinking is known in the Piagetian literature as *figurative,* since it involves the reconstruction and/or evocation of specific physical facts, that is, the shapes of events.

Both de Ajuriaguerra[148,213] and Inhelder[214] had noted that children with language disorders evidence special difficulty in tasks that require figurative thought. Following this suggestion, Johnston and Ramstad rated their experimental tasks according to whether they seem to entail figurative, imagistic, thought.[215,216] Regardless of conceptual domain, the children had greatest difficulty with those problems that invited visual imagery and offered little opportunity for the physical manipulation of materials. Similarly, Kamhi's language disordered children had greatest difficulty with haptic recognition, a task that invites imagery.[217] However, his data did not indicate similar difficulty on two other imagery tasks. And Murphy failed to find group differences in four of her five imagery tasks.[230]

A recent study by Savich suggests that methodological weaknesses were responsible for negative findings in earlier experiments.[231] Murphy had matched her subjects with the Ravens, a nonverbal intelligence test that invites imagery, possibly eliminating the group differences she hoped to study.[230] Kamhi had used imagery tasks that may have been too difficult for his subjects,[217,232] creating a "floor" effect. Savich, matching with the Wechsler and using older subjects, observed performance on five imagery tasks. Her language disordered children were less successful than their age peers on all five. They had trouble predicting the position of a "snail" on a circular path, the position of fold lines on paper squares, the composite shape of geometric forms, and the three-dimensional rotation of block arrays. Johnston and Ellis Weismer also reported performance on a mental rotation task.[233] Their language disordered subjects evidenced longer reaction times with larger rotational arcs, thus proving that they had used imagistic strategies.[234] Even when initial response time was controlled, however, they solved the problems more slowly than did their normal peers.††

Conclusions

At first glance, the search for an underlying deficit in symbolic representation seems to have paid off. Only Levi and Longobardi's§ study of imitative gestures has failed to reveal group differences.[235] Studies of symbolic play and visual imagery indicate that language disordered children indeed have difficulty using nonverbal as well as verbal symbols. Correlations between performance in the two modes have been generally moderate, but significant.[224,228,231,244] Moreover, relative performance levels have been exactly in line with what would be expected for two cognitive systems that share a common attribute, symbolism, but differ in other respects.[236] Verbal abilities are sometimes reported to be in advance of nonverbal symbolic abilities,[80,225,237] sometimes equivalent to them,[226] and other times behind them.[80,217,227,237] Language deficits then could reflect a more basic problem in symbolic function.

Upon reflection, however, these findings are open to at least one alternative explanation. The initial studies of conceptual development pointed to symbolic impairments that *exceeded* deficits in reasoning abilities.[214–217] Subsequent studies have not been designed to address this issue. Until further research is done, it remains possible that the observed symbolic deficits merely reflect some more pervasive cognitive limitation that affects both symbolic and nonsymbolic aspects of mental activity.

Hierarchical Planning

A second hypothesized explanation for language disorder is found in the work of Cromer.[238,239] He postulates a cognitive mechanism responsible for converting "intentions that are not temporally ordered . . . into real time sequences" and vice versa.[239] This hierarchical planning ability, he argues, underlies a number of "superficially sequential activities" including the processing of complex rhythmic or linguistic events. Disability in this aspect of thought would thus hinder performance in both verbal and nonverbal tasks. Kracke had found that language disordered 12 year olds had difficulty noting differences in rhythmic sequences of pulses, presented either auditorily or tactually.[240] Unlike comparison groups of deaf and normal children, her language disordered subjects seemed to process the pulses element by element instead of treating the patterns as wholes.

Cromer used construction and drawing tasks to further study hierarchicalization abilities.[239] Lan-

†† This analysis is not included in the published report.

§ This sign indicates that the subjects in study cited may not fit the operational criteria of language disorder used in this chapter.

guage disordered, deaf, and normal children, aged 8 to 16, were asked to copy a mobile-like figure in two and three dimensions. As an index of hierarchical strategies, Cromer measured their ability to switch from one side of the mobile to the other as they proceeded to draw or build. The language disordered children had great difficulty using such a strategy even when it was demonstrated. They preferred instead to work from one contiguous element to the next without interruption. The deaf and normal children showed no such limitation.

Cromer's notion of a hierarchicalization disability is intriguing, particularly for its short-term memory implications. In both the rhythm and mobile tasks, children must represent perceived events in an economical and powerful fashion, one that reduces memory loads and leaves processing "space" for comparison or motor planning activities. A hierarchicalized representation would meet this demand. However, hierarchical schemes can arise either from low-level perceptual processes or from higher-level conceptual and linguistic knowledge. For example, the relationships between elements in a visual gestalt are perceived, whereas the relationships between the phrases of a complex sentence must be constructed out of interpretations of form and meaning. A single mechanism that could span such different mental systems seems unlikely, but further research may clarify the nature of the mechanism and its dysfunction.

Hypothesis Testing

Until recently,[241] child language theories were virtually unanimous in claiming that children actively analyze and compare linguistic input, forming hypotheses about underlying organizational schemes and evaluating these hypotheses with new linguistic data. Impairment in hypothesis testing abilities was thus a prime candidate for explaining language disorder. Children with such an impairment might be expected to have difficulty learning language patterns and solving analogous nonverbal problems.

Researchers have explored this possibility by observing language disordered children in various concept formation and hypothesis testing paradigms. In a typical experiment, children view a series of cards each portraying two geometric forms. One of the forms represents a target class such as *large* forms or *square* forms. The task is to determine the attribute(s) that characterize this targetted class. On each trial, children pick the form that exemplifies their current solution to the problem. Periodic feedback allows them to evaluate and change their hypotheses.

Four studies of this sort have been reported, with mixed results. Hoskins[242] and Nelson, Kamhi, and Apel[243] found that school-age language disordered children were less adept than their mental or chronological age peers at finding the correct answers. They solved fewer problems or needed more trials to find the solutions. Kamhi, Catts, Koenig, and Lewis[244] and Kamhi, Nelson, Lee, and Gholson,[245] in contrast, report equivocal findings. A few of their language disordered subjects (10 to 20 percent) failed to complete the task. Those who did, tended to require more trials to reach criteria and to be unable to verbalize their hypotheses, but there were no significant group differences.

Methodological variation makes it difficult to evaluate this disagreeement. The studies that indicate some hypothesis testing disability seem to use children with more severe language delays and to present tasks that are more age-appropriate. Interestingly, they also give children verbal feedback that explicitly mentions pertinent attributes, for example, "Yes, the answer is in the picture of the big, black square." Perhaps the normal children in these studies were able to make better use of such cues.

Language disordered children probably do have difficulty in hypothesis testing tasks, but further research is needed to reveal the extent and exact nature of their problems. The interpretive questions are of two sorts. First, the conscious problem solving strategies employed in the cognitive tasks may be qualitatively different from the largely unconscious comparison processes evoked in language learning. Secondly, hypothesis testing ability is clearly a composite skill, entailing many different mental processes. For example, Nelson, Kamhi, and Apel argue that their results implicate poor encoding into short-term memory rather than problems with evaluating the data or maintaining information in storage.[243] If so, hypothesis testing loses its explanatory value. Many cognitive tasks require short-term memory encoding. It remains to be seen whether language disordered children have trouble in all of them.

Conclusions

Taken as a whole, the research on the cognitive abilities of language disordered children presents a convincing picture of substantial impairment. At many ages; across visual, auditory, and tactile stimuli; across many domains of knowledge; in symbolic and nonsymbolic activities; in tasks with little to no explicit verbal demand, language disordered children perform below age expectations. Efforts to identify a mental impairment that could explain both the language delay and the poor performance on nonverbal tasks have thus far been unsatisfactory. Symbolic dysfunction, hierarchical planning disability, and hypothesis testing disability are "middle-level" constructs that refer to complexes of mental processes or schemes. Their explanatory power and their psychological validity have not yet been demonstrated. However, they do force one to think more carefully about the nature of human intellect. Even if future studies lead elsewhere, these hypotheses may prove to have been valuable way stations to an adequate explanation.

The next generation of cognitive studies is likely to focus on more molecular processes, the basic mechanisms that in various combinations participate in all thought. An earlier section considered the work on attention. The studies of hierarchicalization and hypothesis testing now raise similar questions about memory. Is it possible that language disordered children make less use of symbols to store interpretations of events, fail to employ economical chunking strategies, or encode events with little regard for their current cognitive goals? In this final section on intellectual development, the focus turns to research on memory.

Memory

Psychological testing and clinical reports had long pointed to some sort of memory problem in language disordered children.[246] Experimental studies of rapid naming and serial memory have supported this view. Even when they know the terms for object classes, language disordered children are slower to recall and produce them.[247–249] They are also less successful than their age peers in remembering nonverbal auditory or visual stimuli in sequences of three or more elements.[165,167,190,191,250] Although some of these experiments required children to learn the associations between particular stimuli and particular response buttons, this fact does not seem to account for the group differences. When Furth and Pufall presented a similar learning task with simultaneous arrays, the language disordered children performed at nearly normal levels.[190] The essence of their difficulty apparently lay in the short-term memory demands of sequential material.

Other researchers have looked more closely at the various components of memory, trying to pinpoint the problem. For older children and adults, one key to remembering lies in the use of rehearsal strategies to maintain information in temporary storage. Stark, Poppen, and May had noted that their language disordered children made an unusual number of errors in recalling the first word in a series,[251] a fact that seemed to point to poor rehearsal strategies.[252] Tomblin explored this possibility with a more carefully designed experiment using two control groups, one matched to the language disordered children by age (aged 9) and one by short-term memory span (aged 5).[253] He then presented unstructured word strings for recall. No differences occurred in recall patterns between the disordered and younger normal groups, but both of these groups had less success than the older normals in remembering the initial elements of the strings. Since memory span is highly influenced by rehearsal, these findings again implicate poor rehearsal strategies.

Kirchner and Klatzky looked more directly at the rehearsal process itself.[254] Twelve pictured objects were named and shown one at a time, with a 15-second pause after each. Subjects were told to rehearse the sequences aloud during these pauses. Various scores captured the nature of the rehearsal strings as well as the child's eventual success in remembering the entire sequence. The language disordered children were apparently less able to maintain the longer strings via rehearsal. Their rehearsal strings were also more likely to contain words that had not been in any list, but were semantically related to list items. These findings suggest that even when language disordered children use verbal rehearsal, the strategy proves inadequate.

Less work has been done on other components of short-term memory, but findings thus far have indicated problems with scanning speed,[255] masking,[256] and retrieval[257,258]—in short, with every major memory function. If these results are confirmed, the short-term memory deficits of language disordered children would appear to be serious.

However, note that the studies that have looked at particular memory processes have all used verbal tasks. Once again the putative deficits could be the direct result of the language disorder itself. Indeed, the two studies that include a control for language ability report no differences between language-matched groups.[258,259] Even when experimental materials are nonverbal, language may be used to aid memory. In the studies that presented sequences of nonsense figures, pictures, lights, or tones, children may have made private use of labels such as "high," "top," "pointy," thus converting the superficially nonverbal tasks into measures of verbal rehearsal. Such covert verbal rehearsal might also explain findings in two studies by Levy and Menyuk.[260,261] These investigators tested memory for object and event sequences presented either verbally or nonverbally. Language disordered preschoolers were equally deficit in both modes of presentation and made the same sorts of errors in each.

A final scatter of studies cautions against the

view that all short-term memory problems reflect deficits in verbal memory. Wyke and Asso asked disordered 7 year olds to recall the positions of markers within two- and three-dimensional "tic-tac-toe" boards following an 8-second delay.[262] The language disordered children made more errors. Further study of the normal children indicated that they did not rely on verbal rehearsal to perform this task. Similarly, Doehring asked 8 and 10 year olds to point to the spot where a light had flashed.[263] In some trials, there was an 8-second delay, in others a patterned screen was placed over the display to interrupt visual fixation. Neither of these procedures impeded the performance of the language disordered children. Although they identified the target spots less accurately than their peers, this finding was apparently not due to problems with maintaining information in short-term storage. The memory deficits implied by these studies cannot be attributed easily to limitations in verbal processes. Nor can the memory deficits observed in the rhythm, drawing, and construction tasks reviewed earlier.

Further research on short-term memory processes in language disordered children is clearly warranted. Evidence of a general deficit in basic memory processes would have obvious widespread implications for language learning and problem solving of all sorts. However, current memory models remind one of the complexity of this research task. Educators have traditionally viewed memory as a structural feature of the mind that "grows" with maturation and sets limits on what can be learned. This may still be true, but now it seems that remembering in the short-term also depends on what one knows,[264] on what one chooses to attend to,[86] and on one's skill in the active, often conscious, use of storage and retrieval strategies.[196,252,265,266]

These higher level functions complicate research on traditional memory constructs such as "span" or "encoding." Take the recent findings of Ellis Weismer as an example.[267] She presented brief stories to language disordered 8 year olds and later asked them about the story content. Some of the questions focused on information explicitly mentioned in the original story. Other questions concerned inferences that could be drawn from this information. Even when they remembered the information presented in the story, the language disordered children had difficulty answering the questions that required inferences. (See also Crais and Chapman.[268]) This finding would seem to imply reasoning problems beyond any memory deficit. However, the disordered children essentially performed at the level of children in a language-matched control group. This fact suggests that language played some key role in the inferential process and affected the ultimate scope of the information that was stored. Identifying the specific nature of memory dysfunctions is not easy. At the least, future studies will need to describe memory activities according to their conceptual and informational requirements, their verbal or nonverbal nature, their use of automatic or controlled mechanisms,[86] and their functional role within a larger task setting.

Implications for Assessment and Intervention

Cognitive research with language disordered children affirms the presence of intellectual deficits at various ages and across diverse domains. This fact suggests new care in interpreting nonverbal IQ scores. Although performance scales are often considered to be measures of nonverbal intelligence, none samples the entire range of conceivable nonverbal knowledge and/or skills—motor coordination, perceptual processing, conceptual transformation of the perceptual givens, logical reasoning, symbol use and so forth. Moreover, each scale carries certain item biases. For example, the Leiter International Performance Scale is heavily weighted toward perceptual matching tasks through age 8, and children tend to have more succcess with these perceptual items than with items that require conceptual interpretations of the stimuli.[269] With thoughtful item analysis, clinicians may utilize performance scales to identify language disordered children's relative cognitive strengths. At the moment, strengths are most obvious in the area of visual perceptual functions,[270] but further research may identify others. In the meantime, the studies reviewed in this section, as well as reports of diminished performance IQ scores in older language disordered children,[271,272] suggest caution in clinical judgments concerning "normal nonverbal intelligence."

If language disordered children bring intellectual as well as linguistic deficiencies, the implications of this fact for intervention are as complex as the relationships between language and thought—and just as controversial. Studies with normal children have identified aspects of cognitive growth, both conceptual and organizational, that typically precede early referential speech[60,221,273] and the learning of certain relational terms.[59,274–276] Rather than establishing global relationships between language level and cognitive stage, these studies point to specific linguistic discoveries that depend upon specific prior cognitive achievements.[62] Wherever this relationship holds true, language disordered children's cognitive deficiencies may place constraints on the content of language therapy. Clinicians may need to wait for necessary cognitive growth or develop nonverbal training activities that would accelerate such growth. A small but growing body of cognitive training studies can provide useful guidelines for this task.[242,277–281]

The fact that cognitive deficiencies may impede language learning does not imply that the relationships between language and thought go in only one direction. Since language is a powerful tool of intellect as well as its product,[282] cognitive deficiencies may result from language disorder as well as be a contributing cause. As reviewed previously, poor verbal skills apparently can hinder short-term memory processes and thus influence success in all sorts of reasoning tasks. Poor verbal skills may also impede the construction of basic concepts such as social categories[283] or metric quantity.[284] Interventionists may be able to limit these consequences of language disorder by presenting nonlinguistic or visual analogues that can sustitute for the oral language forms. Children who are unable to learn the auditory rote counting sequence, for example, may be able to learn a sign equivalent. And finally, children with poor language skills are at an obvious disadvantage whenever a learning task is presented verbally. Kamhi, Gentry, and Mauer's disordered children took three times longer to learn a problem solving strategy that was taught with words than one that was taught with physical demonstration.[285] Teachers of language disordered children may be able to improve their classroom success by providing visual as well as verbal instruction.

EPILOGUE

The mood of the Stanford Institute was one of cautious optimism. As one discussant voiced it, "[We] consider the developmental language disorder as a developmental lag . . . with the possibility of catching up and even accelerating" (p 27). It seemed then that a child with normal nonverbal intelligence, an intact sensorimotor system, and a healthy affect should have a good prognosis, in spite of early language delays. If such children exist, researchers have had trouble finding them. Instead, children with language disorders seem more likely to manifest pervasive cognitive dysfunction and persistent problems in learning. The relationships between various linguistic, attentional, perceptual, conceptual, reasoning, and memory deficits may be uncertain, but there is little reason to doubt their reality.

What then is the utility of the term "language disorder?" This depends on the job that needs doing. If one needs to *describe* this particular developmental profile, the term "language disorder" is at best inadequate and at worst misleading. Not only does it fail to capture the widespread cognitive impairments evidenced by such children, it also implies that once a child learns to speak the problem is resolved.

If one needs to *explain* this particular developmental syndrome, to denote its primary causal force, the term "language disorder" is again inadequate. Given the thorough integration of language and mind, no single designation can do justice to cause and effect relationships. Imagine the following developmental scenario. A language disordered child enters the world with certain "hard-wired" processing deficiencies. These deficiencies lead directly to early delays in the construction of both nonverbal relational knowledge and language knowledge. The lack of relational concepts further delays language learning; the lack of language skills further delays cognitive growth. And at all points in development, the original processing deficiencies impede the utilization of both verbal and nonverbal schemes. Obviously, no single term can effectively capture this interplay of causal vectors.

What if, however, the goal were not to describe or to explain, but to *illuminate,* to denote the essential key to a puzzle? Then the term "language disorder" serves well, for it points to a particular problem space with known characteristics. Language is a symbolic medium *and* a set of rapidly sequenced auditory events *and* a multilayered system intricate enough to meet the demands of human communication and thought. Language disorders may arise only when dysfunctions exist in each of these areas. If so, the quest for single causes or single remediations is doomed. Language is the complex invention of a complex mind. Clinicians should not be surprised that some children find it difficult to learn nor underestimate their handicap when they do.

REFERENCES

1. Proceedings of the institute on childhood aphasia. San Francisco: National Society for Crippled Children and Adults, 1962.
2. Weiner P. The study of childhood language disorders: nineteenth century perspectives. J Commun Disord 1986; 19:1–47.
3. Miller J, Chapman R, MacKenzie H. Individual differences in the language acquisition patterns of mentally retarded children. Proc Symp Res Child Lang Disord 1981; 2:130–146.
4. Aram D, Ekelman B, Nation J. Preschoolers with language disorders: 10 years later. J Speech Hear Res 1984; 27:232–244.
5. Stark R, Bernstein L, Condino R, Bender M, Tallal P, Catts H. Four-year follow-up study of language impaired children. Ann Dyslexia 1984; 34:49–68.
6. Strominger A, Bashir A. A nine year follow-up of language delayed children. Paper presented to the American Speech Hearing Association, Chicago, 1977.
7. Bloom L, Lahey M. Language development and language

disorders. New York: John Wiley & Sons, 1978.

8. Weiner P. Developmental language disorders. In: Rie H, Rie E, eds. Handbook of minimal brain dysfunction. New York: John Wiley & Sons, 1980:298.

8a. Adams M Sr, Pace S. A descriptive linguistic investigation of language problems in preschool children. Paper presented to the American Speech Hearing Association, Chicago, 1969.

9. Leonard L. What is deviant language? J Speech Hear Res 1972; 37:427–446.

10. Menyuk P. Comparison of grammar of children with functionally deviant and normal speech. J Speech Hear Res 1964; 7:109–121.

11. Morehead D, Ingram D. The development of base syntax in normal and linguistically deviant children. J Speech Hear Res 1973; 16:330–352.

12. Johnston J, Kamhi A. The same can be less: syntactic and semantic aspects of the utterances of language impaired children. Merrill-Palmer Q 1984; 30:65–86.

13. Meline T, Sanders L. Imitation, comprehension, and spontaneous production of main verbs by normal and disordered language children. Paper presented to the American Speech Hearing Association, Houston, 1976.

14. Miller J. Assessing language production in children. Baltimore: University Park, 1981.

15. Johnson N, Mandler J. A tale of two structures: underlying and surface forms in stories. Poetics 1980; 9:51–86.

16. Stein N, Glenn C. An analysis of story comprehension in elementary school children. In: Freedle R, ed. New directions in discourse processing. Vol. 2. Norwood, NJ: Ablex 1979:53.

17. Brewer W. The story schema: universal and culture specific properties. In: Olson D, Torrance N, Hildyard A, eds. Literacy, language, and learning: the nature and consequences of reading and writing. New York: Cambridge University Press, 1985.

18. Clancy P. The development of narrative discourse in Japanese. Papers and reports in child language development. No. 17. Dept. of Linguistics, Stanford University, 1979:41.

19. Mandler J, Johnson N. Remembrance of things parsed: story structure and recall. Cognit Psychol 1977; 9:111–151.

20. Karmiloff-Smith A. Psychological processes underlying pronominalization and non-pronominalization in children's connected discourse. In: Kreiman J, Ojeda A, eds. Papers from the para-session on pronouns and anaphora. Chicago Linguistic Society, University of Chicago, 1979.

21. Liles B. Episode organization and conjunctive accuracy in spoken narratives of normal and language disordered children. Proc Symp Child Lang Disord 1985; 6:148–157.

21a. Roth F, Spekman N. Story grammar analysis of narratives produced by learning disabled and normally achieving students. Proc Symp Child Lang Disord 1985; 6:67–79.

22. Klecan-Aker J. Syntactic abilities in normal and language deficient middle school children. Top Lang Disord 1985; 5:46–54.

23. Liles B. Cohesion in the narratives of normal and language disordered children. J Speech Hear Res 1985; 28:123–133.

24. Graybeal C. Memory for stories in language impaired children. Appl Psycholinguist 1981; 2:269–284.

25. Hedberg N, Fink R. Surface and deep structure characteristics of language disordered children's narratives. Paper presented to the American Speech Hearing Language Association, Washington, DC, 1985.

26. Sleight C, Prinz P. Use of abstract orientations, and codas in narration by language disordered and nondisordered children. J Speech Hear Disord 1985; 50:361–371.

27. MacLachlan B, Chapman R. Communication breakdowns in normal and language/learning disabled children's conversation and narration. Proc Symp Child Lang Disord 1985; 6:55–72.

28. Caro D, Schneider P. Creating referents in text: a comparison of learning disabled and normal adolescents' narratives. Proceedings of the symposium on research in child language development 1982; 3:123–134.

29. Liles B. The production and comprehension of narrative discourse in normal and language disordered children. J Commun Disord 1985; 18:409–427.

30. Johnston J. Narratives: a new look at communication problems in older language disordered children. Lang Speech Hear Services Schools 1982; 13:144–155.

31. Brown R. A first language: the early stages. Cambridge, MA: Harvard University Press, 1973.

32. Johnston J, Schery T. The use of grammatical morphemes by children with communication disorders. In: Morehead D, Morehead A, eds. Normal and deficient child language. Baltimore: University Park, 1976:239.

33. Ekelman B, Aram D. Syntactic findings in developmental verbal apraxia. J Commun Disord 1983; 16:237–250.

34. Ingram D. The acquisition of the English verbal auxiliary and copula in normal and linguistically deviant children. Papers and reports in child language development. No. 4. Committee on Linguistics, Stanford University, 1972:79.

35. Kessler C. Post-semantic processes in delayed child language related to first and second language learning. In: Dato D, ed. Georgetown University roundtable on language and linguistics. Washington, DC: Georgetown University, 1975:159.

36. Steckol K, Leonard L. The use of grammatical morphemes by normal and language impaired children. J Commun Disord 1979; 12:291–301.

37. Chafe W. Meaning and the structure of language. Chicago: University of Chicago Press, 1970.

38. Fillmore C. The case for case. In: Bach E, Harms R, eds. Universals in linguistic theory. New York: Holt, Rinehart & Winston, 1968:1.

39. Schlesinger I. Relational concepts underlying language. In: Schiefelbusch R, Lloyd L, eds. Language perspectives: acquisition, retardation and intervention. Baltimore: University Park, 1974:129.

40. Bowerman M. Early syntactic development: a cross-linguistic study with special reference to Finnish. London: Cambridge University Press, 1973.

41. Slobin DI. Psycholinguistics. 2nd ed. Glenview, IL: Scott, Foresman, 1979.

42. Leonard L, Bolders J, Miller J. An examination of the semantic relations reflected in the language usage of normal and language disordered children. J Speech Hear Res 1976; 19:371–392.

43. Freedman P, Carpenter R. Semantic relations used by normal and language impaired children at stage 1. J Speech Hear Res 1976; 19:784–795.

44. Lee L. A study of normal and atypical semantic development. Unpublished manuscript, Northwestern University, 1976.

44a. Lee L. Linguistic approaches to developmental language disorders. Folia Phoniatr 1974; 26:33–67.

45. Leonard L, Steckol K, Schwartz R. Semantic relations and utterance lengths in child language. In: Peng F, von Raffler Engel W, eds. Language acquisition and developmental kinesics. Tokyo: University of Tokyo, 1978:93.

46. Johnston J, Kamhi A, McDonald J. Patterns of predicate use in language impaired children. Proc Symp Res Child Lang Disord 1981; 2:17–28.

47. Wells G. Language development in the preschool years. Cambridge: Cambridge University Press, 1985.

48. Leonard L, Camarata S, Rowan L, Chapman K. The communicative functions of lexical usage by language impaired children. Appl Psycholinguist 1982; 3:109–125.

48a. Leonard L, Schwartz R, Chapman K, Rowan L, Prelock P, Terrell B, Weiss A, Messick C. Early lexical acquisition in children with specific language impairment. J Speech Hear Res 1982; 25:554–563.

49. Gentner D. On relational meanings: the acquisition of verb meaning. Child Dev 1978; 49:988–998.
50. Chapman K, Leonard L, Rowan L, Weiss A. Inappropriate word extensions in the speech of young language disordered children. J Speech Hear Disord 1983; 48:55–62.
51. Leonard L, Camarata S, Schwartz R. Chapman K, Messick C. Homonymy and the voiced-voiceless distinction in the speech of children with specific language impairment. J Speech Hear Res 1985; 28:215–224.
52. Illerbrun D. The comprehension of spatial adjectives by children with normal and children with deviant language development. Hum Commun 1975; Autumn:27–36.
53. Peach R. Comprehension of relative and contrastive objectives by language disordered children. Paper presented to the American Speech Hearing Association, Chicago, 1977.
54. Ingram D. The acquisition of questions and its relation to cognitive development in normal and linguistically deviant children: a pilot study. Papers and reports in child language development. No. 4. Committee on Linguistics, Stanford University, 1972:13.
55. Lee R, Ashmore L. Receptive and expressive wh-question performance by language-delayed children. J Commun Disord 1983; 16:99–109.
56. Barblan L, Chipman H. Temporal relationships in language: a comparison between normal and language retarded children. In: Drachman G, ed. Salzburger Beitrage zur Linguistik 5: (in press).
57. Nippold M, Fey M. Metaphoric understanding in preadolescents having a history of language acquisition difficulties. Lang Speech Hear Services Schools 1983; 14:171–180.
58. Partyka C, Kresheck J. A comparison of categorization skills of normal and language-delayed children in early elementary school. Lang Speech Hear Services Schools 1983; 14:243–251.
59. Cromer R. The cognitive hypothesis of language acquisition and its implications for child language deficiency. In: Morehead D, Morehead A, eds. Normal and deficient child language. Baltimore: University Park, 1976:283.
60. Edwards D. Sensory-motor intelligence and semantic relations in early child grammar. Cognition 1974; 12:395–434.
61. Ervin-Tripp S. Some strategies for the first two years. In: Dil A, ed. Language acquisition and communicative choice: essays by Susan Ervin-Tripp. Stanford: Stanford University, 1973:204.
62. Johnston J. Cognitive prerequisites: the evidence from children learning English. In: Slobin DI, ed. The cross-linguistic study of language acquisition. Vol. 2. Hillsdale, NJ: Erlbaum, 1985:961.
63. Johnston J, Slobin DI. The development of locative expressions in English, Italian, Serbo-Croatian, and Turkish. J Child Lang 1979; 16:529–546.
64. Liles B, Shulman M, Bartlett S. Judgments of grammaticality by normal and language disordered children. J Speech Hear Disord 1977; 42:199–209.
65. Watson L. Conversational participation by language deficient and normal children. In: Andrews J, Burns M, eds. Selected papers in language and phonology. Vol. II. Evanston, IL: Institute for Continuing Education, 1977:104.
66. Bartak L, Rutter M, Cox A. A comparative study of infantile autism and specific developmental receptive language disorders. Br J Psychiatry 1975; 126:127–145.
67. Caparulo B, Cohen D. Cognitive structures, language, and emerging social competence in autistic and aphasic children. J Am Acad Child Psychiatry 1977; 116:620–645.
68. de Hirsch K. Differential diagnoses between aphasic and schizophrenic language in children. J Speech Hear Disord 1967; 32:3–10.
69. Bartak L, Rutter M, Cox A. A comparative study of infantile autism and specific developmental receptive language disorders: III. Discriminant function analysis. J Autism Child Schizo 1977; 7:383–396.
70. Cantwell D, Baker L, Rutter M. A comparative study of infantile autism and specific developmental receptive language disorder. IV. Analysis of syntax and language function. J Child Psychol Psychiatry 1978; 19:351–362.
71. Dore J. Variation in preschool children's conversational performance. In: Nelson K, ed. Children's language. Vol. 1. New York: Gardner, 1978:397.
72. Halliday M. Learning how to mean. London: Edward Arnold, 1975.
73. Snyder L. Communicative and cognitive abilities and disabilities in the sensori-motor period. Merrill-Palmer Q 1978; 24:161–180.
74. Rowan L, Leonard L, Chapman K, Weiss A. Performative and presuppositional skills in language disordered and normal children. J Speech Hear Res 1983; 26:97–105.
75. Shatz M, Bernstein D, Shulman M. The responses of language disordered children to indirect directives in varying contexts. Appl Psycholinguist 1980; 1:295–306.
76. Brinton B, Fujiki M. A comparison of request-response sequences in the discourse of normal and language disordered children. J Speech Hear Disord 1982; 47:57–62.
77. Bates E. Language and context. New York: Academic Press, 1976.
78. Greenfield P, Zukow P. Why do children say what they say when they say it? An experimental approach to the psychogenesis of presupposition. In: Nelson K, ed. Children's language. Vol. 1. New York: Gardner, 1978:287.
79. Shatz M. Communication. In: Mussen P, ed. Handbook of child psychology. 4th ed. Vol. III. Flavell J, Markman E, vol. eds. Cognitive development. New York: John Wiley & Sons, 1983:841.
80. Skarakis E, Greenfield P. The role of new and old information in the verbal expression of language disordered children. J Speech Hear Res 1982; 25:462–467.
81. Meline T. Referential communication skills of learning disabled/language impaired children. Appl Psycholinguist 1986; 7:129–139.
82. Leonard L. Conversational replies of children with specific language impairment. J Speech Hear Res 1986; 29:114–119.
83. Reichle J, Busch C, Doyle S. The topical relationship among adjacent utterances in productively delayed children's language addressed to their mothers. J Commun Disord 1986; 19:63–74.
84. Rosinski M, Newhoff M. Conversational responsiveness in language disordered children. Proc Symp Res Child Lang Disord 1982; 3:135–144.
85. Ceci S. Extracting meaning from stimuli: automatic and purposive processing of the language-based learning disabled. Top Learn Learn Disabil 1982; 2:46–53.
86. Ceci S. Automatic and purposive semantic processing characteristics of normal and language/learning disabled children. Dev Psychol 1983; 19:427–439.
87. Mackworth N, Grandstaff N, Pribram K. Orientation to pictorial novelty by speech-disordered children. Neuropsychologia 1973; 11:443–450.
88. Brinton B, Fujiki M, Loeb D, Winkler E. Development of conversational repair strategies in response to requests for clarification. J Speech Hear Res 1986; 29:75–81.
89. Gallagher T. Revision behaviors in the speech of normal children developing language. J Speech Hear Res 1977; 20:303–318.
90. Garvey C. The contingent query: a dependent act in conversation. In: Lewis M, Rosenblum L, eds. Interaction, conversation and the development of language. New York: John Wiley & Sons, 1977:63.
91. Gallagher T, Darnton B. Conversational aspects of the speech of language disordered children: revision behaviors. J Speech Hear Res 1978; 21:118–135.
91a. Brinton B, Fujiki M, Channell R. Revision sequences in normal and language disordered children. Paper presented

to the American Speech Language Hearing Association, Washington, DC, 1985.
92. Meline T, Meline N. Facing a communicative obstacle: pragmatics of language impaired children. Percept Mot Skills 1983; 56:469–470.
93. Gale D, Liebergott J, Griffen S. Getting it: children's requests for clarification. Paper presented to the American Speech Language Hearing Association, Los Angeles, 1981.
94. Hoar N. Paraphrase capabilities of language impaired children. Paper present at the Boston University Conference on Language Development, Boston, 1977.
95. Ervin-Tripp S. Sociolinguistics. In: Berkowitz L, ed. Advances in experimental social psychology. Vol. 4. New York: Academic Press, 1969:91.
96. Fey M, Leonard L. Partner age as a variable in the conversational performance of specifically language impaired children. J Speech Hear Res 1984; 27:413–423.
97. Fey M, Leonard L, Wilcox K. Speech style modifications of language-impaired children. J Speech Hear Disord 1981; 46:91–96.
98. Messick C, Newhoff M. Request forms: does the language delayed child consider the listener? Paper presented to the American Speech Hearing Association, Atlanta, 1979.
99. Prinz P. An investigation of the comprehension and production of requests in normal and language disordered children. J Commun Disord 1982; 15:75–93.
100. Prinz P, Ferrier L. Can you give me that one? The comprehension, production and judgment of directives in language impaired children. J Speech Hear Disord 1983; 48:44–54.
101. Leonard L. Speech selection and modification in language disordered children. Top Lang Disord 1983; 4:28–37.
102. Prutting C, Kirchner D. A clinical appraisal of the pragmatic aspects of language. J Speech Hear Disord 1987; 52:105–119.
103. Donahue M. Requesting strategies of learning disabled children. Appl Psycholinguist 1981; 2:213–234.
104. Bates E, MacWhinney B. A functionalist approach to the acquisition of grammar. In: Ochs E, Schieffelin B, eds. Developmental pragmatics. New York: Academic Press, 1979:167.
105. Givon T. Function, structure and language acquisition. In: Slobin DI, ed. The cross-linguistic study of language acquisition. Vol. 2. Hillsdale, NJ: Erlbaum, 1985:1005.
106. Fey M, Leonard L. Pragmatic skills of children with specific language impairment. In: Gallagher T, Prutting C, eds. Pragmatic assessment and intervention issues in language. San Diego: College-Hill Press, 1983:65.
107. Wollner S. Communicating intentions: how well do language impaired children do? Top Lang Disord 1983; 4:1–14.
108. Cunningham E, Siegel L, van der Spuy H, Clark M, Bow S. The behavioral and linguistic interactions of specifically language delayed and normal boys and their mothers. Child Dev 1985; 56:1389–1403.
109. Paul R, Cohen D, Caparulo B. A longitudinal study of patients with severe developmental disorders of language learning. J Am Acad Child Psychiatry 1983; 22:525–534.
110. Liles B, Watt J. On the meaning of "language delay." Folia Phoniatr 1984; 36:40–48.
111. Byers-Brown B. Language vulnerability, speech delay and therapeutic intervention: evidence for distinctive etiologies. Br J Disord Commun 1976; 11:43–56.
112. Ingram T. The classification of speech and language disorders in young children. In: Rutter M, Martin J, eds. The child with delayed speech. Clinics in developmental medicine. No. 43. London: William Heinemann Medical Books, 1972.
113. Linck H, Haberkamp H. Sprachentwicklungsbehinderung-Sprachentwicklungsverzögerung: Versuch einer Abgrenzung. Folia Phoniatr 1976; 28:141–160.
114. Menyuk P. Children with language problems: what's the problem? In: Dato D, ed. Georgetown University roundtable on languages and linguistics. Washington, DC: Georgetown University, 1975:129.
115. Bax M, Stevenson P. Analysis of a developmental language delay. Proc R Soc Med 1977; 70:727–728.
116. Kerschensteiner M, Huber W. Grammatical impairment in developmental aphasia. Cortex 1975; 11:264–282.
117. Trantham C, Pedersen J. Normal language development—the key to diagnosis and therapy for language disordered children. Baltimore: Williams & Wilkins, 1976.
118. Weiner P. A language delayed child at adolescence. J Speech Hear Disord 1974; 39:202–212.
119. Eisenson J, Ingram D. Childhood aphasia: an updated concept based on recent research. Papers and reports in child language development. No. 4. Committee on Linguistics, Stanford University, 1972:103.
120. Lee L. Developmental sentence types: a method for comparing normal and deviant syntactic development. J Speech Hear Disord 1966; 31:311–330.
121. Gardner H. Frames of mind. New York: Basic Books, 1983.
122. Johnston J, Blatchley M, Streit G. Miniature language system learning by normal and language disordered children. Proc Symp Res Child Lang Disord 1985; 6:1–10.
123. Dollaghan C. Fast mapping in normal and language impaired children. Proc Symp Res Child Lang Disord 1984; 5:73–89.
124. Dollaghan C. Child meets word: "fast mapping" in preschool children. J Speech Hear Res 1985; 28:449–454.
125. Peters A. The units of language acquisition. Cambridge: Cambridge University, 1983.
126. Weiss A, Leonard L, Rowan L, Chapman K. Linguistic and nonlinguistic features of style in normal and language impaired children. J Speech Hear Disord 1983; 48:154–164.
127. Aram D, Nation J. Preschool language disorders and subsequent language and academic difficulties. J Commun Disord 1980; 13:159–170.
128. Griffeths C. A follow-up study of children with disorders of speech. Br J Disord Commun 1969; 4:46–56.
129. Hall P, Tomblin B. A follow-up study of children with articulation and language disorders. J Speech Hear Disord 1978; 43:227–241.
130. Schery T. Correlates of language development in language disordered children. J Speech Hear Disord 1985; 50:73–83.
131. Cromer R. The basis of childhood dysphasia: a linguistic approach. In: Wyke M, ed. Developmental dysphasia. London: Academic Press, 1978:85.
132. Gillam R, Johnston J. The development of print awareness in language disordered preschoolers. J Speech Hear Res 1985; 28:521–526.
133. Van Kleek A. Assessment and intervention: does meta matter? In: Wallach G, Butler K, eds. Language learning disabilities in school-age children. Baltimore: Williams & Wilkins, 1984:179.
134. Van Kleek A, Schuele C. Precursors to literacy: normal development. Top Lang Disord 1987; 7:13–31.
135. Dollaghan C. Normal and language disordered children's awareness of verb propositional schemata. Paper presented to the American Speech Language Hearing Association, Toronto, 1982.
136. Dunton S, Fujiki M, Brinton B. Metalinguistic judgement skills in normal and language disordered children. Paper presented to the American Speech Language Hearing Association, San Francisco, 1984.
137. Kamhi A, Koenig L. Metalinguistic awareness in normal and language disordered children. Lang Speech Hear Services Schools 1985; 16:199–210.
138. Kamhi A, Lee R, Nelson L. Word, syllable and sound awareness in language disordered chidren. J Speech Hear Disord 1985; 50:207–212.

139. Keegan T. The ability of language disordered children to judge semantic restrictions in sentences. Paper presented to the American Speech Hearing Association, Houston, 1976.
140. Liles B. Response accuracy and response latency of normal and language disordered children. Folia Phoniatr 1982; 34:265–275.
141. Hall J, Humphreys M. Research on specific learning disabilities: deficits and remediation. Top Learn Learn Disabil 1982; 2:68–78.
142. Gibbs D, Cooper E. Prevalence of communication disorders in a learning disabled population. Paper presented to the American Speech Language Hearing Association, Detroit, 1986.
143. Lieberman R, Moore S, Hutchinson E. What's the difference between language impaired and learning disabled children? Paper presented to the American Speech Language Hearing Association, San Francisco, 1984.
144. Bashir A, Kuban K, Kleinman S, Scavuzzo A. Issues in language disorders: considerations of cause, maintenance, and change. In: Miller J, Yoder D, Schiefelbusch R, eds. Contemporary issues in language intervention. ASHA reports. No. 12. Rockville, MD: Am Speech Lang Hear Assoc, 1983:92.
145. Snyder L. Developmental language disorders: elementary school age. In: Holland A, ed. Language disorders in children. San Diego: College-Hill Press, 1984:129.
146. Scarborough H, Dobrich W. Illusory recovery from language delay. Proc Symp Res Child Lang Disord 1985; 6:90–99.
147. Bishop D, Edmundson A. Language impaired four year olds: distinguishing transient from persistent impairment. J Speech Hear Disord 1987; 52:156–173.
148. de Ajuriaguerra J, Jaeggi A, Guignard F, Kocher F, Manquard M, Roth S, Schmid E. The development and prognosis of dysphasia in children. In: Morehead D, Morehead A, eds. Normal and deficient child language. Baltimore: University Park, 1976:1345.
149. Liles B, Bartlett S. Toward a better description of language disordered children. In: Andrews J, Burns M, eds. Selected papers in language and phonology. Vol. 1. Evanston, IL: Institute for Continuing Professional Education, 1977:1.
150. Wolfus B, Moscovitch M, Kinsbourne M. Subgroups of developmental language impairment. Brain Lang 1980; 10:152–171.
151. Ruder K, Smith M. Issues in language training. In: Schiefelbusch R, Lloyd L, eds. Language perspectives: acquisition, retardation, and intervention. Baltimore: University Park, 1974:565.
152. Ruder K, Smith M, Waryas C. Design strategy for a coherent applied psycholinguistics. In: Ruder K, Smith M, eds. Developmental language intervention: psycholinguistic applications. Baltimore: University Park, 1984:1.
153. McLean J, Snyder-McLean L. A transactional approach to early language training. Columbus, OH: CE Merrill, 1978.
154. Miller J, Yoder D. A syntax teaching program. In: McLean J, Yoder D, Schiefelbusch R, eds. Language intervention with the retarded. Baltimore: University Park, 1972:191.
155. Duchan J. Language assessment: the pragmatics revolution. In: Naremore R, ed. Language science: recent advances. San Diego: College-Hill Press, 1984:147.
156. Reichstein J. Auditory threshold consistency in differential diagnosis of aphasia in children. J Speech Hear Disord 1964; 29:147–155.
157. Rosenthal W. Auditory and linguistic interaction in developmental aphasia: evidence from two studies of auditory processing. Papers and reports in child language development. No. 4. Committee on Linguistics, Stanford University, 1972:19.
158. Holloway G. Auditory-visual integration in language delayed children. J Learn Disabil 1971; 14:204–208.
159. McReynolds L. Operant conditioning for investigating speech sound discrimination in aphasic children. J Speech Hear Res 1966; 9:519–528.
160. Wilson L, Doehring D, Hirsh I. Auditory discrimination learning by aphasic and non-aphasic children. J Speech Hear Res 1960; 3:130–137.
161. Efron R. Temporal perception, aphasia, and déjà vu. Brain 1963; 86:403–424.
162. Hirsh I, Sherrick C. Perceived order in different sense modalities. J Exp Psychol 1961; 62:423–432.
163. Lowe A, Campbell R. Temporal discrimination in aphasoid and normal children. J Speech Hear Res 1965; 8:313–314.
164. Tallal P. Rapid auditory processing in normal and disordered language development. J Speech Hear Res 1976; 19:561–571.
165. Tallal P, Piercy M. Developmental aphasia: impaired rate of non-verbal processing as a function of sensory modality. Neuropsychologia 1973; 11:389–398.
166. Stark R, Tallal P. Perceptual and motor deficits in language impaired children. In: Keith R, ed. Central auditory and language disorders in children. Houston: College-Hill Press, 1981:121.
167. Tallal P, Stark R, Kallman C, Mellits D. A reexamination of some nonverbal perceptual abilities of language impaired and normal children as a function of age and sensory modality. J Speech Hear Res 1981; 24:351–357.
168. Thal D, Barone P. Auditory processing and language impairment in children: stimulus considerations for intervention. J Speech Hear Disord 1983; 48:18–24.
169. McCroskey R, Thompson N. Comprehension of rate controlled speech by children with specific learning disabilities. J Learn Disabil 1973; 6:621–627.
170. Tallal P, Piercy M. Defects of non-verbal auditory perception in children with developmental aphasia. Nature 1973; 241:468–469.
171. Tallal P, Piercy M. Developmental aphasia: rate of auditory processing and selective impairment of consonant perception. Neuropsychologia 1974; 12:83–93.
172. Tallal P, Piercy M. Developmental aphasia: the perception of brief vowels and extended stop consonants. Neuropsychologia 1975; 13:69–74.
173. Frumkin B, Rapin I. Perception of vowels and consonant-vowels of varying duration in language impaired children. Neuropsychologia 1980; 18:443–454.
174. Tallal P, Stark R. Speech acoustic-cue discrimination abilities of normally developing and language impaired children. J Acoust Soc Am 1981; 69:568–574.
175. Leonard L. The nature of specific language impairment in children. In: Rosenberg S, ed. Advances in applied psycholinguistics. New York: Cambridge University Press (in press).
176. Rees N. Auditory processing factors in language disorders: the view from Procrustes' bed. J Speech Hear Disord 1973; 38:304–315.
177. Rees N. Reply to "A different view of auditory processing factors in language disorders." J Speech Hear Disord 1975; 40:414–415.
178. Lubert N. Auditory perceptual impairments in children with specific language disorders: a review of the literature. J Speech Hear Disord 1981; 46:3–9.
179. Rees N. Saying more than we know: is auditory processing disorder a meaningful concept? In: Keith R, ed. Central auditory and language disorders in children. Houston: College-Hill, 1981:94.
180. Stark R, Tallal P. Analysis of stop consonant production errors in developmentally dysphasic children. J Acoust Soc Am 1979; 66:1703–1712.
181. Tallal P, Stark R, Curtiss B. Relation between speech perception and speech production impairment in children with developmental dysphasia. Brain Lang 1976; 3:305–317.
182. Tallal P, Stark R, Kallman C, Mellits D. Developmental dysphasia: the relation between acoustic processing deficits

and verbal processing. Neuropsychologia 1980; 18:273–284.

183. Tallal P, Stark R, Mellits D. The relationship between auditory temporal analysis and receptive language development: evidence from studies of developmental language disorder. Neuropsychologia 1985; 23:527–534.
184. Clark H, Clark E. Psychology and language. New York: Harcourt, Brace, Jovanovich, 1977.
185. Stark R, Bernstein L. Evaluating central auditory processing in children. Top Lang Disord 1984; 4:57–70.
186. Stark J. A comparison of the performance of aphasic children on three sequencing tests. J Commun Disord 1967; 11:31–34.
187. Weiner P. The cognitive functioning of language deviant children. J Speech Hear Res 1969; 12:53–64.
188. Weiner P. The perceptual level functioning of dysphasic children: a follow-up study. J Speech Hear Res 1972; 5:423–438.
189. Furth H. Sequence learning in aphasic and deaf children. J Speech Hear Disord 1964; 29:171–177.
190. Furth H, Pufall P. Visual and auditory sequence learning in hearing impaired children. J Speech Hear Res 1966; 19:441–449.
191. Poppen R, Stark J, Eisenson J, Forrest T, Wertheim G. Visual sequencing performance of aphasic children. J Speech Hear Res 1969; 12:288–300.
192. Tallal P, Stark R, Mellits D. Identification of language impaired children on the basis of rapid perception and production skills. Brain Lang 1985; 25:314–322.
193. Rosenthal W. The role of perception in child language disorders: a theory based on faulty signal detection strategies. Paper presented to the American Speech Hearing Association, Las Vegas, 1974.
194. Norman D. Memory and attention. 2nd ed. New York: John Wiley & Sons, 1976.
195. Brown A, Bransford J, Ferrara R, Campione J. Learning, remembering and understanding. In: Mussen P, ed. Handbook of child psychology. Vol. III. Flavell J, Markman E, vol. eds. Cognitive development. New York: John Wiley & Sons, 1983:77.
196. Kail R, Bisanz J. Information processing and cognitive development. In: Lipsitt L, Spiker C, eds. Advances in child development and behavior. Vol. 17. New York: Academic Press, 1982:45.
197. Otto D, Honck K, Finger H, Hart S. Event related slow potentials in aphasic, dyslexic and normal children during pictorial and letter-matching. Proceedings of the third international congress of event related slow potentials of the brain. Bristol, England, 1973.
198. Edwards M. Developmental verbal dyspraxia. Br J Disord Commun 1973; 18:64–70.
199. Mason S, Mellor D. Brainstem, middle latency and late cortical evoked potentials in children with speech and language disorders. Electroencephalogr Clin Neurophysiol 1984; 59:297–309.
200. Martinius J. Complex visual reaction time measurements under irregular and regular preparatory interval conditions in children with developmental language problems. Acta Paedopsychiat 1984; 50:111–118.
201. Catts H, Condino R, Stark R. Impulsivity in language impaired children. Paper presented to the American Speech Language Hearing Association, Toronto, 1982.
202. Nelson L, Kamhi A, Apel K. Cognitive style differences between language impaired and MA-matched children. Proc Symp Res Child Lang Disord 1986; 7:35–43.
203. Johnston J, Smith L. Dimensional thinking in language impaired children. Paper presented to the Symposium on Research on Child Language Disorders, University of Wisconsin, Madison, 1987.
204. Ludlow C, Cudahy E, Bassick C, Brown G. The auditory processing skills of hyperactive, language impaired and reading disabled boys. In: Katz J, Lasky E, eds. Central auditory processing disorders: problems of speech, language and learning. Baltimore: University Park, 1983.
205. Leonard L. The role of non-linguistic stimuli and semantic relations in children's acquisition of grammatical utterances. J Exp Child Psychol 1975; 19:346–357.
206. Schwartz R, Chapman K, Terrell B, Prelock P, Rowan L. Facilitating word combination in language impaired children through discourse structure. J Speech Hear Disord 1985; 50:31–39.
207. Campbell T, McNeil M. Effects of presentation rate and divided attention on auditory comprehension in children with an acquired language disorder. J Speech Hear Res 1985; 28:513–520.
208. Liles B, Cooker H, Kass M, Carey B. The effects of pause time on auditory comprehension of language disordered children. J Commun Disord 1978; 11:365–374.
209. McGinnis M. Aphasic children: identification and education by the association method. Washington, DC: Volta, 1963.
210. Stark J, Foster C, Giddan J, Gottsleben R, Wright T. Teaching the aphasic child. J Except Child 1968; 12:149–154.
211. Wilbur R. The linguistics of manual language and manual systems. In: Lloyd L, ed. Communication assessment and intervention strategies. Baltimore: University Park, 1976: 423.
212. Uzgiris I, Hunt J. Assessment in infancy. Urbana, IL: University of Illinois, 1975.
213. de Ajuriaguerra J. Speech disorders in childhood. In: Carterette E, ed. Brain function: speech, language and communication. UCLA forum in medical sciences. No. 4. Berkeley: University of California, 1966.
214. Inhelder B. Cognitive development and its contribution to the diagnosis of some phenomena of mental deficiency. Merrill-Palmer Q 1966; 12:299–319.
215. Johnston J, Ramstad V. Cognitive development in preadolescent language impaired children. In: Burns M, Andrews J, eds. Selected papers in language and phonology. Evanston, IL: Institute for Continuing Professional Education, 1977:43.
216. Johnston J, Ramstad V. Cognitive development in preadolescent language impaired children. Br J Disord Commun 1983; 18:49–55.
217. Kamhi A. Nonlinguistic symbolic and conceptual abilities of language impaired and normally developing children. J Speech Hear Res 1981; 24:446–453.
218. Camarata S, Newhoff M, Rugg B. Perspective taking in normal and language disordered children. Proceedings of the symposium on research in child language disorders 1981; 2:81–88.
219. Camarata S, Newhoff M, Rugg B. Classification skills and language development in language impaired children. Austr J Human Commun Disord 1985; 13:107–115.
220. Stark R, Tallal P, Kallman C, Mellits E. Cognitive abilities of language delayed children. J Psychol 1983; 114:9–19.
221. Bates E, Benigni L, Bretherton I, Camaioni L, Volterra V. The emergence of symbols. New York: Academic Press, 1979.
222. Morehead D. Early grammatical and semantic relations: some implications for a general representational deficit in linguistically deviant children. Papers and reports in child language development. No. 4. Committee on Linguistics, Stanford University, 1972:1.
223. Brown J, Redmond A, Bass K, Liebergott J, Swope S. Symbolic play in normal and language-impaired children. Paper presented to American Speech Hearing Association, Washington, DC, 1975.
224. Lovell K, Hoyle H, Sidall M. A study of some aspects of the play and language of young children with delayed speech. J Child Psychol Psychiatry 1968; 9:41–50.
225. Roth F, Clark D. Symbolic play and social participation

abilities of language impaired and normally developing children. J Speech Hear Disord 1987; 52:17–29.
226. Terrell B, Schwartz R. Object transformation: the linguistic aspect of symbolic play? Proc Symp Res Child Lang Disord 1983; 4:127–136.
227. Terrell B, Schwartz R, Prelock P, Messick C. Symbolic play in normal and language disordered children. J Speech Hear Res 1984; 27:424–429.
228. Udwin O, Yule W. Imaginative play in language disordered children. Br J Disord Commun 1983; 18:197–205.
229. Lowe M, Costello A. Symbolic play test. Windsor, Berkshire: NFER, 1976.
230. Murphy V. A comparison of four measures of visual imagery in normal and language disordered children. Master's Thesis, Northern Illinois University, 1978.
231. Savich P. Anticipatory imagery in normal and language disabled children. J Speech Hear Res 1984; 27:494–501.
232. Inhelder B. Operational thought and mental imagery. Monogr Soc Res Child Dev 1965; 30:4–18.
233. Johnston J, Ellis Weismer S. Mental rotation abilities in language disordered children. J Speech Hear Res 1983; 26:397–403.
234. Kosslyn S. Image and mind. Cambridge, MA: Harvard University Press, 1980.
235. Levi G, Longobardi M. Sulla rappresentazione gestuale in bambini disfasici. Neuropsich Infantile 1974; 158:771–793.
236. Cromer R. Reconceptualizing language acquisition and cognitive development. In: Schiefelbusch R, Bricker D, eds. Early language: acquisition and intervention. Baltimore: University Park, 1981:51.
237. Skarakis E. The development of symbolic play and language in language disordered children. Doctoral Dissertation, University of California, Santa Barbara, 1982.
238. Cromer R. Developmental language disorders: cognitive processes, semantics, pragmatics, phonology and syntax. J Autism Dev Disord 1981; 11:57–74.
239. Cromer R. Hierarchical planning disability in the drawings and constructions of a special group of severely aphasic children. Brain Cognit 1983; 2:144–164.
240. Kracke I. Perception of rhythmic sequences by receptive aphasic and deaf children. Br J Disord Commun 1975; 10:43–51.
241. MacWhinney B. The competition model. In: MacWhinney B, ed. Hillsdale, NJ: Erlbaum, 1987:249.
242. Hoskins B. A study of hypothesis testing behavior in language disordered children. Doctoral Dissertation, Northwestern University, 1978.
243. Nelson L, Kamhi A, Apel K. Cognitive strengths and weaknesses in language impaired children: one more look J Speech Hear Disord 1987; 52:36–43.
244. Kamhi A, Catts H, Koenig L, Lewis B. Hypothesis testing and non-linguistic symbolic abilities in language impaired children. J Speech Hear Disord 1984; 49:169–176.
245. Kamhi A, Nelson L, Lee R, Gholson B. The ability of language disordered children to use and modify hypotheses in discrimination learning. Appl Psycholinguist 1985; 6:435–451.
246. Richman L, Lindgren S. Patterns of intellectual ability in children with verbal deficits. J Abnorm Child Psychol 1980; 8:65–81.
247. Anderson J. Initiatory delay in congenitally aphasoid children. Cerebral Palsy J 1965; 26:9–12.
248. Leonard L, Nippold M, Kail R, Hale R. Picture naming in language impaired children. J Speech Hear Res 1983; 26:609–615.
249. Wiig E, Semel E, Nystrom L. Comparison of rapid naming abilities in language-learning-disabled and academically achieving eight year olds. Lang Speech Hear Services Schools 1982; 13:11–23.
250. Bernstein L, Stark R. Speech perception development in language impaired children: a four year follow up study. J Speech Hear Disord 1985; 50:21–30.
251. Stark J, Poppen R, May M. Effects of alterations of prosodic features on the sequencing performance of aphasic children. J Speech Hear Res 1967; 10:849–855.
252. Kail R. The development of memory in children. San Francisco: WH Freeman, 1979.
253. Tomblin J. Some characteristics of auditory memory in children with language disorders. Paper presented to the American Speech Hearing Association, Washington, DC, 1975.
254. Kirchner D, Klatzky R. Verbal rehearsal and memory in language disordered children. J Speech Hear Res 1985; 28:556–564.
255. Sininger Y. Memory scanning speech in normal and language disordered children. Paper presented to the American Speech Language Hearing Association, Cincinnati, 1983.
256. Greyerbiehl D. Attention control deficits within sensory memory in language disordered children. Paper presented to the American Speech Language Hearing Association, Toronto, 1982.
257. Ceci S, Ringstrom M, Lea S. Do language-learning disabled children have impaired memories? In search of underlying processes. J Learn Disabil 1981; 14:159–173.
258. Kail R, Hale C, Leonard L, Nippold M. Lexical storage and retrieval in language impaired children. Appl Psycholinguist 1984; 5:37–49.
259. Craig H, Wiley J. Rehearsal as a strategy in the solution of a short-term sequential memory task by language disordered and normal children. Unpublished manuscript, University of Michigan, 1976.
260. Levy C, Menyuk P. Relation between certain cognitive skills and sentence comprehension in children. Paper presented to the American Speech Hearing Association, Las Vegas, 1974.
261. Levy C, Menyuk P. Developmental language disorders: linguistic and non-linguistic processing. In: Burns M, Andrews L, eds. Selected papers in language and phonology. Evanston, IL: Institute for Continuing Professional Education, 1977:52.
262. Wyke M, Asso D. Perception and memory for spatial relations in children with developmental dysphasia. Neuropsychologia 1979; 17:231–239.
263. Doehring D. Visual spatial memory in aphasic children. J Speech Hear Res 1960; 3:138–149.
264. Chi M. Knowledge structures and memory development. In: Siegler R, ed. Children's thinking: what develops? Hillsdale, NJ: Erlbaum, 1978:73.
265. Brown A. The development of memory: knowing, knowing about knowing, and knowing how to know. In: Reese H, ed. Advances in child development and behavior. Vol. 10. New York: Academic Press, 1975:103.
266. Huttonlocher J, Burke D. Why does memory span increase with age? Cognit Psychol 1976; 8:1–32.
267. Ellis Weismer S. Constructive comprehension processes exhibited by language impaired children. J Speech Hear Res 1985; 28:175–184.
268. Crais E, Chapman R. Story recall and inferencing in language/learning disabled and non-disabled children. J Speech Hear Disord 1987; 52:50–55.
269. Johnston J. Interpreting the Leiter IQ: performance profiles of young normal and language disordered children. J Speech Hear Res 1982; 25:291–296.
270. Wiig E, Berman L. Selection of visual dimensions by aphasic and nonaphasic children. Percept Mot Skills 1972; 34:311–315.
271. O'Grady D, Fogelson M, Tomb M, Willis J. Language disorders in adolescence: a ten year follow-up study of children earlier diagnosed as language disordered. Paper presented to American Speech Hearing Association, Las Vegas, 1974.
272. Eisenson J. Developmental aphasia—a postulation of a un-

itary concept of the disorder. Cortex 1968; 4:184–200.

273. Sinclair H. Sensorimotor action patterns as a condition for the acquisition of syntax. In: Huxley R, Ingram E, eds. Language acquisition: models and methods. New York: Academic Press, 1971:121.
274. Johnston J. On location: thinking and talking about space. Top Lang Disord 1981; 2:17–32.
275. Gitterman D, Johnston J. Talking about comparisons: a study of young children's comparative adjective usage. J Child Lang 1983; 10:605–621.
276. Slobin DI. Cognitive prerequisites for the development of grammar. In: Ferguson C, Slobin DI, eds. Studies of child language development. New York: Holt, Rinehart, & Winston, 1973:175.
277. Butterfield E. Instructional techniques that produce generalized improvements in cognition. In: Mittler P, ed. Frontiers of knowledge in mental retardation: social, educational, and behavioral aspects. Baltimore: University Park, 1981:79.
278. Garkusha Y. An experiment in developing voluntary attention in children with motor-alalia. Sov Psychol 1984; 22:6–88.
279. Inhelder B, Sinclair H, Bovet M. Learning and the development of cognition. Cambridge, MA: Harvard University Press, 1974.
280. Kuhn D. Mechanisms of change in the development of cognitive structures. Child Dev 1972; 43:833–844.
281. Strauss S. Inducing cognitive development and learning: a review of short-term training experiments. The organismic developmental approach. Cognition 1972; 11:329–357.
282. Rees N. Noncommunicative functions of language in children. J Speech Hear Disord 1973; 38:98–110.
283. Rice M, Kemper S. Child language and cognition. Baltimore: University Park, 1984.
284. Saxe G. A developmental analysis of notational counting. Child Dev 1977; 148:512–520.
285. Kamhi A, Gentry B, Mauer D. Analogical learning and transfer in language impaired children. Paper presented at the Symposium for Research in Child Language Disorders, University of Wisconsin, Madison, 1987.

24 Language Disorders in the Adolescent

Arthur M. Guilford, Ph.D.

The acquisition and development of speech and language skills in preschool and young school-age children have been researched extensively. However, there remains a paucity of research relating directly to the language problems evidenced in adolescents. Only in the past several years have clinicians and researchers increased their interest in the area of language disorders in the adolescent years.

Older students with language handicaps have been neglected by the speech-language pathologist in the public schools and in private clinical settings. This neglect may be attributed in part to the lack of training and educational experiences provided to graduate students in speech-language pathology by our university programs. Although I have seen a gradual increase in the emphasis applied to the area of adolescent language disorders in the 1980s, a survey of graduate training programs by Boyce, Godwin, and Larson found that only 50 percent of the training programs in five midwestern states provided formal course work in language assessment or remediation for this group of students.[1] Furthermore, the pervading feeling among many professionals has been that educational habilitative endeavors are most profitable when they are concentrated on young children in the preschool and early school-age years.[2]

Clearly, many children continue to have speech and language problems well beyond the early developmental years. Retrospective studies of children who were identified as requiring speech or language habilitation have revealed that these children may continue to require special educational placements throughout their adolescence and young adulthood. Also, language disorders that continue to persist through the elementary school years may result in lowered academic achievement.[3–5]

Over the past several years, there has been increasing interest in the diagnosis and treatment of adolescents with language disorders. Several states now mandate the treatment of all school-age children between the ages of 3[3] and 21 years. Also, with the passage of PL 94–142 (Education for all Handicapped Children Act), a free and appropriate education is currently being afforded to increasing numbers of adolescents who would have otherwise been denied special services.

Another problem in the diagnosis and treatment of adolescents has been the lack of adequate assessment instruments that provide reliable information on their language skills. Assessment instruments for this age range cannot rely on updated versions of tests that were standardized on much younger children, but must reflect knowledge of normal adolescent behavior.[6] Older students are different from younger ones in many ways. Brown has indicated that older handicapped students have increased mobility beyond the confines of the school setting, require increased behavioral independence, and suffer from increased feelings of failure, thereby resulting in lowered self-esteem.[7] Furthermore, the demands placed on adolescents to conform to the adult model of communicative competency cannot be overlooked.

Differential diagnosis of language delay and disorders involves more than determining etiologies of impairments. Language diagnosis consists of drawing from the different disciplines of linguistics, psycholinguistics, psychology, neuropsychology, special education, speech-language pathology, and audiology and must include the interaction of these disciplines into a holistic diagnostic model. Before beginning the diagnostic process, one must consider what a child needs in order to develop language: (1) adequate hearing, (2) adequate intellectual capacity, (3) emotional stability, (4) communicative awareness sufficient to create the desire to interact and communicate with others, (5) central and peripheral nervous system integrity, and (6) adequate exposure to good language models.[8] Dysfunctions in any of these may contribute to the language disorders evidenced in adolescents.

The Diagnostic and Statistical Manual of Mental Disorders, third edition (DSM III), published by the American Psychiatric Association, has recognized three types of language disorders:[9] (1) failure to acquire language, which is considered rare and is most often the result of severe mental retardation; (2) acquired language disorders, which are usually the result of neurologic disorders or trauma; and (3) delayed or developmentally disordered language acquisition, which include difficulties in receptive or expressive language functions. Further, the DSM III presents the following diagnostic options for development disorders in children:

1. Attention deficit disorder (1) with or (2) without hyperactivity.
2. Developmental reading disorder.
3. Developmental arithmetic disorder.
4. Developmental language disorder of the (1) expressive or (2) receptive type.
5. Developmental articulation disorder.
6. Mixed specific developmental disorder.
7. Atypical specific developmental disorder.

Although these diagnoses are often made early in a child's development, they may persist well into adolescence. Furthermore, speech-language pathologists and special educators no longer accept nor support the belief held previously that children with language disabilities outgrow their deficits or that early diagnosis and treatment guarantee the elimination of the communication deficit.[2,10] Strong support exists for the finding that language deficits evidenced in young children persist into adolescence.[11–13]

It would appear inappropriate to assume that the etiologic factors are identical for all adolescents with language disorders. When one looks closely at language disorders seen in this age group, one sees that they may fall into one or more of the following etiologic categories:

1. Adolescents who were diagnosed as language disordered during the preschool years, but after treatment continue to manifest residual language impairments. These impairments may have been secondary to hearing loss, central or peripheral nervous system dysfunction, inadequate language models, or general interference with any of these processes.
2. Adolescents who were diagnosed as cognitively handicapped as preschoolers or during the early school years and continue to manifest semantic, cognitive, or perceptual-motor deficits in language skills at an older age.
3. Adolescents who were developing normally through the period of primary language development, but suffered a loss or disruption in that development because of physical, emotional, or traumatic causes.
4. Adolescents who were diagnosed as learning disabled either in the elementary school years or in junior high and demonstrate either language problems as a direct cause of the learning disability or the learning disability as a direct cause of the language disorder.

LANGUAGE DISABILITIES

Historically, there has always been an interrelationship between the disciplines of speech-language pathology and learning disabilities, although sometimes many aspects of this relationship appeared unclear and perhaps ill-defined. When one reviews the literature in learning disabilities, it becomes obvious that the field encompasses at least three distinct areas: spoken language, written language, and perceptual-motor processes.[14] Within the area of spoken language, much of the information concerning learning disabilities and spoken language disorders originated from knowledge gained from documentation and knowledge of adults with language disorders; from the medical disciplines; and from the field of deaf education. For example, Gall, Bouillaud, Broca, and Jackson hypothesized the relationship of brain damage to a model of the speech process. Somewhat later, Bastian and Wernicke proposed and developed theoretic models describing detailed relationships of the neurologic correlates of speech and language processes.[14]

In the 1950s, much independent work came together to enhance the knowledge and understanding of childhood language disorders. But even prior to the 1950s, McGinnis was researching and documenting clinical approaches to children with language disorders. Through her work with deaf children, McGinnis was able to document a clinical approach for children who were not deaf, but were unable to acquire language normally.[15] McGinnis developed a treatment approach for severely language handicapped children called the "association method." This method of teaching became widely followed, largely because of the success with the method in the remediation of children with childhood aphasia. McGinnis, Kleffner, and Goldstein reported on two different forms of childhood aphasia, which they labelled expressive aphasia and receptive aphasia.[16] Much of what they described for the expressive aphasic appears to apply to children who under current diagnosis would now be labelled as oral apraxic, that is, poor expressive speech with repeated vocalizations of sounds and poor oral and verbal imitation skills despite the intactness of oral vegetative functions. They described receptive aphasia as occurring in children with hearing and intelligence within normal limits, verbal jargon responses, poor abilities to comprehend verbal information, and discrepancies between their ability to hear and their ability to understand speech. These descriptions, although they have changed over time, became landmarks in the field of childhood language disorders.

Morley did much for the profession of speech-language pathology and the diagnosis and treatment of children with language disorders in both England and the United States.[17] Morley classified children with speech disorders into those with language disorders of which there were four types—(1) aphasia of either the receptive or expressive variety; (2) alexia; (3) agraphia; and (4) delayed development of speech associated with mental retardation, mental illness, or hearing disorders—and those with articulation disorders, which included also a subcategory of articulatory apraxia. One can see in these classifications that the close association between oral and written language for disorders of reading and writing accounts for two of her diagnostic categories for children with language disorders.

In the 1960s, Osgood developed a model of language and was joined later by Myklebust who pioneered differential diagnosis of speech (language) problems in children who had either suffered brain damage and subsequent disruption to their language development or were not developing their language normally. Later in the 1960s, Wepman and Kirk built on Osgood's model of language and proposed modality-specific testing and training for language disordered individuals.

In the mid-1970s, Cruickshank and Hallahan initiated a true multidisciplinary approach to evaluation and remediation of learning disabilities in which they assimilated information from the areas of oral and written language and perceptual-motor development.[14] The interdisciplinary approach to learning disabilities was aided in large part by the passage in 1975 of The Education for All Handicapped Children Act (PL 94–142). This law requires multidisciplinary team assessment for all learning disabled students who present the need for other special educational services. Furthermore, natural interactions between disciplines appear obvious. A screening instrument administered by the reading specialist may reveal problems in written language; a learning disabilities specialist, while administering a diagnostic math test, may observe problems in articulatory proficiency; and a speech-language pathologist, while evaluating language functions, may discover poor sound blending skills in the child. It would be foolish, therefore, to ignore the interdisciplinary nature of this disorder.

Learning disabilities have been defined by the National Advisory Committee on Handicapped Children (NACHC) as disorders in understanding or using spoken or written language. The current federal definition of "specific learning disabilities" states that

> Children with specific learning disabilities exhibit a disorder in one or more of the basic psychological processes involved in understanding or using spoken or written language. These may be manifested in writing, spelling, or arithmetic. They include conditions which have been referred to as perceptual handicaps, brain injury, brain dysfunction, dyslexia, developmental aphasia, etc. They do not include learning problems which are due primarily to visual, hearing, or motor handicaps, to mental retardation, or to environmental disadvantage.[17a]

Although this definition is comprehensive, it is hard to implement because it is nonoperational.[11] Special educators have needed to operationalize the definition to include the presence of (1) significant deficits in perception, integration, and verbal and nonverbal expression, which must be capable of (2) diagnosis through accepted test batteries, and these delays must be demonstrated through (3) discrepancies between expected (intellectual capacity) and realized achievement (quantifiable performance) in one or more of the following: spoken, read, and written language; mathematics; and spatial orientation.[18]

The National Joint Committee for Learning Disabilities (NJCLD) has attempted to strengthen the definition of learning disabilities to include factors not considered in the federal definition of this disorder. Specifically, the NJCLD included in their definition the following:

> Learning disabilities is a generic term that refers to a heterogeneous group of disorders manifested by significant difficulties in the acquisition and use of listening, speaking, reading, writing, reasoning, or mathematical abilities. These disorders are intrinsic to the individual and presumed to be due to central nervous dysfunction. Even though a learning disability may occur concomitantly with other handicapping conditions (e.g. sensory impairment, mental retardation, social and emotional disturbance) or environmental influences (e.g. cultural differences, insufficient/inappropriate instruction, psychogenic factors), it is not the direct result of those conditions or influences (p 336).[19]

Estimates of the prevalence of learning disabilities vary considerably from as low as 1 percent to as high as 30 percent of the population.[11] The United

States Office of Education estimates that between 1 and 3 percent of school-age children are learning disabled.[14] Of these children, from 40 to 60 percent (approximately 2 percent of the schoool-age population) are considered to have a primary language disorder, which includes difficulties in the comprehension, expression, recall, and discrimination of language. Ten to 40 percent of the learning disabled population have been considered to demonstrate articulatory and graphomotor disorders, and 5 to 15 percent of this group demonstrate visual discrimination and visual memory deficits.[11,20]

Children who have been labelled as learning disabled often clearly display deficits in the language areas of phonology, semantics, and syntax. Children's thinking and learning strategies are closely related to their language skills. Therefore a disability in one aspect of learning influences skills in all areas. Wallach and Goldsmith have indicated that the "core of learning disability for some children is at the language-symbolic level, and we consider reading to be a multifaceted language activity of a special nature which strongly relies upon the phonological (sounds), lexical (vocabulary), and comprehension systems already available to the child."[21] Further, the auditory and verbal strategies for learning disabled children may be different from those used by children without learning difficulties.

It has been demonstrated clearly that children with learning disabilities are delayed in learning linguistic relationships, particularly in the areas of spatial, temporal, comparative, and passive functions. These delays, so readily apparent in the language of young children, may persist into adolescence.[11,22,23] Magee and Newcomer found a significant relationship between oral language skills and overall achievement in children diagnosed as learning and reading disabled.[24] They concluded that a child's language performance may be considered as indicative of his or her learning proficiency.

Difficulties with word finding also have been reported to be symptomatic of children with language disabilities.[11,13,23,25,26] These children take a longer length of time to recall low-frequency words in describing objects or events and in completing open-ended sentences. Wiig and Semel have indicated that the difficulties in word finding are likely to result in problems with expressive syntax and word order.[27] Finally, Wiig and Semel and Bryan, Donahue, and Pearl reported that the child with language disorders may have a great need for clarification in conversation and may experience a reduced facility at asking questions, elaborating on a topic, and using conversational rules.[11,28]

Beilen has demonstrated that the ability to perform sophisticated language skills is essential in the acquisition of creative thinking, rationalization, and understanding the logic of academic instruction.[29] Clearly, the more complex the school curriculum, the more comprehensive are the demands on the student to process, comprehend, and produce acceptable language responses. Also, the American Speech-Language-Hearing Association has recognized that language disorders persist into adolescence and may manifest themselves in academic failures as well. It has been stated that the language disordered individual ". . . frequently demonstrates disruption in 1) higher order thinking, in 2) learning and school curriculum, and in 3) managing the language of instruction."[30]

Language is an essential and necessary skill for success in academic, social, and emotional development. Basic diagnosis of the adolescent must incorporate the principles of multidisciplinary assessment. Clinicians must continue to be aware of the fact that language is not an isolated skill, but rather that it is dependent upon complex interactions of academic and experiential learning and language strategy development. Language behavior is not isolated nor easily categorized. Its significance in the child's academic success is easily witnessed when the role of language is considered in the teaching of reading, math, history, geography, and even physical education.[31]

LANGUAGE DEVELOPMENT IN ADOLESCENTS

There is a lack of agreement concerning language development through the adolescent years. That the performance of adolescents changes on tests of vocabulary has long been established, but that language measures, other than vocabulary, change with increasing years is not uniformly agreed upon.[32] Prather presents rather convincing evidence that several current tests for adolescent language disorders do not reveal a change in syntactic skills over increasing years.[33] Prather concludes that while tests for general language functioning may not show differences between the ages of 11 and 18 years, that tests of vocabulary, concepts, and general knowledge of academic content do show differences for these ages. Evidence for her conclusions are drawn from the Clinical Evaluation of Language Function test[34] in that no change in the criterion scores on six of the 13 subtests from the sixth through the twelfth grade occurred. On the remaining seven subtests, the change is from two items to four items only. The subtests that produced the greatest differences were processing relationships and ambiguities, producing word associations, and producing model sentences.

Additional evidence for the lack of language growth in adolescence is demonstrated by Prather in her review of test preformances on the Test of Adolescent Language (TOAL).[35] Prather has indicated that students show less growth of language functions on the subtests for grammar than on the four vocabulary subtests. The age range covered for this test is from 11 to 18½ years. Furthermore, when one examines the language dimensions tested on this measure, the general hierarchy of development that clearly emerges, from first through last, is one of listening, speaking, reading, and writing. The normal period of language development for these last two dimensions appear to extend into the teen years.[33]

Although there is some evidence that no appreciable language growth occurs through the teen years, it should be remembered that the measures on which these results have been based have varied considerably from test to test. Therefore, definitive knowledge of language development in the teen years may remain unreliable until uniformity of test instruments or assessment procedures are developed and normative data become available on larger numbers of adolescents between 11 and 18 years.

Preliminary test results with the Adolescent Language Screening Test[26] (ALST) on 775 students from 11 through 17 years of age have shown somewhat different results than those reported by Prather.[33] Of the total number of students, 567 were considered normal because they had never been identified as requiring special services and were progressing adequately through school with an overall GPA of no less than 2.0 (A = 4.0), and 208 students were identified as requiring special services in the schools, but were without evidence of mental retardation. As seen in Figure 24–1, language changes across the ages when total test performance is considered.

As Figure 24–1 reveals, a gradual increase in the percentage of correct responses occurs across total test performance. Also, it is readily observable that there are differences between total test performance of students identified as requiring the special service of a speech-language pathologist and those requiring a learning disabilities specialist. Furthermore, among the normal students, three distinct groups emerge according to total test performance: group I (11, 12, and 13 years), group II (14 and 15 years), and group III (16 and 17 years). Although the total test mean distribution of scores was not exceptionally large (mean range from 70.0 percent to 83.5 percent), the differences between group means appears relevant (group I mean = 72.0 percent; group II mean = 79.0 percent; and group III mean = 83.2 percent). Clearly the greatest change was in the years between 13 and 14 (group I to group II), with less change between 15 and 16 years (group II to group III).

The difference between ages may be further substantiated when one evaluates the suggested pass-fail criteria, which were established at the first quar-

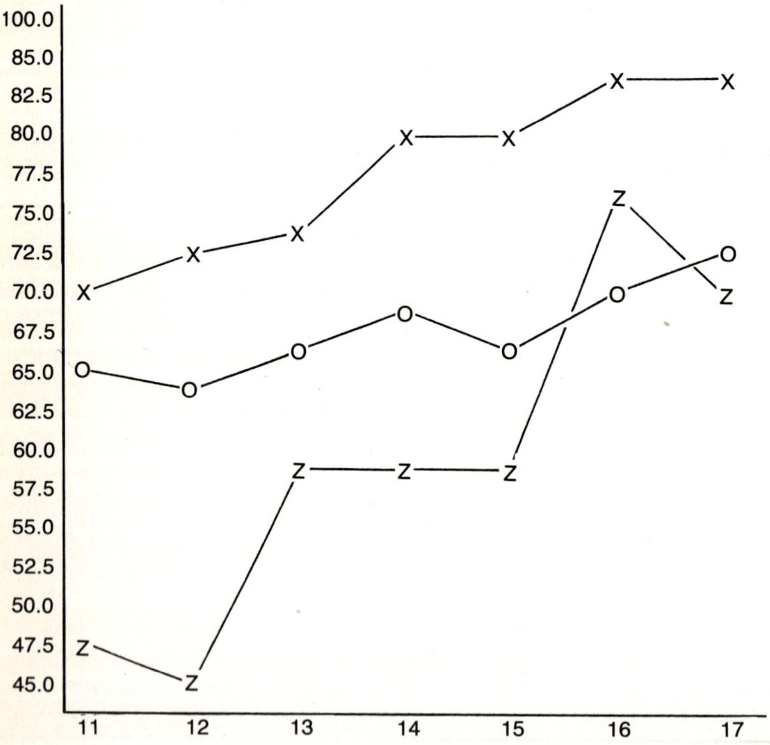

Figure 24–1 Distribution of total test performance on the adolescent language screening test. Abbreviations: X = normal students; O = students requiring speech-language services; Z = students requiring learning disabilities services.

TABLE 24–1 Suggested Pass-Fail Criteria on the Adolescent Language Screening Test

Chronologic Age Group	*Use*	*Content*	*Form*	*Total*
11	5.00	26.00	27.00	62.00
12	5.00	28.00	27.00	62.00
13	5.00	29.00	27.00	64.00
14	6.00	34.00	28.00	71.00
15	6.00	34.00	29.00	71.00
16	7.00	37.00	31.00	78.00
17	7.00	38.00	32.00	78.00

From Morgan DL, Guilford AM. The adolescent language screening test. Tulsa, OK: Modern Education Corporation, 1984:26.

tile of performance for each of the ages. The suggested pass-fail criteria changes across language dimensions and between ages, as seen in Table 24–1. Although the differences in the suggested criteria are more obvious within the language dimension of content, observable differences do occur within the dimension of form. If one were to remove the phonologic data from the area of form, the increase in language performance due to syntactic variation between ages would seem even more remarkable.

Analysis of performance of normal students on subtest 5, sentence formulation, and subtest 6, morphology from the area of form, reveals additional evidence that language functions continue to change throughout the adolescent years. Table 24–2 presents the total correct, means, and combined performance for subtests 5 and 6 for group I (11 to 13 years), group II (14 to 15 years), and group III (16 to 17 years) students.

It is clear from these data that a progression of expressive language as measured by these two subtests occurs. Although the observed changes become less with increasing age, there are quantifiable differences between the performance of these three groups. Results of these two subtests appear to support the idea that morphology changes more dramatically across the adolescent years, although there are certainly observable, though subtle, changes in sentence formulation as well. If the tasks required on these two measures were increased beyond the language screening level, one might find additional language changes.

Epstein has provided thought-provoking information concerning brain growth patterns seen between birth and 16 years.[36–38] Epstein has demonstrated that five major brain growth periods occur that correspond to the following developmental periods: (1) 3 to 10 months, (2) 2 to 4 years, (3) 6 to 8 years, (4) 10 to 12 years, and (5) 14 to 16 years.[37,38] If the first three growth spurts are compared to language developmental landmarks, striking similarities between developmental language changes and these growth spurts are seen. For example, clinicians know that the child shows remarkable prelinguistic development during the first 9 to 10 months of life. These behaviors refine from prelocutionary actions (nonintended) to illocutionary (intended) actions by the time a child reaches approximately 10 months of age. Clinicians are aware also of the rapid changes that take place in the language of children between 2 and 4 years of age. Furthermore, when the test data from instruments standardized on children between $2^1/_2$ years and 8 years are analyzed, strong differences in the language behaviors seen in 6- to 8-year-old children are found. This latter stage would correspond with Epstein's third brain growth period.

Epstein's work becomes even more interesting upon analysis of the three language groups that emerged in the ALST's standardization. Epstein has indicated that at each brain growth stage, the child becomes capable of more complex reasoning skills.[36] Therefore children should make developmental language changes following the spurts in brain growth. If there is a relationship between language and brain growth, then it stands to reason that even in adolescence changes in language could occur surrounding the growth spurts. In fact, this reasoning appears to hold when one considers that a brain growth period occurs at 10 to 12 years and again at 14 to 16 years. Based on my results, adolescents change in their language behaviors between 13 and 14 years, remain stable during 14 and 15 years, and show change again by 16 years of age. Epstein clearly presents compelling evidence that brain growth, reasoning, reading, and language development all occur together.[36] Additional documentation of language changes in adolescence may support the interrelationship of these functions.

TABLE 24–2 Group Performance on Subtests for Sentence Formulation (Subtest 5) and Morphology (Subtest 6) on the Adolescent Language Screening Test

	Sentence Formulation		*Morphology*		*Combined*		
	Σ	$\bar{x}$	Σ	$\bar{x}$	Σ	$\bar{x}$	%
Group I (11–13 yrs)	1493	6.11	1607	6.59	3100	12.70	0.45
Group II (14–15 yrs)	1039	6.83	1361	8.95	2400	15.78	0.56
Group III (16–17 yrs)	1298	7.73	1519	9.04	2817	16.76	0.60

Abbreviations: Σ = total; $\bar{x}$ = mean; % = overall percentage correct of those items.

LANGUAGE ASSESSMENT

Diagnosis is as critical an issue among language disordered adolescents as it is in the preschool group. Historically, all evaluation instruments and identification approaches emphasized the years of 4 to 8 as critical for preschool and elementary school assessment. Little if any emphasis was given to the adolescent with persisting language disorders. However, it must be remembered that oral language performance of secondary students is indicative of the complex language abilities required for academic success.[39]

Assessment with adolescents follows the same testing paradigm as with younger children with communication disorders, with the exception that far fewer standardized test instruments are available to assess adolescents than for younger children. Only since the late 1970s and the early 1980s have speech-language pathologists developed standardized language screening and assessment language measures for the adolescent.

Selected Screening Tests

Currently three screening tests for language disorders have been standardized on the adolescent population. These screening measures are the Clinical Evaluation of Language Functions (CELF) screening tests,[34] the Screening Test of Adolescent Language,[40] (STAL) and the ALST.[26] The purpose of these screening measures is to identify individuals who are at risk for language disorders and to provide a quick measure of the student's performance on the presented language measures. Furthermore, each measure should be reliable and identify individuals who are in need of additional evaluation.

Prior to the development of these screening tests, clinicians had to rely on informal dialogues and monologues with adolescents on their case loads. Questions presented to the student were usually based on family relationships or activities in the school. Due to the informal nature of these questions, analysis of the student's language was difficult at best. Many of these informal measures resulted from the lack of available normative data on language development within this age range. Furthermore, many of these informal assessments lack reliability and validity and at best lead to doubtful test interpretation. The advent of standardized measures for this age group has improved clinical skills in screening and assessing language deficits.

The CELF screening tests were designed to screen for language disorders at two broad grade levels: elementary Level (kindergarten to fifth grade) and advanced Level (fifth to twelfth grade).[34] This screening instrument probes aspects of language comprehension and verbal expression across 48 items at the elementary level and 52 items at the advanced level. The CELF screening tests do not include the elicitation of a spontaneous language sample. They continue to be standardized nationally, and at present 1,405 children have been included in the normative sample. The CELF screening tests are a part of a more comprehensive language assessment instrument, the Clinical Evaluation of Language Function. The authors report adequate to high test-retest reliability over a 6-week period and correlations with the Detroit Test of Learning Aptitude (DTLA) and ITPA for the verbal subtests at the elementary level of 0.62 and 0.49, respectively. In the advanced level, the verbal subtests correlated with the Illinois Test of Psycholinguistic Abilities (ITPA) verbal subtest at 0.46. The estimated time to complete the advanced level of the CELF screening tests is approximately 15 minutes, with estimates for the completion of the elementary level only slightly less.

The STAL was designed for students in grades 6 to 12 and consists of four expressive subtests: (1) vocabulary, (2) auditory memory span, (3) language processing, and (4) proverb explanation.[40] The STAL does not include the elicitation of a spontaneous language sample. There were a total of 425 students in the normal population, with 206 sixth grades and 219 ninth graders represented. All students were obtained from the Phoenix public schools, and there was an approximately equal distribution of subjects between males and females. Test-retest reliability on 30 students was reportedly good, with a correlation of 0.98. Concurrent validity was established through correlations with four subtests from the DTLA (coefficient of correlation = 0.86). The test scores are presented in either raw scores or converted to percentile ranks, and minimum passing scores were recommended for students in grades six to eight and nine to twelve. These scores were derived by taking late sixth grade norms for the first group and late ninth grade norms for the second group. Students in grades seven, eight, ten, eleven, and twelve were not actually tested in the standardization. However, it was concluded that any student regardless of age who fails either the entire test or any one subtest should be considered for additional examination for language functions. The approximate testing time is 7 to 10 minutes for the STAL.

The ALST was developed to screen for language deficits in the dimensions of use (subtest 1, pragmatics); content (subtests 2, receptive vocabulary; 3, concepts; and 4, expressive vocabulary: naming to confrontation, naming to description, and use of lexical items); and form (subtests 5, sentence formulation; 6, morphology; and 7, phonology).[26] The ALST is the only screening test that currently requires the elicitation of a language sample. This language sample is essential to the analysis of pragmatic language behavior. The test was standardized on 775 students at ages 11 through 17 years and included white, black, Hispanic, and other minority students. There were more than 100 students in the normal population at each of the age levels tested. In a recent revision of the test, additional norms are provided for black subjects.[41] All students in the standardization sample had normal hearing, vision, and were selected from public and private schools in urban and rural settings in order to represent a broad cross-section of social and cultural diversity from within the state of Florida. Means and standard deviations for each age level are provided for all students, then subdivided according to the distribution of students requiring special services (speech-language therapy or learning disabilities), and those not requiring special services. Suggested pass-fail criteria scores for use, content, form, and total score by age and race (black or white) were established at the first quartile and are presented in the test manual. Reliability for the total test performance is not reported in the test manual. Validity was established through theoretic justification of similarity with other test items that assess these language behaviors, correlations with CELF,[42] and significant Scheffe *a posteriori* analysis of between mean differences for the clinical and normal groups of students.[43] Currently, this language screening test is the only available one that includes analysis of pragmatic functions. The approximate testing time for this instrument is 8 to 10 minutes.

Selected Language Assessment Instruments

Clinical Evaluation of Language Functions—Diagnostic Battery. The CELF was developed by Semel and Wiig as a language measure for the school-age population between kindergarten and twelfth grade.[34] The CELF has a total of 13 subtests, which are distributed across the dimensions of processing (6 subtests), production (5 subtests), and 2 supplementary subtests. A brief summary of each of the subtests follows.

Processing Word and Sentence Structure. This comprehension subtest uses visual stimuli so that the student matches the sentence spoken by the examiner to one of four presented items.

Processing Word Classes. In this subtest, the student identifies the appropriate category in which two words (out of a field of either three or four) spoken by the examiner best fit. A sample of categories include weather, clothing, and spatial relationships.

Processing Linguistic Concepts. The student receives oral directions in which he or she points to colored lines in the manner described by the examiner.

Processing Relationships and Ambiguities. Grammatic and spatial relationships and ambiguities are explored in which the student answers questions following oral presentation of sentences or metaphors.

Processing Oral Directions. The student is required to respond to oral directions by pointing to figures that vary in color, shape, serial order, and physical location.

Processing Spoken Paragraphs. The student is required to answer questions following the oral presentation of a paragraph by the examiner.

Producing Word Series. In this timed subtest, the student is required to recite automatized material including the days of the week and months of the year.

Producing Names on Confrontation. Rapid naming of visually presented colors, shapes, and colored shapes is required on this timed subtest.

Producing Word Associations. The student is given one minute to name as many foods and animals as possible.

Producing Model Sentences. In this imitation task, the student is required to repeat sentences that are presented orally.

Producing Formulated Sentences. The student is required to self-generate a sentence containing a word given by the examiner.

Supplementary Subtest: Processing Speech Sounds. The student indicates whether or not two words presented are the same or different.

Supplementary Subtest: Producing Speech Sounds. The student's articulatory proficiency is evaluated by having him or her name a picture in a cloze procedure presented by the examiner.

The test requires approximately 60 minutes to administer, although the time may vary dependent upon the ceiling effect within each of the subtests. The CELF covers a variety of language functions that Semel and Wiig have indicated are useful in differentiating students who have language or learning problems from those who are achieving normally academically.[34] Test-retest reliability was reported on only 30 second graders and fell between 0.56 to 0.98 for the subtests. Concurrent validity has been reported by comparing the CELF total to the ITPA verbal (coefficient of correlation = 0.87), CELF production to the ITPA (coefficient of correlation = 0.83), and CELF subtests to selected subtests from the DTLA (coefficients of correlation were in the 50s).

The CELF has undergone several updates since it was initially published in 1980, and these updates are available through Merrill Publishing Company.[44,45] In these updates some pass-fail scores have been revised since it was felt that the original cutoff scores had been placed too low. Currently, the CELF scores are expressed in pass-fail raw scores; percentile ranks for grade levels and standard scores for ages for production and processing total scores; language ages for processing and production total scores; and means and standard deviations for each of the subtests by ages. Spekman and Roth[46] and Stephens and Montgomery[47] have provided excellent critiques of the CELF. These reviews should be considered for more comprehensive and detailed analysis of this test instrument.

Test of Adolescent Language. The TOAL was developed by Hammill, Brown, Larson, and Wiederholt in order to evaluate students between 11 years and 18 years, 5 months.[35] The theoretic model presented by the authors suggests that the TOAL considers features (semantics and syntax), systems (receptive and expressive), and forms (spoken and written). This test is one of the few available for this age range that provides information on students' abilities in written and oral language. For this reason, many special educators in learning disabilities and speech-language pathology have found the TOAL a useful test instrument.

There are a total of eight subtests on the TOAL, and they consist of the following.

Listening Vocabulary. Words with multiple meanings are used in which the student must select the best two pictures that best fit the orally presented definition.

Listening and Grammar. In this task, the student is required to indicate which two of three orally presented sentences have the same meaning.

Speaking and Vocabulary. The student is given a word orally that he or she must use correctly in an oral sentence.

Speaking and Grammar. The student is required to repeat an orally presented sentence immediately following the presentation from the examiner.

Reading and Vocabulary. The student is required to complete a classification task in which he or she first reads three words, then four others and decides which two out of the alternatives belong to the same category as the ones that he or she read first.

Reading and Grammar. The student reads five sentences and decides which two mean approximately the same thing.

Writing and Vocabulary. The student is required to produce a written sentence containing a word that he or she has read.

Writing and Grammar. The student reads several short sentences that must be combined in order to produce one written grammatically correct complex sentence.

Clinicians have often reported that the task demands are fairly high on the TOAL. These demands may result in a high failure among language disabled adolescents since many of the tasks require that the student be able to select two correct items or make other similar choices from a narrow field. Also, for many adolescents, their language deficits are seen more often in the written domains of language, and because of the heavy emphasis of this test on reading and writing, their language scores may be artificially lowered. However, if the clinician is attempting to clarify the interaction between the student's written and oral deficits, then this test may be the ideal one to use.

The TOAL was standardized on 2,723 students from 17 different states within the United States. The scoring of the test consists of scaled scores for each of the subtests, which can be combined and converted to quotients in order to represent composite scores on the test. The scaled and composite scores may be converted to percentile ranks as well. Also, all subtest scores may be combined in order to obtain an "adolescent language quotient" for the entire test performance. Finally, minimal guidelines are given that would allow the examiner to equate the composite and subtest scaled scores to five descriptive categories of superior through poor.

Test reliability was established extensively through the use of internal consistency, interscorer, and test-retest. All of the reported values were high and certainly within acceptable limits. Portions of the TOAL were used for validity measures with all or subtests from various test instruments: Peabody Picture Vocabulary Test (PPVT), DTLA, California Test of Basic Skills (CTBS), and Test of Written Language (TOWL). Overall, these coefficients of correlation fell within the range 0.40 and 0.50, although a few of the coefficients were at the upper end of the scale. Overall, apparently this test instrument was carefully constructed and considered appropriate psychometric validation of the material in the test.[47]

Fullerton Language Test for Adolescents. The age range for the Fullerton language test for adolescents (Fullerton) is from 11 to 18 years and was developed by Thorum.[48] Although a theoretic model for this test is not presented, it was developed to differentiate language disordered from non–language impaired adolescents. The Fullerton consists of eight subtests, which are briefly described as follows.

Auditory Synthesis. This subtest has two parts. In the first, the student is required to synthesize orally produced speech sounds into a meaningful word;

whereas in the second part, the student must synthesize orally produced syllables into a meaningful word.

Morphology Competency. A list of twenty words, which is comprised of many bound morphemes, is given orally to the student who must use the word appropriately in a sentence or phrase.

Oral Commands. The student is required to follow a series of orally presented commands of varying syntactic complexity containing dimensions of size, color, and shape.

Convergent Production. The student is presented with a homonym and is required to either define the word or to use it correctly in a sentence.

Divergent Production. Categorical naming is imposed upon the student within a 20-second time constraint for each stimulus item.

Syllabification. Over a series of 20 items, the student is required to indicate the number of syllables that he or she hears in orally presented words and sentences.

Grammatic Competency. The student evaluates the grammar of a verbally presented sentence and makes appropriate changes to the ungrammatic utterances.

Idioms. The student is required to verbally explain or interpret a series of 20 idioms.

The Fullerton was standardized on 727 students across the age range tested. Included with the white students were small samples of black and Hispanic students as well; however, the distribution of the minorities was not across all age ranges nor was it equally distributed. A ceiling effect occurs rapidly in the Fullerton, and, for this reason, little change is seen in test scores across the age range. This lack of change may reflect a weakness in the test in that items in the subtests do not tap language changes that may be subtly occurring in adolescents. Or this lack of change in language scores may reflect the fact that the Fullerton is too easy for many adolescents; therefore it does not show a distribution of performance across ages. Regardless of the cause, this lack of performance distribution may significantly limit the application of this test.

Thorum reports test-retest and split-half reliabilities on approximately 75 students.[48] Both of these reliability measures were within an acceptable range. Validity is evaluated through content, item, and diagnostic validity. The content and item validity are derived from comparisons with other known language measures, whereas the diagnostic validity is derived from comparisons between test performance of students enrolled in special education and those achieving normally in school. Scores on the Fullerton are based on levels of language performance and include competency level, instruction level, and frustration level. Clinicians may have some difficulty in interpreting these levels and in making meaningful treatment assignments based on the interpretation of the test. Although the Fullerton presents some interesting items, in particular the interpretation of figurative language through the expression of idioms, it does not appear to be as strong diagnostically as either the CELF or TOAL.

Limitations abound in all standardized tests. Many of the tests do not cover all aspects of language, but rather rely on the assessment of specific performances within a language dimension. Other tests are not standardized on populations that are comparable to the ones with which clinicians are working. Therefore, it is often considered prudent to administer more than one language measure in order to best determine the adolescent's language profile and learning strengths and weaknesses. Appendix 1 presents a brief summary of some additional tests appropriate to the evaluation of different dimensions of adolescents' language performance. Clinicians may wish to select carefully from tests given in this table and from others in order to develop a comprehensive test battery for adolescents. It is certainly abundantly clear that speech-language pathologists will continue to develop new tests and refine versions previously standardized as their knowledge base increases for this population. Until such time that speech-language pathologists have begun to address all issues relative to adolescents, they need to rely on a variety of test instruments and other informal sources for their diagnostic information. Only with time and the advent of new technologies will they become truly comprehensive and self-reliant in their diagnostic skills.

LANGUAGE INTERVENTION

The availability of relevant clinical information for the adolescent has increased. Early in the development of this clinical domain, much of what had been suggested for older school-age clients involved abstracting therapeutic materials and approaches from what clinicians had been using with younger children in order to apply these materials to the adolescent. This remedial approach led to high dropout rates among students enrolled in clinical services and so convinced many special educators that the speech-language pathologist was not well trained to work with the variety of problems associated with adolescence.

Fortunately, over the past several years interest in providing appropriate services to and delivery models for older students has increased. In addition, many principals at middle, junior high, and high schools and other administrators have recognized the need for interdisciplinary treatment approaches and have teamed the learning disabilities specialist and the speech-language pathologist in a single classroom in order to address the multiplicity of problems evidenced in students with significant language disorders. This team approach has led to the development of comprehensive curricula, which are able to address both the oral and written aspects of the student's language disorder.

Larson and McKinley have developed a comprehensive service delivery model for adolescents.[49] This multifaceted approach considers many different aspects of the adolescents' language and includes consideration of academic, social and emotional, and vocational skills of students. There are four major components to their service delivery model that are relevant for the speech-language pathologist working with adolescent students.

Information Dissemination. Public relations are an important aspect for the speech-language pathologist if services are to be continued at the secondary level. Special educators, guidance counselors, social workers, and administrators need to be made aware of the role of the speech clinician in working with adolescents. Furthermore, it is important that students become aware that services are available within the school to meet their needs. In addition to the referrals from teachers and other personnel within the school, students should be encouraged to make self-referrals when they are concerned with any aspect of their communicative skills.

Identification. The need for effective identification of language disorders has been discussed previously. Provision of effective screening and follow-up is needed, with appropriate diagnostic procedures when necessary. Also, the speech-language pathologist utilizes formal and informal assessment measures, relying heavily on reports from teachers and parents as to weaknesses and strengths in the student's communicative effectiveness.

Evaluation and Program Planning. At no other time in a student's academic experience does having the student involved actively in the decisionmaking process become more necessary than in the determination of an effective intervention plan. Following a comprehensive diagnostic evaluation from the clinician and other professionals, program implementation must be discussed with the student. Larson and McKinley strongly suggest that if the adolescent is unmotivated, denies the existence of the disorder, or refuses to accept responsibility, then he or she should not be forced into therapy.[49]

Intervention. It is suggested that intervention models at the secondary level include direct and indirect service models. Also, the importance of counseling cannot be overlooked when working with secondary students. The overall importance of pragmatics (language use) is emphasized in the delivery model by Larson and McKinley.[49] Finally, the authors emphasize that intervention, if it is to be effective, must occur with team efforts, for the speech-language pathologist cannot accomplish meaningful communicative goals working independently of the student's environment.

Pragmatic Language Behaviors

It is clear that investigation and treatment of pragmatic language skills have entered the areas of speech-language pathology and language disabilities. Direct observations of social conversational skills, peer-to-peer, and peer-to-teacher interactions have been used as avenues of exploration. Methodologic differences and experimenter interpretation have influenced the results of investigations of students' pragmatic skills. However, there are observations of these behaviors that can be summarized for language disabled adolescents.

1. As a group, language disabled adolescents may be less sensitive to conversational rules and, as a result of this insensitivity, may appear to be hostile listeners and less cooperative than their normal peers.[50,51]
2. Within a conversation, language disabled youngsters are more likely to give ambiguous information within their exchanges than their normal peers. This difference is likely to be related to syntactic deficits and to the language disabled youngsters generalized lack of understanding of many conversational rules.[52]
3. Language disabled children may be less skillful than normal children at understanding nonverbal behaviors.[11] These differences may lead to inappropriate responses and may well contribute to a perception of them as hostile listeners by their peers.
4. Language disabled children are not likely to request clarification when given ambiguous messages by peers.[52] Additional information suggests that among the language disabled group, young girls are even more impaired than boys in their social conversational skills.
5. Language disordered adolescents do not ask as many questions as their non–language disordered peers, and the questions that they ask are less likely to be open ended. This finding may be related to their own feelings of social inadequacy or to a general lack of assertiveness.[53–55]
6. Language disabled youngsters are more likely to agree, less likely to argue, and are generally less persuasive than are their nondisabled peers.[52]

7. As the social situation becomes more demanding and abstract, the language disabled adolescent has an increasingly difficult time responding appropriately in that conversational setting.

8. There is little evidence to support the idea that language disabled adolescents are socially withdrawn. They are often found to take as many peer-to-peer conversational turns, but the quality of their exchanges may vary from the non–language disabled.[52]

9. "Deficits in pragmatic competence, whatever the source, may therefore become part of the cycle of social and educational failure experienced by learning disabled children (p 18).[52]

Wiig and her colleagues have developed a number of treatment approaches for language remediation in adolescents. The particular emphasis of their programs has been on communicative competencies (pragmatic language skills) within this age range. Their series of programs are referred to as the *Let's Talk Social Communication* series (Let's Talk) and include the following: *Let's Talk for Children,*[56] *Let's Talk Inventory for Adolescents,*[57] *Let's Talk Intermediate Level,*[58] and *Let's Talk Developing Prosocial Communication Skills.*[59] Of these series of programs, the *Let's Talk Inventory for Adolescents* (LTIA) is a test that would be useful prior to the use of these clinical materials; however, contained within each of the clinical packets is a communication assessment that may be used for informal analysis. Of the programmed materials, the *Let's Talk for Children* (LTC) would be appropriate either for students having more severe language difficulties or for younger children than would be treated with the *Let's Talk Intermediate Level* (LTIL). The *Let's Talk Developing Prosocial Communication Skills* (LTDPCS) program is appropriate for young adults or children with communication disorders, but who are generally functioning at a more sophisticated language level, for it provides remedial suggestions for more complex variations of similar activities than presented in LTIL.

All of these programs are complete and provide the instructor with many useful materials. Wiig and Bray have indicated that their materials and training packets would be appropriate for use by speech-language pathologists, special educators, English as a second language specialists, and classroom teachers.[58] Also, their materials may be easily adapted for use in vocational, educational, and clinical settings. Since the emphasis of their training materials is on communication competencies, it is recommended that they be used with small groups of three to five students, although they can easily be modified to include a small classroom size.

The LTIL and the LTDPCS utilize the same four language functions as targets for language training. Therefore the difference between these two programs is not in the functions emphasized, but the level of the material within each function. The four functions that are addressed are (1) ritualizing, which includes greetings, calls for attention, requests, and initiating; (2) informing, which includes asking for and telling object names, actions and functions, place and time, and expressing conditions, states, and reasons; (3) controlling, which includes asking and telling about wants and needs, persuading, promising and responding to the promise, giving warnings, and exchanges of information; (4) feeling, which includes the expression of both positive and negative feelings; expressing affection, approval, and disapproval; and promoting socially effective and acceptable verbal conversation.[57,58]

The stimulus materials for all components in the Let's Talk series have been thoughtfully developed and provide the clinician with a rationale for intervention, including explicit definitions of terms and taxonomies used in the programs. In addition, the materials supplied include communication activity cards, designed to stimulate conversation within a particular speech act (e.g., formulating and responding to greetings and farewells) and containing the specific objectives, prerequisite concepts, suggested materials, and appropriate activities for elicitation of the targeted speech acts. The communication activity cards are designed for easy reference by the teacher or clinician and may be placed in a ring binder along with other specific stimulus materials.

Pictured materials include communication situation cards and communication card decks. The communication situation cards are designed to be used with the communication activity cards and are associated with several different speech acts. For each of these colored illustrations, the authors have presented a script that may be followed in order to elicit the targeted speech act. The communication card decks are designed to be used in card games that may provide a variety of activities in which students can use a variety of speech acts. The cards include signs, labels, warnings, place and directions, invitations and suggestions, favors and assistance, and choices.[58] Suggestions for use of these materials are outlined in the manuals for LTIL and LTDPCS. Finally, both sets of materials include progress checklists and detailed instructions for the clinician or teacher. Overall, these materials seem to have been well developed and carefully planned. The speech-language pathologist may find these materials useful when developing pragmatically based programs for adolescents or adults with communication problems. Following adolescents through these training materials and documenting their progress over time will be interesting.

Several other clinical and classroom management approaches using pragmatic models for intervention and teaching have been suggested. For example, Bourgault suggests the use of Halliday's seven pragmatic functions as a basis for intervention and assessment of adolescents' language skills.[60] These functions, described more fully by Halliday[61] and Simon[62,63] include the following:

1. Instrumental: language to satisfy material needs as in stating "I want" or "I need."
2. Regulatory: language that is used to exert control over the behavior of others as expressed in "do this" or "do as I request."
3. Interactional: language that establishes and maintains contact with individuals in the environment who matter to him and is expressed in "we" or "you and me."
4. Personal: language that is used to express the child's own individuality and self-awareness and is often in the form of "look at me" or "here I am."
5. Heuristic: language that is used to explore or to ask about the environment and is often seen in "why" or "tell me why."
6. Imaginative: creative functions of language are observed in play acting and pretending as evidenced in "let's play" or "let's pretend."
7. Informative: language that is used to communicate information not shared by the listener and is expressed in "guess what I did" or "I've got to tell you something."

These functions are combined into classroom goals for pragmatic language function and include activities in speaking, listening, writing, and reading. The classroom curriculum should include an appropriate class plan and personal functions as expressed through language units, which are further delineated into individual educational plans. This plan consists of two parts: academic responsibilities and social responsibilities. Academic responsibilities are further subdivided into form, which refers to the use and mastery of grammatic features, and semantic components and style, which refer to the manner of utterance production.[63]

Bourgault presents an interesting format for teaching pragmatic language skills to adolescents in the classroom setting in that she relies on television programming for the curriculum's "textbook."[60] In a unique approach, she suggests videotaping and analysis of popular television shows for presentation to students in the classroom. These shows are discussed through oral and written language in terms of language function, form, and style. Further, she has developed a series of language exercises that rely on group discussions, team efforts by two or three students, and individualized instruction. She feels that this type of learning experience gives students a more positive experience than the traditional teaching paradigm because it provides success with language in its functional usage of high-interest material.

Cognitive and Thinking Skills

Other methods of instruction with language disabled adolescents have stressed the importance of logical thinking development or cognitive skills enhancement. Alley and Deshler[2] and Schumaker and Deshler have developed and expanded an approach in which the major goal is to teach *how* to learn rather than *what* to learn. Alley and Deshler have defined learning strategies as ". . . techniques, principles, or rules that will facilitate the acquisition, manipulation, integration, storage, and retrieval of information across situations and settings" (p 13).[2] Their learning strategies approach appears to be effective as long as the student has achieved at least a third-grade reading level, if their learning occurs both symbolically and concretely and if they possess at least average intellectual capacities. Furthermore, the tasks used in this method of instruction allow for easy generalization of behaviors into other pragmatically relevant situations. Apparently, the only major drawback to this method of teaching is that some adolescents in need of learning strategies may not meet entrance criteria for the program. For these students, other basic instructional methods would need to be used and once mastered would facilitate a student's move into this program.

Boyce and Larson[65] have developed techniques of teaching strategies for problem solving and thinking skills based on Feuerstein's[66] instructional sequence. Activities that are advocated in this approach include working on cognitive skills at the input, elaboration, and output levels. Thinking skills in which the collection of information occurs are stressed at the input level, whereas utilization of these data is emphasized during elaboration; and finally, output involves the processes of communicating the outcome of the elaboration.[65] Furthermore, they approach the assessment of these areas by considering differences in learning strategies that develop during early or late adolescence and so adjust their assessment procedures accordingly.

The training approach suggested by Boyce and

Larson utilizes group interaction in order to facilitate problem solving. During the input process, questions are presented by the instructor that emphasize the nature of the problem presented. For example, the instructor might ask, "What information have you been given?" or "Can you describe the nature of the problem to be solved?" Following training on the input level, students are led through the elaboration phase in which they are encouraged to discuss the problems at length, pointing out the nature of the problem and even possible alternative solutions. In addition, discussions of actual problem solving processes or plans that the student is going through during the elaboration phase are encouraged. As well, in the output process, students' oral and written language skills are monitored, while the process that the student went through to solve the problem is expanded simultaneously. This treatment approach draws from a variety of other commercially available materials, and it is structured well for the clinician interested in working with adolescents who need training on these processes.

Minimal Speaking Competencies

As more and more treatment approaches are designed for adolescents, it becomes increasingly clear that we need to define and in some instances refine our knowledge of minimal speaking competencies for adolescents. These competencies should clearly involve addressing occupational, social, citizenship, telephone usage, appropriateness of vocal inflection and volume, and interpersonal dialogues as essential to diagnosis and treatment.

Several states have developed minimal competencies for adolescent students, and copies of these may be obtained from departments of education in the various states. Sample states that have developed competencies for students within this age range include Minnesota, Michigan, Illinois, Florida, Arizona, Pennsylvania, and Texas. Certainly development of competencies is as critical for these students as it is for younger ones. Bassett, Whittington, and Staton-Spicer provide a good source of speaking and listening competencies for high school graduates.[67] This list may be a useful starting point for the development of competencies in adolescents.

When one is developing a set of competencies for adolescents, it is important to keep in mind that one must treat oral and written aspects of language also. Clearly there are few children who have suffered through their developmental years with language problems who do not have concomitant written language deficits as well. Effective clinicians are able to treat both oral and written deficits concurrently, while planning effective strategies that enhance all language modalities.

The following list is a summary of many treatment considerations that must be addressed when working with adolescents. Certainly this list is not all inclusive, but it may provide a framework for structuring the development of competencies and of effective treatment plans to implement those competencies.

1. When working with language disordered adolescents, remember that it is best to keep the size of the group small in order to provide group interaction and individualized instruction as well.
2. Establish conversational rules that facilitate group interaction, but teach appropriate conversational strategies used in verbal exchanges. Effective teaching does not just teach the subject, but models acceptable social behaviors and interactions as would be experienced in conversational turn taking.
3. Know the baseline language measures of the students enrolled in your classes. One can only quantify language change when one is aware of the strengths or weaknesses of the students enrolled in the program. One needs to develop appropriate teaching strategies that allow one to teach to the strengths of the student, while simultaneously facilitating growth from their weaknesses.
4. Multimodality approaches often reach more students than limited sensory experiences. For example, when working on an experience, which would include reading, try acting out parts of the passage while simultaneously showing the student written and pictured symbols of the material.
5. Keep in mind that the majority of the students enrolled for language intervention at the adolescent age have had years of failure and disappointments. Keep your instruction upbeat and reinforcing. In the educational systems, reading is erroneously equated with intellectual functioning. Therefore, many students have had years of feeling dumb and inadequate due to their failures to achieve age-appropriate reading levels. Continue to remind them of their accomplishments—not their failures.
6. Mastery of new material is dependent upon the quality of learning rather than the quantity. It is important that instruction be directed to integration and mastery of concepts in order to facilitate cognitive changes.
7. Do not try to speed the learning process more quickly than can be effectively accomplished. Too often one assumes that because a skill is demonstrated that it is therefore learned. Introduction

of new information before true mastery of the previously taught material has been effectively integrated results in failures at more advanced levels of learning. It is better to provide more experience with development of a concept through exposure with multiple interpretations of that concept than to assume mastery too quickly. Overlearning through realistic exposure to development of a concept cannot be all bad.

8. Often it is necessary to address auditory perceptual aspects of language before working on expressive aspects of communication. Be prepared to increase students' abilities to respond to conversation in varying amounts of noise as you attempt to build their realistic coping skills.

9. Consider that the development of a "critical thinker" is essential to your treatment.[68] Remember that critical thinkers are those who can make realistic judgements about multiple aspects of language use. Abstract forms of language must be understood and internalized if effective logical thinking is to emerge.

10. Monitor the development of overgeneralizations and overuse of back-channel communication devices in adolescents because these may actually interfere with the development of cognitive skills.

11. Teach effective arguing and personal position support because these skills assist the students with language disorders to become more self-reliant and effective in modifying the behaviors of others.

12. Teach skills that enable adolescents without adequate reading or writing skills to survive in a competitive adult world. For example, the use of money, understanding spatial relationships of map reading, shopping in a supermarket, recognizing warning and traffic signs, and filling a prescription are often essential to effective treatment of the adolescent.[65]

13. Develop effective learning strategies in your students. These strategies should include techniques, principles, and rules that enable students to learn and to solve problems effectively and independently.

14. Make the therapeutic situation rewarding and reinforcing to regular school curricula. There is no reason to reinvent the wheel; therefore rely on work currently being addressed in the classroom and utilize the same materials in order to enhance the learning potential of the student. However, be careful not to confront students constantly with materials identical to those that have just recently resulted in classroom failures. Use classroom materials, but approach the learning of them in different ways than taught by the teacher. New approaches to the same curriculum should be developed that maximize learning and minimize failure.

SUMMARY

As seen from this discussion, many treatment approaches are currently available for working with adolescents with a variety of communication disorders. I have sampled only a few of the contemporary remedial techniques and procedures; there is certainly not sufficient space within the confines of this material to cover all possible techniques and approaches adequately. For more comprehensive reviews of clinical information concerning adolescents with language and language learning disorders, one may wish to read Wiig and Semel,[11] Wallach and Butler,[69] and Simon.[68] In addition, new materials are being developed and disseminated at a rapid rate. (See Appendix 2 for sample clinical materials.)

It is important to remember that each adolescent must be viewed individually, and appropriate clinical planning must take place first on an individual basis. Although rather generic group language dysfunctions have been summarized, it is certainly important to realize that these are generalizations and not all students possess each of the varieties of disorders described here. Clear similarities do occur between adolescents with language learning disorders, but certainly one should never assume that they represent a homogeneous group.

The adolescent years are often described as tumultuous ones, for they are filled with change, awakening, conflict, and new challenge. These normal processes are difficult under the best of circumstances, but are even more complex given the additional disadvantages of a communication disorder. Although clinicians often clearly focus on all of the negative aspects of the adolescent years, it is important to keep in mind that these years do not have to become devastating ones. Many problems that result from failures in communication may be alleviated through carefully planned and implemented programs for these young adults. True, clinicians may make progress with students more quickly during their early years, but sufficient research is available that supports the fact that language gains in all modalities can be achieved effectively during the adolescent years as well. There are even cognitive changes that occur during the adolescent years, which may actually facilitate our efforts.

Through guidance and counsel, clinicians can encourage and facilitate realistic understanding of the deficits, while simultaneously reinforcing positive accomplishments. Clinical work with adolescents presents challenges, but for many it becomes the most rewarding work of their careers. It is exciting to be on the threshold of discovery of new knowledge concerning the processes of language development and disorders in adolescence.

APPENDIX 1

The following are supplemental tests that may be useful for the comprehensive evaluation of the adolescent with language disorders.

Content Receptive

Ammons Full Range Picture Vocabulary Test. This receptive vocabulary test is standardized between the ages of $2^1/_2$ years and $16^1/_2$ years. This test requires visual stimulation with simultaneous stimulation of a single word. It requires approximately 20 minutes to administer.

Peabody Picture Vocabulary Test—Revised. This receptive one-word vocabulary test is one of the most widely used receptive vocabulary tests among special educators and psychologists. This instrument is standardized between the ages of $2^1/_2$ years and 40 years. The test requires visual identification of line drawn stimulus plates with simultaneous stimulation of a one-word verbal response. The test requires approximately 20 minutes to administer. A basal and ceiling level are established, and the test is highly standardized.

Token Test for Children. Although this test is standardized at the lower end of the adolescent years (3 to 12 years), it may be a useful instrument for receptive language functioning. The stimulus items on this test are large and small geometric forms of varying color. The client is required to make a gestural response after having been presented with a verbal command of varying length and complexity. This test requires approximately 10 to 15 minutes to administer. There is an adult version of this test also, which might be useful for the older adolescent or the adult with continuing or acquired language problems.

Content Expressive

The Word Test. This test is useful only for younger adolescents (12 or under); it may provide information relative to the use of expressive content.[70] The student is required to orally define words, state multiple meanings of words, give antonyms and synonyms, explain semantic absurdities, and make categorical associations. The test administration time is approximately 20 to 30 minutes.

The Boston Naming Test. This experimental test has been standardized on a limited sample of students from kindergarten through to grade five and also on adults between 18 and 59 years.[71] This test is a part of the Boston Diagnostic Aphasia Examination and may prove to be useful in the elicitation and interpretation of students' naming responses. In addition to the latency of response, the students' responses when cuing is used are considered also. This test's standardization is currently being expanded through the University of South Florida, Tampa, FL.

Test of Word Finding. This test of expressive word finding is standardized on children from ages 6 to 12 years. There are a variety of naming tasks, which include picture naming (verbs and categories), sentence, description, and comprehension assessment. Latency and cueing are considered. Approximate testing time is 30 minutes, dependent upon the number of subtests that are given to the child.

Form

Phonology

A wide selection of articulation tests are currently available for the child or adult with phonologic disorders. Presented here is a small selection of the tests that may be appropriate for adolescents.

Goldman-Fristoe Test of Articulation. This articulation test is nicely presented in a self-contained test kit and includes, for the most part, one colored stimulus item per page. This test has been standardized from 2 years to adults. It tests a variety of sounds in initial, medial, and final word positions; and it includes two stories in order to elicit connected responses. The test takes approximately 25 minutes to administer.

Fisher-Logemann Test of Articulation. This articulation test is based on a distinctive feature model and tests a variety of sounds and blends through picture stimulation. There are several small pictures on a page, and the colors are rather limited. The analysis of the articulatory patterns are according to the features of manner, place, and voicing errors. In addition to the pictured stimuli, a sentence articulation test is provided for the older client who can read. Test administration time is approximately 20 to 25 minutes. In addition to the complete test, there is a screening test that would require approximately 5 to 7 minutes to administer.

Templin-Darley Test of Articulation. This has become a classic articulation test for the preschool and early school-age child (2 to 8 years). There are several small pictures on a page, which are not highly colorful; however, this lack of vivid color should not be a problem for older students. It would be appropriate for the adolescents as well; however, the norms on the younger group should not be used.

Several subtests are a part of this test and include screening, blends, diphthongs, and the Iowa Pressure Test (useful for the detection of oronaso resonance difficulties). The test requires approximately 30 minutes to administer if all sections are given.

Phonology: Auditory Discrimination

Flowers-Costello Test of Central Auditory Abilities. This test is useful for children in kindergarten through to grade six and was designed to identify students with central auditory processing deficits, potential learning problems, and to make educational judgements regarding auditory deficits.[73] The test requires administration in a relatively quiet room and can be administered in under 30 minutes.

Goldman-Fristoe Test of Auditory Discrimination. This test of auditory discrimination is one of the most widely used test instruments for the detection of a variety of auditory discrimination problems for the preschool and early school-age child. The test does provide norms from 4 years of age to adults. Test administration time is approximately 20 minutes. The test is highly standardized and may be used in conjunction with the Goldman-Fristoe Diagnostic Discrimination tests I, II, and III (standardized from 3 years, 3 months to 8 years, 7 months).

Tree-Bee Test of Auditory Discrimination. This test of auditory discrimination is standardized from 3 years to adults. This test is fairly easy to administer, and public school clinicians have reported that they like the ease in which this test may be administered and interpreted.

Syntax

Language Assessment Tasks. This test instrument evaluates articulation, voice, syntax, semantics, and communicative function.[74] A language sample is taken and transcribed, and specific sentence generations are used to evaluate syntax. The semantic language function is evaluated through word definition and the use of "wh-" questions. An interview is used to ask teachers about the overall effectiveness of the student's communication. Test administration time is under 30 minutes.

The Reporter's Test. This test, although originally standardized for adult aphasics, has been shown to be useful in the evaluation of content and syntax of children in kindergarten through to grade nine ($4\frac{1}{2}$ years to $16\frac{1}{2}$ years). Standardization for children may be found in an article by Jordan and Hall.[76] The Reporter's Test should be used as a companion test to the Token Test, because it is the expressive of the Token Test. In the use of the Reporter's Test, the relevant aspects of each token and action are identified and labelled by the student. The total test time for both tests has been estimated to be between 20 to 30 minutes.

Use

The majority of the tests within this area have been designed to assess communicative competencies among adolescents or younger children. Most of these instruments require the elicitation of spontaneous language samples or interactional conversations with the examiner. This general area is one of growing concern among special educators working with language disabled adolescents and is most likely an area in which one will find additional tests being published in the next several years.

Communication Competency Assessment Instrument. The purpose of this instrument is to identify students who upon high school graduation may still have difficulties with minimal speaking and listening competencies. This test is quick as the student is requested to speak extemporaneously for 3 minutes (which is later rated by the clinician); then the students are required to listen to a short videotaped lecture and, during an interview, answer questions about the lecture.

Communicative Competence: A Functional-Pragmatic Language Program. This program provides both diagnostic and remedial information appropriate for the young adolescent.[62] The inventory evaluates spontaneous conversational language samples according to form, function, and style. A program for remediation of conversational disorders is provided in the materials.

Let's Talk Inventory. The purpose of this inventory is to elicit communication functions and speech acts that are used in social communication.[57–59] Specifically, this instrument evaluates ritualizing, informing, controlling, and feeling. A programmed approach to language remediation is a companion to this test instrument.

Broad-Based Language Assessments

Illinois Test of Psycholinguistic Abilities. This language test, which is based on an early psycholinguistic model of language, consists of 12 subtests that evaluate various aspects of different language processes.[78] This test has been widely used by special educators, but has limited application to the adolescent group since it is standardized up to 11 years of age only.

Detroit Tests of Learning Aptitude—2. This language test reflects a revision of the original Detroit Test of Learning Aptitude and represents many changes, including a reduction in the total test administration time.[79] There are 11 subtests on this instrument, and they test a wide variety of language processes, including both visual (reading) and oral tasks. The test is standardized for students between 6 years and 17 years of age. Scores are reflected in standard scores, percentile ranks, and composite scores, and the scores reflect strengths and weaknesses in the student's ability to learn.

Test of Language Development—Intermediate. This language test would be appropriate for younger adolescents only since it is standardized from 8 years, 6 months through to 12 years, 11 months.[80] The test consists of five subtests and includes the following: sentence combining, characteristics, word ordering, generals, and grammatic comprehension. Available scores are for spoken language (total test), listening, speaking, semantics, and syntax. Test administration time is approximately 40 minutes.

Woodcock-Johnson Psycho-Educational Battery. This test battery consists of a number of subtests that were designed to evaluate the student's learning potential.[81] This broadly based language test may be useful for identifying young children and adolescents who are experiencing difficulties with both oral and written aspects of language. The standardization was extensive for this test, and clinicians in the schools have reported good diagnostic value.

APPENDIX 2

Clinicians will continue to see an increasing number of commercially available programs for adolescents. In the past 7 to 10 years, a rapid growth has occurred in the number of available materials. The best solution to effective therapy is individually planned intervention strategies to meet the needs of each client enrolled. Sometimes, it becomes expedient to supplement the clinician's own creativity with creative thinking from others. Therefore, sometimes clinicians will want to rely on commercially available materials. This list should not be considered as comprehensive, but it does provide the reader with an overview of a selection of the materials that were not covered in the text of the chapter and are available for use with adolescents.

Cognitive and Thinking Skills

Let's Look at Logic

This approach contains filmstrips, cassettes, and logic cards. The emphasis of this material is to encourage logical thinking and includes such activities as determining if the presented reasoning is correct. Later in the materials, more advanced logic problems are presented.

Problem Solving

This approach is an introduction to problem solving through the use of film strips and other educational materials. Basic strategies are presented which help adolescents deal with human relationships.

Successful Problem Solving

These materials are designed to be useful for students in grades 6 to 12; in addition to being useful for language skills, they reinforce math-oriented problem solving activites. Good verbal interaction could come from these problems if they are approached in the right framework.

Instrumental Enrichment

These materials developed by Feuerstein provide a fine framework for the development of curricula that address a variety of cognitive deficits. In particular, training and activities focus on a sampling from the following: orientation, comparisons, analytic perceptions, categorizations, family relationships, and illustrations.

Classification and Organization Skills

Thirty two activities are arranged in a progressive order of difficulty and include activities such as sorting according to "who, what, where, why, and when." These activities may be useful for the reinforcement of writing tasks in which students would need to organize their thoughts and put them on paper.

Computer Games

This area is being used collectively to indicate that almost all computer word games have some degree of logic and cognitive thinking implied in their execution. Word games in particular may be useful for reinforcing reading skills and basic logic. Expect to see in the next few years a dramatic increase in the number of computer materials available for students within this age group.

Listening and Expressive Skills

Radio Listening

Clinicians can actually develop effective treatment approaches to listening skills by having students listen to old radio programs and reporting on those programs. In addition, they may wish to conduct a radio program and record the program for others in their group to analyze. This activity can be highly motivating.

Teaching Critical Listening

This is a three-step program to develop effective listening skills. Advertisements are used; they are analyzed according to the level at which they appeal, the presence of propaganda devices, and conclusions that may be drawn. This can be a highly contemporary approach to listening skills and can be modified easily to meet current needs.

HELP: Handbook of Exercises for Language Processing

These volumes are designed to improve auditory and language processing skills. The activities in these materials may be useful from 6 years through adulthood and contain useful lists and activities, which can be modified and shaped to meet the needs of the student.

Thematic Language Stimulation

This workbook was originally designed for use with adult aphasics, but it may be useful for adolescents as well. The workbook contains many worksheets that can be reproduced and provides stimulation on a variety of activities based on language, including word categorization and sentence production.

Workbooks for Aphasia

Brubaker has developed a series of workbooks that are useful with language intervention with adult aphasics, but may also be useful for adolescents. The workbooks vary and should be selected according to the needs of the student. Some of the activities need to be modified, but there are excellent definitions, reading, and writing skills emphasized in many of the materials. A recent publication contains thinking skills activities as well.

Communication Skills and Classroom Management

Although this is not a single set of materials to use with adolescents, it is a book that contains a variety of contributed chapters that address the educational and language needs of the language disabled adolescent. Specific information covered in this book include interpersonal behaviors, communicative competencies, and reading and written language activities. There are many valuable suggestions provided in this material.[68]

Semel Auditory Processing Program

The purpose of these training materials is to assist the classroom teacher or specialist to remediate problems that originate from the student's inability to process information in the classroom setting. There are three levels to these materials: the beginning level (3 to 7 years), the intermediate level (7 to 11 years), and the advanced level (11 plus years). The focus of the training materials is on syntax and morphologic rule structure. These materials have been demonstrated by Semel and Wiig to be highly effective in training language disabled adolescents.

Developmental Syntax Program

The focus of these materials is to provide a set of programmed procedures for establishing word formation rules through training in morphologic structure. There are three stages to this training, and these stages include ear training, production, and generalization.

Interactive Language Developmental Teaching

These materials have been available for some time, but include good rationale and procedures useful for young children and adolescents who are experiencing difficulty with syntactic formulations. The narrative materials in the lessons lend themselves easily to modifications dependent upon the student's language needs. Stories are used to elicit targeted responses.

Clinical Language Intervention Program

The purpose of these materials is to facilitate the acquisition and training of specific but selected semantic and syntactic structures. Four major language function areas are featured in the training materials: syntax, semantics, memory, and pragmatics. This training approach was designed to be used with students at the elementary or secondary level and may be modified to meet the needs of students individually.

Functional Communication Competencies

Development of Functional Communication Competencies

Wood has developed materials that are useful in developing communication competencies in students in kindergarten to grade 6 and in grades 7 to 12. This approach is highly reinforcing to the curriculum since it draws heavily from the material covered there. The instructional objectives are to expand the repertory of communication acts, identify and sharpen students' skills in using communication acts, implement communication acts, and teach a system for the evaluation of effectiveness.

Let's Talk

These materials were developed by Sathre, Olson, and Whitney and include activities to increase verbal and nonverbal interpersonal communication skills. In these materials, specific suggestions for classroom management and strategies for teaching interpersonal behaviors are provided. In particular, clinicians may find the sections dealing with social listening skills, self-perception, and honesty in verbal interactions useful when working with language disabled adolescents.

Procedures for Teaching Social Skills

Although this is not a set of materials, it is a term used collectively to apply to a variety of approaches that may be useful in working with language disabled adolescents. Usually several phases to the training are contained in these materials, and they include structured systematic group activities in which rationale, modeling of the skill, and rehearsal of the social skill are emphasized. Generalization of the skill follows; its application variety of settings would occur next, followed by a final phase—error intervention.

REFERENCES

1. Boyce N, Godwin E, Larson V. Communication disorders services: grades 7–12. Unpublished survey, Eau Claire, WI: University of Wisconsin-Eau Claire, Department of Communication Disorders, 1979.
2. Alley G, Deshler D. Teaching the learning disabled adolescent: strategies and methods. Denver: Love Publishing, 1979.
3. Aram D, Nation J. Preschool language disorders and subsequent language and academic difficulties. J Commun Disord 1980, 13:159–170.
4. Griffiths CPS. A follow up study of children with disorders of speech. Br J Disord Commun 1969; 4:46–56.
5. King R, Jones C, Laskey E. In retrospect: a fifteen-year follow-up report of speech-language-disordered children. Lang Speech Hear Serv Schools 1982; 13:24–32.
6. Larson VL, McKinley NL. General intervention principles with language impaired adolescents. Top Lang Disord 1985; 5:70–77.
7. Brown V. Curriculum development resources. In: Mann L, Goodman L, Wiederhold JL, eds. Teaching the learning disabled adolescent. Boston: Houghton-Mifflin, 1978.
8. Richardson SO. Differential diagnosis in delayed speech and language development. Folia Phoniatr 1983; 35:66–80.
9. Task Force on Nomenclature and Statistics. Diagnostic and statistical manual of mental disorders. 3rd ed. New York: American Psychiatric Association, 1980.
10. Wiig EH, Semel EM. Language assessment and intervention. Columbus: CE Merrill, 1980.
11. Wiig EH, Semel EM. Language assessment and intervention for the learning disabled. 2nd ed. Columbus: CE Merrill, 1984.
12. Wiig EH, Roach MA. Immediate recall of semantically varied sentences by learning disabled adolescents. Percept Mot Skills 1975; 40:119–125.
13. Kahn MS. Learning problems of the secondary and junior college learning disabled student: suggested remedies. J Learn Disabil 1980; 13:40–44.
14. Mercer C. Children and adolescents with learning disabilities. Columbus: CE Merrill, 1979.
15. McGinnis MA. Aphasic children: identification and edu-

cation by the association method. Washington, D.C.: Alexander Graham Bell Association for the Deaf, 1963.
16. McGinnis MA, Kleffner FR, Goldstein R. Teaching aphasic children. Volta Rev 1956; 58:239–244.
17. Morley ME. The development and disorders of speech in childhood. Edinburgh: Livingstone, 1957.
17a. The Education of All Handicapped Children Act (PL 94–142), 1975: P. 42478.
18. Johnson SW, Morasky RL. Learning disabilities. Boston: Allyn and Bacon, 1977.
19. Hammill DD, Leigh JE, McNutt G, Larsen SC. A new definition of learning disabilities. Learn Disabil Q 1981; 4:336–342.
20. Denckla MB. Minimal brain dysfunction and dyslexia: beyond diagnosis by exclusion. In: Blau ME, Rapin I, Kinsbourne M, eds. Child neurology. New York: Spectrum, 1981.
21. Wallach G, Goldsmith SC. Language based learning disabilities: reading is a language tool too! J Learn Disabil 1977; 10:178–183.
22. Wiig EH, Semel E. Comprehension of linguistic concepts requiring logical operations by learning disabled children. J Speech Hear Res 1973; 16:616–626.
23. Wiig EH. Language disabilities of adolescents: implications for diagnosis and remediation. Br J Disord Commun 1976; 11:3–17.
24. Magee P, Newcomer PL. The relationship between the oral language skills and academic achievement of learning disabled children. Learn Disabil Q 1978; 1:63–67.
25. German D, Newman J. Word finding difficulties in children with learning disabilities. J Learn Disabil 1979; 12:43–48.
26. Morgan DL, Guilford AM. Adolescent language screening test. Tulsa, OK: Modern Education Corporation, 1984.
27. Wiig EH, Semel E. Productive language abilities in learning-disabled adolescents. J Learn Disabil 1975; 8:578–586.
28. Bryan T, Donahue M, Pearl R. Studies of learning disabled children's pragmatic competence. Topics in language and learning disabilities Aspen: Aspen System Corporation, 1981.
29. Beilin H. Studies in the cognitive basis of language development. New York: Academic Press, 1975.
30. American Speech-Language-Hearing Association. Position statement on language learning disorders. Asha 1982; 24:937–944.
31. Wallach GP, Lee AD. So you want to know what to do with language-disabled children above the age of six. Top Lang Disord 1980; 1:99–113.
32. Dunn LM, Dunn LM. Peabody picture vocabulary test-revised. Circle Pines, MN: American Guidance Service, 1981.
33. Prather EM. Developmental language disorders: adolescents. In: Holland A, ed. Language disorders in children. San Diego: College-Hill Press, 1984:159.
34. Semel E, Wiig EH. Clinical evaluation of language function. Columbus: CE Merrill, 1980.
35. Hammill DD, Brown VL, Larsen SC, Weiderholt JL. Test of adolescent language: a multidimensional approach to assessment. Austin, TX: Services for Professional Educator, 1980.
36. Epstein HT. Some biological bases of cognitive development. Bull Orton Soc 1980; 30:46–62.
37. Epstein HT. Growth spurts during brain development: implications for educational policy and practice. In: Chall JS, Mirsky AF, eds. Education and the brain. Chicago: University of Chicago Press, 1978:343.
38. Epstein HT. Correlated brain and intelligence development in humans. In: Hahn ME, Jensen C, Dudek B, eds. Development and evolution of brain size: behavioral implications. New York: Academic Press, 1979:112.
39. American Speech-Language-Hearing Association. Position statement of the American-Speech-Language-Hearing Association (ASHA) and the National Association of School Psychologists (NASP) on Identification of Children and Youth with Language Learning Disorders. Legislative council handbook LC 20-86. Washington, DC: Asha, 1986.
40. Prather E, Breecher S, Stafford M, Wallace E. Screening test of adolescent language. Seattle: University of Washington Press, 1980.
41. Morgan DL, Guilford AM. Performance of black students on the ALST. Supplement to: Morgan D, Guilford AM. Adolescent language screening test. Tulsa, OK: Modern Education Corporation, 1986.
42. Tomchick P. A comparative analysis of scores achieved on the adolescent language screening test (ALST) and the test of adolescent language (TOAL). Masters Thesis, University of South Flordia, 1984.
43. Morgan DL, Guilford AM, Hollahan KB, Ritterman SI. Development and standardization of a test of adolescent language. FL Lang Speech Hear Assoc J 1982; 3:29–33.
44. Semel E, Wiig EH. Clinical evalution of language function. Update on the CELF. Columbus: CE Merrill, 1982.
45. Semel E, Wiig EH. Clinical evaluation of language function. Update on CELF. Columbus: CE Merrill, 1984.
46. Spekman N, Roth F. Clinical evaluation of language functions (CELF) diagnostic battery: an analysis and critique. J Speech Hear Disord 1984; 49:97–100.
47. Stephens MI, Montgomery AA. A critique of recent relevant standardized tests. Top Lang Disord 1985; 5:21–45.
48. Thorum A. The Fullerton language test for adolescents. Palo Alto, CA: Consulting Psychologists Press, 1980.
49. Larson V, McKinley NL. General intervention principles with language impaired adolescents. Top Lang Disord 1985; 5:70–77.
50. Bryan T, Wheeller R, Felcan J, Henek T. Come on dummy: an observational study of children's communications. J Learn Disabil 1976; 9:661–669.
51. Bryan T, Bryan J. Understanding learning disabilities. 2nd ed. Sherman Oaks, CA: Alfred, 1978.
52. Bryan T, Donahue M, Pearl R. Learning disabled children's peer interaction during a small group problem solving task. Learn Disabil Q 1981; 4:13–22.
53. Dudley-Marling C. The pragmatic skills of learning disabled children: a review. J Learn Disabil 1985; 18:193–199.
54. Torgesen JK. The role of nonspecific factors in the task performance of learning disabled children: a theoretical assessment. J Learn Disabil 1977; 10:27–34.
55. Wong BYL, Wong R. Role taking in normal achieving and learning disabled children. Learn Disabil Q 1980; 3:11–18.
56. Wiig EH, Bray CN. Let's talk for children. Columbus: CE Merrill, 1983.
57. Wiig EH. Let's talk inventory for adolescents. Columbus: CE Merrill, 1982.
58. Wiig EH, Bray CM. Let's talk intermediate level. Columbus: CE Merrill, 1984.
59. Wiig EH. Let's talk developing prosocial communication skills. Columbus: CE Merrill, 1982.
60. Bourgault R. Mass media and pragmatics: an approach for developing listening, speaking, and writing skills in secondary school students. In: Simon C, ed. Communication skills and classroom success. San Diego: College-Hill Press, 1985:241.
61. Halliday MAK. Explorations of the functions of language. London: Edward Arnold, 1973.
62. Simon CS. Suggested strategies for a functional-pragmatic approach to language therapy. Tucson, AZ: Communication Skill Builders, 1980.
63. Simon CS. Communicative competence: A functional-pragmatic approach to language therapy. Tucson, AZ: Communication Skill Builders, 1981.

64. Schumaker J, Deshler D. Setting demand variables: a major factor in program planning for the LD adolescent. Top Lang Disord 1984:22–40.
65. Boyce NL, Larson VL. Adolescents' communication: development and disorders. Eau Claire, WI: Thinking Ink Publications, 1983.
66. Feuerstein R. Instructional enrichment. Baltimore: University Park Press, 1980.
67. Bassett R, Whittington N, Staton-Spicer A. The basics in speaking and listening for high school graduates: what should be assessed? Commun Educ 1978; 27:298–302.
68. Simon CS, ed. Communication skills and classroom success. San Diego: College-Hill Press, 1985.
69. Wallach G, Butler K, eds. Language learning disabilities in school-age children. Baltimore: Williams & Wilkins, 1984.
70. Jorgensen C, Barrett M, Hursingh R, Zachman L. The word test. Moline, IL: Linguisystems, 1981.
71. Kaplan E, Goodglass H, Weintraub S. Boston naming test. Philadelphia: Lea & Febiger, 1983.
72. German D, Allen TX. Test of word finding. DLM Teaching Resources, 1986.
73. Flowers A, Costello MR, Small V. Flowers-Costello test of central auditory abilities. Aspen, CO: Perceptual Learning Systems, 1970.
74. Kellman M, Flood C, Yoder D. Language assessment tasks. Unpublished manuscript, 1978.
75. DeRenzi E, Ferrari C. The reporter's test: a sensitive test to detect expressive disturbances in aphasics. Brain 1978; 85:665–678.
76. Jordan LS, Hall PK. The token and reporter's tests using two scoring conventions: a normative study with 286 grade and junior high students. Lang Speech Hear Serv Schools 1985; 16:227–237.
77. Rubin R. Communication competency assessment instrument. Annadale, VA: Speech Communication Association, 1982.
78. Kirk SA, McCarthy JJ, Kirk WD. Illinois test of psycholinguistic ability. Urbana: University of Illinois Press, 1968.
79. Hammill D. Detroit tests of earning aptitude-2. Austin, TX: Pro-Ed, 1985.
80. Hammill D, Newcomer P. Test of language development-intermediate. Austin, TX: Pro-Ed, 1982.
81. Woodcock R, Johnson MB. Woodcock-Johnson psychoeducational battery. Bingham, MA: Teaching Resources, 1977.

25 Aphasia in the Adult

Malcolm R. McNeil, Ph.D.

A PHILOSOPHICAL PERSPECTIVE

The study of aphasia is undertaken because it is an occult disorder, part of the unknown black box, and as such is a challenge for the academician. For some, the study of aphasia offers potential insight into some basic and universal properties of man and nature. Others regard aphasia as a relatively specific, frequently occurring pathology capable of being caused by discrete central nervous system (CNS) lesions from which brain-behavior relationships can be inferred. For others, aphasia is a symptom of an underlying CNS lesion, which by itself must be dealt with as a life-threatening condition. For still others, it is a condition that interacts with and affects intellectual, emotional, social, and physical health and therefore must be dealt with as a condition affecting the quality of life. For these reasons, philosophers, linguists, psychologists, sociologists, social workers, neurophysiologists, neurologists, neuropsychologists, psychiatrists, audiologists, speech-language pathologists, and many other "-ers" and "-ists" have studied the disorder. The current state of knowledge about aphasia is the result of study by these diverse professionals seeking various kinds of understanding of the condition. In order to synthesize and assimilate the information on aphasia from these divergent disciplines, a broad (multiform) and changeable (protean) approach to the disorder must be taken. A multiform approach is one that recognizes that the problems of aphasia can and must be viewed from as broad a perspective as possible. A protean approach is one that allows and actually demands as much change and flexibility in theory and practice as circumstances warrant and evidence allows.

This chapter will attempt to integrate a number of approaches to the study of aphasia into one, not unbiased, but consolidated view of the essential nature of aphasia and the secondary and associated behaviors that accompany it. The conclusions drawn are believed to be supported by the data available. However, consistent with a protean approach, the constructs and conclusions presented are clearly open to revision or abandonment if contradictory evidence or a new framework for interpreting old data should gain acceptance in the scientific aphasiology community. What follows is a review and discussion of some of the more important constructs that have been applied to the study of aphasia. The constructs chosen for discussion are not exhaustive. Those presented were chosen because they are believed to be those that hold the greatest promise for an eventual understanding of the disorder and those that inform both the theoretical and clinical demands of a theory of aphasia. As a beginning, some definitions of aphasia are reviewed, and a reformulated definition is offered based on the nature of the disorder as discussed in the following sections. A comprehensive review of classification system terminologies is provided in a cross-correlational matrix, with reference to the underlying neuroanatomic and behavioral assumptions on which each classification seems to be based. Other theoretical constructs for the study of aphasia are discussed, including intelligence and memory, and competence versus performance. Illustrations of performance deficits in aphasia are presented through evidence from differing etiologic groups, from analyses of the source for intrasubject variability, from examining how aphasic performance is manipulable, from the notion that aphasia exists on a continuum of normalcy, and from evidence that aphasic persons have preserved metalinguistic abilities. Next, some theoretical issues and the available data on the interrelated conditions of recovery, prognosis, and treatment efficacy are reviewed. Finally, a review of assessment and treatment approaches is presented.

DEFINITIONS

According to Schuell, Jenkins, and Jimenéz-Pabón, speech pathologist, psychologist, and neurologist, respectively,

> . . . aphasia [is] a general language deficit that crosses all language modalities and may or may not be complicated by other sequelae of brain damage.
>
> . . . The language deficit . . . is characterized by reduction of available vocabulary, impaired verbal retention span, and impaired perception and production of messages, perhaps secondary to impairment of the first two dimensions (p 113).[1]

Benson, a neurologist, defines aphasia as "the loss or impairment of language caused by brain damage" (p 1).[2]

Because aphasia can occur coincident with other higher cognitive disorders that share symptomatology and/or are capable of masking the aphasia, definitions of exclusion have been used in combination with inclusional ones. Exclusional definitions include that of Schuell et al: "With generalized or scattered brain damage, there may be further manifestations, such as various forms of dysarthria, confusion, memory loss, or even psychosis. We consider it important to distinguish the latter group of symptoms from aphasia" (p 113).[1]

Darley, a speech-language pathologist, offers the following exclusional definitions:

> Aphasia is not the result of restriction of sensory input . . . Neither is it the result of mental defect. It is true that patients who display generalized intellectual impairment show deterioration of performance on certain language tasks, particularly more difficult ones . . . Their language difficulty, however, is only one aspect of a more comprehensive difficulty in thinking. In dementia the degree of language impairment is roughly proportional to the deterioration evident in other mental functions . . .
>
> . . . Confused patients display reduced recognition and understanding of their environment, faulty memory, unclear thinking, and disorientation in time and space. They may display a language problem, usually the production of irrelevant, confabulatory responses to open-ended, less structured questions and situations. Nevertheless the language they produce is syntactically correct, their words are well chosen, and their responses to specific questions and structured situations may be normal.
>
> Nor is aphasia the result of poor motor control. . . . Aphasia is not the result of a mechanical difficulty in speech production. It is a disorder of language, not of speech.[3]

All of these definitions are clearly influenced by the psychological processes that are believed to be related to language and how language is organized in the brain. The assumptions and constructs underlying the definition that follows are woven throughout the remainder of the chapter. It is offered here as one interpretation of the current state of knowledge in the form of a summary of the major observable behavioral characteristics, psychological processes subsuming these behaviors, and known neuroanatomic substrates supporting the disturbed processes for aphasia.

Aphasia is a multimodality physiologic inefficiency with verbal symbolic manipulations (e.g., association, storage, retrieval, and rule implementation). In isolated form, it is caused by focal damage to cortical and/or subcortical structures of the hemisphere(s) dominant for such symbolic manipulations. It is affected by and affects other physiologic information processing and cognitive processes to the degree that they support, interact with, or are supported by the symbolic deficits.

Many of the concepts supporting this definition are incompletely defined and only partially developed in the physiology and psychology literature. This incompleteness is understandable given their immense complexity; thus it is also understandable why concise statements of higher cognitive processes, including language and its representation in the brain, can be made in only the most general of terms at this time. Although this approach to defining aphasia is dramatically different from (though not inconsistent with) that offered by Benson,[2] any reliance on tenuously defined constructs is justified. Aphasiologists are obligated to entertain rather vague notions such as symbolism, associations, storage and retrieval processes, and linguistic rule implementation processes. Similarly, the type, size, and site of lesion, as well as physiologic and psychological supporting processes such as the relationship between thought and language, are all crucial elements that must be considered in the understanding of the nature of aphasia and in the management of the aphasic person's interpersonal and intrapersonal communication deficits.

A dissection of the definition provided previously offers some critical and fundamental clues to the nature of aphasia. These issues will be discussed following a discussion of classification systems and the neural substrates of aphasia and following a philosophical discussion of approaches to the study of adults with aphasia. They will be discussed along with several important theoretical issues relevant to an understanding of the fundamental nature of the disorder and the people who have it. The issues derived from the definitional dissection include an analysis of (1) the uni- versus multimodality nature of the disorder, (2) the performance versus competence nature of the deficit, (3) the verbal (linguistic) versus nonverbal (nonlinguistic) domain of the disorder, (4) the cortical versus subcortical locus of the damage that results in the disorder, and (5) the universus multidimensional (across cognitive systems) nature of the disorder.

CLASSIFICATION SYSTEMS AND NEURAL SUBSTRATES

Historically, a need for psychological organization, well-defined categorical boundaries, and management paradigms based on a medical model of syndromes has produced grouping of patients who share some common characteristic(s). This commonality could be the presence or absence of particular behaviors (e.g., sound and syllable substitutions in the presence of inordinate difficulty in verbal repetitions), the modalities most or least affected, or the site or etiology of the lesion producing the aphasia. What follows in Table 25–1 is a summary of the major classification systems that have appeared in the literature over the past 120 years. As with the definitions, underlying assumptions about what language is and the way that language is organized in the brain dictated the classification schemata.

In each classification system, a lesion in a particular location was believed to correspond to a particular "type" of aphasia; however, the authors of some classification systems were not clear about the locations of these lesions. In those cases, an attempt has been made to correlate their behavioral descriptions with the same or similar descriptions by other authors who have made clear statements about lesion sites for their types of aphasias. Because of the clarity, currentness, and concurrent validity of the Benson[2] classification system, it is used as a model wherever possible. The principle characteristics of the major types of aphasia from this classification system are presented in Table 25–2.

Marie,[4] Bay,[19] Schuell et al,[1] and Darley[33] have rejected the notion that there are different types of aphasia with differing underlying neuroanatomic and neurophysiologic mechanisms. Marie was so sure of this unitary nature of aphasia that he stated categorically that the aphasias are *one.*[4] As the result of a large factor analytic study, Schuell et al concluded that there is essentially one underlying verbal deficit that all patients share and that is the essence of their aphasia.[1] The other factors, and hence categories of aphasia that were derived, were attributed to aphasia plus complications of perceptual, sensorimotor, or general intellectual deficits. Brown's central language processor model[34,35] was an attempt to relate the multimodality single-dimensional findings of Schuell et al to possible neuropsychological and anatomic substrates. Recent research from a variety of perspectives might also be interpreted as support for the unidimensionality of aphasia (semantics,[36] pragmatics,[37] and discourse[38,39]). However, this evidence is in no way a reflection of unanimity among aphasiologists for this "single aphasia" view.

The notion of a multimodality basis for aphasia is based on the assumption that aphasic behaviors result from damage to the central language processor that is shared by all input and output channels.[40] To entertain a unimodality aphasia is to postulate multiple language competencies that are somehow arranged by input or output modalities. Using the previous definition, aphasic behaviors can and must be found in all modalities, albeit to differing levels of severity. Instances whereby a single modality is effected (as in cases of isolated apraxia of speech pure word deafness, word blindness, and alexia without agraphia) are better considered as entities separate from aphasia. The definitional requirement of a multimodality deficit stands in direct opposition to the assumptions made by Badecker and Caramazza.[41] These authors use patterns of impaired performance to constrain theories of language processing. According to the authors, the essential assumptions that must be made for this to be a reasonable enterprise are ". . . that language processing mechanisms can be affected selectively by brain damage and that the impaired system cannot exploit mechanisms of organization of mechanisms which did not exist prior to the disruption that caused the aphasia" (p 238).[42]

Both of these assumptions—the selective nature of the deficit in terms of the modalities affected or the cognitive and linguistic domains involved—as well as other unaffected cognitive and linguistic processes are not supported by the majority of neurophysiology or aphasiology literature. However, one should note that the other theoretical arguments proposed by these aphasiologists against the use of the current classification systems deserve serious attention by the theorist and the clinician.

The model on which most classification systems are built is a neuroanatomic one (for examples of exceptions, see Brown,[27] Head,[9] and Wepman and Jones[43]) in which centers for specific functions are housed and association areas surround and interact with the centers and other association areas by connecting pathways. A review of any neurolinguistic model makes clear the dependence of the classification systems on the isomorphic relationship between the behaviors and their neural substrates. However, even a cursory inspection of the neurophysiology literature[44–47] suggests that connectionistic models are unsupported by contemporary data on microneuroanatomy and neurophysiology. Indeed, morphologic variations in the brain[48,49] anatomic variations in the functions of specific structures[50,51] and the possibility of remote effects of focal lesions,[13,52] as well as the fact that the "loss of certain performances through damage to their substrata, bring about modifications of other depending performances," (p 9)[13] make connectionistic explanations of asphasia untenable. Others (e.g., Freud[53]) have provided cogent arguments, rationales, and clinical material against such connectionistic models. Criticisms have ranged from the probability of misapplying therapeutic principles because of heterogeneity of subjects within any type of aphasia,[33] to the failure of such classifications to inform neuropsychological and cognitive theories of aphasia,[41,42,54–58] to the classifications systems' invalidity on a linguistic construct level,[59] to the inability of the centers and pathways models to account for the variable performance that is a hallmark of aphasic behavior.[60]

Where then is the validity for the Boston classification system?[2,61] The validity appears to be restricted to clinical neurology and not to clinical speech-language pathology nor to theoretical neuropsychology or cognitive psychology. The validity appears to be found in the correlations between groups of behaviors and sites of lesions determined by autopsy or neuroradiologic studies and appears to be restricted to the utility of the clinical neurologist.[31,50,62–64] What is unclear is whether those factors on which the classifications of aphasia are based are related to disturbed basic sensorimotor processes or whether they describe underlying differences in the symbolic and language deficit per se, which is the common factor from which they can be called aphasic. Nonetheless, several studies have confirmed a neuroanatomic analogue for the different classifications of the Boston system (see Figure 25–1 for a summary of this lesion-aphasia classifications system).

A reconciliation between the theoretical and the neurophysiologic evidence against such a simplisitic brain-behavior relationship and the aphasia test with neuroradiologic data supporting it is not easily effected. However, if one accepts Jackson's[65] idea that "to locate the damage that destroys speech and to locate speech are two different things" because of the factors listed previously such as variability, diaschisis, and interactive processes, then the reconciliation can be made between a construct that is theoretically invalid but clinically useful, even if a "marriage" cannot. It is thus possible in some cases of aphasia (at most, about 60 percent[64]) to classify a patient with standardized behavioral measures and to infer the location of the lesion. Kertesz[66] has devised a diagnostic instrument that forces nearly 100 percent of all aphasic patients into a predetermined class or type. However, the percentage of patients that a particular instrument can classify cannot be used as strong evidence to support the connectionistic model from which the measures were derived.

An important issue related to the classification of aphasic individuals is how and whether the classification of patients is useful. Indeed, to classify or not to classify is a relevant question from several points of view. Most American-trained neurologists, physiatrists, and psychiatrists and a few otolaryngologists receive some training in disorders of higher cognitive functions, including aphasia. With rare exceptions, all are taught to classify Aphasics* in one way or another. Most often the classification involves a grouping of behaviors or possibly an estimate of the severity of the deficit. However, as Duffy[67] has pointed out, patient description or group identity by the severity of deficit is also a classification system that comes with no less theoretical constraints and commitments than the more traditional schemata. Frequently the classification adopted involves the receptive versus expressive dichotomy. Probably equally often, the sensorimotor dichotomy is used. The strong influence of the "Boston school," fathered by the late neurologist Geshwind and adopted by neurologists such as Benson, Brown, Boller, and Kertesz, by psychologists such as Goodglass, Kaplan, Howes, Gardner, Zurif, and Caramazza, by linguists such as Whitaker, Blumstein, and Buckingham, and by speech-language pathologists such as Helm, Holland, Sparks, Naeser, and Martin, has brought about the dissemination and adoption of the "Boston classification" system (see Table 25–2) in many medical schools. It is important to know at least the more common classification systems because speech-language pathologists are often part of a team of professionals who assess, diagnose, and treat the person with aphasia. Under these circumstances, it is critical to the patient's management that the team members be able to communicate with one another on common terminological grounds. In addition, much of the scientific literature is written with respect to classes of aphasic patients, and only through a thorough command of the literature by the professionals involved do aphasic patients receive the scientifically based management that they deserve.

Another, more fundamental issue arises with a decision by the speech-language pathologist to use a classification system to communicate ideas or intentions about his or her patients. Strong theoretical and practical implications accompany the adoption of a particular classification system. Calling a pa-

* The word "aphasic" is best used as an adjective. However, for convenience it is used as a noun throughout this chapter. In order to preserve the dignity of the aphasic *person,* the word "Aphasic" is capitalized throughout. The same is true for Normal and Nonaphasic persons.

TABLE 25–1 Classifications of Aphasia

		Anterior to Rolandic Fissure			*Posterior to Rolandic Fissure*			
Proponent	*Central Language Processor (Represented Diffusely in the Brain)*	*Premotor Cortex*	*Posterior $^2/_3$ 3rd Frontal Convolution*	*General Frontal to Rolandic Fissure*	*Posterior Superior Temporal*	*Parietal Temporal*	*Arcuate Fasciculus*	*Angular Gyrus*
Marie, 1906[4]	Aphasia							
Wernicke, 1885[5]		Transcortical motor	Cortical motor		Cortical sensory		Conduction	
Broca, 1865[6]			Aphemia		Verbal amnesia			
Bastian, 1869[7]			Aphasia		Amnesia	Word blindness		
Pick, 1913[8]	(Amnesic)		Expressive		Impressive			
Head, 1926[9]	Semantic		Verbal		Syntactic			
Weisenberg and McBride, 1935[10]	(Amnesic)		Expressive		Receptive			
Kleist, 1934[11]	(Amnesic)		Word muteness anarthria*		Word deafness		Repetition	
Nielsen, 1938[12]	(Amnesic)	Transcortical motor	Broca's; Subcortical motor		Wernicke's			
Goldstein, 1948[13]	(Amnesic)	Transcortical motor	Central motor Peripheral motor† Peripheral sensory‡		Wernicke's sensory			
Eisenson, 1954[14]	(Amnesic)		Predominantly expressive		Predominantly receptive			
Brain, 1961[15]	(Nominal)		Broca's		Central			
Wepman and Jones, 1961[16]	Semantic		Syntactic		Pragmatic jargon			
Russell and Espir, 1961[17]			Motor		Central	Alexia		
Gloning et al, 1963[18]	(Amnesic)		Motor		Sensory			
Bay, 1964[19]	Pure‡	Echolalia	Cortical dysarthria		Sensory			
Luria, 1964,[20] 1966,[21] 1977[22]	Semantic	Dynamic	Efferent motor		Sensory			
Goodglass et al, 1964[23]				Nonfluent				
Howes, 1964[24]			Type A					
Schuell et al, 1964[1]	Group 1‡ (simple aphasia) group 2		Group 3 minor group 1†		Group 5		Group 4	
Geschwind, 1965[25]		Transcortical motor	Broca's		Wernicke's		Conduction	Anomic
Hécaen and Dubois, 1971[26]	(Amnesic)	Expressive 2	Expressive 1		Sensory 2 Sensory 1		Expressive 3	
Brown, 1972[27]	(Anomic)	Transcortical motor	Agrammatic anarthria†		Semantic		Phonemic	
Lecours, 1974[28]			Broca's 1 Broca's 2		Wernicke's 1 Amnesic (mild Wernicke's)	Wernicke's 2	Conduction	
Adams and Victor, 1977[29]	(Anomic)	Isolation of speech area§	Broca's Pure word muteness†		Wernicke's		Conduction	
Mohr et al., 1978[30]			Big Broca's Little Broca†					
Kertesz and Phipps, 1977[31]	(Anomic)	Transcortical motor Isolation[4]	Broca's		Wernicke's		Efferent conduction	
Hécaen and Albert, 1978[32]	(Amnesic)	Transcortical motor	Pure motor		Sensory	Alexia with agraphia	Conduction	
Benson, 1979[2]	(Anomic)	Transcortical motor Mixedtranscortical§	Broca's Aphemia†		Wernicke's	Alexia with agraphia	Conduction	

* These categories and the lesion site may be akin to lesions affecting the arcuate fasciculus. However, this is not always clear from the authors' descriptions.

† Behavior is akin to modern concept of apraxia of speech and probably involves a more focal lesion than the other categories in this column.

TABLE 25–1 Continued

			Subcortical				*Other*			
Diffuse Parietal	*General Posterior to Rolandic Fissure*	*Anterior Interior Parietal*	*Maries Quadra-lateral Space*	*Thalamus*	*Striatal*	*White Matter*	*Nonlocal-izable/ Diffuse Lesion*	*Bilateral Temporal Lobe*	*Dominant Heschi's Gyrus*	*Occipital Lobe*
Transcortical sensory						Subcortical motor[†]	Total		Subcortical sensory	
								Pure word deafness		
Nominal							Total			
							Expressive Receptive			
						Anarthria[†]				
Transcortical sensory						Subcortical motor				
Transcortical sensory		Central*				Peripheral motor Peripheral sensory	Mixed echolalia			
		Central*					Total or global	Pure word deafness	Pure word dumbness	
		Central* Conduction*						Pure word deafness		
		Sensory*								
Acoustic-Amnestic		Afferent motor*								
	Fluent Type B									
							Group 5			
Transcortical sensory Sensory 3 (attentional disorder)										
Isolation of speech area[§]							Total	Pure word deafness[§]	Pure word deafness[§]	Pure word blindness
Transcortical sensory		Afferent conduction					Global			
Isolation[§] Transcortical sensory								Pure word deafness[§]	Pure word deafness[§]	Pure alexia
Transcortical sensory Mixed transcortical[§]			Aphasia of Marie's quadra-lateral space	Thalamic aphasia	Striatal aphasia	Aphasia from white matter lesions	Global	Pure word deafness[§]	Pure word deafness[§]	Alexia without agraphia

[‡]The "pure" category of Bay is akin to Marie's aphasia, and Schuell's simple aphasia (Group I).
[§]This category fits into two lesion locations and is listed under both.

TABLE 25–2 Speech-Language Characteristics of Various Aphasic Syndromes from the Boston Classification System

Aphasic Syndrome	*Conversational Speech*	*Auditory Comprehension*	*Auditory Speech Repetition*	*Confrontation Naming*	*Reading*		*Writing*
					Aloud	*Comprehension*	
Anomic	Fluent, empty	Good to mild	Good	Severely abnormal	Good or abnormal	Good or abnormal	Good or abnormal
Broca's	Nonfluent	Good	Abnormal	Abnormal	Abnormal	Good or abnormal	Abnormal
Wernicke's	Fluent, paraphasic	Abnormal	Abnormal	Abnormal	Abnormal	Abnormal	Abnormal
Conduction	Fluent, paraphasic	Good	Abnormal	Usually good	Abnormal	Good	Abnormal
Transcortical motor	Nonfluent	Good	Good	Abnormal	Abnormal	Often good	Abnormal
Transcortical sensory	Fluent, paraphasic echolalic	Severely abnormal	Good	Abnormal	Abnormal	Abnormal	Abnormal
Mixed transcortical	Nonfluent with echolalia	Severely abnormal	Good	Severely abnormal	Abnormal	Abnormal	Abnormal

After Benson DF. Aphasia, alexia, and agraphia. New York: Churchill Livingstone, 1979.

tient an agrammatic Aphasic (see the exchange by Caplan[68] and Badecker and Caramazza[41]) or one with Broca's aphasia, or calling all Aphasics simply aphasic without an accompanying adjective (not classifying) implies much about the mechanisms that cause the behaviors, much about what behaviors accompany the dominant classificatory behaviors, much about the site and possible etiology of the lesion, something about prognosis, and for some clinicians, much about treatment (see the series of essays on these issues by Aten, Darley, Duffy, Holland, Ulatowska in the 1983 volume of *Clinical Aphasiology*).

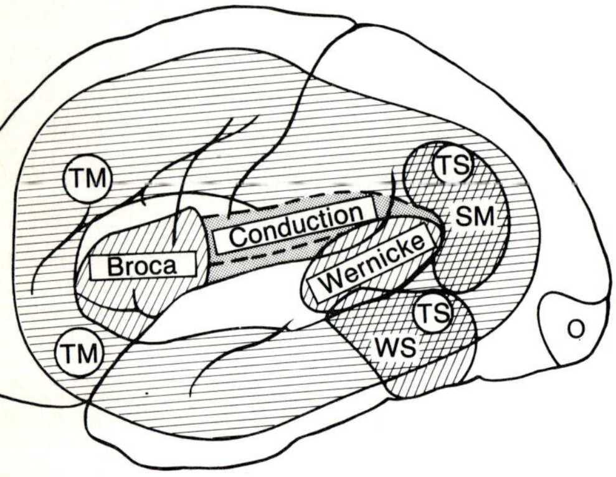

Figure 25–1 Light areas are areas of brain tissue that when infarcted are not expected to result in aphasia. Lesions in the areas with vertical stripes correspond to Broca's (syntactic disorders) and Wernicke's (perceptive and receptive disorders) aphasia. A lesion in the shaded area (arcuate fasciculus) results in conduction aphasia. A lesion in either of the open circles labelled TM results in transcortical motor aphasia. A lesion in either open circle labelled TS results in transcortical sensory aphasia. Mixed transcortical aphasia (isolation of the speech area) results from a lesion encompassing the area with the horizontal stripes. Anomic and global aphasia can result from lesions anywhere in any of the aforementioned areas. Two varieties of anomia also have localizing value. Semantic anomia occurs from lesions in the hatched area SM (semantic disorders), and word selection anomia occurs with lesions in the hatched area WS. Broca's area is also the area for frontal alexia, and parietal-temporal alexia shares the area with SM. Occipital alexia is found in the clear area O. (After Benson DF. Aphasia, alexia, and agraphia. New York: Churchill Livingstone, 1979.)

As a shorthand in communication, it is reasonable that professionals attempt to group aphasic patients who share common symptoms. However, three temptations arise when clinicians classify their patients. The first is a tendency to see behaviors in terms of classification categories, which forces them into a mold even when the behaviors are disparate. The second problem is to ignore sometimes critical assessment in areas that the classification does not cover. (Note that the areas of assessment that form the basis of Benson's classification are only a small part of the information on which most contemporary speech-language pathologists assess and treat.) The third potential problem is related to the other two, but highlights the fact that the physiologic, perceptual, cognitive, linguistic, and communicative abilities and disabilities, and the strategies implemented to overcome the aphasic deficits, are individualized. Thus the dimensions on which the patient is classified do *not* predict these other more salient treatment variables for *any* individual. In other words, within-group variance is likely to be as large or larger than between-group variance for many dimensions on which treatment is based. In summary, if aphasic patients are classified, classification should be done with an awareness of the temptations to see what is not there, to miss what is there, and to ignore individual differences.

APPROACHES TO THE STUDY OF ADULTS WITH APHASIA

Philosophers have been concerned with language and its pathology longer than any other discipline. However, the 19th century neurologists were the ones who delivered aphasiology from utter chaos to the point where research from several diverse perspectives has provided great insight into some aspects of its essential nature. Communication and its impairments have been viewed from mathematical models and human information processing as rule systems, images, schemata, and reverberating circuits.[69] Aphasia has been viewed from a cybernetic perspective. It has been modeled on cerebral reflex constructs and on ontogenetic and microgenetic regression constructs. Jenkins et al proposed slightly different terminology for the framework on which to view communication disorders in general and aphasia in particular. The terminology used is derived from philosophy and logic, but is based in part on the Jacksonian distinction between language used propositionally and language used nonpropositionally. These authors assert that "*how* a proposition is asserted is just as important as *what* is asserted. Similarly, *why* a proposition is formulated is just as important as whether it is true or not" (p 76).[69] The how, what, and why were viewed from two major processes used in the more general communication process—formulation of propositions and instantiation of propositions. Formulation refers to the communicator's psychological needs, attitudes, intents, indicative core (that part of the message or communiqué that has factual importance and is capable of being true or false), and the modes of knowledge or cognition that surround the unasserted mental propositions, independent of any particular linguistic form. The modes of cognition or knowledge were related to knowledge by acquaintance (speculated to be a right [language-nondominant] hemisphere function) and by description (speculated to be a left [language-dominant] hemisphere function). Within this framework, two kinds of communiqués are distinguished—those involving signs and those involving symbols. Instantiation refers to "the manner or mood of assertion or expression which determines how the proposition is made publicly manifest as [a] communique" (p 76).[69] Signal and symbolic communiqués may vary in the manner in which they are made publicly manifest. For example, "a verbal statement can be whispered timidly, or shouted with conviction, spoken rapidly or slowly, slurred or pronounced distinctly, directed at a particular audience or tossed to the wind. The manner of articulation or enactment describes the performance factors involved in the public declaration of the communiqué" (p 79).[69] The

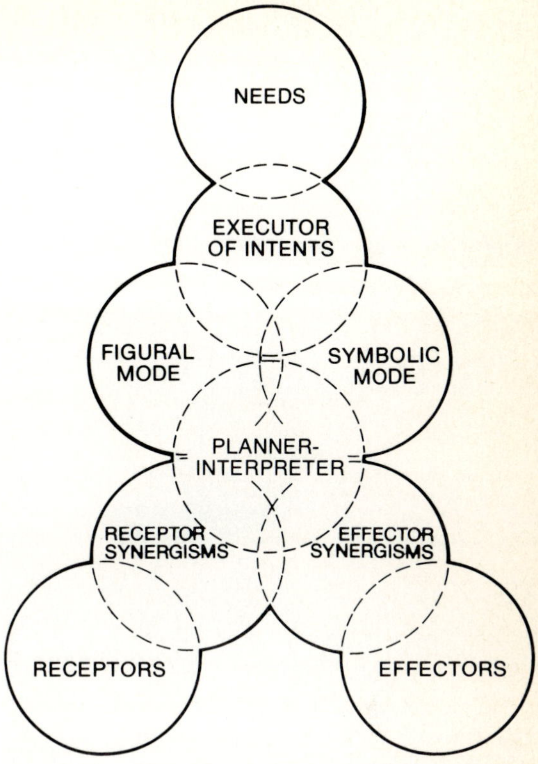

Figure 25–2 Schema for discussing the communication process. (After Jenkins JJ, Jimenéz-Pabón E, Shaw RE, Sefer JW. Schuell's asphasia in adults: diagnosis, prognosis and treatment. 2nd ed. Hagerstown, MD: Harper and Row, 1975:85.)

mood has to do with the producing or receiving end of the communication chain. According to Jenkins et al, the specification of these variables offers a functional description of the communiqué.

Applying these processes to the cognitive and neurophysiologic elements of planning movements, interpreting incoming stimuli, receiving synergisms (preprogrammed subroutines for analyzing incoming messages), sending effector synergisms (preprogrammed sequences of coordinated activities that, once initiated, run automatically to completion), sensory receptors, and neuromotor effectors, Jenkins et al have provided a useful construct for evaluating the level(s) or process(es) disordered in aphasia. This model is illustrated in Figure 25–2. This schema is particularly appealing because it is specific enough to outline areas of direction on which most clinical aphasiologists would agree, but nonspecific enough to allow variations of models within a particular subcomponent of the schema. For example, whether the approach chosen to describe the symbolic operations is from a transformational grammar point of view, from a phrase structure grammar point of view, or from some other construct is unspecified. At this time, having all subcomponents of the model unspecified is necessary because the scientific knowl-

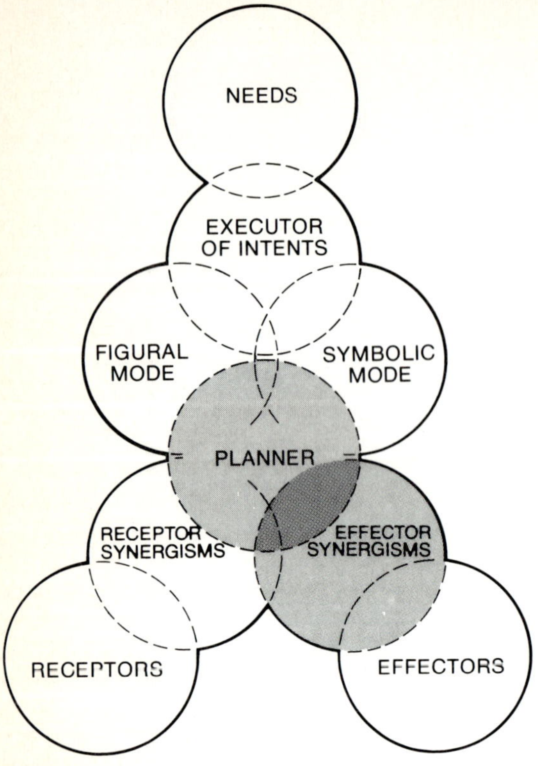

Figure 25–3 Possible schema for apraxia of speech. (After Jenkins JJ, Jimenéz-Pabón E, Shaw RE, Sefer JW. Schuell's aphasia in adults: diagnosis, prognosis and treatment. 2nd ed. Hagerstown, MD: Harper and Row, 1975.)

edge base is inadequate to offer a definitive explanation of them. The schema seems to offer a convenient representation of the more abstract and conceptually more difficult nature of the communicative process and its malfunctions with various neuropathologies. For example, using this construct, Figure 25–3 might illustrate apraxia of speech, whereas Figure 25–4 illustrates a twelfth cranial nerve flaccid dysarthria, neither of which is considered an aphasia. Figure 25–5 illustrates Schuell's conception of simple aphasia, and Figure 25–6 illustrates what will be argued in this chapter to be a better characterization of the loci of these same aphasic deficits.

One other construct deserves mention for its importance in characterizing the general nature of aphasia, as well as in characterizing the clinical management of each individual patient. Aphasia should be viewed from three perspectives: (1) the processes, levels, or functions that are essential disturbances of aphasia; (2) the secondary processes, levels, or functions that are disturbed because of the primary disturbances; and (3) the undisturbed processes, levels, or functions that can be used to facilitate or circumvent the disturbed ones. McNeil and Kimelman[70] have elaborated this trinocular view of aphasia as applied to auditory processing and comprehension and postulated specific cognitive, linguistic, and information processing subsystems that correspond to these three perspectives.

Central to the interactive schema proposed by Jenkins et al[69] and the integrative schema proposed by McNeil and Kimelman,[70] Muma and McNeil [71] have called for more psychosociolinguistic research in aphasia. This type of research calls for an integration of cognition (content), linguistics (form), and communication (use). Flying in the face of strong historic and contemporary approaches, it is proposed here and elaborated in the sections that follow that cognition, including cognitive style (e.g., tempo, divergent versus convergent, analytic and synthetic, and enactive, iconic, and symbolic operations) and some cognitive processes (e.g., rule- versus non-rule-governed learning), are essentially preserved in aphasia. In addition, the linguistic (e.g., semantic, syntactic, morphologic, phonologic, and suprasegmental rules) and communicative (e.g., speech acts, elocutionary force, construction, utilization processes) facets are disturbed secondarily because of the primary disturbances. The primary disturbances appear to consist of such dynamic processes as those attributable to the general consequences of brain damage.[72] These consequences might include such factors as increased fatigability, increased sensory thresholds, decreased speed of reaction, fluctuation

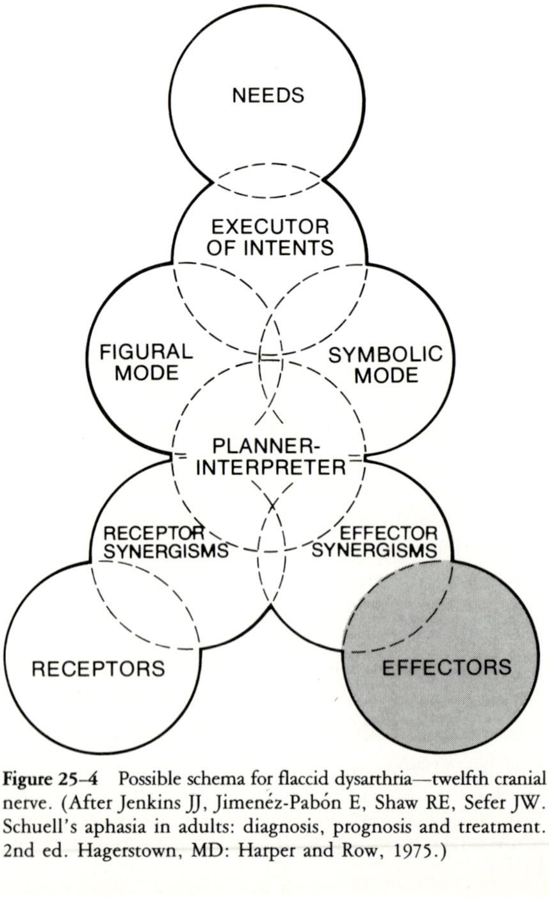

Figure 25–4 Possible schema for flaccid dysarthria—twelfth cranial nerve. (After Jenkins JJ, Jimenéz-Pabón E, Shaw RE, Sefer JW. Schuell's aphasia in adults: diagnosis, prognosis and treatment. 2nd ed. Hagerstown, MD: Harper and Row, 1975.)

of attention and effort allocation, and inertia of neurophysiologic excitation and inhibition.

What follows is a review of two areas of research that have offered considerable insight into the nature of the aphasic person's disorders (intelligence and memory). Following these discussions, a brief discussion of the verbal versus nonverbal nature of the aphasic deficit, the cortical versus subcortical specificity of the aphasia-producing lesion, and the uni- versus multidimensional (across cognitive structures) nature of the deficit will be discussed. Finally, a major portion of the chapter will be discussed within the framework of an important and pervasive theoretical issue in aphasia—loss or competence versus interference or inefficiency.

INTELLIGENCE

Like most of the psychological and physiologic constructs describing aphasia, the way that "intelligence" is conceived defines its relationship with aphasia. Historically, the issue seems to be traceable to Marie[4] (in Zangwill[73]). However, history also reveals that there is no simple answer to the question, do persons with aphasia have a reduced intelligence?[9,13,74,75] With the possibility of as many as 120 factors defining intelligence without a single "g" factor[76,77] (see Basso et al for a contradictory viewpoint[78]) and the possibility of most factors involving verbal symbolization processes, it is not surprising that the question remains answered incompletely. However, the pursuit of these answers is not trivial. In addition to the obvious theoretical importance, Zangwill[73] has suggested that the intellectual status of Aphasics has practical importance for occupational prospects and for such medicolegal issues as testamentary capacity and custody and child support, as well as for offering a prognosis concerning rehabilitation potential and extended care placement.

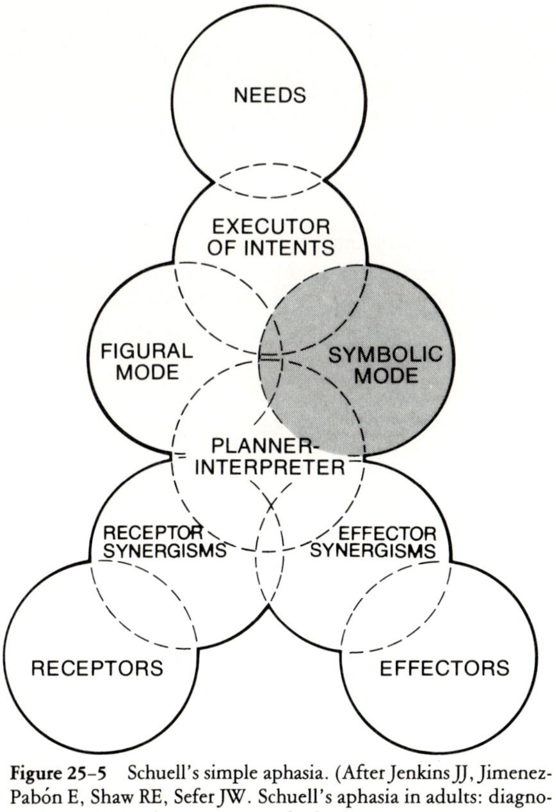

Figure 25-5 Schuell's simple aphasia. (After Jenkins JJ, Jimenez-Pabón E, Shaw RE, Sefer JW. Schuell's aphasia in adults: diagnosis, prognosis and treatment. 2nd ed. Hagerstown, MD: Harper and Row, 1975.)

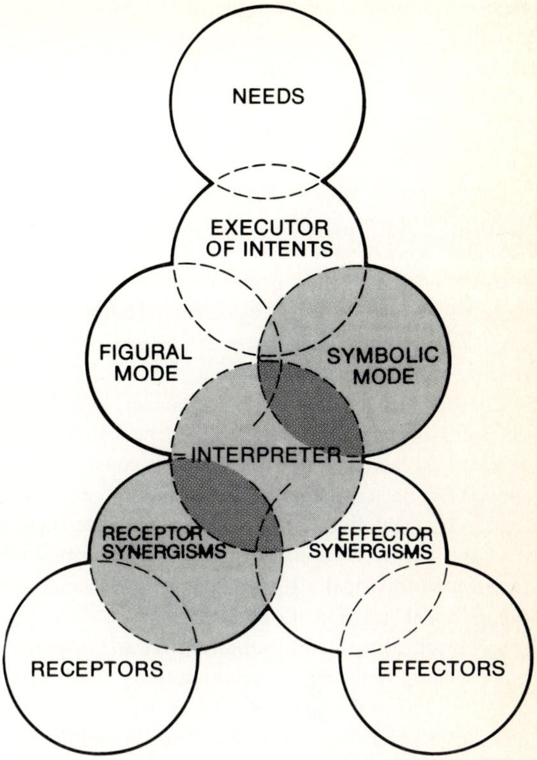

Figure 25-6 Proposed scheme for aphasia. (After Jenkins JJ, Jimenéz-Pabón E, Shaw RE, Sefer JW. Schuell's aphasia in adults: diagnosis, prognosis and treatment. 2nd ed. Hagerstown, MD: Harper and Row, 1975.)

Evidence from tests of "abstraction," in the Goldsteinian[13] sense, which are assessed by nonverbal classification tests, has generally found Aphasics deficient compared to Normals, but not more so than comparable brain-damaged patients without aphasia.[79–81] Similarly, there is no conclusive evidence that Aphasics display a generally reduced intelligence from tests of "drawing" and "modelling"[73] (however, see Bay[19,82] for the exception to this generalization). Standardized intelligence tests divided into verbal and performance (nonverbal) abilities have shown, without exception, a significant and substantive difference between deficits on verbal and nonverbal tests, with poorer performance by Aphasics on verbal tests when compared to nonaphasic brain damaged groups.[10] When compared to Normals, however, the performance (nonverbal) abilities are usually significantly poorer.[83–86] But to what one attributes this performance deficit is critical. In this vein, Alajouanine and Lhermitte[87] reported that of 218 cases of aphasia, only 25 percent had an intelligence quotient (IQ) of less than 80 on a standard IQ test. In these 55 cases, 44 were reported to have constructional apraxia. The apraxia appears to have effectively lowered their performance scores and consequently their full scale quotient. Therefore, one must keep in mind that there are factors other than language or general competence (knowledge or intelligence) that influence performance, and ". . . estimates of intelligence in aphasic patients should be based on 'performance' tests only if constructional apraxia has been satisfactorily excluded."[73] Although the study of intelligence has offered valuable insight into the nature of aphasia, simple correlations between an individual's IQ and his or her social and occupational position do not exist.

"Intelligence" is minimally (if at all) impaired, but reasoning or creative mental activity may appear reduced. This reduction is found inordinately in the domains that are loaded on fast and efficient verbal symbolic operations (e.g., those operations that are more likely required for the practice of medicine or for a professor than those required for an automobile mechanic or a construction worker). With the possible exception of global,[88] total, or Schuell's group V Aphasics who do not show physiologic recovery and are indistinguishable from demented or generally intellectually impaired patients, Aphasics cannot be considered to have reduced "intellectual" abilities (see Collins for a more detailed discussion of intelligence in global aphasia[89]). Further, IQ per se is not sufficient to predict much of anything about the person with aphasia.

If, in general, intelligence functions are insufficient to describe or explain the nature of aphasia or the person with aphasia, then other conceptual models must be constructed for such descriptions and explanations. Other constructs have been proposed from which to describe and explain aphasia in addition to the centers-pathways models and the general intelligence deficit models. A discussion of memory processes in aphasia follows as one possible source for this description and explanation.

MEMORY

Psychological and physiologic models of memory are abundant.[90–93] Although researchers disagree about the exact structure and limits of the various stages or processes of memory, they generally agree, based on a wealth of psychophysiologic evidence, that memory can be subdivided into at least three phases: (1) iconic (visual) or echoic (auditory) memory that lasts only a few milliseconds, (2) short-term memory that lasts only about 30 seconds, and (3) long-term memory that can last nearly indefinitely, particularly if acted upon (accessed or rehearsed) periodically.

Memory is to some extent developmental, and short-term memory is limited in capacity. There are predictable patterns or curves for the storage, transfer, and retrieval of information. These processes and resultant curves are affected by such variables as list length, intertrial interval, anticipated cues or prestimulus set, number of response alternatives, effects of patterns and subpattern sequential properties, modality, linguistic variables, and many others.[94–96]

One important distinction with relevance for aphasia has been found between verbal and nonverbal memory tasks as a function of left- versus right-hemisphere lesion. Milner has devised a number of tasks to test patients with left and right anterior-tip temporal lobe lesions pre- and postoperatively.[97–99] Although these patients are not considered aphasic, the basic finding has been that the left temporal lobe (language dominant) is specialized for short-term verbal memory and is thus disturbed when a lesion occurs. Similarly, the right temporal lobe is specialized for nonverbal short-term memory and is thus disturbed when a lesion occurs. Techniques other than creating lesions, such as dichotic listening[100] and dichoptic watching,[101] have also generally supported the left-verbal and right-nonverbal dichotomy.

Language-dominant hemisphere lesions might be expected to produce verbal memory deficits in persons with aphasia, and that has in fact been confirmed.[102–105] However, these same authors have found reduced memory for nonverbal material as well.[106] A reduced rate and amount of information processed in memory have been speculated as the cause for the verbal memory disorders[1] as well as the nonverbal memory disorders.[107,108]

Iconic Memory

The literature dealing with iconic or echoic memory in aphasia is sparse. A study by Loverso,[109] though designed to investigate the effects of alerting signals on reaction time in Aphasics, provides some information on iconic memory. Loverso demonstrated that Aphasics could respond accurately within the range of exposure duration generally assigned to iconic memory. Even though standard methods for investigating iconic memory (e.g., backward masking) were not used in this study, it provides a preliminary indication that iconic memory operates in the direction of normal. The fact that information is operated upon in short-term memory is also evidence that sensory memory *can* operate in a normal fashion. For example, the serial position study of Locke and Deck demonstrated the normally expected recency effect in their aphasic subjects,[110] compared to the primacy effect. Recency has been attributed to sensory storage.

Short-Term Memory

Short-term memory has been investigated in a variety of ways. Aphasics have been shown to produce significantly fewer digits forward or backward (regardless of the hemisphere of involvement or anterior or posterior lesion site*) than either normal controls or nonaphasic brain damaged patients.[111] Cermak and Moreines[112] found that the Aphasics' retention of verbal (words and letters) material was even more impaired than that of brain-damaged patients who are essentially described by their memory deficits (amnesic patients with Korsakoff's psychosis). When given additional time to rehearse the verbal material, the Aphasics showed improvement, although not to the level of the Normals nor the amnesic patients. In a follow-up study designed to investigate the specificity of the memory loss for verbal material, Cermak and Tarlow[113] verified their earlier findings and those of DeRenzi and Nichelli,[114] Flowers,[115] Schuell et al,[1] Swinney and Taylor,[116] Tzortzis and Albert,[117] and Warrington and Shallice[118] that Aphasics demonstrate a substantive verbal short-term memory deficit. This finding has since been confirmed by Adamovich,[119] Albert,[120] Warren et al,[121] Rothi and Hutchinson,[122] and others. In addition, however, Cermak and Tarlow found that their Aphasics were not different from normal subjects on a nonverbal (picture) memory task, but performed significantly more accurately than patients with Korsakoff's psychosis on this nonverbal task (a finding contradictory to several studies cited earlier).[113] The difference between the two types of material was explained by the Aphasics' inability to overtly[123] or covertly rehearse the verbal material in short-term storage, a process imperative to getting it into long-term memory,[94] and their ability to utilize visual imagery for mediating the nonverbal material (a process not utilized by the patients with Korsakoff's psychosis[124]). Heilman, Scholes, and Watson proposed this nonrehearsal strategy as the basis for the memory deficits in patients with Broca's and conduction aphasia.[125] Rothi and Hutchinson supported this general finding, but only for nonfluent patients.[122] Fluent Aphasics, right-brain damaged, and Normals did show evidence of rehearsal. However, the rehearsal evidenced in the fluent group was insufficient to bring them to the quantitative level of the right-brain damaged or normal groups.

Adamovich reported on the Aphasics' "internal handling of information" or the type of sensory code used for maintaining information in short-term memory.[119] This aspect was investigated by analyzing the "perceptual confusions" of the spoken names of the 26 letters of the alphabet within a recognition paradigm and by analyzing the recall confusions (with imposed response delay) between visually and auditorily presented stimuli. The results were that the Aphasics made about twice as many errors as the Normals on all three tasks. These results were interpreted as evidence for perceptual as well as for memory deficits. Further, the perceptual confusions were similar for both Aphasics and Nonaphasics, both making a preponderance of "sounded like" or "rhymed with" errors. The recall strategies were interpreted as different between the two subject groups. On the one hand, the control subjects made "sound alike" or "rhymed with" errors regardless of the modality, and no differences in the number of errors by modality occurred. On the other hand, the aphasic subjects made "sound alike" errors when the stimuli were presented auditorily, but made "look alike" errors when the stimuli were presented visually. Adamovich suggested that the aphasic subjects in this study did not appear to be using a speech code to store the letters in long-term memory, as the normal subjects were.

Swinney and Taylor studied the strategies of aphasic and normal control subjects used in the search of memory for recently acquired information (short-term memory).[116] This study was accomplished using a paradigm created by Sternberg,[126] which uses the reaction time to items that are correctly recalled to judge the type of search (self-terminating or exhaustive) used in locating a stimulus in lists of various lengths. They found that the normal subjects used a serial exhaustive scan of short-term memory, whereas the aphasic subjects not only were quantitatively slower in their search of short-term memory, but were judged to be qualitatively different as well, using a self-terminating search. Warren et al challenged Swinney and Taylor's findings on the grounds that it was clearly contradictory to previous literature comparing the memory systems of aphasic subjects with normal controls,[121] as well as being erroneous from a statistical standpoint. Warren et al utilized a paradigm similar to that of Swinney and Taylor, but demonstrated some interesting differences as well as some similarities in their results. The aphasic subjects were significantly and substan-

* Albert found that a lesion anywhere in the perisylvian region produces a verbal short-term memory deficit.[120] In addition, posterior lesions create a slight but insignificant increase in total errors or errors of sequencing.

tively slower in their search of short-term memory (less than half as many items searched per second), made more errors (which were not included in the analysis), and showed a significantly longer reaction time than did the control subjects. However, they showed a qualitatively similar linear increase in reaction times as the subset size increased (two, four, or six items) and evidenced the same exhaustive search strategy as the normal subjects.

Lubinski and Chapey also investigated the recall strategies of normal nonaphasic and aphasic subjects.[127] They sought to determine the number of verbal items that could be recalled, their recall organizational abilities, types of errors, clustering or categorizing strategies, effects of repeated trials on memorization ability, and relationships between strategies and traditional tests of aphasia.

Consistent with all other studies, Lubinski and Chapey found that their aphasic subjects recalled significantly fewer items than the normal subjects.[127] In addition, the learning curves were similar for both groups. Although reduced quantitatively, aphasic subjects in this investigation organized items significantly less efficiently during study periods and clustered items significantly less efficiently for facilitating recall than did the normal subjects. Finally, these researchers found ". . . a moderately strong relationship between aphasia severity as expressed in the overall combined verbal and gestural score and aphasic subjects' ability to recall items, organize their study time effectively and cluster their responses." Severity was measured with the Porch Index of Communicative Ability (PICA).[128]

Flowers demonstrated the universal finding that Aphasics are able to recall significantly fewer items from short-term memory than are the Normals,[115] but not fewer than the brain-damaged nonaphasic group. He also demonstrated that all subject groups had approximately the same degrees of proactive interference and proactive interference release. Proactive interference is the process that occurs during a recall task when some aspect of recalling prior items interferes with the recall of subsequent items. Proactive interference release is the process whereby recall is enhanced by items occurring before the test items (priming). Flowers interpreted these findings to indicate that proactive interference does not account for the short-term memory deficits of aphasic patients to an extent greater than its contribution to normal and brain-damaged nonaphasic patients. Like other authors, he suggested that a slow processor may account for the short-term memory deficits.

Caramazza et al investigated aphasic subjects' short-term memory for words in the context of a sentence.[129] Patients were presented orally with a sentence, and, immediately upon the completion of the stimulus, they were given a word from that sentence. The task was to recall the word that followed the probe item in the sentence. This particular task was chosen because it was sensitive to "the structure of the internal representation constructed for the sentence." Given the a priori assumption based on the literature that patients with Broca's aphasia would have more trouble with function words and bound morphemes (e.g., -et, -ed, -est) and patients with Wernicke's aphasia would have more trouble with content words (e.g., nouns and verbs), they predicted that there should be a significant difference between groups in the types of words recalled. Results suggested that there were no differences between the groups on the overall short-term memory capacity for sentence material. In addition, the groups did not differ in their ability to retrieve particular grammatic markers or selective grammatic classes of words within the sentence. Both patient groups had more difficulty retrieving function words than content words.

McNeil and Hageman reported that about 90 percent of their 30 aphasic subjects demonstrated at least one instance of poorer performance as a semantic sentence comprehension task (Revised Token Test commands) increased in length of commands.[130] However, in most instances, sentence type (e.g., prepositional phrases) or a processing inefficiency (e.g., intermittent auditory processing) appeared to account for more of the deficits than memory factors per se.

Two additional factors concerned with short-term memory have been investigated in aphasia. The first is the serial position (recency and primacy) effect, and the second is the short-term memory for temporal sequences (the preservation or loss of order versus loss of number). With regard to the first, there appears to be some discrepancy in the literature as to whether aphasic patients demonstrate better performance at the beginning of a string, fade in accuracy during middle portions, and return to near beginning levels at the end of the string, the way normal subjects do. Flowers found that his aphasic subjects had a steady decrease in performance from the initial to medial to final positions, whereas his brain-damaged nonaphasic and normal subjects both demonstrated the typical "U"-shaped recency and primacy effects.[115] Both Warren et al[121] and Adamovich[119] found a flat serial position effect. Locke and Deck demonstrated a normal serial position curve with primacy better than recency and both substantially better than the medial position, for all subjects, with the following exception.[110] For the aphasic subjects, recall of the initial and the medial position was poorer when the stimulus was one that could not be named easily. This finding appears to have been due to the inability to rehearse the initial item and thereby implicates the necessity of verbal rehearsal in short-term storage of initial position items. As the authors suggest, this finding also demonstrates that "in other experiments, where the stimuli are not preselected for nameability, one cannot expect rehearsal—even where the subject might otherwise attempt it—and the level of recall may be less than his maximum performance."[110]

With regard to the second factor, memory for sequences, the literature is replete with evidence that aphasic patients have great difficulty with short-term memory for sequences, be it auditorily, visually, verbally, or nonverbally, often when the sequence can be recalled in its entirety—though out of sequence.[115,117,120,131,132] Efron[132] and Goodglass et al[133] found poorer serial memory performance in patients with Broca's aphasia compared to other types when the stimuli were delivered auditorily. This finding raises the question as to whether the sequencing deficit is one of storage or one on the output side of retrieval, a question consistent with that raised by Kimura and Archibald.[134]

Long-Term Memory

Long-term memory in persons with aphasia is usually regarded as normal unless the Aphasic is more than simply aphasic, for example, generally intellectually impaired, confused, schizophrenic, or suffering from Korsakoff's psychosis or another neuropathology that characteristically demonstrates long-term memory disorders.[115,135] Schuell et al summarized the state and nature of the long-term memory abilities in persons with aphasia:

> Aphasic patients keep appointments and appear on time, even when the regular hour is changed, if they understand the instructions in the first place. They remember assignments and bring the correct materials with them. They return library books when they are due. If they have to go to the dentist when they are scheduled for the clinic, they stop by and report the change of program.
>
> This is quite different from the behavior of a patient with generalized loss of memory. In this condition, the patient who has just received medication forgets he has had it, and asks for it over and over. He forgets that his wife has just left the hospital, and asks again and again if she is coming to see him. This behavior goes on repetitiously all day long, day after day. When the condition is severe, the patient may not remember he has met the clinician before, although he has spent several hours in his office (p 325).[1]

Reporting a case of paroxysmal aphasia, Lecours and Joanette offer a limpid account of the long-term memory abilities of one aphasic patient:

> Brother John remains capable, throughout long spells, to remember events—linguistic or otherwise—that have occurred previously. He will therefore carry out, in the course of a dysphasic episode, verbal instructions given days or weeks before: without being capable of any linguistic recapitulation, inner or overt, he has thus carried on with instructions such as sampling his own deviant speech on magnetic tapes, attempting to write a few words at peak of spell, alerting a third party in order to have one of us informed of the occurrence of a severe dysphasic episode (p 12).[136]

In order to make the previous generalization tenable, the nature of long-term memory must be operationally defined. As used in this context, long-term memory encompasses the storage of both semantic and episodic information. In a general sense, episodic memory is the representation given to context. It is characterized by a high capacity for entries, permanency, and encoding that occcurs in images, associations, spatial arrays, and time codes. Semantic memory has the same computational structure as episodic memory; however, it is coded by the lexicon and the meaning or semantic relationships constructed among its entries.[137,138] Used in the sense that Schuell et al intended,[1] long-term memory refers to the information stored and not to the process of filing new entries into storage or accessing previously stored entries. It is in fact these filing and retrieving cognitive processes that support semantic memory that are always involved in the Aphasics' understanding and production of language. It was these processes assessed by Risse, Rubens, and Jordan in their study of what they referred to as "long-term memory."[139] In this study, they found that Aphasics with inferior frontal lobe and/or basal ganglia lesions were more severely impaired in both the acquisition and long-term retention of word lists than Aphasics with posterior temporoparietal lesions. Conversely, the patients with the posterior lesions had significantly more difficulty with short-term memory tasks than the Aphasics with anterior lesions. In this study, long-term memory was defined as an item that was recalled spontaneously on two successive trials of the nine-item word list administered immediately after its presentation. Recall of items after 60 minutes of intervening activities was also significantly poorer for the Aphasics with anterior lesions. However, recognition of those same items was not significantly different from the Aphasics with anterior lesions or from a normal control group following a filled 60-minute interval. The point here is that this level of memory is not considered "long term" in the sense of being available for general language use to inform oneself or others. One way to assess the long-term lexical store is through a lexical decision task, whereby the patient is asked to judge whether a word is a real or a novel word (one form of a recognition memory task). In this way, the recognition of a lexical item can provide evidence that a word is within the Aphasic's long-term memory, possibly with less contamination of the cognitive supporting processes than by other assessment procedures. The loosening of or "fuzzy" semantic associations in aphasia, about which aphasiologists have speculated, would then represent an aspect of the retrieval process and not the actual structure of the lexical entries themselves. In fact, evidence shows that the size of the lexicon grows in number of entries in the normal adult population, and this growth continues through the geriatric years. There is little reason to believe that the same growth is not true for the Aphasic if the processes necessary for entering new information into the long-term semantic store are intact or at least operational. In short, there is abundant evidence that the contents of long-term storage systems (both episodic and semantic) remain relatively intact with aphasia-producing lesions.

Several tentative conclusions can be made about the nature of memory processes in aphasia.

1. Although sensory (iconic and echoic) memory does not appear to have been directly studied in Aphasics, some experimental evidence shows that iconic memory is intact.
2. Short-term memory is disturbed in Aphasics to a greater extent than in Normals or brain-damaged Nonaphasics, in terms of total number of units stored and in memory for sequences.
3. Although memory for nonverbal stimuli is usually better than memory for verbal stimuli, both may be impaired in aphasia.
4. The short-term memory deficits appear to be caused by perceptual (e.g., feedback) problems, information processing inefficiencies (e.g., psychophysiologic inertia) as well as rehearsal, naming, and capacity deficits.
5. The style of the search of short-term memory appears to be an exhaustive one like that of Normals; however, individual Aphasics may adopt a self-terminating search strategy.
6. Aphasics appear inefficient at employing top-down clustering and organizing strategies.

VERBAL VERSUS NONVERBAL

While the debate continues among aphasiologists with reference to the specificity of the verbal deficits that define aphasia, the literature continues to mount in support of a coexisting nonverbal symbolic deficit along with the verbal symbolic (linguistic) one. Aphasics have been shown to be disordered in the formation of nonverbally mediated associations,[88,140,141] pantomime expression,[142] pantomime comprehension,[143] nonverbal problem-solving and categorization,[144] and a variety of other cognitive functions, including spatial map orientation and short-term memory for nonverbal material. Although aphasiologists generally agree that Aphasics do not suffer a general intellectual deficit, sufficient evidence makes it necessary to acknowledge these nonverbal deficits and entertain the possibility of a shared underlying mechanism with the verbal deficits.

CORTICAL VERSUS SUBCORTICAL DAMAGE

Since Wernicke,[145] the great majority of model builders have described the cerebral representation of language as consisting primarily of cortical centers and pathways. When subcortical structures were considered, they were included only when the pathways connecting them to the cortex were disrupted. Although these center and pathway models still predominate, their scope has expanded to include a variety of subcortical structures, which, when damaged, create aphasic behaviors indistinguishable in several respects from those produced by cortical lesions. Subcortical structures, currently considered as aphasia-producing when lesioned, include the (1) insula,[146] (2) thalamus,[147] (3) caudate and lenticular nuclei,[148] (4) putamen,[149] (5) globus pallidus,[150] and (6) white matter subserving the frontal, temporal, and parietal lobes.[150]

Whether or not these more recently described aphasia-producing lesion sites continue to be conceptualized on center and pathway models, as the cortical systems have been misconceptualized, remains a matter for further investigation and debate. However, little doubt remains that the hegemony given the cortex as the genesis of all aphasic behavior is in need of, and in the process of, serious revision.

UNI- VERSUS MULTIDIMENSIONAL (ACROSS COGNITIVE AND LINGUISTIC DOMAINS)

Most of the research on aphasia in recent times has attempted to differentiate types of aphasia by the linguistic level that is impaired (e.g., pragmatic, semantic, syntactic, phonologic). The conclusion required from Darley's review of studies attempting to confirm a linguistic-level specific deficit as a basis for aphasic subtypes[151] is that the supportive evidence is extremely weak. Research since Darley's 1982 review[33] has proliferated with the same goals. From this research, one must reach the same equally disappointing conclusion that the current models of linguistic structure do not adequately predict nor explain the experimental findings. Generally speaking, the comprehension abilities of the aphasic person differ along linguistic dimensions quantitatively but not qualitatively.[70] Many studies have failed to differentiate aphasic subtypes at the syntactic level,[152–159] at the semantic level,[36,152,158,160] and at the phonologic and suprasegmental levels.[159,161] Furthermore, given the known interaction of linguistic processes at any information processing level[162] and the general interdependence of linguistic levels (see McNeil and Kimelman[70] for a review of such evidence as it relates to aphasia), it would be surprising if a single linguistic level or process would evidence selective impairment at a competence (linguistic structure) level. That is, any deficits found in any selective linguistic domain, such as color naming deficits, likely yield to an explanation of a true pathway disconnection, to a perceptual or motor disorder, or to a deficit of an underlying cognitive structure that supports that particular linguistic operation. An example of this might include the disturbance of short-term memory proposed by Davidoff and Ostergaard[163] for the color anomia found in one patient.

Although it might be possible for data derived from aphasia to inform theories of language use, as Caramazza has suggested,[54] it is in my judgment unlikely that aphasia informs theories of language structure because the language (the units of linguistic information stored in semantic memory and the rules that govern them) is actually not lost by the presence of aphasia. Rather, the access to the language structures and the deposit of new lexical entries or the association of incoming linguistic information is interfered with in the aphasic person. The section that follows elaborates and clarifies these notions.

LOSS (COMPETENCE) VERSUS INTERFERENCE (PERFORMANCE)*

Are the verbal symbol manipulations on which Aphasics evidence trouble actually lost from their repertoire, or are they only inaccessible but somewhere preserved in the sable collectives of their brain? The evidence needed to answer this comes primarily from five sources: (1) the aphasia can be transitory; (2) the Aphasic's performance is variable; (3) the Aphasic is stimulable; and (4) aphasia seems to reside on an aphasia to normal continuum.

Aphasia can be Transient

Epileptogenic Aphasia

Epilepsy is not a particularly newly discovered etiology for aphasia,[74,164–169] nor is it neglected in the recent literature.[136,170–173] Linebaugh et al proposed two instances in which aphasia may be seizure-related.[174] The first differentiates the patients according to etiology (a known etiology, be it postinfarction epilepsy or cortical irritation by neoplasm), and the second instance occurs in persons with epileptiform discharges without identifiable structural pathology. Although both groups evidence aphasia following a seizure, patients in the second group are without language deficits preceding the fit. However, the important point is that in both groups the aphasic behavior is either heightened or only present during the seizure and returns to a baseline level (preictal deficit level or normal) in a short time. The nature of this interictal aphasia is indistinguishable from other more static lesions producing aphasia.[136] In fact, the signs and symptoms have even been described by means of classic classification terminology.[166] One epileptogenic Aphasic was even reported as evidencing several aphasia "types" (global, Wernicke's, conduction, and amnestic [anomic]) over the course of a single seizure.[136] The transitory nature of these ictal aphasia episodes must be interpreted as evidence that aphasia can be caused by an interference (be it electrical, biochemical, psychical) of verbal symbolic processes and that an abolishment of a center or pathway is unnecessary to cause it.

Migraine-Induced Aphasia

Another paroxysmal disorder, in addition to epilepsy, that can cause aphasia is migraine headache.[175,176] Although well-described behavioral data are sparse in patients with migraine, it appears that aphasia can result from any of Wolff's [177] phases of migraine, including (1) vasoconstriction of intracranial arterioles resulting in cerebral ischemia, (2) vasodilation of the extracranial vessels, or (3) the postvascular phase, where edema may be present.[175] The exact nature of the aphasia evidenced by migraine-producing conditions appears to be indistinguishable from aphasia produced by other lesions. It too is transient.

* The terms "competence" and "performance" are not synonymous with "comprehension" and "production." See the treatises by Bloom 3,[188] Ingram 1,[189] and Chapman [190] for discussions of comprehension versus production. Likewise, when used by linguists the terms "competence" and "performance" sometimes carry a special connotation that is not directly analogous to loss and interference. They are intended, in this discussion, to be synonyms. See the discussion by Lesser [72] for the issues as they relate to aphasia.

Structural Cerebral Lesions

The types of identifiable structural lesions that might cause aphasia can be subdivided into several types. The first type of structural lesion is identifiable only (or primarily) on autopsy, whereas the other types are often identifiable by neuroradiographic techniques of various sorts or by chemical laboratory assay such as cerebral spinal fluid or blood analysis. These types of lesions are classically thought to be transient, and in fact are defined by their transitory nature. These include (1) transient ischemic attack (TIA), (2) lacunar infarcts, and (3) reversible ischemic neurologic deficits (RIND).

TIAs, primarily of the middle cerebral artery distribution of the dominant hemisphere, are known to produce aphasia. The effects of a TIA disappear in less than 24 hours.[178–181] Transient aphasia associated with discrete white matter lesions (lacunar infarcts) accompanying the diagnosis of multiple sclerosis has been reported.[29] RIND resulting in aphasia are expected to resolve within a 3-week period and, like TIAs and lacunar infarcts, are characterized by their transitory nature.

Aphasia produced by intracranial pressure constitutes another etiologic category. Relief of the pressure by the surgical repair of a strategically placed aneurysm, the removal of a meningioma or of an intracerebral neoplasm, the evacuation of a subdural or intracerebral hematoma, or the shunting of a ventricle (for the reduction of hydrocephalus*) can improve or alleviate aphasia. Well-documented speech and language data on the recovery from intracranial pressure-induced disorders are essentially nonexistent in the literature.

Infections (e.g., abscess) and metabolic disturbances (e.g., diabetes) make up another lesion type. If treated expediently, these disorders can be reversed, with resultant reversal of behavioral deficits, including aphasia.

The final lesion types are considered more static lesions† and consist of all other lesions that produce aphasia. Thrombotic and embolic etiologies in the dominant hemisphere language area are common aphasia-producing lesions. However, tumor, hemorrhage, arteriovenous malformation, and closed or penetrating head trauma can also cause aphasia. Even though these area-specific etiologies are considered to produce relatively static behavioral deficits, surgical intervention has been shown to produce rather dramatic and relatively fast improvement of aphasia caused by arteriovenous malformation,[182,183] and of aphasia in patients with a malignant neoplasm.[184] In addition to the instances in which aphasia improves rapidly after insult, the physiologic recovery (spontaneous recovery‡) evidenced by most aphasic patients with "static" lesions, which is not attributable to treatment (either medical [chemoelectrical] or behavioral), is not attributable to relearning the use of verbal symbols and must be considered evidence that aphasia can be transitory, at least in part. The nature of the nonrecovered aphasia will be returned to in the section that follows on patient variability.

Aphasia is Variable

There are an almost infinitely large number of factors that determine whether a person with aphasia receives, recognizes, perceives, comprehends, retrieves, programs, executes, and hence produces a symbolic unit. At any of these operations, performance is variable on repeated trials of equally difficult but different units or even on the same unit. This variability can occur over a period of seconds, minutes, hours, or from day to day. In order for this variability to be detected, four distinctive characteristics of the measuring instrument must be present. (See McNeil and Prescott[185] for a more complete discussion of these issues along with examples of their control in test design.)

First, the test items used to assess any function or set of functions at any single level of difficulty *within* a given subtest must be homogeneous.[186] The stimuli used to elicit a response, the modalities used for receiving the test stimuli, the test instructions, and the responses themselves must be the same from item to item. Similarly, such factors as the amount of response required, the linguistic status, familiarity, and the length of the task must be held constant within any given subtest. This content homogeneity is determined by performing a conceptual evaluation of the tasks. This evaluation must be performed on every possible dimension that has been shown to influence performance on that task (an evaluation of content validity) or that could logically be expected to influence it. This evaluation is usually accom-

* Hydrocephalus would not be expected to produce aphasia in the absence of other disturbed mental functions, and thus the general picture of an improved dementia (including language functions) would be expected.

† Static does not mean that the lesion cannot change in character, but the effects of the lesion are usually considered to be more stable over time.

‡ The term *spontaneous recovery* is the common term used to describe the natural resolution of the aphasia which occurs between 1 month[3] and 6 months[191] after onset. The term is an unfortunate one, because it has a very different meaning in the experimental psychology literature, and it does not accurately reflect the gradual, albeit unaided, recovery of functions.

plished by a statistical determination of the internal consistency of the stimuli and the tasks within each subtest (see Cronback[187] for a further discussion of the importance of, and methods used in determining, internal consistency).

The second requirement of a test used to evaluate variability is that there are an adequate number of homogeneous test items within a given subtest. The exact number of test items that constitutes adequacy for a given task may vary with the severity of the aphasia and the difficulty of the task. However, in most instances, two or three items are clearly not enough, and ten appears to be a maximum number needed for eliciting the variability that is attributed to something other than the task demands.[128,185]

The third requirement for measuring variability is that the instrument (test-retest), the same judge (intrajudge), and different judges (interjudge) are all proven reliable so that if changes on the same task occur from item to item or from day to day, it can be reliably judged to be the result of the patient's performance and not the instability of the test or the testers.

The fourth requirement is that the system used to evaluate performance is valid and sensitive to small amounts and subtle indications of aphasia. Plus-minus (correct-incorrect) scoring methods are, in most instances, inadequate to detect variability in aphasia. Rating scales, category scales, and descriptive methods may prove more appropriate for assessing subtle but important fluctuations in behavior. The multidimensional scoring system developed by Porch[128] and modified by McNeil and Prescott[185] and Marshall[192] appears most appropriate and probably necessary for an accurate measurement of the moment-to-moment variability displayed by persons with aphasia.

Given these characteristics of the tool, it is possible to determine whether the task or how much of the task (be it auditory comprehension, naming, writing, reading, gesturing) is within the patient's repertoire. For example, take ten homogeneous items that are scored with a 15-point multidimensional scoring system. If a score of 15 is what nonaphasic "normal" persons would do on this task, one can call this the target. If the patient can reliably (from test to retest) perform one or more of the test items at a 14-point level (McNeil[60] reported high test-retest reliability for aphasic subjects for this sort of measure), then one can state with some confidence that the ability to perform this task at this difficulty level is within the patient's repertoire. The difference between the target and the highest level performed may be considered the amount *lost*. All scores falling below the top performance level may be considered the deficit that is due to fluctuations within the individual, not attributable to the difficulty of the task per se. One can possibly convert these figures to percentages of deficit, which are then accounted for by either a loss of ability or an inconsistent performance of the task due to some internal state factors. This variability in performance, which is attributable to internal state factors, has been found recently to occur to a rather striking degree.[60] Table 25–3 summarizes this percentage of internal state factor deficit for 30 left hemisphere-damaged Aphasics and for 30 right hemisphere-damaged Nonaphasics on the ten multidimensionally scored subtests of the Revised Token Test. The difficulty of the subtest as indicated by the subtest mean score, was found to correlate reasonably highly with the internal state factor value for most subtests; however, some subtests did not correlate highly at all.[60] This finding was interpreted as evidence that the internal state factor measure is independent of the severity of the deficit. The fact that overall only 12 percent of the deficit that the aphasic group showed was attributable to a loss of ability to perform the task must be considered as substantive evidence that lost ability (auditory comprehension in this instance) plays a small role in making Aphasics perform the way they do. Even at the loss levels reported in these data, the ability to do the task at some reduced level of efficiency is present. Only the most severely (e.g., globally) involved patient does not perform the task at all and then probably only when the behavior is judged on a plus-minus basis. This reduced efficiency appears to be the case across all types of aphasia and across all psycholinguistic operations. One need only look at the standard deviations for groups on any task to note the variability around the mean across or within individuals. For example, patients with Broca's aphasia are not without function words; they may be inordinately impaired in their use compared to another type of Aphasic, but even then, the impairment of function words would not be expected to be present in any consistent manner (See Zurif[193] for possible mechanisms, and Berndt and Caramazza[194] for a review of the syndrome). Likewise, patients with Wernicke's aphasia are not without auditory comprehension on any dimension. They may be inordinately impaired in their use of the auditory system compared to those with Broca's aphasia,[195] and, on some dimensions of auditory comprehension, they are indistinguishable from those with Broca's aphasia, even on the severity continuum.[160]

It should be noted that these are conservative estimates of the amount of deficit that is attributable to internal state factors. It may be that literally 100 percent of the deficit is a performance deficit, and 0.0 percent is actually lost because all of the deficit is judged by performance. If the Aphasic can be induced to perform the task at a normal or target level, then preserved competence can be argued for. Nonetheless, if the Aphasic reliably demonstrates a particular type or level of deficit, as those subjects reported by McNeil[60] they can be considered to be functionally incompetent to that degree. Conversely, to the Aphasic, one would hypothesize that the percentage of internal state factor deficit which the right hemisphere-damaged nonaphasic subjects would show would be even greater than that of the Aphasics, since they are without a frank aphasia or language deficit. This result would be predicted if the construct and tasks were actually measuring something specific to competence and performance in aphasia. The severity of auditory processing deficits evidenced by the right hemisphere-damaged nonaphasic group on these tasks was less than the aphasic group; however, they had significantly more difficulty than the normal subjects.[185] The 98 percent internal state factor deficit (see Table 25–3) offers concurrent validity to support the concept that there is little language loss per se, and the difficulty experienced in this particular task is attributable to a performance—not a competence—deficit.

What is the nature of the nonphysiologically recovered disability—the loss and the performance deficit? The deficit that was characterized as a loss, may in most instances, be characterized as a more severe degree of the performance deficit, but probably not different in quality or mechanism. Like the performance deficit, the loss appears to be an inaccessibility or inefficiency in the basic physiology or in the psycholinguistic and cognitive operations performed in the use of language. Support for this notion comes from the fact that under ideal conditions, some of the functions most severely impaired have been elicited. Jackson described several examples of this,[65] one of which was a lady who, with the following exception, used only the verbal automization "yes, but you know," for 6 months between the onset of her language deficit and her death. When she saw a child in an injurious situation, she yelled "take care." Other aphasiologists have followed Jackson's notions about the educing effects of manipulating automaticity and propositionality[72,196–199] and have described its facilitative effects on even the most difficult speech-language operations. The fact that the material was available for use must be interpreted as evidence that the linguistic units were not lost, but rather inaccessible. Other methods used for the facilitation of performance deficits will be described in the subsequent stimulation and treatment sections.

McNeil[60] has suggested that any mechanism proposed for the explanation of the performance deficit in aphasia must account for several seemingly disparate phenomena.

1. The mechanism must be consistent with a general inefficiency of processing, independent of the hemisphere of damage, presence of aphasia, or even the presence of brain damage (i.e., it should be expected to occur in normal nonbrain-damaged persons).
2. The mechanism must be consistent with an internally generated but environmentally modified mechanism.
3. The mechanism must be intermittently variable, but reliably so.
4. Whatever form this nonaphasic-specific cyclical generator takes, it must be at the base of a psychological process that is capable of being focused or allocated to specific cognitive operations, such as verbal symbolic operations.

Another approach to variability is that which can *invariably* be observed across modalities. If language is stored, housed, and retrieved from a "central language processor," then abilities demonstrated on one modality but not on another can be argued as evidence that that particular linguistic unit or psycholinguistic skill is not lost, but for some reason is inaccessible at that particular time. A review of the profiles on the PICA,[128] which allows cross-modality comparisons, reveals that it is the extremely rare patient who performs without modality variability. For this and other reasons, Weigl and Bierwisch[200] dismissed as absurd the proposition advocated by Whitaker[201] that some linguistic functions or psycholinguistic operations might have their own independent loss of competencies. Whitaker

TABLE 25–3 Percentage of Deficit on Revised Token Test Subtests which are Accounted for by Internal State Factors for Aphasic and Nonaphasic Brain-Damaged Adults

	Revised Token Test Subtests										
Subject Group	*I*	*II*	*III*	*IV*	*V*	*VI*	*VII*	*VIII*	*IX*	*X*	*A*
Left-hemisphere damaged:											
Aphasic	99	98	89	85	84	81	83	72	87	94	87
Right-hemisphere damaged:											
Nonaphasic	100	100	94	96*	99*	96*	95	97*	100*	100	98

* = $p < 0.05$ between groups.

proposed a central language system that, when damaged, produced a competence deficit, and a peripheral language modalities system that, when damaged, produced a performance deficit. Indeed, the importance of establishing a competency loss in aphasia led Whitaker to suggest that since aphasia results from brain damage,[202] the idea that brain damage would not produce a loss of a linguistic ability would imply that language and competence have no representation in the brain. To Whitaker this idea, of course, would be untenable, and would all but eliminate any hope of finding a neural analogue of language in the brain. Two lines of evidence make Whitaker's position rather untenable. First, if aphasia is a multimodality disorder that affects the central language processor, and is defined as such, then the peripheral language modality-specific disorders are not really aphasia per se, but are akin to Schuell's complications of aphasia that often, if not always, accompany it. The subjects on which the variability data were collected in most of the studies reported here, and on the variability data presented from the Revised Token Test, were all multimodality disordered Aphasics. Their performance therefore cannot be construed as evidence for a loss or a competence deficit. Second, if language were represented in the brain more diffusely than current and classic connectionistic neurology has proposed,[45] then isolated lesions that cause aphasia would not be expected to devastate a particular function or operation (be it competence for social acceptability, output, input, phonology, syntax, semantics).[72]

Language competence has also been assessed through a variety of metalinguistic tasks that attempt to determine Aphasics' intuitive knowledge of the language. Like all tasks, these metalinguistic tasks are subject to the same performance variations. Therefore, if a subject does the task, one can say with some assurance that that patient has the knowledge of that particular skill or structure. However, if the task is not performed or is performed incorrectly, little assurance can be given that the patient does not have the knowledge. In addition, metalinguistic judgments are often difficult for normal nonaphasic individuals who can display a normal use of the language for those same structures about which they cannot intuit.

Before describing the third source of evidence for a loss versus interference of language—the manipulability of the Aphasic—discussing the source of the variability seems appropriate. It was stated earlier that the performance deficit appears to be an inefficiency in the system(s). With a goal of describing basic neurophysiologic mechanisms that cause the performance deficit, it seems expedient to search for the source of the inefficiency. One way to approach this task is to review those mechanisms that have been proposed by our aphasiology predecessors to explain nonlanguage performance deficits. Table 25–4 is a summary of many of the nonlanguage (nonaphasic) characteristics of Aphasics frequently mentioned in the literature. Any of these pathologic conditions can mask, be confused with, or simply interact with the other more specific symptoms of aphasia. Thus differential diagnosis and careful appraisal are obviously imperative. However, their further delineation is beyond the scope of this chapter. But more germane to this discussion are the neurophysiological deficits listed in Table 25–4. Some of these "nonaphasic-specific" deficits, which have been mentioned in the literature, deserve special consideration for their potential in explaining the source of performance deficits and hence much of aphasia. They have been described as "nonlanguage deviations in aphasia" by Wepman,[203] as a "generalized reduction in efficiency after brain damage" and "change in dynamic neurophysiological processes" by Lesser,[72] and as the "fundamental disorders in aphasia" by Kreindler and Fradis.[214] What follows is a brief discussion of the first three neurophysiologic deficits with an elaboration of the final three. The other two disturbed processes, variability and reduced efficiency (often mentioned together), are addressed more completely elsewhere in this chapter. However, variability is consistently mentioned in the literature[1,9,210] as a striking if not fundamental feature of aphasia:

> In almost no other disability is as much inconsistency of behavior to be noted (p 32).[203]

> Aphasic patients show great variability and inconsistency of response . . . (p 72).[212]

> An inconstant response is one of the most striking results produced by a lesion of the cerebral cortex. . . . It is not a sufficient test to hold up some object and ask the patient to name it; at one time he may be able to do so, at another he fails completely (p 145).[9]

In fact, Kreindler and Fradis include variability as one of the "fundamental deficits common to all aphasic patients."[214] Although this seems to be true, it is best viewed as a symptom of some neurophysiologic malfunction and not the malfunction per se. Similarly, a reduction of efficiency of many processes seems to characterize aphasia well, but this inefficiency does not account for the variability common to all Aphasics.

Increased performance time is a well-documented characteristic of aphasic performance.[23,109,214] Kreindler and Fradis'[214] summary of their experiments on the

TABLE 25–4 General Sources, Review, and Deliniative Sources (in Parentheses) and Nonaphasic (not Peculiar to Aphasics) Sensory, Motor, Higher Cognitive, and Psychosocial Characteristics that Accompany Aphasia

Literature Source	*"Nonaphasic" Characteristic Sensory*
Lesser[72]	Visual field defects including neglect and hemi-inattention[204]
Jenkins et al[69]	Peripheral hearing disorders[205]
Lesser[72]	
Jenkins et al[69]	Auditory agnosia[206]
Lesser[72]	
Lesser[72]	Word-deafness[25,27]
Lesser[72]	Visual agnosia[207,208]
Jenkins et al[69]	Auditory discrimination
Jenkins et al[69]	Visual discrimination
	Motor
Wepman[203]	Limb paralysis or paresis
Lesser[72]	
Jenkins et al[69]	Apraxia of speech[209,210]
Lesser[72]	
Jenkins et al[69]	Dysarthria[209,211]
Lesser[72]	
Wepman[203]	Psychomotor retardation
	Higher Cognitive
Wepman[203]	Loss of recent and past memory
Wepman[203]	Reduced association of ideas
Wepman[203]	Loss of abstract ability[13]
Wepman[203]	Poor organizing ability
Wepman[203]	Poor judgment
Wepman[203]	Constriction of thought and interest
Wepman[203]	Reduced generalization and categorization ability
Wepman[203]	Reduced ability to inhibit internal emotional forces
Eisenson[212]	which disturbs the action of the intellect (emotional ability)[213]
Wepman[203]	Reduced spontaneity
Wepman[203]	Impulsiveness
Wepman[203]	Inability to correct behavior when recognized as wrong
	Psychosocial
Wepman[203]	Feelings of inadequacy
Wepman[203]	Egocentricity
Wepman[203]	Increased irritability
Wepman[203]	Euphoria
Eisenson[203]	
Wepman[203]	Social withdrawal and seclusiveness
Wepman[203]	Reduced ability to adjust to new situations
Wepman[203]	*Catastrophic reactions[13]
Wepman[203]	Reduced initiative
Jenkins et al[69]	
Wepman[203]	Disinterest in the environment, both physical and human
Wepman[203]	Lack of introspection or self-criticism
Wepman[203]	Automatic verbalization
Wepman[203]	Distrust of own ability
Jenkins et al[69]	Change in attitude toward communication
Eisenson[212]	General depression
Eisenson[212]	Guilt
Wepman[203]	Regressive, infantile behavior
Wepman[203]	Posttraumatic psychotic behavior showing illusions, hallucinations, delusions, and extravagant behavior
Wepman[203]	Anxiety and tension
Eisenson[212]	
Wepman[203]	Changing personality profile (the emergence and submergence of characteristics)
	Basic Neurophysiologic Processes
Goldstein[13]	Increased performance time
Kreindler and Fradis[214]	
Lesser[72]	

TABLE 25–4 Continued

Literature Source	*"Nonaphasic" Characteristic Sensory*
Goldstein[13] Kreindler and Fradis[214] Lesser[72]	Increased perceptual threshold
Kreindler and Fradis[214] Lesser[72]	Disordered temporal nervous processes
Kreindler and Fradis[214] Lesser[72]	Generally reduced efficiency (aphasic → normal continuum)
Wepman[203] Schuell et al[1] Kreindler and Fradis[214] Eisenson[212] Lesser[72]	Variability in performance
Goldstein[13]	Increased inertia (inertness of excitation and inhibition processes—perseveration)
Wepman[203] Kreindler and Fradis[214] Eisenson[212] Lesser[72]	
Wepman[203] Shuell et al[1] Kreindler and Fradis[214] Lesser[72]	Increased fatigability (adaptation and habituation)
Wepman[203] Kreindler and Fradis[214] Jenkins et al[69] Lesser[72]	Disordered attentional processes

* "Catastrophic reaction" is a term used by Goldstein to refer to reactions he observed when patients were faced with a problem that was extremely difficult for them. He said they reacted in the following way: ". . . looks dazed, changes color, becomes agitated, anxious, begins to fumble, his pulse may become irregular; a moment before amicable, he is now sullen, evasive, exhibits temper or even becomes aggressive." This maladaptive behavior is exceedingly rare in aphasics, and the agressive behavior is even more rare. Its frequency and importance have been overrated by Wepman[203] and others.

time taken to initiate a response and the time taken to complete the response provides an accurate summary of other's data as well: ". . . we have been able to establish that the increase in performance latency and duration is common to all aphasics and, interestingly enough, not only in the case of verbal performance, but also in tests where both the stimulus and the response were nonverbal" (p 65).

When the responses were correct, as they often were, these findings could be interpreted as evidence of a general inefficiency. However, these authors reported intermittent variability in the latency of responses (a naming task in this instance) of 2.95, 3.60, 2.58, 2.17, and 1.17 seconds. Inefficiency alone cannot account for this intermittent variability.

Altered perceptual thresholds and altered temporal processes have been documented in aphasic patients on a variety of tasks and across modalities. These disturbed processes include intensity difference limens[215,216] spatial processes in the auditory and visual modalities,[217,218] temporal perception,[132,219–225] temporal resolution,[226–229] auditory duration,[215] and speech and nonspeech rate perception.[230–233]

Increased inertia is a term used by Birch et al[234] to describe the increase in time required by the affected system to process information and recover from the effects of preceding stimulation. Increased inertia is then reflected in the increased latency of responding and in the increased recovery time (a mechanism that could account for part of Kreindler and Fradis'[214] "inability to shift" tasks, and Porch's "slow rise time" and "noise buildup" as described by Brookshire.[224] Kreindler and Fradis[214] described a phenomenon that shares a similarity of title and possible neurophysiologic mechanism with inertia, but implies a difference in behavior. Inertness of excitation and inhibition is the mechanism to which they attribute one of the most frequently noted aphasic deficits: perseveration. In their description of perseveration, they state,

> It [perseveration] appears both during spontaneous speech and during performance of two different short-spaced tasks. In the latter case, the patient's difficulty in shifting from one stimulus and reaction to another is evidenced by his tendency to fix himself upon the first reaction in which he may continue for a long time, regardless of the stimuli used. This [intoxication] bears on both verbal and non-

verbal reactions, proving that perseveration is general in character (p 66).

Perseverations of speech appear to cross linguistic levels, occuring as semantic, syntactic, and phonologic errors[235,236] and across modalities.[1,237] Kreindler and Fradis[214] also suggest that defects in excitation of inhibition mobility account for the consistently found (across many studies by several researchers and across all of their subjects) disorders in reproducing rhythmic (time altered) tapping with a limb and in Aphasics' difficulty in differentiating stimuli. Goldstein[13] suggested an abnormal spread and duration of stimuli within the CNS as the mechanism of perseveration. Wepman[237] and Rochford[236] both suggest moment-to-moment alterations of attention as the source of perseveration. Leichester et al[238] suggested two mechanisms of perseveration—one due to a previously correct and reinforced response and the second due to the patient's use of irrelevant parameters of the stimuli (attention paid to these attributes). Others[65,239–241] have addressed the prevalence and mechanisms of perseveration in aphasia. These studies show clearly that perseveration could account for some patterns of variability. What is not clear is why a perseverative pattern would be broken and then reappear unless a change in the external environment (including any of the number of stimulus parameters) was associated with this change, or unless there was a variable internal factor such as attention to which the change could be attributed.

Increased fatigability, according to Kreindler and Fradis,[214] is ". . . evidenced by the fact that performances suddenly become bad, or by the fact that he has difficulties in carrying out the tasks. . . . One of the reasons of this fatigue is an overstraining of mobility; fatigue is brought about when difficult tasks are too short-spaced" (p 71). They also mention increased fatigue with verbal as compared to nonverbal tasks. Goldstein[13] viewed fatigue as a defense mechanism that could be hastened by placing the patient in situations that elicited catastrophic reactions. Fatigue, then, should manifest itself as a steady decrease in performance level unless the time between stimuli increases (an external variable). One should note that there are two, possibly more, likely explanations for a steady decrease in performance level across successive stimuli. The first is sensory adaptation, which is roughly equivalent conceptually to effector fatigue, except that it occurs on the input side. The second is habituation, which is a response decrement as a result of repeated stimulation. In this instance, the interjection of a novel stimulus returns performance to its previous level without an alteration in response or in stimulus presentation (as long as the rate is below the absolute refractory period of a nerve).* Nonetheless, for whatever mechanism, the behavioral pattern should be one of a decrease in performance without signs of improvement across consecutive trials.

Disordered attentional processes is the final, and possibly the most important, deficit for explaining some aspects of variability in aphasia. Most texts written by authorities on aphasia have included attentional disorders in their list of factors that could give the clinician difficulty in separating the real aphasic behaviors from those extraneous to it,[72,214,237] but have not discussed its importance nor delineated its role in doing so. The reasons for giving such a languid station to attention may be appreciated, given the station that attention holds in cognitive and information processing theory. Titchener's[242] observation on the discovery of attention as a construct in psychology still holds some value for psychologists and aphasiologists today: ". . . the discovery of attention did not result in any immediate triumph of the experimental method. It was something like the discovery of a hornet's nest: the first touch brought out a whole swarm of insistent problems. . . ." Nonetheless, like many of the other constructs dealt with in this chapter, this construct offers some potential insight into the nature of aphasia that other constructs do not. Unlike their predecessors and contemporaries, Kreindler and Fradis[214] recognized the important contribution that attentional disorders might play in aphasia and devoted an entire chapter to the "concentration and mobility of attention in aphasia." The results of their studies with sizable groups of aphasic subjects demonstrated that they were deficient compared to normal control groups, on several visual-verbal (letters and words), visual-nonverbal (pictures and geometric figures), and auditory-nonverbal (environmental sounds corresponding to the words in both verbal tasks) tasks. They found that with the visual modality, focused attention (vigilance) was significantly worse for the aphasic group and greater difference between groups occurred for the verbal than for the nonverbal tasks. Omissions were more frequent for both Aphasics and Normals than were selection errors and more frequent for verbal than for nonverbal tasks. Auditory attention to nonverbal environmental sounds (e.g., dog barking or a bell ringing) revealed that both subject groups produced more errors of omission (not responding by tapping the table when the target sounds appeared in a random list of foils) than of

* See Sharpless and Jasper[244] and Thompson and Spencer[245] for reviews of habituation and the difficulties in applying this term to brain-damaged humans.

selection (tapping the table when a sound other than the target was presented). However, the difference between the normal and aphasic groups was greatest for the selection errors, where the Aphasics produced 14 times as many as the Normals. Results of the verbal tasks revealed that Normals again made more omission than selection errors, but to the same extent for both spoken letters and words. Aphasics also made more omissions but significantly more errors on spoken letters than on words.

On another task of visual-visual and auditory-visual digit matching, the Aphasics took twice as long as the Normals on both tasks. However, the Aphasics showed great variations in latency from item to item, suggesting to the authors[214] "important fluctuations in focused attention."

From their studies, Kreindler and Fradis[214] reached the following two conclusions that are relevant to this discussion: (1) Aphasics have lower speed in working than normal subjects regardless of the form (expressive, receptive, amnestic, total) of their aphasia; (2) Aphasics are impaired in focused attention. This was evidenced by the fact that in all aphasic forms studied, the number of omissions exceeded that of selection errors and by the fact that moment-to-moment fluctuations occurred frequently.

Kreindler and Fradis also attempted to investigate the type of attention required to follow several stimuli in succession within the setting of a given action and required to shift from one activity or stimulus to another (attention mobility). This mobility of attention was assessed with a visual-visual and auditory-visual match. In the visual-visual presentation, the tasks were to place a card with a two-digit number on it on the same number found on a six-column by six-row array of two-digit numbers. In the auditory-visual presentation, the subject pointed to the correct number from the same visual array. Accuracy and latency of response were the dependent variables. Although attention mobility is an important parameter of attention in general, the tasks reported by these authors appear to assess focused attention and are difficult to interpret in the terms outlined by their definition of attention mobility.

Kahneman[243] proposed a theoretical framework in which a central pool of attention, effort, and capacity was shared by all sensory, integrative, and motor operations, across all modalities. Kahneman's model assumes a limited but variable capacity of attention or effort that can be allocated to any task or set of tasks at one time. The amount of capacity allocated is determined by the effort or attention needed. Need is determined moment to moment by feedback about ongoing events. If a task becomes more demanding, attention is allocated to that neural operation so long as capacity is not exceeded. Figure 25–7 is a reproduction of Kahneman's model illustrating the supply of effort as a function of primary task demands. From his review of the literature and from his own research, Kahneman[243] has concluded that it is not cognitive direction nor motivation that determines the capacity allocated, but rather the task demand. If the task is very easy or very difficult, errors occur, and voluntary attempts to allocate more attention to the task will be unsuccessful even when incentives for better performance are provided.

From Figure 25–7, one can see that there is a linear relationship between effort allocation (solid black line) and demand to the point where the demand (dash-dot line) exceeded the supply. At this

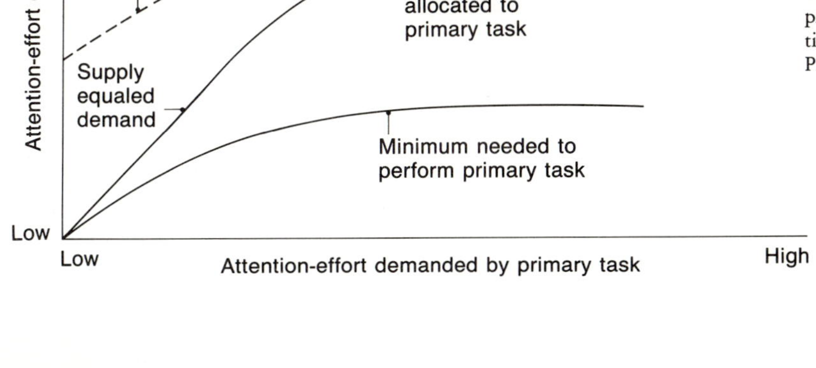

Figure 25–7 Allocation of attention-effort as a function of the demands of the primary task. (After Kahneman D. Attention and effort. Englewood Cliffs, NJ: Prentice-Hall, 1973.)

point, the supply continued to increase slightly to asymptote. One can also see in this figure that there is some spare capacity, most of which is ordinarily (under all but the most unusual and demanding circumstances such as life and death crises) unavailable for use in the primary task. According to Kahneman, *all* life-sustaining and voluntarily directed activities require some part of this central pool of capacity, effort, and attention. It is important to note that capacity (represented by the dashed lines) is variable, and the amount of spare and total capacity is, again, dependent on the demands of the primary task. Therefore, if the primary task demands are low, there is more spare capacity that can be allocated to secondary tasks, but the maximum capacity available is lower than when a more demanding task is called for. The solid dark line below the attention-effort allocation line represents the minimum needed to perform the particular task.

Hageman's[246] review of the literature on attention and on brain damage led him to speculate about the effects of brain damage on Kahneman's attention-effort allocation model. He suggested that when brain damage is present (including aphasia), there is evidence for an overall reduction of maximum capacity, a reduced point on the level of task demand where demand is exceeded by the supply, and a reduced or absent spare capacity. Figure 25–8, a modification of Hageman's proposal, is a representation of this situation; however, this figure deviates from Hageman's in that there is no proposed reduction in the maximum available capacity relative to the level of task demand and no reduced spare capacity. This difference implies two important propositions. First, no real loss of competence occurs, and second, the effort allocation errors would not likely be caused by over-allocation of effort, but would be caused only by undershooting the attention-effort level needed to perform the task (which actually may be more than premorbidly because of general inefficiency in all processing systems due to the brain damage in general). One other point relative to the proposed model must be addressed. If maximum capacity were not reduced, Hageman's model would predict that secondary tasks would be performed without reduced decrement on the primary task because of the amount of spare capacity available. Two factors preclude this. First, the secondary tasks are generally performed inefficiently because of the brain damage. Second, the fact that the capacity is not disturbed is no assurance that under most noncrises or nonclinician-stimulated situations it is available for use. This is another instance in which language competence is presumed and generally unavailable for employment because of the interfering performance factors. With the lowered performance level nearly equaling the task, it is easy to understand why small changes in task demands would cause failure on the task. However, the moment-to-moment fluctuations that occur on a set of items in which little or no change occurs in task demands have still to be dealt with. On the surface, the allocation of attention and effort do not seem to account for these behaviors. However, even in normal nonbrain-damaged individuals, there are continuous fluctuations in all functions including the allocation of attention and effort. On the one hand, the Normal operates at a level high enough above the minimum level to allow up and down variations. On the other hand, the Aphasic has even greater variations in attention and effort

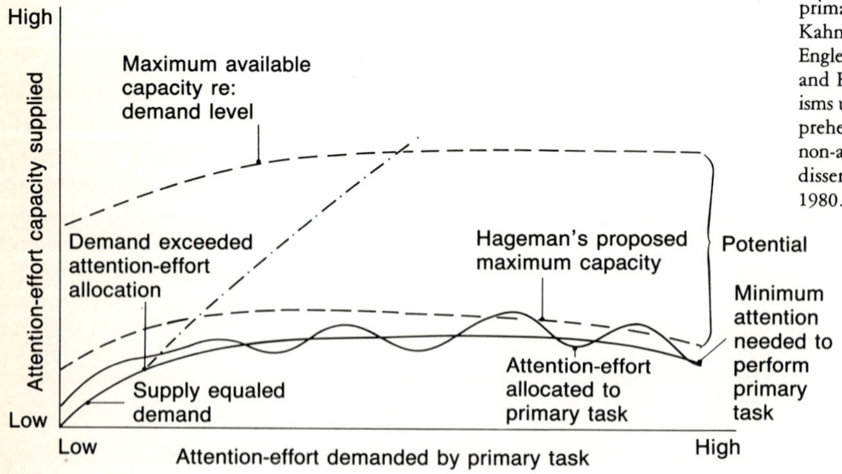

Figure 25–8 Allocation of attention-effort as a function of the demand of the primary task in brain damage. (After Kahneman D. Attention and effort. Englewood Cliffs, NJ: Prentice-Hall, 1973; and Hageman CF. Attentional mechanisms underlying patterns of auditory comprehension in brain-damaged aphasic, non-aphasic and normal listeners. Doctoral dissertation, University of Colorado, 1980.)

allocation and frequently (depending on the specific task demands) and periodically falls below the minimum needed to perform the task. Any call for other service competing with the central pool of attention (almost without regard for the nature of the secondary task) will, in all but the Aphasics with the mildest deficits, interfere with performance on the primary task. This appears to be one possible explanation, or a portion of an explanation, for the high prevalence of the intermittent performance pattern found on sentence level,[130,247] word level, and nonverbal auditory processing tasks,[247] as well as on most other behaviors displayed by patients with aphasia.[214]

McNeil proposed internally generated oscillators as another portion of a possible explanation, in addition to an attention explanation, for the intermittent behaviors.[60] Internally generated oscillators operating on the principle of negative feedback or on the principle of dissipative structures could provide the source for the cyclical behaviors described before. The CNS generates bodily rhythms of various frequencies. Examples of precisely timed biologic rhythms include the cell division cycle, rapid eye movement (REM) sleep cycles, and the menstrual cycle. These cycles are internally generated and can function independently of external influences, or they may be adaptive responses to environmental cycles or external perturbations. There is reason to believe that rhythmic fluctuations underlie all biologic functions including speech, language, and other cognitive functions. Brain damage could diminish an organism's ability to interact appropriately with its environment or could result in the generation of aberrant bodily rhythms.

Oscillations explained as dissipative structures arise from nonlinear systems in which fluctuations are amplified through the organism's interaction with its environment.[248] The more components encompassed within this structure (the organism and its environment), the more interactions that occur, and the more fluctuations away from an equilibrium state result. It is these fluctuations, according to dissipative structure theory, that result from receptivity to perturbations that drive the system to a new average state. Instead of being a mechanism for establishing homeostasis, it is these fluctuations that become the essential elements of such systems. These fluctuations lead not only to cyclical physiologic or behavioral consequences, but also to the formation of new substances in biochemical systems that modify the kinetics of the original system. Dissipative structures have been demonstrated experimentally in biochemical, organic, mineral, biologic, and insect social structures.[248] They have also been proposed to account for much of the variability in human motor performance.[249,250] Although the notion of dissipative structures leads to some potentially important hypotheses about the mechanisms that generate the fluctuations of performance in aphasic persons, there are many factors that need to be established before they can be seriously entertained as an explanatory candidate for the variability that Aphasics have in the use of their language. Perhaps these naturally occurring biologic fluctuations discussed as oscillators or dissipative structures operate on a cognitive system such as attention or resource allocation to create the cyclical variations in verbal behavior that characterize aphasia.

The nature of attention and fluctuating biologic rhythms appears to meet many of the requirements for a mechanism that would explain the disparate phenomena of aphasia mentioned earlier in this chapter. That is, the mechanism must be allocatable in portions or degrees rather than in an all-or-none fashion. It must be present in all individuals independent of the side of hemispheric damage, presence of brain damage, or the presence of aphasia. It must be rapidly variable and under feedback control. Attention is capable of being allocated intermittently, inefficiently, and differentially, either by hemisphere,[251] by cognitive process, or by subcomponent within a cognitive domain (e.g., lexical versus semantic processes within the linguistic domain,[162] or selection versus sequencing within the memory retrieval system). Attention is capable of high-frequency fluctuations[252] and is susceptible to brain damage in nearly any part of the cortex or subcortex,[253] but is probably more susceptible to lesions in and around the classical language areas.[254]

Aphasia is Stimulable

In 1976, Darley[255] reviewed, summarized, and interpreted the available research over the previous 20 years on how the aphasic patient can be stimulated or manipulated to perform at an increased level of accuracy and efficiency. In this erudite review, he quoted the discussion of Schuell et al[1] relative to what it takes to stimulate aphasic patients into operation. Their contentions are well worth reiterating here. Darley,[255] quoting Schuell et al,[1] stated,

> It is our basic premise that an aphasic patient is aphasic because there is a lesion in his brain that interferes with processing of verbal messages. . . . The clinical evidence in aphasia indicates that the language storage system is at least relatively intact . . . but the integrity of previously stored patterns is not a sufficient condition for complex discriminatory and selective behavior. . . . Converging evidence from many lines of research indicates that repeated sensory stimulation is essential for organization,

storage, and retrieval of patterns in the brain, and it would be strange if language patterns operated according to some other principle.

It would seem that sensory stimulation is the only method we have for making complex events happen in the brain . . . the first principle of treatment for aphasia should be the use of intensive auditory stimulation, although not necessarily stimulation through auditory channels alone. . . . We must insure that the stimuli we use get into the brain (p 336–339).

In 1982, Darley[33] expanded his discussion of factors that maximize input to the aphasic person. He reviewed the stimulation methods whereby aphasic patients have been shown to change performance levels because of specific stimulus manipulations. The various categories of stimulus manipulation and the researchers who studied them follow (the categories and the references cited here are not completely consistent with those cited by Darley):

1. Stimulus and contextual characteristics including saliency-redundancy in terms of the loudness of the stimuli,[256] binaural intensity variations of the stimuli,[257] linguistic context,[231] visual perceptual factors,[258,259] modality of presentation,[260] effects of visual and auditory background noise,[261–263] word imagability,[264–266] delayed auditory feedback,[267] and voice channel (live voice versus tape recording).[268,269]
2. Linguistic factors of the stimulus and response, including word frequency,[270,271] syntactic complexity,[272] semantic complexity,[273] grammatic word class,[261] and abstraction level.[274]
3. Stimulus and response length.[233,275]
4. The role of context including prestimulation[269,276–278] and additional simultaneous stimulation.[279,280]
5. Variations in the time dimension, including those that were discussed previously under increased performance time, altered perceptual thresholds, and temporal processes.
6. Scheduling of stimuli presentations, including the benefits of massed versus distributed treatment,[281,282] the methods of sequencing tasks in treatment,[112,283–287] and the scheduling of reinforcement.[288]
7. The importance of attitude.[198,289–292]
8. The content of the therapy, including linguistic unit to be worked on, such as words or words in sentences,[200,285,293,294] content units[295,296] reviewed,[77,199,255,297,298] and how to deal with errors once they arise.[297,299,300]

To Darley's sublime review, a few categories might be added because of their relevance to this discussion. To the stimulus characteristics, Gardner[301] added the notion of operativity, and Gardiner and Brookshire[302] added some literature on the effects of multimodality presentations of the stimulus. Kushner[303] suggested some treatment methods for undesirable social and emotional behaviors in persons with aphasia. Finally, Wepman[304] discussed the importance of self-correction as a prognostic sign in aphasia.

With few exceptions, and then only in those studies designed to illustrate the effectiveness of treatment, these sources have demonstrated that the performance of the aphasic person is manipulable, and this manipulability is not attributable to a relearning of suprasegmental, phonologic, morphologic, syntactic, semantic, or pragmatic rules. Likewise, psychophysiologic reorganization does not account for the ability to appreciate time-altered speech, enlarged print, or real objects as compared to pictures of those objects. Beyond the fact that these studies have illustrated that Aphasics are stimulable, they illustrate that the data are in the Aphasic's repertoire and are not lost, and further proper stimulus and response control can succor those inefficiencies in the systems.

Aphasia to Normal Continuum

Freud[53] and Jenkins et al[69] are among those scholars who have suggested that aphasic persons are qualitatively similar to but quantitatively different from Normals, especially if the Normals are tired, hurried, or dividing their attention. In terms of their reduced available vocabulary and impaired verbal retention span, Jenkins et al state that ". . . aphasics in general make the same kinds of errors but with far greater frequency. In other words, there seems to be evidence that the same cognitive system is involved but is working with much less efficiency" (p 101).

Howes[24] arrived at the same conclusion as Jenkins et al[69] relative to a normal but poorly accessible lexicon.

Shewan and Canter[275] investigated the auditory comprehension of aphasic patients along length and lexical and syntactic complexity. From their results, they suggested that auditory comprehension may be conceived best as a continuum, with Normals representing one pole and patients with Wernicke's aphasia representing the other. They concluded that ". . . the mechanism for understanding language appeared to be much the same for normals and aphasics. However, aphasics seem to operate the mechanism with reduced efficiency" (p 227).

In 1976, Shewan[305] again demonstrated the aphasic to normal continuum with regard to the position of errors on an auditory sentence comprehension task.

In what appears to be the only study of its kind, Hageman[246] attempted to specify further the nature of the aphasic to normal continuum in auditory processing. Using the prevalence of patterns of auditory processing disorders referred to earlier in this chapter as the dependent variables, Hageman attempted to stress the attention-effort capacity of normal nonaphasic subjects with competing auditory processing tasks. The general findings of this study were that the Normals produced significantly better scores than the Aphasics, but the qualitative performances (prevalence of auditory processing pattern type) were nearly identical when the Normals were stressed enough to degrade their performance.

Using a choice reaction-time task to words and nonwords presented auditorily and visually, Jiménez[306] interpreted her findings to show that although the aphasic group performed more slowly than the nonaphasic group, the patterns of performance were similar. Kim[307] reached essentially the same conclusions as Jimenéz on visual and auditory sequencing tasks.

Other researchers have sought to specify the other parameters on which Aphasics perform like Normals, but with a reduced efficiency. These parameters include perceptual speed[308] and several linguistic levels and processes, including semantic and lexical,[24,309,310] pragmatic,[1,119] syntactic,[286,311,312] discourse comprehension,[313–315] and discourse production (story structure and retelling of narratives).[316] In addition, Aphasics have been observed to acquire new material as Normals.[105,106] Many of these authors have suggested from their results that Aphasics operate like Normals when they are stressed or asked to make verbal maneuvers such as word associations. Again, this subtle but important thread that runs through a substantial body of the literature provides evidence that aphasia is not a loss of function, but rather a reduction in efficiency in its employment.

RECOVERY, PROGNOSIS, AND EFFICACY OF TREATMENT

The recovery of function after brain damage is the process by which a particular behavior is reinstated that has been disturbed by the brain injury and most likely involves the utilization of that part of the system that is spared.[317] When brain injury occurs, the potential exists for behaviors (or an absence of behaviors) to arise from any of three sources. First, if a substantial amount of tissue is lost, there is loss of a major function (probably limited to primary sensory and motor functions unless the lesion is extensive) that was in essence housed in that location of the brain. Second, the lesion may produce general (e.g., naming) or secondary (remote) effects on other nondamaged systems. Third, the neural injury may cause the individual to shift behavioral control to unaffected systems.[317]

The most popular explanation for a relatively quick improvement of abilities following the onset of aphasia is physiologic recovery (discussed earlier in this chapter). The explanation for this is that other neural centers specializing in similar functions[318,319] are capable of assuming these "lost" functions (vicariation) or that transformations of the function itself may occur in areas having altogether different functions.[320] This process of reorganization has been suggested as possible, even in the adult human CNS, because of such properties as compensatory and collateral sprouting.[318,319] Several aphasiologists have suggested that the right (language-nondominant) hemisphere is a likely candidate for this assumption of symbolic functions,[320,321] whereas others have suggested that adjacent tissue within the same hemisphere may, or is more likely to, assume the functions,[182,183] possibly with the aid of the language-nondominant hemisphere.

Another possible explanation for the relatively fast return of functions is that there could have been an interfering physiologic state that caused the diminished behavior (e.g., cerebral edema), which resolved and allowed the return of the use of that particular function. In this case, and consistent with the major thesis proposed in this chapter, the function may not have been lost at all because verbal symbolic processes are not stored in discrete locations, but rather are dependent on complex, diffusely organized processes in cortical, subcortical, and possibly nondominant hemisphere substraits. Thus the behavioral defect may be, at least in part, a function of the compensatory strategies that the patient adopts in an attempt to use the function(s) that are interfered with at present.[317] Abundant behavioral and neurophysiologic data from animals (see LeVere[317] for a review), as well as the hierarchy of behavioral deficits used to quantify aphasic deficits on such tools as the PICA[128] and the Revised Token Test,[185,322] seem to substantiate this notion of adapted strategies.

The first issue in recovery is whether or not it occurs. The next issue is what recovers, and, finally, under what circumstance it does or does not recover. Evidence as to whether recovery occurs under any conditions is available. One can state categorically that without additional neurophysiologic or psychological pathology, the majority of aphasic patients can expect some degree of restoration from their symbolic disorders. The physiologic recovery that occurs relatively quickly (2 to 6 months) following the insult, which is not attributed to treatment, has been correlated with a variety of biographical and physiologic patient factors. These same factors have been discussed as important in the determination of candidacy for treatment. Thus it appears that the positive prognostic factors for physiological recovery are those same factors that are related to positive prognoses for treatment. The factors related both positively and negatively to recovery from aphasia are interrelated, are sometimes difficult to quantify, and are documented relatively sparsely in the scientific literature. Both intuition from dedicated clinicians and data from competent researchers provide the sources for these factors. Table 25–5 is a summary of those studies that suggest the positive, negative, or neutral prognostic value of a particular factor. Although the apparent value of each of these factors can be summarized as follows, one must remember that the definitive prognostic value of any variable may not have been established to date.

"Type" of Aphasia

Global aphasia offers a poor prognosis for recovery. However, one must remember that group data may not predict well for an individual. Darley[323] warns us that ". . . no single negative factor is so uniformly potent as to justify excluding a patient from at least a trial of therapy." Presumably, this would encompass type (or severity) of aphasia, in-

TABLE 25–5 Factors Influencing Prognosis and Recovery in Aphasia

Positive Prognostic Value	*Negative Prognostic Value*	*No Prognostic Value*
"Type" of aphasia		
Broca's or expressive [presence of] Weisenberg and McBride,[10] Butfield and Zangwill,[324] Wepman,[203] Longerich and Bordeaux,[325] Messerli et al,[326] Kertesz and McCabe[327]	Schuell et al,[1] Vignolo,[198] Keenan and Brassell[328]	Basso et al[329]
Global [presence of]	Unanimous throughout the literature: Kertesz and McCabe,[327] Schuell et al[1]	
Anomic aphasia [presence of] Kertesz and McCabe[327]		
Familial left handedness in right handers, left handedness or ambidexterity		
Subirana,[330,331] Zangwill,[332] Gloning et al,[333] Luria[320]		
Specific linguistic abilities		
Good writing		Keenan and Brassell[328]
Schuell,[334] Culton,[335] Smith,[107] Porch et al[336]		
Good oral language		
Keenan and Brassell[328]		
Good auditory comprehension		Sarno et al[339]
Keenan and Brassell,[328] Culton,[337] Schuell,[334] Kertesz et al[338]		
Good visual matching		
Hanson and Cicciarelli[340]		
Good reading ability		Keenan and Brassell[328]
Nonlinguistic speech abilities		
High speech stimulability Keenan and Brassell[328]		
Attempted self-correction		
Wepman,[304] Vignolo,[198] Eisenson[341]		
Age		
Youth		Sarno and Levita,[345] Culton,[335] Keenan and Brassel,[328] Kertesz and McCabe,[327] Porch et al[336]
Eisenson,[342] Wepman,[304] Vignolo,[196] Sarno et al,[343] Sands et al,[344] Smith[107]		
Sex		Kertesz and McCabe,[327] Sarno et al[339]
Severity at onset		
Overall severe aphasia	Godfrey and Douglass,[346] Schuell et al,[1] Sands et al,[344] Sarno et al,[339,343] Kertesz and McCabe,[327] Wepman,[203] Hanson and Cicciarelli,[340] Kenin and Swisher,[347] Holland and Sonderman,[300] Porch,[128] Basso et al[348]	

TABLE 25–5 Continued

Positive Prognostic Value	*Negative Prognostic Value*	*No Prognostic Value*
Etiology of aphasia-producing lesion		
Trauma		
Butfield and Zangwill,[324] Frazier and Ingham,[349] Luria,[320] [nonpenetrating]		
Arteriovenous malformation		
McNeil,[183] Kunc,[182] Wertz et al,[350]		
Size and location of lesion		
Small, focal lesions		
General consensus throughout the literature, e.g., Lomas and Kertesz,[351] Kertesz et al,[338]		
Lesions outside the "language areas"		
General consensus		
The initiation of aphasia therapy (efficacy)		
Clinical experience evidence		
Fenelon et al,[352] Luria,[320] Frazier and Ingham,[349] Weisenberg and McBride,[10] Darley,[353] Messerli et al,[326] Eisenson[342]		
Uncontrolled data-based studies		
Butfield and Zangwill,[324] Wepman,[203] Schuell et al,[1] Beyn and Shokhor-Trotskaya,[295] Leischner and Linck,[354] Sands et al,[344] David et al,[355] Dabul and Hanson[356]		Marks et al[357]
Controlled data-base studies		
Perry,[358] Prescott and McNeil,[359] Broida,[360] Wertz et al,[361] Smith,[362] Gloning et al,[363] Vignolo,[198] Basso et al,[329] Hagen,[364] Basso et al,[348] Deal and Deal,[365] Holland,[366] David et al,[355] Shewan and Kertesz,[367] Wertz et al[368]	Sarno et al,[343] Lincoln, Mulley and Jones[369]	
Early initiation of treatment following onset		
Butfield and Zangwill,[324] Wepman,[203] Vignolo,[198] Sands et al,[344] Kertesz and McCabe,[327] Basso et al,[348] Leischner and Linck,[354] Basso et al,[329] Deal and Deal[365]		Wertz et al[368]
Psychosociologic factors		
High regularity of employment		Keenan and Brassell[328]
High occupational status		Sarno et al[339]
High education level	Eisenson[341]	Sarno et al,[339] Basso et al[329]
Poor current living environment		Sarno et al,[339] Stoicheff[289]
Good general health		
Eisenson,[342] Leischner and Linck[354]		Keenan and Brassell[328]
Presence of concomitant sensorimotor deficits	Eisenson,[341] Schuell et al,[1]	
High preillness language proficiency		Sarno et al[339]
High premorbid intelligence	Eisenson[370]	
Wepman,[203] Messerli et al[326]		
Presence of personality deviations	Eisenson,[342,370] Wepman[203,371]	

cluding those with concomitant nonlanguage higher cognitive involvement. Those Aphasics with Broca's aphasia appear to recover differently across studies. Partial account may be paid to the differences in defining subject types across studies and certainly other potent prognostic factors such as severity interact to make comparisons difficult. Nonetheless, the available literature suggests that persons with Broca's aphasia (possibly those with "little Broca's" aphasia[30]) offer a better prognosis than persons with several other aphasic syndromes. Anomic aphasia, almost by definition, is less severe than other syndromes and appears to offer a good prognosis for recovery.[327]

Table 25–6 summarizes the results of Kertesz and McCabe's[327] study on recovery of aphasia by syndrome. From these data, one can see that for those aphasic patients who did evolve, the majority either evolved into an anomic category or recovered completely, irrespective of the classification from which they came. In most cases (with the possible exceptions of the evolution of the Broca's to a transcortical motor aphasia, and the evolution of the Wernicke's to a global aphasia), the evolution suggests a progression to a less severe degree of aphasia. In addition, the higher percentage of subjects who did not change from one syndrome to another might suggest a poorer prognosis for a given syndrome (e.g., Broca's aphasia). However, this would be a fallacious interpretation because the range of severity of all aphasic symptoms can vary within a syndrome to the

TABLE 25–6 Evolution of the Recovery Process in Aphasia

Initial Classification (percent of syndrome remaining unchanged)	*Final Classification Evolved to*	*Percentage Evolved (%)*
Global—N = 22 (77%)	Broca's—N = 2	9
	Transcortical motor—N = 1	5
	Conduction—N = 1	5
	Anomic—N = 1	5
Broca's—N = 17 (76%)	Transcortical motor—N = 1	6
	Anomic—N = 3	18
Conduction—N = 8 (13%)	Anomic—N = 2	25
	Nonaphasic—N = 5	63
Wernicke—N = 13 (46%)	Global—N = 1	8
	Transcortical sensory—N = 1	8
	Anomic—N = 4	31
Isolation—N = 2 (50%)	Anomic—N = 1	50
Transcortical motor—N = 3 (0%)	Anomic—N = 2	67
	Nonaphasic—N = 1	33
Transcortical sensory—N = 3 (0%)	Anomic—N = 1	33
	Nonaphasic—N = 2	67
Anomic—N = 25 (52%)	Nonaphasic—N = 12	48
Summary—N = 93	All classification—N = 40	43
	Broca's—N = 2	5
	Conduction—N = 1	3
	Anomic—N = 14	35
	Global—N = 1	3
	Transcortical motor—N = 2	5
	Transcortical sensory—N = 1	3
	Nonaphasic—completely recovered—N = 20	50

After Kertesz A. Aphasia and associated disorders: taxonomy, localization and recovery. New York: Grune & Stratton, 1979.[373]

same degree that they can vary between syndromes. For example, a patient with Broca's aphasia can range in reading, writing, and talking skills from one so severely affected as to be rendered "severely" noncommunicative to one whose communicative disability might be evident only to him- or herself and then only under unusually stressful conditions. Thus, with the exception of global aphasia, the syndrome type is a poor predictor of severity of involvement, and evolution from one type to another is not synonymous with improvement. Even in "global" aphasia, the prognosis is far from doomed or even prescribed because of the label or the syndrome to which they are assigned.[89]

In actuality, it is highly unlikely that any aphasic individual recovers "completely." If a complete recovery is suggested by test results, it is most likely a function of the insensitivity of the test or the limited range of cognitive-linguistic-communicative skills assessed by the test. Nonetheless, it is apparent from Kertesz and McCabe[327] that a substantial number of Aphasics (approximately 22 percent recovered "completely") can be expected to make substantive improvements following the onset of aphasia. This improvement is particularly likely if they begin with behaviors consistent with transcortical, anomic, or conduction aphasia.

Familial Left Handedness in Right Handers; Left Handedness or Ambidexterity

The available literature suggests that persons who have a familial history of left-handedness, even though they themselves are right-handed, and who become aphasic because of a left-hemisphere insult, have a better prognosis than right-handers without a familial left-handed history. Similarly, left handers and ambidextrous Aphasics offer a better prognosis than right handers. The hypothesized reason offered for this is that language is more lateralized in one hemisphere (usually the left) in the right handers and thus suffers greater interference with a unilateral lesion and less interference in bilaterally organized brains. It also follows then that the nonright handers should suffer aphasia with a lesion in either hemisphere. However, it must be cautioned that there is much less than perfect correlation between handedness and hemispheric dominance for language, and handedness varies greatly depending on how it is measured.[372,372a] Similarly, the establishment of degree of hemisphere dominance for language may vary greatly within the same individual depending on the method of assessment.

Specific Linguistic Abilities

Good writing, oral language, auditory comprehension, and visual matching early after onset have been shown to be of positive prognostic value. Of those functions that have been studied, only high reading ability seems to offer no predictive power. Whether poor linguistic abilities are of equally poor prognostic value has not been established; however, it is likely that that would be the case.

Nonlinguistic Speech Abilities

The ease with which aphasic behavior can be modified shortly after onset was found to be a positive prognostic sign. Similarly, successful and attempted self-initiated corrections of errors have been shown to suggest consistently the ability to detect and change erroneous behaviors, both important abilities involved in the recovery process.

Age

Unless the Aphasic is severely affected and old, age appears to play a small or clinically unimportant role in recovery. Again, age, etiology (younger Aphasics tend to become aphasic by traumatic accidents), and severity appear to interact in ways that make isolation of one biographical variable difficult. Nonetheless, in general, age does not appear to be a potent variable influencing recovery.

Sex

The sex of the individual does not appear to influence recovery, given the data available to date.

Severity at Onset

The more severe the aphasia and the more pronounced the concomitant sensory and motor deficits, the poorer the prognosis. This relationship is potentially the most important variable affecting prognosis. Interpolation from Porch's recovery profiles[374] suggests that patients between the fortieth and sixtieth percentiles on the PICA at 1 month after onset offer the probability of the most recovery at 6 months after onset. This does not mean that patients above or below this level do not offer a favorable prognosis.

Etiology of the Aphasia-Producing Lesion

The literature is sparse with respect to controlled studies comparing recovery and prognosis with various etiologies. Traumatic lesions, particularly those that do not penetrate the cranium, appear to offer a better recovery than penetrating head injuries, including surgery, and other etiologies such as thrombotic or embolic infarcts. Arteriovenous malformations have been suggested to offer a better prognosis than thrombotic, embolic, traumatic, or surgical etiologies. However, the number of subjects on which these data are based is too small for strong conclusions.

Size and Location of Lesions

Given the fact that any lesion must be rather focally located to cause aphasia only, small lesions invariably offer a better prognosis for recovery of speech and language. A large lesion located outside the classic "language areas," as described earlier in this chapter, may offer a better prognosis than a small focal lesion in a critical zone. Thus size and location interact.

Initiation of Aphasia Therapy (Efficacy)

Although there are no all-or-none statements about any factor's influence on recovery, that the evidence is overwhelmingly in favor of the notion that treatment affects recovery is apparent from Table 25–5. No studies have suggested a negative influence on recovery with the initiation of treatment, and several have suggested a positive effect. Few studies have evidenced no effect of treatment. The task remains to define who is and who is not a candidate for aphasia treatment as well as the nature of that treatment, including the type, duration, and frequency. However, one can now say with a great deal of confidence that aphasia treatment is efficacious for most persons with aphasia, and physiologic recovery cannot account completely for the gains made during treatment.

Early Initiation of Treatment Following Onset

Current myth suggests that treatment initiated within the first month following onset is likely to result in significantly better overall recovery than treatment initiated thereafter. Although the data are as yet turbid, it appears that the earlier the treatment is initiated, the better the chance that the treatment positively affects recovery. This myth, though not established as dogma, has some of its basis in the belief that the system might be more malleable soon after onset and that maladaptive behaviors are less likely to arise with the early initiation of treatment. However, it should be noted that there is sufficient evidence to suggest that treatment can be efficacious at any duration after onset, and an extended time after onset alone is not sufficient to deny treatment to a potential patient.

Psychosocial Factors

Those psychosocial factors that the aphasic person brings with him or her from his or her premorbid life would be expected to interfere with his or her life situations, at least to the extent that they would interfere with anyone's. In addition, as Darley has suggested, "The aphasic patient has suffered an amputation of his capacity to interact and communicate with his fellow men. . . . This constitutes a threat not only to his earning capacity but to his identity as an individual and a human being" (p 139).[3] The gravity of this situation may vary greatly from patient to patient, and the extent to which the individual is affected and deals with it effectively is the extent to which it may affect prognosis and recovery. Overall, from the scant literature available, only concomitant sensory and motor deficits and frank personality deviations have been found in the literature unchallenged as negative prognostic factors. High regularity of employment, high occupational status, a poor current living environment, and high preillness language proficiency appear to have no prognostic value.

ASSESSMENT

In the design, construction, and standardization of a test for aphasia both theoretical or conceptual and technical issues must be dealt with. The conceptual problem refers to *how* one views aphasia as well as for what purposes the test is to be administered. How one views aphasia is related to the underlying mechanisms that are believed to cause or be most descriptive of the disorder. If one views aphasia as a *loss* of language (the rules or the actual lexicon), the test or assessment procedures may differ dramatically from those based on a view of aphasia as an interference or inefficiency of language processes. Even if an inefficiency explanation is accepted, the disordered language and communicative systems can be approached from a lower level psychophysiologic model, a cybernetic-information processing model, any number of cognitive models, psycholinguistic models, linguistic models, and pragmatic and communicative models. If aphasia is viewed as a disorder crossing many domains, such as those listed before, then the test instrument or assessment procedures must reflect this multiform nature and assess each component, as well as the interaction among components, in as much isolation as possible. It is revealing the obvious to say that no single test or even battery of tests meets these multiform assessment criteria. However, careful test construction and standardization can aid in the delineation of functions for which a particular test can be used. What follows is a brief discussion of those psychometric characteristics against which all tests or assessment procedures for aphasia must be judged.

The technical problems in aphasia testing include a well-documented process of standardizing the test and a well-defined and standardized administration procedure. Four types of validity and at least three types of reliability must be addressed (preferably by the test's author, prior to its publication).

The standardization of a test for aphasia requires—at a minimum—that the population from which the standardization sample was drawn be clearly defined in terms of those variables that the literature has shown to be important to aphasic performance (e.g., sample size, time after onset, etiology, severity). The task and item instructions that are presented to the subject should be clearly specified in such a manner that they are replicable by two different administrators and by the same administrator on two different occasions without themselves influencing performance. The stimuli should be presented in a specified physical arrangement both within and between subtests so that a variation in performance can be judged to be the result of a change within the patient or the change of task demands, and not the stimuli used to elicit the response (unless, of course, the stimuli are the independent variable for the test or subtest). The procedures used in evaluating each response should be clearly described and sufficiently objective to provide for reliability. If special training is required, it must be specified by the author(s) of the test. Porch[374] described from the literature five methods currently in use for scoring behavioral events in aphasic patients.

1. The descriptive method is the process of noting anything that is deemed important by the tester. It offers the advantage of allowing for the possibility of recording a maximum amount of information with a minimum restriction on the scorer. Interjudge, and even intrajudge reliabil-

ity, is usually poor, and scoring relies solely on the skills and biases of the scorer (which may or may not be a liability, depending on the uses to which the data is put). Recording of response information tends to be cumbersome, and interpretation is usually problematic between scorers.

2. The plus-minus scoring method dichotomizes all responses into categories of correct and incorrect. It provides an easy and reliable way of recording responses and tabulating scores, but sacrifices valuable information about the patient's behavior.
3. Rating scales place responses on a scale of goodness according to a predetermined standard of adequacy. Interpretation of test results is difficult because of the subjectivity of steps such as "good" or "fair."
4. Category scales differ from rating scales in that they are clearly defined descriptions of a single dimension of performance, such as the time or accuracy dimension. However, the different levels within this single dimension still add to a scale of goodness and possess the limitations of rating scales.
5. Multidimensional scales incorporate several dimensions of behavior found in the literature, which are believed to be important components of aphasia, into one hierarchically arranged scale. The hierarchy can be arranged to reflect severity of involvement from various points of view, such as communicative acceptability, loss of neural tissue, or recovery of function. Porch[336] introduced multidimensional scoring to aphasia testing with a 16-point scale assessing the accuracy, responsiveness, completeness, promptness, and efficiency dimensions of behavior. The type of scoring or evaluative system chosen to describe behavior depends on a variety of factors. No clear statement can be made about the value of any scoring system compared to the others that applies to all conditions or purposes of testing. In the most general sense, the following hierarchy is offered as a guide to test scoring, from the least desirable to most desirable methods: (1) descriptive, (2) plus-minus, (3) rating scales, (4) category scales, and (5) multidimensional scales.

If normative data are provided for purposes of comparing subjects to a standard (representative) population, then those criteria for deriving the normative data must be presented for examination.

A test's validity can be addressed from several different but related perspectives. Construct validity is the validation of a test's theory and model and is partially related to the conceptual problem of how one views aphasia. Construct validity is evaluated by investigating what psychological qualities the test actually measures. The examination of construct validity requires both an empirical and a logical attack. If a test were to be consistent conceptually with the nature of aphasia as presented in this chapter, then it would in its construction and interpretation reflect the construct that aphasia is an inefficiency of symbolic processing. Further, this inefficiency can vary in degree across modalities, and disorders of memory, retrieval, and attention allocation may be present, as well as inefficient implementation of linguistic rules. The evaluation system would reflect behaviors believed to represent general inefficiency caused by brain damage, as well as specific inefficiency of the interaction between top-down (e.g., linguistic and general intellectual) and bottom-up (psychophysiologic and information processing) processes in addition to the compensatory strategies that are enacted once the system is damaged.

Predictive validity refers to the degree of confidence with which behaviors at a different setting (external validity) can be predicted by current test data. Content validity refers to the degree to which the content of the test is representative of the class of situations or subject matter about which conclusions are to be drawn. Content validity is assessed by critical evaluation of the claims made by the test designer regarding adequacy of test sampling or representativeness of content in relation to the universe of items adopted for reference. The nature of aphasia demands that the test sample a large enough range of tasks in terms of processes and difficulty level that an accurate description of performance can be obtained from the mildly to severely impaired. As discussed earlier in this chapter, a sufficient number of homogeneous items should be included within each subtest to describe performance accurately and reliably, given the great variability of performance within aphasic individuals.

When the actual task that the Aphasic is to perform is selected, the same general criteria apply as for the stimuli selection. The tasks should be homogeneous within a subtest. For example, the input modality, amount of output, output modality, and mode of response should be held constant within each subtest. As discussed earlier, homogeneity is determined logically and with statistical measures of internal consistency. Intrasubtest task homogeneity allows for intersubtest comparison by changing either the task or the response requirements. The task should be carefully controlled so that it is not culturally biased. If the test is culturally loaded, it should be used only for that population on which it was standardized. Similarly, the tasks should not include unusual linguistic structures or content and should be within the range of intellectual normalcy and should not be influenced by educational factors. If education or another biographical factor is present, separate reference data should be presented to account for the differences between patients.

The final set of requirements for an aphasia test is concerned with establishing a coefficient of stability or reliability. Test-retest reliability refers to the stability of the test from one administration to another. The test must be proven stable so that if change occurs it can be accurately judged to have occurred in the patient and not because of the instability of the test.

Intrajudge reliability refers to the demonstrated stability of the test when scored twice by the same tester. It is necessary to establish this reliability so that instability of the results can be reliably judged to be due to the patient's performance and not to administration or scoring. Interjudge reliability suggests that the test must be able to be scored the same way by two or more different judges so that changes that occur can be judged accurately to have occurred in the patient's performance and not in the scoring differences per se. Given the complexity of multidimensional scoring, it may be that reliability can be obtained only by reviewing a taped administration (video or audio). If this is the case, then a fourth type of reliability (live to video and/or audio) should be provided by the test constructor. The desired value of the different reliability coefficients is dependent upon the exact nature of the test and the purposes for which the data are used. Most contemporary aphasia tests report several types of reliability data, and most reach correlation coefficients approaching or above 0.90. Correlation coefficients below 0.70 may be judged too low since they account for less than 50 percent of the variance between test scores.

Assessment Purpose

The reasons why one might use a test designed for aphasia and related disorders are varied. A test may help in the detection or confirmation of a suspected problem. Tests may be used for the determination of lesion localization. Tests may be used for predicting eventual outcome or for candidacy of treatment. A test may also be used for classifying a patient according to a syndrome (a practice for which little clinical justification or utility can be found). It may be used to specify the degree (severity) of involvement, which may influence the type of treatment (treatment focus) that is utilized. An aphasia test might be used in the measurement of change that accompanies treatment, no treatment, or further neurologic insult (as a dependent measure). A test might also help in the determination of treatment termination criteria. Finally, a test may help in the differential diagnosis of aphasia from other disorders resembling it. Table 25–7 summarizes 18 of the most often used and cited aphasia tests along with an evaluation of their most valid and often utilized purposes.

Of the aphasia tests that are presently commercially available, and are summarized in Table 25–7, no single test meets all of the psychometric requirements outlined previously. Most clinical aphasiologists use a battery of tests, one for detection of subtle or "latent" aphasia, another for classification purposes, another for determining a prognosis, possibly another for focusing treatment, and possibly yet another for measuring the external validity of that treatment. As mentioned earlier, the crucial factors are the theoretical underpinnings on which the test is built and the degree to which the test is psychometrically sound, and thus interpretable, as a well-designed and well-executed experiment is interpretable. Table 25–8 further describes these previously outlined and published tests for aphasia, along with a brief evaluation of the tests' primary limitations and assets. Critical reviews of most of the tests (with the exception, for example of the Communicative Abilities in Daily Living,[377] Reading Comprehension Battery for Aphasia[385] and Revised Token Test[185]) have been published by Brookshire[387] and by Darley.[353] Papers by Darley[151] and Linebaugh[388] effectively contrasted and compared the published aphasia tests in the 1979 Volume of *Clinical Aphasiology*. Evaluations of most of the tests can also be found in the most recent issue of Buros' *Mental Measurements Yearbook*.

Keep in mind that the conceptual framework on which the test is built along with the specific purposes for which the test is given determine the instrument chosen. The PICA and the Revised Token Test[185] may be the most psychometrically sound tools available and possibly the most amenable to quantification. They may therefore be well suited for the measurement of patient change. The PICA and the Minnesota Test for Differential Diagnosis of Aphasia[380] appear to offer the most prognostic information and differential diagnostic information. The Revised Token Test[185] and Word Fluency Measure[386] appear to be among the most sensitive to small amounts of impairment (although the Word Fluency Measure[386] has recently been questioned as an appropriate tool because of its test-retest instability). The Communicative Abilities in Daily Living[377] and Functional Communication Profile[378] may be most predictive of communication outside the clinical setting. The Boston Diagnostic Aphasia Examination[62] and the Western Aphasia Battery[66] appear to be the most valid and reliable for cate-

TABLE 25–7 Assessment Purpose

General Test Battery	*Detect/ Confirm*	*Lesion Localization*	*Predict*	*Classify Syndrome*	*Classify Severity*	*Focus Treatment*	*Measure Change*	*Termination Criterion*	*Differential Diagnosis*
Aphasia language performance scale[375]	X				X	X			X
Appraisal of language disturbance[376]	X				X	X			
Boston diagnostic aphasia examination[62]	X	X		X	X	X			
Communicative assessment in daily living[377]	X				X	X	X		X
Examining for aphasia[14]	X				X	X			
Functional communication profile[378]	X								
Halstead aphasia test form M[379]	X								
Language modalities test for aphasia[16]	X			X	X	X			
Minnesota test for differential diagnosis of aphasia[380]	X		X	X	X	X	X		X
Neurosensory center comprehensive examination for aphasia[381]	X	X		X	X		X		
Orzeck aphasia evaluation[382]	X								
Porch index of communicative ability[128]	X	X	X	X	X	X	X	X	X
Sklar aphasia scale[383]	X				X				
Western aphasia battery[66]	X	X	X	X	X	X	X		X
Special single modality tests									
Auditory comprehension test for sentences[384]	X				X	X	X		
Reading comprehension battery for aphasia[385]	X				X	X			
Revised token test[185]	X				X	X	X		
Word fluency measure[386]	X				X		X		

From McNeil MR. Current concepts in adult aphasia. International Rehabilitation Medicine 1984; 6:128–134.

gorizing types of Aphasics given one model of classification. Most tests give information about the focus of treatment; however, the PICA appears to address this issue with greater care and specification than the other tests. The Reading Comprehension Battery for Aphasia[385] is the only in-depth protocol for assessing reading deficits in aphasia.

TREATMENT

Aphasia treatment has been demonstrated to be efficacious for groups of patients and for individuals. The exact approach to treatment varies with the patient's specific deficits, severity, assets, and psychosocial character. Treatment approaches have been directed at the patient's assumed areas of deficit (e.g., psychological maladjustments, linguistic deficits, perceptual processing deficits) as well as toward the general nature of the treatment and its effect upon the patient (e.g., behavioral treatment, pharmaceutical treatment). Another way to classify the types of treatment approaches is by the relative directness with which the aphasic is facilitated or manipulated by the intervention procedures. In this schema, direct treatment techniques are those that cause a clear neurochemical or neurophysiologic change in the patient. Semidirect techniques are those behavioral procedures that may or may not be highly controlled, but are believed to have an impact on the nervous system through sensory motor and cognitive manipulations. Indirect techniques are those that are so removed from organized sensorimotor and cognitive stimulation that they would not be expected to effect change. The indirect techniques are those that the patient might well encounter in his or her normal routine and, if they are capable of stimulating change in the patient, would have done so in the normal course of living. A fourth and final type of treatment is not designed to facilitate any inefficiency or loss of the system (although they could), but rather to circumvent the deficit. These techniques would be considered compensatory. Table 25–9 presents an outline of the most commonly referenced, and perhaps used, treatment approaches. Some are loosely organized principles, others are specific

TABLE 25–8 Published Tests for Aphasia

Test Name (Abbreviation)	*Primary Limitations*	*Primary Assets*
General assessment batteries		
Aphasia language performance scale (ALPS)[375]	Relies heavily on subjectivity and clinician's expertise for administration and interpretation	Short administration time (20–30 min)
Appraisal of language disturbance (ALD)[376]	Without validity data	Systematically manipulates tasks by modalities
Boston diagnostic aphasia examination (BDAE)[62]	Lack of prognostic and treatment planning information and test length	Diagnosis of presence and type of aphasic syndrome Comprehensive inventory of tasks
Communicative assessment in daily living (CADL)[377]	Poor construct validity	Objective "communicative" assessment with external validity
Examining for aphasia[14]	Without standardization validity or reliability data	Assesses top end of performance scale in depth
Functional communication profile (FCP)[378]	Lack of prognostic and treatment planning information	Rapid administration Easily understood by nonspeech-language pathologists
Halstead aphasia test form M[379]	Without standardization, validity, and reliability data	
The language modalities test for aphasia (LMTA)[16]	Deficient normative, validity, and reliability data Awkward administration using filmstrip	Psycholinguistic model on which it was based
Minnesota test for differential diagnosis of aphasia (MTDDA)[380]	Test length	Comprehensiveness Prognostic value
Neurosensory center comprehensive examination for aphasia[381]	Relies heavily on subjectivity and clinician's expertise for administration and interpretation Without good standardization, validity, and reliability data	Variety of tasks and functions sampled
Orzeck aphasia evaluation (OAE)[382]	Relies exclusively on subjectivity and clinician's expertise for administration, scoring, and interpretation Without standardization, validity, and reliability data	
Porch index of communicative ability (PICA)[128]	Does not stress the top end (linguistic and cognitive) of the top-down bottom-up interactive model (this is also true with most other batteries)	Treatment planning A dependent measure for clinical and research purposes Differential diagnosis Highly quantified
Sklar aphasia scale (SAS)[383]	Limited range of tasks assessed	Concurrent validity with other aphasia tests
Western aphasia battery (WAB)[66]	Lack of prognostic and treatment planning information	Diagnosis of presence and type of aphasic syndrome Shorter than the BDAE
Special Single Modality Tests		
Auditory comprehension test for sentences (ACTS)[384]	Lack of sensitivity to mild impairments	Short administration Well standardized
Reading comprehension battery for aphasia (RCBA)[385]	Without validity and normative data	Assesses a good range of reading operations
Revised token test (RTT)[185]	Test length (30 min)	Highly quantified A good dependent measure for clinical and research purpose Sensitivity to mild deficits
Word fluency measure (WF)[386]	Lack of validity and reliability data	Sensitivity to mild deficits

techniques, and still others are whole programs or packages. Aside from loose generalities, most approaches, techniques, and programs are lacking in established efficacy.

In addition to those variables discussed earlier in the context of evidence that the patient is manipulable or stimulable, and those factors that are shown to influence prognosis and recovery, Darley[389] concluded three important factors relative to treatment.

(1) Intensive therapy has a decisive, positive effect on recovery from aphasia in patients in whom spontaneous recovery has run its course. (2) Beneficial effects are maximized if treatment is started early and is prolonged for a period of several months. . . . (3) The gains that result from aphasia therapy are not confined to changes in lis-

TABLE 25–9 Treatment Approaches, Techniques, and Prognosis Available for Intervention with Adult Aphasic Patients

Type of Therapy	*Sources*	*General Effectiveness on Language Communication*
Direct		
Pharmaceuticals		
Sodium amytal (sedative, hypnotic, anticonvulsant)	Linn and Stein[403]	Favorable
	Linn[404]	Transient improvement
	Billow[405]	Transient improvement
	Bergman and Green[406]	Deleterious effects
	D'Asard[407]	Equivocal—improved on automatic language
Meprobamate (tranquilizer, muscle relaxant, anticonvulsant)	West and Stockel[408]	No effects
Methylphenidate [Ritalin] (stimulant, antidepressant)	Darley et al[409]	No effects
Chlordiazepoxide [Librium] (tranquilizer)	Darley et al[409]	No effects
Triavil [Perphenazine + Amitriptyline] (tranquilizer-antidepressant)	Adamovich[410]	Deleterious effects across all modalities on one patient
Hyperbaric oxygen	Sarno et al[411]	No effects
Supplemental oxygen respiration	Altschuler[412]	Significant improvement in gestural and graphic abilities; no effect on verbal abilities
Thalamic electrical stimulation	Ojemann[413]	Significant positive effects on naming for a few days postoperatively
Hypnosis	Crasilneck and Hall[414]	Increased "motivation for recovery"
Biofeedback* (electromyography)	McNeil et al[415]	Preliminary results—effecacious for controlling tension-anxiety
Relaxation (progressive-general)	Marshall and Watts[299]	Preliminary results—inconclusive
Semidirect		
Stimulation approaches		
Wepman's thought-centered therapy	Wepman[199,237] and Martin[297]	Generally untested
Schuell's stimulation approach	Schuell et al,[1] Duffy,[67,416] Weigel-Crump and Koenigsknecht[294]	Efficacious
Divergent semantic intervention	Chapey[393,417]	Generally untested
Deblocking	Weigl,[196] Weigl and Bierwisch[200]	Generally efficacious
Promoting aphasics' communicative effectiveness (PACE)	Davis and Wilcox[298]	Preliminary studies—efficacious
Self-adjusting therapy	Mysak and Guarino[418,419]	Untested
Environmental language intervention	Lubinski[420]	Untested
Operant conditioning and programmed (machine) therapy	Brookshire,[421] Holland,[422] Goldfarb,[423] Keith and Darley,[424] Keenan[425]	Generally efficacious
Teaching strategies	McNeil and Kozminski[322]	Generally efficacious
Visual action therapy	Helm and Benson[426]	Preliminary results—efficacious with global aphasics
Preventive therapy	Beyn and Shokhor-Trotskaya[295]	Efficacious for preventing telegraphic speech
Home therapy (nonprofessionally administered)	Darley,[3] Boone,[427] Flowers and Danforth,[428] DiSimoni[429,430]	Controversial—generally untested
Compensatory (alternative/augmentative)		
Nonverbal communication	Towey and Pettit[431]	Preliminary results—efficacious with global aphasics
Communication boards	Davis,[432] DiSimoni[429,430]	Untested
Bliss and other nonverbal symbolic communication	Gardner et al,[433] Glass et al[434]	Preliminary results—efficacious with global aphasia
Nonspeech-language initiation program	Carrier and Peak,[435] DiSimoni[429]	Untested
Electromechanical devices	Vanderheiden and Grilley,[436] Vanderheiden[437]	Generally untested

TABLE 25–9 Continued

Type of Therapy	Sources	General Effectiveness on Language Communication
Gestural communication Finger spelling	Eagleson et al[438]	Preliminary results—efficacious for some aphasics
American Indian sign (Amerind)	Skelly,[439] Rao[440]	Generally untested except for apraxia of speech

* Biofeedback and relaxation may be classified better as semidirect techniques. However, like hypnosis, it attempts to influence language and communication through methods other than stimulating language or language processes per se, and in that way might be more direct.

tening, reading, speaking, and writing, but are also observed in attitude, appropriateness of affect, morale, and maintenance of social contact (p 141).

A discussion of these therapies, the theoretical constructs on which they are built, and for whom each is most efficacious is beyond the scope of this chapter. Three excellent sources are recommended for the elaboration of treatment issues in aphasia. The first two are major summaries and overviews of issues and techniques as they relate specifically to the implementation of treatment. The first is *Clinical Management of Neurogenic Communicative Disorders,* edited by Johns.[390,391] The second is *Language Intervention Strategies in Adult Aphasia,* edited by Chapey.[392,393] The third source is a yearly publication from the Clinical Aphasiology Conference, titled *Clinical Aphasiology,* edited by Brookshire, 1972–1988. The articles in *Clinical Aphasiology* vary in topic and approach and are generally of excellent quality in terms of theoretical, technical, and clinical concerns.

From the general efficacy of each treatment listed in Table 25–9, that little is known about what type of therapy is efficacious and for whom is apparent. Regardless of whether neurologists are qualified to be involved directly in the language rehabilitation process per se or not, it is time to turn ourselves to Benson's[394] suggestions: "If we accept that aphasia therapy is of value, attention can be directed to an important aspect: What are the current techniques and can they be improved?" What the current techniques are is clear. If they work, for whom, and if they can be improved remain the clinical aphasiologist's immediate challenges. It is the speech-language pathologist who must accept these challenges. In doing so, he or she must avoid any tendencies toward professional narrow mindedness and any inclinations to ride clinical bandwagons. Although speech-language pathologists are not unique professionals in their susceptibility to these inclinations, neither are they immune to the comforts offered by doing so. However, the effects of such comforts inevitably place tacit but substantial restrictions on their professional growth and clinical effectiveness. Aphasiologists must develop, as Nietzsche[395] suggested in general, a "profound aversion to reposing once and for all in any one total view of the world." They must ". . . refuse to be deprived of the stimulus of the enigmatic" (p 262).

The concepts of parsimony and the reductionism inherent in the scientific method, which calls for integrated precision and control, need not be inconsistent with a multiform approach to aphasia if the consumer of this approach is restricted to the theorist, the researcher, the professor disseminating information, and the beginning student of aphasia. What about the clinician? Is the multiform protean approach appropriate for the practicing clinician faced with the manipulation of attitudes, behaviors, and even neurophysiologic processes? It is appropriate, but only insofar as the clinician is also a theorist or a researcher. It is not appropriate to the clinician, in the traditional clinician's role. It is as Rosenbek[396] suggested in his address to the 1979 Clinical Aphasiology Conference: ". . . The clinicians in this room ought to place themselves firmly into the stream of change, and ought not to move until we have tested and gotten to know what is true and what is false about some little area of treatment" (p 172). He went on to say that those clinicians who achieved this would be easily recognized by their "wrinkled feet." Indeed, the clinical aphasiologist must put into practice only that which has been thoroughly tested and must resist the temptation to integrate new ideas or theories until they are facts. Wrinkled feet are essential for being accountable to ourselves, our professional colleagues and most importantly, to our patients. All other areas of aphasiology require that information be acquired from anywhere and integrated with everything that makes an ounce of sense. Those aphasiologists not wearing the clinician's hat are recognized by their silk smooth soles.

If clinicians are deprived of the comforts of narrow mindedness and the temptations of jumping on perfectly reasonable but untested bandwagons, then their repertoire of clinical tools and techniques might be severely limited. If this is the case, then the validity of the tools and techniques currently in use in the name of treatment require systematic verification. The recent development and proliferation of single subject research studies[397–400] appears to have offered one viable experimental model for determining what is true and what is false about some little area of treatment. Multiple repetition of the single subject design on many different patients[401] or the more traditional group designs[402] allows generalizability once efficacious techniques are found. *However, practicing in the name of treatment what is reasonable but untested cannot be considered efficacious.*

REFERENCES

1. Schuell H, Jenkins JJ, Jimenéz-Pabón E. Aphasia in adults: diagnosis, prognosis, and treatment. New York: Hoeber Medical Division, Harper & Row, 1964.
2. Benson DF. Aphasia, alexia, and agraphia. New York: Churchill Livingstone, 1979.
3. Darley FL. Treatment of acquired aphasia. In: Friedlander WJ, ed. Advances in neurology. Vol. 7. New York: Raven Press, 1975.
4. Marie P. Révision de la question de l'aphasie: la troisième circonvolution frontale gauche ne joue aucun role speciale dans la function du langage. Semin Med 1906; 26:241–247.
5. Wernicke K. (1851). Cited in: Lichtheim L. On aphasia. Brain 1885; 7:433–484.
6. Broca P. Sur le siege de la faculté du langage articulé. Bull Soc Anthropol Paris 1865; 6:337–393.
7. Bastian HC. On the various forms of loss of speech in cerebral disease. British Foreign Medical Chirurg Review 1869; 43:209–236, 470–492.
8. Pick A. Die Agrammatischen Sprachstorungen. Berlin: Springer, 1913.
9. Head H. Aphasia and kindred disorders. Vol. I, II. London: Cambridge University Press, 1926.
10. Weisenburg TM, McBride KE. Aphasia: a clinical psychological study. New York: Commonwealth Fund, 1935.
11. Kleist K. Leitungsaphasie (Nachsprechaphasie). In: Bonhoeffer K, ed. Handbuch der Aertzlichen Erfahrugen im Weltkriege 1914/1918. Leipzig: Barth, 1934.
12. Nielsen JM. The unsolved problems in aphasia: I. Alexia in "motor" aphasia. Bull Los Angeles Neurol Soc 1938; 4:114–122.
13. Goldstein K. Aftereffects of brain injuries in war. New York: Grune & Stratton, 1948.
14. Eisenson J. Examining for aphasia. New York: Psychological Corporation, 1954.
15. Brain WR. Speech disorders. London: Butterworth, 1961.
16. Wepman JM, Jones LV. The language modalities test for aphasia. Chicago: Education-Industry Service, 1961.
17. Russell WR, Espir MLE. Traumatic aphasia: a study of aphasia in war wounds of the brain. London: Oxford University Press, 1961.
18. Gloning I, Gloning K, Hoff H. Aphasia: a clinical syndrome. In: Halpern L, ed. Problems of dynamic neurology. Jerusalem: Hebrew University Press, 1963:63.
19. Bay E. Principles of classification and their influence on our concepts of aphasia. In: De Reuck AVS, O'Connor M, eds. Ciba foundation symposium on disorders of language. Boston: Little, Brown, 1964:122.
20. Luria AR. Factors and forms of aphasia. In: De Reuck AVS, O'Connor M, eds. Ciba foundation symposium on disorders of language. Boston: Little, Brown, 1964:143.
21. Luria AR. Higher cortical functions in man. New York: Basic Books, 1966.
22. Luria AR, Hutton JT. A modern assessment of the basic forms of aphasia. Brain Lang 1977; 4:129–151.
23. Goodglass H, Quadfasel A, Timberlake WH. Phrase length and the type and severity of aphasia. Cortex 1964; 1:133–153.
24. Howes D. Application of the word frequency concept to aphasia. In: De Reuck AVS, O'Connor M, eds. Ciba foundation symposium on disorders of language. Boston: Little, Brown, 1964:47.
25. Geschwind N. Disconnection syndromes in animals and man. Brain 1965; 88:237–294, 584–644.
26. Hécaen H, Dubois J. La neurolinguistique. In: Perren GE, Trim JLM, eds. Applications of linguistics. London: Cambridge University Press, 1971:85.
27. Brown JW. Aphasia, apraxia and agnosia: clinical and theoretical aspects. Springfield, IL: Thomas, 1972.
28. Lecours AR. Le cerveau et le langage. Union Med Can 1974; 103:123–263.
29. Adams RD, Victor M. Principles of neurology. New York: McGraw-Hill, 1977.
30. Mohr JP, Pessin MS, Finkelstein S, Funkenstein HH, Duncan GW, Davis KR. Broca aphasia: pathologic and clinical aspects. Neurology 1978; 28:311–324.
31. Kertesz A, Phipps JB. Numerical taxonomy of aphasia. Brain Lang 1977; 4:1–10.
32. Hécaen H, Albert ML. Human neuropsychology. New York: John Wiley & Sons, 1978.
33. Darley FL. Aphasia. Philadelphia: WB Saunders, 1982.
34. Brown JA. A model for central and peripheral behavior in aphasia. Paper presented to the Academy of Aphasia, Rochester, Minnesota, 1968. In: Perkins WH, ed. Speech pathology: an applied behavioral science. St. Louis: CV Mosby, 1977:132.
35. Perkins WH. Speech pathology: an applied behavioral science. St. Louis: CV Mosby, 1977.
36. Klor BM, Ratusnik DL. Semantic relations in aphasic adults. In: Brookshire RH, ed. Clinical aphasiology conference proceedings. Minneapolis: BRK Publishers, 1980:47.
37. Prinz PM. A note on requesting strategies in adult aphasics. J Commun Disord 1980; 13:65–73.
38. Ulatowska HK. Macaluso-Haynes S, North AJ. Production of narrative and procedural discourse in aphasia. In: Brookshire RH, ed. Clinical aphasiology conference proceedings. Minneapolis: BRK Publishers, 1980:17
39. Ulatowska HK, North AJ, Haynes SM. Production of discourse and communication competence in aphasia. In: Brookshire RH, ed. Clinical aphasiology conference proceedings. Minneapolis: BRK Publishers, 1981:75.
40. Lenneberg EH. Biological foundations of language. New York: John Wiley & Sons, 1967.
41. Badecker W, Caramazza A. On considerations of method and theory governing the use of clinical categories in neurolinguistics and cognitive neuropsychology: the case against agrammatism. Cognition 1985; 20:97–125.
42. Caramazza A. The logic of neuropsychological research and the problem of patient classification in aphasia. Brain Lang 1984; 21:9–20.
43. Wepman JM, Jones LV. Five aphasias: a commentary on aphasia as a regressive linguistic problem. In: Disorders of communication ARNMD 42. Baltimore: Williams & Wilkins, 1964.
44. Mountcastle VB. The view from within: pathways to the study of perception. Johns Hopkins Med J 1975; 136:109–131.
45. Mountcastle VB. An organizing principle for cerebral function: the unit module and the distributed system. In:

Schmitt FW, Worden FG, eds. The neurosciences; fourth study program. Cambridge: MIT Press, 1979:25.
46. Szentagothai J. The "module-concept" in cerebral cortex architecture. Brain Res 1975; 95:475–496.
47. Szentagothai J. Basic circuitry of the neocortex. Exp Brain Res 1976; Suppl 1:282–287.
48. Rubens A. Anatomical asymmetries of human cerebral cortex. In: Harnad S, Doty R, Goldstein L, Jaynes J, Krauthamer G, eds. Lateralization in the nervous system. New York: Academic Press, 1977:503.
49. Whitaker HA, Selnes OA. Anatomic variations in the cortex: individual differences and the problem of the localization of language functions. In: Harnad SR, Steklis HD, Lancaster J, eds. Origins and evolution of language and speech. Ann NY Acad Sci 1976; 280:844–854.
50. Naeser MA, Hayward RW. Lesion localization in aphasia with cranial computed tomography and the Boston Diagnostic Aphasia Examination. Neurology 1978; 28:545–551.
51. Bogen JE, Bogen GM. Wernicke's region—where is it? In: Harnad SR, Steklis HD, Lancaster J, eds. Origins and evolution of language and speech. Ann NY Acad Sci 1976; 280:834–843.
52. von Monakow C. Die Lokalisation im Grosshirn und der Abbau der Funktion durch Kortikaie Herbe. Weisbaden: Bergmann, 1914.
53. Freud S. On aphasia (1891). Translated by Stengel. London: Imago, 1953.
54. Caramazza A. On drawing inferences about the structure of normal cognitive systems from the analysis of patterns of impaired performance: the case for single-patient studies. Brain Cognit 1986; 5:41–46.
55. Shallice T. Case study approach in neuropsychological research. J Clin Neuropsychol 1979; 1:183–211.
56. Marshall JC. What is a symptom-complex? In: Arbib MA, Caplan D, Marshall JC, eds. Neural models of language proccesses. New York: Academic Press, 1982:389.
57. Marshall JC. The description and interpretation of aphasic language disorder. Neuropsychologia 1986; 24:5–24.
58. Schwartz MR. What the classical aphasia categories can't do for us, and why. Brain Lang 1984; 21:3–8.
59. McNeil MR. Current concepts in adult aphasia. Int Rehab Med 1984; 6:128–134.
60. McNeil MR. Aphasia: neurological considerations. Top Lang Disord 1983; 3:1–19.
61. Goodglass H, Kaplan E. The assessment of aphasia and related disorders. Philadelphia: Lea & Febiger, 1984.
62. Hayward RW, Naeser MA, Zatz LM. Cranial computed tomography in aphasia. Radiology 1977; 123:653–660.
63. Naeser MA, Hayward RW. The resolving stroke and aphasia: a case study with computerized tomography. Arch Neurol 1979; 36:233–235.
64. Mazzocchi F, Vignolo LA. Localization of lesions in aphasia: clinical-CT scan correlations in stroke patients. Cortex 1979; 15:627–654.
65. Jackson JH. On the nature and duality of the brain. In: Jackson JH, ed. Selected writings. Vol. II. New York: Basic Books, 1958:129.
66. Kertesz A. Western aphasia battery. In: Kertesz A, ed. Aphasia and associated disorders; taxonomy, localization and recovery. New York: Grune & Stratton, 1979.
67. Duffy JR. Schuell's stimulation approach to rehabilitation. In: Chapey R, ed. Language intervention strategies in adult aphasia. Baltimore: Williams & Wilkins, 1981:105.
68. Caplan D. In defense of agrammatism. Cognition 1986; 24:263–279.
69. Jenkins JJ, Jimenéz-Pabón E, Shaw RE, Sefer JW. Schuell's aphasia in adults: diagnosis, prognosis and treatment. 2nd ed. Hagerstown: Harper & Row, 1975.
70. McNeil MR, Kimelman MDZ. Toward an integrative information-processing structure of auditory comprehension and processing in adult aphasia. Semin Speech Lang 1986; 7:123–146.
71. Muma JR, McNeil MR. Intervention in aphasia: psychosociolinguistic perspectives. In: Chapey R, ed. Language intervention strategies in adult aphasia. Baltimore: Williams & Wilkins, 1981:195.
72. Lesser R. Linguistic investigations of aphasia. New York: Elsevier, 1978.
73. Zangwill OL. Intellectual status in aphasia. In: Vinkin PJ, Bruyn GW, eds. Handbook of clinical neurology. Vol. 4. New York: Elsevier, 1969:105.
74. Jackson JH. On affection of speech from disease of the brain. Brain 1878; I:304–330; 1879; II:203–222, 323–356.
75. Lebrun Y, Hoops R. Intelligence and aphasia. Amsterdam: Swets & Zeitlinger, 1974.
76. Guilford JP. Intelligence—1965 model. Am Psychol 1965; 21:20–26.
77. Meeker MN. The structure of intellect: its interpretation and uses. Columbus: CE Merrill, 1969.
78. Basso A, DeRenzi E, Faglioni P, Scotti G, Spinnler H. Neuropsychological evidence for the existence of cerebral areas critical to the performance of intelligence tasks. Brain 1973; 96:715–728.
79. Reitan RM. Intellectual functions in aphasic and non-aphasic brain injured subjects. Neurology 1953; 3:202–212.
80. Bauer K, Beck D. Intellect after cerebro-vascular accident. J Nerv Ment Dis 1954; 120:379–395.
81. Zangwill OL. Intelligence in aphasia. In: De Reuck AVS, O'Connor M, eds. Ciba foundation symposium on disorders of language. Boston: Little, Brown, 1964:261.
82. Bay E. Aphasia and non-verbal disorders of language. Brain 1962; 85:411–426.
83. Meyers R. Relation of "thinking" and language: an experimental approach using dysphasic patients. Arch Neurol Psychiatry 1948; 60:119–139.
84. Reitan RM. Intelligence and language functions in dysphasic patients. Disord Nerv Sys 1954; 15:1–8.
85. Reitan RM. The performance of aphasic, non-aphasic, and control subjects on the Rorschach Test. J Gen Psychol 1954; 51:199–212.
86. Reitan RM. The significance of dysphasia for intelligence and adaptive abilities. J Psychol 1960; 50:355–376.
87. Alajouanine T, Lhermitte F. Nonverbal communication in aphasia. In: De Reuck AVS, O'Connor M, eds. Ciba foundation symposium on disorders of language. Boston: Little, Brown, 1964:168.
88. Basso A, Faglioni P, Spinnler H. Non-verbal color impairment of aphasics. Neuropsychologia 1976; 14:183–193.
89. Collins M. Diagnosis and treatment of global aphasia. San Diego: College-Hill Press, 1986.
90. Craik FIM, Lockhart RS. Levels of processing: a framework for memory research. J Verbal Learn Verbal Behav 1972; 11:671–684.
91. Craik FIM, Tulving E. Depth of processing and retention of words in episodic memory. J Exp Psychol [Gen] 1975; 104:268–294.
92. Lindsay PH, Norman DA. Human information processing: an introduction to psychology. New York: Academic Press, 1972.
93. Neisser U. Cognitive psychology. Englewood Cliffs, NJ: Prentice-Hall, 1967.
94. Atkinson RC, Shiffrin RM. The control of short-term memory. Sci Am 1974; 62:82–90.
95. Battig WF. An unremembered principle serial-position feature. Am J Psychol 1978; 91:587–605.
96. Simon HA. Complexity and the representation of patterned sequences of symbols. Psychol Rev 1972; 79:369–382.
97. Milner B. Psychological defects produced by temporal lobe

excision. In: The brain and human behavior. Proceedings of the association for research in nervous and mental disease. Baltimore: Williams & Wilkins, 1958:244.
98. Milner B. Laterality effects in audition. In: Mountcastle VB, ed. Interhemispheric relations and cerebral dominance. Baltimore: Johns Hopkins Press, 1962:177.
99. Milner B. Brain mechanisms suggested by studies of temporal lobes. In: Millikin C, Darley FL, eds. Brain mechanisms underlying speech and language. New York: Grune & Stratton, 1967:122.
100. Berlin CI, McNeil MR. Dichotic listening. In: Lass NJ, ed. Contemporary issues in experimental phonetics. New York: Academic Press, 1976:327.
101. White MJ. Hemispheric asymmetries in tachistoscopic information processing. Br J Psychol 1972; 63:495–508.
102. Boller F, DeRenzi E. Relationships between visual memory deficits and hemispheric locus of lesion. Neurology 1967; 17:1052–1058.
103. Boller F, Spinnler H. Visual memory for colors in patients with unilateral brain damage. Cortex 1967; 3:395–405.
104. Carson DH, Carson FE, Tikofsky RS. On learning characteristics of the adult aphasic. Cortex 1968; 4:92–112.
105. Tikofsky RS. Two studies of verbal learning by adult aphasics. Cortex 1977; 7:105–125.
106. Tikofsky RS, Reynolds GL. Further studies of nonverbal learning and aphasia. J Speech Hear Res 1963; 6:329–337.
107. Smith A. Objective indices of severity of chronic aphasia in stroke patients. J Speech Hear Disord 1971; 36:167–207.
108. Weinstein S. Deficits concomitant with aphasia or lesions of either cerebral hemisphere. Cortex 1965; 1:154–169.
109. Loverso FL. The effects of alerting signals on left brain damage (aphasic) and normal subject accuracy and response time to visual stimuli. Doctoral Dissertation, University of Colorado, 1980.
110. Locke JL, Deck JW. Retrieval failure, rehearsal deficiency and short term memory loss in the aphasic adult. Brain Lang 1978; 5:227–235.
111. Black FW, Strub RL. Digit repetition performance in patients with focal brain damage. Cortex 1978; 16:12–21.
112. Cermak LS, Moreines J. Verbal retention deficits in aphasic and amnesic patients. Brain Lang 1976; 3:16–27.
113. Cermak LS, Tarlow S. Aphasic and amnesic patients' verbal vs. nonverbal retentive abilities. Cortex 1978; 16:32–40.
114. De Renzi E, Nichelli P. Verbal and non-verbal short-term memory impairment following hemispheric damage. Cortex 1975; 11:341–354.
115. Flowers CR. Proactive interference in short-term recall by aphasic, brain-damaged nonaphasic and normal subjects. Neuropsychologia 1975; 13:59–68.
116. Swinney DA, Taylor OL. Short-term memory recognition search in aphasics. J Speech Hear Res 1971; 14:578–588.
117. Tzortzis C, Albert ML. Impairment of memory for sequences in conduction aphasia. Neuropsychologia 1974; 12:355–366.
118. Warrington E, Shallice T. The selective impairment of auditory verbal short-term memory. Brain 1969; 92:885–896.
119. Adamovich BL. A comparison of the processes of memory and perception between aphasic and non-brain-injured adults. In: Brookshire RH, ed. Clinical aphasiology conference proceedings. Minneapolis: BRK Publishers, 1978:327.
120. Albert ML. Short-term memory and aphasia. Brain Lang 1976; 3:28–33.
121. Warren LR, Hubbard DJ, Knox AW. Short-term memory scan in normal individuals and individuals with aphasia. J Speech Hear Res 1977; 20:497–509.
122. Rothi LJ, Hutchinson EC. Retention of verbal information by rehearsal in relation to the fluency of verbal output in aphasia. Brain Lang 1981; 12:347–359.
123. Goodglass H, Denes G, Calderon M. The absence of covert verbal mediation in aphasia. Cortex 1974; 10:264–269.
124. Cermak LS, Reale L, DeLuca D. Korsakoff patients' nonverbal vs. verbal memory: effects of interference and mediation on rate of information loss. Neuropsychologia 1977; 15:303–310.
125. Heilman KM, Scholes R, Watson RT. Defects in immediate memory in Broca's and conduction aphasia. Brain Lang 1976; 3:201–209.
126. Sternberg S. Memory scanning: mental processes revealed by reaction time experiments. Am Sci 1969; 57:421–457.
127. Lubinski R, Chapey R. Constructive recall strategies in adult aphasia. In: Brookshire RH, ed. Clinical aphasiology conference proceedings. Minneapolis: BRK Publishers, 1978:338.
128. Porch BE. Porch index of communicative ability. Vols. I, II. Palo Alto, CA: Consulting Psychologists Press, 1967.
129. Caramazza A, Zurif EB, Gardner H. Sentence memory in aphasia. Neuropsychologia 1978; 16:661–669.
130. McNeil MR, Hageman CF. Auditory processing deficits in aphasics evidenced on the Revised Token Test: incidence and prediction of across subtests and across item-within subtest patterns. In: Brookshire RH, ed. Clinical aphasiology conference proceedings. Minneapolis: BRK Publishers; 1979:47.
131. Albert ML. Note: auditory sequencing and left cerebral dominance for language. Neuropsychologia 1972; 10:245–248.
132. Efron R. Temporal perception, aphasia and déjà vu. Brain 1963; 86:403–424.
133. Goodglass H, Gleason JB, Hyde M. Some dimensions of auditory language comprehension in aphasia. J Speech Hear Res 1970; 13:595–606.
134. Kimura D, Archibald Y. Motor functions of the left hemisphere. Brain 1974; 97:337–350.
135. Butters N, Samuels I, Goodglass H, Brady B. Short-term visual and auditory memory disorders after parietal and frontal lobe damage. Cortex 1970; 6:440–459.
136. Lecours AR, Joanette Y. Linguistic and other psychological aspects of paroxysmal aphasia. Brain Lang 1980; 10:1–23.
137. Tulving E. Episodic and semantic memory. In: Tulving F, Donaldson W, eds. Organization of memory. New York: Academic Press, 1972.
138. Loverso FL. Rehabilitation of language-related memory disorders in aphasia. In: Chapey R, ed. Language intervention strategies in adult aphasia. 2nd ed. Baltimore: Williams & Wilkins, 1986:239.
139. Risse GL, Rubens AB, Jordan LS. Disturbances of long-term memory in aphasic patients: a comparison of anterior and posterior lesions. Brain 1984; 107:605–616.
140. De Renzi E, Pieczuro A, Vignolo L. Ideational apraxia: a qualitative study. Neuropsychologia 1968; 6:41–52.
141. Faglioni P, Spinnler H, Vignolo L. Contrasting behavior of right and left hemisphere-damaged patients on a discriminative and semantic task of auditory recognition. Cortex 1969; 5:366–389.
142. Duffy JR, Watt J, Duffy RJ. Deficits of nonverbal communication in aphasic patients: a test of some current causal theories. In: Brookshire RH, ed. Proceedings of the clinical aphasiology conference. Minneapolis: BRK Publishers, 1978:153.
143. Pickett L. An assessment of gestural and pantomimic deficits in aphasia patients. Acta Symbolica 1974; 3:69–86.
144. Prescott TE, Loverso FL, Sellinger M. Differences between normal and left brain damaged (aphasic) subjects on a nonverbal problem solving task. In: Brookshire RH, ed. Clinical aphasiology. Minneapolis: BRK Publishers, 1984:235.

145. Wernicke C. Der aphasische Symptomenkomplex. Breslau: Cohn & Weigart, 1874.
146. Damasio H, Damasio AR. The anatomical basis of conduction aphasia. Brain 1974; 103:337–350.
147. Cohen JA, Gelfer CE, Sweet RD. Thalamic infarction producing aphasia. Mt. Sinai J Med 1980; 47:398–404.
148. Wallesch C, Kornhuber HH, Brunner RJ, Kunz T, Hollerbach B, Sugar G. Lesions of the basal ganglia, thalamus, and deep white matter: differential effects on language functions. Brain Lang 1983; 20:286–304.
149. Naeser M, Alaxander MP, Helm-Estabrooks N, Levine HL, Laughlin S, Geschwind N. Aphasia with predominantly subcortical lesion sites. Arch Neurol 1982; 39:2–12.
150. Knopman DS, Selnes OA, Nicum N, Rubens AB, Yock D, Larson D. A longitudinal study of speech fluency in aphasia: CT correlates of recovery and persistent nonfluency. Neurology 1983; 33:1170–1178.
151. Darley FL. The differential diagnosis of aphasia. In: Brookshire RH, ed. Clinical aphasiology conference proceedings. Minneapolis; BRK Publishers, 1979:23.
152. Gardner H, Denes G, Zurif E. Critical reading at the sentence level in aphasia. Cortex 1975; 11:60–72.
153. Goodglass H. Studies on the grammar of aphasics. In: Goodglass H, Blumstein S, eds. Psycholinguistics in aphasia. Baltimore: Johns Hopkins University Press, 1973:183.
154. Goodglass H, Berko J. Agrammatism and inflectional morphology in aphasia. J Speech Hear Res 1960; 3:257–267.
155. Goodglass H, Blumstein SE, Gleason JB, Hyde MR, Statlender S. The effect of syntactic encoding on sentence comprehension in aphasia. Brain Lang 1979; 7:201–209.
156. Goodglass H, Hunt J. Grammatical complexity in aphasic speech. Word 1958; 14:197–207.
157. Odell KH. Comparison between auditory and reading comprehension in aphasic adults. Masters Thesis, University of Wisconsin, Madison, 1983.
158. Parisi D, Pizzamiglio L. Syntactic comprehension in aphasia. Cortex 1970; 6:204–215.
159. Pizzamiglio L, Appicciafuoco A, Rozauno C. Recovery of comprehension in aphasic patients. In: Lebrun Y, Hoops R, eds. Recovery in aphasics. Atlantic Highlands, NJ: Humanities Press, 1976:163.
160. Pizzamiglio L, Appicciafuoco A. Syntactic comprehension in aphasia. J Commun Disord 1971; 3:280–288.
161. Blumstein S, Goodglass H. The perception of stress as a semantic cue in aphasia. J Speech Hear Res 1972; 15:800–806.
162. Arvedson J. Effect of lexical decisions on auditory semantic judgments using divided attention in adults with left and right hemisphere lesions. Doctoral Dissertation, University of Wisconsin, Madison, 1986.
163. Davidoff JB, Ostergaard AL. Colour anomia resulting from weakened short-term colour memory: a case study. Brain 1984; 107:415–431.
164. Jackson JH. The selected writing of John Hughling Jackson. Vol. 2. London: Hodder & Stoughton, 1931. Reprinted New York: Basic Books, 1958.
165. McRoberts RG, Hens JS. Petit Mal and aphasia: a contribution to the problem of epilepsy and the convulsive state. Transactions Am Neurolog Assoc 1929; 55:567.
166. Winkler EG, Freiman GV, Lieberman SS. Astrocytoma of the left temporal lobe: contribution to the problem of psychopathology of epileptic personality disorder and to the problem of semantic aphasia. Am J Psychiatry 1951; 108:343.
167. Landau WM, Kleffner FR. Syndrome of acquired aphasia with convulsive disorder in children. Neurology 1957; 7:523–530.
168. Salmon A. An unusual receptive aphasia as a manifestation of temporal-lobe epilepsy: report of a case treated by surgery. N Engl J Med 1957; 257:313.
169. Serafetinides EA, Falconer MA. Speech disturbances in temporal lobe seizures. Brain 1963; 86:333–346.
170. DeFasquet EG, Gaudin ES, Bianchi A, De Mendilpharsu SA. Prolonged and monosymptomatic dysphasic status epilepticus. Neurology 1976; 26:244–247.
171. Gascon G, Victor D, Lombroso C, Goodglass D. Language disorder, convulsive disorder and electroencephalographic abnormalities. Arch Neurol 1973; 28:156–162.
172. Hamilton NG, Matthews T. Aphasia: the sole manifestation of focal status epilepticus. Neurology 1979; 29:745–748.
173. Porrazzo SA, Mayersdorf A. The measurement of interictal speech and language disturbances in temporal lobe epilepsy. In: Brookshire RH, ed. Clinical aphasiology conference proceedings. Minneapolis: BRK Publishers, 1976:110.
174. Linebaugh CW, Coakley AS, Arrigan AF, Racy A. Epileptogenic aphasia. In: Brookshire RH, ed. Clinical aphasiology conference proceedings. Minneapolis: BRK Publishers, 1979:70.
175. Chao D. Paroxysmal disorders. In: Carter S, Gold AP, eds. Neurology of infancy and childhood. New York: Appleton-Century-Crofts, 1974:132.
176. Lhermitte F, Gautier JC. Aphasia. In: Vinken PJ, Bruyn GW, eds. Handbook of clinical neurology. Vol. IV. Disorders of speech, perception, and symbolic behavior. Amsterdam: North-Holland 1969:84.
177. Wolff HG. Headache and other pains. New York: Oxford University Press, 1948:268.
178. Whisnant JP, Gardner JC, Taylor WF. Natural history of transient ischemic attacks. In: Toole JF, Mossy J, Janeway R, eds. Seventh conference on cerebral vascular disease. New York: Grune & Stratton 1971:161.
179. Baker RN. Prospective study of transient ischemic attacks. In: Toole JF, Mossy J, Janeway R, eds. Seventh conference on cerebral vascular disease. New York: Grune & Stratton, 1971:166.
180. Fields WS, Remington RD, Meyer JS. Progress report of the joint study of extracranial arterial occlusion: controlled study of surgical treatment of transient ischemic attacks. In: Toole JF, Mossy J, Janeway R, eds. Seventh conference on cerebral vascular disease. New York: Grune & Stratton, 1971:170.
181. Kuller LH. Formal discussion (of cerebral vascular insufficiency [TIA]). In: Tool JF, Mossy J, Janeway R, eds. Seventh conference on cerebral vascular disease. New York: Grune & Stratton, 1971:175.
182. Kunc Z. Surgery of arteriovenous malformations in the speech and motor-sensory regions. J Neurosurg 1974; 40:293–303.
183. McNeil MR. Prediction and pattern of recovery from aphasia with arteriovenous malformation. In: Brookshire RH, ed. Clinical aphasiology collected proceedings. 1972–76. Minneapolis: BRK Publishers, 1978:71.
184. Pettit JM, McNeil MR, Soloman JR. Right hemisphere dominance for language: evidence before and after surgical removal of a malignant tumor. Paper presented to the International Neuropsychology Society, New York. INS Bull 1978; December:15.
185. McNeil MR, Prescott TE. Revised Token Test. Baltimore: University Park Press, 1978.
186. Porch BE. The use of homogeneous subtest items in assessing aphasia. Paper presented at the Annual Convention of the American Speech and Hearing Association, Chicago, 1971.
187. Cronback LJ. Essentials of psychological testing. New York: Harper & Row, 1970.
188. Bloom L. Talking, understanding, and thinking. In: Shiefelbusch RL, Lloyd LL, eds. Language perspectives—acquisition, retardation and intervention. Baltimore: Uni-

versity Park Press, 1974:285.
189. Ingram D. The relationship between comprehension and production. In: Shiefelbusch RL, Lloyd LL, eds. Language perspectives—acquisition, retardation and intervention. Baltimore: University Park Press, 1974:313.
190. Chapman RS. Discussion summary—developmental relationship between receptive and expressive language. In: Shiefelbusch RL, Lloyd LL, eds. Language perspectives—acquisition, retardation and intervention. Baltimore: University Park Press, 1974:335.
191. Luria AR. Restoration of function after brain injury. New York: Macmillan, 1963.
192. Marshall RC. Heightening auditory comprehension for aphasic patients. In: Chapey R, ed. Language intervention strategies for adult aphasia. Baltimore: Williams & Wilkins, 1981:297.
193. Zurif EB. Language mechanisms: a neuropsychological perspective. Am Sci 1980; 68:305–311.
194. Berndt RS, Caramazza A. A redefinition of the syndrome of Broca's aphasia: implications for a neuropsychological model of language. Appl Psycholinguist 1980; 1:225–275.
195. Boller F, Vignolo LA. Latent sensory aphasia in hemisphere-damaged patients: an experimental study with the Token Test. Brain 1966; 89:815–829.
196. Weigl E. The phenomenon of temporary deblocking in aphasia. Zeitschr Phonet Sprachwissenschaft Kommunikations-Forschung 1961; 14:337–361.
197. Luria AR, Simernitskaya EG. Note: interhemispheric relations and the functions of the minor hemisphere. Neuropsychologia 1977; 15:175–178.
198. Vignolo LA. Evolution of aphasia and language rehabilitation: a retrospective exploratory study. Cortex 1964; 1:344–367.
199. Wepman JM. Aphasia: language without thought or thought without language? Asha 1976; 18:131–136.
200. Weigl E, Bierwisch M. Neuropsychology and linguistics: topics of common research. Found Lang 1970; 6:1–18.
201. Whitaker HA. Linguistic competence: evidence from aphasia. Glossa 1970; 4:46–53.
202. Whitaker HA. On the representation of language in the human brain. Edmonton: Linguistic Research, 1971.
203. Wepman JM. Recovery from aphasia. New York: Ronald Press, 1951.
204. Friedland RP, Weinstein EA. Hemi-inattention and hemispheric specialization: introduction and historical review. In: Weinstein EA, Friedland RP, eds. Hemi-inattention and hemisphere specialization. Advances in neurology. Vol. 18. New York: Raven Press, 1977:1.
205. Ludlow CL, Swisher LP. The audiometric evaluation of adult aphasics. J Speech Hear Res 1971; 14:535–543.
206. Goldstein MV. Auditory agnosia for speech (pure word deafness): a historical review with current implications. Brain Lang 1974; 1:195–204.
207. Fredericks JAM. The agnosias: disorders of perceptual recognition. In: Vinken PJ, Bruyn GW, eds. Handbook of clinical neurology: disorders of speech perception and symbolic behavior. Vol. 4. Amsterdam: North-Holland, 1969:207.
208. Teuber HL. Postscript: some needed revisions of the classical views of agnosia. Neuropsychologia 1965; 3:371–378.
209. Darley FL, Aronson AE, Brown JR. Motor speech disorders. Philadelphia: WB Saunders, 1975.
210. Rosenbek JC. Treating apraxia of speech. In: Johns DF, ed. Clinical management of neurogenic communicative disorders. Boston: Little, Brown, 1978:191.
211. Rosenbek JC, LaPointe LL. The dysarthrias: description, diagnosis, and treatment. In: Johns DL, ed. Clinical management of neurogenic communicative disorders. Boston: Little, Brown, 1978:251.
212. Eisenson J. Adult aphasia: assessment and treatment. New York: Appleton-Century-Crofts, 1973.
213. Halstead WC. Brain and intelligence. Chicago: University of Chicago Press, 1948.
214. Kreindler A, Fradis A. Performances in aphasia: a neuro dynamical diagnostic and psychological study. Paris: Gauthier-Villars, 1968.
215. Needham EC, Black JW. The relative ability of aphasic persons to judge the duration and intensity of pure tones. J Speech Hear Res 1970; 13:225–230.
216. Baru AV, Kareseva TA. The brain and hearing. New York: Consultants Bureau, 1972.
217. Swisher LP, Hirsh IJ. Brain damage and the ordering of temporally successive stimuli. Paper presented to the Annual Meeting of the Academy of Aphasia, Denver, 1971.
218. Brookshire RH, Lommel M. Perception of sequences of visual, temporal and auditory spatial stimuli by aphasic, right-hemisphere damaged, and non-brain damaged subjects. J Commun Disord 1974; 7:155–169.
219. Edmondson HS. The Seashore measures of musical talents as a prognostic guide in language rehabilitation for persons with aphasia. Doctoral Dissertation, University of Michigan, 1953.
220. Edwards AE, Auger R. The effects of aphasia on the perception of precedence. Proceedings of the Convention of the American Psychological Association, 1965; 207–208.
221. Brookshire RH. Visual and auditory sequencing by aphasic subjects. J Commun Disord 1972; 5:259–269.
222. Brookshire RH. Recognition of auditory sequences by aphasic, right-hemisphere-damaged, and non-brain-damaged subjects. J Commun Disord 1975; 8:51–59.
223. Niccum NE. Auditory temporal discrimination by aphasic subjects. Master's Thesis, University of Minnesota, 1974.
224. Brookshire RH. Auditory comprehension and aphasia. In: Johns DL, ed. Clinical management of neurogenic communicative disorders. Boston: Little, Brown, 1978:103.
225. Snelbecker GE, Fullard W, Reiling A, Love C. Auditory information processing by normal and CVA hemiplegic adults. Percept Motor Skills 1974; 38:855.
226. Ebbin JB, Edwards AE. Speech sound discrimination of aphasics when intersound interval is varied. J Speech Hear Res 1967; 10:120–125.
227. Sheehan JC, Aseltine S, Edwards AE. Aphasic comprehension of time spacing. J Speech Hear Res 1973; 16:650–657.
228. Albert ML, Bear D. Time to understand: a case study of word deafness with reference to the role of time in auditory comprehension. Brain 1974; 97:373–384.
229. Liles BZ, Brookshire RH. Effects of pause time on auditory comprehension of aphasic subjects. J Commun Disord 1975; 8:221–236.
230. Gordon MC. Some effects of stimulus rate and complexity on perception and retention in brain-damaged patients. Cortex 1970; 6:273–286.
231. Gardner H, Albert ML, Weintraub S. Comprehending a word: the influence of speech and redundancy on auditory comprehension in aphasia. Cortex 1975; 11:155–162.
232. Campbell TF, McNeil MR. Effects of presentation rate and divided attention on auditory comprehension in children with an acquired language disorder. J Speech Hear Res 1985; 28:513–520.
233. Weidner WE, Lasky EZ. The interaction of rate and complexity of stimulus on the performance of adult aphasic subjects. Brain Lang 1976; 3:34–40.
234. Birch HG, Belmont I, Karp E. Delayed information processing and extinction following cerebral damage. Brain 1967; 90:113–130.
235. Buckingham HW. Avakian-Whitaker H, Whitaker HA. Linguistic structures in stereotyped aphasic speech. Linguistics 1975; 154:5–13.
236. Rochford G. A study of naming errors in dysphasic and demented patients. Neuropsychologia 1974; 9:437–443.

237. Wepman JM. Aphasia therapy: a new look. J Speech Hear Disord 1972; 37:203–214.
238. Leichester J, Sidman M, Stoddard L, Mohr JP. The nature of aphasic responses. Neuropsychologia 1971; 9:141–155.
239. Jauhiainen T. Phonemic analysis of perseveration: a case report. Proceedings of the XVIth international congress of logopedics and phoneatrics. Basel: Karger, 1976:240.
240. Helmick JW, Berg CB. Perseveration in brain-injured adults. J Commun Disord 1976; 9:143–156.
241. Allison RS, Hurwitz LJ. On perseveration in aphasia. Brain 1967; 90:429–447.
242. Titchener EB. Lectures on the elementary psychology of feeling and attention. New York: Macmillan, 1908.
243. Kahneman D. Attention and effort. Englewood Cliffs, NJ: Prentice-Hall, 1973.
244. Sharpless A, Jasper H. Habituation of the arousal reaction. Brain 1956; 79:655–680.
245. Thompson RF, Spencer WA. Habituation: a model phenomenon for the study of neuronal substrates of behavior. Psychol Rev 1966; 73:16–43.
246. Hageman CF. Attentional mechanisms underlying patterns of auditory comprehension in brain-damaged aphasic, non-aphasic and normal listeners. Doctoral Dissertation, University of Colorado, 1980.
247. Norris WE. A comparison of patterns of auditory processing deficits between sounds and words in aphasic patients. Master's Thesis, University of Colorado, 1980.
248. Prigogine I. Order through fluctuation: self-organization and social system. In: Jantsch E, Waddington CH, eds. Evolution and consciousness: human systems in transition. Reading, MA: Addison-Wesley, 1976:93.
249. Kelso JA, Holt KG, Kugler PM, Turvey MT. On the concept of coordinative structures as dissipative structures. II. Empirical lines of convergency. In: Stelmach GE, Requin J, eds. Tutorials in motor behavior. Amsterdam: North-Holland, 1980.
250. Kugler PM, Kelso JA, Turvey MT. On the concept of coordinative structures as dissipative structures. I. Theoretical line. In: Stelmach GE, Requin J, eds. Tutorials in motor behavior. Amsterdam: North-Holland, 1980:3.
251. Friedman A, Polson MC, Dafoe CG, Gaskill SJ. Dividing attention within and between hemispheres: testing a multiple resource approach to limited-capacity information processing. J Exp Psychol [Human Percept Perform] 1982; 8:625–650.
252. McNeil MR, Odell K, Campbell TF. The frequency and amplitude of fluctuating auditory processing in aphasic and nonaphasic brain-damaged persons. In: Brookshire RH, ed. Proceedings of the clinical aphasiology conference. Minneapolis: BRK Publishers, 1982:220.
253. Lenneberg EH. Epilogue: language, speech and speakers. Neurosci Res Prog Bull 1974; 12:619–636.
254. Skinner JE, Yingling CD. Central gating mechanisms that regulate event-related potentials and behavior: a neural model for attention. In: Desmedt JE, ed. Attention, voluntary contraction and event-related cerebral potentials: progress in clinical neurophysiology. Vol. I. Basel: Kager, 1977:30.
255. Darley FL. Maximizing input to the aphasic patient: a review of research. In: Brookshire RH, ed. Clinical aphasiology conference proceedings. Minneapolis: BRK Publishers, 1976:1.
256. McNeil MR, Darley FL, Olsen WO, Rose DE. Effects of intensity variations on auditory processing in aphasia. I. Equal intensities at each ear. Audiology 1983; 22:560–581.
257. McNeil MR, Darley FL, Rose DE, Olsen WO. Effects of intensity variations on auditory processing in aphasia. II. Different intensities at each ear. Audiology 1983; 22:582–615.
258. Benton AL, Smith KC, Lang M. Stimulus characteristics and object naming in aphasic patients. J Commun Disord 1972; 5:19–24.
259. Corlew MM, Nation JE. Characteristics of visual stimuli and naming performance in aphasic adults. Cortex 1975; 11:186–191.
260. Goodglass H, Barton MI, Kaplan EF. Sensory modality and object naming in aphasics. J Speech Hear Res 1968; 11:488–496.
261. Weinstein S. Experimental analysis of an attempt to improve speech in cases of expressive aphasia. Neurology 1959; 9:632–635.
262. Wertz RT, Porch BE. Effects of masking noise on the verbal performance of adult aphasics. Cortex 1970; 6:399–409.
263. Siegenthaler BM, Goldstein J. Auditory and visual figure-background perception by adult aphasics. J Commun Disord 1967; 1:152–158.
264. West JF. Imaging and aphasia. In: Brookshire RH, ed. Clinical aphasiology conference proceedings. Minneapolis: BRK Publishers, 1977:239.
265. West JF. Heightening the action imagery of materials used in aphasia treatment. In: Brookshire RH, ed. Clinical aphasiology conference proceedings. Minneapolis: BRK Publishers, 1978:261.
266. Faber M, Aten JL. Verbal performance in aphasic patients in response to intact and altered picture stimuli. In: Brookshire RH, ed. Clinical aphasiology conference proceedings. Minneapolis: BRK Publishers, 1979:177.
267. Stanton JB. The effects of delayed auditory feedback on the speech of aphasic patients. Scott Med J 1958; 3:378–384.
268. Boller F, Cole M, Vrtunski PB, Patterson M, Kim Y. Paralinguistic aspects of auditory comprehension in aphasia. Brain Lang 1979; 7:164–174.
269. Green E, Boller F. Features of auditory comprehension in severely impaired aphasics. Cortex 1974; 10:133–145.
270. Rochford G, Williams M IV. The effects of word frequency. J Neurol Neurosurg Psychiatry 1965; 28:407–413.
271. Goodglass H, Hyde MR, Blumstein S. Frequency, picturability and availability of nouns in aphasia. Cortex 1969; 5:104–119.
272. Goodglass H, Gleason JB, Bernholtz NA, Hyde MR. Some linguistic structures in the speech of a Broca's aphasic. Cortex 1972; 8:191–212.
273. Gainotti G, Caltagirone C, Ibba A. Semantic and phonemic aspects of auditory language comprehension in aphasia. Linguistics 1975; 154:15–29.
274. Siegel GM. Dysphasic speech responses to visual word stimuli. J Speech Hear Res 1959; 2:152–160.
275. Shewan CM, Canter GJ. Effects of vocabulary, syntax, and sentence length on auditory comprehension in aphasic patients. Cortex 1971; 7:209–226.
276. Waller MR, Darley FL. The influence of context on the auditory comprehension of paragraphs by aphasic subjects. J Speech Hear Res 1978; 21:732–745.
277. Weigl E, Bierwisch M. Neuropsychology and linguistics. In: Goodglass H, Blumstein S, eds. Psycholinguistics and aphasia. Baltimore: Johns Hopkins University Press, 1973:10.
278. Brookshire RH. Effects of prompting on spontaneous naming of pictures by aphasic subjects. Hum Comm 1975; 3:63–71.
279. McDearmon JR, Potter RE. The use of representational prompts in aphasia therapy. J Commun Disord 1975; 8:199–206.
280. Podraza BL, Darley FL. Effects of auditory prestimulation on naming in aphasia. J Speech Hear Res 1977; 20:669–683.
281. Pizzamiglio L, Roberts M. Writing in aphasia: a learning

study. Cortex 1967; 3:250–257.

282. Helmick JW, Wipplinger M. Effects of stimulus repetition on the naming behavior of an aphasic adult: a clinical report. J Commun Disord 1975; 8:23–29.

283. Brookshire RH. Visual discrimination and response reversal learning by aphasic subjects. J Speech Hear Res 1968; 11:677–692.

284. Engmann DL, Brookshire RH. Effects of simultaneous and successive stimulus presentation on visual discrimination by aphasic patients. J Speech Hear Res 1970; 13:369–381.

285. Brookshire RH. Effects of task difficulty on the naming performance of aphasic subjects. J Speech Hear Res 1972; 15:551–558.

286. Brookshire RH, Nicholas LE. Verification of active and passive sentences by aphasic and nonaphasic subjects. J Speech Hear Res 1980; 23:878–893.

287. Porch BE. Therapy subsequent to the PICA. In: Chapey R, ed. Intervention strategies in adult aphasia. Baltimore: Williams & Wilkins, 1981:283.

288. Brookshire RH. Effects of delay of reinforcement on probability learning by aphasic subjects. J Speech Hear Res 1971; 14:92–105.

289. Stoicheff ML. Motivating instructions and language performance of dysphasic subjects. J Speech Hear Res 1960; 3:75–85.

290. Toubbeh JE. Clinical observations on adult aphasia. J Commun Disord 1969; 2:57–68.

291. Darley FL. Impairment of communication ability in patients with cerebrovascular accidents. Mayo Clin Proc 1967; 42:648–652.

292. Skelly M. Aphasic patients talk back. Am J Nursing 1975; 75:1140–1142.

293. Brookshire RH. Effects of trial time and intertrial interval on naming by aphasic subjects. J Commun Disord 1971; 3:289–301.

294. Weigel-Crump C, Koenigsknecht RA. Tapping the lexical store of the adult aphasic: analysis of the improvement made in word retrieval skills. Cortex 1973; 9:411–418.

295. Beyn ES, Shokhor-Trotskaya MK. The preventive method of speech rehabilitation in aphasia. Cortex 1966; 2:96–108.

296. Hatfield FM. Rehabilitation of language. Speech Pathol Ther 1964; 7:68–77.

297. Martin AD. An examination of Wepman's thought centered therapy. In: Chapey R, ed. Language intervention strategies in adult aphasia. Baltimore: Williams & Wilkins, 1981:141.

298. Davis GA, Wilcox MJ. Incorporating parameters of natural conversation in aphasia treatment. In: Chapey R, ed. Language intervention strategies in adult aphasia. Baltimore: Williams & Wilkins, 1981:169.

299. Marshall R, Watts M. Relaxation training: effects on the communicative ability of aphasic adults. Arch Phys Med Rehab 1976; 57:464–467.

300. Holland AL, Sonderman JC. Effects of a program based on the token test for teaching comprehension skills to aphasics. J Speech Hear Res 1974; 17:589–598.

301. Gardner H. The contribution of operativity to naming capacity in aphasic patients. Neuropsychologia 1973; 11:213–220.

302. Gardiner BJ, Brookshire RH. Effects of unisensory and multisensory presentation of stimuli upon naming by aphasic subjects. Lang Speech 1972; 15:342–357.

303. Kushner D. Techniques for changing uncooperative behaviors: some case studies and considerations. In: Porch BE, ed. Clinical aphasiology conference proceedings. Albuquerque, NM; V.A. Hospital, 1974:55.

304. Wepman JM. The relationship between self-correction and recovery from aphasia. J Speech Hear Disord 1958; 23:302–305.

305. Shewan CM. Error patterns in auditory comprehension of adult aphasics. Cortex 1976; 12:325–336.

306. Jimenéz BC. Reaction times of aphasic and non-aphasic adults identifying words and nonwords. Paper presented to the Annual Convention of the American Speech and Hearing Association, Chicago, 1977.

307. Kim YC. Deficits in temporal sequencing of verbal material: the effects of laterality of lesion. Brain Lang 1976; 3:507–515.

308. Conrad K. New problems of aphasia. Brain 1954; 77:491–509.

309. Schuell HR. Paraphasia and paralexia. J Speech Hear Disord 1950; 15:291–306.

310. Rinnert C, Whitaker HA. Semantic confusions by aphasic patients. Cortex 1973; 9:56–81.

311. Crocker JR. Language competence of aphasic adults. Paper presented to the Annual Convention of the American Speech and Hearing Association, New York, 1970.

312. Ludlow CL. The recovery of syntax in aphasia. Paper presented to the Academy of Aphasia, Albuquerque, 1973.

313. Brookshire RH, Nicholas L. Comprehension of directly and nondirectly stated main ideas and details in discourse by brain-damaged and non-brain-damaged listeners. Brain Lang 1984; 21:21–36.

314. Nicholas L, Brookshire RH. Consistency of the effects of rate of speech on brain-damaged adults' comprehension of narrative discourse. J Speech Hear Res 1986; 29:462–470.

315. Wegner M, Brookshire RH, Nicholas L. Comprehension of main ideas and details in coherent and noncoherent discourse by aphasic and nonaphasic listeners. Brain Lang 1984; 21:37–51.

316. Ernest-Baron CR, Brookshire RH, Nicholas L. Story structure and retelling of narratives by aphasic and non-brain-damaged adults. J Speech Hear Res 1987; 30:44–49.

317. LeVere TE. Recovery of function after brain damage: a theory of the behavioral deficit. Physiol Psychol 1980; 8:297–308.

318. Cotman CW, ed. Neuronal plasticity. New York: Raven Press, 1978.

319. Kerr FWL. Structural and functional evidence of plasticity in the central nervous system. Exp Neurol 1975; 48:16–31.

320. Luria AR. Traumatic aphasia. The Hague: Mouton, 1970.

321. Pettit JM, Noll JD. Cerebral dominance in aphasia recovery. Brain Lang 1979; 7:191–200.

322. McNeil MR, Kozminsky L. The efficacy of five self-generated strategies for facilitating auditory processing. In: Brookshire RH, ed. Clinical aphasiology conference proceedings. Minneapolis: BRK Publishers, 1980:268.

323. Darley FL. Treat or neglect? Guest editorial. J Am Speech Hear Assoc 1979; 21:628–631.

324. Butfield E, Zangwill O. Re-education in aphasia: a review of 70 cases. J Neurol Neurosurg Psychiatry 1946; 9:75–79.

325. Longerich MC, Bordeaux J. Aphasia therapeutics. New York: Macmillan, 1954.

326. Messerli P, Tissot A, Rodriguez J. Recovery from aphasia: some factors of prognosis. In: Lebrun Y, Hoops R, eds. Neurolinguistics 4, recovery in aphasics. Amsterdam: Swets & Zeitlinger, 1976:124.

327. Kertesz A, McCabe P. Recovery patterns and prognosis in aphasia. Brain 1977; 100:1–18.

328. Keenan JS, Brassell EG. A study of factors related to prognosis for individual aphasic patients. J Speech Hear Disord 1967; 32:148–153.

329. Basso A, Faglioni P, Vignolo LA. Etude controlée de la re-education du langage dans l'aphasie: comparison entre aphasique traites et nontraites. Rev Neurol 1975; 131:607–

614.
330. Subirana A. The prognosis in aphasia in relation to the factors of cerebral dominance and handedness. Brain 1958; 81:415–425.
331. Subirana A. Handedness and cerebral dominance. In: Vinken PJ, Bruyn GW, eds. Handbook of clinical neurology. Vol. 4. Disorders of speech perception and symbolic behavior. Amsterdam: North-Holland, 1969:248.
332. Zangwill OL. Cerebral dominance and its relation to psychological function. Edinburgh: Oliver & Boyd, 1960.
333. Gloning I, Gloning K, Haub G, Quatember R. Comparison of verbal behavior in right-handed and non-right-handed patients with anatomically verified lesions of one hemisphere. Cortex 1969; 5:43–52.
334. Schuell H. Aphasic difficulties understanding spoken language. Neurology 1953; 3:176–184.
335. Culton GL. Reaction to age as a factor in chronic aphasia in stroke patients. J Speech Hear Disord 1971; 36:563–564.
336. Porch BE, Collins M, Wertz RT, Friden TP. Statistical prediction of change in aphasia. J Speech Hear Res 1980; 23:312–321.
337. Culton GL. Spontaneous recovery from aphasia. Ph.D. Dissertation, University of Denver, 1968.
338. Kertesz A, Harlock W, Coates R. Computer tomographic localization, lesion size, and prognosis in aphasia and nonverbal impairment. Brain Lang 1979; 8:34–50.
339. Sarno MT, Silverman M, Levita E. Psychosocial factors and recovery in geriatric patients with severe aphasia. J Am Geriatr Soc 1970; 18:405–409.
340. Hanson WR, Cicciarelli AW. The time, amount and pattern of language improvement in adult aphasics. Paper presented to the American Speech and Hearing Association Convention, Las Vegas, 1974.
341. Eisenson J. Aphasia: a point of view as to the nature of the disorder and factors that determine prognosis for recovery. Int J Neurol 1964; 4:287–295.
342. Eisenson J. Prognostic factors related to language rehabilitation in aphasic patients. J Speech Hear Disord 1949; 14:262–264.
343. Sarno MT, Silverman M, Sands E. Speech therapy and language recovery in severe aphasia. J Speech Hear Res 1970; 13:607–623.
344. Sands E, Sarno MT, Shankweiler D. Long-term assessment of language function in aphasia due to stroke. Arch Phys Med Rehab 1969; 50:202–207.
345. Sarno MT, Levita E. Natural course of recovery in severe aphasia. Arch Phys Med Rehab 1971; 52:175–179.
346. Godfrey CM, Douglass E. The recovery process in aphasia. Can Med Assoc J 1959; 80:618–624.
347. Kenin M, Swisher LP. A study of pattern of recovery in aphasia. Cortex 1972; 8:56–68.
348. Basso A, Capitani E, Vignolo LA. Influence of rehabilitation on language skills in aphasic patients: a controlled study. Arch Neurol 1979; 36:190–196.
349. Frazier CH, Ingham SD. A review of the effects of gunshot wounds of the head: based on the observation of two hundred cases at U.S. General Hospital No. 11, Cape May, NJ. Arch Neurol 1920; 3:17–40.
350. Wertz RT, Messert B, Collins M, Rosenbek JC, Kao CC. Right-hemisphere language dominance in a case of left-hemisphere arteriovenous malformation. J Speech Hear Disord 1977; 42:106–112.
351. Lomas J, Kertesz A. Patterns of spontaneous recovery in aphasic groups: a study of adult stroke patients. Brain Lang 1978; 5:388–401.
352. Fenelon J, Dissez A, Crouigneau C, Arne L. Reeducation de l'aphasie. Experience d'un service de reeducation. Bordeaux Med 1969; 2:2557–2570.
353. Darley FL, ed. Evaluation of appraisal techniques in speech and language pathology. Philippines: Addison-Wesley, 1979; 189–246.
354. Leischner A, Linck HA. Neure Erfahrungen mit der Behandlung von Aphasien. Nervenarzt 1967; 38:199–205.
355. David RM, Enderby P, Bainton D. Progress report on an evaluation of speech therapy for aphasia. Br J Disord Commun 1979; 14:85–88.
356. Dabul B, Hanson WR. The amount of language improvement in adult aphasics related to early and late treatment. Paper presented to the annual convention of the American Speech and Hearing Association, 1975, Washington, DC.
357. Marks M, Taylor M, Rusk HA. Rehabilitation of the aphasic patient: a summary of three years' experience in a rehabilitation setting. Arch Phys Med Rehab 1957; 38:219–226.
358. Perry P. The comparative effectiveness of language training and spontaneous recovery in improving the spoken language vocabulary comprehension of adult aphasics. Paper presented to the Annual Convention of the American Speech and Hearing Association, Washington, DC, 1975.
359. Prescott TE, McNeil MR. Measuring the effects of recovery of aphasia. Paper presented to the Clinical Aphasiology Conference, Albuquerque, 1973.
360. Broida H. Language therapy effects in long term aphasia. Arch Phys Med Rehab 1977; 58:248–253.
361. Wertz RT, Collins MJ, Weiss D, Kurtzke JF, Friden T, Brookshire RH, Pierce J, Holtzapple P, Hubbard DJ, Porch BE, West JA, Davis L, Matovitch V, Morley GK, Resurreccion E. Veterans Administration cooperative study on aphasia: a comparison of individual and group treatment. J Speech Hear Res 1981; 24:580–594.
362. Smith A. Diagnosis, intelligence, and rehabilitation of chronic aphasia: final report. Ann Arbor: University of Michigan Department of Physical Medicine and Rehabilitation, 1972.
363. Gloning K, Trappl R, Heiss WD, Quatember R. Prognosis and speech therapy in aphasia. In: Lebrun Y, Hoops R, eds. Recovery in aphasics. Amsterdam: Swets and Zeitlinger, 1976:57.
364. Hagen C. Communication abilities in hemiplegia: effect of speech therapy. Arch Phys Med Rehab 1973; 54:454–463.
365. Deal JL, Deal LA. Efficacy of aphasia rehabilitation: preliminary results. In: Brookshire RH, ed. Clinical aphasiology conference proceedings. Minneapolis: BRK Publishers, 1978:66.
366. Holland AL. The usefulness of treatment for aphasia: a serendipitous study. In: Brookshire RH, ed. Clinical aphasiology conference proceedings. Minneapolis: BRK Publishers, 1980:240.
367. Shewan CM, Kertesz A. Effects of speech and language treatment on recovery from aphasia. Brain Lang 1984; 23:272–299.
368. Wertz RT, Weiss DG, Aten JA, Brookshire RH, Garcia-Bunuel L, Holland AL, Kurtzke JF, LaPointe LL, Milianti FJ, Brannegan R, Greenbaum H, Marshall RC, Vogel D, Carter J, Barnes NS, Goodman R. Comparison of clinic, home and deferred language treatment for aphasia. Arch Neurol 1986; 43:653–658.
369. Lincoln NB, Mulley GP, Jones AC. Effectiveness of speech therapy for aphasic stroke patients. Lancet 1984; 1:1197–1200.
370. Eisenson J. Aphasics: observations and tentative conclusions. J Speech Hear Disord 1947; 12:290–292.
371. Wepman JM. A conceptual model of the processes involved in recovery from aphasia. J Speech Hear Disord 1953; 18:4–13.
372. Chapman LJ, Chapman JP. The measurement of handedness. Brain Cognit 1987; 6:175–183.
372a. Schacter SC, Ransil BJ, Geschwind N. Associations of handedness with hair color and learning disabilities. Neu-

ropsychologia 1987; 25:269–276.

373. Kertesz A, ed. Aphasia and associated disorders: taxonomy, localization and recovery. New York: Grune & Stratton, 1979.

374. Porch BE. Multidimensional scoring in aphasia testing. J Speech Hear Res 1971; 14:776–792.

375. Keenan JS, Brassell EG. Aphasia Language Performance Scale. Murfreeboro, TN: Pinnacle Press, 1975.

376. Emerick L. Appraisal of Language Disturbance. Marquette, MI: Northern Michigan University Press, 1971.

377. Holland AL. Communication Abilities in Daily Living: A Test of Functional Communication for Aphasic Adults. Baltimore, University Park Press, 1980.

378. Sarno MT. The Functional Communication Profile. New York: Institute of Rehabilitation Medicine, 1969.

379. Halstead WC, Wepman JM, Reitan RM, Heimburger RF. Halstead Aphasia Test, Form M. Chicago: University of Chicago Industrial Relations Center, undated.

380. Schuell H. The Minnesota Test for Differential Diagnosis of Aphasia. Minneapolis: University of Minnesota Press, 1965.

381. Spreen O, Benton AL. Neurosensory Center Comprehensive Examination for Aphasia. Victoria, BC: University of Victoria, 1969.

382. Orzeck AZ. Orzeck Aphasia Evaluation. Los Angeles: Western Psychological Services, 1964.

383. Sklar M. Sklar Aphasia Scale. Beverly Hills: Western Psychological Services, 1966.

384. Shewan CM. Auditory Comprehension Test for Sentences. Chicago: Biolinguistics Clinical Institutes, 1979.

385. LaPointe LL, Horner J. Reading Comprehension Battery for Aphasia. Tigard, OR: CC Publications, 1979.

386. Borkowski JG, Benton AL, Spreen O. Word fluency and brain damage. Neuropsychologia 1967; 5:135–140.

387. Brookshire RH. Introduction to aphasia. Minneapolis: BRK Publishers, 1973.

388. Linebaugh CW. Assessing the assessments: the adequacy of standardized tests of aphasia. In: Brookshire RH, ed. Clinical aphasiology conference proceedings. Minneapolis: BRK Publishers, 1979:8.

389. Darley FL. A retrospective view: aphasia. J Speech Hear Disord 1977; 42:161–169.

390. Johns DF, ed. Clinical management of neurogenic communicative disorders. Boston: Little, Brown, 1978:103–128, 191–242, 251–310.

391. Johns DF, ed. Clinical management of neurogenic communicative disorders. 2nd ed. Boston: Little, Brown, 1985:179–242.

392. Chapey R, ed. Language intervention strategies in adult aphasia. Baltimore: Williams & Wilkins, 1981:105–154, 169–222, 249–264, 283–346.

393. Chapey R, ed. Language intervention strategies in adult aphasia. 2nd ed. Baltimore: Williams & Wilkins, 1986:66–80, 239–250, 284–294, 345–359.

394. Benson DF. Aphasia rehabilitation: editorial. Arch Neurol 1979; 36:187–189.

395. Nietzsche R. The will to power. In: Kaufmann W, ed. New York: Vintage Books, 1967.

396. Rosenbek JC. Wrinkled feet. In: Brookshire RH, ed. Clinical aphasiology conference proceedings. Minneapolis: BRK Publishers, 1979:163.

397. Thompson CK, Kearns KP. An experimental analysis of acquisition, generalization and maintenance of naming behaviors in a patient with anomia. In: Brookshire RH, ed. Clinical aphasiology conference proceedings. Minneapolis: BRK Publishers, 1981:35.

398. Davis GA. The clinical application of withdrawal, single-case research designs. In: Brookshire RH, ed. Clinical aphasiology conference proceedings. Minneapolis: BRK Publishers, 1978:11.

399. Warren LR. Research design: considerations for the clinician. In: Chapey R, ed. Language intervention strategies in adult aphasia. 2nd ed. Baltimore: Williams & Wilkins, 1986:66.

400. Thompson CK, Byrne M. Across setting generalization of social convention in aphasia: an experimental analysis of "loose training." In: Brookshire RH, ed. Clinical aphasiology conference proceedings. Minneapolis: BRK Publishers, 1984:132.

401. Tonkovich J, Peach RK. Once is not enough: some thoughts on replication in functional analysis research in aphasia. In: Brookshire RH, ed. Clinical aphasiology. Minneapolis: BRK Publishers, 1981:121.

402. Wertz RT. Rosenbek JC. Group designs for the study of aphasia. In: Brookshire RH, ed. Clinical aphasiology conference proceedings. Minneapolis: BRK Publishers, 1978:1.

403. Linn L, Stein M. The use of sodium amytal in the treatment of aphasia. Bull United States Army Med Depart 1946; 5:705–708.

404. Linn L. Sodium amytal in treatment of aphasia. Arch Neurol Psychiatry 1947; 58:357–358.

405. Billow BW. Observation on the use of sodium amytal in the treatment of aphasia. Med Rec 1949; 162:12–13.

406. Bergman P, Green M. Aphasia: effects of intravenous sodium amytal. Neurology 1951; 1:471–475.

407. D'Asard MJ. An experimental investigation of effects of sodium amytal on communication of aphasic patients. Doctoral Dissertation, University of Southern California, 1955.

408. West R, Stockel D. The effect of meprobamate on recovery from aphasia. J Speech Hear Res 1965; 8:57–62.

409. Darley FL, Keith RL, Sasanuma S. The effects of alerting and tranquilizing drugs upon the performance of aphasic patients. In: Brookshire RH, ed. Clinical aphasiology conference proceedings. Minneapolis: BRK Publishers, 1977:68.

410. Adamovich BL. The effect of triavil on language abilities of aphasic patients (abstr). Asha 1980; 22:762.

411. Sarno MT, Sarno JE, Diller L. The effect of hyperbaric oxygen function in adults with aphasia. J Speech Hear Res 1972; 15:42–48.

412. Altschuler SL. The effects of supplemental oxygen respiration on hemiplegic aphasic adults. In: Porch BE, ed. Clinical aphasiology conference proceedings. Albuquerque, NM: V.A. Hospital, 1974:21.

413. Ojemann GA. Subcortical language mechanisms. In: Whitaker H, Whitaker HA, eds. Studies in neurolinguistics. Vol. I. New York: Academic Press, 1976:103.

414. Crasilneck HR, Hall JA. The use of hypnosis in the rehabilitation of complicated vascular and post-traumatic neurological patients. Int J Clin Exp Hypnosis 1970; 18:145–159.

415. McNeil MR, Prescott TE, Lemme ML. An application of electromyographic biofeedback to aphasia/apraxia treatment. In: Brookshire RH, ed. Clinical aphasiology conference proceedings. Minneapolis: BRK Publishers, 1976:151.

416. Duffy JR. Schuell's stimulation approach to rehabilitation. In: Chapey R, ed. Language intervention strategies for adult aphasia. 2nd ed. Baltimore: Williams & Wilkins, 1986:187.

417. Chapey R. Divergent semantic intervention. In: Chapey R, ed. Language intervention strategies in adult aphasia. Baltimore: Williams & Wilkins, 1981:155.

418. Mysak ED, Guarino CG. Self-adjusting therapy. In: Chapey R, ed. Language intervention strategies in adult aphasia. Baltimore: Williams & Wilkins, 1981:209.

419. Mysak ED, Guarino CG. Self-adjustment therapy. In: Chapey R, ed. Language intervention strategies in adult aphasia. 2nd ed. Baltimore: Williams & Wilkins, 1986:284.

420. Lubinski R. Environmental language intervention. In:

Chapey R. Language intervention strategies in adult aphasia. Baltimore: Williams & Wilkins, 1981:223.
421. Brookshire RH. Probability learning by aphasic subjects. J Speech Hear Res 1969; 12:857–864.
422. Holland AL. Case studies in aphasia rehabilitation using programmed instruction. J Speech Hear Disord 1970; 35:377–390.
423. Goldfarb R. Operant conditioning and programmed instruction in aphasia rehabilitation. In: Chapey R, ed. Language intervention strategies in adult aphasia. Baltimore; Williams & Wilkins, 1981:249.
424. Keith R, Darley RL. The use of a specific electric board in rehabilitation of the aphasic patient. J Speech Hear Disord 1967; 32:148–153.
425. Keenan J. A method for eliciting naming behavior from aphasic patients. J Speech Hear Disord 1966; 31:261–266.
426. Helm N, Benson FD. Visual action therapy for global aphasia. Paper presented to the Academy of Aphasia, Chicago, 1978.
427. Boone DR. A plan for rehabilitation of aphasic patients. Arch Phys Med Rehab 1967; 48:410–414.
428. Flowers CR, Danforth LC. Rationale and development of a step-wise auditory comprehension improvement program administered to aphasic patients by family members. In: Brookshire RH, ed. Clinical aphasiology conference proceedings. Minneapolis: BRK Publishers, 1979:196.
429. DiSimoni FG. Therapies which utilize alternative or augmentative communication systems. In: Chapey R, ed. Language intervention strategies in adult aphasia. Baltimore: Williams & Wilkins, 1981:329.
430. DiSimoni F. Alternative communication systems for the aphasic patient. In: Chapey R, ed. Language intervention strategies in adult aphasia. 2nd ed. Baltimore: Williams & Wilkins, 1986:345.
431. Towey M, Pettit JM. The treatment of global aphasia through a communication competence approach (abstr). Asha 1980; 22:701.
432. Davis A. Linguistics and language therapy: the sentence construction board. J Speech Hear Disord 1973; 38:205–214.
433. Gardner H, Zurif EB, Berry T, Baker E. Visual communication in aphasia. Neuropsychologia 1976; 14:275–292.
434. Glass A, Gazzaniga M, Premack D. Artificial language training in global aphasics. Neuropsychologia 1973; 11:95–103.
435. Carrier J, Peak T. Non speech language initiation program. Lawrence, KS: H H Enterprises, 1974.
436. Vanderheiden G, Grilley K, eds. Non-vocal communication techniques and aids for the severely physically handicapped. Baltimore: University Park Press, 1975.
437. Vanderheiden G, ed. Non-vocal communications resource book. Baltimore: University Park Press, 1978.
438. Eagleson H, Vaughn G, Knudson A. Hand signals for dysphasia. Arch Phys Med Rehab 1970; 51:111–113.
439. Skelly M. American Indian gestural code. New York: Elsevier North-Holland, 1979.
440. Rao PR. The use of Amer-Ind code with aphasic adults. In: Chapey R, ed. Language intervention strategies in adult aphasia. 2nd ed. Baltimore: Williams & Wilkins, 1986:360.

Voice Disorders

26 Voice Disorders in the Child

Thomas S. Johnson, Ph.D.
Dee R. Child, M.S.

The problem of voice disorders in children has a significant place in clinical practice for the speech-language pathologist. Studies regarding the prevalence of voice disorders in childhood indicate that between 60 and 90 children per 1,000, or 6 to 9 percent,[1] have voice problems. Many vital issues may be raised concerning the relative importance of the symptoms which may be present in the vocal disturbances of childhood. Many of these issues continue to be unresolved without the substantiation of scientific investigation. Many questions about the importance, evaluation procedures, and management processes of voice disorders in children remain unanswered. Some of these questions are: How important in the priority system are voice disturbances in children? What are the long-term effects of voice problems on the psychosocial development and personality of the child? How should children's voice problems be treated? and, How may clinical progress be measured and monitored during management? These are difficult issues with a complex array of factors determining the ultimate outcomes. In this chapter we attempt to put those issues in perspective with the focus on current literature and practice as well as to present our own clinical biases.

HISTORICAL PERSPECTIVE

The evaluation and treatment of voice disorders has had a long and curious development, with its roots primarily in vocal music and with some adaptation from early medical science. The history of voice therapy in children and adults has been influenced greatly by this strong connection with the musical and theatrical arts and the subsequent effects on contemporary practices of therapy. Concurrent, sometimes controversial philosophies have grown from clinicians advocating a more symptomatic approach to vocal behavior and those who held that voice disturbance was reflective of basic personality disturbance. Hence, a wide variety of therapy and management approaches have emerged, some of which have seemed foreign and strange to practicing speech-language pathologists. Symptomatic treatments were generally adapted from general speech, vocal music, and theater, whereas psychiatric medicine and clinical psychology contributed personality theories and therapies. The belief held by a number of early writers, that the voice is the "mirror of the emotions" and that it plays an important role in revealing information about the fears, anxieties, and emotional struggles of the individual,[2,3] contributed significantly to the early development of clinical practice for the management of voice problems. This significance has been largely neutralized by the more recent symptomatic focus advocated by Boone,[4–6] Wilson,[1,7,8] Perkins,[9–11] and Wilson and Rice.

Moore,[13] in his excellent and thought-provoking treatise on the major issues in voice disorders, reviewed 50 years of research and practice and compared then contemporary textbook writings in voice disorders with several classic publications of earlier years. His discussion concluded:

> Four features stand out in the recent publications: (1) voice disorders are described in greater detail and reflect an increased understanding of basic problems, but the problems are the same; (2) more attention is paid to specific vocal disorders such as laryngectomy; (3) there is a greater variety of therapeutic techniques; and (4) the major emphases in therapy remain as before: training in breath control (where indicated), relaxation and reduction of lar-

yngeal tension, training in listening, articulatory adjustments, and special techniques. These are applied to deviations in pitch, intensity, and quality (including the resonance disorders). Obviously, not much change in the basic clinical practices appears to have occurred over the years (p 156).

In 1985, Johnson[14] wrote that it was striking that Moore's conclusion could be drawn again several years later from a review of recent titles in the field. Even ten years after Moore's reflective writing, we find that the situation has still not changed significantly. Again, greater amounts of descriptive material have been made available; additional attention has been given to special problems (especially the neuropathies and spastic dysphonia); however, the major emphases with respect to management procedures remain essentially the same with the addition of some functional compilations and kit-formatted materials.[15–18] The continuing lament remains the lack of published empirical data validating these clinical methodologies.

Current evaluation and therapeutic practices have been comprehensively described in recent years by Aronson,[19] Boone,[6] Cooper and Cooper,[20] Green,[21] Moncur and Brackett,[22] Prater and Swift,[23] and Stemple.[24] The specific applications to clinical management and evaluation of children's voice problems have been addressed comprehensively by Wilson,[1] Leith and Johnston,[25] and Filter.[26] Their writings all have great value to the clinician who is faced with making day-to-day decisions on clinical management. The procedures and practices are described efficiently and effectively from a practitioner's viewpoint. We regard five references[1,6,11,25,75] as being the most important clinical literature addressing the vocal disturbances of childhood.

Scientifically, the big disappointment with clinical methodology in childhood voice disorders continues to be a significant lack of research or clinical data applied to validate the described and prescribed clinical methodologies. Research on the clinical effectiveness of voice therapy procedures remains regrettably sparse.[13,14,26,28,29] The overwhelming majority of evaluative and treatment procedures described in the literature have not been subjected to rigorous clinical research and contain few reports of precise data collection or even case-study presentations substantiating their effectiveness.[30] Contemporary voice clinicians continue to work with little or no validating data regarding current practices in voice evaluation and management. In addition, the clinical compilation of normative performance data on perceptual and acoustic measurement procedures has been agonizingly slow though the potential of new technology is perhaps the most exciting part of contemporary developments in voice disorders.[14,28,31,32]

CURRENT PRACTICES: ETIOLOGIC VARIABLES

One important issue already alluded to was the question, How important in the priority system are voice disturbances in children? This issue determines the extent of concern for the identification and treatment of the vocal disturbances of childhood. The answer to this question is not an easy one, especially when the long-term effects of these problems are not known, particularly with the most common "benign" childhood problems secondary to vocal use, abuse, and misuse. Many anecdotal reports indicate that some children with long-term "benign" problems, such as nodules, polyps, and thickened cords (i.e., the hyperfunctional group), have an increased frequency of vocal disturbances continuing into adulthood. Perhaps a reduced vocal quality capability in these individuals could have been improved if treated properly during childhood. More likely and more importantly, however, is the possibility that a strong clinical sensitivity to childhood vocal disturbances will identify the rare child who may contract severe disease with vocal disturbance as one of its symptoms. Perkins[9] described the speech-language pathologist as the best-trained critical listener who is in a position to be the first to identify a potential symptom of disease (e.g., hoarseness). Hence, Perkins' thoughtful statements[9] may be the best reason to place childhood vocal disturbance as a priority concern for speech-language pathologists. In addition, the evidence from our colleagues who study nonverbal communication indicates that the total effect of one's communication may depend as much as 38 percent on the vocal aspects of communication.[33] Thus, if it is desirable to provide an "equal opportunity" for all to succeed in society, that provision should also include an equal opportunity to develop a fully communicative and quality vocal product to effectively use the language and communication of commerce in that society. Because a vocal disturbance might influence as much as 38 percent of an individual's total effect of communication on those with whom he or she interacts, we could conclude that vocal disturbance merits definitive attention in childhood.

Fortunately, childhood vocal disturbances are not commonly a symptom of more serious disease; however, the prevalence of such uncommon cases in many caseloads should cause professionals much caution and concern regarding these symptoms. The vocal symptom known as hoarseness (vocal roughness) is in every way a "life-threatening" symptom and should not be ignored nor easily discounted. In fact, the speech-language pathologist would be well served to be clinically sensitive to all the early diagnostic signs and symptoms of laryngeal disease as clearly compiled in sources such as Brewer[34] or Wood and Northern.[35] Hoarseness (vocal roughness) is a frequently occurring vocal symptom that can signal a wide range of potential medical-physiologic concerns. These concerns may include simple inflammatory laryngitis of non-specific origin, the hyperfunctional group (such as nodules, polyps, thickened cords, and contact ulcers), hyperkeratosis, leukoplakia, laryngeal carcinoma, vocal fold paralysis, tuberculosis, syphilis, papillomatosis, and a variety of other common systemic disorders, such as lupus and rheumatoid arthritis.

This range of potential diseases all with a presenting symptom of hoarseness (vocal roughness) or other vocal disturbances should cause the speech-language pathologist to consider carefully the potential etiological variables associated with disturbances of the voice in childhood as well as in adulthood.

To determine the etiologic variables currently discussed in the literature, we completed a systematic review of the most recent (1981–1987) literature. Sources for the review included relevant periodical journals, textbooks on voice disorders, chapters within general textbooks in communication disorders and otolaryngology, and other available published and unpublished materials including theses and dissertations. As we reviewed each original source, we summarized and recorded basic information into a computer data base. The resulting information was compiled, analyzed, and summarized. Initially, we attempted to review recent literature relating specifically to different etiologic factors influencing voice disorders only in children. However, because of the relatively small amount of literature specific to childhood voice disorders, we completed a broader analysis of voice disorders in all age groups, assuming that the etiologic variables would also generally (though to a lesser extent) apply to children. The literature reveals numerous etiologic factors influencing voice disorders, and, in most cases, lists them under more general categories of function or dysfunction. Table 26–1 lists the specific etiologic variables and the general categories of function and dysfunction identified in the systematic review.

The wide variety of etiologic variables that may be responsible for producing vocal disturbances in childhood should encourage the speech-language pathologist to consider carefully the evaluative process and to be sure to include medical examination and clearance as a necessary component of that process. Medical clearance should be sought prior to any consideration for a program of voice therapy to rule out the many possibilities of vocal symptoms resulting from undiagnosed disease in need of medical-physiologic treatment. Medical textbooks in laryngology generally recommend indirect laryngoscopy for all patients presenting a chronic hoarseness or other vocal disturbances as symptoms.[35–38]

Symptoms: Chronic and Transient

One difficult, pragmatic task in the management of childhood vocal disturbances is to differentiate a chronic vocal disturbance from a more transient problem. Childhood is a period marked by a high frequency of transient, respiratory tract problems with concommitant vocal symptoms. The chronicity of these problems needs to be determined during an extended evaluative period by the speech-language pathologist. DeWeese and Saunders[36] write that "any patient who is hoarse longer than two weeks deserves a careful inspection of the larynx'' (p 106). Bryce[39] expands this concept stating that:

> Hoarseness which is temporary occurs so commonly that it tends to be disregarded. Unfortunately, very often a more serious disease is misdiagnosed as laryngitis, and thus its diagnosis is delayed. It is essential to realize that hoarseness resulting from acute inflammatory disease of the larynx does not persist, although it may recur. It has been emphasized for many years that the symptom of hoarseness that persists beyond three weeks without an accompanying respiratory inflammation must be investigated fully. This can be done by simple, indirect laryngoscopy (p 24).

In our experience, some speech-language pathologists hesitate to recommend or refer children for laryngeal examination for a variety of reasons. These reasons range from economic considerations for the client or the parents to feelings of professional inadequacy or insecurity about making such referrals. Some speech-language pathologists are "disappointed" when children who are referred for laryngeal examination return with a finding of "no observable pathology" from the laryngologist. They appear almost relieved when the physician finds a vocal pathology which seems to "validate" their own diagnostic-referral concern and professional worth. Actually, the best finding for such children is the negative result. This finding simply indicates that the child is at an early stage in the potential development of vocal dysfunction and an intervention program designed to prevent further development of the dysfunction should be implemented. Such an intervention might be focused on the interruption of the hyperfunctional cycle by reducing identified contributing factors to the vocal disturbance.

TABLE 26–1 Etiologic Variables Associated with Vocal Disturbance

Specific Etiologic Variable	*General Category of Function/Dysfunction*
abnormal pharynx	organic
absence of epiglottis	organic
accidents	mechanical laryngeal trauma
adenoidectomy	organic
allergies	functional
assault from blunt objects	mechanical laryngeal trauma
assimilative nasality	resonance
bilateral vocal cord paralysis	peripheral neuropathy
cerebral palsy	primary disorder related
chemical burns	burn-related laryngeal trauma
chronic laryngitis	laryngeal pathologies
cleft palate	primary disorder related
closed head injuries	central neuropathy
congenital cyst	organic
congenital laryngeal web	organic
congenital stenosis	organic
congenital structural anomalies	congenital
congenital subglottis hemangiomas	congenital
contact ulcer	autogenous laryngeal trauma
conversion aphonia	laryngeal pathologies
conversion behaviors	personality related
conversion voice disorders	functional
coughing	abuse
deafness	primary disorder related
deformities of cricoid cartilage	organic
delayed mutation	functional
dislocation of laryngeal cartilages	mechanical laryngeal trauma
disorders of cerebellar system	neurogenic, myopathic, apraxic
disorders of extrapyramidal system	neurogenic, myopathic, apraxic
disorders of lower motor neuron, myoneural junction	neurogenic, myopathic, apraxic
disorders of upper motor neuron	neurogenic, myopathic, apraxic
dysarthrias of multiple motor systems	neurogenic, myopathic, apraxic
elevated loudness	autogenous laryngeal trauma
elevated pitch	autogenous laryngeal trauma
endotracheal intubation	mechanical laryngeal trauma
environmental stress	personality related
essential tumor	central neuropathy
excessive talking	autogenous laryngeal trauma
excessive throat clearing	autogenous laryngeal trauma
faulty learning	functional
faulty tongue posture	resonance
faulty voice habits	functional
fractures	mechanical laryngeal trauma
frequent colds	medically related
glandular conditions	functional
glossectomy	medically related
granulomas	structural
hard glottal attack	autogenous laryngeal trauma
harmonal disorder	medically related
hearing loss	
hypernasality	resonance
hyponasality	organic
hysterical aphonia	functional
identity conflict	personality related
imitation	functional
improper endoscopic exam	mechanical laryngeal trauma
inappropriate loudness	abuse
inappropriate pitch	abuse
inappropriate rate	abuse
inappropriate resonation	abuse
inappropriate respiration	abuse
incomplete mutation	functional
indwelling nasogastric tubes	mechanical laryngeal trauma
intubation granuloma	mechanical laryngeal trauma

TABLE 26–1 Continued

Specific Etiologic Variable	*General Category of Function/Dysfunction*
keratosis	autogenous laryngeal trauma
laryngeal cancer	laryngeal pathologies
laryngeal disease	organic
laryngeal trauma	organic
laryngectomy	medically rated
laryngoesophageal cleft	organic
laryngomalacia	organic
leukoplakia	autogenous laryngeal trauma
limited carcinoma	structural
loud talking	abuse
loudness	functional
malignant tumors	organic
mandibulectomy	medically related
mental retardation	
multiple sclerosis	
mutational falsetto	functional
Myasthenia Gravis	
nervous disorder	medically related
neurologic loss of volition control of phonation	neurogenic, myopathic, apraxic
neurological disorders	primary disorder related
palatal	medically related
papilloma	organic
Parkinsons disease	central neuropathy
penetrating injuries	mechanical laryngeal trauma
personality disorders	functional
physiologic disease	organic
pitch deviations	functional
polyps	autogenous laryngeal trauma
premenstrual and menstrual problems	functional
prolonged endotracheal intubation	organic
prolonged mutation	functional
pseudobulbar palsy	central neuropathy
psychological	functional
psychoneurosis	functional
quality	functional
respiratory illness	medically related
scoliosis	
short palate	organic
shouting	abuse
Shy-Drager Syndrome	neurologic diseases
singing	autogenous laryngeal trauma
sinus disorders	medically related
spasmodic dysphonia	functional
speak in abusive manner—folds are weak	autogenous laryngeal trauma
stomach disorder	medically related
strained vocalizations	autogenous laryngeal trauma
stridency	resonance
structural disease	organic
systemic illness	organic
thermal burns	burn-related laryngeal trauma
throat clearing	abuse
too-high tracheostomy	mechanical laryngeal trauma
traumatic laryngeal web	mechanical laryngeal trauma
underdevelopment of 1 vocal cord	organic
unilateral vocal cord paralysis	peripheral neuropathy
upper respiratory conditions	functional
velopharyngeal insufficiency	primary disorder related
ventricular dysphonia	functional
ventricular phonation	laryngeal pathologies
vocal abuse	organic changes—abuse & misuse
vocal cord paralysis	laryngeal pathologies
vocal fatigue	autogenous laryngeal trauma
vocal misuse	organic changes—abuse & misuse
vocal nodules	autogenous laryngeal trauma
yelling	abuse

Categories of Etiologic Variables

Typically, the etiologic variables of voice disorders are grouped into more general categories which are then divided into more specific subcategories. Wilson[1] classified the causes of voice problems in children into four categories: (1) organic; (2) organic changes resulting from vocal abuse and misuse; (3) function; and (4) factors contributing to the voice problem. Wilson further divided these categories into more specific disorder groups. For example, under the organic category, etiologic variables are grouped under (1) structural anomalies; (2) paralysis of any one or several of the nerves supplying the larynx; (3) growths in or around the larynx; and (4) trauma to the larynx. Additionally, he listed resonance problems and neurologic, developmental, and hearing problems as other etiologic variables affecting voice problems.

Other authors have classified the causes of voice disorders under somewhat different headings, but with generally similar groupings of conditions. Pannbacker[40] divided the cause of voice problems into three general categories: (1) organic, resulting from structural or physiologic disease; (2) psychogenic or functional, caused by psychoneurosis, personality disorders, or faulty habits of voice usage; and (3) indeterminate or undetermined cause such as spastic dysphonia. Stemple[24] uses the general categories: (1) vocal misuse—inappropriate respiration, phonation, resonation, pitch, loudness, and rate; (2) medically related etiologies—surgeries, chronic illnesses, or disorders; (3) primary disorder etiologies—anatomic, physiologic, and neurologic that have vocal symptoms secondary to primary problem; and (4) personality-related etiologies—stress, conversation behaviors, and identity conflict. Wilson and Starr[41] placed subjects into categories: (1) structural, subjects with disorders that effect laryngeal mass and function; (2) peripheral neuropathy, subjects with unilateral and bilateral vocal fold paralysis; (3) central neuropathy, subjects with closed head injuries; and (4) functional, subjects with no known laryngeal pathology but with deviations in pitch, loudness, or quality.

In summary, the etiologic variables of vocal disturbance in childhood seem to fall within one of the following broad categories: vocal abuse, physiologic base, neurogenic base, and functional. We use these categories to describe management in the remainder of this chapter.

CLINICAL PROCESSES IN VOICE EVALUATION

Before a successful remediation program for any type of childhood voice disorder is possible, a thorough voice evaluation and examination is necessary. Voice evaluation and management must be carefully linked to each other in the clinical decision making process. Further, continuous assessment during management programs is now recognized to be extremely important in effective voice therapy.[27]

Stemple[24] suggested that:

> The primary objective of the diagnostic voice evaluation is to discover the etiological factors specific to the development of the voice disorder. Speech pathologists use their knowledge of laryngeal anatomy, physiology, pathologies of the laryngeal mechanism, and common etiological factors in a systematic evaluation designed to determine these specific causes.
>
> Secondary objectives of the diagnostic evaluation include education and motivation of the patient and the establishment of credibility and trust in the speech pathologist (p 89).

The School Setting

In the school situation, voice screening is the usual initial step for discovering children with voice disorders. The speech-language pathologist in the schools is in an excellent position to develop effective voice-screening procedures for the early identification of such children.[6] A combination of the usual school screening activities with a well-designed voice clinic using a full "team-approach" to voice management can be a highly successful model for the early identification, evaluation, and follow-up for children with vocal disturbances.[42–46] The voice clinic in the school setting combines the resources of the laryngologist, speech-language pathologist, school nurse, and other professionals to intervene effectively in childhood voice disturbances. In three reports regarding the development and results of school voice clinics, Miller and Madison[45,47] reported that of the 249 students (ages pre-2 years through 12 years) attending those particular school voice clinics, 40 percent were diagnosed as having nodules, 12 percent had chronic laryngitis, 9 percent had thickened cords, 29 percent had concommitant medical problems, two cases had contact ulcers, and one case had vocal cord paralysis. The voice clinic model provides an effective way within the school setting to deal with the issues of chronic versus transient problems and to provide adequate follow-up to children with voice disturbances with little cost or delay.[45–47]

The Team Approach

The literature suggests that a more thorough assessment of voice disorders in children is accomplished through a team approach including a laryngologist, a speech-pathologist, nurses, and other consultive professional personnel. A team approach concept allows consideration of all possible etiologic variables of the voice disturbance. This approach also increases the likelihood that children with voice problems will receive comprehensive and coordinated care from the time the problems are first discovered through examination, consultation, treatment, and follow-up.[1] The team responsibilities reflect an important professional role for each specialist. The laryngologist is responsible for examining the laryngeal mechanism for medical-physiologic pathology, for determining the laryngeal mechanism for medical-physiologic pathology, for determining the need for surgical or medical intervention, and for providing medical clearance for potential therapy. The speech-language pathologist is responsible for identifying the symptomatic range of vocal disturbance, evaluating the communicative effect and priority, and for establishing improved vocal functioning through various therapies.[24] Murry[48] stated that:

> The laryngologist provides essential information about the structures of the larynx, but it is the speech pathologist who must identify the behavioral parameters that contribute to the production of dysphonia. Therefore, the assessment procedure must attempt to identify behavior characteristics of the patient and his voice which cause the voice to deviate from accepted norms (p 478).

The medical examination should include an examination of the head and neck, including a laryngoscopic evaluation of the larynx, which may be accomplished with mirror laryngoscopy or with the new endoscopic techniques.[49] The use of fiberoptic endoscopy adds important new documentation and educational capability to the team in the evaluative process. Most practitioners concur that a thorough evaluation including a medical examination of the voice is essential prior to the beginning of voice treatment.

The evaluation process allows the voice clinician to determine what management steps should be taken with the patient. If voice therapy is found to be necessary, the evalution assists the clinician in developing a therapy plan and in predicting the prognosis of the patient's outcome.[6]

Models of Evaluation

A variety of evaluative formats or models for the accurate assessment of voice disorders in children are discussed in the literature.

Aronson[19] suggested that the evaluating clinician should: (1) obtain a case history; (2) administer a voice evaluation; (3) interpret findings; and (4) make clinical decisions. Aronson also recommended that the speech-language pathologist should rate esthetic and intelligibility factors in contextual speech, should measure sustained vowel /a/ prolongation, should assess coughing and sharp glottal attack, should determine and analyze pitch range, should measure the vocal endurance, should perform a motor speech examination, should assess musculoskeletal tension, should test for pain in larynx, should observe the elevation of larynx and hyoid bone, should examine voice improvement, should measure optimum pitch, and should perform a rating of the voice using a voice profile.

Stemple[24] recommended evaluating the medical and social history of the problem, administering an oral-peripheral examination, and a voice evaluation. The voice evaluation suggested by Stemple includes subjective measures of voice quality; measures respiration; assesses phonation (e.g., hard glottal attacks, glottal fry, and breathiness), resonation, pitch, loudness, rate, laryngeal strength and tone; and identifies the type of vocal abuses that occur. Impressions of the evaluation are then summarized, a prognosis is made, and recommendations are outlined.

Murry[48] prescribed a similar evaluative process including complete case history, respiratory evaluation, peripheral oral examination, phonatory evaluation, resonance and loudness assessments, clinical impressions, and the summary and recommendations.

Boone's model of voice evaluation includes a case history format used in the evaluation of children[15] which seeks input from the child, teacher, and parent. The format includes the description of the problem, causal information, onset data, variability of the symptoms, voice usage, and abuse and misuse behaviors. Although the focus of the evaluation is upon the larynx and respiratory systems, an examination of facial structures, mouth, dentition, tongue, teeth, hard and soft palate, pharynx, and nasal cavities is also recommended. In the voice evaluation itself, Boone recommended the observation and detailed measurement of respiratory adequacy as a primary part of the voice evaluation because the vocal folds are activated for phonation by the air stream passing through the closed glottis. Hence, Boone's model of vocal assessment includes a thorough examination including measures of lung volume (vital capacity, tidal volume, inspiratory reserve, and expiratory reserve); air pressure measures; air flow measures (s:z ratio, phonated /a/); motions of the torso; type of breathing patterns, pitch measures (frequency range, optimal pitch, habitual pitch, and variations in pitch and loudness); and measurements of voice quality. Boone emphasized the importance of the speech-language pathologist in becoming an essential observer as these types of assessments are made and in striving to describe observed behavior rather than merely labeling the behavior. He suggested that voice rating scales assist the clinician in separating the various processes contributing to voice disturbance into separate components. Johnson[27] suggested that voice clinicians need to be excellent observers and that they focus on three levels: respiration, phonation, and resonation. The behavior observations made at each of these levels are important keys to the entire voice evaluation process.

Prater and Swift[22] suggested an evaluative structure including:

1. Case history, objective judgement of severity of dysphonia (by listening to the patient read or speak).
2. Determination of esthetic quality of the voice and intelligibility (by audio or videotaping a sample of the patient's voice).
3. Description of the patient's vocal fold structure and function from a laryngologist.
4. Respiratory capabilities (e.g., termination of speech coincides with termination of exhalation, sustained vowel production, sustained /s/and /z/ productions, endurance of sustained speech production).
5. Type of respiration pattern (clavicular, thoracic, diaphragmatic-abdominal breathing).
6. Muscle coordination for respiration.
7. Phonatory and respiratory efficiency (Maximum phonation time (MPT), estimated MPT, sustained s/z production, mean flow rate, phonaton quotient).
8. Strength of glottal closure.
9. Pitch range, optimal pitch, habitual pitch, and other pitch qualities.
10. Loudness.
11. Voice quality (breathiness, harsh, hoarseness, and vocal fry).
12. Resonance quality (hypernasality, hyponasality, denasality, effeminate voice quality, and cul-de-sac resonance).
13. Vocal endurance.
14. Sites of vocal hypertension.

Filter[26] prescribed a process consisting of case history; perceptual description (pitch, loudness, severity, tension, and hypernasality); evaluation of associated behaviors (breathing, muscular tension, ability to carry a tune, articulation, pitch discrimination, pitch variability, imitation of pitch, loudness, rate, prosody, self-ratings of tension, and anxiety); assessment of additional data regarding speech anxiety, vocal abuse, breathing, and duration of vowels; and measurements of variability.

Leith and Johnston[25] suggested that the childhood voice evaluation should consist of:

1. General data collection: auditory classification (subjective voice measures), collection of historical information, observation of general motor skills, oral-peripheral examination, and hearing test.
2. Competence and performance evaluation: respiration (breathing patterns and checking action); phonation (vocal fold approximation from open and from closed position, duration of vocal fold vibration, contrast of vocal fold vibration, and stability of vocal fold vibration); laryngeal adjustments (pitch level, pitch changes, loudness level, loudness change, and pitch-loudness interaction); and resonance coupling.
3. Integrated vocal analysis to determine if a voice problem exists and, if so, in what aspect of vocal production.
4. Environmental guidance of vocal behaviors: assessing the influence on vocal production by changes in internal and external environment.
5. Decisionmaking: deciding if the client has a handicapping voice disorder and, if so, what type of treatment to provide.

One of the most comprehensive evaluation system models is that proposed by Wilson.[1] Wilson recommended the use of several voice profiles in assessing the childhood voice. He discussed 10 profiles of the Buffalo III Voice Profile system and suggested that they form the basis for the first step in examination and analysis of the voice. The speech-language pathologist selects from a list the voice profiles which are suitable and applicable for the child: (1) voice screening, (2) group behavior, (3) voice, (4) voice abuse, (5) speech anxiety, (6) resonance, (7) hearing impaired voice, (8) voice recording, (9) voice diagnostic, (10) voice therapy progress. All the profiles except the diagnostic summary and voice recording are based upon a five-point profiling scale that has three main features: (1) a severity ranking of the problem; (2) the possible impairment caused by the problem; and (3) examination and voice therapy intervention strategies. The severity ratings include: (1) normal voice, (2) mild severity, (3) moderate severity, (4) severe, and (5) very severe. The speech-language pathologist, the patient, teachers, and parents each use specific profiles for observing and rating the child's voice in various settings. The Buffalo III Voice Profile rates 12 major components of voice including laryngeal tone, pitch, loudness, nasal resonance, oral resonance, breath supply, muscles, voice abuse, rate, speech anxiety, speech intelligibility, and overall voice rating. In addition to the appropriate voice profiles, the evaluation of pitch, loudness, quality, resonance, and vocal abuse is also made. If vocal abuses are discovered, they are described and evaluated and intelligibility is assessed. Wilson also recommended the measurement of frequency range, fundamental frequency, loudness, voice quality, maximum phonation time, s:z ratio, breathing habits, posture, and evaluation of velopharyngeal competency.

Wilson[42] and Wilson and Rice[12] described the Wilson Voice Profile, a rating scale profile system that is used frequently to describe various dimensions of vocal performance. The profile includes a seven-point overall severity scale, a rating of pitch, a rating of vocal cord openness or closure, and ratings of resonance cavity, constancy, intensity, and vocal range. The Wilson profile system is a useful scaling procedure to describe important vocal features; however, it does not provide a system that is highly sensitive to clinical change. Several investigations have assessed the judgement reliability of the profiling system[50–52] and have found good interjudge reliability for most of the parameters. The major advantages of the Wilson profile are its wide visibility, acceptance, and use among clinical practitioners and the excellent audio and video training materials available for use in practice.

Objective Evaluation

Johnson[27] advocated the development of an objective voice evaluation procedure based on the work of Michel and Wendahl,[28] Beckett,[53] and other investigators in voice science. Reed[29] indicated that the most fundamental need for voice research was to replace the vague terminology with measurable observations sensitive enough to allow the results to be interpreted by other investigators. More recently, Filter[26] reviewed much of the work completed in the voice evaluation area over the past several years. He described current case-history procedures, screening procedures, perceptual description formats, associated behaviors, and additional data. Michel and Wendahl's landmark discussion[28] concerning correlates of voice production suggested 12 measurable parameters to be considered for investigation. These 12 correlates form a basic set of measurable features of the voice, which, when investigated fully, could constitute a beginning measurement battery that might be used to assess the adequacy of laryngeal or vocal functioning. Michel and Wendahl[28] proposed "to present voice as a multidimensional series of measurable events, implying that a single phonation can be assessed in many different ways" (p 267). The 12 correlates they proposed were vital capacity of the lungs, maximum duration of controlled sustained blowing, modal frequency level, maximum frequency ranges, maximum duration of sustained phonation, volume-velocity flow during phonation, glottal waveform, sound pressure level, jitter of the vocal signal, shimmer of the vocal signal, effort level (vocal), and transfer function of the vocal tract. Reed,[29] in discussing and adapting Michel and Wendahl's correlates, subsequently suggested six parameters that could serve as initial efforts to address the major concepts of voice quality: volume-velocity airflow, jitter, shimmer, effort level, electromyographic studies, and rise-fall time.

Since the 1960s, data from voice science laboratories have emerged signaling interest in the development of objective measurement parameters of the voice. An exhaustive review of the laboratory work is outside the scope of this chapter; however, much excellent basic laboratory work has yielded important information regarding the measurement of laryngeal function. Central to this work is that of Koike and colleagues,[54–57] Isshiki and associates,[58–63] Iwata and von Leden,[64] and Yanagihara and associates.[65–67] These data are effectively summarized by Hirano.[31]

In another landmark article, Beckett[53] suggested that several of the specific measures derived from the voice science laboratory could be applied clinically to patients with respirometric or voice disturbances. Additionally, he suggested that the respirometer was an effective, reliable means of obtaining those data clinically without the extensive and expensive instrumentation used in the voice science laboratory. Beckett proposed seven aerodynamic measures that could have diagnostic or clinical value. They included one-stage vital capacity (VC), phonation volume (PV), phonation time (PT), maximum predicted phonation time (MPT), mean flow rate (MFR), vocal velocity index (VVI), and phonation time-maximum predicted phonation time ratio (PT/MPT).

Johnson and associates began in 1970 to apply such data-gathering techniques on an experimental basis to clinical populations of voice disordered individuals, as well as to subjects without voice disorders. Initially, they conducted a series of studies that made use of precision measurement in combination with behavior modification techniques in persons with voice disorders.[68–73] These investigations culminated with the publishing of the Vocal Abuse Reduction Program (VARP)[74,75] as an effective data-based clinical voice management program (see later discussion). The cited thesis studies were single-subject investigations of the effectiveness of VARP. With the establishment of this program as an effective, replicable, and predictable clinical procedure, it became possible to use several experimental measurement procedures, as suggested by the work of Michel and Wendahl[28] and that of Beckett[53] for monitoring data as voice therapy progressed during VARP intervention. Two investigators, Thompson[76] and Smee,[77] demonstrated the feasibility of using experimental measurement procedures for monitoring client progress during voice management. This monitoring was done by tracking the measures over the course of treatment with several individual subjects, VARP being used as the intervention procedure. Although feasibility for the therapeutic tracking use of the procedure was demonstrated, the amount of information known about unimpaired performance on the individual measurements was minimal, and guideposts for interpreting the meaning of changes in those measurements were limited. Subsequently, investigators began to study the use of these measures on the performance of varying age groups of children and adults without voice disorders.[78–83] The results of these investigations were summarized by Hammond[84] and again later by Johnson.[85] The measurements included in the battery selected for study were vital capacity (VC), phonation volume (PV), phonation time (PT), phonation time ratio (PTR), maximum flow rate (MFR), phonation quotient (PQ), vocal velocity index (VVI), and phonation volume-vital capacity ratio (PV/VC). As indicated previously, these measures were originally derived from the voice science literature and were adapted for use as suggested by the work of Beckett[53] and Michel and Wendahl.[28] Preliminary data and further information on this battery of clinical measurements were discussed by Johnson.[14,85]

Precision assessment in screening or voice therapy with laryngeal disorders was also advocated by Davis.[86] He suggested that acoustic analysis is preferable to auditory preceptual methods and stated that,

> Acoustic techniques for voice analysis are based on the source of the signal and the method of analysis. One source is direct signals (e.g., radiated sound pressure and throat contact signals); the other source is indirect signals (e.g., glottal or residual signals derived from using inverse filtering techniques). For each of these sources, the signals may be analyzed in the time domain (e.g., to determine mean fundamental frequency or mean perturbation) or in the frequency domain (e.g., to determine long-term average spectral slope or energy distribution [p 80]).

Other authors have also expressed a disenchantment with a reliance on subjective-perceptual judgements in voice evaluation. Several authors have examined the difficulty with perceptually based judgements in the evaluation of voice problems. Results of a study of 64 children (ages 5 to 15 years) with voice problems indicated that perceptual judgment alone was not reliable to diagnose children with nodules.[52] Blaustein and Bar[87] studied 161 school-aged children, ages 4 to 14 years (74 males, 84 females) who received vocal assessments. Their results indicated that perceptual judgments were not accurate among listeners and concluded that a more objective measurement method was needed.

Hirano's compilation[31] of clinical examination parameters provides an indepth consideration of contemporary attempts to objectify the voice evaluation process. In the examination of phonatory ability, Hirano suggested seven primary parameters of voice to be evaluated. The seven are: (1) maximum phonation time (sustained production of /a/); (2) frequency range of phonation; (3) speaking fundamental frequency; (4) vocal register; (5) intensity range of phonation; (6) fundamental frequency–intensity profile; and (7) glottal efficiency.

Wilson and Starr[41] seriously challenged some of Hirano's reliance on the objective measurements and suggested that it is unlikely that such measures as glottal efficiency or air flow measures alone are effective ways by which to identify laryngeal dysfunction related to laryngeal pathology. They emphasized the need to combine these data with other information including subglottal air pressure information and information on vocal fold movement to produce useful identification data.

All the "objective measurement" procedures just discussed are at early stages of development and definitive data are not available for reliable and dependable clinical usage. However, important and basic investigations on this work continue. Eckel and Boone[88] alluded to the clinical usefulness of objective measurement in monitoring client progress in their discussion of a 19-year-old university singer with bilateral nodules. Other investigators have similarly investigated various measurement procedures as possible correlates of laryngeal function. Gordon, Morton, and Simpson[89] measured maximum phonation time for several vowels and reported greatly reduced times in persons with laryngeal pathologies. They also reported increased air flow rates during phonation in these patients. Boone[5] discussed the use of s/z as an indicator of vocal fold pathology among voice clients. He reported that vocal folds with pathology appear to function less efficiently, resulting in a decrease in glottal resistance and increased airflow with shortened phonation times. Tait, Michel, and Carpenter[90] studied children with normal voices, aged 5, 7, and 9, and found that they produced s:z ratios close to 1.0, with /z/ duration being typically slightly longer than the /s/. Eckel and Boone[89] concluded that s/z used alone or in conjunction with other measures appeared to be an excellent indicator of poor laryngeal function resulting from glottal margin lesions. Inglis[79] and Lee[80] also studied s/z in their investigations and found them to be clinically sensitive indicators of laryngeal function. Several investigators have reported data on the maximum duration of sustained phonation (phonation time) using sustained vowels[8,78,91–96] and have suggested its clinical utility.

Smitheran and Hixon[97] investigated a clinical method for estimating laryngeal airway resistance during vowel production and suggested that their procedure may be useful in discriminating between persons with normal laryngeal function and those with disordered laryngeal function. The procedure takes advantage of measuring oral pressure and airway opening flow by use of a specially designed utterance that alternates voiceless stop-plosives and voiced vowels. Oral pressure is obtained with an oral catheter, one end being placed in the oral cavity and the other coupled to a differential air pressure transducer. Airway opening flow is channelled through an anesthesia mask covering the mouth and nose. Flow from the mask is sensed by a pneumotachometer, also coupled to a separate air pressure transducer. The resultant conditioned data are recorded on a storage oscilloscope and a thermal recorder. The preliminary data gathered with the system supported the reliability and validity of the method as a way of estimating laryngeal airway resistance during vowel production. The authors cited exploratory clinical evidence to support the sensitivity of the method in detecting differences between persons with and without vocal pathology. This experimental procedure also appears to have great potential for use not only in discriminating between normal and disordered laryngeal functioning, but also in the periodic tracking of clinical progress.

The results of these investigations suggest that a variety of noninvasive clinical measures are available to the clinician as potentially valuable sensors of clinical progress. Though many research data remain to be gathered to establish their ultimate scientific validity, initial investigations have demonstrated their usefulness, relative simplicity, and convenience in clinical management.

Instrumentation

To gather these "more objective" data, some sophisticated instrumentation may ultimately be required. Davis' work[86] used digital computer techniques to extract vocal function data from the acoustic speech signals. Hirano assisted in the development of a "Phonatory Function Analyzer"* to gather some of his data on air flow, intensity, fundamental frequency, and phonation time. Significant new voice analysis instrumentation is now available that undoubtedly will contribute greatly to research and development in the objective measurement of vocal function.

Three additional instruments merit special mention. The Visi-Pitch† can accurately extract cycle-to-cycle fundamental frequency and can display each cycle in real-time. The Voice Identification PM Series Pitch Analyzers‡ are microprocessor controlled and can extract precise acoustic information about both fundamental frequency and intensity. The third instrument is a new digital spectrograph,† which allows for detailed spectrum analysis with new high-speed components. These high-technology instruments have the capability of greatly increasing our basic knowledge about the parameters of the human voice and will provide additional valuable clinical tracking capability to the voice therapy process. A thorough consideration of these potentially significant advances awaits data from continuing investigations. In addition, the application of these procedures to childhood voice disturbance adds additional challenges to the continued research and development in this arena.

The implication of increasing objectivity of vocal measurement is that clinicians will no longer be able to justify a lack of precision on the basis that such measures of the voice are too difficult to obtain in the clinic or are not available. Measurement and objectivity will continue to be an increasing necessity in the clinical evaluation process surrounding voice disorders. Voice clinicians must take responsibility for finding and implementing reliable and sensitive clinical measures of vocal function within their clinical settings. The question regarding such measurement and objectivity is no longer "if," but rather "how."

The preceding summary of models and procedures for voice evaluation contain many common elements. In childhood voice disturbance, it seems that the ideal evaluation would include the resources of both a laryngologist and a speech-language pathologist in concert using the data from (1) a thorough case history; (2) a complete laryngoscopic examination; (3) perceptual assessments of pitch, intensity, and quality; (4) a battery of objective aerodynamic and acoustic measurements; (5) examination of abuse and environmental variables; and (6) recordings of the voice over time.

* Nagashima Medical Instruments, 24-1, Hongo 5-chome, Bunkyo-Ku, Tokyo 113, Japan.

† Kay Elemetrics, 12 Maple Avenue, Pine Brook, New Jersey, 07058.

‡ Voice Identification, Inc., P.O. Box 714, Somerville, New Jersey 08876.

CLINICAL PROCESSES IN VOCAL MANAGEMENT

The literature concerning the management of childhood voice problems presents a wide range of therapeutic approaches. These approaches seem to be widely applicable within the state of knowledge about vocal function and the physiologic processes that contribute to it. Certain principles can guide the therapeutic activities within a reasonable rationale and framework.

Management Phases and Models

Wilson[1] suggested that the management of voice problems proceed through four phases: (1) introduction to voice therapy; (2) analyzing the voice; (3) changing voice use; and (4) establishing good voice. This phasing model of management is a good fundamental structure within which to consider therapy for childhood voice problems.

In the introductory phase, Wilson specified that the major objectives included reviewing adjunct examinations, making audio- or videotape recordings, reviewing the child's problem with the child, discussing the therapy program, and obtaining a "Voice Notebook" for the child.

The second phase, analyzing the voice, includes a complete voice analysis adapted to the type of problem presented by the child, as described earlier in this chapter. Wilson specified his Buffalo III Voice Profile System for the analysis phase which, as described previously, includes 10 separate profiles used to rate vocal characteristics and to aid in the establishment of the goals of therapeutic process.

The third phase, changing voice use, uses Wilson's 10-step Voice Therapy Outline. In addition, "good voice" rules are presented to the client and a program to eliminate vocal abuse is conducted. Specific vocal behaviors are approached as specified therapy targets including laryngeal tones, oral and nasal resonance, loudness, pitch, rate, speech intelligibility, and the prosodic factors of speaking. A variety of voice projects are suggested to promote the generalization and daily use of new vocal communication patterns.

The final phase, establishing the good voice, is intended as a habituation phase where permanent carryover of the newly established vocal patterns is sought. Reducing vocal hypertension and obtaining a balanced muscular tonus are also worked on during this phase.

Wilson wrote "The goal of all voice therapy is to help children learn to use their voices effectively so they speak with a pleasing voice quality, with properly balanced resonance, and with appropriate voice pitch level, loudness, and inflection" (p 15).

Stone and Casteel[98] suggested that the curriculum for teaching new vocal communication patterns should have two facets. One should be with the mechanics or techniques for teaching normal laryngeal function and the other should be with teaching the client responsibility in using the new function.

Murry[48] proposed that specific goals in the treatment of voice disorders might be divided into seven categories: (1) improving vocal hygiene; (2) reducing or eliminating internal and external sources of vocal abuse and excessive vocal loudness; (3) developing a relaxed, easy phonation; (4) increasing the stability of the respiratory and phonatory systems; (5) reducing situational stresses; (6) establishing appropriate pitch and intonation characteristics; and (7) improving the patient's ability to monitor his vocal output in all speaking situations.

Leith and Johnston[25] suggested that the general course of treatment should be initially to get the new vocal behavior to occur. Next, the new behavior should be shaped gradually to the appropriate form for normal vocal production or to the limits imposed by any possible intervening factor, such as a medical or structural problem. Finally, the new vocal behavior should be stabilized and generalized.

Johnson[75] recommended a basic three-step treatment model for children with chronic hoarseness resulting from vocal misuse or abuse (hyperfunction). The model includes: (1) a systematic reduction of vocal misuse-abuse behavior (the Vocal Abuse Reduction Program); (2) the establishment of good vocal quality (vocal facilitative approaches); and (3) the extension-generalization of good vocal quality to all situations.

Management Within Categories of Voice Disorders

Another way to consider the management procedures in childhood voice disorders is within the four categories specified earlier in this chapter; namely those disorders with a psychological base, a physiologic base, a neurologic base, or a vocal abuse or hyperfunctional base. Each of these categories has process and procedural variables unique to the disorder base.

Psychological Base

Disorders with a psychological base in childhood are fairly infrequent, but include conversation disorders, personality-related disorders, certain pitch disturbances, and functional aphonias.

Aronson[19] suggested that the treatment model for conversation disorders include: (1) patient education (teaching the child and parent about the cause of the vocal dysfunction); (2) direct voice therapy to reestablish the voice; (3) catharsis and counseling to discuss feelings about the return of the voice with encouragement to use it fully; and (4) referral for further psychotherapy, if applicable.

Stemple[24] in discussing personality-related disorders recommended medical examination, diagnostic examination, direct manipulation of the voice, and counseling to determine why the vocal disturbance was present and to determine if additional counseling is necessary.

Wilson[1] discussed the general problem of improper pitch in childhood and suggested that the treatment of such disorders should include a program of listening training followed by the teaching of the correct pitch level and appropriate pitch variability. Wilson also recommended his 10-step voice therapy outline for pitch. Some of these disorders in children represent potential psychoemotional problems which need special care.

Treatment for mutational falsetto according to Aronson[19] should include the evoking and identification of a low-pitched voice, which is then shaped into regular speech. Similarly, Wilson[1] recommended that the treatment of disturbed vocal mutation should be accomplished through listening training and by developing an awareness of differences, teaching gross and fine discriminations, and followed by the production of a lower pitch.

Functional aphonia is a somewhat different type of psychological voice disorder, but the treatment is similar to other disorders within this general classification. Again, the problem is not seen frequently in childhood, but, if encountered, the therapy processes are adaptable from the adult literature. Successful voice therapy for functional aphonia must begin by having the clinician explain the problem to the client using a physiologic description of the aphonia. The description avoids implying that the client could choose to phonate. Instead, describing to the child what is actually happening (i.e., keeping the vocal cords apart) should make it clear that the clinician knows what the problem is. The clinician then suggests to the client that "We will do things in therapy that will bring the cords together again to produce normal voice." Next, the clinician should evaluate whatever nonverbal phonations the child may have in his coughing, grunting, laughing, and crying repertoire, and then describe them to the child as normal phonatory activities "where the vocal cords are getting together well to produce these sounds." These nonverbal phonations should then be gradually shaped into the habitual usage of speech.[6] Murray, Carr, and Jacobs[99] have reported on the successful use of these procedures with youth whose ages range from 11 to 15 years.

Physiologic Base

Disorders with a physiologic base include a wide array of problems that have a structural genesis or a malfunctioning physiology. Included in this category are many problems of resonance, respiratory insufficiency, functional laryngitis sicca, ventricular phonation, and the voice problems of hearing impairment. In the vocal remediation of children who demonstrate physiologic disorders, the primary disorder should be treated first and voice therapy is usually a secondary consideration, if considered at all in the treatment. The therapy for these disorders includes compensatory voice intervention and the strengthening or gaining of greater efficiency with the remaining intact physiology.

One important physiologic disorder of childhood is the problem of resonance. We do not discuss this category of problem in significant detail here as it is considered elsewhere in this volume (see Chapter 18). Boone[6] suggested that any attempts at voice therapy for these problems be deferred until the evaluation of the problem and attempts at correction of the physiologic condition have been completed. Methods for working with resonance include the altering of tongue position, changing of loudness, ear training, establishing a new pitch, careful explanation of the problem to the patient, providing specific feedback, voice placement techniques, and respiration practice procedures.[6]

When voice therapy for resonance disorders is indicated, Wilson[1] specified that the goals for therapy should be: (1) to improve the oral–nasal resonance balance to reduce or eliminate hypernasality; (2) to improve articulatory precision and increase the level of speech intelligibility; (3) to eliminate specific problems in loudness, pitch, and rate; (4) to modify or eliminate voice abuse and improve laryngeal tone; (5) to eliminate facial grimaces and nares constrictions; (6) to develop a program of physical exercises for breath pressure and muscular tension, breath direction, speech organ activation, and velopharyngeal closure; and (7) to improve oral–nasal resonance balance to reduce or eliminate hyponasality.

Stemple[24] suggests identification of the problem, ear training, articulation therapy, pitch and loudness modification, non-speech phonation, and negative practice to manage resonance problems.

Respiratory problems would constitute another

dimension of physiologic-based problems. Most of the current literature recommends the proper identification of the specific problem, providing ear training, and attempting to maximize the usable respiratory capacities of the voice in efficient voice production. Boone's facilitative approaches are especially helpful in establishing correct and efficient respiratory usage.

Stone[100] presented a suggested regime for dealing with clients who have a type of laryngitis sicca syndrome in which the main physiologic difficulty is a lack of glandular secretions and mucosal lubrication available in the laryngeal region. The symptoms also include a frequent dry persistent cough or throat-clearing behavior to remove thick viscid secretions or tenacious mucous from the vocal folds. Stone recommended a multidimensional approach to this problem in addition to the medical treatment prescribed, including the decreasing of exposure to tobacco, marijuana, and alcohol; eliminating caffeine from the diet, and reducing milk products; increasing the intake of liquids to include a recommended dosage of eight glasses of water per day; the use of mucolytic agents; tongue-tip up breathing; reduction of exposure to potential environmental irritants, such as hair sprays, perfumes, deodorants, cleaning compounds, industrial fumes, and exhaust; and the reduction of use, abuse, misuse of the voice in general. Ballinger[37] discussed the medical treatments commonly employed for this condition. The frequency of childhood occurrences of this problem is unknown.

Ventricular phonation is treated by a searching process for finding true vocal fold vibration, which should provide the client with a more satisfactory voice than that produced by the ventricular folds. This process is achieved by using such facilitative approaches as inhalation-exhalation phonation.[6] Wilson[1] suggested that the most useful technique for eliminating ventricular phonation and transferring phonatory effort to the true cords is listening training combined with direct teaching of an improved voice. Again, instances of this disorder in childhood are rare.

Some authors also included hearing impairment as a physiologic-based voice disorder. Therapeutic management of voice problems with these children has been addressed by Boone[6] and Wilson[1] in considerable detail and we do not attempt to summarize those methods in this chapter.

Neurologic Base

The overall management of voice problems related to neural innervation requires medical and neurologic management as well as the short- and long-term participation of the speech-language pathologist. These disorders include vocal fold paralysis, neuropathies, dysarthrias, tremor, and the spastic dysphonias. The incidence of such problems in childhood is infrequent and hence, the procedural aspects of management are not summarized in any detail in this context. The work of Aronson[19] is of great value to the clinician regarding these specific disorders.

Vocal Abuse or Hyperfunctional Base

Data from several recent studies[1,43–46,101,102] indicate that the childhood vocal disturbances identified most frequently are ones related directly to vocal abuse. Johnson[14] concluded that 85 to 90 percent of the voice problems of childhood are related to vocal abuse or misuse or to disorders that are considered to be "hyperfunctional" in nature. These disorders include vocal nodules, vocal polyps, thickened vocal folds, contact ulcers, and some forms of simple laryngitis.

The concept of vocal hyperfunction includes any behaviors that result in excessive muscular tension in the vocal tract. This excessive tension may come from any of the variety of vocal behaviors that induce tension into the vocal tract at any level (respiratory, phonatory, or resonatory). The laryngeal mechanism is largely a muscular system and functions in the same way as other muscular systems in the body in relation to hyperfunctional usage. To use the analogy of running and the muscular system of the legs, an individual could abuse or misuse the leg muscles in several ways: either by running too long, too hard, or in an abnormal fashion, or by putting too much stress on one leg or the other. Any of these activities could lead to a hyperfunctioning leg-muscle system. The analogy holds true also for use of the vocal musculature. Additionally, prolonged hyperfunctioning of a muscle system fatigues the muscles to the degree that they finally become unable to produce a normal degree of muscle tone, and the condition of hypofunction sets in. As hypofunction increases, the muscular effort also increases, adding more hyperfunctional usage to the system and fatiguing the muscles even more. Thus the condition increases in severity in a vicious spiral. Likewise, in laryngeal functioning, prolonged hyperfunctional use of the voice fatigues the vocal musculature to the degree that the muscles are unable to produce a normal degree of muscle tone, and a degree of hypofunction sets in. This hypofunction causes the vocal musculature to work even harder at producing appropriate phonation and in doing so, adds more hyperfunctional behavior, thus further fatiguing the musculature. More effort is added, and the condition worsens. This combined process of hyper- and hypofunctioning is an interesting phenomenon in the larynx, especially because the hyperfunctional behavior can also lead to the formation of organic-structural changes (such as nodules, thickened cords, and polyps) on the margins of the vocal folds. Such charges complicate the process and consequently affect the level of effort required for vocal fold functioning because of the increased mass of the folds generated by the presence of these vocal pathologies and an increased difficulty in approximating the margins of the vocal folds for phonation.

Several additional factors may interplay in this process of hyperfunction to produce a "hyperfunctional voice problem." These factors are susceptibility factors and relate to predisposing characteristics of the person with hyperfunctional vocal behavior. The combination of these susceptibility factors with hyperfunctional behavior (i.e., use, abuse, and misuse) of the laryngeal mechanism can result in the formation of laryngeal pathologies and can produce vocal symptoms (Fig. 26–1). Susceptibility factors include histologic differences in the basic cellular makeup of the individual laryngeal mechanisms, the presence of an invading bacterial or viral organism, the physical conditioning history of the individual's laryngeal mechanism, and other such factors that could increase an individual's susceptibility to the development of laryngeal problems. In Figure 26–2 we present hypothetical examples of the combination of susceptibility factors and hyperfunctional behaviors in a general hyperfunctional equation relationship.

In Example 1, the individual has not conditioned his or her voice properly and then overuses the voice in singing, resulting in laryngeal inflammation and vocal disturbance. This example is representative of frequently seen cases in which students majoring in vocal music come to college with little vocal training or experience and throw themselves completely into vocal performance and practice with little thought about the need to condition the vocal musculature. This situation is analogous to the nonrunner who decides to run in a marathon race with little thought beforehand about a long and intensive program of physical conditioning. In children, it would be analogous to the child who is described as being vocally aggressive and who constantly talks, loud talks, yells, and screams.

Example 2 represents the frequently seen school child who seems not to yell or scream any more than his or her peers, but whose larynx has developed a set of vocal nodules. Histologic differences may be present in the individual larynx and it is our hypothesis that such physiologic differences may ultimately account for one child developing nodules whereas another does not, although their levels of vocal usage are strikingly similar. Examples 3 and 4 provide additional hypothetical examples of how the hyperfunctional cycle can work to cause vocal problems.

The modification of hyperfunctional problems necessitates interrupting the hyperfunctional cycle and reducing the amount of potential hyperfunctional behavior, which, along with the susceptibility factors, has produced the vocal pathology. The clinician must remain aware and conscious of the sus-

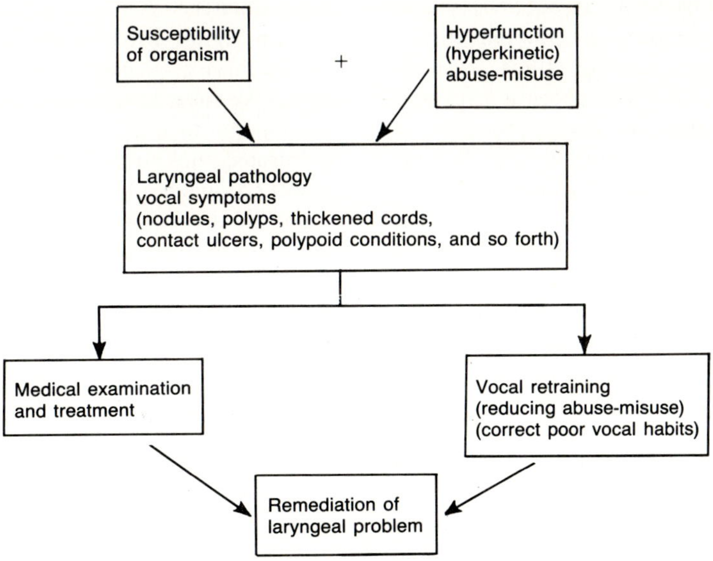

Figure 26–1 Process for the development and treatment of disorders with a hyperfunctional base.

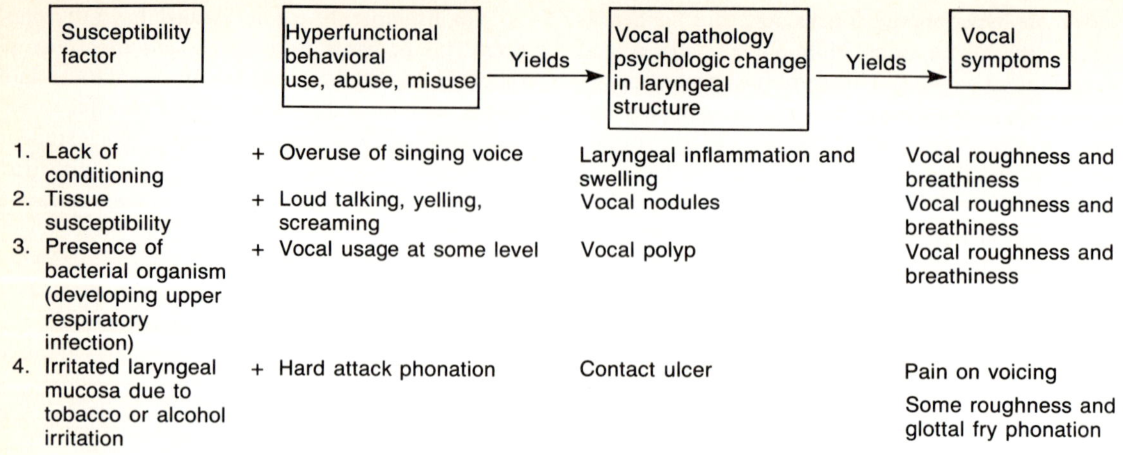

Figure 26–2 The hyperfunctional equation with four hypothetical examples of how it works.

ceptibility factors in planning and carrying out appropriate therapy procedures and, in some instances (e.g., lack of conditioning), build components into the total therapeutic plan to handle such factors.

The technology of applied behavior analysis suggests that behaviors be precisely defined so that they can be observed and counted readily. In attempting to interrupt the hyperfunctional cycle and to reduce the amount of potential hyperfunctional behavior, the clinician needs to pinpoint carefully which of the client's behaviors is primarily responsible for the voice problem. Once the contributory behavior or behaviors are pinpointed precisely, and a baseline of those behaviors is obtained over a selected time, then the clinician must select a strategy to reduce the rate of occurrence of those behaviors. Respective pinpointed hyperfunction-producing behaviors associated with these problems include behaviors involved in phonation, respiration, and resonation. Specific examples in children include yelling, loud talking, coughing, throat clearing, strained phonation, hard attack phonation, pharyngeal tightness, inappropriate tongue carriage, restricted mouth opening, speaking on expiratory reserve air, and inadequate breath support.

In 1976, the lead author published a data-based program, the Vocal Abuse Reduction Program (VARP), based on seven years of supportive single-subject design research.[74] This program used a self-control management strategy from applied behavior analysis with a sensitive data collection procedure in the form of daily behavioral charting to produce a replicable, valid therapeutic procedure for affecting the reduction of hyperfunctional voice behaviors. The VARP also gave the clinician the opportunity to monitor progress continuously over the course of therapy by viewing the daily behavior records of vocally abusive behaviors. The VARP is a clinical management program that pinpoints vocal abuse and misuse behaviors for each client with such behaviors resulting in the formation of laryngeal pathologies (i.e., nodules, polyps, contact ulcers, and thickened cords), systematically and precisely reduces the pinpointed vocal abuse behaviors in specific high-probability situations or periods, and reduces or eliminates the abuse-generated laryngeal pathology and makes possible the establishment of normal voice quality. The VARP is described in detail by Johnson[75,103]

Figure 26–3 presents an example of the daily behavior chart obtained when the VARP is used. The record indicates the rate of occurrence of abuse and misuse behaviors in selected periods, which are gradually increased in length as control is obtained in each situation. The data themselves represent data collected by the client, who counts his or her own abuse and misuse behaviors with the assistance of a wrist counter.

In Figure 26–3 we present "yells" and "loud talk" behaviors occurring during specified situations over a 12-week management program with VARP. During the first 2 weeks, the behaviors were self-monitored only during the morning recess period at school (20 minutes of monitored time). During weeks 3 and 4, the monitoring time was extended to include afternoon recess (totaling 35 minutes of monitored time). The magnitude of change during these first 4 weeks range from 1.7 behaviors per minute (or 34 yells–loud talks in 20 minutes) on the first data day to 0 yells–loud talk behaviors in 35 minutes on the final day of week 4. The rate of yelling and loud talking behavior may be seen to decelerate markedly during this period as a consequence of self-monitoring those behaviors. In week 5, the monitored time is further extended to include a 35-minute lunch period (total monitored time, 70 minutes), with 3 days at the end of the week of no recorded yells or loud talk behaviors. In weeks 6 and

7, the period is again extended to include after school until 6:00 PM, bringing the total monitored time to 220 minutes. Again, three days of no yells or loud behaviors appear at the end of week 7. The monitored time was then extended to include the entire day during weeks 8 through 12, with resulting low rates of yells and loud talk behaviors, including several full days during which no self-observed loud talk and yell behaviors occurred. On the third day of week 8, the client was seen by the laryngologist, who reported no remnant of the moderately large bilateral nodules. Rechecks by the examining laryngologists on the dates indicated at the top of the chart revealed no reoccurrence of the nodules. Interestingly good vocal quality did not return completely until week 10.

Intervention with VARP has been studied systematically in a series of similar single-subject research projects at Utah State University. These successful systematic replications of VARP intervention have demonstrated the effectiveness and predictability of the VARP procedure.

Certainly, other methods can reduce hyperfunctional voice behaviors effectively; however, no reported procedures have the data base and predictive capability of the VARP. For example, Wilson and Rice[12] and Boone[15] both described abuse-reduction programs but presented no clinical data to support the procedures' effectiveness.

The recent interest in behavioral approaches to the study of the voice management process suggests some basic management principles:

1. Voice and voice disorders are not mysterious problems requiring unusual procedures to manage them effectively. Fundamental clinical processes are the same as those appropriate for other communication disorders.

2. Voice and its associated features are behaviors. Hence, voice and the parameters relating to its physiology and pathology are not exempt from the principles of behavior. Most voice problems spring from hyperfunctional action of the vocal mechanism, and these behaviors can be modified by applied behavior analysis procedures.

3. Some voice disorders have primarily an or-

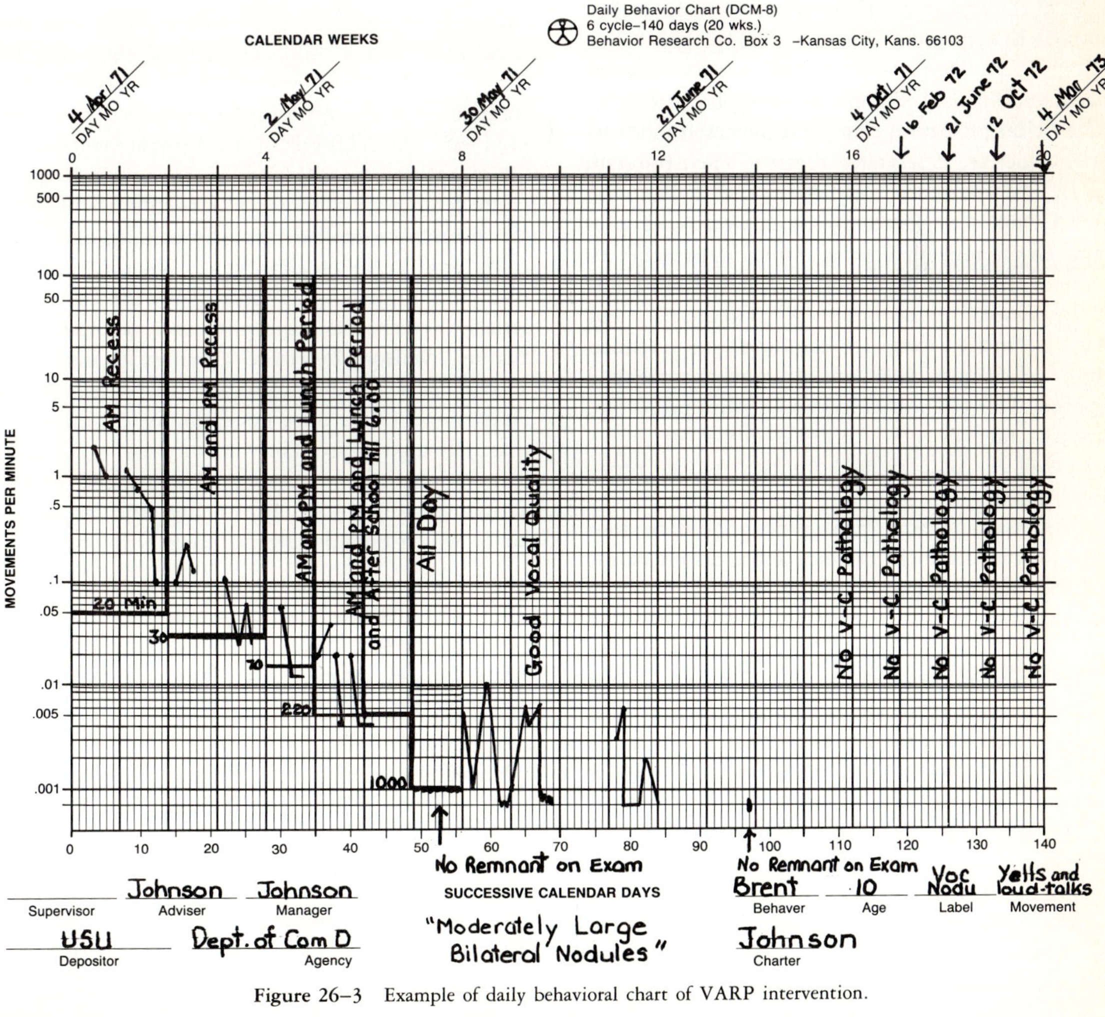

Figure 26–3 Example of daily behavioral chart of VARP intervention.

ganic basis. Even so, the therapeutic and evaluative procedures used to facilitate a better voice can take advantage of what is known about the modification of behavior. This fact has been largely neglected in the voice therapy literature.

4. The use of careful stimulus programming, control, and precise consequence management is as facilitative in voice therapy as it is in other areas of speech-language pathology.

These principles suggest that there are many potential applications of applied, behavioral analysis technology to voice problems in both children and adults, whether hyperfunctional in nature or of an organic origin. At present, little material exists in the voice literature regarding these potential applications.[104] In his review of instructional programs in the field, Mowrer lamented the lack of such developed programs for the treatment of voice disorders. Additionally, Johnson,[27] Moore,[13] and Reed[29] have all addressed the serious lack of research data addressing fundamental therapeutic management questions. The recent report by Drudge and Phillips[105] was cited by both Mowrer[104] and Reed[29] as an example of the type of research that is seriously needed in voice therapeutics. Their 31-step program was designed to accomplish four major goals: elimination of vocal abuse, easy initiation of phonation, increased clear phonation time, and increased loudness without increase in laryngeal tension. Their program was criterion referenced, and they presented data on three clients who successfully completed the program. Other behavioral programmed approaches to the management of voice problems have been studied by Smee,[77] Coachbuilder,[106] Greiner,[107] and Vance.[73] Briefly, these studies used the extended length and complexity of utterance therapy strategy[108] to program for pitch disorders and quality problems. Data presented in these studies indicated the effectiveness of the programmed approach to the problems studied.

Aronson suggested that there should be four phases in the treatment of voice abuse disorders: (1) an informational phase in which the structure and function of the larynx is explained; (2) an auditory discrimination phase in which the clinician compares normal voices to those having dysphonia as a result of vocal abuse; (3) a vocal production phase in which the clinician assists the client in finding situations in which vocal abuse is most likely to occur and trains the child to reduce vocal loudness and glottal attacks; and (4) a parent counseling phase.[19]

Boone[6] recommended that hyperfunctional therapy begin with the identification of vocal abuse and misuse followed by systematic attempts to decrease the occurrence of the abuse-misuse behaviors. The voice clinician should then search with the patient for the best voice the patient is able to produce by using various therapy techniques which Boone called facilitating approaches.

Stone and Casteel[98] recommended three objectives to vocal abuse therapy: (1) to elicit laryngeal function with the absence of excessive muscle activity that has become associated with habitual phonation; (2) to shape relaxed laryngeal function into behavior that results in normal vocal production; and (3) to institute a stimulus-response pattern of normal behavior in a nonthreatening-to-threatening hierarchy of speaking situations. Their intervention model includes a progression from a sustained sound through dialogue in those different situations using the appropriate voice. Relaxation techniques also are taught and progression in vocal skills development is charted.

Wilson's continuing work[1] with specific reference to children's voice problems is extremely well done. The most recent edition of his textbook contains a wealth of management and evaluation procedures and materials. We recommend this book for all clinicians who work with the vocal disturbances of childhood. Wilson[1] suggested six goals for voice therapy with children and recommended that they be adapted to each child's laryngeal dysfunction. According to Wilson, some children may require all six goals to a therapy program whereas others may need less. The goals are: (1) to eliminate voice abuse; (2) to balance muscular tonus; (3) to teach appropriate loudness; (4) to teach desirable use of pitch; (5) to teach controlled rate of speaking; and (6) to teach production of clear voice. Wilson described many techniques and provided many innovative materials to teach and accomplish each of these goals. Further, Wilson[1] described a variety of interesting approaches adapted to childhood including: (1) the establishment of a voice notebook for the client; (2) materials used to explain the voice and voice problem; (3) ideas for discussing vocal hygiene; and (4) an innovative voice therapy outline, such as the one below which provide clinical imagery for the child:

1. I know the rule about my voice.
2. I can tell when other people use their voices incorrectly.
3. I can tell when other people use their voices correctly.
4. I can tell when I use my voice incorrectly.
5. I can tell when I use my voice correctly.
6. I know the places where I use my voice incorrectly.
7. I know the places where I use my voice correctly.
8. I can use my voice correctly some of the time.
9. I can use my voice correctly most of the time.
10. I can use my voice correctly all the time.

In addition, Wilson recommended the teaching of

listening training (i.e., awareness of differences in others, gross discrimination of differences in others, fine discrimination of differences in others, and listening to one's own voice); teaching negative practice; charting; and establishing a program of reinforcement. Stone,[100] Boone,[6] and Johnson[75] indicated the importance of the client becoming aware of the types of abusive behaviors being produced. Once the abusive situations are isolated, the clinician is urged to obtain baseline measurements of the number of times the vocal abuse is observed during a particular time. High-probability periods must be determined for each client and the specific abusive behavior must be monitored during each period. It is important that the client accept responsibility for the type of behavior exhibited.

Once the vocal hyperfunctional behaviors are being monitored and controlled, Boone[6] suggested that various facilitative techniques be implemented. A voice therapy facilitating technique is that technique which, when used by a particular client, enables the client to readily evoke a unit of good voice behavior. Once discovered, the facilitating technique and the resulting phonation become the symptomatic focus for therapy. Boone recommends choosing from 25 facilitating approaches in voice therapy: alteration of tongue position, biofeedback, change of loudness, chant talk, chewing approach, digital manipulation, ear training, elimination of abuses, elimination of hard glottal attack, establishment of new pitch, explanation of problem, feedback, gargle approach, hierarchy analysis, inhalation phonation, masking, negative practice, open-mouth approach, pitch inflections, place the voice, pushing approach, relaxation, respiration training, voice rest, and yawn-sigh approach. These facilitating approaches are described both in Boone's text and in his recent voice program kits.[15,16]

Stemple[24] recommended the following model in treatment of vocal abuse in children: (1) identify the abuses: shouting, loud talking, vocal noises, and throat clearing; (2) describe the effect the abuses have on the voice: use pictures, diagrams, and drawings; (3) define specific occurrences of the abusive behaviors; and (4) modify the behavior (teach child HOW to shout), modify or eliminate vocal noises, nonplay shouting, throat clearing, and strengthen laryngeal muscles.

There is little difference in the kind of voice therapy given for the differing kinds of dysphonia related to vocal hyperfunction. In the treatment of vocal polyps, Greene[21] and Stone[100] both recommended vocal rest and voice therapy focused on consultation about abusive behaviors. For hard glottal attack, Stemple[24] recommended teaching the client to produce a soft glottal attack or an easy onset by initiating phonation with /h/. This therapy is followed by using vowels to generate normal phonation and then progressing through conversational speech. Wilson[1] suggested in working with patients who have excessive loudness, to teach loudness listening training. This training is accomplished by teaching the patient to develop an awareness of excessive loudness or softness in speech intensity and then proceeding to gross and fine discrimination. Wilson also suggested the use of his 10-step Voice Therapy Outline for Loudness designed to focus the correct perception of loudness, to specify appropriate places to use loudness, and to establish the correct use of loudness.

Medical-Surgical Considerations

Sometimes surgical intervention may be considered for the elimination of laryngeal pathology secondary to vocal abuse in children. In children, surgery should not usually be considered for the hyperfunctional group of disorders because of the large incidence of recurrence and the risk of surgical injury to the larynx, and because voice therapy can effectively manage virtually all of them. The therapy of choice in children and adults who have vocal pathology secondary to hyperfunction is vocal reeducation rather than surgical removal of the pathology. This conservative philosophy regarding the management of childhood disorders currently prevails throughout the field of laryngology. The well-informed speech-language pathologist should be assertive in seeing that children are given appropriate treatment prior to any serious consideration of vocal surgery. Such an advocacy position is both professionally appropriate and ethically sound when one truly understands the nature of these vocal problems.

Prevention: The Future

Prevention of vocal abuse is a developing alternative to vocal abuse reduction therapy. It is believed that systematic approaches to vocal management and education can accomplish much with the hyperfunctional disorders of voice in children. Nelson and Schneiderman[109] developed such an educational program, which was used as a preventative program with 155 second and third graders. Educating students in the prevention or control of vocal abusive behaviors may directly reduce the future need for specific voice therapy of this type. Prevention strategies are particularly appropriate for the hyperfunctional group of voice disorders because the basic causes of these problems are well known and are preventable to a significant degree. Certainly, in the future the application of "best practices" in the care, health, and hygiene of the vocal mechanism should reduce the number of new cases of voice disorders.

Although knowledge of treatment in the area of psychological, physiologic, and neurologic disorders is of great importance, understanding and operating effective treatment methods dealing with vocal abuse and hyperfunction in children must be considered paramount because of the significantly higher incidence of this type of disorder in children. Therefore, the most frequently used models of voice treatment in children are those that directly manage hyperfunctional vocal behaviors accompanied by a facilitative program of proper vocal hygiene and care.

SUMMARY

One of the difficulties in the preparation of a chapter of this magnitude is the realization that one cannot do justice to the entire scope of the subject matter. Neither is it possible that a single chapter on a topic area such as this one can be expected to give the reader even a basic foundation of skill competence in work with childhood voice disturbance without the addition of the experiential base. Brodnitz[30] has lamented the lack of depth of the preparation of new professionals in speech-language pathology, especially with reference to voice disorders. His reflective and long-term perspective on the state of the art of the profession is significant in terms of the inadequate preparation most new professionals receive in the area of voice. Brodnitz criticized the current model of professional preparation in university settings where a basic conflict seems to exist between the demands of "academe" and the practical aspects of professional competence in the speech-voice clinic. He cited the differences between the experience base of medical school physicians with the same base of university professors in speech-language pathology. He wrote that,

> Leading physicians are constantly surrounded by patients for whom they are responsible. Surgeons stand daily in the operating room where they constantly check on the results of their own techniques and try out others used by colleagues. Specialists of internal medicine discuss on daily rounds all forms of medical pathologies with staff, interns, and residents.
>
> Chiefs of departments of speech and voice pathology have much less opportunity for such constant experience with patients of their own, particularly with voice cases. They have to be generalists in the whole field of speech, voice, language, and hearing. Faculty meetings, the fight for budgetary needs, administrative tasks, and courses of their own take up much of their time . . . Quite a few excellent professors of speech-language pathology have admitted to me how few patients with voice disorders they or even their associates handle every year. Still they have to give courses about the treatment of voice disorders with which they have little personal experience (p 26).

A similar lament could be echoed with regards to graduate practicum experiences with voice problems, which often only barely reach a specified certification minimum.

Further, Brodnitz found from his unique perspective as a physician-phoniatrist, that the current periodic journals in the communicative disorders discipline do not facilitate the publication and dissemination of clinical data on practical approaches for treating various conditions of the voice. He contrasted this finding with the medical specialty journals in which the physician "often finds detailed case-by-case reports about practical approaches for treating various conditions. New suggestions by one author are soon tried out in other medical centers and critically analyzed, results are reported, or new variations are introduced" (p 26). The lack of such dissemination organs in the profession is regrettable and is a barrier to the progress of clinical practice.

Speech-language pathologists must take these as well as other valid observations and concerns about their current professional preparation and practice and effect changes which will bring about an increased professional competence in the identification, evaluation, and management of voice disorders in both children and adults. Brodnitz suggested that communicative disorders is in the situation in which medicine was 50 years ago. He wrote,

> At that time, medical students were trained as 'generalists.' The vast majority of them became general practitioners who handled all kinds of diseases with the help of a smaller number of highly trained specialists. Now things have changed, with the majority of medical students becoming specialists, experts in special fields. What happened to medicine should also happen in speech-language pathology. A graduate student should have greater exposure to a special branch of diagnostics and therapy (p 26).

Specialization in voice disorders may ultimately become a reality in the credentials of competent professionals in speech-language pathology. The advent of such a change would of necessity bring many changes in professional preparation including, we hope, substantially more clinical practicum experiences with voice-disordered children and potentially specific centers for training these "voice specialists." Only then can the significant advances in voice research and treatment finally begin to surge beyond the observations of redundancy as described by Moore,[13] Reed,[29] Johnson,[14] and Brodnitz.[30]

REFERENCES

1. Wilson DK. Voice Problems of Children (3rd ed). Baltimore: Williams & Wilkins, 1987.
2. Brodnitz F. Vocal Rehabilitation (4th ed). Am Acad Opthalmol Otolaryngol, Rochester, 1971.

3. Moses P. The Voice of Neurosis. New York: Grune & Stratton, 1954.
4. Boone DR. The Voice and Voice Therapy (1st ed). Englewood Cliffs: Prentice-Hall, 1971.
5. Boone DR. The Voice and Voice Therapy (2nd ed). Englewood Cliffs, Prentice-Hall, 1977.
6. Boone DR. The Voice and Voice Therapy (3rd ed). Englewood Cliffs, Prentice-Hall, 1983.
7. Wilson DK. Voice Problems of Children (1st ed). Baltimore: Williams & Wilkins, 1972.
8. Wilson DK. Voice Problems of Children (2nd ed). Baltimore: Williams & Wilkins, 1979.
9. Perkins W. Speech pathology: an applied behavioral science. St Louis: CV Mosby, 1971.
10. Perkins W. Quantification of vocal behavior: A foundation for clinical management of voice. In: Bless D, Abbs J, eds. Vocal fold physiology contemporary research & clinical issues. San Diego: College-Hill Press, 1983.
11. Perkins WH, ed. Current therapy in communicative disorders: voice disorders, New York: Thieme-Stratton, 1985.
12. Wilson FB, Rice M. A programmed approach to voice therapy. Austin: Learning Concepts, 1977.
13. Moore GP. Have the major issues in voice disorders been answered by research in speech science? A 50 year retrospective. J Speech Hear Disord 1977; 42:152–160.
14. Johnson TS. Voice disorders: The measurement of clinical progress. In: Costello JM, ed. Speech Disorders in Adults. San Diego: College-Hill Press, 1985.
15. Boone DR. The Boone voice program for children. Tigard, OR: CC Publications 1980.
16. Boone DR. The Boone voice program for adults. Tigard, OR: CC Publications 1982.
17. Mueller P. Vocal re-education therapy. New Richmond: Whitehaven, 1980.
18. Polow N, Kaplan ED. Symptomatic voice therapy (2nd ed). Tulsa: Modern Education Corporation, 1980.
19. Aronson A. Clinical voice disorders, an interdisciplinary approach (2nd ed). New York: Thieme, 1985.
20. Cooper M, Cooper MH. Approaches to vocal rehabilitation. Springfield: CC Thomas, 1977.
21. Greene M. The voice and its disorders. Philadelphia: JB Lippincott, 1980.
22. Moncur JP, Brackett IP. Modifying vocal behavior. New York: Harper & Row, 1974.
23. Prater R, Swift R. Manual of voice therapy. Boston: Little, Brown, 1984.
24. Stemple J. Clinical voice pathology: theory and management. Columbus: CE Merrill, 1984.
25. Leith W, Johnston R. Handbook of voice therapy for the school clinician. San Diego: College-Hill Press, 1986.
26. Filter M. In: Filter M, ed. Phonatory disorders in children, Springfield: CC Thomas, 1982.
27. Johnson TS. A precision approach to hyperfunctional voice problems. Logan: Utah State University, 1974.
28. Michel JF, Wendahl R. Correlates of voice production. In: Travis LE, ed. Handbook of speech pathology and audiology. New York: Appleton-Century-Crofts, 1971.
29. Reed CG. Voice therapy: a need for research. J Speech Hear Disord 1980; 45:157–169.
30. Brodnitz F. Academe and the clinic. Asha 1986; 28, 12, 25–26.
31. Hirano M. Clinical examination of voice. Disorders of human communication, Vol 5, New York: Springer-Verlag, 1981.
32. Baken R. Clinical measurement of speech and voice: an introduction. San Diego: College-Hill Press, 1986.
33. Mehrabian A. Communication without words. Psychol Today 1968; 2:52–58.
34. Brewer D. Early diagnostic signs and symptoms of laryngeal disease. Laryngoscope 1975; 85:499–515.
35. Wood R, Northern J. In: Jafek B, ed. Manual of otolaryngology: a symptom-oriented text. Baltimore: Williams & Wilkins, 1979.
36. DeWeese DD, Saunders WH. Textbook of otolaryngology. St Louis: CV Mosby, 1973.
37. Ballinger J. Diseases of the nose, throat, ear, head, and neck (13th ed). Philadelphia: Lea & Febiger, 1985.
38. Gould W, Lawrence V. Surgical care of voice disorders. disorders of human communication, Vol 8, New York: Springer-Verlag, 1984.
39. Bryce DP. Differential diagnosis and treatment of hoarseness. Springfield: CC Thomas, 1974.
40. Pannbacker M. Classification systems of voice disorders: a review of the literature. Language Speech Hear Serv in Schools 1984; 15:169–174.
41. Wilson K, Starr F. Use of the phonation analyzer as a clinical tool. J Speech Hear Disord 1985; 50:351–356.
42. Wilson FB. The voice disordered child: a descriptive approach. Lang Speech Hear Serv Schools 1972; 4:14–22.
43. Leeper HA Jr, Leonard JE, Iverson RL. Otorhinolaryngologic screening of children with vocal quality disturbances. Int J Pediatr Otorhinolaryngol 1980; 2:123–131.
44. Wing DM, Johnson TS, DeVoe S, Pearson M. Vocal abuse reduction program: a Montana pilot project for the management of children's voice disorders. Final report, Montana VARP Project, Montana Office of the Superintendent of Public Instruction, September 1975.
45. Miller S, Madison C. Public-school voice clinics, part II: a working model. Language Speech Hear Serv in Schools 1983; 14:260–265.
46. Madison C, Meadors D, Miller S. A survey study of a public school voice clinic program. Language Speech Hear Serv in Schools 1984; 15:275–280.
47. Miller S, Madison C. Public-school voice clinics, part I: a working model. Language Speech Hear Serv in Schools 1983; 14:51–57.
48. Murry T. Phonation: Assessment. In: Lass N, McReynolds L, Northern J, Yoder D, eds. Speech, language and hearing pathologies of speech and language, Vol II. Philadelphia: WB Saunders, 1982.
49. McFarlane S, Lavorato A. The use of video endoscopy in the evaluation and treatment of dysphonia. J Commun Disord 1984; 8.
50. Starr CD, Wilson FB. Reliability considerations of a voice profiling system. Human Commun 1976; 1:47–56.
51. Moody DK, Montague J, Bradley B. Preliminary validity and reliability data on the Wilson voice profile system. Language Speech Hear Serv in Schools 1979; 10:231–239.
52. Filter M, Poyner R. A descriptive study of children with chronic hoarseness. J Communic Dis 1982; 15:461–482.
53. Beckett RL. The respirometer as a diagnostic and clinical tool in the speech clinic. J Speech Hear Disord 1971; 36:235–241.
54. Hirano M, Koike Y, von Leden H. Maximum phonation time and air usage during phonation. Folia Phoniatr 1968; 20:185–201.
55. Koike Y. Vowel amplitude modulations in patients with laryngeal diseases. J Acoust Soc Am 1968; 45:839–844.
56. Koike Y, Hirano M. Significance of vocal velocity index. Folia Phoniatr 1968; 20:285–296.
57. Koike Y, Hirano M, von Leden H. Vocal initiation: acoustic and aerodynamic investigations of normal subjects. Folia Phoniatr 1967; 19:173–182.
58. Isshiki N. Regulatory mechanism of voice intensity variation. J Speech Hear Res 1964: 7:17–29.
59. Isshiki N. Vocal intensity and air flow rate. Folia Phoniatr 1965; 17:92–104.
60. Isshiki N, Okamura H, Morimoto M. Maximum phonation time and air flow rate during phonation: Simple clinical tests for vocal function. Ann Otol Rhinol Laryngol 1967; 76:998–1007.
61. Isshiki N, Okamura H, Tanabe J, Morimoto M. Differ-

ential diagnosis of hoarseness. Folia Phoniatr 1969; 21:9–19.
62. Isshiki N, von Leden H. Hoarseness: aerodynamic studies. Arch Otolaryngol 1964; 80:206–213.
63. Isshiki N, Yanagihara N, Morimoto M. Approach to the objective diagnosis of hoarseness. Folia Phoniatr 1966; 18:393–400.
64. Iwata S, von Leden H. Phonation quotient in patients with laryngeal diseases. Folia Phoniatr 1970; 22:117–128.
65. Yanagihara N, Koike Y. The regulation of sustained phonation. Folia Phoniatr 1967; 19:1–18.
66. Yanagihara N, Koike Y, von Leden H. Phonation and respiration. Folia Phoniatr 1966; 18:323–340.
67. Yanagihara N, von Leden H. Respiration and phonation. Folia Phoniatr 1967; 19:153–166.
68. Beck MA. The remediation of vocal nodules in school children: a therapeutic program. Master's Thesis, Utah State University, 1976.
69. Hunsaker JC. Behavior modification and functional voice disorders. Master's Thesis, Utah State University, 1970.
70. Parrish ML. A therapeutic program for the remediation of vocal nodules in children. Master's Thesis, Utah State University, 1972.
71. Pierce GL. An analysis and reduction of breathiness with accompanying inspiratory speech. Master's Thesis, Utah State University, 1974.
72. Rothwell R. A therapeutic program for the remediation of hyperfunctional voice disorders in adults. Master's Thesis, Utah State University, 1974.
73. Vance SE. A therapeutic approach to an extended length of utterance program for extension and generalization of appropriate vocal quality production. Master's Thesis, Utah State University, 1976.
74. Johnson TS. Vocal abuse reduction program. Logan: Utah State University, 1976.
75. Johnson TS. Vocal abuse reduction program (VARP). San Diego: College-Hill Press, 1985.
76. Thompson CG. The feasibility of using respirometer measurements as a monitoring agent of laryngeal functioning during vocal nodule rehabilitation. Master's Thesis, Utah State University, 1976.
77. Smee JS. An analysis of contact ulcer reduction using the vocal abuse reduction program and vocal quality program. Master's Thesis, Utah State University 1974.
78. Child DR. Maximum phonation time: optimum number of trials and normative performance on fourth grade children. Master's Thesis, Utah State University, 1979.
79. Inglis JM. Obtaining normative data on vocal parameters in a group of adult speakers. Master's Thesis, Utah State University, 1977.
80. Lee RL. Phonation and respiratory production in cheerleaders. Master's Thesis, Utah State University, 1978.
81. Taylor TJ. Air flow parameters in college-age individuals. Master's Thesis, Utah State University, 1980.
82. Williams K. Performances of elementary school aged children on respirometric and phonatory measures. Master's Thesis, Utah State University, 1977.
83. Williams SW. A comparative analysis of the Collins P-900 9 liter respirometer and the dropper compact spirometer. Master's Thesis, Utah State University, 1979.
84. Hammond J. A precision approach to evaluation and therapy in voice. Master's Thesis, Utah State University, 1981.
85. Johnson TS. Voice disorders: The measurement of clinical progress. In: Costello JM, Holland AL, eds. Handbook of speech and language disorders. San Diego: College-Hill Press, 1986.
86. Davis S. Acoustic characteristics of laryngeal pathology. Darby J, ed. Speech evaluation in medicine. New York: Grune and Stratton, 1981.
87. Blaustein B, Bar A. Reliability of perceptual voice assessment. J Communicative Dis 1983; 16:157–161.
88. Eckel FC, Boone DR. The s/z ratio as an indicator of laryngeal pathology. J Speech Hear Disord 1981; 46:147–149.
89. Gordon MT, Morton FM, Simpson IC. Airflow measurements in diagnosis, assessment and treatment of mechanical dysphonia. Fol Phoniatrica 1978; 30:166–174.
90. Tait NA, Michel JF, Carpenter MA. Maximum duration of sustained /s/ and /z/ in children. J Speech Hear Disord 1980; 45:239–246.
91. Coombs J. The maximum duration of phonation of /a/ in normal and hoarse voiced children. Master's Thesis, Portland State University, 1976.
92. Kushner D, Michel J. Maximum phonation times in 100 adults. Paper presented Ann Conv Am Speech Hear Assoc, San Francisco, 1978.
93. Lewis K. The maximum duration of phonation /a/ in children. Master's Thesis, Portland State University, 1977.
94. Mele L. Maximum phonation time in children four and five years of age. James Madison University, 1981.
95. Norwood ED. Variability in test-retest of maximum duration of sustained /a/ in children. Master's Thesis, Portland State University, 1978.
96. Ptacek PH, Sander EK. Maximum duration of phonation. J Speech Hear Disord 1963; 29:171–182.
97. Smitheran JR, Hixon TJ. A clinical method for estimating laryngeal airway resistance during vowel production. J Speech Hear Disord 1981; 46:138–146.
98. Stone R, Casteel R. Restoration of voice in nonorganically based dysphonias. In: Filter M, ed. Phonatory voice disorders in children. Springfield: CC Thomas, 1982.
99. Murray S, Carr M, Jacobs V. Functional aphonia in the child and adolescent. Language Speech Hear Serv in Schools 1983; 14:260–265.
100. Stone R. Management of childhood dysphonias of organic bases. In: Filter M, ed. Phonatory disorders in children. Springfield: CC Thomas, 1982.
101. Warr-Leeper GA, McShea RS, Leeper HA Jr. The incidence of voice and speech deviations in a middle school population. Language Speech Hear Serv in Schools 1979; 10:14–20.
102. Reich A, Mason J, Polen S. Phonation-time measures in third-grade girls with normal voice quality. Language Speech Hear Serv in Schools 1986; 17:262–269.
103. Johnson TS. Treatment of vocal abuse in children. In: Perkins WH, ed. Current therapy of communicative disorders: voice disorders. New York: Thieme-Stratton, 1984.
104. Mowrer DE. Methods of Modifying Speech Behaviors (2nd ed). Columbus: CE Merrill, 1982.
105. Drudge MKM, Phillips BJ. Shaping behavior in voice therapy. J Speech Hear Disord 1976; 41:398–411.
106. Coachbuilder DP. Programming all exercises for the development of pitch. Master's Thesis, Utah State University, 1972.
107. Greiner G. A programmed therapy approach to pitch disturbances of the voice. Master's Thesis, Utah State University, 1973.
108. Ryan BP. Programmed therapy for stuttering in children and adults. Springfield: CC Thomas, 1974.
109. Nelson H, Schneiderman C. Classroom program for the prevention of vocal abuse and hoarseness in elementary school children. Language Speech Hear Serv in Schools 1983; 14:121–127.

27 Voice Disorders in the Adult

Charles G. Reed, Ph.D.

Voice production serves many functions and exerts a profound influence on our lives. Adults utilize voice to express basic wants and needs, communicate socially, and earn a livelihood. Perkins has suggested voice contributes significantly in interpersonal communication.[1] Voice is an essential element to articulatory and prosodic linguistic functions. Perhaps equally as important, voice can convey nonlinguistic functions of speaker identity, personality, emotion, somatic conditions, and aesthetic information. Adult voice disorders can range from mild hoarseness to complete voice loss from a total laryngectomy. The negative impact upon social and vocational functions can be significant and vary according to the degree of impairment and vocal need.

This chapter will address normal and abnormal voice physiology and the relationships to perceptual features of voice disorders. Normal processes are covered in depth in Section 1 and are only briefly summarized here. The primary focus will be on laryngeal voice disorders and etiologies. Fundamental issues of voice classification and definitions will be reviewed, and specific assessment strategies and rehabilitation procedures will be presented. Finally, issues regarding our knowledge of adult voice disorders will also be discussed.

NORMAL VOICE PRODUCTION

Van den Berg proposed the myoelastic-aerodynamic theory to explain the production of vocal sound as a sensitive interaction between the exhaled airstream and the mass-tension of the vocal folds.[2] In essence, the theory suggests that as the vocal folds approximate in the midline, exhaled air from the lungs creates subglottal pressure greater than the resistance of the folds and displaces them in a lateral direction. The opening phase of the cycle allows a decrease in air pressure and increases vocal fold elasticity. The combined forces of increased fold elasticity and of the Bernoulli effect from air flowing through the narrow glottis return the vocal folds to the midline, until the cycle repeats itself.

Moore[3,4] and Moore, Hicks, and Abbott[5] have discussed factors related to normal and abnormal voice production; the interaction and variation of five basic factors of vibration influence phonation. Air flow and subglottal pressure set the vocal folds into motion. Elasticity, or stiffness and tension, of the vocal folds affects resistance to movement and speed of recovery, whereas length, mass, and compliance affect elasticity of the vocal folds. If all other factors are equal, a long fold vibrates at a lower frequency than a shorter fold, and more force is required to move and stop a larger mass than a smaller one. Variable compliance of the vocal folds also influences vibration: a structure with greater compliance, or less resistance to displacement, moves more easily than a less compliant one.

Variable interaction of the aforementioned basic factors yields perceptual vocal factors of pitch, loudness, and quality. Normal vibration of the vocal folds should be relatively regular, repetitive, and have synchronous lateral and medial movements with a period of vocal fold contact. The sound generated by the laryngeal source is modified by resonance of the supraglottic vocal tract.

Pitch or frequency of vocal fold vibration is related to vocal fold adjustment of mass, elasticity, and length. When the folds are shortened, their cross-section becomes thicker, thereby reducing their elasticity and so producing a lower frequency of vibration that results in a lower pitch. When the folds are elongated, they become thinner, reducing their cross-section and increasing their elasticity. Consequently, the frequency of vibration is increased, resulting in a perception of higher pitch. Isotonic contraction of the vocal folds can also raise the pitch by increasing elasticity of the folds and their frequency of vibration. The general mass of the vocal folds also affects pitch.

Voice loudness is determined by sound pressure pulses related to the volume and velocity of airflow through the glottis. An increase in expiratory force increases the amplitude of the vocal folds, and they return to the midline more quickly and remain in approximation longer. Thus, increases in the amplitude of the sound waves are perceived as a louder sound. Variations in the sensitive interaction between subglottal pressure from expiratory force and glottal resistance yields differences in loudness.

Moore has offered a succinct definition: "Quality is the auditory impression created by the complexity of the sound wave" (p 2).[4] The definition suggests that the perception of voice quality is the result of vibratory patterns of the sound source and its resonance characteristics. Each individual possesses a unique laryngeal structure and resonating cavity to create the variations in voice perceived as "voice quality." Within an individual, the opening, closing, and closed phases of the vibratory cycle can vary, as can the resonance characteristics, in order to alter the essential sound of the voice.

PHYSIOLOGIC CORRELATES OF PERCEPTUAL FEATURES

The laryngeal sound source has been assumed primarily responsible for phonation disorders. Consequently, a series of experiments has been conducted to examine the vibratory patterns of normal and pathologic vocal folds.[6–9] Ultrahigh-speed pictures were selected to examine each vibratory cycle separately. The movements of each vocal fold during the opening, closing, and closed phases of a cycle were plotted and examined across time. Normal vocal fold movements display relatively synchronous, repetitive lateral and medial movements with complete glottic closure.[6,9]

Moore and Thompson analyzed the number of ultrahigh-speed film frames and the acoustic wave length for consecutive cycles of two hoarse speakers.[8] Both measures displayed cycle-to-cycle random variability, which distinguished hoarseness from normal voice. The speaker judged to be the most hoarse exhibited the greatest cycle-to-cycle variability.

Von Leden, Moore, and Timcke examined the vibratory patterns of pathologic larynges including unilateral vocal fold paralysis, localized edema, sessile polyp, and bilateral nodules.[7] The pathologic conditions reviewed as a group demonstrated considerable diversity; the vocal folds may meet for varying periods of time or remain apart throughout the complete cycle. The investigators concluded that normal vibratory patterns are not common in the pathologic larynx, and rapid changes in the vibratory pattern typically occur. Growths on the vocal folds may prolong approximation at the site of the lesion, but prevent complete approximation in the adjacent sections of the folds, thus creating a breathy voice quality.

Moore, Hicks, and Abbott have summarized the physiologic attributes of harshness and hoarseness.[5] Harsh voice quality was described as the opposite of breathiness. The vocal folds remain approximated a disproportionate length of time of the vibratory cycle because of reduced subglottal air pressure or excessively tight glottal closure. Speaking in a low pitch with vocal fry also characterizes harshness. Harshness may occur with or without the presence of vocal fold pathology.

Moore, Hicks, and Abbott reported that "roughness" from random variations in the periodicity or intensity of consecutive sound waves was the distinguishing feature of hoarseness.[5] The authors have provided a succinct statement about the physiology of hoarseness:

> Any disease or condition in the larynx that changes the size, stiffness, or surface characteristic of one or both vocal cords, or that causes excessive squeezing of one cord against the other, may create the conditions for hoarseness. Enlargements due to tumor or edema, reductions resulting from surgery or atrophy, flaccidity subsequent to neural involvement, or functional hypercontraction of the adductory muscles represent the kinds of changes to which reference has been made (p 713).

In general, any condition that alters the repetitive, synchronous vibration of the vocal folds causes hoarseness.

The vocal fold vibratory patterns generate the characteristic laryngeal sound quality. Pathologic changes in the vocal folds or less than optimal use of the mechanism may alter the vibratory patterns sufficiently to create a perceptual voice disorder.

CLASSIFICATION AND DESCRIPTION OF VOICE DISORDERS

Aronson has proposed that voice disorders are traditionally classified according to three categories: etiology, kinesiology, and perceptual features.[10] The etiologic view classifies the signs and symptoms by the ultimate cause or theory. For example, a neurologic disease may cause a unilateral vocal fold paralysis that precipitates abnormal voice signs such as hoarseness. The kinesiologic category classifies voice disorders by the firmness of vocal fold closure. Laryngeal voice disorders are usually considered to range between degrees of "hypofunction" and "hyperfunction" and are typically determined by listening to behavioral parameters of voice. The perceptual system is an attempt to describe voice by means of the auditory impressions of the listener. For example, "harsh, hoarse," are terms often used to describe laryngeal voice disorders. The categories are not always mutually exclusive, and many clinicians combine the essential features of the systems. Each classification system will be reviewed in the subsequent sections of this chapter.

Etiologic Classification

Brodnitz differentiates organic from functional voice disorders according to the primary cause of the vocal abnormality.[11] In organic voice disorders, the structural change, such as nerve damage, leukoplakia, or papilloma, is the primary event causing the voice disorder. Conversely, functional disorders describe any voice disorder in which the primary causative factor is improper function. For example, because nodules and polyps are caused by voice abuse and misuse, that is, improper function, the voice disorder is still considered functional.

Aronson expresses similar criteria to differentiate organic from functional voice disorders.[10] The disorder is considered organic if it is caused by a structural, physiologic, or systemic illness. Aronson suggests "functional" is a common synonym for "psychogenic," which is caused by psychoneuroses, personality disorders, or faulty voice usage. The psychogenic voice disorders may occur with a normal larynx or with secondary laryngeal pathology, such as a vocal nodule or a contact ulcer.

Other writers have quetsioned the usefulness of separating voice disorders into organic or functional categories. Perkins has rejected the view that "functional" suggests normal structures but improper learning, whereas "organic" narrowly means structural change in an organ.[1] Perkins considered it an incongruous dichotomy to suggest functional voice disorders are caused by learning, thereby implying that organic changes, such as vocal nodules, are not also the result of improperly learned voice habits. Perkins felt etiology is relatively unimportant for voice therapy.

Boone has also objected to the etiologic organic and functional dichotomy.[12] Traditionally, an otolaryngologist describes the voice disorder as functional if there is no structural deviation. However, Boone has observed that

> It is usually impossible to separate the organic voice problem from the functional one. For example, continuous faulty abuse and misuse of the vocal cords may lead to the development of vocal nodules. The structural or organic problem results from the functional misuse, and to separate the functional from the organic in such cases makes little sense (p 44).[12]

Similar to Perkins' view noted before, Boone has also suggested that there are no separate voice therapy techniques for organic and functional etiologies.

Kinesiologic Classification

The basic concept of describing laryngeal voice disorders by the degree of vocal fold approximation has had wide appeal. This approach has had significant impact upon voice diagnosis and appraisal. It explains the etiologies of various voice disorders and serves as a component of the perceptual systems. Froeschels introduced the terms "hyperfunction" and "hypofunction."[13]

Brodnitz described hyperfunction as excessive muscular tension in the vocal tract and stated: "The vast majority of functional voice disorders begin with excessive use of muscular force" (p 51).[11] Hyperfunction is considered to cause abnormal voice quality with normal appearing vocal folds, but it is also responsible for pathologic changes in the folds such as noninfectious laryngitis, nodules, polyps, and contact ulcers. Other authors have agreed with his assessment.[1,3,4,10,12] Brodnitz has also reported that "Hypofunction appears to be the end stage of prolonged hyperfunction" (p 52).[11] "Phonasthenia" and "myasthenia laryngis" are also terms used to denote hypofunction or weakening of the thyroarytenoid muscles.

Boone has offered a concise definition of hyperfunction: "Excessive muscular contraction and force of movement in respiration, phonation, or resonance can be labeled as vocal hyperfunction" (p 4).[12] He has suggested that voice disorders should be approached by considering the phonatory process and parameter of voice affected. Phonation changes are primarily affected by changes in mass and size and degree of vocal fold approximation. Boone reported that "most functionally caused dysphonias are related directly to under- or overadduction of the vocal folds and to alterations in air flow" (p 45).[12] Vocal fold growths, such as nodules and polyps, alter mass and size of the vocal folds and affect fold approximation.

Implicit in the kinesiologic classification system are the concepts of vocal abuse and misuse. Abuse of the voice mechanism includes excessive talking, yelling, coughing, and throat clearing; smoking; and drinking alcoholic beverages. Voice misuse involves improper use of the mechanism such as initiating phonation too abruptly, excessive firmness of vocal fold approximation, and speaking too loudly or at an inappropriate pitch level. Voice abuse and misuse are generally considered responsible for many benign growths of the larynx such as nodules, polyps, and contact ulcers.

Perceptual Classification

The perceptual classification system described voice disorders based on what is heard by the listener. To be considered a disorder, an individual voice is judged and compared against a standard of normalcy. Moore has presented a traditional definition that recognizes group differences and essential voice parameters: "When an individual speaks habitually with a voice that differs in pitch, loudness, or quality from the voices of others of the same age and sex within his cultural group, he is considered to have a voice disorder" (p 535).[3] The voice parameters of pitch, loudness, and quality must be judged in relation to whether the individual is male, female, child, or adult. A normal voice should exhibit adequate pitch and loudness flexibility for inflection and emphasis, and the quality should be pleasant. Pitch disorders are usually judged to be too high or low for the individual's age and sex; the habitual loudness level may be judged too loud or soft.

Agreement between listeners on the descriptions of complex voice quality disorders is usually more difficult than judgements about pitch and loudness. Perceptual definitions of voice quality often intertwine auditory impressions with kinesiologic assumptions about voice production. Each term for laryngeal disorders may comprise several perceptual elements.

Fairbanks has presented three traditional definitions to describe the perceptual features of laryngeal voice disorders.[14] "Harsh" quality is characterized by aperiodic noise, or "roughness," as its distinguishing feature. Excessive laryngeal tension and low pitch are present perceptually. Abrupt initiation of phonation and low voice loudness may also be noted. The result is an unpleasant voice quality that gives the impression of excessive vocal effort. By contrast, "breathy" voice quality exhibits an audible escape of air during phonation, limited voice intensity, and the tendency for voice initiation to be aspirate. Fairbanks considered breathiness to be the result of insufficient firmness of glottal closure for a given airflow. "Hoarseness" combines the features of harshness and breathiness, though one feature may predominate.

Many clinicians combine the features of each classification system when attempting to describe voice disorders. They may refer to the voice disorder as "functional" if no pathologic changes of the mechanism occur or as "organic" if tissue change occurs. The voice may also be described as "tense," suggesting that a perceptual feature reflects a kinesiologic condition. Clinically, the value of each approach must be judged on its ability to provide useful direction for diagnostic and rehabilitation endeavors.

PATHOLOGIC CHANGES OF THE VOCAL FOLDS

Ballenger has described several common pathologic conditions of the vocal folds related to voice abuse and misuse.[15] The speech pathologist has a role in the effects of these disorders, and an understanding of their characteristics is important in order to achieve correct appraisal and remediation choices. Specific guidelines will be presented in subsequent sections of this chapter.

Chronic Simple Laryngitis

Mechanical trauma from voice abuse and misuse can cause the vocal folds' mucosa to become diffusely reddened with evidence of small dilated blood vessels. The margins of the vocal folds appear rounded, and the folds flabby. Alcohol as a vasodilating agent and tobacco smoke can also contribute to laryngitis. Respiratory tract infections produce purulent material that contacts the larynx and so causes laryngitis. However, infectious laryngitis requires medical help rather than voice therapy.

Vocal Nodules

Ballenger described vocal nodules as a form of localized chronic laryngitis.[15] Nodules consist of a small mass of inflammatory tissue at the juncture of the anterior and middle thirds of the vocal folds. Nodules are usually bilateral, but may be unilateral. Early, beginning nodules tend to be soft and reddish with normal squamous epithelium and underlying edema. More mature nodules are firm, with fibrosis and hyalinization with a thickened epithelium.

Vocal Polyps

Typically, polyps are unilateral and occur at the same point of the vocal fold as nodules. They are localized lesions that may be sessile (broadly based) or pedunculated and so extend from a narrow base. Polyps appear as larger, exaggerated forms of beginning nodules, but tend to be more vascular. More mature polyps display some fibrosis and hyalinization. Polyps are considered to occur from a brief duration of vocal strain. Persistent vocal abuse and/or heavy tobacco smoking may cause "diffuse vocal polyposis" or polypoid degeneration. Edematous material extends diffusely throughout Reinke's space and along the margins of the vocal folds.

Contact Ulcer

The mucosa along the medial border of the posterior third of the glottis becomes damaged, creating a small superficial ulceration that exposes the arytenoid cartilage. The ulceration may be unilateral or bilateral, and it results from the forceful approximation of the arytenoid cartilages during phonation. Continued mechanical trauma produces raised, inflamed granulation tissue around the ulcer. Contact ulcer occurs almost exclusively in adult males who are typically considered to be aggressive with a low pitch and hard glottal attack. The patient may complain of pain in the neck radiating to the ear, a persistent urge to clear the throat, and throat tickle. Boone has also reported that esophageal reflux from diaphragmatic or hiatal hernia may be related to contact ulcer.[12]

Vocal Fold Paralysis

A pathologic condition of the folds not related to voice abuse and misuse is vocal fold paralysis. Central or peripheral nerve damage affects the intrinsic laryngeal muscles, but paralyzed folds vibrate if they are in a position to be activated by the airstream. The type of paralysis refers to what the affected folds are unable to do, either adduct or abduct. The paralysis may be unilateral or bilateral, but unilateral adductor paralysis is the most common. The voice is usually breathy and rough. Abductor paralysis is a rare condition in which the paralyzed fold remains in the midline position, producing a relatively normal voice but mild dyspnea. Damage to the superior laryngeal nerve causing cricothyroid muscle paralysis is also rare as an isolated lesion. The affected fold tends to atrophy, and the voice is hoarse with a reduced ability to vary pitch. The period of spontaneous recovery and maximum compensation is generally considered not to extend beyond 6 to 9 months. Excellent, complete reviews of paralyzed vocal folds have been offered by Aronson[10] and Ballenger.[15]

Myasthenia Laryngis

Ballenger has described a condition of the aged larnyx characterized by hypotonia of the laryngeal muscles.[15] Indirect laryngoscopy typically reveals bowing of the membranous portion of the vocal folds. Honjo and Isshiki reported aged men tend to have vocal fold atrophy and/or edema and a higher pitch than young men.[16] Aged women tend to have vocal fold edema and slight hoarseness and a lower pitch than young women.

VOICE ASSESSMENT

Successful patient care begins with a cooperative relationship between the speech pathologist and referral sources. The speech pathologist may have initial contact with the voice patient, but should not conduct treatment without the patient receiving an evaluation by the otolaryngologist. The otolaryngologist should communicate his or her findings clearly to the speech pathologist, with a complete description of laryngeal structures and functions. Pathologic changes of the larynx, including size and composition of growths, are reported as well as related medical conditions, such as allergies. A team effort between the speech pathologist and otolaryngologist provides the best evaluation and rehabilitation approach; specific examples will be offered in subsequent sections of this chapter.

The speech pathologist's assessment procedures involve collecting data to provide a comprehensive description of the disorder and related conditions. The information allows the speech pathologist, in a cooperative effort with the otolaryngologist, to assign a label, propose a prognosis, and plan rehabilitation. Basic adult case history information, including health history, applicable to all types of patients and a standard speech mechanism examination should be conducted for voice patients and has been described elsewhere.[17,18] For the purpose of brevity, the presentation of material in this chapter will be restricted to procedures specific to voice disorders.

Voice History

Specific voice history questions have been offered by others.[3,4,12,17] The initial questions seek the patient's complaint or description of the voice disorder and related anomalies. Many patients express more concern about and wish relief from the somatic feelings[19] related to the voice disorder than the actual sound of the voice. The patient's description reveals his or her general attitude and degree of concern about the disorder; the patient's descriptive language also indicates his or her insight into the disorder and interpretation of the otolaryngology results.

The chronologic history of the disorder provides important information. Specifying the time of onset and whether the disorder developed suddenly or gradually often reveals the patient's attitude toward the disorder, prognosis, and nature of the disorder. A voice disorder that existed for a long time before the patient sought help suggests the patient has not been concerned. Poor patient motivation and/or learned behavior of long duration offer an unfavorable prognosis. The developmental course of the disorder is explored thoroughly. Occurrence and remissions of the disorder are usually indicative of nonpathologic changes in the vocal folds. Patients with pathologic changes of the vocal folds typically report an abnormal voice that does not periodically return to normal, but may gradually worsen. Voice disorders that develop gradually and fluctuate in response to voice abuse are common of functional dysphonias and growths of the vocal folds.

Sudden onset within a few minutes or hours, especially if the voice disorder is severe, should be explored carefully. Sudden onset could suggest allergy, extreme vocal abuse, inhalation of toxic fumes, or psychogenic etiology. Events concurrent with the beginning of the voice disorder are investigated carefully. The patient may have had other physical reactions indicative of a response to an environmental agent or emotional conflict. Aronson has reported patients may have three common reactions to exploration of emotional issues.[10] One reaction may be initial steadfast denial in which the clinician should abandon pursuit of the issue, but return to it later in the session or during a subsequent session. If a voice-related interpersonal conflict exists, there is a high probability that the patient will confirm it later. The second response is a patient who is aware of the possible relationship between emotional conflict and the voice disorder and is willing and occasionally eager to discuss it. The third circumstance is the patient who vigorously denies associated emotional problems because none exists or because poor insight or high resistance is prevalent. It is also determined if the patient had surgery or perhaps a precipitating illness that may have resolved, but the dysphonia remained.

The patient's description of voice variability often provides clues about the etiology and therapy direction. Some patients report that their voice remains consistent. However, the typical voice patient that engages in voice abuse and misuse reports that his or her voice is better in the morning and becomes worse throughout the day with voice use. A sufficient period of voice rest often improves the voice. By contrast, a patient with allergy and postnasal drip during sleep experiences his or her worst voice in the morning, and it gradually improves during the day.

The clinician asks the patient if there are situations in which the voice is better or worse and determines if consistent patterns of relationships emerge. The clinician inquires if particular events or conditions precede voice patterns of variability. For example, seasons or daily weather conditions may affect the voice, and general fatigue or emotional stress may contribute to changes in the voice.

Asking the patient to describe vocal demands during a routine week and weekend day often assists discovery of and affect relationships between voice abuse and voice deterioration. The patient describes the voice use required by the job and also how much speaking occurs in the home. The frequency and type of social and recreational activities are also explored. The basic purpose of this inquiry is to gain general insight into how voice abuse may contribute to the disorder. A more thorough, careful exploration of possible voice abuse is conducted in therapy.

The family constellation and living conditions are determined by standard adult case history procedures. However, this basic information should be supplemented if the patient's voice is similar to anyone else's in the family. Interactions of the family unit may precipitate voice abuse and affect others. Vocal competition and demands are ascertained. The responses of relatives and friends to the patient's voice often reveals possible reinforcement for the disorder or disturbing adverse reactions. The patient's reaction to others' comments and his or her judgement about the impact of a better voice indicate his or her expectations and desire to change.

A voice-related medical history includes who the patient has consulted about the voice problem; the consultant's findings and recommendations are obtained. If remedial efforts were conducted, the clinician determines by whom, what the results were, and why therapy ceased. Serious illnesses, head and neck injuries or surgery, and medication history are explored, especially if they occurred coincident with the voice disorder. Allergies or metabolic disturbances may also contribute to a voice disorder.

Written reports of significant conditions are requested from appropriate professionals, and referrals made when warranted. The patient's tobacco and alcohol use may also have etiologic importance. Finally, the patient's description of accompanying somatic feelings,[19] such as throat pain, dryness, or the need to clear the throat, is discussed.

The voice clinician can combine the history information from the patient interview, physician's reports, and hospital medical chart to formulate a complete history of the voice disorder. The information provides a partial description of factors related to the occurrence and development of the voice disorder. Combined with the voice description discussed in the next section, a prognosis, recommendations, and a rehabilitation plan can be proposed.

Voice Description and Appraisal

Basic approaches that can be used in any clinic to describe voice quality, pitch, and breath support for voice will be presented in the following sections. Instrumentation that can provide better accuracy and quantification of the measures will also be discussed. A clear, concise analysis and presentation of the information assists the otolaryngologist and patient regarding treatment decisions.

Voice Quality

Each voice patient should have an individual baseline audiotape recording, with pretreatment tasks, and periodic reevaluation recordings. The patient's name and the date should be stated at the beginning of each recording. The voice tasks should include sustaining the vowel /a/, counting from one to 20, reading standard material such as *The Rainbow Passage,*[14] and 3 minutes of monologue. Samples of pitch and loudness manipulation may also be recorded for later analysis and to serve as a permanent record.

The traditional terminology used to describe laryngeal voice quality was reviewed earlier. However, the terms are broad, imprecise, and require a combination of perceptual features. The terms also have different meanings between clinicians, thus yielding poor reliability. I prefer the system designed by Wilson and Broda-Masiuk[20] to describe the audible features of voice. The voice profile (Fig. 27–1) offers precise perceptual components for the listener. The clinician can listen to a voice sample and judge perceptually the presence or absence and prominence of each voice profile component. Wilson and Broda-Masiuk present audio training tapes that yield high inter- and intralistener reliability. Rather than use a broad, nondescript term such as "harshness," the clinician can communicate the more precise presence of each voice component to the patient and other professionals. The ability to recognize and specify individual perceptual features also assists therapy planning and evaluation.

Just below the patient identity information in the upper right-hand corner in Figure 27–1 is a "Voice Rating." This category is essentially a voice severity rating scale from "1," indicating the disorder is barely perceptible, to "7," meaning it interferes significantly with communication. The relative severity rating of each voice, in conjunction with other information, affects decisions about prognosis and remediation. Wilson and Broda-Masiuk provide audiotaped voice samples that reflect different points on the scale.

The "Laryngeal Cavity" segment reflects perceptual judgements on the firmness of vocal fold closure and pitch. The horizontal line "A" represents a continuum of vocal fold closure. A −4 rating indicates that the folds are totally open and that the patient can produce little, if any, friction noise for communication. The next point along the continuum, −3, represents narrowing of the glottis, causing friction noise to produce a whisper. The presence of breathiness, −2, is characterized by friction from excessive airflow, indicating less than normal vocal fold approximation. Breathiness also usually causes a reduction in loudness. Optimal vocal fold approximation yielding a normal voice is rated 1. The +2 represents a voice characterized by excessive tension and sometimes accompanied by an increase in loudness. The +3 rated voice exhibits extreme tension with erratic or aperiodic vocal fold closure patterns, with occasional vocal arrests. An individual with these voice characteristics would be diagnosed as spastic dysphonia.

The vertical line "B" reflects perceptual ratings of pitch in relation to an individual's age, sex, and social impact. Extreme pitch deviation is indicated if the speaker presents uncertain sexual identity based on acoustic cues alone. For example, if a male's pitch is so high he may be mistaken for a female during telephone conversations he would receive a +3 pitch rating. Conversely, if a female's pitch falls within the male range, she would receive a −3 rating. The +2 and −2 ratings indicate the pitch is judged above or below normal, but not sufficiently to cause social anxiety.

The "Resonating Cavity" section is a rating scale for resonance perceptual features. On the vertical line "C," −2 represents denasality or lack of nasal resonance of normally nasalized sounds, and 1 means normal nasal resonance. Assimilation nasality, +2, is excessive nasal resonance of vowels only when they

Voice Profile

Name: ____________________ Age: ____________________ Sex: ____________________

B.D.: ____________________ Date: ____________________ Ref. source: ____________________

Address: ____

Phone: ____________________

(circle one)
Voice rating: 1 2 3 4 5 6 7

Laryngeal cavity	Resonating cavity		Loudness	
Pitch	Nasality	-2	1	+2
high	hypernasal	soft		loud
B	C			
+3	+4			
+2	+3			
	+2			
A open -4-3-2 1+2+3 closed	-2 1+2		Vocal range	
-2	-2	-2	1	+2
-3	hyponasal	monotone		variable pitch
low				

Indicate presence or absence of acoustic features by (✓)

	Yes	No
Intermittent diplophonia	______	______
Diplophonia	______	______
Audible inhalation	______	______
Pitch breaks	______	______
Erratic phrasing	______	______
Immature resonance	______	______

Comments: ____

____

____

____
Clinician

Marking system

Primary feature X
Intermittent feature (int)
Secondary feature/e.g. +2
Noted feature/e.g. +2

Figure 27–1 Voice profile. (From Wilson FB, Broda-Masiuk D. Voice disorders. Bellingham, WA: Voice Tapes, 1987:19.)

follow nasal consonants. A +3 rating indicates the nasalization of vowels, regardless of phonemic context, and slight nasality of consonants. A +4 rating represents nasality of all phonemes with frequent consonant distortion caused by nasal emission and inability to impound oral air adequately. On the horizontal line, −2 indicates slightly denasal back-throat resonance, and +2 indicates frontal resonance with nasalization characteristic of the "effeminate" voice.

To the right of "Resonating Cavity," loudness should be rated as soft, normal, or loud and vocal range as monotone, normal, or excessive variable pitch. The presence or absence of other vocal characteristics may be noted on the lower half of the profile. A marking system is presented, which allows the clinician to indicate the relative prominence of each feature noted.

Pitch Appraisal

Special approaches are required to determine habitual pitch, pitch range, and optimal pitch. Pitch manipulations may be analyzed live or later from an audiotape recording. The parameters of pitch may be measured by the clinician's ability to match the patient's voice to an appropriate note from a pitch pipe or piano or to a frequency produced by a tone generator. Equipment is also available to display a voice sample as cycles per second (Hz).

Habitual, or modal, pitch is the pitch used most frequently while speaking. Moncur and Brackett have offered relatively simple but effective methods for determining habitual pitch.[21] Their first approach suggests having the patient read a passage while the clinician listens carefully to the general pitch level. The clinician hums a pitch that seems approximate to the patient's average pitch; the clinician should also hum a pitch that sounds higher or lower to confirm that the average pitch determined is accurate. The clinician prolongs humming the approximation of the patient's level and matches it with a pitch pipe, piano, or tone generator to determine the note or frequency that reflects the patient's habitual pitch. If the clinician cannot hum the patient's pitch because their ranges are too dissimilar, for example, a female clinician and a male patient with a very low pitch, the humming step can be eliminated, and the patient's pitch can be matched directly with the pitch pipe or piano.

Another method suggested by Moncur and Brackett is averaging key words.[21] The clinician listens to the patient and softly imitates his or her pitch patterns. The clinician prolongs the vowel of words that seem to characterize the patient's modal pitch pattern and matches the pitch level with a pitch pipe or piano. This step is repeated to obtain the values for several words; then the average pitch level of the samples taken is determined. Boone has offered a similar approach by recommending the approximate pitch of seven or eight voice samples from a tape recording be determined, and the pitch level that occurs most often is the modal pitch.[12]

If the patient's inflection patterns create difficulty, then estimating the habitual pitch, a method suggested by Fairbanks,[14] may be helpful. The patient reads the *The Rainbow Passage* while gradually compressing his or her pitch range until chanting in a monotone pitch, which the clinician may match with a pitch pipe or piano.

The fundamental frequency values of adult males and females have been studied and may be compared to measures obtained by clinicians. Hollien and Shipp investigated the mean speaking fundamental frequency of 175 males ranging in age from 20 to 89 years.[22] The authors noted a trend of lowering fundamental frequency through adulthood and middle age, which reversed in later ages of life. Specifically, the speaking fundamental frequency values by decade were 120 Hz for the 20- to 29-year-old group, 112 Hz for the 30 to 39 year olds, 107 Hz for the 40 to 49 year olds, 118 Hz for the 50 to 59 year olds, and 112 Hz for the 60 to 69 year olds. The fundamental frequency increased to 132 Hz for the 70 to 79 year olds and 146 Hz for the 80 to 89 year olds. By contrast, Kelley[23] observed that the mean fundamental frequency decreases in adult females as age increases.[23] The mean fundamental frequency for 20 to 29 year olds was 227 Hz, but remained 214 Hz for each decade from 30 to 59 years of age. The mean fundamental frequency decreased to 209 Hz for 60 to 69 year olds, 206 Hz for 70 to 79 year olds, and 197 Hz for 80 to 90 year olds.

The patient's pitch range is also determined live or from an audiotape of his or her performance. The clinician models the task and instructs the patient to begin at his or her typical pitch and say "ah" in decreasing steps to the lowest note he or she can produce, and the clinician matches the patient's final note with a pitch pipe or piano. When the lowest note has been determined, the patient begins again at his or her typical pitch and produces "ah" in increasing steps to his or her highest note, including falsetto, which the clinician matches with a pitch pipe or piano. It is often helpful to have the patient take a breath just before producing his or her lowest and highest notes and prolong them, yielding a longer sample for the clinician to match. It is easier for some patients to glide up or down the scale rather than by steps.

Hollien, Dew, and Philips have presented normative data on the phonational frequency ranges of 332 adult males and 202 adult females, ages 18 to 36.[24] The mean phonational frequency range exceeded three octaves or 38 semitones for males and 37 semitones for females. The mean values for the lowest and highest phonation frequencies were 78 and 698 Hz for males and 139 and 1108 Hz for females. However, the authors reported that the data exhibited substantial standard deviation, and individual ranges varied from approximately 1.5 to 4.5 octaves.

Optimum pitch is generally considered to be a pitch level produced most efficiently with the least amount of effort by the laryngeal mechanism. However, Moncur and Brackett[21] have questioned the validity of optimal pitch, and Boone[12] has cautioned that "It is doubtful, however, that optimum pitch represents any exact cycles-per-second value. Optimum pitch is more often found in two or three notes somewhere at the bottom of the individual's pitch range, several notes higher than the lowest possible pitch production" (p 97). It does seem reasonable to assume that speaking at an inappropriate pitch requires unnecessary strain and effort. Ideally, optimum and habitual pitch should be the same. However, the concept of optimum pitch is probably invalid for pathologic larynges.

Fairbanks has presented a standard method of determining optimum pitch.[14] The patient's pitch range from the lowest note to the highest, including falsetto, should be assessed by the method described earlier. The total number of whole notes is counted; optimum pitch for males is one-fourth of the way up from the bottom of the complete pitch range, but for females, it is one or two notes lower than the one-fourth level.

Fairbanks has also offered a graphic means (Fig. 27–2) of establishing optimum ("natural") pitch. The

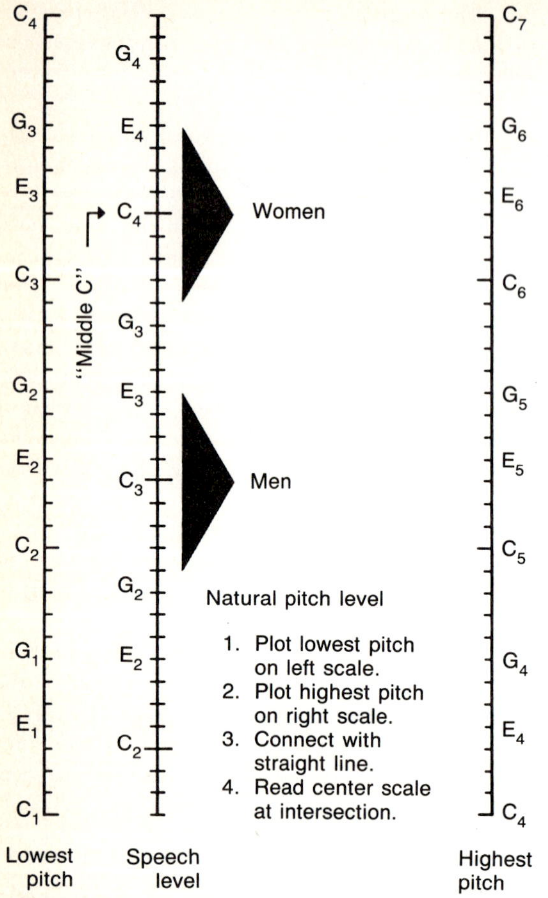

Figure 27–2 Comparison of pitch levels on the musical scale. (From Fairbanks G. Voice and articulation drillbook. New York: Harper & Row, 1960.)

lowest and highest notes are plotted on the appropriate ordinances and connected by a straight line. Where the line intersects the central scale should be the individual's optimum pitch.

An instrument particularly useful for obtaining pitch values is the Visi-Pitch by Kay Elemetrics Corporation. The Visi-Pitch can determine the highest and lowest fundamental frequency in order to establish the pitch range and the average fundamental frequency of a voice sample for habitual pitch. Pitch contours and perturbation measures are also observable. The data can be presented by oscilloscopic display, digital writeout, and hardcopy. Two models of the Visi-Pitch can interface with an Apple II computer to provide diskette storage of data, graphics, or statistics.

Respiration Appraisal

Efficient breath support for voice requires adequate movement of air effortlessly, a quick and quiet inhalation, and responsive control of exhalation. Three types of breathing patterns for voice have been described by Boone.[12] "Clavicular" breathing is an inefficient method in which the patient elevates the shoulders on inhalation, straining the neck accessory muscles to elevate the upper thorax. Elevation of the clavicles and neck muscle strain is visually evident. The preferred type of breathing for voice has been referred to as "diaphragmatic abdominal" by Boone[12] and "central control" by Moncur and Brackett.[21] During inhalation, abdominal and lower thoracic expansion is noticeable with slight secondary movement of the upper thorax. Moncur and Brackett have observed that "central control will tend to reduce the need for upper thoracic control (expansion of upper rib cage) and do much toward eliminating unwanted tension in the neck" (p 128). Boone has reported that most voice patients utilize "thoracic" breathing for voice, a pattern of midthoracic expansion during inhalation that lies somewhere between upper thoracic clavicular movement and lower thoracic diaphragmatic abdominal movement.

The type of breathing for voice can usually be observed visually. However, if loose fitting or bulky clothing interferes with observation, the clinician may place a hand on the patient's abdomen so that lower rib and abdominal expansion can be felt while the patient converses or reads prose. A hand placed on the upper thorax can also indicate the degree of movement in this area. During expiration for voice, the diaphragmatic abdominal area should relax gradually. Respiratory efficiency can also be judged by noting how many words the patient says per exhalation.

Boone has also suggested several common faults of respiration that may be observed.[12] The patient may exhale air before initiating phonation, leaving inadequate air supply for normal phrase length. The patient may also continue to speak when he or she has practically exhausted his or her air supply. Other patients may take an inadequate inspiration of air, thus reducing expiratory force and vocal loudness. As well, a singer or lecturer may place an unnecessary focus on breathing by attempting a "big" breath, perhaps with clavicular breathing, which he or she cannot control efficiently during expiration.

Eckel and Boone have reported a simple method of assessing the patient's respiratory and phonatory efficiency, the s to z ratio.[25] They investigated 28 dysphonic subjects with laryngeal pathology, 36 dysphonic subjects without laryngeal pathology, and 86 normal speakers. Each subject was instructed to take a deep breath and sustain /z/ and then /s/ for as long as possible at a comfortable pitch and loudness level. They were given two trials for both phonemes, and the longest duration for each was the subject's score. The /s/ value was divided by the /z/ score to produce an s to z ratio. The normal speaking and dysphonic patients without laryngeal pathology produced similar ratios, approximately 1.0, indicating voiceless expiration time closely matched phonation time. In contrast, dysphonic patients with laryngeal pathology produced, 95 percent of the time, s to z ratios in excess of 1.4. The data suggest additive mass along the glottal margin affects vocal fold approximation efficiency, thus decreasing glottal resistance and increasing airflow and reducing phonatory duration time. The s to z ratio is a useful measure that could be repeated periodically to determine change across time.

Instrumentation has been designed to provide a variety of useful respiration measures. The clinician should obtain baseline values that can be compared to periodic measures throughout voice therapy. A wet spirometer consists of an inverted tube placed in a larger tube containing water. Air blown into the inverted tube causes it to rise in the water of the larger tube in proportion to the quantity of air exhaled by the patient. The elevation of the inverted vessel is expressed as milliliters. To obtain vital capacity, the patient is asked to inhale deeply and exhale as completely as possible into the spirometer's mouthpiece. In adult males, the vital capacity ranges from 3,500 to 5,000 ml. Tidal volume is the amount of air inhaled and exhaled during a normal breathing cycle. Normal average tidal volume for adult males is 750 ml and for adult females 339 ml. Inspiratory reserve volume, or complemental air, is the maximum amount of air that can be inspired beyond tidal inspiration and averages about 1,500 ml for adults. Expiratory reserve volume, or supplemental air, is the amount of air that can be expired beyond tidal expiration. The average volume is similar to inspiratory reserve volume for adults, approximately 1,500 ml.

Lung volume capacity is not typically a problem for voice patients unless they have emphysema or other chronic pulmonary disease. More important for most voice patients is information on the coordination of abdominal and thoracic movements during speech. The pneumograph records breath support movements. Straps are placed around the patient's thorax and abdomen, and then rubber tubes, coupled to a pressure transducer, are attached to each end of the straps; expansion of the thorax and abdomen creates a negative pressure in the tubes, which through the pressure transducer results in a graphic recorder writeout of movement patterns.

A pneumotachograph is an instrument that measures volume-velocity airflow through the glottis. Normal phonation of a vowel in the modal register yields approximately 100 ml per second of air through the glottis.[26] However, patients with unilateral vocal fold paralysis, tumors, or large benign lesions exhibit high airflow rates between 209 and 700 ml per second.[27] Vocal fold paralysis or obstructing lesions prevent normal vocal fold closure, resulting in higher airflow through the glottis.

Glottal resistance is an important measure that is reflected as a ratio between subglottal pressure and airflow. The traditional method of determining subglottal pressure requires (1) a tracheal puncture with a needle in order to place a polyethylene tube in the trachea[26,28] and (2) a pneumotachograph (through which airflow is recorded) attached to an anesthesia mask. The polyethylene tube and pneumotachograph are connected to differential pressure transducers in order to determine subglottal pressure and airflow.

Smitheran and Hixon have devised a noninvasive method of estimating glottal resistance that compares favorably with the traditional method, but is more easily determined in the clinic.[29] The authors base their method on the concept that for an instant during the production of voiceless plosives, oral pressure and tracheal pressure are identical. Consequently, they measured oral pressure with a polyethylene tube positioned in the oral cavity during production of the /pi/ syllable at a rate of 1.5 syllables per second. Airflow was determined in the traditional manner. Smitheran and Hixon felt glottal resistance data would be a useful measure for functional, hyperfunctional, and hypofunctional voice disorders and neurologic voice disorders.

The clinician should have obtained the following information upon completion of the appraisal period: (1) a complete description of the patient's laryngeal structures, functions, and pathologic changes, provided by the otolaryngologist; (2) the patient's voice concerns and relevant history, including reports from other appropriate professionals; (3) a speech mechanism evaluation; and (4) a clear description of the patient's vocal parameters. Examination of the information allows the clinician, in cooperation with the otolaryngologist, to discuss recommendations with the patient.

Recommendations

Recommendations may need to be deferred if more information is required from other professionals. However, if sufficient information has been obtained, the clinician should consider three essential questions:

1. Is there a disorder?
2. Is there a problem?
3. What is the potential for change?

If the patient's voice is within the normal range for his or her age and sex, he or she does not have a voice disorder, and so therapy is not warranted. The patient may have a voice disorder, but it may not be a problem for him or her, that is, have sufficient negative impact that the patient is motivated to change his or her voice. The clinician should explain that the patient has a voice disorder, but it is ultimately the patient's choice whether or not to receive therapy.

The patient may have a significant voice disorder and consider it a problem he or she desires resolved, but may have poor potential for change by voice therapy alone. The need for a clear description from the otolaryngologist of laryngeal pathologic changes and related medical conditions was emphasized earlier. The condition of the larynx indicates whether or not surgery is required before voice therapy.

With a cooperative, motivated patient, chronic simple laryngitis, small fibrotic nodules, soft nodules, small polyps, and contact ulcers can be reversed with voice therapy. However, large fibrotic nodules, larger polyps, and contact ulcers with extensive granulation require surgery followed by voice therapy. The patient and surgeon should be aware that the dysphonia may persist after surgery[30,31] and still require voice therapy.

The patient may have pathologic laryngeal changes that can be eliminated without surgery. The clinician presents a basic outline of the rehabilitation plan including appropriate medical attention, voice abuse reduction, correction of voice misuse, or some combination thereof. It should be explained that the reduction in pathologic conditions is dependent upon the patient's ability to reduce voice abuse and misuse.

Most patients choose voice therapy hoping to prevent surgery. However, other patients recognize their potential for change without surgery is negligible and would involve more adjustment than they are willing to consider. These patients typically use their voice in their profession an inordinate amount of time and perhaps under stressful conditions. Surgery followed by voice therapy may reduce the occupational voice disability.

In summary, recommendations are dependent upon whether the patient has a voice disorder or not and, if so, the extent of laryngeal pathologic change and the likelihood of having ancillary medical conditions, such as allergies or sinusitis, resolved. Potential for change is also affected by patient motivation and ability to adjust work and/or social vocal demands.

VOICE REHABILITATION

Choosing and implementing rehabilitation procedures involves establishing a philosophy of voice therapy and understanding treatment options. This section of the chapter will describe specific approaches for eliminating voice abuse and misuse and how to extend better voice to natural environments. Distinctive techniques for special problems, including patients who had a laryngectomy, will also be discussed.

Philosophy

The voice clinician should base his or her rehabilitation approaches upon an underlying philosophy. Therapy procedures should not be conducted without a clear rationale for choosing them. Several voice authorities have offered rehabilitation principles worthy of consideration.

Brodnitz felt the goal of vocal rehabilitation is to return vocal production to a total and unified function.[11] Vocal functions should not be manipulated independently, but by techniques that treat vocal function as an integrated gestalt. Brodnitz indicated it was impossible to isolate and treat dysfunction in a single or pair of muscles. Consequently, Brodnitz advocated the chewing method because it reduced hyperfunction in an integrated manner at the laryngeal level and throughout the vocal tract. Functional dysphonia and disorders from organic changes in the vocal folds are treated similarly because voice abuse and misuse are the etiologic bases for both types of disorders. Systematic voice practice was advocated in order to extend improved voice production through more complex practice levels.

Perhaps Perkins has provided the most accepted philosophy of voice therapy: "The notion that voice is produced most hygienically when it is produced most effortlessly appears to have universal agreement" (p 507).[32] He elaborated on this concept by suggesting that ". . . the mark of the optimally produced voice, hygienically, acoustically, and aesthetically, is the ability to vary vocal effort proportional to the needs of pitch, loudness, voicing, and vocal mode while keeping constriction minimal" (p 520). Perkins recommended a system of operant therapy be applied to specified vocal dimensions. However, like Brodnitz, Perkins advocated therapy procedures that integrated the voice dimensions holistically into a unified optimal vocal performance. Perkins felt therapy should be based on functional analysis of vocal behavior; therefore etiologic behaviors are irrelevant. However, he recognized the following about pathologic changes of the vocal folds: ". . . optimal vocal functioning is limited to varying degrees, determinable only by behavioral assessment, as long as any of these conditions prevail" (p 523).

Moore addressed organic voice disorders of three types.[3] The first type was voice problems from vocal abuse that produced myasthenia laryngis, thickened vocal fold tissue, vocal nodules, contact ulcer, or chronic laryngitis. The second type involved vocal deviations subsequent to surgical intervention that provides an essentially normal larynx, and third, voice problems from endocrine imbalance or anemia despite medical treatment. Moore coined an excellent term, "restorative therapy," to describe the basic goal of therapy for these disorders. Moore suggested the clinician utilize psychological, environmental, and physiologic procedures to ". . . establish a method of voice production in which the natural rejuvenating processes can occur, since normal structures tend to reestablish themselves when given the opportunity; and to develop vocal habits that can be used effectively to meet the ordinary demands of living'' (p 561). In essence, restorative therapy for organic disorders is designed to allow vocal structures to heal by eliminating voice abuse and misuse.

According to Moore, the psychological approach includes considering the patient's attitude.[3] The patient must understand that habitual abuse and misuse of the voice will continue the disorder, and the best vocal usage possible must be maintained. The patient is not expected to implement the therapy regimen conscientiously unless the clinician has clearly explained rehabilitation goals and rationale. More extensive psychological counseling should be enacted by the speech pathologist or other appropriate professionals when indicated. The environmental approach recognizes that the communication demands of work, home, and recreational situation must be addressed for therapy to be successful. The phsyiologic aspects of therapy involve voice rest to promote healing followed by training the patient to phonate in a relaxed easy manner.

Aronson has offered some common principles of voice therapy.[10] Progression from abnormal to normal voice requires the patient's conscious, volitional response to instructions. Auditory discrimination and feedback are crucial to successful therapy because tactile and proprioceptive feedback is diminished in phonation. Although the fundamental principles for a specific disorder do not vary, therapy must still be tailored to each individual. However, Aronson emphasizes that voice disorders should not be considered exclusively from a learning theory perspective, and voice disorders resulting from emotional stress should not be treated as only a mechanical problem. Hyperfunctional or musculoskeletal tension voice disorders involve excessive laryngeal muscle tension as a reaction to the stress of life and either acute or chronic anxiety.

Boone has espoused "symptomatic" voice therapy,[12] and he suggested

> In general, however, voice therapy approaches do not distinguish between functional and organic problems. That is, for example, the patient with functional dysphonia, with or without the development of vocal nodules, will basically require the same general kind of voice therapy, a program designed to reduce abuse-misuse and to use the voice as easily as possible (p 61).

Instead, the clinician analyzes how the phonatory processes of mass and size and approximation are affected and relates these observations to the perceptual dimensions of loudness, pitch, and quality. The clinician must then utilize techniques that facilitate the patient's best voice along the perceptual dimensions of loudness, pitch, and quality. The patient's best voice becomes the target model, or symptomatic focus of therapy, to be practiced systematically. The patient's best voice production, or target model to be practiced, becomes his or her therapy goal. Boone emphasizes that there must be a continuous search in every clinical session for the patient's best voice. The patient may become more capable of producing better voice, and so the target model changes accordingly. However, although Boone did not advocate a differential approach for functional and organic disorders, he did recognize obstructive masses ". . . may prevent the patient from achieving a ''good-sounding'' voice, no matter what he or she does'' (p 61).

The philosophies reviewed previously share common themes, but differ somewhat in emphasis. Voice disorders that require management by a speech pathologist demand reduction of vocal abuse and misuse. Patients with hyperfunctional voice disorders especially need to learn a more optimal manner of phonation in order to achieve acceptable voice quality. The authors previously quoted also recognize that the patient's psychological state is important, but differ in their view of the clinician's level of responsibility.

There are three broad approaches to vocal rehabilitation. The first approach involves medical treatment including psychiatric. The second approach is voice abuse counseling, which may require short-term total voice rest. Third, techniques to reduce voice misuse are fundamental to voice therapy. Depending upon the patient's needs, a single approach or combination thereof may be required. Each of these approaches will be reviewed, with emphasis on voice abuse and misuse techniques. The interested reader should note that Wilson and Broda-Masiuk[20] and Boone[33] have offered excellent detailed programs for adult rehabilitation.

Medical Rehabilitation

Specific examples of laryngeal pathologic conditions that require medical treatment prior to voice therapy were presented in the assessment section of this chapter. However, Moore, Hicks, and Abbott have delineated several etiologies of voice disorders that may require medical treatment.[5]

1. Pathologic conditions of the vocal folds from voice misuse or abuse, such as vocal nodules or polyps, may require surgery.
2. Acute anxiety and emotional turmoil may contribute to vocal hyperfunction without observable pathologic changes.
3. Diseases and growths, including infections, paralyses, and benign and malignant tumors, require medical attention.
4. Mechanical and chemical irritants affecting the mucosa: fumes, allergens, stomach reflux, and subtances causing noninflammatory edema, such as glandular imbalance, may cause a voice disorder.
5. Congenital anomalies and destruction of laryngeal tissue by surgery, trauma, or disease may also require medical care.
6. Systemic disorders such as anemia or metabolic disturbances contributing to chronic fatigue may cause a voice disorder.

Explanation of the Disorder

Voice therapy should begin with presenting an explanation of the disorder to the patient. The perceptual features of the voice are described, and the reasons why the particular sound occurs are explained. For example, if the patient exhibits breathiness, it is necessary to indicate that the vocal folds are not achieving adequate closure perhaps because of paralysis or obstructing growths such as fibrotic nodules. If the voice sounds tense, the clinician explains that the patient is using too much effort to phonate and is approximating the folds with excessive force. If this results in pathologic changes of the vocal folds, the patient is told that fold tissue cannot withstand this type of phonation without an adverse reaction. The role of voice abuses such as yelling, loud and/or excessive talking, and throat clearing are expounded upon. How these behaviors contribute to the patient's complaint about uncomfortable somatic feelings should also be presented. Any helpful analogy, such as nodules and calluses, is given.

Explanation of the disorder removes anxiety of the "unknown" and enhances motivation—important psychological aspects. Perhaps equally as important, explaining the disorder serves as a foundation for the therapy approach rationale. For example, the need to reduce vocal abuses to allow healing becomes obvious.

Voice Abuse Counseling

Voice disorders are often the result of personality and/or job choice. The typical hyperfunctional voice patient is a gregarious individual who enjoys socializing and talking. He or she is often energetic and speaks louder than necessary. He or she may also choose a vocation that involves extensive verbal interaction with others, for example, sales persons, lecturers, or managers. If the voice disorder is to be reduced or eliminated, voice abuse counseling is critical for such individuals whether they have a normal larynx or pathologic changes of the vocal folds. I agree with Boone[12] who stated:

> It appears to require only a minimal amount of vocal abuse each day to maintain a dysphonia or to develop and maintain a laryngeal pathology . . . the elimination or reduction of vocal abuse will often be remarkably effective in eliminating the dysphonia and its accompanying laryngeal pathology. For any voice patient with approximation or mass-size problems of the vocal folds, vocal abuse, if present, should be eliminated or at least reduced (p 139).

Eliminating the mechanical trauma from vocal abuse is an excellent "restorative therapy"[3] technique to help rejuvenate the vocal folds. Reduction of the vocal fold pathology or rest for normal appearing folds enhances the ability of voice misuse facilitation techniques to achieve a further reduction in the dysphonia.

An extreme method of eliminating vocal abuse is to impose total voice rest. This is a short-term solution subsequent to surgery for laryngeal growths in order to allow healing. The surgeon prescribes the amount of voice rest, from 2 days to 2 weeks, depending upon the size of the pathology removed. Voice rest is also helpful for periods of infectious or voice abuse caused by laryngitis. A brief 2 to 3 days of voice rest can improve the success of voice misuse facilitation techniques. However, voice rest should be used sparingly. Aronson has cautioned it should only be used briefly subsequent to surgery.[10] Aronson reported voice rest could contribute to a psychogenic voice disorder by suggesting a concern about the ability to phonate.

A general list of voice abuses may be presented to a patient and refined over time to account for his or her individual needs. The physiologic rationale for eliminating the abuses is explained. Many voice patients must learn to use the voice quietly and to maintain a low loudness level while speaking. Low loudness phonation is preferable to whispering because the patient may unintentionally modify the normal whisper to a deleterious "stage whisper." The patient must be cautioned not to yell, talk louder than normal conversational level, or talk in noisy environments that require a louder voice in order to be heard. The patient may need to reduce the amount of talking to no more than necessary. If the patient's vocation, such as sales manager, demands a certain amount of talking, he or she must determine speaking priorities. There are situations in which the patient must talk; therefore he or she may need to restrain his or her speaking in less critical situations. The patient may also be in a position of authority to delegate some speaking responsibility to others.

Other voice abuses that patients may need to control include coughing or clearing the throat, common behaviors of hyperfunctional voice patients. Tobacco smoke is an irritating agent for the larynx and also drys the vocal folds' membranes. Alcohol is a vasodilating agent often consumed in noisy environments that facilitates loss of inhibitions resulting in more and louder talking than usual.

Many of the aforementioned vocal abuses are easily identified and reduced through counting and graphing their occurrence. However, these therapy activities compose only the elementary stage of successful voice abuse counseling. The challenge involves examining each individual's vocal demands and assisting the implementation of favorable modifications. It is difficult for a patient to recall his or her speaking situations with sufficient accuracy to be helpful, and most clinicians do not have enough time to observe the patient adequately. However, a modified version of the "Speaking-Time Log"[17] can be utilized to determine the patient's verbal patterns of daily life, that is, how much he or she talks, in what situations, to whom, and the effects on the larynx. The patient records on a piece of paper from left to right the following information: (1) the time of day to the nearest hour, (2) a brief description of the speaking situations, (3) an estimate of the speaking time in minutes, and (4) a rating of the voice and/or somatic feelings on a five-point scale. The patient completes the log for 2 or more week days, a weekend day, and reports if each day was relatively "typical" to indicate if the data are a representative sample. If he or she reports his or her verbal activities involve frequent anxious or aversive speaking situations, he or she also rates the "reaction" to each situation on a five-point scale.

The diary provides useful information. A baseline record of minutes talked and course of voice deterioration is determined. Perhaps the most important use of the diary is the daily record of each patient's unique voice use. Patterns of repetitive circumstances that precipitate improved or deteriorated voice are usually evident. The clinician examines the information carefully and explores with the patient possible adjustments he or she can employ to enhance the favorable circumstances and to counteract the adverse ones. The patient's work and social schedule may be adjusted to reduce talking and stressful situations. For example, business managers can often delegate some speaking responsibilities to others and, perhaps, serve a consulting role in business meetings. Information derived from the diary suggests implementation of procedures beyond the usual admonition to talk less and more quietly. For example, a patient who was president of a family-owned corporation had diary entries that revealed his voice seriously deteriorated only after board meetings. By the patient's report, confirmed by audiotape recordings of the sessions, the meetings were usually stressful and aggressively competitive with all participants speaking loudly and frequently interrupting each other. The board members agreed to establish parliamentary procedures and other rules of conduct that reduced the verbal aggression, and the patient's voice improved quickly.

Correction of Voice Misuse

Patients with hyperfunctional voice disorders must learn to produce phonation more efficiently with less effort. They often use excessive adductory force during phonation, which may produce or maintain pathologic changes or contribute to functional dysphonia. They may also speak at an incorrect pitch, use inadequate breath support, or produce asynchronous fold vibration.

Boone has presented an excellent description of 25 voice "facilitating approaches," many of them appropriate in correcting voice misuse.[12] The effectiveness of each technique varies with individual patients. Each technique should be analyzed by its ability to improve the voice. Systematic application of the techniques assists judging their effectiveness. For example, each technique is attempted ten times, and each response is judged and tabulated "correct" if it facilitates improved voice and "wrong" if favorable change does not occur. Percent of correct responses reveals the most successful technique. Alternating the habitual (disordered) voice with the voice achieved by a facilitation technique may be necessary in order to judge voice change. If two facilitation techniques achieve similar results, they should be alternated for ten responses each in order to assist comparison. If effectiveness remains similar, then the least complicated technique should be chosen. The following is a brief presentation of several effective facilitation techniques.

Imitation of Breathiness

Breathy phonation is an excellent technique for eliminating excessive vocal fold tension and can serve a "restorative" function. Moore has stated:

> Breathiness, purposely produced, keeps the vocal cords from striking each other as vigorously as in other types of phonation, and the closed phase of the vibratory cycle is shortened, thereby reducing the time in which the cords are in contact. The relaxed breathy-voice production also

reduces the pressure between the arytenoid cartilages, which is particularly advantageous with contact ulcers (p 563).[3]

Breathy phonation reduces stress on pathologic conditions of the vocal folds better than "normal" vocal fold approximation. Vocal folds that appear normal on indirect laryngoscopy often produce improved voice subsequent to a few days of breathy phonation. It is often easier for a patient with a tense voice to gradually approximate normal from the opposite extreme (breathy) of the patient's typical (tense) voice. The simplest method of facilitation is for the clinician to model breathy phonation during /a/ or counting from one to five; the patient is asked to imitate the examples. The breathiness should be continuous throughout the phonation. Reducing loudness, perhaps to a whisper, and gradually increasing the loudness may help achieve breathy phonation. A similar concept is to teach an aspirate initiation of phonation by saying words that begin with /h/ then gradually "fade" the /h/ until the vowels are initiated with a soft, breathy attack. Air wastage from breathiness usually requires increased breath support for compensation.

Yawn-Sigh

The yawn-sigh approach is excellent for reducing vocal hyperfunction. Perkins has suggested the approach is effective because the yawn is a respondent behavior that inhibits vocal constriction and provides proprioceptive contrast to excessive tension.[32] The yawn relaxes the pharynx by stretching and lengthening the muscles.

The clinician explains to the patient that a yawn is a slow inspiration with a wide mouth opening. The activity is demonstrated, and then the patient is asked to yawn and note the feeling in the vocal tract. Another yawn is demonstrated and is followed by a slow exhalation sigh with soft phonation. Breathy, relaxed phonation usually results. Sometimes it helps to instruct the patient to keep the low loudness level, but to begin phonation at a higher pitch and gradually glide down the scale. With this combined approach, there is often a point during the downward pitch glide in which the voice sounds better than by either technique alone. When the better voice is heard, the patient can be signaled to stop the downward pitch glide and to maintain phonation at that level. After several productions of good phonation, the yawn is replaced by normal, quick inspiration followed by a prolonged, gentle sigh with soft phonation. Successful accomplishment of good phonation without the yawn is extended to include quiet production of words and phrases, perhaps containing the initial /h/. The sigh is faded to gradually approximate more normal, less breathy phonation. Finally, the patient just imagines the relaxed feeling while speaking.

Chewing

The chewing approach of Froeschels is a highly regarded method of reducing vocal hyperfunction.[13] Brodnitz suggested the chewing approach functioned holistically to reduce hyperfunctional tension of the vocal folds and resonators and adjusted pitch to a more natural level.[11] Perkins felt chewing facilitated better voice because it was a respondent behavior,[32] and Moore explained: "The chewing movements are less complex than those used in speaking, and by overriding the ordinary speech adjustments they reduce the habitual patterns of hypertension that may have been established" (p 143).[4]

To implement the technique, the clinician explains that the patient is using voice with excessive tension, and the rationale described previously is presented. The clinician gives verbal instructions and demonstrates each step. It may also be helpful to have the patient observe him- or herself in a mirror. The patient performs closed mouth chewing movements with free movements of the tongue and exaggerated jaw excursions. Next, the patient does the exaggerated chewing movements with an open mouth. Verbal feedback about the patient's performance and adequate practice for an easy chewing motion are provided. After successful completion of these steps, the patient employs the exaggerated, open mouth chewing motions and adds very soft phonation. Brodnitz reported that if the tongue is motionless on the floor of the mouth, a monotonous "Yam-Yam" results.[11] Brodnitz emphasized that free movements of the tongue are essential for success. A relaxed, improved voice should be heard. Good voice must be achieved at each step before advancing to the next. While continuing the chewing movements and soft phonation, the patient counts slowly from one to ten. Brodnitz recommends that the previously described procedure be repeated many times during the day for a minute each time. Frequent repetition of the sequence assists carry-over to the next steps. The patient then practices reading and conversation with the chewing motions. Finally, the patient gradually reduces the chewing movements to normal speech patterns until ultimately he or she "just thinks" of chewing.

Appropriate Pitch

Hyperfunctional voice patients commonly speak at an incorrect pitch level that requires more effort than necessary. The habitual pitch should approximate the optimal pitch except for voice disorders from additive mass of the vocal folds, which typically lowers the pitch. Reduction of the mass from surgery or improvement in voice abuse and misuse habits often restores the normal pitch automatically. Patients with functional voice disorders may use an inappropriately high or low pitch habitually. Establishing an appropriate pitch usually reduces hyperfunction.

Many voice patients can change their pitch voluntarily through instruction and demonstration by the clinician. During the demonstration, the patient is asked to change his or her pitch in steps from one pitch level to another by a series of /a/, "do, re, mi," or counting. The patient may also be asked to glide up or down the pitch scale during the production of /a/. The clinician signals when the target pitch is achieved, and the patient continues his or her response at that pitch level. The patient's phonation is recorded, and he or she matches his or her own best pitch on subsequent attempts. If the patient cannot change pitch voluntarily, the yawn and sigh approach, the chewing method, or extending the pitch from a cough or throat clear may be effective. Graphic and digital feedback from the Visi-Pitch displays pitch accuracy to the clinician and patient. The target pitch is extended from vowels to single words, phrases, sentences, paragraphs, and conversation. Prior to each subsequent level response, it is often helpful to produce /a/ at the target pitch for reference purposes.

Respiration

Few voice patients require direct respiration training. Reduction of laryngeal hyperfunction and simple instruction on the need for more or less respiratory inspiration is adequate "training" for most patients. The respiration faults described in the assessment section of this chapter can often be remediated through discussion and feedback. Anderson has offered a succinct statement of the requirements of breath support for speech: ". . . (1) an adequate movement of air with a minimum of effort; (2) an inhalation that can be accomplished quickly and silently; (3) a sensitive and responsive control over the outgoing breath; and (4) a minimum of interference with the voice-producing mechanism in the throat" (p 35).[34] He suggests breath control is more sensitive and flexible if the primary activity is in the central portion of the body, directly under the arch of the ribs in the abdominal area. There should be no more than slight secondary movement of the upper thorax.

The patient is instructed to sit or stand and to place hands on waist with the thumbs behind and fingers firmly across the abdomen. The patient inhales slowly and produces a prolonged exhalation while attending to the feel of lower thoracic expansion. Next, the speed of inhalation is increased while maintaining the prolonged exhalation. While continuing to feel lower thoracic breathing movements phonation is introduced by extending /a/ comfortably. Boone has suggested any patient that can hold an extended vowel for 20 seconds has good breath control for voice.[12] The patient practices counting on exhalation, increasing the number if he or she can do so comfortably. Reading material for breath support from voice and articulation drillbooks may be utilized followed by conversation practice.[14,21,34] During each step, the patient may use his or her hands to assist monitoring respiration movements, but the tactile feedback is eliminated when no longer needed.

Auditory Training

To progress through the therapy regimen, it is crucial that the patient be able to recognize favorable and unfavorable vocal responses. The patient must learn to recognize differences in voice production, to change poor responses consistently, and to replicate correct behavior. An individual monitors his or her voice production and the clinician must emphasize feedback primarily through the auditory system. The ultimate success of the voice facilitation techniques discussed before are dependent upon the patient's ability to monitor and recognize their influence on the voice.

Initial instruction includes a discussion of the patient's abnormal voice parameters. Tape recorded playback of others' or, preferably, the patient's voice samples demonstrating different severity levels of the voice parameters are presented while the clinician describes the characteristics. The patient's typical voice productions may be compared to voice responses during facilitation techniques. Subsequently, tape recorded voice samples are presented to the patient, and he or she describes them with the clinician offering feedback on the patient's judgements. Next, the vocal response to each of the facilitation techniques is recorded on a loop tape recorder for quick playback, and again the patient judges his or her response followed by clinician evaluation. Favorable target voice productions are saved on the tape loop for the patient to try and match. Although specifically discussing pitch training, Boone could have applied the following statement to modeling any voice parameter: "There appear to be distinct advantages in using patients' own voices as the model, in that they already have had the experience of producing the sound they are trying to duplicate" (p 144).[12] The patient attempts to match the auditory model and, after sufficient success, to produce the target voice without the aid of the model. During the last two steps, the patient judges his or her productions live without playback.

It was suggested earlier that voice facilitation techniques be attempted systematically in order to judge their effectiveness. The clinician may also manipulate the variables of pitch, loudness, and gradual increase of vowel intensity while applying facilitation techniques. Combinations of techniques are often more effective than single approaches. Slow head rotation in a wide circle preceding chewing or yawn-sigh may enhance the techniques. Manipulating pitch or including imitation breathiness during chewing or adding /h/ words to the yawn-sigh are examples of effective combinations.

Carry-Over

When an acceptable voice has been achieved through vocal abuse counseling and facilitation techniques, the correct response is gradually shaped to become more complex. Concurrently, the antecedent stimuli that evoke the response are extended so that the response occurs under a variety of similar conditions to achieve generalization or carry-over. The systematic shaping process is an effective approach, but has received less attention for voice than for many other disorders. A review of the principles will assist carry-over procedures.

Costello presented an excellent review of systematic programmed instruction with examples of adequate and inadequate applications.[35] The components of programmed instruction are stimulus, response, consequence and schedule, and criterion. The function of antecedent stimuli is to evoke a particular response, and systematic selection of stimuli is important for carry-over to occur. Costello has stated: "During the course of a program the stimuli change so that the control of correct responding is altered from highly supportive conditions at the beginning of the program to minimal cues commensurate with those occurring in the natural environment at the end of the program" (p 7). The terminal response, which is the goal of the entire program, is specified initially. The program is then designed to require responses that gradually increase in length and complexity while becoming more similar to the terminal response. For effective learning to occur, the program should provide at least 60 to 80 percent correct responses at each step.[36] The effectiveness of the program is evaluated at each step by detailed data collection. Immediately following a response, functional positive or negative consequences are applied on a prearranged schedule. Few errors should occur in a carefully constructed program. Programs also specify pass criteria for advancement to the next step and fail criteria so that alterations are made in the program to improve performance. Selection of criteria is arbitrary, but Costello suggested the pass criterion could be 90 percent correct in a specified number of trials or 30 consecutive correct responses. Fail criterion could be 10 consecutive incorrect responses or less than 80 percent correct responses for three consecutive sessions.

Drudge and Philips[37] have described a program of rehabilitation for three patients with vocal nodules and hoarse voice that has many of the characteristics presented by Costello.[35] The authors utilized the yawn-sigh and breathy attack (/h/) facilitation techniques to establish easy initiation of phonation and clear phonation. They designed a 31-step program that gradually shaped the behavior, increasing complexity and length into spontaneous speech. Initially, the patient was required to produce a fraction of a second of clear phonation with the yawn-sigh, which was then extended from 4 to 6 to 8 seconds. The initial /h/ was followed by vowel sounds to facilitate gentle approximation of the vocal folds. The next step required production of words with easy initiation and clear phonation.

Phrases and sentences were repeated with clear phonation, then 30-second and 1-minute reading passages were required. From reading, the patient progressed to 30 seconds then to 1 minute of conversational responses. Finally, the patient had to maintain clear phonation outside the clinic in difficult speaking situations. Correct responses were reinforced on a variable schedule and client behaviors charted. The criterion for advancement to the next step varied, but was presented as a ratio, for example, 8:10 and 50:60.

The concept of gradually extending the length and complexity of the response is sound. However, many patients have difficulty maintaining the response in life situations. Having the patient conduct a hierarchy analysis helps bridge the gap between the clinic and other environments.[12] The daily diary concept, discussed earlier under Voice Abuse Counseling, is an excellent approach for identifying difficult environmental situations. By this point in therapy, the patient should be an excellent judge of his or her voice. The patient rates his or her voice, and perhaps emotional response, to the situation on a five-point scale. A hierarchy of situations from best to worst voice is established. The patient performs "contracts" (assignments) in which the number of practice attempts and amount of time in each is specified. The patient rates his or her voice in each and progresses through the hierarchy from the easiest rated through the most difficult situations based upon established criteria for advancement. Continuous data collection by the patient enhances evaluation of performance revision, when necessary, of the hierarchy.

Special Disorders

Four special voice disorders are referred to speech pathologists from otolaryngologists. These disorders present different problems to the voice clinician and require special techniques.

Ventricular Fold Phonation

Ballenger has referred to this disorder as "dysphonia plicae ventricularis."[15] During phonation, the vocal folds may be slightly abducted, and the ventricular folds approximate toward the midline and produce a low-pitched, monotonous, hoarse voice. Ventricular fold phonation may be in response to pathology of the vocal folds or with a normal mechanism.

The chewing and yawn-sigh approaches may facilitate phonation with the true vocal folds exclusively, but I have had the best success with the "inhalation phonation" technique described by Boone.[12] Following an explanation of the disorder, the clinician demonstrates a relatively prolonged phonation on inhalation, which the patient then imitates several times. Next, the clinician instructs the patient to produce another inhalation phonation and then match the same high-pitched voice on a prolonged exhalation. It is usually critical that the latency between inhalation phonation and exhalation phonation be short. After several successful matches, the patient produces another inhalation and exhalation phonation, but this time glides from the high pitch to a more appropriate pitch during exhalation. Then the inhalation phonation is eliminated, and the patient is asked to produce the high pitch then glide down to the appropriate pitch. Finally, the patient initiates the appropriate pitch and prolongs an /a/, then counting, phrases, sentences, paragraphs, and conversation.

Falsetto

The voice disorder in which postpubescent males maintain their preadolescent pitch has been referred to as "functional falsetto," "mutational falsetto," or "puberphonia." Some males may have lowered their pitch partially but not completely into the normal adult male range. Indirect laryngoscopy reveals a normal adult male larynx capable of producing a more normal low pitch. Aronson has reported the etiology is probably psychogenic with a stronger feminine than masculine self-identification or neurotic need to reject adulthood.[10] Other explanations are possible.

Functional falsetto can usually be treated successfully, and the patients are typically very grateful. A surprising number of patients can imitate the clinician who begins in falsetto and gradually steps or glides down until an appropriate pitch is achieved. This technique is so simple and straightforward that it is worth several attempts if the first effort is not successful. The clinician signals the patient when he reaches the target pitch and has him prolong an /a/. The patient's performance is tape recorded, and, after several successes, a sample of his target pitch is played back so that he can match it without starting at the falsetto. Beginning with throat clearing or a cough that is immediately blended into an extended /a/ is also a useful approach. The target pitch is gradually programmed from /a/ to more complex stimuli. The patients are typically reluctant to use the new pitch in many situations, and patience, encouragement, and a hierarchy analysis is important for success. After the patient can converse with the clinician with the target pitch, he performs prearranged practice "contracts" with other clinic personnel, voice patients, strangers, then perhaps an accepting, understanding friend. The primary goal is to extend the use of the new pitch gradually to situations in which the patient should have a high probability of success. Presence of family members is often the most difficult situation for the patient to confront with the new voice.

Conversion Aphonia

Aphonia is a voice disorder often referred to as "functional aphonia" or "hysterical aphonia" to denote loss of phonation with normal vocal fold structure and function. Aronson has described aphonia as a psychogenic conversion indicating loss of voluntary muscle control as a consequence of environmental stress or interpersonal conflict.[10] Voice loss is considered a defense mechanism against an environmental threat. The patient speaks in a whisper, but may produce a normal /ee/ during indirect laryngoscopy and coughs or laughs normally.

Aronson has reported that 80 percent of aphonic patients are female.[10] They may have a previous history of aphonia or dysphonia from which they have recovered. Conversion aphonia often begins with an upper respiratory infection or flu that creates laryngitis and hoarseness. Coincident with or subsequent to the laryngitis, the hoarseness worsens to aphonia. The onset of aphonia may occur suddenly, within minutes or hours.

The majority of patients with functional aphonia achieve normal voice through behavioral techniques (to be described). However, if the patients' emotional stability appears questionable or if they have not produced at least brief episodes of normal phonation after several sessions, they may be considered for referral for psychiatric evaluation. Approaching the disorder in a confident, straightforward manner is important. Boone has stressed that the clinician should not imply the patient could phonate normally if he or she wanted to, but, instead, present the disorder behaviorally by indicating that the patient is keeping the vocal folds apart and techniques will be utilized to bring the folds together again.[12] Whenever the patient achieves a normal voice, or a closer approximation, the clinician explains that the folds are coming together better. Next, the patient produces a throat clear or cough, which typically produces phonation. After several successful throat clears or coughs, the patient is asked to extend the nonverbal phonation immediately into a prolonged /a/. The /a/ may be extended into syllables, words, and counting. After numerous correct responses and much encouragement, the patient is asked to produce /a/ without being preceded by the nonverbal phonation. A hierarchy analysis is utilized in a manner suggested for functional falsetto. The response is firmly established at each step before advancing to the next, especially for nonclinical situations. Other techniques that facilitate normal phonation include inhalation phonation, chewing, yawn-sigh, and pushing.

Spastic Dysphonia

Adductor spastic dysphonia is a severe voice disorder characterized by a combination of vocal symptoms, which may include extreme medial compression of the vocal folds, hard glottal attacks, vocal arrests, roughness, and breathiness. The primary impression presented by these patients is the great effort expended while talking.

Izdebski, Dedo, and Boles compiled a comprehensive case history profile of 200 patients with spastic dysphonia.[38] The authors reported a 2:1 ratio of women to men, and the average age at onset was 43 years. Infectious illnesses and stress were the most frequent circumstances occurring at the time of onset. The patients with spastic dysphonia reported more illnesses throughout their lives and neurologic disorders in family members than a control group. However, the study did not reveal a factor or cluster of factors, including the traditional view of stress, that could be interpreted as unequivocally related to spastic dysphonia.

Shipp, Izdebski, Reed, and Morrissey conducted an acoustic analysis of voice and an electromyographic study of intrinsic laryngeal muscles of a single subject.[39] The subject exhibited vocal roughness, diplophonia, and occasional vocal arrests that interfered with fluency. The interarytenoid and thyroarytenoid muscles displayed sudden increased activity just prior to the vocal arrests, suggesting vocal fold hyperadduction that inhibited vibration. The subject's left recurrent laryngeal nerve was temporarily blocked by an injection of 3-ml lidocaine (1 percent) solution, thereby producing a unilateral vocal fold paralysis that relieved the spastic dysphonia voice symptoms and muscle activity. The authors interpreted these results as suggesting the origin of the disorder is neither psychogenic nor within the laryngeal muscles or their peripheral nerves. A more likely locus is the brain stem.

Dedo and Shipp[40] and Shipp[41] have described a method of surgery and voice therapy for spastic dysphonia that achieves a success rate of 85 to 90 percent. Evaluation procedures include the patient's sustaining /a/ at a comfortable pitch level, in falsetto, and at the lowest modal frequencies possible; reading *The Rainbow Passage;*[14] and producing spontaneous speech. The patients with spastic dysphonia are free of voice tension and vocal tremor while sustaining /a/ at falsetto, whereas patients with essential voice tremor continue to exhibit vocal tremor. It is also important to differentiate adductor spastic dysphonia from the relatively rare intermittent abductory dysphonia, which is characterized by sudden unvoicing of one or more syllables following voiceless consonants while maintaining normal phonation the remainder of the time. If abductor dysphonia is suspected, the patient reads the all-voiced sentence, "Early one morning a man and a woman were ambling along a 1-mile lane running near Rainy Island Avenue" and the voiced and voiceless sentence, "He saw half a shape mystically cross a simple path at least 50 or 60 steps in front of his sister Kathy's house." An individual with intermittent abductory dysphonia reads the all-voiced sentence normally, but exhibits abnormal vocal symptoms during the voiced and voiceless sentence. These patients are not surgical candidates.

For those who may benefit from surgery, the surgeon could block the recurrent nerve presurgically on one side with 1-percent lidocaine in order to demonstrate to the patient what effects permanent paralysis of the recurrent nerve could have on voice. Preoperative counseling by the speech pathologist is important. The patient is told that there is no guarantee of "normal" voice postoperatively because there is variation in the final position of the paralyzed fold. However, there is a high probability of relief from the excessive laryngeal tension. The patient may experience reduced loudness, breathiness, and some hoarseness and must also be prepared for typical radical shifts in vocal quality the first two postoperative days and not to be alarmed. Family members are also told what to expect.

The surgeon performs a small horizontal incision in the anterior neck just above the manubrial notch typically on the left side, and approximately a 25-mm segment of the recurrent laryngeal nerve is excised. The desired result is a paralyzed vocal fold in the paramedian position approximately 1 to 2 mm from the midline. It is important to visit the patient the evening of the surgical day to reassure him or her that the lack of vocal control is to be expected for a few days.

Preoperatively, the patient tends to cope with his or her vocal symptoms by lowering the fundamental frequency to the lowest 10 percent of the pitch range, and, postoperatively, he or she typically continues the habitual pattern. To counteract this behavior, the patient is asked to sustain an /u/ vowel in falsetto and utilize a glissando maneuver to the lowest frequency. If pitch breaks or aphonic breaks are noted, the patient must maintain a pitch level above this point while practicing sustaining vowels, counting, and reading. The target pitch can gradually be lowered without breaks until it is well within the normal range, but it is not allowed to drop to the previous habitual level.

The patient is also counseled to maintain a relatively low loudness level and reduce respiratory force in order to counteract the previous tendency to overcome the excessive laryngeal tension by excessive respiratory effort. The central breathing approach, described earlier, is utilized to achieve easy, effortless breath support. The patient is also taught to maintain slightly breathy phonation. These approaches reduce the probability that hyperadduction spastic dysphonia vocal behavior will occur.

Laryngectomy

A total laryngectomy is a devastating event for the patient and his or her family. They must adjust to physical problems, concerns about maintaining employment, social activities, and fears of cancer recurrence and death. Loss of oral communication and the resultant isolation is also a major concern. The remainder of this section of the chapter will address the primary approaches to alaryngeal communication.

Preoperative Counseling

The laryngectomee's rehabilitation requires a good professional relationship and communication between the speech pathologist and the otolaryngologist. A team approach, including other professionals and the primary health care physician, greatly enhances patient care. The speech pathologist should conduct preoperative counseling for all patients and their families; he or she needs to ascertain that the otolaryngologist has told the patient that he or she will have a total laryngectomy before initiating counseling. The clinician reads the medical chart and consults with the nurses and physician about the patient's and spouse's reactions, coping abilities, and obtains medical, social, and vocational information. Sufficient time is allowed so that the session is not rushed and a subsequent follow-up session can be scheduled.

The three primary goals of preoperative counseling include emphasizing support offered by the rehabilitation staff, giving information, and answering questions. A caring attitude can be suggested early in the session by inquiring about the patient's history and lifestyle. It is beneficial to determine if the patient has family members and friends who live nearby and can offer support. The patient is asked about social and recreational interests, vocation, and intentions of returning to work. The information is useful later in the session.

The remainder of the session is primarily devoted to giving information and answering questions. Pre- and postoperative anatomy and physiology regarding communication function is reviewed. The clinician explains that air flows from the lungs through the trachea and serves as a power source when it passes through the larynx and causes the vocal folds to vibrate as a sound source. The sound continues up the throat where it is articulated for speech. This simple explanation serves as a foundation for discussion of postoperative communication changes and alaryngeal options.

The clinician explains that the surgery will remove the larynx and the patient will breathe through the stoma and not the nose and mouth. He emphasizes that the sound source will be removed and the respiration or power source disconnected from the vocal tract. A primary task of the session is to ascertain that the patient and family realize that the patient will not have a voice after the operation. The physician has typically discussed these details, but it is helpful to be redundant and to emphasize the voice loss.

The previous information is followed by the assurance that other means of oral communication are available after the operation and a speech pathologist will assist the patient when he or she is medically able. The three basic means of alaryngeal communication are described briefly: artificial larynx, esophageal speech, and voice prostheses. The patient should not be overwhelmed with details, which are more appropriate for postoperative discussion. The speech pathologist indicates success cannot be guaranteed, but there is a high probability that one or more of the options will yield functional communication. Physical changes after the operation are reviewed, such as the patient's appearance in immediate postoperative care and a diminished sense of taste and smell.

Support is offered again by reviewing the information shared at the beginning of the session and relating it to the patient's future in an encouraging manner. It may be that the patient may be able to return to his or her job, interact with family and friends, and still be able to enjoy many of the same social and recreational activities. If the patient and family wish, written information and a visit from a laryngectomee is provided. It is important to choose a visiting laryngectomee that shares your rehabilitation philosophy and does not have a strong bias against any of the alaryngeal communication options. The session is completed by emphasizing three primary points:

1. The patient can live an essentially normal life.
2. After the operation, the patient will not have a voice and will not be able to speak as he or she does currently.
3. Other means of communication are available.

Another session is scheduled before the operation to answer any additional questions the patient may have.

Postoperative Counseling

Salmon and Goldstein have succinctly expressed a proper approach: "Given adequate knowledge, the laryngectomized person has the right to choose his method or methods of alaryngeal communication (p IX).[42] Unless medical reasons contraindicate one or more of the options, each is explained, and advantages and disadvantages discussed. The clinician begins by reviewing preoperative anatomy and physiology. This review is followed by an explanation of how pulmonary air serves as a power source and how vibrating muscle tissue (the vocal folds) serves as a sound source.

Artificial larynges are classified and discussed according to their power source (battery or pneumatic) and placement (external or intraoral). Examples of the artificial larynges (to be discussed) used in my clinic are presented in Figure 27–3. The Servox Speech Aid is described as a battery-powered external placement device, which can also be used intraorally with the oral connector. The Cooper-Rand Electronic Speech Aid is a battery-powered intraoral device. The Tokyo is a pneumatic artifical larynx that utilizes air from the stoma to vibrate a stretched rubber membrane within the metal housing and introduces the sound intraorally through the rubber tube.

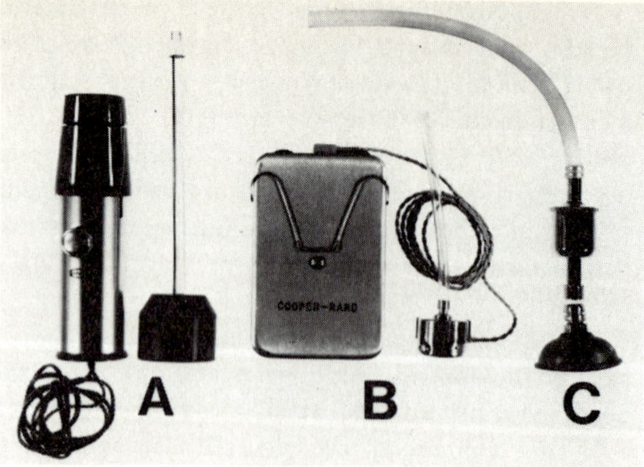

Figure 27–3 Artificial larynges. *A*, Servox Speech Aid. *B*, Cooper-Rand Electronic Speech Aid. *C*, Tokyo.

Pictures of the head and neck showing the configuration of the trachea and esophagus are helpful in describing esophageal speech. The clinician explains that the patient learns to inject air in the mouth down into the esophagus, trap the air, and expel it up the throat, and the sound is articulated for speech. The air serves as a power source, which causes the pharyngoesophageal muscle tissue to vibrate as the sound source. The sound may resemble a belch initially, but is refined with longer sound duration into functional speech.

Voice prostheses are presented as the third alaryngeal option.[43,44] The American V. Mueller voice restoration stem (Fig. 27–4) is the primary prosthesis used in my clinic. The clinician explains that the surgeon creates a midline tracheoesophageal puncture 3 to 5 mm below the superior margin of the tracheostoma. A No. 14 French catheter remains in the puncture site for at least 48 hours until the speech pathologist fits the proper length voice prosthesis. The voice prosthesis serves as a one-way valve that allows pulmonary air to enter the esophagus, but prevents tracheoesophageal puncture stenosis and aspiration of liquids and food. A picture (Fig. 27–5) may be utilized to demonstrate that when the tracheostoma is occluded by the thumb or tracheostoma valve,[45] pulmonary air is directed through the airflow port and valve slit into the esophagus. The air serves as a power source, and the pharyngoesophageal muscle tissue vibrates as the sound source articulated for speech.

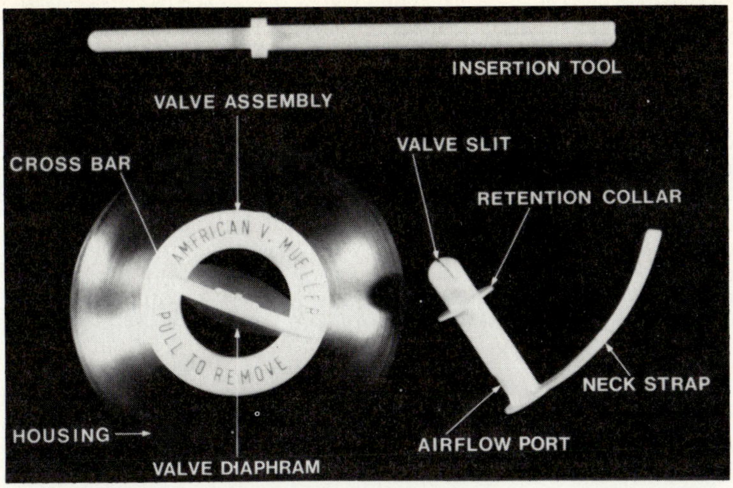

Figure 27-4 The American V. Mueller voice restoration system.

Salmon reported that laryngectomees and their spouses expressed a need for written information.[46] A chart (Table 27–1) is presented and discussed. The term "potential" advantages and disadvantages is stressed because preferences and concerns vary among patients. Gardner[47] and Salmon's[48] reviews of the classic literature suggested only 60 to 65 percent of laryngectomees acquire functional esophageal speech, which is closer to my experience than more recent data[49,50] suggesting approximately 25 percent learn functional esophageal speech. Diedrich and Youngstrom have reported it requires 6 to 12 months to acquire esophageal speech that can be "reasonably understood."[51] Blom, Singer, and Hamaker reported 94 percent of their patients achieved good to superior tracheoesophageal speech 4 days following initial placement of the voice prosthesis.[52] Other studies have compared voice and prosody,[53] intelligibility and acceptability[54–59] between alaryngeal methods of communication. Following discussion of the written information, a videotape demonstrating each alaryngeal method is shown.

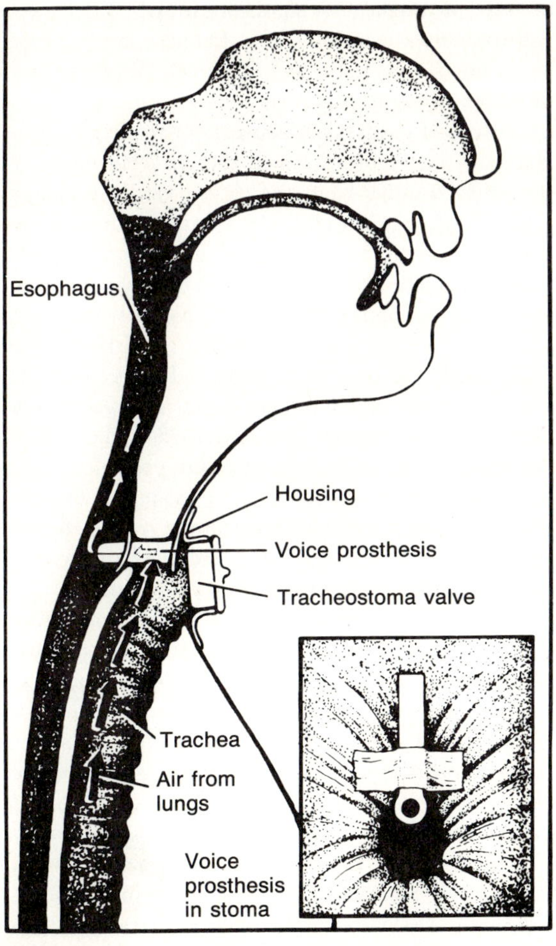

Figure 27-5 A cross-section of the American V. Mueller voice restoration system in use.

Artificial Larynx. A complete review of types and utilization of artificial larynges has been presented by Salmon and Goldstein.[42] Initially, determination of the best placement and a comparison of intraoral and external placement devices is required. Placement of the tube is in the corner of the mouth and along the inner margin of the upper first and second molars. External devices are tried systematically on both sides of the neck and the midline above the stoma. A radical neck dissection often contraindicates effective use on the involved side. The clinician places the device and asks the patient to count from one to five when the device is activated. Careful listening determines the best device and placement. A mirror is used to teach the patient correct placement with the nondominant hand. With external placement the patient must visually observe and feel the device's location; the patient must listen for extraneous noise that occurs when the angle of the device does not allow the vibrator to be flush against the neck. Following successful placement, the patient learns to activate the device when he or she begins articulation and to deactivate the instrument with cessation of articulation. Counting and

TABLE 27–1 Alaryngeal Methods of Communication: Potential Advantages and Disadvantages

	Advantages	*Disadvantages*
Artifical larynges	Provides means of early communication Can be learned in short time Functional intelligibility Adequate loudness Relatively normal speaking rate and pause time	Device is visible Requires use of at least one hand Requires some maintenance and additional cost (batteries, repairs) Quality of voice is somewhat mechanical
Esophageal speech	No devices are required Both hands are free Functional intelligibility	Approximately 40% cannot learn this method Acquiring functional speech can take 6 months to 1 year Low voice pitch Low loudness Somewhat reduced speaking rate and length of phrases; increased pause time
Voice prostheses	Can be learned in short time Functional intelligibility Functional loudness Approximates normal speech rate, phrase length, and pause time	Additional surgery is required Requires some maintenance (cleaning and taping) Additional cost to replace device Requires use of one hand unless tracheostoma valve is utilized Low voice pitch

deactivating the device after every fifth number assists learning. The patient speaks with a slightly slower than normal rate with exaggerated articulation and equal duration of each syllable. Slash marks are placed at appropriate points in reading material for deactivation of the instrument. Reading material without markers and conversation is then practiced while attending to the slow rate, exaggerated articulation, and equal duration syllables. The principles of programming for carry-over are appropriate for artificial larynx use.

Esophageal Speech. Instruction for esophageal speech suggests two broad approaches to air intake: inhalation and injection.[47,51] The inhalation method instructs the patient to open his mouth and inhale quickly ("sniff"), which creates negative pressure within the esophagus. The pressure differential between the esophagus and higher atmospheric pressure in the oropharyngeal area causes air to flow into the esophagus. A second method involves consonant injection in which the patient attempts exaggerated production of voiceless plosives (/p/, /t/, /k/), affricates (/tʃ/), or clusters (/st/, /sk/, /sp/) combined with vowels. Diedrich and Youngstrom reported that patients may achieve air intake with an individual method, but emphasize that most esophageal speakers use combinations of methods.[51] They suggest patients attempt the methods in a successive manner in the order presented.

The key to having the patient appear and sound as normal as possible is to keep effort at a functional minimum. There should not be extraneous head and body movements during speech attempts. The injection movement must be small, aided by inhalation, and done with the least amount of tension to reduce or eliminate the audible "klunk." Latency between air intake and expulsion must be brief with relatively slow expulsion of pulmonary air in order to reduce stoma noise and improve initiation and duration of esophageal sound.

Voice Prosthesis. The patient inhales a moderate amount of breath, then the clinician occludes the patient's stoma while the patient exhales and says "ah" or counts. Initially, the clinician can achieve better occlusion and proper digital pressure more readily than the patient. If voice is not achieved, the prosthesis is removed briefly to reduce air resistance and the process is repeated. When consistent voice is achieved, the patient is instructed to occlude the stoma with the nondominant hand flat against the chest and arm relaxed against the side. The pad of the thumb with the lightest pressure possible is preferred for occlusion. To inhale a moderate amount of air, the patient is instructed to remove the thumb slightly from the stoma. Minimum excursion enhances accurate respositioning of the thumb.

The patient must initiate exhalation smoothly with a gradual application of power to keep muscular tension low. Instructions to produce voice "as softly as you can," then "a little louder" until a comfortable loudness level can be achieved also reduces unnecessary effort. The patient may need to be reminded to inhale when he or she needs to and not to attempt to speak when he or she is literally "out of breath." The clinician monitors the voice quality and reinforces the least tense productions. Voice is practiced in a hierarchy of increasing stimulus response complexity for effective carry-over. I have presented an expanded discussion of prosthesis patient selection, fitting, and rehabilitation.[60]

SUMMARY

The focus of this chapter has been clinical. A brief discussion of normal voice production and physiologic causes of abnormal voice was followed by a description of voice disorders and pathologic changes of the vocal folds. It was felt this information would serve as a useful foundation for voice assessment and rehabilitation procedures. Case history and appraisal results of voice were related to possible recommendations. The discussion of rehabilitation received the greatest emphasis and included philosophy, physician's role, voice abuse counseling, correction of voice misuse, and carry-over considerations. Unique approaches for special voice disorders and the patient with a laryngectomy were also presented. Additional references for the interested reader were included throughout the chapter.

An overview of the chapter suggests a major issue for the future is better continuity between voice science, assessment, and rehabilitation for voice disorders. Moore presented a 50-year retrospective of speech science and voice disorders and felt that more basic study of voice and voice production should be clinically oriented.[61] Voice terminology is an obvious area needing refinement. For example, Perkins reviewed nine texts and reported that 27 terms were used to describe voice quality.[1] Furthermore, the terms proliferated from a variety of origins with inadequate correspondence of meaning between listeners. Michel and Wendahl expressed concern that "knowledge" about voice too often rests on uncritical assumption rather than empirical evidence.[62] The authors suggested the inexact terminology should be replaced with an approach necessary for more objective voice assessment and as a sensitive indicator of rehabilitation effects across time. Michel and Wendahl stated that ". . . the first step in the study of voice must be the determination of pertinent, measurable parameters. Pertinent in that changes in these variables will have a perceptible effect, and be measurable to quantify and correlate the changes with the effects" (p 467).

Physiologic and acoustic measures utilized for voice science provide accurate, precise measures of vocal events for assessment and rehabilitation. Ludlow and Hart[63] and others[64–69] have presented examples and discussion of such clinicial measures. Widespread use of computers and further development of software make measurement accessible to more clinics. Although group designs are appropriate for many topics of research, single-subject experimental designs are particularly useful for examining treatment effectiveness with individual patients.[70–73] I have presented examples of clinical issues worthy of investigation and suggested specific research strategies.[74]

REFERENCES

1. Perkins WH. Vocal function: a behavioral analysis. In: Travis LE, ed. Handbook of speech pathology and audiology. New York: Appleton-Century-Crofts, 1971:481.
2. van den Berg J. Myoelastic-aerodynamic theory of voice production. J Speech Hear Disord 1958; 1:227–243.
3. Moore GP. Voice disorders organically based. In: Travis LE, ed. Handbook of speech pathology and audiology. New York: Appleton-Century-Crofts, 1971:535.
4. Moore GP. Organic voice disorders. Englewood Cliffs, NJ: Prentice-Hall, 1971.
5. Moore GP, Hicks DM, Abbott TB. Defects of speech and language. In: Ballenger JJ, ed. Diseases of the nose, throat, ear, head and neck. 13th ed. Philadelphia: Lea & Febiger, 1985:692.
6. Timcke R, von Leden H, Moore GP. Laryngeal vibrations: measurements of the glottic wave: Part I. The normal vibratory cycle. Arch Otolaryngol 1958; 68:1–19.
7. von Leden H, Moore GP, Timcke R. Laryngeal vibrations: measurements of the glottic wave. Part III. The pathologic larynx. Arch Otolaryngol 1960; 71:16–35.
8. Moore GP, Thompson CL. Comments on the physiology of hoarseness. Arch Otolaryngol 1965; 81:97–102.
9. Moore GP. Observations on laryngeal disease, laryngeal behavior and voice. Ann Otol Rhinol Laryngol 1976; 85:553–564.
10. Aronson AE. Clinical voice disorders. New York: Thieme-Stratton, 1980.
11. Brodnitz F. Vocal rehabilitation. Rochester, MN: American Academy of Ophthalmology and Otolaryngology, 1965.
12. Boone DR. The voice and voice therapy. Englewood Cliffs, NJ: Prentice-Hall, 1983.
13. Froeschels E. Hygiene of the voice. Arch Otolaryngol 1943; 38:122–130.
14. Fairbanks G. Voice and articulation drillbook. New York: Harper & Row, 1960.
15. Ballenger JJ, ed. Diseases of the nose, throat, ear, head and neck. Philadelphia: Lea & Febiger, 1985.
16. Honjo I, Isshiki N. Laryngoscopic and voice characteristics of aged persons. Arch Otolaryngol 1980; 106:149–150.
17. Darley FL, Spriestersbach DC, eds. Diagnostic methods in speech pathology. New York: Harper & Row, 1978.
18. Nation JE, Aram DM. Diagnosis of speech and language disorders. St. Louis, MO: CV Mosby, 1977.
19. Brewer DW. Early diagnostic signs and symptoms of laryngeal disease. Laryngoscope 1975; 85:499–515.
20. Wilson FB, Broda-Masiuk D. Voice disorders. Bellingham, WA: Voice Tapes, 1987.
21. Moncur JP, Brackett IP. Modifying vocal behavior. New York: Harper & Row, 1974.
22. Hollien H, Shipp T. Speaking fundamental frequency and chronologic age in males. J Speech Hear Res 1972; 15:155–159.
23. Kelley A. Fundamental frequency measurement of female voices from twenty to ninety years of age. Unpublished manuscript, Greensboro: University of North Carolina, 1977.
24. Hollien H, Dew D, Philips P. Phonational frequency ranges of adults. J Speech Hear Res 1971; 14:755–760.
25. Eckel FC, Boone DR. The s/z ratio as an indicator of laryngeal pathology. J speech Hear Disord 1981; 46:147–150.

26. Isshiki N. Regulatory mechanism of voice intensity variation. J Speech Hear Res 1964; 7:17–29.
27. Yanagihara NY, von Leden H. Respiration and phonation. Folia Phoniatr (Basel) 1967; 19:153–166.
28. Shipp T, McGlone R. Laryngeal dynamics associated with voice frequency change. J Speech Hear Res 1971; 14:761–768.
29. Smitheran J, Hixon T. A clinical method for estimating laryngeal airway resistance during vowel production. J Speech Hear Disord 1981; 46:138–146.
30. Baker B, Fox S, Baker C, McMurry G. Persistent hoarseness after surgical removal of vocal cord lesions. Arch Otolaryngol 1981; 107:148–151.
31. Wolfe V, Ratusnik D. Vocal symptomatology of postoperative dysphonia. Laryngoscope 1981; 91:635–643.
32. Perkins WH. Vocal function: assessment and therapy. In: Travis LE, ed. Handbook of speech pathology and audiology. New York: Appleton-Century-Crofts, 1971:505.
33. Boone DR. The Boone voice program for adults. Tigard, OR: CC Publications, 1982.
34. Anderson VA. Training the speaking voice. New York: Oxford University Press, 1961.
35. Costello JM. Programmed instruction. J Speech Hear Disord 1977; 42:3–28.
36. Boone DR, Prescott TE. Content and sequence analysis of speech and hearing therapy. Asha 1972; 14:58–62.
37. Drudge MK, Philips BJ. Shaping behavior in voice therapy. J Speech Hear Disord 1976; 41:398–411.
38. Izdebski K, Dedo H, Boles L. Spastic dysphonia: a patient profile of 200 cases. Am J Otolaryngol 1984; 5:7–14.
39. Shipp T, Izdebski K, Reed C, Morrissey P. Intrinsic muscle activity in a spastic dysphonia patient. J Speech Hear Disord 1985; 50:54–59.
40. Dedo HH, Shipp T. Spastic dysphonia: a surgical and voice treatment program. San Diego: College-Hill Press, 1980.
41. Shipp T. Treatment of spastic dysphonia following surgery. In: Perkins WH, ed. Current therapy of communication disorders: voice disorders. New York: Thieme-Stratton, 1983:81.
42. Salmon SJ, Goldstein LP, eds. The artificial larynx handbook. New York: Grune & Stratton, 1978.
43. Singer MI, Blom ED. An endoscopic technique for restoration of voice after laryngectomy. Ann Otol Rhinol Laryngol 1980; 89:529–533.
44. Panje WR. Prosthetic vocal rehabilitation following laryngectomy: the voice button. Ann Otol Rhinol Laryngol 1981; 90:116–120.
45. Blom ED, Singer MI, Hamaker RC. Tracheostoma valve for postlaryngectomy voice restoration. Ann Otol Rhinol Laryngol 1982; 91:576–578.
46. Salmon SJ. Pre- and postoperative conferences with laryngectomized and their spouses. In: Keith RL, Darley FL, eds. Laryngectomee rehabilitation. Houston: College-Hill Press, 1979:379.
47. Gardner WH. Laryngectomee speech and rehabilitation. Springfield, IL: CC Thomas, 1971.
48. Salmon SJ. Factors that interfere with acquiring esophageal speech. In: Keith RL, Darley FL, eds. Laryngectomee rehabilitation. Houston: College-Hill Press, 1979:501.
49. Schaefer SD, Johns DF. Attaining functional esophageal speech. Arch Otolaryngol 1982; 108:647–649.
50. Gates GA, Ryan W, Cooper JC, Lawlis GF, Cantu E, Hayashi T, Lauder E, Welch RW, Hearne E. Current status of laryngectomee rehabilitation: I. Results of therapy. Am J Otolaryngol 1982; 3:1–7.
51. Diedrich W, Youngstrom K. Alaryngeal speech. Springfield, IL: CC Thomas, 1966.
52. Blom ED, Singer MI, Hamaker RC. A prospective study of tracheoesophageal speech. Arch Otolaryngol Head Neck Surg 1986; 112:440–447.
53. Robbins J, Fisher HB, Blom EC, Singer MI. A comparative acoustic study of normal, esophageal, and tracheoesophageal speech production. J Speech Hear Disord 1984; 49:202–210.
54. Kalb MB, Carpenter MA. Individual speaker influence on relative intelligibility of esophageal speech and artificial larynx speech. J Speech Hear Disord 1981; 46:77–80.
55. Clark JG, Stemple JC. Assessment of three modes of alaryngeal speech with a synthetic sentence identification (SSI) task in varying message-to-competition ratios. J Speech Hear Res 1982; 25:333–338.
56. Tardy-Mitzell S, Andrews ML, Bowman SA. Acceptability and intelligibility of tracheoesophageal speech. Arch Otolaryngol 1985; 111:213–215.
57. Williams SE, Watson JB. Differences in speaking proficiencies in three laryngectomee groups. Arch Otolaryngol 1985; 111:216–219.
58. Merwin GE, Goldstein LP, Rothman HB. A comparison of speech using artificial larynx and tracheoesophageal puncture with valve in the same speaker. Laryngoscope 1985; 95:730–734.
59. Doyle PC, Flower RM, Danhauer JL, Reed CG. Consonant intelligibility in esophageal, tracheoesophageal, and dual-mode talkers. Paper presented at the Annual Convention of the American Speech-Language-Hearing Association, Washington, DC, 1985.
60. Reed CG. Surgical-prosthetic techniques for alaryngeal speech. Commun Dis 1983; 8:109–124.
61. Moore GP. Have the major issues in voice disorders been answered by research in speech science? A 50-year retrospective. J Speech Hear Disord 1977; 42:152–160.
62. Michel JF, Wendahl R. Correlates of voice production. In: Travis LE, ed. Handbook of speech pathology and audiology. New York: Appleton-Century-Crofts, 1971:465.
63. Ludlow C, Hart MO, eds. Proceedings of the conference on the assessment of vocal pathology. Vol. 11. Rockville, MD: ASHA Reports, 1981.
64. Kitzing P, Lofqvist A. Evaluation of voice therapy by means of photoglottography. Folia Phoniatr (Basel) 1979; 31:103–109.
65. Kitojima K. Quantitative evaluation of the noise level in pathologic voice. Folia Phoniatr (Basel) 1981; 33:115–124.
66. Rontal E, Rontal M, Jacob HJ, Rolnick MI. Quantitative and objective evaluation of vocal cord function. Ann Otol Rhinol Laryngol 1983; 92:421–423.
67. McHenry MA, Reich AR. Effective airway resistance and vocal sound pressure level in cheerleaders with a history of dysphonic episodes. Folia Phoniatr (Basel) 1985; 37:223–231.
68. Klingholz F, Martin F. Quantitative spectral evaluation of shimmer and jitter. J Speech Hear Res 1985; 28:169–174.
69. Askenfelt AG, Hammarberg B. Speech waveform perturbation analysis: a perceptual-acoustical comparison of seven measures. J Speech Hear Res 1986; 29:50–64.
70. McReynolds LV, Kearns KP. Single-subject experimental designs in communicative disorders. Austin, Texas: Pro-Ed, 1983.
71. McReynolds LV, Thompson CK. Flexibility of single-subject experimental designs. Part I: review of the basics of single-subject design. J Speech Hear Disord 1986; 51:194–203.
72. Kearns KP. Flexibility of single-subject experimental designs. Part II: Design selection and arrangement of experimental phases. J Speech Hear Disord 1986; 51:204–213.
73. Connell PJ, Thompson CK. Flexibility of single-subject experimental designs. Part III: Using flexibility to design or modify experiments. J Speech Hear Disord 1986; 51:214–225.
74. Reed CG. Voice therapy: a need for research. J Speech Hear Disord 1980; 45:157–169.

Special Populations and Communication

28 Reading and Writing Disorders in the Learning Disabled Student

Mary Ross Moran, Ph.D.

The 1980s opened with the inclusion of reading and writing within the American Speech-Language-Hearing Association's (ASHA) definition of language. Special educators have interpreted that addition as an acknowledgment that reading and writing instructors are members of the language intervention team, a major step toward collaborative service delivery by speech-language pathologists and special education teachers. Although primary intervention in both reading and writing continues to be delivered to handicapped learners by special educators or language arts specialists, speech-language pathologists increasingly express interest in more refined knowledge of reading and writing disorders, especially as they are manifested by the population labelled "learning disabled."

Why should speech-language pathologists be concerned about the learning disabled population? For three reasons. First, a definition of learning disabilities based upon language appears in federal guidelines for education of handicapped learners. Second, the populations served by practitioners and studied by researchers overlap across speech-language pathology and learning disabilities. Third, the number of clinical and public school clients who are labelled "learning disabled" has grown markedly during the 1980s: the likelihood of this label being attached to a client has increased each year.[5]

Beyond the oral language data provided by their own professional literature, what might speech-language pathologists want to know about learning disabled children and youth before engaging in collaborative planning for these clients? Because identification of learning disabled students remains controversial, this discussion opens with alternative definitions and criteria for eligibility. Subtype research is next summarized in an attempt to answer the question of how many learning disabled students are language impaired. Current assessment practices for reading and writing are examined, followed by some common profiles of strengths and deficits. Optional strategies for management of reading and writing disorders are described within the context of a continuum of services.

IDENTIFICATION OF LEARNING DISABLED STUDENTS

The consensus of current professional discussion is that the learning disabled population is heterogeneous. Students to whom the label has been assigned are proving to be as different from one another as from normally achieving learners. Attempts to describe a learning disabled population still command professional attention 25 years after the term was coined.[1] In a survey of experts, "arriving at a conceptual and operational consensus of just what constitutes a learning disability" was cited by 59 percent of respondents as the most fundamental concern facing the field.[2]

The definition incorporated into the regulations governing the Education for All Handicapped Children Act states that the term applied to ". . . disorders (1) in one or more of the basic psychological processes involved in (2) understanding or in using language, spoken or written, which may manifest itself in an imperfect ability to listen, think, speak, (3) read, write, spell or to do mathematical calculations. (4) The term includes such conditions as perceptual handicaps, brain injury, minimal brain dysfunction, dyslexia and developmental aphasia. (5) The term does not include children who have learning problems which are primarily the result of visual, hearing or motor handicaps, of mental retardation, or of environmental, cultural or economic disadvantage."[3]

Four years into the implementation of the federal regulations, a restatement of definition was published by the National Joint Committee on Learning Disabilities (NJCLD), comprising representatives of six national professional organizations. This group identified a series of problems associated with the federal definition—demands for homogeneity among students so classified, age limitations based upon the term "children," overinterpretation of the presumed neurologic origin of the disorder, and failure to acknowledge multiple handicaps. The revised definition said that "*Learning disabilities* is a generic term that refers to a heterogeneous group of disorders manifested by significant difficulties in the acquisition and use of listening, speaking, reading, writing, reasoning or mathematical abilities. These disorders are intrinsic to the individual and presumed to be due to central nervous system dysfunction" (p 336).[4]

In the mid 1980s, the definition was still being revised, this time by a parent-support organization—the Association for Children and Adults with Learning disabilities (ACLD). Again the emphasis shifted, this time to include the life span, nonverbal abilities, social and vocational manifestations, and a range of intellectual functioning. "*Specific learning disabilities* is a chronic condition of presumed neurological origin which selectively interferes with the development, integration, and/or demonstration of verbal and/or nonverbal abilities. *Specific learning disabilities* exists as a distinct handicapping condition in the presence of average to superior intelligence, adequate sensory and motor systems, and adequate learning opportunities. The condition varies in its manifestations and in degree of severity. Throughout life the condition can affect self-esteem, education, vocation, socialization, and/or daily living activities" (p 1).[5]

OVERLAP WITH LANGUAGE IMPAIRMENT

Some of the clauses in the 1981 and 1985 definitions could clarify the relationship between learning disabled and language impaired school-age clients. The NJCLD designation of a heterogeneous group of disorders should combine with the ACLD criterion of average intellectual functioning to allow professional persons to view some language impairment as one subtype of learning disability (alongside learning disabled subtypes based upon attentional, memory, perceptual, motor, or social disabilities).

The language disorders associated with learning disabilities could be usefully described as those manifested in the presence of average nonverbal IQ and sensory integrity. Such a conceptualization could help to sort out the learners appropriate for joint intervention by speech-language pathologists and learning disabilities specialists.

However, the more precise definitions have appeared too late to influence confounding practices arising from implementation of the federal mandate. Federal regulations continue to provide the bases for state and local eligibility criteria for services.[1,6] Anecdotal reports of learning disabled students being inappropriately over- or under-referred to speech-language pathologists, and inconsistent practices in assigning professional responsibilities, are caused partly by the definitions.

In the 1977 federal regulations, "speech impaired" was defined as "a communication disorder, such as stuttering, impaired articulation, *a language impairment* or a voice impairment, which *adversely affects* a child's *educational performance*" [emphasis added].[3] Since definitions for both learning disabilities and speech impairments cover language disorders leading to educational performance problems, some degree of overlap or redundancy is inevitable. Speech impairment may be considered as a primary handicapping condition or as a condition secondary to another handicapping category, in which case language intervention is provided as a related service. Therefore the extent to which language impairment is classified as a primary handicap or as a related condition varies from state to state, in accordance with each state's category designations, eligibility criteria, and especially the age range of handicapped children served. In a survey of learning disabilities experts, 55 percent of respondents stated that they would not identify a student as learning disabled before the age of 6 years; 24 percent said 6 to 7 years.[7]

As an example of how client age affects classification, Snyder has claimed that those children considered language impaired at the preschool level invariably become reclassified during school years.[8] "When language-disordered children enter elementary school, they often come to be associated with different labels: learning disabled, language and learning disabled, reading-disabled or even dyslexic" (p 130).[8] Such reclassification is consistent with interpretations of language impairment as identifiable in preschool and of learning disability as reserved for school-age children.

The extent of overlap between categories can be resolved with empirical research. In the meantime, sample descriptions in research reports on language performance of school-age children suggest that readers must be cautious in generalizing findings to either the learning disabled or the language impaired population. Research reports may omit statements of (1) whether or not subjects labelled "learning disabled" included those receiving language therapy as a related service, or (2) whether or not those labelled "language impaired" included subjects identified by the school as learning disabled.

Terminology may also present an impression of *identity* between language disability and learning disability. For example, Wren defined "the concept of a language learning disability . . . a disturbance in processing oral language. . . ." (p ix).[9]

Learning disabilities specialists would not argue with that identification of one kind of specific learning disability related to the ability to process auditory information. Indeed, such a subtype has been identified repeatedly, as is discussed in another section of this chapter. No problem would arise if the modifier "language" or "auditory" consistently preceded the words "learning disabilities." However, subsequently in the preface and in chapter subtitles, Wren used the generic term "learning disabilities" without qualification or limitation to auditory or language learning disabilities.[9] The effect is to make it appear that the generic term "learning disabilities" is synonymous with an oral language processing disorder. Such application of the term does not represent common usage among learning disabilities specialists and offers potential for misunderstanding across the disciplines.

INCREASED PREVALENCE OF STUDENTS LABELLED LEARNING DISABLED

The problem of whether or not and to what extent learners are served by speech-language pathologists or learning disabilities specialists is compounded as the numbers of identified learning disabled students increase. Prevalence increased more than 100 percent in the first 5 years of the federal mandate; more than two in five handicapped children are labelled "learning disabled."[1] The growth rate led to renewed interest in the concept of a discrepancy formula as a means to establish minimum entry criteria for learning disabilities services.

State eligibility guidelines that include a discrepancy formula require demonstration of a gap between observed academic performance and that expected on the basis of measured intellectual functioning. In other words, a student is not considered learning disabled unless the IQ is at least average and significantly higher than achievement scores.

Typically, a discrepancy formula compares an individual measure of intellectual functioning, such as the Wechsler Intelligence Scale for Children Revised,[10] with an individual survey test of academic achievement, such as the achievement portion of the Woodcock-Johnson Psycho-Educational Battery.[11] According to Reynolds, an appropriate formula uses standard scores rather than grade or age equivalents; takes into account the regression of achievement upon IQ as a function of imperfect correlation between the two tests; and is applied to only one pair of scores since multiple comparisons result in significant findings by chance.[12] Furthermore, a discrepancy formula must not be the sole criterion for placement or failure to provide services.

State application of a discrepancy formula might affect language impaired students in two ways. First, services for the learning disabled may be denied to those whose levels of intellectual functioning are globally depressed by a language disorder so that the discrepancy between ability and achievement is minimal. Second, younger children are less likely to demonstrate the required discrepancy.[13] For example, McKinney found that only 40 percent of first and second graders referred for language disabilities met discrepancy criteria in their state.[14]

While discrepancy formulas were being tested to control the prevalence of students labelled learning disabled, the figure for this category at mid-decade remained just above 4 percent of the student population nationwide.[1,15] Another line of research has explored identification of subgroups of reading and learning disabled students as a means to match specific characteristics with specialized instruction.

LEARNING DISABILITY SUBGROUPS

Heterogeneity of the learning disabled population has hampered efforts to develop generalizable research. Practitioners have not known which, if any, of the results from intervention studies could be generalized to other samples. A body of studies known as subtype research seemed to offer promise of organizing reading disabled or learning disabled students for intervention experiments using differentiated instruction. Such studies provide some insight into numbers of reading and learning disabled students who exhibit language impairment.

However, samples selected for subtype studies present a number of interpretation problems. Early studies selected reading disabled subjects from clinical populations; therefore, whether those subjects are or are not classifiable as learning disabled is open to question, since a reading disability has multiple causes including motivational and instructional variables. Furthermore, even those later studies that drew subject samples from the learning disabled groups identified by schools share the problem of diverse identification procedures across schools. In addition, failure of most researchers to investigate the characteristics of normal learners in the same settings weakens the interpretation of learning disabled subtypes, since identified groups might be subtypes of all, not just learning disabled learners.

What is the contribution of subtype results if some of the studies and interpretations are flawed? Although programmatic subtype research has not yet produced rigorous data to support differentiated instruction,[14] it is worth examining because it suggests that there are some learning disabled students who are—and some who are not—language impaired.

Review of more than a dozen years of subtype research reveals that four subgroups have recurred. According to McKinney's summary, the first is characterized by either a generalized language impairment or a specific auditory information-processing disorder, accompanied by intact visual-perceptual and motor skills;[14] this group has been reported in various studies as 13 percent to 41 percent of samples. A second subgroup demonstrates specific visual and/or motor impairments with no evidence of generalized or specific language disorders; prevalence is reported ranging between 24 percent and 34 percent of samples. A third reliable subgroup shows mixed perceptual and linguistic impairments; often characterized as the most severely handicapped, this group ranges from 8 percent to 23 percent of the samples studied. A fourth reliable subgroup is made up of students classified as disabled readers or learning disabled who show no generalized or specific deficits on testing; McKinney ascribes problems to attention or behavior disorders, motivational factors, or psychological processes not measured by researchers to date.[14]

Two distinct approaches to subtyping are represented in the body of studies. One approach, usually labelled "a clinical inferential" method, utilizes descriptive profile analysis to infer subtypes from visual examination of a battery of test results. Another uses multivariate statistical procedures to derive empirical distinctions between subgroups.

The inferential method has been associated primarily with studies that drew reading disabled students from clinical populations. For example, Boder[16] explored Johnson and Myklebust's[17] proposed conceptual dichotomy into auditory and visual types of disabled readers. She analyzed reading and spelling performance of reading disabled students, classifying 93 percent of her sample into three subtypes. Her dysphonetic sample (67 percent) read words at sight using a gestalt approach, but did not apply phonetic analysis. A dyseidetic type (10 percent) laboriously sounded out words, but could not recognize them at sight. A third subset called "alexic" (23 percent), the most severely disabled readers, were both dysphonetic and dyseidetic. Boder's work led to other inferential subtype classifications of disabled readers; those studies are not reviewed because subjects cannot be identified as learning disabled.

The multivariate statistical approach was used in more recent studies that examined learning disabled samples from school populations. Studies reported by Satz and Morris used cluster analysis first to identify a group of learning disabled subjects and then to reveal five subtypes among the identified learning disabled students: (1) global language impairment (30 percent), (2) language fluency disorder (16 percent), (3) mixed global language and perceptual impairment (11 percent), (4) visual and perceptual-motor impairment (26 percent), and (5) no neuropsychological impairment (13 percent).[18]

In contrast to Satz and Morris's samples selected by the researchers, subjects employed by Lyon and colleagues were labelled by their schools as learning disabled, met federal criteria as handicapped, and were receiving special education services. One study by Lyon and Watson of learning disabled and achieving adolescents yielded six subtypes through cluster analysis: (1) combined auditory and visual deficits (11 percent), (2) combined linguistic and perceptual-motor deficits (13 percent), (3) expressive language deficits (13 percent), (4) visual-perceptual deficits (34 percent), (5) auditory sequencing deficits (13 percent), and (6) normal diagnostic profile (17 percent).[19] A subsequent study by Lyon, Stewart, and Freedman of younger learning disabled and achieving subjects revealed that the visual-perceptual and auditory-verbal subtypes were associated with the younger subjects, whereas the language comprehension deficits were more characteristic of the older subjects.[20]

A longitudinal project undertaken by McKinney and associates employed first and second graders identified as learning disabled by their schools matched by sex and race to randomly selected, normally achieving students from the same regular classroom.[21] Over a 3-year period, a series of language, cognitive, and task and social behavior measures were applied. These programmatic studies differed from those described before in that these attempted to assess (1) behavioral status, as reported by both regular and learning disabilities teachers in addition to neurologic and language characteristics measured by psychometric procedures; (2) stability of subtypes over time; and (3) the ability of subtype membership to predict academic outcomes.

Subjects in seven identified subtypes did not differ in academic performance during the first year. However, over the next 3 years of schooling, the subtype groups became differentiated. Those in normal and withdrawn subtypes showed achievement progress as measured by a survey instrument; the attention deficit, conduct problems, and global-behavior problem groups showed declining rates of progress over 3 years, although McKinney documented similar time spent in services for learning disabled students over that period.

A related longitudinal study placed learning disabled and normally achieving children into five groups—overachievers, target achievers, underachievers, slow learners, and disabled achievers—and followed their progress for 3 years. Although the results are flawed by the use of age-equivalent scores instead of interval-data standard scores for comparison, this study contributed a procedure for comparing all low achievers in order to learn whether or not learning disabled students become more disabled over time while normally achieving students remain stable.

Apart from the studies generally known as subtype research, other investigators have attempted to identify learning disabled subgroups by using hypotheses about specific learning characteristics. Programmatic research on selected variables has been conducted at the federally funded Institutes for Research in Learning Disabilities.

In Virginia, attention disorders have been intensively studied by Hallahan and his colleagues. Their results have led researchers to describe learning disabled students as passive learners and to ascribe the strategy-deficient, inactive pattern to the inability to stay on task.[23] An attention deficit hypothesis has persisted as an explanation of a reliable subgroup of learning disabled students, despite criticisms of methodology and interpretations.[24]

In related investigations, Torgeson and his colleagues have conducted a series of studies on memory processes in attempts to account for the failure of learning disabled students to become actively engaged in an instructional interaction with teachers and materials. Across more than a dozen experiments, learning disabled subjects with memory deficits were compared with learning disabled children without memory deficits and with normally achieving learners. Results showed that memory deficits were constant over tasks and materials and were not subject to modification by incentives or mnemonic strategies.[25] Torgeson later concluded that differences between learning disabled and nonlearning disabled readers were primarily due to the rate of access to verbal information in long-term memory; however, the limited information base of nonreaders was cited as a confounding variable.[26]

Social skills of learning disabled adolescents have been studied extensively at the Kansas Institute for Research in Learning Disabilities. Characteristics on which the learning disabled groups were rated significantly lower than the nonlearning disabled groups included accepting negative feedback, initiating conversation, following instructions, giving negative feedback, giving positive feedback, negotiation, and problem solving. Only one characteristic—resisting peer pressure—discriminated a learning disabled group from a delinquent group.[27]

At the Chicago institute, the social status of learning disabled students has been investigated for deficits of behavior, social perceptiveness, nonverbal communication, and language skills, resulting in some conclusions indicting the learning disabled child's pragmatic skills.[28,29] Although Dudley-Marling has criticized the programmatic studies on methodologic grounds,[30] some trends in the relationship between pragmatic skills and academic underachievement emerge from the studies.

A dissent from attempts to develop homogeneous subgroups has come from the Minnesota Institute for Research in Learning Disabilities, which has studied identification issues. Results of programmatic studies led this research group to conclude that learning disabled and nonlearning disabled underachievers overlap to such an extent that "there are no characteristics that students labelled LD evidence that are not demonstrated with equal frequency by NLD students" (p 79).[31] Of course, the researchers were describing results of what they considered inappropriate processes of identifying learning disabled students as subjects for intervention.

What can be concluded from attempts to develop typologies? The data indicate that at least one language subtype recurs among heterogeneous groups classified as reading disabled or learning disabled; however, subtypes across studies are too varied to illuminate the relationship between learning disabilities and language impairment. Furthermore, "significant gaps exist in our knowledge about the nature and development of various LD subtypes, and their relationship to academic performance and instructional outcomes. . . . Subtype research demonstrates the limitations of single-deficit theories and shows that classification based on a single attribute does not account for the majority of the variance in LD samples, nor does it in any way deal with the different patterns of strengths and weaknesses displayed by LD children" (p 57, 61).[14]

ASSESSMENT OF READING AND WRITING

Measurement of academic performance and instructional outcomes has changed over recent years. According to Shuy, two paradigm shifts in linguistics affected analysis of reading and writing as well as oral language: "the first was the creation of sociolinguistics in the late sixties; the second was the focus on units of analysis larger than the sentence, or discourse analysis, in the seventies"(p 78).[32]

Shuy summarized the contributions of sociolinguistics as a new concern with subjective, functional, variable, dynamic reading and writing in social context as opposed to the older view of objective, formal, universal, static language considered apart from its context. A concomitant trend toward analyzing larger chunks of data led to replacement of sentence-level linguistics with discourse analysis in both reading and writing. Yet Shuy contended that in the mid 1980s, "Efforts to apply pragmatics to reading and writing have only begun."[32]

The trends identified by Shuy are seen in assessment practices in both reading and writing over the past decade. Reading assessment has moved from a recoding through a psycholinguistic decoding to a cognitive emphasis. Writing measures have shifted from an indirect syntactic focus based on a hierarchical view of discrete reading and writing skills to direct holistic procedures based on an interactive theory of acquisition of reading and writing.

Evaluation of reading or writing for learning disabled students begins with the same practices applied to any apparent underachievers: learning disabilities specialists attempt to determine (1) the extent of the discrepancy between cognitive potential and reading or writing performance; (2) diagnostic patterns of strengths and deficits on which to base a program plan; and (3) the contributions (as far as can be ascertained) of attentional, memory, motivational, and anxiety factors in performance.

Emphases upon specific tasks depend upon concepts of reading and writing; that is, methods of determining readers' and writers' strengths and deficits vary with operational definitions of reading and writing and with the theories or models to be followed in instruction. Of course, the types of instruments used are dictated by the purposes of the evaluation. For instructional planning purposes, a few common patterns of both reading and writing can be described.

Reading Assessment

Directors of a reading program might view reading according to varied definitions included in Harris and Hodges' dictionary of terms.[33] Definitions and related theories arrange themselves along a continuum.

Definitions and Theories

The two extreme positions on the continuum define reading as either (1) association of a sound representation with its corresponding visual image in order to permit recognition of words already established in the oral vocabulary and thus draw meaning from the symbols or (2) a central thought process utilizing prior knowledge to select, predict, compare, and confirm hypotheses in order to put meaning into printed symbols.[34]

The first definition is associated with recoding theories featuring phonics instruction. The second corresponds with cognitive theories, which associate reading success with retrieval of prior life experiences along with the ability to apply metacognitive strategies to comprehension of printed text. In the center is a position identified with psycholinguistic decoding theories linking reading skills to prior semantic and syntactic oral language competence.

Recoding theories hold that reading begins with the smallest units—letters or words. The reader's first task is to translate print to sound as a means of access to the oral language system and to obtain meaning. Graphic characters are converted into phonemic counterparts (initial and final consonant clusters, /th/, /ch/; vowel digraphs, /ou/, /ie/; diphthongs, /oi/, /ai/), which are then blended and matched with previously learned vocabulary and syntax stored in memory. Recoding also includes the use of contrasting word-shape clues ("tap" and "pat" differ in extensions above and below lines; "Charles" and "Christmas" are similar, but differ in length) and memorization of nonphonetic sight words ("though," "rough"); however, these are supplementary to the phonetic transcription.

A recoding position does not equate reading with word calling. Comprehension is the goal, but it is dependent upon precise code breaking. According to Chall, unlocking the code is a step that readers must take, at least temporarily, on the way to the automatization of word recognition, which underlies fluency and more mature reading behaviors.[35] The assumption is that printed symbols are processed through the auditory system and the oral language of readers.

At a middle position on the continuum, the work of Goodman[36] and Smith[37] represents a synthesis of recoding skills and language competence. According to this decoding model, readers simultaneously use three types of cues in progressing toward meaning. Graphophonic information, drawn from sight recognition and word analysis, provides clues to the text. However, readers do not need to decode all the words in a text in order to grasp the meaning. Rather, they make use of their knowledge of semantic associations and syntactic slots to predict which words would make sense in a particular position in a sentence. They then repeatedly test their predictions as they read ahead. Semantic cues are used to reorganize concepts during the act of reading; predictions are either confirmed or disconfirmed as individually decoded words alter and refine the sense of the total text. Basic knowledge of verb slots and noun slots enables readers to use syntactic clues to provide useful synonyms consistent with meaning if the graphophonic cues do not permit precise translation to the oral vocabulary. Goodman stated that this interaction between decoding skills and underlying language competence made possible a series of educated guesses.[36] A major assumption underlying this model is that reading is an active process dependent not only upon semantic and syntactic competence but also upon readers' initiative and problem-solving skills.

Going beyond both recoding and decoding theories, cognitive theories hold that meaning resides neither in recognizing words already in the oral vocabulary nor in predicting text by means of oral competence. Meaning is seen as a construction based upon the readers' cognitive expectations. Readers place minimal reliance on graphophonic, semantic, or even syntactic clues. Instead, they impose meaning on what they read by setting up expectations based on schema they bring to reading from prior life experiences. "Schemata are constructs that are applicable to general cognitive activity or information processing. They are similar to concepts but can apply to a wider variety of phenomena" (p 29).[38] Rumelhart has equated a schema with a play—it has a plot and a cast of characters.[39] For example, a basal reader story about a birthday party is dependent for comprehension upon readers knowing from experience that such a party includes eating cake and opening gifts brought by guests. The underlying assumption is that reading not only is interactive, but is more dependent upon prior knowledge than upon recoding skills or oral language competence.

Ideally, all three of these theories combine in the design of a complete reading assessment. In practice, many learning disabilities specialists have been trained to favor one type of assessment over the others. Some evaluators emphasize recoding skills, using a bottom-up approach by measuring subskills and then presenting connected text for a comprehension profile only at the levels at which readers can first recode words in isolation. Such evaluations feature grapheme and phoneme correspondence, phonetic word families presented for substitution of initial consonants (man, can, fan), blending tasks (/c/ + /a/ + /t/ = cat), and pronunciation of flashed words in isolation (presented at $^1/_2$ second each) followed by untimed presentation of the words not read automatically. This procedure demonstrates the extent to which readers can recode unfamiliar words if given time to do so. Recoding approaches to assessment typically emphasize oral reading of connected text, so that mispronunciations can be marked for phonetic analysis in order to discover possible misunderstandings of phonic generalizations.

Psycholinguistic decoding assessment also emphasizes oral reading of connected text, which permits miscue analysis following precise recording of omissions ("He ________ home"), insertions ("He the went home"), and especially substitutions ("He wagon home"). Analysis of substitution patterns reveals which features of the written text readers notice.

Cognitive assessment emphasizes comprehension of text. Emphasis is upon silent reading of connected text, followed by unaided recall (without the examiner asking specific questions) and summarization (in the reader's own words) of what was read. The paraphrase is then examined to determine how well the reader drew inferences from given (old) information in order to acquire new information from the text. Reading may be followed by an inquiry designed to evaluate the reader's strategies for gaining meaning from print materials.

Purposes

Differing reasons for assessing reading govern selection of varying evaluation procedures. In general, norm-referenced tests are used for administrative purposes to determine eligibility for programs. A standard score or percentile rank may predict the extent to which a reader can be expected to participate in the mainstream reading program. Results of group measures such as the Iowa Tests of Basic Skills[40] or the reading tests of the Stanford Achievement Tests series[41] might alert teachers to a reading problem. Group-administered achievement tests can indicate the need to take a closer look at reading skills, but they cannot confirm reading as a cause of failure, since factors such as attention, following directions, and other task behaviors that might interfere with achievement cannot be appropriately monitored during group tests.

Therefore an individually administered measure such as the reading cluster of the Woodcock-Johnson Psycho-Educational Battery[11] or the Woodcock Reading Mastery Tests Revised[42]—each of which measures both word recognition and comprehension—must be administered in order to document reading problems as a specific area of difficulty. The former provides a reading cluster score made up of letter and word identification, word attack, and passage comprehension—a cloze task in which silent reading is followed by insertion of a sensible word to fill a blank. The latter provides five reading clusters that evaluate, respectively, readiness, basic skills, comprehension, full-scale total reading, and short-scale total reading. Measures missing from both these widely used norm-referenced tests are aided or unaided checks of comprehension of paragraph length passages and estimates of reading rate.

Although it is sometimes misapplied as a reading measure, the individually administered Wide Range Achievement Test Revised (WRAT)[43] cannot be used to evaluate reading because it does not measure comprehension of connected text.

For diagnostic purposes, to discover patterns of reading problems, and to make an informed decision about how much time to devote to reading in a resource room or special class, teachers prefer to use criterion-referenced skill tests, informal inventories, and cloze tasks over classroom materials. Criterion-referenced skill tests include measures like the Brigance Diagnostic Comprehensive Inventory of Basic Skills,[44] which provides measures of discrete recoding skills such as basic sight recognition (automatic naming of high frequency words), phonic analysis (sounding consonants, vowels, diphthongs, and blends), and structural analysis (placing prefixes, suffixes, and infixes to modify words). Brigance tests cover multiple grade levels, and they provide details that can be used to formulate instructional objectives for decoding skills. But the tests are not useful for determining comprehension of passages; the format provides no means to record or interpret results of oral reading of connected text, nor is a second passage provided for silent reading.

Informal inventories offer better opportunities to measure connected reading. However, inventories are limited by the need to establish grade levels through readability formulas, which are based upon the assumption that sentence length and vocabulary, rather than complexity of sentence structure and inference load, influence reading difficulty.

Published inventories like the Ekwall Reading Inventory,[45] the Classroom Reading Inventory,[46] and the Classroom Reading Placement Inventory[47] offer two to four passages at each grade level, usually one or two paragraphs in length. Grade levels for sequenced passages have been established by readability formulas based upon word length, sentence length, and frequency of occurrence of vocabulary items.[48] Comparable passages at each grade level allow a teacher to use one for silent reading and another for oral reading. If the learner is below grade six, both oral and silent reading are typically measured; for middle school and secondary students, testing is usually limited to silent reading.

Informal inventories estimate three reading levels.[49] The independent level describes the grade of materials at which readers can process text with 98 to 100 percent word recognition and 90 to 100 percent comprehension without teacher assistance. The immediate instructional level is established at the grade at which readers can decode with 90 to 97 percent accuracy and comprehend at 70 to 90 percent accuracy; this range estimates the appropriate materials to be used for classroom instruction. The potential instructional or listening capacity level is the grade at which students can obtain 70 percent accuracy on a comprehension task on a passage above the immediate instructional level, which the examiner has read aloud.

By grade four, normally achieving readers' decoding skills have nearly caught up to their oral language skills. If the independent level is grade three, then the immediate instructional level is grade four and the listening capacity level is grade five; such a profile indicates that semantic and syntactic oral language skills are at a level just slightly higher than word-recognition skills. This represents a normal pattern. Teachers can set a realistic goal of bringing the instructional reading level up to the listening capacity level by working on decoding skills and by modeling for students a variety of strategies to take advantage of established semantic and syntactic oral language skills.

In addition to, or instead of, using published informal reading inventories for elementary students, teachers can develop their own based upon adopted reading series. This is done by presenting selected passages from the beginning, middle, and end of the reading books spanning the student's nominal grade. For example, a low-achieving third-grade student might be presented with passages from first, second, third, and fourth grade reading books. Again, passages are presented for oral, silent, and listening capacity comprehension checks, and three reading levels are established. The advantage of a teacher-made informal inventory is that it provides a measure of performance on the materials actually used for reading instruction: the teacher need not estimate the relationship between test performance and classroom functioning. Furthermore. a teacher-made test can be designed to include a higher number and more types of comprehension questions than are typically included in published inventories, so that more detailed information is provided.

A cloze task is another means to gain a curriculum-based measure of readers' abilities to deal with classroom materials, but it can be extended to include texts other than graded materials used for reading instruction. Teachers select a science, social studies, or other text that students are expected to read in class, make a photocopy of one or more pages (100 to 250 words, graduated upward with testees' grade levels) and then white out every eighth, seventh, or fifth word (graduated downward with testees' grade levels) after the title and the first sentence. Students under grade six read the passage aloud and secondary students read it silently, supplying orally a word that would make sense in each blank space.

If readers can supply an acceptable insertion for 40 percent to 60 percent of the blanks, the material is appropriate in difficulty for presentation with teacher assistance (instructional level).[49] If the percentage correct is below that range, a lower level of the adopted series or supplementary subject matter material is substituted as a more appropriate text. Such informal methods as criterion-referenced tests, inventories subjected to miscue analysis, and cloze tasks, in combination, provide the detailed pattern information necessary to plan instruction.

Reading Profiles

Some typical patterns of classroom reading problems recur among learning disabled students. Common profiles derived from clinical experience with inventories, cloze tasks, and oral miscue analysis can indicate generalized language impairment as well as specific reading disability.

On informal inventories, normally achieving readers usually score a grade or two higher on a listening capacity task because their receptive language skills allow them to grasp syntactic clues and meanings of words read by the examiner that they may not yet be able to decode for themselves from the visual symbols. Among indicators of a general language lag, an important piece of evidence is that the potential instructional level is the same as the immediate instructional level. For example, if both those levels emerge as grade four on an informal inventory, readers demonstrate that their receptive oral language skills are no higher than their decoding skills in reading.

The cloze task (based upon the curriculum) is another means to gather evidence about a generalized language disorder. Readers with underlying oral language competence substitute words from the appropriate form, class, or function category; that is, adverbs are placed in adverb slots and prepositions in preposition slots in sentences. Interclass substitutions (noun for verb, adjective for noun) are a red flag for syntactic problems. Furthermore, inappropriate vocabulary items, especially similar sounding words with a different meaning ("checking" for "catching"), should alert teachers to the possibility of a generalized language problem or a word-finding difficulty.

Other kinds of profiles come from such techniques as oral miscue analysis.[36] The types of cues being overused or underused, regardless of whether a substitution altered meaning, and relative percentages of specific qualitative patterns exhibited by readers offer evidence of their decoding skills and underlying language competence. For example, readers who are overly dependent upon graphic cues and do not monitor their reading against their own oral vocabulary are likely to make substitutions featuring nonsense words such as these:

tarnd paggy
She trained the puppy

In contrast, readers who have strong semantic and syntactic skills, but weak phonics abilities might substitute these sensible but inaccurate words by guessing from context:

taught dog
She trained the puppy

Readers who lack the ability to respond to syntactic cues and do not monitor for sense might make real-word interclass substitutions:

tennis partly
She trained the puppy

These examples indicate how a reading or learning disabilities specialist can use reading assessment results to supplement the speech-language pathologist's findings to confirm or disconfirm a generalized language disorder. It is critical for instructional planning purposes to sort out whether readers demonstrate problems across oral language and reading or exhibit a specific reading disability in the presence of intact oral language skills. Implications are illustrated in the section on Management of Reading and Writing Problems.

Writing Assessment

Options available to measure writing have a shorter history than do choices for reading. Shuy pointed out that when new directions for literacy research were explored in 1973, "The major focus was on reading, with little attention to writing" (p 83).[32]

In the intervening years, writing has attracted growing interest in the general education curriculum, but improvements in methods of measuring writing skills have lagged behind shifts in models for written language.[50,51]

Definitions and Theories

School writing for many years has been viewed as a product to be evaluated only in its completed form.[52] Over the past decade, writing has come to be defined in terms of the process writers engage in as they carry out the task; however, process measures are in the early stages of development.[53]

Writing evaluation has also been influenced by a general shift in research interest to larger units of discourse. In the past, the focus of product evaluation was a set of discrete skills that measured agreement with grammatical and stylistic conventions of written language, often considered at the sentence level. Writing testers of large groups over the past decade have come to focus on measurement of the entire written product as a global communicative unit rather than as a collection of component skills. At the same time, those responsible for individualized writing instruction continue to attempt to describe components of the written product that can be separately analyzed and, presumably, isolated for emphasis in instruction.

Product definitions describe writing as the final edited version that is submitted to the teacher, who is seen as audience and examiner. According to these views of writing, student performance is acknowledged, but the competence that may underly the strategies by which the paper was produced is not examined. Analysis of cognitive or metacognitive strategies employed to select form or content are not considered within this model of writing. Product measures are either indirect—based upon contrived samples presented for correction or insertion—or direct—based upon spontaneous or elicited samples formulated and transcribed by an individual writer. Direct evaluation may be holistic—assigning a single score for overall quality—or analytic—assessing separate scores for selected components.

Process definitions describe writing on the basis of the cognitive strategies employed in its execution, rather than on the basis of outcomes. Flower and Hayes described the cognitive process of writing as encompassing highly embedded acts, such as preplanning, drafting, revising, and editing, through which writers shift back and forth as they set and reset writing goals, learning as they write.[54] These stages are viewed as recursive rather than linear: they comprise the tasks in which beginning and mature writers have been found to differ.[50] Central to process definitions is the discovery of appropriate form and content for authentic audiences other than the teacher. Examples of process evaluation are found in reviews of research reports.[53]

Gillam and Johnston presented two contradictory theories of writing development.[55] One theory views the development of written language as dependent upon prior establishment of oral language skills. According to this theory, written language is recoded into the known oral language, which is the foundation underlying both reading and writing. This theory was espoused by Fries[56] and Bloomfield.[57] Myklebust,[58] an early researcher of writing by disabled readers, also advocated the recoding view, which conceptualizes reading and writing as secondary skills.

A contrasting theory views oral and written language as interactive rather than sequential, with the two related skills domains sharing overlapping schema with reading. According to this theory, early literacy in both reading and writing have the potential to improve oral language because the three skills develop simultaneously and reinforce one another. According to researchers working with normally developing beginning writers, the interactive view better describes how language learners make use of their oral communicative competence.[59] Features of early writing related to oral language include invented phonetic spellings; those factors related to reading include the tendency to employ written syntax in imitation of that used in instructional materials for beginning readers.[60]

An evaluator's position in regard to how writing develops tends to influence practices. A recoding theorist may not evaluate writing at all if reading is demonstrated at very low levels of achievement. An interactionist would be likely to ask a subject to speak, read, and write about the same topic and compare performance across the three sets of competencies.

Purposes

For administrative purposes—determining whether learning disabled students qualify as disabled in written language and are therefore eligible for services—indirect procedures are now typically employed by learning disabilities specialists. Unfortunately, results of indirect measures do not offer information about writing, but only about conformity with conventions. Therefore much of the decisionmaking is flawed with regard to qualifying learning disabled students on the basis of disabilities related to written expression. Direct writing samples subjected to holistic evaluation would constitute a more appropriate evaluation procedure; but since available holistic procedures do not yield standard scores that could be placed into a discrepancy formula, it is not likely that they will be adopted for this purpose.

To derive the detailed information needed to plan for individualized instruction, analytic direct evaluation is preferable to holistic rating, which does not offer indications of where or why the writing is breaking down.[61] Analytic procedures are time-consuming, but they can lead to short-term objectives for instruction.[62]

Types of Evaluation

Assessment practices associated with product views of writing include indirect measures of writing skills; that is, students' abilities to produce original text are inferred from nonwriting tasks in which testees merely select or insert an appropriate correction into a contrived passage written by a teacher or publishing staff. Examples of these discrete tasks are seen in the Brigance Diagnostic Inventory of Essential Skills,[44] in the word usage and style subtests of the Test of Written Language,[63] and in the dictation and proofing subtests of the Woodcock-Johnson Psycho-Educational Battery.[11] Though such items are commonly labelled in interpretation sections of test manuals with terms such as "writing" or "written expression," they do not demand formulation of any connected text by the testee. Instead, such indirect procedures measure conformity with conventions of standard American English grammatical usage or spelling[64] and do not predict in any way how a given student will apply the tested skills when asked to formulate language into connected written discourse.[61] Indirect measures can be viewed as estimates of general proficiency in recognition or correction of school language, but they are not writing tests.[65]

Product concepts of writing also encompass direct measures, in which original text is composed and at least two samples from each writer are examined. Direct products can be evaluated holistically or analytically. Holistic rating involves an impressionistic reaction to a first reading by assigning a numerical value for overall quality. It does not attempt to account for relative contributions of individual components such as a T-unit (one independent clause plus its embedded or subordinated dependent clauses)[66] or sentence construction, topic sentences, or specific rhetorical devices.[67] Examples of holistic scoring include procedures used for the National Assessment of Educational Progress and the essay tests used for College Board examinations.[68] These procedures feature agreement by a group of raters on a set of anchor papers against which essays to be scored are compared. Each paper is then read by at least two raters (three in cases of disagreement), and a composite single score is assigned to represent the global quality of the paper.

Analytic evaluation involves measuring component subskills such as the formulation of complex T-units, organization of T-units into sentences and paragraphs, use of unifying techniques such as transition terms, and extent to which the overall product meets the form, content, and audience-accommodation demands of a specific discourse type. Examples of varied approaches to analytic evaluation of groups of papers are provided in a publication of the Wisconsin Writing Project.[69] Examples of analytic systems designed for disabled writers are those developed by Poteet[70] and Moran.[71] Each system selects limited components from among the dozens of identifiable skills, describes those components differently, and places varying relative emphasis upon composing and aspects of transcription involving grammar, spelling, and mechanics.

Users of analytic measures do not deny that writing involves a complex interacting skills network; the goal is to understand a coherent communicative unit rather than discrete skills. But analytic scoring allows evaluators to isolate selected components for closer investigation of how those parts are combined by writers undertaking specific assignments. The basic distinction between holistic and analytic scoring is whether the procedure results in a single overall rating for a paper or a group of scores for separate components.

One position in the professional literature holds that holistic rating offers better opportunities to emphasize the communication as a seamless whole, whereas analytic scoring tends to focus upon discrete components of the task at the expense of the overall impression.[67] A counterargument contends that holistic rating also places covert emphasis upon specific subskills, but because those biases are not identified openly, their contribution to the rating outcome cannot be ascertained.[61]

Writing Profiles

Empirically derived descriptions of the writing skills of learning disabled subjects are all based upon product examination. Furthermore, most studies of learning disabled writers have focused upon formal aspects of writing rather than substantive composition competencies. Response to contrived tasks in which students merely inserted or corrected elements of sentences are not reviewed. Studies of writing by reading disabled students, such as the pioneering work of Myklebust,[58] are not reviewed because it is not known whether any of his subjects were learning disabled.

Using Myklebust's procedures, Poteet compared elicited writing samples of learning disabled students, identified by their schools, and achieving students and then compared their writing performances to their oral responses for the same picture stimulus.[72] Although the learning disabled writers showed some strengths in ideation and organization, results indicated the achievers had significant superiority in mechanics and approximately double the written productivity. However, the productivity of the learning disabled students on the oral task was comparable to that of the achievers, thus indicating specific differences between oral and written performances on similar tasks.

Strengths in ideation as well as in ability to formulate complex structures were identified by McGill-Franzen, who subjected a single sample by a single learning disabled adolescent to multiple analyses of early and late developing syntactic structures.[73] She found that both average words per T-unit and the presence of late developing structures compared favorably with findings among normally developing writers. However, she also found that low total productivity, run-on sentences and fragments, and multiple misspelled words obscured the writer's many composing strengths.

Using computer analysis of samples, Morris and Crump compared learning disabled writers with normally developing writers matched for age and IQ range.[74] When samples were analyzed for syntactic density, significant differences favored the nonlearning disabled group on this measure of subordination and embedding. Type-token ratio was greater for the nonlearning disabled writers at every age level, indicating limited variety in word types among the learning disabled writers. However, T-unit length, a measure of productivity, did not differ significantly between groups in this sample.

Employing part of a preliminary version of an analytic scoring system, later expanded to include content measures,[71] I compared three groups (identified by the researcher) aged 14 through 16—achievers, low achievers, and learning disabled students—across written and oral language samples over the same topics.[75] Written samples demonstrated significant differences that favored achieving adolescents over learning disabled students on mean morphemes per T-unit, a measure of productivity, but not on percentage of complex T-units, a measure of structural mastery. The learning disabled writers used all the same word classes as did the achievers, but the frequency of occurrence was lower in the learning disabled samples. The only significant difference between the written samples by learning disabled writers as compared to those of the low achievers was a lower spelling percentage correct.

Comparison of oral samples revealed no significant differences in productivity or complexity across the three groups:[76] learning disabled speakers used the same word classes in similar proportions and employed the same percentages of complex structures as did achievers. Demonstrated oral language competence was not reflected in written language, just as Poteet had found, indicating that writing is for some learning disabled students a specific disability rather than a reflection of generalized language disorder.

Limited studies of learning disabled writers have thus tended to find reduced productivity and variety, plus multiple errors across conventions of spelling and punctuation of sentences. However, strengths have been shown in complexity of syntactic structures as measured by T-units. Since reported studies have tended to focus analysis at the sentence level, little is known about the ability of learning disabled writers to organize larger units of discourse.

On the basis of clinical assessment and from experience, some typical patterns have emerged among learning disabled students. The most pervasive substantive skill that learning disabled writers appear to lack is the ability to anticipate what the reader would have to be told in order to grasp the intended written communication. Learning disabled writers of all ages tend to start their messages in the middle of things—for example, with a pronoun lacking a referent—as if the reader ought to be able to know what they mean to write about. This failure to distinguish given or shared information between writer and reader from new information to be conveyed is typical of learning disabled students' inability to shift to a reader's point of view.

A second common substantive problem occurs when learning disabled students are asked to write expository or persuasive prose as opposed to narrative discourse. Apparently because of their lack of experience in the nonnarrative modes,[52] many writers attempt to use narrative schema imposed on factual reports or argumentation. The result is a mismatch between demands of the task and the forms selected to do the job. For example, a learning disabled student might prepare a laboratory report limited to descriptions of his own sequential actions and omitting any results of the experiment. Or in a paper intended to persuade a school administrator to rescind a dress code, such students may simply recount their own experiences with the code without presenting any objective arguments against it.

A pattern detectable among learning disabled writers is a tendency to repeat stereotyped phrases or clauses. Five consecutive T-units may be written in the same clause type. For example, if the first one reads, "Soccer is exciting," the chances are high that subsequent clauses will duplicate the subject plus copula plus predicate adjective pattern throughout that sample.

Product analysis usually confirms lower productivity among learning disabled than among achieving writers. Learning disabled students produce considerably less original text in writing sessions. Productivity problems can be seen in the overall length of the text and also in the length of individual T-units, which are typically shorter, as measured by words or morphemes, than those produced by achieving writers at comparable reading levels.

The major factor in T-unit length is the tendency of learning disabled writers to join relatively unelaborated noun and verb phrases; that is, optional free modifiers such as adjectives, adverbs, prepositional phrases, and clausal complements are less frequent. These structures do occur in the repertoires of learning disabled writers just as they do among achieving writers, but the proportions are lower. The result is an impression of skeletal propositions lacking precision or descriptive vividness. This type of telegraphic writing is often in direct contrast with the writers' abilities to elaborate upon the same statements in oral discussions. When questioned about this discrepancy, learning disabled students have said that they do not attempt to write more because they cannot spell the words. Apparently, a voluntary inhibition of productivity is operating at a conscious level for some learning disabled writers.

Typically, there is a discrepancy between the learning disabled students' strengths in their capacity to *formulate* T-units and their weaknesses in their ability to *mark* those T-units with conventional sentence boundaries. Achieving writers know how to mark their T-units with an initial capital letter and end punctuation; whereas learning disabled writers either mark fragments as sentences ("Except for country music.") or omit capitalization and end punctuation, thereby resulting in run-on sentences ("country music is better than rock it has more melody it also tells a story"), which are more frequent than fragments missing either subject or predicate.

A pervasive characteristic of learning disabled writers that is often misinterpreted is their tendency to omit words other than subject or predicate, insert redundant function words, and substitute similar-sounding but inappropriate vocabulary items. The example, "Football is game that that scores countdowns," demonstrates all three types of these common practices—an omission, a duplication, and an inaccurate vocabulary choice. Unless such products are carefully analyzed, they can present an impression of syntactic disorder; in fact, the essential parts of the independent clause are usually present, but some teachers inaccurately call these productions fragments because they are disjointed and difficult for readers to comprehend. Most of these lapses can probably be attributed to attentional deficits rather than to problems at syntactic levels, as shown by learning disabled writers' tendencies to make suitable changes without direction after the problem is pointed out.

Closely related and perhaps also due to attention problems is a tendency to take more time to copy a passage than to write it spontaneously in the first place. This phenomenon occurs with regularity among learning disabled writers, and it offers an explanation for their strong resistance to substantive revision or rewriting of their productions.

One of the most persistent differences between learning disabled writers and either achieving or low achieving nonhandicapped writers occurs in spelling performance. Indeed, spelling that omits entire syllables ("ced" for "children") is a frequent anecdotal report from teachers of learning disabled students when referring them for clinical evaluation, and papers with more than half the words misspelled are frequent.

Spelling is listed as a separate category of disability under federal regulations, and it also distinguishes learning disabled writers from other low achievers.[75] However, spelling is often inappropriately assessed by the use of indirect measures—multiple choice or oral dictation of words in isolation. These methods contaminate spelling with reading recognition and auditory processing; they should be avoided in favor of direct evaluation of student written connected text.

The sparse assessment data available to describe writing characteristics of learning disabled students has, of course, placed limitations on instructional programs. Development of writing instruction has been identified as a high priority for learning disabled students.

MANAGEMENT OF READING AND WRITING PROBLEMS

Reading and writing profiles offer implications for team intervention, suggesting which personnel should be assigned and what types of instruction should be provided. However, profiles are useful only if differential instruction is provided to match varying needs. In other words, relative emphases in instruction must accord with assessment findings. For example, reading instruction differs depending upon whether students demonstrate oral language impairment plus reading problems or, instead, manifest a specific reading disability without evidence of generalized language disorder.

Differentiated Instruction

A generalized language problem associated with failure to progress in reading may be indicated by listening capacity scores equal to instructional reading level. Instruction might be approached by concentrating first on concept and vocabulary building, along with varied oral practice featuring formulation of meaningful connected clauses in an interactive structure. Lessons incorporate modeling provided by the teacher reading to students as the students look at the text to associate oral and graphic representations. Writing is introduced early to reinforce the concept of words and clauses as meaningful units. Instructors also offer opportunities for actual life experiences in order to build understanding of the world as a prerequisite to comprehension and production of written text. A combined oral and written language program is ideally delivered by a speech-language pathologist and a reading instructor working cooperatively to provide a variety of meaningful language experiences prior to and accompanying intensive formal reading instruction.

If assessment results show weak graphic and phonic associations accompanied by mild sensorineural hearing loss or generalized consonant-discrimination problems, phonics instruction may be deleted from the reading program. Instead, instruction in sight vocabulary is intensified by means of configuration (word shapes) cues and multisensory visual, tactile, kinesthetic methods in sequential, rather than simultaneous, presentation.

If oral language skills appear to be appropriate and the problem is determined to be a specific reading disability, instruction balances decoding and comprehension procedures so that readers have a variety of strategies to apply when they do not recognize words or draw meaning from a passage. Mildly disabled readers may require no more than modified developmental reading instruction with more trials and increased opportunities in order to practice a variety of strategies under supervision. Others, perhaps the largest group of disabled readers, need intensive corrective instruction in the specific skills that they have not mastered despite exposure to developmental instruction; this group might be characterized by their application of a single approach to all unknown materials rather than varying their word-attack and comprehension strategies. A small number of disabled readers are severely handicapped and must be offered intensive, one-to-one special instruction, perhaps over a period of years.

D'Alonzo has pointed out that special academic instruction in reading and writing may constitute only one of four reasonable approaches to appropriate instruction for learning and behavior problems.[78] He listed (1) tutorial procedures (learning specific skills or content), (2) strategies for gaining information (learning how to learn), (3) compensatory methods (learning through alternative systems to bypass disabilities), and (4) counseling (learning to live with the problem). Approaches (3) and (4) acknowledge that a few learning disabled students may never reach functional literacy in reading and writing and must be taught to compensate throughout their life spans and to practice assertiveness and negotiation in order to persuade others to meet their needs. According to D'Alonzo, nonacademic approaches to assisting learning disabled students become more important as students progress through school.[78] However, among academic problems, those associated with teaching reading and writing remain foremost in collaborative planning between the speech-language pathologist and the learning disabilities specialist.

Management Emphases

Review of professional literature reveals multiple studies of a variety of reading approaches applied to learning disabled subjects. Reading instruction appears to be well represented in the curricula for learning disabled students at all levels, though the emphases vary. According to Lyon, 60 percent to 80 percent of learning disabled students are placed in special programs for reading instruction.[79]

In contrast, writing instruction for learning disabled students does not appear to be widespread as part of a resource-room program, nor has writing practice in mainstream classes been assigned much instructional time. Applebee found that writing of a paragraph or more consumed only 3 percent of class time in all subjects and 10 percent in English classes.[52] Elementary programs have also been criticized by Graves for their failure to provide writing practice.[80] As for the learning disabled students, ". . . few teachers engage such children in this [literary] activity regularly" (p 280),[74] and "Many . . .continue to be constrained by an undefined [writing] curriculum" (p 258).[77] Many secondary learning disabled students interviewed about their experience with writing practice reported having participated in no writing instruction at all.[81]

What type of reading and writing curriculum might a learning disabilities specialist provide? Definitions and theories of reading and writing that govern the aforementioned assessment practices also inform management practices. Programs for learning disabled students tend to focus on skills instruction, holistic integration of reading and writing, or direct teaching of metacognitive strategies.

Skills Instruction

Reading

The underlying principles for the teaching of reading from the bottom up as suggested by Stetson[34] are the following:

1. Subskills of word recognition and comprehension are identifiable and sequential, with higher level skills dependent upon mastery of prerequisites.
2. Comprehension is dependent upon accurate and fluent word recognition; therefore automatic decoding skills have first priority.
3. Prerequisite skills not yet established are drilled and practiced to mastery through a series of specific discrete instructional objectives.

The goal of skills instruction is to develop word recognition to the point that it is so automatic that readers need not attend to decoding, but may be free to focus on the content of the printed message.

Skills instruction typically includes some use of basal reading series adopted for the district. Although learning disabled students seldom use graded basals during instruction in resource rooms, they are usually expected to function at some level in the adopted basal reader in the mainstream class. Therefore learning disabilities teachers may draw a sight vocabulary list from the adopted basal series to preteach the lexicon students must manage in the regular classroom. Such a grouping might be supplemented with lists of high frequency nouns, verbs, adjectives, and adverbs; nonphonetic function words such as articles, prepositions, conjunctions; or sets of survival words associated with public signs and meeting daily nutritional and safety needs.

Learning disabilities teachers may select a more systematic supplement to the basal system, such as a direct instruction procedure to teach decoding skills with drill and practice over repetitive lessons.[82] Direct instruction methods offer the advantage of more trials per learner per skill than are delivered through basal systems, and they provide the highly structured lessons that allow learning disabled students to predict the format of each day's lesson so that new interaction patterns with the instructor do not have to be acquired each day. However, disadvantages of routine scripted instruction may include fatigue and loss of attention, as well as a possibility that material may become meaningless upon daily repetition and regular review.

Any number of supplementary materials and procedures might be combined in skills instruction. Linguistic reading packages based upon substitution of initial consonants to create word families, or programmed materials to teach phonics generalizations or vocabulary, might be part of the daily routine. Prominent features of skills lessons are worksheets and drills at the chalkboard to reinforce textbook lessons with immediate application. Table 28–1 lists identifiable skills that are presumed, in skills theory, to be subject to direct teaching.

Again, these skills might be presented in many ways. Reid and Hresko described conventional approaches to reading as including basal readers; supplemental phonics programs; linguistic readers using phonetically regular word families; alternative systems using a contrived alphabet or inserting pictures into text; direct instruction methods employing scripts and numerous opportunities for programmed responses; language experience approaches using stories dictated by students as reading materials; and multisensory approaches employing various combinations of visual, auditory, tactile, and kinesthetic stimuli simultaneously or sequentially.[83] Gearheart presented a classification of reading approaches according to the source of the first words students learn.[84] Words selected by the students are used with language experience and other individualized reading programs that do not attempt to control vocabulary, but instead urge readers to learn words meaningful to them. High frequency words are incorporated into basal readers, structured reading kits, and high-interest, low-vocabulary readers—all of which control vocabulary difficulty and sentence length. Words with consistent letter-sound patterns are used in phonics programs, linguistic readers, and modified alphabets—all of which teach regular structures until they are mastered before introducing exceptions. These lists are illustrative of many available in standard texts on methods for teaching students with learning disabilities.

In addition to the traditional aforementioned methods, Reid and Hresko described a psycholinguistic approach.[83] Based upon the work of Goodman[36] and Smith,[37] it presents skills instruction at the level of silent comprehension, bypassing translation to sound on the assumption that meaning is derived directly from print. Instruction is based upon application of graphic, syntactic, or semantic cues that allow readers to process text without using spoken language to mediate between print and interpretation. This method features movement between surface and deep structure and emphasizes

TABLE 28–1 Identifiable Skills Subject to Direct Teaching

Word Recognition	*Comprehension*
Automatic naming of high frequency words	Immediate recall of overt, literal material
Had, did, was, went, girl, boy, mother, father	What was the boy's name?
Automatic naming of nonphonetic function words	Delayed recall of overt, literal material
The, but, from, your	Similar question following on intervening task
Phonics analysis/synthesis	Drawing inferences about unstated details
An + oth + er = another	What time of year do you think this happened?
Structural (morpheme/affix) analysis	Predicting outcomes
Over-coat, un-cover-ed, tran-scrip-tion	At the halfway point, ask "What will happen next?"
Context (semantic and syntactic) analysis	Formulating conclusions
"Nurse" decoded from earlier word "doctor"	What did the boy learn from what happened?
Noun inferred from presence of "the"	Recognizing an overt main-idea statement
	Find the sentence that tells what the passage is mainly about
	Inferring an unstated main idea.
	In your own words, give me a sentence that tells what this passage is mainly about
	Relating generalizations to stated support
	What are the reasons for believing . . . ?
	Distinguishing fact/fiction or fact/inference
	Did this really happen or is it made up?
	What points do we know for sure?
	Which ones might two people disagree about?
	Retelling a passage in sequence without aid
	Tell me, in order, what you just read
	Summarizing main points of a passage without aid
	Tell me the main ideas of what you read

reading practice over drills and exercises. Skills specifically taught by this method include scanning, selecting cues, predicting graphic representations, searching memory, formulating tentative hypotheses about meaning, testing passages against sense, and regressing to point of error when interpretation violates sense. Application of these instructional methods has shown that, as readers improve in rapid silent comprehension, attempts to read orally show decreasing accuracy; therefore oral reading is used neither for instruction nor for evaluation of progress. Instead, aided and unaided comprehension tasks provide progress records.

Writing

According to Applebee, skills instruction in writing continues to be featured in school language art programs.[52] Many of those programs are based upon grammar, on the assumption that indirect instruction such as generalizations related to syntax, punctuation, or capitalization is automatically transferred to writing tasks requiring formulation of novel sentences. The weight of instructional literature strongly argues against attempts to improve writing through this type of program;[85] nevertheless, drills featuring contrived samples of writing are included in many discussions of methods of teaching writing to learning disabled students.

Of course, approaches based upon grammar and using contrived samples are only one possible skills approach. Siegel, Jensen, Chittenden, and Wall described four sequences for teaching writing developed by them for successive levels of instruction and for both achieving and basic writers.[86] Their work offers a synthesis of models for teaching writing and provides a general overview of instructional responsibilities. Giordano first reviewed functional and academic writing tasks and then gave specific suggestions for instruction of learning disabled writers.[87] Although his work emphasizes error instead of writers' strengths, it also presents some developmental sequences and a scope chart incorporating higher level composing skills.

Table 28–2 lists some of the interrelated but identifiable writing skills that might be isolated and emphasized sequentially in a skills instruction program. Drawing from such a list for skills instruction might include sentence-building activities beginning with the students' own spontaneous clauses and then moving into sentence-combining practice in order to increase the complexity and variety of T-units and sentences. Moving up the skills hierarchy, when sentence formulation and variety have been demonstrated to criterion, models of formula paragraphs might be introduced for copying, followed by paraphrase and imitation activities. When three or four paragraph types have been mastered, transition terms might be employed to teach ways of achieving unity. Varied audiences might be described or selected by students to provide opportunities to modify vocabulary and degree of formality. Finally, three to five discourse types might be practiced with varying purposes for writing and with different audiences described to govern each assignment.

Skills approaches have the advantage of allowing instructors to concentrate upon one or two components toward sequential mastery of a complex process instead of requiring students to master everything at once. A disadvantage is the artificial segmentation of skills that must be ultimately coordinated into a fluent whole if reading is to be a meaningful activity; some students remain fixated at the lowest skills levels and become word-by-word or overanalytical phonics-based readers, with resulting breakdown in comprehension.

Holistic Integration of Reading and Writing

Holistic techniques attempt to combine reading and writing (typically along with speaking and listening) in a unified instructional program. These approaches are based upon the principle that language competencies are interrelated and reinforce one another if tasks are presented to incorporate more than one language skill within a single activity or over a given lesson. McNutt listed four components to be interwoven and integrated into daily instruction: (1) foundation oral language experiences such as brainstorming, storytelling, and field trips; (2) choral reading and group writing in loose, cooperative groupings; (3) independent and teacher assisted individualized reading and writing; (4) teacher to student and student to student discussions of what has been read and written.[88] The emphasis is upon taking advantage of natural language interactions and using the students' own reading and writing experiences as materials for class lessons. Direct instruction is minimized, contrived samples of the writing of others is avoided, and students are encourged to interact verbally with one another and with the teacher throughout the instructional period.

An example of a holistic approach provided by Gearheart is a language experience lesson in which students' dictated oral stories or reports are written down by the teacher, typed, and presented as reading instructional materials and then revised on paper by students as a writing activity.[84] Gearheart further described how to move students through a concrete to abstract progression, building upon known oral language skills. In this sequence, students first orally describe concrete experiences and then write their descriptions, moving from labels to add descriptors based upon size, color, and other features. Next, students write descriptions of remembered objects and events and/or add imagined features to picture stimuli. A third step requires keeping a diary or journal to record sequences of events. A fourth stage incorporates experiences explained in figurative language and a variety of discourse types.

Perhaps the most comprehensive presentation of an integrated language arts program is that of Moffett and Wagner.[89] Based upon the concept that the student is the center of the instructional approach, the work presents an entire curriculum, kindergarten through one postsecondary year, featuring

TABLE 28–2 Interrelated but Identifiable Writing Skills that Might Be Isolated and Emphasized Sequentially in a Skills Instruction Program

Organization	*Coherence*	*Audience Accomodation*	*Conventions*	*Discourse Types*
Clause Independent, dependent introductory, complementary T-unit Simple—one independent clause; complex—one independent plus one or more introductory, complementary, embedded Sentence types Simple, complex, compound-complex Paragraph types Enumerative, sequential, comparison-contrast	Local Semantic connections—transitions between sentences Global Semantic connections—transitions for overall unity	Given or new information Clear exposition, context; placement of new information in independent clauses, given in dependent clauses Appropriateness of appeals Diction and tone selected for purpose and relationship	Sentence boundary markers Initial capital letter and end punctuation Spelling Phonetic and nonphonetic words Internal punctuation, capitalization Commas, apostrophes, quotation marks; proper nouns Compliance with format guidelines Paragraph indentations, margins, salutations, heads	Expressive Describe how you feel when you. . . . Descriptive Describe the appearance and other features of. . . . Expository Describe the steps in. . . . Compare the actions in. . . . Narrative Tell what happened when you or a friend. . . . Persuasive Offer a set of reasons why. . . . Argue for or against. . . .

oral discussion followed by free writing and student selection of writing assignments.

Advantages of holistic approaches for learning disabled students center on the opportunities to plan redundancy and review across all language modalities. For example, the same vocabularies can be used for oral discussion of word meanings, sight reading, handwriting practice, spelling, and formulating T-units, both orally and in writing, followed by student recognition of words in context by reading their own written products. A holistic approach grasps natural opportunities to teach and uses the interaction of situation, students, materials, and the excitement of the moment to facilitate learning.

Disadvantages center on the lack of structure as perceived by some teachers and some learning disabled students. Teachers are more dependent upon their own resources to coordinate instruction across multiple materials, and some find the planning burdensome. Some learning disabled students who require a great deal of external structure do not repond favorably to impromptu lessons with varying formats that require frequent shifts of focus or task and flexibility in interactions.

Direct Teaching of Metacognitive Strategies

The human organism has been described as composed of representational and executive systems. According to Reid and Hresko[83] and Gearheart,[84] the former system as explicated by cognitive psychologists incorporates conscious and automatic perception and associative memory; the latter is a higher order control mechanism that both monitors and directs behavior to edit and modify activities. Emphasis upon the representational system in instruction has given way to a variety of methods of improving students' employment of executive functions in learning.

One approach toward this end is cognitive behavior modification. As described by Meichenbaum, this procedure consists of global and task specific sequences, begins with task and learner analysis, and uses overt verbalizations and self-regulatory tasks.[90] The emphasis is upon cognitive change through active, conscious application of self-treatment procedures including instruction, monitoring, recording, and reinforcement. Wong described how such procedures could be applied to teaching reading and other academic competencies.[91] Harris and Graham used self-control procedures to improve learning disabled students' composition skills.[92]

Heuristics based upon cognitive theories have been applied to both reading and writing at the Kansas Institute for Research in Learning Disabilities. First used with adolescent learning disabled students, instruction in learning strategies has been adapted for younger learning disabled students as well. Strategies were developed to overcome a combination of characteristics of textbooks, which are not designed for easy comprehension,[93] and heavy demands placed on students by classroom procedures and expectations.[94] Strategies have been devised to lead students step by step through varied textbook formats to help them make use of organizational cues provided in the text. For example, a procedure called "multipass" leads students into a series of data collection passes through a text.[95] The strategy has been adapted for listening to taped materials that are accompanied by color coded textbooks.[96] Other specific strategies are designed to teach paraphrasing, self-questioning, limited sentence and paragraph writing, and specific study skills.

Based upon a sequence of specific steps covering pretest, description, modeling, rehearsal, guided practice, independent practice, posttest, feedback, and generalization,[97] learning strategies provide for learning disabled students the executive planning that they do not appear to engage in spontaneously. Furthermore, since learning strategies require students to ask themselves questions, organize, and summarize content as they study, they are forced to become participants in the lesson. Many of the available strategies incorporate key words, charts, or other brief, vivid cues repeated throughout the lesson in order to keep students on task. Although validation studies to date are limited to those conducted by the Institute researchers, their results support the learning strategies model as an effective method to help learning disabled adolescents read and write in mainstream classrooms.

Advantages of direct instruction in learning strategies are the orderly sequential clues for attention disordered students and active engagement in ongoing monitoring for passive learners. Disadvantages center on the high reading levels required to follow written instructions, generally fourth grade or above, or the need to memorize sequential steps by repeated listening. Entry skills must be verified prior to instruction.

Beyond the academic focus of skills, holistic, or strategy procedures, nonacademic management plans have been described by Torgeson[98] to improve memory, by Hallahan and Sapona[99] to focus attention, and by Hazel, Schumaker, Sherman, and Sheldon[100] to teach social skills.

Continuum of Program Options

Before appropriate instructional programs can be implemented, the reading and writing interventions available in a specific district must cover the entire continuum of needs. Provisions should be available for discrete and multiple problems, including specific reading disability, specific writing disability, a combination of the two, or any combination of one or both with an oral language disorder.

Again, a specific *reading* disability is indicated if there is a significant (usually two standard deviations) discrepancy between expected performance based on the *verbal* IQ and a norm-referenced measure of comprehension of connected reading, confirmed by clinical diagnostic data from criterion- and curriculum-referenced assessment procedures. In the absence of norm-referenced direct writing measures, a specific *writing* disability is more difficult to document, but performance on a direct holistic measure of composition considerably below the level of the students' *verbal* IQ peers should permit informal comparative documentation preferable to indirect measures. If both reading and writing performances are significantly lower than *verbal* IQ, both would be classified as disabilities. However, if the *verbal* IQ plus reading or writing are depressed to approximately the same degree with the *performance* IQ two standard deviations higher, the evidence does not support a specific reading or writing problem, but rather a generalized language problem to be confirmed or disconfirmed in consultation with a speech-language pathologist who has evaluated oral language samples.

All these possibilities require a range of services across general and special education. A first consideration must be that many students who read below nominal grade level are not disabled; that is, instructional reading level may be below nominal grade but commensurate with performance IQ. Unless IQ and adaptive behavior are low enough to qualify for services under the category of mental retardation, such youngsters should be served within the general education instead of the special education programs.

A second caution is that students who do demonstrate specific reading or writing disability may be failing for reasons other than a handicapping condition. They should be served first by a reading or language arts specialist in general education as a preassessment intervention to determine whether they can respond to remedial, as opposed to special, education. Many reading or writing problems—those associated with lack of systematic, continuous, appropriate instruction or arising from attentional or motivational problems—respond positively to one to one instruction, but do not necessarily require special education.

Third, reading and writing problems accompanied by evidence of generalized language disability (high performance IQ and significantly lower verbal IQ and listening capacity) should be served by a team including a speech-language pathologist and either a reading or language arts specialist or learning disabilities specialist.

Fourth, those reading or writing discrepancies that satisfy eligibility criteria for placement in learning disabilities programs should be further scrutinized in order to determine whether the pattern of test results shows the kinds of strengths (high verbal IQ and listening capacity) that tend to rule out generalized language disorder. If so, reading or writing instruction is delivered by the learning disabilities specialist, in consultation with regular classroom teacher(s) with whom the student is simultaneously placed.

IMPLICATIONS FOR RESEARCH AND CURRICULUM DEVELOPMENT

In a study of the terms used in definitions and the eligibility criteria employed by states, McNutt found that a language component was included in the definition of learning disabilities by 87 percent of the 50 states responding.[6] She further found that states "are slowly moving toward definitions that are more in concert with the Federal definition." If this is the case, the later, broader definitions of learning disabilities may not assist in clarifying the extent of overlap between learning disabilities and language impairments. Apart from the effects of definitions and eligibility criteria, however, a growing body of research reveals that students classified by researchers or by school systems as learning disabled demonstrate heterogeneous disorders including language, attentional, memory, and social problems, manifested in a variety of configurations by individual learning disabled students.

Although oral language disorders have not been universally identified among learning disabled students, 60 percent to 80 percent display reading disabilities[79] and an unknown percentage demonstrate specific disabilities in written language. Thus the association of learning disabilities with at least one of three types of language problems is well documented. Whether students displaying those language problems are considered a subset of the speech impaired category or a subset of the learning disabled category, professional personnel in schools and clinical settings assume obligations for both research and curriculum development.

Research Needs

Implications for research in learning disabilities center on alternatives to ineffective attempts to select school-age children eligible for services under this category of exceptionality. Professional journals continue to debate proposed technical and policy solutions;[12] the term "learning disabled" (used for the population to be served by practitioners and studied by researchers in attempts to guide practices) remains inadequately defined.

The most promising solution suggested to date could be applied to the approximately 85 percent of handicapped students whose impairments are too subtle to make categorical classification obvious.[6] The suggestion is that the label be applied to all mildly handicapped students and that markers of various types be attached to identify subgroups for scientific experiments in differentiated interventions. Thus, for one intervention study, a group is identified with variables A, B, C; for another investigation, a group is described with markers D, E, or A, F, and G.[101] The advantages would be open acknowledgment of the heterogeneity of the population, an end to circular research based upon students identified by the system, and the beginning of opportunities to sort out those characteristics that might be amenable to intervention from those that may be resistant to change for the life span.[102] The trade-offs exacted from researchers would include longer-term commitments to subject samples, in order to permit fuller descriptions, and willingness to engage in programmatic interventions instead of single study approaches, since response to instruction over time could be expected to sort out meaningful subgroups more effectively than any combination of psychometric measures.

If groups subjected to a series of systematic, repeated intervention experiments were described in detail in regard to phonologic, semantic, morphologic, syntactic, and pragmatic oral competencies, decoding and comprehension reading profiles, and both composing and transcribing characteristics of written language, then programmatic intervention results could be analyzed to determine which combinations of markers appeared to facilitate favorable responses to which types of interventions. The advent of curriculum-based assessment offers opportunities to describe reading and writing in detail for pre- and posttest measures without relying upon norm-referenced tests, which lack content validity.[103]

Curriculum Needs

As evidenced by the effects of state competency tests, curriculum is affected by the measures selected to document student growth.[103] Therefore, professional efforts devoted to development of curriculum-based assessment procedures and on new models of reading and writing will have considerable impact on how those competencies are taught.

In the reading field, methods of measuring comprehension strategies should take precedence. For example, a high priority might be replacement of lists of specific comprehension questions by other means of determining the students' grasp of the entire communicative unit. Another need is for procedures capable of evaluating how prior knowledge about content is used and how executive cognitive cues such as advance organizers are employed. Such measures could identify differences between successful and unsuccessful readers. Analysis of those differences could then inform development of direct comprehension learning strategies.

Among written language measures to be developed, a high priority is a holistic direct evaluation procedure that could result in some type of comparison across time and against verbal and performance IQ. This comparison would make it possible to document individual needs and growth in writing competency. Without adequate means to document strengths and deficits over an instructional period, writing instruction does not assume appropriate emphasis in individualized educational programs.

A major instructional need is to consolidate teaching of oral, reading, and writing competencies into meaningful language experiences instead of fragmented therapy and lessons. Although there is merit in focusing upon specific competencies for short-term emphasis (because no one can teach everything at once), much more thought and effort might be devoted to the integration of the three language skills over long-term instruction. Speech-language pathologists, language arts specialists, and reading specialists can join with learning disabilities specialists to develop language programs encompassing oral language, reading, and writing for appropriate review and reinforcement across professional contributions.

SUMMARY

Students with learning disabilities manifest reading and writing disorders that may or may not be accompanied by oral language delay or impairment. As the label "learning disabled" is applied to more and more mildly handicapped students, the identification of learners who qualify for special education under federal and state guidelines remains controversial. Furthermore, distinctions between language disorders and learning disabilities are rendered more difficult by overlap in categorical definitions.

Nevertheless, subtype studies have consistently disclosed that one group of learning disabled students demonstrate a generalized language disorder, but other groups exhibit specific reading or writing problems despite oral language competence. The speech-language pathologist and the learning disabilities specialist, in collaboration, serve the students in the former group. The learning disabilities specialist, in consultation with teachers of mainstream language arts or English classes, works with the latter group. Still other students who demonstrate reading or writing disabilities yet do not qualify for special services are referred to remedial programs in the general education curriculum.

Assessment of reading and writing competence is undergoing a shift from focus on word recognition and compliance with writing conventions to increased emphasis on reading comprehension and composition content. Reading instruction and evaluation vary with theoretical positions ranging from recoding based on phonics, through psycholinguistic decoding using semantic and syntactic cues, to cognitive strategies employing conceptual schema along with self-questioning to construct meaning. Group or individual norm-referenced tests screen students for administrative purposes, but program planning requires the more detailed data offered by informal inventories or measures of response to curriculum materials. Learning disabled readers exhibit predictable profiles of relative strengths and weaknesses.

Writing instruction currently emphasizes process over product, and incorporates direct evaluation of multiple samples of original text composed for varied purposes and different authentic audiences. Limited assessment data relating to writing characteristics of learning disabled students reveal strengths in composition along with recurring patterns of deficits in productivity and compliance with conventions.

The management of reading and writing problems depends upon planning differentiated instruction to match the specific patterns demonstrated by groups of learners. Reading approaches include emphasis on word recognition skills, psycholinguistic cues, or cognitive strategies. Collaborative intervention by the speech-language pathologist and the learning disabilities specialist implies team planning of meaningful oral and written language experiences rather than fragmented lessons delivered in isolation. Although traditional programs have emphasized reading at the expense of writing instruction, integrated approaches offer promise of providing more adequate writing practice for learning disabled students. Holistic instruction in listening, speaking, reading, and writing permits instructors and students to take advantage of natural language opportunities. Reading and writing competencies—presented in tables—can be isolated for purposes of emphasis over short-term instruction but must be consolidated into complex reading and writing performance to meet classroom and life demands.

If reading and writing evaluation and intervention are to meet the needs of learning disabled students, further research and curriculum development must be pursued. A promising research practice is detailed description of subjects' oral language, reading, and writing characteristics, in acknowledgment of the heterogeneity of learning disabled students, so that practitioners might know how to generalize findings to specific groups of students. Development of better measures of reading comprehension and direct writing products could lead to improved progress data and foster curriculum development in these areas.

Although contributions vary among speech-language pathologists and learning disabilities specialists, these professional persons share responsibility for at least one subset of students. Whether those students are considered a subgroup of the "speech impaired" or "learning disabilities" category depends upon interpretations of federal and state guidelines, but appropriate services imply collaborative intervention along with joint research and curriculum development.

REFERENCES

1. Kavale K, Forness S. The science of learning disabilities. San Diego: College-Hill Press, 1985.
2. Adelman H, Taylor L. The future of the LD field: a survey of fundamental concerns. J Learn Disabil 1985; 18:423–427.
3. Office of Education. Procedures for evaluating specific learning disabilities. Federal Register 1977; 42:65082–65085.
4. Hammill D, Leigh J, McNutt G, Larsen S. A new definition of learning disabilities. Learn Disabil Q 1981; 4:336–342.
5. ACLD Board of Directors. Definition of the condition, specific learning disabilities. ACLD Newsbriefs 1985; 158:1–3.
6. McNutt G. The status of learning disabilities in the states: consensus or controversy? J Learn Disabil 1986; 19:12–16.
7. Tucker J, Stevens L, Ysseldyke J. Learning disabilities: the experts speak out. J Learn Disabil 1983; 16:6–14.
8. Snyder L. Developmental language disorders: elementary school age. In: Holland A, ed. Language disorders in children. San Diego: College-Hill Press, 1984:129.
9. Wren C. Language learning disabilities. Rockville, MD: Aspen, 1983.
10. Wechsler D. Wechsler intelligence scale for children revised. Cleveland: Psychological Corporation, 1974.
11. Woodcock R, Johnson M. Woodcock-Johnson psycho-educational battery. Allen, TX: DLM, 1977.
12. Reynolds C. Critical measurement issues in learning disabilities. J Spec Educa 1985; 18:451–475.
13. Leigh J. CLD position statements. Learn Disabil Q 1986; 9:245–247.
14. McKinney J. Research on conceptually and empirically derived subtypes of specific learning disabilities. In: Wang

M, Walberg H, Reynolds M, eds. The handbook of special education; research and practice. Oxford: Pergamon Press, 1985:47.
15. Chalfant J. Issues in determining eligibility: a national overview. In: Mellard D, DeLoach T, eds. A synopsis of conference proceedings. Lawrence, KS: Institute for Research in Learning Disabilities, 1985:8.
16. Boder E. Developmental dyslexia: a diagnostic approach based on three atypical reading-spelling patterns. Dev Med Child Neurol 1973; 15:663–687.
17. Johnson D, Myklebust H. Learning disabilities; educational principles and practices. New York: Grune and Stratton, 1967.
18. Satz P, Morris R. Learning disability subtypes: a review. In: Pirozzolo F, Wittrock M, eds. Neuropsychological and cognitive processes in reading. New York: Academic Press, 1981:109.
19. Lyon R, Watson B. Empirically derived subgroups of learning disabled readers: diagnostic characteristics. J Learn Disabil 1981; 14:256–261.
20. Lyon R, Steward N, Freedman D. Neuropsychological characteristics of empirically derived subgroups of learning disabled readers. J Clin Neuropsychol 1982; 4:343–365.
21. McKinney J, Feagans L. Academic and behavioral characteristics: longitudinal studies of learning disabled children and average achievers. Learn Disabil Q 1984; 7:251–265.
22. Short E, Feagans L, McKinney J, Appelbaum M. Longitudinal stability of LD subtypes based on age- and IQ-achievement discrepancies. Learn Disabil Q 1986; 9:214–225.
23. Hallahan D, Reeve R. Selective attention and distractibility. In: Keogh B, ed. Advances in special education. Vol. 1. Greenwich, CN: JAI Press, 1980:141.
24. Fleisher L, Soodak L, Jelin M. Selective attention deficits in learning disabled children: analysis of the data base. Except Child 1984; 51:136–141.
25. Torgeson J. The use of rationally defined subgroups in research on learning disabilities. In: Das JU, Mulcahy R, Wall A, eds. Theory and research in learning disabilities. New York: Plenum Press, 1982:111.
26. Torgeson J. Memory processes in reading disabled children. J Learn Disabil 1985; 18:350–355.
27. Schumaker J, Hazel S, Sherman J, Sheldon J. Social skill performances of learning disabled, non-learning disabled and delinquent adolescents. Learn Disabil Q 1982; 5:388–397.
28. Bryan T, Donahue M, Pearl R, Sturm C. Learning disabled children's conversational skills. Learn Disabil Q 1981; 4:250–259.
29. Bryan T, Donahue M, Pearl R. Learning disabled children's peer interactions during a small-group problem-solving task. Learn Disabil Q 1981; 4:13–22.
30. Dudley-Marling C. The pragmatic skills of learning disabled children: a review. J Learn Disabil 1985; 18:193–199.
31. Ysseldyke J, Thurlow M, Graden J, Wesson C, Algozzine B, Deno S. Generalizations from five years of research on assessment and decision making: the university of Minnesota Institute. Except Educa Q 1983; 4:75–93.
32. Shuy R. Changing linguistic perspectives on literacy. In: Orasanu J, ed. Reading comprehension from research to practice. Hillsdale, NJ; Erlbaum, 1986:77.
33. Harris T, Hodges R. A dictionary of reading and related terms. Newark, DE: International Reading Association, 1981.
34. Stetson E. Introduction to written receptive language. In: Phelps-Gunn T, Phelps-Terasaki D, Stetson E. Remediation and instruction in language. Rockville, MD: Aspen, 1983:129.
35. Chall J. A decade of research on reading and learning disabilities. In: Samuels S, ed. What research has to say about reading instruction. Newark, DE: International Reading Association, 1978.
36. Goodman K. Reading, a psycholinguistic guessing game. In: Singer H, Ruddell R, eds. Theoretical models and processes of reading. Newark, DE: International Reading Association, 1976:259.
37. Smith F. Understanding reading. New York: Holt, Rinehart, and Winston, 1978.
38. Hasenstab M, Laughton J. Reading, writing, and the exceptional child. Rockville, MD: Aspen, 1982.
39. Rumelhart D. Understanding and summarizing brief stories. In: LaGerge D, Samuels S, eds. Basic processes in reading; perception and comprehension. Hillsdale, NJ: Erlbaum, 1977:265.
40. Hieronymus A, Lindquist E, Hoover H. Iowa tests of basic skills. Chicago: Riverside, 1982.
41. Gardner E, Rudman H, Karlsen B, Merwin J. Stanford achievement test series. 7th ed. Cleveland: Psychological Corporation, 1984.
42. Woodcock R. Woodcock reading mastery test-revised. Circle Pines, MN: American Guidance Service, 1987.
43. Jastak J, Wilkinson G. Wide range achievement test-revised. Wilmington, DE: Jastak, 1984.
44. Brigance A. Comprehensive diagnostic inventory of basic skills. N. Billerica, MD: Curriculum Associates, 1983.
45. Ekwall E. Ekwall reading inventory. Boston: Allyn and Bacon, 1979.
46. Silvaroli N. Classroom reading inventory. 4th ed. Dubuque, IA: Brown, 1982.
47. Sucher F, Allred R. Classroom reading placement inventory. Oklahoma City: Economy, 1981.
48. Rush T. Assessing readability: formulas and alternatives. Read Teacher 1985; 39:278–283.
49. McLoughlin J, Lewis R. Assessing special students. Columbus: CE Merrill, 1985.
50. Graser E. Teaching writing; a process approach. Dubuque, IA: Kendall/Hunt, 1983.
51. Moran M. Options for written-language assessment. Focus Except Child 1987; 19:1–10.
52. Applebee A. Contexts for learning to write. Norwood, NJ: Ablex, 1984.
53. Faigley L, Cherry R, Jolliffe D, Skinner A. Assessing writers' knowledge and processes of composing. Norwood, NJ: Ablex, 1985.
54. Flower L, Hayes J. A cognitive process theory of writing. College Compos Commun 1981; 32:365–387.
55. Gillam R, Johnston J. Development of print awareness in language-disordered preschoolers. J Speech Hear Res 1985; 28:521–526.
56. Fries C. Linguistics and reading. New York: Holt, Rinehart, and Winston, 1963.
57. Bloomfield L. Language. New York: Holt, Rinehart, and Winston, 1963.
58. Myklebust H. Development and disorders of written language. New York: Grune and Stratton, 1973.
59. Clay M. What did I write? Auckland: Heinemann Educational Books, 1975.
60. Read C. What children know about language: three examples. Lang Arts 1980; 57:144–148.
61. Charney D. The validity of using holistic scoring to evaluate writing: a critical overview. Res Teach Engl 1984; 18:65–81.
62. Moran M. Objectives for writing instruction. Top Lang Disord 1987; 7(4).
63. Hammill D, Larsen S. Test of written language. Austin, TX: Pro-Ed, 1983.
64. Odell L. Measuring changes in intellectual processes as one dimension of growth in writing. In: Cooper C, Odell L, eds. Evaluating writing. Urbana, IL: National Council of Teachers of English, 1977:107.
65. Lloyd-Jones R. Primary trait scoring. In: Cooper C, Odell L, eds. Evaluating writing. Urbana, IL: National Council of Teachers of English, 1977:33.

66. Hunt K. Syntactic maturity in school children and adults. Monogr Soc Res Child Dev 1970; 35(134):1–44.
67. White E. Holisticism. College Compos Commun 1984; 35:400–409.
68. Myers, M. A procedure for writing assessment and holistic scoring. Champaign, IL: National Council of Teachers of English, 1980.
69. Smelstor M, ed. A guide to evaluating students' writing. Madison: Wisconsin Writing Project, 1978.
70. Poteet J. Informal assessment of written expression. Learn Disabil Q 1980; 3:88–98.
71. Moran M. Analytic profile of composing and transcribing. Kansas City, MO: Mss Press, 1987.
72. Poteet J. Characteristics of written expression of learning disabled and non-learning disabled elementary school students. Diagnostique 1979; 4:60–74.
73. McGill-Franzen A. Beyond illiterate, what can you say? Learn Disabil Q 1979; 2:76–80.
74. Morris N, Crump D. Syntactic and vocabulary development in the written language of learning disabled and non-learning disabled students at four age levels. Learn Disabil Q 1982; 5:163–172.
75. Moran M. A comparison of formal features of written language of learning disabled, low-achieving and achieving secondary students. Research report 34. Lawrence, KS: Institute for Research in Learning Disabilities, 1981.
76. Moran M. A comparison of formal features of oral language of learning disabled, low-achieving, and achieving secondary students. Research report 35. Lawrence, KS: Institute for Research in Learning Disabilities, 1981.
77. Roit M, McKenzie R. Disorders of written communication: an instructional priority for LD students. J Learn Disabil 1985; 18:258–259.
78. D'Alonzo B. Educating adolescents with learning and behavior problems. Rockville, MD: Aspen, 1983.
79. Lyon R. Identification and remediation of learning disability subtypes. Learn Disabil Focus 1985; 1:21–35.
80. Graves D. Balance the basics; let them write. New York: Ford Foundation, 1978.
81. Moran M. Learning disabled adolescents' responses to a paragraph-organization strategy. Pointer 1983; 27:28–31.
82. Gersten R, Woodward J, Darch C. Direct instruction: a research-based approach to curriculum design and teaching. Except Child 1986; 53:17–31.
83. Reid D, Hresko W. A cognitive approach to learning disabilities. New York: McGraw-Hill, 1981.
84. Gearheart B. Learning disabilities: educational strategies. St. Louis: CV Mosby, 1985.
85. Hillocks G. Research on written composition. Urbana, IL; National Conference on Research in English, 1986.
86. Siegel G, Jensen J, Chittenden L, Wall J. Sequences in writing, grades K-13. Berkeley: Bay Area Writing Project, 1980.
87. Giordano G. Teaching writing to learning disabled students. Rockville, MD: Aspen, 1984.
88. McNutt G. A holistic approach to language arts instruction in the resource room. Learn Disabil Q 1984; 7:315–320.
89. Moffett J, Wagner B. Student-centered language arts and reading, K-13. Boston: Houghton-Mifflin, 1976.
90. Meichenbaum D. Teaching thinking: a cognitive-behavioral approach. In: Interdisciplinary voices in learning disabilities and remedial education. Austin, TX: Pro-Ed, 1983:1.
91. Wong B. Issues in cognitive behavioral interventions in academic skill areas. J Abnorm Child Psychol 1985; 13:425–442.
92. Harris K, Graham S. Improving learning disabled students' composition skills: self-control strategy training. Learn Disabil Q 1985; 8:27–36.
93. Brown A, Armbruster B, Baker L. The role of metacognition in reading and studying. In: Orasanu J, ed. Reading comprehension from research to practice. Hillsdale, NJ: Erlbaum, 1986:49.
94. Schumaker J, Deshler D. Setting demand variables: a major factor in program planning for the LD adolescent. Top Lang Disord 1984; 4:22–40.
95. Schumaker J, Deshler D, Denton P, Alley G, Clark F, Warner M. Multipass: a learning strategy for improving reading comprehension. Learn Disabil Q 1982; 5:295–304.
96. Schumaker J, Deshler D, Denton P. An integrated system for providing content to LD adolescents using an audiotaped format. In: Cruickshank W, Klieban J, eds. Early adolescence to early adulthood. The best of ACLD. Syracuse: Syracuse University Press, 1984:79.
97. Alley G, Deshler D. Teaching the learning disabled adolescent; strategies and methods. Denver: Love Publishing, 1979.
98. Torgeson J. The relationship between memory and attention in learning disabilities. Except Educa Q 1981; 2:51–59.
99. Hallahan D, Sapona R. Self-monitoring of attention with learning disabled children: past research and current issues. J Learn Disabil 1983; 16:616–620.
100. Hazel S, Schumaker J, Sherman J, Sheldon J. Application of a group training program in social skills and problem solving skills to learning disabled and non-learning disabled youth. Learn Disabil Q 1982; 5:398–408.
101. Mann L, Davis C, Boyer C, Metz C, Wolford B. A retrospective analysis of child service demonstration centers' compliance with the federal definition of learning disabilities. J Learn Disabil 1983; 16:14–17.
102. Keogh B. Classification, compliance and confusion. J Learn Disabil 1983; 16:25.
103. Eaves R. Educational assessment in the United States. Diagnostique 1985; 10:5–35.

29 Speech and Language Disorders Related to Hearing Impairment

Mary Joe Osberger, Ph.D.
Linda J. Hesketh, M.S.

Estimates of the incidence of hearing impairment in children range from 1 to 2 per thousand to 50 per thousand.[1] The incidence of hearing impairment in children is difficult to determine because a variety of definitions may be used to define the impairment. The figures indicating the higher incidence reflect the inclusion of children with mild and moderate hearing losses. These children are often excluded from national surveys because they may not be enrolled in special educational settings or be receiving special services.

The management of hearing-impaired children presents a challenge to both professionals and parents. Because the effects of a hearing loss are manifested in deficits in speech and language, as well as in auditory skills, professionals in a variety of disciplines are usually involved in the development and implementation of intervention programs. These professionals include audiologists, speech-language pathologists, educators (both regular classroom teachers and teachers of the hearing impaired), psychologists, and physicians. The range of professionals has increased since the introduction of Public Law 94-142. Education of hearing-impaired children in the "least restrictive environment" has resulted in a dramatic increase in the number of these children who are enrolled in public school settings. Prior to that time, most hearing-impaired children were educated in schools for the deaf, which were staffed primarily by teachers of the hearing impaired. The integration of hearing-impaired children into the public school setting has eliminated the need for large residential schools in many states and has permitted children increased contact with their families and their normal-hearing peers.

The growing number of hearing-impaired children in public schools has heightened awareness of the needs of this heterogeneous population. In the past, emphasis was placed on meeting the needs of children with severe and profound hearing losses because they were perceived as having the greatest need for special services. In contrast, children with mild or moderate hearing losses often were neglected; thus they received inadequate support services.[2] We now know that children who are hard of hearing are susceptible to significant language problems that can interfere with reading ability and academic success.

FACTORS AFFECTING THE DEVELOPMENT OF COMMUNICATIVE SKILLS

Terminology

First, it is necessary to define some common terminology. "Hearing impaired" is the generic term used to describe any child whose hearing thresholds fall outside the normal range of hearing (i.e., 0 to 20 dBHL).[3] As more information has become available about the auditory capabilities of hearing-impaired individuals, the terms "deaf" and "hard of hearing" have undergone redefinition throughout the years. Here, we have adopted the approach of Boothroyd[4] and have defined these terms based on the ability of the individual to use audition to understand speech, if necessary, with amplification. In this sense, "hard of hearing" is used to describe an individual who uses hearing as the primary mode for speech perception, speech monitoring, and language acquisition. Information perceived through the visual modality (i.e., through speechreading or a manually coded English system) may supplement information, which is perceived through audition. The term "deaf" describes an individual whose hearing loss is so severe that the auditory channel cannot be used as the primary one to perceive and monitor speech or to acquire language. In this case, *auditory* information is used to supplement information perceived through vision or touch.

Children who are hard of hearing and have a mild hearing loss (15 to 30 dBHL) develop speech and language skills spontaneously. Included in this category are children who have unilateral hearing losses. Some of these children might evidence delays in language acquisition, but more data are needed to establish under what conditions the delays occur and the extent of such delays. With appropriate intervention, the language problems of these children can usually be resolved. For children with hearing loss of a moderate degree (31 to 60 dBHL), conversational speech is not completely audible, thereby resulting in delays in speech and language acquisition. With hearing aids, audibility of speech is completely restored, thereby permitting them to use their good auditory discrimination abilities. With appropriate intervention, the communicative problems of these children can be minimized or eliminated.

Children with severe hearing losses (61 to 90 dBHL) do not hear conversational speech normally, and thus they do not develop functional communicative skills without intervention. Speech can become fully audible with appropriate amplification, but they may still demonstrate difficulty in discriminating between speech features. These individuals can usually acquire many speech and language skills through the auditory modality. Functionally, some children with severe losses may perform more like "deaf" children, who depend on visual information to learn speech and language.

Speech is not fully audible to children with profound losses (91 dBHL or greater), even with appropriate amplification. This limitation, combined with very reduced auditory discrimination abilities, makes it difficult for these children to learn speech and language primarily through the auditory modality. Within each of the hearing-loss categories, children do demonstrate large differences in their speech perception abilities. For this reason, it is unwise to predict a child's potential for acquisition of spoken language on the basis of hearing thresholds alone. Variables that may account for some of the large individual differences are discussed below.

Age of Onset of Hearing Loss

The age of onset of a hearing loss exerts a strong influence on the effects that it will have on a child's communicative skills. Obviously, a child who has a congenital hearing loss is at greater risk for delays in speech and language development than is the child who acquires a hearing loss after some period of normal auditory experience. Traditionally, a hearing loss that occurs before speech and language are developed is called "prelingual," whereas the term "postlingual" is used to describe a hearing loss that occurs after these skills are developed. The difficulty with this binary classification system is that it implies there is a definable age at which speech and language development are complete. The developmental literature has identified ages at which the major milestones in speech and language are acquired by normally developing children, but refinements in these skills probably continue until at least adolescence.[5,6] Further, there are large individual differences in developmental rates among children. Skills may not be mastered and fully integrated into a child's communication system for several years after their emergence is first noted. These skills, in particular, seem to be susceptible to the effects of sudden deafness during childhood.

Aspects of the intervention program vary depending on the child's age at the time of hearing-loss onset. For children with a congenital hearing loss or an onset during the first year or so of life, emphasis should be placed on the *development* of nearly all the skills of interest. In contrast, management of the child who experiences a significant hearing loss after 5 or 6 years of age, focuses on maintaining, or regaining, skills already learned, with attention to those aspects of speech language that have not yet been developed. Management of children who are still in the formative years of speech and language (i.e., between 2 and 6 years of age) when their hearing loss develops will vary depending on the needs of each child.

Age of Identification of Hearing Loss

A factor that interacts with the effect of age of onset of deafness on the child's communicative skills is the degree of hearing loss, but the exact relationship between these two variables has not been studied systematically. The age of identification of a child's hearing loss is closely related to the severity of the loss. The more severe the loss, the more delayed the child's speech development, the more obvious the child's reduced auditory responsiveness, the sooner the parents will come to suspect there is a problem. Children with mild, moderate, or high-frequency impairments usually go undetected until they reach school.[7] Most parents regard hearing loss as "all" or "none", and the notion of a partial impairment is unfamiliar to them. Consequently the hard-of-hearing child's inconsistent responses to sound and delays in language development often are attributed to intellectual or behavior problems.

Additional Handicaps

Other handicapping conditions can coexist with a sensorineural hearing loss and serve to exaggerate the effects of the hearing impairment on developmental processes. Some problems such as mental retardation, physical disabilities, or reduced visual acuity, may be relatively easy to diagnose. In contrast, deficits in visual processing, visual-motor coordination, or memory, which also have been found to occur in hearing-impaired children, are more difficult to identify.[8] Further, skills in these areas typically are not assessed in the hearing-impaired population unless the child is evaluated by a multidisciplinary team.[8] It has been conservatively estimated that roughly 25 percent of all hearing-impaired children have a handicap in addition to hearing impairment,[9,10] with "learning disability" being the one most frequently cited.

Communication Methodology

To appreciate some of the issues surrounding speech and language development in hearing-impaired children, it is necessary to discuss some aspects of the communication methodologies that are used with them. The method used to communicate with (and educate) hearing-impaired children has been a source of great controversy since the 1800s. Historically, there have been disagreements regarding whether or not children should be educated using an "oral" or a "manual" approach. Use of an oral or auditory-oral approach requires that the child use his or her residual hearing and speechreading to learn to comprehend and produce spoken language. The rationale for this approach is that development of those skills necessary to communicate with the "hearing world" occur only if the child is given repeated practice and experience with these skills. Some oral philosophies emphasize the use of auditory skills to perceive spoken language,[11,12] whereas others stress the use of speechreading as well as audition.[13] Until the mid 1960s, most programs used an oral approach to educate hearing-impaired children, at least through the elementary school years. Practices varied among schools regarding the use of signs with older students. There was a greater likelihood that signs would be used in residential schools, particularly because this was the primary mode of communication between the students who lived there. Signs were generally not used while speaking, and it appears that American Sign Language, or some modification of it, was the system used most often in these situations. Because speech was not used while signing, it was referred to as "manual" communication.

American Sign Language (ASL) is based on the French sign language, and it was brought to the United States in 1816 by Thomas Gallaudet. It is considered a language because it has it's own grammar and vocabulary.[14] It cannot be written, but can be represented by pictures. Because the word order and grammar differ from English, it is not possible to speak English and sign ASL at the same time.

It is important to keep in mind that at this time, most children with severe or profound hearing losses attended schools for the deaf as either day or residential students. Children with moderate hearing losses or less were usually mainstreamed into regular classrooms with some resource support. The development of improved hearing aids over the years has resulted in successful management of many hearing-impaired children using an auditory-oral type of approach, especially if the child's aided auditory thresholds fall within the range of conversational speech for frequencies from 500 through 4,000 Hz.

With time it became apparent that a large portion of children had not developed the oral skills necessary to become competent oral communicators by the time they were ready to graduate from high school. Even more troublesome were the severely reduced language and academic skills of this population. Even those children who learned to talk intelligibly often failed to acquire language skills commensurate with those of their normal-hearing peers. The solution to this problem seemed obvious and led to the use of sign for all children, even those in parent-infant and preschool programs. However, the use of ASL did not seem appropriate to educators because the ultimate goal of signing was to provide a visual representation of English. This led to the development of several manually coded English systems.[15–17] These systems use the same word order as English, thereby permitting the signer to speak and sign at the same time. Because the child receives spoken as well as signed English, the method became known as Total Communication (TC). At the same time, the child is expected to speak when she or he signs. The systems are heavily inflected and also represent pronouns and function words. Fingerspelling is used with these systems just as it is used with ASL. In the 1960s, one of these systems, Signed English,[18] was implemented with preschoolers at Gallaudet College. Since that time, there has been a steady increase in school programs using Total Communication and a decrease in the number of oral programs.

However, it has become apparent over the years that the use of TC has not been the hoped for panacea for alleviating the language problems of hearing-impaired children, especially for those children with profound hearing losses. Studies continue to demonstrate that the profoundly hearing-impaired child acquires only fourth-grade reading skills even though exposed to manual English throughout most of his or her education.[8]

The next step to take in improving communication methodology is less obvious than when children experience limited success with an oral approach. As a first step, it is necessary to examine why a child's language skills have not developed satisfactorily with manually coded English systems. There appear to be several reasons. First, English is an auditory language and no matter what visual system is used to represent it, to decode the written English, the child must ultimately learn the sound-symbol system. Perhaps we have not done an adequate job in helping the child apply his knowledge of signed English to learn how to read. Many people assume that this is the responsibility of the classroom teacher. If, however, the speech-language pathologist plays a major role in the child's language intervention program, then she or he must be aware of the linguistic skills that the child needs for successful *academic* performance as well as for communicative competence.

Second, studies have shown that both teachers and parents fail to become proficient users of manually coded English.[19–20] Some common problems in their use is failing to use a one-to-one sign-word correspondence, dropping morphological markers, and omitting function words.[21] Teachers often fail to use idioms or figurative language with children because of the limitations of the sign systems. Data collected by Moeller and Luteke-Stahlman[22] indicate that the mean length of the preschool child's signed utterances exceed those of their parents. Moreover, many of the children in TC programs have failed to reach their potential in the development of auditory-oral skills. In many programs, hearing aid usage is poor, and there is insufficient emphasis and training on the development of speech production skills. In practice, many of these programs might be more appropriately labeled as "manual" rather than Total Communication.

Some educators are encouraging the use of ASL in the classroom to teach children certain concepts about language, which might aid in their acquisition of English. For example, to teach the concept of "plural," the ASL plural sign could be used (which is "book" signed repeatedly to convey the notion of more than one). Once the child has the concept of "plural," then the manually coded English representation of "books" can be presented. This innovative use of signs appears to have potential application in improving the language skills of profoundly hearing-impaired children. A concern is that people using ASL in this manner might not pair it with the English representation, thereby resulting in nothing more than the use of pidgin signs (the use of ASL signs in English word order with many of the grammatical structures of ASL and English omitted). If this were to happen, then there would be little likelihood of observing any significant change in the language abilities of hearing-impaired children.

Another communication option is the use of Cued Speech,[23] a system composed of basic hand shapes that are formed at four different locations around the mouth. Each hand shape corresponds to three or four consonant sounds that are differentiated from one another through speechreading. It is not clear how effective this method is for promoting the acquisition of spoken language, but data are available that indicate that it aids in speech perception tasks.[24] Clinical experience has shown the use of cues to be helpful during speech production training, irrespective of whether the child communicates orally or with Total Communication. If the target sound is not visible, the use of cues helps the child focus on the target sound. The approach is particularly helpful if the child has some knowledge of phonics.

Decisions involving the selection of communication methodology are often difficult ones to make. Often, selection of an option is dictated by the programing that is available to the child. When there is a choice to make, a wide range of diagnostic information is needed to make a thoughtful decision. Too often, the decision is based only on audiometric information. Evaluations of the child's speech, language, and *functional* auditory skills need to be performed.[25] In addition, other factors such as the learning style of the child and the attitudes of the parents about the different methodologies should be taken into consideration.

Effect of Hearing Loss on Parent-Child Interactions

The parents play a key role in a hearing-impaired child's intervention program, especially during the infant and preschool years. The presence of a severe or profound hearing loss can disrupt aspects of adult-child interactions. Research findings in the normal developmental literature show that adults speak to infants in special ways; this is because infants react to the conversational attempts of adults, and adults interact with infants as if they were conversational partners long before children are language users.[26] Further, there is evidence to suggest that the speech presented to infants has characteristics that differ from those found in adult-adult interchanges. The most prominent feature of this type of speech is use of a high fundamental frequency (Fo) and large changes in intonation, which are tied to linguistic aspects of the message.[26]

There is evidence to suggest that normal adult-child interactions are affected when the child is hearing impaired. Studies have shown that normal-hearing caregivers of hearing-impaired children tend to be more physically manipulative, more dominant, and more verbally controlling than the caregivers of children with normal hearing.[27] The presence of a hearing loss also alters the linguistic input that the caregiver provides. Normal-hearing mothers of hearing-impaired infants have been observed to control the topic, failing to observe the child-directed discourse convention that typically occurs with young children. It is easy to understand how this might happen if the child is so severely delayed in speech and language development that the caregiver must assume almost complete responsibility for conversational maintenance. That is, the normal turn-taking routines are reduced or absent with the adult being the only active partner in the "conversation." Also, the characteristics of the mother's speech, which are so salient to infants (i.e., changes in fundamental frequency), may not be perceptible to the child with a hearing loss. If the mother is not reinforced by the child for whom these special speech patterns are intended, then it is likely that use of them will be extinguished. If this happens, the other linguistic modifications and accommodations that accompany the speech patterns might also be affected. Assuming that adult-child interchanges serve some prelinguistic function, it is easy to see how severe delays in language development can begin during early childhood in the hearing-impaired.

The intervention goal with parents is to teach them how to be facilitators of communication development in natural contexts. Before this can happen, however, it is necessary to assess the manner in which the parents interact with their child. Facilitative interaction is critical not only during the years of infancy, but throughout childhood. Direct teaching in this area might be needed for some parents if the normal patterns of dyadic interaction have been affected by the presence of a hearing loss.[28]

COMMUNICATIVE SKILLS OF HEARING-IMPAIRED CHILDREN

The effects of a hearing loss on the development of communicative skills is both varied and complex. All things being equal, the more severe the hearing loss and the earlier the onset, the greater the effects on developmental processes. Effective intervention programs need to consider *all* the skills directly affected by the presence of a hearing loss, that is, auditory, speech, and language. These areas are discussed separately for organizational purposes. This organization is not meant to imply that these skills develop independently of one another or that they should be addressed independently in an intervention program.

Speech Perception Abilities of Hearing-Impaired Children

A person's ability to understand speech depends on the acoustic features of the speech signal, the amount of linguistic information available, and the quality and quantity of previous auditory experiences. Most of the speech perception research has examined the ability of adults with acquired sensorineural hearing loss to perceive the acoustic characteristics of speech. Nonsense syllables have been used as the stimuli, presented at varying intensity levels or in the presence of background noise. In general, the frequency of perceptual errors increases as the hearing loss increases.[29,30] The pattern of errors varies according to the configuration of the loss as long as nonsense syllables are used as the stimuli.[31] The performance patterns can be explained by the acoustic information available in the listener's frequency region of residual hearing. For example, listeners with flat or rising losses have difficulty distinguishing nasal consonants (the acoustic cues for these phonemes are in the low-frequency region), whereas people with sloping high-frequency losses have difficulty perceiving sibilance (frication).[31]

Listeners with moderate and severe hearing losses are able to perceive consonant voicing and manner of articulation distinctions (e.g., /ba/ vs /pa/; /ba/ vs /ma/; or /ba/ vs /za/), but they have a great deal of difficulty in distinguishing place of articulation (e.g., /ba/ vs /da/ vs /ga/).[32] Vowel errors are infrequent in adults with acquired hearing losses (unless the loss is in the severe to profound range) because the acoustic cues that distinguish these sounds are in the frequency region where residual hearing is present.[22] For this reason, most nonsense syllable tests for adults assess the discrimination and identification of consonant sounds.

Unlike adults, children with moderate to severe sensorineural hearing losses often have difficulty distinguishing one vowel from another. Confusions may involve vowels with high-frequency second formants (e.g., /i/ vs /I/), or they may involve confusions between front and back vowels that have similar first frequency formants (e.g., /i/ vs /u/). Erber[33,34] found that children with severe losses not only had trouble distinguishing place of articulation, but also often confused consonants with differing manners of articulation (e.g., /ba/ vs /va/). The severely hearing-impaired children in Erber's study were able to distinguish nasal vs. nonnasal consonants (e.g., /ma/ vs /ba/), although their labeling of /m/ and /n/ was not always correct.

A study by Boothroyd[29] provided new information on the acoustic speech characteristics perceived by children with severe to profound sensorineural hearing losses. The results showed that the average pure-tone hearing levels (in dBHL)[3] at 500, 1,000, and 2,000 Hz, up to which a given phonemic contrast could be recognized were: (1) 75 dB for consonant place; (2) 85 dB for initial consonant voicing; (3) 90 dB for initial consonant continuance; (4) 100 dB for vowel place; (5) 105 dB for syllabic pattern, and (6) greater than 115 dB for vowel height.

The work of Boothroyd is significant because it demonstrates that children formerly labeled as "deaf" (i.e., with hearing losses of 90 dB or greater) constitute a heterogeneous group with respect to auditory capabilities. It is important to recognize that the performance of children with losses of 115 dB and greater probably reflects perception of the speech signal on the basis of vibrotactile rather than auditory sensation. If the child is responding on the basis of tactile sensation, he or she is able to perceive time and intensity changes of speech, but not the rapid shifts in frequency domain that are needed to understand words.[33] Thus, timing patterns (e.g., number of syllables, stressed versus unstressed syllables) and the greater intensity with which low vowels (i.e., /a, ae, ɔ/) are produced than high ones (i.e., /i, I, u/) are perceptible by "feeling" the pattern rather than hearing the stimuli. According to Erber,[34] vowel classification on the basis of intensity cues is much less precise in word or sentence contexts where syllable stress can modify the relative intensities and durations of the segments.

Research has shown that information perceived via the auditory and visual channels can complement one another to improve speech recognition.[33,34] People with moderate and severe hearing losses, including children, use visual information to supplement auditory information. In contrast, children with profound losses rely primarily on visual cues to perceive speech; this results in only slightly higher performance with combined auditory-visual cues than only visual.

Even though it is not reasonable to assume that all children with profound, or even severe, hearing losses can be taught to hear and discriminate every component of speech, it appears that a large proportion of these children can learn to make use of a number of acoustic cues with which to understand many aspects of spoken language. Until the child is given adequate training, it is impossible to determine the limitations that the hearing handicap has imposed on the auditory mechanism for speech processing.

Speech Production Abilities of Hearing-Impaired Children

The speech of hearing-impaired talkers has been the subject of numerous research studies. Both perceptual (listener judgments and transcription) and instrumental (acoustic and physiologic) analyses techniques have been used. The majority of data have been collected on speech samples subjected to phonetic transcription and subsequent error analysis. Some data are available on the acoustic and physiologic correlates of these production patterns. Both perceptual and instrumental analyses have been used to describe segmental and suprasegmental aspects of hearing-impaired children's speech as well as intelligibility. Only a brief review of this literature is provided (see Osberger and McGarr[35] for a comprehensive overview) in terms of suprasegmental production patterns, followed by segmental patterns, and intelligibility data. This organization is not meant to imply that these aspects of speech production develop or occur independent of one another.

Suprasegmental Production Patterns

These production patterns involve characteristics of speech that extend over units composed of more than one phonetic segment. Included in this category are characteristics of timing, intonation, and stress assignments.

Prolongation of speech segments may result in the perception of speech as slow and labored,[36] thereby distorting the rhythm of the utterance and causing temporal distortions at the segmental level. In the latter case, hearing-impaired children have been shown to distort the relationship between vowel duration and the voicing characteristic of the following consonant.[37] The proportional shortening of unstressed vowels and syllables relative to stressed ones is smaller, on the average, in the speech of hearing-impaired children than in the speech of children with normal hearing.[36] Correction of the temporal relationship between stressed and unstressed syllables has been shown to result in small improvements in intelligibility.[38,39] Appropriate prepausal lengthening may not be present in hearing-impaired children's speech, which cues the perception of phrase and sentence boundaries.[36] Another manifestation of poor timing control is reduced coarticulation of speech sounds.[40] It appears as if profoundly hearing-impaired children learn to produce the phonemes of English as unmodified targets rather than as segments that vary in production as a function of context. Acoustically, this problem reflected in the abnormal duration of segments and distorted frequency transitions.[41]

Intonation and pitch problems are frequent in the speech of the hearing impaired and reflect poor laryngeal control in these speakers.[42,43] Acoustically, fundamental frequency (Fo) is too high or too low. This problem is probably caused by the average vocal-fold tension being too high or too low.[44] Improper adjustment of vocal-fold posture can result in an Fo contour that is overly sensitive to adjustments in the speech of these individuals.[45] Relatively few studies have examined the Fo characteristics of intonation contours produced by hearing-impaired speakers,[35,36] probably because this aspect of speech is difficult to quantify without reference to the linguistic context. In fact, quantitative descriptions of intonation in the speech of normal-hearing talkers are still being developed. Common problems involving intonation are insufficient variation in Fo throughout and utterance, excessive and inappropriate variations in Fo, and failure to produce a terminal fall in pitch at the end of a phrase.[30,42]

Segmental Production Patterns

The most extensive work in this area has been conducted by Levitt and his colleagues.[30,46,47,48] Broad phonemic transcriptions were performed on sentences containing words with a sample of all English phonemes, which were produced by a group of hearing-impaired children with hearing losses ranging in severity from moderate to profound. This research has shown a remarkable consistency in error patterns across different groups of children. Further, the largest difference between children was in the frequency of errors with type of error varying to a much smaller extent. Levitt and Stromberg[47] have analyzed error patterns in terms of the articulatory features involved. Even though the underlying articulatory maneuvers must be inferred from the data, the analysis scheme provides a very useful way of analyzing segmental production skills. The segmental errors in the speech of the hearing-impaired are reviewed using the data and classification scheme of Levitt and Stromberg. It should be kept in mind that many of the types of errors that they described have been identified by other investigators in different populations of children.

With respect to vowels, Levitt and Stromberg[47] found that omission of the target vowel did not occur frequently. The most common error involved substitution of one vowel for another with the tense-lax substitution of front vowels (i.e., /i/ and /I/) the most frequent. The next most frequent type of substitution involved "near neighbors" in the articulatory vowel quadrilateral (e.g., /I/ and /E/), followed by substitutions to a more schwa-like vowel. The frequent use of schwa-like vowels results in vowel neutralization, which is a term frequently used to describe vowel production by the hearing impaired. Acoustic descriptions of hearing-impaired children's vowel productions have been restricted to studies involving speakers with profound hearing losses. The classic work in this area has been performed by Monsen,[49] who described the acoustic manifestation of vowel neutralization as overlapping F1–F2 frequency plots for the different vowels. As a consequence, the phonologic space for vowels, defined by the minimum and maximum values for the first two formants, is reduced. This reduced phonologic space has been attributed to a relative immobility of the second formant, with F2 remaining relatively stable around 1,800 Hz for all vowels, and to a restricted range of the first formant. Monsen has postulated that the relatively greater distortion in the F2 dimension reflects the abnormal auditory feedback that the hearing-impaired speaker receives, the relative invisibility of tongue movements that reflect changes in F2, or both. Stevens[42] and his colleagues have suggested that inadequate posturing of the articulatory, laryngeal, and respiratory structures can lead to production of vowels with a narrow range of F2 movement. They postulate that hearing-impaired speakers maintain a relatively backed position of the tongue because the muscles that maintain the static tongue-body position remain tensed as part of an overall deviant speech posture. Consequently, the tongue body does not undergo much displacement in the front-back direction during speech production. This results in a restricted range of movement of the second formant from one vowel to another. Other posturing problems can lead to abnormalities in vowel characteristics which include indistinct resonances, additional resonances (due to nasalization), or irregularities in the output spectrum.

The error-classification system used by Levitt and Stromberg[47] to describe consonant production consists of six basic groups of errors: omissions, asynchrony, constriction errors, placement errors, glottal substitutions, and unidentifiable substitutions. Omission of consonants occurred in the word-final position most often with relatively infrequent occurrence in the word-medial and word-initial position. Consonants produced in the middle of the mouth were omitted most often, followed by consonants produced in the back of the mouth. Consonants produced in the front of the mouth were omitted infrequently. The lower rate of front consonant omission is often attributed to the high visibility of their articulatory movements. Another issue is that the articulators, which are highly visible, also are more constrained in their movements (i.e., the lips), thus reducing the number of errors that can be made with them. Another common notion is that the frequency of errors increases as the place of production moves further back in the mouth. If this were true, then production of alveolar and palatal sounds should be better than velar. As noted above, velar sounds are less prone to error than are alveolar ones. Alveolar sounds might be in error more often because there are many sounds with this place of production, thus requiring relatively high articulatory precision to differentiate between them. In contrast, there are only three velar sounds in English that the child must learn to produce and distinguish.

After omission errors, the next most common type of error reported by Levitt and Stromberg involved constriction, specifically that of over-constriction. These errors presumably occurred because the constriction of the vocal tract was too great, thereby resulting in the substitution of a stop for a continuant sound, such as a fricative. Errors involving under-constriction of the vocal tract did not occur frequently, but when they did they were seen most often in the form of the fricative /h/ substitution for /k/ or /g/.

Asynchrony errors involving voicing were frequent with the voiced cognate substituted for the voiceless cognate for stop consonants. The relative frequency of this type of substitution was nearly equal for the fricatives. The voiced-voiceless confusion in hearing-impaired children's speech has been well-documented in acoustic[50,51] and physiologic studies.[52,53] The latter studies suggest that the source of these problems is a failure to coordinate respiration, laryngeal valving, and supralaryngeal movements.

Asynchrony errors involving velar control also were common.[47] These errors resulted in a nasal consonant being substituted for a stop or vice versa. The substitution of /b/ for /m/ was especially frequent. Errors of this type occur because the speaker fails to coordinate movements of the velum with other articulatory gestures, a problem that Stevens et al[42] attribute to postural inadequacies.

Levitt and Stromberg[47] found that errors in placement were relatively infrequent. That is, the speakers tended to have the correct placement for the articulatory target but the manner of the consonant was not produced correctly. This pattern of errors illustrates the difficulty that hearing-impaired speakers have in coordinating gestures to achieve the desired target. Glottal stops were most often substituted for stops and affricates. This error type, as well as that of unidentifiable substitutions, occurred with greater frequency in the speech of the most unintelligible talkers in the study. Stevens et al attribute the use of glottalization to posturing difficulties. In particular, they observed that profoundly hearing-impaired speakers used a glottal constriction to reduce the amplitude of sound between syllable nuclei rather than using supralaryngeal movements to valve the airstream for amplitude reduction. The severely reduced intelligibility of these speakers is no surprise when a maneuver such as this is used to mark the end of syllables.

Intelligibility

Research has shown a systematic relationship between degree of hearing loss and intelligibility. All things being equal, the greater the loss, the more unintelligible the child's speech will be.[30,54] The exception to this trend occurs when the hearing loss enters the profound range of impairment. In this case, there appears to be no clear-cut relationship between hearing level and speech intelligibility: some children develop intelligible speech and some do not. Thus, the presence of a profound hearing loss does not in itself predict unintelligible speech.

As the number of segmental errors increases in a child's speech, intelligibility decreases.[30] High negative correlations have been reported for the total number of vowel errors and consonant errors and intelligibility.[30,55] Monsen[54] found that the ability to distinguish /t/ versus /d/ with appropriate VOT values, a wide vowel space, as determined by the difference in formant values between /i/ and /ɔ/, and proper acoustic distinctions between nasals and glides accounted for 73 percent of the variance in intelligibility scores among children. These data should not be interpreted to mean that control of the suprasegmental aspects of speech are not important. In fact, children who have good segmental production skills are likely also to have good control of the suprasegmental aspects of speech. At the suprasegmental level, errors resulting in an incorrect temporal relationship between stressed and unstressed syllables, and errors involving poor phonatory control have been found to have a negative effect on intelligibility.[30,38,43]

The largest body of data on the intelligibility of hearing-impaired children's speech is based on write-down procedures that require panels of listeners to write down what they think the child has said. The samples are then scored for the percentage of words understood by the listeners. In addition to the speaking proficiency of the talker, a number of variables have been found to affect scores on these measures. Intelligibility is affected by the syntactic complexity of the material[56,57] and the complexity of the word-form (i.e., polysyllabic), as well as the articulatory targets (i.e., consonant clusters).[56] These effects are more noticeable for unintelligible than intelligible talkers. Monsen observed an interaction between listener experience and the degree of intelligibility of the talkers, with listener experience having the greatest effect on the intelligibilty scores of the least intelligible talkers. In contrast, McGarr[58] found that the experienced listeners always achieved higher scores than did inexperienced ones. Other factors that Monsen[56] found to be related significantly to intelligibility scores were: repetition of the utterance, the presence of context, and the visibility of the talker.

Language Skills of Hearing Impaired Children

Current theories of language acquisition suggest that hearing-impaired children must acquire language rules and knowledge in the following three related areas to be competent communicators: form (syntax), content (semantics), and function (pragmatics).[59] The receptive and expressive language skills of hearing-impaired children are discussed here using this framework.

Form

The majority of information on hearing-impaired children's language abilities has been collected in the area of syntax and/or form. Most of this research was conducted in the late 1960s and early 1970s when there was strong interest in applying syntactic models, such as transformational grammar, to study language. Children who are hard of hearing demonstrate delays in the acquisition of syntax, but not to the same extent as do children with profound hearing losses. Schoolage hard-of-hearing children usually have no difficulty acquiring the basic rules of English, but they may have significant difficulty in understanding and producing complex grammar rules such as those involving relative clauses or the passive voice.[60,61] These problems may not interfere with routine communication but they may affect reading comprehension and academic performance.

Profoundly hearing-impaired students encounter great difficulty in learning English syntax. Unlike hard-of-hearing students, most of the research in this area has shown that hearing-impaired students acquire only those structures necessary to comprehend and generate the simplest English sentences.[8,62,63] The forms that are the most difficult are those that do not adhere to a simple subject-verb-object order. Verb forms, inclusion of function words, and use of pronouns also are troublesome for profoundly hearing-impaired children.[64,65] In a study involving profoundly hearing-impaired students in a residential setting, the syntactic skills of the students, on average, approached the developmental level of a 6 to 7 year old.[8] Another discouraging finding of this study was that, on average, the profoundly hearing-impaired students reached a plateau in learning English grammar and showed no further improvements in this aspect of language (or semantic development) after 12 to 13 years of age. In fact, as the children got older, the performance differences between them and children with normal hearing increased. Similar delays in the acquisition of syntax and the plateau in learning have been reported by Engen and Engen[66] in another large sample of hearing-impaired children. The inability of these children to comprehend complex syntactic structures poses serious problems for reading. In fact, data obtained by Quigley, Power, and Steinkamp[67] indicate that beginner reading materials, designed for normal-hearing students, contain complex syntactic structures that are beyond the linguistic competence of many hearing-impaired children. The superficial knowledge of the organization and function of English also has been shown to have a dramatic effect on hearing-impaired students' ability to use language to aid memory[68,69] and to understand the implications of discourse organization.[70]

The delays in syntax acquisition displayed by hearing-impaired children demonstrate that they are unable to extract the underlying rules of the language by mere exposure to it. This is not surprising in view of their dependence on learning language through the visual modality. Many of the morphological markers and words that cue a change in word order, or denote the presence of a pronoun, or a clause, are likely to be missed when reading signs or speechreading, especially if they are not familiar forms to the child. These markers also are the ones most likely to be dropped by nonproficient signers.[19] Those children who have little residual hearing and who must depend almost exclusively on visual input to learn language are most likely to have the greatest difficulty in extracting the underlying rules of English.

Content

The word knowledge of hearing-impaired children differs from that of their normal-hearing peers with respect to their command of literal word meanings and the breadth of their lexicon.[71] Even children with mild hearing losses have been shown to demonstrate significant delays in vocabulary development.[7] One major reason for the limited vocabulary skills of hearing-impaired children appears to be their dependence on direct teaching of the meaning of the words that they learn, a situation in marked contrast to that of the child with normal hearing who acquires the majority of word meanings vicariously. This also appears to reflect the dependence of these children on the visual system for learning an auditory language such as English. The reduced lexical skills of these children are reflected in their restricted knowledge of synonyms and their difficulty in recognizing relationships between words. The latter problem results in inefficient organization of lexical information and is evidenced in their lack of understanding of the concept of shared attributes or basic classification principles.[8,71] It appears as if they memorize the meaning of isolated words using no conceptual framework to organize their lexical knowledge. This places severe limitations on their ability to store and retrieve information efficiently.

Words take on varied meanings in context and hearing-impaired children have particular difficulty in determining new meanings in this situation.[71] Further, they often have difficulty understanding nonliteral language, such as, puns,[72] metaphors, and some aspects of humor. Their knowledge of the world is often tied to the "here" and "now," which often interferes with their ability to learn abstract uses of words and to perform verbal reasoning tasks.[71]

Hearing-impaired students demonstrate developmental gaps in their word knowledge.[8,71] Basic concepts and words that are acquired during the preschool years are often missed. For this reason, a hearing-impaired child's performance on vocabulary measures cannot be assumed to be commensurate with the developmental language level corresponding to the level of performance. Also, it appears that concepts that are perceived easily through vision (e.g., size) are acquired earlier than other functional concepts (e.g., pronouns, position).[8,71]

Function

Relatively few studies have examined the pragmatic skills of hearing-impaired children. Clinical experience and the limited data available indicate that this is an area in which hearing-impaired children demonstrate significant difficulty. Curtiss, Prutting, and Lowell[73] observed that profoundly hearing-impaired preschoolers used a range of pragmatic intentions, but they did so primarily through nonverbal means (i.e., gestures). The pragmatic functions used most often were labeling and naming, acknowledgment, and demand which are some of the earliest used by children with normal hearing.

The delayed pragmatic skills of hearing-impaired children are evident in discourse situations. McKirdy and Blank[74] found that dyads with profoundly hearing-impaired children used significantly fewer conversational turns than dyads with hearing children. The majority of communication initiations by the hearing-impaired children were in the form of a specific demand for a response, whereas the children with normal hearing also responded when there was no explicit demand to do so. The hearing-impaired children were observed to give more inappropriate and ambiguous responses when higher levels of abstraction were required to answer a question. They also were able to perform on a higher level when they initiated communication than when they were required to respond to their partner's initiations.

Clinical observation has revealed a number of difficulties that hearing-impaired children demonstrate in discourse situations.[71] Because of problems in question comprehension, hearing-impaired children may fail to follow the rules for turn-taking and topic-negotiation. Further, the child may not understand the notion of presupposition and use restricted and elaborated codes inappropriately. The child's syntax problems may be the source of his or her difficulty in following topic-shifts in a conversation. This is particularly evident if the cl.ild is delayed in the development of conjunctions. If the child has formulation and sequencing problems, these difficulties will be apparent in discourse situations. Many hearing-impaired children have not learned appropriate clarification and repair strategies to use when they do not understand what has been said to them. Often, there will be a complete breakdown in communication because the child has not learned to ask for repetition of an utterance directed to him or her. Thus, the available research and clinical data suggest that hearing-impaired children must be taught directly the rules that govern conversations, just as they are taught semantic relationships and the rules of word order and morphological usage.

ASSESSING THE COMMUNICATIVE SKILLS OF HEARING-IMPAIRED CHILDREN

Auditory Skills

Assessment of the child's ability to use his or her residual hearing to understand speech is essential to developing an effective intervention program. It is important to emphasize that large individual differences exist in the speech perception abilities among persons who have a similar degree and configuration of hearing loss. Thus, the data relating degree of hearing loss and speech perception abilities should be used as a guide in selecting assessment procedures and planning an intervention program and not as a predictor of performance. In addition, the degree of hearing loss cannot predict reliably the child's potential to learn to process speech auditorily.

Formal Tests

The tests most commonly used are those administered by audiologists as part of the child's audiologic evaluation. These most often consist of monosyllabic word tests using an open-response format such as the Northwestern University-Children's Perception of Speech (NU-CHIPS) test[75] or a closed-response set formant such as the Word Intelligibility by Picture Identification (WIPI).[76] Performance on these and other measures will be influenced by the child's degree of hearing loss, age, receptive language skills, and previous auditory training experiences. These tests yield a performance score but provide limited information that will help in the formulation of an intervention program.

A test, which has been standardized on hearing-impaired children 4 to 12 years of age with varying degrees of hearing loss, is the Test of Auditory Comprehension (TAC).[77] It consists of 10 subtests, ordered in a hierarchy of task complexity, ranging from discrimination between environmental sounds and speech to comprehension of stories in the background of competing speech messages. A zero signal-to-noise ratio is used, which makes the results of the test particularly informative for mainstreamed children who must listen under similar conditions in regular classrooms. The child's performance on this test can be used to help develop an intervention program using the training curriculum (Auditory Skills Curriculum),[78] which was developed by the same group of clinicians. One problem with the TAC is that it takes more time to administer than monosyllabic word tests; this might make its use impractical in some audiology clinics.

A procedure that can be used to assess the auditory skills of children with limited residual hearing is the Minimal Auditory Capabilities (MAC) Battery.[79] This test was originally developed for use with persons with profound, postlingual hearing losses who were hearing aid or cochlear implant users. Because it employs a written/read response format, it is limited to use with children who can read and perform the response task. The MAC Battery consists of 13 auditory tests and 1 speechreading test. The auditory tasks range from identification of intonation and stress patterns of English to recognition of words and sentences. Preliminary data are available on the performance of profoundly hearing-impaired adults with postlingual hearing loss.[79]

Informal Procedures

A child's age, language skills, or degree of hearing loss may make it impractical to administer monosyllabic word tests or the other measures described above. In this case, informal procedures can be used. Although some of the measures may be administered in a sound-treated booth, this is not necessary if testing is carried out for the purpose of obtaining informal, diagnostic information for planning an intervention program.

Erber[34] has developed an assessment approach that is based on the range of speech stimuli and auditory response tasks that occur during communication. The progression of speech stimuli, from simple to complex, is as follows: speech elements, syllables, words, phrases, sentences, and connected discourse. Any type of speech stimulus can be used in one of the following response-task paradigms, progressing from easy to difficult: detection, discrimination, identification, and comprehension. An informal assessment procedure, the Glendonald Auditory Screening Procedure (GASP)[34] focuses on three types of stimuli and response tasks: phoneme detection, word identification, and sentence comprehension. Erber recommends that the procedures be used in a face-to-face situation so that the clinician can employ adaptive (i.e., diagnostic) teaching techniques to develop appropriate intervention strategies. If, for example, the child gives an incorrect response when the stimulus is presented auditorily, then visual cues, tactile cues, or both can be added to determine if this improves performance.

The Phoneme Detection task requires the child to respond when isolated vowels and consonants (fricatives, affricates, nasals) are presented. Control trials are included in which no speech sound is presented. Inclusion of the control trails provides a means for estimating validity of the detection data. A high false-positive rate would suggest invalid data—possibly indicating that the child did not understand the task. The phoneme detection data can be compared to the audiometric data to determine if the results are reasonably consistent. In addition, detection data are clinically useful in considering auditory feedback capabilities for speech-sound production.

The Word Identification stimuli are divided into the following four sets: monosyllables, trochees, spondees, and three-syllable words. Through a picture-pointing response, estimates can be made as to whether the child's responses are based on segmental features of speech (correct identification of words) or if they are based on suprasegmental features (i.e., syllable number and stress). In the latter instance, the child is able to differentiate words between categories but not within a category. Children who perceive only the time and intensity patterns of speech should be able to identify stress pattern and syllable number (i.e., perform within category discrimination). Because these patterns of speech are also discriminable on the basis of vibrotactile sensation,[34] it cannot be assumed that performance is based on auditory perception. In contrast, identification of words correctly within each of the categories, requires the use of spectral cues, which implies perception on the basis of auditory sensation. Thus, the results of this type of test can help the clinician establish whether the child has residual auditory function. Children who can identify words are presumably "hearing" them whereas children who identify only stress pattern or syllable number may be "feeling" the distinctions. Results from the Word Identification subtest can be used to formulate a therapy approach with emphasis placed on tasks based on suprasegmental features (e.g., identification of phrases on the basis of rate, pitch, duration cues), or segmental features (e.g., comprehension of connected discourse).

The Sentence Comprehension subtest codes responses to ten questions according to presentation strategies used to cue comprehension: (1) auditory only; (2) auditory with emphasis on words or sounds; (3) auditory and visual; (4) gestures and (5) number of presentations. For children using total communication, it is often clinically useful to present incorrect items adding sign. Correct responses with signed input suggest the child's difficulty was due to the auditory demands rather than to language difficulties.

Hard-of-hearing children between the ages of three and four are typically able to respond correctly to most items on the GASP. Children with profound losses vary in their ability to respond appropriately. Factors that can account for the variation in performance include the ability to make use of available acoustic information, prior auditory training, and linguistic development. The child's linguistic development is important because it affects his or her ability to predict messages from the distorted auditory signal that is received.

A second tool for assessing speech perception based on auditory or vibrotactile cues is the Auditory Numbers Test (ANT).[80] The ANT is not as comprehensive as the GASP, but it can be used with younger profoundly hearing-impaired children (e.g., 3 years old) provided the child has basic number concepts. The test format requires the child to point to the number of ants based on detection of syllable number. For example, "one-two-three" is presented to elicit a response to three. Following the pattern-perception phase, spectral perception is assessed by saying the number only (e.g., "three"). If the child is responding based on pattern perception, he or she always indicates "one" to any of the numbers presented. Spectral perception is indicated by correct responses to individual numbers.

These tests are useful for establishing initial training objectives. The Word Identification subtest on the GASP and the ANT are helpful for estimating spectral versus pattern perception. It is important to note that results obtained with some children may initially suggest pattern perception only. However, after a period of systematic auditory training, retest results suggest spectral perception abilities. Until a child is given adequate training, it is impossible to determine the limitations that the hearing handicap has imposed on the auditory mechanism for speech processing.

Speech Production Skills

Because the speech problems of hearing-impaired children stem from inadequate control at nearly all levels of production, comprehensive assessment is crucial in this area. Ideally, the process should consist of physiologic analyses to identify the underlying source of the problems, acoustic measures to describe the speech characteristics in objective terms, and perceptual measures to determine what listeners actually hear in the child's speech. Unfortunately, physiologic and acoustic measures are not practical in most clinical situations, and the majority of assessment techniques that are available require perceptual analyses. Therefore, procedures that are suggested here are limited to those involving this form of analysis. Application of these procedures is assumed to be preceded by an oral-peripheral examination to identify gross structural and functional abnormalities.

Suprasegmental Skills

Assessment of suprasegmental (and segmental) skills should examine the child's ability to (1) monitor speech production via his or her residual hearing, and (2) produce the features of interest in a phonetic and phonologic context. Information relative to speech monitoring abilities can be obtained by observing the child's ability to produce targeted speech patterns on the basis of an auditory model only. The child's performance on selected tasks administered during the assessment of auditory skills, described in the previous section, also should be helpful. Production of motor speech patterns is examined in the phonetic level evaluation whereas the phonologic evaluation examines the child's ability to use these speech patterns in a systematic and meaningful way. Presumably, skills must be established at the phonetic level before they are used phonologically. Once established at the phonetic level, there is automatic transfer to the phonologic level, at least in the speech of normally developing children. Clinical observation suggests that the more hearing the child has, the greater the likelihood that automatic transfer will occur.[81,82] Systematic teaching often is required before the transfer from one level to the next occurs in the speech of profoundly hearing-impaired children.[81,82]

The procedure that is used more often to assess phonetic skills is the Phonetic Level Evaluation developed by Ling.[12] This is an imitation task, which requires the child to produce nonsense syllables with variations in duration, pitch, and loudness. Ideally, imitation is performed using only auditory cues. This provides the clinician with an opportunity to evaluate the child's ability to perceive and produce speech features through his or her residual hearing. If the child is unable to perform the production task, then additional cues (i.e., visual and/or tactile) are provided to determine if the incorrect production is due to a problem at the production level or the perception level. The child's productions are judged as correct, inconsistent, or incorrect with no indication of what problems occur when an incorrect or inconsistent production is made.

A problem with this test is that the child is required to produce speech changes that do not necessarily occur in spoken English. For example, changes in fundamental frequency (i.e., pitch) and intensity (i.e., loudness) occur together in normally produced speech to signal contrastive stress. The reason this happens is due to the physiologic changes that affect both of these aspects of speech at the same time. Thus, to perform an extensive evaluation (and subsequent training) of a child's ability to produce pitch and loudness changes independent of one another does not seem to be the best use of the clinician's or the child's time. Rather, evaluation of a child's ability to produce nonsense syllables with stress and intonation changes typical of spoken English appears to provide more relevant diagnostic information. Because no formal tests have been developed to assess these skills, informal procedures will have to be developed, such as those described by Osberger.[81] These procedures consist of production of nonsense syllables within a phrase structure. In particular, the child is asked to produce short phrases with a falling intonation contour or with changes in duration, pitch, and loudness to signal contrastive stress.

Unfortunately, Ling does not describe in any detail an evaluation technique to evaluate suprasegmental skills at the phonologic level. What ultimately happens is that these skills are not examined in the speech of most hearing-impaired children. As a consequence, clinicians consider the child's performance on the Phonetic Level Evaluation (i.e., production of isolated syllables with changes in duration, pitch, loudness) as representing changes in the suprasegmental aspects of speech. Informal procedures can be developed to assess suprasegmental skills at the phonologic as well as phonetic level. For example, once nonsense syllable sequences are developed to assess the stress and intonation patterns of English (as described above), the child's ability to produce these same patterns in phrases and sentences, using language that is meaningful to him or her, can be examined. Some children, especially those with more residual hearing, may be able to produce suprasegmental features in a phonologic context, but not a phonetic one.[82] It is important that this skill be identified so that unnecessary training is not devoted to nonsense syllable drill.

Attempts should be made to elicit productions from the child that will help to identify other abnormalities in production that occur frequently in the speech of the hearing impaired. Insertion of glottal stops and intrusive sounds between syllables is attributable to poor timing and reduced coarticulation skills. The clinician should have the child produce words with high and low vowels to identify possible vowel-related pitch problems. Exaggerated jaw and lip movements should also be noted.

Segmental Skills

Phonetic level skills are assessed commonly with the Phonetic Level Evaluation.[12] At the segmental level, the child is required to produce vowels in isolation and to produce single syllables containing all the consonants of English with [i], [a], and [u]. The syllables are then repeated and alternated to assess the child's coarticulation skills. Productions are elicited on an imitative basis using auditory cues only. This test provides a useful way to assess phonetic level skills; however, many clinicians terminate assessment after this measure is administered and fail to examine the child's phonologic skills.

Assessment of phonologic skills can be performed on a spontaneous speech sample (which can be the same sample elicited for language analysis) or the corpus can consist of the child's production of words using picture articulation tests. The clinician may need to modify aspects of the picture articulation testing to obtain all the information necessary to formulate an intervention program. One limitation of picture articulation tests is that they only sample production of consonants that are elicited in one word. The word may not be within the child's vocabulary, thereby resulting in elicitation of the production through imitation. Also, clinical experience suggests that many hearing-impaired children's articulation skills are lexically bound. That is, they learn how to produce the articulatory targets in restricted words (and phonetic contexts) because they are common words, which are well rehearsed in the child's speech. For example, the child might be able to say the word "dog" intelligibly, but is unable to produce [d] and [g] in other words. Further, articulation skills may be different when a target phoneme is produced in a word that is embedded in a sentence rather than when the word is produced in isolation.[58]

Intelligibility

There are few procedures to assess intelligibility in a clinical setting. In most research situations, a write-down procedure has been employed where a panel of listeners is asked to write down what they think a child is saying. This is a valid and reliable procedure, but it is not practical in most clinical settings. The procedure that has been used most often is a rating of intelligibility on a 1 to 5 scale.[83] This procedure can be administered in a relatively short period of time, but there are questions as to the reliability and validity of the procedure.[84]

A different approach is the use of forced-choice tests to evaluate intelligibility. The Speech Intelligibility Evaluation (SPINE) evaluates a child's ability to produce selected phonetic distinctions of English. The listener must decide, with a forced-choice format, which of four possible words the child has produced. The phonetic distinctions were selected on those that have been found to have a significant effect on intelligibility.[85] The test is relatively quick to administer and it provides quantitative information about the intelligibility of the child's speech. A limitation of the test is that it uses a written-read format, which restricts the range of children with whom it can be used. Also, to obtain improved scores over time requires substantial changes in the child's speech production abilities. Thus, the test appears most useful for obtaining performance data rather than using a measure to monitor change in skills.

A similar procedure has been developed by Boothroyd[86] and is referred to as the Speech Pattern Contrast test (SPAC). Use of this test provides information on the child's ability to produce the segmental features of vowel height, vowel place, and consonant place, voicing, and continuance in the initial and final positions of monosyllabic words.

Assessment Philosophy

Comprehension and production skills should be assessed in hearing-impaired children because they demonstrate deficits in both areas. Assessment of comprehension skills is particularly important because a hearing-impaired child's language problems stem from an inability to *perceive* spoken language in a normal fashion. A battery of formal and informal tests should be used to ensure that a range of linguistic skills are assessed in form, content, and function. Previous publications have suggested specific tests that are appropriate for use with hearing-impaired children.[8,71] In this chapter, the application of such measures with hearing-impaired children is presented. Informal assessment procedures most often are used within the context of diagnostic teaching. Information on these procedures is presented in the following section on Intervention.

The reasons for performing a language assessment are varied. One reason is to obtain a measure of *performance* on various linguistic tasks. When this is the objective, formal tests, which have been standardized on a population of children, are the best procedures to use. Most of the available tests have been standardized on children with normal hearing. Some clinicians have the notion that only tests standardized on hearing-impaired children should be used with this population. Even though there may be instances where it is desirable to compare the performance of a child relative to his or her hearing-impaired peers, more frequently the goal is to determine the delays and "deviancies" in a child's language abilities relative to normally developing children. If the tests are administered using total communication, then results should be interpreted with caution. This does not mean, however, that useful performance data cannot be obtained with these procedures.

If the intent is to measure a child's proficiency

in ASL, designs to assess English language skills are not appropriate. However, experience has shown that clinicians and teachers often assume that hearing-impaired children are using ASL when in fact they are using a pidgin sign system. It may be helpful to assess the language skills of these children with formal measures to determine their knowledge of English. Even if a child's primary language is ASL, valuable information can be obtained with respect to proficiency with English from the administration of tests standardized on children with normal hearing. In other words, use of such measures need not be viewed as "penalizing" the child for deficiencies in English language use, but rather they are used to obtain diagnostic information needed to develop intervention goals to promote English language acquisition. One caution in interpreting test results is that hearing-impaired children have been shown to demonstrate gaps in their knowledge. Thus, if a hearing-impaired child's score is consistent with a particular developmental level, it cannot be assumed that the hearing-impaired child's language abilities are the same as those of the normal-developing children on whom the test was standardized.

The information obtained from standardized measures also can be used to examine the child's performance over time. Even though a child may still demonstrate delays in language, relative to his or her normal-hearing peers, examination of test scores from one year to the next may show that he or she has made progress in language development. If comparison of a child's performance to hearing-impaired peers is desired, and there are no standardized data on the tasks of interest, the teacher or clinician can administer tests to a group of hearing-impaired children in their school. The average performance of the children can be calculated and then the scores of each child can be compared to the average of the peer group. If a child's performance falls below (e.g., 1 standard deviation) the mean then learning problems, in addition to those imposed by the handicap, might account for the below average performance.[7] On the other hand, if a child scores above the mean, then an accelerated language and academic program might be indicated. This application of formal tests provides *diagnostic* information for intervention planning and is not meant to replace the use of standardized data.

Formal measures can be used in a variety of ways to obtain diagnostic information. In these instances, scores are not reported, but test items are used as probes to identify areas of strength and weakness. However, if the clinician exposes the child to a number of the items on the test, the items cannot be used at a later time to obtain performance data on this same measure. If testing at a later date is planned, then analogous items that assess the same concepts can be developed for diagnostic teaching. During administration of formal tests, task analysis can be performed by the clinician to obtain information about a child's learning style.[71] Some behaviors to note include the following abilities: to attend to a structured task, to problem solve, to use prompts and multisensory cues, and to retrieve information. Impulsive behavior, low frustration level, and word-finding problems also should be noted.

The clinician needs to be aware of the nonlinguistic strategies that the child might use in testing situations. Because a hearing-impaired child's cognitive skills might exceed linguistic skills, it is important to determine if the child is using linguistic or nonlinguistic strategies during the process of evaluation (and during intervention). This can become problematic during testing because the delayed language skills of the hearing-impaired child often necessitate administration of tests designed for use with younger children with normal hearing. In this situation, a hearing-impaired child might be able to take advantage of certain nonlinguistic cues that a younger child, for whom the test was developed, would not know or use.

Language Sampling

Many of the language problems of hearing-impaired children are best assessed from analysis of spontaneous language samples. Obtaining both narrative and conversational segments is recommended. Analysis of the narrative segment yields information on syntactic complexity, descriptions, sequencing a series of events, and cause and effect explanations. From a conversational analysis, the child's skills as an initiator and responder can be assessed. Conversational samples are useful for developing hypotheses about comprehension of syntactic and semantic features. It also is important to assess the ability to take turns around a topic, and use of clarification strategies when he or she doesn't understand.

Procedures for eliciting, recording, transcribing and analyzing spontaneous language samples are discussed in detail in Miller.[87]

Sampling considerations with the hearing-impaired population include elicitation of the sample by a person familiar with the child's signs and/or speech. If an unfamiliar person is involved, it is likely that the child would compensate for poor speech or sign intelligibility by modification or simplification of language. A second sampling issue is that of using video recording. For children using a manual or a total communication system, video taping is necessary for accurate transcription and provides a means to record utterances from all speakers (not just the child). Speaker interaction is helpful for analyzing the child's comprehension and his or her role as a responder. Utterances from all speakers should be coded for modality-use: verbalization, sign, vocalization, or combinations of them. Interaction of syntactic complexity and presentation modality may affect the child's response behaviors.

As described in Miller,[87] quantitative and qualitative analyses can be performed on the language sample. Mean length of utterance (MLU) can be calculated for both oral and total communication samples. However, caution is advised, in using normative data that correlates age with MLU, especially for samples collected from children who use total communication. Assumptions made about syntactic development from MLU cannot be applied to samples in manually coded English because increases in mean length of signed utterances frequently reflect increases in content and free functors rather than grammatical morphemes.

INTERVENTION PROCEDURES

Auditory Skills

Auditory management goals and procedures begin during informal assessment and diagnostic teaching when the child's strengths and weaknesses are determined. At this time, cues, feedback, and modifications in the acoustic environment, which are helpful for the child, are explored. The areas of focus for auditory management include the amplification system; use of residual hearing for speech, language, academic, and communication purposes in therapy settings and in the classroom; and examination of acoustic environment.

Amplification Issues

Listening and visual checks of the hearing aid are critical to increasing the percentage of functioning systems. All school personnel having regular interaction with the child, and all family members should be trained to inspect the hearing aid. Data have revealed that at any given time in the school day 30 to 70 percent of the children's hearing aids are not working properly.[88–92] Hearing-aid monitoring should not be the responsibility of only one person (e.g., audiologist or teacher). Diefendorf and Arthur[93] instituted a parent focused hearing-aid monitoring program. Results of their program revealed a decrease in malfunction rate from 30 percent before training to 5 percent after training with most of the problems continuing to be weak or dead batteries. Their study also showed that a visual and listening check failed to identify electroacoustic problems less than 1 percent of the time. Results from this study and that of Lotterman, Kasten and Majerus[94] suggest that listening checks should be performed at the end of the day. Reduced battery voltage is more likely to be detected at the end of the day than in the morning after a period of "no load" being placed on the battery.

It also is important to perform listening checks at the beginning of the day and before auditory training sessions. These listening checks should be performed with a listening scope or personal earmold. Clicks, distortion, or weak volume should be noted. The five-sound test[95] is useful for listening across the frequency range. A visual inspection of the aid reveals the presence of moisture in the tubing, worn or frayed cords, or a cracked case. For further information on hearing aid monitoring see Diefendorf and Arthur,[93] Hanners and Sitten,[96] and Riedner.[91]

It is recommended that the child be involved in the monitoring program. With practice, a typical 3 to 4 year old can remove and insert the battery, use a battery tester, inspect the tubing, and remove moisture, if present. In our experience, a child can independently insert the earmold in his or her ear by 4 to 4½ years of age. Showing the child a visual display of the results of the daily hearing-aid check helps to increase motivation and participation in the monitoring program.

Classroom Observations

Observational data are crucial for determining how the child uses his or her residual hearing in daily environments. Among observations to make about the child are the ability to (1) participate in class discussions, (2) grasp concepts presented through auditory-verbal modality, (3) learn new words and predict meaning from context, (4) understand directions, (5) take lecture notes, and (6) respond to auditory failure. The child's ability to use auditory skills for speech development and monitoring also should be noted. Behaviors to observe include the ability to pronounce new words and to monitor the loudness level of speech. Any difference in the child's performance in quiet and noisy situations should be noted.

Manipulation of the Acoustic Environment

Environmental modifications include improving the signal-to-noise ratio by reducing the noise, increasing the level of the signal, or both. Studies have shown that hearing-impaired listeners require more favorable signal-to-noise ratios to understand speech than do listeners with normal hearing.[97,101] The average sound pressure levels (SPL) in the classroom have been measured at 60 to 70 dB SPL.[97,98] Signal:noise (S:N) ratios in these settings are frequently no better than +5 dB.[97] Classroom noise is of two general types, constant and fluctuating. Constant noise comes from fans, air conditioners, or spill over from adjacent classrooms. Fluctuating noise is from hallway noise, chairs moving, or speech. Reverberation, the prolongation of sound after the source has ceased vibrating, is another form of noise, which affects understanding of speech. Reverberation is reduced when absorbent materials (carpeting, drapery, cork boards, acoustic tiles, or over-stuffed chairs) replace hard reflective surfaces (ceramic tile, linoleum, wooden walls and ceilings, blackboards, and wooden or metal chairs).

FM systems are an effective means for achieving a good S:N ratio. These systems have a microphone/transmitter worn around the teacher's-speaker's neck and a receiver/hearing aid worn by the child. The receiver can be wired to snap-on transducers and earmolds or used with personal hearing aids either through direct attachment or through the aid's telecoil via an induction loop worn around the child's neck. A study by Ross, Giolas, and Carver[101] revealed mean word discrimination scores obtained in classroom listening conditions to be 36 percent better with the FM system than with the child's usual amplification condition.

Intervention with an FM system requires routine charging of the system batteries, monitoring the FM system, and switching microphone input according to the listening conditions. FM systems typically allow listening to the teacher-speaker via the FM signal. This provides the best S:N ratio condition.

A second listening condition is the FM signal and/or environmental microphone. This gives a poorer S:N ratio, but allows the child to hear other speakers and his or her voice for speech monitoring. Use of an environmental microphone is especially useful for class discussions; lecture or small-group instruction is best in the FM signal only condition.

In addition to using an FM system to improve S:N ratio and making modifications in the acoustic properties of the environment, seating arrangements relative to the speech and noise source can contribute to improved listening conditions. In a classroom setting, seating should be arranged to have the major noise source to the side of the child and signal straight ahead.

FM systems and acoustic engineering can provide a significant improvement in the environment. Many modifications can occur to create an optimal acoustic environment at home and at school. However, frequently the child will need to listen in poor conditions. Intervention focusing on developing auditory skills in noise is recommended. Structured training should include listening in noise. Using tape recorded competing signals allows a means for altering the S:N ratio and the spatial arrangement of the signal and noise typical of the child's environment.

Application of Auditory-Skills Intervention Principles

Integration of auditory speech and language goals provides the most effective intervention program. This includes auditory-only practice with stimuli selected for speech and language intervention. When first teaching a language or speech skill, presenting multiple cues to the child (e.g., auditory, visual via speechreading, gesture, or sign) assists initial skill acquisition. Auditory only or auditory and speech reading practice is frequently helpful at all stages of development from initial performance levels through generalization. Use of a procedure such as the GASP,[34] described previously, provides information for formulation of specific intervention goals. Difficulties on this measure suggest those tasks that should be focused on in therapy. Application of this technique is demonstrated below. The application of speech and language intervention principles is also demonstrated with this child.

SK age 7, has a profound bilateral mixed hearing loss of unknown etiology and of unknown age of onset; although his adoptive parents suspect the onset to be shortly after birth. Figure 29–1 shows his responses to pure-tone stimuli. Due to foster home placements and occupation-related moves by his adoptive parents, intervention programming has been inconsistent.

SK communicates primarily through sign. He has a history of malfunctioning hearing aids and inconsistent cooperation with wearing the aids. Recently, he has had surgical intervention to repair a perforated tympanic membrane.

Results of testing from the GASP are shown in Table 29–1. Intervention focused on (1) increased consistency of hearing aid use, (2) increased identification and comprehension of suprasegmental features, and (3) increased perception of segmental speech features.

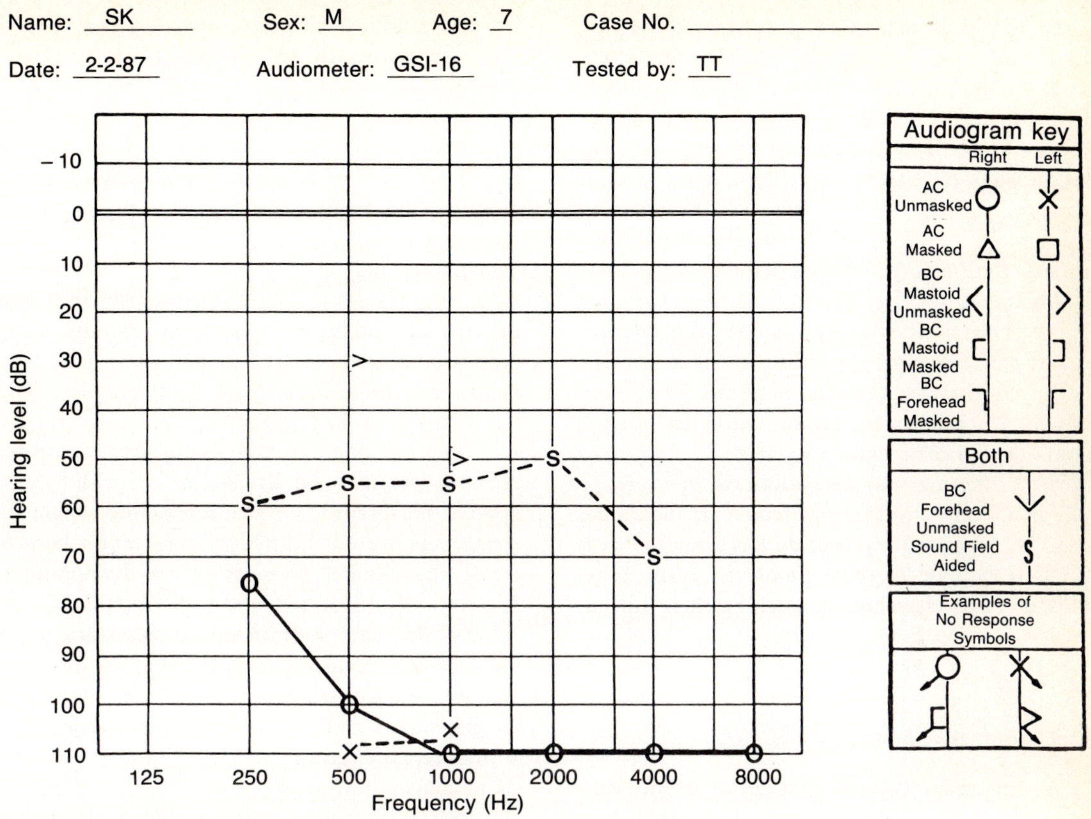

Figure 29–1 SK's audiogram.

A list of daily phrases used at home was gathered from the parent. These phrases were analyzed in terms of similarity and dissimilarity on the basis of duration, intonation pattern, and rate. Examples of phrases included "put the plates on the table," "hurry, the bus is coming!" "wash your face," "time to eat." Training focused on correct identification of the phrases based on suprasegmental cues. During training sessions, the phrases were presented by the parent using live-voice or on an audio-tape card. Within a few sessions, SK was able to identify consistently the phrases on the basis of key segmental features (e.g., recognition of /e/ cued him to the correct identification of "wash your face"). At home, the parents used these phrases with auditory or auditory-visual (i.e., speechreading) presentation. They reported positive responses to increasing the range of alternatives ("put the mustard on the table," "put the milk on the table," "put the sugar on the table").

During practice sessions, SK spontaneously imitated the intonation patterns. Intonation contours and syllabic maintenance were not previously present in his spontaneous or imitated speech production.

Speech Production Skills

A major problem in developing an intervention program to improve the speech skills of hearing-im-

TABLE 29–1 SK's Performance on the GASP

Subtest	*Performance*
Detection	
Vowels	All vowels detected except /i/
Consonants	Nasals, liquids, glides detected; no fricatives or affricates
Word identification	
Identification	3/18 (17%)
Categorization	14/18 (78%)
Sentence comprehension	
Auditory only	0/10 (0%)
Auditory plus speechreading	0/10 (0%)
Auditory plus signs	9/10 (90%)

paired children is that most professionals who are charged with the responsibility of delivering these services are inadequately trained to do so.[102] Often, individual time designated for speech and language training is devoted to language issues only, with little or no attention directed toward improving speech (or auditory) skills. Further, activities to promote the carry-over of speech skills to meaningful contexts are often missing in the classroom.

Another difficulty is that budget constraints often preclude most school programs from offering adequate support services in this area. It is not unusual to find that one clinician may serve 30 or more children. A child may receive individual speech training only once or twice a week for a brief period of time or training may be performed with groups of children. Some children may receive no individual training in speech development during periods of their education. Because of these problems, many hearing-impaired children are not reaching their full potential in oral skill development.

Selecting Intervention Goals

An important issue in developing an intervention program is establishing realistic expectations. The more severe the hearing loss, the greater the likelihood that many features of speech will have to be taught directly to the child. Children who are hard of hearing, and even many who have severe hearing losses require less focused training and drill than children with profound losses. However, the degree of hearing loss should not be used to set limits on the child's potential to develop intelligible speech. Even though there is a close relationship between production and perception skills, it is evident that hearing-impaired children learn to produce many aspects of speech that they do not hear.[30] That is, it cannot be assumed that the only modality that the child uses for speech learning and monitoring purposes is the auditory one. On the other hand, the majority of children with profound hearing losses do not develop "normal" sounding speech. The goal of therapy with these children is development of functional speech skills. It is most useful to view intelligibility as spanning a continuum rather than representing a single level of performance. Some children's speech skills develop to the point where they are able to communicate orally with a wide range of people, whereas functional speech usage for other children means that they can be understood by a limited number of people in restricted contexts.

Several different approaches may be used to select training objectives, each of which relies on careful scrutiny of the assessment results. Training objectives identified with each type of approach might not differ very much. One approach is to analyze the test results in terms of those skills that need to be developed using a prescribed training sequence. An example of this is use of the results from the Phonetic Level Evaluation, which selects objectives based on a specific training program.[12] At the phonetic level of training, the skills and subskills are well defined by Ling, thereby making it relatively easy to use the results of the Phonetic Level Evaluation to plan an intervention program. Because Ling's evaluation procedures are less defined for phonologic skills, it is more difficult to select training objectives for this area of work.

Another approach is to examine the assessment results in terms of the diversity of each child's sound system. For example, a goal for a child whose consonant repertoire is limited to stops might be to increase the number of contrasts by developing the fricative feature or the oral-nasal distinction. Another child may be omitting all word-final consonants so that focus of therapy might be to increase the number of contrasts in the post-vocalic position. At the suprasegmental level, the goal might be to introduce Fo contrasts to signal phrase boundaries or to convey contrastive stress.

Selecting training objectives also might be based on correcting those errors that appear to have the greatest effect on the intelligibility of the child's speech.[38] For example, if a child has extreme variations in pitch, this problem might be corrected not only for the purpose of helping the child produce a more pleasant sounding voice but to assist in achieving greater control and coordination of respiratory, laryngeal, and articulatory gestures. This will more than likely lead to improved production of other aspects of speech including segmental features.

Training Strategies

The majority of speech training programs that have been developed for use with hearing-impaired children are descriptive in nature, and they lack empirical data that demonstrate the effectiveness of the proposed procedures. Some available data show that certain features of speech can be improved in the speech of profoundly hearing-impaired talkers when intense and systematic training procedures are applied.[81,103–105]

The training program that is used most often is the one developed by Ling. His approach employs a highly structured and systematic scheme that develops speech skills using residual hearing to the fullest possible extent. Two major principles that underlie Ling's speech training program are as follows: (1) speech skills are developed in the hearing-impaired child in the same order as they occur in the child with normal hearing; (2) speech should be taught within a dynamic framework, focusing on the rapid and precise movements required to produce intelligible speech. The assessment procedures described above reflect the strategies of the training program. That is, speech is developed at the phonetic and phonologic levels. Motor-production skills are first developed in nonsense syllables, progressing from isolated syllable production to strings of repeated and alternated syllables. Once production at the phonetic level has been mastered, the skills are assumed to transfer to phonologic use. The program also contains a suggested order of training for the segmental and suprasegmental features of speech.

Since it was introduced, Ling's[12] training program has been used by a large number of professionals. Unfortunately, it also has been misused by a number of these people. There are many positive aspects to the program that have wide application to the development of speech production skills in hearing-impaired children. The program, however, is a developmental one and is most appropriate for use with young hearing-impaired children (infants and preschoolers). Aspects of the program also have application to remedial speech training with older students, but not without modification. For example, if it is determined that erratic variations in pitch should be corrected in the speech of an adolescent, some of the teaching strategies in Ling's program can be applied during training. To begin at Stage One of Ling's program to develop suprasegmental skills in an adolescent is inappropriate. No doubt many school-age hearing-impaired students have been subjected to hours of nonsense syllable drill with little or no change in their speech. Correction and or development of some patterns in the speech of these children might not be realistic.

The application of Ling's teaching program has resulted in most clinicians and teachers initiating training with nonsense-syllable drill with little or no attention paid to phonologic use. Osberger[81] found that drill work on strings of nonsense syllables produced with differing voice patterns (duration, intensity, loudness) did not train the children to produce the suprasegmental features of English. For example, a child might have been able to produce a syllable with a low, mid, and high-pitched voice, but this skill in and of itself did not guarantee that the child would be able to produce the subtle changes in fundamental frequency typical of spoken English. This is not to say that use of nonsense syllables is never appropriate. Rather, the clinician should be aware of what the use of nonsense syllables is really training the child to do.

Modified procedures have been described by Osberger[81] to develop duration patterns needed to convey changes in stress. Work on loudness, or intensity, was restricted to helping the child learn to use appropriate voice levels based on the context in which speech was being used (e.g., a whisper in the library, and a loud voice or shout when calling to a friend down the street). Suggested training goals for pitch control are directed toward helping the child learn to produce the various intonation contours of English. The skills were developed first using nonsense syllables within a phrase structure. After these were mastered by the children, the same patterns were applied to phrases containing vocabulary and language that were familiar. This approach allows the clinician to integrate speech and language goals and to develop auditory skills if speech is elicited from the child using only auditory cues.

Dunn and Newton[82] have developed a model for speech development in hearing-impaired children, which incorporates practice on phonetic and phonologic skills concurrently. With this approach, emphasis is placed on learning motor production skills within the context of words rather than nonsense syllables to promote the integration of motoric, auditory, and linguistic skill. This approach appears to have application to a wide range of hearing-impaired children. However, for those children who have very limited speech skills, use of nonsense syllables to establish basic production patterns appears unavoidable.

Integration of Speech, Language, and Auditory Skill Development

Many clinicians have the notion that speech training only consists of structured training sessions geared toward development of specific features of speech. Work on generalization of these skills usually consists of drills with key phonemes and words inserted in phrases and sentences. Insufficient attention is usually directed toward developing conversational speech skills. Development of these skills can also be incorporated into speech training sessions. It is an important feature of training for children of all ages because it helps them to develop effective communication strategies and pragmatic use of language.

An approach to developing pragmatic use of speech skills is use of connected discourse tracking.[106] The tracking technique was originally developed to assess and train speech reception skills,[107] but it has been used to train speech production skills as well. A team of two people is required; one person serves as the sender, and the other individual serves as the receiver. The sender reads successive segments from a prepared text (e.g., a simple story), and the receiver must repeat verbatim what has been said. If the segment is not understood correctly, the sender can use various verbal strategies to aid the receiver's comprehension such as repeating the missed segment, rephrasing, and exaggerating segments. Performance is measured in number of words of text repeated correctly per unit of time. This performance measure can be used both as an index of efficiency of communication and to quantify progress over time. Applied as a speech training procedure, the hearing-impaired child is required to read the text to the clinician. If used to train speechreading and auditory skills, the clinician can read the text to the child.

Use of the tracking technique for speech training with a small group of profoundly hearing-impaired children has demonstrated the feasibility of using this method in speech training sessions.[106] The children enjoyed the task and appeared highly motivated to participate. Some of the students were surprised that their speech could be understood without the use of signs. They developed greater awareness of some of the articulation errors in their speech and self-corrected them. The children also learned to use various repair and clarification strategies when they were not understood. These strategies included chunking, repetition, paraphrasing, defining, or spelling missed words. Learning these strategies was a substantial achievement for some of the students.

A modification of this approach requires the child to communicate with others using speech only in situations where the potential for both learning and success are high. The difficulty of the situation (for both the child and the listener) can be varied systematically along three dimensions: the listener, the situation, and the content of the message. A relatively easy situation would employ a listener who is familiar with the child's speech. Communication would occur in a familiar situation with predictable comments, and the child would be required to transmit only the gist of the message to the listener. For a child who is successful at this level, the difficulty of the task could be increased by decreasing the amount of experience that the listener has in hearing the speech of the child, decreasing the contextual and situational cues, and increasing the level of the content to be delivered (i.e., conveying key words and phrases in the message). During the conversation, the child is required to understand what is said by the other person, which helps to develop the use of speechreading and auditory skills at the same time as speech and language skills. This technique can be applied in training sessions as well as in classroom or home situations.

Application of Speech Training Principles

SK's performance on the Phonetic Level Evaluation revealed that he was able to vary the duration and loudness of his vocalizations but not the pitch. Elicitation of the consonants and vowels was accomplished via fingerspelling and written cues as SK was unsuccessful in producing the targets using only audition and vision (speechreading). He was able to produce /a, u/ and /aI/ and /b, f,/ and /h/ correctly, and /m/ inconsistently in single and repeated consonant-vowel (CV) syllables. His spontaneous speech consisted of vocalizations with no recognizable sounds of English that were not produced in a one-to-one correspondence with signed productions. The vocalizations were continuous with no evidence of even syllable boundaries.

The goals of speech training were to increase range of pitch change in his voice, to produce variations in duration of phonation to approximate syllable number, to produce vocalizations on different loudness levels, to produce /b/ and /f/ in consonant-vowel-consonant (CVC) words. Activities were designed to stimulate vocal variations in relation to or dependent upon a specific event. Examples of the activities are: hiding an object (toy lion figure) in the room and using vocal intensity to give cues to the seeker as to its location (e.g., loud voice = object farther away, soft voice = object closer); using pitch to indicate the color of pegs desired for a "Lite-Brite" picture; changing duration of vocalization in response to the movement of a string being pulled by SK through the clinician's fingers. During training sessions, an auditory model was provided by the clinician in addition to visual, gestural, and tactile cues.

To stimulate sound production, drill with direct imitation of the clinician's model was employed. Visual and auditory cues were used to stimulate sound production. Sounds were practiced in syllables and words through repeated drill games (e.g., "concentration" or board games). Word pairs that differed in the initial consonant (e.g., bunny versus funny) were used to stimulate auditory and visual (speechreading) awareness of the cues associated with each sound. At the end of 3 months of training, SK was able to vary his pitch correctly in nonsense syllables and in meaningful situations (e.g., he used three different pitch levels when retelling the story of Goldilocks and the Three Bears). He was able to control the overall loudness of his voice on demand. He was also producing approximations of the number of syllables in utterances (e.g., the short phrases used to develop auditory skills).

Correct production of /b/ in CVC words increased from 30 percent accuracy in direct imitation (auditory and visual cues) to 80 percent accuracy after 3 months of training. The CVC productions at the end of training were not elicited via imitation but rather in response to questions (e.g., "What does a dog eat?" "bone"). Prior to training, SK could produce /f/ in CV syllables with about 80 percent accuracy in direct imitation. At the end of the training period, he was able to produce /f/ in a select group of CVC words in response to a question about 80 percent of the time. SK also learned to produce pairs of words that were identical except for the initial sounds (e.g., /b/ or /f/) in direct imitation using visual and auditory cues with 60 percent accuracy.

Language Skills

Probes and Diagnostic Teaching

Task and error analyses from formal tests and hypotheses from language sample analysis should be used for developing probes in which stimulus and response variables are systematically manipulated to reveal more closely a child's strengths and weaknesses, concept understanding, or confusion. When designing probes, careful attention needs to be given to the directions, cues and prompts, materials used and response format. The clinician should have a clear idea of the desired or correct response. Probes that do not have an adequate number of trials or an unspecified target response are of limited usefulness in planning effective intervention programs. Criterion-reference data are often a helpful guide for choosing stimuli and for response specification.[108]

Given the language problems of hearing-impaired children, probes and diagnostic teaching are frequently designed to identify factors that might facilitate the development of form, content, and function of language.

Form

Probes of form may focus on the child's ability to use clinician expansion, modeling, or contrastive drill for production of grammatical morphemes or syntactical structures. Strategies helpful for comprehension of these morphemes and structures often include visualization with objects or actions, or pairing simplified or chunked utterances with syntactically complex utterances. For example, "Neither the boy nor the girl came to the party" could be presented as, "the boy did not come. The girl did not come."

Frankmann, Herman, MacKain, and Oyer[109] explored strategies for training comprehension of passive voice in hearing-impaired children. Findings suggested differences in generalization between two orders of training with the nonreversible, reversible, agent-deleted order being better than agent-deleted, nonreversible, reversible order.

Content

Results from the Definitions subtest on the Test of Oral Language Development-Primary,[110] the Word Test,[111] and subtests from the Woodcock-Johnson Psycho-Educational Battery[112] may suggest that the need for diagnostic teaching to develop in-depth word knowledge. Three teaching strategies to promote development of this skill are semantic mapping, semantic feature analysis and contextual analysis.[113]

A semantic map (Fig. 29–2) is a visual tool to categorize and show relationships between words. The clinician can use the map to promote classification skills and discuss attributes. When used interactively, the clinician or child can introduce categories and describe attributes. Independent map development can reflect the child's depth of word knowledge and word relationships, and provide a basis for intervention.

Figure 29–3 shows an example of semantic feature analysis. This tool illustrates similarities and differences of words within a category. Discussion of features often results in providing new information to the child; information that can be linked to previous knowledge or experience. Comparing and contrasting categorical items can facilitate complex sentence development (e.g., palaces and apartments are alike because they are both places for people to live) as well as promote word knowledge.

Contextual analysis is a critical skill for hearing-impaired children. These children often receive partial information because of auditory-speech perception deficits, ambiguities from signed input, and/or an inadequate linguistic framework. In cases where a key word is unfamiliar, contextual analysis can often result in discovery of word meaning. Johnson, Toms-Bronowski, and Pittelman discuss three clue types for contextual analysis: direct explanation, appositive, and contrast.[113] Direct explanations are simplified definitions (e.g., annoyed implies being up-

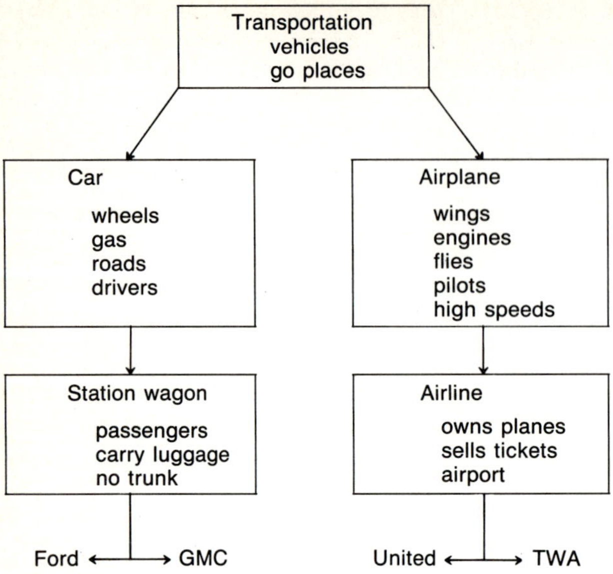

Figure 29-2 Example of a semantic map.

set or bothered by something). Appositives are words or clauses restating the previous text (e.g., he was quite annoyed, or irritated, to have the mosquitoes buzzing and biting all night). Contrast cues explain the opposite meaning of the term (e.g., when the annoying mosquitoes left, the people could again enjoy the park). The clinician may want to probe the child's predictive skills using a cloze procedure (e.g., the soccer team scored another ________). The cues or context which help with completion can then be identified and discussed. Sentences providing elaborate context or descriptive explanations can be used for predicting word meaning (e.g., ants and bees at a picnic are annoying).

Function

Results from language sample analyses, the Preschool Language Assessment Inventory (PLAI)[114] and Test of Problem Solving (TOPS),[115] can be helpful for identifying areas of language function needing further focus. Observation and probes of language function are useful for investigating the child's skills in discourse, clarification, expressing a repertoire of functions, and sequencing and content organization.

Observational data from parent-child and teacher-child interactions help to determine if the child's general environment is one that facilitates communicative interaction. Starck and Spitz[116] have identified several facilitators and nonfacilitators for adult-child interaction. Adult use of descriptions, models, expansions, open-ended questions, pause time, and turn-taking were found to enhance communication. Nonfacilitators included questions that did not elicit more or new information, directives, exact repetitions without pause time for a child's response, non responsiveness to the child's verbal or nonverbal behavior, and empty positive reinforcers (e.g., "good job").

In addition to adult input, a child's discourse skills depend on comprehension of questions at various levels of abstraction.[74] Blank, Rose, and Berlin[114]

	Has Wheels	Uses Gas	Uses Wind	Enclosed	For Emergency
Pickup	X	X		X	
Fire engine	X	X		X	X
Glider			X	X	
Motorcycle	X	X			
Canoe					
Sailboat			X		
Helicopter		X		X	X

Figure 29–3 Example of semantic feature analysis.

use four levels of abstraction (1) matching perception, (2) selective analysis of perception, (3) reordering perception, and (4) reasoning about perception. As discussed previously, hearing-impaired children have difficulty responding to and initiating utterances of increased abstraction.[74] Blank et al[114] provide several examples helpful for the integration of question abstraction into language learning activities. In addition to level of abstraction or question form, other factors may affect a child's ability to comprehend and respond to discourse demands. For example, the child may not understand that a question has been asked and a response is expected. For the child with normal hearing, intonation cues and altered stress patterns mark questions. For the hearing-impaired child, decoding sign, extralinguistic cues consisting of facial expression and pause while extending the final sign, can signal that a question has been asked.[114] A signed question mark also serves to mark questions. Infrequent use of these markers has been noted during parent-child interaction.[117] Semantic and syntactic constraints also figure prominantly in a child's ability to answer questions. Moeller, Osberger, and Eccarius[117] suggest several prompts for promoting question comprehension: refocus child and repeat; model with related content; analogous examples; visualization; and relevant yes/no comparison. Analysis of prompt effectiveness is useful for determining factors affecting question comprehension.

Successful conversation depends on requesting clarification when incomplete information is given or part of the message is not understood. Observational data and contrived situations are useful for analyzing a child's use of clarification. Moeller et al[117] have developed a checklist procedure to analyze a child's use of clarification strategies. It focuses on four levels of clarification: (1) failure to seek clarification; (2) verbal or nonverbal indication of nonunderstanding; (3) acknowledgment of input and indication of inability to answer; and (4) specific request for clarification. They also recommend observation in three contexts: discussion of a familiar topic; discussion of a new topic; and contrived pragmatic violation (i.e., a situation in which the clinician omits critical information).

In addition to requesting clarification, the child needs to provide clarification when he or she is not understood. Observational data collected with familiar and unfamiliar listeners are often helpful for determining the child's revision behaviors. That is, does the child repeat the previous response verbatim, or make semantic or syntactic revisions when no clarification is requested. A study by Hughes and James[118] revealed that, in general, school-age profoundly hearing-impaired children revised their original utterance in response to a listener's request for clarification. Failure to make revisions was usually associated with poorer grammatical skills.

Strategies for communicative enhancement that revolve around comments on the "here and now," basic needs, and social routines have been explored for use in interactions with hearing-impaired children. One strategy or tool for promoting social interaction is sociodramatic or interactive play.[119,120] Unlike free play, sociodramatic play is goal oriented and is designed to stimulate interactive language. The clinician serves as a facilitator providing prompts and ideas for interaction. Both child and clinician assume roles using a script. Initially, familiar events are represented with realistic props (e.g., shopping or McDonalds sequence). Gradually the props, event, familiarity, and facilitator role are reduced and language and cognitive demands are increased. Two levels of assessment are helpful for planning interactive play: (1) level of social participation; and (2) cognitive level. DeMaio[119] discusses the following six categories of social participation: unoccupied behavior, onlooker behavior, solitary-independent play, parallel play, associative play, and cooperative play. The first three levels are considered unsocial and the last three social. The social levels are differentiated by increased material exchange and the purpose, or goal, of play. Parallel play is defined as the child playing independently but choosing materials and activities similar to other children. No attempt is made to exchange materials. In associative play, the child engages in activities with other children and shares materials, but there is no group purpose. Cooperative play is organized with specific purposes and with participants having defined roles. Based on Piaget's work,[121] scales for assessment of symbolic play have been developed.[122,123] Results of these assessments are useful for integrating symbolic representation with social levels of behavior. It is important to note that these levels of play interact and that a child in preoperational development may have play behaviors ranging from solitary play, which is dramatic in nature to parallel play with intentional manipulation of objects for creating structures. Examples of interactive play procedures are presented in the case example below and in Moeller and McConkey[120] and Yoshinaga-Itano and Downey.[124]

Application of Language Intervention Principles

The following case information on 7-year-old SK should highlight some of the issues presented in language assessment and intervention.

From a nonstandard presentation of the Test of

Auditory Comprehension of Language-Revised (TACL-R),[125] it was noted that SK had difficulty understanding clauses with pronominal referents (the girl said we're eating popcorn); question forms (who is by the table?); negatives (it's not a cup); passive voice (the boy is chased by the dog), and conjunctions (the lady is eating a banana and the man is drinking milk). Analysis of the narrative language sample revealed a mean length of utterance of 5.0 morphemes. SK's syntactical structures were characterized by article + noun + verb + prepositional phrase; noun + auxiliary + present progressive verb, and noun + adjective. Prepositions were used consistently, whereas the use of articles and auxiliary forms was inconsistent. Plurals, possessives, past tense, and copular forms were omitted. Most of SK's utterances related to the "here and now"; he described salient points and relayed the sequence and emotional detail of the pictured story. SK consistently used greetings and polite forms. He clarified statements by rephrasing or requesting the clinician to consult with his parents. He would fail to seek clarification, although puzzled looks and "I don't know" responses were observed at times. Conversation and interactive play showed limited verbal and nonverbal interaction with the clinician. Parental report showed a tendency to play alone even though an older sibling with good signing skills created an environment in which interactive play was possible. Initial attempts by the clinician to facilitate interactive play revealed SK's difficulty in assuming a role and developing a theme. His tendency was to "fly away" wanting to be chased. Based on the error analysis of the TACL-R and limited conversation, comprehension of question forms and level of abstraction was probed. At concrete levels (i.e., matching perception and selective analysis of perception),[114] SK could answer yes/no questions consistently. He was inconsistent in answering what, what-doing, or where questions. His inconsistency appeared to reflect a vocabulary deficit. His responses were gestures or "I don't know" and he only occasionally gave related responses, such as "where" answers for "what" questions. With increased abstraction (using language to predict, reflect on, and integrate ideas and relationships), SK typically provided no response. It was hypothesized that increased abstraction, syntactic complexity, and vocabulary deficits contributed to his difficulty at this level.

Therapy focused on expansion of expressive and receptive language skills through interactive play. Specific objectives were (1) to engage in cooperative play through continued interaction of a sociodramatic dialogue with the clinician; (2) assume a role to dramatize a script from everyday experiences; (3) respond to clinician questions relating to interactive play (e.g., why is the baby crying?)

Fisher-Price toys (hospital, McDonalds), kitchen and restaurant props, toy shopping cart, and toy telephones were used to represent everyday scripts. (SK had recently been in the hospital for minor surgery, hence the hospital props). The clinician prompted interactive play using self talk, verbalization or sign of own activities; parallel talk, verbalization or sign of SK's activities; modeling, verbalization or sign of common scripts while playing (time for dinner! come and eat!); expansion, repeating SK's utterance in correct grammatical form (SK: baby cry. Clinician: the baby is crying.); expatiation, broadening the content of SK's utterances and expressing relationships (SK: Baby cry. Clinician: The baby is crying because she is hungry).

Initially, SK did not understand assuming a role of a Fisher-Price figure (e.g., mom, dad, boy) and did not respond to initiations made by the clinician's figure. After repeated attempts during a 15-minute period, SK responded with his figure nonverbally. The format was changed to more real-life props associated with restaurant and shopping scripts, with the hope that manipulating abstraction level would positively affect SK's responsiveness. Within three 15-minute play periods over a 1½-week time span, SK was able to sustain cooperative play. Data collected during the sessions showed 13 initiations of dialogue and a 90 percent response rate to the clinician over the 15-minute play segment. SK's interaction revealed information about his world knowledge. When the clinician in her role as customer said to the waiter (SK) that her pretend hamburger was cold, he took it to the kitchen area; placed it in the imaginary microwave, pushed buttons, waited, removed it, and returned it to the clinician saying it was now hot. While role playing paying the bill, SK brought money to the customer with the bill. When the customer left a tip under the plate, SK truly thought the play money was real money and that it was for him.

Recommendations for continued therapy include increased question comprehension during interactive play (Why are you going to the doctor? Are you sick? Do you need a check-up?) In addition, facilitative strategies continue to be assessed for their effectiveness in promoting linguistic development. Level of abstraction during interactive play should be increased through gradual reduction in realistic props.

SUMMARY

The pervasive effects of a hearing loss on the development of communicative and linguistic skills in a child requires an integrated approach to assessment and intervention. At the same time, the heterogeneity of the hearing-impaired population necessitates a rehabilitative program designed to meet the needs of each child. An integral part of the intervention process is to help the parents learn to cope with the consequences of a hearing loss on their child's development of speech and language skills and to assist them in becoming good facilitators of communication development.

Effective management of hearing-impaired children requires knowledge of their auditory, speech, and language skills, as well as knowledge of normal developmental processes. Existing data have revealed differences in the speech perception abilities of children with varying degrees of hearing loss. This information is useful in selecting appropriate assessment and intervention procedures. Further, more recent research suggests that some children with profound hearing losses may have no residual auditory function. Children with mild or unilateral losses, who at one time were believed to experience no educationally significant delays because of their handicap, are receiving increased attention, especially in the classrooom setting. Effective management of all hearing-impaired children requires careful monitoring of the child's amplification systems, observation of the child's auditory responsiveness in the classroom, creation of an optimal acoustic environment, and identification of specific auditory skills to be developed.

The presence of a hearing loss can affect all aspects of speech development especially if the hearing loss is of a severe degree or greater. Numerous segmental and suprasegmental errors have been described in the hearing impaired, which are caused by poor control and coordination of maneuvers at all levels of speech production. The errors appear to interact in a complex manner to reduce the intelligibility of the speech of these children. Assessment procedures should address segmental and suprasegmental skills as well as intelligibility. Some commercially available tests are appropriate to assess some aspects of their speech production whereas other production skills need to be assessed with informal procedures.

Development of effective intervention strategies to improve the speech skills of hearing-impaired children require attention to motor production skills and integration of these skills to linguistically meaningful contexts. The greater the hearing loss, the less likely that motor production skills will transfer automatically to phonological use. Direct training of these skills might be necessary. It is crucial that children be required to use both auditory and speech skills in situations outside the individual therapy setting. Today, most children are in total communication programs that provide little opportunity for this to happen. Thus, the clinician must work closely with their classroom teacher to facilitate the development of functional communicative skills in everyday communicative settings.

The language problems of the hearing impaired are reflected in their lack of knowledge and use of form, content, and function. Because of the nature of their handicap, comprehension deficits will always be present. Deficits in language acquisition affect the child's performance in academic settings as well as in communicative situations. Relatively few studies have examined the comprehension abilities of hearing-impaired children or their functional use of language. Assessment of language skills should address comprehension and production skills by means of utilizing a battery of formal and informal measures. Intervention strategies relay heavily on the use of diagnostic teaching to identify areas of strength and weakness. Language intervention goals should not be addressed in isolation, but rather within a broad developmental framework. Emphasis should be placed on developing cognitive and linguistic skills. Auditory and speech skills should be viewed as integral to the language acquisition process and closely aligned with communication goals.

Implications for Future Research

Technological advances in engineering and computer science have potential impact on the management of hearing-impaired children. Digital signal processing techniques are being applied to hearing aid design, which holds promise for improving the characteristics of the signal delivered to the listener. Research examining the speech perception abilities of the hearing-impaired will undoubtedly provide a better understanding of the effects of hearing loss on auditory processing of speech. For those children who are totally deaf, the development of devices such as cochlear implants or tactile aids may prove to be important aids for the development of auditory-oral skills. Advances in digital speech processing also have important implications with respect to the speech production skills of the hearing impaired. Acoustic analyses can quantify the distortions in their speech and provide inferences about the underlying causes. Development of practical procedures to assess and to train directly the physiologic aspects of production patterns in the hearing impaired is an area of need. Of particular interest, is the development of computer assisted training procedures.

Research on language skills in the hearing impaired, which is based on models of normal language acquisition, has just begun. Relatively little is known about the effects of hearing loss on mother-child interactions and the early stages of language development. Few descriptive data are available on the pragmatic skills of hearing-impaired children, and there are few, if any, practical procedures that can be applied in a clinical situation to assess discourse and other pragmatic skills.

The increase in the number of clinicians and researchers who are interested in the hearing-impaired population suggests that a wealth of new information on this population will continue to be generated.

Acknowledgment. The assistance of Jenny Villwock in collecting the clinical data on SK is gratefully acknowledged.

REFERENCES

1. Davis J, Hardick EJ. Rehabilitative audiology for children and adults. New York: John Wiley & Sons, 1981.
2. Davis J, ed. Our forgotten children. Minneapolis: University of Minnesota Press, 1977.
3. American National Standards Institute. Specifications for audiometers (ANSI S3.6, 1969). New York: ANSI, 1970.
4. Boothroyd A. Hearing-impairments in young children. Englewood Cliffs: Prentice-Hall, 1982: 115–143.
5. Kent RD. Anatomical and neuromuscular maturation of the speech mechanism: evidence from acoustic studies. J Speech Hear Disord 1976; 19:421–447.
6. Gleason GB, ed. The development of language. Columbus: CE Merrill, 1985.
7. Davis JM, Elfenbein J, Schum R, Betler RA. Effects of mild and moderate hearing impairments on language, educational, and psychosocial behavior. J Speech Hear Disord 1986; 51:53–62.
8. Osberger MJ. Language and learning skills of hearing-impaired students Asha Monogr 1986:23.
9. Gentile A, McCarthy B. Additional handicapping conditions among hearing-impaired students, limited states: 1971–72, Series D: No. 14. Washington: Gallaudet College Press, Office of Demographic Studies.
10. Power DJ, Quigley SP. Problems and programs in the education of multiply disabled deaf children. Urbana: University of Illinois Press, Institute for Research and Exceptional Children, 1971.
11. Pollack D. Educational audiology for the limited hearing infant. Springfield, IL: CC Thomas, 1970.
12. Ling D. Speech and the hearing-impaired child. Washington: Alexander Graham Bell Association for the Deaf, 1976.
13. Calvert D, Silverman R. Speech and deafness. 2nd ed. Washington: Alexander Graham Bell Association for the Deaf, 1983.
14. Wilbur RB. American sign language. Baltimore: University Park Press, 1979.
15. Bornstein H. Signed English: a manual approach to English language development. J Speech Hear Disord 1974; 39:330–343.
16. Gustason G, Pfetzing D, Zawolkow S. Signing exact English. Rossmoor, CA: Modern Signs Press, 1972.
17. Anthony D. Seeing essential English manual. Anaheim: Anaheim Union School District, 1971.
18. Bornstein H, Saulnier K, Hamilton L. Signed English: a first evaluation. Am Ann Deaf 1980; 125:467–481.
19. Crandall K. Inflectional morphemes in the manual English of young hearing-impaired children and their mothers. J Speech Hear Res 1978; 21:372–386.
20. Marmor G, Petitto L. Simultaneous communication in the classroom: how well is English grammar represented? Sign Lang Stud 1979; 23:99–136.
21. Newton L. Linguistic environment for the deaf child: a focus on teacher's use of nonliteral language. J Speech Hear Res 1985; 28:372–386.
22. Moeller MP, Luteke-Stahlman B. Personal communication, 1987.
23. Cornett O. Cued speech parent training and follow-up training program. Washington: Bureau of Education for Handicapped, 1972. (DHEW publication No. 96).
24. Nichols G, Ling D. Cued speech and the reception of spoken language. J Speech Hear Disord 1982; 25:262–269.
25. Brookhouser PE, Moeller MP. Choosing the appropriate habilitative track for the newly identified hearing-impaired child. Ann Otol Rhinol Laryngol 1986; 95:51–59.
26. Sachs J. Prelinguistic development. In: Gleason GB, ed. The development of language. Columbus: CE Merrill, 1985:37–60.
27. Cross T, Johnson-Morris J, Nienhuys T. Linguistic feedback and maternal speech: comparison of mothers addressing hearing and hearing-impaired children. First Lang 1980; 1:163–189.
28. Kenworthy OT. Caregiver-child interaction and language acquisition of hearing-impaired children. Top Lang Disord 1986; 6:1–11.
29. Boothroyd A. Auditory perception of speech contrasts by subjects with sensorineural hearing loss. J Speech Hear Res 1984; 27:134–144.
30. Smith CR. Residual hearing and speech production in deaf children. J Speech Hear Res 1975; 18:795–811.
31. Bilger R, Wang M. Consonant confusions in patients with sensorineural hearing loss. J Speech Hear Res 1976; 19:718–748.
32. Owens E, Benedict M, Schubert E. Further investigation of vowel items in multiple-choice speech discrimination testing. J Speech Hear Res 1971; 14:841–847.
33. Erber NP. Auditory, visual, and auditory-visual recognition of consonants by children with normal and impaired hearing. J Speech Hear Res 1972; 15:364–371.
34. Erber NP. Auditory training. Washington: Alexander Graham Bell Association for the Deaf, 1982.
35. Osberger MJ, McGarr N. Speech production characteristics of the hearing impaired. In: Lass N, ed. Speech and language: advances in basic science and research. New York: Academic Press, 1982:221.
36. Stevens KN, Nickerson RS, Rollins AM. On describing the suprasegmental properties of the speech of deaf children. In: McPherson D, Davids M, eds. Advances in prosthetic devices for the deaf: a technical workshop. Rochester: National Technical Institute for the Deaf, 1978: 134–155.
37. Monsen RB. Durational aspects of vowel production in the speech of deaf children. J Speech Hear Res 1974; 17:386–398.
38. Osberger MJ, Levitt H. The effect of timing errors on the intelligibility of deaf children's speech. J Acoust Soc Am 1979; 66:1316–1324.
39. Maassen B, Povel D. The effect of segmental and suprasegmental corrections on the intelligibility of deaf speech. J Acoust Soc Am 1985; 78:877–886.
40. Monsen RB. General effects of deafness on phonation and articulation. In: Hochberg I, Levitt H, Osberger MJ, eds. Speech of the hearing impaired: research, training, and personnel preparation. Baltimore: University Park Press, 1983:23.
41. Monsen RB. Second formant transitions of selected consonant-vowel combinations in the speech of deaf and normal-hearing children. J Speech Hear Res 1976; 19:279–289.
42. Stevens KN, Nickerson RS, Rollins A. Suprasegmental and posture aspects of speech production and their effect on articulatory skills and intelligibility. In: Hochberg I, Levitt H, Osberger MJ, eds. Speech of the hearing impaired: re-

search, training, and personnel preparation. Baltimore: University Park Press, 1983:35.

43. McGarr NS, Osberger MJ. Pitch deviancy and intelligibility. J Commun Disord 1978; 11:237–248.
44. Angelocci A, Kopp G, Holbrook A. The vowel formants of deaf and normal-hearing eleven to fourteen year old boys. J Speech Hear Disord 1964; 24:156–170.
45. Bush M. Vowel articulation and laryngeal control in the speech of the deaf. Doctoral Dissertation, Massachusetts Institute of Technology, 1981.
46. Monsen RB. Acoustic qualities of phonation in young hearing-impaired children. J Speech Hear Res 1979; 22:270–288.
47. Levitt H, Stromberg H. Segmental characteristics of the speech of the hearing impaired: factors affecting intelligibility. In: Hochberg I, Levitt H, Osberger MJ, eds. Speech of the hearing impaired: research, training, and personnel preparation. Baltimore: University Park Press, 1983:53.
48. Gold T. Speech production in hearing-impaired children. J Commun Disord 1980; 13:397–418.
49. Monsen RB. Normal and reduced-phonological space: the production of English vowels by deaf adolescents. J Phonetics 1976; 4:189–198.
50. Irvin BE, Wilson LS. The voiced-unvoiced distinction in deaf speech. Am Ann Deaf 1973; 118:43–45.
51. Monsen RB. The production of English stop consonants in the speech of deaf children. J Phonetics 1976; 4:29–42.
52. Mahshie J, Conture E. Deaf speakers' laryngeal behavior. J Speech Hear Res 1983; 26:550–559.
53. McGarr N, Lofqvist A. Obstruent production by hearing-impaired speakers: interarticulator timing and acoustics. J Acoust Soc Am 1982; 72:34–42.
54. Monsen RB. Toward measuring how well hearing-impaired children speak. J Speech Hear Res 1978; 21:197–219.
55. Hudgins CV, Numbers FC. An investigation of the intelligibility of the speech of the deaf. Genetic Psychol Monogr 1942; 25:289–392.
56. Monsen RB. The oral speech intelligibility of hearing-impaired talkers. J Speech Hear Disord 1983; 48:286–296
57. Carney AE. Understanding speech intelligibility in the hearing impaired. Top Lang Disord 1986; 6:47–59.
58. McGarr NS. The intelligibility of deaf speakers to experienced and inexperienced listeners. J Speech Hear Res 1983; 26:451–458.
59. Bloom L, Lahey M. Language development and language disorders. New York: John Wiley & Sons, 1978.
60. Wilcox J, Tobin H. Linguistic performance of hard of hearing and normal-hearing children. J Speech Hear Res 1974; 17:286–293.
61. Davis J, Blasdell R. Perceptual strategies employed by normal hearing and hearing-impaired children in the comprehension of sentences containing relative clauses. J Speech Hear Res 1975; 18:281–295.
62. Kretschmer R, Kretschmer L. Language development and intervention with the hearing impaired. Baltimore: University Park Press, 1978.
63. Quigley S. Steinkamp M, Power D, Jones B. Test of syntactic abilities. Beaverton, OR: Dormac, 1978.
64. Pressnell L. Hearing-impaired children's comprehension and production of syntax in oral language. J Speech Hear Res 1973; 16:12–21.
65. Brannon J, Murry T. The spoken syntax of normal, hard of hearing and deaf children. J Speech Hear Res 1966; 9:604–610.
66. Engen E, Engen T. Rhode Island test of language structure manual. Baltimore: University Park Press, 1983.
67. Quigley S, Power D, Steinkamp M. The language structure of deaf children. Volta Rev 1977; 79:73–84.
68. Fremer J. Recognition memory for approximations to English in deaf and hearing subjects at three age levels. Doctoral Dissertation. New York: Columbia University, 1971.
69. Odom P, Blanton R. Phrase-learning in deaf and hearing subjects. J Speech Hear Res 1967; 10:600–605.
70. Kretschmer R, Kretschmer L. Pragmatics: development in normal-hearing and hearing-impaired children. In: Subtelny J. Speech assessment and speech improvement for the hearing impaired. Washington: Alexander Graham Bell Association for the Deaf, 1980.
71. Moeller MP, McConkey AJ, Osberger MJ. Evaluation of the communicative skills of hearing-impaired children. Audiology 1983; 8:113–128.
72. Fruchter A, Wilbur R, Fraser B. Comprehension of idioms by hearing-impaired students. Volta Rev 1984; 86:7–20.
73. Curtiss S, Lowell EL, Prutting CA. Pragmatic and semantic development of young children with impaired hearing. J Speech Hear Res 1979; 22:534–552.
74. McKirdy LS, Blank M. Dialogue in deaf and hearing preschoolers. J Speech Hear Res 1982; 25:487–499.
75. Katz DR, Elliott L. Development of a new children's speech discrimination test. Paper presented at the Convention of the American Speech-Language-Hearing Association, Chicago, Nov 18–21, 1978.
76. Ross M, Lerman J. A picture identification test for hearing-impaired children. J Speech Hear Res 1970; 13:44–53.
77. Office of the Los Angeles County Superintendent of Schools. Test of Auditory Comprehension. North Hollywood: Foreworks, 1979.
78. Office of the Los Angeles County Superintendent of Schools. Auditory Skills Curriculum. North Hollywood: Foreworks, 1979.
79. Owens E, Kessler D, Raggio M, Schubert E. Analysis and revision of the minimal auditory capabilities (MAC) battery. Ear Hear 1985; 6:280–287.
80. Erber NP. Use of the auditory numbers test to evaluate speech perception ability of hearing-impaired children. J Speech Hear Disord 1980; 45:527–532.
81. Osberger MJ. Development and evaluation of some speech training procedures for hearing-impaired children. In: Hochberg I, Levitt H, Osberger MJ, eds. Speech of the hearing impaired: research, training, and personnel preparation. Baltimore: University Park Press, 1983:333.
82. Dunn C, Newton L. A comprehensive model for speech development in hearing-impaired children. Top Lang Disord 1986; 6:25–46.
83. Subtelny JD, Whitehead R, Orlando N. Description and evaluation of an instructional program to improve speech and voice diagnosis of the hearing impaired. Volta Rev 1980; 82:85–95.
84. Schiavetti N, Metz D, Sitler R. Consruct validity of direct magnitude estimation and interval scaling of speech intelligibility: evidence from a study of the hearing impaired. J Speech Hear Res 1983; 26:30–35.
85. Monsen RB. A usable test for speech intelligibility of deaf talkers. Am Ann Deaf 1981; 126:845–852.
86. Boothroyd A. Evaluation of speech production of the hearing impaired: some benefits of forced-choice testing. J Speech Hear Res 1985; 185–196.
87. Miller J. Assessing language production in children. Baltimore: University Park Press, 1981.
88. Coleman RF. Is anyone listening? Lang Speech Hear Services Schools 1975; 6:102–105.
89. Gaeth JH, Lounsbury E. Hearing aids and children in elementary schools. J Speech Hear Disord 1966; 31:283–289.
90. Jones PA. Annual inspection of personal hearing aids of Clarke School students, 1972–73. Unpublished manuscript, Clarke School for the Deaf. Northampton, MA, 1973.
91. Riedner ED. Monitoring of hearing aids and earmolds in an educational setting. J Am Aud Soc 1978; 4:39–43.
92. Zink GD. Hearing aids children wear: a longitudinal study of performance. Volta Rev 1972; 45–51.

93. Diefendorf A, Arthur D. Monitoring children's hearing aids: re-examining the problem. Volta Rev 1987; 89:17–26.
94. Lotterman SH, Kasten RN, Majerus DM. Battery life and nonlinear distortion in hearing aids. J Speech Hear Disord 1967; 33:274–278.
95. Ling D, Ling AH. Aural habilitation: the foundations of verbal learning. Washington: Alexander Graham Bell Association for the Deaf, 1978.
96. Hanners BA, Sitten AB. Ears to hear: a daily hearing aid monitor program. Volta Rev 1974; 76:530–536.
97. Sanders DA. Noise conditions in normal school classrooms. Except Child 1965; 31:344–353.
98. Ross M. Hard of hearing children in regular schools. Englewood Cliffs: Prentice-Hall, 1982.
99. Erber NP. Auditory and audiovisual reception of words in low-frequency noise by children with normal hearing and by children with impaired hearing. J Speech Hear Res 1971; 14:496–512.
100. Gengel RW. Mean intelligibility functions of nine sensorineural hearing-impaired subjects for vowels and consonants. In: Stark RE, ed. Sensory capabilities of hearing-impaired children. Baltimore: University Park Press, 1974.
101. Ross M, Giolas T, Carver PW. Effects of three classroom listening conditions on speech intelligibility. Am Speech Hear Assoc 1973; 4:72–76.
102. Hochberg I, Levitt H, Osberger MJ. Improving speech services to hearing-impaired children. Asha 1980; 22:480–486.
103. Osberger MJ, Johnstone A, Swarts E, Levitt, H. The evaluation of a model speech training program for deaf children. J Commun Disord 1978; 11:293–313.
104. Monsen RB, Shaughnessy DH. Improvement in vowel articulation of deaf children. J Commun Disord 1978; 11:417–424.
105. Osberger MJ. Training effects on vowel production by two profoundly hearing-impaired speakers. J Speech Hear Res 1987; 30:241–251.
106. Osberger MJ, Johnson DL, Miller JD. Use of connected discourse tracking to train functional speech skills. Ear Hear 1987; 8:31–36.
107. DeFilippo C, Scott BR. A method for training and evaluating the reception of ongoing speech. J Acoust Soc Am 1978; 63:1186–1192.
108. Vetter DK. Designing informal assessment procedures. In: Yoder D, Kent R, eds. Decision making in speech-language pathology. Toronto: BC Decker, 1988:193.
109. Frankmann JP, Herman SE, MacKain KS, Oyer HJ. Methods of training deaf children to comprehend the passive voice. J Speech Hear Res 1979; 22:247–258.
110. Newcomer P, Hammill D. Test of language development-primary. Austin, TX: PRO-ED, 1982.
111. Jorgensen C, Barrett M, Husingh R, Zachman L. The word test. Moline, IL: LinguiSystems, 1984.
112. Woodcock R, Johnson MB. Woodcock-Johnson Psycho-Educational Battery. Boston: Teaching Resources, 1977.
113. Johnson DD, Toms-Bronowski S, Pittelman SD. Vocabulary development. Volta Rev 1982; 85:11–24.
114. Blank M, Rose SA, Berlin LJ. The language of learning: the preschool years. New York: Grune & Stratton, 1978.
115. Zachman L, Jorgensen C, Huisingh R, Barrett M. Test of problem solving. Moline, IL: LinguiSystems, 1984.
116. Starck MJ, Spitz RL. Teaching communication facilitators: a classroom model. Paper presented at Am Speech Lang Hear Assoc Convention, San Francisco, 1984.
117. Moeller MP, Osberger MJ, Eccarius M. Cognitively based strategies for use with hearing-impaired students with comprehension deficits. Top Lang Disord 1986; 6:37–50.
118. Hughes MC, James SL. Deaf children's revision behaviors in conversations. J Commun Disord 1985; 18:227–243.
119. DeMaio LJ. Establishing communication networks through interactive play: a method for language programming in the clinic setting. Semin Speech Lang 1984; 5:199–211.
120. Moeller MP, McConkey AJ. Language intervention with preschool deaf children: a cognitive/linguistic approach. In: Perkins W, ed. Hearing disorders. New York: Thieme-Stratton, 1984.
121. Piaget J. Play, dreams, and imitation in childhood. New York: WW Norton, 1962.
122. Lowe M, Costello AJ. Symbolic play test. Windsor, England: NFER Publishing, 1976.
123. Westby CE. Assessment of cognitive and language abilities through play. Lang Speech Hear Services Schools 1980; 3:154–168.
124. Yoshinaga-Itano C, Downey DM. A hearing-impaired child's acquisition of schemata: something's missing. Top Lang Disord 1986; 7:45–57.
125. Carrow-Woolfolk E. Test of auditory comprehension of language. 2nd ed. Indianapolis: Bobbs-Merrill, 1985.

30 Communication Disorders in the Aging

Mariana Newton, Ph.D.

DEMOGRAPHIC CHANGES

Explosion and Implosion

Although most would agree that reaching the age of 65 years is not a definition of old, the aged have been defined, for many purposes (e.g., demographics, retirement, Medicare, social security) as persons who have attained the age of 65 years or older. The aged are the fastest growing age group in the United States.[1] In 1980, 11.3 percent of the population was 65 or older; by the year 2030, that group is expected to comprise over 20 percent of the population.

In order to understand better the growth of segments within the aging population, a practice has evolved of dividing the aged into three subgroups: the young-old are those aged 65 to 74 years; the old-old are aged 75 to 84 years; the very old are 85 years or older. Table 30–1 reflects the population projections from the years 1980 to 2030 and the percentage of that population in segments of the aging population.

In addition to the rapid increase in the aged population, the most significant trends include a huge jump between the years 2010 and 2025 due to the aging of the "baby boom" and changes in life expectancy for both the young and the very old, thus resulting in disproportionate increases in the very old segment. This latter circumstance is referred to as the aging implosion.

The life expectancy of women is greater than men. In 1983, the male-female ratio of those 65 or older was 2:3 and for those 85 or older, the ratio was 2:5. The life expectancy has increased about the same for males and females, but the differences in ratios result from different life expectancies at birth. Caucasians have a slightly longer life expectancy than blacks. The primary reason for increases in life expectancy and reductions in death rates is an age-specific reduction in cardiovascular deaths related to technological advances, cultural emphasis on wellness, and better long-term care.[2]

THEORIES OF DEVELOPMENT AND CHANGE IN THE AGING

Biologic Models

As science and technology delve deeper and deeper into the microstructures and functions of the human organism, one of the fundamental questions in gerontology attracts more attention. Do nonreproducing cells have attributes of potential immortality or does time alone impose self-limitations? That is, are the causes of death intracellular or extracellular.[3] Another biologic theory of aging contends that aging is the result of a increased and/or disordered immunogenetic diversification, which results in confusion of cells.[4] This confusion would create a situation analagous to the rejection phenemonon seen toward transplanted organs from their new host. A third theory questions the possibility that time patterns are programmed into individual organisms genetically.[5]

TABLE 30–1 Growth of the Population Aged 65 and Over, By Selected Age Groups, 1980–2030

Year	Population (thousands)	Percentage of Population			
		Young-old	Old-old	Very old	Total (65 + years)
1980	226,505	6.9	3.4	1.0	11.3
1990	249,731	7.2	4.1	1.4	12.7
2000	267,990	6.6	4.6	1.9	13.1
2010	283,141	7.2	4.3	2.4	13.9
2020	296,339	10.0	4.8	2.5	17.3
2030	304,330	11.3	6.9	2.9	21.1

From U.S. Bureau of the Census. America in transition: an aging society. Current population reports, September, 1983; Series P-23, No. 128. Base data from U.S. Bureau of the Census. Decennial censuses of population, 1900–1980 and Projections of the population of the United States: 1982–2050 (Advance Report), Current population reports, October 1982; Series P-25, No. 922, as cited in and adapted from United States Office of Technology Assessment. Technology and aging in America, OTA-BA-264. Washington, DC: U.S. Congress, 1985.

Psychological Models

The broadest theoretical view among psychological models is that aging is comprised of a series of more or less discrete stages. This theory is a continuation of the parentally-popular, if not scientific, stage theory in child development. Other theories are more process-oriented in conceptualizing aging and are more likely to highlight the heterogeneity of the population. Trend models include three types: increment, stability, and decrement. In childhood, the increment model is applied more often; certain characteristics increase with age. In old age, the decrement model is used; biologic losses result in loss of function.[6] The regression hypothesis, one decrement model that has been used in the study of language, holds that the dissolution of language occurs as a mirror image of the evolution of language. The decrement model is often divided into (1) losses which are irreversible, and (2) losses with compensation.[6] Compensible losses are those for which there are gains to offset losses to regain stability. An extension of this model would hold that for some losses, there may be gains that more than offset the losses. A loss of job to retirement is compensated for, for some at least, with more free, flexible time.

The above models are conceptual in nature and quite narrow and specific. There really is no unifying, general theory of aging.[7] Instead, as in biology and psychology, students of communication and aging are problem and data oriented, around a collection of hypotheses proposed to explain specific aspects of speech, language, and hearing in the aged. As Ulatowska noted, we are pretheoretical![8]

Trend and process models have dominated research on communication changes in the aging. Although a life-long model of communication is yet to be developed, the initial explorations in hearing and speech production have generally followed a trend model, with an effort to relate trends to biologic observations. The most recent investigations of language changes in normal aging and senility have been more process oriented, which reason suggests is the most appropriate direction.

RESEARCH ISSUES

Period and Longitudinal Studies

Period and longitudinal studies represent some important distinctions in studies of aging. Period studies are cross-sectional; events (data) recur across a population within a specified time. The data are analogous to a snapshot picture of a group. Period studies generate age differences between subjects or groups of subjects. Longitudinal studies follow experiences or behaviors of a specific group over time. Such data are analogous to a movie. Period studies permit the observation of age differences, a comparison of two people or groups of different ages. Longitudinal studies address age changes, or what happens as people get older. Age differences do not always reflect age changes.

Age and Cohort Effects

In both longitudinal and point studies, one of the variables is age. A second variable is cohort. A birth cohort includes people born within a specific period of time, often 5- to 10-year intervals. Changes that are related to the time of birth, for example, historical events, social and cultural changes, economic conditions, are cohort effects. For example, suppose we wish to study average income of audiologists of various ages, we sample incomes of audiologists in decile segments, from 20 year olds up to 70 year olds, and we average the incomes in each decile group. The point data would probably show gradually increasing income to middle age and then a gradual reduction in income up to retirement. These data, however, are misleading. In fact, a longitudinal study of the income of audiologists would most likely show gradually escalating incomes throughout their working life. The difference is attributable to cohort effects. The 50 and 60 year olds started work earlier than younger subjects, when salaries were lower. Hence, even though they have had a steady rise in income, their salaries are less than younger men who started work more recently, at a higher salary and with bigger raises each year. A comparison of the cross-sectional data with longitudinal data reveals the cohort effects.

Synthetic Designs

Age-specific cross-sectional data over several years, or a cross-sectional sequence, is used to approximate cohort experience. This sequence would include two or more cross-sectional studies, using the same age segments, executed at two or more times. A longitudinal sequence would involve two or more longitudinal studies using two or more cohorts.

A combination of cross-sectional and longitudinal sequences was developed by Schaie.[9,10] The study begins with a cross-sectional study using several cohorts. After a period of years, these subjects are retested, thus providing some longitudinal data on several cohorts, or a longitudinal sequence. At the same time, a new group of subjects is added, using the same cohorts, making a second cross-sectional study. The measurement of the second group after the same interval of time as with the first group constitutes the second longitudinal sequence. Groups can be continually added, each time enlarging the cross-sectional group as well as increasing the longitudinal data. In this way, synthetic longitudinal data, with no cohort effects are obtained without taking as much risk relative to the representativeness of the sample and the availability of subjects for repeated measures.

Sampling Problems

Although longitudinal studies have many advantages, they also have some sampling problems. Getting and keeping a representative sample over a long period of time is the chief problem. Aged volunteers for research studies are usually people with more money, more education, and more access to cultural advantage than those who do not volunteer. Men volunteer more than women, whites more than blacks. These characteristics of volunteer subjects make representativeness of the sample difficult. However, volunteers are often active in various social networks, which makes finding them as subjects much easier. Once they have been found, the problem is keeping them for repeated measures over a long period of time. People move, become ill, develop research-confounding conditions, become disinterested, and (particularly in the very old segment) die.

The selection and assignment of subjects by chronologic age reveals only the passage of time since their birth. Chronologic age is useful for identifying population groups, but it is a poor descriptor of those within the groups. Aging is a gradual process; people do not suddenly become old after a certain amount of time. Voluminous anecdotal and research evidence in every discipline attests to the incredible individual variability within the population over 65 years of age, and even within smaller stratifications of the chronologically aged. However, on the other hand the biologic characteristics that would make more homogenous groups have yet to be determined.

Measurement Obstacles

In addition to the complexities of sampling, some general characteristics of the aging organism and personality are a challenge to the researcher or clinician. One pervasive characteristic is the generalized slowing of the aged—slowing in movement, adaptation, processing, deciding, reacting, and responding.[11] Moreover, some elderly people fatigue more with less activity than do younger individuals. These two factors, plus those that follow, confuse the interpretation of their communication behavior.

Cautiousness. Cautiousness may account for some variance in test performance (e.g., elevated hearing thresholds). Refusal of the aging to respond to or to participate in certain tasks has been attributed to an "unconfident strategy,"[12] related to anxiety or fear of failure. Older subjects have been observed in a number of studies to avoid making responses, which involved risk-taking or which might result in error.[13,14,15,16,17] Contradicting these findings, Yanz and Anderson, investigating response criteria on speech-recognition tasks, concluded that decision criteria did not distinguish young versus elderly listeners.[18] Further, Gordon-Salant found that elderly subjects do employ different decision criteria in speech recognition tasks, but their criteria are less conservative than those of younger subjects.[19] Gordon-Salant noted that a high degree of confidence in one's own responses may encourage the elderly person to guess extensively during speech recognition tasks. In daily communication, guesses may lead the elderly to respond as if they have understood a message, when in fact they have not, thereby impairing communication efficiency further.

Disengagement. Older people tend to withdraw or become relatively more introverted. Cumming and Henry argued that disengagement was a natural, normal process, an almost certain "stage" of development.[20] Later attention focused on the societal forces that played on the degree of engagement of the elderly. Subsequent reseach identified age, health (physical and mental), personality, social role, types of activity, and the availability of a confidant as important factors.[15]

Rigidity. Stereotyped response patterns are resistant to change. These factors are difficult to assess in the elderly because personality factors, life-long habits, education, intelligence, and cultural factors may influence them.[15] Clinically, older individuals may require more time for adaptation to new environments, people, and activities.

Depression. Loss of peers and spouse, health problems, economic restrictions, reduced feelings of self-worth and of being needed, social isolation, family relationships and attitudes, and relocation trauma may contribute to attitude and behavior.[15] Conversely, the positive aspects of these factors may prevent depression and may contribute to a healthier personality in some aged persons.

Health and medication. Chronic illness is a major problem for the aged. Because of age, they are vulnerable to many conditions, which are not common in younger persons. Poor health consumes much of the elders' time, thought, money, and patience.

Related to health status is drug consumption. Even though the elderly make up approximately 12 percent of the population, they consume up to 30 percent of all medications.[21] Often as many as six to ten different drugs are taken together. Adverse drug reactions are not uncommon; the effects of drugs on communication are not always known, but are not unlikely either.

NEUROBIOLOGIC CHANGES

A number of changes in gross anatomy have been seen in the brains of the aged: (1) brain weight decreases with age[22] by 11 percent between 25 and 96 years of age.[23] Five percent of this loss occurs by age 70, 10 percent by age 80, and 20 percent by age 90 years.[24] In addition, decrease in brain volume relative to skull capacity occurs as a function of age.[22] Changes in outward appearance of the brain with age include narrowed gyri, widened sulci, shrunken appearance, thickening of the meninges, atrophy of the corpus callosum, shrinking of the basal ganglia, distended ventricles, and an increase in cerebrospinal fluid.[22]

Microscopic anatomic changes in the central nervous system have been documented. The decrease in number of small central nervous system neurons with advancing age is particularly important not only because of fewer number, but also because small fibers have a relatively slower conduction rate than larger fibers.[25] Changes in the proportion of slow conductors (small fibers) to fast conductors (large fibers) may cause "blurring" of discrimination of complex stimuli (see discussion below).

Related to the loss of fibers is the reduction of neuron density in the cerebral cortex with advancing age.[25] The greatest cell loss in superior temporal gyrus, with lesser reductions in the precentral gyrus, area striata, inferior temporal gyrus, and post central gyrus.[25]

Neuron loss occurs in peripheral nervous system too. The greatest loss occurs through a reduction in the number of larger fibers.[26] Included in this area is the reduction of neurons within the auditory and speech production mechanisms.

Aging has a more serious influence on the less primitive aspects of the nervous system.[27] That is, later evolved structures, such as the cortex, are more vulnerable to senescence than are more primitive structures, such as the vegetative centers of the brain.

Why is the nervous system so vulnerable to deterioration with aging? The nervous system consists of exclusively postmitotic neuronal elements. That is, every neuron present in the old person was present at that person's birth.[28] Some parts of the nervous system, such as axons and dendrites, are relatively permanent.[29] The cells of the central nervous system which are lost do not regenerate nor are lost cells replaced by the division of remaining cells. Hence, an accumulated loss of nervous system cells results. The older you are, the more you have lost, without replacement.[28]

A certain advantage of a degree of permanence of the nervous system allows the human brain to retain information over a period of time and to add new information to a growing fund of knowledge. If the elements of the nervous system were constantly replaced, what hope would there be for lasting memories?

On the other hand, one of the consequences of keeping neural elements in service for a long time (as opposed to retirement and replacement) is that some deterioration is probable. Some parts simply wear out; they will not be replaced. Some parts will be damaged. The cells of the central nervous system are highly vulnerable to oxygen supply; even minor deprivations of oxygen cause damage or death of nervous system cells. Aging is accompanied by cardiovascular insufficiencies, for example, constriction of the blood vessels, less efficiency in the heart as a pump, and reduction in efficiency of gaseous exchange in the lungs. Moreover, there is an increased tendency for pigment deposits (lipofuscin) in cells of the aging brain.[22,30] Common thought is that the concentration of lipofuscin affects the physiologic capabilities of the neurons and may result in the death of such cells.[30] Even though, in the beginning, the brain has an enormous stockpile of neurons—many more than needed at any given time—the reserve is gradually diminished with age.[31,32]

In summary, the vulnerability of the nervous system to deterioration results from normal attrition related to wear and tear on relatively permanent elements, nervous system damage and reduced plasticity, and damage related to specific diseases of the nervous system.

Differential Aging

There is a growing body of information regarding differential aging of the cerebral hemisphere. Several have employed dichotic listening tasks, with mixed results. Some have reported an increasing right-ear advantage with increasing age;[33] others argue that left-hemisphere lateralization does not increase as a function of age.[34,35] Support for the latter view of no increase in lateralization with age is provided by studies using visual tasks.[34,36,37]

Behavioral observations suggest more degradation with increasing age of many cognitive functions associated with the right hemisphere compared to functions associated with the left hemisphere.[38–40] A study to test this hypothesis showed that right-ear stimulations resulted in markedly faster reaction times to the verbal stimuli, indicating that the left hemisphere was dominant for this group of geriatric subjects.[41] The authors suggest that the linguistic processing mechanisms of the right hemisphere become more vulnerable to and, therefore, are inhibited by the dominance of the left hemisphere. Obler, Woodward, and Albert did not find such differences.[37] They tested 96 right-handed people 25 to 80 years of age on verbal and nonverbal matching tasks, presented tachistoscopically. They found age-related slowing, but no systematic age-related changes in lateralization were apparent.[37]

COGNITIVE PROCESSES

Intelligence

Studies of intellectual functioning in old age have generally focused on the analysis of performance on standardized intelligence tests, such as the Wechsler Adult Intelligence Scale and the Stanford-Binet Test of Intelligence.[42] Schaie and Geiwitz argue that intelligence tests are not "age fair" because intellectual competence in old age is very different from that in younger years.[6] The traditional tests are well suited to measure progress through stages of knowledge acquisition,[43] but not adequate to assess the ability to solve relevant problems, strategies of information processing, and relevant intellectual integrity.[6] Moreover, the early cross-sectional studies used an IQ score for data; every group had an average IQ of 100, by definition. Because this ratio uses chronologic age as the divider, the fact that younger subjects had to achieve a much higher raw score than older people to reach an IQ of 100 is masked. Schaie and Geiwitz note that if raw scores were compared across age groups, younger subjects would have the highest average score and the scores would systematically decline with increasing age.[6] The interpretation of these tests was that intelligence systematically declined as age increased.

Schaie and Geiwitz note another problem with the early, cross-sectional tests.[6] These tests measured differences in scores for different age groups. A longitudinal study, however, revealed no decline in IQ with age; in fact, it showed an increase.[44] The outcome differences between the cross-sectional and longitudinal studies are due to cohort effects, for example, quality of education and quality and availability of nutrition and medical care.

Two features of the scores of the elderly on standardized intelligence tests have been noted repeatedly: (1) some subtest scores decline with age and others do not; and (2) scores on performance subtests are much poorer than on the full-scale test. The poor scores may be explained in part by the speed factor in performance tests.

Education has proved to be an important factor in intelligence test experiments. Birren and Morrison discovered that educational level has much more to do with performance on the intelligence tests than age.[45] Considering the impact of education and the cross-sectional nature of studies of intelligence in the aged, the presence of cohort effects may even exaggerate the differences in education between younger and older subjects.

Health of the subjects also has a significant impact on test scores. Botwinick and Birren compared test results on a group of aged persons in excellent health with a group of elderly persons who constituted a typical representation of persons without incapacitating health problems.[46] In this study, healthier subjects performed better on the intelligence tests.

Miller contends that "fluid" intelligence (adaptability to new situations, learnability of new ideas, ability to establish new relationships) is more susceptible to aging than crystallized abilities (learned intellectual skills).[47] What about problem-solving skill, creative thinking, and development of new ideas—all "fluid" intelligence abilities. Evidence suggests that fluid intelligence measures are the most vulnerable to decline with age.[15,42,48–50]

Other researchers have focused on the qualitative thought development during later stages of the life span in a Piagetian construct. The hypothesis has been that intellectual functions in the aged would be represented in the Piagetian construct—in reverse of what is seen in developing children. This thinking is encouraged by Piagetian theory, which holds that the attainment of logical operations, abilities during childhood and adolescence, is a durable achievement and that once these cognitive abilities have been mastered, they are maintained through the remainder of the life-span.

Several investigations have assessed the status of Piagetian task performance in normal populations of old people.[10,51–53] These studies consistently report less than optimal performance by the aged on various operations measures. Papalia et al studied 48 subjects ranging in age from 64 to 85 years.[54] These subjects were given various Piagetian conservation of substance, weight, and volume tasks. The main finding of the investigation indicated that conservation of substance, weight, and volume is an intact ability for a significant proportion of the subjects in the sixth, seventh, and eighth decades of life. This is a cross-sectional study, but even so the data suggest that there is some qualitative intellectual change in older people, and it contradicts the Piagetian notion that once these abilities are developed in young life, they are maintained throughout the life-span. In another study, Papalia also noted age differences in performance for substance, weight, and volume conservation, but that the ability to conserve number was intact for the old as well as the young.[51] Lower levels of volume conservation performance in older persons has also been found.[53] Elderly subjects performed less well than young adult groups on Piaget's conservation of surfaces test.[52] It also seems that more complex ones such as weight and substance conservation reveal age-related decrements. These findings support the notion of an orderly cognitive decline in later life, in the reverse order of acquisition.[51,52]

One of the controversial findings in these studies has to do with the influence of education on performance. A strong education-performance relationship was observed in the study by Papalia, Salverson, and True,[54] which is contradictory to the findings of Papalia, Storck et al, and Sanders et al.[51–53] Here again, the cohort effects may not be separable from main effects, without measurements over time.

MEMORY

Models of Memory

Until recently, a linear model guided investigations of human memory. In this linear model, neural changes known as engrams are thought to be registered first in sensory memory, from which peripheral and attentional engrams are transferred to short-term memory. Short-term memory requires conscious awareness and has a limited capacity, or life. Through rehearsal, information from short-term memory can be stored in long-term memory. In the linear model, memory problems arise when storage capacity is insufficient, rapid decay occurs, transfer fails, or various combinations of these. The brain is organized so that various regions of the neocortex simultaneously carry out these operations.

A hypothetical view of memory has emerged, which holds that information storage is tied to specific processing areas involved in learning. That is, memory is stored as changes in the same neural system involved in perception and processing of information to be learned.[55] In addition to short- and long-term memory, additional divisions, based on distinctions in memory processes, are made in long-term memory: declarative memory (facts, episodes, lists, routes—episodic and semantic) and procedural (performance practice).

Memory Loss

Minimal or no differences in short-term memory are seen in the aged even though memory loss is one of the most common complaints.[56] Both speed and accuracy of retrieval are maintained in old age in processes involving automatic activation of information.

However, secondary, or long-term memory, does not hold as well.[56] Age-related decrements have been found with different stimuli and various presentation modalities.[57] Given the nature of the linear model, questions arise about the responsibility of memory store capacity and transfer attributes in these differences. There is cumulative agreement that the age-related problems are in information encoding and retrieval.[56]

Within long-term memory processes, age-related declines occur in episodic memory. There is disagreement about problems related to age in semantic memory. Earlier studies[58] and priming experiments[59] have yielded no differences with age, but generative naming task studies do show differences because, according to Craik such tasks involve retrieval processes that require more effort, thus slowing down the process.[60]

MOTOR SYSTEMS

The most notable difference in motor performance of the aged is a generalized slowing of behavior, as previously mentioned. Reaction times of adults to auditory and visual stimuli increase up to the age of 20 years and then undergo a steady decline.[61,15] Interestingly, voice onset times are not slower, but they are more variable.[62,63]

Several factors account for some variability in slowed responses. Botwinick and Thompson noted that increased reaction times may be related to athletic process.[64] Young athletes had better reaction times than young nonathletes. Spiriduso proposed that lifestyles, especially physical activity, may have more to do with reaction time than aging.[65] Frequently-performed motor activities are less vulnerable to aging effects than those activities engaged in less frequently.[66] Botwinick and Thompson observed that the slowness in reaction time of the aging can be reduced or eliminated with practice.[64]

What would account for decreased reaction time? Acuity problems are more frequent in the old and may prevent adequate sensory stimulation for response. Increased stimulus intensity reduces age-related differences in reaction time.[15] But sensory impairments are not pervasive enough to account for the prevalence of motoric slowness. More likely, central deficits account for the greatest portion of psychomotor slowness in the elderly. Welford suggested four changes in the central nervous system, which would influence psychomotor performance as a function of age: (1) reduction in the number of functional neuron cells reduces signal strength and processing capacity; (2) increase in random neural activity—or noise—in the aging brain; (3) longer "after effects" of neural activity, which "echo" or blur the brain's processing of subsequent signals; (4) diminished arousal levels, which reduce optimum activity levels from those of younger persons, and which result in overall reduction of signal strength and functional capacity.[67]

SENSORY PROCESSES

A general decline in the sensory and perceptual functions occurs in humans with advanced age. The age of onset and the rate and course of the declines vary among and within various sensory modalities. Four reasons account for most sensory loss, in general. They are as follows:

1. The central nervous system receives less information or distorted information upon which to act because of non-neural anatomic changes in the sensory systems
2. Degeneration through loss of neural units in the sensory systems extends from peripheral mechanisms to brain stem and cortex
3. The effects of various losses in each of the sensory systems on the integration of sensory information may be much larger than an addition of the losses
4. Related to the integration or lack of integration, older people may have a certain inflexibility in responding and a reduced ability to change their minds or to be open to unexpected sensations. Moreover, such nonsensory factors as cognition, memory, and personal attitudes may influence the ability of the organism, as a whole, to cope.

Several conjectures about the responsiveness of the elderly to sensory testing exist. One suggestion is that reduced sensory system sensitivity may exacerbate the general caution of elders in responding to stimuli, requiring greater stimulus intensity "to be certain" of or to have confidence in the presence of stimuli before responding.[12,15] In a number of studies, older subjects have been observed to avoid making responses that involve risk-taking or that might result in error.[14,16,17]

On the other hand, many older people are reluctant to admit to deterioration in function since this admission contradicts their denial of advancing age. It is again noteworthy that Yanz and Anderson, when investigating response criteria on speech-recognition tasks, concluded that decision criteria did not distinguish young versus elderly listeners,[18] and that Gordon-Salant found that elderly subjects do employ different decision criteria in speech recognition tasks, but their criteria are less conservative than that of younger subjects.[19] Gordon-Salant noted that a high degree of confidence in their own responses may encourage elderly people to guess extensively during speech recognition tasks. In daily communication, guesses may lead the elderly to respond as if they have understood a message, when in fact they have not, thereby impairing communication efficiency further.

Changes in sensory processes related to aging are important in understanding communication changes and disorders in the aging. Sensory loss and changes affect the efficiency and accuracy of sensory information reception and perception. Although the relationships of hearing and oral communication are readily acknowledged, vision is important in the perception of linguistic stimuli and in the perception of the communicative signal as a whole—approximately 65 percent of which is nonverbal.[68] The sensory systems involved in touch, taste, and smell are less essential to communication, although touch, pressure, and proprioception are important feedback systems for the production aspects of speech.

Vision

Decreased acuity, increased light requirements, slower adaptation to light changes, and difficulties in color perception are among the most notable changes in vision related to aging. Little change in visual acuity related to age from 15 to 50 years have been reported.[15,26,69,70] However, substantial losses in acuity occur from age 50 to 70 years[15] because pupil size decreases with age, thus allowing less light to the retina.[71] Since less light enters the eye, the aged require more illumination—almost twice the illumination of younger persons.[6,15,26,72–74] In addition, their accommodation to light decreases with advancing age.[72] The thresholds for adaptation to darkness decrease as a function of age;[75,76] there is disagreement about the rate of adaptation to darkness.

Light contrast discrimination and color vision are different in older people. The yellowing of the lens of the eye with age changes its spectral quality, making blue and green more difficult to discern than red and yellow.[6,15,26,72,74,77] Also, fusion threshold for a flickering light has been shown to deteriorate with advancing age[15,26,72] because of the thickening of the lens and reduction in pupil size, which reduces the amount of light to the retina from a given source.

A number of studies indicate that marked changes in visual perception occur with advancing age. Older subjects show less flexibility in their visual perceptual judgments, adhering more rigidly to first impressions.[78,79] In addition, older subjects have more difficulty than younger subjects in extracting information from a complex visual presentation, for example, extracting data from a matrix, or from hidden figures, identifying overlapping capital letters.[80,81,82]

Hearing

Hearing impairment in the aging was first thought to involve only the peripheral auditory system.[83] Now it is known that all parts of the auditory system are vulnerable to effects of aging.[84–88]

Differences in the external ear related to aging, although interesting, are not directly related to decrements in auditory function. However, stiffness of the middle ear system, thickening of drum in subjects with chronic arthritis, ossification and increased rigidity in the ossicular chain[85,89] and general atrophy in muscles of middle ear and ligaments[89,90] may result in some decrease in hearing acuity and distortion in the hearing mechanism.[83] General atrophy of the organ of Corti[91,92] and loss of hair cells[91,93–96] are differences in the old which are not seen in the young. These differences may be related to metabolic changes in the hair cells, which are coincident with a decrease in enzymatic activity.[94] Change in stiffness of basilar membrane[86,97,98] and atrophy and rupture of basilar membrane[98] have also been related to hearing impairment in the aged.

Atrophy of the stria vascularis, described in the aged, is significant because the stria vascularis is a source for production of endolymph and a source of DC potential important in processing in the inner ear.[86,97] Therefore, atrophy of the stria vascularis is thought to be a major factor in presbycusis. Additional evidence for this relationship comes from the observation that changes in the composition of endolymph sometimes appear concurrently with presybycusis.[99]

In the inner ear, loss of ganglion cells in the spiral ganglion have been reported,[91,97,100] although the loss must be near 75 percent before significant changes in hearing threshold occur.[101] Narrowing of the internal auditory meatus, attributable to progressive reduction of supportive tissue,[102] compresses fibers of auditory nerve, leading to atrophy.[103] There appear to be fewer fibers in the cochlear division in 44 to 60 year olds than in younger persons.[103] Such nerve degeneration results particularly in auditory discrimination problems, rather than affecting acuity.[84,93]

Structural changes in the brain stem and auditory cortex are difficult to document. However, loss of neurons in the whole nervous system is widely verified,[24] and some differences in various parts of the auditory brain stem and cortex have been associated with aging.[87,100] The emerging evidence of central as well as peripheral involvement in hearing impairment in the aging comes from behavioral and electrophysiologic studies of central auditory function.[88,104–106]

HEARING IMPAIRMENT

Prevalence

Age. The prevalence of hearing impairment markedly increases with age. From 2 percent in children under 17 years of age, the prevalence increases to 12 percent in those aged 45 to 64, to 24 percent of the young-old, and to 39 percent of those 75 years of age or older.[107] At present, more than 7 million elderly persons have significant hearing impairments. Hearing loss is more prevalent among the poor, the institutionalized, and men. At the rate of expected population increase into the next century, the hearing impaired elderly will number in excess of 10 million.[2]

Gender. There is a difference of opinion regarding gender differences in age-related hearing impairment. Males show sensitivity decrements at an earlier age than females; relatively large differences occur in the third decade of life.[108] Hearing loss is greater in higher frequencies, especially in males.[108] Katsarkas and Ayukawa reported no gender difference.[109]

Residence. Percentage of institutionalized elderly with hearing impairment is generally higher than observed in similar aged noninstitutionalized elderly.[110–114] Incidence of hearing loss in nursing home residents varies widely, from 20 percent[110] to 97 percent.[115] Variability may be due to the varied nature of patients in nursing homes, the definition of hearing loss, and the procedures used to assess hearing.

Cardiovascular health. Hearing loss and an increase in blood pressure occur with aging in healthy persons in the United States.[116] The Mabaan tribe in Southeast Sudan, who live in a very quiet, almost silent atmosphere, and who eat almost no meat or saturated fat, do not smoke, are not obese, age more slowly and live longer than Americans, have significantly more acute hearing at all ages (10 to 70 years) than people of corresponding ages who live in industrial areas in the United States and who are exposed to excessive noise.[117] Rosen and colleagues hypothesize that the Mabaans probably have low generalized atherosclerosis and greater elasticity of the small arteries. While many older persons in the United States not exposed to excessive noise have an air-bone gap (12 dB or greater), the Mabaans experienced an air-bone gap 50 percent less than Americans of comparable age and only reached the 12 dB gap at 75 years of age, compared to 55 years of age for Americans.[118] In another experiment in which hospital patients formerly on a high cholesterol diet were changed to low cholesterol, the experimental group (low cholesterol), aged 50 to 59 years, had better hearing and a smaller air-bone gap than those 10 years younger in the control group. Rosen concluded that the correlation of otologic and hearing findings with the high incidence of cholesterol and coronary heart disease suggests that, if for no other reason, the reduction in cholesterol is advantageous to hearing in old age![119]

Presbycusis

Presbycusis is the term used to denote hearing loss related to aging. Four or five types of presbycusis have been identified: (1) sensory presbycusis, in which there is epithelial atrophy, involving all cochlear structures and leading to an abrupt hearing loss in the high frequencies; (2) neural presbycusis, characterized by atrophy and/or loss of neurons in the auditory pathway;[86,100] (3) metabolic presbycusis, from atrophy of the stria vascularies, leading to a fairly uniform hearing loss for pure tones; (4) mechanical presbycusis, resulting from stiffening of the basilar membrane, which in turn leads to increased hearing loss as frequency gets higher.[86] A fifth type, sociocusis, is related to lifelong exposure to noise.[120,121]

Decrease in pure tone acuity, especially for high frequencies is the most common characteristic of hearing impairment related to advanced age.[122–125] Kirikae et al reasoned that since histologic examination reveals a diminution of the number of nerve fibers in the auditory pathway, conduction of high frequency tones is more affected than low frequency because the number of fibers conducting high frequencies originally is lower than the number conducting low frequencies.[100]

Tinnitus often accompanies sensorineural hearing loss.[126] The prevalence of tinnitus increases with age, and is more common in women than in men.[127] Speech discrimination (listening) problems are exacerbated by tinnitus in one third of persons with tinnitus.

AUDITORY COMPREHENSION

Discrimination

Speech discrimination is a problem in those with presbycusic losses.[93,128–131] The decline in discrimination is also a function of age.[125]

Since presbycusis involves hearing for high frequency sounds more than for low frequency, speech discrimination is poorest for those consonants having high frequency components (e.g., voiceless fricatives and anterior plosives). In addition, consonants carry much less acoustic energy than vowels. These two factors are primarily responsible for difficulty presbycusic listeners have in discriminating phonetically similar words and in comprehending words with high frequency consonants carrying a large informational load. The problem is exacerbated in a noisy environment; the noise masks the weaker consonants.[93,132,133] This circumstance has been referred to as phonemic regression.[134]

Speech discrimination decreases with age, particularly after age 60, in both quiet and noise conditions.[135,136] Why?

"Blurring" may interfere with discrimination, especially for complex stimuli, such as speech. Because there is a greater loss of small nerve fibers than large fibers in the aging central nervous system,[24] the number of small nerve fibers becomes disproportionately small compared to the available large neurons. Moreover, smaller nerve fibers are slower conductors of impulses than are larger fibers. This difference in the rate of conduction is even greater with increasing age.[67,137] These two circumstances of the aging nervous system—fewer small nerve fibers and slower conduction in them—may result in a "blurring" effect because fibers of different sizes, number, and conduction rates with a single nerve trunk or bundle would cause impulses to be spread out in time and strength as they reach auditory cortical centers for perception.

"Neural noise"[136] results from an increase in the loss of neural cells[84] and/or increased random neural activity.[138,139]

"Activation" or "arousal" resulting from lowered synaptic resistance or some other yet unknown factor may cause the neurons to be unusually responsive to stimulation. This overarousal is helpful to a point, but in the presence of a string of rapidly successive stimuli, as in speech, the first stimulus causes a large number of neurons to fire,[140,141] thus resulting in the cells being in a refractory period when the rest of the stimuli are presented to the nervous system for response.[142]

Aging nervous systems may have longer neural "aftereffects" following stimulation,[136] thereby creating an effect something like the effect of playing the piano with the sustaining pedal held down. Perseverative aftereffects (i.e., difficulty in changing sensory-perceptual sets) have also been proposed as interferences with speech discrimination.[67]

Questions have been raised about whether neural noise, arousal and increased aftereffects are the result of age or may be more peripheral phenomena. Further, if there are age changes in these phenomena, the discrimination problems they may produce can be counteracted by increased attention, interest, motivation, and/or memory on the part of the listener.[136]

Other manifestations of presbycusis include difficulty in discrimination of time-distorted speech, using compressed or expanded stimuli;[143–148] variable alterations in loudness[149,150] and pitch perception.[151]

Hearing Handicap

While various formal measures of hearing acuity and speech recognition and discrimination are used clinically to assess the hearing of the aged, these measures are not always good predictors of the degree of impairment that the listener experiences in everyday communication situations. Speech discrimination in quiet is highly predictable from pure tone hearing thresholds; but relatively little listening is done in quiet. Several tests have been devised to assess the effects of hearing impairment on communicative function. The Speech-In-Noise Test (SIN) was a better predictor of hearing communication performance than any of the traditional audiometric measures.[152]

Weinstein and Ventry studied the audiometric correlates of hearing handicap as measured by the Hearing Handicap Inventory for the Elderly (HHIE).[153] Pure tone sensitivity for the better ear was most highly correlated with the HHIE. Word recognition accounted for no more than 20 percent of the variance in HHIE scores. There is considerable individual variability in the emotional and social response to hearing impairment, especially in those with mild hearing losses. The variability plus the fact that audiometric data can account for less than 50 percent of the variance in hearing handicap suggest that hearing handicap in the elderly will be measured more accurately by self-report than by inference from audiometric data.

SPEECH PRODUCTION

Articulation

Articulation in the Healthy Aged

Ryan and Burk found that imprecise articulation of consonants and slow rate of articulation were predictive of perceived age of their 40 selected male speakers.[154] They suggested that persons who are judged to be older on the basis of articulatory imprecision and slowness may be speakers who are mildly dysarthric on a "dysarthria continuum."

Ptacek et al found uniformly slower diadochokinetic rates for older adults compared to younger subjects.[155] The rates for the younger subjects were consistent with previously published normative data for young adult speakers. Some of the difference in the performance of older subjects may be due to difficulty in eliciting maximum rates. The authors attributed this difficulty to poor motivation and comprehension of the task. Contrarily, lack of maximum effort may be related to the cautiousness with which older people sometimes respond and the importance to the aging of accuracy over speed.

Sixty subjects (30 male, 30 female), aged 50 to 80 years, were examined for nasalance, as an indicator of articulatory control, during the reading of four passages containing varying frequencies of nasal consonants.[156] The results indicated that there were no systematic increases in nasalance as a function of age. On one passage which contained no nasal sounds, subjects aged 66 to 80 years had more nasalance than those in younger groups. The difference was due to significantly greater nasalance values for females. The authors suggest that, consistent with findings in other populations, slower rates of speech in older persons may result in discontinuities in velopharyngeal closure, which could account for increased nasalance. However, the conclusion is suspect because (1) gender differences are not accounted for, and (2) systematic increases in nasalance as a function of age are denied.

Pathology-Related Changes

There are many neuropathologies that have a deleterious consequence to speech production. Several such diseases typically have their onset in adulthood. Cardiovascular disease is the greatest single cause of speech and language disability in the elderly. A slow progressive impedance in circulation or an acute incident, a cerebrovascular accident (CVA), results in neural tissue death, which can result in motor speech and language impairments (see Chapter 31 for a full discussion).

Amyotrophic lateral sclerosis (ALS) is a progressive, degenerative disease of the nervous system, which has its onset in the fourth or fifth decade. This disease involves both upper and lower motor neurons and markedly shortens the life-span to approximately 3 years beyond medical diagnosis. The motor speech involvement results eventually in unintelligible speech. Before that time, however, speech is very slow and hypernasal, with marked hyperkinetic laryngeal valving and inadequate respiratory support, which results in short, choppy phrasing.

Parkinson's disease also has its onset in adulthood, usually after 50 years of age. The articulatory symptoms in Parkinson's disease have been summarized.[156a–159] Problems in articulatory and vocal tract control are characteristic. In a descriptive study of the misarticulations of Parkinson's patients, about 45 percent of the 200 Parkinson's patients exhibit some misarticulations. Analysis of these highly consistent errors revealed that manner errors predominated; stop-plosives, affricates, and fricatives were the most affected. The articulatory errors reflected inadequate close constriction of the vocal tract at the point of articulation, or articulatory undershoot.[160] Labial rigidity and the hypokinesia of Parkinson's syndrome are correlated. It appears that the rigidity causes a generalized hypokinesia.[161] This hypokinesia is also reflected in slow diadochokinetic rates.[162]

Prosodic disturbances (monotone voice) are seen in patients with Parkinson's disease. Training, in both comprehension and production, produced improvement in prosody; the motor aspects of prosody were complicated by difficulty in the recognition of prosodic errors.[163]

Voice

Age Recognition and Perception of the Aging Voice

Several studies have demonstrated the ability of untrained listeners to make age discriminations from recorded voice samples, thereby suggesting that some variation in acoustic information, directly or indirectly related to physiologic change in the larynx, occurs with increasing age. Ptacek and Sander investigated the ability of 10 untrained listeners to differentiate "over 65 years of age" and "under 25 years of age" on the basis of voice in three listening conditions: (1) a prolonged vowel, (2) a reading sample played backwards, and (3) a reading sample played forward.[164] The listeners correctly identified 78 percent of the prolonged vowel samples, 87 percent of the reading samples played backwards, and 99 percent of the reading samples played forward. Shipp and Hollien asked 25 listeners to make direct age estimations from voice recordings.[165] These estimations were averaged and correlated (+0.88) with actual chronological ages of 175 male speakers, aged 20 to 89 years. Ninety-eight college students were asked to guess the ages of 32 male and female speakers, aged 17 to 68 years.[166] The correlation between actual chronological age and mean guessed age was 0.93. Elderly women are not as accurate as young women in estimating age from voice.[167]

Listener judgments of age based on voice are conservative; a regression toward the mean reflects a tendency of listeners to "center" their judgments. That is, the listeners underestimated the ages of the oldest speakers and overestimated the ages of the youngest speakers.[165,166] This finding suggests that the process of age estimation from voice involves primarily the identification of those in the middle of the age range, guessing those who fall just outside of that range to be slightly below or slightly above the range. That is, perhaps it is the mature voice that is most distinguishable perceptually.

To what perceptual features of the voice do listeners associate with increasing age? Ryan and Burk studied both perceptual and acoustic correlates in aging males.[154] They found that perceptual variables correlated better with age than individual acoustic measures and, hence, were more predictive. Particularly, perception of vocal tremor, laryngeal tension, and air loss were significant. Ryan and Burk suggest that listener perceptions may reflect primary physiologic changes in the structure and/or function of the voicing mechanism, or that they may reflect coping strategies that the speaker employs to compensate for insufficiency or variability in the fine motor control or in the driving respiratory control for phonation that are perceived by listeners.[155] On the other hand, Blonksy et al using cinefluoroscopic examinations of neuromuscular control during speech and swallowing, found no hoarseness, lingual dysfunction, labial dysfunction, voice tremor, or dysfluency in 10 normal geriatric controls, aged 60 to 75 years.[168] Horii and Ryan found an unusually large correlation (r = 0.63) between measured fundamental frequency and the perception of chronological age.[169] Moreover, on those subjects on which listeners didn't agree well, there was an absence of a correlation between fundamental frequency and perception of age. The authors concluded that these latter speakers had acoustic characteristics that are inconsistent with the "perceptual norm" for their age.

Ryan and Capadano and Hartman and Danhauer asked their listeners to identify features they listened to while judging speakers' ages.[166,170] Pitch, volume, clarity, and rate of speech were identified most often.

The perceptual features that correlate well with perceived age or that are identified as important by listeners may not be singularly important. Instead, they may be components of an amalgamation of features which, when heard together, are meaningful with regard to age. The listener may be responding directly to the vocal features, or it may be that in identifying the important characteristics, they are responding stereotypically to their perceptions of the subjects' ages.[166] Further, these features that have been identified by judges are important paralinguistic variables; studies of age-dependent differences in paralinguistic cues have not been found.

Acoustic Changes

Several acoustic changes have been documented. Their relative importance in listener judgments of age by voice is undetermined. Ryan found that vocal intensity increased with age in males, 40 to 80 years of age, with significant increases in the 70- to 80-year-old group.[171] All of Ryan's subjects had normal hearing. Ryan suggested that feedback mechanisms of the respiratory and phonatory mechanisms may be less sensitive and thus require greater effort to produce adequate sensory feedback information. This additional effort would result in an increase in vocal intensity.

Higher average fundamental frequencies and greater fundamental frequency variability in aging males has been reported, [169,172–174] a finding not supported anatomically.[175] On the basis of analysis of fundamental frequency during reading, McGlone and Hollien found that there were no differences between various age groups of women (65 to 94 years).[176] Ryan and Burk found only a weak correlation of mean fundamental frequency and no relationship of fundamental frequency variability with perceived age.[154] Benjamin found a significantly lowered fundamental frequency related to age.[177] These studies reported average group data for chronological age groups. The discrepancies among the studies may reflect the significant variability now recognized in physiologic aging within chronological age groups.[178,179]

Spectographic analysis of speakers over a recording period as long as 29 years revealed that the frequency position of formants and the pitch of voiced sounds shift to a lower frequency as an adult speaker ages.[180] These authors also found that the ability to control the pitch frequencies of vocal sound decreased with increasing age, which may be the phenomenon judged perceptually as vocal tremor. Wilcox and Horii and Benjamin found significantly increased fundamental frequency perturbation.[177,181] Also, the total pitch range is significantly lower for older male and female adults (65 to 79 years) as compared to younger adults (under 40 years of age).[164]

Most of the studies to date investigating listener perceptions and acoustic changes in the voice related to aging are referent to subjects' chronological age. Hence, inferences are drawn about the physiologic changes in the voice reflected in listener perceptions and acoustic changes without consideration of variances in physiologic aging within specific age groupings.[174] Ramig and Ringel found significant differences in vocal acoustics for individuals within the same chronological age span (65 to 75 years), but in good and poor physiological condition.[178] The acoustic differences were attributed to differential degeneration of the vocal mechanism consistent with general body physiology. In a subsequent study, Ramig studied vowel spectral noise in persons of different chronologic ages and varying general physiologic condition.[182] The magnitude of vowel spectral noise was correlated to a significant degree with physiologic aging; correlations with chronological aging were not significant. Hence, Ramig concluded that physiologic condition is a significant variable in the study of acoustic characteristics of the aging voice.

Neurologic changes and changes in the respiratory, phonatory, and articulatory structures and function have been cited as causal in explaining observed acoustic changes in the voice as a function of aging. Skeletal changes, reduced tissue elasticity, and muscular atrophy and weakness are thought to be related to reduced fine motor control of phonatory and articulatory behavior.[175,183] Studies of voice onset time as a representation of fine motor control in the phonatory system revealed no differences in mean voice onset time as a function of age in either men or women.[62,63] However, the variability within subjects and groups was greater with increased age[62] and voice onset time varies with vowel context.[63]

Disorders of the Voice

Phonatory abnormalities of Parkinson's patients have been described by Logemann and her colleagues and reflect, as does articulation and prosody, the hypokinesia and rigidity typical of this disease.[184] Parkinson's patients have a relatively slow fundamental frequency of the voice and no tremor.[185] These symptoms appear to reflect rigidity in the phonatory posture of the larynx and are correlated with the symmetry of trunk and limb rigidity in most Parkinson's patients.[186]

Rhythm, Rate, and Fluency

Reduced overall speaking rate in oral reading as a function of age in males has been reported.[171,173,187] The results on speaking rate in impromptu speaking as a function of age are conflicting.[171,173] As noted above, Ryan and Burk reported that a slower rate of articulation was an important predictor of perceived age, which would result in a reduced number of words per minute.[154] Several possible explanations might account for a reduced rate of speaking due to interword or intraword delays: (1) coping behavior for age-related changes in speech production rate, facility, accuracy; (2) change in timing and precision of neurologic and neuromuscular signal and responses in speech production; and (3) related to a general marked slowing of responses[188] and slowing of central information processing mechanisms.[61,189] In the latter situation, changes in function of peripheral mechanisms would be secondary to changes in central processing centers.

Adult onset dysfluency is usually associated with trauma or vascular disease. Patients with Parkinson's disease or supranuclear palsy have been reported to have stuttering-like behavior. In these cases, onset was slow and an early symptom of the disease. The stuttering behavior consisted of repetitions and prolongations on initial syllables on both small grammatical and substantive words. More dysfluency occurred in self-formulated speech. Positive adaptation effects and the absence of secondary behaviors and fear reactions are characteristic.[163]

LANGUAGE

Vocabulary Comprehension and Use

The findings on vocabulary in the aged vary. On a task of defining words in response to the word, no age effect is detected.[190,191] Scores on the Peabody Picture Vocabulary Test are even across decades.[192,193] Analysis of written vocabulary in journals and letters of two subjects up through their fifties revealed increases in vocabulary with aging.[194] A study using free word associations also showed an age effect,[195] but the data appear to reveal more cohort effects than vocabulary changes. The two subjects mentioned above, whose vocabulary increased for a time, showed decreases in written vocabulary after 60 years of age.[194] An age effect was obtained on task of naming the word in response to a definition of that word; both accuracy and stimulus-response latency were reduced as a function of age.[195a]

However, on a task of defining the word in response to the word, the aged were not different from younger subjects.[195a] The difference in the two tasks is a matter of going from conceptual to lexical versus lexical to conceptual; poorer performance of the aged in going from conceptual to lexical may reflect difficulty in accessing the lexical store.

Sentence Comprehension

Measures of verbal learning and vocabulary, using single words, do not assess the semantic-syntactic abilities required for decoding sentences, which transcends the ability required for understanding single words.

Studies of sentence comprehension in the aged have produced mixed results as well.[57] Speed and accuracy are again factors in performance. When quickness of response is required, an age effect is shown; on accuracy measures, age effects are less often seen. In addition, those studies that show an age effect on sentence comprehension utilize, for the most part, tasks involving low probability and low predictability, both semantically and syntactically.[57,195b,196] Comprehension of relativized sentences remains stable in subjects up to 60 years of age. Older subjects made more errors and more serious errors (multiple errors within a sentence) in sentence comprehension.[16]

Because of limitations in information processing, redundancy is used to facilitate fast and accurate comprehension. Redundancy rules express how one language component implies another. Rules promote comprehension by providing organizational information to both speakers and listeners. Redundancy includes phonological rules governing probability of occurrence of letter combinations, grammatical rules, which organize and inform, and semantic rules of probability of word combinations and sequences. According to Craik, older people do not use rules of redundancy as well as younger subjects.[197] On the contrary, Fullerton and Smith found that older adults use grammatical redundancy more than young subjects to discern and encode important information in sentences.[198]

Poorer performance in sentence comprehension occurs when listeners must engage in cognitively effortful encoding processing. Encoding voice information is an example of cognitively effortful processing, which is age sensitive. Improved performance in intentional voice encoding was traded for a decrement in sentence recall in older adults. Generalization of this principle would suggest that the engagement of the aged in tasks requiring effortful encoding results in generally diminished total processing capacity.[199]

Discourse Comprehension

Comprehension of discourse in the aged has been investigated by Ulatowska and various colleagues.[200,201] These investigators advised that the various results of other comprehension studies were due, in part, to the error of extracting for study various features of the cognitive-linguistic complex from their functional environments. The results of the studies demonstrate age effects on story recall and probe questions and were interpreted to point to the fruitfulness of semantic and pragmatic studies to develop life-span psycholinguistics.

Generative Naming

Spreen and Benton found that the performance of elderly persons was not as good as younger subjects.[201a] However, given sufficient time, older people may be able to name as many items, with fewer repetitions, as younger persons.[201a] Two explanations for this contrast come to mind: (1) the general slowing of behavior in the old affects the rate at which naming occurs, but improves accuracy; or (2) older persons intent on accuracy (quantity) threatened by ideational limitations sacrifice some speed.[57]

Sentence and Discourse Production

Using measures of sentence length in spontaneous speech, the performance of elders is not different from younger subjects.[202] In some instances, the length of utterances is greater for older speakers.[191,203,204] The often-heard accounts of loquaciousness in the aged may be informal awareness of the observed longer, more elaborate, but less precise utterances of the aged.

The oral and written descriptions of younger, middle-aged, and older subjects of the Cookie-Theft picture were analyzed and compared.[205] Younger subjects used more fragments and incomplete sentences; the 60-year-olds used more words and more embedded sentences, but fewer total sentences and fewer themes.[206] The investigators likened the performance of the 60-year-olds to performances of Wernicke's aphasia patients in that they more frequently modified nouns and their verb-to-noun ratio was higher. Analysis of 105 additional written descriptions of the Cookie-Theft picture revealed that subjects in the three oldest decades (fifties, sixties, and seventies) also used full sentences and more words per sentence than younger subjects. However, the written descriptions of the oldest group (70-year-olds) looked more like that of the youngest group (30-year-olds) in terms of the use of complete sentences and number of words per sentence. The number of themes was greater as a function of age and the number of words remained constant across ages, in contrast to the results in the first study.[191]

Older persons produce fewer propositions in narratives and fewer steps in procedural discourse. In addition, they have more instances of referential ambiguity in all types of discourse. Older subjects produced a greater number of pronouns and reduced the number and variety of noun types and proper nouns.[8] These differences suggest a general cognitive-linguistic decline with advancing age, which is not accounted for on the basis of education or other cohort effects. Semantic content and processing appear to be particularly vulnerable. Ulatowka and her colleagues note that the strength of the cognitive and linguistic relationships are not apparently as great as was anticipated.[200]

Syntax has been thought to be generally well-preserved in the normal aged,[207] and even in the dementias.[208] But recent studies challenge that view, finding age-related differences in verb tense and agreement, possessives, and grammatical complexity through analysis of spoken and written language samples.[57,209]

Pragmatics

Functions of Communication and Competence

An investigation to assess competence in independent living utilized several measures of cognition (Block Design and Similarities subtests of the WAIS and the Associate Learning subtest of the Wechsler Memory Scale) and three qualitative ratings of discourse (procedural and narrative).[210] The quality of the discourse was rated on a 5-point scale, with particular judge attention to such characteristics as relevance, clarity, and informativeness of subjects. In this population of 27 adults (18 women and 9 men) ranging in age from 65 to 87 years, higher levels of competence were associated with functioning in more demanding environments and functioning in a variety of roles in various organizations and activities in the community. Also, performance on the cognitive measures was related to both competence and the quality of the discourse, with competence and discourse quality also significantly correlated. The study affirms the long-held belief that communicative abilities were a major part of competence and independence.

Studies of pragmatic functions and interactional strategies may yield information that will help to distinguish those language changes which are induced by social factors. Ulatowska et al cite the possible trade off of social relationships and communicative efficiency and effectiveness.[200] Patterson and Newton studied turn-taking breakdown and repair strategies in elderly women's conversations with interactants of varying ages.[211] Intrusive interruptions by the older women were the most frequent type of breakdown; repair was accomplished most often by the older women, through yielding to the partner. The authors questioned the ability of older adult women to give, read, and react to turn-yielding cues.

Communication Environments

An investigation of perceptions of elderly and chronically ill patients regarding the spoken communication that occurs in a long-term care facility addressed numerous questions.[212] How much do the patients talk? Who are their communication partners? Where do they talk? What topics do they talk about? Do patients want to talk and do they enjoy talking? What factors affect communication? What suggestions do patients have for improving the communication atmosphere? The authors used a focused semi-standardized interview of 24 patients. A common observation is the limited amount of spoken communication in long-term care facilities. Residents sit quietly in their rooms or lined up along a hallway. There is little communication, although patients are capable of communicative interactions. Patients reported their perceptions: (1) there is an average amount of communication, but they themselves spoke very little; (2) patients avoid talking to their roommates, "gossipers," "bores," antagonists, and to the speech impaired; (3) desired partners would be friendly, good at conversation, and intelligent; (4) others in the environment are not similar enough to them to talk to; (5) their talk is about trivia, health and medication, home and family, hospital activities, personal interest, "anything," food and eating, and "nothing"; (6) they talk for companionship and releasing emotions and to transmit information about themselves and their needs; (7) most of their communication takes place in public areas, but public areas should, in their view, be avoided as a talking place; (8) their communication has little value, but they like to talk and want to talk; (9) they would like to talk to staff, but desire is not reciprocal; (10) communication is influenced by personal characteristics, staff characteristics, interests and activities, health, rules operating on their floor, and factors associated with institutional living; (11) communication would be improved if they could choose their own roommates, have a "talking room" for private conversations, and have cocktail hours!

DEMENTIA

Demographics

Between 1.2 and 4 million Americans are impaired by dementia.[2] The wide variance in prevalence is likely due to varying diagnostic criteria applied regionally and historically. Indeed, dementia is often confused with other ailments and is not confirmed except through postmortem examination.

There are many etiologies of dementia. They are generally categorized into two categories: primary neurologic disease and systemic diseases. Some dementias are common primary neurologic diseases, for example, Alzheimer's disease and arteriopathic dementia. Some are treatable, for example, normal pressure hydrocephalus, tumors, subdural hematomas, alcoholic dementia. A third category includes Korsakoff's psychosis, Huntington's chorea, Creutzfeld-Jacob disease, and Pick's disease. There are a number of systemic diseases of other organ systems which result in neurologic deficits. The first symptoms of the disease may be seen as neurologic dysfunction, even though the nervous system is secondarily involved.

The most common cause of dementia is Alzheimer's disease, accounting for 50 to 75 percent of all dementias, and affecting 20 percent or more of those over 80 years of age. Treatable dementias, 20 percent of all dementias, include those related to drug side-effects or abuse, depression, endocrine disturbances, infections, nutritional deficiency, metabolic disorders, trauma, and toxicity. Approximately 15 to 20 percent of all dementias are related to cardiovascular disease (e.g., stroke, multiple mini-strokes), some of which are treatable and others of which are not. The distinction between treatable and irreversible dementias is clinically critical, for obvious reasons.

Diagnostic Criteria

Dementia is characterized by the following five diagnostic criteria: (1) loss of intellectual abilities sufficient to interfere with social functioning; (2) memory impairment; (3) no indication for brain damage as a cause of impairment; (4) no indication for delirium or intoxication; and (5) at least one of the following: impairment of abstract thinking; impairment of judgment; aphasia, apraxia, agnosia; and, a personality change.[213] Given that cognitive, memory, and thought impairments are mandatory for diagnosis and considering that communication is inextricably linked to them, the conclusion that communication impairments are characteristic of dementia is believable. What is the nature of those impairments?

Speech Production

Phonological rules are well preserved in mild and moderate dementia patients, and even in some severely demented individuals.[214–216] Demented persons can recognize and correct phonological errors, even though the meaning of the utterance may escape them.

Morphology

Rules of morphology are maintained. Like phonology, they are automatic structural components of the language.

Syntax

Usually, syntax is automatic too. But syntax can be brought to consciousness. Syntactical forms that affect meaning cause the probability of misuse in demented patients to increase.[217] Semantic errors which cause illogical utterances are more likely to be overlooked by the demented.[214–216]

Semantics

Semantic knowledge is knowledge of meaning and reference. It is the knowledge of concepts and temporal or situation context. It is the knowledge that is used to recognize the ambiguous and the illogical. Content and semantic variety is much greater than variety of form or structure; hence, it is also less predictable.

Bayles and Kazniak, in an extensive review and analysis of the literature and of their own studies, argue that the communication is impaired in persons with dementia because ideation is impaired and that ideation is impaired because of particular impairment of content and processes of semantic memory, of which episodic memory is a part.[57] These impairments account for the often cited emptiness in the meaning and reference of the utterances of the demented.[191,218]

The evidence is extracted from various disciplines.[57] Most of the evidence describes differences by categories of the severity of dementia. Hence, frequent comparisons are made between groups of subjects with mild, moderate, or severe dementia. In addition to tests of the theoretical premises, Bayles and Kazniak identify measures and behaviors which distinguish dementias of different etiologies and those which distinguish dementias from normal aging and from conditions confused with dementia.

The following four areas of evidence for deterioration of the content of semantic memory are analyzed: (1) decrements in confrontation and generative naming; (2) progressively diminishing vocabulary; (3) reduced abilities to comprehend and produce pantomime; and (4) disintegration of word associations. Both confrontational and generative naming abilities distinguish severity groups of demented subjects.[219–221] Generative naming deficits identify more accurately mildly demented patients than do confrontation naming tasks, based on accuracy of response[222] and quickness of response.[223] Mildly demented patients make more "in-class" errors associated with the stimulus; in more severely demented persons, meaningful associations of stimulus to response become increasingly vague.[57,218,220,224]

Both receptive and expressive vocabulary are impaired in demented patients. Greater impairments are seen in more severely demented persons.[57,225,226] Moderately and severely demented persons have a diminished ability to comprehend and produce pantomime (e.g., name an item after its use is mimed or pretend to use an object after it is named).[57] Further, the relevancy of word associations, except for syntigmatic associations, distinguishes the severity groups of demented persons.[227]

The evidence for deterioration in semantic processes includes the performance of demented persons on tasks of reading comprehension, linguistic reasoning, and ideation. Many demented patients are fluent readers, but comprehension accuracy distinguishes severity groups.[57,228–230] Lexical disambiguation is least affected in dementia, but structural and logical disambiguation tasks clearly distinguish normals from mild dementia patients and mild from moderate dementia patients.[57] Demented persons often correct phonological or syntactical errors in sentences, but rarely correct semantic errors.[214,216] Poor performance on generative naming tasks and disordered, noninformative oral and written discourse distinguish the demented by severity groups and from normals.

The extensive examination and analysis of data leads to some logical clinical applications for the identification and evaluation of persons with senile dementia. In this regard, several areas of examination appear to be clinically critical: confrontational and generative naming, receptive and expressive vocabulary, word associations, structural and logical disambiguation, correction of semantic errors in sentences, and written and oral discourse.[57] Since form holds longer and content yields early in the course of dementing diseases,[57] particular attention in clinical analyses should be paid to content, rather than to form.

Pragmatics

When dementia is severe, affected individuals use fewer perlocutionary acts and diversity is reduced in illocutionary acts. Only utterance acts may be used in severe dementia. Bayles and colleagues asked dementia patients to describe four common objects.[223] The number of informational units was greatest for normals and was lower for each increasingly severe group. Also, the frequency of perseverative responses increased as a function of severity of dementia. Repetition of ideas was more common than sound, word, or phrase repetition or the use of interjections and fillers. Demented patients also produce fewer ideas in written discourse with a less diverse vocabulary than normals. Total word output does not always diminish;[223] that observation may be related to multiple word explanations when lexical access is impaired. Pragmatic aspects of communication have not been addressed as extensively as other aspects; pragmatic comprehension and performance is very difficult to quantify because of the intimate and complex relationships among various aspects of language and the many factors affecting language. Those very complexities and the evidence of marked disturbances in the cognitive-linguistic functions persuade an expectation of diversity of the types as well as the effectiveness of communicative acts.

Dementia Contrasted

Interetiologic (Alzheimer's disease, Parkinson's disease, and Huntington's disease) comparisons and contrasts of performance of demented patients revealed more similarities than differences, especially in moderately and severely impaired groups. That is, severity of dementia predicted performance better than did etiology.[57]

Bayles and Kazniak also addressed distinctions between cortical and subcortical dementias, a classification preferred by some.[57] By definition, there are anatomic and physiologic differences. Motor systems are usually normal in cortical dementias, except in the last stages; subcortical dementias are characterized by dysarthria, abnormal posture and gait, movement disorders, and slow movements. Dysarthria is common in both Parkinson's disease and Huntington's chorea. Persons with subcortical involvement are more often depressed; mood is normal in cortical dementias. With subcortical dementia, patients have difficulty remembering; in cortical dementias, learning new information is difficult. Both cortical and subcortical dementias are characterized by remarkable impairments in the cognitive-linguistic complex. Differences in cognition are more a matter of severity, with the cortical dementia patients most severely disturbed. This classification would include the vascular disease dementias in the cortical group; hence, aphasia is characteristic of some of those patients. W. R. Miller described poor performance of depressives on various measures of learning and memory.[231] From that, the question arises about diagnostically differentiating between depressives and dementias. Distinction is important since the course would be quite different and certainly the treatments would be different. Lack of motivation related to depression, rather than basic memory deficits, could account for the poor performance of depressives. Miller and Lewis, using a signal detection method, examined the recognition memory of depressed or demented elderly.[232] The depressed patients performed more like the normal controls, whereas the demented patients were remarkably different. The depressed subjects were much less willing to guess, employing strict decision criteria. Whitehead reported that depressed persons attach importance to nonspecific task attributes, which leads to variability in performance on various tasks.[233] The reasons for caution on the part of depressives is not clear. Lowered motivation or the aversiveness of wrong guesses are two possibilities.

Comparisons and contrasts of communication impairments in dementia with those in aphasia is beyond the scope of this chapter. Controversies have centered around the use of the term "aphasia" to describe the language and speech impairments in dementia. At the core of the discussions is the fact that aphasias are usually produced by focal lesion and dementias are usually produced by diffuse lesions. From a clinical standpoint, the differentiation between aphasia and language disturbance in dementia is complicated by the observation that some aphasic patients (i.e., patients with focal lesions), also have some generalized cognitive linguistic degeneration and, conversely, some patients with dementia also have more specific, focal-like communicative disorders. Bayles and Kazniak contrast the performance of aphasic and dementia patients on a variety of measures, illustrating the cognitive-linguistic features which distinguish each.[57]

EVALUATION AND FACILITATION OF COMMUNICATIVE COMPETENCE

Several general observations about communication in the aging guide the consideration of intervention strategies. Most healthy elderly people remain communicatively competent throughout their lives. Various changes in particular aspects of communication do change; some changes are a function of age and others occur in spite of it. But, even in the midst of changing social, cultural, economic, and familial milieus, those changes are barely noticeable and are not problematic. The remarkable ability and effort of an aging, but healthy, organism to preserve communicative competence until death shows the importance of communication for life.

Communication competence in the aging is threatened most by diseases to which the aging are particularly vulnerable and from which they may escape death, but not the dependence and/or isolation resulting from communicative impairment. Sensory impairments, speech production disorders, and, most of all, disintegration of the cognitive-linguistic complex can be devastating, not only to the individual, but to every aspect and domain of the larger society. Quite literally, when one is robbed of communication, all lose.

Emanating from these observations are certain principles of communication facilitation in the aged. First, the focus of any such facilitation should not be limited to the old, but should include families and larger networks of which older people are a part. Communication change or impairment not only disturbs the homeostasis of the aged individual, but also that of the family. Moreover, in the family lie external resources that can be brought to bear in the absence of sufficient internal resources of the aged. In addition to the usual mechanisms of health care delivery, extended families, churches, support groups, social and civic organizations, retirement centers, and the myriad of community agencies constitute a rich reservoir of opportunity and assistance.

Further, given the interactional nature of communication as a process, reason dictates that facilitation should be centered on interactions and their many contexts. The traditional service delivery model, where the patient goes to the service, may not be appropriate. Instead, taking the service to the patient may help to solve transportation and fatigue problems, but also affords opportunities for communication facilitation in natural, meaningful environments. The increasing use of home care is an important option in service delivery, which reduces problems inherent in office-based service delivery. Speech-language pathology services for the aged are particularly suited for, and even enhanced by, delivery in more natural environments.

Trends in residential patterns of the elderly suggest another opportunity for service delivery to the elderly. Retirement centers, life-long care facilities, nursing homes, day care centers, and other group environments afford opportunities for facilitated group interactions and for the training of personnel and visitors (including families) in functional, facilitative strategies.

Communication facilitation goals and strategies for the aged must be functional. There are few studies on the efficacy of speech therapy for aphasic patients. Some are not particularly favorable or have demonstrated mixed results.[234] Several have reported more positive results.[235–237] However, in all of the studies one of the most important factors in success appears to be the functionality of the treatment. Aphasic patients perform better and make better progress with relevant material (familiar everyday happenings, matters of immediate concern) in auditory comprehension, speech repetition, naming, and reading comprehension.[238–242] A study of the efficacy and long-term effects of group functional therapy revealed that functional communication therapy in a group did produce measurable results on communicative activities of daily living. Those scores were maintained 6 weeks after termination of therapy.[243]

The facilitation of communication success in the aged occurs in three domains: physical, personal, and social. The physical environment is easily adjusted, but often neglected. Because of sensory impairments in the aged, the lighting and acoustics need special attention. Rooms need to be well lit. Faces of interactors need to be visible and lit, with no backlighting. Background noise is disturbing to the hearing impaired and to the disoriented; a quiet environment is conducive to hearing and listening. Small conversational groupings permit an ideal two to three feet distance between conversants and allow interactors to orient to the better ear of the hearing impaired elderly.[244] A degree of privacy for conversations, also minimizes visual and auditory distractions and encourages more intimate communication.

Some facilitative strategies address the personal needs of an aged individual. For example, rehabilitation programs for the hearing-impaired elderly are individually determined. Such a program might include medical and/or surgical treatment, amplification with custom ear molds, and a comprehensive program of aural rehabilitation. Assistive listening devices may assist hearing-impaired elderly persons in noisy rooms and in groups of talking people, for example, church, club meetings, lectures, concerts, and businesses. Still other devices provide alerting signals, enhance telephone communication, and amplify sound from the television or radio.

For the person who is impaired in speech production, a therapeutic program to improve the intelligibility of speech may be most appropriate. In severe circumstances, speech may need to be augmented through formal or informal gestures or through a speech aid (e.g., speech and language board or speech synthesizer). The personal needs of an elderly individual should dictate the appropriateness of any facilitative measure.

Common to all circumstances is the need for every individual who experiences some communicative difficulty, be it a minor inconvenience or a severe impairment, to acknowledge their needs to others. Acknowledging the handicap or the communication difficulties makes the communication interactor feel more positively toward the communicatively impaired. Encouraging and training the communicatively impaired to acknowledge their communicative difficulties and suggest ways in which the interactor can be helpful to the interaction puts the interactor at ease.[244,245]

While communication facilitation in the physical and personal domains is important, the greatest obstacles to communication success and satisfaction lie in the social domain. Talk is not valued equally everywhere. Some societies favor loquaciousness, others taciturnity. Moreover, communication is a multichannel activity; several behavioral modes operate simultaneously to convey messages (e.g., dress, posture, words, distance, gestures, crying, noise-making, and looking). Different places have different rules for communication. Sigman described the rules in a nursing home, which dictated that to be in a certain room, patients had to wear a particular type of clothing (no nightclothes), and communicative interaction was offered or withheld, depending on location and dress.[246] Attitudes toward the aging and expectations for behavior are communicated through conversational behavior. That is, for example, the topics of conversation, how long and how many turns each partner gets, and the responsiveness of interactors to the communicative initiative and expressions of the aging reveal the collective ideology of an institution (e.g., a nursing home), as well as the individual attitudes of interactors.

The essence of communication facilitation in the social domain is to relinquish control and to be responsive. Communication is facilitated when questions to which the answers are already known are not asked and when mindless activities to pass time do not occupy the aged. Perschbacher describes an application of reminiscence in a nursing home, which involved the teaching of history to a third grade class through the oral histories of the old.[247] An extensive cognitive-communication facilitation program was implemented in a nursing home through conversation and discussion groups, reading, writing, artistic endeavors and performance, and formal and informal enrichment.[248]

An integral part of the programs identified above, and of all communication facilitation programs, is the encouragement of helpful interactor communicative behavior. Some skills are generically helpful and can be taught to caregivers, volunteers, and families—for example, speaking slowly and clearly, without shouting, paraphrasing instead of repeating exactly, or orally emphasizing new topics to call attention to topic change.

Several manners of responding, developed primarily in the field of gerontology, reflect the importance of active, attentive listening. Responsive interactant behavior is particularly helpful in encouraging the aged to initiate and maintain communication effort. Several strategies have been used successfully. Orientation therapy aims to redirect errant thinking to present reality of time, place, and events.[249] Validation therapy leads to improvement of behavior patterns in speech, continence, self-stimulation, contentment, and awareness of external reality.[249] Validation techniques require the assumption that all behavior has meaning and that even when thinking is flawed by error or disorientation the underlying feelings and content survive. Interactants pursue the communicative interaction in spite of errors by recognizing, valuing, and supporting the patients' feelings in whatever time or place is real to them, even though it may not correspond to present reality.[249]

Validation can be used individually or in group sessions. In groups, it is important that group members have some homogeneity with regard to the degree of disorientation. The conversation in group therapy centers around conflicts and problems, with the leader exploring meaning and the feelings that correspond. Validation therapy encourages the patient to work out unresolved social and emotional conflicts, to relive past pleasures, to restimulate sensory memories, and to relieve boredom and stress by retreating from painful feelings or memories. Validation is a companion method of responding to patient behavior, not an alternative method.

A contrast of the responses of the interactant is illustrative of the different kinds of responses required of each.

Patient: I just saw my daughter here in the bathroom.

Orientation Therapy: You are in your bedroom. Your daughter isn't here right now. Today is Tuesday. Your daughter will come here tomorrow.

Validation therapy: Would you like your daughter to come here to see you?

Remotivation responsiveness uses more emotionally neutral themes. The goals here are not to problem solve, but to kindle enthusiasm for previously-done tasks, celebrations, or special activities (e.g., holidays, clothing, cooking). Life review therapy (reminiscing) focuses on listening and understanding the patient's memories for events, activities, and people. Life review has positive psychotherapeutic value. Individuals reflect on their lives in order to resolve, reorganize, and reintegrate the past with the present.[250] The principles of life review and validation therapies have not been systematically tested, but seem to have some value in facilitating the communication, through recall and rehearsal of semantic and episodic memory.

The majority of the aged show changes in communication behavior consequent to aging, but these changes infrequently affect their ability to carry on meaningful, productive lives. Some aged individuals fall prey to disease, which results in impairments of neuromotor or cognitive-linguistic foundations for communicative competence. Whatever the circumstance, the role of the speech-language pathologist and audiologist is to address the physical, personal, and social barriers to successful, satisfying communication. It is a formidable and rewarding challenge.

FUTURE RESEARCH DIRECTIONS

Among the most urgent research needs are studies designed to identify and describe age-related changes in communication. As contrasted with those identifying age-related differences in communication, such studies require longitudinal study. There are a number of research problems associated with longitudinal studies, not the least of which in the aging population is the problem of subject attrition. However, synthetic designs, such as that proposed by Schaie,[9,10] minimize risks related to sample representativeness and subject availability for repeated measures, while reducing cohort effects.

By its varied nature, communication is particularly susceptible to cohort effects. Hence, age-related differences in various aspects of communication behavior are difficult to interpret. The differences may not be due solely to aging, but rather to various other factors that characterize cohort groups. Several examples are readily apparent. Marked social changes have occurred over a period of years. Educational values and opportunities are different now than in the educational years of the old. The use of tobacco and other irritants to the mechanisms for vocal support and production have changed; gender and geographical location are critical variables in these changes. Dietary practices may be an important cohort factor, especially given the changes in dietary practices related to cholesterol in the past 20 years. Changes in environmental stress and in stress-related coping mechanisms may have an impact on communication. Older people were treated medically differently than younger people; effects of medical and pharmaceutical treatment in earlier days on voice and neurologic structure and function of old people may produce communication differences related to cohorts that are not solely consequential to aging. Studies of communication change over time in the aged would facilitate separation of age effects from cohort effects. Such a separation is critical to inferential, and then to empirical, understanding of physiologic and other correlates of communicative behavior.

Are communication changes in normal aging similar to those seen in older people who have diseases, e.g., Alzheimer's disease, cerebrovascular disease, but not as severe or more slowly progressing? Are any differences between the normally aging and the pathologically aging qualitative or quantitative? Some researchers suggest that neurologically, the same features seen in the brains of Alzheimer's patients (e.g., neurofibrillary tangles, senile plaques, granulovacuolar degeneration) are also seen, but to a lesser degree, in some normally aging persons. Moreover, normally aging persons often complain of relatively minor memory impairment; more severe memory impairment is a major feature of dementia. Specific, seemingly focal impairments in isolated aspects of communication characterize some normally aging persons, whereas obvious focal lesions related to cerebrovascular accidents produce more grave language and speech disorders. Performance of normally aging persons on various test batteries show some distinction between normally aging subjects and younger subjects. Performance also more clearly distinguishes severity groups of Alzheimer's patients and patients with Alzheimer's disease, and with other diseases and conditions to which the aged are particularly vulnerable. However, these studies are essentially studies of differences between groups. Studies of changes in communicative behavior over time, particularly in normals, are few. Bayles and Kazniak[57] expect to report in the near future the results of a 5-year longitudinal study on communication behavior in demented patients. Their data will be particularly useful, both methodically and as a springboard for future studies of the normally aging and of those with neuropathies associated with aging.

Communication is a complex, interactive process. While much of the initial research on communication differences and changes in the aging has focused on a singular aspect of communication and, until recently, primarily on hearing and speech and language production, the future must address communication processes of aged in natural, interactive environments. Ulatowska et al[200] advise focus on semantic and pragmatic aspects of complex discourse in order (1) to increase understanding of age-related changes in communication; (2) to develop of a lifespan psycholinguistic; and (3) to advance knowledge of the relationships of cognition and language.

In addition to the communication behavior, the natural communication environments of the aged deserve considerable research attention. The influence of a variety of environmental variables on communication efficiency and effectiveness deserves address. Such variables include, but are not limited to (1) communication partners' perceptions of and attitudes toward the aged; (2) facilitative communication techniques used by the old and their caregivers, families, and other communication partners; and (3) acoustic, illumination, proximity and aesthetic characteristics in frequently used communication spaces.

REFERENCES

1. Brotman H. Population projects: part I. Tomorrow's older population (to 2000). Gerontologist, 1977; 17:203–209.
2. Technology and aging in America. United States Office of Technology Assessment. OTA-BA-264. Washington, DC: United States Congress, 1985.
3. Sobel H. Aging theory: cellular and extracellular modalities. In: Kastenbaum R, ed. Contributions to the psychobiology of aging. New York: Spring Publishing, 1965:57.
4. Walford RL. Immunology and aging. In: Kastenbaum R, ed. Contributions to the psycho-biology of aging. New York: Springer, 1965:81.
5. Jarvik LF. Chromosomal changes and aging. In: Kasterbaum R, ed. Contributions to the psycho-biology of aging. New York: Springer, 1965:87.
6. Schaie KW, Geiwitz J. Adult development and aging. Boston: Little, Brown, 1982.
7. Birren JE, Renner VJ. Research on the psychology of aging; principles and experimentation. In: Birren JE, Schaie KW, eds. Handbook of the psychology of aging. New York: Van Nostrand Reinhold, 1977:3.
8. Ulatowska HK, ed. The aging brain: communication in the elderly. San Diego: College Hill Press, 1985.
9. Schaie KW. A general model for the study of developmental change. Psychol Bull 1965; 64:92–107.
10. Schaie KW. Quasi-experimental research designs in the psychology of aging. In: Birren JE, Schaie KW, eds. Handbook of the psychology of aging. New York: Van Nostrand Reinhold, 1977:39.
11. Welford AT. Motor performance. In: Birren JE, Schaie KW, eds. Handbook of the psychology of aging. New York: Van Nostrand Reinhold, 1977:450.
12. Rabbitt P. An age decrement in the ability to ignore irrelevant information. J Gerontol 1965; 20:233–238.
13. Wallach MA, Kogan N. Aspects of judgment and decision making: interelationships and changes with age. Behav Sci 1961; 6:23–36.
14. Rees JN, Botwinick J. Detection decision factors in auditory behavior of the elderly. J Gerontol 1971; 26:133–136.
15. Botwinick J. Aging and behavior. New York: Springer, 1973.
16. Feier CD, Gerstman LJ. Sentence comprehension abilities throughout the adult life span. J Gerontol 1980; 35:722–728.
17. Marshall L. Auditory processing in aging listeners. J Speech Hear Disord 1981; 46:226–240.
18. Yanz JL, Anderson SM. Comparison of speech perception skills in young and old listeners. Ear Hear 1984; 5:134–137.
19. Gordon-Salant S. Effects of aging on response criterion in speech recognition tasks. J Speech Hear Res 1986; 29:155–162.
20. Cumming E, Henry WE. Growing old: the process of disengagement. New York: Basic Books, 1961.
21. Ouslander JG. Drug therapy in the elderly. Ann Intern Med 1981; 95:711–722.

22. Brody H, Harman D, Ordy JM, eds. Clinical, morphologic, and neurochemical aspects in the aging nervous system. New York: Raven Press, 1975.
23. Appel FW, Appel EM. Intracranial variation in the weight of the human brain. Hum Biol 1942; 14:48–68.
24. Ordy JM, Brizee KR. Neurobiology of aging. New York: Plenum, 1975.
25. Brody H. Organization of the cerebral cortex. III. A study of aging in the human cortex. J Comp Neurol 1955; 102:511–556.
26. Corbin KB, Gardner ED. Decrease in number of myelinated fibers in human spinal roots with age. Anat Rec 1937; 68:63–74.
27. Birren JE. The psychology of aging. Englewood Cliffs: Prentice-Hall, 1964.
28. Strehler BL. Introduction: aging and the human brain. In: Terry RD, Gerson S, eds. Aging 1975; 3:1–22.
29. Raisman G. What hope for repair of the brain? Ann Neurol 1978; 3:101–106.
30. Brizzee KR, Johnson FA. Depth distribution of lipofuscin in cerebral cortex of albino rat. Acta Neuropath (Berl) 1974; 16:205–209.
31. Lawrence S, Stein DG. Recovery after brain damage and the concept of localization of function. In: Finger S, ed. Recovery from brain damage, research and theory. New York: Plenum, 1978:369.
32. Stein DG, Firl AC. Brain damage and reorganization of function in old age. Experimental Neurol 1976; 52:157–167.
33. Clark L, Knowles J. Age differences in dichotic listening performance. J Gerontol 1973; 28:173–178.
34. Nebes RD, Madden DJ, Berg WD. The effect of age on hemispheric asymmetry in visual and auditory identification. Exp Aging Res 1983; 9:87–91.
35. Borod JC, Goodglass H. Lateralization of linguistic and melodic processing with age. Neuropsychologia 1980; 18:79–83.
36. Byrd M, Moscovitch M. Lateralization of peripherally and centrally masked words in young and elderly people. J Gerontol 1984; 39:699–703.
37. Obler LK, Woodward S, Albert ML. Changes in cerebral lateralization in aging. Neuropsychologia 1984; 22:235–240.
38. Botwinick J. Intellectual abilities. In: Birren JE, Schaie KW, eds. Handbook of the psychology of aging. New York: Van Nostrand Reinhold, 1977:500.
39. Goldstein E, Shelly C. Does the right hemisphere age more rapidly than the left? J Clin Neuropsychol 1981; 3:65–78.
40. Riege WH, Metter EJ, Williams MV. Age and hemisphere asymmetry in nonverbal factual memory. Neuropsychologia 1980; 18:707–710.
41. Rastatter MP, Lawson-Brill CL. Reaction times of aging subjects to nonaural verbal stimuli: some evidence for a reduction right-hemisphere linguistic processing capacity. J Speech Hear Res 1987; 30:261–267.
42. Horn J. Organization of data on life-span development of human abilities. In: Goulet LR, Baltes PB, eds. Life-span developmental psychology: theory and research. New York: Academic Press, 1970:424.
43. Humphries LG, Parsons CK. Piagetian tasks measure intelligence and intelligence tests assess cognitive development: a reanalysis. Intelligence 1979; 3:369–382.
44. Owens WA. Age and mental ability: a second adult follow-up. J Educ Psychol 1966; 57:311–325.
45. Birren JE, Morrison DF. Analysis of the WAIS subtests in relation to age and education. J Gerontol 1961; 16:363–369.
46. Botwinick J, Birren JE. Intellectual abilities. In: Birren JE, Schaie KW, eds. Handbook of the psychology of aging. New York: Van Nostrand Reinhold, 1977:580.
47. Miller E. Abnormal aging: the psychology of senile and preseniledementia. New York: John Wiley & Sons, 1977.
48. Botwinick J. Cognitive processes in maturity and old age. New York: Springer, 1967.
49. Horn J. Intelligence: why it grows, why it declines. Transaction 1967; 5:23–31.
50. Horn J. Organization of abilities and the development of intelligence. Psychol Rev 1968; 75:242–259.
51. Papalia DW. The status of several conservation abilities across the life-span. Hum Dev 1972; 15:229–243.
52. Sanders S, Laurendeau M, Bergeron J. Aging and the concept of space: the conservation of surfaces. J Gerontol 1966; 21:281–285.
53. Storck PA, Looft WR, Hooper FH. Interrelationships among Piagetian tasks and traditional measures of cognitive abilities in mature and aged adults. J Gerontol 1972; 27:461–465.
54. Papalia DW, Salverson SM, True M. An evaluation of quantity conservation performance during old age. Int J Aging Hum Dev 1973; 4:103–104.
55. Squire LR. Mechanisms of memory. Science 1986; 232:1612-1619.
56. Poon LW. Differences in human memory with aging: nature, causes, and clinical implications. In: Birren JE, Schaie KW, eds. Handbook of the psychology of the aging. New York: Van Nostrand Reinhold, 1985:427.
57. Bayles KA, Kazniak AW. Communication and cognition in normal aging and dementia. Boston: College Hill Press, 1987.
58. Perlmutter M. What is memory aging the aging of? Dev Psychol 1978; 14:330–345.
59. Byrd M. Age differences in the retrieval of information from semantic memory. Exp Aging Res 1984; 10:29–33.
60. Craik F. Age differences in remembering. In: Squire LR, Butters N, eds. Neuropsychology of memory. New York: Guilford, 1984:3.
61. Welford AT. Psychomotor performance. In: Birren JE, ed. Handbook of aging and the individual: psychological and biological aspects. Chicago: University of Chicago Press, 1959.
62. Sweeting PM, Baken RJ. Voice onset time in a normal aged population. J Speech Hear Res 1982; 25(1):129–134.
63. Neiman GS, Klich RJ, Shuey EM. Voice onset time in young and 70-year-old women. J Speech Hear Res 1983; 26:118–129.
64. Botwinick J, Thompson I. Practice of speeded response in relation to age, sex, and set. J Gerontol 1967; 22:72–76.
65. Spiriduso W. Reaction and movement time as a function of age and physical activity level. J Gerontol 1975; 30:435–440.
66. Smith K, Green D. Scientific motion study and aging process in performance. Ergonomics 1962; 5:155–164.
67. Welford AT. Performance, biological mechanisms and age: a theoretical sketch. In: Welford AT, Birren JE, eds. Behavior, aging and the nervous system. Springfield, IL: Charles C Thomas, 1965:3.
68. Hymes D. Language in culture and society. New York: Harper & Row, 1964.
69. Weale RA. On the eye. In: Welford AT, Birren JE, eds. Behavior, aging, and the nervous system. Springfield, IL: Charles C Thomas, 1965:307.
70. Corso JF. Sensory processes and age effects in normal adults. J Gerontol 1971; 26:90–105.
71. Birren JE, Casperson RC, Botwinick J. Age changes in pupil size. J Gerontol 1950; 5:216–221.
72. Weiss AD. Sensory functions. In: Birren JE, ed. Handbook of aging and the individual: psychological and biological aspects. Chicago: University of Chicago Press, 1959.
73. Cristarella MC. Visual function of the elderly. Am J Occup Ther 1977; 31:432–440.

74. Fozard JL, Wolf E, Bell B, McFarland RA, Podolsky S. Visual perception and communication. In: Birren JE, Shaie KW, eds. Handbook of the psychology of aging, New York: Van Nostrand Reinhold, 1977:497.
75. Birren JE, Shock NW. Age changes in rate and level of visual dark adaptation. J Appl Physiol 1950; 2:407–411.
76. Domey RG, McFarland RA, Chadwick E. Dark adaptation as a function of age and time: II. A derivation. J Gerontol 1960; 15:267–279.
77. Storandt M. Psychologic aspects. In: Steinberg FV, ed. Care of the geriatric patient. 6th ed. St. Louis: CV Mosby, 1983:417.
78. Botwinick J, Robbin JS, Brinley JF. Reorganization of perception with age. J Gerontol 1959; 14:85–88.
79. Heath HA, Orbach J. Reversibility of the necker cube: IV response of elderly people. Percept Mot Skills, 1963; 17:625–626.
80. Clay HM. An age difficulty in separating spatially contiguous data. J Gerontol 1956; 11:318–322.
81. Axelrod S, Cohen LD. Senescence and imbedded figure performance in vision and touch. Percept Mot Skills 1951; 12:283–288.
82. Bondy M. The identifying of overlapping capital letters by subjects of different age. Proceedings of the 7th International Congress of Gerontology, Vol. 6. Vienna: Viennese Medical Academy, 1966.
83. Davis H. Abnormal hearing and deafness. In: Davis H, Silverman R, eds. Hearing and deafness. New York: Holt, Rinehart & Winston, 1978:87.
84. Hinchcliffe R. The antomical locus of presbycusis. J Speech Hear Res 1962; 27:301–310.
85. Crabbe F. Presbycusis. Acta Otolaryngol [Suppl] 1963; 183:24–26.
86. Schuknecht HF. Further observations on the pathology of presbycusis. Arch Otolaryngol 1964; 80:369–382.
87. Hansen C, Reske-Nielsen E. Pathological studies in presbycusis. Arch Otolaryngol 1965; 82:115–132.
88. Otto WC, McCandless GA. Aging and the auditory site of lesion. Ear Hear 1982; 3:110–117.
89. Rosenwasser H. Otitic problems in the aged. Geriatrics 1964; 19:11–17.
90. Covell W. Histological changes in the aging cochlea. J Gerontol 1952; 7:173–177.
91. Schuknecht H. Presbycusis. Laryngoscope 1955; 65:402–419.
92. Jorgensen M. Changes of aging in the inner ear. Arch Otolaryngol 1961; 74:56–62.
93. Pestalooza G, Shore I. Clinical evaluation of presbycusis on the basis of different tests of auditory function. Laryngoscope 1955; 65:1136–1163.
94. Gacek R. Degenerative hearing loss in aging. In: Fields W, ed. Neurological and sensory disorders in the elderly. New York: Stratton International Medical Book, 1975.
95. Dayal VS, Shattachargga TK. Comparative study of age-related cochlear hair cell loss. Ann Otol Rhinol Laryngol 1986; 95:510–519.
96. Soucek S, Michaels L, Frohlich A. Evidence for hair cell degeneration as the primary lesion in hearing loss of the elderly. J Otolaryngol 1986; 15:175–183.
97. Crowe S, Guild S, Polvogt L. Observations on the pathology of high tone deafness. Bull Johns Hopkins Hosp 1934; 54:315–379.
98. Schuknecht HF. The effect of aging on the cochlea. In: Graham B, ed. Sensori-neural hearing processes and disorders. Boston: Little, Brown, 1967:393.
99. Goodhill V, Guggenheim P. Pathology, diagnosis and therapy of deafness. In: Travis L, ed. Handbook of speech pathology and audiology. New York: Appleton-Century-Crofts, 1971:279.
100. Kirikae I, Sato T, Shitara T. A study of hearing in advanced age. Laryngoscope 1964; 74:205–220.
101. Schuknecht H, Woellner R. Experimental and clinical study of deafness from lesions of the cochlear nerve. J Laryngol 1955; 69:75–97.
102. Krmpotic-Nemanic J. A new concept of the pathogenesis of presbycusis. Arch Otolaryngol 1971; 93:161–166.
103. Rasmussen A. Studies of the VIIIth cranial nerve of man. Laryngoscope 1940; 50:67–83.
104. Feldman R, Reger S. Relations among hearing, reaction time, and age. J Speech Hear Res 1967; 10:479–495.
105. Welsh LW, Welsh JJ, Healy MP. Central presbycusis. Laryngoscope 1985; 95:128–136.
106. Stach BA, Jerger JF, Fleming KA. Central presbycusis: a longitudinal case study. Ear Hear 1985; 6:304–306.
107. Ries PW. Hearing ability of persons by sociodemographic and health characteristics. Vital and health statistics. United States Department of Health and Human Services, National Center for Health Statistics. DHHS publication No. (PHS) 82-1568, series 10, No. 140, Hyattsville, MD, 1982.
108. Rowland M. Basic data on hearing levels of adults, 25–74, U.S. United States Department of Health and Human Services, National Center for Health Statistics. 1971–75, USDHEW publication No. (PHS) 80-1663, series 11, No. 215, Hyattsville, MD, 1980.
109. Katasarkas A, Ayukawa H. Hearing loss due to aging (presbycusis). J Otolaryngol 1986; 15:239–244.
110. Wunderlich G. Characteristics of residents in institutions for the aged and chronically ill. National Health Survey, Series 12:2, Washington, DC: Department of Health, Education, and Welfare, 1965.
111. Bloomer H. Communication problems among aged county hospital patients. Geriatrics 1960; 15:291–295.
112. Alpiner J. Audiological problems of the aged. Geriatrics 1963; 18:19–26.
113. Chafee C. Rehabilitation needs of nursing home patients: a report of a survey. Rehabil Lit 1967; 28:377–382.
114. Schow RL, Nerbonne MA. Hearing levels among elderly nursing home residents. J Speech Hear Disord 1980; 45:124–132.
115. Miller J, Ort R. Hearing problems in a home for the aged. Acta Otolaryngol 1965; 59:33–34.
116. Lasser RP, Master AM. Observation of frequency distribution curves of blood pressure in persons aged 20–106 years. Geriatrics 1959; 14:345.
117. Rosen S, Plester D, El-Mofty A, Rosen HV. High frequency audiometry in presbycusis: a comparative study of the Mabaan tribe in the Sudan with urban populations. Arch Otolaryngol 1964; 79:1–32.
118. Glorig A, Davis H. Age, noise, and hearing loss. Trans Am Otologic Soc 1961; 49:262–280.
119. Rosen S. Hearing studies in selected urban and rural population. Trans N Y Acad Sci 1966; 29:9–21.
120. Glorig A, Nixon J. Hearing loss as a function of age. Laryngoscope 1962; 72:1562–1610.
121. Corso J. Presbycusis, hearing aids, and aging. Audiology 1977; 16:146–163.
122. Bunch CC. Age variations in auditory acuity. Arch Otolaryngol 1929; 9:625–626.
123. Bunch CC. Further observations on age variations in auditory acuity. Arch Otolaryngol 1931; 13:170–180.
124. Steinberg JC, Montgomery HC, Gardner MB. Results of the world's fair hearing test. J Acoustical Soc Am 1940; 12:291.
125. Goetzinger C, Rousey C. Hearing problems in later life. Med Times 1959; 87:771–780.
126. Tyler RS, Baker LJ. Difficulties experience by tinnitus sufferers. J Speech Hear Disord 1983; 48:150–154.
127. Leske MC. Prevalence estimates of communicative disorders in the U.S.: Language, hearing, and vestibular disorders. Asha 1981; 23:229–237.
128. Schuknecht H, Igaraski M. Pathology of slowly progres-

sive sensorineural deafness. Trans Acad Ophthalmol Otolaryngol 1964; 68:222–242.
129. Harbert F, Young I, Menduke H. Audiologic findings in presbycusis. J Aud Res 1966; 6:297–312.
130. Punch J, McConnell F. The speech discrimination function of elderly adults. J Aud Res 1969; 9:159–166.
131. Corso J. Auditory perception communication. In: Birren J, Schaie KW, eds. The psychology of aging. New York: Van Nostrand Reinhold, 1977:535.
132. Sataloff J, Vassallo L. Hard-of-hearing senior citizens and the physician. Geriatrics 1966; 21:182-185.
133. Klotz REE, Kilbane M. Hearing in an aging population. Preliminary report. N Engl J Med 1962; 266:277–280.
134. Gaeth JH. A study of phonemic regression in relation to hearing loss. Doctoral dissertation, Northwestern University, XVI, 1948. As cited in: Smith R, Prather W. Phoneme discrimination in older persons under varying signal-to-noise conditions. J Speech Hear Res 1971; 14:630–638.
135. Blumenfeld VG, Bergman M, Millner E. Speech discrimination in an aging population. J Speech Hear Res 1969; 12:210–217.
136. Smith R, Prather W. Phoneme discrimination in older persons under varying signal-to-noise conditions. J Speech Hear Res 1971; 14:630–638.
137. Birren JE, Botwinick J. Age differences in finger, jaw and foot reaction time to auditory stimuli. J Gerontol 1955; 10:429–432.
138. Crossman ERFW, Szafran J. Changes with age in the speed of information intake and discrimination. Experientia [Suppl] 1956; 4:128–135.
139. Gregory RL. Increase in "neurological noise" as a factor in aging. In: Proceedings. IV. Congress of the International Association on Gerontology 1959; 1:314.
140. Freeman GL. The facilitative and inhibitory effects of muscular tension upon performance. Am J Psychol 1933; 45:17–52.
141. Freeman GL. The optimal muscular tensions for various performances. Am J Psychol 1938; 51:146–150.
142. Welford AT. Social, psychological and physiological gerontology—an experimental psychologist's approach. In: Williams RH, Tibbitts C, Donahue W, eds. Processes of aging. Vol. 1. New York: Atherton Press, 1963.
143. Calearo C, Lazzaroni A. Speech intelligibility in relation to the speed of the message. Laryngoscope 1957; 67:410–419.
144. deQuiras J. Accelerated speech audiometry, an examination of test results. Tanndorf J, trans. Trans Beltone Institute Hear Res Chicago: Beltone Institute of Hearing Research, 1964, No. 17.
145. Sticht T, Gray B. The intelligibility of time compressed words as a function of age and hearing loss. J Speech Hear Res 1969; 12:443–448.
146. Schon T. The effects of speech intelligibility of time-compression and expansion on normal hearing, hard of hearing, and aged males. J Aud Res 1970; 10:263–268.
147. Konkle D, Beasley D, Bess F. Intelligibility of time-altered speech in relation to chronological aging. J Speech Hear Res 1977; 20:108–115.
148. DiCarlo L, Taub H. The influence of compression expansion on the intelligibility of speech by young and aged aphasic (demonstrated CVA) individuals. J Commun Disord 1972; 5:299–306.
149. Jerger J, Shedd J, Harford E. On the detection of extremely small changes in sound intensity. Arch Otolaryngol 1959; 69:200–211.
150. Goetzinger C, Proud G, Dirks D, Embrey J. A study of hearing in advanced age. Arch Otolaryngol 1963; 73:662–673.
151. Konig E. Pitch discrimination and age. Acta Otolaryngol 1957; 48:475–489.
152. Davignon D, Leshowitz B. The speech in noise test: a new approach to the assessment of communication cability of elderly persons. Int J Aging Hum Dev 1986; 23:149–160.
153. Weinstein B, Ventry IM. Audiometric correlates of the hearing handicap inventory for the elderly. J Speech Hear Disord 1983; 48:379–384.
154. Ryan W, Burk K. Perceptual and acoustic correlates of aging in the speech of males. J Commun Disord 1974; 7:181–192.
155. Ptacek PH, Sander EK, Maloney WH, Jackson CCR. Phonatory and related changes with advanced age. J Speech Hear Res 1966; 9:353–360.
156. Hutchinson JM, Robinson KL, Nerbonne MA. Patterns of nasalance in a sample of normal gerontologic subjects. J Commun Disord 1978; 11:469–481.
156a. Canter GJ. Speech characteristics of patients with Parkinson's disease. III. Articulation, diadochokinesis, and overall speech adequacy. J Speech Hear Disord 1965; 30:217–224.
157. Darley FL, Aronson AE, Brown JR. Differential diagnostic patterns of dysarthria. J Speech Hear Res 1969; 12:246–269.
158. Grunwell P, Huskins S. Intelligibility in acquired dysarthria—a neurophonetic approach: three case studies. J Commun Disord 1979; 12:9–22.
159. Sarno M. Speech impairment in Parkinson's disease. Arch Phys Med Rehabil 1968; 49:269–275.
160. Logemann JA, Fisher HB. Vocal tract control in Parkinson's disease: phonetic feature analysis of misarticulations. J Speech Hear Disord 1981; 46:348–352.
161. Hunker CJ, Abbs JH, Barlow SM. The relationship between Parkinsonian rigidity and hypokinesia in the orofacial system: a quantitative analysis. Neurology 1982; 32:749–754.
162. Kruel E. Neuromuscular control examination (NMC) for parkinsonism: vowel prolongations and diadochokinetic and reading rates. J Speech Hear Res 1972; 15:72–83.
163. Kuller WC. Dysfluency (stuttering) in extrapyramidal disease. Arch Neurol 1983; 40:175–177.
164. Ptacek P, Sander E. Age recognition from voice. J Speech Hear Res 1966; 9:273–277.
165. Shipp T, Hollien H. Perception of the aging male voice. J Speech Hear Res 1969; 13:703–710.
166. Ryan E, Capadano H. Age perceptions and evaluative reactions toward adult speakers. J Gerontol 1978; 33:98–102.
167. Linville SE, Korabic EW. Elderly listeners' estimates of vocal age in adult females. J Acoust Soc Am 1986; 80:692–694.
168. Blonsky R, Logemann J, Boshes B, Fisher H. Comparison of speech and swallowing function in patients with tremor disorders and in normal geriatric patients: cinefluorographic study. J Gerontol 1975; 30:299–303.
169. Horii Y, Ryan W. Fundamental frequency characteristics and perceived age of adult male speakers. Folia Phoniatr 1975; 33:227–233.
170. Hartman D, Danhauer J. Perceptual features of speech for males in four perceived age decades. J Acoust Soc Am 1976; 59:713–715.
171. Ryan W. Acoustic aspects of the aging voice. J Gerontol 1972; 27:265–268.
172. Mysak ED. Pitch and duration characteristics of older males. J Speech Hear Res 1959; 2:46–54.
173. Mysak ED, Hanley T. Vocal aging. Geriatrics 1959; 14:652–656.
174. Hollien H, Shipp T. Speaking fundamental frequency and chronologic age in males. J Speech Hear Res 1972; 15:155–159.
175. Mueller PB, Sweeney RJ, Baribeau LJ. Senescence of the voice: morphology of excised male larynges. Folia Phoniatr 1985; 37:134–138.

176. McGlone R, Hollien H. Vocal pitch characteristics of aged women. J Speech Hear Res 1963; 6:164–170.
177. Benjamin BJ. Frequency variability in the aged voice. J Gerontol 1981: 36:722–726.
178. Ramig LA, Ringel RA. Effects of physiological aging on selected acoustic charcteristics of voice. J Speech Hear Res 1983; 26(1):22–30.
179. Ramig LA. Effects of physiological aging on speaking and reading rates. J Commun Disord 1983; 16:217–226.
180. Endres W, Bambach W, Flosser G. Voice spectrograms as a function of age, voice disguise, and voice imitation. J Acoust Soc Am 1970: 49:1842–1848.
181. Wilcox KA, Horri Y. Age and changes in vocal jitter. J Gerontol 1980; 35:194–198.
182. Ramig LA. Effects of physiological aging on vowel spectral noise. J Gerontol 1983; 38(2):223–225.
183. Honjo I, Isshiki N. Laryngoscopic and voice characteristics of aged persons. Arch Otolaryngol 1980; 106:149–150.
184. Logemann JA, Fisher HB, Boshes B, Blonsky E. Frequency and cooccurrence of vocal tract dysfunctions in the speech of a large sample of parkinson patients. J Speech Hear Disord 1978; 43:47–57.
185. Paulson GW. Benign essential tremor: features that aid in diagnosis. Postgrad Med 1982; 71:105–107.
186. Hanson WR, Metter EJ. DAF speech rate modification in Parkinson's disease: a report of two cases. In: Berry WR, ed. Clinical dysarthria. San Diego: College Hill Press, 1983:231.
187. Oyer HJ, Deal LV. Temporal aspects of speech and the aging process. Folia Phoniatr 1985; 37, 109–112.
188. Griew S. Information transmission and age. In: Williams R, Tibbits C, Donahue W, eds. Processes of aging; social and psychological prospectives. New York: Atherton Press, 1963.
189. Birren JE. The significance of age changes in speed of perception and psychomotor skills. In: Anderson JE, ed. Psychological aspects of aging. Washington: American Psychological Association, 1956:97.
190. Fox C. Vocabulary ability in later maturity. J Educ Psychol 1947; 38:482–492.
191. Obler LK, Albert ML. Language and aging: a neurobehavioral analysis. In: Beasley DS, Davis GA, eds. Aging: communication processes and disorders. New York: Grune & Stratton, 1981:107.
192. Dunn LM, Dunn LM. Peabody picture vocabulary test (revised). Circle Pines, MN: American Guidance Service, 1981.
193. Bayles KA, Tomoeda CK, Boone DR. A view of age-related changes in language function. Dev Neuropsychol 1985; 1:231–264.
194. Smith M. Relation between word variety and mean letter length of words with chronological and mental ages. J Gen Psychol 1957; 56:27–43.
195. Riegel K. Changes in psycholinguistic performances with age. In: Talland G, ed. Human aging and behavior. New York: Academic Press, 1968:239.
195a. Bowles NL, Poon LW. Aging and retrieval of words in semantic memory. J Gerontol 1985; 40:71–77.
195b. Borod JC, Goodglass H, Kaplan E. Normative data on the Boston diagnostic aphasia examination, parietal lobe battery, and Boston naming test. J Clin Neuropsychol 1980; 2:209–215.
196. Obler L, Nicholas M, Albert ML, Woodward S. On comprehension across the adult life span. Cortex 1985; 21:273–280.
197. Craik F. Short-term memory and the aging process. In: Talland GE, ed. Human aging and behavior. New York: Academic Press, 1968:131.
198. Fullerton AM, Smith AD. Age-related differences in the use of redundancy. J Gerontol 1980; 35:729–735.
199. Kausler DH, Puckett JM. Adult age differences in memory for sex of voice. J Gerontol 1981; 36:44–50.
200. Ulatowska HK, Cannito MP, Hayashi MM, Flemming SG. Language abilities in the elderly. In: Ulatowska HK, ed. The aging brain: communication in the elderly. San Diego: College Hill Press, 1985:125.
201. Ulatowska HK, Hayashi MM, Cannito MP, Fleming SG. Disruption of reference. Brain Lang 1986; 28:24–41.
201a. Spreen O, Benton A. Neurosensory center comprehensive examination for aphasia. Victoria, BC: Neurology Laboratory, Department of Psychology, University of Victoria, 1969.
202. Gordon K, Hutchinson J, Allen C. An evaluation of selected discourse characteristics among the elderly. Research laboratory report. Pocatello, ID: Department of Speech Pathology and Audiology, Idaho State University.
203. Obler L, Albert M, Goodglass H, Benson D. Aging and aphasia type. Brain Lang 1978; 6:318–322.
204. Smith M. Linguistic constancy in individuals when long periods of time are covered and different types of material are sampled. J Gen Psychol 1955; 56:27–43.
205. Goodglass H, Kaplan E. The assessment of aphasia and related disorders. Philadelphia: Lea & Fibiger, 1972.
206. Obler LK. Narrative discourse style in the elderly. In: Obler LK, Albert ML, eds. Language communication in the elderly. Lexington, MA: Heath, 1980:75.
207. Nebes RD, Andrews-Kulis MS. The effect of age on the speed of sentence formation and incidental learning. Exp Aging Res 1976; 2:315–331.
208. Halpern H, Darley FL, Brown JR. Differential language and neurologic characteristics in cerebral involvement. J Speech Hear Disord 1973; 38:162–173.
209. Kynette D, Kemper S. Aging and the loss of grammatical forms: a cross-sectional study of language performance. Lang Commun 1986; 6:65–72.
210. North A, Ulatowska H. Competence in independently living older adults: assessment and correlates. J Gerontol 1981; 36:576–582.
211. Patterson L, Newton M. Turn taking convensions in dyads involving aged persons. Paper presented at the Annual Convention of the American Speech-Language-Hearing Association, Detroit, 1986.
212. Lubinski R, Morrison EB, Rigrodsky S. Perception of spoken communication by elderly chronically ill patients in an institutional setting. J Speech Hear Disord 1981; 46:405–412.
213. American Psychiatric Association. Diagnostic and statistical manual of mental disorder. 3rd ed. DSM III. Washington, DC: American Psychiatric Association, 1980.
214. Bayles KA, Boone DR. The potential of language tasks for identifying senile dementia. J Speech Hear Disord 1982; 47:210–217.
215. Irigaray L. Le language des dements. The Hague: Mouton, 1973.
216. Whitaker H. A case of the isolation of the language function. In: Whitaker H, Whitaker H, eds. Studies in neurolinguistics. Vol. 2. New York: Academic Press, 1976:1.
217. Schwartz MF, Marin OSM, Saffran EM. Dissociations of language function in dementia: a case study. Brain Lang 1979; 7:277–306.
218. Obler LK, Albert ML. Language in aging. In: Albert ML, ed. Clinical neurology of aging. New York: Oxford, 1984:245.
219. Beasley DS, Davis GA, eds. Aging: communication processes and disorders. New York: Grune & Stratton, 1981.
220. Bayles KA, Tomoeda CK. Confrontation naming impairment and dementia. Brain Lang 1983; 19:98–114.
221. Kirshner HS, Webb WG, Kelly MP. The naming disorder of dementia. Neuropsychologia 1984; 22(1):23–30.
222. Bayles KA, Tomoeda CK. Confrontation and generative naming abilities of dementia patients. In: Brookshire RH, ed. Proceedings of the clinical aphasiology conference. Minneapolis: BRK Publishers, 1983:304.

223. Bayles KA. Communication in dementia. Paper presented at the University of Texas at Dallas Callier Annual Bruton Lecture Series, An International Symposium on the Aging Brain—Biological, Cognitive and Linguistic Considerations, Dallas, TX.
224. Schmitt FA, Mitchell DB. Naming speed, retrieval efficiency, and facilitation in dementia of the Alzheimer's type. Paper presented at the annual meeting of the International Neuropsychological Society, Houston, TX, 1984.
225. deAjuriaguerra J, Tissot R. Some aspects of language in various forms of senile dementia (comparisons with language in childhood). In: Lenneberg EH, Lenneberg E, ed. Foundations of language development: vol. 1. New York: Academic Press, 1975:323.
226. Bayles KA. Effects of dementing illness on communicative function. Paper presented as part of symposium to the International Neuropsychological Society, San Diego, California.
227. Gewirth LR, Shindler AG, Hier DB. Altered patterns of word association in dementia and aphasia. Brain Lang 1984; 21:307–317.
228. Schwartz MF, Saffran EM, Marin OSM. Fractionating the reading process in dementia: evidence for word specific print-to-sound associations. In: Coltheart M, Patterson K, Marshall JC, eds. Deep dyslexia. London: Routledge and Kegan Paul, 1980:259.
229. Warrington EK. The selective impairments of semantic memory. Q J Exp Psychol 1975; 27:635–657.
230. Bayles KA. Management of neurogenic communication disorders associated with dementia. In: Chapey R, ed. Language intervention strategies in adult aphasia. Baltimore: Williams & Wilkins, 1986:462.
231. Miller WR. Psychological deficit in depression. Psychol Bull 1975; 82:238–260.
232. Miller E, Lewis P. Recognition memory in elderly patients with depression and dementia: a signal detection analysis. J Abnorm Psychol 1977; 86:84–86.
233. Whitehead A. The pattern of WAIS performance in elderly psychiatric patients. Br J Social Clinical Psychol 1973; 12:435–436.
234. Sarno MT, Silverman M, Sands E. Speech therapy and language recovery in severe aphasia. J Speech Hear Res 1970; 13:607–623.
235. Hagen C. Communicative abilities in hemiplegia: effect of speech therapy. Arch Phys Med Rehabil 1973; 54:454–463.
236. Wertz RT, Collins MJ, Weiss D, Kurtzke JF, Friden T, Brookshire RH, Pierce J, Holtzapple P, Hubbard DJ, Porch BE, West JA, Davis L, Matovitch V, Morley GK, Resurreccion E. Veterans administration cooperative study on aphasia: a comparison of individual and group treatment. J Speech Hear Res 1981; 24:580–594.
237. Basso A, Capitani E, Vignolo LA. Influence of rehabilitation on language skills in aphasic patients. Arch Neurol 1979; 36:190–196.
238. Scheull H. Auditory impairment in aphasia: Significance and retraining techniques. J Speech Hear Disord 1953; 18:14–21.
239. Brookshire R. Auditory comprehension and aphasia. In: Johns D, ed. Clinical management of neurogenic communicative disorders. Boston: Little, Brown, 1978:103.
240. Schlanger P, Schlanger B. Adapting role-playing activities with aphasic patients. J Speech Hear Disor 1970; 35:229–243.
241. Holland A. Comment on "Spouses' understanding of the communication disabilities of aphasic patients." J Speech Hear Disord 1977; 42:307–311.
242. Wallace GL, Canter GJ. Effects of personally relevant language materials on the performance of severely aphasic individuals. J Speech Hear Disord 1985; 50:385–390.
243. Aten J, Calicuiri M, Holland A. The efficacy of functional communication therapy for chronic aphasic patients. J Speech Hear Disord 1982; 47:93–96.
244. Matkin ND, Hodgson WR. Amplification and the elderly patient. Otolaryngol Clin North Am 1982; 15:371–386.
245. Blood G, Blood I. A tactic for facilitating social interaction with laryngectomees. J Speech Hear Disord 1982; 47:416–419.
246. Sigman S. Conversational behavior in two health care institutions for the elderly. Int J Aging Hum Behav 1985; 21:137–154.
247. Perschbacher R. An application of reminiscence in an activity setting. J Gerontol 1984; 24:343–345.
248. Feier CD, Leight G. A communication-cognition program for elderly nursing home residents. Gerontologist 1981; 21:408–416.
249. Jones GMM. Validation therapy: a companion to reality orientation. Can Nurse 1985; 80:20–22.
250. Chubon S. A novel approach to the process of life review. J Gerontol Nurs 1980; 6:343–347.

31 Speech and Language Disorders Associated with Various Neuropathologies

John D. Tonkovich, Ph.D.

Neurologic damage in individuals effects a number of motor, sensory, and other behavioral changes, which may or may not include communication disorders. The damage may be focal or diffuse, reversible or irreversible. It may result from a single neurologic episode or several or may be progressive and degenerative. When they exist, speech and language sequelae of neuropathologies are determined by a number of factors, including the nature of the damage, the location of the damage, and the extent of the damage, as well as the premorbid communicative abilities of the individual.

Stroke or cerebrovascular accident (CVA) is the most commonly occurring neuropathology, and it is recognized primarily, though not exclusively, as a disorder of aging. Stroke incidence figures led Metter[1] to infer that for a population of 230 million people at any given time, approximately one million will be living after suffering a stroke, while 250,000 to 500,000 will suffer a stroke annually, and 125,000 to 250,000 will subsequently die from stroke-related causes. The aphasias associated with CVAs affecting the left hemisphere have a long, rich history of investigation and description, and these communicative disorders have been addressed in Chapter 25. The motor speech disorders or dysarthrias, which often result from CVA have also been studied extensively. For a complete description of these disorders see Chapters 18 and 19. Communicative disorders resulting from unilateral damage to the right cerebral hemisphere have gained attention from speech-language pathologists only since the mid-1970s. These communicative disorders, which seem to reflect the combined interactive effects of impairments of the cognitive and linguistic systems, constitute one of the primary focuses of this chapter.

Following cerebrovascular accident, the next most commonly occurring neuropathology results from head trauma. Because of the high incidence of closed head injuries, primarily as a result of motor vehicle accidents, and increased survival rates over the last several decades, attributable to improved health care technology, closed head injury survivors and their resultant communicative impairments have been the focus of speech-language rehabilitation efforts. Once again however, interest in these communicative impairments has only occurred primarily since the 1970s. Like the right hemisphere damaged patients, closed head injured patients display communicative impairments which are typified by cognitive and linguistic deficits. These communicative impairments will also be addressed in this chapter. Since many of the speech-language intervention techniques for right hemisphere damaged and closed head injured patients target some of the same behavioral skill areas, treatment techniques for both groups are discussed at the end of this chapter, following extensive description of each group separately.

Motor speech disorders associated with progressive, degenerative neuropathologies such as Parkinson's disease, multiple sclerosis, amyotrophic lateral sclerosis, Huntington's chorea, and Friedreich's ataxia, are described in Chapter 19. For a description of the communicative disturbances associated with dementia, see Chapter 30.

RIGHT HEMISPHERE COMMUNICATIVE DISORDERS

Communicative disorders associated with unilateral damage to the right cerebral hemisphere went largely unnoticed and untreated until the middle 1970s. Whereas other neurobehavioral sequelae associated with right hemisphere damage had been identified and described long before that time, speech-language pathology intervention for CVA patients was limited to those who exhibited aphasia and/or dysarthria. That right hemisphere damaged patients were overlooked by speech-language pathologists was no coincidence. Several factors were responsible for this lack of attention to right hemisphere based communicative disorders.

Physicians, by and large, were not likely to refer right hemisphere damaged patients for speech-language pathology services unless these patients displayed overt symptoms, such as dysarthria and/or hemispatial visual neglect, that interfered with communicative aspects of reading and writing. Right hemisphere damaged patients, after all, tended to have good, though copious sentence formulation skills. They showed auditory comprehension within functional limits and no evidence of word-retrieval disorders. In short, these individuals could not be described as being aphasic. While such patients had some difficultics using language appropriately in context, speech-language pathologists were not accustomed to working on communicative disorders which were not deficits in language structure. Right hemisphere damaged patients tended to have good language structure, but impaired language function.

Occasionally, right hemisphere damaged patients were referred for speech-language pathology services because of dysarthric speech. These few individuals had "slurred speech," characterized primarily by consonant imprecision in the context of respiratory, phonatory and/or resonance dysfunction. Most right hemisphere damaged patients however, demonstrated well preserved speech sound production, even though noticeable aberrations in prosodic aspects of speech production (e.g., stress, intonation, inflection) existed for a number of these patients. Speech-language pathologists generally were unaccustomed to treating prosodic aspects of speech in the absence of articulatory impairments, and so prosodic disturbances associated with right hemisphere damage were ignored.

Because a number of right hemisphere damaged patients show an indifference toward or denial of their symptoms, a condition known as anosognosia, they probably were not able to detect any change in their own communicative abilities. Patients themselves then did not seek speech-language pathology advice, partly because of lack of awareness of communicative deficits and mostly because they could talk.

Developments in fields such as sociology, linguistics, and sociolinguistics in the late 1960s and early 1970s provided the impetus for a change in the way communicatively impaired right hemisphere damaged patients were managed. A trend toward understanding how language is used in context became popularized in research investigations as individuals became enthralled with the so-called pragmatic aspects of language. As the interest and fascination with these pragmatic aspects grew and developed in the field of speech-language pathology in the 1970s and early 1980s, a new role emerged for speech-language pathologists. Not only could communicative disorders reflecting structural language deficits be identified, described, and managed, but those reflecting functional language deficits became identifiable, describable, and manageable as well. One of the pragmatic aspects of language that underwent description and investigation was the role of prosody in communicative interactions, and subsequently speech-language pathologists also became more interested in the prosodic deficits that stemmed from right hemisphere damage.

Thus, there is a relatively short history of clinical speech-language pathology interventions with right hemisphere damaged patients. Because of this short history, speech-language evaluation procedures generally have not been standardized, and treatment procedures have not been subjected to rigorous scientific and experimental scrutiny. Nonetheless, in the following sections of this chapter, a description of communicative problems and related disorders which affect communication skills of right hemisphere damaged patients will be provided. Next, a review of evaluation procedures which have been developed for detecting these disorders will be presented. Speech-language treatment procedures for managing right hemisphere communicative disorders are discussed later in the chapter.

Right Hemispheric Functions

That functional distinctions between the two cerebral hemispheres exist was first hypothesized a number of years ago. John Hughlings Jackson in 1874 proposed the functional differentiation of the left and right hemispheres.[2] He speculated that the left hemisphere mediated verbal actions, whereas the right hemisphere mediated more perceptual phenomena such as visual recognition of objects. Cummings noted that while Jackson's notion underlies many current theories about hemispheric specialization, it was not widely appreciated in its time[3]; it only gained acceptance in the second half of the twentieth century, when split-brain studies provided substantiation for the validity of Jackson's early notion.

The left hemisphere and right hemisphere both participate in intellectual and communicative functions such as auditory comprehension, reading comprehension, and arithmetic operations, but research has been interpreted to suggest that each cerebral hemisphere makes an individual contribution to the resulting cognitive achievement. Much of the information gathered about functional specialization of the two hemispheres has come from several sources. First, studies of split-brain patients, in whom the corpus callosum has been surgically severed, has provided an opportunity for the functions of the two hemispheres to be examined separately.[4,5,6] There has also been investigation of patients with agenesis of the corpus callosum, a rare congenital condition in which the corpus callosum is inadequately developed or absent.[7,8,9] Observations of patients with unilateral lesions to each hemisphere have been the source of additional information. Finally, investigations involving normal subjects, in which auditory dichotic or visual high-speed tachistoscopic presentations of stimuli are utilized, have provided additional data.[10,11,12] A review of these data has prompted investigators to dichotomize the functions of the two hemispheres (Table 31–1). In general, whereas the left hemisphere is believed to process verbally, linguistically, logically, and analytically, the right hemisphere is assumed to be primarily responsible for managing stimuli visuospatially, imaginatively, and holistically. Although these functional distinctions between the two hemispheres are generally well accepted, Gardner cautioned that:

> a disconnected region may behave differently than a region still connected to destroyed tissue; in addition, brains whose hemispheres have been disconnected may differ from brains in normally developed individual, who . . . unlike the epileptics . . . have not had to develop alternative pathways for accomplishing critical functions (p 367).[13]

For these reasons, the discussion which follows is limited to right hemisphere communicative disorders resulting from acquired unilateral lesions to that hemisphere.

Lezak proposed four classes of intellectual functions: receptive functions, memory and learning, thinking, and expressive functions.[14] Receptive functions refer to an individual's abilities to acquire, process, classify, and integrate information. Memory and learning are the means by which this information is stored and recalled. Thinking refers to the mental organization and reorganization of information. Expressive functions are the means through which information is acted upon or communicated. Using this framework as a basis for discussing impairments secondary to right hemisphere damage, an examination of communicative and communication-related behaviors follows.

TABLE 31–1 Some Dichotomies Proposed to Characterize the Functions of the Two Cerebral Hemispheres

Left Hemisphere	*Right Hemisphere*
Verbal	Nonverbal, visuospatial
Sequential	Simultaneous
Temporal	Spatial
Logical, analytic	Holistic, synthetic
Serial	Parallel
Difference detecting	Similarity detecting
Digital	Analogic
Rational	Intuitive
Segmental	Spatial, global
Symbolic or propositional	Visual or imaginative

Adapted from Springer SP, Deutsch G. Left brain right brain. San Francisco: WH Freeman, 1981, and from Cummings JL. Hemispheric specialization: a history of current concepts. In: Burns MS, Halper AS, Mogil SI, eds. Clinical management of right hemisphere dysfunction. Rockville, MD: Aspen Systems Corporation, 1985.

Receptive Functions

Receptive functions may be conceptualized as lying along a continuum that begins with sensation, the stimulation of sensory modalities (i.e., visual, auditory, tactile), and ends with perception, a phenomenon whereby sensory impressions are integrated into psychologically meaningful data for memory. Two classes of sensation disorders have been reported for right hemisphere damaged patients, and a variety of perceptual disorders, primarily in the form of recognition disorders (agnosias), have been identified and described.

Two varieties of sensation disorders associated with right hemisphere damage are hemianopsia and hemianesthesia. Left homonymous hemianopsia, in which the patient sees only those images to the right of midline, may result from damage to fibers of the primary visual cortex mediated by the right hemisphere. Unilateral left-sided hemianesthesia, or loss of tactile sensations in the left side of the body may also result from right hemisphere damage.

In contrast, a variety of perceptual disorders have been reported for right hemisphere damaged individuals. In these persons, sensory systems are intact, but the perceptions of sensory inputs are disrupted. Table 31–2 summarizes types of perceptual disorders which may be associated with right hemisphere damage. These perceptual deficits may be viewed as representing five major categories of disorders: unilateral (left) attentional disorders, mental attentional activation disorders, visuospatial agnosia, auditory agnosia, and tactile agnosia.

Unilateral attentional disorders are not uncommon sequelae to right hemisphere lesions. Patients may show a tendency to neglect stimuli presented to the left side of space, in spite of adequate sensory processing capabilities. Neglect is more commonly associated with right hemisphere lesions than left hemisphere lesions, and it generally lasts longer and is more severe. Myers noted that a neglect syndrome may be observed in right hemisphere damaged patients, and that the symptoms associated with this syndrome vary as a function of size and site of lesion.[15] In functional terms, patients with left hemispatial neglect may not attend to the left side of printed text or to a person addressing them from the left side. They may not eat the food placed on the left side of their plates. They may extinguish left sided stimulation, when, for instance, they are touched on both sides of the body. In its most severe form, patients may show a lack of awareness of impaired limbs, and may treat them derisively.[16] It is also not uncommon for these individuals to display anosognosia or denial of illness.

Numerous attempts to account for the neglect syndrome in right hemisphere damaged patients have converged on the notion of an integrated cortical network involved in the distribution of directed attention to extrapersonal space.[15,17,18,19] This network involves three interconnected cortical regions (the dorsal portion of the inferior partietal lobule, the dorsolateral frontal lobe or frontal eye fields, and the anterior cingulate gyrus), and these in turn are connected to the brain stem reticular formation. Myers drawing from the work of Mesulam distinguished between two neglect syndromes, parietal neglect and frontal neglect:

> Parietal neglect: A disturbance in the distribution of attention such that there is a failure to attend and respond to stimulation presented in extra-personal or ego-centric contralateral space.
>
> Frontal neglect: A disturbance in the inner representation of motor programs for the exploration and manipulation of contralateral space (p 448).[15]

Because lesion size is not typically discrete and because adequate spatial representation and adequate searching and scanning are mutually dependent, Mesulam noted that parietal and frontal neglect do not exist in isolation.[19] This notion is supported by other perceptual deficits commonly associated with right hemisphere damage.

Mental attentional activation disorders arise from patients' inabilities to demonstrate awareness of stimulus saliency. Patients may show external distractibility, failing to identify accurately elements of the figure-ground relationship, with excessive attention to extraneous (typically auditory and/or visual) stimulation. Patients may also fail to complete tasks accurately because of an internal distractibility, which impairs the ability to attend to those tasks. Other symptoms may include impaired recognition on scanning tasks[20] and poor eye contact during conversational interchanges.[21]

A variety of visual and visuospatial agnosic disturbances may also occur in right hemisphere damaged patients. Object agnosia may occur in which patients are unable to perceive and discriminate identical objects. Prosopagnosia, or the inability to recognize familiar faces, such as friends and family members, can occur. While typically attributable to bilateral lesions of posterior hemispheres,[22,23] the symptom has been noted in patients with unilateral right-sided lesions.[24,25] Defects of recognition of unfamiliar faces also have been reported for right hemisphere damaged patients by Malone et al, who stated that discriminations of familiar and unfamiliar faces involve mutually exclusive central nervous system mechanisms.[26] Given this finding, it is possible for a patient to have difficulty recognizing familiar, but not unfamiliar, faces and vice versa. Constructional apraxia stemming from right parietal lesions may be observed in right hemisphere damaged patients on

TABLE 31–2 Perceptual Deficits Associated with Right Hemisphere Damage

Source	*Examples*
Unilateral (left) attentional disorders	Hemispatial neglect (visual, auditory, tactile)
	Extinction to double simultaneous stimulation
	Hemisomatognosia
	Anosognosia with denial of illness
Mental attentional activation disorders	External distractibility
	Internal distractibility
	Visual scanning defects
	Poor eye contact
Visuospatial agnosia	Object agnosia
	Prosopagnosia
	Constructional apraxia
	Apraxia for dressing
	Spatial acalculia
	Topographic disorientation
Auditory agnosia	Deficient discrimination of vocal parameters
	Phonagnosia
	Affective agnosia
Tactile agnosia	Astereognosis

visuoconstructive tasks, such as puzzle assembly and block design, and on visuographic tasks, such as copying and drawing. Apraxia for dressing, inability to dress, is sometimes observed in right hemisphere damaged patients. This condition is believed to reflect deficits in body schema and spatial relations and not motor impairment.[27] Another symptom that may be observed is spatial acalculia, in which patients are unable to perform "pencil and paper" arithmetic tasks as a result of poor alignment of numbers on the page. Topographic disorientation is another symptom that may occur, and it is typified by loss of environmental familiarity and orientation, even in familiar surroundings.[28,29]

Auditory agnosic disturbances have also been reported for patients having unilateral right hemisphere lesions. Among these disturbances are deficits in the discrimination of vocal parameters such as pitch, intensity, tempo, tone, tonal patterns and timbre; phonagnosia, or pathologic recognition of voices;[30] and affective agnosia, in which patients fail to comprehend the affective prosodic aspects of speech without impairment of propositional language comprehension.[31,32] Tactile agnosic disturbances, in the form of astereognosis, may also occur. In this condition, patients are unable to discriminate objects via the tactile modality.

To summarize, a number of deficits in receptive functions may occur in right hemisphere damaged patients. Although some deficits are directly related to sensory impairment (e.g., hemianopsia and hemianesthesia), most receptive deficits occur in the context of intact sensory systems. The neurologic mechanisms underlying these latter deficits often appear to be related to attentional deficits arising from parietal and frontal neglect. Patients with these deficits are unable to integrate salient elements of external sensory stimuli with adequate and appropriate internal motor plans for acting upon those stimuli.

Memory and Learning Functions

Two types of memory and learning functions, which have been reported in right hemisphere damaged patients, are nonverbal amnesia and reduplicative paramnesia.[16] In the former condition, patients display recall of nonverbal visual material. In the latter condition, sometimes referred to as environmental reduplication,[33] patients insist that a current unfamiliar environment (e.g., the hospital) is located closer to a more familiar, significant environment (e.g. the patient's home).

It is often difficult to parcel out the nonverbal amnesia of right hemisphere damaged patients because of inherent difficulties with the tasks that purport to identify the phenomenon. For instance, two tests that have been administered to right hemisphere damaged patients are Rey's Auditory-Verbal Learning Test (AVLT)[34] and its companion pictorial version Lezak's Pictorial Verbal Learning Test (PVLT).[35] These tests are designed to measure immediate memory span, to reveal learning strategies, and to measure retention following an interpolated activity. On the AVLT, there are five presentations with recall of a 15-word list, one presentation of a second 15-word list, and a sixth recall trial. Retention is examined from 30 minutes to days later. Words are presented at the rate of one per second. On the PVLT, picture stimuli are used instead of auditory stimuli, and picture cards are turned at the rate of one per second. Patients with right-sided lesions retained auditorily presented information on the AVLT better than pictorial information on the PVLT,[35,36] implying difficulty with nonverbal visual material. The extent to which verbal mediation was involved, however, confounds this implication, as the stimuli included some fairly common nouns such as "house" and "book."

Additional evidence for poor memory for visual stimuli has been provided by tests of memory for designs. On these tests, patients are exposed to abstract line drawings for 5 to 10 seconds, followed immediately, or after a brief delay, by a drawing trial in which the patients are required to reproduce what they remember. Such tests are highly sensitive to right hemisphere brain damage,[35] and right hemisphere damaged patients (regardless of lesion site) have been reported to show more impaired reproductions than left hemisphere damaged patients. Despite confounding variables such as hemispatial inattention and visuospatial disturbances, Delaney, Wallace and Egelko demonstrated that while on immediate recall such tests did not discriminate between patients with right- and left-sided lesions, right hemisphere damaged patients performed significantly poorer on recall of the figures after a 30-minute delay than did left hemisphere damaged patients or normal control subjects.[37] These data offer support for the notion of nonverbal amnesia.

Reduplicative paramnesia has been reported in some right hemisphere damaged patients.[33,38,39] It has typically been noted in patients having a combination of right parietal and bilateral frontal injuries or in patients in acute confusional states subsequent to right parietal damage.[16] Again, this symptom complex is not exclusively a memory deficit although poor visual memory contributes to the symptoms. Additional contributions to this confabulatory state have been attributed to factors such as impaired spatial perception and a lack of awareness in the dissonance in responses.

In summary, memory and learning deficits specifically related to the visual modality have been reported for right hemisphere damaged patients. The phenomena of nonverbal amnesia and reduplicative paramnesia reflect the interactions between deficient visual memory and other symptoms associated with right hemisphere damage.

Thinking Functions

Any number of thinking functions may be impaired in patients subsequent to right hemisphere damage. These functions often play a significant role in and have substantial impact upon communicative behaviors. The thinking functions that may be impaired may be conceptualized as falling into one of the following three broader categories: deficient abstraction; disorders of ordering, organization, and planning; and impaired reasoning.

There is a tendency for many individuals subsequent to right hemisphere damage to perform mental operations in a concrete rather than abstract mode. This results in literal interpretations of more figurative notions and consequently may affect the ways in which these individuals comprehend and use language.

Some right hemisphere damaged patients have demonstrated this behavior in the interpretation of proverbs and idiomatic expressions. Benton reported that patients with right frontal lobe disease performed more poorly than patients with left frontal lobe disease on a multiple-choice version of Gorham's Proverbs Test.[40,41] This test contains 40 proverb items, each with four choices of possible answers. Only one of the choices is abstract and appropriate, with the other three being concrete interpretations or total misinterpretations. Winner and Gardner investigated metaphoric sentence comprehension in aphasic and right hemisphere damaged subjects.[42] Subjects were required to match a metaphoric sentence (e.g., he has a heavy heart) to its appropriate interpretation as depicted in one of four pictured choices. Aphasic subjects performed this task significantly better than right hemisphere damaged subjects, who most often selected choices depicting the literal interpretation of the metaphor. An additional finding of this investigation was that when right hemisphere damaged subjects were asked to explain the meaning of the metaphors they tended to give accurate interpretations and appeared unaffected by discrepancies between their explanations and their inaccurate picture choices. Myers and Linebaugh investigated comprehension of common idiomatic expressions such as "face the music" in right hemisphere damaged, left hemisphere damaged (aphasic), and control subjects.[42a] Subjects were presented with two-sentence stories, each ending with a common idiom. The outcome of the story could be determined with correct (figurative) interpretation of the idiom. Five response categories varied according to literal vs. accurate depiction of the idiom and incorrect vs. correct context of the story events. A final foil depicted the opposite outcome of the story. Right hemisphere damaged subjects performed the task significantly more poorly than aphasic and control subjects. Further, although they selected the correct context significantly more often than the incorrect one, they selected the literal depiction of the idiom significantly more often than the accurate one.

Deficits in abstraction at the single word level have also been noted in right hemisphere damaged subjects. Gardner and Denes studied connotative (nonliteral, interpretative) versus denotative (literal) aspects of words such as "rose" in right hemisphere damaged and left hemisphere damaged (aphasic) subjects.[43] The denotative task of the study required subjects to point to one of four picture choices when presented with the spoken stimulus word, and in general, right hemisphere damaged subjects performed this task adequately. The connotative task required subjects to point to one of two sets of geometric forms or expressive lines which best represented the connotative meaning of the stimulus word. Two of the six right hemisphere damaged subjects refused several times to do the connotative task altogether, and the right hemisphere damaged subjects who completed the task performed it more poorly than the aphasic subjects, who managed the connotative task surprisingly well.

Deficits in abstraction in right hemisphere damaged patients may also be manifested in their overpersonalization of external events.[44,45] In other words, when asked to expound on a broad general topic, patients may tend to provide tangential egocentric, personalized remarks in their response. For example, Boyarsky reported that a right hemisphere damaged patient responded to the stimulus "tell me why you think there can or cannot be peace on earth" with comments such as "I think we're having big problems because my limited involvement with the Russians . . ." and "I guess I do have some lingering racial prejudice, but I never have enforced it."[46] These remarks did not add anything substantively to the patient's response, but reflected concrete, egocentric patient behaviors. Similarly, Tonkovich reported the response of a right hemisphere damaged patient to the question "what do you think of President Reagan's policies regarding the American farmers?" The patient's response was "President Reagan's policies regarding farmers? Don't ask me. I haven't been on a farm in years."[47] This overpersonalized response reflects the patient's inability to form abstract opinions about extrapersonal entities.

Overpersonalization may also be noted in responses of right hemisphere damaged patients to idiomatic interpretation tasks. Burns, Halper and Mogil suggested that these overpersonalized comments often represent past experiences of the patient such as "Like the storm in '72" in response to the idiom "it's raining cats and dogs" and "that's my problem, I'm always tripping" in response to the idiom "look before you leap."[20]

Because humor appreciation involves interpretation of linguistic nuances and subtleties, it is not surprising that right hemisphere damaged patients may have difficulty with humor. This difficulty is sometimes seen as a loss of inhibition as patients tell "off color" jokes, but more often it is manifested in a failure to recognize humor. Wapner, Hamby and Gardner investigated humor in right hemisphere damaged and control subjects.[48] Subjects were presented with the body of a joke and then asked to choose the accurate punchline from four choices. Choices for the punchline were either: (1) appropriate and funny; (2) appropriate and straightforward; (3) sad; or (4) nonsequitur endings that did not follow logically from the body of the joke. Right hemisphere damaged subjects selected nonsequitur endings three times more often than controls. When questioned about their choices, right hemisphere damaged subjects typically confabulated some illogical relationship between their nonsequitur choice and the joke.

Other evidence for deficient abstraction skills in right hemisphere damaged patients relates to difficulty integrating complex ideational materials to interpret the moral of a story. A second component of the previously mentioned Wapner, Hamby, and Gardner study was designed to ascertain whether right hemisphere damaged patients would have difficulty abstracting the moral of a fable-like story.[48] Further, to probe whether difficulties with this task were due to impairments in appreciation of linguistically presented narratives or in narratives per se, subjects were presented stories in both linguistic (oral-auditory) and nonlinguistic (film) versions. The film version was a 7-minute silent film *The Fence,* which depicted a conflict between two neighbors and its eventual resolution. An oral text corresponding to the film was presented and/or a companion story, *The Silver Hammer,* matched in length, complexity, and other story-grammatical features served as the oral-auditory version. Immediately after stories were presented, patients were asked questions probing for the moral of the story and given a multiple choice if they were unable to correctly identify the moral. Right hemisphere damaged patients had difficulty inferring the moral of the story, providing the correct moral only 50 percent of the time. Incorrect responses were typified by patients simply repeating the plot or providing a literal response. Common literal responses for *The Fence* included "keep trash in your own yard" and "never grow a house in front of a flower" instead of a correct moral such as "do unto others as you would have them do unto you." The dissociation between an incorrect choice and a patient's confabulated relationship is exemplified in the following excerpt from one patient, when given four proverbs and asked to choose the one most representative of *The Fence:*

> People who live in glass houses shouldn't throw stones . . . [the man] threw a lot of stones and his house collapsed . . . but he didn't live in a glass house! He lived in a brick house, and he had windows and doors (p 23).[48]

A variety of disorders of ordering, organization, and planning have been noted in patients with right hemisphere damage. These may take a number of forms and may result in disruption of functional activities of daily living. For example, patients may show distorted relationships for placement of written materials relative to visual space, and may consequently write on the table top after they pass the right-hand margin of a page. They may show difficulty with the sequencing of dressing activities, and/or they might demonstrate impractical planning for maintaining personal independence in activities such as cooking, grooming, and driving. Although patients often retain abilities to perform isolated steps of these types of activities, the sequencing and integration of the steps into a meaningful activity are disrupted.

In terms of verbal expression, right hemisphere damaged patients often exhibit difficulties organizing discourse succinctly and meaningfully. These difficulties are often exemplified in the excessive verbosity or copious verbal output in conversational speech which characterized many right hemisphere damaged patients. As an example, Boyarsky's patient's response to the topic of peace on earth included the following copious excerpt:

> . . . As a consequence, I see in my own thinking, many of these things cropping up in the years to come that I think would always have a factor on true peace on earth, unfortunately. I hope for my own kids and grandchildren's sake that it does come about. But I have to admit that I am not sold on the idea that it ever will. I hope that my prophecy is wrong. I hope that there is peace

on earth sometime and hopefully in the not too distant future. 'Cause it isn't pleasant to live under the aspect of the . . . some nut pushing a button and wiping us all out under a nuclear holocaust. But, I think I've covered the subject the best I can (p 7).''[46]

Empty phrases such as "I see in my own thinking" and "I have to admit that" offer substantively little to the discourse, and the patient seemed to have trouble making a point succinctly. This conversational behavior is not common in most nonbrain-damaged normal speakers, who show much greater facility with planning and organizing discourse.

The results of two additional components of the Wapner, Hamby and Gardner study point to additional evidences for impairments in organization, ordering, and planning.[48] A story arrangement task was administered to right hemisphere damaged and control groups. The task required subjects to arrange randomly ordered sentences presented on individual cards into a coherent narrative. The stories were constructed so that ordering was dependent upon subjects' processing of and sensitivity to spatial information, temporal information, or categoric information. The three informational constructs were performed by right hemisphere damaged subjects with roughly the same patterns of difficulty demonstrated for left hemisphere damaged (aphasic) and control groups. All groups were most successful when ordering temporal elements and least successful with categoric elements. Right hemisphere damaged patients were more markedly impaired both in integrating the elements of a story and in appreciating its "narrative form" on the story arrangement task. They performed the task significantly worse than nonbrain-damaged subjects and with about the same accuracy levels as aphasic subjects.

Another task was constructed to determine how subjects integrated story elements relative to different contents. One story dealt with a farmer and his hired hand who wouldn't fix a leaking barn; a second was about a grocer who was robbed; and the third described a little girl who stowed away on a fire engine just before a fire broke out. Permutations of these three stories were provided by adding one of three types of elaboration elements: spatial elements (e.g., "the large moving van concealed the front of the police station"); emotional elements stated explicitly (e.g., "the little girl began crying") or implicitly (e.g., "her heart pounded as she crept in"); and noncanonical (bizarre) elements (e.g., "the farmer decided to give the hired hand a raise"). A fourth story that included all three types of elaboration elements was also presented. After each of the four stories was presented, subjects were required to retell the story in detail and to answer a set of questions about particular elements that required integration into the narrative. When subjects failed to answer questions accurately, they were provided with four choices and asked to select the most appropriate response. Right hemisphere damaged patients used embellishments in their retold stories three times more often than aphasic or normal control subjects. The authors noted that patients most likely to embellish their stories had large anterior right hemisphere lesions. Some of the embellishments noted challenged the basic theme of the stories (e.g., one patient who said "no kid could sneak on a fire engine"). Other embellishments consisted of additions to or changes in the story. Nine of the 16 right hemisphere damaged subjects confabulated in their story retelling. The authors stated that the findings from right hemisphere damaged subjects suggested that these patients had difficulty treating the story as a separate fictive entity, allowing personal memories and associations, differences of opinions, and asides to surface in their stories. These disjointed associations and descriptions reflect poor organization of verbal output relative to the integration of salient details and contribute to copious output.

Yet another thinking function which has been demonstrated to show impairment in right hemisphere damaged individuals is reasoning. Burns, Halper and Mogil noted that on high-level symbolic reasoning tasks, right hemisphere damaged patients might need assistance with focusing and maintaining attention.[20] It is not uncommon for patients to give minimal attention to salient features of a reasoning task and/or focus far too much attention on insignificant and nonsalient features. Since the right hemisphere is believed to be primarily responsible for integrative functions, it is not surprising that the results of a number of studies have shown that right hemisphere damaged patients perform logical reasoning and verbal abstraction tasks poorly.[48,49,50] The aforementioned studies of Winner and Gardner in which right hemisphere damaged patients showed a tendency to select literal choices for depicted metaphors and of Wapner, Hamby and Gardner in which these patients showed a tendency to confabulate illogical relationships between their nonsequitur responses and joke stimuli, afford additional evidence for impaired reasoning.[42,48]

In summary, patients with right hemisphere damage may show a variety of impairments of thinking functions. Reasoning and abstraction are often impaired, and patients consequently have difficulty integrating salient information and ordering, organizing, and planning. Functional implications of thinking function impairments are copious verbal output, increased literal-mindedness, failure to appreciate humor, and an inability to use logic appropriately to solve problems.

Expressive Functions

Two primary expressive functions have been reported to be disrupted in right hemisphere damaged individuals. One of these functions reflects a disturbance in pragmatic aspects of communication, as many patients show deficits in using language appropriately in context. The second of these functions involves impairment in the comprehension and/or production of affective prosody.

A variety of pragmatic communication disturbances has been reported in right hemisphere damaged patients.[20,21,45] The most notable violation of conversational rules results from patients' copious verbal output. Patients consequently take conversational turns, which are disproportionately too long, and topic maintenance is often affected simultaneously. Patients may be prone to make remarks that are tangential to the topic being discussed or may have difficulty changing topics or initiating new topics in conversational interchanges. Additional pragmatic disturbances may be noted when patients use vague or improperly placed pronouns or other indefinites to refer to entities not clearly identifiable to their conversational partners. This frequently results from patients' distorted presuppositions or apparent lack of awareness of information they share with their conversational partners. Patients may also show difficulty with backchannel communiction devices (e.g., nonverbal agreement, feedback from facial expression) which serve to keep conversations flowing smoothly between conversational partners. Previously mentioned deficits such as embellishments, irrelevant information, and faulty reasoning may also serve to impede conversational success for these patients.

A number of reports of prosodic irregularities in right hemisphere damaged patients point to the notion that they are often impaired in the comprehension and/or use of emotionally-driven prosody to convey affective states.[16,32,51,52] Patients with these prosodic irregularities consequently may have impairments in determining the emotional or affective states of their conversational partners and/or in adequately conveying their own emotional or affective states.

Tucker, Heilman and Watson tested the ability to discriminate affective speech on the basis of same/different discriminations and the ability to repeat emotionally "neutral" sentences such as "fish can jump out of the water" in patients with right parietal lesions, conduction aphasic patients with left parietal lesions, and non-neurologic control subjects.[32] Patients with right parietal dysfunction performed significantly poorer than aphasic subjects on discriminating emotional tones of anger, happiness, sadness, and indifference. Patients with right parietal dysfunction also performed the evocative task of producing prosodic representations of these four emotional tones significantly poorer than the nonaphasic control subjects. Ross used the term "aprosodia" to refer to this disability and provided some fairly convincing evidence that patients with anteriorly placed right hemisphere lesions tended to have difficulty with the production of emotionally-driven prosody (motor aprosodia), whereas those with posteriorly placed right hemisphere lesions had difficulty comprehending emotionally driven prosody (sensory aprosodia).[52] The impairment of prosodic aspects of speech renders right hemisphere damaged patients ineffective in communicative situations, in that affective state recognition and production establishes the underlying mood of conversational interchanges.

To summarize, right hemisphere damaged patients may display a variety of impairments that have direct impact on their ability to function in verbal activities of daily living. Receptive functions, memory and learning functions, thinking functions, and expressive functions may all be diminished, and these factors serve to increase the likelihood that right hemisphere damaged patients will be unsuccessful in their communicative endeavors. It cannot be denied that the communicative disturbances noted in right hemisphere damaged patients reflect underlying cognitive impairments, nor that the complex interactions between cognitive and linguistic systems form the basis for these disorders. Because speech-language pathologists have not had a rich history in examining cognitive variables as they related to communicative disorders, assessment of the communicative disorders associated with right hemisphere damage poses some unique clinical challenges.

EVALUATING COMMUNICATIVE SKILLS IN RIGHT HEMISPHERE DAMAGED PATIENTS

A comprehensive protocol useful for evaluating the communicative impairments in right hemisphere damaged patients is the RIC Evaluation of Communication Problems in Right Hemisphere Dysfunction (RICE).[20] Five components are included in the protocol: Behavioral Observation Profile; Visual Scanning and Tracking; Tasks for Assessment and Analysis of Writing; Rating Scale of Pragmatic Communication Skills; and Metaphorical Language Test. This protocol was intended to supplement commercially available standardized assessment tools, and it was not standardized on a population of right hemisphere damaged patients. Components of the RICE consist mainly of subjective rating scales, although the authors of the protocol attempted to use numerical values and objective indices of behavioral limitations whenever possible.

Components of RICE

Behavioral Observation Profile

The Behavioral Observation Profile, involves observing the patients' communicative behaviors in a variety of contexts. These contexts include a one-to-one interview with the patient in a quiet, nondistracting environment; a one-to-one interview in a distracting environment; and a three-way interview with a family member or second professional. Nine behaviors are targeted for observation and evaluation: attention, eye contact, awareness of illness, orientation to place, orientation to time, orientation to person, facial expression, and topic maintenance. Each of these parameters is scored on a five-point scale, where a score of 1 represents the greatest amount of impairment, and a score of 5 an appropriate level of communicative behavior. Behavioral descriptors are provided for three of the five scores for each parameter. For example, for the attention parameter, a score of 1 is described as "inattentive," a score of 3 is described as "attentive and responsive part of the time (50 percent)", and a score of 5 is described as "fully responsive." The numerical values for parameters under each condition are totaled and the three totals are averaged arithmetically. The resulting score, ranging from 9 to 45, is compared with a predetermined severity rating scale (Table 31–3). Despite methodology which misuses statistical procedures, the Behavioral Observation Profile provides salient diagnostic information.

Visual Scanning and Tracking

A second component of the RICE is Visual Scanning and Tracking. Four "subtests" include scanning for large, widely spaced letters; scanning for small, closely spaced letters; scanning for large, widely spaced words; and scanning for small, closely spaced words. It should be noted that large letters are 1/8 inch high and "widely spaced" ranges from 5/16 to 1/2 inch in this context. For each subtest, the patient is required to scan horizontal arrays of letters or words to find target letters or words, which have been provided at the left-hand side of the row. The number of errors and time to complete each subtest are recorded, although these data are not summarized further. In conjunction with other measures, this component of the RICE can demonstrate left hemispatial inattention in some right hemisphere damaged patients.

Assessment and Analysis of Writing

Tasks for Assessment and Analysis of Writing, the third component of the RICE, was designed specifically for detecting problems with written spatial organization. Three tasks are included. The first task involves having the patient copy the alphabetically-balanced sentence "The quick brown fox jumps over

TABLE 31–3 Severity Ratings on the Behavioral Profile of the RICE.[20]

Arithmetic Average of Scores Obtained in Three Contexts	*Severity Rating*	*Patient Description(s)*
9–15	Severe	Marked deficits in attention, orientation, and communicative interactions
16–23	Moderately severe	Generally, marked deficits in attention, orientation, and communicative interactions, with some appropriate behaviors retained
24–31	Moderate	Functional communication in simple familiar contexts, with some difficulties in attention, eye contact, awareness of deficits, orientation, and/or affect
32–39	Mild	Appears to function adequately in most situations, with specific deficits noted in distracting settings or through structured assessment
40–45	Minimal to normal	Communicates in full range of contexts although subtle integrative deficits may persist

After Burns MS, Halper AS, Mogil SI. Clinical management of right hemisphere dysfunction. Rockville, MD: Aspen Systems Corporation, 1985.

the lazy dog." The second task requires the patient write and spell correctly ten single words that are dictated. Finally, the patient is required to provide a written description of an action picture or recent event or a letter to a family member in at least 100 words. The three tasks are scored relative to the following 11 parameters: visuospatial disorganization; left-sided neglect; omissions of letters; perseveration of strokes and/or letters; ambiguous sentences; run-on sentences; incomplete sentences; grammatical errors; phonetically based spelling errors; and visually based spelling errors. Each parameter is rated along a five-point continuum, where a score of 1 represents the most impairment and 5 the least impairment. Scores for each parameter are added together, although no additional data analysis occurs with the total score.

Rating Scale of Pragmatic Communication Skills

The fourth RICE component is the Rating Scale of Pragmatic Communication Skills. Four sections designed to measure patients' nonverbal communication behaviors, conversational skills, use of linguistic context and narrative discourse organization are included in this component. Table 31–4 highlights specific parameters utilized in this component. Each parameter is scored along a five-point continuum. These parameters are scored relative to conversational speech elicited from the patient. Intonation, facial expression, and eye contact are scored as they were on the Behavioral Observation Profile. Gestures and proxemics (body posture changes relative to conversation) are scored. Conversational skills measures include conversational initiation, turn-taking and verbosity. Linguistic context parameters include topic maintenance, which is scored as it was on the Behavioral Observation Profile; turn-taking, which reflects how a patient responds to and uses nonverbal signals (such as pausing and eye contact) to signal conversational turns; and referencing skills, which involve determining how well patients use pronouns and other referents to previous information within a dialogue (anaphora) and upcoming information within a dialogue (cataphora). Narrative organization involves asking the patient to retell a joke or short story. The specific parameters of organization and completeness are also scored. Individual scores are totaled for the Rating Scale of Pragmatic Communication Skills, although it is unclear what this total score means.

TABLE 31–4 Communicative Parameters of the Rating Scale of Pragmatic Communication Skills from the RIC Evaluation of Communication Problems in Right Hemisphere Dysfunction[20]

Nonverbal communication	Intonation Facial expression Eye contact Gestures and proxemics
Conversational skills	Conversational initiation Turntaking Verbosity
Use of linguistic context	Topic maintenance Presupposition Referencing skills (anaphora and cataphora)
Organization of a narrative	Organization Completeness

Metaphorical Language Test

Finally, a Metaphorical Language Test is included in the RICE protocol. On this test, the patient is required to explain five proverbs (e.g., "a stitch in time saves nine") and five idioms (e.g., "it's raining cats and dogs") from an auditory stimulus. Instead of a rating scale for these items, a checklist is used. Parameters of the checklist are the following descriptions: completely incorrect; literal interpretation; partially correct; perseverative response; and normal abstract interpretation. Curiously, only the number correct is scored for this component. The checklist parameters, apart from signalling error responses, in no other way contribute to patients' overall scores on the RICE.

The RICE represents a preliminary attempt to sample a number of communicative behaviors in right hemisphere damaged patients, yet it may not be extensive enough to uncover all of a patient's communicative impairments and concomitant functional limitations. Burns, Halper and Mogil therefore recommend a number of supplemental tests which may be administered.[20] A partial listing of commercially available diagnostic tests which may be suitable for right hemisphere damaged patients is presented in Table 31–5. One additional assessment battery, the Ross Information Processing Assessment, although primarily intended for use with closed head injured patients, utilized right hemisphere damaged patients in its preliminary standardization data.[53] It may provide additional useful diagnostic information, and is discussed later in this chapter.

COMMUNICATIVE DISORDERS IN CLOSED HEAD INJURY

The incidence of closed head injury in the United States has been estimated to be approximately

TABLE 31–5 Supplemental Diagnostic Tests Which May be Suitable for Use in the Evaluation of Right Hemisphere Damaged Patients.

Test	*Measures*
Adult Basic Learning Examination (ABLE) Levels I, II and III[54]	Auditory vocabulary, reading comprehension, spelling, arithmetic computations, problem solving
Boston Diagnostic Aphasia Examination Acalculia Subtest[55]	Mathematical skills
Detroit Tests of Learning Aptitude[56]	Pictorial absurdities, verbal absurdities, auditory attention span, social adjustment, orientation, memory for designs, likenesses and differences
Developmental Test of Visual-Motor Integration[57]	Integration between visual perception and motor behavior
Developmental Test of Visual Perception[58]	Various visual perceptual parameters
Gates-MacGinitie Reading Tests: Survey D, E and F[59]	Reading vocabulary and comprehension
Iowa Silent Reading Tests: Levels 1, 2, 3[60]	Vocabulary, reading comprehension, directed reading, and reading efficiency
Metropolitan Reading Instructional Tests: Elementary, Intermediate, and Advanced I[61]	Various reading parameters
Motor-Free Visual Perception Test[62]	Spatial relationships, visual discrimination, figure-ground, visual closure, and visual memory
Ross Test of Higher Cognitive Processes[63]	Abstract and critical thinking skills
Stanford Achievement Test-Listening Comprehension Test: Intermediate I, II, Advanced[64]	Ability to retain details and organize content of orally presented information
Visual-Verbal Test[65]	Abstract conceptual similarities and conceptual shift
Watson-Glaser Critical Thinking Appraisal[66]	Inferencing ability, recognizing assumptions, making deductions, drawing conclusions, and evaluating arguments
Woodcock Reading Mastery Tests[67]	Letter and word identification, word attack, and word and passage comprehension

Adapted from Burns MS, Halper AS, Mogil SI. Clinical management of right hemisphere dysfunction. Rockville, MD: Aspen Systems Corporation, 1985.

400,000 per year.[68] Of this number, an estimated 30,000 to 50,000 individuals are left with residual physical and/or intellectual impairments which prevent them from returning to a "normal" life.[69,70] Because most head injuries are caused by highway motor vehicle accidents and since children and young adults constitute the largest proportion of survivors of these accidents rehabilitation efforts have become increasingly important as these individuals tend to have relatively normal life expectancies.[71,72]

For the purposes of discussion in this chapter, closed head injury will refer to nonpenetrating traumatic injuries of the head, which result in cerebral dysfunction. This is to distinguish closed head injuries from penetrating head injuries (such as occur as a result of missile wounds), which also occur traumatically and result in primarily focal damage. In closed head injury, damage is often diffuse and widespread, rather than focal, and may occur with or without alteration of consciousness. While closed head injuries in younger individuals most often result from motor vehicle accidents, they are more commonly associated with falls in geriatric individuals.

Closed head injuries are caused by a blunt blow to the head, which results in the brain being set into motion within the skull at the moment of impact. The force of the blow is distributed to all parts of the brain, and motion of the brain substance causes damage to the cerebral tissue. A variety of consequenses may be associated with this motion. Primary damage can occur on impact from compression, tension, and shearing of the brain tissue,[73] and lesions may be multifocal or diffuse. Secondary damage may result from cerebral edema, increased intracranial pressure, and hematomas.[74]

Several major problems have existed relative to the investigation of rehabilitation efforts with closed head injured patients, and consequently there has been a paucity of research on treatment outcomes for these individuals.[75] One methodological problem that cannot be accounted for easily in research designs is the heterogeneity of the population of closed head injured individuals with respect to distribution of lesions and severity of lesions. Another problem which exists is that closed head injured patients tend to exhibit a long course of recovery following injury, so that it is often difficult to distinguish between spontaneous recovery and the recovery which comes about as a result of intervention efforts. In addition, it is difficult to allocate randomly a control population to a nontreatment group.[68] Additional limitations are imposed by heterogeneity in the closed head injured population with respect to pretraumatic intelligence, educational levels, vocational levels, personality, and coping styles, and also in posttraumatic care, support systems, and emotional and behavioral reactions of the patient.[74] Despite these difficulties in investigating closed head injury, it is generally well accepted that a large percentage of closed head injured patients are left with residual communicative impairments following injury. Studies generally support that speech-language pathology interventions may be helpful. In the following sections, a description of the types of communicative impairments associated with closed head injury is provided, with reference to the cognitive and cognitive-language processes which appear to underlie these impairments. Prognostic and recovery information about closed head injured patients is provided, as well as methods for evaluating the communicative skills of these patients.

Types of Disorders

While many closed head injured patients have difficulties with communication, most of them are not "aphasic" in the sense of traditional aphasic syndromes. Heilman, Safran and Geschwind noted that only two percent of consecutive hospital admissions for closed head injury could be categorized into traditional aphasic syndromes, the most common types being anomic aphasia, followed by Wernicke's aphasia.[76] Sarno, Buonaguro, and Levita reported that on the basis of test results of 125 closed head injured postcoma patients, 19 could be classified as having fluent aphasia, 13 had nonfluent aphasia, and five had global aphasia.[77] When Wernicke's aphasia is noted in acute stages following closed head injury, it may be transient, and comprehension may be restored as a hematoma resolves or is removed surgically.[78] Sarno reported that virtually all of the 69 patients consecutively admitted to a rehabilitation facility, although not exhibiting traditional aphasic syndromes, presented "subclinical" aphasic deficits characterized chiefly by impairments of confrontation naming, word fluency, and auditory comprehension of complex commands.[79]

Ylvisaker and Szekeres advocated a broader definition for the deficits associated with closed head injury, and identified the cognitive-language deficits as those "impairments of language use or of language learning that are reflective of more general cognitive deficits" (p 475).[74] These include disorganized discourse, inefficient integration of large amounts of language, weak verbal learning, and inadequate use of language for reasoning and problem solving. Because the array of speech, language, and cognitive deficits associated with closed head injury varies widely among patients as a function of site of lesion and extent of damage, it is often difficult to parcel out whether the underlying deficit observed in a patient's communicative behavior is attributable to speech, language or cognitive bases. Therefore, for the purposes of this chapter, the generic term "cognitive-communicative deficit" is used to describe the communicative impairments observed in closed head injured patients.

A wide variety of cognitive-communicative impairments have been noted in closed head injured patients. Initially, many patients may be mute for anywhere from several days to years. Following this period, a number of conditons may arise. A commonly occurring clinical picture has been referred to as language of confusion.[80,81] This symptom cluster may be characterized by reduced recognition of, understanding of, and responsiveness to the environment; faulty memory; impaired reasoning; unclear thought processes; temporal and spatial disorientation; irrelevancy; and inapproriate maladaptive behaviors.[72] Simultaneously, patients often display concomitant learning and memory deficits such as anterograde amnesia and retrograde amnesia. Anterograde amnesia refers to difficulty learning new information and skills posttraumatically, whereas retrograde amnesia reflects an inability to remember pretraumatic events.

When damage incurred involves the brain stem, patients may exhibit flaccid dysarthric speech, with or without concomitant dysphagia. Damage to upper motor neurons, the cerebellum, and/or the extrapyramidal system may give rise to a variety of mixed dysarthric conditions.

Most often, and not surprisingly, the communicative behaviors of closed head injured patients are not unlike those observed in right hemisphere damaged patients. Closed head injured patients are likely to show attentional deficits, caused by disinhibition, hyperactivity, and distractibility, and may have difficulty sustaining or shifting attention.[68] They are likely to show perceptual difficulties in recognizing features and relationships among features; memory and learning difficulties; impairments in organization relative to analyzing, classifying, integrating and sequencing; difficulties in deductive, inductive, and analogical reasoning; impairments in problem solving and judgment; reduced deficit awareness; confabulation; and strained and often unsuccessful conversational interactions secondary to disinhibition, reduced awareness of social conventions and rules, inappropriateness, and impulsivity.[82]

As previously mentioned, classical aphasic syndromes in closed head injured patients are typically rare, with anomic aphasia and Wernicke's aphasia being the most predominant types. However, aphasic deficits in auditory comprehension, word retrieval, world fluency, sentence repetition, reading and writing may vary from patient to patient, usually as a function of the locus and extent of damage to the left hemisphere. Apraxia of speech, associated with left frontal lesions, is not typically noted in head injured patients.[72]

Some fairly common neurobehavioral sequelae associated with closed head injury likely have some additional impact on patients' communicative behaviors. Many closed head injured patients sustain bilateral damage to the frontal lobes, which typically impairs affective behavior. Possible outcomes of bifrontal injury include abulia, characterized by a lack of initiative or spontaneity in desired or automatic motor tasks;[72] personality alterations, often with respect to control of anger; and euphoria or irritability inconsistent with the patient's actual mood.[83]

In summary, a broad range of cognitive-communicative impairments is represented in the closed head injured population. There are no easily identifiable symptom clusters which typify impairments in these individuals, but rather overt behavioral manifestations of neurologically-based speech, language, cognition, and behavioral impairments.

Prognosis for Recovery from Closed Head Injury

It is difficult to account for recovery of functions in individuals following closed head injury, but some preliminary investigations have provided evidence for several prognostic factors which might be considered. Lezak noted that the recovery of actual function in closed head injured patients appears to vary widely from patient to patient relative to the nature of the function, task complexity, and severity of injury, although there are some consistent trends in the posttraumatic course of these patients.[14] Investigators, by and large, have been unable to control variables such as type of damage, extent of impairment, age, types of treatment, and tests used to measure progress in their studies of recovery following closed head injury, and consequently it has been difficult to clearly interpret and extract prognostic variables from the data. Nonetheless, investigations of recovery from closed head injury have focused on age at onset, coma, medical complications, posttraumatic amnesia, cognitive variables, and behavioral and psychological variables.

Age at onset of closed head injury has been believed to be an important prognostic variable. LeMay and Geschwind proposed the following timetable for recovery: maximum recovery in children under 5 years of age following closed head injury might take decades; individual 20 to 40 years of age continued to improve for 5 to 6 years following onset; individuals 40 to 60 years of age continued to improve for 2 years following injury; and individuals over age 60 generally achieved maximum potential in 9 months following injury.[84] Levin reported that older head injured patients performed more poorly on more difficult memory tasks of the Wechsler Adult Intelligence Scale (WAIS) than younger head injured patients.[78] Lezak however, investigating recovery of memory and learning functions following closed head injury, found no significant differences in test performance between those under age 25 and those older than 25.[14]

The duration of coma has been proposed by many to be the best prognostic indicator of functional recovery from closed head injury. Generally, the longer the duration of the coma, the less satisfactory the recovery. Lezak investigated two groups of patients (1) those who were unconscious for less than 2 weeks after injury, and (2) those who were unconscious for 2 weeks or more.[14] The latter group performed more poorly on every learning and memory task in the study than the former group. Brooks et al, in an investigation of recovery noted that patients who were in a coma for 3 months or less had a better prognosis for independent living than those who had been in a coma for 4 months or longer following injury.[85]

Brooks et al also noted prognostic implications for medical complications following head injury.[85] Patients who experienced intracranial mass lesions (i.e., epidural, subdural, and intracerebral hematomas; focal edema) that required surgical decompression and modification had a poorer prognosis for recovery, especially relative to motor activity, than those who did not. Additional medical complications that have been cited as poor prognostic recovery indicators include anoxia, increased intracranial pressure, intracranial hemorrhage, elevated or reduced blood pressure, hyperthermia, and presence of seizures.[68,86,87,88]

Other studies of recovery from head injury have focused on duration of posttraumatic amnesia, or that period subsequent to injury during which the patient lacks continuous memory for ongoing events in daily life. Bever, speculating on the outcomes of several studies, suggested that the longer the period of posttraumatic amnesia, the more severe the residual deficits from closed head injury.[89] Patients who experienced posttraumatic amnesia of less than 1 hour tend to have mild deficits, whereas those whose posttraumatic amnesia lasted longer than 4 weeks would be left with extremely severe deficits. Mandleburg, reporting on WAIS performance following closed head injury, noted that the duration of posttraumatic amnesia had no bearing on eventual cognitive level outcomes.[90] Long periods of posttraumatic amnesia were significantly correlated with impaired memory function, but not with changes in personality or development of mental illness subsequent to head injury. Mandleburg also reported severe residual brain injury when the posttraumatic amnesia lasted longer than 24 hours.

Cognitive variables have been implicated in the results of several other studies of closed head injury recovery. Using two groups of closed head injured patients, Adamovich and Henderson noted that patients less than 6 months postinjury differed from patients at least 6 months postinjury qualitatively in their error responses on an antonym-generating task.[91] The latter group performed significantly better than the former group on memory tests, visual and verbal sequencing tasks, problem solving, and task-specific insight, but not on recall tasks. This suggests that different cognitive functions recovered at different rates. Additional support for this notion was offered by Groher, who reported that closed head injured patients in his recovery study showed the most improvement on expressive and receptive language tasks and on memory tasks during the first month after regaining consciousness, with only gradual improvements noted in the following 4 months.[92]

A variety of behavioral and psychological variables have also been postulated as prognostic indicators, although few, if any, have been substantiated by research findings. Good prognostic indicators have been associated with pretraumatic personality characteristics such as self-motivation, goal-directedness, and strong will. Pretraumatic personality factors believed to be poor prognostic indicators have included emotional and psychological instability, substance abuse (particularly alcohol and drugs), poor work and school history, and general lack of motivation to succeed.[68]

Although studies of recovery relative to prognostic variables in closed head injured patients have provided some interesting findings, it is apparent that there is a high degree of variability in results, and most prognostic indicators to date are tentative at best. While recovery of function varies widely among closed head injured patients relative to specific function, certain trends regarding course of recovery have been suggested. These trends appear to account for the majority of patients.

Neurologic Recovery Following Coma

The most common characteristic of severe closed head injury is loss of consciousness, from which five general recovery phases have been identified. The depth and duration of each phase varies from patient to patient, and not all patients progress through each phase.[72] These phases are as follows:

1. Coma—marked by paralysis of all cerebral functioning
2. Semicomatose—patient begins to withdraw to painful stimuli
3. Stuporous—patient is restless, mute, and responsive to simple commands
4. Confused—responses are disoriented
5. Conscious—patient recovers orientation, retention, and insight.

For those patients who are in a coma following head injury, the Glasgow Coma Scale (Table 31–6) is widely used by health care professionals because it quantifies and objectifies the coma status with results that are consistently reproducible.[93] A numerical value that ranges from no response through normal response is assigned to each of three behavioral responses: eye opening, motor performance, and ver-

TABLE 31–6 Glasgow Coma Scale

Response	*Status*	*Score*
Eye opening	Spontaneous	4
	To verbal command	3
	To pain	2
	None	1
Best motor response to verbal command, to painful stimulus	Obeys	6
	Localizes	5
	Withdraws	4
	Abnormal flexion	3
	Extension	2
	None	1
Best verbal response	Oriented; converses	5
	Confused conversation	4
	Inappropriate words	3
	Incomprehensible sounds	2
	None	1
TOTAL		3–15

Adapted from Jennett B, Bond M. Assessment outcome after severe brain damage: practical scale. Lancet 1975; 1:480.

bal performance. In quantitative terms, coma is defined as a total score of eight or below, and patients whose total scores fall within a score below four usually die. Those who are believed to be rehabilitation candidates have scores ranging from four to 15.[94] The hierarchies for each response area appear to represent the hierarchies of function recovery by closed head injured patients.

A widely used clinical tool for assessing and documenting the behavior of closed head injured patients is the Rancho Los Amigos Levels of Cognitive Functioning.[95] The scale corresponds to the course of recovery from coma described above, and is presented in Table 31–7. According to Hagen, the purpose of this type of evaluation is to establish the presence and pattern of change in such basic neurobehavioral dichotomies as follows:

1. Response to external stimuli versus no responses
2. Gross undifferentiated response to stimuli versus differentiated response to stimuli
3. Differentiated response to stimuli, but no continued response after withdrawal of stimuli versus differentiated and sustained response after withdrawal of stimuli
4. Sustained response to stimuli, only if stimuli brought to patient versus sustained response on basis of patient's self-directed behavior
5. Inappropriate versus appropriate responses to stimuli, whether externally presented or self-initiated (p 258).[73]

This behavioral scaling technique is intended to be utilized by all disciplines interacting with the patient, especially for patients at and between levels II and VII. Systematic observations of the patient's behavioral response in terms of type, nature and quality afford insights into determining the level at which the patient is functioning in the hierarchy of cognitive purposes. Further, the Rancho Los Amigos Scale, can provide information regarding (1) the patient's most typical cognitive level to anticipate the patient's highest level of functioning at any given point in time, (2) patient's responses below his or her most consistent level of functioning, thus alerting caregivers to alterations in the environment that need to be made to ensure the highest level of cognitive and communicative functioning possible; and (3) the emergence and stabilization of behaviors occurring at the next highest cognitive level, thus

TABLE 31–7 Rancho Los Amigos Scale Levels of Cognitive Functioning

Level		*Response*
I	None	Unresponsive to all stimuli
II	Generalized	Inconsistent and nonpurposeful, nonspecific reactions to stimuli Responses are limited and stereotyped
III	Localized	Inconsistent but specific reactions to stimuli May respond to simple commands (e.g., "close your eyes") in an inconsistent, delayed manner
IV	Confused Agitated	Bizarre, nonpurposeful behavior relative to environment. Attention span is short. Patient lacks short term recall
V	Confused Inappropriate Nonagitated	Fairly consistent responses to simple commands; responses to more complex commands are nonpurposeful, random or fragmented Performs previously learned tasks but is unable to learn new ones
VI	Confused Appropriate	Behavior is goal-directed but dependent upon external input for direction Responses are appropriate to situation with incorrect responses due to memory difficulties
VII	Automatic Appropriate	Responses appear appropriate and oriented to setting Carry-over for new learning is present, but slow; insight, judgment, and problem solving are poor
VIII	Purposeful Appropriate	Correct responding, carry-over of new learning No supervision needed May continue to show abstract reasoning difficulties, poor tolerance for stress, and poor judgment

Adapted from Hagen C, Malkmus D. Intervention strategies for language disorders secondary to head trauma Presented to the American Speech-Language-Hearing Association, Atlanta, 1979.

alerting caregivers to modify treatment plans accordingly.

While the Ranchos Los Amigos Levels of Cognitive Functioning Scale is sometimes criticized because of its subjective ratings, it has reasonable interrater reliability as a tool and a fairly high degree of test-retest reliability. Gouvier et al although advocating the use of the Disability Rating Scale[96] for monitoring recovery from severe head injury, demonstrated that the Levels of Cognitive Functioning had a mean Spearman rho correlation coefficient of 0.89 for three independent raters, with correlation coefficients for pairs of raters which ranged from 0.87 to 0.94.[97] The Spearman rho correlation coefficient for test-retest reliability was 0.82. The Levels of Cognitive Functioning Scale was also shown to have good concurrent validity and substantial discharge concurrent validity when compared with other measures, though it was not particularly effective in terms of predictive validity relative to patient status at discharge. Nonetheless, the Levels of Cognitive Functioning Scale affords good opportunities for describing the recovery stages of closed head injured patients.

Assessing Communicative Skills of Closed Head Injured Patients

Few protocols for assessing cognitive-communicative abilities of closed head injured patients have been developed especially for speech-language pathologists. Many of the test batteries employed in clinical practice utilize measures that have no normative data or measures that were standardized on populations other than closed head injured patients.

The Ross Information Processing Assessment (RIPA) represents a preliminary step toward remedying some of the previous problems associated with assessment of closed head injured patients by speech-language pathologists.[53] Standardization data were obtained from test administrations to normal subjects and right hemisphere damaged patients, as well as closed head injured patients at or above Level V.

The RIPA was designed to:

> . . . verify and quantify the verbal information processing deficits in closed head injury subjects and to establish specific severity ratings of overall and individual abilities. Periodic retesting provides objective data for quantifying improvement in function of information processing (p 1).[53]

The RIPA consists of 10 subtests, each containing 10 items. It can be administered in approximately 40 minutes, and provides three types of scores: (1) raw scores; (2) diacritical scores; and (3) percentile rankings. A summary of each of the RIPA's subtest areas, and raw and diacritical scoring aspects of the test battery are presented in Table 31–8.

One particular feature of the RIPA is the consideration of qualitative aspects of patient responses in addition to quantitative test scores. These diacritical scores provide valuable insights into efficiency of communicative attempts. Another significant aspect of the RIPA is that it provides percentile rankings corresponding with raw numeric scores for each subtest, thereby providing the examiner with a meaningful and objective profile of patient impairments and the relative severity of each. The RIPA also purports to provide sufficient patient data to develop and implement a treatment plan, although supplemental testing often might be warranted.

No other standardized battery of tests for assessing cognitive-communicative functions in closed head injured patients has been developed. Adamovich, Henderson, and Auerbach, however, provided details of a pilot battery designed to diagnose and assess cognitive processing in head injured patients. Subtest areas are provided in Table 31–9.[68]

Arousal and alerting tasks of this battery are designed to test abilities to respond at a reflexive level, and include ringing a bell near the patient and attempting to elicit a rooting reflex. Tasks in the perceptual or low level selective attention component are designed to test information integration at the sense organs relative to internal or stored representations of the stimulus. Tasks in this component include assessment of visual and auditory tracking, environmental sound recognition, shape recognition, and word recognition in the context of an auditorily presented paragraph in a "quiet" condition and in background noise. A variety of tasks designed to test patients' abilities to differentiate two or more stimuli are provided in the discrimination component of the battery. Visual discrimination tasks requiring the patient to identify color, shape, and size variables both individually and in combination are provided. Auditory discrimination tasks require patients to match an auditorily presented word with its printed correlate, presented among four other visual and/or auditorily similar foils. Picture and object discrimination tasks involve having the patient orally name pictured objects and then write names of pictured objects. Discrimination of sentences includes having patients match one of two visually presented sentences such as "she picked up the dog" and "she picked at the dog" with appropriate picture stimuli. Two-step discrimination requires patients to signal each time they hear a number followed by a color in an auditorily presented list of color, number, and object words.

The orientation component of the battery tests patients' orientation to person, place, and time. The organization subtest is designed to measure patients'

TABLE 31-8 Features of the Ross Information Processing Assessment[53]

Subtests		Scoring: Raw Scores	Scoring: Diacritical Scores
I	Immediate memory Patient required to repeat numbers, words, and sentences of increasing length	3—Correct response 2—Partially correct response 1—Error response or denial 0—Unintelligible or no response	c—confabulation d—denial or refusal dl—delay e—frank effort i—irrelevant p—perseveration pc—partially correct or incomplete r—repetition sc—self-correction t—tangential
II	Recent memory Patient required to recall specific newly acquired information about his/her environment and daily activity		
III	Temporal orientation (recent memory) Patient asked questions related to time		
IV	Temporal orientation (remote memory) Patient asked questions related to time, which require remote recall of temporally sequenced and associated stimuli		
V	Spatial orientation Patient asked spatial orientation questions which require organization, categorization and sequencing		
VI	Orientation to environment Patient required to answer questions relative to awareness and perception of the environment		
VII	Recall of general information Patient required to recall general information in remote memory		
VIII	Problem solving and abstract reasoning Patient required to complete tasks which require the use of problem-solving and reasoning strategies		
IX	Organization Patient required to recall category members within a 1-minute time limit and to recall a category type given three category members		
X	Auditory retention and processing Patient required to answer multiunit yes/no questions containing temporal, spatial, and comparative information		

skills in dealing with discrete actions or components which must be grouped or sequenced according to the priority of each component using a learned strategy, and it includes categorization, closure, and sequencing tasks. Categorization tasks include sorting pictures by class and by function, describing salient features of common objects, and describing similarities and differences of word pairs such as "newspaper-magazine." Closure tasks include those requiring patients to fill in missing letters of stimuli

TABLE 31-9 Subtest Areas Designed to Diagnose and Assess Cognitive Processing in Closed Head Injured Patients[68]

Arousal and alerting	*Orientation*	*Recall*
Perception or low level selective attention Tracking Sound Recognition Shape Recognition Word Recognition Word Recognition in Noise Discrimination Visual Auditory Pictures/Objects Sentences Two Step Discrimination	Organization Categorization Closure Sequencing	High level thought processes Convergent Thinking Deductive Reasoning Inductive Reasoning Divergent Thinking Multiprocess Reasoning

such as h__t to form real words and those requiring patients to identify words which are presented in a sound-by-sound manner auditorily. Sequencing tasks include having patients visually sequence shapes according to size, letters to form words, sentences to form a paragraph, and steps within an event.

Immediate, delayed (short-term), and free recall are assessed in the recall subtest. These tasks include immediate and delayed recall of similar words, delayed recall of related sentences, delayed recall of words with interference, a word fluency measure, the following of multistep oral commands, and recall of paragraphs presented visually and auditorily. The authors advise that responses to these tasks are intended to be evaluated relative to a number of parameters, including the number of items recalled versus the number given, the type of stimuli presented (e.g., linguistic versus nonlinguistic, related versus unrelated), the mode of stimulus presentation (e.g., visual versus auditory), and apparent strategies utilized (e.g., verbal description, visual imagery, categorization, rehearsal, use of associations, temporal or spatial orientation, and primacy and recency).

High level thought processes subtests are designed to assess high level problem solving, reasoning, and judgment. These include tasks involving convergent thinking, deductive reasoning, inductive reasoning, divergent thinking, and multiprocess reasoning. Convergent thinking tasks assess skills in recognizing and analyzing relevant information in order to identify the main point of short stories. Deductive reasoning tasks assess abilities to draw appropriate conclusions for specific situations. Inductive reasoning tasks include requiring patients to provide the antonyms of words such as "spoiled" and to complete simple analogies (e.g., girl is to bed as baby is to ________). Divergent thinking tasks require patients to generate sentences depicting two different meanings of homographic words such as shoulder, to explain the meanings of idioms and proverbs, and to recognize auditorily presented absurdities. The multiprocess reasoning subtest includes tasks designed to assess skills with insights regarding performance of situation-specific tasks (e.g., going on a shopping trip) and with amounts of information needed to solve deductive reasoning problems.

While the aforementioned battery of Adamovich, Henderson, and Auerbach shows great promise as a tool for assessing cognitive-communicative impairments in closed head injured individuals, it is incomplete.[68] Few exemplars are probed in each cognitive skill level area, and little direct attention is given in the battery to specific abilities to comprehend and use language. Additional shortcomings relate to the fact that most tests in the battery are too difficult and beyond the capabilities of head injured patients at lower levels of cognitive functioning and may not be taxing enough to detect subtle residual deficits occurring in individuals with mild closed head injuries.

A variety of supplemental tests, many of them neuropsychological diagnostic tests, may be utilized to provide more in-depth assessment of specific cognitive skill areas. Some commonly used tests are listed in Table 31–10. Hagen cautioned that most cognitive abilities cannot be directly assessed until patients reach level VII, automatic-appropriate on the Rancho Los Amigos Scale.[95] For this reason, and due to the lack of any other standardized measures, informal assessment and observations of patient behavior, especially relative to the Rancho Los Amigos Scale, are perhaps the best available methods for evaluating patients at lower levels of cognitive functioning.

Patients who sustain mild closed head injuries pose yet another diagnostic problem for clinicians. Mild head injuries are actually more common than severe ones, and patients are usually hospitalized for less than 48 hours.[72] Since cerebral injury is mild in these individuals, it generally resolves quickly. Rimel noted that some of these mildly head injured patients are left with substantial disabilities.[94] They complain of headaches, dizziness, irritability, insomnia, concentration problems, memory problems, changes in temperament, and/or emotional disposition. These problems pose serious threats to employment, emotional, and social status, and assessment of the nature and degree of impairment is often elusive. Holzer et al noted that this cluster of symptoms referred to as the posttraumatic syndrome, has been especially significant in those patients having pretraumatic behavioral or psychological disorders.[72] While even skillful speech-language pathologists may have difficulty assessing the cognitive-communicative needs of mildly impaired closed head injury patients, many of these patients may benefit from training in goal-setting, planning, and developing compensatory strategies for impaired communicative behaviors and situations. Nonetheless, psychological or psychiatric evaluation of this group of patients is indicated.

In summary, a variety of measures for assessing cognitive-communicative behaviors in closed head injured patients are available, although most formal measures are geared toward patients at higher levels of cognitive functioning. Patients who show greater degrees of cognitive impairment are best assessed through informal measures and observation. Those with subtle residual cognitive deficits are more difficult to assess, and will likely benefit from psycho-

TABLE 31–10 Some Commonly Used Tests for Measuring Cognitive Abilities in Closed Head Injured Patients

Cognitive Abilities Tested	*Tests*
Attention, discrimination, temporal sequencing, retention span	ITPA[8]
	Visual Sequential Memory subtest
	WAIS[99]
	Digit Span subtest
	Detroit Tests of Learning Aptitude[56]
	Auditory Attention Span for Unrelated Words and Related Syllables subtest
	Visual Attention Span for Objects and Letters subtest
	Developmental Test of Visual Pereception[58]
	Southern California Figure-Ground Visual Perception Test[100]
	Luria's tests for Perception and Reproduction of Pitch Relationships and Reproduction of Rhythmic Structure[101]
	Goldman-Fristoe-Woodcock Sound-Symbol Tests[102]
	Goldman-Fristoe-Woodcock Test of Auditory Discrimination[103]
	Nonverbal Test of Cognitive Skills[104]
Immediate and recent memory	Wechsler Memory Scale[105]
	WAIS[99]
	Digit Symbol subtest
	Goldstein-Scheerer Stick Test[106]
	Benton Revised Visual Retention Test[107]
	Luria's Mnestic Tests[101]
	Goldman-Fristoe-Woodcock Auditory Memory Tests[108]
	Nonverbal Test of Cognitive Skills[104]
Categorization, association, integration, synthesis	Color Form Sorting Test[109]
	Detroit Tests of Learning Aptitude[56]
	WAIS[99]
	Block Design subtest
	Object Assembly subtest
	Picture Arrangement subtest
	Ross Test of Higher Cognitive Processes[63]
	Nonverbal Test of Cognitive Skills[104]

Adapted from Hagen C. Language disorders in head trauma. In: Holland AL, ed. Language disorders in adults: recent advances. San Diego: College-Hill Press, 1984.

logical or psychiatric evaluation in addition to evaluation by speech-language pathology.

TREATMENT OF COGNITIVE-COMMUNICATIVE DEFICITS

Sensory Stimulation for Patients with Decreased Responsiveness

For closed head injured patients at low levels of cognitive functioning (levels I, II, and III), a variety of procedures for providing multimodality sensory inputs have been advocated.[72,73] The effectiveness of such stimulation techniques has not been established, and clinicians may engage in these activities solely on the basis of blind faith. Still, these sensory stimulation procedures are widely used in clinical practice with low-functioning closed head injured patients.

The goals of providing external multisensory stimulation to these patients purportedly are to prevent sensory deprivation and heighten attention, to enhance patient comprehension of simple commands, to establish consistency of response in a rudimentary way, and to elicit appropriate responses, which can ultimately be channeled into other adaptive skill areas. Some specific stimulation techniques by modality are listed in Table 31–11.

Advocates of multisensory stimulation suggest that each team member provide stimulation tasks for brief periods throughout the day, once the patient has received medical clearance for such activities. Prior to stimulation, clinicians should provide an introductory explanation of the procedure, even though the patient may give the impression of not comprehending what is said. Patients generally should be allowed to respond following presentation of a stimulus, before the clinician attempts to stimulate again with the same stimulus or a novel stimulus. Often, when patients respond to such stimulation, it is some gross motor reaction and is typically latent. Gradually, response consistency might be shaped, and clinicians may try to promote response generalization, by moving from stimuli that elicit a strong response toward those stimuli which do not elicit such strength.

There is considerable controversy about sensory stimulation techniques and their benefit during coma and early postcoma states. Proponents of these procedures generally believe that although they do not cause recovery, they serve to heighten and give direction to the recovery process. Nonetheless, the fact that they have not been subjected to rigorous, scientific investigation should be considered when implementing these procedures.

Techniques to Establish Attention and Concentration

Several procedures for establishing attention and concentration skills have been described, and although these may be appropriate for right hemisphere damaged and closed head injured patients, there is little evidence to support their effectiveness. Adamovich, Henderson and Auerbach stated that attention was a secondary focus of all treatment tasks and that tasks should be implemented which gradually extend the length of time the patient is capable of maintaining attention.[68] Further, they advocated implementing the treatment goal of promoting shifting attention from one item or task to another. Burns, Halper and Mogil proposed a treatment hierarchy for attending behaviors which began with focusing patient attention in a distraction-free environment.[20] Specific tasks recommended included getting patients to establish eye contact with a conversational partner, visual gaze to a treatment activity, and a pointing response to a treatment activity, and to shift eye contact away from the treatment activity toward the conversational partner.

TABLE 31–11 Some Common Sensory Stimulation Techniques Used with Low Functioning Head Injured Patients

Modality	*Stimuli Presented*
Auditory	Fast, loud, irregular rhythms (e.g., bells; horns)
	Music (radio, tape recording)
	Tape recording of family members' voices
	Clapping, snapping fingers
Visual	Colorful items (mobiles, photographs, paintings)
	Photographs (of patient, family members, friends, clinicians)
	Television
Olfactory	Noxious odors (e.g., dilute ammonia, vinegar, garlic)
	Pleasant scents (e.g., extracts, spices, colognes/perfumes)
	Food items (e.g., popcorn, ground coffee, banana, orange)
Tactile	Assorted textures (e.g., terry cloth, velcro, carpeting, feathers, sandpaper)
	Bathing (e.g., face cloth, soap, water)
Gustatory	Extracts (e.g., peppermint, vanilla)
	Fruit juices
	Vinegar
Vestibular	Tilt-table, rocking bed or chair to provide swinging motions

Adapted from Holzer ML, Stiassny DA, Senner-Hurley F, Lefkowitz NG. Brain trauma. In: Logigian MK, ed. Adult rehabilitation: a team approach for therapists. Boston: Little, Brown, 1982.

Because patients often lack the capability of sustaining attention during treatment activities, Haarbauer-Krupa et al advocated the use of compensatory strategies to assist patients with concentration.[105] Such strategies might take the form of external aids such as using a timer or alarm watch to focus patient attention for specified time periods; organizing the work environment to eliminate distractions; and using a written or pictorial task plan with built-in periods for resting and reinforcement. Other strategies for increasing attention and concentration skills might focus on establishing internal procedures for patients to use. In establishing these procedures, clinicians may require that patients set increasingly demanding goals for themselves, including sustained work time. Other internal procedures might involve training patients to generate self-cues such as "am I wandering?" and "what am I supposed to do?" to keep them on task.

Two treatment tasks recommended by Adamovich, Henderson, and Auerbach may also prove useful for remediation of attention and concentration difficulties.[68] Patients may benefit from tracking tasks that require them to follow specific auditory and/or visual stimuli. They may benefit similarly from tasks that require them to draw within boundaries.

Patients with unilateral visual neglect may benefit from compensatory aids from reading and writing. Such aids might consist of having a red line drawn vertically at the left- or right-hand margins to draw patient attention to stimuli in the neglected field. When providing these compensatory aids, clinicians may find it useful to encourage patients simultaneously to self-generate cues such as "I need to look all the way to the left."

Despite a few anecdotal reports of patients using the previously mentioned techniques for attention and concentration, systematic investigation of these intervention techniques has not yet occurred.

Techniques for Improving Perception

Several techniques for improving patient perceptual skills have been described. These have included having patients: (1) develop recognition for environmental sounds; (2) complete visual scanning, tracking, and cancellation tasks; (3) turn their heads to compensate for visual field defects; (4) organize writing and arithmetic tasks spatially; and (5) draw within boundaries. Haarbauer-Krupa et al advocated encouraging patients to give feedback to their conversational partners as necessary (e.g., "please slow down"; "please repeat that") and to request longer time for viewing and reading tasks as necessary. Further, the elimination of extraneous visual distractors from the treatment environment is advocated.[105]

To improve perceptual skills in closed head injured patients, Adamovich, Henderson and Auerbach suggested the use of computer-assisted training.[68] There is some controversy among clinicians regarding the use of computer-assisted training for these patients however. Haarbauer-Krupa et al stated that there is little evidence to support that microcomputer training, in and of itself, significantly improves real-life performance of functional skills.[105]

Techniques to Improve Memory and Recall

Treatment strategies to aid recall of information have been described extensively, although by and large, the efficacy of these strategies has not been firmly established. The use of external memory aids has been advocated,[20,105] particularly the use of memory books or logbooks, in which salient information about ongoing daily activities is documented. Patients are encouraged to carry these books with them throughout the day and to refer to them for assistance in recalling recent information. Rehearsal is a strategy that has also been described extensively. Patients are encouraged to use both covert (silent) and overt (vocalized) rehearsal to aid them with memory functions.

Other techniques and strategies, which have been described for improving memory and recall functions, include training patients to use mnemonics such as rhymes and acronyms;[20,68,105] and verbal descriptions, categorization of information, temporal and spatial ordering, and use of primacy and recency benefits.[68]

Haarbauer-Krupa et al suggested that at retrieval, patients should be encouraged to reconstruct the environment in which information was received.[105] They also encouraged training patients to use self-questioning strategies (e.g., "Do I understand?"; "Do I need to ask a question?") in order to ensure that sufficient information was received.

A common technique advocated for aiding patient memory and recall is the use of visual imagery.[20,68,105] Several varieties of visual imagery strategies may be used including; (1) conventional images, which associate and relate interacting pairs of items (e.g., Mary Brown is married and has brown hair); (2) absurd images, which make a novel or ridiculous connection with an item (e.g., Mr. Lee with a Sara Lee pie on his face); (3) exaggerated images, which create an image of an item in exaggerated form (e.g., speech pathologist with a loud voice); (4) out-of-proportion images, which encourage visualization of an aspect of an item as larger or smaller than natural (e.g., the audiologist with huge ears); (5) out-of-place images, which require visualization of an item in an unexpected place (e.g., to remember to complete homework, tape it over the television screen).[20]

Studies of the effects of visual imagery in training memory and recall functions in patients have been few in number and each with only a few subjects. Glasgow et al reported that the use of simple visual imagery to associate face-name pairs was helpful to one of two closed head injured patients, but not to a second patient, who benefited from oral rehearsal.[110] Some generalization of the visual imagery strategies to the home environment was noted by these investigators about one of the patients, but the generalization noted was facilitated by the patient's frequent reference to reminder cards while at home. The effects of imagery training on recall functions were also investigated by Crovitz, whose findings for one closed head injured patient were that recall was critically dependent on cues provided by the examiner and not on patient-generated cues.[111] Further, data from this investigation showed no convincing evidence of generalization to daily activities.

Techniques to Improve Integration Skills

A variety of tasks designed to encourage patients to integrate important contextual information for judgment and problem-solving skills has been described, again mostly without confirming research data. These tasks have included having patients (1) recognize auditorily presented and visually presented absurdities; (2) solve inductive and deductive reasoning problems, using strategies employing features such as cause-effect relationships, analogies, and relevancy; (3) provide alternate solutions to a single problem to demonstrate increased cognitive flexibility; (4) plan sequences and steps necessary for the completion of everyday tasks; (5) perceive relationships (e.g., familial, part-whole, categorical, similarities and differences); (6) interpret imagery representations (e.g., cartoons, visual and auditory representations of metaphors, similes, and idioms);

(7) interpret and appreciate humor (e.g., puns, ambiguities, cartoons, political satire); (8) demonstrate convergent thinking skills, as in determining the main point or moral of a story; (9) outline and/or role play situation-specific behaviors (e.g., "What would you do if you received a number of harassing phone calls?"); and (10) use microcomputer programs designed expressly for the improvement of problem solving and/or reasoning skills.[20,45,68,105]

Haarbauer-Krupa et al also advocated the encouragement of patient-generated strategies to assist them in integrating salient information.[105] Patients may be trained to use self-questioning strategies to generate alternatives (e.g., "What else could I do?"); to scan the environment for appropriate cues regarding appropriateness and inappropriateness (e.g., a "no smoking" sign); and to identify specific times and places for behaviors which are appropriate in certain situations.

Techniques to Improve Organizational Skills

Tasks purportedly designed to enhance patient ability to organize information efficiently have been provided in the literature as well. These have included having patients (1) group words or pictures according to category or theme; (2) complete closure, sequencing and figure-ground tasks, as well as tasks involving the assimilation of fragmented stimuli; (3) retell or generate stories and narratives; (4) set priorities in completing steps in a process; (5) give directions to others; (6) outline visually or auditorily presented verbal material; and (7) use self-rehearsal as a facilitating strategy for organization.[20,68,105]

Techniques to Improve Pragmatic Communication Skills

Haarbauer-Krupa et al advocated the use of a number of patient strategies for adoption in conversational situations.[105] The strategies that patients may be encouraged to use include: (1) noting the topic being discussed in any conversation; (2) self-questioning about the main point or topic being discussed; (3) alerting others before shifting topics; (4) watching others for visual feedback about whether patients are being understood; and (5) setting limits of time or an allowable number of sentences in any one conversational turn.

Burns, Halper, and Mogil suggested a variety of treatment activities for improving pragmatic skills, including: (1) drills designed to improve stress and intonation; (2) training about the appropriate use of nonvocal cues such as eye contact and facial expression in conversational interchanges; (3) practice in the identification of conversational postulate violations; (4) training in the use of discourse cohesion devices (e.g., anaphoric and cataphoric referencing); and (5) practice in generating dialogue skills.[20]

To summarize, treatment activities for right hemisphere damaged and closed head injured patients have been well established, but critical research support regarding the efficacy of such interventions is painfully absent. This latter notion prompted Myers to challenge clinicians carefully to document treatment progress and to share results of clinically based research with colleagues to enhance sophistication in knowledge about treatment outcomes.[112] For a more complete description of specific techniques described in this section of the chapter, the reader is referred to Myers;[45] Adamovich, Henderson, and Auerbach;[68] Burns, Halper, and Mogil;[20] Haarbauer-Krupa et al;[105] and Tonkovich.[47]

SUMMARY

Clinical management of right hemisphere damaged and closed head injured patients by speech-language pathologists has a brief history relative to the history of speech-language pathology involvement with other communicative disorders. In pioneering efforts, clinicians have faced the challenge of intervening with the unique cognitive-communicative impairments of these two populations by developing diagnostic methods and treatment strategies. The blatantly absent empirical data to support these clinical management procedures point to serious immediate and future needs.

First, standardized diagnostic protocols with excellent test-retest reliability, consistency, and validity need to be established for sensitively diagnosing the cognitive-communicative impairments in these populations and for measuring behavioral changes over time. Next, scientific scrutiny of clinical techniques must establish their effectiveness so that speech-language pathologists can justify their role in the rehabilitation of these data. More empirical data in the form of group and single-subject research designs is necessary to accomplish this goal. While right hemisphere damaged and closed head injured patients have demonstrable needs regarding communicative behavior, speech-language pathologists cannot afford to continue "blind faith" management procedures.

REFERENCES

1. Metter EJ. Medical aspects of stroke rehabilitation. In: Chapey R, ed. Language intervention strategies in adult aphasia. Baltimore: Williams & Wilkins, 1986:141.
2. Jackson JH. On the nature of the duality of the brain. In: Taylor J, ed. Selected writings of John Hughlings Jackson. London: Hodder & Stoughton, 1982:119.
3. Cummings JL. Hemispheric specialization: a history of current concepts. In: Burns MS, Halper AS, Mogil SI, eds. Clinical management of right hemisphere dysfunction. Rockville, MD: Aspen Systems Corporation, 1985:1.
4. Milner B, Taylor L. Right hemisphere superiority in tactile pattern-recognition after cerebral commisurotomy. Neuropsychologia 1972; 10:1–15.
5. Sperry RW. Lateral specialization in the surgically separated hemispheres. In: Schmitt FO, Worden FG, eds. The neurosciences. Third study program. Cambridge: Massachusetts Institute of Technology Press, 1974.
6. Zaidel E, Zaidel DW, Sperry RW. Left and right intelligence: case studies of Raven's progressive matrices following brain bisection and hemidecortication. Cortex 1981; 17:167–186.
7. Jeeves MA. Psychological studies of three cases of congenital agenesis of the corpus callosum in man. In: CIBA Foundation study group no. 20, eds. Functions of the corpus callosum. London: Churchill, 1965:63.
8. Bogen JE. The callosal syndrome. In: Heilman KE, Valentstein E, eds. Clinical neuropsychology. New York: Oxford University Press, 1979:128.
9. Van der Vlugt H. Aspects of normal and abnormal neuropsychological development. In: Gazzaniga MS, ed. Handbook of behavioral neurobiology, vol 2, neuropsychology. New York: Plenum Press, 1979:107.
10. Kimura D. Cerebral dominance and the perception of verbal stimuli. Can J Psychol 1961; 15:166–171.
11. Kimura D. Left-right differences in the perception of melodies. Q J Psychol 1964; 16:355–358.
12. Bryden MP, Ley RG. Right hemispheric involvement in imagery and affect. In: Perecman E, ed. Cognitive processing in the right hemisphere. New York: Academic Press, 1983:41.
13. Gardner H. The shattered mind. New York: Vintage Books, 1974.
14. Lezak M. Recovery of memory and learning functions following traumatic brain injury. Cortex 1979; 15:63–72.
15. Myers PS. Right hemisphere communication impairment. In: Chapey R, ed. Language intervention strategies in adult aphasia. Baltimore: Williams & Wilkins, 1986:444.
16. Cummings JL. Neurological syndromes associated with right hemisphere damage. In: Burns MS, Halper AS, Mogil SI, eds. Clinical management of right hemisphere dysfunction. Rockville, MD: Aspen Systems Corp, 1985:7.
17. Heilman KM, Bowers D, Speedie L, Coslett HB. Comprehension of affective and nonaffective prosody. Neurology 1984; 34:917–921.
18. Heilman KM, Valenstein E, Watson RT. Neglect and related disorders. Semin Neurol 1984; 4:209–219.
19. Mesulam MM. A cortical network for directed attention and unilateral neglect. Ann Neurol 1981; 10:309–325.
20. Burns MS, Halper AS, Mogil SI. Clinical management of right hemisphere dysfunction. Rockville, MD: Aspen Systems Corporation, 1985.
21. Senner-Hurley F, Lefkowitz NG. Stroke: speech-language rehabilitation. In: Logigian MK, ed. Adult rehabilitation: a team approach for therapists. Boston: Little, Brown, 1982:275.
22. Cohn R, Neumann MA, Wood DH. Prosopagnosia: a clinicopathological study. Ann Neurol 1977; 1:177–182.
23. Meadows JC. The anatomical basis of prosopagnosia. J Neurol Neurosurg Psychiatry 1974; 40:395–403.
24. Hecaen H, Angelergues R. Agnosia for faces (prosopagnosia). Arch Neurol 1962; 7:92–100.
25. Whitely AM, Warrington EK. Prosopagnosia: a clinical, psychological and anatomical study of three patients. J Neurol Neurosurg Psychiatry 1977; 40:395–403.
26. Malone DR, Morris HH, Kay MC. Prosopagnosia: a double dissociation between the recognition of familiar and unfamiliar faces. J Neurol Neurosurg Psychiatry 1982; 45:820–822.
27. Wall N. Stroke rehabilitation. In: Logigian MK, ed. Adult rehabilitation: a team approach for therapists. Boston: Little, Brown, 1982:225.
28. Paterson A, Zangwill OL. A case of topographical disorientation associated with a unilateral cerebral lesion. Brain 1945; 68:188–212.
29. Hecaen H, Tzortzis C, Rondet P. Loss of topographic memory with learning deficits. Cortex 1980; 16:525–542.
30. van Lancker DR, Canter GJ. Impairment of voice and face recognition in patients with hemispheric damage. Brain Cognit 1982; 1:185–195.
31. Heilman KM, Scholes R, Watson RT. Auditory affective agnosia. J Neurol Neurosurg Psychiatry 1975; 38:69–72.
32. Tucker DM, Watson RT, Heilman KM. Discrimination and evocation of affectively intoned speech in patients with right parietal disease. Neurology 1977; 27:947–950.
33. Ruff RL, Volpe BT. Environmental reduplication associated with right frontal and parietal lobe injury. J Neurol Neurosurg Psychiatry 1981; 44:382–386.
34. Rey A. L'examen clinique en psychologie. Paris: Presses Universitaires de France, 1964.
35. Lezak MD. Neuropsychological assessment. 2nd ed. New York: Oxford University Press, 1983.
36. Davis ME, Binder LM, Lezak MD. Hemispheric side of damage and encoding capacity. Presented to the International Neuropsychological Society, Mexico City, 1983.
37. Delaney RC, Wallace JD, Egelko S. Transient cerebral ischemic attacks and neurological deficit. J Clin Neuropsychol 1980; 2:107–114.
38. Benson DF, Gardner H, Meadows JC. Reduplicative paramnesia. Neurology 1976; 26:147–151.
39. Fisher CM. Disorientation for place. Arch neurol 1982; 39:33–36.
40. Benton AL. Differential behavioral effects in frontal lobe disease. Neuropsychologia 1968; 6:53–60.
41. Gorham DR. A proverbs test for clinical and experimental use. Psychol Rep 1956; 1:1–12.
42. Winner E, Gardner H. The comprehension of metaphor in brain damaged patients. Brain 1977; 100:717–729.

42a. Myers PS, Linebaugh CW. Comprehension of idiomatic expressions by right-hemisphere damaged adults. In: Brookshire RH, ed. Clinical aphasiology conference proceedings. Minneapolis: BRK Publishers, 1981:254.

43. Gardner H, Denes G. Connotative judgments by aphasic patients on a pictorial adaptation of the semantic differential. Cortex 1973; 9:183–196.
44. Lemon P, Burns M, Lehner L. Communication deficits associated with right cerebral damage. Presented to the American Speech-Language-Hearing Association, Atlanta, 1979.
45. Myers PS. Treatment of right hemisphere communication disorders. In: Perkins WH, ed. Language handicaps in adults. New York: Thieme-Stratton, 1983:57.
46. Boyarsky M. Communicative competence of right brain damaged individuals in narrative discourse. Presented to the American Speech-Language-Hearing Association, Washington, DC, 1985.
47. Tonkovich JD. Managing pragmatic communication defi-

cits associated with right hemisphere damage. Semin Speech Lang 1987; in press.
48. Wapner W, Hamby S, Gardner H. The role of the right hemisphere in the apprehension of complex linguistic materials. Brain Lang 1981; 14:15–33.
49. Hier DB, Kaplan J. Verbal comprehension deficits after right hemisphere damage. Appl Psycholinguist 1980; 1:279–294.
50. Foldi NS, Cicone M, Gardner H. Pragmatic aspects of communication in brain-damaged patients. In: Segalowitz S, ed. Language functions and brain organization. New York: Academic Press, 1983:131.
51. Ross ED, Mesulam MM. Dominant language functions of the right hemisphere? Arch Neurol 1979; 36:144–148.
52. Ross ED. The aprosodias. Arch Neurol 1981; 38:561–569.
53. Ross DG. Ross information processing assessment. Tigard, OR: CC Publications, 1986.
54. Karlsen B, Madden R, Gardner E. Adult basic learning examination (ABLE): levels I, II, and III. New York: Psychological Corporation, 1971.
55. Goodglass H, Kaplan E. The assessment of aphasia and related disorders. Philadelphia: Lea & Febiger, 1983.
56. Baker HJ, Leland B. Detroit tests of learning aptitude. Austin: PRO-ED, 1967.
57. Beery KE, Buktenica NA. Developmental test of visual-motor integration. Chicago: Follett, 1967.
58. Frostig M. Developmental test of visual perception. Chicago: Follett, 1963.
59. MacGinitie WH. Gates-MacGinitie reading tests: survey D, E, F. 2nd ed. Chicago: Riverside Publishing Co., 1978.
60. Farr R. Iowa silent reading tests: levels 1, 2, 3. New York: Psychological Corporation, 1973.
61. Farr R, Prescott GA, Balow IH, Hogan TP. Metropolitan reading instructional tests: elementary, intermediate, and advanced I. New York: Psychological Corporation, 1978.
62. Colarusso RP, Hammill DD. Motor-free visual perception test. Novato, CA: Academic Therapy Publications, 1972.
63. Ross JD, Ross CM. Ross test of higher cognitive processes. Novato, CA: Academic Therapy Publications, 1976.
64. Gardner EF, Rudman HC, Karlsen B, Merwin JC. Stanford achievement test—listening comprehension test: intermediate I, II, advanced. New York: Psychological Corporation, 1982.
65. Feldman MJ, Dragow J. Visual-verbal test. Los Angeles: Western Psychological Services, 1981.
66. Watson G, Glaser EM. Watson-Glaser critical thinking appraisal. New York: Psychological Corporation, 1980.
67. Woodcock R. Woodcock reading mastery tests. Circle Pines, MN: American Guidance Service, 1973.
68. Adamovich BB, Henderson JA, Auerbach S. Cognitive rehabilitation of closed head injured patients: a dynamic approach. San Diego: College-Hill Press, 1985.
69. Anderson DW, McLaurin RL, eds. Report on national head and spinal cord injury conducted for NINCDS. J Neurosurg Suppl 1980:S1–S43.
70. Kalsbeek WD, McLaurin RL, Harris BSH, Miller J. The national head and spinal cord injury survey. J Neurosurg 1980; 53:513–531.
71. Fields JH. A study of the epidemiology of head injury in England and Wales. London: Department of Health and Social Security, 1976.
72. Holzer ML, Stiassny DA, Senner-Hurley F, Lefkowitz NG. Brain trauma. In: Logigian MK, ed. Adult rehabilitation: a team approach for therapists. Boston: Little, Brown, 1982:297.
73. Hagen C. Language disorders in head trauma. In: Holland AL, ed. Language disorders in adults: recent advances. San Diego: College-Hill Press, 1984:245.
74. Ylvisaker M, Szekeres SF. Management of the patient with closed head injury. In: Chapey R, ed. Language intervention strategies in adult aphasia. Baltimore: Williams & Wilkins, 1986:474.
75. Benton AL. Behavioral consequences of closed head injury. In: Odom GL, ed. Central nervous system trauma research status report. Washington: NINCDS, NIH, Public Health Service, 1979.
76. Heilman KM, Safran A, Geschwind N. Closed head trauma and aphasia. J Neurol Neurosurg Psychiatry 1971; 34:265–269.
77. Sarno MT, Buonaguro A, Levita E. Characteristics of verbal impairment in closed head injured patients. Arch Phys Med Rehabil 1986; 67:400–405.
78. Levin HS. Aphasia in closed head injury. In: Sarno MT, ed. Acquired aphasia. New York: Academic Press, 1981:311.
79. Sarno MT. Verbal impairment after closed head injury: report of a replication study. J Nerv Ment Dis 1980; 168:685–692.
80. Halpern H, Darley FL, Brown JR. Differential language and neurologic characteristics in cerebral involvement. J Speech Hear Disord 1973; 38:162–173.
81. Wertz RT. Neuropathologies of speech and language: an introduction to patient management. In: Johns DF, ed. Clinical management of neurogenic disorders. Boston: Little, Brown, 1978:1.
82. Szekeres SF, Ylvisaker M, Holland AL. Cognitive rehabilitation therapy: a framework for intervention. In: Ylvisaker M, ed. Head injury rehabilitation: children and adolescents. San Diego: College-Hill Press, 1985.
83. Hecaen H, Albert ML. Disorders of mental functioning related to frontal lobe pathology. In: Benson DF, Blumer D, eds. Psychiatric aspects of neurologic disease. New York: Grune & Stratton, 1975:217.
84. LeMay M, Geschwind N. Asymmetries of the human cerebral hemispheres. In: Caramazza A, Zurif E, eds. Language acquisition and language breakdown. Baltimore: Johns Hopkins University Press, 1978:311.
85. Brooks DN, Aughton ME, Bond MR, Jones P, Rizvi S. Cognitive sequelae in relationship to early indices of severity of brain damage after severe blunt head injury. J Neurol Neurosurg Psychiatry 1980; 43:529–534.
86. Gazzaniga MS, Hillyard SA. Language and speech capacity of the right hemisphere. Neuropsychologia 1971; 9:273–280.
87. Whitaker HA, Ojemann GA. Lateralization of higher cortical functions: a critique. Ann NY Acad Sci 1977; 299:459–473.
88. MacKay D. Cognitive behavior therapy. Br J Hosp Med 1982; 27:242–247.
89. Bever TG. Cerebral asymmetries in humans are due to the differentiation of two incompatible processes: holistic and analytic. Ann NY Acad Sci 1975; 265:252–262.
90. Mandleburg IA. Cognitive recovery after severe head injury: WAIS verbal and performance IQs as a function of post traumatic amnesia and time from injury. J Neurol Neurosurg Psychiatry 1976; 29:1001–1007.
91. Adamovich BB, Henderson JA. Cognitive deficits post traumatic head injury: diagnostic and treatment implications. Presented to the American Speech-Language-Hearing Association, Cincinnati, 1983.
92. Groher M. Language and memory disorders following closed head trauma. J Speech Hear Res 1977; 20:212–223.
93. Jennett B, Bond M. Assessment outcome after severe brain damage: practical scale. Lancet 1975; 1:480–484.
94. Rimel R. Epidemiology and recovery patterns in adult head trauma. Presented at the Third Annual Conference, Head Trauma Rehabilitation—Coma to Community, San Jose, 1980.
95. Hagen C, Malkmus D. Intervention strategies for language disorders secondary to head trauma. Presented to the Amer-

ican Speech-Language-Hearing Association, Atlanta, 1979.
96. Rappaport M, Hall KM, Hopkins K, Belleza BS, Cope DN. Disability rating scale for severe head trauma: coma to community. Arch Phys Med Rehabil 1982; 63:118–123.
97. Gouvier WD, Blanton PD, LaPorte KK, Nepomuceno C. Reliability and validity of the disability rating scale and the levels of cognitive functioning scale in monitoring recovery from severe head injury. Arch Phys Med Rehabil 1987; 68:94–97.
98. Kirk SA, McCarthy J, Kirk WD. Illinois test of psycholinguistic abilities. Champaign: University of Illinois, 1968.
99. Wechsler D. Wechsler adult intelligence scale. New York: Psychological Corporation, 1955.
100. Ayres AJ. Southern California figure-ground visual perception test. Los Angeles: Western Psychological Services, 1966.
101. Christensen AL. Luria's neuropsychological investigation. New York: Spectrum, 1985.
102. Goldman R, Fristoe M, Woodcock RW. Goldman-Fristoe-Woodcock sound-symbol tests. Circle Pines, MN: American Guidance Service, 1974.
103. Goldman R, Fristoe M, Woodcock RW. Goldman-Fristoe-Woodcock test of auditory discrimination. Circle Pines, MN: American Guidance Service, 1970.
104. Johnson GO, Boyd HF. Nonverbal test of cognitive skills. Columbus: Charles E Merrill, 1981.
105. Haarbauer-Krupa J, Henry K, Szekeres SF, Ylvisaker M. Cognitive rehabilitation therapy: late stages of recovery. In: Ylvisaker M, ed. Head injury rehabilitation: children and adolescents. San Diego: College-Hill Press, 1985:311.
106. Goldstein K, Scheerer M. Goldstein-Scheerer stick test. New York: Psychological Corporation, 1945.
107. Benton AL. The revised visual retention test. New York: Psychological Corporation, 1963.
108. Goldman R, Fristoe M, Woodcock RW. Goldman-Fristoe-Woodcock auditory memory tests. Circle Pines, MN: American Guidance Service, 1974a.
109. Weigle E, Goldstein K, Scheerer M. Color form sorting test. New York: Psychological Corporation, 1945.
110. Glasgow RE, Zeiss RA, Barrera M Jr, Lewinsohn PM. Case studies on remediating memory deficits in brain-damaged individuals. J Clin Psychol 1977; 33:1049–1054.
111. Crovitz HF. Memory retaining in brain-damaged patients: the airplane test. Cortex 1979; 15:131–134.
112. Myers PS. Right hemisphere impairment. In: Holland AL, ed. Language disorders in adults: recent advances. San Diego: College-Hill Press, 1984:177.

32 Speech and Language Differences and Disorders of Multicultural Populations

Orlando L. Taylor, Ph.D.

Speech and language behaviors are generally considered to be disordered when they deviate sufficiently from a norm to interfere with communication, call attention to themselves, or cause the user to be maladjusted.[1] In the United States, the norm is usually defined as the phonologic, semantic, grammatic, pragmatic, and discourse features of the English language that are used by the "standard makers." Generally, these persons are white, middle to upper class, and well educated.

Since the 1960s, with the rise of popularity in the disciplines of sociolinguistics and ethnography of communications, scientists and practitioners have increasingly recognized the fact that "normal" for a given speaker is determined by his or her culture with the particular type of language used within these cultural constraints controlled by language interactions among several social factors. Therefore, pathologic communication within a specified group of speakers can be measured only against the language norms for their community or culture. The major social and cultural factors that affect language use are education, socioeconomic status, gender, age, region, race or ethnicity, peer group association and/or identification, and first language and/or cultural community.

Because of the differences that can occur within a language, there is a distinct possibility that a perfectly normal speaker of a particular dialect of a language is inaccurately labeled as having a *pathology* of language when, indeed, there is only a *difference* in language use. For example, in some normal varieties (dialects) of English spoken in the United States, a sentence such as "He be sick" is a perfectly normal sentence to refer to a male who is constantly or habitually ill. However, if a speech-language pathologist only knows a standard American English dialect, he or she may incorrectly think the utterance means a male person *is* sick at the moment. Its use in a formal situation might call attention to itself, and repeated negative reactions to its use might cause the speaker to at least become "sensitive" about its use.

In the previous example, attention should be drawn to two important themes that will recur throughout this chapter. First, the word "dialect" is used merely to mean a variety of a language. It is not used pejoratively, as is frequently the case with lay persons, to mean a nonstandard or nonprestigious way of speaking. Second, improper application of the classic definition of speech-language pathology can result in the inaccurate labelling of normal communicative behavior as pathologic.

Discussions of language variation invariably lead to a discussion of standard English. Contrary to popular belief, standard English is not one way of speaking, nor is it a way of speaking that is intrinsically a better way of speaking the English language. The concept of a "standard" in any language is an outgrowth of a number of political, social, educational, and economic factors. Usually, the dialects spoken by the politically, socially, economically, and, especially, educationally powerful and elite come to gain sufficient prestige to become the standard variety of the language. These standard forms become tantamount to official versions of the language that hold currency in education and commerce, even when no official language, has been designated by the national government.

There are several varieties of standard English spoken in the United States, virtually all of which are identified with specific regions of the country or with certain identifiable racial, ethnic, or language groups. Although these varieties of standard English may contain differences in such dimensions of language as phonology, semantics, pragmatics, and discourse, particularly in informal situations, the varieties share a common set of grammatic rules. According to writers such as Wolfram and Fasold, societal attitudes on language prestige are most prevalent in the grammatic dimension of language (syntax and morphology).[2]

In this chapter, three major topics will be explored: (1) social and cultural factors that influence language acquisition and behavior, (2) linguistic descriptions of major nonstandard varieties of American English, and (3) application of sociolinguistic data and theory to the practice of speech-language pathology.

LANGUAGE AS A MANIFESTATION OF CULTURE

Culture may be defined as the set of perceptions, behaviors, values, preferences, world views, technologies, social organizations, and interpersonal interactional patterns used by members of a specified group to ensure the acquisition and perpetuation of what they consider to be a high quality of life. In short, cultures represent the strategies and codes of personal conduct that humans develop to interact with physical and social environment. Cultures are arbitrary and changeable. They overlap with one another, yet contain internal variations. As well, culture exists at different levels of conscious awareness for its individual members.

Language is the use of verbal and nonverbal markings used by humans throughout the world to codify culture. In a very real sense, language is perhaps the most overt representation of culture. Through its use, ideas are formed, permuted, synthesized, and communicated among the members of a culture and preserved for perpetuity. Language has both a structural element (a phonology, syntax, vocabulary) and a communicative, or use, element. The communicative element includes the rules governing discourse, conversations, and functional devices used by speakers of a language to achieve specific purposes.

This intimate linkage between language and culture may be schematized as shown in Figure 32–1.

SOCIAL AND CULTURAL FACTORS THAT INFLUENCE LANGUAGE ACQUISITION AND BEHAVIOR

Basic Concepts and Terminology

As stated, social and cultural factors influence all dimensions of language. In heterogeneous societies such as the United States, the interplay among social and cultural factors results in linguistic variation within the national or official language.

To date, the sociolinguistics, the pragmatics, and the ethnography of communication have provided the major frameworks for the exploration of linguistic variation. Sociolinguistics studies the structure and use of language in its social and cultural context. Pragmatics investigates language use in interactional communicative settings, employing the speech act as the fundamental unit of analysis. The speech act incorporates the intentional, semantic, and grammatic properties of utterances.

There are several important concepts that have been associated with the study of linguistic variation. Saville-Troike writes:[3a]

> The ethnography of communication provides a synthesizing focus that concentrates on the patterning of communicative behavior as it constitutes one of the subsystems of culture, as it functions within the holistic context of the culture of a group, and as it relates to patterns in other component systems. This perspective first and foremost takes language as a socially situated cultural form, while at the same time recognizing the necessity to analyze the linguistic code itself and the cognitive processes of its speakers and hearers. To accept a lesser scope for the study of communication is to risk reducing it to triviality and to abandon any possibility of understanding how language actually functions in the lives of individuals and cultural groups.
>
> The subject matter of the ethnography of communication is best illustrated by two of its most general questions: What does a speaker need to know to communicate appropriately within a particular speech community? And how does he or she acquire this knowledge? Such knowledge, together with whatever skills are needed to make use of it, is termed "communicative competence"[4a] The requisite knowledge includes not only rules for commu-

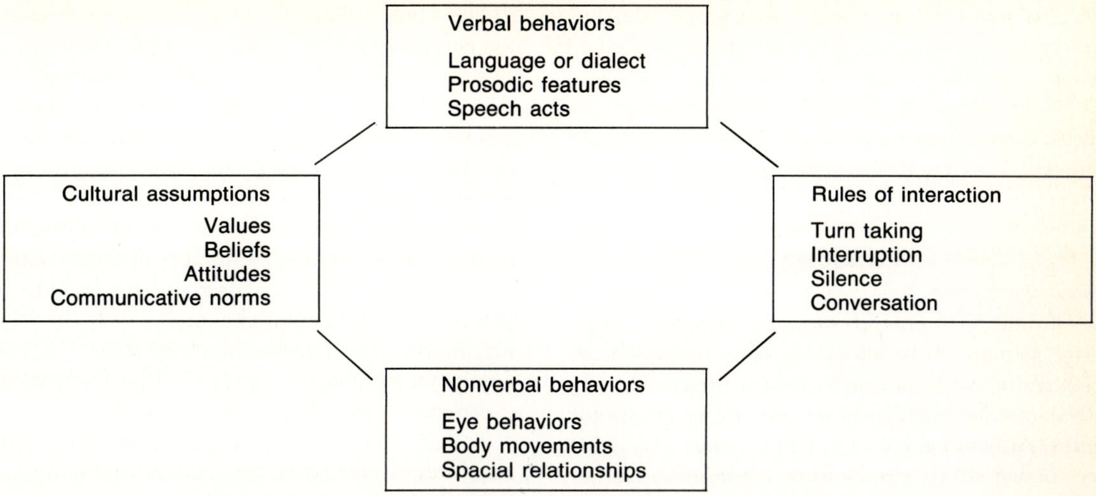

Figure 32–1 A schema of the intimate linkage between language and culture.

nication (both linguistic and sociolinguistic) and shared rules for interaction, but also the cultural rules and knowledge that are the basis for the context and content of communicative events and interaction processes. The primary aim of this approach is to guide the collection and analysis of descriptive data about the ways in which social meaning is conveyed, constructed, and negotiated.

Communicative competence is represented by a set of conversational postulates or rules for interaction. Examples of conversational postulates would be such rules as "whisper in church" and "speak standard English in formal situations." A speech community is any human aggregate whose members regularly and frequently interact by means of a shared set of verbal symbols and who possess shared knowledge of the rules for the production and interpretation of speech used by members of that group, for example, Southerners, inner city blacks, Chicanos, Americans, or teenagers.[3,4,4a]

The range of linguistic codes existing in a speech community or spoken by an individual member is called the "linguistic repertoire."[5] It may include a standard language, a regional dialect, and a local dialect; or it may be described as a formal style, a colloquial style, or an occupational jargon.[5] The extensiveness of one's linguistic repertoire is related to such factors as motivation, exposure, social status, social mobility, and occupation. The ability to move effectively from one code to another in social situations is referred to as code switching.[6,7]

The linguistic repertoire of a speech community may consist of several mutually intelligible dialects or varieties of the language spoken in that community that are subject to structural, stylistic, and social variation. Note that a dialect is merely any way of speaking a language, ranging from the most nonstandard to the most standard. Stylistic variation concerns speech that fits the occasion, whether it be formal (e.g., a public lecture) or informal (e.g., a casual conversation with a friend). The standard dialect is one of several styles within a speech community.[8] It is the formal, public, prestigious variety of a language that is favored by the "establishment" and supported by its major social institutions.[9]

A vernacular or colloquial variety of a language is more informal, casual, and intimate. It is not used in writing nor in school. Social variation occurs when communicators interact with each other. Thus a specific linguistic structure may assume various communicative functions or values depending upon the intent of the speakers. For instance, an interrogative sentence such as "Do you have a match?" is not always intended as a question, but may also be used to request a match or to command someone to light one's cigarette. Selection of a specific linguistic structure, then, is dependent upon a speaker's perception of the social situation and his or her communicative intention.

Finally, sociolinguistic variables identify the nonlinguistic dimensions of the social context that influence the selection of a particular language variety, for example, the speaker, listener, audience, topic, setting. These variables are hierarchically ordered or stratified within a speech community. Social indicators in language show a regular distribution within a given socioeconomic, ethnic, sex, or age group, in that they are used by each individual in that group in more or less the same way in any context. Language markers demonstrate the same social distribution as indicators and, in addition, reflect stylistic differences in casual versus careful speech. Language stereotypes are markers that are considered to be characteristic of a particular speech community, but need not represent actual usage. Each of these variables is discussed in some detail by Bell,[10] Labov,[10a] and Penalosa.[11]

With these concepts and terms in mind, let us discuss the major social and cultural factors that influence language behavior and acquisition.

Ethnicity

Ethnic background typically influences language patterns. Although race is often confused with ethnicity, it should be remembered that race is largely a biologic designate and, as such, many ethnic (or culture) groups exist within a single race. The point here is that ethnic influences on communicative behavior is neither biologic nor genetic. Instead, they are related to the transmission and/or preservation of cultural attitudes and values associated with a particular ethnic group. Some linguistic forms are characteristic of certain ethnic or cultural groups to the extent that when they are used, they immediately mark the speaker as either being from that group or having had a great deal of interaction with the group. For example, individuals using the sentence "He be sick" to refer to a male person who is habitually ill reveal previous or present membership in a working-class black American community or at least some interaction with or knowledge of a community of this type. It should be noted that some biologically black, English speaking groups (e.g., Barbadians) are not described as using this particular form.

Several researchers have stressed the importance of ethnic differences in their writings on language variation (Rosten on Yiddish communities;[12] Pearce-Hopper and McMahon on native Americans;[13] Castaneda et al[14] and Penalosa[11] on Chicanos; Labov on Jewish, Italian, and Polish communities;[15] and Brandes and Brewer on Appalachian, black, Chicano, and Yiddish communities[16]). Although there are clearly identifiable ethnic markings in American English, it must be stressed, however, that ethnic group membership alone does not preclude one from acquiring or using a number of other language codes.

Social Class, Education, Occupation

Historically, linguistic differences have served to identify and separate social classes. In closed societies, members of the servant class do not typically imitate the speech of the aristocracy.[5] In open societies, there is usually more social mobility and intermingling among classes, although certain nonmainstream groups may remain socially isolated owing to factors such as segregation or geography. In addition, Hollingshead has argued that social class status and mobility are highly correlated with educational achievement and occupation.[17] Because of the social variable, the lower-class individual's linguistic repertoire may not include the standard dialect spoken by the more learned and elite members of his or her society.

Researchers have attributed many dimensions of language variation to a number of social class influences. The chief social factors have included (1) poverty and home environment,[18–20] (2) child-rearing practices and maternal teaching styles,[18,21–23] (3) family interactional patterns,[18,24,25] (4) travel and experience,[18] and (5) code-switching.[26–28]

Bernstein has emphasized social class differences regarding access to certain communicative codes.[29] He suggests that the lower classes use a more restricted, context-dependent code with particular meanings and that the upper classes use a more elaborated, context-independent code with universal meanings. The implication is that lower-class children would have difficulty in schools where the elaborated code is required. The problem with Bernstein's theory is that it has a built-in bias toward the middle-class communication style in that it implicitly assumes that it, and not the style of the lower class, is "normal." Such measures as mean length of utterance embrace some of the notions contained in Bernstein's theory and, as such, are implicitly biased against low-income speakers. It may indeed be the case that all children have access to so-called elaborated codes, but may choose not to use them in certain situations. Future research in the area of pragmatics might provide insights into this topic.

Region

Regional dialects are closely tied to social dialects, but are generally defined by geographic boundaries. There are at least ten regional dialects recognized in the United States, including Southern, Eastern New England, Western Pennsylvania, Appalachian, Central Midland, Middle Atlantic, and New York City.[30] A map reflecting these dialect regions is shown in Figure 32–2. Wardhaugh notes that the distribution of linguistic forms is related to such factors as (1) geographical features (e.g., mountains, climate, and water); (2) trade routes (e.g., influence of outsiders); (3) settlement patterns (e.g., cultural and ethnic backgrounds of settlers); (4) religion (e.g., Amish of Pennsylvania or Mormons of Utah); and (5) politics (power relationships in the region).[9]

In general, regional dialects are marked by specific linguistic patterns. Few native-born Ameri-

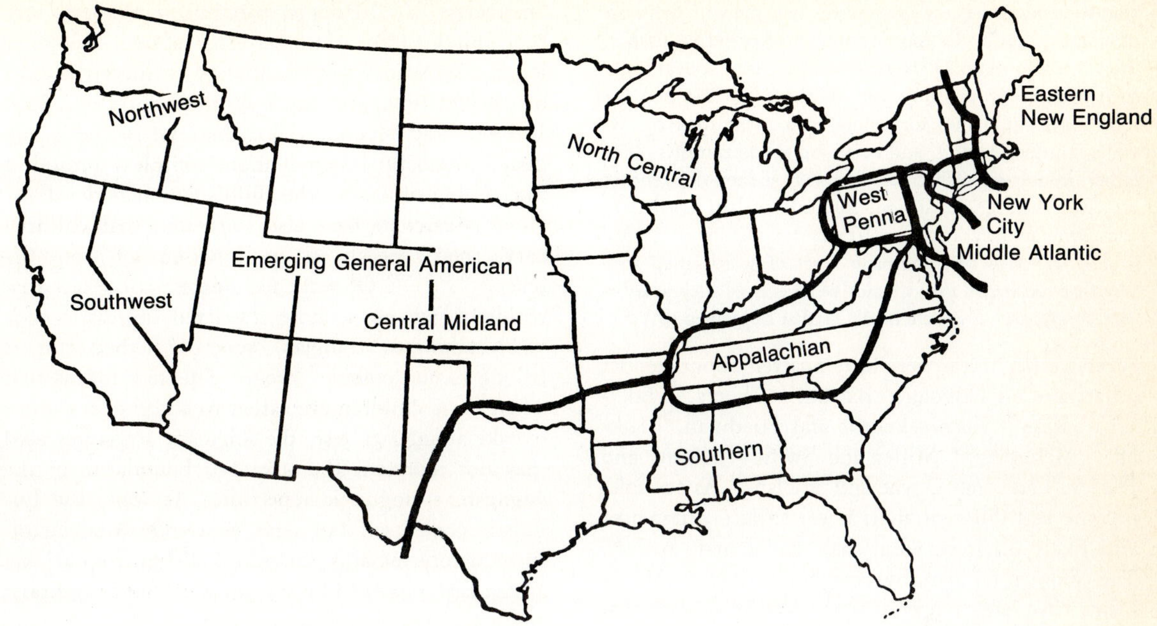

Figure 32–2 Map of major American English speech varieties. (From Nist J. A structural history of English. New York: St. Martin's Press, 1966:371.)

cans, for example, would have difficulty recognizing a stereotyped Southern, New York City, or Boston dialect. Wardhaugh suggests that regional dialects may be recognized by a variety of linguistic characteristics.[9] For example, the speech of a particular geographical region might be marked by a particular vowel quality in a certain set of words, the absence of a particular expected phoneme in still another set, the use of certain names for objects, and extensions of a syntactic feature.

Edwards argues that the maintenance of a regional dialect in a particular speaker may be related to such factors as local pride, local activities, or a deliberate rejection of wider affiliations.[5] Individuals may give up regionalisms to further occupational, political, or social aspirations. Some regional dialects are viewed negatively by outsiders or by upper-class members of the same region. Some speakers have compromised by using regional dialects locally or in intimate situations and a more nonregionalized standard dialect away from home or in formal situations. Since there are regional standards that approximate the general standard, many persons, of course, have not found it necessary to abandon their regional dialects.

Gender

Hardly anyone would fail to recognize a speaker as being male or female. A major difference in the speech of men and women results from contrasting physical and psychological characteristics of the voice, such as pitch and intonation. The male voice is generally lower owing to longer, thinner vocal cords, although some social programming is probably present in determining a male's selection of a "masculine" voice. Women are also influenced by social definitions of voice usage. For instance, Wardhaugh argues that women typically vary their intonation patterns more extensively than men to signal endearment, excitement, "mothering," and pleasure.[9] Again, these variations are probably related more to culture than to biology.

There are differences related to the use of taboo words.[31] For instance, certain forms are often considered inappropriate for women to use, for example, curse words and off-color jokes, but are used by men as a sign of masculinity and toughness. Trudgill also notes that men tend to use more nonstandard forms than women since women tend to value the status and appearances associated with standard language usage.

Speaking more explicitly, Wardhaugh makes the following observations concerning the difference between the "characteristic language uses of men and women":

> [Women] tend to be more precise and "careful" in speaking: for example, they are more likely than men to pronounce the final *-ing* forms with a *g*, to say *fighting* rather than *fightin'*. In general they take more "care" in articulation. This behavior accords with other findings that

women tend to be less innovative than men in their use of language and to be more conscious of preferred usages. They are also more likely than men to use "appeal tags" such as isn't it? or don't you think? . . . Women use more different names for colors than men: mauve, lavender, turquoise, lilac, and beige are good examples. Men either do not use such color words or, if they do, tend to use them with great caution. Intensifiers such as *so, such,* and *quite,* as in *He's so cute, He's such a dear,* and *We had a quite marvelous time* comprise a set of words used in a way that most men avoid; emotive adjectives such as *adorable, lovely,* and *divine* are hardly used at all by men (p 128).[9]

Several other researchers have written about gender differences in language: Barron,[32] Cherry,[33] Edelsky,[34] Key,[35] Koenigsknecht and Friedman,[36] Lakoff,[37] McCarthy,[38] Miller and Swift,[39] Thorne and Henley,[40] and Van Duyne and Scanlan.[41] As sex roles become less differentiated, fewer surface differences will likely occur between male and female speech. The Women's Liberation and Equal Rights Movements have already opened up to women jargons that were previously dominated by men.

Situation or Context

Language may vary according to the situation and context in which it is spoken.[5,42–44] Several important situational and contextual variables may influence all dimensions of language behavior. The most important of these variables are setting, location, occasion, participants, topic, purpose, and spatial positions of participants. In addition to these variables, there are still other dimensions of the situation or context variable.

Dyadic interactions. These interactions involve a speaker and hearer, an addressor and addressee, a sender and receiver, and sometimes a third participant, for example, an audience observing the interaction. The speaker's role in the dyadic interaction, as well as his or her background and status, help determine language usage.

Role relationships. These relationships can be contrasted in terms of such dyads as parent and child, employer and employee, doctor and patient, husband and wife, clinician and client, actor and audience, and child and stranger. Some occupational roles, for instance, require a more formal code. For example, a patient or client is comfortable when a doctor or lawyer or therapist speaks formally in routine situations, but may appreciate a more intimate tone in a crisis situation. An employer's choice between formal and informal code may signal dissatisfaction or closeness with the employee. Several researchers have identified a special form of address used by parents to children often called baby-talk or "motherese."[45–48] Parents, particularly mothers, vary their pitch, intonation patterns, speech, sentence length, structure, and vocabulary to meet the cognitive and linguistic needs of their children. Both Bruner[49] and Moerk[50] claim that the mother's language gradually becomes more complex through a fine-tuning process as the child's language develops. Some researchers have also suggested that children vary their speech as a function of the listener.[6,26,45,51–54] Of particular interest is the fact that children may use a more restricted linguistic code when talking to strangers, especially if the strangers belong to an "outside" group. This fact means that when some children are called to a clinician's office to take a language test, the linguistic structures used may not represent the advanced boundaries of the youngster's linguistic repertoire. As well, the linguistic code itself can serve as a contextual factor: introductory remarks; an eulogy differs from a joke; a standard phrase differs from a colloquial phrase; and a poem differs from a speech.

Age

Differences in speech relative to the age of the speaker and listener have been commonly referred to as age-grading.[2,9] Anyone knowledgeable about child language acquisition is aware of the fact that children's language patterns change with cognitive and social growth. As children change, so does their language. People accept single word utterances from a 1-year-old child, anticipate simple sentences from a 3-year-old child, and expect adult-like syntactic structures from a 6-year-old child.

During the formative years, caretakers have a primary influence on the child's language usage.[49,50] However, the research reports are somewhat conflicting and limited concerning the importance of peer and sibling influence during the language acquisition period.[50] Some investigators have implied that children whose primary language models are siblings and peers do not develop language as quickly as other children.[55–57] Other investigators have argued for the importance of siblings and peers in the acquisition of vocabulary and other language skills.[58,59]

Wolfram and Fasold have stressed the importance of peer influence on language during adolescence.[2] They report that adolescents learn a "local dialect that is primarily that of [their] immediate peers." Teenagers generally speak a special jargon that identifies them as belonging to that particular age group. Typically, peer pressure prevails over parental norms during adolescence. Some parents express concern over peer influences, even prior to adolescence. They complain that "My child picked that language up from kids at school or from the children at the playground."

Language is a fairly good indicator of a person's age. The language pattern of a senior citizen, for instance, is different from that of a younger adult, which, in turn, varies from that of a teenager, and so on. Language patterns that violate age constraints tend to draw attention to the speakers—"That boy talks like an old man" or "That lady sounds like a teenager." Similarly, peer-influenced language draws attention to itself. Finally, "baby-talk" spoken to someone other than young children or an intimate friend would be very noticeable. Obviously the effects of age-grading on language use are important.

First Language Community or Culture

Individuals whose native language or culture is different from the official language and culture of a society typically acquire the official language with distinct vestiges remaining from their first language. Such persons are considered to be bilingual in that they presumably control parts or all of two languages. (In recent years, the term "bidialectal" has been coined to refer to persons who control parts or all of two dialects.)

Bilingual persons typically code-switch from one language to another, depending upon the social situation.[10] In the process of code-switching, the first language may interfere with the production of linguistic structures in the second language. For example, a Mexican-American might mix English and Spanish words in the same sentence: "May I have coffee con leche?" Or morphologic "errors" might be made, for example, deletion of plural, possessive, and/or verb endings. Phonology and syntax in the second language may also be affected by the first language. For example, English sounds such as /v/, /tʃ/, and /I/ do not occur in Spanish, and with respect to word order, adjectives follow nouns rather than precede them. (More examples of Spanish influences on English are presented in Tables 32–2 and 32–3.)

Several factors influence a bilingual's code-switching efficiency, including those factors that have been mentioned already such as age, education, and situation. Also, the frequency with which one hears and interacts within the second language code and the nature of instruction in the second language typically determine one's skill in the use of a second language.[60] As well, if one comes to use a second language more than a first language, facility in the native language might be lost if it is not reinforced at home.

As can be surmised from this discussion of the social and cultural factors that influence language, no one variable operates independently of other variables. The language pattern used during any speech event is dependent upon the interactional influence of several factors such as age and sex of speaker and addressee, ethnic and social background, occasion, and setting. Therefore, no one sample of a person's speech taken from an isolated situation can be considered representative of the individual's complete linguistic repertoire. Although it is possible to identify one's typical speech pattern, that pattern cannot be considered the only speech variety available to that person. It is particularly important in the clinical situation that the clinician recognize the individual's potential for language variation. That which is spoken or learned in a diagnostic or therapy situation is not necessarily the same language spoken at home or in the community.

DESCRIPTIONS OF SELECTED DIALECTS OF AMERICAN ENGLISH

As discussed in the introduction to this chapter, varieties (dialects) exist within every language. These varieties are related to the social and political history of its speakers. In the United States, the varieties of English spoken are related to (1) the languages brought to the country by various cultural groups, for example, speakers of English, Polish, Chinese, Wolof; (2) the indigenous native American languages spoken in the country; (3) the cultural mix of the various communities and regions where the cultural groups settled; (4) the political and economic power wielded by the various cultures that settled in the regions; and (5) the migration patterns of the cultural groups within the country.

In many parts of the southern United States, for instance, the original languages spoken were typically some type of English brought from the southern portion of Great Britain, indigenous native American languages, and a number of languages brought from West Africa, for example, Wolof, Mende, and Fulani. The political and social power base was held by the British settlers; thus their language came to assume power in education and commerce. However, the language of these persons was likely influenced by the languages spoken by the Africans and native Americans. As a result, a particular type of English emerged in the region, which may be called Southern English. Of course, within the South, there are regional differences. Furthermore, the language of the more educated members of the European community gained prominence in schools and business.

It is a well-documented fact that the American

society, like most societies, is socially stratified. Social stratification refers to a hierarchical ordering within a society that delineates social classes. According to Trudgill, social classes are aggregates of individuals with similar social and/or economic characteristics.[31] An individual's social class influences his or her entire way of life, particularly the language that he or she uses. Therefore, one's social class has a great deal of influence on the type and style of language that one uses. This language is referred to as social-class dialect. Generally, in most large societies, particularly where there are many peoples from various cultural, national, religious, ethnic, and racial backgrounds, social dialects evolve. In the United States, several social dialects are in common use. These dialects are coexistent with identifiable speech communities.

Within each speech community, linguistic variations occur, each of which is influenced by the social variables discussed earlier—age, gender, socioeconomic class, education, and region. Again, note that these variables are *not* biologic, although certain speech communities are coexistent with biologic (racial) groups, for example, the black community in the United States. Also, the social variables do not exist as mutually exclusive entities. Instead they interact in such a way as to permit the generation of specified sets of utterances in a given speaker.

Many speakers are knowledgeable and sensitive to the linguistic expectations of many audiences; therefore they are capable of code-switching to different dialects—even dialects that are not indigenous to their speech communities—when the situation dictates. This interaction between structure and function might be an important pragmatic consideration of sociolinguistics generally and dialectology in particular. For example, a gifted black speaker might use one dialect variety when communicating with working-class blacks (vernacular black English), another when communicating with educated blacks (standard black English); and still another when communicating with working-class Southern whites (southern white nonstandard English).

Specialists in communication disorders must keep language variations in mind when defining, diagnosing, and treating communication pathologies. A failure to take such considerations into account can result in confusing dialect variation with communication pathology and in "treating" a legitimate language difference when second dialect instruction, at most, is indicated.

There are several fine descriptions available on commonly spoken dialects (American English dialects,[2,61,62] and black English[63–65]) in the United States. Although readers should familiarize themselves with available literature on language variations that exist in the communities in which they reside or have professional responsibility, some of the common dialects of English are summarized next.

Black English

Perhaps the most controversial and most written about dialect of American English is "black English," variously referred to as "black dialect," "black English vernacular," and "ebonics." Writings on this subject began to emerge in the sociolinguistic literature in the late 1960s and early 1970s in the writings of such scholars as Baratz, Stewart, Dillard, Labov, Wolfram, and Fasold. Much of the research was conducted under the sponsorship of the Center for Applied Linguistics in Washington, D.C.

Black English, as used in much of this research, may be defined as the set of phonologic, grammatic, and pragmatic rules used by working-class black people, especially for communication in informal situations within the speech community. These linguistic features, like those of any other dialect, are presumed to be explained on the basis of social and historical facts, not biologic differences. Further, speakers of black English are presumed to be knowledgeable of other dialects of English, notably standard English, as demonstrated by their comprehension of other dialects and the obvious overlaps with other dialects. With respect to this latter point, linguistic analyses of transcripts of black English speakers reveal that the overwhelming majority of the utterances of such speakers conform to the rules of general American speech.[66] Observations of this type reveal a fundamental characteristic of a dialect in any language; that is, dialects of a language are not mutually exclusive.

The major characteristics of black English, as described by the myriad of writers on the subject, have been summarized by Williams and Wolfram.[67] Their summary is presented in chart form in Table 32–1.

Careful review of the 29 linguistic rules presented in Table 32–1 shows considerable overlap between black English and several other dialects, notably Southern English and Southern white nonstandard English. Because of this overlap, the communication pathologist needs to be careful not to assume that a particular linguistic feature used by a black person is a feature of black English. Because blacks in the United States have a strong historical link with the Southern states—through the linkage with slavery—an expectation of a considerable overlap between black English and numerous dialects spoken in that region is both reasonable and obvious.

There are several theoretical positions advanced

TABLE 32–1 Major Phonologic and Grammatic Characteristics of Black English (B), Southern English (S), Southern White Nonstandard English (SWNS), and Appalachian English (A)

Features	*Descriptions*	*Examples*	*B*	*S*	*SWNS*	*A*
Consonant cluster reduction (general)	Second of two consonants in word final position belonging to the same base word deleted	tes (test)	x		x	
	Addition of past tense {-ed} morpheme produces consonant cluster, which is reduced	rub (rubbed)	x		x	
	Plural formations of reduced consonant cluster assume phonetic representations of sibilants and affricates	desses (desks); tesses (tests)	x		x	
The /θ/ phoneme	/f/ for /θ/ between vowels and in word final position	nofin (nothing); Ruf (Ruth)	x			
The /ð/ phoneme	/v/ for /ð/ between vowels and in word final position	bavin (bathing); bave (bathe)	x			
The /r/ and /l/ phonemes	Omitted after a vowel	sistuh (sister);		x		
	Absent preceding a consonant	hep (help);		x		
		"I be there at eight" (I'll be there at eight)	x	x		
The /b/, /d/, and /g/ phonemes	Devoicing at the end of a syllable	but (bud) with vowel length maintained	x			
	Deletion of /d/ when followed by a consonant	ba' boy (bad boy)				
Vowel nasalization	Final consonants dropped at the end of stressed syllables, with preceding vowel nasalized (usually not present in unstressed syllables, e.g., mailman)	mæ̃' (man); ru' (run)	x			
	No contrast between vowels /I/ and /E/ before nasals	pin (pin, pen); tin (tin, ten)		x		
Unstressed initial syllables	Unstressed initial syllables deleted	'member (remember); 'posed to (supposed to)		x	x	x
Retention of intrinsic /h/	/h/ phoneme retained in initial position before vowels	hit (it); hain't (ain't)				x
Vowel glides	Vowel glides /ay/ and /oy/ pronounced as separate vowels	sahd (side); bouh (boy)		x		
	Absence of vowel glide when followed by a voiced sound or pause	absent in side, boy; present in kite, fight		x		
	/ow/ produced as /ɚ/	holler (hollow); winder (window)				x
"ire" sequences	Reduction of glides to single vowels	tar (tire);				x
		far (fire)				x
Miscellaneous	/str/ becomes /skr/	skring (string);	x		x	
	/ask/ becomes /aks/	skreet (street)	x			
Past tense forms	Past tense morpheme {-ed} not pronounced because of consonant cluster reduction rule	finish (finished); crack (cracked)	x			
Completive aspects with "done"	"done" plus a past form denotes an action started and completed in the past	"I done tried."	x			
Remote time construction with "been"	"Been" denotes an action having taken place in the distant past	"I been had it there for about 3 years."	x			
Third person singular present tense marker	{-s} absent	"He walk."	x			
	Third person forms "has" and "does" absent	"She always do silly things."	x			
	Hypercorrect addition of {-s}	"I walks."	x			
Future	Use of "gonna"	"She gonna go."	x		x	
	Reduction of "gonna" to 'ngna, 'mana, 'mon, and 'ma	"I'ngna go."	x		x	
		"I'mana go."	x		x	
		"I'mon go."			x	
		"I'ma go."	x			
Invariant "be"	"Be" used to describe an object or event distributed intermittently in time	"While I be good."	x			

TABLE 32–1 Major Phonologic and Grammatic Characteristics of Black English (B), Southern English (S), Southern White Nonstandard English (SWNS), and Appalachian English (A) *(Continued)*

Features	*Descriptions*	*Examples*	*B*	*S*	*SWNS*	*A*
A + verb + ing	"a" prefixed to certain verbs with the (-ing) participial form	"He woke up ascreaming."		x	x	
Absence of forms of the copula (to be)	Absence of "is" in forms where it can be contracted	"He a man."	x			
	Absence of "are" where it can be contracted	"You good."	x			
Double modals	Concurrence of certain modals such as might, could, might should	"It liketa scared me to death."	x		x	x
Intensifying adverbs	Use of intensifiers, e.g., "right," "plumb," to refer to completeness	right large; plumb foolish	x		x	x
Negation	Use of ain't for have/has, am/are, didn't	"He ain't go home." (He didn't go home)	x			
Multiple negation	Placement of a negativized form of the verbal auxiliary before the main verb of a phrase having a negative marker	"Couldn't nobody do it."	x			
	Placement of a negative form the noun phrase in a previously negative statement	"Nobody didn't do it."	x			
	Negative concord across clause boundaries	"There wasn't much I couldn't do." (There wasn't much I could do)	x			
Possessive	Absence of final (-s) possessive marker	"The girl hat."	x			
Plural	Absence of suffices (-s or -es)	"She took five book."	x			
	Absence of plural suffices to reference weights and measures	Two pound; three foot			x	x
	Regular plurals with irregular nouns	Two foots; two deers	x		x	
Relative clauses	Relative pronoun deletion	"That's the dog bit me." (That's the dog that bit me)	x		x	x
Questions	Same interrogative form for direct and indirect questions	"I wonder was she walking?"	x		x	x
Existential "it"	Use of "it" for "there"	"It's a store in the corner."	x		x	
	Use of "they" for "there"	"They's copper heads in here."			x	x
Pronouns	Use of objectives as subjects	"Him ain't playing."	x			
	Nominative or objective cases of personal pronouns used for possessives	"James got him book."	x			
	Use of nonreflexive pronouns with a direct object	"I cut me a limb off a tree."		x		

After Williams R, Wolfram W. Social dialects: differences vs. disorders. Washington, DC: American Speech and Hearing Association, 1977.

to explain the features of black English described in Table 32–1. The most popular, and perhaps the most tenable, of these theories is the creolist theory.

Briefly stated, the creolist position holds that black English is an outgrowth of a complex history of language hybridization involving several African languages and four main European languages—Portuguese, Dutch, French, and English. According to Dillard, one of the foremost creolists, these hybrids developed in Africa, as well as on American plantations, in the form of pidgins and creoles. According to DeCamp, pidgin languages develop when peoples speaking different languages come in contact with each other and have a need to find a common language, usually for purposes of commerce.[68] Typically, pidginization is carried out by speakers of nondominant cultural groups who are in direct contact with a dominant group that speaks another language. At the outset of its development, a pidgin is usually informal, consisting of single-word utterances and many gestures.

Over time, usually within a century, this rather simplistic language system becomes more formal in that vocabulary items selected primarily from the dominant language are embedded in a phonologic and grammatic system derived from the nondominant language. When this process occurs, together with its acceptance as a native language, the language is referred to as creole language. Eventually, as the speakers of creole languages become more assimilated into the dominant culture, creole languages tend to converge toward the standard language through an intermediate stage referred to as decreolization.

There are some problems with the creole theory of black English. For instance, it tends to view the language as being European based rather than African based. Despite problems of this type, the creolist position of black English at least provides a historical orientation to the analysis and understanding of black American speech.

Several researchers dispute the validity of the concept of black English. Some of the objections are based on semantics. Others are based on the argument that to claim a single variety of speech accurately describes a population as culturally and geographically diverse as American blacks is untenable. Still others reject the notion of black English on the grounds that its descriptions are limited to the speech of the working classes and deny the existence of equally black but more educated forms of speech spoken by the black middle class. Finally, writers such as Kochmann,[69] Labov,[64] and Smitherman[70] would argue that the focus on the study of the structure of language, rather than on the use of language as a communicative tool, has prevented scholars from appreciating the full essence of black communicative behavior. Such oral traditions as proverbs, rhetorical style, and verbal contests are totally ignored by the formal, structural analyses of contemporary linguistics.

The current author is among a small group of scholars which have attempted to define black English in such a way as to take into account the language and communicative behaviors of the full range of black people in the United States.[71] In this model, this black English is defined as the totality of speech spoken by blacks in the United States, ranging from the standard (standard black English) to the nonstandard (nonstandard black English). The model is sufficiently broad to take the situation or context variable into account, as well as the rules pertaining to both language structure and language use in the interactive or communicative sense.

Spanish-Influenced English

It is a well-known fact that one's acquisition of a new language is influenced by the phonology and grammar of one's native language. Because of this phenomenon, it is possible to identify several sources of linguistic interference when a person of one language community attempts to acquire a second language, especially when that language contains elements that are not present, or at least not significant, in the native language.

Because of the number of persons with Hispanic background in the United States, Spanish-influenced English is perhaps the best example of language interference in this country. Since numerous persons of Hispanic ancestry populate many of the nation's urban areas, particularly in the Northeast and Southwest, communication pathologists in these areas should familiarize themselves with the phonologic and syntactic interferences of Spanish on English listed in Tables 32–2 and 32–3. A knowledge of these interferences reduces the probability of confusing language variation with pathology.

All of the interferences summarized in Tables 32–2 and 32–3 are caused by differences between Spanish and English. For example, Spanish has a five-vowel phonemic system—i, e, a, u, o—whereas most

TABLE 32–2 Example of Spanish Interference on English Phonology

Features	*Environments*	*Examples*
The /š/ phoneme	/č/ for /š/ in all positions	chair (share); watch (wash)
The /z/ phoneme	/s/ for /z/ in all positions	sip (zip); racer (razer)
The /n/ phoneme	/ŋ/ for /n/ in the word final position	siŋ (sin)
The /v/ phoneme	/b/ for /v/ in all positions	bat (vat); rabble (ravel)
The /θ/ phoneme	/t/ or /s/ for /θ/ in all positions	tin or sin (thin)
The /ð/ phoneme	/d/ for /ð/ in all positions	den (then); ladder (lather)
The /I/ phoneme	/iy/ for /I/ in all positions	cheap (chip)

TABLE 32–3 Examples of Spanish Interference on English Syntax

Features	*Environments*	*Examples*
Forms of "to be" (copula)	Absent in present progressive	"He getting hungry."
Pronouns	Absent in subjects of sentences	"Carol left yesterday. I think is coming back tomorrow."
Third person (-s)	Absent in third person verb agreements	"He talk fast."
Past (-ed)	Absent in past tense inflections	"He walk fast yesterday."
Go with to	Future markings	"He go to see the game tomorrow."
No for don't	Imperatives	"No do that."
the for possessive pronoun	With body parts and personal objects	"I hurt the finger."
Present tense markings	Progressive environments	"I think he come soon."
Locative adverbs	Place near verb	"I think he putting down the rifle."

English dialects have the same five vowels (although not exactly equivalent) with tense versus lax contrasts and three dipthongs.

Cultural Issues in Pragmatic and Discourse Behavior

In addition to differences in surface-structure features of language across cultural diversity, variations typically occur in other dimensions of language, including pragmatics and discourse.

In the area of pragmatics, a body of literature is emerging that suggests that if one disregards surface-structure features of language, universal patterns of acquisition emerge among children from culturally and linguistically diverse backgrounds. (Stockman reports a similar observation in the area of semantics, noting their studies of the action, state, location, and possession categories, which show that normally developing nonstandard speakers build their surface linguistic forms on the same kind of semantic base as standard speakers.[71a]) Specifically, Peters[71b] reports that irrespective of socioeconomic status, children use the same basic speech acts at a given age in interacting with familiar persons and with strangers.

Although researchers such as Labov and Wolfram have refuted claims made about deficiencies in the language of lower-class children, much of their refutation has been based on theoretical assumptions and structural grounds. Pragmatic data dispel some of the myths about deficiencies in the language of lower-socioeconomic children, particularly those from ethnic and racial minorities. Some differences in pragmatic behavior do exist, however, mainly with respect to the frequency of occurrence of specific categories. However, these differences are not of the magnitude that historical reports have led one to believe. Indeed, pragmatic data force one to review a number of claims pertaining to differences between lower-socioeconomic children and their middle-socioeconomic counterparts.

Discourse narratives represent a major dimension of communicative behavior that is subject to cultural differences. One of the primary ways in which humans in all societies organize and make sense of their experiences is through the use of narratives.[72,73] The ability to tell stories about "this happened and so that happened" develops early and rapidly in childhood with little or no formal training:

> In all societies, either one or several speakers can create a narrative, and members of each sociocultural group recognize and produce narratives in predictable coherent organized patterns of structure and content. In some societies, narratives appear in a wide array of genres, ranging from literary forms to accident reports. For mainstream middle-class members of most Western societies, the term narrative is often synonymous with story, but in some sociocultural groups, such fictional narratives may be relatively rare, while other narrative forms abound.[74]

However, like other aspects of language and communication universals, the manifestation of narrative behavior is culture bound. Several investigators have claimed that children from various sociocultural groups within the United States vary with respect to their communicative strategies, just as they do with respect to their surface-structure features of language.[75–78] These communicative strategies are probably correlated with different approaches to conceptualization, social interaction, and problem solving.

Tannen claims that these various communicative strategies range along a cultural continuum anchored by "oral strategies" at the one end and "literate strategies" at the other.[79,80] Oral cultures tend to have such traditions as oral narratives and poetry, whereas literate cultures have such traditions as essays and essay-influenced speech.[81–85]

Of course, all individuals have a certain degree of control over both ends of the continuum. At the same time, some cultures apparently have a greater propensity for extending farther into one end or the other than other cultural groups. For example, some authors claim that lower- and working-class children are more likely to come to school with little mastery of the literate style of communication (the school's preferred style) than their middle-class counterparts.[75,76] Apparently, the topic-centered (literate) cognitive style is greatly dependent upon the extent to which stories are read to children from books. Because of the standard English preferences for the literate style, children who do not use the literate style are typically the recipients of negative teacher attitudes, lowered teacher expectations, and fewer opportunities for oral participation in classrooms.

Michaels claims that two basic narrative styles are used by humans, topic centered (literate-strategy narratives) and topic associating (oral-strategy narratives).[76] She makes no attempt to judge which of these two styles produce better stories. However, the characteristics of the topic-centered style appear to be similar to the criteria used by teachers and other professionals in determining what is and is not "a good story."

Table 32–4 summarizes the major characteristics of topic-centered (literate-strategy) narratives and topic-associating (oral-strategy) narratives as described by Michaels. In general, the characteristics of topic-centered narratives are (1) a linear presentation of a tightly structured discourse on a single topic or series of closely related topics with no major shifts in perspective; (2) a temporal orientation or thematic focus; (3) a high degree of thematic coherence and a clear thematic progression that begins with temporal grounding, a statement of focus, introduction of key agents, and some indication of spatial grounding; and (4) an orientation, which is followed by elaboration on the topic, and finishes with a "punch-line" resolution.

The stories presume little shared knowledge between speakers and listeners, thus requiring precise detail. The topic-centered style appears to be the one most commonly used by Anglo middle-class children. For instance, Michaels reports that 96 percent of a group of middle-class white children she observed used topic-centered stories.[76] By contrast, only 34 percent of her working-class black children used topic-centered stories. No definitive data are available on the frequency of occurrence of topic-centered stories by middle-class black children or by middle-class children from other ethnic groups. However, what is known is that the topic-centered style is not only the preferred style in the classroom, but also the expected style. An example of a topic-centered story is presented in Table 32–5.

TABLE 32–4 Two Types of Narrative Strategies

Literate-Strategy Narratives TOPIC CENTERED	*Oral-Strategy Narratives* TOPIC ASSOCIATING
Tightly structured discourse on single topic or series of closely related topics Lexically explicit referential, temporal, and spatial relationships No major shifts in perspective, temporal orientation, or thematic progression High degree of thematic coherence and a clear thematic progression Begin with temporal grounding, a statement of focus, introducing key agents, and some indication of spatial grounding Orientation is followed by elaboration on the topic The child marks syntactically complete, independent clauses with special sharing time intonation (high rising tone with vowel elongation) that means "more to come" and demarcates the clause as an information unit Finishes with a punch-line sort of resolution, signaled by a markedly lower pitch or falling tone Stories tend to be short and concise	A series of associated segments that may seem anecdotal in character, linked implicitly to a particular topical event or theme, but with no explicit statement of an overall theme or point Although these stories start with time, person, and place, temporal orientation, location, and focus often shift across segments—these shifts are marked by shifts in pitch contours and tempo, often accompanied by a formulaic time marker Relationship between parts of the narrative have to be inferred by the listener Temporal indicators (yesterday, last night, tomorrow) occur more than once The special sharing time intonation is used not to mark continuity, but to highlight discontinuity, marking the separation of narrative segments and shifts in temporal orientation, location, or focus The stories may give the impression to those who have no control over the style of having no beginning, no middle, no end—thus no point Tend to be longer and seem to be not concise

From Michaels S. "Sharing time": Children's narrative styles and differential access to literacy. Lang Soc 1981; 10:423–442.

TABLE 32–5 An Example of a Topic-Centered Story

Um . . . tomorrow/my sister's gonna have her birthday party: /

it's gonna be at Arlington Boys' Club/

'cuz they have a swimming poo:l/

and we're gonna rent it/
'n . . . so we can use it/

and . . and . . . there's gonna be a lot of . . . people/
and so my sister/

we're gonna have . . b-be able to use the game roo:m/
and . . my mom said . . . she left all her bathing suits/

down the Cape/so she's gonna have to go buy one/
and my mom said/um . . . um . . it's a heating swimming pool
and she'll be in there a:ll/ . . a:ll da:y//

Abbreviations: / = non-final phrase boundary ("more to come");
// = final phrase group;
. . = short pause;
. . . = measurable pause;
: = vowel elongation;
↗ = formulaic intonation pattern to mark "sharing time" talk, i.e., high rising tone with vowel elongation, sharp pitch modulation, and slow rhythmic tempo. A "calling" contour as in "dinner time." Accounts for 60% of all tonal contours in White children's narratives, and 37% of tonal contours in Black children's narratives.

After Michaels S. Influences on children's narratives. Newsletter Lab Comp Hum Cog 1983; 5(2):30.

In contrast, topic-associating stories tend to be a series of associated segments that are linked implicitly to a topic, event, or theme, but with no explicit theme or point. They typically start with a set of background statements, then shift across segments, with the shifts being marked by pitch and tempo indicators. The various segments are typically implicitly linked to a topical event or theme, even though temporal orientation, location, and focus of segments often shift from one segment to the other. The linkage among the various segments are left for listener inference inasmuch as there is a presumed shared knowledge between speakers and listeners. Because of this latter presumption, these stories tend to contain less detail than topic-centered narratives. At the same time, their focus on a number of themes result in longer presentations.

Topic-associating stories are throught to be used more often by working-class children, especially working-class black children. They seem to be perfectly acceptable, understandable, and frequently used by persons who come from oral cultures, but appear to have no point to persons from those cultures that seem to prefer and use a more topic-centered orientation to narratives. An example of a topic-associating story is presented in Table 32–6.

Michael reports further that white listeners tend to describe topic-associating stories as "a terrible story"; "incoherent"; "hard to follow" or "mixed-up"; and "doesn't connect." Moreover, they tend to pick topic-associating stories as typical of students who would have less academic success than children who produced topic-centered stories. Some refer to predicted reading problems for topic-associating children, as well as "language problems," "family problems," and "emotional problems."

By contrast, black listeners tend to find topic-associating stories easy to understand, well-formed, interesting, and containing "lots of detail and description." Many black informants in the Michael study labelled these stories as the best they heard. All commented on the nonlinear quality of the stories, but none appeared to reject the strategy. Moreover, black listeners were more likely to give positive ratings to both topic-associating and topic-centered stories than white listeners.

Although the current research on cultural dimensions of discourse generally, and narratives in particular, are preliminary at best, there seems to be ample reason to claim that these topics are essential to a comprehensive understanding of normal and disordered communication.

TABLE 32–6 An Example of a Topic Associating Story

on George Washington's birthday/

I'm goin'/ice:/ my gran:dmother/

we never um/haven't seen her since a long ti:me/

and/ . . . and she lives right (n) nea:r u:s/
and/ . . . she:/ and she's gonna/
I'm gonna spend the night over her house/

and/ . . . every weekend/ she comes to take me/

like on Saturdays and Sundays/awa:y/from ho:me
and I spend the night over her house/

and one day I spoi:led her di:nner/

. . . um and we was having um/we was/um
she paid ten dollars/
and I got eggs/ . . . and stuff/
and I didn't even eat anything//

Abbreviations: / = non-final phrase boundary ("more to come")
// = final phrase group
. . = short pause
. . . = measurable pause
: = vowel elongation;
↗ = formulaic intonation pattern to mark "sharing time" talk, i.e., high rising tone with vowel elongation, sharp pitch modulation, and slow rhythmic tempo. A "calling" contour as in "dinner time." Accounts for 60% of all tonal contours in White children's narratives, and 37% of tonal contours in Black children's narratives.

After Michaels S. Influences on children's narratives. Q Newsletter Lab Comp Hum Cog 1983; 5(2):30.

APPLICATION OF SOCIOLINGUISTIC DATA AND THEORY TO THE PRACTICE OF SPEECH-LANGUAGE PATHOLOGY

Sociolinguistic data and theory may be used by the speech-language pathologist in a number of ways.

Attitudes. Perhaps the most important implication of recent sociolinguistic data and theory has to do with attitudes toward language variation. Specifically, a careful analysis of the literature should help the speech-language pathologist to view language variety as a normal phenomenon and not necessarily as an indicator of communication pathology. This outlook is viewed as a critical first step for developing speech and hearing programs compatible with the types of language likely to be heard in various communities in the United States.

Definitions. The next important implication of recent sociolinguistic research relates to the definitions of pathologic speech. Traditional definitions of speech disorders have typically categorized speech as being pathologic if it deviates sufficiently from a rather rigid, monocultural, middle-class set of linguistic norms. Contemporary sociolinguistics provides a theoretical orientation and data base for defining pathology from the perspective of language norms generated by various speech communities. Where existing data are inadequate to permit a cultural orientation to defining and diagnosing communication pathology, clinicians and scholars can utilize elicitation and analytic procedures of the type described by the various researchers discussed in this chapter.

Tests. Communication pathologists rely heavily on standardized tests to determine the presence or absence of communication disorders. Most tests in current use in speech-language pathology are based on linguistic presuppositions consistent with Northern Midland standard English. For this reason, many of these tests, when administered and scored according to prescribed norms, yield data that unfairly penalize speakers of nonmainstream dialects and give the inaccurate impression of a communication disorder when, in fact, no disorder exists.

For example, a test that views the pronunciation of the word "toothbrush" as "toofbrush" as indicative of an articulation error, as opposed to a dialect difference, causes the administrator to make a faulty speech judgement. Similarly, the test that penalizes a subject for saying "he from Chicago" (as opposed to "he's from Chicago") because it is not a grammatic sentence fails to consider the fact that dialects of English may have different rules for constructing sentences of similar underlying meaning. Indeed, such tests may cause the administrator to inaccurately conclude that a subject is 1 to 2 years retarded in language acquisition (and possibly mentally retarded) when, in fact, the subject may be ahead of the linguistic expectations for his or her speech community.

I am among those authors who have discussed, in some detail, sociolinguistic dimensions in standardized tests.[71] Drawing upon my work with researchers in several related disciplines, I list seven distinct sources of possible bias in tests:

1. Social situational bias—violation of a situation or context rule for the test taker.
2. Value bias—mismatch between values presumed in test items and the values of the test taker.
3. Phonologic bias—mismatch between phonologic rules presumed in a test item and the phonologic rules of the test taker.
4. Grammatic bias—mismatch between grammatic rules presumed in a test item and the grammatic rules of the test taker.
5. Vocabulary bias—mismatch of lexical items and their use between test maker and test taker (may include underlying cognitive mismatches).
6. Pragmatic bias—mismatch between rules of communicative interaction of the test maker and test taker.
7. Directions or format bias—confusions or misunderstandings created for test taker by the use of unfamiliar or ambiguous directions and/or test formats.

Taylor, Payne, and Anderson[86a] state that prior to the collection of assessment data from any individual, the assessor must engage in preassessment, assessment, and a number of assessment activities that involve cultural considerations.

At the preassessment level, these activities include:

1. Familiarization with cultural, social, and cognitive norms of the individual's community.
2. Familiarization with linguistic and communicative norms of the individual's speech community.
3. The selection of appropriate unbiased standardized and criterion-referenced tests.
4. Preparation of culturally appropriate natural elicitation procedures.

At the assessment level, culturally valid procedures must be employed to obtain a sample of the client's communicative behavior. Three essential elements of this process involve:

1. The administration of unbiased evaluation procedures.
2. The collection of idiosyncratic sociocultural and communicative behaviors.
3. The elicitation and observation of spontaneous communicative behavior in a variety of settings.

With respect to culturally valid tests, Vaughn-Cooke[86b] suggests that the following six basic principles should be employed in the selection of appropriate instruments for persons from a given population:

1. The test should be based on valid assumptions about language.
2. The test should be able to account for language variation.
3. The test should be based on a developmental model.
4. The results of the test should provide principled guidelines for language intervention.
5. The test should be able to provide an adequate description of some aspect of the child's knowledge of language.
6. The test should reflect the latest developments in linguistic theory.

Following the collection of data from formal tests and natural language samples, the speech-language pathologist must then engage in several post-assessment, culturally based activities. They are (1) scoring and error analysis of data from structured and spontaneous elicitations, (2) consideration of peer and/or community definitions of communication pathology, and (3) peer and/or community corroboration of test and natural data.

Teaching Standard English as a Second Dialect

Although some would reject the notion that speech-language pathologists should be involved in teaching standard English as a second dialect under any circumstance, the American Speech-Language-Hearing Association permits such involvement if the clinician is knowledgeable about (1) the learner's first dialect as a rule-governed linguistic system, (2) contrastive analyses procedures, and (3) the impact of language attitudes on language behavior.

The research literature has provided strong support to the notion that negative language attitudes and inadequate knowledge of linguistic systems of various learners can result in low educational achievement and negative self-concepts. This literature also formed the basis of several court cases, legislative initiatives, and policy statements from educational agencies. One of the most celebrated of these cases involved a suit filed against the Ann Arbor Michigan School Board by a group of nine parents of children whose indigenous dialect was "black English vernacular." In this case, the judge specifically cited teacher ignorance of issues related to language variation and negative teacher attitudes.

The most impressive evidence that has been cited to account for the current failures with respect to teaching standard English to nonstandard speakers revolves around the philosophy, assumptions, and traditional classroom methodologies as employed in language arts education. This evidence suggests that traditional methodologies have failed primarily because they have been prescriptive and corrective and that they have focused excessively on language structure rather than on communicative competence. Moreover, the instructional methodologies have not been culturally based, and they have made little use of indigenous, nonstandard dialects, probably because of linguistic naiveté or negative attitudes toward language variation.

I have devised an instructional strategy for teaching standard English that takes into account the learner's indigenous language system.[87] My model is based on modern sociolinguistic theory and established principles of second language teaching. It requires

1. Considerations of the effect of language attitudes on language teaching and learning.
2. The principles of linguistic contrastive analysis.
3. Extensive practice of specific structures of standard English in a variety of listening and production activities.

Central to this model is the notion that standard English instruction does not require the denigration or elimination of the learner's indigenous language system. It recognizes that the selection of language codes is situationally based, and, for this reason, students need to retain their home dialect for use in the situations where its use is appropriate. Several basic tenets underpin a culturally based approach to teaching standard English as a second dialect.[87]

A Communicative Rather than Structural Focus. In addition to a knowledge of structural linguistic rules, effective communication within a given dialect requires knowledge for engaging in conversations (turn taking, interruptions); producing monologues and dialogues; articulating such intentions as informing, stating feelings, ritualizing; and producing nonverbal rules to accompany conversation.

Concern for Structure, Situation, and Thought. Structure refers to the various forms of usage appropriate for different communicative acts, phonetic and grammatic differences, differences between speaking and writing, and the linguistic characteristics of standard English. Standard English as a second dialect instruction requires the combination of direct instruction with an abundance of opportunities to hear and practice the various patterns of the targeted language in such activities as choral reading, conversations and discussions with standard English speakers, and Readers' Theater and dramatic activities.

Situation refers to the setting, the audience, and the purpose associated with a communication act. The learner must be able to determine the type of communication that would be most appropriate to a given situation. For example, standard English may be more appropriate for formal situations, whereas nonstandard English may be more appropriate in more informal situations.

Thought relates to the content of a given communication act. Thought typically occurs in the person's primary language or dialect (i.e., the one with which he or she comes to school). Cummins suggests that children who acquire a second language after a first language is reasonably well established must be given every opportunity for his or her cognitive skills to continue development in the first language.[88] In time, a second language system can be taught as an overlay to the cognitive system established in the first language. To do otherwise, Cummins adds, is to thwart both the cognitive and linguistic development in the first language, thereby eroding the foundations needed for further language and academic learning.

A Linkage to "Products." Language and communication do not exist in a vacuum. Therefore, standard English as a second dialect (SESD) programs must link instruction to short- and long-range "products," that is to tangible purposes such as interviews, plays, dialogues during field trips, puppet shows, interpretative reading, or brainstorming for a writing activity.

A Linkage to a Developmental Teaching Model. The acquisition of a second dialect proceeds, through an orderly process, from the introduction of a particular aspect of language through to its mastery. This developmental model schematizes the steps through which the learner must proceed when learning a new linguistic system, while preserving his or her indigenous system for use in appropriate situations and appropriate tasks (Figure 32–3). The model has the following eight steps or stages.

Positive Attitude Toward One's Own Language. The development of positive attitudes and self-evaluations of the learner's indigenous language system is fostered through lessons on such topics as the historical development of various dialects and on language diversity within the United States.

Awareness of Language Varieties. Exposure to a variety of forms of languages and dialects spoken in the United States in stories, poems, records, tapes, or video recordings of various speakers in a variety of situations is encouraged. At this stage, the specific elements of likenesses and differences are not emphasized.

Recognizing, Labeling, and Contrasting Dialects. The recognition of specific differences in fea-

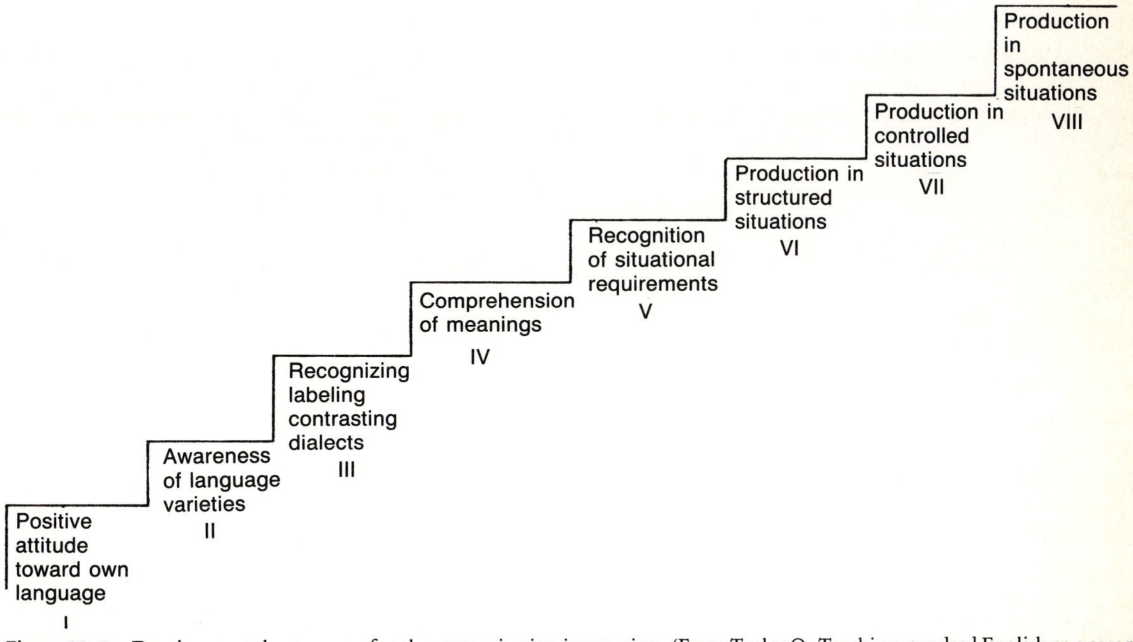

Figure 32–3 Developmental sequence of oral communication instruction. (From Taylor O. Teaching standard English as a second dialect. In: Taylor O, ed. Treatment of communication disorders in culturally and linguistically diverse populations. San Diego: College-Hill Press, 1986:153.)

tures of various languages and dialects is developed, and associations of specific features with each linguistic system are made.

Comprehension of Meanings. The recognition of differences in meanings (and intentions) associated with translation from one language or dialect to another is developed.

Recognition of Situational Language Requirements. The selection process for specific language, dialect, and communicative requirements of various situations and audiences is taught.

Production in Structured Situations. Practice in production of successive approximations of a targeted dialect is provided.

Production in Controlled Situations. Practice in production of a targeted dialect without a model, for example, role-playing or retelling a story, is provided.

Production in Spontaneous Situations. Production of appropriate language and communicative behavior in real life situations, in which spontaneous productions are required, is taught.

SUMMARY

In this chapter, some basic concepts pertaining to language and culture have been explored, some of the common varieties of American English described and sociolinguistic data and theory linked to the field of communication disorders. Although research in these areas is realtively new and incomplete, it has already begun to change many traditional approaches to defining, diagnosing, and managing communication disorders. Finally, an approach is presented to teach standard English as a second dialect.

REFERENCES

1. Van Riper C. Speech corrections. Englewood Cliffs, NJ: Prentice-Hall, 1978.
2. Wolfram W, Fasold RW. The study of social dialects in American English. Englewood Cliffs, NJ: Prentice-Hall, 1974.
3. Gumperz JJ. The speech community. In: Giglioli PP, ed. Language and social context. Baltimore: Penguin Books, 1972.

3a. Saville-Troike M. Anthropological considerations in the study of communication. In: Taylor, ed. Nature of communicative disorders in linguistically and culturally diverse populations. San Diego: College-Hill Press, 1986:47.

4. Hymes D. Foundations of sociolinguistics: an ethnographic approach. Philadelphia: University of Pennsylvania Press, 1974.

4a. Hymes D. On communicative competence. Paper presented at the Research Planning Conference on language development among disadvantaged children. Yeshiva University, 1966.

5. Edwards AD. Language in culture and class. London: Heinemann Educational Books, 1976.
6. Gleason JB. Code switching in children's language. In: Moore TE, ed. Cognitive development and the acquisition of language. New York: Academic Press, 1973.
7. McCormack WC, Wurm SA, eds. Language and man: anthropological issues. The Hague: Mouton 1976.
8. Haugen E. Dialect, nation, language. In: Pride JB, Holmes J, eds. Sociolinguistics. Baltimore: Penguin Books, 1972.
9. Wardhaugh R. The contexts of language. Rowley, MA: Newbury House Publishers, 1976.
10. Bell RT. Sociolinguistics: goals, approaches and problems. London: BT Batsford, 1976.

10a. Labov, W. Sociolinguistic patterns. Philadelphia: University of Pennsylvania Press, 1972.

11. Penalosa F. Introduction to the sociology of language. Rowley, MA: Newbury House Publishers, 1981.
12. Rosten L. The joys of yiddish. New York: McGraw-Hill, 1968.
13. Pearce-Hopper L, McMahon J. A study of language deficits in reservation and urban Indian children groups. Paper presented at the Annual Convention of the American Speech-Language-Hearing Association, Atlanta, GA, Nov. 1979.
14. Castaneda A, James RL, Robbins W. The educational needs of minority groups. Lincoln: Professional Educators Publications, 1974.
15. Labov W. The social stratification of English in New York City. Washington, DC: Center for Applied Linguistics, 1966.
16. Brandes PD, Brewer J. Dialect clash in America: issues and answers. Metuchen, NJ: Scarecrow Press, 1977.
17. Hollingshead AB. Two factor index of social position. New Haven: Yale University Press, 1965.
18. Lawton D. Social class, language and education. London: Routledge & Kegan Paul, 1968.
19. Williams F, ed. Language and poverty. Chicago: Markham, 1970.
20. Anastasiow NJ, Hanes ML. Language patterns of poverty children. Springfield, IL: Charles C Thomas, 1976.
21. Bee HL, Van Egeren LF, Strissguth AP, Nyman BA, Leckie MS. Social class differences in maternal teaching strategies and speech patterns. Dev Psychol 1969; 1:726.
22. Brandis W, Henderson D. Social class, language and communication. Beverly Hills: Sage Publications, 1970.
23. Snow C, Arlman-Rupp A, Hassing Y, Jobse J, Jootsen J, Vorster J. Mother's speech in three social classes. J Psycholinguist Res 1976; 5:1–20.
24. Rosch E. Style variables in referential language: a study of social class difference and its effect on dyadic communication. In: Freedle RO, ed. Discourse processes: advances in research and theory. Vol. I. Norwood, NJ: Ablex, 1977:141.
25. Adlam DS. Code in context. London: Routledge & Kegan Paul (with the assistance of Geoffrey Turner and Lesley Lineker), 1977.
26. Gay J, Tweney RD. Comprehension and production of standard and black English by lower-class black children. Dev Psychol 1976; 12:262–268.
27. Meissner JA, Apthrop H. Nonegocentrism and communication mode switching in black preschool children. Dev Psychol 1976; 12:245–249.
28. Van der Geest T, Gerstel R, Appel R, Tervoort B. The child's communicative competence. The Hague: Mouton, 1976.
29. Bernstein B. Socialization: with some reference to educability. In: Bernstein B, ed. Class, codes and control: theoretical studies towards a sociology of language. London: Routledge & Kegan Paul, 1971:143.
30. Nist J. A structural history of English. New York: St. Martin's Press, 1966.

31. Trudgill P. Sociolinguistics: an introduction. New York: Penguin Books, 1974.
32. Barron NM. Grammatical case and sex role: language differences in interaction. Doctoral dissertation. University of Missouri Press, 1970.
33. Cherry L. The preschool teacher-child dyad: sex differences in verbal interaction. Child Dev 1975; 46:532–535.
34. Edelsky C. The acquisition of communicative competence: recognition of linguistic correlates of sex roles. Merrill-Palmer Q Behav Dev 1976; 22:47–59.
35. Key MR. Linguistic behavior of male and female. Linguistics 1972; 88:15–31.
36. Koenigsknecht RA, Friedman P. Syntax development in boys and girls. Child Dev 1976; 47:1109–1115.
37. Lakoff R. Language and woman's place. Lang Soc 1972; 2:45–79.
38. McCarthy D. Some possible explanations of sex differences in language development and disorders. J Psychol 1953; 35:155–160.
39. Miller C, Swift K. One small step for genkind. In: DeVito J, ed. Language: concepts and processes. Englewood Cliffs, NJ: Prentice-Hall, 1973:171. (Reprinted from the New York Times Magazine, April 16, 1972.)
40. Thorne B, Henley N. Language and sex: difference and dominance. Rowley, MA: Newbury House Publishers, 1975.
41. Van Duyne HJ, Scanlan D. Gender difference in the development of the regulatory function of language. J Genet Psychol 1976; 128:17–26.
42. Hymes D. Models of the interaction of language and social life. In: Gumperz JJ, Hymes D, eds. Directions in sociolinguistics: the ethnography of communication. New York: Holt, Rinehart & Winston, 1972:35.
43. Fielding G, Fraser C. Language and interpersonal relations. In: Markova I, ed. The social context of language. New York: John Wiley & Sons, 1978:217.
44. Ochs E, Schieffelin BB, eds. Developmental pragmatics. New York: Academic Press, 1979.
45. Farwell CB. The language spoken to children. In: Papers and reports on child language development, No. 5. Stanford University, Committee on Linguistics, April 1973:31–62.
46. Ferguson C. Baby talk in six languages. Am Anthropol 1964; 66:103–114.
47. Ferguson C. Baby talk as a simplified register. In: Papers and reports on child language development. No. 9. Stanford University, Committee on Linguistics, April, 1975.
48. Snow C. Mother's speech to children learning language. Child Dev 1972; 43:549–565.
49. Bruner J. Learning the mother tongue. Hum Nature 1978; (Sept):42–49.
50. Moerk EL. Semantic and pragmatic aspects of early language development. Baltimore: University Park Press, 1977.
51. Ervin-Tripp S. Wait for me, roller skate! In: Ervin-Tripp S, Mitchell-Kernan C, eds. Child discourse. New York: Academic Press, 1977:165.
52. Mitchell-Kernan C, Kernan KT. Pragmatics of directive choice among children. In: Ervin-Tripp S, Mitchell-Kernan C, eds. Child discourse. New York: Academic Press, 1977:189–208.
53. Shatz M, Gelman R. The development of communication skills: modification in the speech of young children as a function of the listener. Monogr Soc Res Child Dev 1973; 38.
54. Shatz M, Gelman R. Appropriate speech adjustments: the operation of conversational constraints on talk to two-year-olds. In: Lewis M, Rosenblum L, eds. Interaction, conversation, and the development of language. New York: John Wiley & Sons, 1977.
55. Davis EA. The developments of linguistic skill in twins, singletons with siblings and only children from age 5 to 10 years. Institute of Child Welfare. Monograph Series No. 14, 1937.
56. Luria AR, Yudovich FI. Speech and the development of mental processes in the child. London: Staples Press, 1959.
57. Sutton-Smith B, Rosenberg BG. The sibling. New York: Holt, Rinehart & Winston, 1970.
58. Bar-Adon A. Primary syntatic structures in Hebrew child language. In: Bar-Adon A, Leopold WF, eds. Child language: a book of readings. Englewood Cliffs, NJ: Prentice-Hall, 1971.
59. Rubin KH. Social interaction and communicative egocentrism in preschoolers. J Genet Psychol 1976; 129:121–124.
60. Hatch ER. Second language learning. In: Bilingual Education: Current Perspectives. Arlington: Center for Applied Linguistics, 1977:60.
61. Allen HB, Underwood GN. Readings in American dialectology. New York: Appleton, 1971.
62. Bailey RW, Robinson JL. Varieties of present-day English. New York: Macmillan, 1973.
63. Dillard J. Black English. New York: Random House, 1972.
64. Labov W. Language in the inner city: studies in black English vernacular. Philadelphia: University of Pennsylvania Press, 1972.
65. Burling R. English in black and white. New York: Holt, Rinehart & Winston, 1973.
66. Lomon B. Conversations in a Negro American dialect. Washington, DC: Center for Applied Linguistics, 1967.
67. Williams R, Wolfram W. Social Dialects: Differences vs. disorders. Washington, DC: American Speech and Hearing Association, 1977.
68. DeCamp D. The study of pidgin and creole languages. In: Hymes D, ed. Pidgnization and creolization of languages. London: Cambridge University Press, 1971:13.
69. Kochmann T. Rappin' and stylin' out in the black community. Champaign, IL: University of Illinois Press, 1971.
70. Smitherman G. Talkin and testifyin: the language of black America. Detroit: Wayne State University Press, 1986.
71. Taylor OL. Black English and what to do about it: some black community perspectives. In: Williams RL, ed. Ebonics: the true language of black folks. St. Louis: Institute of Black Studies, 1979.
71a. Stockman I. Language acquisition: the black child. In: Taylor O, ed. Nature of communication disorders in culturally and linguistically diverse populations. San Diego: College-Hill Press, 1986:117.
71b. Peters C. A pragmatic investigation of the speech of selected black children. Doctoral Dissertation. Howard University, 1983.
72. Hymes D. Narrative form as a "grammar" of experience: native Americans and a glimpse of English. J Educ 1982; 164:121–142.
73. White H. The value of narrativity in the representation of reality. J Crit Inquiry 1980; 7:5–27.
74. Heath SB. Cross-cultural aspects of narratives. Top Lang Disord 1986.
75. Heath SB. What no bedtime story means: narrative skills at home and school. Lang Soc II 1982; 49–76.
76. Michaels S. 'Sharing time': children's narrative styles and differential access to literacy. Lang Soc 1981; 10:423–442.
77. Michaels S, Collins J. Oral discourse styles: classroom interaction and the acquisition of literacy. In: Tannen D, ed. Coherence in spoken and written discourse. Norwood, NJ: Ablex, 1984:219.
78. Reed CE. Teaching teachers about teaching writing to students from varied linguistics, social and cultural groups. In: Whiteman MF, ed. Writing: the nature, development and teaching of written communication. Hillsdale, NJ: Lawrence Erlbaum, 1981.
79. Tannen D. Oral and literate strategies in spoken and writ-

ten narratives. Language 1982: 58(1):1–21.

80. Tannen D. Implications of the oral/literate continuum for cross-cultural communication. In: Alatis J, ed. Current issues in bilingualism: Georgetown University roundtable on languages and linguistics, 1980. Washington, DC: Georgetown University Press, 1981.
81. Hymes D. "In vain I tried to tell you": essays in native American ethnopoetics. Philadelphia: University of Pennsylvania Press, 1981.
82. Bennett AT. Discourses of power, the dialects of understanding the power of literacy. J Educ 1982; 165:53–74.
83. Scollon R, Scollon S. Narrative, literacy, and face in interethnic communication. Norwood, NJ: Ablex, 1981.
84. Scollon R, Scollon S. The literate two-year old: the fictionalization of self. Working papers in sociolinguistics. Austin, TX: Southwest Regional Laboratory, 1979.
85. Sherzer J. Kuna ways of speaking: an ethnographic perspective. Austin, TX: University of Texas Press, 1983.
86. Michaels S. Influences on children's narratives. Newsletter Lab Comp Hum Cog 1983; 5(2):30–34.

86a. Taylor O, Payne K, Anderson N. Distinguishing between communication disorders and communication differences. Semin Speech Lang 1987; 8(4):415–428.

86b. Vaughn-Cooke B. Improving language assessment in minority children. Asha 1983; 25(9):29–34.

87. Taylor O. Nature of communication disorders in culturally and linguistically diverse populations. San Diego: College-Hill Press, 1986.
88. Cummins J. Bilingualism and special education: issues in assessment and pedagogy. San Diego: College-Hill Press, 1984.

33 Effective Communication for the Severely Handicapped Child

David E. Yoder, Ph.D.
Francisco Villarruel, M.S.

Over the years, society has gone through a major change in attitudes and acceptance of severely handicapped children and youth. With each new phase, however, one can identify additional barriers that must be overcome to provide adequate assessment and intervention services.

The increase in services for severely handicapped children and youth has been based upon four major assumptions. First, the recognition that severely handicapped children and youth can improve their level of functioning if they are given the proper opportunity, and in some cases, the proper technology. The philosophical basis of this first assumption is derived, in part, from the second, which is an increase in services for severely handicapped children and youth: that is, an increased acceptance and development of the perspective of individualization. Although "diagnostic" labels are still popular, professionals have come to view severely handicapped children and youth as being unique persons, with unique problems, who demonstrate unique challenges for educational, vocational, and rehabilitation professionals.

Third, services are on the increase because of the increase in and provision of educational, medical, rehabilitative, vocational, and legal rights for severely handicapped individuals. The development of many of these services can be attributed to the legal mandates (e.g., Public Law (PL) 94–142, the Rehabilitation Act of 1973), which specifically address the needs of the severely handicapped. These mandates resulted in an increase in funded research, funds for the development of innovative curricula, and the establishment of educational and vocational centers for the severely handicapped.

Finally, changes in our attitudes toward the severely handicapped may be related to an increased emphasis on the prevention of developmental disabilities and secondary handicaps. Social service agencies have provided invaluable services in an effort to educate "high-risk mothers" about proper nutrition and medical care to prevent birth complications such as prematurity. Screening programs have also been developed which can detect causative medical disorders such as phenylketonuria (PKU). For children born with handicaps, research and development of early intervention programs, which focus upon the provision of infant stimulation and parent education, are also available.

This chapter attempts to outline some major barriers and solutions to providing communication competencies for severely handicapped children and youth. Two major sources (or barriers) are considered (Fig. 33–1), which function to interfere with the acquisition and development of functional communicative competence for severely handicapped children and youth: intrapersonal and interpersonal barriers. The perspective maintained is that the change agents can serve as the major force in the remediation of these barriers. This perspective is based upon two assumptions. First, that communication interactions are a multidimensional, multichannel phenomena in which the interactants' behaviors are coordinated across temporal dimensions, and influenced by the interactants themselves.[1] Second, that changes in one part of the system or in the barriers which are encountered by the severely handicapped child or youth may change other parts, which in turn could affect the total system.[2]

DEFINING THE SEVERELY HANDICAPPED: A PROBLEM WITH CURRENT TERMINOLOGY

What constitutes a condition of a person that can be described as severely handicapped? This is a question that researchers, teachers, and clinicians have attempted to resolve for many years.[3–7] Unfortunately, there has been no resolution to this question. The term "handicapped" is used to describe children who deviate from the average or norm in (1) mental/cognitive characteristics, (2) sensory abilities, (3) neuromotor or physical characteristics, (4) social behavior, (5) communication abilities, or (6) multiple combinations of the differences listed above.

Perhaps the most widely accepted definition of severely handicapped was developed by the Bureau for Education of the Handicapped (BEH). According to this definition:

> Severely handicapped children are those who because of the intensity of their physical, mental, or emotional problems, need educational, social psychological and medical services beyond those which are traditionally offered by regular and special education programs, in order to maximize participation in society and self-fulfillment. Such severely handicapped children may possess severe language or perceptual-cognitive deprivations and evidence a number of abnormal behaviors including failure to attend to even the most pronounced stimuli, self-mutilation, manifestations of durable and intense temper tantrums, and the absence of even the most rudimentary forms of verbal control. They may also have extremely fragile physiological conditions (Sec 121.2).[8]

Dollar and Brooks suggest that this definition includes, but is not limited to, children classified as deaf-blind, multiply handicapped, autistic, cerebral palsied, neurologically impaired, brain-damaged, schizophrenic, and mentally retarded.[4]

Samples of other definitions for severely handicapped are listed in Table 33–1. Developed for differing classification and consequent treatment and funding purposes, these definitions differ from one another in focus. For example, the definition as proposed by the Bureau of Education for the Handicapped is based upon an exclusion principle, and is oriented toward educational placement of severely handicapped children and youth rather than describing what is meant by the term severely handicapped. Conversely, the definition of the Rehabilitation Act of 1973 views severely handicapped persons in terms of their employment potential. From yet another perspective, Sontag, Smith and Sailor describe severely handicapped children from the perspective of how various deficits may impair functional skills.[7]

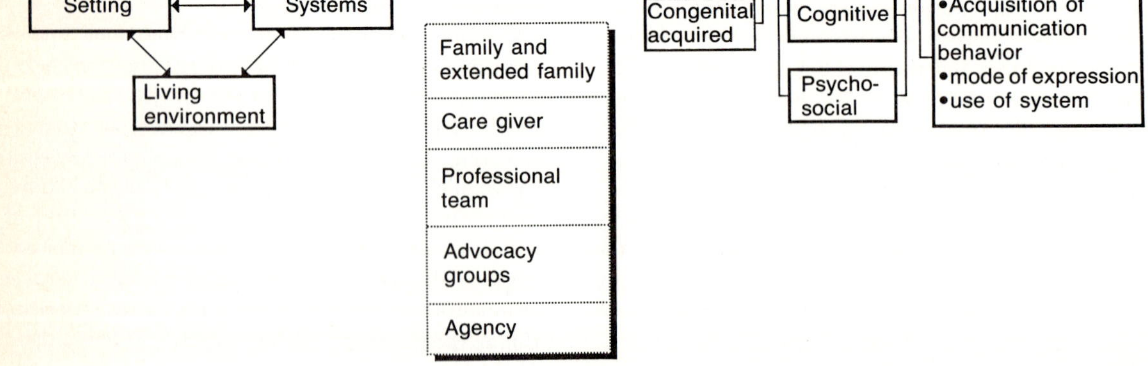

Figure 33–1 Service delivery barriers affecting the development of functional communicative competence.

TABLE 33–1 Definitions of Severely Handicapped

Organization	*Definition*
PL 94–142[8] US	Multihandicapped means concomitant impairments (such as mentally retarded-blind, mentally retarded-orthopedically impaired, etc, the combination of which causes such severe educational problems that they cannot be accommodated in special education programs solely for one of the impairments. The term does not include deaf-blind children
Rehabilitative Services Administration (1973)	. . . [The severe disability] that physical or mental impairment which seriously limits the functional capabilities (mobility, communication, self-care, self-direction, work tolerance, work skills) of a handicapped individual to the extent that the person is unable, to a substantial degree, to cope with the physical, or mental demands of gainful employment and whose rehabilitation normally requires multiple services (restorative, compensatory training, selective placement) over an extended period of time
Southeastern Regional Coalition (SERC) (1979)[6]	The severely handicapped individual is defined for educational purposes as (1) having serious primary disabilities that are cognitive (e.g., −4 standard deviations below a normal IQ on a standardized test of intelligence such as the Revised Stanford-Binet Test of Intelligence) and/or behavioral (e.g., Autistic or childhood schizophrenic), (2) having the high probability of additional physical and/or sensory handicaps, and (3) requiring significantly more resources than are provided for the mild and moderately handicapped in special education programs (p 39)
Wisconsin Administrative Code	Severe mental retardation is determined by an individual with scores −4 to −5 standard deviations below the mean on a measured intelligence scale A multiple handicapped child is one who has 2 or more handicapping conditions leading to an EEN* which may require programming considerations and are determined by an M-team composed of specialists trained, certified and experienced in the teaching of children with the EEN.*
Sontag, Smith, and Sailor[7]	. . . children who are divergent in degree, not in kind . . . form an extremely heterogeneous group, comprising not only the organically impaired, but also those whose serious emotional disturbances, deafness, blindness, or severe orthopaedic impairments render them functionally retarded. When we speak of the severely/profoundly handicapped, we are referring not simply to the severely mentally retarded, but to a population of multihandicapped persons, including the severely emotionally disturbed, the severly health-impaired, and so on (p 5)

* EEN = exceptional educational need, a generic term for children with special educational needs, including speech-language, in Wisconsin State Statute 115.

Unfortunately, rather than clarifying our views, the myriad of definitions for severely handicapped persons has only served to cause confusion on the part of service providers and funding agencies, thus posing barriers to serving this population. The barriers are twofold. First, it is clear that the definitions presented do not adequately account for the vast individual differences within this population. Problems resulting from various severe handicapping conditions (e.g., visual impairments, mental retardation) are not additive in nature, but should actually be viewed as synergistic, due to the dynamic interaction of the handicaps. This means the severely handicapped individuals cannot be treated as a homogeneous group. Second, potential for diverse interactions among intrapersonal variables (see Fig. 33–1) further contributes to heterogeneous groups within severely handicapped populations.[9]

The implications of viewing severely handicapped individuals as a homogeneous group directly affects the provision of educational and supportive services. With continued funding cutbacks across the national, state, and local levels, both direct and indirect program support for the disabled will be more difficult to secure and maintain. In essence, the possibility of groups of severely handicapped individuals with similar etiologies being denied funding may be forthcoming. In the event that this occurs, parents may be required to secure alternative educational and funding sources. The problem with this, however, is that the organizations that provide services for the severely handicapped are also experiencing funding cutbacks. In a recent publication, Cherow, Matkin, and Trybus list over 117 professional societies, associations, special interest organizations and agencies that provide services to handicapped individuals.[10] As a result, parents, educators, professional service groups (e.g., Association for Retarded Citizens, The Association for Severely Handicapped), and communities are forced to accept less desirable alternatives to services and to focus their attentions instead on the maintenance of the current services.

Two additional barriers, which have historically been overlooked, and which may affect appropriate service delivery to the severely handicapped are (1) societal and individual cultural and ethnic groups' views of handicaps and (2) the distinction between rural, urban, and "large city" differences. As a society, we have become more willing and better able to deal with severely handicapped children. For example, there have been established within communities across the United States, various support groups, which can provide assistance and guidelines to parents on managing their child's problems (e.g., Association for Children with Down Syndrome, Association for Retarded Citizens, Association for the Aid of Crippled Children). Further, public and state legislation (e.g., PL 94–142) has resulted in increased education services provided to severely handicapped children and youth. This does not imply, however, that total acceptance or support for handicapped children exists.

Differences in the cultural acceptance of handicapped individuals within our society may be pronounced, ranging from a willingness to eventually accept the disability and seek professional assistance, to denial and familial embarrassment. For example, economically disadvantaged families may not be willing, or feel that they are able, to seek the advice or assistance of professionals. Another example of this phenomenon are certain Asian populations, who are seemingly less accepting of their child's handicap, viewing it as a source of embarrassment, and consequently are not willing to seek professional assistance. Instead, they tend to keep the handicapped child "hidden" within the confines of their own home, choosing instead to provide for the child to the best of their abilities. Subsequently, professionals must be sensitive to cultural and parental perspectives of severe handicapping conditions in the identification, assessment, and ecological management of the severely handicapped child's communication program.

The distinction between rural, urban, and city differences, although seemingly trivial, is in fact an important consideration and major barrier in respect to opportunities for environmental stimulation, assessment, and service delivery systems. Within the urban settings, such as typical "small" cities or university towns, there appears to be ample opportunity for assessment, and even low-cost educational opportunities. Often found within these areas are educational opportunities or university supported educational and service facilities that contribute to the overall program quality of service provided for handicapped persons and their families. Within large cities (e.g., Chicago, New York), parents may have difficulty choosing among the plethora of clinics providing services and, at the same time, experience difficulty in transportation to and from these clinics.

Rural residents are posed with different problems and/or opportunities from those encountered by urban dwellers. In rural and remote areas, the distance to clinical service centers may be extreme, both for assessment and educational or remedial services. Service delivery systems for rural populations are further hampered due to the low incidence of handicapped individuals residing within these areas. In these settings, it may not be considered "cost-effective" for the educational system to hire additional teaching and support staff. The burden may then fall upon the parents, who are forced to seek the best opportunities for their children, oftentimes at their own expense. When rural school districts are able to secure professional services, an added burden may be placed on professionals who must travel to these rural settings. For example, they may be unable to transport easily the necessary programs and assistive devices (e.g., computers, augmentative communication systems, etc.) to be used for stimulation, teaching, or intervention.

Although federal guidelines have been valuable in establishing minimum requirements that must be met in the services delivered to severely handicapped children, they have not removed all of the barriers to service delivery. PL 94–142 mandates educational services to all handicapped children from 3 through 21 years of age. However, states are not required to provide services to infants and preschoolers, nor are ample federal or state funds available for such services.

As a result of lack of funding legislation and funding cutbacks, early intervention programs have been difficult to implement, in spite of their reported value. According to Appell, early intervention is critical for the young severely handicapped child, as well as for the caregivers, in order to prevent dysfunctional interactions and overwhelming deprivation.[11] Waiting until severely handicapped children are 3 years of age, however, may only serve to contribute to and increase feelings of incompetence for both the infant and the caregiver.

The concept and significance of early intervention has gained much attention and support over the years. Appell has argued that the rationale for early intervention programs for the severely impaired include the following:

1. An infant born biologically intact can develop to full genetic potential if the environment is normal
2. An infant born biologically intact demonstrates developmental attrition, that is, failure to achieve the genetic potential, if environmentally deprived
3. An infant born with biologic deficits, such as deafness, blindness, brain injury, or some combination thereof, is at risk of developmental at-

trition equal to or greater than biologic insult. The rationale for intervention programs for such children is a belief that compensatory or alternative programs for such children may prevent or minimize the attrition.[11]

Parents and educators must become more aware of advocacy groups, which can not only direct them, but assist them in securing the most comprehensive and quality services for their severely handicapped children. Taken together, these conjoined forces may help to alleviate barriers to providing quality services for young severely handicapped children (Fig. 33–2).

The change agent team can also become advocates for services for the severely handicapped child. The team's influence upon the settings, systems, and living environments can bring about changes in the types of services provided by agencies. Furthermore, they can also influence changes in the policies which govern the provision of services.

Attempts to secure the most comprehensive service delivery systems across various communities may never be overcome on the federal level. If, however, the focus is generalized to the local and state levels, the problems may be more manageable. The major issue inherent in providing adequate services for severely handicapped children then becomes one of an integrated approach. Although the number of professionals involved within the service delivery team can vary, as can their respective involvements, this integrated approach would create rich opportunities, shared insights, and an ecological approach to communication management. One means of implementing this approach, which could effectively overcome this barrier, would be the creation of a comprehensive service delivery system, enacted by state laws, creating a legal mandate for community services. This would include aspects of diagnosis, evaluation, management teams, personal care, day care, respite care for the handicapped child, parent and family education, vocational and rehabilitative training for independent work, family and individual counseling, protective and legal services, community based programming, transportation, and research and development for curriculum development and training.

FROM IDENTIFICATION TO ECOLOGICAL ASSESSMENT AND MANAGEMENT

Given the number and variety of definitions used to describe severely handicapped children and youth, it is not surprising that confusion exists in the areas of identification and assessment of both the person

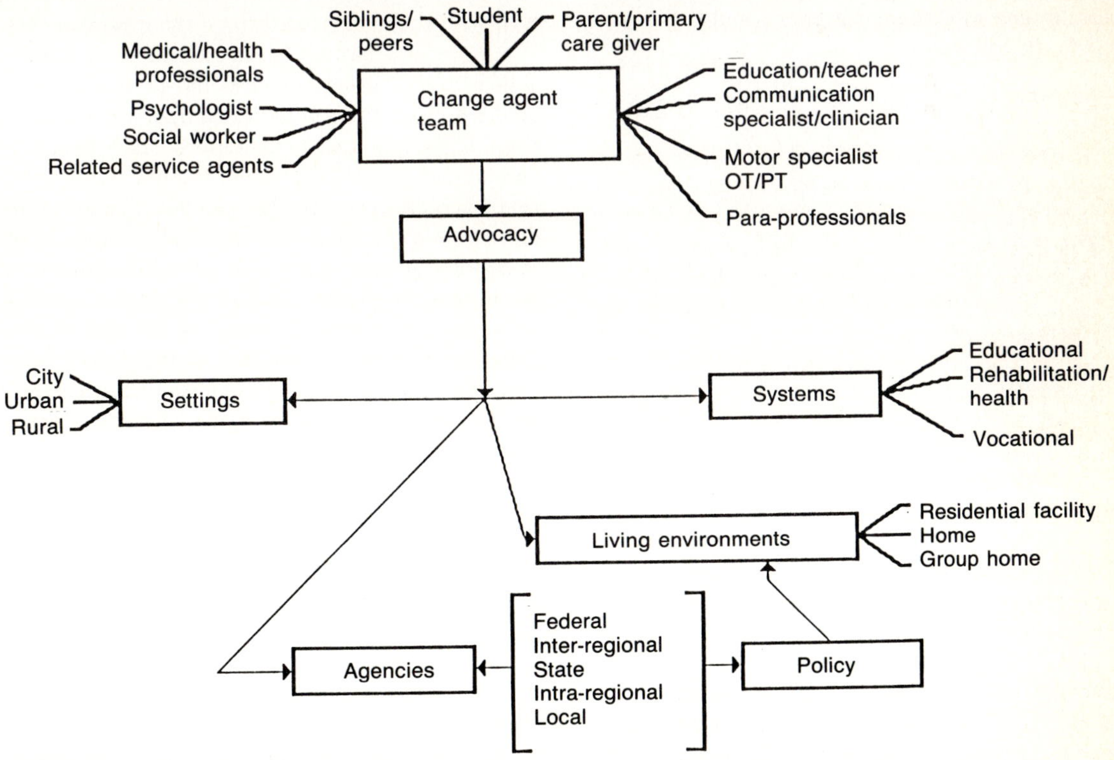

Figure 33–2 Ecological management: an interpersonal service delivery approach.

needing the service and the service delivery system itself. In order to secure adequate financial programming support, parents and educators must be aware of and address the following three issues related to assessment before proceeding with intervention:

1. What criteria should be used in identifying children and youth with severe handicaps?
2. What criteria should be used in assessing the adequacy of programs for severely handicapped persons? and
3. How might educational assessment of severely handicapped children and youth differ from other assessments of children and youth needing special education programs?

Let us look at the issues of identification and assessment of severely handicapped children and youth.

Identification

Using the BEH definition as the theoretical framework for the following discussion, three characteristics of severely handicapped individuals may be defined as follows: (1) they must have a "severe" or "intense" handicap, (2) they need an educational program requiring greater resources than are normally provided by traditional programs, and (3) they need programs that focus on skills necessary for greater independent functioning and self-fulfillment. Identification and assessment batteries should therefore include the following:

1. Methods of measurement of the individual's current level of functioning
2. Items that are sequential and in a logical hierarchy to provide entry level considerations in curriculum development
3. A description of the testing conditions under which the person performed at an optimal level so that optimal learning environments may also be established, and
4. An identification of criteria used for acceptable performance.[4]

The BEH definition of severely handicapped, however, fails to encompass several variables, which we believe are important to an accurate description of the functional capacities of the severely handicapped individual. For example, there is no description of single versus multiple impairments, nor of the severity or residual abilities of the individual. No provision is made for other health factors that might affect the individual's behavior and performance (e.g., diabetes, arthritis, etc.). Nor is age of onset taken into consideration. Therefore, it becomes important for the assessment team to be cognizant of how these variables might interact to influence the functional capabilities of the individual.

Assessment of Communication Skills

Assessing the communication skills of severely handicapped children and youth is an extremely complex and difficult task. It requires the use of many methods and procedures to generate the individual data necessary to plan eventual communication teaching programs. Problems are compounded by the fact that as the severity of the handicapping condition increases, the number of available valid and reliable assessment tools decreases. Additionally, the assessment task is complicated by the low frequency response rate of severely handicapped students to stimuli and by their general low level of attention and interest.

Some major barriers exist, which confront us relative to communication skill assessment. One such barrier relates to lack of appropriate assessment tools. Clinicians and teachers work with specific time constraints and large case loads, and therefore it is necessary to use those procedures that can provide us the maximum amount of information about the student's communication abilities in the most efficient manner. However, it is widely known that doing quick assessments of communicative behavior with severely handicapped persons is next to impossible, even with the tools needed to do the measurements.

A second barrier relates to the student's inability to use usual response modes during standardized tests, due to physical and/or sensory problems. Assessment tool modifications which have been developed for physically handicapped or sensory impaired persons (such that they require a response mode different from pointing with the hand, saying a word, or making an X in a box) are not only difficult, if not impossible, to find, but are also looked upon by our educational systems as a less than adequate method of measuring the true abilities of the person being evaluated. In all cases, the clinician or teacher must use additional ingenuity to adapt assessment stimuli input for the sensory impaired student. An additional problem with modifying tests is that the modified mode (e.g., scanning, encoding) may place additional cognitive and/or motor demands on the student and thus underestimate the child's true abilities. Add sensory and motor problems to limited cognitive abilities and we have a *difficult-to-assess student*.

According to Sheehan,[12] one of the major goals of assessment measures is to predict specific developmental patterns and to diagnose and suggest intervention strategies for the handicapped and at-risk population. The assumption underlying assessment is that a meaningful evaluation is a necessary prerequisite to an appropriate and functional intervention strategy. Thus, the emphasis of planning a comprehensive assessment is to foster this design of a functional intervention program based on the need for severely handicapped persons to perform real-life activities.[13–18]

Selecting Functional Assessment Tools

Though previously stated, the objective of any behavioral assessment is to obtain a valid estimate of the severely impaired child's developmental strengths and weaknesses. To accomplish this successfully, the assessment team must judiciously select an assessment scale appropriate for the child's developmental level, handicapping condition, and available response modes. In order to meet these objectives, the assessment team must take into consideration several parameters.

When restricted to using traditional assessment tools, Fewell outlines several critical factors to be considered in instrument selection, including (1) the purpose for testing; (2) the use of the data; (3) the examiners; (4) the children to be assessed; (5) those who are to receive the results; and (6) the fiscal and material resources available for the testing.[19] In addition, it is imperative that the assessment team consider the philosophy of the assessment-curriculum packages. By their very nature, different scales have different outcome measures. Therefore, when using several instruments to assess handicapped children, the assessment team must be certain to select instruments whose outcome data will be compatible. Traditionally, three basic paradigms have been used in assessing the developmental skills of children under the age of 3 years: direct testing, naturalistic observation, and interviews. The advantages and disadvantages of each of these approaches follows.

Direct Testing

Direct testing methods generally use one of three types of tests: *norm-referenced, criterion-referenced,* or *curriculum-referenced tests.* Although each of these approaches are unique, they all yield one or two scores describing the child's status in terms of deviation from age of expectancy or deviation from the mean performance of other children of the same age. The major assumption underlying the use of these tests is that certain standards, including the use of predetermined administration procedures, are maintained in any test situation.

Norm-referenced Tests. Norm-referenced tests can be used as either a screening instrument (e.g., *Denver Developmental Screening Test*[20]) or as a diagnostic instrument (e.g., the *Bayley Scales*[21]). The use of these types of instruments has had wide-spread popularity. Proponents of norm-referenced instruments suggest that they are extremely helpful in educational planning. By the same token, recent research has revealed that norm-referenced scales, in particular the *Bayley Scales,* may overestimate the true level of functioning as a result of out-dated norms,[22] or may underestimate the level of functioning because scales were normed on samples excluding children with physical or cognitive handicaps.[12] Another disadvantage of using norm-referenced tests is that many of the items included on these scales are inappropriate for use with handicapped children because they are above any level of functioning which may be achieved by severely handicapped children (Table 33–2)

Criterion-referenced Tests. The primary purpose of criterion-referenced tests is to indicate the child's mastery of specific skills within a specific behavioral domain. These lists are usually organized across several domains (e.g., cognitive, language, fine and gross motor). A child's status is described in terms of the skills mastered with each of the domains. Subsequently, an age level, which is normally based on the mean age of children mastering the skill, is assigned to each skill. The major advantage of criterion-referenced assessments is that they are more closely tied to curriculum than norm-referenced assessment instruments, and in some cases, are synonymous with curriculum. The major disadvantage of criterion-referenced tests is that they do not provide sufficient information to determine why a specific skill was not performed by the child (see Table 33–2).

Modification of Standardized Tests

McLean and Snyder-McLean, and Wasson, Tynan and Gardiner have suggested several modifications of normed and criterion referenced standardized tests which can be used with severely handicapped children.[23,24] McLean and Snyder-McLean argue for the use of modifications since the purpose of assessment is "to obtain the most representative picture possible of the child's current level of functioning" (p 126).[23] Such modifications include repeated and simplified instructions, additional cues such as gesturing or modeling, modifying the required mode of response, adapting or changing stimulus materials, and reinforcing correct answers. Although these modifications invalidate the typical scoring procedures and standard interpretations, the information obtained may be valuable in determin-

TABLE 33-2 Barriers of Using Norm-referenced and Criterion-referenced Assessments with Severely Handicapped Individuals*

Barriers — *Norm-referenced Assessments*	*Explanation*
Age appropriateness	Materials that are appropriate for infants and young children are generally not appropriate for older, severely handicapped individuals. The lack of age appropriate stimuli may make testing situations unmotivating Test items developed for infants assume an infantile level of motoric functioning. Many items found in cognitive or communicative subscales that are appropriate for preambulatory infants become singularly inappropriate when administered to an ambulatory child or a large, physically robust person
Adaptations	Adaptations defeat the purpose of the norm-referenced test, which is intended to compare the performance of individuals under very carefully documented conditions
Lack of sensitivity	The number of items per subscale are generally few, providing insufficient sensitivity to distinguish between children who develop relatively slowly. Furthermore, these subscales are not likely to provide the indepth information required by the professional team interested in one domain of the child's development to construct specific interventions
Confounding of skill areas	Many norm-referenced tests are confounded by items between subscales, i.e., items from any given subscale are likely to tap skills from other developmental areas
Corrections for prematurity	Use of a corrected age may minimize discrepancies between the subject and CA Cohorts, preventing the unnecessary labeling of the infant as developmentally disabled. Correction for gestational age, however, implies that biological factors are the predominant influences on behavior in the early months of life. Conversely, basing scores on an infant's chronological age implies that maturational or environmental factors are the predominant influences on behavior during this period of development.
Criterion-referenced Assessments	
Procedural weaknesses	Many criterion-referenced tests consist of a checklist of pertinent behaviors which exist or don't exist. Test stimuli and the range of acceptable responses are seldom specified and procedures may not be provided for testing those items which do not occur spontaneously
Lack of reliability and validity data	
Lack of scoring standards	Some assessments provide only for visual profiles, others provide no method of deriving a score from test performance
Ordinality and educational implications	When items from different tests are arranged according to the sequence of acquisition observed in the development of nondisabled children, their ordinality becomes highly questionable. Issues of ordinality become problematic when assessment data are tied closely to instructional consequences. If a child fails an item on a criterion-referenced test, that item may be assumed to constitute an appropriate instructional objective. If the item does not represent either a functional and age-appropriate behavior in and of itself or a demonstrated prerequisite to other functional behaviors, such a conclusion is not warranted

* Rowland, Charity M. Personal communication, Teaching Research Div., Oregon State System of Higher Educ. Monmouth, OR, 1985.

ing instructional strategies. If used with an assessment battery that is developmentally based, these modifications may help identify subsequent programming, which is logical and sequentially based, for the attainment of higher level skills. Dubose points out, however, that once these adaptations and modifications are made, norm-referenced comparison becomes dubious.[5]

Another frequently-given reason for modification of standardized assessments is that these instruments generally do not include a fair or sufficient number of behavioral items within the particular behavioral domain for severely handicapped persons. In attempting to address the fact that severely handicapped children generally do not develop the degree of behavioral complexity or competency that characterizes normal development—and which is assessed in standardized assessment tools—clinicians may be inclined to choose parts of one instrument and parts of another, with the hope that this will provide them with the most comprehensive summary of the child's level of functioning. The methodologic hazard encountered by this type of reasoning is twofold. First, this procedure is not psychometrically sound because the norms for most tests are computed on an overall basis rather than on an item basis. Thus, the use of only selected items invalidates the use of standardized norms. The second hazard with this approach is related to the violation of the underlying philosophy of the specific assessment battery. In other words, some assessment tools (e.g., Bayley, Vineland) are sequenced developmentally, thereby suggesting that skills addressed early on are prerequisites for higher-level skills. When taken out of sequence, the particular items are invalidated with respect to their content validity.

Curriculum-referenced Scales

Curriculum-referenced tests actually fall under the rubric of criterion-referenced measures because performance on an item is compared to a standard of mastery or sequence of skills, rather than compared to other children. An example of a curriculum-referenced scale is the *Early Communication Skills Curriculum* (ECSC).[25] The ECSC is designed to facilitate the social and communicative skills of profoundly handicapped or severely developmentally delayed individuals functioning below 12 to 15 months developmentally. The teach-test-teach paradigm of this curriculum allows for the assessment not only of the level of functioning, but also for periodic probes of maintenance and generalization of skills.

Observational Methods

A second traditional method for gathering information about children is through naturalistic observation. The essence of this procedure is the recording of behaviors as they occur in a variety of settings. Naturalistic observations have several advantages. Foremost among them is that they sample the child's typical behavior, thus allowing for the assessment of many important skills not covered in testing situations (e.g., peer interaction, inappropriate behavior). By their very nature, observational methods assume a within-subject (single-subject) design. The major advantage of this approach is that it is well suited to explore the effectiveness treatment variables targeted for intervention. The major misconception of this approach is that it is not systematic. Because of the inherent complexities with single-subject experimental designs, the reader is referred elsewhere for a review of the issues and assumptions underlying this approach.[26,27]

Parental Interviews

A third procedure for gathering information is through the use of parent interviews, either structured and formal, or unstructured and informal. An example of an interview scale is the *Wisconsin Behavior Rating Scale* (WBRS).[28] The WBRS incorporates an educational model that perceives sensorimotor deficits as characteristic of handicapped persons and focuses on the development of their abilities.[29] Other interview scales included the AAMD *Adaptive Behavior Scale*[30] and the *Vineland Social Maturity Scale*.[31] The primary advantage of interview techniques is its efficiency. Using the primary caregiver as an informant, interview scales may obtain information which is not always included on formal assessment instruments. By the same token, the major disadvantage of informant scales is the fact that the primary caregiver may overestimate the child's true level of functioning.

The development of these scales has several inherent advantages over the more traditional assessment scales. First, these scales attempt to measure skills which are not only considered to be "functional" (i.e., skills that enable a child to interact in the environment), but also which are potential programming targets. Moreover, because the items included on these scales were carefully delineated in respect to their content validity, there exists an allowance for the discrimination of the slow and gradual progress typical of severely handicapped persons.

A second advantage of these scales is the administration procedures. Specifically, the behaviors evaluated within these scales are assessed either through observation of children within their natural environments, or from an informant (e.g., the primary caregiver). When direct testing is required, it is intended to test target behaviors that were not displayed during an observational period or when there is a degree of uncertainty.

A third advantage of these types of scales is their reliability with respect to the "criterion for competent performance" for children with various impairments. In other words, the required responses within the communication domain would be different for a child with sensory and motoric impairments. As an example, in assessing the child's ability to respond to its name, an examiner would observe the child's behavior when the child's name is called or signed. For a child with deaf-blindness, the examiner would be permitted to produce the child's sign name in his/her hand—after it had been established that the child was not merely responding to random tactile stimulation. For a motor impaired child, similar procedures would be followed. The criterion of performance, though, would require eyes be turned toward the source of the sound or with cessation or increase in the child's activity.

Although there are several inherent advantages, there also exists one major disadvantage. Specifically, these scales are not intended, nor are they adequate as a primary means of assessment. The intervention team must use other instruments to corroborate and support their clinical findings.

Functional Assessment: An Alternative Approach

As has already been mentioned, one of the major assumptions made by the "diagnostic programmer"[17] asserts that sufficient information can be extracted from the use of traditional scales to develop a curriculum for intervention. We must recall, however, that what is not conveyed by traditional resources is how development and performance will be different when children are disabled. From the preceding discussion, it is readily apparent that the traditional assessment strategies are not adequate for persons with severe handicaps. Specifically, traditional strategies are primarily concerned with the identification of traits, aptitudes, and medical diagnostic criteria associated with the etiology of the impairment. Although this information is important, it fails to provide information relative to the individual's adaptation to various situations and environments. What is truly needed, then, is a basic understanding of individual differences so that examiners can formulate expectations and plan assessment strategies that are less likely than standard procedures to penalize the impaired child, and can make decisions about the child's learning and coping skills.[13,17,32]

The current trend involves the development of functional assessment systems to augment traditional assessment strategies.[13,14,17,32] The use of behavioral evaluations and observations has increased dramatically in recent years, and has grown out of the literature which has recommended the use of functional evaluations.[13] The behavioral information gathered can be used as a basis for planning, for indications of progress, or for a means of comparison with respect to other persons within the child's environment. According to Halpern and Fuhrer, functional assessment is "the measurement of purposeful behavior in interaction with the environment, which is interpreted according to the assessment's intended uses" (p 3).[16] We would extend this definition to include the measure of dynamic characteristics of the individual, including activities, skills, performance, environmental conditions, and needs. The basic use of a functional assessment, then, is to serve as a guide to (1) assessment, (2) planning, (3) implementation, (4) monitoring, and (5) the evaluation of intervention.

Figure 33–3 presents an outline, which can be used in examining the parameters of functional communication competence and subsequently guide the clinician's efforts to develop a curricular approach for an intervention program. The rationale behind this approach combines observational methods, with intended references to formal assessments, which describe and define in specific and objective terms those skills within the severely handicapped person's repertoire that allow him or her to participate in a wide variety of integrated community environments. Rather than entering with set agenda assessment strategies, this approach is consistent with Miller's recommendation that prior to the formal evaluation period, the assessment team attempt to answer these three questions:

1. Why are we assessing the child?
2. What are we going to assess?
3. How are we going to assess the child?[33]

It should be noted that this model is also embedded within a framework of ecological assessment. The ecological assessment, as presented here, encompasses two perspectives. First, the severely handicapped student is seen as possessing a behavioral ecology to the extent that changes in one behavior may affect other behaviors. Thus, it is imperative that an attempt be made to delineate the possible communicative functions of aberrant behavior.[34,35] The major advantage of these naturalistic observations is the assertion that they sample the child's typical behaviors, thereby allowing for the observation and subsequent evaluation of many important skills, which may not be directly assessed in formal assessment instruments (e.g., nonverbal and verbal aspects of communication, interaction style, independence). Second, naturalistic observations permit the systematic analysis of behaviors and the contexts in which they do not occur.

Our model of functional assessment includes a task analysis approach. The task analysis approach is not concerned with either causation or cognitive theories of development, but rather is based upon the principles of behavioral psychology. This behavioral approach to assessment focuses upon the resulting behavior of the child when presented with a specific stimulus. Thus, the focus of the assessment is precisely to identify the skills that the child exhibits and those that the child needs to learn in order to function at the highest level of independence possible.

INTRAPERSONAL BARRIERS AFFECTING THE DEVELOPMENT OF FUNCTIONAL COMMUNICATION SKILL

It has been suggested that language development depends on the convergence of cognitive, affective, and linguistic processes rather than being an ability which emerges independent of these factors.[36–38] Moreover, language is considered, foremost, a tool for communication within some social context.[39]

Language deficits or disorders appear to be one of the major handicapping conditions associated with severely handicapped individuals. According to Ingalls, a deficit in language skills is perhaps the single most important characteristic that distinguishes

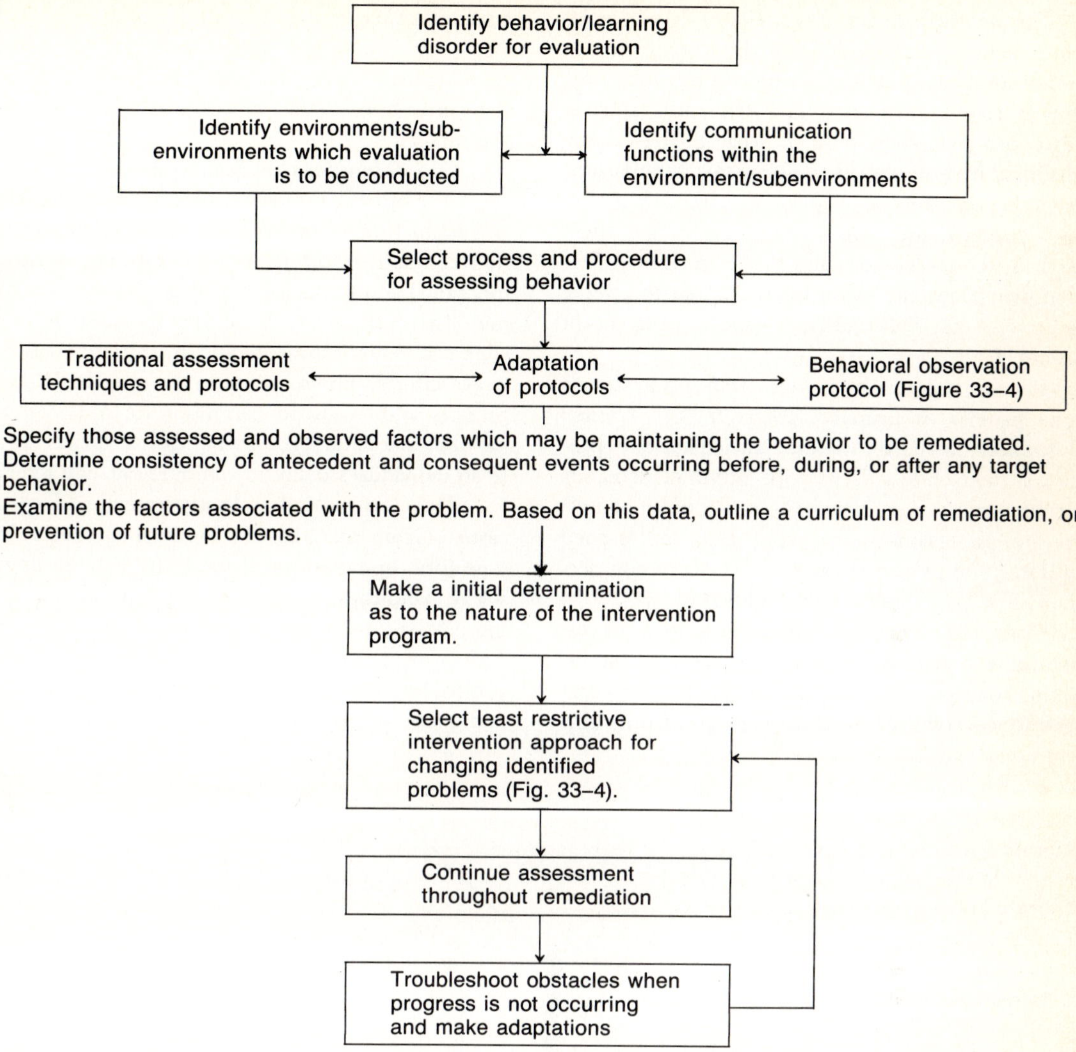

Figure 33–3 A schema for identifying the parameters of functional communication. (Adapted from Karan OC, Berstein GS, Harvey JR, Bates PE, Renzaglia A, Clees T. An extended evaluation model for the severely handicapped. AAESPH Rev 1979; 4(4): 374.)

a mentally retarded person from a nonretarded person.[40] Considering the importance of language in human interaction, it seems logical that the lack of communication skills may adversely affect other aspects of the individual's life.

The severity of the disability may limit the child's active physical exploration of the environment. According to Seligman, this results in motivational, cognitive, and emotional disturbances, that is, the motivation of the organism to initiate responses drastically decreases; the heightened negative emotional state undermines the ability to perceive a successful outcome to responding, and consequently further opportunities for learning are avoided.[41] The impact on cognition may affect the child's ability to (1) sense information (stimuli) from the environment (sensory information); (2) recognize information as something that has been experienced in some form previously, which requires selectivity as well as organization (perception); (3) store this information (memory); and (4) retrieve it for use in making decisions.[42,43]

The concept of learned helplessness can also be used to explain the difficulties experienced by severely handicapped individuals in language development. Fouts, Couch and O'Neil suggest that:

> the inability to speak creates a tremendous loss of control over one's environment, producing a situation analogous to that of learned helplessness. Consequently, these children should be passive and indifferent with regard to communication behaviors, and this passivity should generalize to situations not involving communication. Furthermore, these children should demonstrate lower overall motivation and greater emotionalism when compared to normal children (p 219).[44]

During early infant interactions, "the consistency, timing, and quality of the caregivers responses create expectancies about control and competence" (p 7)[45] Inconsistent or absent early caregiver interactions may contribute to what Siegel-Causey and Guess have described as iatrogenic retardation, which they consider as a form of learned helplessness.[46] Siegel-Causey and Guess suggest that these less-than-rich interactions and lower levels of expectation may contribute to the child's failure to achieve cognitive, psycholinguistic, and neuromotor milestones.

Prizant suggests that too often professionals blame parents or primary caregivers for "learned helplessness" because they may anticipate and provide for their child's needs with minimal demands for communication.[47] However, well-intentioned efforts by professionals may contribute to learned helplessness to an even greater extent. Common detrimental practices include the following:

Compliance and Respondent Training. Some degree of "behavioral control" is necessary for conceptual growth and acquisition of communicative knowledge, but at what point does this result in passivity and lack of initiation. What is the long-term cost of an "easily managed" or well-behaved student if the ability to initiate communicative interactions and to express basic needs is discouraged.

Cue-dependent or Situation-specific Learning. Too often communication programming efforts and evaluation of such efforts occur in highly limited contexts resulting in the learning of limited functional communication ability. Inherent in communicative growth is the ability to use such knowledge across environments and to initiate communicative efforts. Environments that offer both opportunities and needs to communicate must be provided so that natural cues rather than artificial cues lead to an individual's desire to communicate and interact.

Developmentally Inappropriate Expectations. Given that the development of speech is an unrealistic immediate goal for many individuals with severe handicaps, it must be recognized that communicative intent can be expressed through a wide variety of presymbolic means including, but not limited to, gestures, picture boards, object boards, and gaze. Demands for developmentally inappro-

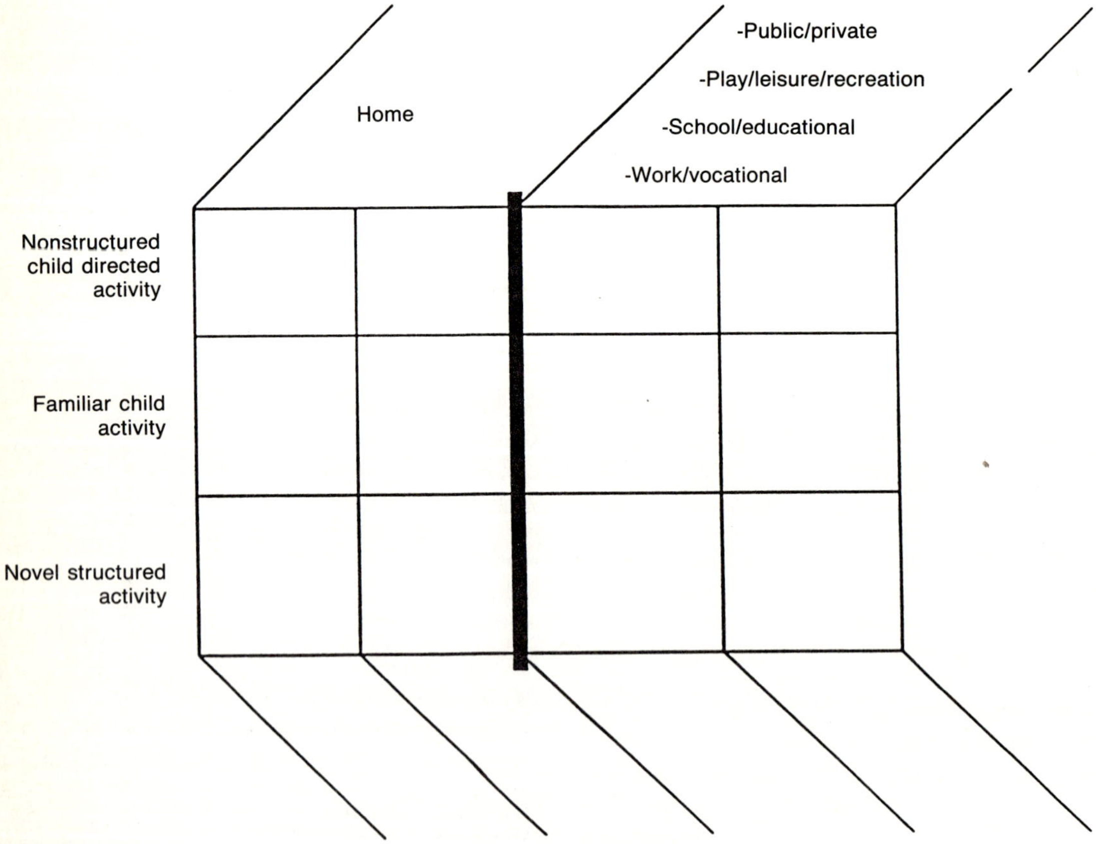

Figure 33-4 Behavioral observation protocol.

priate communication (e.g., use of a symbol system for a presymbolic individual) may result in frustration for all involved, and may actually result in communication breakdowns rather than enhance communicative competence. Furthermore, those interacting with individuals must be able to adjust their language and interactive style to facilitate mutually satisfying communicative and social interactions.

Any attempt to ameliorate learned helplessness and foster communication development must focus primarily upon the environment. Yoder suggests that we must provide experiences which facilitate cognitive and communicative behavior.[48] Such experiences include social environments that provide touching, holding, hugging, physical contact, and communication with the infant; physical environments that provide visual and auditory stimuli, which the infant can control, and a variety of prospective interactants with the severely handicapped child (for the sake of preventing parental and caregiver "burn-out," as well as for the purpose of providing a variety of intrapersonal stimulation for the child). This notion is based upon the research of Yarrow, Klein, Lomonaco and Morgan, who suggest that early cognitive and communication development can be significantly related to the level of stimulation, intensity of expression of positive affect, active kinesthetic stimulation, and variety in the inanimate environment of the child.[49]

As is illustrated within Figure 33–5 the dynamic interaction of intrapersonal variables affect not only the child's knowledge base, but also the ability to effect changes within the environment. Keogh and Reichle suggest severely handicapped children may be viewed as differing in their apparent propensity to learn, their degree of motor impairment, which can influence their ability to produce voluntary discrete responses, and in their degree of participation.[50] The greater the individual variation across these dimensions, the more likely children are to require some level of organized instruction before they are able to acquire and utilize a functional repertoire of communicative behaviors.

Prior to intervention, however, an evaluation of the individual's ecological needs and opportunities must be assessed (Fig. 33–6). The goal of this assessment is to foster the design of functional intervention, based on the objective for the severely

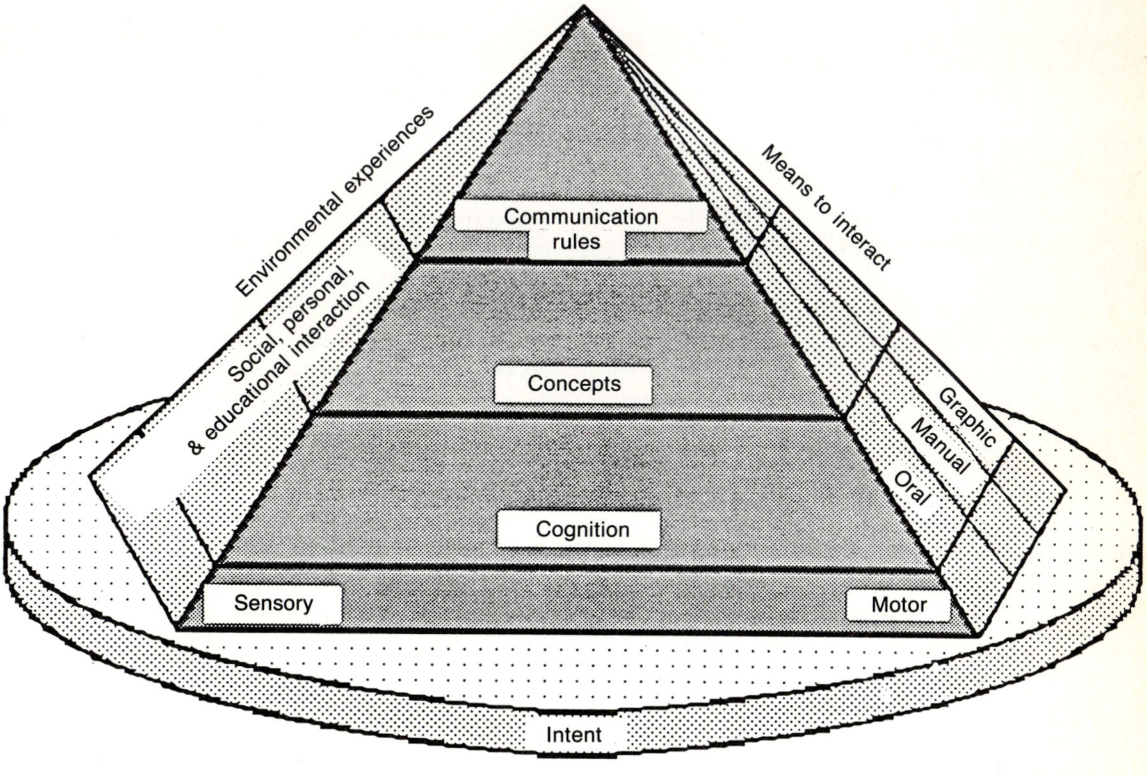

Figure 33–5 Requisities for communicative competence.

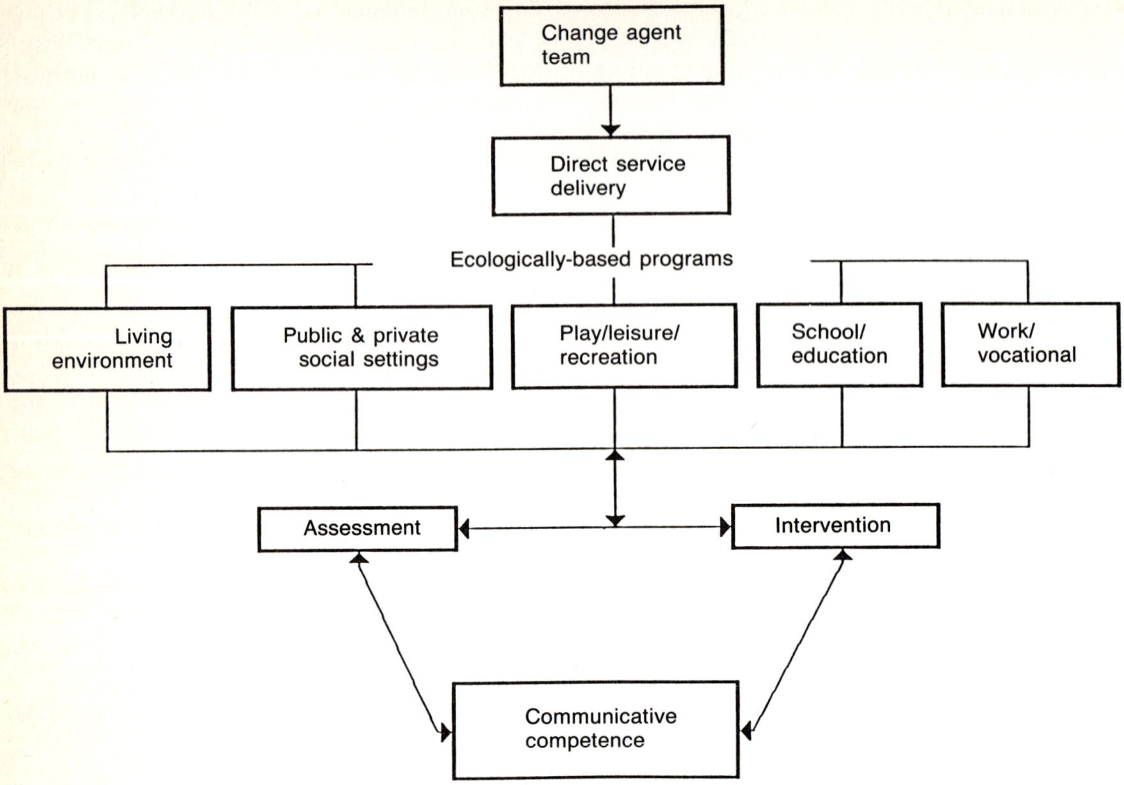

Figure 33–6 Community based programming: an interpersonal delivery approach.

handicapped child to initiate and successfully perform real-life activities.[13,15]

COMMUNICATION MANAGEMENT (INTERVENTION) WITH YOUNG SEVERELY HANDICAPPED CHILDREN AND YOUTH

Upon the identification of a handicapping condition, decisions of when and what type of intervention programs (if any at all) are warranted. The basic goal of language intervention is to increase children's communication efficiency within the context of social interaction. Early intervention programs are frequently introduced for the young severely handicapped child, with the major emphasis attempting to foster the growth of behaviors intended to accelerate the rate of development, acquisitions of new behaviors, and an increased level of independent functioning. Another major emphasis of early intervention programs is to prevent the development of secondary handicaps.

Early intervention programs can serve two major purposes. First, they can provide indirect services to both the family and the child. Specifically, parents of handicapped children, who frequently need assistance and guidance in providing care for their handicapped child, may require emotional support and respite care. The provision of respite care, if available, can provide parents the opportunity to meet their own, and other familial needs. Furthermore, parents who may not have been prepared for the problems of parenting per se, let alone the problems of parenting a handicapped child, may know little about securing supportive services for their child or themselves. With early identification, professionals can advise parents of the types of services that may be available within the given community.

As depicted in Figure 33–2, this approach considers parents and professionals as advocates for services. Through support groups and professional agencies, parents and educators not only secure the necessary educational and fundamental supportive funds for the handicapped child, but also bring about a community awareness. All too frequently, communities have been either unwilling or unable to provide services to severely handicapped children and youth. As mentioned previously this is often rural areas, where a severely handicapped child may be the only one within the entire community, and perhaps even the school district, to have a severe handicapping condition. What then is the solution to this barrier?

As has already been mentioned, making certain that parents are aware of the various agencies and legal rights, which both they and their child have, can, perhaps, be viewed as the initial step. Just as important, however, is caregiver and family education about communication development through social interaction. Parents and family members may know little about the procedures for providing appropriate care or fostering the development of their child through interaction strategies. All too frequently, parents and family members attempt to compensate for the child's handicap by attempting to anticipate the needs of the child, therefore, interfering with the development of intentional communication. As a result, severely handicapped children may acquire a degree of learned helplessness as discussed earlier, becoming overly dependent on the environment to anticipate desires, needs and emotions. To be effective, parent and family education must occur early in the child's life.

The education of the family and community is intended to contribute to the establishment of responsive environments. The significance of a responsive environment may lie in severely handicapped children learning that their behaviors can affect the environment. Environmental interactions allow infants gradually to build a more sophisticated knowledge base of the world by selecting information and fitting it to their current structured organization or understanding of the environment and the world. Subsequently, this may encourage infants to interact even more with their environment, thus facilitating other learning.

For the young severely handicapped child, intervention may have its greatest impact at a very young age. The concepts of cause and effect, control over the environment, and differentiated behaviors, which signal the caretaker that the child is in need or desires something, may be reinforced and taught. Early stimulation programs, as a part of their hidden curriculum, also have the advantage of helping to reinforce and educate the infant to the realization that there are other individuals with whom the infant can interact.

Second, the intervention strategy, or curriculum approach chosen for the severely handicapped child also requires serious consideration. The philosophy of different approaches can vary significantly, and serves as the basis for the skills and goals of the content. A dichotomy, which is helpful in reviewing curricula approaches, is based on the following perspective: should severely handicapped students be treated as slowly developing persons who can (or should) replicate the normal growth process, or should goals and objectives be constructed through analysis of the functional requirements of present and future environments? Historically, intervention programs have waited for the attainment of either sensorimotor stage V or VI before the initiation of formal programs. The basis of this argument is derived from the perspective that early social interactions between infants and their primary caregivers have been suggested to provide a basis for the development of communication.[39] Furthermore, Bates suggests that before children can develop interpersonal communication skills, they must satisfy the following:

1. Be aware that others around them are using a system of communication
2. Discover roles of precommunicative give and take
3. Discover shared symbols that may be used to indicate and demand
4. Discover shared symbols that indicate individual referents, and
5. Learn the meanings for these symbols in isolation and later in strings.[51]

However, recent research has suggested that for children not at sensorimotor stage V or VI, a preferred intervention effort is to structure a beginning communication strategy so as to embrace the fundamental need to attend to the severe cognitive and perceptual deficits of children, while teaching a generalized immediately useful requesting skill.[50,52] Specifically, this approach with a severely handicapped child or youth attempts to reinforce and expand upon the behaviors which are considered to be communicative in nature. The theory behind this approach is to facilitate the acquisition of the concept that the behaviors of the severely handicapped infant or youth can affect environmental changes.

Bricker and Carlson suggest that a broad-based approach to early language intervention with severely handicapped children is warranted.[53] They suggest that such an approach should include attending to the development of social, affective, and sensorimotor behaviors. Mahoney also supports this position, arguing that the context of language intervention needs to encompass all aspects of the child's social milieu: "The ethological approach would develop an intervention program based upon the principle that language evolves from the social interaction and nonverbal communication systems which exist between language-learning children and their primary language models" (p 145).[54] Other researchers have supported this notion by designing and advocating that a social-ecological approach to early language intervention be used.[23,25,50,55–57]

A socio-ecological approach to language intervention is based upon one major assumption. The primary change agent is the individual who is most familiar with the child (e.g., parent or other primary caregiver). The role of the interventionist is to assist this individual in acquiring the necessary skills to become an effective change agent. The introduction and utilization of curricula approaches are intended to provide guidelines for the construction of communication-rich environments, which may be highly attractive and motivating to the child. Furthermore, the curricula approaches are designed to encourage the change agent to be responsive to the child, rather than anticipating the needs of the child or attempting to train and elicit specific responses from the child. Further support is given to this approach by Bricker and Carlson who suggest that:

> To limit the context of intervention to only professional staff defies logic from two perspectives. First, the primary caregiver, usually the mother, is the one individual with whom the infant spends the most time. If the mother remains ignorant of how to arrange the environment and respond to her child, this greatly reduces the number of opportunities that could be used to foster the development of appropriate communicative behavior. Second, through bonding and attachment the primary caregiver is usually the infant's most salient social reinforcer. To ignore this relationship is to ignore a powerful reinforcer for building communicative skills (p 42).[53]

The instructional philosophy advocated by this approach is further imbedded within two perspectives. First, attempts to arrange the environment in a highly attractive manner are intended to captivate the child's attention and interest. Second, and perhaps more important, caregivers may create environments which can be used within an evaluative framework (Fig. 33–7) to monitor the maintenance and generalization of the trained behaviors,[58] and to continually reassess the needs of the child.

Prizant suggests that within and across handicapping conditions individual differences is the rule rather than the exception.[47] Dimensions of individual differences may include (a) learning or cognitive style, (b) individuals who are active versus passive communicators, (c) individuals who are emotionally well-adjusted versus individuals who develop emotional problems secondary to their primary disabilities, and (d) differences in life experiences and communicative needs.

Blanket programmed approaches too often do not consider these differences, yet they remain prevalent. The ineffectiveness of packaged approaches must be recognized when evaluated within the criterion

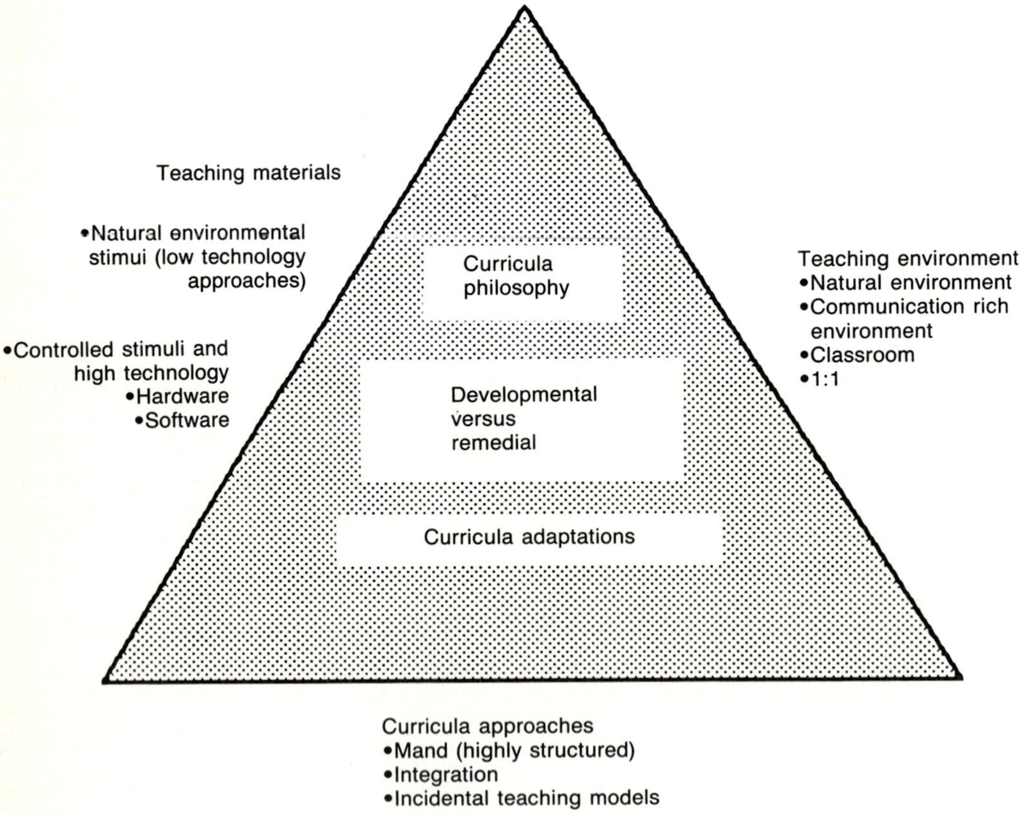

Figure 33–7 Management approaches used in the development of functional communication competence.

of functional communication ability. For professionals who have come to rely on such approaches for communication training, a shift of orientation is necessary. For future professionals, recognition of individual differences and incorporation of this knowledge into program planning is an essential part of their training. Future research needs to consider how such individual differences may bear on communication assessment and programming.

A major impediment to teaching functional communication skills in the classroom lies in the organizational and administrative constraints on what teachers must instruct and what they must do. Often a major emphasis in special education classrooms focuses upon the teaching of classification schemas, matching objects, sight-word recognition, sensorimotor exploration, toileting, alphanumeric recognition (and if possible, production), and the construction of syntactic and grammatical sentences. It is not surprising then, that this "instructional environment" only minimally contributes to socio-ecological communicative competence.

Instruction within natural environments has been discussed in various places.[13,15,59] This approach espoused and found effective for severely handicapped adolescents and young adults, arranges the environment to teach students chronological age-appropriate functional skills in natural environments (see Fig. 33–7). We have used the nonmutually exclusive curricular domains shown on Figure 33–8 both to assess and teach functional communication skills to severely handicapped children and youth. Use of these domains has been found by us to be useful in identifying functional communication behavior needed for everyday functioning within the various environments in which handicapped and nonhandicapped persons live. Assessing a person's knowledge of communication across the various domains places the teacher and clinician in a position of establishing an "honest and appropriate communication need," not based on linguistic developmental norms, but on a set of behaviors for which the students indicate a need.

Communication

- Living environment
- Public & private social setting
- Play/leisure/recreation setting
- School/education environment
- Work/vocational setting

Figure 33–8 Five nonmutually exclusive natural environmental domains.

A primary focus of a program to establish functional communication skills within the natural environment is to answer questions related to how a student communicates and under what conditions communication can and does occur (Table 33–3). We know that the communication behaviors and needs demonstrated by the severely handicapped person are varied and changing. Depending upon the severity of the cognitive, sensory and motor ability, the communication behaviors of severely handicapped individuals may range from no spoken language to highly unintelligible speech. Other severely handicapped individuals may possess adequate motor skills to use manual sign systems. Still other severely handicapped individuals may have need for an expressive system of graphic symbols on a communication board, book, or chart.

Perhaps the most realistic and necessary approach to teaching functional communication behavior to the severely handicapped infant or youth can be drawn from the needs of the individual across several natural environments. This notion is based on the hypothesis that students can acquire communication behavior commensurate with, but not in excess of, their cognitive abilities. Because of the pervasive nature of communication break-downs with the severely handicapped person, and because of the ubiquitous nature of communication in daily living, it is necessary to deal with communication skill development within the context of the student's learning and living environment. That is why communication teaching must be discussed within the context of the natural environment. Establishing communicative competence is the goal for every student, regardless of how handicapped that person may be. One cannot, however, apply the rules of communicative discourse of the normal developing child to severely handicapped persons and expect to reach the goal of "communicative competence" (Fig. 33–9). On the other hand, if we treat communicative competence as a "relative" behavior rather than an "absolute," dependent upon the individual's potential for acquiring such, then most severely handicapped persons can succeed.

Technology: Barrier or Solution?

Severely physically handicapped infants and toddlers are usually motorically limited in the amount of interaction that they can have with their environment. This may limit learning, thus causing secondary handicaps and creating an even more handicapped individual. Goldenberg raises the question as to the level of motor interaction necessary to obtain the sensorimotor experiences needed by severely

TABLE 33-3 Some Basic Considerations in Evaluating the Functional Communication Needs of Severely Handicapped Children and Youth

- Does the child exhibit the desire to communicate?
  - Indicate behavior (how) desire is demonstrated
- Is there opportunity to communicate and interact with others?
  - Discuss with whom and in what way this takes place
- Are the child's communication attempts recognized and acted upon by others in the environment?
  - Show how this is done and what reciprocal behavior the child may engage in when there is a successful communication interaction
- What are the modes the child uses to communicate?
  - Has the child been taught to communicate or express his wants/needs in this manner, or has it come about spontaneously (self taught)?
- What potential modes for communication are available to the child which may improve functional communication?
  - Eye gaze; gestures; sign system; picture book, etc
- List the communication functions which the child currently uses
  - e.g., Requests; intentions
- What is the prognosis for oral communication?
  - See Shane and Bashir*
- Who serves as the primary message receiver?
  - Parent; caregiver
- How do the physical and social environments in which the child will primarily use the communication system affect the system chosen for use
  - Is the system primarily for school; work; home, etc.
- What are the educational and vocational goals for the child?
  - How the family considered special programming relative to vocational/work potential

* Shane HC, Bashir AS. Election criteria for the adoption of an augmentative communication system: preliminary considerations. *J Speech Hear Dis* 1980: 45:408–444.

motor handicapped individuals for cognitive development.

Goldenberg suggests that active control over the environment may not be necessary, and that handicapped individuals may be able to receive feedback from their surroundings in some other form. As a means of acquiring this information, Goldenberg suggests that microcomputer technology provides the means to maximize children's ability to interact with their environment, as well as providing a means to evaluate systematically the consistency and accuracy of those interactions.

The process of developing functional communication and effective interaction skills in severely handicapped children has been aided recently by the use of technology. The development of various alternative and augmentative communication systems has been successfully used with a number of severely handicapped individuals. Research in the area of nonelectronic and electronic communication aids has focused upon the development of assessment, prescription, and management strategies, and are reviewed elsewhere.[61–64]

Communication competence
Knowledge of:
When to speak (communicate)*
When not, and
As to what to talk (communicate)* about
With whom
Where, and
In what manner.

*Modifications by DE Yoder, 1985.

Figure 33-9 Defining communicative competence. (From Hymes D. Introduction. In: Cazden C, John V, Hymes D, eds. Functions of language in the classroom. New York: Teachers College Press, 1972; and Hymes D. On communicative competence. In: Pride JB, Holmes J, eds. Sociolinguistics. Baltimore: Penguin Books, 1972.)

Vanderheiden suggests that technology can also be used as an environmental control device.[65] The premise of this approach is to facilitate the learning and acquisition of co-occurrences and the notion that the individual can control or bring about change in the environment.

As was previously mentioned, severely handicapped infants and children may be overly passive, and therefore considered to have acquired a degree of learned helplessness. As such, severely handicapped infants and youth are generally not aware of the fact that their behaviors can bring about environmental change and feedback. The significance of being aware that their behavior can bring about change is valuable in the acquisition of cognitive and communicative competence. It is important that young severely handicapped infants and children acquire the competence or knowledge that they have the ability to detect and utilize co-occurrences. This competence, embedded in the changing concept of infants in general, has particular importance for developing process-oriented cognitive curriculums for handicapped infants. Brinker and Lewis discuss three basic types of co-occurrences, consisting of (a) two events that occur together in the environment, (b) two events that occur together with the organism, or (c) an event in the organism that co-occurs with an event in the environment.[66] According to Brinker and Lewis, the success or failure in detecting and remembering co-occurrences has important implications for subsequent development. They suggest that the successful detection and recall of co-occurrences has a positive effect upon motivational, affective, and cognitive structures.

The cognitive-developmental approach assumes that severely handicapped persons are capable of perceiving, interpreting, and evaluating contingencies in their respective environment. Recent efforts to investigate the phenomenon of the handicapped infants' ability to perceive environmental stimuli changes within these stimuli, and their ability to control the presentation of these stimuli has been aided by the introduction of microprocessors. Although still in its infancy, this research has provided valuable insight—particularly within the realm of Piagetian stage development and the potential to train handicapped infants within and between these stages—thus suggesting that the early introduction of social and environmental contingency awareness can contribute to the development of communicative competency.

The development of a generalized expectancy to control the physical and social worlds is a potential problem for handicapped infants.[60,66,67] Various handicapping conditions can deprive an infant of contingency experiences through one of the following mechanisms:

1. Medical involvement that decreases the opportunity for social interaction
2. Parental attitudes and feelings that may reduce the number of concurrence that the parents provide
3. The limited response repertoire of handicapped infants that generally makes both social and object co-occurrence less likely
4. The ability to detect and remember co-occurrence that may be limited for some handicapped children
5. A complex process of infant-environment transactions that progressively reduces the frequency of social co-occurrences.

Of the three kinds of co-occurrences, the type that may not be affected as dramatically by handicapping conditions is that involving internal events. The handicapped infant may be forced to rely on internal co-occurrences to consistently experience control over the environment. For example, Field found that developmentally-matched handicapped children differ from nonhandicapped children in that the former exhibited more behavior directed to self and less behavior directed to teachers and peers.[68] Furthermore, within the handicapped population, chronologically older children, who were developmentally matched to a younger handicapped population, showed less behavior directed to others.

It has been suggested that the detection of co-occurrences is dependent upon the young child's sensory abilities.[66,69] Specifically, Brinker and Lewis suggest that the association of two events to be detected rests on some form of short-term memory.[66] Another cognitive process advocated by Brinker and Lewis and Lewis and Goldberg as necessary for the detection of co-occurrences is the ability of the individual to maintain the information of co-occurrences over long periods of time.[66,69] Lewis and Goldberg and McCormick and Noonana suggest that the co-occurrences act on the individual in four ways. First, co-occurrences orient the child to attend to the environment. Second, they arouse the child and help to modulate its state. Third, the detection of co-occurrences leads to a positive affective tone. Fourth, through the operation of memory, they become elements for subsequent intentional actions and ultimately for the development of mental structure.[69,70]

In order to (a) account for the casual nature of the responsiveness-attention relationship and (b) to investigate whether responsiveness other than of a social nature is effective, Brinker and Lewis studied three handicapped infants.[67] Subjects included a low birth-weight premature infant whose chronological age was 3 months after correction for her prematurity, a 4-month-old female Down syndrome infant, and a 6-month-old Down syndrome male child. Using an Apple IIe, the computer was programmed to cycle through a series of consequences, depending upon the child.

For the children within this study, the microcomputer was programmed to cycle through three different consequences, switching after 2 minutes with each one if the criterion was met. The consequences for the infants included (a) a tape recording of the Sesame Street theme song, (b) activation of a battery powered train, and (c) presentation of a black and white drawing of a child's face. Movement of a predetermined limb with sufficient force resulted in a 4-second presentation of one of these consequences. Changing from one consequence to another occurred when fewer than four limb movements per minute occurred.

Infants who received contingent stimulation rather than noncontingent stimulation were expected to differ in at least three ways: (a) they would learn to pull the string to elicit a contingent consequence; (b) they would be more alert and interested and would therefore stay longer in the experimental setting before becoming fussy; and (c) they would be happier as a consequence of the contingency between behavior and the picture onset.

After brief periods of experimental intervention, these children learned to control consequences in their environment and also systematically to vary their behavior to explore specific contingencies. In Piagetian terms, they had developed procedures characteristic of secondary circular reactions.

The results of this study support the Lewis and Goldberg notion that contingent stimulation has cognitive, attentional, and motivational effects[69] and supports the other findings relating contingent stimulation to IQ scores. Although alert and cognitively advanced infants may elicit more environmental stimulation and responsiveness,[71] these data also support the notion that contingent environments may facilitate the cognitive development through its motivational, attentional, and affective features.

In a similar series of experiments, Behrmann and Lahm have been developing a systematic approach to teaching computerized environmental interactions.[72] The initial phase of their research project examines the parameters (motor, language, and cognitive developmental levels) for using the microcomputer to establish cause-effect relationships. Eight levels of use, ranging from the establishment of a cause-effect relationship to the use of a menu-driven program for initiating environmental interactions with multiply handicapped children between the ages of 6 and 12 months, were included.

Based on the research findings of Behrmann and Lahm, it appears that infants and toddlers understood the cause-effect relationship between the computer screen and the control switch. It also appears that their response times were adequate and consistent. Of the five mildly handicapped children who participated in this study, two met the criterion of responding in 5 seconds or less, 80 percent of the time over three or four sessions. Two other children were close to that criterion but were showing a deterioration of response time. The fifth child, although never close to criterion, showed the same deterioration of response time. The researchers interpreted these results by hypothesizing that the five children apparently understood the task, while the deterioration in performance was attributed to a loss of interest, with other aspects of the testing environment becoming more interesting to the child.

Subjectively, these studies suggest that lower functioning groups of handicapped children appear to understand the cause-effect relationship between the computer screen and their control switch, which is, at minimum, the prerequisite for using a computer system to control the environment functionally. However, these data indicate that children may have difficulty reaching a criterion response time of 5 seconds or less. It also appears that their response time can become adequate and consistent. The noted variance across handicapped infants in their ability to respond within set criterion times raises questions about expected levels of performance and response times that are realistic for severely multihandicapped children. However, after looking at the two distinct groups of handicapped children discussed in these studies, it becomes evident that there exists a need for empirical investigations to answer the question of what is an appropriate response, and how might training facilitate the acquisition of consistent and accurate responding.

According to Dickson what was once conceived as a solution to increasing communication skills within the classroom has, in fact, created an additional barrier for teachers.[73] Specifically, curricula which emphasize communication skills often require teachers to structure and organize activities. These additional time constraints place additional demands upon the teachers, and may result in the modifications of the curricula to accommodate the limited time.

Dickson suggests that given the pressures on schools to achieve multiple objectives, including social and communication skills, the creation of learning activities that offer rich opportunities for acquiring skills may be a viable solution to this problem. Dickson suggests that these activities may take the form of entire classroom activities, or learning centers deliberately structured for creating interaction between children.[73]

Within these structured environments, Dickson proposed the development and use of computerized software, which may facilitate academic learning and social interaction.[74] Used in this way, the computer can create a powerful educational tool, creating challenging, stimulating environments in which to learn.

The computer, therefore, can be used across a variety of situations which could significantly contribute to the severely handicapped student's learning environments and strategies. Traditionally, the computer has been used in education as a learning and instructional aid. The advantage of using the microcomputer in this manner is that it possesses the potential to interact with the user. It is able to present a stimulus, accept a response, evaluate the response, present appropriate feedback and reinforcement, record responses, and then move to the next instructional segment. This type of computer use, however, is not particularly conducive to exploratory learning.

Geoffrion and Goldenberg, Goldenberg, and Weir have reported effective gains resulting from Logo programming with severely cerebral-palsied children.[60,75,76] In these studies, children have demonstrated the ability to comprehend and express concepts that require spatial-environmental knowledge, as well as planned patterns of movement through the environment. The value of these exploratory learning programs (i.e., LOGO) is that they reinforce the concept of control over the environment in a motivating game-like format.

In summary, the microcomputer may be used as a powerful learning tool and communication aid for severely handicapped children. As a communication aid, microcomputers can make a unique contribution to language intervention with severely handicapped children, facilitating individual participation in both oral and written language. Meyers has suggested the following types microcomputer-based intervention designed to promote the acquisition and development of language and literacy skills:

1. A beginning communication device and language acquisition aid for severely physically handicapped toddlers
2. An augmentative communication device and language development tool for toddlers with delayed speech
3. A beginning reading and writing tool for handicapped pre-schoolers
4. A communicative device and language development tool for normal school-age children
5. A literacy development and remedial literacy tool for school-age handicapped children.[77]

The philosophy of microcomputer intervention with severely handicapped persons focuses upon normalizing the experiences of handicapped children rather than normalizing the behavior of these individuals. Unfortunately, longitudinal research and funds are necessary to further investigate the role of microcomputers as a habilitation tool with severely handicapped children.

TOWARD SOLUTIONS

Many factors have combined to stimulate efforts to improve the design and the delivery of assessment and intervention programs focused on the social and communicative skills of children and youth with severe handicaps. The obvious keystone for such efforts is the Federal laws that mandate appropriate and needed education services in least restrictive environments for all children. Undergirding and supplementing these laws, however, are philosophical, and moral motivations within our society, which insist that no person should be denied efforts to maximize his or her individual potential for participating in all dimensions of that society.

Some of the many barriers to the attainment of the ideal have been discussed. There are, however, many individuals and groups that have mounted efforts both to identify and to overcome these barriers. There is an obvious need to coordinate these efforts that now appear to be focused in four primary groups. One such group includes the professional associations that represent various academic and service disciplines that are active in the design and implementation of the intervention programs and services for children with severe handicaps. Another group active in these efforts is the collective of Federal agencies charged with the responsibility to support the research and development processes that will produce the intervention programs needed for the task. Also heavily involved in these efforts are the state and local agencies that are charged with the responsibility to assure that the needed educational services are delivered to those handicapped children who require them. The fourth readily identifiable group involved in the efforts to attain appropriate and adequate services for children and youth with severe handicaps is that collective made up of consumers of such programs and services—the children and youth who have severe handicaps and their families.

Important and relevant activity to suggest some solutions to the barriers and concerns discussed in this chapter grew out of the OSEP/TADS Symposium.[78]

The product of that Symposium provided a series of consensus statements about the provisions of quality intervention services to children and youth with severe handicaps. It also provided statements about goals and objectives that should direct efforts to attain such ideal services.[79]

The major points to be discussed here begin with a definition of "functional communication," which can be used to guide the development of appropriate assessment and treatment goals for persons with severe handicaps. This definition is followed by a discussion of major points made in the consensus statements from the symposium. These include statements relevant to (1) the ecological targets and contexts of intervention; (2) the delivery of such instruction; and (3) the needs of personnel offering such instruction.

A Definition of "Functional Communication"

The definition of "functional communication" arrived at in the Symposium was as follows:

1. The ability to communicate for a variety of purposes relevant to the individual's life experience
2. The ability to use a variety of means (e.g., verbal and/or nonverbal) to accomplish these purposes effectively

3. The ability to initiate and maintain social interactions as a critical dimension of communication (p III–2).[78]

This definition reflects a strong representation of the pragmatic dimensions of language and, as such, departs from past perspectives primarily focused on the linguistic-form dimension of language. Overall, then, the emphasis is on communication goals as opposed to language goals. The definition's specific reference to various modes of communication does not ignore the form component of communication. Rather, it insists that both the form and function dimensions of language be well represented in the intervention goals set forth for children and youth with severe handicaps.

Ecological Targets and Contexts for Intervention

The Symposium participants adopted the following consensus statement: "Communication programs for children and youth who are severely handicapped shall be provided within, and functionally oriented in the home, school, recreational, leisure, and vocational environments" (p III–4). They further state that: "These programs for the communication skills of severely handicapped children and youth shall be evaluated within each of these environments" (p III–4).[78] These statements function to operationalize and extend elements of the definition of functional communication. They demonstrate the view that such interventions are directed toward attaining communicative repertoires that will be useful in a broad range of environments. Further, they insist that evaluation of intervention successes be made on functional criteria—i.e., the targeting and attainment of communicative repertoires that are useful in various, normalized environments. These goals represent both important products and processes in communication intervention. As noted, they emphasize the attainment of both communicative form and function. They also point the way for identifying and attaining such products through the identification, analysis, and educational use of a variety of desireable environmental contexts for severely handicapped children and youth.

The Delivery of Instruction in Communication

The OSEP/TADS Symposium participants offered the following consensus statement regarding the delivery of instructional services in the communication domain:

> The delivery of instruction and services for communication skills to severely handicapped children and youth shall incorporate the knowledge, skills, and experiences of a variety of individuals such as parents, teachers, peers, speech-language pathologists, occupational therapists, physical therapists, audiologists, nurses, physicians, and employers (p III–4).[78]

Although such a far-ranging statement may be somewhat threatening to professionals in various academic and service disciplines, the basis upon which it was framed must be carefully examined. This statement appears to be based on three major realities in this difficult educational domain. The first reality is that the communicative needs of persons with severe handicaps must attain a density of programming that is quite beyond that which is reasonable for any one professional, or any one discipline, to provide. No one person can possibly offer enough intervention time to meet the needs of such children adequately. Further, no single professional discipline is represented in each and all of the environments in which communicative goals are sought and in which intervention contexts are provided. Thus, it must be made possible for many professionals (and nonprofessionals) to contribute to the improvement of the communicative skills of children and youth with severe handicaps. Second, and related to the first, is a realization that it is not effective to make one profession or discipline solely responsible for meeting the communicative needs of severely handicapped persons because, then, approaches often become narrow and begin to exclude other needed resources in both personnel and substance. Rather than vesting responsibility in one profession or discipline, all professionals and significant others must contribute to intervention programs in communication. As one faces the realities involved in meeting the needs of children with severe handicaps, one can see that only the richest program of multiple intervention participants is really fair to the children themselves. Such perspectives naturally assume multidisciplinary approaches that are coordinated and complementary. If multidisciplinary efforts are fractionated and parochial, effective intervention is essentially doomed.

The third basis for the Symposium participants' advocacy for a multidisciplinary approach to the communicative needs of children with severe handicaps is that if total responsibility is given to only one person or one discipline there is a high potential that other people and other disciplines that are important and highly visible in the children's environment will feel justified in not offering communicative training to such persons. There is no one who is knowledgeable about the need for responsiveness to the communicative behaviors of children with severe handicaps who can conscientiously ignore the usefulness of other persons in the intervention effort. Thus, parents and professionals in all academic and service disciplines can be, and should be, expected to contribute to the improvement of communicative skills among the severely handicapped student population.

Needs of Personnel Offering Instruction to Children with Severe Handicaps

Beyond the statement regarding the need for multidisciplinary and parental efforts for delivering intervention programs in communicative skills, the participants in the OSEP/TADS Symposium offered several statements regarding the need for substantive training of these personnel. The following four statements are pertinent to this issue. They are, as follows:

> Competencies necessary for personnel delivering services to children and youth who are severely handicapped must be identified;
>
> Preservice and continuing education programs, based on identified competencies, should be developed for personnel in communication skill programs for children who are severely handicapped;
>
> Personnel who work with severely handicapped children and youth shall be trained to incorporate communication skills into the curricula and to share responsibility for teaching these skills;
>
> Families of children and youth with severe handicaps should be provided instruction in ways to assist in the development and enhancement of communication skills (p III–7).[78]

The preceding statements all testify to the notion that the various multidisciplinary team members should *share* a common philosophical and substantive base for delivering communicative skill training to severely handicapped children. If we recall the definition about what constitutes functional communication and ecological validity in such treatment, we can see that it is the intent that all team members should share a basic body of knowledge that will allow them to function in a cooperative and complementary manner. This is, of course, a rather radical and demanding position. It means that *all* disciplines must commit to and implement the study of the communicative process at levels appropriate to children and youth with severe handicaps. Speech-language practitioners must extend their learning about communicative behaviors beyond linguistic language forms in the oral mode and be fully knowledgeable about prelinguistic communicative behaviors and the variables functional in their acquisition. Similarly, special educators specializing in providing service to the severely handicapped can no longer be satisfied with a few gross and arbitrary language goals to be 'trained' in mass-trial procedures one-on-one. Rather, all professionals and nonprofessionals working with severely handicapped children and youth must understand the basic processes by which social interaction repertoires and communicative behaviors emerge and are maintained and expanded.

Such shared knowledge bases should function to minimize obstacles to interdisciplinary efforts. Professionals with a common knowledge base should be able to work in complementary fashion with confidence that the child is being well served. Most disputes at the direct service level appear to occur in conditions where there are serious professional differences in the philosophy and goals for intervention.

Many of the participants in the OSEP/TADS Symposium reported on direct experience with multidisciplinary team efforts generated from common philosophical and substantive bases. These reports indicated that such experiences have, generally, been highly positive. More often than not, teams that shared common goals and philosophies tended to focus on the important needs of their child constituents. An appreciation of these needs and the work needed to satisfy them rather quickly dispelled disciplinary egocentrism. Though of course, this might not always be the case, it appears to be an appropriate target.

Other statements from this Symposium emphasized that State and local education agencies need to assure that appropriate substantive training and other supports will be made available to such multidisciplinary teams.

Two additional statements speak to the need for substantive training for all persons working in this educational domain. These read, as follows:

> Individuals who prepare speech-language pathologists should be provided opportunities and incentives to enhance their knowledge and skills in the area of effective communication programming for children and youth with severe handicaps; and
>
> Preservice preparation programs for speech-language pathologists should include information about, and experience with, children and youth with severe handicaps.

These specific statements reflect a concern that many professors in speech-language pathology and audiology preparation programs have no experience with severely handicapped children and thus, too often, professional preparation programs in speech-language and hearing do not prepare their professional personnel adequately for this ever-growing clinical and research constituency. While such indictments are punishing to the speech-language and hearing discipline, there are data that confirm that many speech-language and hearing professionals feel unprepared to meet the needs of persons with severe handicaps.[80]

There must also be more substantive training in *communication* skills of severe and profoundly handicapped persons for academic and service disciplines whose primary curricula are focused on other substance, such as special education and physical therapy. It makes for some improved symmetry for speech-language and hearing professionals to make concomitant efforts to assure that their knowledge of communicative systems is inclusive of knowledge important to the child with severe handicaps. The specification of the knowledge bases needed by each discipline cannot be adequately covered in this chapter, but rather, is available in a rapidly growing literature within the disciplines represented in the overall educational and therapeutic efforts being directed toward the population of persons with severe handicaps.

A wide range of professionals who are active in the provision of educational services to children and youth with severe handicaps are continuing to examine and discuss the barriers to attaining adequate intervention for the amelioration of the serious communication problems that are usually attendant to severely handicapped children and youth. These professionals continue to endorse an a priori assumption that educational services for these children must be provided in least restrictive environments; utilizing both professionals and parents; and marked by procedures and materials, which were age-appropriate in the sense that they do not cause such children ". . . to appear infantile, (or) devoid of personal preferences . . ." (p III–5).[78]

The following statements provide clear directions for efforts to provide quality communication treatment for children and youth with severe handicaps. These directions to be identified in four generalizations summarize the products of the OSEP/TADS Symposium. These generalizations are as follows:

1. The model for communication intervention should be one that focuses on the social functions of communication and recognizes a wide range of conventional and nonconventional means for attaining these functions
2. The delivery of communication intervention services should utilize professionals of many disciplines and should emphasize a role for parents
3. Improved substantive training in communication and language should be assured for all the professionals and nonprofessionals in the service chain for severely handicapped children
4. Professionals specializing in speech-language and hearing should be assured better education in applying current knowledge in that domain to the communicative problems of children with severe handicaps
5. Professionals in educational and therapeutic disciplines other than speech-language pathology and audiology also should be assured better education in the substance of communication and language that relates to the needs and status of children with severe handicaps.

Finally, the operationalization of these views will demand the full participation of all professional associations whose members are involved with severely handicapped children. The need for full Federal and State government involvement in these efforts is also required. Specifically, there is the need for State agencies to assure adequate inservice training and appropriate service delivery systems, and for Federal agencies to support the development of adequate and appropriate training in all pertinent academic disciplines, as well as support for demonstrations of idealized intervention programs aimed at the communication needs of children with severe handicaps.

SUMMARY

Developing communicative competence for most of us has been an easy and nonthought-giving process. To develop such competence for the severely handicapped child and young handicapped child and young persons has for the most part been extremely difficult, if attained at all. The barriers, which most severely handicapped persons face personally, have to do with problems in cognition, sensory avenues, and motor ability. Added to the personal concerns are environments that frequently are less supportive. These take on many different forms: from a parent who doesn't care to one who cares "too much"; from local education systems (LES), which provide a service, but of questionable quality, to LESs that leave no service unprovided and are of the best quality; from state systems that provide minimal funds to those that provide amply (never too much). There are policy issues that continue to threaten service delivery at all levels, and funds appear never to be sufficient. The barriers of poor assessment tools, intervention strategies and too few professionals trained to provide communication skills to severely handicapped, all add up to bring even the strongest among us to feel defeated.

There is hope. The changes that have come about in the past 15 years for the support of severely handicapped can be measured in many ways. Policy changes at the Federal level have assisted. Development of curricular materials and the education of personnel to serve severely handicapped persons is on the increase. New strategies for intervention, assessment, and advocacy have been encouraging. Technology continues to bring new focus on what can be accomplished for the welfare of severely handicapped persons. Though we can become discouraged by the barriers and hopeful with some of our solutions, we must also be continually pushing for MORE.

The future relative to providing the services necessary for developing communicative competence with severely handicapped persons lies not with any one agency, professional group of persons, parents, or paid advocates. The provision of the necessary service lies in the collective efforts of all agencies, policy makers, educators, institutions, parents, and the like. We must not only continue to seek out the service barriers and attempt to resolve them, but we must also be visionary and futuristic in our approach. While technology may be one of our more current and useful resources for providing communication strategies for the severely handicapped, let us not be seduced into believing it is going to answer our problems.

We have yet to take one more large and aggressive step to assisting in the services needed, and that, we believe, is to market the needs of the severely handicapped child and youth. It would be worthwhile exercise for all of us to explore how we might market the needs of the severely handicapped at the local, the state, and the regional level. With good marketing efforts, we believe there would eventually be an awareness of what the severely handicapped person may need of us, and also how severely handicapped persons can become more a part of the community from which we have too frequently excluded them. By providing the severely handicapped person a communicative system we will eventually allow them to "speak" for themselves—and what could be a stronger advertisement for the service, which we will have provided, than that?

NOTES

1. Portions of this chapter were presented at the symposium on Children and Youth With Severe Handicaps: Effective Communication. Washington D.C.: Office of Special Education Programs (OSEP) and Technical Assistance Development System (TADS), 1985.

2. The revised version of the WBRS will have norms for each of the subpopulations, residing within the community and within residential settings. Furthermore, the alternative items for severely handicapped children and youth (e.g., deaf-blind) will be incorporated within the scale, rather than as separate sections.

3. Dickson WP, Martin CA, Villarruel F. Using a microcomputer to create social interactions among handicapped and nonhandicapped children in a mainstream preschool. Working paper. 1985.

4. The major portion of the discussion in the section titled Toward Solutions is taken from a report of the ASHA/TASH Joint Committee on Persons with Severe Handicaps entitled Improving Communication Intervention for Children and Youth with Severe Handicaps. James E. McLean, Committee Chair and primary author, 1987.

REFERENCES

1. Higginbotham DJ, Yoder DE. Communication within natural conversational interaction: implications for severely communicatively impaired persons. Top Lang Disord 1982; 2:1–19.
2. Karen OC, Berger C. Developing support networds for individuals who fail to achieve competitive employment. In: Rush FR, ed. Competitive employment: service delivery models, methods, and issues. Baltimore: Brookes Publishing, 1986.
3. Baker DB. Severely handicapped: toward an inclusive definition. AAESPH Review 1979; 4:52–65.
4. Dollar SJ, Brooks C. Assessment of severely and profoundly handicapped individuals. Except Educ Q 1980; 1:87–101.
5. Dubose RF. Identification. In: Snell ME, ed. Systematic instructions of the moderately and severely handicapped. Columbus, OH: Merrill-Palmer, 1979.
6. Fewell RR, Cone JD. Identification and placement of severely handicapped children. In: Snell ME, ed. Systematic instructions of the moderately and severely handicapped. 2nd ed. Columbus, OH: Merrill-Palmer, 1983.
7. Sontag E, Smith J, Sailor W. The severely/profoundly handicapped: Who are they? Where are they? J Spec Educ 1977; 11:5–11.
8. Bureau for Education of the Handicapped. Office of Education. Federal Register 40, 1975.
9. Flathouse VE. Identifying needs and resources in the delivery of instructional services. In: Campbell B, Baldwin RV, eds. Severely handicapped/hearing impaired students: strengthening service delivery. Baltimore: Brookes Publishing, 1982.
10. Cherow E, Matkin ND, Trybus RJ. Hearing-impaired children and youth with developmental disabilities. Washington, DC: Gallaudet College Press, 1985.
11. Appell MW. Early education for the severely handicapped/hearing impaired child. In: Campbell B, Baldwin RV, eds. Severely handicapped/hearing impaired students: strengthening service delivery. Baltimore: Brookes Publishing, 1982.
12. Sheehan R. Infant assessment: a review and identification of emergent trends. In: Bricker DD, ed. Intervention with at-risk and handicapped infants: from research to application. Baltimore: University Park Press, 1982, 47–61.
13. Brown L, Branston MB, Hamre-Nietupski S, Pumpian I, Certo N, Gruenewald L. A strategy for developing chronological-age-appropriate functional curricular content for severely handicapped adolescents and young adults. J Spec Educ 1979; 13(1):81–90.
14. Falvey MA. Community based curriculum: instructional strategies for students with severe handicaps. Baltimore: Brookes Publishing, 1986.
15. Gruenewald L, Schroeder J, Yoder DE. Consideration for curriculum development and implementation. In: Campbell B, Baldwin V, eds. Severely handicapped/hearing impaired students: strengthening service delivery. Baltimore: Brookes Publishing, 1982.
16. Halpern AS, Fuhrer MJ. Functional assessment in rehabilitation. Baltimore, MD: Brookes Publishing, 1982.
17. Karen OC, Berstein GS, Harvey JR, Bates PE, Renzaglia A, Clees T. An extended evaluation model for the severely handicapped. AAESPH Rev 4 4:374–398.
18. Wehman P, Hill JW. Preparing severely handicapped youth for less restrictive environments. Assoc Severely Handic 7:33–39.
19. Fewell RR, Sandall SR. Developmental testing of handicapped infants: a measurement dilemma. Top Early Childhood Spec Educ 6(3):86–99.
20. Frankenberg WK, Dodds JB, Fandal AW, Kazuk E, Cohrs

M. Denver Developmental Screening Test (DDST). LADOCA Project & Publishing Foundation, 1975.
21. Bayley N. The Bayley Scales of Infant Development. New York: Psychological Corporation, 1969.
22. Campbell SK, Siegel E, Parr CA, Ramey CT. Evidence for need to renorm the Bayley scales of infant development based on the performance of a population-based sample of 12-month-old infants. Top Early Childhood Educ 1986; 6:83–96.
23. McLean JE, Snyder-McLean LK/A transactional approach to early language training. Columbus, OH: Merrill Publishing, 1978.
24. Wasson P, Tynan T, Gardiner P. Test adaptations for the handicapped. Austin, TX: Educational Service Center, Region 20, 1982.
25. Higginbotham DJ, Mathey-Laikko P, Reichle JE, Lippert J, Yoder DE. Early Communication Skills Curriculum (ECSC). Madison, WI: Central Wisconsin Center for Developmental Disability, 1984.
26. Kratochwill T. Single subject research—strategies for evaluating change. New York: Academic Press, 1978.
27. McReynolds LV, Kearns K. Single-subject experimental designs in communicative disorders. Austin, TX PRO-ED, 1983.
28. Song A, Jones S, Lippert J, Metzgen K, Miller J, Borrca C. Wisconsin Behavior Rating Scale. Madison, WI: Central Wisconsin Center for the Developmentally Disabled, 1980.
29. Song A, Jones S, Lippert J, Metzgen K, Miller J, Borreca C. Wisconsin behavior rating scale: measure of adaptive behavior for the developmental levels of 0 to 3 years. Am J Ment Defic 1984; 88:401–411.
30. Nahira K, Foster R, Shellhass M, Leland H. AAMD Adaptive Behavior Scale. Washington, DC: AAMD, 1974.
31. Doll EA. Vineland Social Maturity Scale. Circle Pines, MN: American Guidance Service, 1965.
32. Brown L, Falvey M, Vincent L, Kaye N, Johnson F, Ferrara-Parrish P, Gruenewald L. Strategies for generating comprehension, longitudinal and chronological age appropriate individual educational plans for adolescent and young adult severely handicapped students. J Spec Educ 1980; 14(2):199–215.
33. Miller JF. Assessing children's language behavior: a developmental approach. In: Schiefelbusch RF, ed. Bases of language intervention. Baltimore: University Park Press, 1978.
34. Donnellan AM, Mirenda PL, Mesaros RA, Fassbender LL. Analyzing the communicative functions of abberant behavior. J Assoc Severely Handicapped 1984; 9(3):201–202.
35. Schuler AL, Goetz C. The assessment of severe language disabilities: communicative and cognitive considerations. Anal Interv Develop Disabil 1981; 1:333–346.
36. Bricker DD, Carlson L. Issues in early language intervention. In: Schiefelbusch RL, Bricker DD, eds. Early language: acquisition and intervention. Baltimore: University Park Press, 1981:477.
37. Miller JF, Chapman RS, Branston MB, Reichle J. Language comprehension in sensorimotor stages V and VI. J Speech Hear Res 1980; 23:284–311.
38. Thoman EB. Affective communication as the prelude and context for language learning. In: Schiefelbusch RL, Bricker DD, eds. Early language: acquisition and intervention. Baltimore: University Park Press, 1981.
39. Bruner J. The ontogenesis of speech acts. J Child Lang 1975; 2:1–19.
40. Ingalls RP. Mental Retardation. New York: John Wiley, 1978.
41. Seligman M. Helplessness. San Francisco: WH Freeman, 1975.
42. Fabricius WV, Wellman HM. Memory development. J Children Contemp Soc 1983; 16:171–187.
43. Flavell JH, Wellman HM. metamemory. In: Kail RV, Hagen JW, eds. Perspectives on the development of memory and cognition. Hillsdale, NJ: Erlbaum, 1977.
44. Fouts RS, Couch JB, O'Neil CR. Strategies for primate language training. In: Schiefelbusch RL, Hollis JH, eds. Language intervention from ape to child. Baltimore: University Park Press, 1979.
45. Lewis ML, Brooks-Gunn J. Toward a theory of social cognition: the development of self. In: Uzgiris I, ed. Social interaction and communication during infancy. San Francisco: Jossey-Bass, 1979.
46. Siegel-Causey E, Guess D. Early development of prelinguistic communication. In: Bullis M, ed. Communication development in young children with deaf-blindness: literature review I (Contract No. 300–83–0237). Manmouth, OR: Oregon State System of Higher Education, Deaf-Blind Communication Skills Center, 1985.
47. Prizant BM. Reactions to Yoder & Villarruel Paper. Proceedings from OSEP/TADS Symposium on Children and Youth with Severe Handicaps-Effective Communication. Washington, DC, 1985.
48. Yoder DE. Communication systems for nonspeech children. New Direc Exceptional Children 1980; 2:63–78.
49. Yarrow L, Klein R, Lomonaco S, Morgan G. Cognitive and motivational development in early childhood. In: Friedlander B, Sterrit G, Kirk G, eds. Exceptional infant, Vol. 3. New York: Brunner-Mazel, 1975.
50. Keogh WJ, Reichle J. Communication intervention for the "difficult-to-reach" severely handicapped. In: Warren SF, Rogers-Warren AK, eds. Teaching functional language. Baltimore: University Park Press, 1985.
51. Bates E. Language and context: the acquisition of pragmatics. New York: Academic Press, 1976.
52. Reichle JE, Yoder DE. Communication board use in severely handicapped learners. Lang Speech Hear Services Schools 1985; 16(3):146–157.
53. Bricker D, Carlson L. An intervention approach for communicatively handicapped infants and young children. New Direc Exceptional Children 1980; 2:33–48.
54. Mahoney GJ. Ethological approach to delayed language acquisition. Am J Ment Defic 1975; 80:139–148.
55. Halle JW. Teaching functional language to the handicapped: an integrative model of natural environment teaching techniques. J Assoc Severely Handicapped 1982; 7:29–37.
56. McDonald J. Language through conversation: a model for intervention with language delayed persons. In: Warren SF, Rogers-Warren AK, eds. Teaching functional language. Baltimore: University Park Press, 1985.
57. Mahoney GJ, Weller EL. An ecological approach to language intervention. New Direc Exceptional Children 1980; 2:17–32.
58. Warren SF, Rogers-Warren AK. Teaching functional language: an introduction. In: Warren SF, Rogers-Warren AK, eds. Teaching functional language. Baltimore: University Park Press, 1985.
59. Donnellan A, Falvey M, Pumpian I, Baumgart D, Schroeder J, Brown L. A strategy for evaluating educational programs for students with autism and other handicapping conditions (draft). Madison, WI: Madison Metropolitan School District, 1980.
60. Goldenberg EP. Social technology for special children. Baltimore: University Park Press, 1979.
61. Musselwhite CR, St. Louis KW. Communication programming for the severely handicapped: vocal and non-vocal strategies. San Diego: College-Hall Press, 1982.
62. Romski MA, Sevick RA, Joyner SE. Nonspeech communication systems: implications for language intervention with mentally retarded children. Top Lang Disord 1984; 5(1):66–81.
63. Schiefelbusch RL, ed. Nonspeech language and communication: analysis and intervention. Baltimore: University Park Press, 1980.
64. Blackstone S. Augmentative communication. In: Lass N, Northern J, McReynolds L, Yoder DE, eds. Handbook on

speech, language & hearing. Philadelphia: BC Decker, 1987.
65. Vanderheiden GC. Practical application of microcomputers to aid the handicapped. Comput 1981; 1:54–61.
66. Brinker RP, Lewis M. Discovering the competent handicapped infant: a process approach to assessment and intervention. Top Early Childhood Spec Educ 1982; 2:1–6.
67. Brinker RP, Lewis M. Making the world work with microcomputers: a learning prosthesis for handicapped infants. Except Child 1982; 48:163–70.
68. Field T. Self, teacher, toy, and peer-directed behaviors of handicapped preschool children. In: Field T. ed. High-risk infants and children: adult and peer interaction. New York: John Wiley, 1980.
69. Lewis M, Goldberg S. Perceptual-cognitive development in infancy: a generalized expectancy mold as a function of mother-infant interaction. Merrill-Palmer Q 1969; 15:81–100.
70. McCormick L, Noonan MJ. A responsive curriculum for severely handicapped preschoolers. Top Early Childhood Spec Educ 1984; 4:79–96.
71. Lewis M, Rosenblum L. The effect of the infant on its caregiver: the origins of behavior. New York: John Wiley, 1974.
72. Behrmann MM, Lahm L. Critical learning: multiply handicapped babies get on-line. In: Behrmann MM, Lahm L, eds. Proceedings of the National Conference on the Use of Microcomputers in Special Education. Reston, VA: The Council for Exceptional Children, 1984.
73. Dickson WP. Creating a communication-rich classroom. In: Wilkinson LC, ed. Communicating in the classroom. New York: Academic Press, 1982.
74. Dickson WP. Thought-provoking software: juxtaposing symbol systems. Educ Researcher 1985; 14:30–38.
75. Geoffrion LD, Goldenberg EP. Computer-based exploratory learning systems for communication-handicapped children. J Spec Educ 1981; 15:325–331.
76. Weir S. Logo and exceptional children. Microcomput 1981; 84:76–82.
77. Meyers LF. Using contribution of microcomputers to language intervention with handicapped children. Semin Speech Lang 1984; 5:23–24.
78. Office of Special Education Programs (OSEP) and Technical Assistance Development System (TADS). A symposium: children and youth with severe handicaps—effective communication. Washington, DC, 1985.
79. McLean JE. Improving communication intervention for children and youth with severe handicaps. Committee report, Personal communication, ASHA/TASH. Joint committee on persons with severe handicaps. 1987.
80. Larkins P. Serving the deinstitutionalized mentally retarded and developmentally disabled population—what are the issues? Asha 1986; 28(11):43–45.

34 Augmentative Communication

Sarah W. Blackstone, Ph.D.
E. Lucinda Cassatt-James, M.A.

Communication underlies the power and pleasure of the human experience, providing each individual with a vital human link. One cannot express feelings, request assistance, state opinions, tell a joke, access information, create poetry, or meet basic needs without the ability to communicate. Language expressed through speech is perhaps our most commonly used communication medium. It helps us organize thoughts, express knowledge and ideas, and control each day's experiences. Of course, speech is not our only means of expression. In fact, more than 60 percent of our messages are conveyed through other means, such as gestures, facial expressions, body posture, and tone of voice.[1]

Augmentative communication is a relatively new area of clinical practice within the field of communication sciences and disorders that addresses the needs of individuals who have severe difficulty speaking. It refers to all forms of human communication that supplement or enhance speech. According to Vanderheiden and Yoder, everyone uses augmentative aids, symbols, and techniques to accomplish a variety of daily communication tasks.[2] Special augmentative aids, symbols, and techniques provide ways for individuals with severe speech-language impairments to produce messages that are recognizable and interpretable by both partners in an interaction.

For all speakers, ideas and messages are expressed via a multicomponent system of communication.[2] This system is comprised of speech as well as a variety of the traditional and special augmentative communication components listed in Table 34–1. The extent to which augmentative communication is employed by an individual depends upon the situation and the demands of the communicative task, the skills of the individual who must execute the task, the aids or techniques employed, and the partner's familiarity with them.

HISTORICAL PERSPECTIVE

In the 1960s and 1970s, some speech-language pathologists and teachers were introducing language boards and manual signs to individuals who could hear, but were physically handicapped, aphasic, mentally retarded, and autistic.[3–7]

Recently, awareness of the augmentative communication area and the availability of these clinical interventions has increased dramatically. Reasons for this rapid growth can be found both within and outside the field of communication sciences and disorders. For example, PL 94–142 (Education for All Handicapped Children Act), passed in 1975, requires states to provide an "appropriate education" within a "least restrictive environment" to school-age children. A more recent law (PL 99–457) provides additional money to encourage states to extend educational opportunities to preschool children. As a result, groups of previously unserved, multihandicapped children have been brought to the attention of professionals in educational settings. It became obvious that children who could not express what they knew could not be tested, respond to questions, participate in class discussions, or complete homework assignments, thus resulting in communicative dissonance (i.e., a dissociation between communication needs and capabilities).[8] In short, they could not benefit from their educational experience. To address the needs of these individuals, speech-language pathologists, teachers, and other professionals began to employ a range of augmentative symbols, aids, strategies, and techniques that

TABLE 34–1 Examples of Augmentative Aids, Techniques, and Symbols

Standard—used by all individuals
Aids: paper and pencil, typewriters, telephones, and computers
Techniques: vocalizations, gestures, facial expressions, head nods
Symbols: alphabet, pictures, line drawings
Special—used by speech- and writing-impaired individuals
Aids: Etrans, language boards and books, speech aids, electronic communication aids, speech synthesizers, adapted computers, switch technologies
Techniques: direct selection, scanning, encoding, manual signs
Symbols: Picsyms, Blissymbolics, special symbol sets

enable severely speech-language impaired children to participate in the educational process.

For adults, the Rehabilitation Act Amendments of 1986 (PL 99–506) place emphasis on individuals with severe handicaps. Such individuals are defined as persons "who have a severe physical or mental disability which seriously limits one or more functional capabilities (such as mobility, communication, self-care self-directions, interpersonal skills, work tolerance or work skills) in terms of employability." The law promotes supported employment (i.e., competitive work in integrated work settings) for individuals with severe handicaps. In addition, the law places increased emphasis on the rehabilitation engineering needs of individuals with severe handicaps. This rehabilitation includes the development and use of augmentative communication systems.

Severe handicaps, rehabilitation engineering, and supported employment opens new avenues for individuals with severe communication disorders who need augmentative communication assistance. Passage of the Rehabilitation Act Amendments of 1986 undoubtedly will affect the growth of augmentative communication in the adult population.

Another factor that affected the growth of augmentative communication was the increased sophistication and decreased cost of computer technologies that could meet a broader range of communication needs for individuals with disabilities, including conversation, writing, graphics, computer access, and telecommunications. Today, the interface problem between human and machine is solved, largely through the utilization of switches, software, and keyboard emulators that permit even the most severely physically impaired to access computers. More than 50 computer-based communication aids are commercially available. Thus individuals can choose from among a variety of features to address specific communication needs.

Within the health-care industry and in some educational settings, a functional approach to disability is being adopted that involves professionals from several disciplines working together. A functional emphasis is important because in most cases, individuals with severe speech impairments are permanently disabled and require life-long management.[9] An interdisciplinary effort is required because of the complexity of issues involved in augmentative communication interventions. The role of professionals in the augmentative communication area is not to "cure" the problem because, unfortunately, "speech cures" are often not possible. Rather, the goal of augmentative communication interventions is to provide compensatory means that enable individuals to function by lessening the impact of limited speech on their daily experiences and opportunities.

The purpose of this chapter is to provide an overview of the augmentative communication area. It begins with defining augmentative communication and its role in the communication of typical as well as impaired speakers. Following this discussion, an overview of the population who uses augmentative aids and techniques and current service delivery approaches is provided. The next section of the chapter attempts to organize aspects of treatment that must be considered by providing an approach to intervention that accounts for the individual client, the augmentative communication components, the context, and the communication tasks in which the client is involved. The development of conversational skills is highlighted. In the final section, we share our perceptions of research areas that need to be addressed to insure the continued effectiveness of augmentative interventions.

THE POPULATION

An estimated two million hearing people in the United States are unable to speak so that others can understand them.[10] An even greater number are unable to write without assistance. The etiologies of severe expressive communication disorders can be congenital or may be acquired at any point in a person's life, from birth to death. Speech problems may improve, remain essentially unchanged, or worsen over time. They are generally permanently disabling, but may also be temporary.

Most severe speech impairments are the result of neurologic problems. Congenital and acquired conditions that affect the central nervous system have associated speech and language impairments. The pattern of neurologic abnormality and the effect on speech vary according to the site and extent of the lesion and the resulting disruption to the central nervous system. Damage to the cortex may affect cognitive, language, motor, and sensory and perceptual systems. Obviously, the greater the damage to the cortex, the more severely impaired and multihandicapped an individual is likely to be. For example, individuals with a primary diagnosis of cerebral palsy, mental retardation, Huntington's chorea, aphasia, and severe head injuries have a high incidence of speech as well as cognitive, language, motor, and other disorders. Conversely, damage to subcortical areas, such as the brain stem and spinal cord, may leave cognition and language intact, whereas motor and sensory deficits that interfere with speech production may be severe.

Some neurologic conditions result in writing impairments only. Augmentative communication teams often have experience addressing the needs of these individuals, as well. Severe writing impairments often exist secondary to motor (e.g., high spinal cord injury that leaves an individual able to speak, but unable to move the upper extremities) or sensory problems (e.g., individuals who are blind). Many individuals who are speech impaired are also writing impaired as a result of multihandicapping conditions.

In addition to neurologic abnormalities, augmentative communication interventions are applied to individuals with medical conditions and/or structural problems involving the face, head, and neck that preclude or interfere with speech production. For example, speech aids and communication aids may be recommended after surgical interventions (i.e., glossectomy or laryngectomy) or because of temporary or permanent tracheostomies.

The problems experienced by individuals with severe speech impairments are the result of either congenital or acquired conditions. These factors are discussed next.

Congenital Conditions

Congenital conditions, by definition, are not progressive and occur during a period of active brain growth. Thus, although the disability is permanent, children with congenital disabilities can and should be expected to make progress year after year. Of course, the extent to which each individual becomes an independent, functional citizen depends on the quality and quantity of interventions provided and on the nature and severity of the disabling condition. Because habilitative services are now mandated within the educational system for children and youth, theoretically, at least, individuals with congenital impairments should be able to reach their functional potential.

Unfortunately, children born with a congenital disability may be limited not only by their handicapping condition(s) (e.g., cerebral palsy, autism, mental retardation, blindness and deafness, severe developmental speech and language disorders), but also by the limitations that are often placed upon them as they grow up.[11] For example, a physically impaired child who is unable to crawl or walk cannot explore the environment or easily play with other children. Similarly, a child with no speech cannot ask simple questions, make mistakes, and/or practice social skills in school or in the community. Without early and consistent intervention, these children are likely to be deprived of appropriate social and learning opportunities.

As adults, some individuals with severe congenital impairments live independently; however, most do not. In part, this lack of independence reflects the severe nature of their problems and multihandicapping conditions. Many times, however, it also reflects the lack of or limited experiences and educational opportunities that adults with severe disabilities have during childhood. Behavioral problems, poor communication skills, poor work habits, restricted experiences, and limited educational achievement preclude many from participating in leisure, vocational, and even social interactions. This lack of opportunity for interaction is particularly true for those who live or have lived in institutions. "Passivity" or "learned helplessness" is a well-described pattern of behavior.[12] It means that the individual develops a passive reaction to the environment because of repeated experiences of being in a passive, helpless state. It is a difficult pattern to change, particularly in adults. In reviewing the augmentative communication literature, we found that the term "learned helplessness" is used to describe nonspeaking individuals with congenital disabilities who are also physically impaired and/or who possess concomitant, significant cognitive limitations. Whether those with acquired speech impairments exhibit similar behaviors is unknown.

Many adults with less severe cognitive and physical handicaps are also prevented from living independently and from securing employment because of their severe communication impairments. Often, their communication system is intelligible to only a limited number of partners. In other cases, they do not have the needed vocabulary that would allow them to carry out tasks at their job sites, communicate during emergencies, or interact with their fellow employees. Unlike children, adults with congenital impairments often have limited access to services or recourse if these services are not provided. Many adult centers offer only day-care programs with little functional training or structured activities provided.

Acquired Conditions

Those individuals who suddenly lose their ability to speak must be viewed from a different perspective than those who are born with a disability. Acquired speech impairments are generally related to three different etiologies: traumatic injury or insult to the brain, degenerative neurologic disease processes, or surgical interventions. In traumatic injuries (whether internally sustained, as in a stroke, or externally imposed, as in a head injury), the event causing impairment occurs suddenly, and improvements can be expected in varying degrees over a number of years. Conversely, with degenerative conditions, speech deteriorates gradually, and expectations for improvement are rare. The third group of individuals with acquired conditions are those whose production of speech is interrupted because of structural problems associated with surgical interventions (e.g., laryngectomy, tracheostomy, glossectomy). Although this group, like the traumatically injured, experiences a sudden loss of speech and an abrupt need for augmentative communication, like those with progressive disorders, they often face the possibility of a recurrence of their disease.

Traumatic Injuries and Insults

Individuals who sustain traumatic injuries experience an unexpected disruption to life as they have known it. Often, these individuals wake up in a hospital and gradually learn that they have been injured or had a stroke that has left them unable to communicate. They remember what it was like to have "normal speech," which makes it difficult to adjust to their handicapping conditions. Many times, the traumatically injured have difficulty accepting special communication aids and techniques, particularly if they make them "look" (e.g., use of a light pointer or a head stick) or "sound" (e.g., a speech synthesizer) different. Even those with mild impairments may become depressed and frustrated. In most cases, however, improvement is possible, thus providing motivation for rehabilitation. Progress can continue over many years, although the most dramatic gains generally occur within the first year. Most persons gradually readjust their lives to accommodate their disabilities. Critical to their rehabilitation is the support they receive from persons in the home, school, community, and/or work. They also receive support from many professional services throughout the course of their recovery.

Like those with congenital impairments, individuals with traumatically acquired communication disorders often have concomitant impairments. The degree of impairment varies depending upon the amount of brain or structural damage the individual incurs. Individuals with damage to the cortex (as observed in head injuries and strokes) often have motor, language, sensory, and cognitive deficits. In many cases, new learning may be difficult or impossible, although some previously acquired skills may be retained. For example, individuals may recall their multiplication tables by rote, but be unable to multiply numbers to complete a homework assignment. The functional profile of these individuals is often uneven. Many times their orientation and behavior vary from day to day. Families and professionals unfamiliar with the variable profiles of the brain injured find this inconsistency in performance and the differences between new and old learning patterns confusing.

When considering augmentative communication interventions, one needs to take impaired learning skills and physical and language disabilities into consideration. On the one hand, it is often contraindicated to select aids and techniques that require the brain-injured child or adult to learn a new way of doing something (e.g., Morse code), until the person demonstrates a capacity to learn new information and to recall it over time. On the other hand, some residual reading and spelling skills may mean the person can use the alphabet functionally on a communication board to create at least some novel messages.

Individuals with lesions only to subcortical areas are less likely to have accompanying language and cognitive problems. For example, persons who have a brain stem stroke or tumor (pontine glioma) experience motor impairments that may affect the bulbar musculature (i.e., larynx, face, lips, tongue, and palate) supplied from the pons and medulla. Those with spinal cord injuries may have functional speech, but no means to complete written communication.

Individuals may also require augmentative aids and/or techniques temporarily. For example, in intensive care units of hospitals, patients are often intubated and have tracheostomies (i.e., they are temporarily unable to speak or write). Gestures, alphabet boards, simple manual signs, and call signals are often their only modes of communication. Dowden reported that these techniques are preferable to electronic aids in acute care settings because they are familiar, readily available, and do not require extensive staff and family training.[13] They allow communication to continue while speech is temporarily interrupted or until a more permanent augmentative aid or technique can be recommended.

Degenerative Conditions

Children and adults with deteriorating neurologic or medical conditions gradually lose their ability to speak and, in some cases, to move, understand, think, and remember. The time frame for this gradual loss of skills can range from a few months to more than 30 years. To intervene appropriately, professionals who work with these individuals need to understand the cause and course of the disease and the prognosis.

Although progressive disease conditions rarely occur in childhood, some examples of degenerative diseases that do affect children include dystonia musculorum deformans and muscular dystrophy, which affect the motor system, and the inborn errors of metabolism and storage diseases, which affect all brain functions.

Progressive neurologic diseases, like congenital and traumatic conditions, may affect upper and/or lower motoneurons. For example, in amyotrophic lateral sclerosis, the anterior horn cells of the spinal cord deteriorate, causing a dissociation between the central nervous system and the peripheral nervous system with a resulting loss of motor function. When the deterioration occurs (as it often does) high in the cord, the innervation of cranial nerves critical to the production of speech and other oral motor functions is affected (i.e., cells that innervate the bulbar musculature in the brain stem). Paralysis results, causing gradually worsening dysarthria and dysphagia. Since the deterioration affects spinal cord neurons only, these individuals remain intact cognitively and lose only motor function. Writing is gradually precluded because the degeneration nearly always affects the use of the upper extremities. Augmentative interventions can be effective in meeting this group's communication needs. The need for special aids and techniques continues to increase as the disease progresses.

In other degenerative conditions (e.g., multiple sclerosis, Parkinson's disease, acquired immunodeficiency syndrome), a more pervasive deterioration of the central nervous system occurs (i.e., cognitive function may deteriorate as well). As with all augmentative interventions, the application of aids and techniques must account for the individual's present and future communication needs. As dementia increases, individuals may continue to require assistance communicating, but they exhibit less interest in interacting with the environment, and gradually augmentative interventions become less effective. Thus the need for augmentative interventions may decline as the disease progresses.

Postsurgical Conditions

Individuals who require augmentative communication interventions as a result of the surgical removal of tissue and organs underlying speech production generally have medical conditions that directly threaten life (e.g., cancer). Some individuals may be able to use speech aids (e.g., electrolarynx), whereas others (those who have complete laryngectomies and glossectomies) require communication aids. Although rare, severe speech impairments may also occur secondary to brain damage to speech areas sustained during surgical procedures. For example, 10 to 20 percent of those with the genetically inherited torsion dystonia or dystonia musculorum deformans who undergo a thalamotomy in an attempt to improve motor function lose their ability to speak as a result of the operation.[14]

Professionals who work with this group deal not only with the life-threatening conditions that originally necessitated surgery (e.g., cancer), but also with the effects on individuals of a sudden loss of speech. Thus intervention considerations may be similar to those experienced by individuals with traumatic insults and degenerative disease processes.

Severe speech and writing impairments are conditions that can occur at any point in an individual's life. Many times the impairment is a result of neurologic problems although medical difficulties and structural conditions can also result in severe expressive communication impairments. These individuals can benefit from augmentative interventions. The next section provides an overview of service delivery in this area of practice.

SERVICE DELIVERY

Team Approach

Clinical services are provided to individuals requiring augmentative communication interventions in all types of clinical settings (i.e., schools, hospitals, rehabilitation centers, private clinics, university clinics, residential institutions, and the client's home). Because of the complex nature of their clients' problems, an interdisciplinary team is generally required to address adequately the needs of these individuals. The most important members on the team are the individual with limited speech and the individual's primary caregivers. Professionals on the team are from multiple disciplines and include those with knowledge and skills necessary to (1) assess the individual's cognitive, language, motor, and sensory skills and abilities; (2) analyze communication tasks that need to be accomplished; (3) select and recommend augmentative communication aids and techniques; (4) describe and identify contextual variables that could contribute to the success or failure of intervention; (5) train individuals to use augmentative aids and techniques effectively to meet their communication needs under various conditions; and (6) provide the follow-up and reassessment necessary to insure a life-long management approach to intervention. Augmentative communication teams also have access to and knowledge about the range of equipment and materials available to meet the communication needs of these individuals.

David Crystal identified four major areas that professionals practicing in augmentative communication need to be knowledgeable about.[15] These are

1. Adult language models.
2. Normal development (language, cognitive, motor) and developmental disabilities.
3. Technology and materials.
4. Interaction characteristics of persons employing augmentative communication.

Because of the type of expertise required, speech-language pathologists often play a leadership role on augmentative communication teams. The American Speech-Language-Hearing Association (ASHA) published a position statement defining the role of the speech-language pathologist and the scope of practice.[16] More recently, the Augmentative Communication Committee at ASHA prepared a list of clinical competencies underlying these practices. Among the competencies included are a knowledge of normal and disordered nonverbal and verbal communication processes; familiarity with both the adult and developmental models of language, language disorders, and speech motor dysfunction; understanding the interaction characteristics of augmentative and natural speakers; and skills in the application of the technologies and materials available (symbol systems, communication aids, computers, switches, and so on). Another important competency involves employing effective training strategies to insure that aids, symbols, techniques, and strategies are used effectively to enhance communication in a variety of settings. Speech-language pathologists also maintain dialogues with families, manufacturers of aids and devices, and other professionals on the team (e.g., occupational therapists, physical therapists, special educators, vocational rehabilitation counselors, rehabilitation engineers, psychologists, social workers). Therefore they should be familiar with (1) team management skills, (2) family dynamics, (3) various features of communication aids and modification options, (4) human-matching and machine-matching interfacing techniques, (5) seating and positioning to facilitate communication, (6) mobility issues, (7) funding issues, and (8) integrating augmentative communication into the client's daily social, academic, vocational, and leisure activities.

Some teams are composed of professionals who work part-time in the area of augmentative communication. Others see only individuals who require augmentative interventions. Depending upon the setting, availability, and expertise of staff, teams may provide services to the spectrum of clients with congenital and acquired conditions, or they may specialize. For example, teams in educational settings and rehabilitation hospitals sometimes work exclusively with one population (i.e., children who are autistic and happen to live within a particular school district). Or a team may specialize in providing sophisticated technologies to severely physically handicapped individuals. In general, most augmentative communication teams attempt to provide services to all those within the community who require them.

The configuration of the augmentative team changes over time. This change reflects a life-long management concept and the changing communication needs and capabilities of individuals over time. During childhood, for example, augmentative teams are often made up of parents, teachers, speech-language pathologists, and occupational or physical therapists. Later on, the speech-impaired individual participates more actively on the team along with vocational counselors and, perhaps, employers and group home staff. When individuals become disabled as adults, physicians often play a central role. In short, augmentative communication teams need to remain flexible and utilize consultative services from various disciplines to meet the needs of their clients.

Service Delivery Models

How best to deliver services and provide equipment to individuals with severe expressive communication disorders is not yet clear. Not only are the needs diverse, but also professionals with expertise in augmentative communication are in short supply. Services are required in all regions of the country and in urban, suburban, and rural settings.

We know that augmentative communication interventions require professionals with a high level of expertise, equipment that is often expensive and not readily available, and the daily support of the client and persons who live, play, and work with clients. As a result, augmentative programs are generally time consuming and thus expensive to operate when compared to other areas of practice.

Three basic approaches to augmentative communication service delivery are currently in use:

Center-Based Model. All individuals are treated at a central location or locations. Special equipment is available on site, and competent professionals can evaluate, prescribe, and provide inservice training to communication partners. Augmentative programs that are center-based attempt to involve families and other professionals from the community (e.g., teachers, employers, clinicians) in all phases of intervention.

Community-Based Model. Professionals provide services and equipment to individuals at their residence, educational or vocational setting, and in the community. In this model, augmentative assessment and interventions are conducted by professionals within the environment where clients usually communicate.

Combination Model. Certain features of the center- and community-based models are combined. Often, evaluations are done at a central site with intervention programming provided either by itinerant team members or by professionals who have been trained by the team (either at the center or in the individual's community). An increasing number of center-based programs are providing itinerant services through satellite programs or mobile vans in an attempt to raise the level of professional expertise in the client's community.

Although the efficacy of these models has not been documented, common sense suggests that some are well suited to meet the needs of rural communities, whereas others may work well in an urban or suburban environment. For example, an individual who is severely physically handicapped and lives on a farm can expect to travel to a center, hopefully within the state, for a comprehensive augmentative communication evaluation, particularly if sophisticated technologies are required. However, professionals who refer this individual should inquire about whether the center has a mechanism in place to address the inservice training needs of the community.

Clinical experience and follow-up reports continue to suggest that there are many cases in which augmentative communication interventions are not being used as professionals in this area would have hoped.[17–19] Researchers feel that most failures are probably due to either inappropriate or inadequate assessment and selection of augmentative components or to inadequate and/or sporadic training in the use of recommended aids and techniques and a lack of follow-up. The success or failure of intervention reflects the models of service delivery employed as well as the commitment and expertise of the individuals and team involved. Apparently, persons most likely to benefit from recommended interventions attend school, work, and live within a community that is both aware and supportive of augmentative communication. Harris wrote that augmentative aids (and techniques) cannot be viewed as panaceas that naturally develop a client's absent communication skills.[18] Once an aid is delivered or a technique is taught, the process of developing or rekindling communication begins.

FRAMEWORK FOR INTERVENTION

The purpose of this section is to (1) provide a framework that describes the process of communication by means of augmentative aids and techniques and (2) within this framework, discuss variables that are pertinent to augmentative communication assessment and intervention practices.

Traditional models of communication describe rules and conventions for communication via a spoken medium. Normally, conversational exchanges are reported to occur at a rate of between 120 and 190 words per minute.[20] Using speech, natural speakers have unlimited access to language, as well as to the range of gestures, facial expressions, and body postures that augment the sending and receiving of messages. Although not included in the traditional speaker and listener model of communication, the importance of these nonverbal and traditional augmentative forms is recognized.

Because individuals with limited speech use special augmentative aids and techniques as their primary means of conveying messages, traditional conversational models are inappropriate. Since they do not provide a framework within which intervention can occur, application of traditional models of communication might well view augmented communication as a deficient or delayed process. Unimpaired speakers who are asked to use augmentative aids and techniques under experimental conditions quickly stop using strategies that work well during spoken conversation (e.g., use of complex syntactic forms, reiteration, and rephrasing of messages) and begin to use strategies that result in effective and efficient exchange of information, feelings, and so on (e.g., telegraphic comments). Communication under these conditions is a different process. In fact, one of the major differences between conversations that occur using speech and those using augmentative aids or techniques is the rate with which messages are generated. During interactions between individuals who use communication aids and their partners, the rate of message transfer is often slow, occurring at one-twentieth the normal speed. As a result, the form, use, and content of expressive language used, even by linguistically competent individuals, is different.

Kraat states that "interventions that do not take into account the differences between individuals who use augmentative components and those who speak, or that assume that aids and techniques can accomplish what normal speech and language interactions do, are based on erroneous assumptions."[11] Therefore a framework of communication that assists in understanding augmentative communication must incorporate a system of rules and conventions that are unique to the communicative modes being used, the individuals who use them, the purpose of the interaction, and the context, as well as principles of traditional models of communication.

Figure 34–1 depicts the framework for augmentative intervention used in this chapter. An interactive approach to augmentative communication intervention includes consideration of the individual augmentative components (both linguistic and nonlinguistic), communicative context (physical, social, and temporal), and communication tasks. For purposes of this discussion, each component is considered independently; however, it is important to understand that each of these variables directly influences the other. The dynamic nature of these interrelationships must therefore be considered when designing and implementing intervention programs.

The Individual

The previous section illustrated the heterogeneous nature of the population that uses augmentative aids and techniques. In no other area of practice within the communication disability field are the characteristics of the clients so vast and varied, and in no other area of practice are so many aspects of the individual likely to be considered when planning assessments and intervention programs. Although it is impossible to characterize the sensory, physical, cognitive, communicative, learning, and personality traits or discuss the educational and vocational opportunities of the population as a whole, some generalizations can be made that may assist the reader in developing an understanding of these individuals. The augmentative aids and techniques used, the environments encountered, and the communicative tasks engaged in are all influenced by the

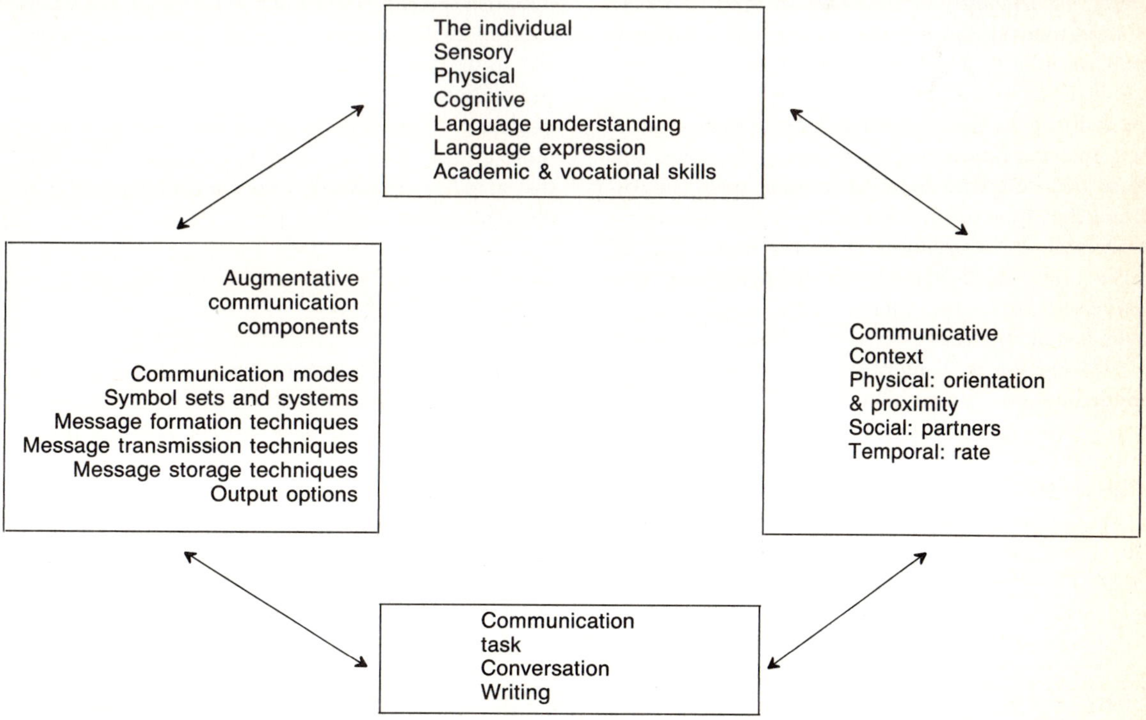

Figure 34–1 Illustration of the dynamic interrelationships among the critical aspects of intervention programming in augmentative communication.

characteristics of the individual. The individual is the focal part of the intervention model.

To fully describe the characteristics of the individual, a comprehensive interdisciplinary assessment is required. Professionals may observe the individual communicating, interview caregivers, and administer criterion-referenced and standardized tests. Complete background information from schools and medical records provide estimates of current functional levels and document previous interventions as well. The team identifies the individual's potential strengths and weaknesses, which then can be verified during the initial assessment. In addition, omissions in available data and discrepancies between reporting sources can be noted. A complete discussion of assessment is beyond the scope of this chapter; however, some considerations are reviewed. The reader is referred to Blackstone,[8] Goossens' and Crain,[21,22] Yorkston and Karlan[23] for more information about assessment.

Sensory Abilities

The individual's ability to see and hear must be ascertained in order to plan augmentative interventions that are meaningful. An individual's visual acuity and perception helps to determine the types of graphic symbols that can be used. Similarly, auditory acuity, which affects the understanding of speech and language, determines what kind of modes of expressions an individual can use (e.g., whether speech synthesis is an option). Since many individuals who benefit from augmentative interventions are multihandicapped, varying degrees of hearing and/or visual impairments are common. However, for those with severe to profound hearing losses and/or blindness whose primary disability is sensory-based, augmentative communication teams rarely play a major role. Audiologists, ophthalmologists, and teachers of the hearing and visually impaired generally provide specialized services to these individuals.

Assessment of Sensory Abilities. Audiologists, ophthalmologists and optometrists should complete acuity assessments. Occupational therapists and psychologists may assess visual perceptual abilities, and audiologists and speech-language pathologists may determine auditory perceptual capabilities. Tactile and kinesthetic assessments may also be indicated for some clients. Neurologists and physical and occupational therapists often assess these areas.

Physical Abilities

Most individuals who use augmentative aids and techniques exhibit some degree of motor impairment. For many, speech motor impairment is the underlying cause of the speech difficulty (e.g., dysarthria and apraxia). For others, motor difficulties may be an associated symptom of a complex condition (e.g., severe mental retardation or severe learning disability). Often, the motor problem involves not only the speech musculature, but also upper and lower extremity function, so that mobility and independence in daily activities are also compromised.

Physical interventions are critical in augmentative communication practices. In fact, augmentative aids and techniques are recommended only after major consideration is given to the person's motor skills and to other aspects of physical management. For example, adequate head control and reliable and consistent alternating head movements might be necessary if an individual is to use two switches to operate a communication device. If independent mobility is a goal, then additional consideration must be given to selecting an electronic communication aid that permits the individual to drive an electric wheelchair.

Assessment of Physical Abilities. Evaluation of the physical abilities of the individual is completed by specialists familiar with motor functioning and disabilities. Traditionally, occupational and physical therapists evaluate mobility, seating, and positioning and suggest special handling techniques and use of specific control sites on the body to accomplish specific motor tasks (e.g., pointing and activating switches reliably). Physicians may participate in the management of the program by prescribing and monitoring the effects of drug therapies. If available, rehabilitation engineers or other professionals with technical backgrounds assess the ways that enable professionals to use technology with individual clients.

Cognitive Abilities

Most clinicians agree that the majority of severely speech-impaired individuals with congenital etiologies exhibit cognitive and/or learning differences. Even individuals with intellectual potential within the normal range often possess significant variability in their cognitive profiles.[24]

Although there is little available information describing the cognitive abilities of individuals who use special augmentative aids and techniques, a recently published study of the demographic distribution of severely speech-impaired students in eastern Washington revealed that at least one-half of the individuals were mentally handicapped.[25] Only a small percentage experienced more mild cognitive or learning difficulties.

Regardless of intellectual potential, individuals with congenital impairments often possess a limited knowledge of the world, largely as a result of limited experience.[11] This limited knowledge may affect concept development, knowledge of cause-effect relationships, and the development of social skills.

As discussed, individuals with acquired disabilities may also have cognitive limitations as part of their disabling condition. The degree of impairment will depend upon the nature and extent of neurologic damage and the individual's premorbid function.

Assessment of Cognitive Abilities. To obtain a comprehensive assessment of the cognitive ability of individuals with severe speech impairments is difficult using currently available tools. Traditionally, assessments are carried out using standardized intelligence tests, such as the Weschler Intelligence Scale for Children-Revised. However, these rarely can be applied to this population unless adaptations are made. Some psychologists use nonverbal tests of intelligence and apply them to the hearing, nonspeaking population (although the tests are not standardized on this group). Examples of such tests include the Columbia Test of Mental Maturity, the Uzgiris-Hunt Scales of Infant Development, and the Leiter, which was standardized on individuals with severe hearing impairments.

Language Understanding

Like general intelligence, the language profiles of the nonspeaking population often show uneven patterns of development. Berninger and Gans studied the language skills of nonspeaking individuals of average intelligence (ages 40, 16, and 9) and found at least age-appropriate understanding of orally presented paragraphs,[24] a skill considered critical to understanding connected discourse. However, other receptive skills (e.g., single word recognition, auditory discrimination) were more variable. Professionals may also use augmentative strategies with severely language-impaired individuals to facilitate the development or return of language skills, even in clients who speak.

Assessment of Language Understanding. The need to detect uneven patterns of development in receptive language is particularly important to the development of intervention programs for this population. Understanding of connected discourse and recognition of single-word vocabulary, knowledge of syntax and grammar, verbal conceptualization, and memory influence the design of an individual's communication system as well as the success with which it is employed. Clinically, there are a number of tests of receptive language abilities that can be adapted for use with the severely speech-language-impaired individual by spatially rearranging stimulus items or presenting information in a yes or no or multiple choice format.

Expressive Language Abilities

Information on the expressive skills (use, content, and form of language produced) of severely speech-impaired individuals is based on data obtained from a limited number of natural studies.

Use. Light, Parnes, and Collier examined the communicative use of language in preschool physically handicapped children under two conditions: (1) a free play activity with caregivers and (2) a series of structured elicitation activities.[26] They found that all subjects expressed a range of communicative functions. However, they also noted that structured activities with a trained communication partner elicited a greater variety of communicative functions than activities with a familiar but untrained one. Similarly, Calculator and Luchko described an adult with intact cognitive abilities (age 24) who, after a multistep training program, used a communication board for a variety of different purposes.[27]

How individuals use communication aids to establish and maintain discourse has also been examined.[28,29] As a group, they are described as rarely initiating conversation, preferring instead to respond to the conversational overtures of their partners. In fact, conversational turns are often taken only when the individual is obliged to do so (i.e., when partners make a specific request that requires a response). Conversational repair strategies also appear to be limited. Not only do these individuals experience a greater number of conversational breakdowns during interchanges, but they are also less effective at using techniques to effect a repair.

Content. The content of messages produced by individuals who use augmentative aids and techniques has received limited attention. Crystal reported that normal children produce approximately 37,000 words in a single day, of which 10 percent are different from one another.[15] In contrast, the vocabulary used by individuals who depend on communication aids, or who sign, is limited.

Form. A number of observations have been made about the communication forms used by persons with severe speech impairments. They are telegraphic (e.g., "want go Grandma"), and appear to vary greatly, and depend upon the communication partner. Researchers have found that subjects use a combination of communication forms to express their ideas and feelings and depend upon standard, as opposed to special augmentative techniques (even when they are available), to express themselves. For example, Calculator and Dollaghan found that subjects often preferred gestures and vocalization over their communication aids, even when the former was ineffective at conveying their messages.[30] Light, Parnes, and Collier reported that their preschool subjects used vocalization, gestures, and eye gaze to request objects and events and used communication aids to provide specific information and clarify messages.[29]

Partners play a major role in determining the form of messages when communication aids and techniques are used. The following example illustrates that although the user of the communication aid (B) can spell and is capable of generating complete sentences, he does not most of the time. His mother (M) assumes major responsibility for constructing the message during the conversation.

M: Who do you want to win the baseball game?
B: (points to) "O" on communication board
M: The Orioles?
B: (nods and smiles)
M: (smiles) Why do you want the Orioles to win?
B: (points to) "BECAUSE" on communication board
M: Because?
B: (gestures to self) (points to) "P" "I" "T" on board
M: Oh! (smiles) You have family in Pittsburgh and they always tease you about the Orioles, right?
B: (laughs and nods head) Yeah!

The truncated form of the message permits a more rapid and naturally paced interactional exchange. The conversation is possible only because the dyad (mother and son) shares many common experiences. A stranger would not be able to predict and construct messages based on such limited linguistic information.

Assessment of Expressive Language. In assessing an individual's ability to express content using language forms and to engage in discourse with others, one should use both natural and eliciting contexts. Collecting an adequate sample of the individual's expressive output can be difficult, however, even when speech is not limited. Most clinicians do not feel it is possible to assess adequately the expressive language capabilities of individuals who require augmentative communication until the individual can spell. Thus the assessment focuses on what is "typically" done by the individual within the natural environment to express meaning and intention and how to improve the individual's ability to communicate effectively.

When assessing discourse skills (i.e., the ability to initiate, maintain conversational exchanges, and repair conversational breakdowns), one should consider the ability to use both linguistic and nonlinguistic components in a variety of different contexts. For a comprehensive picture of discourse abilities, performance in natural contexts as well as facilitative, eliciting situations are addressed. In addition, interviews with and observations of primary communication partners interacting with the client are helpful in defining the individual's expressive language profile.

Academic and Vocational Skills

Not surprisingly, individuals with limited speech and variable cognitive and language profiles often experience academic difficulties. Many educators and speech-language pathologists report that even those severely speech-impaired clients with normal or near-normal intelligence encounter educational difficulties at some point during their school careers. Berninger and Gans' research[24] has documented that the reading levels of cognitively intact subjects is not as high as would be expected given their cognitive abilities and language levels.

Limited written language and spelling skills have a particularly detrimental effect on individuals who must communicate using special augmentative aids and techniques. Without literacy skills, individuals remain limited in the vocabulary they can generate and the number of special augmentative techniques and communication aids they can use. Only if the individual is a competent speller can independence in communication be achieved.

Overall, data on performance in various academic subjects is limited. However, researchers do know that many adults with congenital disabilities have had limited educational opportunities and have severely limited academic skills. To date, few severely speech-impaired persons attend college or maintain full-time jobs. Whether this is a result of physiologic learning disabilities or ineffective teaching methods and techniques remains unclear. However, with the increasing use of technology within the classroom and improved teaching strategies, future investigations may be better able to establish relationships between the population's academic achievement and their cognitive and language profiles.

The development of efficient work study habits and independence in the learning process are clinically related communication tasks. The development of such skills must occur early on in an individual's learning career. The absence of required class assignments and homework and limited opportunities for participating in group activities often contribute to a passive learning style on the part of the student and lowered expectations on the part of the teacher. Technology is obviously an important tool to developing students' independence in learning. However, adjustments to teaching style and curriculum modifications are equally important.

With the increased use of technology in the classroom and workplace, improved teaching strategies, and incentive programs for hiring the handicapped, more severely speech-impaired persons should be able to achieve their academic and vocational potential. Technologic support allows students and workers to rely on themselves to organize assignments, complete tasks, develop effective study and work skills, and develop independence. Individuals should have access to communication within the learning and work environment as well as during leisure activities and at home. Although providing low- and high-tech communication aids to those who need them can be costly, not providing needed equipment is ultimately more costly in terms of wasted human resources.

Assessment of Academic and Vocational Skills. Academic achievement is typically assessed by means of standardized or criterion-referenced measures to determine a "grade-level" performance. Many of these tests can and are adapted for use with the severely speech and language impaired. Following assessment, educational placement should be based on the individual's cognitive profile and academic achievement, not on orthopaedic problems or unintelligible speech. For example, a student with a physical disability but normal intelligence and age-appropriate academic skills should be placed in regular education with the necessary equipment and support services. A youngster who is cognitively impaired and uses a voice output aid can attend classes with other students who have similar learning profiles.

Vocational achievement is typically assessed with regard to "productivity" measures on a set of tasks required by a supervisor. Performance scales based on a task analysis and periodic reviews can be used to monitor vocational achievement. Prevocational assessments vary according to the task required to complete specific jobs. However, good communication skills and work habits underlie success on any job. Without augmentative communication interventions, few severely speech- and writing-impaired individuals are able to succeed in the workplace.

Personality Characteristics

Reactions to and acceptance of augmentative communication as an alternative or supplement to speech varies among individuals. Clinical experience suggests that persons who are exposed to augmentative aids and techniques at an early age are more apt to view them as viable options to spoken communication and to incorporate them into their communication system. Clinicians also generally feel that the amount of residual speech (but not necessarily the intelligibility of that speech) and the ability to use traditional augmentative methods have a significant impact on acceptance. Individuals who are successful communicators using vocalizations and gestures, even with a limited number of partners (e.g., family, classroom teacher), often do not recognize the need to use special augmentative strategies with unfamiliar partners and so may resist them. Although individuals with acquired disabilities may initially have more difficulty accepting the use of aids and techniques, in most cases, they eventually understand that they are necessary if they want to communicate effectively.

Assessment of the Individual

Subsequent to obtaining information about the individual's sensory, physical, cognitive, language, and personality characteristics as well as educational and vocational skills, it is possible to answer the following assessment questions.

1. What, if any, are the individual's sensory deficits?
2. What are the individual's gross and fine motor capabilities? How reliable are his or her movements? Is fatigue a factor in program design? Does he or she have independent mobility?
3. What is the individual's cognitive profile (as compared to his or her developmental level or premorbid condition)?
4. What does the person understand about the world (e.g., general knowledge, social skills)?
5. Is the individual's linguistic system intact? If not, what is his or her profile of linguistic abilities?
6. What articulatory and gestural repertoire does the person use for communicative purposes? What is the potential in this area?
7. Does the individual produce intelligible utterances? Under what circumstances? With whom?
8. What is the form and content of the individual's messages? What symbols are preferable to and for this person? Under what circumstances? With whom?
9. What are the individual's current and future academic and vocational goals? What are his or her communication needs?
10. What are the attitudes of the individual, family, and others about augmentative communication interventions?

Augmentative Communication Components

The success of augmentative interventions depends upon the extent to which the use of augmentative components meets the communication needs of the individual. Vanderheiden and Lloyd list specifications for a functional communication system that includes the ability to (1) meet a full range of communicative functions and tasks; (2) allow interaction with all communication partners in any environment; (3) permit efficient and effective communication while maximizing conversational control; (4) permit expression of increasingly complex ideas and messages as the user grows and develops; (5) be integrated and accepted into the user's social and physical environments; (6) interface with existing seating systems, environmental controls and teaching aids; and (7) be purchased and maintained without financial hardship.[31]

Most individuals use a variety of speech and augmentative components to accomplish communication tasks. The extent to which special and standard components are used is determined by the individual and his or her communication needs. In Figure 34–2, the communication systems of three individuals are diagrammed. Example A is a normal speaking child, age 10 years, who uses a combination of speech and standard augmentative components (e.g., gestures, home computer, paper and pencil, crayons). Example B illustrates the communication system of an adult, age 43 years, who is severely speech- and writing-impaired. This individual uses an electronic communication aid, a language board, some manual signs and a few gestures, and vocalizations to communicate at home and during leisure activities. Because of severe physical disabilities, special augmentative components constitute a major portion of this person's communication system. In Example C, the system of a severely mentally retarded youngster, age 6 years, who functions at a developmental level of 12 months is depicted. This child relies primarily on gestures and vocalizations to communicate as would be expected in a 1-year-old infant. Speech has not developed (and

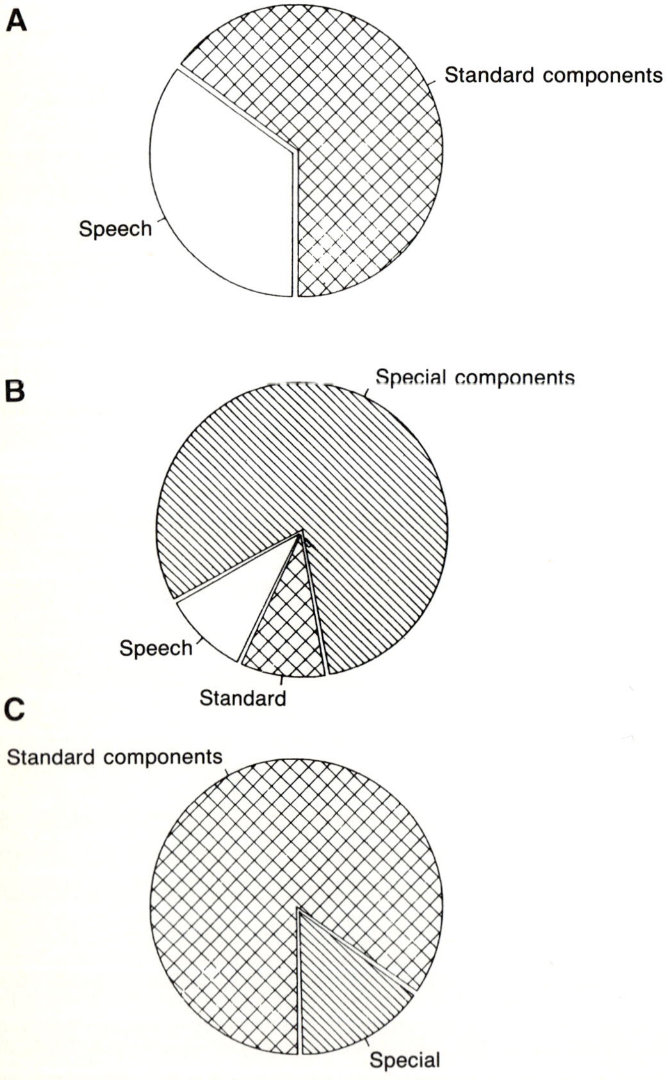

Figure 34–2 Diagrams of the communication systems of three individuals. *A*, This example is of a normally developing 10-year-old child. *B*, This example is of a 43-year-old woman with severe speech and writing impairments. *C*, This example is of a 6-year-old boy with severe mental retardation.

because of motor and cognitive problems is unlikely to). Augmentative communication intervention has provided this child with a few manual signs, which he uses to request food, ask for assistance, and ask for a favorite toy.

Augmentative communication components include the modes of communication utilized, the types of symbol sets and systems employed, and the means by which messages are formed and transmitted.

Communication Modes

Components of each individual's communication system are often described as unaided and aided communication. Unaided communication does not require any tool outside the body. It includes vocalization, eye gaze, informal and idiosyncratic gestures, and manual signs. Aided communication refers to the use of devices, which are typically divided into "high-tech" and "low-tech" communication aids. Communication aids include telephones, typewriters, pencils, and crayons (i.e., any communication method used to transmit a message), as well as manual communication books, dedicated communication devices, and specially adapted computers and switch technologies. "High tech" refers to devices and related peripherals that require electrical or battery power for operation. In contrast, "low tech" refers to aids that do not require electrical nor battery power, such as clinician-made communication boards.

Symbol Sets and Systems

Messages are expressed through symbols. The symbols used in augmentative communication are probably the most important component of an individual's communication system and one of the most difficult areas to deal with during intervention. Individuals with speech impairments rarely have access to a sufficient number of symbols, and their communication partners are often unfamiliar with the symbols used or have difficulty understanding them when they are produced or selected by the speech-impaired person.

The various available symbol sets and systems are often classified as either closed or open systems. Closed symbol sets are those that have a finite number of lexical items (e.g., Picsyms, Rebus), whereas open sets offer an infinite number of vocabulary choices (e.g., traditional orthography). Obviously, open symbol systems are preferable because they permit individuals unrestricted access to language.

Symbols are also classified in terms of their dynamic and static properties.[31] Dynamic symbols are symbol sets and systems that are produced by the individual (e.g., manual sign language). Static symbols are permanently available to the user through a display or set of stored options. A communication board using pictures or Blissymbols employs a static symbol system. Selection of one or more symbol sets or systems for use in augmentative communication requires careful consideration of variables such as the client's mental age, linguistic skills, communication needs, and communication partners. Vanderheiden and Lloyd provide a summary listing and review of a variety of symbol systems currently in use.[31]

Message Formation Techniques

Individuals generate messages using production- and/or selection-based techniques.[31] Symbols independently produced to create a message (e.g., gestures, signs, and speech) are production-based. Most unaided augmentative communication employs production-based techniques. Individuals choosing symbols from a preidentified set (e.g., symbols on a communication aid) in order to formulate and communicate a message use a selection-based technique.

Persons who use augmentative communication aids generate messages using selection-based techniques. The specific techniques employed depend upon the individual's motor control and ability to understand the selection technique. There are three ways in which an individual selects messages: direct selection, encoding, and scanning. All three techniques are used with electronic and nonelectronic communication aids.

1. Direct selection requires that the individual select symbols (in a single movement) by pointing either with a part of the body (e.g., hands, eyes) or an adaptive device (e.g., head pointer, light pointer).
2. Encoding is a multistep process used by severely motor-impaired individuals to select two or three symbols from a discrete set of symbols (e.g., dot and dash configurations, as in Morse code, or picture symbols, as in semantic compaction and/or Minsymbols). The "code" corresponds to the desired message.
3. In scanning, symbols are presented one at a time. The individual selects the desired symbol when it is highlighted. Scanning can be accomplished by the individual's communication partner or by an electronic aid.

When an individual is unable to access equipment (e.g., a severely physically impaired person or a visually impaired individual who cannot use a keyboard), the difficulty can be overcome by employing special equipment, such as keyboard emulators (e.g., firmware cards) and control interfaces (e.g., switches, speech recognizers), that, together, can permit use of most commercially available software. Some individuals use adapted keyboards that have been modified in shape or function but still retain many characteristics of a traditional keyboard. In other instances, an individual may employ specially designed switches (i.e., joy stick, paddle switch, optical head pointer) that can be activated by different parts of the body to control a scanner. These control interfaces may be used to operate a variety of different types of communication aids.

The success with which an individual uses production- and/or selection-based techniques depends upon cognitive, language and physical abilities, the purpose of the message, and the context in which it is presented. As illustrated in Figure 34–2, individuals employ a variety of techniques, selecting those combinations that best meet their needs.

Message Transmission Techniques

In spoken communication the cognitive skills and/or linguistic abilities of the individual are directly reflected in the on-line generation of messages. This direct reflection is often not the case when individuals employ augmentative symbols, aids, and techniques. Many times, the communication aid does not provide the user with the symbols or the time to produce grammatically and syntactically accurate messages. Or the individual has not learned or been exposed to the symbols that facilitate expression.

Individuals who have access to a range of symbols and are competent users of a language system often prefer to forego grammatical and syntactic accuracy in order to achieve speed and efficiency in message transmission. For example, during conversations, individuals may prefer to communicate only key words, first letters, or general topics, expecting the partner to predict his or her meaning. Word and/or sentence prediction strategies used by familiar partners are also available with some electronic communication aids that use special communication software. Speed of transmission and message complexity can also be enhanced by the use of stored messages that can be retrieved quickly.

Message Storage Techniques

There are numerous ways to store and retrieve messages. All require the use of computer technologies (i.e., aided techniques). The simple way is to provide a one-to-one correspondence between the symbol and the message. For example, 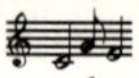 is the Picsym that stands for "music." In this method, the single word "music" is stored in memory under the symbol for "music". In the "holophrastic" method, a single symbol is used to stand for an entire message. In this instance, the message "I'd like to hear some music" might be stored under the music Blissymbol. To increase the number of available messages to which the individual has access, many communication devices permit multiple messages to be stored in different "levels" or "pages" of memory. This type of storage permits organization of messages according to different topics or different contexts. For example, one level may contain messages related to favorite toys and games, whereas a second might refer to classroom reading activities.

Messages can also be stored and retrieved under sequences of multiple symbols. When the user enters a particular combination of symbols, the message corresponding to that exact sequence is recalled. Symbols under which messages can be stored and retrieved may be numbers (numeric encoding) or letters (logical letter encoding, abbreviation expansion). In other instances, an individual might sequence a series of pictures (minsymbols) on a dedicated communication aid to produce messages. This procedure is referred to as semantic encoding.[32]

Output Options

The symbol output generated from low-tech communication aids and manual signs requires that the communication partner translate graphic symbols or manuals signs and gestures. High-tech, portable communication aids offer a variety of output options for the user, with artificial speech and hardcopy printout being the most common outputs for communication aids. At present, two methods of generating speech are commonly used: synthesized speech and digitized speech. Communication devices using synthesized speech generate artificial speech based on the rules of pronunciation of the particular culture. Currently, the low-cost synthesized speech used in communication aids sounds mechanical and lacks intonation and inflectional qualities. In contrast, digitized speech, which is human speech that has been digitally stored in memory,[31] sounds more human. However, digital recording requires high memory capacity to store information. Thus the more technically sophisticated the system is, the more expensive it is.

In addition to speech output, many electronic communication aids provide hard copy or printed copies of messages. A temporary record is provided by a correctable display, and a built-in or external printer allows permanent recording. Some communication aids can also be used as data entry terminals, thus providing a data output option.

Assessment Considerations of Augmentative Components

The development of an appropriate augmentative communication system is a complex and lengthy task. In most cases, an attempt is made to develop a system that is comprised of residual speech, both low- and high-tech aids, and unaided techniques, such as the use of voice and gestures. The augmentative components that make up each person's system are unique and based on individual needs, goals, and capabilities. It is the sensory, physical, cognitive, linguistic, academic and vocational performance and personality characteristics of an individual that underlie and define the possible options that can be used to meet communication needs and goals.

Because of the complexity of the assessment task and the many issues involved in determining the possible components of an individual's communication system, it is critical that professionals with knowledge and skills in the augmentative field who are familiar with a range of available aids and techniques participate in the assessment process. This participation often requires someone with technical expertise. Blackstone describes a method for organizing data obtained about the individual that focuses on the team and utilizes their knowledge about features of various aids and techniques.[8]

As part of the assessment process and prior to making final recommendations, performance evaluations should be conducted. During a performance evaluation, data are collected on the client's actual use of augmentative components. In some cases, in-depth evaluations are conducted during a field test that lasts from 2 to 6 weeks. In other cases, performance evaluations are carried out as part of an intensive 1- or 2-day assessment. Field tests are conducted in real environments and, if possible, should be completed when expensive equipment is being considered.

The information gathered by the augmentative communication team about the individual's potential for using various augmentative aids and techniques provides answers to the following assessment questions:

1. What speech and augmentative components can the individual effectively employ? Are certain components of the individual's potential communication system usable in some situations and not others?
2. How abstract a symbol set or system can the individual understand? What size should the symbols be? How many? How should they be placed on a display? What should the size and orientation of the display be?
3. What production- and/or selection-based techniques can the individual use to generate messages?
4. Does the client need high-tech equipment? If so, how will he or she access it? Do positioning or fatigue factors affect performance?
5. How can the client store, retrieve, and produce messages utilizing available symbols?
6. What types of outputs are required for successful performance in a variety of environments?
7. Are portability and durability important selection factors? How reliable is the equipment? Who will be responsible for maintaining it?
8. Is funding available for material and equipment purchases?
9. Do the communication system components address short-term communication needs? Can components be expanded to meet the user's predicted long-term communication needs?

A major goal of augmentative communication assessments is to select system components that provide a *best match* or *fit* for each individual. In the past, selection of communication aids or techniques was misconstrued as the primary goal in the augmentative communication area. However, researchers have learned that the primary goal must be the successful application of system components in real communication environments.

The Communicative Context

Cassatt-James[28] and Light, Parnes, and Collier[29] found that the context in which communication occurs can facilitate or have a detrimental effect on the quantity and quality of interactions between individuals who use augmentative aids and techniques and their partners. The identification and description of contextual parameters are important aspects of intervention. Three types of contexts are considered in this discussion: physical, social, and temporal.

Physical Context

Various parameters of the physical context affect the communicative success of individuals who use augmentative aids and techniques. First is the physical orientation of communication partners. In conversations between speaking partners, face-to-face orientation is typical. Participants are able to understand the meaning of a message not only from the linguistic information provided, but from other paralinguistic and nonverbal cues as well. However, unless speech or signed output is used, face-to-face contact between partners is frequently impossible for individuals using communication aids. In fact, partners generally must position themselves behind or next to the communication aid user in order to interpret the message.

Second, proximity to one's communication partner is also a critical variable in communicative interchanges. For example, nonelectronic aids do not allow transmission of messages over distances. With the exception of vocalization, unaided techniques require that the listener be able to make visual contact with the speaker. Although typical speakers frequently converse across rooms and over the telephone, these options are often unavailable to individuals who use nonelectronic communication aids. However, communication over distance is possible for individuals who can easily produce some intelligible speech or if a communication aid with audible signalers and/or speech output is used.

A third important consideration of the physical environment is the degree to which individuals are able to be mobile. Independent mobility, even for children as young as $2^1/_2$ years, results in increased self-confidence and physical and psychological independence.[33] For example, a preschooler who is taught to control an electric wheelchair can explore the neighborhood and learn about what's going on in the world. A high school student who is able to move independently to the computer room at school is able to take advantage of learning opportunities afforded by high technology equipment and is able to complete homework and generate written assignments using school computers.

Fourth, environments that are accessible provide individuals with opportunities to learn, develop independence, and interact with a greater number of communication partners. For example, a high school that is wheelchair-accessible allows a greater number of severely speech-impaired individuals to meet and interact with typical peers in "a least restrictive environment."

Social Context

A major focus in augmentative communication has been on the social context because communication partners play such a critical part in the successful application of augmentative aids and techniques. Researchers have observed that individuals rarely interact with their peers.[11,18,30] Instead, elementary-age children and young adult subjects were found to converse with their teachers, caregivers, and other adults. Characteristics of conversational interaction between users of augmentative techniques and their speaking partners are discussed in the next section, The Communication Task.

Temporal Context

The temporal properties of the context in which communication occurs are particularly important when one or more of the participants use augmentative aids and techniques. As discussed previously, rate of communication among severely speech-impaired individuals and their partners is significantly different from that of speaking persons. Whereas typical speakers produce as many as 200 words per minute, individuals who use augmentative aids and techniques express an average of only six words per minute. Generating written language is also a slow process for those with physical impairments. Even with current advances in technology, individuals experience a reduction in the speed with which they can take notes and complete written assignments. To facilitate conversation, clients and their communication partners are taught strategies to increase their rate of message exchange. Some developers of high-tech aids build in features that improve both the speed of message formation and transmission for both conversation and written communication tasks.

Assessment of the Communicative Context

Environmental assessments provide a systematic means of defining the parameters of the context in which individuals need to communicate. The characteristics of individuals, along with the characteristics of the environments within which they participate help the augmentative communication team recommend potential aids and techniques as well as identify those contexts that must be considered in the intervention process. A comprehensive assessment of the individual within a variety of contexts provides answers to the following questions:

1. What environments does the individual participate in?
2. Does the individual need to communicate across distances?
3. How does the individual travel between environments?
4. How many communication partners does the in-

dividual have? What are the physical, cognitive, language, and academic characteristics of these partners?
5. Is the individual communicating in dyadic situations? In group activities?
6. Is the individual required to communicate quickly in any contexts?

The Communication Task

Within each context, individuals may wish to engage in a range of communication tasks, including conversation and writing. Conversational tasks include those communicative interactions that one normally accomplishes using speech (expressing basic needs, chatting on the phone with a friend, participating in a group discussion, telling a joke). Written tasks include activities such as note taking, making a grocery list, and word processing.

Conversation

Conversations between nonspeaking individuals and their partners are markedly different from the symmetrical and transactional discourse patterns of speaking adults. Identification and maintenance of discourse topics, patterns of turn taking, and conversational repair strategies are a few of the altered interactional patterns observed. Individuals with severe expressive communication impairments tend to respond to the conversational turns of others rather than initiate communication attempts independently. Researchers report that less than 15 percent of the turns of individuals who use communication aids are comprised of initiations.[28,29] Severely speech-impaired persons also are unskilled in establishing and maintaining discourse topics. For the most part, partners assume primary responsibility for the execution of the discourse. Not only do they typically choose the topic of conversation, but they frequently insure its continuation as well. For example, Light, Collier, and Parnes report that caregivers of physically handicapped preschool children use turnabouts to insure the latter's continued participation in the discourse.[26] In contrast, individuals with severe speech impairments rarely produce conversational acts that require the occurrence of a subsequent turn by their listeners. As noted before, their conversational turns typically consist of contingent responses to the previous speaker's turns.

Another characteristic described by researchers and clinicians is the lack of conversational control that individuals with augmentative aids and techniques exert during conversations. This lack of control reflects the failure to establish and maintain conversational topics, participate in turn taking, and secure the continuation of the discourse through the use of turn soliciting strategies. To achieve a more equitable balance of power during conversation, strategies and procedures to facilitate the severely speech-impaired individual's independence in communication are used. A review of some of these procedures can be found in the next section, Strategies to Improve Conversational Competency.

Writing

Little is known about the written language abilities of severely speech-impaired individuals. The sophistication of the content of their written language, the accuracy of their grammar, and the complexity of their sentence structure is not well described. These skills are probably most deficient in individuals with congenital disabilities because they often have limited practice in writing due to physical limitations.

Data are limited on the spelling abilities of individuals who employ graphic symbols. Berninger and Gans evaluated spelling skills in three cognitively intact, severely speech-impaired persons with cerebral palsy and found that all three performed below age level. Interestingly, however, spelling skills actually appeared to be more developed than reading skills. The researchers caution that better achievement in spelling may have been "the consequence of the experience these subjects had in using electronic communication devices and microcomputers for linguistic communication" and should not be interpreted to mean that these individuals "do not make spelling errors . . . and do not have great difficulty with spelling vowel sounds."(p 49)[24]

Individuals with severe speech impairments who possess adequate composition and spelling skills have access to an independent and unrestricted means of communication. Regardless of whether individuals use dedicated communication aids or off-the-shelf computers, graphic print capabilities permit generation of text, math, note taking, and drawing.

Writing competency underlies conversational competency in the severely speech-impaired population. Without the ability to spell accurately and generate connected written discourse, these individuals can never truly become independent in communication. Intervention programs in augmentative communication must therefore consider the development of writing proficiency. Each client's potential for developing skills in the area of written language must be addressed and facilitated. Although many individuals do not become fluent in written discourse, in many cases they can learn a variety of component skills that can be used to enhance their ability to express themselves through both conversation and graphic mediums.

Assessment of the Communication Task

Intervention programs in augmentative communication generally focus on two aspects of communicative competency: conversation and written language.

Study of the conversational skills of an individual requires systematic observation of performance during dyadic interchanges as well as group discussions. Even though no standardized evaluation procedure has been validated for use with this population, several assessment protocols have been employed on a limited empirical and clinical basis. All of these procedures require videotaped samples of interactive behavior that are later transcribed and coded according to various discourse parameters. Clinicians feel that the subtle yet complex communicative behavior that is expressed via traditional as well as special augmentative aids and techniques is best examined by means of a permanent visual record.

Written language skills can be assessed most efficiently if an individual uses an electronic communication aid or a computer. Procedures developed for assessing the abilities of the mainstream population can easily be adapted for these individuals.

For conversational tasks, assessment data may provide answers to the following questions:

1. How successful is the individual at gaining the attention of the listener?
2. How skilled is the individual at securing, maintaining, and relinquishing conversational turns?
3. How cooperative are the partners at maintaining the discourse? What strategies are employed?
4. How effective are the partners at repairing conversational breakdowns? What types of repair strategies are employed?
5. How well does the individual monitor the intelligibility of his or her message?
6. Does the individual modify his messages according to the background knowledge and skills of the conversational partner?

For writing text and other graphic-related tasks, assessment data can provide information about:

1. What are the written communication needs of the client?
2. What is the individual's potential for the development of functional written language abilities? What long-term goals can be identified?
3. Are specific intervention strategies and techniques required to maximize written language expression?
4. How proficient is the individual in specific written language skills including composition, spelling, grammar, and syntactic complexity?
5. How sophisticated are the individual's self-checking and proofing skills?

Intervention Planning

Critical to intervention planning is information about the individual, augmentative components that are or could be used, the contexts within which individuals communicate, and the communication tasks that need to be accomplished. Assessment data are the basis for recommendations and, if equipment is needed, for written prescriptions for communication devices. Intervention goals are derived from these data as well. Kraat listed three general areas that augmentative communication goals typically may address:[11] (1) improving daily functional communication and interaction; (2) serving as a bridge to the development of natural speech and spoken language comprehension; and/or (3) determining whether language skills can be acquired using augmentative components.

However, the goals and objectives for each individual are more specific to the communication tasks that must be accomplished. In the next section, the development of conversation competency is highlighted.

STRATEGIES TO IMPROVE CONVERSATIONAL COMPETENCY

Communicative competency refers to the knowledge and skills that underlie expression through speech (e.g., face-to-face conversation and telecommunications), as well as writing (e.g., notes, term papers, reports) and computer use (e.g., word processing, data entry). Although writing and related communication tasks are critical to the ultimate success of an individual's communication efforts, conversational competency is the primary focus of most augmentative communication intervention programs and a goal in language intervention.

Conversational competence can be defined as the ability to

1. Convey a range of ideas and attitudes.
2. Converse for a variety of conversational purposes.
3. Interact with a number of communication partners.

4. Use forms that permit maximum speed and efficiency.
5. Use rules of discourse appropriate to the situation.

To achieve conversational competency, an individual must have access to the language of the culture and must be able to use socially acceptable conventions and rules to express it.

Developing the skills to be a competent conversationalist in persons using augmentative aids and techniques is a difficult and challenging task. Clinicians often express concern about the lack of functional use of augmentative communication components by these individuals. These concerns have been substantiated by follow-up studies.[34] Formal training is required if clients are to benefit from recommended augmentative aids and techniques. This section focuses on the skills that are required (as listed previously) and on strategies that can be employed by clinicians to facilitate the development of conversational competencies in these individuals.

Convey a Range of Ideas and Attitudes

Conveying a range of ideas and attitudes is difficult because individuals who use augmentative aids and techniques frequently have limited language content because they often communicate via a closed symbol set that offers a restricted number of vocabulary options. Even if they employ an open symbol system such as orthography, some restriction in language topics can occur because of the individual's difficulty in spelling unusual or difficult words. Additionally, vocabulary displays that are made available to clients are generally selected by individuals who are unlikely to be aware of their ideas or attitudes. One way to illustrate the difficulty in vocabulary selection is to ask a friend to select vocabulary for you to use on a communication board using a picture symbol set. Then try to use it at home with your family to carry on a conversation.

The more open the symbol system, the less often an individual encounters vocabulary restrictions. This principle is extremely important from an intervention standpoint. It supports the notion that programs should strive to develop the potential in each client for recognizing and using increasingly more abstract symbol sets and systems. In addition, it suggests the need to develop adequate spelling skills in this population. Even simple sound-letter correspondence knowledge allows an individual to use strategies such as initial letter or sound cueing. Phonetic spelling permits spelling with familiar communication partners. Accurate spelling not only eliminates the problem of closed vocabulary sets, but also allows the individual access to a greater range of sophisticated communication aids and techniques.

Strategies for Increasing the Ability to Convey Ideas and Attitudes

Intervention strategies that attempt to increase an individual's ability to converse on a variety of topics by expanding available vocabulary can be taught. The strategies employed depend upon the age and developmental level of the client. Suggestions for intervention include the following:

1. Training clients to use a multicomponent communication system (i.e., if a message cannot be conveyed using one mode, such as a communication aid, the client is taught to use one or more other modes, such as gestures, mime, or manual signs).[28]

2. Developing a client-centered vocabulary that stresses the selection of symbols with high communicative value. In this way, vocabulary items included on the display have a high probability of being used by the individual. Van Tatenhove describes five different methods for selecting vocabulary: environmental inventory, dialoguing, shadowing, role playing, and video or audio recording.[35] See also Kraat[11] and Yorkston, Dowden, and Marriner.[36]

3. Updating vocabulary regularly; delete outdated items and add new ones as needed.

4. Providing vocabulary for and encouraging the use of general topic clues (e.g., the individual points to a symbol that says "I'm talking about a special holiday," expecting the partner to guess Thanksgiving).

5. Teaching the client to use initial letter or sound cues (e.g., "the first letter is _____; the word begins with the _____ sound") if vocabulary items are missing.

6. Encouraging the client to combine available symbols in novel ways as a way to cue conversational partners. For example, a child might point to the symbols "woman black hat" to describe the witch he or she saw at his or her school Hallowe'en party.

7. Developing multiple vocabulary displays that reflect the kinds of lexical items required for specific activities. For example, high school students might use one overlay for a biology class and another for a psychology class. A preschooler might have one communication board for use in the housekeeping corner and another for use during arts and crafts activities. The design, construction, and implementation of context-specific communication aids is described in detail by Cook[37] and Schippits.[38]

8. Including specific vocabulary expansion

messages that request the listener to guess what the message is (e.g., messages such as "I'll try to spell it"; "I'll give you some clues"; and "Please guess").

9. Selecting symbol systems that include specific symbol strategies that can be used to expand the number of vocabulary elements available to the user. For example, students who use Blissymbols might have the symbol for "opposite" and one member of each polar opposite on their communication board. If they have the symbol for "hot" but need the symbol for "cold," they simply point to "hot, opposite."

10. Alerting the listener when a particular vocabulary item is unavailable during the conversation, (e.g., "the word is not on my board" or signing "I don't know the sign").

Converse for a Variety of Conversational Purposes

Although vocabulary restrictions contribute to the difficulty individuals have in accomplishing conversational tasks, the nature of the augmentative components employed also makes it difficult to express a wide range of speech acts. For example, requesting a drink of water if you are unable to speak can be frustrating unless you are near a drinking fountain, have a communication symbol available to depict the need, or are with someone who can interpret your speech or gestures.

Although individuals with limited speech have the potential to produce a wide range of speech acts,[26,28] in practice they typically produce only yes or no responses or provide information requested by others. This restricted use of language may be related to several factors, including (1) the individual's communication style, (2) the individual's lack of experience using a range of speech acts, (3) the aspects of the social context, and (4) the limitations of the symbol systems or sets employed.

Strategies to Expand the Variety of Speech Acts

Intervention strategies should strive to develop the functional use of language for a variety of different purposes. Suggestions for intervention include the following:

1. Providing a range of vocabulary options that can be used to express a variety of speech acts. Since a number of communicative functions (e.g., statements, requests for information) cannot be expressed easily by means of nonlinguistic forms (e.g., gestures, facial expressions), symbols should be available.

2. Structuring and manipulating aspects of the context to elicit certain types of speech acts (e.g., setting up role playing situations to provide the opportunity to practice telling a joke).

3. Using familiar routines in the natural environment to provide opportunities for the client to use specific types of communicative functions. This strategy can be accomplished by first completing a task analysis of daily situations within the individual's experience. Then the analysis can be used to target events within which to stimulate the expression of different speech acts (e.g., requesting assistance, greeting, and stating an opinion).

4. Using scripts to elicit a range of speech acts. Structured situation-specific activities, such as bathing a baby doll or interviewing a teacher for the school paper, can be outlined, delineating the dialogue of the conversational partner and the projected messages of the client. When the scripts are completed, the speech-language pathologist and client practice until the client is successful in participating in the activity and produces the appropriate communicative intents.

5. Generalizing the speech acts learned to other routines and events. Once the use of a variety of communicative functions is established in structured, eliciting contexts, use a systematic process to generalize these behaviors to novel situations in the natural environment.

Interact Effectively with Communication Partners

The social contexts within which speech-impaired individuals communicate frequently do not facilitate the conversational competencies of individuals who use augmentative communication. A major reason cited is the interactive behaviors of communication partners. Partners have been described as ignoring or failing to interpret communication attempts unless those attempts are made by means of a formal system (e.g., a communication aid).[30] Researchers have also suggested that partners often do not provide enough time for individuals to respond. Partners that provide feedback on an ongoing basis during the conversation to insure its maintenance help to reduce the occurrence of communication failures; however, many pretend they understand a message when they have not.

The extent to which partners are able to understand messages produced by individuals who use augmentative aids and techniques often depends upon their background knowledge of the individual. The more familiar partners are with the individual's personality, life style, likes, and dislikes, the better able they are in interpreting each communication attempt.

Strategies for Teaching Partners to Become Facilitating Agents

One of the most critical aspects of intervention is the training of communication partners. The role of partners in the success or failure of a communication exchange has been discussed in depth.[11,39] Intervention suggestions to facilitate the partner's role include the following:

1. For aided communication, providing instructions on the language board or communication aid that describe how to converse via the client's system. Instructions should state how to use the formal aid as well as how the client indicates yes or no, communicates using idiosyncratic gestures, and so on.
2. Providing didactic sessions for communication partners to explain the components of the individual's augmentative system and how the individual uses it for different purposes in different contexts. Modeling system use and observing how the partner interacts with the individual can be used to provide constructive feedback.
3. Implementing training activities in a variety of real environments that include a range of partners to be trained, particularly the individual's peers.
4. Developing the partner's background knowledge of experiences, interests, and habits of the individual. This knowledge helps the partner to predict messages and repair conversational failures.
5. If appropriate, developing a mechanism that allows information sharing among partners in different environments about special events in the individual's life. Wasson describes a procedure for facilitating information exchange among partners.[40]
6. Expanding the number of communication partners to which the individual has access by providing individuals with independent mobility. Utilize augmentative components, such as electronic devices, that promote independence in communication. Always be sure that communication aids include symbols that are familiar to a range of partners or use speech output, if appropriate.
7. Being an advocate in the community for clients who use augmentative communication by promoting awareness and acceptance of various aids and techniques. Dashiell, Hanson, Hinchliffe, Hunt, and Botti provide a detailed description of how to integrate individuals who use augmentative aids and techniques into the community.[41]

Use Forms that Permit Maximum Speed and Efficiency

Individuals who use communication aids or who sign rarely use the grammatic and syntactic forms of spoken language, particularly when maximum speed and efficiency in communication are desirable. In an effort to more closely approximate the flow of natural conversation, many communicatively competent individuals prefer to use a more telegraphic method of information exchange. In other cases, however, individuals must forego grammatic and syntactic accuracy because the symbol sets they use do not lend themselves to the generation of well-formed English sentences.

Strategies to Enhance Maximum Speed and Efficiency

Fortunately, a variety of techniques exist that enhance speed and efficiency in conversation. Some of these strategies include the following:

1. Speaking in telegraphic utterances with friends.
2. Using high-tech communication aids that have message storage capabilities. This type of aid permits individuals to use correct grammatic and syntactic forms quickly and accurately and to prestore generic phrases.
3. Considering the use of communication software that assists message construction by (1) allowing lengthy messages to be stored and retrieved using abbreviated codes (semantic encoding, logical letter encoding) and (2) logically predicting vocabulary choice and/or word using semantic and syntactic rules.
4. Promoting rapid and efficient exchanges of information using coconstruction of messages. For example, to convey information rapidly, an individual who uses a communication aid might produce telegraphic utterances that the partner translates into a full message. The utterances may consist of key words or perhaps only the initial letters of each word in the message. Coconstruction can include (1) filling in missing elements (e.g., a child points to the symbols "I, go, car" and the parent expands the message by saying, "You want to go in the car") and (2) predicting the message (for partners who are familiar with the interests and experiences of the individual) when given a limited number of cues or a telegraphic message. For example, a teenager points to the symbols "$, record" and the letter sequence "U, 2" and his friend predicts the message, "You want to go to the Waxy Maxy record store and get the new U2 album."

5. Teaching the individual how to effectively combine different modes of communication to express a message more rapidly. For example, an individual might combine gestures (e.g., looking at the refrigerator) with one or two symbols (e.g., "cold") to indicate the desire for a cold drink.

Although such techniques have proved to be effective strategies for improving the speed of message transmission, they have not contributed to the congenitally impaired individual's learning of the rules of grammar and syntax. If communication aids and manual signs are to be used effectively as academic tools, such skills, particularly as they relate to written language, are critical. Intervention programs need to address speed and efficiency in conversation as well as grammatic and syntactic accuracy in written tasks.

Use the Rules of Discourse Appropriate to the Situation

Discourse involves turn taking—the ability to secure, maintain, and transfer a conversational turn. As discussed previously, individuals who use augmentative aids and techniques are deficient in this skill area. Even though they do assume turns when obliged to do so (i.e., when their conversational partners make specific requests of them), they rarely initiate turns independently.

Individuals need techniques to gain attention, initiate a communication topic with familiar and unfamiliar partners, maintain the topic over several turns, and repair conversational breakdowns. Some suggestions for facilitating discourse maintenance are included next.

Strategies to Initiate and Establish Conversation

Intervention efforts are often directed toward improving the client's ability to initiate and participate in conversations with speaking individuals as well as nonspeaking and other handicapped peers. For individuals with severe speech impairments to initiate conversations in all situations, a number of parameters need to be considered. First, these individuals must be able to secure the attention of potential communication partners in all situations, including at a distance and under noisy conditions. Second, the conversational topic must be established. Intervention strategies include the following:

1. Using vocalizations or gestures to gain attention. Or, if an individual is severely vocally or physically impaired, battery-operated call signals or other similar devices can be used.

2. Using conversational topic-initiating symbols, such as "Hey, I have some great news!", "Do you have some time now?"; and "There's something I need to discuss with you." These symbols are placed on the communication displays and used by the individual to gain the attention of and orient potential listeners to the upcoming conversation.

3. Providing symbol messages to indicate the need to change topics (e.g., "I'd like to discuss something else now").

Strategies for Increasing Relevant and Worthwhile Conversations

Being a good conversationalist involves more than simply gaining a listener's attention. The ability to make relevant and worthwhile contributions to the discourse topic may be a difficult task for the individual with limited speech. Some intervention ideas include the following:

1. Providing clients with a wide range of experiences, including exposure to activities and events that are of interest to individuals of similar ages and developmental levels.

2. Planning (and encouraging families to plan) novel activities and surprise occurrences regularly in order to provide individuals interesting topics about which to converse.

3. Insuring that vocabulary symbols related to these activities are available to the individual.

Strategies to Develop Skill in Conversational Turn Taking

A competent conversationalist is able to initiate and maintain a topic of conversation over several interchanges. The conversational partner can play a major role in facilitating improved turn taking skills in individuals who use augmentative aids and techniques by doing the following:

1. Actively facilitating the individual's initiation behavior by using an expectant time-delay technique. For example, the conversational partner can simply wait for the individual to initiate a response or use a quizzical facial expression or other similar behaviors to cue the individual. The goal is to provide adequate time for the individual to respond.

2. Employing task interference strategies to elicit turns. In this procedure, the partner either directly or indirectly interferes with the successful execution of an activity, which causes the individual

to initiate some type of response (e.g., seek assistance or comment on the interruption of the task). For example, the partner might provide a student with only some of the art materials required to complete a craft activity or provide cleansers but no sponges for a janitorial task.

3. Insuring continuation of turn taking by using turnabouts.[42] Turnabouts are turns that maintain continuation of the discourse by responding to the previous speaker's turn, thus connecting it to the preceding discourse, while also requiring its own response, thus connecting it to the succeeding discourse. For example, a student with a communication aid might point to the symbol "lemonade" to which the communication partner would respond "You want some lemonade. Okay, do you want ice in it?" The partner has maintained the topic of conversation by responding to the initiation and by producing a question to which the student must respond.

4. Scheduling training sessions that allow the individual to practice conversational skills in supportive situations. Role-play interactions with a variety of different partners in a number of different scenarios. Vary the conversational partners present.

5. Developing the individual's sensitivity to the feedback cues provided by his or her listeners by teaching individuals to recognize confusion, feigned understanding, and lack of interest in listeners.

6. Insuring that the individual's communication aid contains symbols that allow regulation of the discourse (e.g., "Please give me time to finish my message" and "It will take me a while to form my message. Please be patient").

7. Teaching all participants in the discourse to elicit and use feedback cues throughout the construction of a message. For example, if a student uses an eye-gaze number encoding system by producing a three-digit code for the phrase "Please reposition my headrest," the partner should repeat each number of the code to insure his or her understanding. The accuracy of the partner's repetition is then confirmed or negated by the user.

Strategies to Facilitate Conversational Repairs

Conversational breakdowns often occur when individuals who use augmentative communication try to converse. Intervention strategies must be taught so that repairs can be made and communication can continue. Strategies should teach the individual and partners when and how to repair breakdowns. Examples include the following:

1. Using different repair strategies depending upon the situation and the conversational partner. For example, the individual might repeat the message, rephrase the message using additional content and form cues, or alter the type of communication mode employed.

2. Including symbol repair strategies on a language board (e.g., "I think you misunderstood me" and "Let me try and explain again"). Providing practice in the use of these symbols.

3. Teaching conversational partners to employ efficient questioning techniques and to use contextual cues and background knowledge to predict or guess the message.

General Procedural Considerations

Selecting Activities

The activities and materials used to develop conversational skills are related directly to the age and functioning level of the individual. However, in all instances, consideration must be given to selecting activities that promote conversational interaction. The importance of materials and activity selection to the interactional patterns of children has been demonstrated by Odom and Strain.[43] They found that play activities and materials can either promote or discourage interaction and that the effects were different for different groups. That activities and materials selected are of interest to the individual is also important. If needed, complete an interest inventory in order to learn about the likes and dislikes of a particular individual.

Implementing Instructional Programs in the Natural Environment

Ideally, training in conversational competency should occur across multiple natural settings and social contexts. Examples of conversational environments that may be considered include the home, neighborhood activities, organized recreational and social activities, routine structured school and vocational contexts, unstructured community-based leisure activities, transportation, in-home and outside emergency situations, and telephone communications.

Involving Partners and Clients in Intervention

Activities designed to develop conversational competency should be client- and partner-directed.

Procedures that address the client can be oriented toward developing two of the most important skills the individual who uses augmentative aids and techniques requires: contextual sensitivity and adequate self-monitoring skills. Because of the uniqueness in communication style and the atypical way that communication occurs, individuals, whenever possible, must learn to evaluate the skills of partners, the demands of the communicative task, and the parameters of the physical environment that affect performance, as well as how best to accomplish a task given the augmentative components available. To teach these skills, the client must become an "active learner" and will ultimately need to assume responsibility for his or her communication successes and failures. Although this goal is unrealistic for young children, it is a goal to work toward. Even very young children can be reinforced when they demonstrate sensitivity to contextual variables, for example, trying to get a parent's attention by kicking, failing, switching modes and vocalizing, and succeeding.

Partner-directed interventions teach procedures based on language training principles, such as expectant time delay and task interference strategies, learning theory principles (e.g., prompts, shaping, reinforcement, and modeling), developmental teaching principles (such as expansions and expatiations), incidental teaching strategies, and social skill training packages using peer facilitators.

RESEARCH NEEDS

Augmentative communication is a relatively new area of clinical practice. As a result, many of the assumptions that underlie current thinking and methodologies are not derived from data-based studies. Much work needs to be done, especially if researchers are to determine what factors characterize and can be used to predict a successful outcome.

This section suggests areas of research needs that relate to the individual, the augmentative components used to enhance communication, and the interventions that are employed to insure that communicative tasks can be accomplished in various settings.

The Population

There is a diverse population with a broad range of communication needs that can benefit from augmentative communication interventions. Because etiologies differ, intervention approaches with congenitally impaired individuals and those with degenerative, traumatic, or surgically caused disabilities are not the same. To identify the best approach for determining a life-long management plan for these individuals, it would be helpful to know how disability groups compare, since many teams serve as resources to all who require augmentative communication within their community.

Unfortunately, the amount of data-based information that describes the exact nature of the population is extremely limited. Demographic studies are needed to better describe age ranges, disability types, problems encountered, and geographic locations. Research is also needed to answer questions about the clinical course of various client groups over time. For example, clinicians need to know what kinds of augmentative interventions individuals with multiple sclerosis need over the course of their disease. When do clinicians intervene, with whom, and how often? What are the effects on language development and/or remediation of various symbol sets and systems, encoding techniques, other rate enhancement strategies, and type of output? Research also needs to define characteristics of "good versus poor" conversationalists.

Because of the diversity of the population, large controlled studies are difficult to carry out. Therefore to answer the questions listed before as well as others relating to the population, descriptive studies and single-subject designs should be employed.[44]

Another issue that must be addressed is related to advocacy for clients. In recent years, society has become increasingly aware of the fact that children who do not have a means of expression cannot receive an appropriate education and that adults who are unable to carry out a range of communication tasks (e.g., converse, write, access computers, use the telephone) are unlikely to function independently in society. This awareness is reflected in federal and state laws and by the increasing availability of third-party support for equipment and clinical services. However, much remains to be done. To properly integrate individuals with severe communication impairments into society, the individuals themselves, their families and friends, and the professionals who work with them must make local communities and governments aware of their needs. Data are needed to support advocacy statements about the need for and success of augmentative communication services and devices.

Augmentative Components

To communicate effectively, an individual must have a multicomponent communication system, and every component of that system must be integrated into all aspects of the individual's life. The effectiveness of each component depends upon the needs, abilities, and circumstances of each individual. However, teaching a person the mechanics of a communication aid or accessing technique does not result in the effective use of that aid or technique. Although special augmentative aids and techniques provide tools that enhance communication, strategies are needed to make these tools effective. Some of these were discussed in the previous section.

Speech-language pathologists also know little about which augmentative communication components or features of augmentative components are likely to be more acceptable and effective with an individual. The application of augmentative components does not necessarily create a "desire" to communicate in individuals with severe speech impairments, nor does it insure the development of communication competencies. Research on human factors in the augmentative communication area has not been conducted.[44] Multiple studies need to be completed to determine which components or features of components can be applied, under what circumstances, and with what disabling conditions. The following are some of the research questions that remain unanswered.

1. What are the effects (and the effectiveness) of speech technologies (speech synthesis and speech recognition)?
2. What are the effects (and the effectiveness) of various encoding and scanning techniques? At what developmental levels can individuals use these techniques for effective communication.
3. What are the effects of machine prediction and other rate enhancement strategies on conversational fluency and efficiency (i.e., ability to produce messages)?
4. What are the effects of various features of aids or techniques on communication partners, on conversational exchanges, on users, on the production of written text?
5. What are the effects of various accessing techniques (e.g., switches) on body posture, and rate and volume of messages produced?
6. Does the use of various augmentative components fatigue the user, and to what extent does this affect the user's performance?
7. What are the optimal performances possible using available communication aids, techniques, and strategies? These questions can be asked of both normal and disabled groups.
8. What aids (or features of aids) are the most desirable to users?
9. In the perception of users, what works, with whom, and under what circumstances? What objective information supports these perceptions?
10. How should the mechanics of communication aids (computers, language boards, manual signs) be taught?

The Communicative Context

Communication partners must be actively involved in all aspects of intervention because their patterns of communication dramatically affect the interaction with individuals who use aids and techniques. Thus research is needed to define the characteristics of "good" versus "poor" communication partners. Additional studies are required to show the effects of independent mobility on communication (e.g., message generation, opportunities, the development of conversational skills). Finally, it is necessary to know more about how to integrate augmentative communication components into all aspects of an individual's life.

The Communication Task

The communication patterns of individuals who use augmentative components must be studied if speech-language pathologists are to help them carry out the diverse communication tasks that are required in different environments. Communication skills can be taught. Strategies that address the development of conversational competency were discussed in a previous section of the chapter. However, many unanswered questions remain:

1. What lexicons do individuals with various types of communication aids use for conversation?
2. What strategies provide the greatest flexibility to individuals who use restricted vocabularies? How should these strategies be taught?
3. How should individuals with severe speech impairments be taught literacy skills?
4. How should these individuals be taught other academic skills?
5. How should the generative use of symbols be taught?
6. What conversational control strategies are effective under what circumstances?

Service Delivery

With increasing information about the need for intervention and the clinical management process, service delivery systems are likely to expand in the area of augmentative communication. What service delivery models are most effective in producing a successful outcome? Information that suggests when to intervene, with whom, and how often will be helpful in developing effective and reliable service delivery models. Efficacy studies also are needed to determine which service delivery models work best under which conditions. And what are the most cost-effective ways of delivering services to various groups under various demographic circumstances.

SUMMARY

This chapter provides an overview of augmentative communication, one area of clinical practice within the field of communication sciences and disorders. To summarize the importance of this area for those individuals with severe speech impairments and to remind professionals whose mission it is to develop and remediate communication skills, Daniel Webster's statement about the value of communication says it best:

> If all my possessions were taken from me, with one exception, I would choose to keep the power of communication. For by it, I would soon regain all the rest.

Acknowledgment. The preparation of this chapter was supported in part by Contract No. 300–85–0139 from the Special Education and Rehabilitative Service Branch, United States Department of Education, Washington, D.C. We wish to thank Deborah Bruskin for her helpful comments.

REFERENCES

1. Birdwhistell R. Background to kinesics. ETC 1955; 13:10–18.
2. Vanderheiden G, Yoder D. Overview. In: Blackstone SW, Bruskin DM, eds. Augmentative communication: an introduction. Rockville, MD: American Speech-Language-Hearing Association, 1986:1–28.
3. Creedon M. Language development in nonverbal autistic children using a simultaneous communication system. Paper presented to the Society for Research in Child Development, Philadelphia, March, 1973.
4. Dixon C. Some thoughts on communication boards. Cereb Palsy J 1986; 26:12–13.
5. McDonald E, Schultz A. Communication boards for cerebral palsied children. J Speech Hear Disord 1973; 38:73–88.
6. Shaeffer B. Spontaneous language through signed speech. In: Schiefelbusch R, ed. Nonspeech language and communication: analysis and intervention. Baltimore: University Park Press, 1980:421.
7. Sklar M, Bennett D. Initial communication chart for aphasics. J Assoc Physical Mental Rehabil 1956; 10:43–43.
8. Blackstone S. Augmentative communication: a clinical management process model. In: Bernstein L, ed. The vocally impaired. New York: Academic Press, in press.
9. Cohen C. Total habilitation and life-long management. In: Blackstone SW, Bruskin DM, eds. Augmentative communication: an introduction. Rockville, MD: American Speech-Language-Hearing Association, 1986:447.
10. Diggs C. Leadership training in augmentative communication. Proposal submitted to the United States Department of Education, Personnel Preparation. Rockville, MD: American Speech-Language-Hearing Association, 1983.
11. Kraat A. Developing intervention goals. In: Blackstone SW, Bruskin DM, eds. Augmentative communication: an introduction. Rockville, MD: American Speech-Language-Hearing Association, 1986:197.
12. Segelman M. Helplessness: on depression, development, and death. San Francisco: WH Freeman, 1981.
13. Dowden P. Augmentative interventions in intensive care units. In: Blackstone SW, Bruskin DM, eds. Augmentative communication: an introduction. Rockville, MD: American Speech-Language-Hearing Association, 1986:321.
14. Cooper IS. Involuntary movement disorders. New York: Harper & Row, 1969.
15. Crystal D. Keynote address. Paper presented at the meeting of the International Society of Augmentative and Alternative Communications, Cardiff, Wales, October, 1986.
16. American Speech-Language-Hearing Association, Ad Hoc Committee on Communication Processes and Non-speaking Persons. Committee position paper. Asha 1981; 23:267–272.
17. Kraat A. Training augmentative communication use: clinical and research issues. In: Galyas K, Lundman M, Lagerman U, eds. Communication for the severely handicapped. Bromma, Sweden: Swedish Institute for the Handicapped, 1982.
18. Harris D, Harris D. Communication interaction processes involving nonvocal physically handicapped children. Top Lang Disord 1982; 2(2):21–37.
19. Beukelman D, Yorkston K, Pabelte M, Naranjo C. Frequency of word occurrence in communication samples produced by adult communication aid users. J Speech Hear Disord 1984; 49(4):360–367.
20. Foulds R. Communication rates for nonspeech expression as a function of manual tasks and linguistic constraints. Proceedings of International Conference on Rehabilitation Engineering. Toronto, 1980.
21. Goossens' C, Crain S. Intervention resource manual. Lake Zurich, IL: Don Johnston Developmental Equipment, 1986.
22. Goossens' C, Crain S. Augmentative communication assessment resources. Lake Zurich, IL: Don Johnston Developmental Equipment, 1986.
23. Yorkston K, Karlan G. Assessment procedures. In: Blackstone SW, Bruskin DM, eds. Augmentative communication: an introduction. Rockville, MD: American Speech-Language-Hearing Association, 1986:163.
24. Berninger V, Gans B. Language profiles in nonspeaking individuals of normal intelligence with severe cerebral palsy. Augmentative Alternative Commun 1986; 2(2):45–50.
25. Matas JA, Mathy-Laikko P, Beukelman DR, Legresley K. Identify the nonspeaking population: a demographic study. Augmentative Alternative Commun 1985; 1(1):17–31.
26. Light J, Collier B, Parnes P. Communicative interaction between young nonspeaking physically disabled children and their primary caregivers. Part II—Communicative function. Augmentative Alternative Commun 1985; 1(3):98–107.
27. Calculator S, Luchko C. Evaluating the effectiveness of a communication board training program. J Speech Ear Disord 1983; 47:281–287.
28. Cassatt-James EL. Establishing the use of multimodalities using the communicative interaction assessment procedure. In: Blackstone SW, Bruskin DM, eds. Augmentative communication: an introduction. Rockville, MD: American Speech-Language-Hearing Association, 1986:307.
29. Light J, Collier B, Parnes P. Communicative interaction between young nonspeaking physically disabled children and their primary caregivers. Part I—Discourse patterns. Augmentative Alternative Commun 1985; 1(2):74–83.
30. Calculator S, Dollaghan C. The use of communication boards in a residential setting: an evaluation. J Speech Hear Disord 1982; 47:281–287.

31. Vanderheiden G, Lloyd L. Communication systems and their components. In: Blackstone SW, Bruskin DM, eds. Augmentative communication: an introduction. Rockville, MD: Asha 1983:471.
32. Baker BR. Mindspeak: a semantic compaction system that makes self-expression easier for communicatively disabled individuals. Byte 1982; Sept:186–202.
33. Paulsson K, Christofferson M. Psychosocial aspects of technical aids: How does independent mobility affect the psychosocial and intellectual development of children with physical disabilities? In: Trefler E, Kozola K, Snell E, eds. Selected readings on powered mobility for children and adults with severe physical disabilities. Washington: RESNA, 1986:27.
34. Culp DM, Ambrosi DM, Berniger TM, Mitchell JO. Augmentative communication aid use—a follow-up study. Augmentative Alternative Commun 1986; 1(2):19–24.
35. Van Tatenhove G. Training caregivers and facilitators to select vocabulary. In: Blackstone SW, Cassatt-James EL, Bruskin DM., eds. Intervention strategies in augmentative communication. Rockville, MD: American Speech-Language-Hearing Association, in press.
36. Yorkston K, Dowden P, Marriner N. Personal correspondence.
37. Cook S. Using topic specific miniboards to allow individuals who use communication aids to initiate communication with school staff members. In: Blackstone SW, Cassatt-James EL, Bruskin DM, eds. Intervention strategies in augmentative communication. Rockville, MD: American Speech-Language-Hearing Association, in press.
38. Schippits S. Developing miniboards to facilitate interaction in the community. In: Blackstone SW, Cassatt-James, EL, Bruskin DM, eds. Intervention strategies in augmentative communication. Rockville, MD: American Speech-Language-Hearing Association, in press.
39. Blackstone S. Training strategies. In: Blackstone SW, Bruskin DM, eds. Augmentative communication: an introduction. Rockville, MD: American Speech-Language-Hearing Association, 1986:267.
40. Wasson P. Messaging and reporting. In: Blackstone SW, Bruskin DM, eds. Augmentative communication: an introduction. Rockville, MD: American Speech-Language-Hearing Association, 1986:411.
41. Dashiell S, Hanson J, Hinchliffe M, Hunt J, Botti C. Procedures for mainstreaming students who use communication aids. In: Blackstone S, Cassett-James L, Bruskin D, eds. Augmentative communication: implementation strategies. Rockville, MD: American Speech-Language-Hearing Association; in press.
42. Kaye K, Charney R. Conversational asymmetry between mothers and children. J Child Lang 1981; 8:35–49.
43. Odom S, Strain P. Classroom-based social skills instruction for severely handicapped preschool children. Top in Early Childhood Educ 1984; 4(3):97–116.
44. Mathy-Laikko P, Yoder D. Future needs and directions in augmentative communication. In: Blackstone SW, Bruskin DM, eds. Augmentative communication: an introduction. Rockville, MD: American Speech-Language-Hearing Association, 1983:471.

35 Communication Problems in the Autistic Client

Barry M. Prizant, Ph.D.

In 1943, Leo Kanner, a child psychiatrist, published an article entitled "Autistic Disturbances of Affective Contact."[1] In this work, Kanner provided detailed and insightful descriptions of 11 patients who, in his opinion, had a unique cluster of symptoms including a severe disturbance in social relatedness, an insistence on preservation of sameness, and a significant impairment of language and communication. Kanner also noted that this clinical syndrome was characterized by an onset within the first 2 years of life, distinguishing it from childhood psychoses of later onset. These first descriptions of children having infantile autism marked the onset of nearly half a century of clinical and experimental enquiry about this perplexing syndrome.

Autism is now recognized as a lifelong developmental disability that occurs in approximately five of every 10,000 births and is four times more common in males than in females. A full range of cognitive functioning is associated with the autistic syndrome, with an estimated 60 percent having IQ scores below 50, 20 percent with scores between 50 and 70, and the remaining 20 percent above 70. A small percentage exhibit superior intellectual abilities. This wide range of intellectual functioning is reflected in the range of communication abilities and disabilities observed in autism. Autism may occur with no specific medical etiology, but is most often associated with pre- and postnatal conditions such as viral infections, metabolic disturbances, and epilepsy.[2]

Kanner's[1,3] early emphasis on language, social, and communicative impairments is reflected in recent conceptualizations of the syndrome.[4] However, much controversy has raged over the years about diagnosis and the very nature of the autistic syndrome. Ornitz indicated that behavior observed in autism falls into three general categories: disturbances in relating to people and objects (disturbances in social and cognitive abilities), disturbances in communication and language, and disturbances in sensory modulation and motility (disturbances in sensorimotor and perceptual functioning).[5] Major diagnostic schemes make reference to most, if not all, of these categories of disturbance (Table 35–1).

DIAGNOSIS AND SYMPTOMATOLOGY

Autism is, by definition, a syndrome identified by observable behaviors or patterns of behavior. Most diagnostic schemes demonstrate significant overlap in criteria cited; however, the differences in wording of specific criteria or the inclusion or omission of criteria all influence the diagnosis. Major categories of symptomatology will be reviewed briefly, with a more in-depth consideration in the subsequent section on theories of primary deficit.

Social and Affective Impairments

The word "autism," referring to a preoccupation with self, reflects Kanner's focus on the isolation and "aloneness" he observed in his original patients.[1] Subsequently, persons with autism have been described as being "in a world of their own" and unable to form emotional attachments. Descriptions of the social and affective impairments differ across diagnostic schemes, which may have a profound im-

TABLE 35-1 Major Diagnostic Schemes

Kanner's first description (1943)
Lack of responsiveness to other human beings*
Insistence on preservations of sameness in environment*
Onset of disorder in first two years of life
Delay in acquisition of speech and abnormalities of language
DSM III—American Psychiatric Association (1980)
Onset before 30 months of age
Pervasive lack of responsiveness to other people (autism)
Gross deficits in language development
If speech is present, peculiar speech patterns such as immediate and delayed echolalia, metaphorical language, and pronominal reversal
Bizarre responses to various aspects of the environment, e.g., resistance to change, peculiar interest in or attachments to animate or inanimate objects
Absence of delusions, hallucinations, loosening of associations, and incoherence as in schizophrenia
National Society for Children and Adults with Autism (1984)
Disturbances in the rate of appearance of physical, social, and language skills
Abnormal responses to sensations; any one or a combination of senses or responses are affected: sight, hearing, touch, balance, smell, taste, reaction to pain, and the way a child holds his or her body
Speech and language are absent or delayed, whereas specific thinking capabilities may be present
Abnormal ways of relating to people, objects, and events
Rutter (1978)
Onset before the age of 30 months
Impaired social development out of keeping with the child's intellectual level
Delayed and deviant language development
Insistence on sameness
Stereotypic behaviors
Abnormal preoccupations
Resistance to change

*Primary criteria.

pact upon the diagnosis. For example, the Diagnostic and Statistical Manual, third edition (DSM III), includes "a pervasive lack of responsiveness to other people" as a criterion,[6] whereas Rutter cited "impaired social development out of keeping with intellectual level."[7] Evidence for improved social relatedness in development as well as variability in social functioning in autism has led researchers to reject the extreme implications of the DSM III terminology.[8]

Language and Communication Impairments

Rutter noted that impairments in language and communication reflect processes of delay as well as deviance.[7] That is, persons with autism show delays in the acquisition of language and communication skills as well as characteristics that cannot be accounted for by developmental delay. Immediate and delayed echolalia, perseverative language, and idiosyncratic use of language are often cited as deviant language forms. Asynchronies in development across emerging skills related to language and communicative behavior may also reflect patterns that are different from developmental delay. These issues will be considered in greater depth later in this discussion.

Insistence on Sameness

Kanner and Rutter emphasized the insistence on sameness as manifest in resistance to change, abnormal and compulsive preoccupations, and the presence of stereotypic behaviors.[1,7] Many persons with autism appear to need structure and predictability to an extreme degree, as evidenced by their reactions of distress in response to violation of established routines and by their inflexibility in relating to people and objects, limited range of interests, and development of repetitive behaviors. It has been suggested that insistence on sameness either reflects a compensatory attempt to make sense of the world[9] or results from a relatively inflexible cognitive style that may underlie many aspects of behavior observed in autism.[10]

Abnormal Responses to Sensations

Many persons with autism appear to overreact or underreact to various forms of sensory stimulation. An individual may demonstrate extreme reactions to seemingly benign auditory or tactile stimulation, yet show little or no response to pain or seemingly noxious stimulation in various forms. Furthermore, many behaviors suggest an attempt to either shut out stimulation (e.g., hands over ears, screaming) or to increase auditory, tactile, or vestibular stimulation (e.g., repetitive tapping, rocking, flapping, or spinning).

The diagnosis of autism remains controversial because of the wide range of symptomatology cited in diagnostic schemes. In reaction to this state of affairs, recent reconsiderations have placed the greater emphasis on social and communicative impairments as the necessary and sufficient criteria for a diagnosis of autism, with often observed associated features, including abnormal sensory responses, insistence on sameness, and abnormal motility patterns, not considered necessary for diagnosis. Furthermore, it has been suggested that the age of onset criterion of 24 or 30 months included in most diagnostic schemes be eliminated.[4,11]

The degree of emphasis given to any of the impairments discussed before depends upon one's underlying beliefs about the nature of autism. Theories of "primary deficit" fall into two general categories based on hypothesized psychogenic (environmental) or biologic (constitutional) etiology.

PSYCHOGENIC THEORIES

In general, psychogenic theories assume that a child was normal at birth and that pathologic personality characteristics of the parents cause severe disturbances in emotional and social development. Autism is viewed as a disorder encompassing the entire range of ego functioning; therefore researchers believe that speech, language, and communication problems are one result of the child's severe social withdrawal and emotional disturbance.

Bettelheim provided the most detailed and controversial psychogenic theory of autism in his book, *The Empty Fortress: Infantile Autism and the Birth of Self.*[12] He attributed autistic behavior to a child's denial of self in defense against a world perceived as hostile and threatening. He cited pathologic parental characteristics (especially maternal) as leading to under- or overstimulation, preventing the child from acting on the environment during critical periods of development. Thus the child is deprived of experiences necessary for developing a concept of self. Bettelheim cited autistic children's "misuse" of pronouns (pronominal reversal) as support for his theory. Bettelheim noted that autistic children often use "you" or "he" instead of "I" when referring to self and claimed that the avoidance of "I" was due to an absence of awareness of self or denial of self.

Other psychogenic theorists have suggested that autism may be due to a general lack of stimulation,[13] a lack of parental warmth,[14] or the "double-bind" attitude of the mother (superficial warmth combined with severe coldness and rejection).[15] However, little support has been found for psychogenic hypotheses. Rutter indicated that in systematic investigations, environmental stresses were not found to be more common for autistic children than for normal children, and no particular deviant patterns of family interaction were found.[16] Most importantly, parents of autistic children were found to be similar in emotional health and parenting practices when compared to parents of other children with disabilities and parents of normal children. Some theorists have proposed "nature-nurture" theories of autism, hypothesizing a biologic predisposition to the syndrome that is triggered by some form of psychological trauma.[17] However, these theories have been refuted by the same lack of evidence as the pure psychogenic theories were as well as by increasing evidence for neurophysiologic involvement.[18]

BIOLOGIC THEORIES

Theories with specified or assumed biologic bases have included varying degrees of emphasis on cognitive impairments,[19,20,21] perceptual disturbances,[22] language impairments,[23] and socioaffective disturbances.[24] Some theories attempt to explain the wide range of symptomatology in autism such that specific deficits (e.g., a language impairment or a perceptual disturbance) are believed to underlie or result in the varied behavioral symptomatology associated with the syndrome, including deviant language behavior, social aloofness, stereotypic motor patterns, and so-called bizarre responses to the environment.

Until recently, researchers espousing specific theories about the nature of autism most often did not address the complex developmental interdependencies among the processes of perception, cognition, social cognition, language and communication, and affect. Some theories of "primary deficit" have been rooted in specific hypotheses about etiologic factors, most often implicating damage or dysfunction in the structures of the central nervous system at either cortical or subcortical levels. Major theories of the nature of autism that assume a biologic basis will now be reviewed with particular emphasis on how the hypothesized primary deficit is presumed to affect the development of language and communication.

Perceptual and Sensorimotor Theories

The two major perceptual or sensorimotor theories of autism are those of "stimulus overselectivity"[25] and "perceptual inconstancy."[22] The theory of stimulus overselectivity states that "the children respond to only part of a relevant cue, or even to a minor, often irrelevant feature of the environment, without learning about the other relevant portions of that environment."[25]

Koegel, Egel, and Dunlap noted that learning language and rules of social interaction requires the processing and integration of multiple stimulus cues;[26] thus overselective responding may account for social and communicative problems in autism. This theory has been criticized on two major points: first, stimulus overselectivity may be a phenomenon characteristic of generalized cognitive impairment and may not be specific to autism,[27] and second, early social deficits observed in the first few months of life in many children diagnosed later as autistic could not be explained by this theory.

The theory of perceptual inconstancy described autistic children as being unable to perceive objects and environmental experiences as remaining the same from time to time, resulting in an inability to relate current perceptions to past experience.[22] More specifically, autistic children were described as experiencing shifting states of arousal to environmental stimulation, fluctuating from hypersensitivity to overinhibition or obliviousness. This inability to modulate sensory input and motor output (later referred to as sensorimotor inconstancy[28]) was attributed to a pathoneurophysiologic process in the brain stem and the diencephalic structures responsible for the gating of sensory input. Ornitz indicated that disturbances of relating to people, cognition, and communication are consequences of inconstancy of perception due to the faulty modulation of sensory input.[5]

Cognitive Theories

Cognitive theories of autism implicated problems in higher order functions of memory processing, rule induction, and concept formation. Rimland proposed a theory of cognitive impairment in which autistic children are unable to attach meaning to incoming sensations.[19] In spite of their relatively good rote memory and intact sensory functions and motor skills, Rimland believed that a basic inability to attach meaning to experience and to form concepts resulted in impaired social and personality development. Severe language and communication problems are the result of impoverished social attachments and a fragmented concept of "self," initially caused by the inability to attach meaning to experience. Rimland hypothesized subcortical damage or dysfunction (in the reticular activating system) as causing the cognitive impairment and thus posited the first detailed biogenic theory of autism in an era when psychogenic theories were prevalent.

Hermelin and O'Connor performed a variety of experiments with autistic children and matched controls in order to investigate the autistic children's abilities to use meaning and to generate rules to aid in memory processing of incoming verbal and visual stimuli.[29] Their results indicated that autistic children performed as well as or better than controls with normal intelligence and mental retardation in memorizing and repeating meaningless stimuli. However, they performed less well when memorization and recall could be enhanced by using meaning in the stimulus display (e.g., grouping words by semantic category) or by inducing rules by which the stimuli were presented (e.g., temporal patterns in the presentation of letters). Hermelin and O'Connor concluded that the basic disturbance in autism was "an inability to create structures governed by complex and flexible rules." They found that most often their autistic subjects used a rote memorization strategy to retain information or imposed idiosyncratic and stereotypic structures. They claimed that this tendency could account for the problems in language and social interaction and for the presence of repetitive stereotypic behaviors. More recently, Hermelin and O'Connor reviewed studies of autistic children's difficulties in recognizing, interpreting, and producing signals related to emotional and affective states.[30] They revised their earlier hypothesis from implicating specific cognitive functions to postulating an impairment in both cognitive and affective processes, which interact to produce an "abnormally functioning logico-affective state."

Using a broad definition of cognition, Rutter argued that a cognitive deficit constitutes the core of autism and may underlie many features of the syndrome.[21] He cited a functional interdependence between the development of cognition, conation (volition, motivation), and affect (feelings, emotions), but stated that affect and conation depended upon cognitive capacities "of one type or another." Thus Rutter saw the inability to deal with social and emotional cues as one aspect of impaired cognition. Some researchers have acknowledged the significance of the cognitive dysfunction in autism, but have suggested that the linguistic impairment is prominent and may account for other symptomatology. Churchill presented the most extreme language-based position.[23] He proposed that a central language disorder may be a necessary and sufficient cause of autistic behavior and that the difference between autism and other central language disturbances (i.e., developmental aphasia) is the severity of involvement. Rutter reported similarities between autistic children and those with developmental receptive language disorders, and he stated that although an aphasic type of disorder may be a central element in the development of some cases of autism, it is not an adequate explanation of other behavioral disturbances.[16] In recent years, disturbances of language and communication have remained central to a diagnosis of autism, but have come to be viewed as a consequence of primary cognitive and/or social dysfunction.[21,30,31]

Social and Affective Theories

Most early theories citing a primary social or affective dysfunction were psychogenic in nature. Kanner spoke of a constitutional deficit in his first description of the syndrome, but later implied a strong psychogenic component in describing cold and impersonal parental characteristics.[1,32] Recently, theories of the nature of autism assuming a constitutional etiology have returned to a focus on social and affective dysfunction. Volkmar noted that the social disabilities are "a major, if not the major, defining characteristic of the syndrome."[33] Fein and colleagues concluded that the social and affective deficits in autism are primary and can account for problems in language, communication, and symbolic play because the development of these abilities depends largely on social relatedness.[31]

Recent research has attempted to describe more specifically the nature of the social and affective impairments. Hobson compared autistic children to normal and retarded children and found a significant impairment in the autistic children's abilities to match drawings and photographs of facial expressions of emotion to videotaped gestures and vocalizations characteristic of those emotions.[24] He indicated that autistic individuals are unable to "sense the meaning of expressions of emotion." Differences or deficits in the use of eye contact,[34] facial recognition,[35] nonverbal and verbal social communication,[30] and social imitation[36] have been cited as evidence for a primary social and affective dysfunction. Social and affective problems also have been found to remain a prominent feature in follow-up studies regardless of the level of cognitive functioning.

SPEECH, LANGUAGE, AND COMMUNICATIVE SYMPTOMATOLOGY

Speech, language, and communication problems are pervasive in the autistic syndrome, as is suggested by their inclusion in all major diagnostic schemes. These problems are apparent in verbal and nonverbal behavior, in prelinguistic and linguistic communication, and in both receptive and expressive modalities. Furthermore, social cognitive abilities correlated with language acquisition and precursors to language form, content, and use are typically affected.[37] These impairments do not reflect simple delays in development; asynchronies across development domains and so-called deviant characteristics are readily observed. Characteristics of speech, language, and communication will now be reviewed along with a consideration of other abilities believed to be closely related to communication development.

Mutism

Hingtgen and Bryson reported the prevalence of mutism (lack of speech) in autistic children to range from 28 percent to 61 percent across nine studies.[38] Schuler and Donnellan-Walsh distinguished between total muteness and functional muteness, with the former characterized by a total lack of vocalization (communicative or self-stimulatory) and the latter characterized by some presence of vocalization, but not used meaningfully in social exchange.[39] For those individuals who are said to acquire some speech, it is often not clear whether recognizable speech production (which may include production of words not used for communication) or communicative language is the criterion used.

The lack of speech development in mute autistic individuals may be attributed to a number of factors. The severity of cognitive deficiency (severe to profound retardation) in an estimated 50 percent may account for a large proportion, considering the strong correlation between speech and language development and measured intelligence.[18] However, the fact that some mute autistic individuals learn to use nonspeech symbolic communication systems suggests specific motor speech involvement. Clinical experience with mute autistic children demonstrating apraxic and dysarthric symptomatology provides some support for this; however, there is a great need for systematic investigation.

Anecdotal reports of autistic children who acquire and then lose speech are common in clinical practice and in published literature. Kurita found that, in a sample of 246 Japanese children diagnosed as autistic, 97 (37.2 percent) lost meaningful words prior to 30 months of age (mean chronologic age, 18 months) as documented by clinical records and parental questionnaires.[40] Three of the children were using two- to three-word sentences with the remainder at a single-word stage at the time of speech loss. Thirty-one children (32 percent) regained meaningful words; for 29 children, this recovery occurred at least a full year after the reported loss. The remaining 66 (68 percent) had no meaningful speech at the time of follow-up, which occurred an average of 38 months after speech loss (mean chronologic age, 5.2 years). Kurita suggested that the speech loss was one manifestation of an underlying regressive change resulting from multiple causative and predisposing factors and that this course of development may represent a clinical subtype of autism.

Pragmatic Behavior—Prelinguistic and Nonverbal Intentional Communication

A number of studies have examined prelinguistic communicative behavior of children with autism. Curcio used questionnaires, direct observation, and specific tasks to gather information about intentional communication in 12 nonverbal autistic children.[41] He found that the children most frequently used protoimperatives (prelinguistic requests for objects or action) with a notable absence of protodeclaratives (prelinguistic acts bringing attention to self or to objects to establish joint reference). The means of communication varied from the use of eye contact accompanied by gestures to physical manipulation. Wetherby and Prutting studied autistic and language-age matched children at prelinguistic and emerging language stages and found that the autistic children showed a much higher proportion of intentional communicative acts for behavioral regulation (e.g., requests, protests) with a virtual absence of acts for attracting or directing adult attention, whereas the normal subjects demonstrated acts for a full range of communicative purposes.[42]

Because of these findings, Wetherby suggested that autistic children may demonstrate a distinctive pattern of early communicative development.[43] Early acts serve relatively nonsocial communicative purposes of behavioral regulation (e.g., requests, protests) with more social purposes, such as bringing attention to the self or directing another's attention to an object or event, appearing later in development. This "ontogeny of communicative functions" is in contrast to the relatively synchronous development of communicative functions demonstrated by normally developing children and other language impaired children.[44]

Kanner's original descriptions of language behavior in autism included many references to its idiosyncratic and unconventional nature.[1,3] Only recently has the possible communicative value of unconventional nonverbal behavior in autism been considered. Ricks recorded the vocalizations of young autistic children and normal toddlers in situations of request, frustration, surprise, and greeting.[45] He found that all the children produced vocalizations specific to each condition. However, when he asked mothers to identify their own child and the situation based on the recordings, he found that mothers of normal children could reliably identify the situations, but could not distinguish the vocalizations of their children from those of the other normal children. In contrast, the mothers of the autistic children could reliably identify their own child and situation, but none of the other mothers could identify the situation on the basis of the vocalizations of the other autistic children. Because of these findings, Ricks suggested that autistic children develop idiosyncratic rather than conventional vocalizations, which may have communicative value only for those who know them well.

Researchers are now looking more carefully at so-called deviant and aberrant behaviors in terms of their possible communicative value. Iwata and colleagues demonstrated that self-injurious behavior was displayed at higher frequencies during high-demand situations for developmentally delayed subjects and may have served a terminating function.[46] Wetherby and Prutting found self-injurious behavior to be used as a means of protest in three young autistic children,[42] and Carr and Durand discussed aggression, tantrums, and self-injury as possible forms of communication in developmentally delayed and autistic individuals.[47] Not all problem behaviors can be interpreted as intentional forms of communication. These behaviors may be considered along a continuum of intentionality from relatively automatic unintentional emotional reactions to fear, frustration, or anxiety, to intentional expressions indicating protest. Movement along this continuum may reflect an individual's increasing knowledge of the effect of his or her behavior on others.[48] These findings are important, considering the high incidence of problem behavior in autism. They provide clinicians with alternative approaches to procedures intended only to eliminate such behavior, without a consideration of the functions served.

Speech and Vocal Characteristics

There have been few investigations of speech articulation or phonologic characteristics of those acquiring speech. Boucher found that her autistic subjects had superior articulation when compared to dysphasic and retarded controls,[49] and Bartolucci, Pierce, Streiner, and Eppel found the same types of phonologic errors as in retarded controls.[50] However, clinical experience suggests significant problems in speech articulation for some individuals possibly due to apraxic or dysarthric involvement.

Another area in need of further study is the discrepancy in speech production between echolalic speech and creative language in children demonstrating both patterns. Prizant found superior articulatory abilities in much of the echolalic speech of four young autistic children as compared to language-age appropriate phonologic patterns in their emerging creative language, suggesting that some forms of echolalic speech are not limited by the same productive constraints as true language production.[51]

Goldfarb, Goldfarb, Braunstein, and Scholl found problems "in virtually every aspect of voice and speech, including volume, pitch, voice quality, rate, phrasing, fluency, stress, intonation and inflection, and articulation," in the speech of 25 schizophrenic (autistic) children; however, no single pattern of problems could be discerned.[52] Baltaxe and Simmons reviewed studies of prosody (i.e., intonation, stress, and timing) in the speech of autistic children.[53] They noted that research did not support anecdotal reports of global abnormalities in prosodic features. Patterns that distinguished the autistic children from the normal and some of the aphasic controls included a range of fundamental frequency that was too narrow or too wide and an inaccurate marking of linguistic information through prosodic features. They indicated that an inability to use prosodic features in speech perception and linguistic comprehension may account for the linguistic chunking observed in the production of echolalia.

Morphology and Syntax

In general, studies of expressive syntax and morphology have found either no significant differences when autistic children were compared to retarded and language impaired controls or patterns of delay when autistic children were compared to normal controls. Of nine morphemes examined in the language samples of autistic and dysphasic children, Cantwell, Baker, and Rutter found differences only in the use of the third person present tense morpheme.[54] Bartolucci, Pierce, and Streiner found significantly more omissions of grammatic morphemes when their autistic subjects were compared to normal controls, but no differences in comparison to the mentally retarded subjects.[55]

Swisher and Demetras reviewed studies of expressive syntax in autistic children as compared to normal, retarded, and language impaired children and concluded that autistic children are delayed when compared to normal controls, but not when compared to children with a specific language impairment or mental retardation.[56] One problem with the literature on the language structure of autistic children is the distinct separation made between levels of language analysis (i.e., phonology, morphology, syntax, pragmatics). For example, so-called deviant language characteristics such as perseverative and metaphorical language and echolalia, considered to be pathognomonic of the syndrome,[3] are either not addressed in studies of language structure or are eliminated during analysis of language samples. One must question whether a somewhat "laundered" view of linguistic structural ability in autism is being presented when the data analyzed may not be fully representative of the full range of productive patterns.

Echolalia

Echolalia, the repetition of speech produced by others, was the focus of Kanner's interest in the language of autistic children.[1,3] The prevalence of echolalic behavior in verbal autistic individuals has been estimated to be 75 percent or greater,[57] and its significance is substantiated by the role it plays in the diagnosis of autism[58] and prognosis for further communicative growth.[59] The two general categories of echolalia that can be distinguished most clearly are immediate echolalia, referring to utterances produced immediately or a brief time after the model utterance, and delayed echolalia, referring to utterances repeated at a significantly later time. Despite their common name, the two categories of echolalia probably involve distinct forms of memory processing. The production of delayed echolalia appears to involve the retrieval of information from long-term memory, whereas immediate echolalia appears to involve reflex-like echoic short-term memory.[60] The term "mitigated echolalia" has been used to refer to immediate and delayed echolalic utterances that reflect some change from the original utterance in segmental or suprasegmental structure.

Some researchers (e.g., Lovaas[61]) have dismissed echolalia as aberrant and socially nonfunctional and therefore in need of eradication; whereas others (e.g., Fay,[62] Shapiro[63]) have discussed echolalia as a strategy to maintain social contact in the face of a severe comprehension deficit (see Prizant for a review of opposing theories[64]). On the basis of Schuler's[65] proposal that immediate and delayed echolalia probably represented a continuum of behavior, Prizant and Duchan[66] and Prizant and Rydell[67] performed videotaped analyses of echolalic behavior in an attempt to document this continuum. Prizant and Duchan derived seven functional categories of immediate echolalia based on the analysis of 1,009 echolalic utterances of four autistic boys. The categories represented utterances produced interactively and noninteractively and with and without evidence of comprehension and underlying communicative intent. Prizant and Rydell performed similar analyses on 387 delayed echolalic utterances and derived 14 functional categories. As with immediate echolalia, the delayed echolalic utterances showed variability in the exactness of repetition, the degree of comprehension of the repeated utterance(s), and the presence or absence of underlying communicative intent. These findings highlighted the importance of considering echolalic behavior as an integral part and reflection of autistic children's developing social cognitive, communicative, and linguistic competence, rather than simply dismissing such behavior as deviant.[68]

Pragmatic Behavior—The Social Use of Language

Researchers widely agree that the most striking problems and developmental discrepancies are apparent when considering the communicative competence of verbal autistic individuals. On the basis of their linguistic ability alone, these autistic individuals would appear to have the requisite skills to be competent communicators. However, the "pragmatic revolution" has taught us that effective communication is determined as much by social cognitive knowledge as by linguistic competence, and as noted earlier, social cognition has been implicated as an area of primary deficit in autism. Pragmatic studies fall into three categories: communicative functions or intentions, discourse and conversational behavior, and language adjustments or stylistic variation.[69,70]

Studies examining communicative functions and intentions in the prelinguistic and echolalic behavior of persons with autism were reviewed earlier, and they will not be reiterated here. A few studies have concerned this issue in verbal individuals. Cunningham compared the language of autistic and retarded children and found that the autistic children used more demands and requests.[71] Watson, Martin, and Schaeffer found that their autistic subjects requested attention and commented much less frequently when compared to studies of normally developing children, and when they looked at all modes of communication, these authors found that autistic children requested objects and actions most frequently.[72] Wetherby hypothesized that the more social functions of communication are those requiring the establishment of joint attention and joint reference and should be more difficult for autistic children to acquire.[43] Thus the more instrumental (less social) functions involving behavioral regulation are observed first in the prelinguistic communication and later in the verbalizations of autistic individuals, a pattern distinct from normal development.[44] However, functions of language that serve to direct attention or establish joint reference are not necessarily absent, but may be acquired by autistic individuals at higher levels in language development. On the basis of their analyses, Watson and colleagues hypothesized that there may be two distinct groups of autistic children, one that is motivated to establish mutual reference, thus having a better prognosis for further linguistic and communicative growth, and one that does not have this motivation, thus having a poorer prognosis.[72]

Conversational and discourse analysis examines the interactive use of language in reference to the interdependencies among utterances across conversational turns. Specific abilities required to be a competent conversationalist include introducing and maintaining topics in an appropriate manner, providing new and relevant information, talking enough but not too much to fill a conversational role, and responding when spoken to. Research and anecdotal accounts suggest that individuals with autism may be impaired in all these dimensions. Dewey and Everard summarized the conversational characteristics of "near normal" autistic adolescents following a survey of 50 parents:[73] autistic adolescents talk too much when exceedingly interested in a topic without realizing that the listener may not be interested; they are sometimes unaware that someone is speaking to them; they seem to be uncertain whether they have said too little, enough, or too much in a given situation; and in general, they lack the reciprocity expected in conversational interaction. Cunningham suggested that autistic children lack empathy or the ability to apprehend a listener's state of mind,[74] a notion recently discussed by Hermelin and O'Connor[30] and Paul.[75]

Hinerman and Channell compared the conversational abilities of seven autistic children and seven normal controls matched for mental age in a task requiring the children to "carry on" a conversation between two toy people.[76] Results indicated that the autistic children introduced the same number of topics as controls; however, they required significantly more prompts (from their mothers) to keep the conversation going and had significantly fewer topic reintroductions, fewer exchanges, fewer total utterances, and fewer utterances per topic. Tager-Flusberg also found that autistic children maintained a topic for significantly fewer turns than normal controls.[77] Paul and Feldman cited difficulties in topic identification and provision of the appropriate amount of information as the major conversational difficulties of their highly verbal subjects.[78] Tager-Flusberg[77] and Paccia-Cooper, Curcio, and Sacharko[79] found that autistic children differed from normal children in that they initiated conversations less frequently and were less likely to respond to others' conversational bids. Tager-Flusberg found that autistic children did not differ from normal controls in making topic-relevant remarks; however, Paccia-Cooper and colleagues noted that the autistic children responded inappropriately to adult questions three times more frequently than controls.

The ability to adjust language use on the basis of situational differences and listener needs is another area of difficulty for verbal autistic individuals. Baltaxe and Simmons compared language patterns of German and American adolescents with autism and noted that "the most prevalent violation of situational constraints" for all subjects was their inability to shift from formal to less formal styles of conversation.[80] This inability was noted more specifically in the German subjects who confused polite and familiar pronominal forms. Baltaxe added that her five autistic adolescent subjects had difficulty with speaker and hearer role relationships and foregrounding and backgrounding information.[81] In a study of four younger verbal autistic children, McCaleb and Prizant found that all subjects introduced old information as frequently as new information in conversational exchanges.[82] Langdell found that autistic children were less competent than retarded controls in adjusting language to provide more explicit information to persons not familiar with an event as opposed to persons familiar with an event.[83] Furthermore, he found that the autistic subjects were less likely to understand nonverbal cues provided by a listener as indicating that more information was needed. However, Paul and Cohen found that their autistic subjects were as likely to respond to requests for clarification as their subjects with mental retardation matched for nonverbal mental age, but their responses were less specific and less likely to add relevant information.[84]

The domain of pragmatic ability is vast, and clearly the development of such competence is interrelated with the development of knowledge of social conventions, knowledge that others have intentions and distinct points of view, and knowledge and/or use of the behaviors, both verbal and nonverbal, that serve to augment, clarify, and regulate communicative interactions and social exchange.

Cognition and Language Development

Prizant proposed that the cognitive style observed in autism, characterized by a specific profile of learning strengths and weaknesses, may provide some insight into the observed role of echolalia and patterns of language acquisition.[10] He noted that relatively intact abilities (e.g., rote memory, visual and spatial judgement) may be accounted for by a "gestalt" or holistic processing style. Frequently noted disabilities (e.g., acquisition of a rule-governed linguistic system, rule-induction in nonlanguage domains) are associated with tasks demanding analytic, sequential processing. Gestalt language patterns (i.e., immediate and delayed echolalia) observed in autism appear to be the result of an inability to induce linguistic rules. For individuals who acquire language, initial forms tend to be primarily echolalic, with subsequent movement to a more flexible rule-governed linguistic knowledge.[85] Prizant noted that similar styles of language acquisition have been observed by researchers studying normal children,[86] and these styles may reflect movement from a primarily gestalt approach to language acquisition to a more analytic approach involving early memorization of unanalyzed language "chunks," with subsequent analysis and segmentation.

As to why this style may be observed, Dawson, Finley, Phillips, and Galpert hypothesized that, early in language development, autistic children may rely on strategies associated with the right hemisphere.[87] These authors and Wetherby[88] suggested that a shift from right to left hemisphere processing may occur in development, possibly accounting for the shift from gestalt forms to more analytic forms. Further research based on neurophysiologic data as well as longitudinal observations of language acquisition in autism is needed to confirm these hypotheses. However, an understanding of these strategies provides specific direction for assessment and intervention efforts.

COMMUNICATION ASSESSMENT AND ENHANCEMENT: PHILOSOPHICAL UNDERPINNINGS

In research and clinical practice, professionals involved in speech, language, and communication assessment and enhancement efforts for persons with autism represent a variety of disciplines including behavioral and developmental psychology, special education, child psychiatry, and speech-language pathology. In practice, speech-language pathologists began to have a significant impact in the mid to late 1970s as a result of three factors: their rapidly developing expertise in severe language and social communicative impairments, the increased emphasis on language and communication problems in autism, and the widespread recognition of autism as a disorder of social, cognitive, and communication development rather than as an emotional disturbance.

The diversity of disciplines that have been involved in speech, language, and communication issues is reflected in the variety of approaches to assessment and intervention. In some cases, different approaches suggest diametrically opposed procedures and/or goals in enhancing communication. For example, traditional behaviorally oriented programs have emphasized compliance training by teaching that imitation of bodily movements or compliance to commands is a necessary prerequisite to communication training. More recent approaches, which have been derived from research and theory on normal social and communication development, emphasize the importance of focusing on initiated and spontaneous communication at early stages of intervention.

For assessment and intervention efforts to be consistent and efficient, it is essential that they be rooted in a theoretically sound philosophy. Most recent practices are based upon eclectic approaches drawn from behavioral, cognitive, and developmental psychology with a strong emphasis on the principles of social and communication development. The philosophical underpinnings of assessment and intervention approaches advocated in this chapter will now be discussed briefly (for more in-depth considerations, see Prizant and Schuler[89] and Prizant and Wetherby[69]). These underpinnings will form the basis for more detailed discussions, presented later in this chapter, on communication assessment and enhancement for persons at different levels of communicative competence. The philosophical underpinnings include, first, understanding communication ability and growth from a systems perspective; second, applying knowledge of cognitive style and developmental discontinuity in autism to assessment and intervention efforts; third, applying principles of normal communication and social development; and fourth, focusing on skills and abilities that will have an impact upon an individual's independence, that is, a functionalist approach.

A Systems Perspective

The acquisition of communicative competence is the result of synergistic growth in social, cognitive and communicative domains. Assessment and intervention efforts that isolate specific skills (e.g., speech articulation) may contribute little to understanding problems or developing communicative competence unless ability in all these areas are considered. In general, the focus of assessment and enhancement efforts should be, first, the means used for communication, second, the functions served by intentional communicative acts, and, third, the appropriateness of these acts to the social conventions of the communicative context.

Communicative means refers to the behavior through which one expresses communicative intentions and may include conventional acts such as vocalizations, gestures, words, or any combination thereof. Relatively unconventional means to communicate are often observed in autism and may include idiosyncratic gestures, echolalia, metaphorical language (i.e., words with private reference), and even aberrant behavior such as aggression or self-injury. Communicative function refers to the purposes served by communicative acts: for example, requests, protests, comments. Communicative intent, a notion closely tied to function, refers to what one intends to communicate. In the most basic sense, communication is successful when a communicative act serves its intended function.

Social appropriateness refers to the extent to which communicative behavior follows accepted social conventions. The degree of social acceptability of communicative means depends upon how conventional or understandable communicative acts are to others and whether communicative attempts take into account the needs of the listener. Another important dimension of social acceptability is adherence to the conventions of conversational behavior including appropriate initiations, topic maintenance, and terminations. Both verbal and nonverbal behavior must be considered in reference to the dimensions of means, functions, and social acceptability, and all three dimensions must be considered in assessment and communication enhancement endeavors.

Cognitive Style and Developmental Discontinuity

As discussed earlier, persons with autism demonstrate a characteristic profile of abilities and disabilities that one should take into account in communication assessment and enhancement. Relative abilities include an excellent rote memory for visual and auditory information and relatively intact abilities in visual and spatial judgement and pattern recognition. Many autistic individuals develop "idiot savant" characteristics or exceptional abilities in musical skills and calculating skills.[90] Relative disabilities typically include an impaired development of verbal and nonverbal communication and social skills and a severe impairment in socioaffective competencies, that is, comprehending the feelings and intentions of others and expressing emotions in a conventional manner. Another major area of disability is in dealing with symbolic and abstract information, especially involving topics outside the specific interests and preoccupations of the individual involved.

Unless knowledge of developmental discontinuity is applied to communication assessment and enhancement, the communicative behaviors of persons with autism are difficult to understand, and they may be misjudged because of the presence of apparent abilities. For example, because of their excellent rote memory, many persons with autism who develop speech are able to memorize phrases and reproduce them at a later time, thus leading to a superficial picture of linguistic competence. The presence of delayed echolalia may lead co-interactants to use language at levels of complexity beyond an individual's language comprehension ability, thus resulting in communication breakdowns. Similarly, hyperlexia, or precocious mechanical reading skills developed by many autistic persons, may lead clinicians or educators to overemphasize the skill as true linguistic competence. This spurious ability may not result in greater competence in daily routines unless the focus is on helping individuals to understand the conceptual meanings for use in functional activities.

Applying Normal Developmental Information

In the 1960s and 1970s, behavior modification approaches dominated the literature in speech and language training for persons with autism.[91] The best known work in this vein is that of Lovaas[61,92] and his colleagues, who applied the basic principles of operant conditioning as espoused by Skinner.[93] Lovaas was able to demonstrate that some, but not all, autistic children could be taught rudiments of speech and language behavior including sound imitation, object labelling, and appropriate responses to specific questions. However, there has been some concern about the traditional behavioral emphasis on language form rather than function[94] and the de-emphasis on individual differences in learning style and developmental levels across social, cognitive, and communicative functioning.

Researchers and clinicians applying traditional approaches either did not consider the emerging developmental literature on communication and language, because of their belief that learning theory was an adequate model to explain development, or dismissed developmental information on the grounds that it could not be applied to autistic individuals. In recent years, there has been some reconciliation between behavioral approaches and developmental models, largely based on the adoption of developmental information by clinicians emerging from a traditional behavioral orientation.[94,95]

Literature on normal social communicative development began to have a major impact upon assessment and intervention for language impaired children in the early 1970s.[96,97] Owing to the dominance of behavioral approaches with autistic children at this time, communication assessment and intervention efforts based on developmental principles did not take hold until the early 1980s. Since that time, speech-language pathologists have come to play a central role in these efforts.[98,99] The application of developmental literature has provided not only a theoretically sound framework for communication assessment and enhancement, but also insight into the nature of social and communicative impairments characteristic of the autistic syndrome.[100,101] The principles of social communicative development that have had the greatest impact upon assessment and treatment follow.

Preverbal Intentional Communication

The development of preverbal intentional communication is a necessary precursor to the later development of communicative language.[102,103] A major shortcoming of traditional behavioral approaches was the emphasis on speech training regardless of an individual's level of social, cognitive, or communicative functioning.[91] As pragmatic models of language acquisition were introduced,[104] the developmental notion of communicative intent began to have an influence on assessment and intervention with language impaired children. The basic premise is that intentional communicative acts develop prior to the emergence of first words and that children first learn about the instrumental power of communication by observing the impact of their prelinguistic gestures and vocalizations upon the behavior of others. Furthermore, communicative intent was defined by the presence of a plan to affect the behavior of others through active signalling—not by the conventionality of the signals used. Thus more primitive and unconventional forms of behavior (e.g., physical manipulation, idiosyncratic gestures, aggression, echolalia) used to affect others' behavior achieved the status of intentional communication.[48]

As applied to communication in autism, the major effect of this literature was to emphasize that persons with autism do attempt to communicate; however, their attempts may be difficult to read because of their idiosyncratic and unconventional form.[10,43] Thus analyzing the communicative intent of behavior has come to be an essential part of assessment practices. In intervention, the increasing focus on communicative intent and function has led clinicians to view symbolic and presymbolic nonspeech communication systems as acceptable alternatives or augmentations to speech.

Communication and Language Skills

Communication and language skills develop within the context of reciprocal social interactive exchanges.[105] The traditional approach to communication training in autism is that of discrete-trial training, emerging out of behavioral approaches of the 1960s and 1970s.[61] Carr summarized the features characteristic of discrete-trial training:[94]

1. Teaching episodes are initiated by the adult.
2. The adult chooses the location—often isolated from the natural context for language use.
3. The adult chooses the entire content of the teaching episode.
4. A teaching episode typically consists of many (i.e., massed) training trials.
5. Correct responding is often followed by arbitrary reinforcers.
6. The method is typically employed to help the child acquire new language forms.

Prizant criticized this approach for a number of reasons.[98] First, it violates the basic tenets of the social-interactive basis of language and communicative development by putting individuals in a primarily respondent role. It is highly unlikely that initiated spontaneous communication results from this methodology, considering the situationally specific and somewhat inflexible learning style observed in autism. Second, because natural motivations for communication are not considered and reinforcement may not relate directly to the communicative act, problems in generalization to more natural contexts are common. And third, it is unlikely that individuals learn about the dialogic nature and social conventions of communicative exchange if they are exposed primarily to highly contrived interactions that bear little resemblance to more spontaneous and natural interactions. The developmental literature on discourse and conversation emphasizes that successful communication must involve reciprocity, mutual negotiation, and active participation. Behavioral interventionists have recently come to recognize the problems of discrete-trial methodologies as applied to communication development and have begun to advocate more natural social-interactive frameworks for communication enhancement.[106–108]

Focus on Communicative Needs Relevant to Life Routines

The level of communicative competence achieved by persons with autism is closely related to measures of outcome.[109] Furthermore, there is preliminary evidence that the development of communicative abilities is directly related to the reduction of socially unacceptable and aberrant behavior.[47,110] Therefore communicative competence may be a primary determinant of the extent to which an individual can participate actively in daily activities and routines in a variety of social contexts.

Communication assessment and enhancement efforts must directly address the issue of functionality. That is, do assessments provide information about current competencies that enable active participation as well as identify disabilities that hinder such participation? Do intervention efforts target knowledge and abilities that are likely to have an immediate as well as future impact upon independent functioning? Unless the answers to these questions are in the affirmative, it is likely that these are nothing more than academic exercises of little value to all involved.

COMMUNICATION ASSESSMENT

Approaches

The ultimate goal of language and communication assessment is to develop a current communicative profile that provides information relevant to communication enhancement efforts. The pervasiveness of language and communication impairments in autism demands that the assessment process be efficient in identifying functional communication needs. Efficiency can be achieved by gathering information from a variety of sources through informal and formal procedures.

Formal procedures include standardized tests, developmental scales, and structured interview protocols, the latter typically used with informants who are familiar with the person being assessed. These procedures tend to be more specific as to the areas being assessed and the procedures and materials used in gathering the information. For standardized instruments and developmental scales, the information obtained through formal assessments is compared to normative data collected from groups of children. The use of more formal procedures places some restrictions on the clinician and, for a number of reasons, may be of limited value if used alone.

First, procedures for administration of formal instruments may have to be modified to the extent that assumptions underlying their use are violated. Assumptions may include, for example, that one administers the test within a specified time period and follows specific procedures. Procedural modifications, which often are necessary owing to the attentional and behavioral problems experienced by persons with autism, may make the use of normative data invalid. Second, there is increasing evidence that persons with autism may demonstrate different sequences and strategies in the acquisition of communicative and linguistic abilities,[10,43] raising some question about the inflexible use of developmental data for assessment purposes. Most formal instruments are based on models of normal development and compare performance to that of normal children. Third, most currently available language assessment instruments assess aspects of language structure in receptive and/or expressive modalities (e.g., phonology, vocabulary, morphology, and syntax). Although this information is important, persons with autism demonstrate the most severe deficits in language use, even when knowledge of structure is relatively intact.[77] Thus assessment of structural linguistic knowledge may yield limited information about communicative competence in natural social interactive exchanges. And fourth, because formal assessment instruments typically are based on models of normal language development or on the performance of normally developing children, they do not account for the unique language symptomatology in autism such as immediate and delayed echolalia, perseverative language, and metaphorical language. Recent literature suggests that these so-called deviant language characteristics may serve important communicative and cognitive functions and thus should be addressed in the assessment process.

Informal approaches include observations of communicative behavior in less structured and more natural interactions. One may gather information by observing individuals in common daily routines in order to generate hypotheses about communicative abilities and disbilities relative to different contexts. One may obtain more specific information by setting up situations designed to test these hypotheses. Informal approaches also include gathering information from informants in semistructured interviews. The primary strength of informal approaches is the provision of ecologically valid information considering the variability in communicative functioning observed in autism across social contexts. One drawback when compared to more formal approaches is the amount of time needed to collect representative samples of language and communicative behavior. Regardless of the level of communicative functioning, the judicious selection of formal procedures used in conjunction with informal approaches can provide information for deriving the most comprehensive profile of language and communicative abilities.

Content

A thorough assessment should provide information about an individual's abilities in three major domains: language behavior (or communicative behavior for individuals not using language), social interactive behavior, and, when relevant, language-related cognitive abilities. Regardless of the level of communicative functioning, there are a number of assessment issues that must be addressed. These generic assessment issues will now be presented followed by a discussion of specific assessment concerns at different levels of cognitive, communicative, and linguistic functioning.

Generic Issues

Assessing Communicative Needs

Efforts to enhance communicative competence of persons with autism must focus on functional abilities that will make an impact upon independent living and quality of life. Ideally, these communicative abilities should enable a person to indicate personal preferences, make decisions, plan for future activities, and engage actively in social exchanges. One can determine specific communicative needs by observing an individual in typical environments with a variety of partners and by gathering information from familiar persons (e.g., caregivers, siblings, teachers) about future environments and current sources of frustration because of communicative limitations. Falvey provides a detailed discussion of the use of ecological inventories that may be used to gather this information systematically.[111]

Assessing Comprehension

Assessment of language comprehension is one of the most challenging and important undertakings with autistic individuals. It is challenging because inconsistent responses to language are typical and may be due to lack of motivation in responding, problems in attending in busy environments, or lack of comprehension. On the one hand, few individuals with autism develop the metalinguistic awareness to request clarification or to indicate that they do not understand, including many at more sophisticated levels of linguistic competence. On the other hand, some individuals develop fairly sophisticated nonlinguistic comprehension strategies similar to those discussed by Chapman[112] and may spuriously appear to be competent in linguistic comprehension. With these cautions in mind, efforts at assessment of linguistic comprehension may utilize both formal and informal procedures appropriate for individuals with language impairments. However, results should always be tempered by the knowledge of inconsistent response patterns observed in autism. (See the article by Lord for a discussion of the complexities of assessing language comprehension in autism.[113])

Assessing Communicative Intent

Prizant and Wetherby provided a detailed discussion of the assessment of communicative intent of persons with autism.[48] Communicative intent was defined as the ability to use expressive signals in a preplanned manner in order to affect the behavior or attitudes of others. The assessment of communicative intent should result in acquiring three types of information: first, the variety or range of functions or intents expressed; second, the level of communicative intent relative to the specific functions; and third, the variety of communicative means used in expressing intent.

Range of Functions or Intents Expressed. Some persons, typically very young children or those with profound cognitive impairments, may not demonstrate any behavior that appears to be intentionally communicative. In these cases, behaviors that may serve a communicative function based on others' imputing of intent should be documented. For example, the visually guided reach of a young child that is interpreted as a request may provide a fertile context for developing intentional requesting behavior.

Three general functional categories that have been documented in the preverbal communicative behavior of normally developing children include behavioral regulation, social interaction, and joint attention. As noted earlier, there is preliminary evidence to suggest that, in autism, behavioral regulatory acts may predominate early in development.[43] Nevertheless, assessment of the range of functions expressed is important for intervention planning and for documenting progress. There are many categorical frameworks that have been used for delineating specific intents or functions of communication with autistic persons.[42,66,67,72,98,114] Categorical systems should be chosen on the basis of their comprehensiveness as well as their ease of use in clinical situations.

Assessing Level of Communicative Intent. McLean and colleagues[115] outlined three general levels of intent based on the work of Bates.[104] Prizant applied this framework to communicative behavior of persons with autism (Table 35–2).[116]

The first level includes perlocutionary communication, which is preintentional and prelinguistic. That is, an individual is not yet directing signals toward others to affect their behavior in preplanned ways; however, intentionality may be attributed to their behavior by others. Examples of perlocutionary behaviors include vocalizations in response to physiologic states, orienting to visual or auditory stimuli in the environment, and even preintentional forms of echolalia.[66]

The second general level of communicative intent, illocutionary communication, includes those individuals who are beginning to communicate intentionally through nonverbal and prelinguistic means. Two sublevels of illocutionary communication, primitive and conventional, differentiate individuals who are using primarily primitive and idiosyncratic signals intentionally from those using more conventional preverbal communicative signals. Examples of primitive illocutionary communication include physical manipulation of others and idiosyncratic vocalizations (understood by familiar people). Examples of conventional illocutionary communication includes conventional gestures for requesting, giving, and showing and conventional vocalization patterns. Some forms of echolalia, especially delayed echolalia, may be used to express communicative intent and still be considered prelinguistic if there is no evidence that rule-governed linguistic behavior underlies its production. The extent to which echolalic productions may be considered primitive or conventional illocutionary communication depends upon how "readable" the signals are to others.

The characterization of communication in autism as idiosyncratic and unconventional pertains to individuals at illocutionary levels as well as at linguistic levels. Thus it is not uncommon to observe extended periods of primitive illocutionary communication prior to the emergence of more conventional forms. Clinical observations suggest that some individuals may even begin using language for communication before conventional illocutionary communication is observed (e.g., pointing or showing behaviors), a distortion of the normal developmental sequence. It may be hypothesized that the severe social cognitive impairment, especially as manifest in limited social imitative skills and joint referencing, inhibits the acquisition of conventional communication, which is learned through involvement in and observation of social interaction. Additionally, conventional forms that may not be acquired until later in development (e.g., pointing and showing behaviors) often are used for joint referencing, a com-

TABLE 35-2 Range of Functioning Represented by Each Level of Communicative Behavior*

Level of Communicative Intent	*Description*	*Behaviors Observed*
Level One		
Proactive perlocutionary (preintentional)	Child actively explores environment Does not direct vocal or gestural signals to others Does not anticipate specific social outcomes contingent upon his or her behavior No evidence of linguistic comprehension	Stereotypic manipulation of objects Orients to visual and auditory stimuli Child may be mute or may produce a variety of vocalizations not directed to others If child is echolalic, the verbal repetition is not produced with communicative intent (i.e., only nonfocused echoing or turn-taking echoing Inconsistent responding to others' speech
Level Two		
Primitive illocutionary (early intentional)	Child begins to direct signals to others expecting specific outcomes Communicative behaviors are concrete or subtle and may be idiosyncratic to "child-significant other" dyads Child shows some persistence in signalling behavior until goal is reached or may become frustrated or distressed if goal is not reached Only evidence of what may appear to be linguistic comprehension occurs in the context of common daily routines involving single-word comprehension with referents in context	Physical manipulation of adults' hands to perform specific tasks Shifting gaze between adult and goal Moving adult physically (e.g., pushing) to initiate action (e.g., leaving the room) Vocalizations may be used in conjunction with physical manipulation If child is echolalic, verbal repetitions may begin to be used with intent (e.g., yes-answer, protest) with accompanying behaviors clarifying intent
Conventional illocutionary (prelinguistic, intentional)	Child has clear concept of communication Child uses conventional and symbolic gestural and vocal means to affect others' behaviors and achieve specific outcomes Prelinguistic communicative signals are interpretable by a wider range of people Child demonstrates greater persistence if communicative goals are not met Increased evidence for linguistic comprehension possibly including simple multiword utterances with referents in context and a few common object labels with referents out of context	Child produces signals consistently in expressing intent Signals may include symbolic point-gestures for requesting, giving, showing, or even pantomime Vocalizations may be characterized by more conventional intonational patterns (e.g., protest, requesting) Some phonetically consistent forms may function as "protowords" and may be used meaningfully, but only in specific contexts If child is echolalic, immediate and delayed echolalia may be used for a wide variety of functions; however, language is still repeated in whole units or "unanalyzed chunks" and may still be situationally constrained in use
Level Three		
Emerging locutionary (intentional, emerging linguistic)	Child is beginning to demonstrate consistent use of linguistic forms for communication (words or signs) Use of such forms is not limited only to specific situational contexts (decontextualized use) Forms are conventional and, therefore, meanings are understood However, certain conventional forms may be used in idiosyncratic ways, accounting for "metaphorical language" Gestural, vocal, and gaze behaviors may serve to clarify child's intent and remain a major part of communicative repertoire Child demonstrates increased linguistic comprehension of single-word and simple multiword utterances with referents in and out of immediate context	Child uses words or signs spontaneously to accomplish specific goals (at least five to ten different words) Words begin to represent classes or concepts; e.g., "cookie" is used to request different cookies in different situations Echolalic children begin to acquire single words and/or begin to demonstrate mitigation (linguistic rule-governed change) in echolalic productions Child demonstrates greater flexibility in functional use of echolalia relative to the situation

TABLE 35–2 Continued

Level of Communicative Intent	*Description*	*Behaviors Observed*
Level Three *(Continued)*		
Locutionary (intentional, linguistic)	Language is a primary means of transmitting and receiving information Linguistic expressive and receptive knowledge extends beyond early multiword utterances, including use and comprehension of grammatical morphemes, various simple sentence types, and possibly complex sentences (for higher level individuals) Language is used consistently to relate information and events temporally and spatially distant from the immediate context Problems exist in comprehension of nonliteral forms of language such as idioms and sarcasm; however, there are no significant problems in comprehension of language relating to familiar events and relatively nonabstract topics	Child initiates and responds to verbal interaction (however, some children may be electively mute, depending upon familiarity of situation and co-interactants) Utterances are primarily creative, but residual echolalic behavior may occur, signalling a lack of comprehension or serving rehearsal or self-regulatory functions Child demonstrates primary problems in use of language, especially pertaining to social conventions in conversation, taking the listener's perspective and repairing breakdowns

*Reprinted with permission from Prizant BM. Assessment and intervention of communicative problems in children with autism. Commun Disord 1984; 9:127–142.

municative function that may be acquired later by autistic individuals.[43]

The third and last general level, locutionary communication, includes those individuals who use or are beginning to use a productive language-based system for communication (i.e., oral language or sign language). Two sublevels of emerging locutionary (emerging language) and locutionary (linguistic) communication differentiate individuals who have acquired a basic single-word vocabulary of at least five to ten words, but who are still communicating primarily through preverbal means, from those who are using language as a primary means of communication and are able to produce and understand multiword utterances. Only a minority of individuals with autism acquire true productive language and typically function at higher cognitive levels.

A few points must be kept in mind when identifying the level of communicative intent. First, these levels are not mutually exclusive; they represent a continuum of behavior and may be used as a heuristic framework to characterize primary levels of expressive communication. Second, echolalic speech may be observed at all three levels and should not necessarily be interpreted as evidence of communicative and/or linguistic competence. Echolalia should be considered as a form of illocutionary communication only when there is independent evidence of communicative intent, and it should be considered locutionary communication only when there is evidence of rule-governed linguistic changes (i.e., mitigated echolalia). Third, the level of communicative intent may vary greatly with the communicative function expressed. Wetherby suggested that autistic children may acquire one function at a time, and progress to more sophisticated means of expression for a specific function, before acquiring other communicative functions, which then follow the same progression. Children who use complex language for requesting, but who use prelinguistic or even aberrant means to protest or bring attention to self, exhibit this pattern of developmental discrepancy. Wetherby also suggested that characterizing communicative growth on a function by function basis may be more fruitful than on overall developmental levels across communicative functions.[43] However, further evidence is needed to support these observations.

Range of Communicative Means Used to Express Intent. The third dimension to consider is the behavior used to express intent. As discussed earlier, a wide range of conventional and unconventional behaviors, as well as verbal and nonverbal behaviors, may be considered. Donnellan and colleagues[114] and Prizant and Schuler[89] presented lists of potential communicative means, including prelinguistic and nonverbal behavior—such as aggression, gaze, gestures, vocalizations, and partial re-enactments of situations—and verbal behavior, such as spoken or signed utterances at different levels of complexity. A careful description of communicative means and the functions they serve provides direction for intervention regardless of an individual's level of communicative competence.

Assessing Socially Interactive Behavior

At all levels of communicative competence, an accurate assessment of social interactive behavior also is essential for planning intervention. By definition, autistic individuals demonstrate impairment in social interactive behavior out of keeping with their intellectual level.[58] Yet the stereotype of individuals who are totally isolated, withdrawn, or in a world of their own is no longer considered credible. Furthermore, researchers are now emphasizing that the social impairment may be attributed largely to a lack of knowledge of social conventions rather than simply an unwillingness to engage in social interaction.[117] Thus social behavior has become an important domain of assessment and intervention efforts.[118,119]

Assessment concerns include an individual's initiation strategies, including mode of initiations, responses to others' initiations, gaze behavior and the use of gaze for communication, action and vocal turn-taking, body posture and orientation, proxemic behavior (the use of space in communication), and, if present, the use of nonverbal or linguistic strategies to maintain interaction or to repair communication breakdowns. The purpose of this assessment is to identify the factor or factors (other than expressive or receptive impairment) that may contribute to either communicative competence or impairment. (See the articles by Prizant and Schuler,[120] Duchan,[121] and Higginbotham and Yoder[122] for a more in-depth consideration of these issues.)

Assessment of an individual's abilities in the generic assessment domains of communicative needs, communicative intent, comprehension, and socially interactive abilities and strategies provides a wealth of information leading to effective communication enhancement efforts. However, there are specific assessment concerns relative to persons at different levels of functioning that need to be considered.

Concerns at Prelinguistic Levels

In addition to determining the level of intent, communicative means relative to specific prelinguistic communicative functions, and comprehension, information should be obtained about social and cognitive abilities believed to be related to language. A profile of abilities across these domains is used in decisionmaking regarding the introduction of nonspeech communication systems. Social and cognitive skills to be assessed may include level of vocal and gestural imitation, schemes for relating to objects (functional object use and symbolic play schemes), causality, and means-ends behavior. Additional considerations include evidence of motor speech impairment (e.g., oral muscular weakness, drooling, limited or undifferentiated vocalizations) and degree of fine motor coordination for pointing or signing. A complete occupational therapy assessment may be helpful.

Individuals who demonstrate significant gaps between expressive abilities and social cognitive and receptive skills (with the latter being more advanced and at least at a 12- to 18-month level) may be candidates for a symbolic or quasisymbolic system (e.g., sign language, picture communication board). Those who demonstrate receptive and social cognitive abilities commensurate with expressive skills (below a 10- to 12-month level) may be better able to learn to use more primitive gestural means (e.g., natural gestures, physical manipulation). Current intentional communicative means, if any are observed, are an important consideration in this regard. Schuler discusses criteria for introducing an augmentative or alternative system or a verbal system.[123] Rigid application of such criteria is ill-advised; however, there is still much to be learned about the effectiveness of different systems with persons with autism.[123,124]

Concerns at Emerging Language Levels

Individuals at this level are beginning to show evidence of the acquisition or capacity for the acquisition of a conventional symbolic system for communication. For these individuals, the first concern is that of specific expressive language delays caused by problems in motor speech planning and execution, which can be observed most readily as an individual acquires a basic vocabulary. As discussed, this issue is important at prelinguistic levels, and it remains crucial at emerging language levels where speech intelligibility may be affected. The symptomatology most suggestive of these problems is the concurrence of a lack of intelligible speech with significantly greater receptive language and cognitive ability. Oral posturing or groping articulatory movements may be observed, suggesting attempts at speaking. Such symptomatology may suggest apraxic involvement. Excessive drooling, poor tongue mobility, a history of feeding problems, and labored speech production when speech is present suggest possible dysarthric involvement.

Judgements of motor speech problems typically depend upon oral motor or speech imitation tasks, with active participation on the part of the affected individual. Unfortunately, for many persons with autism, making these judgements is confounded by interactional problems, poor eye contact, a possible lack of compliance, and difficulty with volitional imitative tasks. As discrepancies between expressive abilities and receptive and cognitive abilities increase, the risk of behavioral problems due to frustration increases. Thus these individuals are prime candidates for alternative or augmentative communication because of their greater sociocognitive competence and the potential for precluding the development of disruptive behavior. There is a paucity of research and clinical reports on motor speech involvement in autism. For assessment and intervention, clinicians would need to rely on the available literature.[125,126]

Many individuals with autism demonstrate few problems in speech production and may display articulatory proficiency that far exceeds comprehension of the forms produced. Assessment of echolalic behavior is important because it provides insight into emerging linguistic competence. An analysis of echolalic behavior provides two types of information: first, an individual's knowledge of communicative function and, second, an individual's progress in linguistic and communicative growth over time. Functional analyses of echolalic behavior provide information about the range of functions an individual is learning to express, even if the means of expression is through immediate and delayed echolalia. As discussed earlier, echolalia may range from primitive and relatively automatic repetition of speech to clearly intentional use of repetition to accomplish specific goals. Dimensions to consider in functional analysis include interactiveness and comprehension of utterances produced and specific nonverbal behavior that may help to determine the presence or absence of underlying intent.[64,68] Specific intervention strategies for echolalic behavior depend to a large extent upon the results of these analyses.

Over time, changes in echolalic behavior relative to the emergence of rule-governed linguistic behavior can be used as an index of emerging linguistic competence. As discussed, Baltaxe and Simmons and Prizant hypothesized that, for echolalic individuals, growth in expressive language abilities is predicated on the segmentation of echolalic "chunks" along with the acquisition of early semantic and syntactic structures, resulting in greater creativity and flexibility in language production.[10,57] For cognitively lower functioning individuals, little change may be noted in echolalic behavior for extended periods of time, whereas individuals at higher cognitive levels may move through echolalic stages more rapidly. In either case, assessment efforts should take into account the form and function of echolalic utterances along with the production of creative utterances in documenting the sophistication of expressive linguistic abilities.

Concerns Beyond Emerging Language Levels

As noted earlier, the most striking disability faced by autistic individuals who have acquired language is inappropriate social usage across communicative contexts and partners. More specifically, knowledge of conventions of conversational behavior tends to be limited or applied in an inflexible manner. Lund and Duchan noted that, to engage successfully and in a socially acceptable manner in conversations, individuals must follow conventions for initiating or opening conversations, for exchanging information about a topic or topics, and for terminating conversations.[127] A complexity of verbal and nonverbal signals are typically used to regulate conversations, but may be limited or absent in autism.

Assessment efforts should identify the sources of interactional and conversational breakdowns in daily interactions. Frameworks for the analysis of conversational behavior derived by Lapidus and Prutting and Kirchner may be helpful in identification of these sources.[37,128] Lapidus divided her analysis into verbal and nonverbal domains. Verbal behaviors assessed include turn-taking, initiating conversation, maintaining conversation, recognizing breakdowns and strategies for repairing breakdowns, acquisition of metalinguistic knowledge, use of politeness forms, and strategies for termination interaction. Nonverbal behaviors assessed include the use of gestures, eye gaze, facial expression, head nods, posture, proximity, bodily contact, head and body orientation, and paralanguage. Owing to the likelihood that many problems will be noted to contribute to ineffective communication, the major sources of breakdowns must be identified. In some cases, the presence or absence of behavior may not be as significant as a lack of flexibility in adjusting communicative attempts to the differing demands of different situational contexts. Therefore assessment must account for situational demands.

A thorough assessment of speech, language, and communicative behavior of persons with autism does not differ significantly from assessment of other persons with language impairment. For this reason, assessment practices may be guided by recent literature.[115,127,129] However, a familiarity with the specific patterns of communicative behavior in autism is essential because of the presence of unconventional communicative forms and extreme developmental discrepancies across different areas of functioning. Once a profile of communicative ability and disability is derived, specific goals and procedures for enhancing communicative competence may be derived. However, assessment is an ongoing process rather than an episodic exercise. As an individual's communicative abilities and needs change, so must goals and procedures to meet those needs.[120,130]

COMMUNICATION ENHANCEMENT

Principles

Attempts at communication enhancement should be guided by basic principles to assure efficiency and effectiveness. First, the focus must be on functional communication, defined as (1) the ability to communicate for a variety of purposes relevant to an individual's life routines, (2) the ability to use a variety of means (verbal and/or nonverbal) to accomplish those goals, and (3) the ability to establish and maintain social interaction as an essential part of communication.[131]

Second, communication enhancement is a team effort in which clients, families, speech-language pathologists, special educators, and other professionals all play a role. Caregivers and other family members are crucial to this effort because they are most familiar with the needs and abilities of the person involved. Both behavioral and developmental approaches now emphasize parent training and participation.[132,133]

Third, the recent convergence of behavioral and developmental approaches has provided a constructive dialogue and has enriched strategies for enhancing communication.[69] Sound behavioral principles of intervention (e.g., the use of natural reinforcers, prompting, and shaping) combined with developmental information (e.g., emergence of intentional communication, sequence of language acquisition) and social and pragmatic strategies should all be utilized to improve intervention efforts.

Fourth, the careful selection of alternatives and augmentations to speech based on matching client characteristics, system requirements, and communicative needs provides all individuals with an opportunity to participate in communicative interactions at a developmentally appropriate level.

Fifth, recognition of the cognitive style and associated learning strengths of many persons with autism (e.g., visual-spatial skills, rote memory) suggests alternative approaches to helping individuals to communicate and to understand life routines. For example, the use of time boards or picture schedules helps to concretize abstract temporal concepts. Conversely, an understanding of limitations associated with autism, such as situation-specific learning and a tendency to apply rote memorization strategies with limited comprehension, obligates clinicians to focus on conceptual underpinnings of language and communication, on initiated and spontaneous communication rather than just rote responding, and on generalization of abilities to natural interactions.

Sixth, because successful communication and language use involve mutual participation and negotiation, a clinician's self-evaluation of language and social interactive style may provide information about sources of breakdowns as well as communicative effectiveness. Helping others to adjust their language and socially interactive behavior is a crucial component of communication enhancement. Duchan provides specific suggestions for analyzing and "fine-tuning" interactive exchanges,[121,134] and Prizant and Schuler provide guidelines for adjusting language and communicative behavior.[120]

With these principles in mind, clinicians need to be creative and resourceful in working with others to create contexts or modifying current life routines to facilitate language and communicative growth. Communication is a reflection of knowledge of people, objects, and events specific to an individual's experience. Limited cognitive and social cognitive knowledge inherent to the autistic syndrome results in impoverished communicative ability. Thus it is not enough to concentrate solely on communicative acts; attempts must be made to help individuals "make sense" of communicative exchanges as they occur in and across daily routines while realizing that, for some individuals, their understanding of events may differ markedly from yours.[134] Snyder-McLean and colleagues,[135] Halle,[106] Hart,[107] and Prizant[98] discuss the importance of structure and predictability as well as strategies to facilitate communication in natural environments.

Communication enhancement efforts must be guided by the establishment of specific goals derived from assessment. Goals will differ depending upon developmental level, chronological age, and communicative profile and needs. However, it is possible to identify general goals based on the level of communicative competence. The following discussion presents potential goals at different levels and is not meant to imply an invariant sequence. If relevant, goals may be targeted simultaneously within or across levels based on communicative needs. Schuler and Prizant[120,130] provide more specific information about communication enhancement at preverbal and verbal levels.

Goals for Persons at Preverbal Levels of Communication

Developing Anticipation of Events and Establishing Contingency. Young children or individuals at lower cognitive levels may appear socially aloof and be focused on self or exploration of inanimate objects. This goal addresses the need to structure early social routines to develop anticipation of external predictable events and actions. The shift from self-orientation to other-orientation allows for the development of the concept of external agent; that is, other persons can be a source of action. Developing a concept of self and others as agent, an important precursor to intentional communication, depends to a large extent upon the ability to distinguish one's own actions and results of those actions from the actions of others. Through the development of predictable joint action routines and others' responding contingently to any behavior that may be interpreted as communicative, an awareness of self as agent and other as agent can be established. Stillman and Battle discussed the "Van Dijk" approach, a strategy originally derived for deaf and blind children that is applicable for children with autism at this level of communication.[136] Adaptations would be necessary for chronologically older persons, but the same principles are applicable. Dawson and Galpert[100] and Tiegerman and Primavera[137] discuss strategies for enhancing early socially interactive capacities with autistic children.

Establishing a Consistent Means of Expressing Intent. As noted, first expressions of communicative intent may be idiosyncratic, inconsistent, and unconventional. This goal focuses on the need for a reliable means to request objects or actions, or to protest. At early levels, physical manipulation, natural gestures, or the use of concrete representations such as objects may serve as communicative means that may later be replaced by more conventional and explicit forms through prompting and shaping. Situations must be engineered to elicit initiated and goal-directed behavior to help individuals develop a concept of communication and the means to express intent.

Expansion of Range of Intents. Effective communication goes beyond the ability to regulate others' behaviors. Limitations in strategies to establish joint reference or to communicate for social interaction rather than for regulatory purposes are characteristic of early communication in autism. Efforts to broaden the range of intents is important for social and communicative growth. Modeling and prompting behavioral acts to serve other than regulatory functions within social routines may help in reaching this goal. However, keep in mind that more social forms of communicative intent may be more difficult to acquire by persons with autism.[43]

Replacing Unacceptable Communicative Means with Socially Acceptable Forms. Many persons with autism affect others' behaviors through the use of aberrant means such as aggression, self-injury, or screaming. These behaviors function to reject, protest, terminate interactions, or even to request assistance. An important early goal is to help an individual express the same intents in an acceptable manner, which may preclude the further development of problem behaviors. Communicative means should be relevant to an individual's developmental level and may include a push-away gesture, head shake, pointing to "no" on a communication board, or signing "no" or "help."

Because of the physical danger of intervening when a person is very upset, initial priorities are for the safety of the person involved and others in the immediate environment. Communicative interventions should occur at the onset of early signs of problems (e.g., bodily tension, expressions of frustration) or should be staged by building in opportunities to reject or protest in regular routines throughout the day. Carr and Durand and Smith discuss these issues in greater detail.[47,110]

Acquisition of More Conventional and Explicit Forms to Express Intent. Primitive means to express intent are limited in that interpretation depends largely upon contextual cues and previous experience with the person involved. As the expression of intent becomes firmly established, an individual must acquire and use more conventional forms (e.g., conventional gestures for indicating, requesting, showing) and more explicit forms (e.g., pictures, signs) to communicate to a wider audience. Procedures of modeling, prompting, and shaping facilitate movement from primitive levels of communication to greater communicative effectiveness.

Ability to Communicate Intent Across Environments and Persons. Early communicative acts are typically context-specific, with limited spontaneous generalization across settings or persons. Because of the learning style of persons with autism, generalization or decontextualization must be "built in" by creating opportunities and needs to communicate the same intent with different persons in different settings. Coordination across different environments (e.g., home, school, workplace) is essential.

Ability to Persist in or Repair Communicative Attempts. Common problems for individuals at this level are their lack of persistence in expressing intent and their lack of strategies in repairing breakdowns. These abilities are important because of the inevitable occurrence of communication problems. Through modeling and prompting, interactive partners must help individuals develop the ability to persist in signalling or shift to an alternative communicative means if an initial attempt is unsuccessful. Building persistence and repair strategies can be done most effectively in highly motivating activities.

Ability to Combine Communicative Means or Shift from One Means to Another. Redundancy in signalling contributes to communicative effectiveness. Unfortunately, many persons with autism use limited signals in communicating intent such as gestures or vocalization used in isolation. For individuals who are demonstrating clear expression of intent, attempts should be made to elicit vocalizations or word approximations in the context of intentional communication. To increase control of volitional vocalization when problems are noted, vocal turn-taking games and imitative exercises may be useful.

Goals for Persons at Emerging Language Levels of Communication

Ability to Consistently Direct Attention to Self Prior to Communicating. Calling or directing attention to self is a goal that may be targeted prior to emerging language stages, but it becomes especially crucial when a person is beginning to use a language-based system. This ability is the first step toward conversational competence because it indicates knowledge of the need to establish mutual attention prior to communicating. It is not uncommon for persons with autism to attempt to communicate through speech, signing, or even a communication board prior to securing attention. The resulting breakdown may discourage further attempts and be counterproductive to communication enhancement efforts. Strategies for directing attention to self may include vocalizing, calling a person's name, using a buzzer, or approaching a person. Selection of strategies varies depending upon factors such as volitional control of speech or vocalizations or the ability to learn others' names.

Acquisition of a Core Functional Vocabulary with Subsequent Expansion. Words targetted in a first lexicon must be chosen on the basis of their functionality, range of application, and potential for expansion into multiword utterances. In addition, words selected should express communicative intentions currently expressed through preverbal means. Families need to be actively involved in selecting early vocabulary to assure carry-over into the home environment. Lahey and Bloom provided guidelines for vocabulary selection that may be helpful in this regard.[138]

Expansion of Intents Expressed Through Verbal and Nonverbal Means. More social forms of intent such as commenting, requesting information, and providing information enable an individual to participate more actively in social interaction, as well as acquire information about his or her experiences. As with preverbal levels, expansion of intents often must be targetted specifically owing to the tendency for persons with autism to use language primarily to serve regulatory functions.

Ability to Combine Words, Signs, and Pictures Creatively to Express Relational Concepts. Once a core vocabulary is established (approximately ten to 15 words used functionally), the next expressive linguistic goal is movement to multiword utterances that allow for more explicit communication. Expression of a variety of semantic relations through speech, signing, or the communication board enables an individual to communicate a wider variety of meanings concerning objects, people, actions, locations, and attributes. Watson discussed a number of semantic relations and functions included as part of a language curriculum for autistic children.[139] Bloom and Lahey provided a detailed consideration of semantic issues in language intervention.[140]

Ability to Produce Intelligible or Unambiguous Communicative Acts. Whereas establishment of effective communicative means was the focus at preverbal levels, refinement of means becomes paramount at emerging language and language levels. Thus efforts should be made to teach greater precision in pointing to a communication board or producing intelligible signs or speech. To test a person's intelligibility in speaking or signalling, it is helpful to ask someone unfamiliar with the individual to interact with him or her for a short period of time. Social validity checks of this kind help to provide objective information on changes in communicative behavior.

Increased Flexibility in Communication Across Persons and Situations. As an individual acquires the linguistic knowledge to communicate more effectively, efforts must continue to provide opportunities for successful communication with many persons across varied contexts. In educational programs, interaction with normal peers provides the opportunity to spend time with good language models as well as develop friendships. Programs with a variety of staff should plan a rotation to allow for varied communicative experiences. Regularly scheduled community activities as part of the educational program or family routine also provides for different communicative opportunities with different communication demands.

More Conventional and Flexible Use of Echolalia to Express Intent. For individuals who demonstrate patterns of echolalia, movement from relatively rigid and nonfunctional forms at early preverbal levels should progress to clearly intentional and functional use with evidence of rule-governed changes. Unconventional forms of delayed echolalia need to be replaced with more conventional forms. Prizant discussed the importance of simplifying the language modeled for persons with autism and of specific strategies for responding to echolalic utterances in order to increase functional usage and conventionality of these forms.[64]

Eventual Segmentation of Gestalt Forms with Rule Induction Allowing for Greater Flexibility and Creativity in Language Production. As an individual progresses through emerging language stages and acquires more sophisticated linguistic knowledge, a gradual reduction in the use of immediate and delayed echolalia is to be expected owing to increased comprehension, a greater ability to formulate novel utterances, and the segmentation of echolalic "chunks" into smaller constituents. Once again, recasting of echolalic forms into simpler utterances along with efforts to enhance linguistic knowledge through action-based interventions (synchronizing language production with action patterns) are primary strategies to help individuals "break the code."

Goals for Persons Beyond Emerging Language Levels

Acquisition of More Sophisticated Linguistic Knowledge Allowing for Expression of Complex Relations. Increased comprehension and production of more sophisticated linguistic forms (e.g., grammatic morphemes, question and negative forms, complex sentences) can be targetted by following principles of intervention with language impaired individuals.[140] However, these efforts must address the issues of functionality, generalization of abilities across persons and contexts, and pragmatic issues such as appropriate use of forms in different situations. Focusing solely on form is no longer justifiable for individuals who demonstrate severe limitations in the social use of linguistic knowledge.

Ability to Convey Information Consistently About Past and Future Events. A hallmark in the acquisition of communication skills is the ability to relate information about the "not here and now." This ability provides the foundation for reflecting on past experiences and planning for future experiences. Visual supports such as picture schedules or language experience stories can be used to facilitate communication about past and future events. Daily schedules should be discussed and reviewed routinely in order to model language use as a tool to anticipate future events and recount completed activities.

Use of Language Skills for Other Than Communication. The cognitive style of persons with autism may allow for more efficient processing of information through the visual-spatial modality. Visual-spatial processing strengths are apparent in many persons with autism who have been reported to use or understand written language prior to oral language. In addition to the use of picture or word schedules, language skills may contribute to activities such as reading, collecting and documenting objects of interest, or even writing stories. For individuals with greater abilities, specific expertise may be developed around highly motivating topics and provide for constructive leisure time activities.

Knowledge and Use of Nonverbal and Paralinguistic Behavior and Acquisition of Conversational Skills and Strategies. For persons who use language as a primary means of communication, breakdowns may still occur because of limited knowledge and limited adherence to social conventions of verbal and nonverbal behavior, which serve to regulate conversational interaction. On the basis of the identification of problems in conversation through informal assessments, situations can be designed to address these problems directly. For example, Lapidus used structured social groups with adolescents and adults to improve social interaction and conversational skills.[42] General conversational conventions such as the use of eye contact, topic maintenance, appropriate use of gestures, as well as more specific problems encountered by individuals, are addressed. Participants are asked to make judgements about their own and others' behavior in role playing and more natural interactions. Videotaped interactions may be used to facilitate such activity. Donnellan and Kilman combined principles of behavioral, developmental, and functional approaches in suggesting the use of social groups to teach social skills.[118] There is a potential danger in teaching conversational behaviors outside the context of conversational episodes. Training isolated behaviors out of context is not likely to result in appropriate usage unless the purpose of the behavior is seen as contributing to effective ongoing interaction. Thus the purpose or the goal of the interaction should be emphasized along with the specific behavior to be acquired. Regularly scheduled activities with a clear group goal such as cooking may provide the motivation and context to practice these skills.

Ability to Recognize Communication Breakdowns and Utilize Appropriate Repair Strategies. A difficult but important goal for persons at this level is the ability to recognize when communication breakdowns occur and to utilize appropriate repair strategies. Developing such metacommunicative knowledge requires the ability to reflect back on one's own behavior. The extent to which this is possible varies with the individual and the specific cause of the breakdown. For example, it may be more difficult dealing with breakdowns that occur because an individual provides too little information (need for listener perspective-taking), but easier to improve behavior demanding less complex judgements (appropriate use of eye contact). In some cases, the acquisition of relatively simple strategies, such as saying "I don't understand," to request clarification may provide an alternative to a breakdown in the interaction. Although progress in this area may be slow because of the social cognitive impairment, improvement in this ability has the potential for greatly increasing communicative effectiveness.

Acquisition of Vocabulary and Knowledge of Communicative "Scripts" Relevant to Specific Activities. The use of language and conversational routines in many daily activities follows formats that are relatively predictable. For example, making a telephone call or ordering food in a fast food restaurant requires specific vocabulary and knowledge of the conversational exchange, but once acquired, these skills are likely to be applicable to a wide variety of similar contexts. These types of functional activities should be identified in assessments of communicative needs and practiced in realistic contexts. If helpful, role playing may be used to help establish these skills prior to or along with the use in natural contexts. The ability to participate actively in such exchanges contributes significantly to an individual's independent functioning and should be targetted at all levels.

SUMMARY

Communication impairments associated with the autistic syndrome are now recognized as central in understanding the nature of autism, as well as in planning and providing effective educational and treatment programs. In this chapter, issues in diagnosis and theories of primary deficits were presented to highlight the prominent position played by communication and language problems throughout the history of the study of autism. An overview of speech, language, and communication problems experienced by persons with autism demonstrated the pervasiveness of these impairments at all levels of functioning. Moreover, the great range of problems demands that each person be approached as an individual; to talk about "autistic communication" as if this term provides a clear description of a person's specific abilities and disabilities and needs is misleading.

Assessment procedures must be flexible enough to identify these individual differences yet provide comprehensive information relative to receptive and expressive language abilities, communication and social interaction skills, and, when relevant, language-related cognitive skills. Approaches to intervention should be rooted in a firm philosophical foundation that, in this chapter, is eclectic in nature, drawing from developmental, behavioral, and functional approaches. Goals for individuals at various levels of ability are derived from individual needs, information about developmental sequences, and an understanding of the specific communication problems and learning characteristics of persons with autism. Currently, researchers and clinicians from many theoretical orientations are coming together in attempts to understand communication problems in autism, and to construct effective models of intervention. This breakdown of theoretical and disciplinary boundaries serves to benefit persons with autism and their families. Speech-language pathologists play a central role in working with persons with autism and undoubtedly will continue to contribute to research and treatment efforts.

Acknowledgments. I wish to thank Drs. Judith Duchan, Adriana Loes Schuler, and Amy Wetherby for a decade of professional collaboration, stimulation, and friendship. Many ideas presented in this manuscript are a direct reflection of their creativity and concern for persons with autism. Thanks also to Dr. David Yoder for his generous support and friendship.

REFERENCES

1. Kanner L. Autistic disturbances of affective contact. Nerv Child 1943; 2:217–250.
2. National Society for Children and Adults with Autism. Definition for the syndrome of autism. Washington, DC: NSAC, 1984.
3. Kanner L. Irrelevant and metaphorical language in early infantile autism. Am J Psychiatry 1946; 103:242–245.
4. Cohen DJ, Paul R, Volkmar FR. Issues in the classification of pervasive and other developmental disorders: towards DSM IV. J Am Acad Child Psychiatry 1986; 25:213–220.
5. Ornitz E. Neurophysiology of infantile autism. J Am Acad Child Psychiatry 1985; 24:251–262.
6. American Psychiatric Association. Diagnostic and statistical manual of mental disorders. 3rd ed. Washington, DC: American Psychiatric Association, 1980.
7. Rutter M. Diagnosis and definition of childhood autism. J Autism Dev Disord 1978; 8:139–161.
8. Volkmar FR, Cohen DJ, Paul R. An evaluation of DSM III criteria for infantile autism. J Am Acad Child Psychiatry 1986; 25:190–197.
9. Morgan S. The unreachable child. Memphis: Memphis State University Press, 1981.
10. Prizant BM. Language acquisition and communicative behavior in autism: toward an understanding of the "whole" of it. J Speech Hear Disord 1983; 48:296–307.
11. Denckla M. New diagnostic criteria for autism and related behavioral disorders—guidelines for research protocols. J Am Acad Child Psychiatry 1986; 25:221–224.

12. Bettelheim B. The empty fortress: infantile autism and the birth of self. New York: The Free Press, 1967.
13. O'Gorman G. The nature of childhood autism. London: Butterworths, 1970.
14. Eisenberg L, Kanner L. Early infantile autism—1943–1955. Am J Orthopsychiatry 1956; 26:556–566.
15. King PD. Early infantile autism: relation to schizophrenia. J Am Acad Child Psychiatry 1975; 14:666–682.
16. Rutter M. The development of infantile autism. Psychol Med 1974; 4:147–163.
17. Tinbergen N, Tinbergen E. Autistic children: new hope for a cure. London: George Allen, 1983.
18. DeMyer MK, Hingtgen J, Jackson R. Infantile autism review: a decade of research. Schizophr Bull 1981; 7:388–451.
19. Rimland B. Early infantile autism. Englewood Cliffs, NJ: Prentice-Hall, 1964.
20. Rutter M. Language disorder and infantile autism. In: Rutter M, Schopler E, eds. Autism: a reappraisal of concepts and treatment. New York: Plenum Press, 1978:85.
21. Rutter M. Cognitive deficits in pathogenesis of autism. J Child Psychol Psychiatry 1983; 24:513–531.
22. Ornitz EM, Ritvo ER. Perceptual inconstancy in early infantile autism. Arch Gen Psychiatry 1968; 18:76–98.
23. Churchill D. The relation of early infantile autism and early childhood schizophrenia to developmental language disorders of childhood. J Autism Dev Disord 1972; 2:182–197.
24. Hobson P. The autistic child's appraisal of expression of emotion. J Child Psychol Psychiatry 1986; 27:321–342.
25. Lovaas OI, Koegel R, Schreibman L. Stimulus overselectivity in autism: a review of recent research. Psychol Bull 1979; 86:1236–1254.
26. Koegel R, Egel A, Dunlap G. Learning characteristics of autistic children. In: Sailor W, Wilcox B, Brown L, eds. Methods of instruction for severely handicapped students. Baltimore: Paul H Brookes, 1980.
27. Gersten R. In search of the cognitive deficit in autism: beyond stimulus overselectivity model. J Spec Educ 1980; 14:47–63.
28. Ornitz EM. The modulation of sensory input and motor output in autistic children. In: Schopler E, Reichler RJ, eds. Psychopathology and child development. New York: Plenum Press, 1976:115.
29. Hermelin B, O'Connor N. Psychological experiments of autistic children. Oxford: Pergamon Press, 1970.
30. Hermelin B, O'Connor N. Logico-affective states and nonverbal language. In: Schopler E, Mesibov G, eds. Communication problems in autism. New York: Plenum Press, 1985:283.
31. Fein D, Pennington D, Markowitz P, Braverman M, Waterhouse L. Toward a neuropsychological model of infantile autism: are the social deficits primary? J Am Acad Child Psychiatry 1986; 25:198–212.
32. Kanner L. Problems of nosology and psychodynamics of early infantile autism. Am J Orthopsychiatry 1949; 19:416–426.
33. Volkmar FR. Issues in social-relatedness in autism. Paper presented at the NIMH Workshop on Autism, Brown University, 1985.
34. Mirenda P, Donnellan A, Yoder D. Gaze behavior: a new look at an old problem. J Autism Dev Disord 1983; 13:397–409.
35. Langdell T. Recognition of faces: an approach to the study of autism. J Child Psychol Psychiatry 1978; 19:255–268.
36. Dawson G, Adams A. Imitation and social responsiveness in autistic children. J Abnorm Child Psychol 1984; 12:209–226.
37. Lapidus D. Developing communication and language skills in autism. Unpublished manual, 1985.
38. Hingtgen J, Bryson C. Recent developments in the study of early childhood psychoses: infant autism, childhood schizophrenia, and related disorders. Schizophr Bull 1972; 5:8–54.
39. Schuler AL, Donnellan-Walsh A. Speech and language characteristics of autistic children. In: Teaching makes a difference (teacher's manual). Santa Barbara: Santa Barbara County Schools, 1976:141.
40. Kurita H. Infantile autism with speech loss before the age of thirty months. J Am Acad Child Psychiatry 1985; 24:191–196.
41. Curcio F. Sensorimotor functioning and communication in mute autistic children. J Abnorm Child Psychol 1978; 8:181–189.
42. Wetherby AM, Prutting C. Profiles of communicative and cognitive-social abilities in autistic children. J Speech Hear Res 1984; 27:364–377.
43. Wetherby AM. Ontogeny of communicative functions in autism. J Autism Dev Disord 1986; 15:295–315.
44. Wollner S. Communicating intent: how well do language impaired children do? Top Lang Disord 1983; 4:2–14.
45. Ricks D. Vocal communication in pre-verbal, normal and autistic children. In: O'Connor N, ed. Language, cognitive deficits and retardation. London: Butterworths, 1975.
46. Iwata B, Dorsey M, Slifer K, Bauman K, Richman G. Toward a functional analysis of self-injury. Anal Interven Dev Disabil 1982; 2:3–20.
47. Carr E, Durand V. The social-communicative basis of severe behavior problems in children. In: Reiss S, Bootsin R, eds. Theoretical issues in behavior therapy. New York: Academic Press, 1985:219.
48. Prizant BM, Wetherby AM. Intentional communicative behavior of children with autism: theoretical and practical issues. Aust J Hum Commun Disord 1985; 13:21–59.
49. Boucher J. Articulation in early childhood autism. J Autism Dev Disord 1976; 7:177–187.
50. Bartolucci G, Pierce S, Streiner D, Eppel P. Phonological investigation of verbal autistic and mentally retarded subjects. J Autism Dev Disord 1976; 6:303–316.
51. Prizant BM. The functions of immediate echolalia in autistic children. Ph.D. Dissertation. Buffalo: State University of New York, 1978.
52. Goldfarb W, Goldfarb N, Braunstein P, Scholl H. Speech and language faults of schizophrenic children. J Autism Child Dev Disord 1972; 2:219–233.
53. Baltaxe CAM, Simmons JQ. Prosodic development in normal and autistic children. In: Schopler E, Mesibov G, eds. Communication problems in autism. New York: Plenum Press, 1985:95.
54. Cantwell DP, Baker L, Rutter M. A comparative study of infantile autism and specific developmental receptive language disorder: IV. Analysis of syntax and language function. J Child Psychol Psychiatry 1978; 19:351–362.
55. Bartolucci G, Pierce S, Streiner D. Cross-sectional studies of grammatical morphemes in autistic and mentally retarded children. J Autism Dev Disord 1980; 10:39–50.
56. Swisher L, Demetras M. The expressive language characteristics of autistic children compared with mentally retarded or specific language-impaired children. In: Schopler E, Mesibov G, eds. Communication problems in autism. New York: Plenum Press, 1985:147.
57. Baltaxe CAM, Simmons JQ. Disorders of language in childhood psychosis: current concepts and approaches. In: Darby J, ed. Speech evaluation in psychiatry. New York: Grune and Stratton, 1981:285.
58. Rutter M. Diagnosis and definition of childhood autism. J Autism Dev Disord 1978; 8:139–161.
59. Howlin P. The effectiveness of operant language training with autistic children. J Autism Dev Disord 1981; 11:89–105.
60. Fay WH. Verbal memory systems and the autistic child. Semin Speech Lang 1983; 4:17–26.
61. Lovaas OI. The autistic child: language development through

behavior modification. New York: John Wiley and Sons, 1977.
62. Fay WH. On the echolalia of the blind and of the autistic child. J Speech Hear Disord 1973; 38:478–489.
63. Shapiro T. The quest for a linguistic model to study the speech of autistic children: studies on echoing. J Am Acad Child Psychiatry 1977; 16:608–619.
64. Prizant BM. Echolalia in autism: assessment and intervention. Semin Speech Lang 1983; 4:63–78.
65. Schuler AL. Echolalia: issues and clinical applications. J Speech Hear Disord 1979; 44:411–434.
66. Prizant BM, Duchan JF. The functions of immediate echolalia in autistic children. J Speech Hear Disord 1981; 46:241–249.
67. Prizant BM, Rydell PJ. An analysis of the functions of delayed echolalia in autistic children. J Speech Hear Res 1984; 27:183–192.
68. Schuler AL, Prizant BM. Echolalia in autism. In: Schopler E, Mesibov G, eds. Communication problems in autism. New York: Plenum Press, 1985:163.
69. Prizant BM, Wetherby AM. Enhancing communication: from theory to practice. In: Dawson G, ed. Autism: new perspectives on diagnosis, nature, and treatment. New York: Guilford Press, 1988.
70. Watson L. Pragmatic problems in autism. In: Layton T, ed. Language and treatment of autistic children. New York: CC Thomas, 1987:89.
71. Cunningham M. A comparison of the language of psychotic and non-psychotic children who are mentally retarded. J Child Psychol Psychiatry 1968; 9:229–244.
72. Watson L, Martin J, Schaeffer B. Form, content and function of the spontaneous communication of autistic students. Aust J Hum Commun Disord 1986; 14:91–102.
73. Dewey M, Everard M. The near normal autistic adolescent. J Autism Dev Disord 1974; 4:348–356.
74. Cunningham M. The five-year study of the language of an autistic child. J Child Psychol Psychiatry 1966; 7:143–154.
75. Paul R. Communication in autism. In: Cohen D, Donnellan A, eds. Handbook of autism and pervasive developmental disorders. New York: John Wiley & Sons, 1987:61.
76. Hinerman P, Channell R. Conversational abilities of autistic individuals. Aust J Hum Commun Disord 1986; 14:103–108.
77. Tager-Flusberg H. Pragmatic development and its implications for social interaction in autistic children. Proceedings of the annual conference of the National Society for Autistic Children, Boston, 1981.
78. Paul R, Feldman C. Communication deficits in autism. Paper presented at Columbia University Institute on Autism, New York, 1984.
79. Paccia-Cooper J, Curcio F, Sacharko G. A comparison of discourse features in normal and autistic language. Paper presented at sixth annual Boston University conference on language development, Boston, 1981.
80. Baltaxe CAM, Simmons JQ. Language patterns of German and English autistic adolescents. In: Mittler P, ed. Proceedings of the International Association for the Study of Mental Deficiency. Baltimore: University Park Press, 1977:223.
81. Baltaxe CAM. Pragmatic deficits in the language of autistic adolescents. J Pediatr Psychol 1977; 2:176–180.
82. McCaleb P, Prizant BM. The encoding of new versus old information in autistic children. J Speech Hear Disord 1985; 30:230–240.
83. Langdell T. Pragmatic aspects of autism. In: Park D, ed. Proceedings of the annual conference of the National Society for Children and Adults with Autism. Washington, DC: NSAC, 1981.
84. Paul R, Cohen D. Responses to contingent queries in adults with mental retardation and pervasive developmental disorders. Appl Psycholinguistics 1984; 5:349–357.
85. Ricks D, Wing L. Language, communication, and the use of symbols in normal and autistic children. J Autism Dev Disord 1975; 5:191–221.
86. Peters A. The units of language acquisition. Cambridge: Cambridge University Press, 1983.
87. Dawson G, Finley C, Phillips S, Galpert L. Hemispheric specialization and the language abilities of autistic children. Child Dev 1986; 57:1440–1453.
88. Wetherby AM. Possible neurolinguistic breakdown in autistic children. Top Lang Disord 1984; 4:19–33.
89. Prizant BM, Schuler AL. Facilitating communication: theoretical foundations. In: Cohen D, Donnellan A, eds. Handbook of autism and pervasive developmental disorders. New York: John Wiley and Sons, 1987:289.
90. Rimland B. Inside the mind of the autistic savant. Psychol Today 1978; 69–80.
91. Bryen D, Joyce D. Language intervention with the severely handicapped: a decade of research. J Spec Educ 1985; 19:7–39.
92. Lovaas OI. Teaching developmentally disabled children. The "me" book. Baltimore: University Park Press, 1981.
93. Skinner BF. Verbal behavior. New York: Appleton-Century-Crofts, 1957.
94. Carr E. Behavioral approaches to language and communication. In: Mesibov G, ed. Communication problems in autism. New York: Plenum Press, 1985:37.
95. Koegel R, Johnson J. Motivating language use in autistic children. In: Dawson G, ed. Autism: new perspectives on diagnosis, nature and treatment. New York: Guilford Press, in press.
96. McLean J, Yoder D, Schiefelbusch R, eds. Language intervention with the retarded: developing strategies. Baltimore: University Park Press, 1972.
97. Schiefelbusch R, Lloyd L, eds. Language perspectives—acquisition, retardation, and intervention. Baltimore: University Park Press, 1974.
98. Prizant BM. Speech-language pathologists and autistic children: what is our role? Part II. Working with parents and professionals. Asha 1982; 24:463–468.
99. Peck C, Schuler AL. Classroom-based language intervention for children with autism: theoretical and practical considerations for the speech and language specialist. Semin Speech Lang 1983; 4:93–103.
100. Dawson G, Galpert L. A developmental model for facilitating the social behavior of autistic children. In: Schopler E, Mesibov G, eds. Social behavior in autism. New York: Plenum Press, 1986:237.
101. Prizant BM, Wetherby AM. Communicative intent: a framework for understanding social-communicative behavior in autism. J Am Acad Child Psychiatry 1987; 26:472–479.
102. Bates E. On the evolution and development of symbols. In: Bates E, Benigni T, Bretherton I, Camaioni L, Votera V, eds. The emergence of symbols: cognition and communication in infancy. New York: Academic Press, 1979:1.
103. Harding C. Acting with intention: a framework for examining the development of the intention to communicate. In: Feagans L, Garvey C, Golinkoff R, eds. The origins and growth of communication. Norwood, NJ: Ablex, 1984:123.
104. Bates E. Language and context: the acquisition of pragmatics. New York: Academic Press, 1976.
105. Bruner J. From communication to language: a psychological perspective. In: Markova I, ed. The social context of language. Chichester: John Wiley & Sons, 1978:17.
106. Halle J. Arranging the natural environment to occasion language: giving severely language delayed children reasons to communicate. Semin Speech Lang 1984; 5:185–199.
107. Hart B. Naturalistic language training techniques. In: Warren S, Rogers-Warren A, eds. Teaching functional language. Baltimore: University Park Press, 1985:63.

108. Peck C. Increasing opportunities for social control by children with autism and severe handicaps: effects on student behavior and perceived classroom climate. J Assoc Persons Severe Handicaps 1985; 4:183–193.
109. Lotter V. Follow-up studies. In: Rutter M, Schopler E, eds. Autism: a reappraisal of concepts and treatment. New York: Plenum Press, 1978:475.
110. Smith M. Managing the aggressive and self-injurious behavior of adults disabled by autism. J Assoc Persons Severe Handicaps 1985; 4:228–232.
111. Falvey M. Community-based curriculum: instructional strategies for students with severe handicaps. Baltimore: Paul Brookes, 1986.
112. Chapman R. Comprehension strategies in children. In: Kavanagh J, Strange P, eds. Language and speech in the laboratory, school and clinic. Cambridge: MIT Press, 1977:308.
113. Lord C. Autism and the comprehension of language. In: Schopler E, Mesibov G, eds. Communication problems in autism. New York: Plenum Press, 1985:257.
114. Donnellan A, Mirenda P, Mesaros R, Fassbender L. Analyzing the communicative functions of aberrant behavior. J Psycholinguist Res 1984; 9:201–212.
115. McLean JE, Snyder-McLean L, Sack S, Decker D. A transactional approach to early language training—a mediated in-service training program. Columbus: CE Merrill, 1983.
116. Prizant BM. Assessment and intervention of communicative problems in children with autism. Commun Disord 1984; 9:127–142.
117. Howlin P. The assessment of social behavior. In: Rutter M, Schopler E, eds. Autism: a reappraisal of concepts and treatment. New York: Plenum Press, 1978:63.
118. Donnellan A, Kilman E. Behavioral approaches to social skill development in autism: strengths, misapplications and alternatives. In: Schopler E, Mesibov G, eds. Social behavior in autism. New York: Plenum Press, 1986:213.
119. Olley J. Social aspects of communication in children with autism. In: Schopler E, Mesibov G, eds. Communication problems in autism. New York: Plenum Press, 1985:311.
120. Prizant BM, Schuler AL. Facilitating communication: language approaches. In: Cohen D, Donnellan A, eds. Handbook of autism and pervasive developmental disorders. New York: John Wiley and Sons, 1987:316.
121. Duchan J. Autistic children are non-interactive: or so we say. Semin Speech Hear 1983; 4:53–61.
122. Higginbotham DJ, Yoder DE. Communication within natural conversational interaction: implications for severe communicatively impaired persons. Top Lang Disord 1982; 2:1–19.
123. Schuler AL. Selecting augmentative communication systems on the basis of current means and functions. Aust J Hum Commun Disord 1985; 13:102–120.
124. Kiernan C. The use of nonvocal communication techniques with autistic individuals. J Child Psychol Psychiatry 1983; 24:339–376.
125. Parsons CL, Crary MA, eds. Aust J Human Commun Disord 1984; 12.
126. Aram DM. Assessment and treatment of developmental apraxia. Semin Speech Lang 1984; 5:2.
127. Lund N, Duchan J. Assessing children's language in naturalistic contexts. Englewood Cliffs, NJ: Prentice-Hall, 1983.
128. Prutting C, Kirchner D. Applied pragmatics. In: Gallagher T, Prutting C, eds. Pragmatic assessment and intervention issues in language. San Diego: College-Hill Press, 1983:29.
129. Miller J. Assessing language production in children. Baltimore: University Park Press, 1981.
130. Schuler AL, Prizant BM. Facilitating communication: prelanguage approaches. In: Cohen D, Donnellan A, eds. Handbook of autism and pervasive developmental disorders. New York: John Wiley and Sons, 1987:301.
131. Prizant BM, Schuler AL. Definition of functional communication. In: Proceedings of the conference on effective communication for severely handicapped children and youth. Washington, DC: Office of Special Education and Rehabilitative Services, 1985:III-20.
132. Manolson A. It takes two to talk. Toronto: Hannen Early Language Resource Center, 1985.
133. Harris S, Boyle T. Parents as language trainers of children with autism. In: Schopler E, Mesibov G, eds. Communication problems in autism. New York: Plenum Press, 1985:207.
134. Duchan J. Language intervention through sensemaking and fine tuning. In: Schiefelbusch R, ed. Communicative competence: assessment and language intervention. Baltimore: University Park Press, 1986.
135. Snyder-McLean L, Solomonson B, McLean JE, Sack S. Structuring joint action routines: a strategy for facilitating communication in the classroom. Semin Speech Lang 1984; 5:213–228.
136. Stillman RD, Battle CW. Developing prelanguage communication in the severely handicapped: an interpretation of the Van Dijk method. Sem in Speech Lang 1984; 5:159–170.
137. Tiegerman E, Primavera L. Imitating the autistic child: facilitating communicative gaze behavior. J Autism Dev Disord 1984; 14:27–38.
138. Lahey M, Bloom L. Planning a first lexicon: which words to teach first. J Speech Hear Disord 1977; 42:340–349.
139. Watson L. The TEACCH communication curriculum. In: Schopler E, Mesibov G, eds. Communication problems in autism. New York: Plenum Press, 1985:187.
140. Bloom L, Lahey M. Language development and language disorders. New York: John Wiley & Sons, 1978.

36 Dysphagia and Disorders of Speech

JoAnne Robbins, Ph.D.

Speech-language pathologists have been involved in the management of children with disorders of oral feeding and swallowing since the first half of the 20th century, when oral motor disorders of speech and swallowing of children with cerebral palsy were initially being managed.[1] Feeding and prespeech oromotor therapy were presumed necessary prior to emergence of normal speech patterns in later childhood. Since that time, advances in medical technology facilitated survival of greater numbers of premature infants who cannot suck and may demonstrate neurodevelopmental disorders. On the other end of the continuum, prolongation of the adult life span has increased the number of individuals surviving with neuromuscular, pulmonary, or gastrointestinal disorders, as well as people with head and neck cancer. Many of these individuals demonstrate oral, pharyngeal, laryngeal, and respiratory control problems affecting both communication and swallowing. Thus, in the latter half of the 20th century, many more speech-language pathologists are choosing to become increasingly involved in evaluation and management of children and adults with disordered swallowing secondary to neurologic and structural abnormalities.

This chapter will present an overview of dysphagia for the speech-language pathologist. First, a definition of dysphagia is provided. Then normal swallowing and the nature of disordered swallowing, evaluation techniques, and management approaches are presented. Finally, the relationship of dysphagia to speech disorders is discussed.

DEFINITION

Dysphagia is a swallowing disorder characterized by difficulty in oral preparation for swallowing and/or for moving material from the mouth to the stomach. Subsumed in this definition are the problems in positioning food in the mouth and in the oral manipulation preceding swallowing, including sucking and chewing.[2]

NORMAL SWALLOWING

Anatomy

The oropharyngeal tract, comprising the three peripheral morphologic features (oral cavity, pharyngeal cavity, and larynx), has three functions: respiration, deglutition, and speech production. For the purpose of speech production, these morphologic features are termed the "vocal tract." When their function is considered during swallowing, the same morphology is termed the "upper aerodigestive tract." Thus normal speech and swallowing both depend on the integrity of many of the same head and neck anatomic structures. However, the normal juxtaposition of particular pharyngeal structures create spaces or pockets that are not relevant to the process of speech production, but are integral to the understanding of dysphagia and its diagnosis and remediation.

The first of these spaces is the vallecula, which is shown in Figure 36–1. The vallecula is the space formed by the juxtaposition of the base of the tongue and the epiglottis.

The other important space is the pyriform sinus, shown in Figure 36–2. The pyriform sinus, also known as the pyriform fossa, is formed by the attachment of the inferior constrictor fibers to the thyroid cartilage.

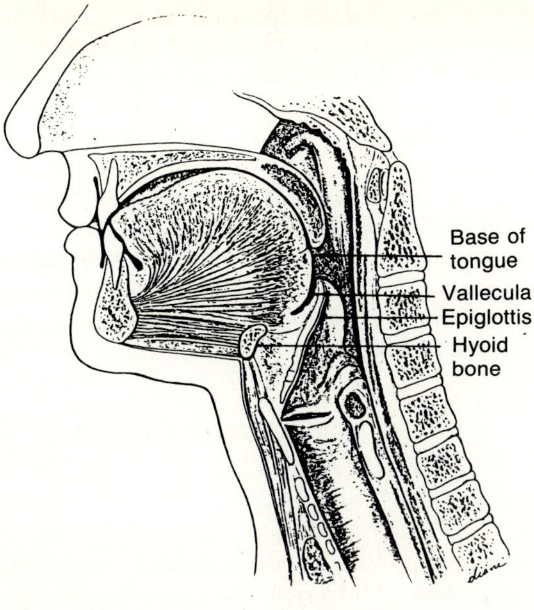

Figure 36–1 The vallecula is the space formed by the juxtaposition of the base of the tongue and the epiglottis.

The vallecula and the pyriform fossa sometimes are referred to as the pharyngeal recesses. They are important spaces for swallowing because in the presence of abnormal oropharyngeal motor events, food may be "pocketed" in these spaces. Upon resumption of breathing after swallowing is completed, the material lodged in these pharyngeal recesses may be inhaled into the airway. Throughout this chapter, the penetration or inhalation of material below the level of the true vocal folds will be termed "aspiration." Recurrent aspiration leads to pneumonia.

Phases

The process of deglutition has been described in terms of phases. One conceptualization is a division into four phases.[3] The first of these is the oral preparatory phase, during which food is manipulated in the mouth, masticated if necessary, and pulled together into a cohesive bolus. The second is the oral phase when the tongue propels the bolus posteriorly until the pharyngeal phase is initiated. During the pharyngeal phase the bolus is propelled through the pharynx. Finally, esophageal peristalsis facilitates passage of the bolus through the esophagus into the stomach during the esophageal phase of swallowing. The initial two phases of swallowing (preparatory and oral) are under voluntary control,[3,4] and the latter two phases, pharyngeal and esophageal, are more automatic in nature.[5,6]

Although the various phases of swallowing have been conceptualized as separate, it must be understood that any division of a functionally integrated system is somewhat artificial. Normal swallowing is a rapid, dynamic process that is a functional composite of many structures and their movements. Nonetheless, division of swallowing into phases permits an organized approach that may facilitate better understanding of the process. Accordingly, the phases, structures, and physiology are presented throughout this chapter in a sequence that reflects the progression of events during swallowing: the volitional phases involving lips, tongue, jaw, and velum are first considered, followed by the events that occur as a function of the automatic pharyngeal phase involving velopharynx, larynx, pharynx, and cricopharyngeus. Since the esophagus is composed primarily of nonstriated muscle that is not amenable to the speech pathologist's behavioral methods of remediation, the esophageal phase will receive little attention in this chapter. The speech pathologist involved in work on dysphagia is encouraged to consult the appropriate colleagues (i.e., radiologist, gastroenterologist) for evaluation and treatment of the esophagus.

NEUROPHYSIOLOGY OF SWALLOWING

Sensorimotor control of a system that is as widely distributed spatially (from the lips anteriorly to the

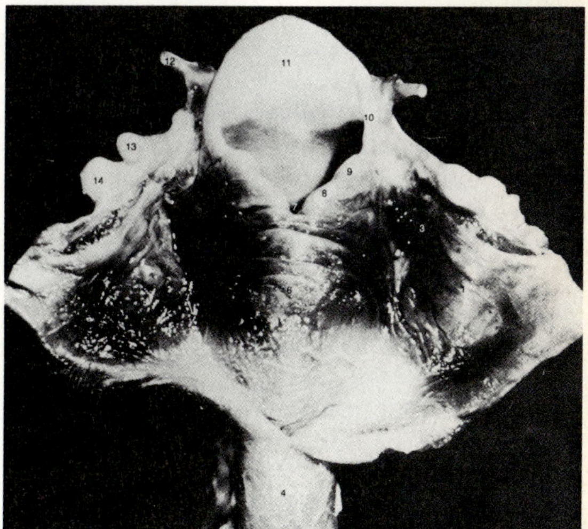

Figure 36–2 The periform sinuses are pharyngeal recesses formed by the attachment of the inferior constrictor fibers to the thyroid cartilage. (Reprinted by permission from Kahane J, Folkins J. Atlas of speech and hearing anatomy. Columbus: CE Merill, 1984:82.)

velopharynx superiorly and the esophagus inferiorly) and equally diverse structurally as is swallowing, requires the coordinated activity of neural mechanisms distributed across both cranial and spinal nervous systems. These neural elements include peripheral nerves and their central nuclei and neural centers, capable of coordinating, integrating, and sequencing the volitional and automatic activities involved in swallowing.[7]

Volitional Phases

The muscles of mastication produce a complex pattern of movement during the oral preparatory phase. As shown in Table 36–1, the volitional actions of the jaw, lips, and tongue are controlled by the trigeminal nerve, aided by motor commands of the facial nerve to break down the food mechanically and to incorporate saliva into the bolus. Duration of bolus formation is variable, depending on the type of food. Volitional tongue movements, controlled by the hypoglossal nerve, transport the bolus to the posterior tongue, which marks the end of the oral phase. Oral phase duration is approximately 1 second, slightly shorter for liquids, slightly longer for other material.

The impact of the volitional tongue action and the characteristics of the bolus on the mucosa of the anterior faucial arches, the palate, pharynx, and epiglottis stimulate sensory components of the glossopharyngeal, vagus, and perhaps trigeminal nerves to initiate the automatic transport of the bolus through the pharynx. The sensory information from these nerves is coordinated by the nucleus tractus solitarii. The tactile information is integrated by the nucleus ambiguus and nucleus dorsalis nervi vagi. These motor nuclei then initiate an involuntary peristaltic wave of muscle contraction preceded by muscle relaxation, which transports the bolus as it descends from the pharynx through the esophagus into the stomach.[7]

Automatic Phases

The sensory and motor components of the pharyngeal phase of swallowing, as shown in Table 36–1, are combined and coordinated by a dominant swallowing center, or central pattern generator (CPG) most likely located within the medullary reticular formation.[4,5] This center ensures the accuracy of bilateral motor activity and proper sequencing of the muscles involved in swallowing.[8] The CPG also precludes competing muscle activity, such as respiration, from interfering with the required pattern of activity, and it ensures that once initiated, the complex motor acts of the pharyngeal phases of swallowing are completed without interruption. A CPG implies that the oral phases of swallowing are voluntary, whereas the pharyngeal and esophageal phases are more automatic. The automatic phases are released by specific patterns of lingual action or posturing during the oral preparatory and oral phases in conjunction with tactile, taste, and temperature characteristics of the bolus exciting groups of receptors in the oropharynx. The pharyngeal phase duration is approximately 1 second.

THE UPPER AERODIGESTIVE TRACT AS A SERIES OF VALVES

The upper aerodigestive tract may be conceptualized as a series of valves, acting to control the passage of a bolus by confining it to a specific pathway and by directing the bolus along the appropriate route in a precisely timed series of events. As shown in Figure 36–3, the valves of the upper aerodigestive swallowing mechanism include the lips, tongue, velopharynx, larynx, and cricopharyngeus. In normal swallowing, the various valves close anterior, posterior, and lateral pathways, or side pockets, so that food does not divert from the intended tract to inappropriate tracts.

Oral Phase Valves

During the oral phases of swallowing, a labial seal produces a valve that prevents material from escaping the oral cavity anteriorly. In addition to the piston-like role of the tongue in moving material through the oral cavity, lingual contact with anterior hard palate and lateral lingual contact with the palatal arch prevents material from falling into the anterior and lateral sulci. The soft palate descends and the tongue dorsum elevates, thereby forming a posterior seal separating the oral and pharyngeal cavities, as shown in Figure 36–4. This linguavelar valve prevents the bolus from entering the pharynx prior to initiation of the pharyngeal phase of swallowing. This valve, forming a barrier between the cavities thus preventing escape of the bolus, is of utmost importance because the airway is open and unprotected prior to initiation of the pharyngeal phase.

Pharyngeal Phase Valves

The pharyngeal phase of normal swallowing is characterized by the actions of three valves in ad-

TABLE 36–1 Cranial and Spinal Nerve Sensory and Motor Innervation for the Phases of Swallowing

	Oral		*Pharyngeal*		*Esophageal*	
Nerve	*Sensory*	*Motor*	*Sensory*	*Motor*	*Sensory*	*Motor*
Trigeminal (fifth)	General sensation; anterior $^2/_3$ tongue, face, buccal, and nasal mucosa	Bolus manipulation and mastication, mandible, myelohoideus, digastric (anterior belly), anterior velar bulging; tensor palatini, palatoglossus				
Facial (seventh)	Taste; anterior $^2/_3$ tongue parasympathetic secretory fibers to salivary glands	Lips and posterior tongue elevation, stylohyoideus, styloglossus, digastric (posterior belly)				
Glossopharyngeal (ninth)	General sensation and taste; posterior $^1/_3$ tongue, mucous membranes of velopharynx		Elicits pharyngeal phase	Stylopharyngeus and superior constrictor		
Vagus (tenth)		Diaphragm active until pharyngeal phase	Elicits pharyngeal phase; membranes of pharynx, larynx, bronchi, esophagus	Velopharyngeal closure and pharyngeal peristalsis, pharynx, larynx, soft palate, nonstriated esophagus		Diaphragm
Spinal Accessory (eleventh)				With vagus to muscles of larynx, velopharynx, pharyngeal constrictors		
Hypoglossal (twelfth)		Tongue shape, all intrinsic and extrinsic tongue muscles except palatoglossus and geniohyoideus	→	→		
C1–3				With hypoglossal to hyoid strap muscles	→	→
T5–6						Preganglionic sympathetic to lower esophagus

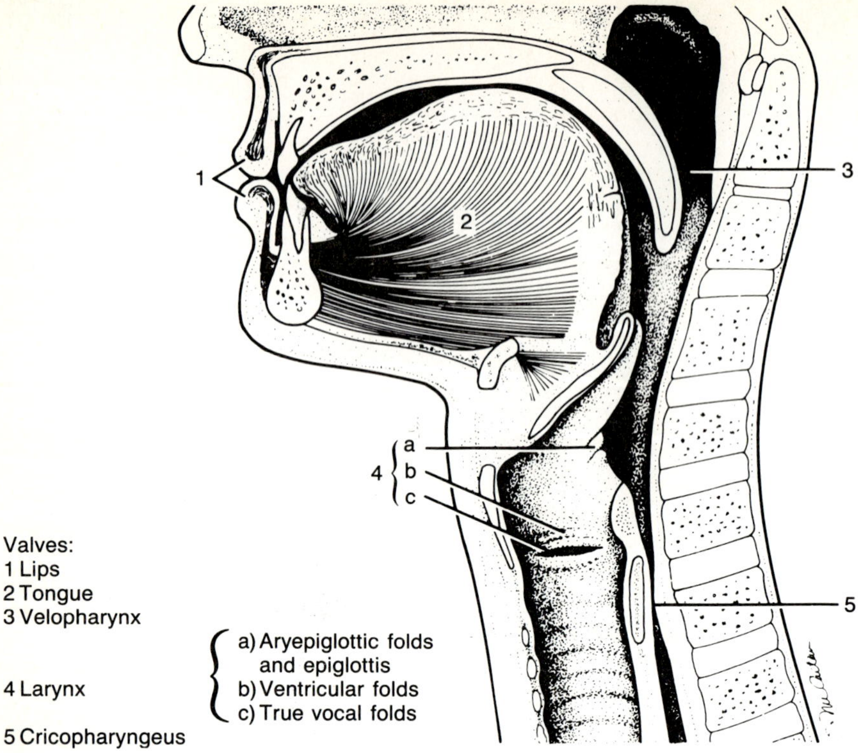

Figure 36–3 The valves of the upper aerodigestive swallowing mechanism. (From Robbins J. Swallowing in ALS and motor neuron disorders. Neurol Clin North Am 1987; 5:213.)

dition to peristalsis. Peristalsis is the sequential contraction of muscles that facilitates passage of the bolus through the cavity. During pharyngeal peristalsis, three pharyngeal valves function to direct passage of the bolus to the esophagus while simultaneously preventing it from entering the nasopharynx and the lower airway.

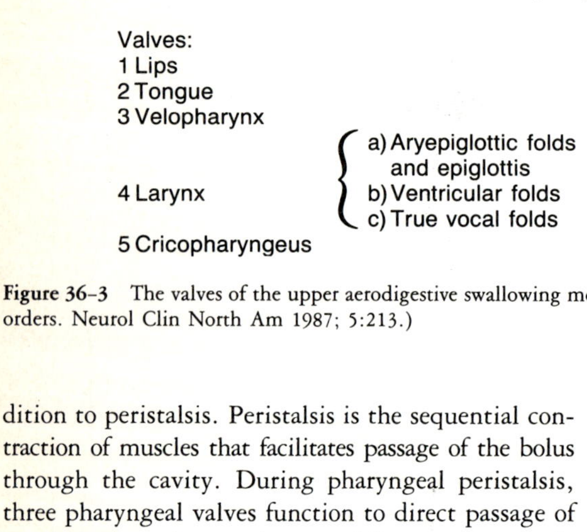

Figure 36–4 Velar lowering and posterior tongue elevation forms a seal separating the oral and pharyngeal cavities. (From Robbins J. Swallowing in ALS and motor neuron disorders. Neurol Clin North Am 1987; 5:221.)

The first valving action during this automatic phase is velopharyngeal closure, produced in part by elevation and retraction of the soft palate, which not only opens the pharynx in advance of the bolus, but also forms a valve through contact with the lateral and posterior pharyngeal walls, to prevent entrance of material into the nasal cavity.

The second major valving action of the pharyngeal phase is that of the larynx, which affords airway protection. As part of this more automatic phase of swallowing, the larynx is drawn upward and forward, tucking under the base of the tongue, while the epiglottis tips posteriorly and inferiorly to cover the laryngeal opening. However, the major protection of the airway is provided by three levels of sphincteric closure: aryepiglottic folds, false vocal folds, and the true vocal folds.

The pharynx joins the esophagus at a juncture termed the "pharyngoesophageal segment," also known as the upper esophageal spincter. This lower boundary of the pharynx and upper boundary of the esophagus is controlled by the action of the cricopharyngeus (lower portion of inferior constrictor), which functions as a valve. Unlike the four valves above this point, the cricopharyngeal valve is generally closed; it remains in a state of tonic contraction until a bolus approaches. Then the cricopharyngeus relaxes to let the bolus pass into the esophagus, after which it resumes its tonic contractile state.

CAUSES

Virtually all diseases or processes (i.e., head and neck cancer, congenital abnormalities) that disturb the peripheral morphologic features of the mouth, pharynx, larynx, and esophagus or the central and peripheral nervous systems underlying the function of these features may produce dysphagia. Table 36–2 is a nonexclusive list of the neuropathologic causes and of the sites that may be associated with swallowing disorders. The same neuropathologies may also underlie speech disorders. Table 36–3 presents congenital, immunologic, genetic, and iatrogenic etiologies of dysphagia. These etiologies may also underlie dysarthric speech. Swallowing disorders occur in all age groups, from newborns to the elderly, and may result from a variety of medical conditions.

The underlying condition generally causes changes in range, force, timing, accuracy, or direction of movement. Such changes have direct implications for the five valves and two major propulsive forces (lingual and pharyngeal peristalsis) described earlier.

ASSESSMENT

The Multivalvular Approach

The multivalvular approach to oropharyngeal motor function during swallowing evolved from the notion that separate assessment of different speech motor subsystems is necessary to develop an optimal program of component-focused rehabilitation.[9,10] Since the underlying morphologic features of swallowing are those involved in speech production, it is probable that, at least in part, the neural control mechanisms for speech and swallowing are the same. Thus the multivalvular approach is appealing and easily adapted for dysphagia assessment. This approach is particularly attractive for evaluation of individuals in

TABLE 36–2 Possible Neurogenic Etiologies of Speech and Swallowing Problems

Cause	*Site*
Upper motoneuron disorders	
Vascular	Thromboembolism in any area of the brain (stroke)
	Cerebral hemorrhage in any area of the brain
Infectious	Meningitis: meninges
	Encephalitis: brain stem, cerebrum
Traumatic	Closed head injury
	Neurosurgical intervention in central nervous system
Autoimmune	Multiple sclerosis: central myelinated tracts
Metabolic	Wilson's disease: basal ganglia, cerebellum
Neoplastic	Intracranial tumors
Degenerative	Cerebral palsy (spastic, ataxic, choreoathetotic)
	Huntington's chronic progressive chorea: basal ganglia
	Parkinson's disease: basal ganglia, substantia nigra of midbrain
	Friedreich's ataxia: widespread central nervous system involvement
	Multisystem degeneration:
	Progressive supranuclear palsy
	Shy-Drager syndrome
	Olivopontocerebellar atrophy
Lower motoneuron disorders	
Infectious	Poliomyelitis; anterior horn cells in brain stem, spinal cord
Traumatic	Closed head injury to peripheral nervous system
	Spinal cord injury
	Neurosurgical intervention in peripheral nervous system
Autoimmune	Guillain-Barré syndrome: peripheral nervous system
	Myasthenia gravis: myoneural junction
	Inflammatory myopathies: striated muscle
Metabolic	Thyroid hypofunction
Degenerative	Muscular dystrophy: striated muscle
	Thoracic masses
Upper and lower motoneuron disorders	
Degenerative	Amyotrophic lateral sclerosis: corticospinal tracts, corticobulbar tracts
	Anterior horn cells in brain stem and spinal cord, motoneurons

After Robbins JA. Swallowing and speech production in the neurologically impaired adult. In: Logemann J, ed. Relationship between speech and swallowing. New York: Thieme, 1985:337.

TABLE 36–3 Congenital, Immunologic, Genetic, and Iatrogenic Etiologies of Swallowing Problems

Congenital	*Immunologic*	*Genetic*	*Iatrogenic*
Cerebral palsy	Arthritis	Down's syndrome	Radiation therapy
Cleft palate	Dermatomyositis	Cystinosis	Chemotherapy
Phenylketonuria	Sjögren's syndrome	Treacher Collins syndrome	Postsurgery
Dysautonomia	Systemic lupus erythromatosis	Huntington's chorea	Medication reaction
Other neuromuscular disorders (e.g., myotonic dystrophy)	Scleroderma		

From The role of the speech-language pathologist in the evaluation and treatment of dysphagia. Asha 1987: 7.

whom dysphagia is secondary to head and neck cancer or neurogenic etiology.

In the postsurgical head and neck cancer group, tumor and sufficient surrounding tissues are removed or resected to assure a reasonable cure rate, and reconstructive efforts are made in an attempt to restore the anatomic and physiologic relationships to as close to normal as possible. In so doing, the anatomic relationships within the upper aerodigestive tract are modified, often reducing efficiency of one or more of the valves and/or propulsive mechanisms depending on the extent of the surgery and the success of the reconstructive efforts. The value of separate assessment of the different motor subsystems is clearly evident when dysphagia is secondary to end-organ impairment.

This approach is also particularly appealing in evaluating potential lower motoneuron disorders where differences in subsystem impairments might be present due to select damage in some cranial nerves and not others. The conduction of multiple valvular assessment in oropharyngeal deficits of suprabulbar origin is also necessary. Individuals with conditions such as amyotrophic lateral sclerosis, Parkinson's disease, or congenital or acquired spasticity do not have equivalent degrees of impairment across all oropharyngeal or limb motor subsystems. Many progressive neuromotor diseases are first observed in a single part of the body and then in other parts over the course of the disease.

PRESWALLOWING PROCEDURES

History

Specific information is required prior to initiation of assessment of the integrity of the valving and propulsive components of the oropharyngeal tract. This information is obtained by gathering historic facts from the individual's chart if he or she is an in-patient in a hospital setting, from a file or record if he or she is in a school or residential institution, or from the client if he or she is a reliable reporter. If the patient is unable to communicate information (i.e., too young, unintelligible with no effective augmentative method) or is unreliable (i.e., dementia) a person familiar with the client should accompany him or her to the evaluation or be contacted to serve as an informant. The following information should be obtained:

1. A knowledge of medical diagnosis or evaluation and its implications for dysphagia diagnosis and intervention.[2] For example, dysphagia secondary to stroke may have a more favorable prognosis and different treatment plan than dysphagia resultant from a progressive disease such as amyotrophic lateral sclerosis.
2. A knowledge of the client's level of alertness and language comprehension relative to the potential for safe oral intake.[2]
3. A knowledge of the client's current nutritional, dietary, or hydration status, as well as the type and method of intake, including a knowledge of special nutritional, dietary, or hydration concerns. The clinician's primary concern must be for the nutritional status of the patient. For example, if a patient is maintained on oral feedings when the speech-language pathologist is consulted, but is reported as becoming progressively dehydrated, it may be appropriate to recommend and discuss with the patient's physician the placement of a nasogastric tube or intravenous line in order to supplement fluid intake.
4. A knowledge of the client's respiratory status, including the presence and type of tracheostomy tube (cuffed, uncuffed, fenestrated) and any existing pulmonary disease.[2] Tracheostomy tubes are generally placed when the airway is obstructed above the level of the vocal folds, or when the upper airway could potentially be obstructed (i.e., edema following surgery). A cuffed tracheostomy tube is preferable when there is a potential for foreign material to enter the patient's airway. When inflated, the cuff contacts the tracheal wall, preventing air from passing upward and preventing material above the larynx from passing down the trachea and bronchi. Thus

identification of a cuffed tracheostomy tube in a patient provides initial information on the presumed severity of dysphagia.

5. A knowledge of the general medical status of the client, including respiratory and medical history, drug history, surgical record.[2] If the patient has a history of chronic pulmonary disease or recurrent pneumonia, the treatment plan is more conservative. Drug history is important information regarding possible underlying neurologic etiology for the dysphagia. For example, patients with tardive dyskinesia secondary to psychotropic medication may demonstrate dysphagia. During the evaluation and management of postsurgical patients, it is important to ascertain from the surgeon the extent of the resection and the exact nature of the reconstruction. Anatomy and anatomic relationships may differ significantly after surgery. Further, the possible underlying neurogenic implications of the surgery are an important consideration.

Oropharyngeal Examination

Assessment of the integrity of the anatomy of the mouth, pharynx, and larynx should be part of the dysphagia evaluation. In addition, assessment of neuromuscular and sensory function of the lips, tongue, velopharynx, and larynx provides important information prior to swallowing evaluation.

Anatomy

Observations of the lips, tongue, faucial arches, palate, soft palate, uvula, and neck should be made in terms of structure (i.e., relative size, symmetry, palatal height, and width). Any abnormalities such as scarring in the oral cavity or neck, atrophy, asymmetries, or fasciculations should be noted.

Motor Examination

The oropharyngeal motor examination should include evaluation of range, force, rate, and accuracy of movements of the lips, tongue, soft palate, and larynx during speech and nonspeech activity, as well as swallowing.[3,11] Examples of some tasks directed at achieving this goal for the lips,· tongue, velopharynx, and larynx follow.

Lips. The lips may assist in maintaining food in mouth.

Nonspeech. Observe lip closure during rest and during a saliva swallow. Observe maintenance of lip closure while head posture is changed.

Speech. Round the lips for /u/ production, and retract them for /i/ production. Alternate /u and i/ as rapidly as possible to obtain a diadochokinetic rate. Also, observe lip closure for production of /m*a*/, and obtain a diadochokinetic rate.

Swallowing. Observe maintenance of lip closure while chewing or moving the mandible. Observe lip closure around a straw or an eating utensil. The examiner may pull on the utensil in order to assess the force, instructing the patient to make an attempt in holding the utensil in his or her mouth by only using a lip seal.

Tongue. The tongue may assist in chewing, bolus formation, and food transit through the oral cavity. Anterior and posterior function should be assessed.

Nonspeech. Tongue protrusion, lateralization to corners of lips, elevation, depression, lateral protrusion into cheeks, and reaching into anterior and lateral sulci should also be evaluated. The patient should also be asked to slide the tongue along the palatal vault from the alveolar ridge anteriorly to the soft palate as if sweeping food from the palate.[3,11] Nonspeech posterior tongue function is difficult to observe.

Speech. Assess the production of diadochokinetic rates for /t*a*/. Assess the production of /k*a*/. Diadochokinetic rates and a sentence containing a number of back velar stop phonemes are used to determine completeness of linguopalatal contact.

Soft Palate. The soft palate prevents nasal reflux of food and permits elicitation of the gag reflex.

Nonspeech. The gag reflex should be elicited by contacting the base of the tongue or posterior pharyngeal wall. A strong contraction of the pharyngeal wall and soft palate should be observed. It should be emphasized that there are no data to support a relationship between the presence of the gag reflex and normal swallowing.[3,12]

Speech. Loud production of /*a*/ for several seconds facilitates examination of soft palate function.[3,11] Rapid repetition of /*a*/ permits further assessment of velar elevation and retraction.[3] Speech assessment should also include repetition of a sentence constructed with nonnasal stops and fricatives for evaluation of nasal resonance and emission.

Larynx. The larynx provides airway protection.

Nonspeech. One important laryngeal function is assessed by having the patient cough. Evaluate the force of the cough for expectorating material from the airway. Neurologically impaired individuals may produce phonation while attempting to cough, and they may also demonstrate longer duration of the "coughing" attempt. Unfortunately, by requesting the patient to cough, the function is not truly reflexive and so does not indicate whether the patient will respond spontaneously if foreign material enters his or her airway. Asking the patient to elevate and lower pitch assesses the function of the cricothyroid muscle and intrinsic vocal cord musculature, thereby testing the superior laryngeal nerve innervation of the cricothyroid. Since the pharyngeal phase of swallowing may be released by the superior laryngeal nerve, as may the cough reflex, an inability to change pitch may imply reduced sensitivity around and within the larynx.

Speech. Voice quality should be assessed. A hoarse voice may be an indicator of reduced laryngeal closure during swallowing. A direct relationship between a hoarse voice and laryngeal valving problems during swallowing is not always the case. However, hoarse voice quality in conjunction with symptoms of dysphagia requires careful laryngeal examination by an otolaryngologist. Finally, assessment of the larynx as a valve for speech production is achieved by diadochokinetic rates of the syllable /h*a*/, listening for clear voice on the vowel and voicelessness on production of the /h/.[3] Additionally the S/Z ratio[13] is useful in assessing laryngeal valving independently of respiratory support.

Oral sensation. Assessment of light touch and temperature (cold versus warm) provides information on areas of reduced sensitivity. Various points along the tongue (lateral and anterior to posterior), buccal mucosa, and faucial arches may be touched lightly with the head of a small laryngeal mirror, as shown in Figure 36–5 (size #00 or #000). For touch, the mirror is kept at room temperature. For temperature sensitivity, it may be dipped into a cup of ice for 5 seconds or briefly run under warm water.

SWALLOWING ASSESSMENT

A variety of diagnostic approaches to swallowing are available to the speech-language pathologist. These range from manual assessment, which is the "laying on of the hands," to more sophisticated techniques, including videofluoroscopy, manometry, ultrasound, and scintigraphy. In order to gain the most information from the swallowing evaluation, it is helpful to organize and interpret the findings of the history taking and oropharyngeal examination.

Interpretation and Application of Historic Information

The client's level of alertness is important for selection of the appropriate diagnostic method. The fluoroscopic method requires performance of swallowing within a few seconds of the request to swallow because ionizing radiation is used. Also some of the methods require the patient to sit in a specified chair, which may be difficult for patients who are wheelchair bound and cannot easily transfer. Also patients must maintain a certain posture, usually sitting upright and relatively still, until testing is completed. Appropriate positioning may be difficult for individuals with movement disorders or hemiparesis.

For the patient with impaired language comprehension, practicing the selected swallowing protocol prior to testing generally is helpful. The most effective set of instructions may be determined for each patient's capabilities.

When a patient has a cuffed tracheostomy tube, the examiner should consult with the doctor for permission to deflate the cuff during swallowing evaluation. It is important to have the patient suctioned immediately after cuff deflation so that material above the cuff does not enter the airway. During swallowing evaluation the tracheostomy tube should be manually closed to simulate oropharyngeal pressures as close to normal as possible.

Surgical information is helpful in determining food placement for the swallowing examination. For instance, the patient with a unilateral resection of

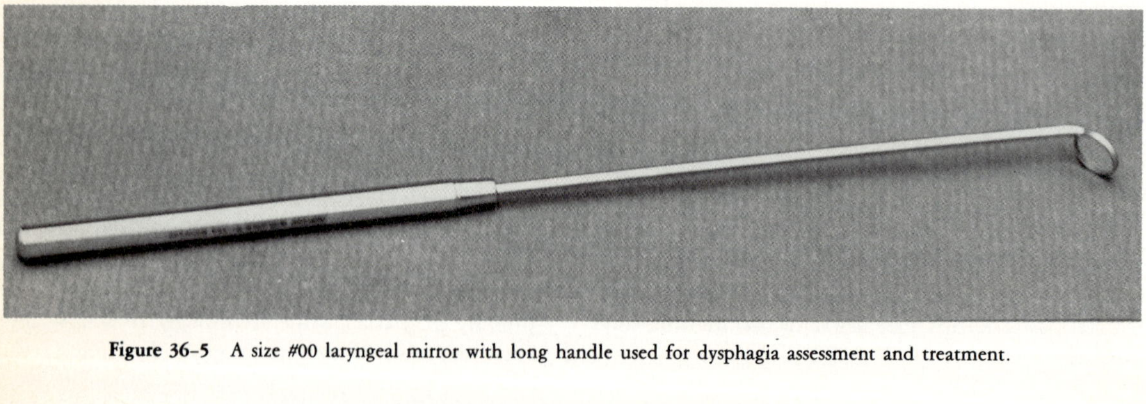

Figure 36–5 A size #00 laryngeal mirror with long handle used for dysphagia assessment and treatment.

the oral cavity may swallow more successfully if the material is placed on the contralateral side.

Finally, if the patient's respiratory status is compromised, the clinician should determine, through consultation with the physician, whether or not the patient can tolerate any material entering the airway during the testing or during therapy. Pulmonary function testing may be obtained by the physician prior to the testing of swallowing. Although no guidelines exist about the amount of aspiration (entrance of foreign material into the airway below the level of the tune vocal cords) a patient can tolerate before developing pneumonia, many physicians find pulmonary function test results helpful in making this decision.

Interpretation and Application of Oropharyngeal Information

Information gained from the oropharyngeal examination allows the swallowing therapist to determine the best posture, position, and consistency of food to be used during the swallowing evaluation. For instance, if a patient demonstrated reduced anterior lingual control, most likely for him or her to propel the food to the back of the oral cavity will be difficult. If the patient has demonstrated no indication of reduced airway protection during swallowing, the clinician may place the food on the posterior tongue to bypass the impaired anterior portion and may also instruct the patient to tilt his or her head backward when he or she is ready ot initiate swallowing, thereby using the momentum of the postural adjustment and gravity to propel the food into the pharynx. For this patient, a thin fluid consistency (i.e., liquid) may be selected to begin the swallowing evaluation. Thus, by interpreting and applying information from a previous examination, a preparatory set may be constructed to facilitate success and to diminish risk during the swallowing examination.

General Rules for Swallowing Evaluation

Amount of Material

Use small amounts of material, insufficient to block the airway. The small amounts also minimize trauma if material enters the lungs. Approximately 2 ml ($^1/_2$ teaspoon) of liquid and 2 ml of semisolid material are used. If mastication is assessed, a solid (usually a cookie) of approximately 1.5 cm is used.

Organizing Observations

During the assessment, analyze events in terms of oral phases and pharyngeal phase. Also analyze events in terms of valving efficiency and propulsive forces.

Assess Therapy Techniques

Some of the methods used to assess swallowing are also helpful in assessing various therapy strategies. That is, variations in posture, food placement, consistency, and instructions may be made during the evaluation.

Manual Swallowing Evaluation

Prior to instructing the patient to swallow, the clinician places his or her hand lightly on the submandibular and neck region with the fingers in strategic locations for assessment of phase durations and range of motor events (Fig. 36–6). The index finger is positioned immediately behind the mandible, the middle finger at the hyoid bone, the third finger at the top of the thyroid cartilage, and the fourth finger at the bottom of the thyroid cartilage. When the patient swallows, the clinician can assess tongue movement with the index finger in the submandibular region. The second finger perceives hyoid movement; the third and fourth fingers assess laryngeal movement during the pharyngeal phase. Computing the time elapsed from the initiation of laryngeal motion to initiation of maximum lingual movement provides a rough estimate of the oral phase of swallowing.[3] Duration of initiation of laryngeal elevation to laryngeal return to rest provides a rough estimate of pharyngeal phase duration.

The major advantage of this technique is that it can be done where the patient is most comfortable, and it requires minimal positioning of the patient and minimal alertness and language comprehension.

The major limitations are (1) if initiation of the pharyngeal phase is delayed, the clinician cannot determine the events occurring during that delay time; (2) bolus movement into and through the pharynx cannot be determined; and (3) entrance of material into the airway is unknown because patients with superior laryngeal nerve damage may not cough spontaneously. In this case, a gurgly voice is an important indicator of aspiration. In summary, a gross estimate of oral phase time is provided, but pharyngeal phase information is unclear.

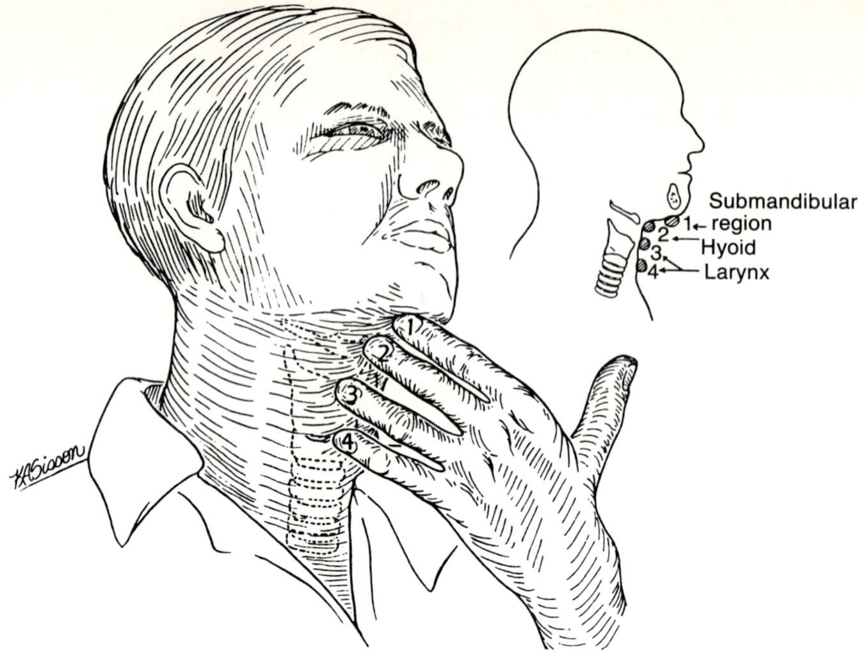

Figure 36–6 Positioning of the fingers during the manual swallowing assessment. (From Logemann J. Evaluation and treatment of swallowing disorders. San Diego: College-Hill Press, 1983:121.)

Videofluoroscopy (Modified Barium Swallow)

Dynamic imaging of the oral cavity, pharynx, and esophagus is done with fluoroscopy. The fluoroscopic image was recorded on movie film earlier in this century (cinefluoroscopy), and it is currently recorded on videotape (videofluoroscopy). Although videofluoroscopy does require ionizing radiation, the amount of exposure is significantly reduced from that of cinefluoroscopy. This technique allows frame-by-frame analysis of all phases of swallowing. Because swallowing is a rapid process with oral phase and pharyngeal phase durations of approximately 1 second each in normals, slow-motion analysis facilitates diagnosis of abnormal movement patterns underlying dysphagic symptomatology. Most video recorders can be connected to the fluoroscopic equipment in a radiology department so the fluoroscopic image is recorded on videotape.

The major advantages of videofluoroscopy are (1) accurate durational information if interfaced with a videocounter timer, (2) provision of slow-motion replay for accurate analysis of movements, (3) permission of visualization of all five valves, including cricopharyngeus, (4) visualization of pharyngeal phase events, (5) determination of amount and etiology of aspiration, and (6) permission of assessment of treatment strategies (i.e., posturing, food consistency).

Disadvantages include (1) exposure to roentgenograms, (2) difficulty in positioning certain patients, depending on available equipment, and (3) hospital setting and noise of equipment may frighten children.

Simultaneous Manometry and Videofluoroscopy

Manometry provides information on the pressure patterns in the pharynx and esophagus during swallowing. The patient swallows a pressure-sensitive tube of small diameter, which may be inserted into the esophagus orally or nasally. Upon swallowing, the manometric catheter measures pressure changes that reflect change in muscle tone. For dysphagia diagnosis, this method is most often used to measure pressure changes that reflect cricopharyngeal or upper esophageal sphincter opening. When manometry is performed in conjunction with videofluoroscopy, the pressure wave forms can be viewed in the context of the valves and movement events simultaneously in the pharynx.

The advantages of this technique, when used in conjunction with videofluoroscopy are that (1) it permits frame-by-frame analysis of the temporal relationship between the pressure changes and oropharyngeal movement parameters and coordination of pressure events with structural movement in the pharynx and (2) it provides direct evidence of pressure change, particularly in the upper esophageal sphincter.

Disadvantages are that (1) it may be difficult to insert the catheter in patients with stricture or hyperactive gag reflex, (2) it may give discomfort to the patient, and (3) manometry *alone* only provides a series of waves and does not relate pressure change to function of a structure (valve) or to a time sequence in relationship to passage of the bolus.

Ultrasound

Pulse-echo ultrasound uses high-speed sound waves to image movements of the tongue and the oral phase of swallowing. A transducer is placed submentally, and the beam is aimed cephalad toward the tongue. A small scanning head can be turned around the patient contact point so that the tongue can be scanned in either the sagittal or the coronal plane. The image is displayed using a video format. Much of the soft tissue anatomy of the tongue and floor of the mouth can be identified on the ultrasound image.

Advantages of ultrasound are that (1) it can image the soft tissue structures and (2) it is noninvasive and harmless.

A major disadvantage is that ultrasound is limited to evaluating the oral phase of swallowing because of its inability to transmit through bone and air.

Scintigraphy

Scintigraphy is an imaging modality that records the passage of a radionuclide bolus through the upper aerodigestive tract. Initially, the method was used to assess emptying of the stomach, and, more recently, it has been employed to study esophageal transit times. It is occasionally used for the study of oral and pharyngeal transit as well.

The major advantages of this technique are that (1) it provides accurate quantitative analysis of bolus flow and transit times, (2) it can provide quantified information on the residue of the bolus in the oral, pharyngeal, and esophageal cavities or in the trachea, and (3) it provides quantification of the amount of material aspirated.

Its major disadvantage is that it does not provide descriptions of the anatomy or detailed motion of the structures.

Findings of the Swallowing Evaluation

The swallowing therapist should be able to determine the underlying movement abnormalities in terms of range of motion, duration, and coordination causing the dysphagic symptoms. A methodical approach to analysis of findings is most helpful. Defining disorders according to phase and impairment of specific valving mechanisms and timing relationships within phases is suggested. Descriptions of bolus transit provide additional information for developing treatment strategies.

Aspiration, defined as the entrance of material below the level of the true vocal cords, is the most life-threatening result of oropharyngeal movement dysfunction. Recurrent aspiration may lead to pneumonia. The events that may underlie the occurrence of aspiration are identifiable during swallowing assessment with videofluoroscopy. Events underlying aspiration may occur during either the oral or pharyngeal phase of swallowing or during a delay in the transition between phases. The causes are attributable to various disordered movement parameters (i.e., force, range, timing, direction, accuracy) of the valving structures or propulsive mechanisms. An additional etiology of aspiration is reduced sensitivity of oropharyngeal areas (i.e., faucial pillars, vallecula) from which the automatic phase of swallowing is elicited. Specific causes of aspiration will serve as examples for discussion of possible findings of the swallowing assessment and appropriate management procedures.

ETIOLOGIES OF ASPIRATION

Oral Phase

Dysfunction of two oral phase valving components, posterior tongue and velum, may result in aspiration of material. That is, if the linguavelar valve is not effected to form a barrier between the oral and pharyngeal cavities during the oral phase of swallowing, material may descend into the pharynx prior to initiation of the pharyngeal phase of swallowing. Premature entrance of material into the pharynx permits penetration of material into the open airway. The airway is not yet protected by the automatic laryngeal excursion and vocal fold adduction, which only occurs as a function of "triggering" of the pharyngeal phase of swallowing. The result of premature entrance of material into the pharynx may be aspiration before swallowing.

Phase Transition

A delayed initiation of the pharyngeal phase of swallowing may also cause aspiration before swallowing. One cause of the delay may be a reduced sensitivity of the posterior lingual area and faucial pillars. In normals, the glossopharyngeal and vagus nerve receptors are stimulated by sensory information (i.e., temperature, taste) from these oral regions. The sensory input is then conveyed to the CPG, which releases the pharyngeal phase of swallowing. When oral sensitivity is reduced, pharyngeal response to the sensory information may be delayed. In this case, material may rest at the base of the tongue or in the vallecula. During the delay time, this material may fall into the open airway causing aspiration before swallowing.

Pharyngeal Phase

Dysfunction of the laryngeal valve is one cause of aspiration during the pharyngeal phase of swallowing. Incomplete vocal fold adduction during the pharyngeal phase of swallowing permits material to enter the airway while the pharyngeal phase is in progress. Thus the result of incomplete laryngeal valving is aspiration during swallowing.

Aspiration after swallowing may be due to cricopharyngeal dysfunction. If the cricopharyngeal valve does not open completely (i.e., unilateral paresis), then pooling occurs in the pyriform sinuses, the pharyngeal recesses above the cricopharyngeus. After swallowing is completed, residual material in the pharynx may spill into the larynx and enter the airway when breathing is resumed.

MANAGEMENT

The swallowing therapist must make two major decisions prior to initiating treatment. One is the choice among compensatory, rehabilitative, or medical treatments. The other decision, which is closely related to the first, is whether or not the patient will receive food by mouth prior to and during treatment.

Method of Nutritional Intake

The selection of appropriate swallowing therapy goes hand in hand with the swallowing therapist's decision as to how the patient will maintain or improve his or her nutritional status. The therapist must determine whether the client will receive food by mouth (oral feeding) or if it is safer for the client to receive nutrition via tube feedings. With regard to dysphagia management, "safety" is achieved by the elimination of two life-threatening processes: recurrent aspiration and weight loss accompanied by malnutrition. The clinician's recommendation about the manner of food intake is based on two pieces of information obtained during swallowing assessment. These are the frequency and amount of aspiration and the duration of swallowing. Any patient who is aspirating significantly (more than 10 percent of all substance types) and consistently, or who is taking an unacceptably long time to eat, is considered a candidate for a nonoral feeding technique to at least supplement nutritional intake. An unacceptably long eating time is a subjective perception made by the patient. Some patients find 30 minutes unacceptably long for consumption of a meal, whereas other individuals endure 60 to 90 minutes per meal in order to continue oral eating. Thus the decision to implement nonoral (tube) feeding should be made by the clinician in conjunction with the patient and/ or the patient's family.

If the decision is made in favor of tube feeding, then the type of tube placement must be selected (surgical versus nonsurgical). In general, if the patient's swallowing disorder is thought to be short-term in nature (3 months or less), a nasogastric tube is the method of choice. A nasogastric tube is passed nasally through the pharynx and esophagus into the stomach.

If swallowing rehabilitation is anticipated to take longer than 3 months, surgical tube placement is more appropriate. Surgically placed feeding tubes include pharyngostomy, esophagostomy, jejunostomy, or gastrostomy. The choice of surgical tube placement depends on the state of the patient's digestive system and the physician's preference.

TREATMENT

Compensatory Treatment

Compensatory treatment implies the use of external factors or new combinations of intact behaviors to override the effects of the impaired movement parameters. When compensatory management is implemented, food is generally introduced early in treatment. Compensatory techniques in dysphagia management include postural adjustment, supraglottic swallow, food placement, and diet modification. A wide range of postural adjustments, food placement strategies, and diet modifications are available. Representative examples in each category will be discussed in this section. Selecting the appropriate strategy, or combination of compensatory treatments, depends on the diagnosed disordered parameters of swallowing. An appropriate example for each type of compensatory strategy for remediation of the various etiologies of aspiration previously discussed is provided in the following section.

Postural Adjustment

In the previous section, impaired linguavelar valving was used to demonstrate an oral phase etiology of aspiration. One appropriate management of that disorder is compensatory in nature. That is, specific postural adjustment can override the loss of the barrier between oral and pharyngeal cavities. The patient would be instructed to tilt his head forward during placement of food in the mouth and during mastication or bolus formation. In this manner, gravity is used to preclude premature entrance of material into the pharynx. When ready to swallow, tilting the head backward capitalizes on gravity to facilitate propulsion of the bolus into the pharynx. The "head back" posture is limited to individuals with intact airway protection.

The client with unilateral cricopharyngeal paresis, described in the previous section as aspirating after swallowing, would benefit from a different postural adjustment. The findings of the videofluoroscopic assessment of this individual's swallowing pattern would indicate pooling of material on one side of the pharynx, above the cricopharyngeus. Instructing this patient to turn the head to the impaired side (i.e., look over the shoulder in the direction of impairment) would close off the weak channel, thus facilitating propulsion of the bolus through the intact pharyngeal channel. This postural adjustment would result in reducing the amount of residual material, thereby eliminating aspiration.

Supraglottic Swallow

An alternative or supplemental approach to the problem of premature entrance of food into the pharynx, as demonstrated in the client with insufficient linguavelar valving, is the supraglottic swallow. The supraglottic swallow is a series of movements that provides airway protection prior to initiation of the pharyngeal phase of swallowing. The steps are (1) hold breath, (2) place food in mouth, (3) swallow, (4) cough to deflect material on vocal cords, and (5) breathe. The supraglottic swallow is the volitional imposition of an otherwise automatic swallowing behavior, vocal fold adduction.

Food Placement

A good example of the compensatory technique of food placement is provided by the individual with unilateral sensory deficit or an oropharyngeal hemiparesis. In these cases, the individual would be instructed to avoid the impaired side and to place food on the intact side.

Diet Modification

There are no absolute rules for diet modification. However, the client with reduced pharyngeal peristalsis generally swallows liquids and soft materials more successfully than solids or crumbly granular items. The client who aspirates is least successful with thin liquids or crumbly granular items that may break apart.

REHABILITATIVE TREATMENT

Rehabilitation therapy implies the retraining of a disordered movement parameter or behavior. Exercise repetition or practice is an essential aspect of this approach. Unlike compensatory management, the patient receiving rehabilitative therapy is often receiving nourishment via nonoral means (tube feedings). Food is not introduced in treatment until significant progress in swallowing has been demonstrated, and the risk of aspiration, weight loss, or malnourishment is minimized or eliminated. The three major rehabilitative approaches in dysphagia management are (1) oromotor exercises, (2) vocal fold adduction exercises, and (3) thermal sensitization.

Oromotor Exercises

Various oromotor exercises can be used in dysphagia therapy. Selection of the appropriate exercise or combination of exercises is based on determination of the valve that is impaired and the specific disordered movement parameter.

Let us return to the example in the previous section of the client who demonstrates aspiration before swallowing due to impaired linguavelar valving. Most likely, this client demonstrates reduced posterior lingual elevation that precludes formation of an efficient barrier between the oral and pharyngeal cavities. Exercises to increase range of posterior lingual elevation include (1) elevating the back of the tongue as far as possible, hold for 1 second, release and (2) production of the linguavelar plosive /k/ in isolation and in lists of words with final /k/, exaggerating that phoneme. The range of motion exercises should be practiced approximately ten times in one session. Ten sessions per day are suggested. A possible exception to vigorous practice of oromotor exercises is if a neuromotor impairment underlying the dysphagia is secondary to a degenerative disease (e.g., amyotrophic lateral sclerosis) in which a fatigue factor must be considered.

Vocal Fold Adduction

If laryngeal incompetence during swallowing cannot be managed quickly with the compensatory techniques of postural adjustment or supraglottic swallow, then a sequence of laryngeal adduction exercises must be initiated.

The client practices holding his or her breath as tightly as possible while pushing down or pulling up on the chair in which he or she is seated. Then the client is instructed to push with only one hand while simultaneously producing a clear voice. Next, the client repeats /*a*h/ with hard glottal attack.[3] This is an example of a series of exercises that should be repeated three times to a session, five to ten sessions per day. The client monitors improvement of vocal fold adduction by listening to the clarity of voice quality. These exercises are often necessary for neurogenic and postsurgical etiologies (particularly supraglottic laryngectomy) of dysphagia.

Thermal Sensitization

Delayed initiation of the pharyngeal phase of swallowing is a commonly observed feature of dysphagic swallowing patterns.[3,14–16] A widely used therapy designed to sensitize or stimulate the response consists of cold stimulation to the base of the anterior faucial arches. Theoretically, with this procedure, the sensitivity of the CPG is heightened so the automatic pharyngeal phase initiates immediately in relationship to the end of the volitional phases.

Thermal sensitization is provided by use of a chilled laryngeal mirror (#00 and #000, as shown in Figure 36–5). This particular instrument is used because the long handle facilitates the clinician's access to appropriate placement, and metal retains temperature. The swallowing therapist strokes one and then the other anterior faucial pillar. Light contact is repeated five to ten times. The purpose of the exercise is to heighten the sensitivity of the area that triggers the pharyngeal phase so that when food or liquid is presented and the patient attempts voluntary swallowing, the pharyngeal phase follows immediately. If the patient is not receiving oral feeding, the clinician instructs the patient to swallow dry after stimulation. If the patient can tolerate small amounts of material, the swallowing therapist may introduce 2 ml of cold water at the anterior faucial pillars, using a straw as a pipette. The therapist assesses the transition time between oral and pharyngeal phases with light finger placement under the mandible and on the neck, as shown in Figure 36–6. If the oral phase duration is assessed as longer than 1 second, the pharyngeal response is delayed. In certain patients, progress may be slow, with restoration of feeding taking a number of months. During the interval, tube feedings maintain the patient's nutritional status.

MEDICAL, SURGICAL, AND PROSTHETIC TREATMENT

Various nonbehavioral training alternatives are available that may result in remediation of particular valving dysfunctions underlying dysphagia. Discussion of several of the more commonly used procedures follows.

Intracordal Injection

Neurologic damage or amount of tissue resected may preclude vocal fold closure even after vocal fold adduction exercises have been attempted for a sufficient period of time. Intracordal injection of Teflon or collagen has corrected glottal incompetence for swallowing as well as speech production in various groups of neurologically impaired adults including cerebrovascular accident (CVA), amyotropic lateral sclerosis, and Parkinson patients.[17–19]
[19] This technique has also been reported to improve swallowing as well as speech production in patients who had head and neck surgery, particularly patients with partial laryngectomy whose remaining tissue in the larynx is insufficient to adduct and protect the airway.[3,19]

Cricopharyngeal Myotomy

Cricopharyngeal myotomy involves slitting the cricopharyngeal muscle from top to bottom to permanently relax the upper esophageal sphincter. It has been reported successful in patients with Parkinson's disease,[20] amyotrophic lateral sclerosis,[21] and oculopharyngeal dystrophy[22,23] who demonstrate oropharyngeal dysfunction. The success of myotomy is negligible in patients who demonstrate difficulty propelling the bolus through the oral and pharyngeal cavities to the upper esophageal sphincter. Myotomy only "relaxes" the sphincter at the bottom of the pharynx. It does not improve transit to that point. Additionally, it appears the suprahyoid musculature must effect anterior and superior excursion of great enough magnitude to provide a necessary mechanical pull that opens the upper esophageal sphincter wide enough to permit bolus passage.[24]

Palatal Reshaping Prosthesis

A palatal reshaping prosthesis benefits some patients who cannot achieve tongue-to-palate contact.[25] The palatal vault is designed to accommodate lingual function. For instance, if anterior lingual elevation is reduced, the anterior palate is dropped; if posterior lingual elevation is limited, the posterior palate may be dropped. If a hemiparetic tongue is the problem, then the longitudinal half of the palate on the affected lingual side is lowered. The prosthesis is designed to maximize residual lingual tissue or neuromotor control for swallowing, as well as speech production.

THE TEAM APPROACH

Dysphagia management usually involves a team of professionals. Management generally requires coordinated services from several specialists. As stressed throughout this chapter, adequate nutrition is the foremost consideration during the course of dysphagia treatment. Therefore the swallowing therapist must have close interaction with particular team members to insure maintenance of adequate nutrition while working on improvement of the patient's swallowing. Treatment should proceed in close cooperation with the client's physician and relevant team members. The team varies depending on the client's needs and may include an attending physician, client, dentist, dietician, educator, engineer, family member, gastroenterologist, neurologist, nurse practitioner, occupational therapist, otolaryngologist, pediatrician, psychiatrist, pulmonologist, radiologist, speech-language pathologist, social worker, and surgeon. Whereas some of the services provided by the team may be consultative or limited, others require on-going intensive treatment. The dysphagia team is often coordinated by the speech-language pathologist.

THE RELATIONSHIP BETWEEN SPEECH DISORDERS AND DYSPHAGIA

As discussed earlier, the anatomy for speech production and swallowing includes the same peripheral morphologic features: oral cavity, pharyngeal cavity, and larynx. These three physical entities make up the vocal tract as well as the upper aerodigestive tract (the esophagus is also included in the latter, but not the former). Consideration of the neural mechanisms controlling speech and swallowing demands an understanding of different behaviors mediated by some neural mechanisms that are the same for the two behaviors.

Deglutition is controlled by volitional and reflexive neural mechanisms. That is, the oral preparatory and oral phases of swallowing are voluntary in nature, whereas the pharyngeal phase of swallowing is automatic, frequently referred to as "reflexive" in much of the literature.[3,16] In contrast, the neural control of speech is overwhelmingly volitional.[4,7] Therefore the initial phases of swallowing are under voluntary control, just as is speech. Clinical observation[16,26] and animal experiments[27] have shown that if the lateral precentral gyrus of the cerebral cortex is damaged, subjects have to tip their heads backward in order to initiate swallowing. Since behaviors controlled by the cerebral cortex are usually considered to be more voluntary than those mediated by brain and spinal reflexes, these data support the idea that some aspects of swallowing are under control of the voluntary nervous system. Thus it appears that the neural controls for speech and the volitional phases of swallowing may be similar and may involve some of the same neural mechanisms.

The events of the more automatic pharyngeal phase of swallowing are controlled by the CPG, which is located in the medullary reticular formation. The existence of such a center implies a "hard-wired" neural circuit that produces the synchronized events of the pharyngeal phase.

In fact, researchers have observed that when oral phase valving structures are intact for the function of speech production, generally they also function adequately for swallowing. When oral structures do not adequately valve the airstream for normal speech production, those same valves generally do not perform their function adequately for normal bolus manipulation during the volitional phases of swallowing.[26,28,29] A good example of this is the findings of myself, Levine, and Logemann who studied speech production and swallowing in patients with left and right cortical cerebrovascular accident (CVA).[26] The presence of verbal apraxia correlated highly with "swallowing apraxia" in the left CVA group.

Yet valving mechanisms that are not intact for the oral phases of swallowing and speech production may, in fact, effect an efficient seal during the more automatic phases of swallowing. The best example of such seemingly paradoxical behavior is the velopharynx, which in normals effects the valving of the airstream during speech production and valves the passage of food during the volitional oral phases as well as the automatic pharyngeal phase of swallowing.

Findings of speech and swallowing movement patterns analyses obtained from the videofluoroscopy recordings of more than 30 subjects with amyotrophic lateral sclerosis have been reported.[28,30] Some subjects with bulbar involvement demonstrated minimal velopharyngeal movement with ineffective valving of the airstream during speech production of nonnasal phonemes and an inability to form the linguavelar valve during the volitional phases of swallowing. However, these same subjects demonstrated effective velopharyngeal elevation and retraction for velopharyngeal closure during the pharyngeal phase of swallowing. The concurring dysarthria characterized by minimal velar retraction and elevation resulting in hypernasality and the impaired linguavelar seal during the oral preparatory swallowing phase indicates a relationship underlying speech production and the voluntary swallowing behaviors. However, the intact velopharyngeal closure during the pharyngeal phase of swallowing reveals the different neural mechanisms underlying that automatic phase. It seems to follow that successful therapy for the valves involved in the oral phases of swallowing simultaneously improves the function of those valves for speech production and swallowing. There is less likelihood that treatment of pharyngeal phase valving mechanisms improves both functions in this neurogenic population.

The most predictable concurrence of speech production and swallowing impairment is found in postsurgical patients with head and neck cancer. Since valving of the airstream for speech production and valving of the bolus pathway in swallowing depends on intact anatomy, the correlation between speech and swallowing deficits appears to be most direct in patients with head and neck cancer who have anatomic disorders somewhere along the oropharyngeal tract.[29] For instance, a partial glossectomy may result in decreased range of lingual motion. The patient may be unable to shape the tongue around a bolus and hold it against the palate or to control the airflow on fricatives and on the release of stop consonants.

For this type of patient with head and neck cancer, exercise programs may improve bolus control and control of airflow. However, a deficit may remain because of insufficient tongue tissue. This deficit may be effectively compensated for with a palate reshaping prosthesis that lowers or fills in the areas of the palate where the tongue cannot reach.[25] Thus combined rehabilitative therapy and prosthetic management would simultaneously improve speech production and swallowing.

The relationship between speech and swallowing is fairly well established in patients with head and neck cancer and other populations with end-organ damage. Despite the frequent concurrence of speech and swallowing disorders in neurologically impaired individuals, limited information is available regarding the relationship between the two functions. The significance of the coexisting disorders, in terms of their neurologic substrates, is unclear. However, research efforts in this area are increasing, and patterns of concurring dysfunction in relation to the site of lesion, trauma, or disease process are beginning to emerge.

The impact of treatment programs on the two functions is even less well understood. Nonetheless, reported cases of acquired dysphagia and dysarthria have demonstrated that rehabilitative or medical and/or prosthetic treatment of one function carries over to the other function, effecting simultaneous improvement of speech production and swallowing.[15,29,31]

The wide interest of speech-language pathologists in swallowing disorders indicates that increasing numbers of clinicians are treating this disordered behavior in various populations ranging from infants to the elderly. It is imperative that clinicians carefully document treatment procedures and results in quantified terms. In this manner, the field of speech-language pathology can begin to clarify the relationship between impaired speech production and dysphagia.

SUMMARY

An overview of dysphagia for the speech-language pathologist was presented in this chapter. A discussion of normal swallowing included anatomy, phases, and neurophysiology underlying the volitional oral preparatory and oral phases of swallowing, as well as the more automatic pharyngeal phase. Approach to diagnosis and management is based on viewing the oropharyngeal tract as a series of valves and propulsive mechanisms.

Assessment was divided into preswallowing procedures and direct swallowing assessment procedures. Preswallowing procedures included a discussion of history-taking and the oropharyngeal motor and sensory examination. A variety of available methods for direct assessment of swallowing were presented and their advantages and limitations evaluated. Methods discussed included manual (hands-on) assessment, videofluoroscopy, manometry, ultrasound, and scintigraphy.

Potential diagnostic findings were presented in terms of aspiration, which is the most life-threatening result of oropharyngeal dysfunction. Possible etiologies of aspiration were discussed with regard to the phases of swallowing and dysfunction of specific oropharyngeal valving mechanisms.

Method of nutritional intake was presented as the first major management decision facing the swallowing clinician. Guidelines for selection of oral versus tube feeding were presented, followed by a discussion of the differences between surgical and nonsurgical methods of tube feedings. Selection of the appropriate therapy was presented as the second major decision facing the clinician. Compensatory, rehabilitative, and medical treatment approaches were described, and applicable examples of specific techniques were provided. A multidisciplinary team approach was recommended.

The final section of this chapter discusses the relationship between dysphagia and speech disorders. It concluded with a call for documentation of clinical procedures for dysphagia management and for quantification of treatment effects by clinicians.

Supported by grants NS 24427 and NS 20167 from the National Institute of Neurological and Communicative Disorders and Stroke.

REFERENCES

1. Westlake H. A system for developing speech with cerebral palsied children. Chicago: National Society for Crippled Children and Adults, 1951:7.
2. Engstrom DH, Fleming SM, Johns D, Larkins PG, Logemann J, Perlman AL, Robbins J, Sonies B, Weinberg B. Ad Hoc Committee on Dysphagia Report, Asha 1987; 29:57–58.
3. Logemann J. Evaluation and treatment of swallowing disorders. San Diego: College-Hill Press, 1983.
4. Larson C. Neurophysiology of speech and swallowing. In: Logemann J, ed. Seminars in speech and language. Vol 6. New York: Thieme, 1985:275.
5. Miller AJ. Deglutition. Physiol Rev 1982; 62:129–184.
6. Doty RW. Neural organization of swallowing. In: Code CF, ed. Handbook of physiology: alimentary canal. Washington, DC: American Physiology Society IV, 1968.
7. Kennedy JG, Kent RD. Anatomy and physiology of deglutition and related functions. In: Logemann J, ed. Seminars in speech and language. Vol 6. New York: Thieme, 1985.
8. Roueche JR. Dysphagia: an assessment and management program for the adult. Minneapolis: Sister Kennedy Institute, Abbot-Northwestern Hospital, 1980.
9. Hardy JC. Suggestions for physiological research in dysarthria. Cortex 1967; 3:128–156.
10. Netsell R, Daniel B. Dysarthria in adults: physiologic approach to rehabilitation. Med Rehabil 1979; 60:502–508.
11. Dobie R. Rehabilitation of swallowing disorders. Am Fam Physician 1978; 27:84–95.
12. DeJong R. The neurologic examination. New York: Hoeber Medical Division, Harper & Row, 1967.
13. Eckel FC, Boone DR. The s/z ratio as an indicator of laryngeal pathology. J Speech Hear Disord 1981; 46:147–150.
14. Robbins JA, Logemann JA, Kirshner H. Swallowing and speech in Parkinson's disease. Ann Neurol 1986; 19:283–287.
15. Robbins JA. Swallowing and speech production in the neurologically impaired adult. In: Logemann J, ed. Relationship between speech and swallowing. New York: Thieme, 1985: 337.
16. Veiss S, Logemann J. The nature of swallowing disorders in CVA patients. Arch Phys Med Rehabil 1985; 66:372–375.
17. Hirano M. Surgical treatment of disorders in the pharyngeal stage of deglutition. Proceedings of symposium Atvalizacao en Endoscopia Peroral, Editora Manole LDTA, 1980: 131–141.
18. Butcher RB. Treatment of chronic aspiration as a complication of cerebrovascular accident. Laryngoscope 1982; 92:681–685.
19. Session D, Zill R, Schwartz J. Deglutition after conservation surgery for cancer of the larynx and hypopharynx. Otolaryngol Head Neck Surg 1979; 87:779–796.
20. Palmer E. Dysphagia due to cricopharyngeus dysfunction. Am Fam Physician 1974; 9:127–131.
21. Lebo C, Sangu K, Norris F. Cricopharyngeal myotomy in amyotrophic lateral sclerosis. Laryngoscope 1976; 86:862–868.
22. Dayal, T, Freeman J. Cricopharyngeal myotomy for dysphagia in oculopharyngeal muscular dystrophy. Arch Otolaryngol 1976; 102:115–116.
23. Duranceau C, Letendre J, Clermont R, Levesque H, Barbeau A. Oropharyngeal dysphagia in patients with oculopharyngeal muscular dystrophy. Can J Surg 1978; 21:326–329.
24. Mendelsohn MS, McConnell FMS. Function in the pharyngoesophageal segment. Laryngoscope 1987; 97:483–489.
25. Wheeler R, Logemann J, Rosen M. Maxillary reshaping prosthesis: effectiveness in improving speech and swallowing of post-surgical oral cancer patients. J Prosthet Dent 1980; 43:313–319.
26. Robbins, JA, Levine RL, Logemann J. Swallowing after cortical CVA: right vs. left hemisphere differences. Asha 27, 1985:114.
27. Larson CR, Byrd KE, Garthwaite CR, Luschei ES. Alterations in the pattern of mastication after ablations of the lateral precentral cortex in rhesus macaques. Exp Neurol 1980; 70:638–651.
28. Robbins JA. Swallowing in ALS and motor neuron disease. Neurol Clin 1987; 5:213–230.
29. Logemann D. The relationship between speech and swallowing in head and neck surgical patients. In: Logemann J, ed. Relationship between speech and swallowing. New York: Thieme, 1985.
30. DePaul R, Abbs J. Manifestations of ALS in the cranial motor nerves: dynametric, neuropathologic, and speech motor data. Neurol Clin 1987; 5:231–250.
31. Harris B, Murray T. Dysarthria and aphagia: a case study of neuromuscular treatment. Arch Phys Med Rehabil 1984; 65:406–412.

37 A Clinical Science Approach to Treatment

Phil J. Connell, Ph.D.
Leija V. McReynolds, Ph.D.

It is sometimes interesting to speculate how a person not familiar with the issues and methods that interest social, behavioral, and cognitive scientists would view the state of the clinical science of speech-language pathology. The crucial question that could be asked of this outsider is, "How convincing is the scientific evidence that supports our clinical work?" After reviewing all the evidence that could be gathered in support of the efficacy of our clinical efforts, would this outsider be impressed with the scientific foundation of our practices or surprised by the lack of empirical support?

We are not optimistic that the outsider's answer would be entirely positive given the current state of the clinical science of speech-language pathology. Our concern stems mostly from the perception that the development of new clinical procedures has greatly outpaced efforts to test their effectiveness. The result is an imbalance between science and practice; an imbalance that is too large to ignore. The situation is similar to having a catalogue of medicinal drugs that provides no basis for distinguishing good drugs from better ones, or even good from bad. The purpose of this chapter is to propose an approach to clinical work that would give an individual clinician the opportunity to gather evidence that could be used to make such distinctions on a procedure by procedure, case by case basis. The evidence generated by this approach can be of sufficient quality to answer satisfactorily the questions of an outsider and, at the same time, have sufficient scientific rigor to satisfy the questions of professional colleagues.

The basic approach that will be proposed in this chapter is that clinicians conduct clinical activities as clinical experiments. It will be argued that the question asked of the hypothetical outsider is the kind of question that speech-language pathologists should be asking themselves routinely. In order to answer such a question, clinicians must make use of as many opportunities as possible to compare the effects of their treatment to the learning that would be expected from no treatment at all and ultimately to the effect of other treatments. To perform routinely treatment research of this type requires a commitment to research, a knowledge of the scientific method, a certain degree of skepticism, and a belief that what is obvious may not be true. The immediate benefit of such an approach would be an increase in the amount of clinical research being performed, thus increasing the understanding of the principles that underlie the treatment of speech and language disorders. The long term benefit is that the profession can raise itself to a higher level of acceptability and dignity, and, as importantly, the clients whom the profession serves will be better guaranteed of having the best treatment available.

This chapter is divided into two major sections. The first section will provide a rationale for the contention that some clinical activities be performed as clinical experiments. Although there are many theoretic positions that have had an impact on clinical work, only two major theoretic positions have had a significant influence in recent years: behaviorism and cognitivism. These positions have been used to support claims about the content, sequence, and procedure of various treatment programs designed to teach people to communicate more effectively. This section will demonstrate that, although these theories have to be taken into account when evaluating treatment in disorders, treatment research is nonetheless possible and necessary. The issues discussed are, in some cases, most applicable to treatment that replaces developmental learning, that is, language, articulation, learning disability, and hearing impairment as defined in the speech-language pathology literature. The discussion will be applicable also to issues in other disorders as well (e.g., stuttering and voice) to the extent that treatment of these disorders is an application of theories of learning and cognition.

The second section will provide a description of the methodology for clinical experimentation—single-subject experimental designs. Taking such an approach to clinical work not only requires a knowledge of the mechanics of experimental design, but also a knowledge of logic that underlies its purely procedural aspects. Once the logic is mastered, adapting designs to the problems and issues that they address becomes possible, thereby obtaining more valid tests of the effect of treatments on individuals.

THE REASON FOR DIFFERENT TREATMENT APPROACHES

The problem that every clinician faces routinely in clinical practice is how to construct a treatment plan that will be effective for an individual client. There seems to be no limit to the ways one can approach this problem as can be seen from even the most cursory review of the treatment literature.[1–3] This diversity in treatment approaches reflects, to a certain extent, the variety of conceptions held about the nature or etiology of communication problems. More than likely, though, the diversity is motivated by basic and deep-seated beliefs concerning the nature of learning and cognition. For example, the difference between one person's belief that a language error such as the omission of the plural morpheme results from an auditory processing deficit and another person's belief that such omissions result from merely a failure to learn a perceivable morpheme may have no ramifications for treatment. In both scenarios, it may be appropriate to provide the client with imitation drills to obtain production of the morpheme in sentences.[4,5] But if one believes that language learning is a cognitive event in which a child examines language data and forms hypotheses that are subsequently tested, then the use of imitation might be excluded as a possible treatment approach.[6,7] The exclusion or inclusion of certain approaches because of their presumed coherence with a theoretic model is obviously more the product of one's beliefs about learning than one's beliefs about cause. However, the effect of one's beliefs is perhaps less acknowledged because such issues are not viewed as being appropriate for the therapeutic application of science.[8] Regardless of the origin of one's clinical practices, it is important that all treatment procedures be submitted to empirical study so that their effect be known and recognized by the clinical community. As the clinical science of speech-language pathology progresses, determination of the relative effectiveness of groups of procedures will be important, regardless of their theoretic orientation, so that an informed selection can be made among them.

It will undoubtedly be found as this process of comparison proceeds that not all procedures can be compared to one another with equal ease. One factor that influences how difficult it is to compare certain procedures is the extent of the difference in the theoretic assumptions underlying them. Perhaps the most well-known difference is the one between those who ascribe to theories of learning that might be called "cognitive" and those who ascribe to theories that might be called "behavioral." The phenomena described by cognitive theories are mental phenomena such as rules, categories, and concepts; the most well-known theories of cognition and language are of this type. In contrast, the phenomena described by behavioral theories are observable acts (responses) and the environmental conditions that surround and control them; the well-known radical operant theory is of this type. The difference in assumptions of those who hold these theories is obvious. If one believes that learning is a mental operation, then the observable acts that might correspond to learning become mere products of mental conditions and, by themselves, unimportant to a description of the mental process of learning. But if one believes that learning is a physical operation in which acts and events are associated, then the mental conditions that might underlie this operation become speculative, for the present time at least.

The result of having two such different sets of assumptions is that treatments that derive from these positions are unlikely to ever be compared directly. The issues that differentiate the positions are assumed as nonempirical primitives of the respective theories and cannot themselves be evaluated through the normal hypothesis testing process. That is, differences in deep-seated beliefs about the nature of learning, differences that cannot themselves be evaluated by empirical means, make it difficult to confirm or disconfirm hypotheses about the comparative effectiveness of treatment procedures that bridge these two theoretic positions. And so given the influence of assumptions on the selection of appropriate measurement procedures, this analysis leads to the generalization that the best way to determine the effectiveness of a treatment is to use a paradigm in which a particular treatment is evaluated within its own theoretic framework. This does not mean that under no circumstances can treatments from different theoretic perspectives be compared, but that the compromises that would have to be made in order to bring certain treatments in line with one another might distort one or both of them to the extent that a valid comparison would be impossible. We will have more to say about treatment comparison in the sections that follow. These discussions will involve the methods available for across-treatment comparisons, but not the validity of such comparisons. Their validity would have to be established prior to applying these methods through argumentation or through evidence that would support the representativeness of each of the teaching procedures compared. Suffice it to say at this point that even though certain treatments are not compared easily, evaluation of the effectiveness of a treatment against a no treatment condition is always possible. Such comparisons form the cornerstones for the development of a clinical science.

THE ARTIFICIAL SEPARATION BETWEEN THERAPY AND SCIENCE

There are two movements in clinical science that are working to separate empirical treatment evaluation from clinical practice. The first is the belief that treatment evaluation can be performed to some extent by comparing treatment to theory.[9,10] This type of evaluation is certainly valuable in that it determines the extent to which a treatment may be viewed as an implementation of certain theoretic assumptions, and hence the extent to which the outcome of a treatment reflects upon the validity of the assumptions. But rather than absolving clinicians from the responsibility for performing empirical treatment evaluation, the recognition of theoretic frameworks actually compels clinicians to develop empirical measurement strategies for the kind of learning that is assumed to be the result of treatment. All theoretic frameworks are in need of confirming or disconfirming data, and the assessment of clinical applications can provide one source. For example, data on the effectiveness of a teaching procedure that is an application of a learning process hypothesized to occur in normal language acquisition would bear directly on the acceptability of the hypothesis and the theoretic assumptions that underlie it. The second movement in clinical science that appears to promote the separation between clinical research and clinical practice is the position that research and therapy are incompatible activities.[11] Two arguments are central to this position. The first is that research is concerned with broader issues of clinical science, whereas clinical work is concerned solely with the welfare of a particular client. It is assumed that a clinician's first responsibility is to use methods that are effective for a particular case, whereas the researcher's responsibility is to uncover unambiguous relationships among variables important to understanding learning in general. It is easy to understand how these two responsibilities can conflict. And the second argument is that if therapy was conducted as a research project, the experimental atmosphere would detract from its effectiveness. For example, the experimental atmosphere would remove the aspects of clinical instinct that may be beneficial to a client. It also might remove the clinician's optimistic demeanor, thus making the client less willing to learn.

In order to evaluate these arguments, we again refer to the medicinal drugs analogy alluded to earlier. An analogous situation would be the following: a rapidly expanding catalogue of drugs of unknown effect (at least in the eyes of science) exists that physicians must choose from in order to provide treatment for patients suffering from various ailments. (It should be evident that this situation is like that of 19th century medicine.)

In this situation, the first argument would be that physicians would not be under any obligation to evaluate the effect of the drugs because their job (and their training) is to treat patients—not to test drugs. The rationale for such a practice would be that physicians are not prepared to deal with the broader issues of science that are entailed in the examination of the effect of drugs on the human body. Thus, even though many drugs might not work (as proved to be the case in 19th century medicine), physicians would not be advised to test the effectiveness of drugs on individual patients because they lack the skills needed to perform such tests. Clearly such a restriction against clinical experimentation in these circumstances is unwarranted.

The second argument could be stated as the following: because physicians inspire their patients to believe that the treatment they are undergoing will be effective, placing a physician into an experimental atmosphere removes this effect and thereby reduces the overall effect of treatment. Again, given the circumstances, the concern for maintaining these secondary avenues of treatment seems unjustified in the knowledge that some of the primary avenues might be ineffective.

Although a certain amount of truth exists in each of these positions, it is not clear that separating science from treatment had any benefit for 19th century patients. Two questions need to be asked: Who would physicians have hurt if they applied a common sense test to determine whether a medicine was effective? And, more importantly, how many patients would have been helped if the common sense procedures were replaced by more precise experimental procedures, especially with the hindsight that most of the medicines of the era were ineffective? It is at least possible that medical treatment would have improved at a faster rate than it did had a climate of experimental evaluation been fostered by the medical establishment of the time. Similarly, we would like to hasten the development of the clinical science of speech-language pathology by fostering this same type of clinical climate among speech-language clinicians.

Even though this analogy to speech-language pathology may not be perfect, clinicians must face the inevitable fact that all their procedures cannot work equally well; that some procedures are superior to others; and that some may only seem to work, but, in reality, are successful only because of the influence of some extraneous set of factors. If a climate can be established that motivates clinicians to be more concerned with the effectiveness of their treatments, then clinicians can begin identifying ineffective procedures and discarding them. We may be a long way from finding the most effective procedures possible for each kind of communication disorder, but we should be able to rid ourselves of ineffective procedures rather quickly.

CREATING AN IDEAL CLINICAL RESEARCH ENVIRONMENT

If clinicians are to make a commitment to clinical research, then they need to confront two problems. The first is obtaining skills for performing good clinical research. Information on what skills need to be obtained is presented in the next section. The second is how to use these skills in clinical practice, that is, how to perform clinical research within the confines of a typical clinical situation. Some general suggestions are offered to make the transition from a primarily service model of treatment to a service and research model.

The basic problems facing a clinical researcher are (1) implementation of the caliber of experimental controls needed to evaluate treatment in the relatively uncontrolled environment of a therapy program and (2) implementation of rather sterile procedures in a situation where clients need psychological and emotional support. A clinical researcher must be sensitive to the human concerns inherent in therapy situations while being ever mindful of the threats to experimental concerns that such concerns can impose; thus differences between the problems encountered by clinical researchers and nonclinical researchers arise. Clinical researchers may not have the range of options that other researchers enjoy in implementing experimental control, but they can maintain a sufficient amount of control as long as they are aware of the biases that can influence a client's progress. For example, clinicians routinely encounter the need to recruit parental assistance as part of a treatment program for a young child or they sometimes need to counsel older clients to persuade them to perform better. Either of these activities could be viewed as a biasing influence on a test of the effectiveness of a certain treatment procedure. As will be shown later in the discussion on certain design options, controlling for such an influence is possible by experimentally separating the effect of the bias from the possible effects of the treatment.

The reality of the situation is that two competing forces in research on the evaluation of treatment always occur. The first force is the responsibility to the client's learning. Any activity that increases the likelihood of learning must be implemented. Thus activities that evaluate treatment cannot be removed entirely from the therapeutic situation in which they are imposed without the situation becoming more research oriented than therapy oriented. The second force is the responsibility to maintain control over treatment so that it can be experimentally evaluated. Thus treatment activities cannot be so uncontrolled as to make an evaluation impossible. The only option is to create a compromise solution that allows the two motives to be addressed simultaneously.

First, the experimental controls imposed by the clinician need to be such that they do not significantly interfere with the process of treatment. Some sacrifices may have to be made in the interest of obtaining a valid measure of effect, but the controls and measurement techniques selected should allow the clinician the leeway needed to perform treatment in a way that is most beneficial to the client at all times. Second, this clinical flexibility must not be so great as to make it impossible to determine whether aspects of the treatment are effective or aspects of the clinical process that are not directly related to the treatment per se are responsible for the learning. For example, it would be necessary to rule out the possibility that the clinician's persuasive skill was totally responsible for the change that might occur. This problem could be approached by monitoring two or more behaviors of each client and using each behavior as a control for the change in another by means of a multiple-baseline design (to be described in the next section). We believe that there are designs that make such compromises possible and practical, and that the effectiveness of therapy and the validity of the treatment evaluation will not suffer.

The kinds of procedures suggested in the next section to accomplish this task are similar in many ways to the process of therapy as it is usually applied in many clinical settings. Individual contact with a client over an extended time interval is the basic requirement for implementation of single-subject experimental designs. This similarity to clinical activities makes the insertion of experimental methods into therapy less traumatic on both the clinician and the client. As will be seen, many of the practices of clinical experimentation are no more time-consuming than carefully prepared therapy. The main difference is that the clinician who performs a form of clinical research when doing therapy has a sense of responsibility to the profession in addition to the responsibility to the client.

DETERMINING WHAT TO EVALUATE: DESCRIPTION

During the course of a day, speech-language pathologists treat a number of clients with a variety of communication disorders. As alluded to previously, each client and each problem requires an individualized treatment plan directed at eliminating the client's specific problem. In order to plan the treatment, the clinician uses information from various sources.

Perhaps the primary source is the diagnostic evaluation conducted prior to planning treatment. Results from standardized and nonstandardized tests and procedures are considered in conjunction with the case history, referral statement, and interview with the client. Compiling information from these activities provides a clear profile of the disordered behavior and allows for the selection of a target for treatment.

Definition of the problem is strongly influenced by the clinician's perception or interpretation of the information obtained during the evaluation, and so, treatment goals are dependent to a large extent on the clinician's individual viewpoint on the nature of the disorder and on his or her conceptualization of how learning proceeds, as discussed earlier. The speech-language pathologist's approach is probably often a function of the academic training program from which his or her degree was obtained. That is, the viewpoint of the instructors forms the basis for the views of the clinician.

For clinicians who have been employed for a number of years, the original conceptualizations have probably been tempered or modified by experiences in providing treatment to many clients. Over time, the speech-language pathologist has changed treatments or parts of treatment as a function of informal observations of client progress. These observations have provided evidence that some treatments, or some components of treatments, appear to be more successful than others. In some instances, the clinician might have an indication of what makes the treatment successful or not successful, but more often cannot identify the responsible variables. This is principally because so many variables are present simultaneously or so many events are occurring at the same time and because the client may have had previous sessions of treatment that had an effect on the behavior undergoing treatment in any particular session. Because so much is happening, identification of the most influential variables is impossible. In addition, clinical activities often change during a session because the client does not appear to improve or progress as well as the clinician expected, and, in order to improve progress, the clinician tries another procedure that may hold more promise than the original planned procedures.

All of the factors mentioned in the preceding paragraphs preclude reaching verifiable conclusions about which treatments or treatment components are most efficient and effective. Yet, from informal observations, a clinician often has indications that a particular treatment seems to be effective, whereas other particular treatments are not. These subjective conclusions are difficult to support without objectively obtained data, that is, documentation of effectiveness is impossible as long as the clinician uses subjective or intuitive evidence to support the conclusions.

However, documentation can be made more objective, and, with appropriate procedures, the variables responsible for successful treatments can be identified. All this is possible within the confines of clinical activities and without serious disruption of treatment to specific clients. Not only is it possible, it is also a useful endeavor for the clinician personally and for other interested groups as well: for example, colleagues, administrators, and members of other disciplines. Perhaps the most important reason for obtaining objective evidence for effective and ineffective treatments is that only through such controlled evaluations can the profession of speech-language pathology develop a scientific base for its intervention, that is, be a clinical science.

Obtaining objective evidence for treatment effectiveness consists of two primary steps. In the first step, written descriptions of clinical activities are used to identify potentially powerful variables for eventual controlled evaluation. In the second step, the identified variables are submitted to controlled evaluation in an experimental study.

Formulating Descriptions of Treatment

As noted earlier, speech-language pathologists engage in a variety of treatments during the course of a day, or week, or month. Not all of the treatments or components are equally effective. Therefore, the clinician needs to obtain information on which treatments or components appear to be worthy of a controlled evaluation, those that seem to promise to be the most effective and efficient, and those that appear to have little or no effect. Procedures for identification of potential variables require operational definitions of each aspect of the treatment, objective measurements of the behavior under treatment, and consistent recordings of the changes in the behavior throughout the treatment from the beginning to the end. Thus description is an essential prerequisite to experimentation. Procedures that lead to valid and reliable descriptions will be explained briefly.

Operational Definition

Operational definitions are basic to all scientific activities. Operational definitions consist of careful, detailed specifications of the operations that need to be completed in order to make an event, a stimulus, a procedure, and a response observable and measurable in an objective manner. An operational definition leaves nothing to the imagination; it explains all the relevant aspects in detail so that no two people can disagree on what is observed. The use of operational definitions in research studies, be they descriptive or experimental, is necessary in order to establish the basic components of research: validity, reliability, and replicability.

For the same reason, operational definitions are important to descriptions of treatments. Unless all relevant aspects of the treatment are described carefully, other clinicians will be unable to administer them. Unspecific descriptions or definitions leave room for individual interpretations by others, and, as a result, the treatment may be modified inappropriately when replicated. A modification, in turn, may result in a less effective treatment or may result in a more effective treatment than the original one described. In either case, the validity of the results as a replication is questionable.

Although speech-language pathologists are accustomed to defining and describing treatments, the definitions and descriptions are seldom complete or specific enough to qualify as operational definitions. This is partly due to the fact that the clinician can fill in any gaps that arise because she or he is directly engaged in the treatment and knows what is to be done. Unfortunately, other clinicians might fill in the gaps in a different way, which would change the treatment. Thus, although definitions are supplied, if they can be modified by others because of such gaps, they are not operational definitions.

However, learning to define treatments operationally is a skill that can be readily acquired with practice. It is sometimes time-consuming, but without such skills, clinical activities remain idiosyncratic and ambiguous. A brief example should demonstrate the difference between definitions that are commonly accepted as complete and an operational definition. The difference illustrates the risks encountered if operational definitions are not used in the description of treatments.

Let us assume one of the steps in a treatment is an imitative one in which the child is learning to name pictures of objects. A usual definition of the procedure would be as follows:

> The clinician presents the picture to the child, models the name of the picture, and asks the child to imitate the model. When the child imitates the name correctly, the clinician presents the child with a reinforcer.

This definition is a reasonable one, and most clinicians would consider it clear and complete. But could the procedure be replicated exactly as it was presented by the clinician who administered and described it?

Not really. For example, would another clinician know if the picture was placed on a table or held in the clinician's hand? Would the second clinician know what to do if the child did not respond or responded incorrectly? Must the child produce each sound in the object's name accurately, or can the child's articulation be distorted or inaccurate on any sound? Other questions can be raised concerning the definition, such as, what is the "reinforcer" and how is it presented? How long will training last? Must the child reach a learning criterion before treatment is terminated? If so, what is the criterion?

It seems tedious to go into such specific details, but without them, the procedure cannot be duplicated—not by other clinicians and, in all likelihood, not by the clinician who administered and described it in the first place. If the procedure cannot be duplicated by anyone, then it cannot be identified for descriptive purposes and certainly not for eventual evaluation for effectiveness. Descriptive data on the procedure cannot be obtained because measuring or recording observations is impossible if one does not know what to look for.

And so operational definitions form the foundation from which a clinical science can emerge. Without them, we cannot know what is taking place in treatment, and if we do not, we cannot isolate variables that can contribute to effective treatments and principles. Needless to say, all aspects of the treatment need to be defined operationally as noted previously. The aspects to be defined operationally include the stimuli presented, the procedures used to present them, the responses produced, and the manner in which the responses are recorded.

Objective and Consistent Measurement

Operational definitions are particularly advantageous to the development of objective measures of behavior undergoing treatment. By specifying the procedures used to evoke the response from the client and describing in detail the form of correct and incorrect responses, the clinician knows precisely when the response of interest occurs and how it should be scored and recorded. In fact, if operational definitions are used, they practically dictate the kind of measure most suitable for describing progress in treatment. Naturally, the measure to be used depends on the behavior being treated and the parameters of the response that need to be scored. Several kinds of measures are available, and they are clearly described in a number of texts.[12–14] Among the measures most frequently employed are rate measures, frequency measures, trial scoring, interval and time sampling, and duration measures. Speech-language pathologists may choose a measure most suitable to the behavior treated from among the measures just listed or may develop their own measures.[15] Trial scoring and response duration are described in this section because they seem particularly suitable for the treatment of communication disorders. For detailed descriptions of other measures, the reader may wish to refer to one or more of the sources cited previously.

Trial Scoring. A frequently used measure in articulation and language intervention is trial scoring. Much of our training is on a trial by trial basis: a stimulus is presented, and a response is produced by the client. If the correct and incorrect responses have been defined operationally, each response can be scored as correct or incorrect, and a frequency count of correct and incorrect responses can be tallied. By graphing the data from each session, using time or sessions on the abscissa and the score for each session on the ordinate, a clinician can observe progress from one session to the next.

Response Duration. Another measure that may be suitable to treatment of stuttering and voice problems is a duration measure. In this measure, the clinician records the duration of a response, for example, the duration of a stuttering episode or the duration of periods of fluency in a stutterer's speech. In treatment of voice, the clinician may wish to train longer periods of vocalization for esophageal speech, in which case duration is an appropriate measure. Duration measures may be objectively recorded by the use of a stopwatch or electric timer. Duration measures may be combined with trial by trial scoring or event recording; the form of the data is dictated by the form of the response that is selected to be trained.

Consistent Recording

Whatever measures are used, it is essential that data on the response be taken during each treatment session. Consistency is important. In order to make decisions about the course of treatment and options available in clinical research, the clinician needs to determine if a pattern emerges across sessions of treatment; an accurate pattern can only be identified if the responses are recorded each day. In addition, the data need to be graphed each day in order to observe if any dramatic changes in behavior occur or if no changes occur.

Speech-language pathologists have been trained to measure and record events in treatment sessions, that is, they are particularly efficient in taking data during intervention. But they are probably less efficient in knowing what the data tell them, and how it can be used to best advantage. One way it can be used is to identify potentially strong and weak treatment variables and to select variables that seem worthy of further investigation in a controlled manner. The next section will present some experimental designs for this evaluation. Using experimental designs, of course, is the second step in the establishment of a scientific base for interventions and the development of a clinical science. The designs that are emphasized are single-subject experimental designs. They have been selected because they were developed just for the purpose of evaluating treatments and treatment variables in a controlled manner; thus they are especially suited to clinical environments.

SINGLE-SUBJECT DESIGN

There are two primary methodologies for establishing cause and effect relations between variables in experimental studies. The more conventional approach is the methodology of group designs in which at least two groups of subjects are formed. One group is the experimental group and the other the control group. The control group serves to account for extraneous variables that might confound the effect of the treatment variable. In group designs, the experimental group is administered the treatment, whereas the control group is not. Any extraneous variables that might be operating on the experimental group during treatment are also operative on the control group, but if changes in the behavior of interest occur only for the experimental group, then it is likely that extraneous variables did not interfere with the treatment effect.

The second approach to experimental evaluation of functional relationships between variables is known as single-subject experimental methodology. It is less commonly used in research and is not as widely known to researchers and clinicians. In this approach to experimental research, the subject serves as his or her own control, and formation of groups is unnecessary. Single-subject methodology is described in this chapter because it is considered a more suitable vehicle for evaluating treatment variables than group designs, primarily because it was designed specifically to explore treatments and treatment variables; thus it is less disruptive to clinical activities and client services. The description in this chapter is limited to basics of the approach, but a number of texts and articles can be consulted for a fuller treatment of the logic, rationale, and the characteristics of each design.[12–14,16–20] Before the basic designs and components within designs are described, the logic and rationale of the designs will be briefly explained.

Logic and Rationale

The purpose of all experimental studies is to isolate the effect of the treatment (the independent variable) on the behavior (the dependent variable) that is being treated. The experimental study is a controlled evaluation of the independent variable. In order to isolate the effect of the treatment under study, it is necessary to take into consideration all the other events, stimuli, and activities in which the client (subject) is engaged because all of these factors are also acting on the behavior; simultaneous with the administration of treatment, the client is influenced by individuals who live with him or her or by teachers in classrooms if the client is a child. If the client is an adult in a hospital, many interactions are occurring that may be affecting the behavior in treatment. In the clinic, these factors and others can interact with the treatment so that it is difficult to know if changes in behavior are the result of the treatment being administered or of the other events operating in the environment of the client. Because of these extraneous, confounding variables, experimental studies are designed carefully to rule them out so that the effectiveness of the treatment can be isolated for evaluation. As mentioned earlier, in group designs, extraneous variables are assumed to be operating at all times, and, to account for them, a control group is formed to determine if the variables are responsible for the learning observed in the experimental group.

In single-subject experimental designs, extraneous variables are also assumed to be operating and need to be accounted for and controlled. Rather than forming a control group, the control is shifted to the subject in that the subject goes through no treatment and treatment phases, that is, the subject participates in all conditions of the experiment. The rationale for doing this is that extraneous variables, if present, are present in the no treatment phase as well as the treatment phase. If the behavior changes only when treatment is administered, and not during the no treatment phase, then the variables are not influencing the behavior nor confounding the effect of the treatment.

Basic Design Components

The two kinds of conditions in single-subject designs are labelled with the letters A and B. A stands for the no treatment (baseline) conditions, and B for the treatment conditions. In the A phase, the behavior of interest is observed and recorded, but no treatment is administered; whereas, in the B phase, the behavior is observed and recorded during treatment. To determine if the treatment has had any effect, above and beyond the effect of extraneous variables, the occurrence of the behavior in the A and B phases is compared. However, one A phase and one B phase is not sufficient to constitute a controlled evaluation of the effect of treatment because there is no evidence to rule out the presence of other events that may have been introduced simultaneously with treatment and that might be responsible for any behavioral changes in the B phase. To account for this possible confounding by extraneous variables, single-subject designs usually incorporate several A and B phases.

Several designs are capable of evaluating the effect of treatment in a controlled fashion. The two basic designs will be described first, and additional designs will be explained briefly. For detailed descriptions, the reader is referred to the numerous books and articles cited earlier.

ABAB Design

The ABAB design is illustrated in Figure 37–1. The first A phase is the baseline in which the

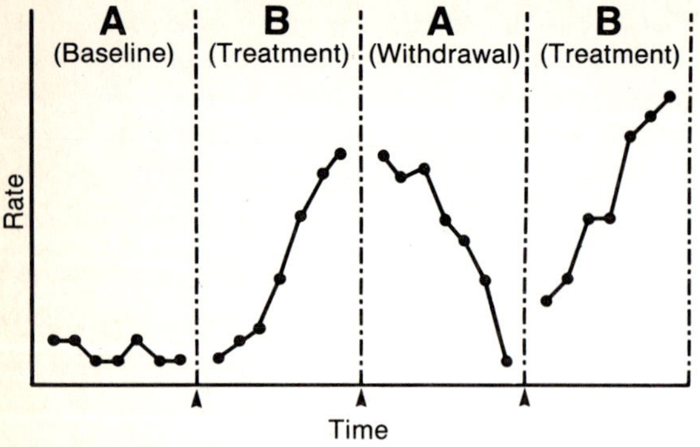

Figure 37–1 The form of an ABAB withdrawal design with alternation of no treatment and treatment phases.

behavior to be treated is measured prior to the introduction of treatment. Usually measurement in this baseline phase continues until the occurrence of the behavior shows stability. When stability is observed, the treatment is introduced in the B phase. After a designated period of treatment, a second A phase is introduced. In the second A phase, the behavior is measured again, but no treatment is administered. The second A phase is similar to the first A phase. If the behavior returns to a level similar to the level in the first A phase, the control needed to show that extraneous variables are not responsible for behavioral changes has been achieved. If extraneous variables had been responsible for the changes observed in the B phase, then these changes would have continued when treatment was no longer present in the second A phase. However, if the behavior returned to the level observed in the first A phase, then it can be safely concluded that the treatment was probably responsible for changes in the treated behavior. To demonstrate control, inclusion of the second B phase is not necessary, but investigators are usually more comfortable ending a study with the client in treatment and with the behavior showing the appropriate occurrence. When the second B phase is initiated, the behavior once more shows the effect of treatment. In essence then, differences in performance between both A phases and both B phases provide evidence of treatment effectiveness and demonstrate that other variables were not responsible for the changes observed during treatment. Evidence for the effectiveness of treatment is shown if the dependent variable shifts from one phase to the next as indicated by the arrows in Figure 37–1.

Variations in ABAB

The ABAB designs may include withdrawals or reversals in the second A phase. In a withdrawal design, the treatment is withdrawn to determine if the behavior reverses to baseline level. However, when an investigator suspects that the behavior is too stable after it is acquired to revert to baseline level with withdrawal of treatment, a reversal can be implemented. In a reversal, a behavior incompatible with the behavior trained in phase B may be trained in order to show that, when treatment is administered to form another behavior, the response trained in B reverts to baseline level again. Two procedures are available to accomplish the reversion. In one procedure the baseline response may be retrained; in the other procedure, a behavior unrelated to the behavior trained may be reinforced.

An example of retraining baseline behavior is shown in a study by Elbert and McReynolds[21] in which children with /s/ errors participated. During the baseline, the children produced /θ/ or another substitution when the /s/ was elicited. In the B phase, the children were trained to produce /s/ correctly. In the second A phase, the children were trained to produce their old error substitution /θ/ again, and, in the final B phase, they learned to produce the correct /s/ sound once more. An example of an ABAB in which incompatible behavior was reinforced during the second A phase is a study in which a child is trained to smile at a moderate rate during the B phase, that is, the child was still frowning on approximately 30 percent of the trials. In the A phase, the consequent event is shifted to the frowning behavior. And so each time the child frowns in the second A phase, a reinforcer is presented. Thus a behavior that is incompatible with smiling is trained until the frequency of the frowning is increased to a predesignated level. In the second B phase, reinforcement is shifted to smiling again to show that the treatment is responsible for the smiling behavior.

Multiple-Baseline Design

A design that is often used in single-subject studies is the multiple-baseline design shown in Figure 37–2. In a multiple-baseline design, measurements are made on more than one behavior, or in more than one setting, or across more than one individual. For example, in the A phase, the measurements are applied to more than one behavior in a multiple-baseline, across-behaviors design. After baselines on the two or more behaviors have stabilized, treatment is introduced for the first behavior, and the baseline measurement is continued on the second behavior. Thus, in Figure 37–2, two behaviors (two language constructions, for example) are measured in the A phase prior to introduction of

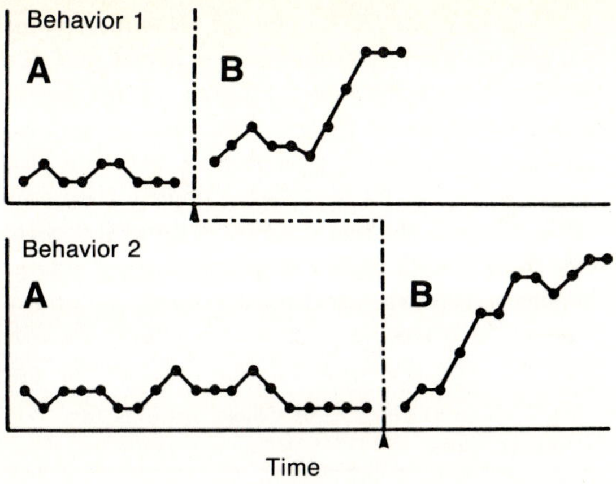

Figure 37–2 A multiple baseline, across behaviors design showing the two experimental phases (*A* and *B*) and an extended baseline phase (*A*) for the second behavior.

treatment. When treatment on the first behavior (one of the language constructions) is introduced in the B phase, the second construction continues to be measured in the extended A phase. At a designated point in the treatment of the first behavior, the same treatment is applied to the second language structure in the B phase for the second behavior.

A hypothetical example of a multiple-baseline design study would be the evaluation of a specific treatment for teaching a child to produce prepositions in the presence of appropriate pictures depicting spatial relationships, for example, "on" and "behind." The baseline would be obtained on the child's production of both prepositions when the pictures are presented. Assuming that the child does not produce either preposition during the baseline, the investigator decides that if each picture is presented three times and incorrect responses continue to be obtained, treatment will be initiated on one of the prepositions. Thus treatment is administered to teach the child to produce "on" to the appropriate pictures. During the treatment for "on," the baseline is continued for the "behind" preposition. Treatment for "on" is presented in the B phase of the top graph in Figure 37–2. When the child has reached training criterion on the "on" preposition, training is shifted to the "behind" preposition; progress in acquiring "behind" is shown on the bottom half of the graph in Figure 37–2.

Control in multiple-baseline designs resides in the second behavior (setting or individual, depending on which design is chosen): as the first behavior is being treated and changes are observed, no changes occur on the second behavior that is not receiving treatment. It is not until treatment is applied to the second behavior that the behavior shows changes. Thus, if extraneous variables had been responsible for the changes observed in the first behavior during treatment of that behavior, changes in the second behavior would also have been observed because extraneous variables were operating on both during treatment of the first behavior. However, if the second behavior changes only when treatment is applied, then the treatment was likely responsible for behavioral change. The arrows in Figure 37–2 show where experimental control is demonstrated and treatment effectiveness is supported by objective evidence.

Variations of the Multiple-Baseline Design

As mentioned, several versions of the multiple-baseline design are possible. In a multiple-baseline, across-settings design, the baseline is first measured in all the selected settings (e.g., therapy room, hospital ward, hallway). When the behavior is stable in all settings during the baseline, treatment is initiated in the first setting (e.g., therapy room). During treatment in the first setting, the baseline is continued in the other two settings. When training has been completed in the first setting, it is applied to the behavior in the second setting. The baseline in the third setting is continued. When training is completed in the second setting, it is shifted to the third setting. A similar sequence across different subjects constitutes a multiple-baseline, across-subjects design.

In some respects, multiple-baseline designs are more complex to implement than are ABAB designs, although they are preferred designs in intervention research. When a multiple baseline is applied across behaviors or settings, counterbalancing is required to control for order effects. To rule out the effect that training on the first behavior might have on the second behavior, counterbalancing the order of training is necessary. Some subjects are initially taught on the second behavior and subsequently the first behavior. In the example of the preposition study, four subjects would receive treatment. Two subjects would learn "on" first and "behind" second. The training order would be reversed for the other two subjects. They would first learn "behind" and subsequently learn "on."

Other Single-Subject Designs

A number of other designs have been developed to obtain answers to questions concerning the effectiveness of treatments. The kinds of questions that are frequently posed and the designs suitable for exploring them are depicted in Table 37–1.[18] The theme developed by Kearns is that the particular question posed by a clinician may be explored in a number of ways with more than one design, and the design eventually chosen is determined on the basis of practical, ethical, and behavioral considerations. As can be seen in the table, a number of designs are available. Detailed descriptions of the designs are offered in the texts listed earlier. Only brief descriptions are provided in the present chapter.

The basic ABAB and multiple-baseline designs have already been described. As explained in Table 37–1, the multiple-probe design is a variation of the multiple-baseline design. It is actually designed to handle questions about intervention programs that contain a number of steps. For example, a language treatment program might contain three successive steps starting with imitation, proceeding to reading, and finally requiring the spontaneous production of responses in the presence of minimal cues. The cli-

TABLE 37–1 Evaluation Strategies, Research Questions, Design Options, and Considerations for Single-Subject Experimental Designs

Evaluation Strategy	*Clinical Research Question*	*Selected Design Options*	*Basic Considerations*
Treatment–no treatment comparison	Does treatment, with all of its components, result in improved performance relative to no treatment?	Withdrawal and reversal designs ABAB BAB ABA	Is the therapeutic effect likely to reverse following the withdrawal of treatment?
		Multiple-baseline designs (MB) across behaviors across settings across subjects	Are functionally independent behaviors or settings available? Are homogeneous subjects available?
		Multiple-probe technique (variation of MB)[22]	Are functionally independent behaviors available? Are long or continuous baselines impractical?
Component assessment	Relative to a treatment package, to what degree do separate components of treatment contribute to improvement?	Interaction (Reduction) BC-B-BC-B BC-B-BC-A-BC-B-BC	Can the components be examined alone and in combination with the treatment package? Can replication be obtained across subjects?
	Does the addition of a component to a treatment package facilitate treatment effectiveness?	Interaction (Additive) B-BC-B-BC B-BC-B-A-B-BC-B	Can the components be examined alone and in combination with the treatment package? Can replication be obtained across subjects?
Treatment–treatment comparison	What is the relative effectiveness of two or more treatments?	Alternating treatments design	Can treatments be rapidly alternated for each subject?
		Replicated crossover design[23]	Are multiple subjects or target behaviors available? Can treatment be "crossed over?" Are nearly equal phase lengths possible?
Successive level analysis	Does treatment result in acquisition of successive steps in a chaining sequence?	Multiple-probe technique	Are steps in the treatment sequence independent? Are earlier steps prerequisite to acquiring later steps?
	Does treatment effectively modify a single, gradually acquired behavior?	Changing criterion design	Will changes in the dependent variable correspond to changes in the criterion level? Will the dependent variable stabilize at successively more stringent criterion levels?

From Kearns K. Flexibility of single-subject experimental designs. Part III: design selection and arrangement of experimental phases. J Speech Hear Disord 1986; 51:205.

nician might wish to know if each step is necessary as a prerequisite to obtaining the response in the next step or if one of the steps could be eliminated. For example, the step in which the response is read by the subject may be unnecessary for learning spontaneous production. To discover if each step is necessary, the experimenter would probe the behavior required in each step. When training is completed on step 1, imitation, the behavior is probed in reading before further training is administered. In addition, the response required in step 3 is probed. If a reading response is produced accurately after imitation training, it is evidence that step 2, teaching the response to a written form, is not necessary and so the client can proceed to step 3 directly after imitation training. That is, all three steps are not essential.

The interaction design is also directed at obtaining evidence for the necessity of all components in a multiple-component intervention program. For example, suppose a treatment for stuttering consists of three components: prolongation, rate management, and reinforcement. The clinician might wish to learn if all three components contribute to treatment effectiveness or if the same results could be obtained if one or more of the components were eliminated. To determine the role played by each component, the experimenter might use the interaction design. Applying this design, the treatment might start with the complete three component program, then only one of the components might be presented for a set time to determine if effectiveness is decreased when the other two components are removed. After a designated period of training of one component, the entire three component package is readministered. If stuttering decreases to the same degree during treatment of one component as during the treatment of three components, the clinician might question the need for all three components in treating stuttering.

The two kinds of interaction designs described in Table 37–1 show how the experimenter may use a design in which the complete program is administered initially and components are withdrawn for individual evaluation or a design in which the individual component is administered alone and then placed in the context of the entire treatment package. Other variations of the interaction design are available depending on the questions posed by the clinician. For example, if the clinician wishes to evaluate a combination of two of the components in a four component program, the two components could be withdrawn simultaneously.

A particularly useful design for comparing treatments is the alternating treatments design in which two different treatments are administered for one behavior in an alternating fashion. The relative effectiveness of the two treatments is demonstrated on a session by session basis by displaying data on the behavior change under two conditions. If the behavior always improves more when one of the treatments is administered, it is possible to conclude that the two treatments are not equally effective.

The final design to be described is the changing criterion design that can be used to increase or decrease the occurrence of a behavior according to a criterion set by the experimenter. For example, if a behavior is initially occurring at a very low rate and the clinician wishes it to occur much more often, a design to facilitate the increase is used. Thus, after baseline, the experimenter determines the rate at which the behavior should occur before reinforcement is provided. Usually, the experimenter sets a realistic rate as the criterion. When the behavior is occurring at the set criterion level, the experimenter sets a more stringent criterion; the behavior now has to occur more often in order to meet the contingency for reinforcement. Gradually, the experimenter sets more stringent criterion levels until the behavior approaches the rate desired by the experimenter.

Controls for the various designs are in some ways different, but in each case, except for the multiple-baseline, across-subjects design, the subject serves as his or her own control. For example, in the changing criterion design, if the rate of the behavior matches and stabilizes at each of the criterion levels set by the experimenter, control is exhibited because the behavior conforms to each criterion change. In the interaction design, the basic ABAB form is maintained, and in the multiple-probe design, the form is similar to the control used in the multiple-base line design.

OTHER DESIGN FACTORS

The function of the designs described is primarily to control for extraneous variables in order to assure internal validity of the studies. In other words, the controls are used to substantiate that the study accomplishes what it intends to accomplish: that it allows the isolation of the effect of the treatment from the effect of all the other variables operating during the treatment. The designs are particularly suitable for that purpose and provide a sophisticated method for evaluation of the treatments. However, the design alone is insufficient to provide convincing scientific evidence for the effectiveness or ineffectiveness of treatments. Other components of the studies need to be taken into consideration. These will be described briefly.

Operational Definitions

The need for operational definitions has already been explained in the previous section. It only needs to be reiterated here that operational definitions of all components of the experiment must be used if internal validity is desired. Without operational definitions, it is impossible to understand the procedures, the behaviors studied, or the scoring. Operational definitions are essential for other reasons: among them, the need for replication and obtaining measures of reliability.

Reliability

In most intervention studies, the treatment is provided by a human, the responses are produced by a human, and the accuracy of the responses is judged through a human perceptual system. Often when the response is a communication behavior, such as articulation, language, voice, or dysfluency, and an instrument cannot be used to record and score the behavior, human judgements are needed. Because the responses are judged by humans, it is essential that more than one judge determines the accuracy of a behavior. If only the experimenter judges the correctness of the subject's response, the experimenter's bias or other factors may possibly influence his or her judgement. Therefore it is necessary to obtain independent judgements of the subject's responses in order to provide evidence that the experimenter's judgements were reliable. Thus reliability in intervention studies must be established if the results are to be accepted with confidence. There are a number of ways to compute reliability, but the most popular is point to point computation. This method requires that each response is scored by two independent observers, and scores are compared for agreement and disagreement. The percentage of agreement is computed by dividing the number of agreements by the total number of agreements and disagreements. Excellent discussions of factors considered in reliability computation can be found in books by McReynolds and Kearns,[14] Kazdin,[13] and Barlow and Hersen.[12]

A Clinical Application

The application of single-subject designs to clinical work requires the consideration of two separate but related questions. The first is, "What treatment needs to be evaluated?" The obvious answer is that all treatments ought be evaluated, but, in reality, such an enterprise would be impossible given the kinds of time and manpower constraints that exist in most clinical environments. Given that a selection must be made, the best grounds for identifying a candidate would seem to be subjective impressions of effectiveness. Treatments that have appeared to be successful on a variety of clients over an extended period of time would be of less interest than treatments that have had inconsistent or only moderate levels of success. This does not mean that treatments that are perceived as successful should not be evaluated in order to verify, or in some cases, remove the perception they enjoy. Rather, such an approach would select those treatments that could have the greatest impact on client learning should the evaluation process uncover methods that might improve the treatment. Following the evaluation of these treatments, other more successful treatments could be evaluated and improved. And once a treatment has been identified, the next question that must be answered is, "What kind of design would be appropriate to apply in order to evaluate the treatment?" Kearns provides a thorough analysis of the kinds of factors that must be considered when selecting a design.[18] These factors include the kind of question that is asked of the treatment and the nature of the skill that the treatment is designed to teach. For example, one has to determine before selecting a design whether the treatment will be compared to other treatments or to a baseline condition. Some designs are incapable of making within-subjects comparisons of two or more treatments, but are fully capable of making within-subjects comparisons of treatment and baseline periods. One also has to determine before selecting a design whether or not the skill to be taught is dependent on other skills and whether or not comparable skills exist that could be used for control. The importance of this factor will be made clear in the following example.

Perhaps the best way to show how these factors interact to constrain the kinds of designs that can be selected to evaluate a treatment is to describe briefly the decision process involved in selecting a design for a recent study performed by one of us.[24] The purpose of the study was to examine the acquisition of semantic roles by comparing the effectiveness of two procedures used to teach them: procedures that emphasized the comprehension of language versus procedures that emphasized the production of language. Although this purpose is more theoretic than clinical in that the major goal was to better understand the acquisition of a narrow domain of language (semantic roles), the procedures would not have been that appreciably different if the purpose had been merely to determine whether comprehension teaching or production teaching was more effective. Thus this study can serve as an example of how treatment research might be approached from a clinical perspective.

The first factor that was taken into account in the process of selecting a design was the fact that a comparison between the two treatments was needed. This necessity obviously required that both treatments be applied and, in keeping with the logic of single-subject methodology, that they both be applied to single subjects.

The second factor that was taken into consideration was the nature of the skill to be learned. In this case, semantic role was selected because of the research interests of the experimenter and not because it presented an ideal tool for evaluating a treatment. The fact is that the selection of semantic role limited the kinds of designs that might have been used to evaluate teaching. For example, reversal designs would not have been appropriate because semantic role learning would probably be resistant to reversal. There is evidence from many sources in literature on normal development that indicates that once a child learns semantic roles, they are used to express relations between many different entities and across many situations. Thus evidence of extensive generalization would by itself preclude the use of a design whose experimental control is based in part on a successful reversal of learning.

The use of a multiple-baseline, across-behaviors design would also be precluded by the nature of semantic role acquisition. Semantic roles appear to be the first step in the process of sentence acquisition and their learning is not equivalent in any obvious sense to learning elements such as words during the same developmental period. The establishment of some equivalency between or among behaviors is necessary in order to justify the use of one or more behaviors as a control for the learning of others. The selection of behaviors that are not part of a developmental sequence, such that one is typically learned before the other, is also necessary. Sequences imply that learning one element has some consequence on learning another. Such a relation would not be appropriate for a design in which experimental control is derived in part from the assumption that certain behaviors are independent, as is the case with multiple-baseline, across-behavior designs.

The design that was selected is one that took these two factors into account. It is best understood by examining the data presented in Figure 37–3. The design actually was not fully developed until after the study had progressed well past the half-way mark. This aspect of single-subject designs makes them particularly suitable for intervention research. Better than any other type of design, these designs have the capability of being modified during a study in reaction to developments that arise once a study is underway.

Experimental control was exerted in this experiment by a composite of three separate multiple-baseline, across-subjects designs. Each of these designs offered a different aspect of control for the evaluation and comparison of the two treatment methods. The first design (left panel) controlled for the influence of extraneous variables on the effects attributed to production teaching. As can be seen in the panel, subjects 1 and 2 demonstrated production of semantic roles only after treatment had been initiated. During those intervals in which no treatment was offered, performance did not change appreciably, indicating that treatment was the causative factor for the change. The second design replicated the first design in part, in that production treatment was applied to two children in sequential manner. The result of this replication was the same: both children learned to use semantic roles only during the treatment periods. The second experimental function of this design was to evaluate the effect of comprehension teaching. It is in this aspect that the

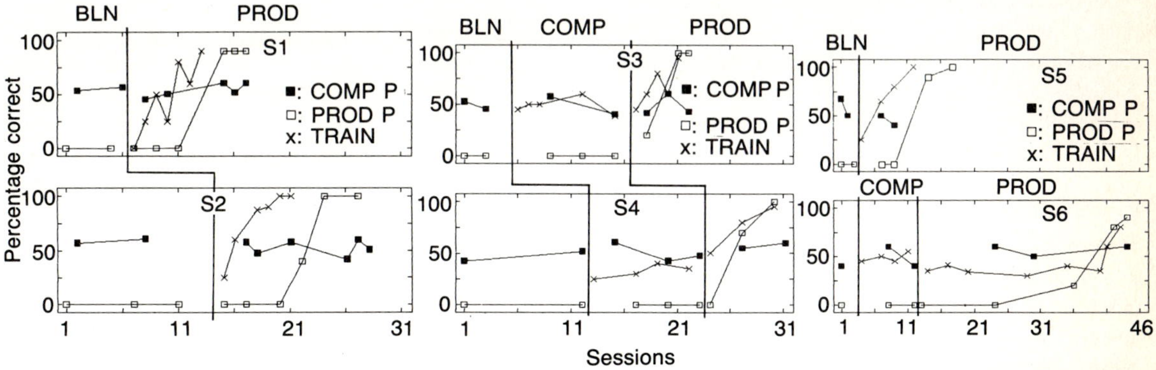

Figure 37–3 Subjects 1 and 2's comprehension probe (COMP P), production probe (PROD P), and training (TRAIN) responses during baseline (BLN), comprehension (COMP), and production (PROD) training; Subjects 3 and 4's comprehension probe (COMP P), production probe (PROB P), and training (TRAIN) responses during baseline (BLN), comprehension (COMP), and production (PROD) training; Subjects 5 and 6's comprehension probe (COMP P), production probe (PROB P), and training (TRAIN) responses during baseline (BLN), comprehension (COMP), and production (PROD) training.

flexibility of single-subject designs was utilized. Although some evidence in previous research indicated that there may be a difference between comprehension and production teaching, none indicated that comprehension teaching would be totally ineffective. The complete lack of effectiveness meant that a different approach had to be taken in order to evaluate the two procedures. What was planned as an across-subjects comparison was changed to a within- and across-subjects comparison in order to prove that the failure to learn through comprehension training was the result of an ineffective approach rather than a poor learner or a learning goal that was beyond the learner's capability. As can be seen in the second panel, learning only occurred when subjects 3 and 4 received production teaching and not when they received comprehension teaching.

The third design merely added replication to the two previous ones. As can be seen in the third panel, production teaching was the only effective procedure although there was some variability in how effective production teaching was (compare subject 6 to the other five subjects).

Types of Flexibility

The flexibility exhibited in this study is a particularly attractive aspect of single-subject designs. There are two kinds of flexibility.

One kind allows for exploring individual variability and modifying treatments to suit individual characteristics and behaviors of clients. For example, if an experimenter decides to use three clients to evaluate a particular treatment and finds that only two of the clients respond appropriately to treatment, the experimenter is free to explore modifications of the treatment that may prove to be more successful with the third client. Speech-language pathologists are familiar with individual variability in clients' responses to treatment. Under controlled conditions, the modifications can be explored and documented. If the unresponsive client responds to the modified treatment, then the investigator has found a treatment for clients who have characteristics similar to the unresponsive client. For a review of this form of flexibility, see Connell and Thompson.[16]

Another kind of flexibility is possible if the experimenter is familiar with the designs available to answer specific questions.[18] Often one design to explore a complex clinical question is risky because of the effect of the treatment. For example, it is possible that a client trained to discriminate between two speech sounds in the confines of an ABAB design will not, or cannot, be brought to baseline level in the second A phase of the experiment. If the investigator foresees such an event, he or she can possibly combine the ABAB with a multiple-baseline, across-behaviors design, for example, by teaching a second discrimination involving two more speech sounds. Then if the second A condition turns out to be unsuccessful, the investigator can fall back on the multiple-baseline design and continue to obtain valid data on the effect of the discrimination training. Possible design combinations in the treatment of communicative disorders are discussed in the texts and articles previously referenced.

SUMMARY

Returning to the image of the hypothetical outsider, it would seem better to be able to tell him or her that the clinical science of speech-language pathology does not yet have conclusive data on all of our treatment practices, but many practicing members of the profession are committed to obtaining such data, than to admit only that the data are not available as of yet. By fostering a clinical tradition for a commitment to experimentation, the profession can raise itself to a higher level of acceptability and dignity, and, more importantly, the clients whom the profession serves will be better guaranteed of having the best treatment available. It is the responsibility of each member of the profession to improve the state of the clinical science of speech-language pathology.

REFERENCES

1. Costello J, ed. Speech disorders in children. San Diego: College-Hill Press, 1984.
2. Perkins W, ed. Current therapy of communication disorders: phonologic-articulatory disorders. New York: Thieme-Stratton, 1983.
3. Winitz H, ed. Treating articulation disorders: for clinicians by clinicians. Baltimore: University Park Press, 1984.
4. Lucas E. Semantic and pragmatic language disorders. Rockville, MD: Aspen Systems Corporation, 1980.
5. Wiig E, Semel E. Language disabilities in children and adolescents. Columbus: CE Merrill, 1976.
6. Courtright J, Courtright I. Imitative modeling as a theoretical base for instructing language disordered children. J Speech Hear Res 1976; 19:655–663.
7. Courtright J, Courtright I. Imitative modeling as a language intervention strategy: the effects of two mediating variables. J Speech Hear Res 1979; 22:389–402.
8. Perkins W. Functions and malfunctions of theories in therapies. Asha 1986; 28:31–33.
9. Johnston J. What is language intervention? The role of theory. In: Miller J, Yoder D, Schiefelbusch R, eds. Contemporary issues in language intervention. Rockville, MD: American Speech-Language-Hearing Association, 1983:52.
10. Kamhi A. Review of language handicaps in children. Asha 1985; 27:4.

11. Siegel G, Spradlin J. Therapy and research. J Speech Hear Res 1985; 50:226–230.
12. Barlow D, Hersen M. Single-case experimental designs. New York: Pergamon Press, 1984.
13. Kazdin A. Single-case research designs: methods for clinical application. New York: Oxford Press, 1982.
14. McReynolds L, Kearns K. Single-subject experimental designs in communicative disorders. Austin: Pro-Ed, 1983.
15. Parsonson B, Baer D. The analysis and presentation of graphic data. In: Kratochwill T, ed. Single-subject research: strategies for evaluating change. New York: Academic Press, 1978:101.
16. Connell P, Thompson C. Flexibility of single-subject experimental designs. Part III: using flexibility to design or modify experiments. J Speech Hear Disord 1986; 51:214–255.
17. Johnston J, Pennypacker H. Strategies and tactics of human behavioral research. Hillsdale, NJ: Erlbaum, 1980.
18. Kearns K. Flexibility of single-subject experimental designs. Part II: design selection and arrangement of experimental phases. J Speech Hear Disord 1986; 51:204–214.
19. Kratochwill T, ed. Single-subject research: strategies for evaluating change. New York: Academic Press, 1978.
20. McReynolds L, Thompson C. Flexibility of single-subject experimental designs. Part I: basics of single-subject designs. J Speech Hear Disord 1986; 51:194–204.
21. Elbert M, McReynolds L. An experimental analysis of misarticulating children's generalization. J Speech Hear Res 1978; 21:136–150.
22. Horner RD, Baer DM. Multiple-probe technique: a variation on the multiple baseline. J Appl Behav Anal 1978; 11:189–196.
23. Barlow DH, Hayes SC, Nelson RO. The scientist practitioner: research and accountability in clinical and educational settings. New York: Pergamon Press, 1984.
24. Connell P. Acquisition of semantic role by language-disordered children: differences between production and comprehension. J Speech Hear Res 1986; 29:366–374.

Section 3
HEARING DISORDERS

Jerry L. Northern, Ph.D.

38 Audiologic Manifestations

Janet M. Zarnoch, M.A.
Jerry L. Northern, Ph.D.

The purpose of this chapter is to provide useful information on the nature, etiologies, and manifestations of hearing disorders. Descriptions of typical audiometric configurations and impedence findings associated with various types of ear disease are provided. In addition, electronystagmography (ENG) test results are discussed when applicable.

THE NATURE OF HEARING LOSS

Hearing loss can be generally categorized as conductive or sensorineural; a mixed disorder combines both types of hearing loss. When auditory dysfunction exists, but peripheral hearing mechanisms are within normal limits, the hearing impairment is categorized as a central auditory disorder.

Conductive impairment occurs when there is a problem in the external ear canal, tympanic membrane, or middle ear cavity that interferes with the transmission of sound along the normal physiologic air-conduction pathway. Causes of conductive hearing loss include cerumen or foreign objects in the external auditory canal, otitis media, otosclerosis, and congenital abnormalities. Medical intervention can usually ameliorate such a hearing loss. Conductive hearing loss may occasionally resolve spontaneously, although some residual of the pathologic condition frequently remains for long periods of time and may cumulate with the next episode. Conductive impairment is characterized by a hearing loss for air-conducted sounds, whereas sounds conveyed to the inner ear directly by bone conduction are relatively unaffected.

Early identification of conductive hearing impairment often allows resolution of the disease process in its elementary states. The degree of hearing loss is considered significant when it interferes with general communicative processes. Adults with mild hearing loss can perceive conversation fairly normally until the hearing loss exceeds 25 dB hearing level. In children, however, even a mild hearing loss can be detrimental. Preliminary evidence indicates that some children with histories of chronic otitis media tend to be significantly delayed in speech and language skills, academic achivement, and general cognitive development.[1] Although specific cause-effect relationships are still under investigation, apparently early audiologic and otologic identification and management are needed, even in cases of relatively mild hearing impairment.

Sensorineural hearing loss occurs when the sensory cells of the organ of Corti within the cochlea or the fibers of the auditory nerve are damaged. Common causes include aging, viral and bacterial infections, ototoxicity, exposure to excessive noise, congenital abnormality, and head trauma. The sensorineural audiogram is characterized by equivalent air-conduction and bone-conduction thresholds. Sensorineural hearing loss may be missed in the routine medical physical examination since the external auditory canal and tympanic membrane appear normal. Such hearing loss is nearly always irreversible. Treatment consists of auditory rehabilitation through hearing aids, lip reading instruction, and auditory training. Hearing impaired children generally require special education to aid development of speech and language. Early identification of sensorineural hearing loss is extremely important. Undetected hearing loss in children not only leads to difficulty in the development of normal speech and language, but may also cause learning and behavioral problems.

An additional consideration is whether the hearing loss is unilateral or bilateral. The child with total deafness in one ear and normal hearing in the other may function well in many situations. Traditionally, unilateral hearing loss was thought to impose little or no detriment to speech and language development. However, it now appears that some children with unilateral deafness tend to be delayed in their language development and academic skills.[2] Thus children with unilateral hearing loss should receive regular audiologic monitoring so that parents and school personnel may be advised of the need for preferential seating or, in some cases, fitting of an appropriate hearing aid. Obviously, careful attention must be given to the hearing in the remaining good ear.

In addition to indicating the nature of a hearing loss, the degree of hearing loss must also be specified. This designation is usually made on the basis of each ear's pure tone average (in dB) for air-conduction thresholds at 500 Hz, 1,000 Hz, and 2,000 Hz. Common descriptive terms used to categorize hearing levels include "normal" (0.0 to 15 dB), "borderline normal" (16 to 25 dB), mild loss (26 to 45 dB), moderate loss (45 to 65 dB), severe loss (66 to 85 dB), and profound loss (86 dB and over). Borderline categories of hearing impairment are often described with a combination of terms such as "mild-to-moderate."

Clearly, the vast number of causes of hearing disorders cannot be covered in one chapter; only the more commonly encountered disorders will be discussed. In cases in which a particular type of disease or syndrome is alluded to or only mentioned briefly, reference will be made to a detailed source of information on the topic. For those readers who are not familiar with the parameters of impedance audiometry and/or ENG, the descriptive paragraphs presented next should be helpful.

ELECTRONYSTAGMOGRAPHY

ENG is a clinical test of vestibular function, but it evaluates the status only of the semicircular canals and not the utricle and saccule. In actuality, only indirect vestibular information is gained from ENG because the measurements obtained result from the effect of the semicircular canals on the ocular muscles.[3] Therefore, the use of ENG presupposes an intact oculomotor system.

ENG is an electrical recording of eye movements based on the corneoretinal potential. The eye functions as an electrical dipole, with the cornea maintaining a positive charge and the retina a negative charge. If electrodes are placed around the eyes, the voltage change in the corneoretinal potential caused by eye deflection can be amplified and recorded (Fig.38–1). It should be noted that electrodes record eye movements only in the plane of

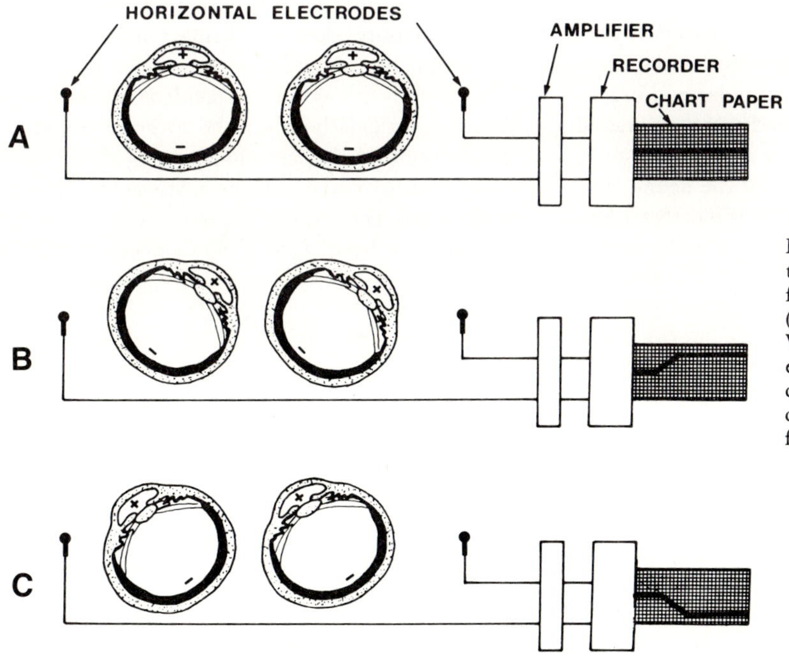

Figure 38–1 A schematic diagram of the corneoretinal potential. The eye functions as an electrical dipole (cornea—positive; retina—negative). When electrodes are placed at the outer canthus of each eye, the voltage change in the corneoretinal potential caused by eye deflection can be amplified and recorded.

the electrode pair. Hence, if electrodes are placed at the outer canthus of each eye, only horizontal eye movements are recorded. Similarly, for electrodes placed above and below the eye, only vertical eye movements are recorded.

The specific type of eye movement recorded through ENG is nystagmus. Nystagmus is a rhythmic back-and-forth movement of the eyeball. Nystagmus that arises from the vestibular system always has a slow and a fast phase. The slow phase is a slow conjugate deviation of the eyes to the right or left and is initiated directly by the vestibular system. The fast phase, initiated by a central mechanism, is the quick return of the eyes to the midline.

Nystagmus is typically referred to as right beating or left beating, and it is named for the direction of the fast phase. Thus, if the eyes drift slowly to the left (slow phase), the quick return (fast phase) is to the right and the result is a right beating nystagmus. Because the fast phase of nystagmus is much easier to observe, the nystagmus is named for it, despite the fact that the slow phase is the vestibular portion of the nystagmus. Figure 38–2 illustrates the difference between right beating and left beating nystagmus as recorded on chart paper with ENG.

The ENG evaluation is carried out in a darkened room and takes approximately 1 hour to complete. The ENG test battery consists of a series of ocular, positional, and bithermal caloric tests, the results of which are viewed as a whole. Certain abnormal findings are suggestive of peripheral vestibular dysfunction, whereas other abnormalities suggest the central nervous system (CNS) as the site of the lesion. When speaking in terms of peripheral versus CNS site of lesion, the following differentiation is made: peripheral refers to the vestibular end-organs and/or the vestibular portion of the eighth cranial nerve up to the point where it enters the brain stem, and central (or CNS) refers to any of the neural connections beyond that point. Keep in mind that ENG results do not diagnose anything, but only supply additional information to that obtained from the history, physical examination, audiograms, roentgenograms, and other laboratory studies.

Normal patients should be able to perform the ocular tests (i.e., calibration, gaze, pendulum tracking, and optokinetic) without difficulty. The optokinetic portion of the ocular test series is the only place where nystagmus is the normal response. Calibration, gaze, and pendulum tests should not show evidence of nystagmus in the normal patient. However, drugs and alcohol must be ruled out if a nystagmus does present itself in an otherwise normal patient.

Positional testing follows the ocular tests. The patient is placed with eyes closed in a series of positions for at least 30 seconds per position. To overcome any central suppression of positional responses, the patient is given mental alerting tasks, such as counting backward from 100 by ones, throughout the sequence of positions tested. Nystagmus that is identified during positional testing is classified as positional in nature. Although experts in the field disagree somewhat, most agree that normal patients should not display a positional nystagmus.

Spontaneous nystagmus is sometimes confused with positional nystagmus. The difference between the two is that positional nystagmus is brought about by changes in head and/or body position. Positional nystagmus can be present in only one or two positions, vary in intensity, change direction from one position to the next, and disappear completely with repeated positioning. But spontaneous nystagmus is present constantly regardless of position. It does not vary in intensity, does not change direction, and does not fatigue nor disappear with repeated positioning. Spontaneous nystagmus is evident during ocular testing, particularly when the eyes are deviated in the direction of the fast phase.

The final portion of the ENG is the bithermal caloric test. The patient is placed in a supine position with the head elevated 30 degrees, thus placing

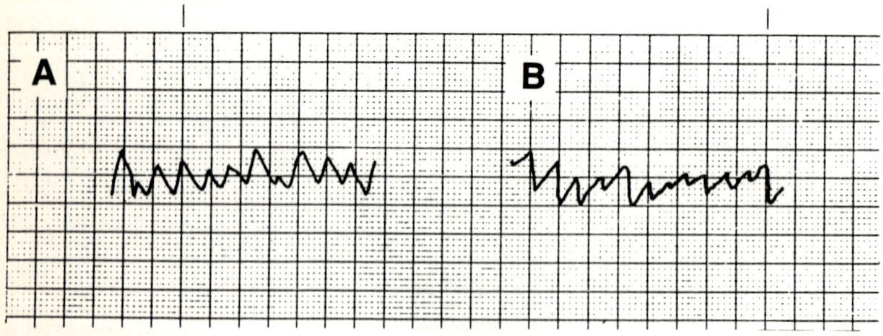

Figure 38–2 Examples of *A*, right beating nystagmus and *B*, left beating nystagmus. When the fast phase is an upward pen deflection, as in *A*, the nystagmus is said to beat to the right. And when the fast phase is a downward pen deflection, the nystagmus is said to beat to the left.

the horizontal semicircular canal in a vertical position for maximal thermal stimulation. Each ear is irrigated with warm (44°C) and cold (30°C) water for 30 to 40 seconds, with a 5 minute rest period between each of the four irrigations. During each irrigation, the patient must close his or her eyes and perform a mental alerting task for the same reason as stated during positional testing. The patient's ability to suppress his or her caloric nystagmus response through visual fixation is evaluated during at least two of the four responses (one from each ear). This evaluation is accomplished by having a patient open his or her eyes during the peak caloric response and fixate on an object for approximately 10 seconds. He or she then closes his or her eyes for the remainder of the recording of the caloric response.

The warm (44°C) irrigations produce nystagmus that beats toward the irrigated ear, that is, right warm produces a right beating nystagmus, and left warm produces a left beating nystagmus. The reverse is true for the cold (30°C) irrigations, that is, right cold produces a left beating nystagmus, and left cold produces a right beating nystagmus. A convenient way to remember this concept is "COWS" (cold-opposite; warm-same).

For each of the four caloric responses, the slow phase velocity is measured in degrees per second for the three strongest nystagmic beats occurring over a 10-second period, and then averaged. The result is four separate values that are used to make two comparative measurements: (1) a comparison between the right and left ear responses to determine if a unilateral weakness (or canal paresis) exists and (2) a comparison between all right beating and all left beating responses to determine if a directional preponderance of right or left beats is present.

Normal caloric responses should be symmetrical between the ears. If there is a difference of 20 percent or greater between the right and left ear responses, a "unilateral weakness" is present. A unilateral weakness is consistent with a lesion in the vestibular end-organ or in the primary vestibular nerve fibers. A significant unilateral weakness is the most concrete finding that an ENG can yield. It not only identifies the site of the lesion as peripheral in origin, but also lateralizes the dysfunction to the right or left ear.

When all four caloric responses are severely depressed or absent, a "bilateral weakness" is present. A bilateral weakness can occur in CNS disease and also in certain peripheral vestibular lesions, such as ototoxicity, bilateral Meniere's disease, bilateral acoustic tumors, and bilateral temporal bone fracture.

A "directional preponderance" occurs when there is a difference of 30 percent or more between the two right beating caloric responses and the two left beating ones. A directional preponderance is a nonlocalizing finding and has little clinical significance.

The ENG test battery is used widely in the clinical evaluation of persons complaining of dizziness, dysequilibrium, vertigo, and other forms of imbalance. The advantages to employing the ENG procedure are numerous: (1) by measuring the slow phase velocity of nystagmus, quantitative measurements of vestibular function are obtained; (2) it can provide objective documentation of a patient's subjective complaints; (3) it can be used to monitor vestibular function in high-risk patients, such as those receiving gentamicin or streptomycin; (4) it evaluates the vestibular function of each ear independently, through bithermal caloric irrigations; and (5) it permits recording of the nystagmus with the patient's eyes closed, which may have been missed due to visual fixation if the patient's eyes were open.[4]

However, ENG is not without its limitations. It is a lengthy, expensive test that causes discomfort to some patients. It is affected by most CNS-active drugs, for example, tranquilizers, antihistamines, soporifics, analgesics, alcohol and cannot be utilized with confidence on very young children. Although ENG is rapidly becoming an integral part of the neurotologic evaluation, the various procedures included in the routine ENG evaluation still lack adequate standardization.

IMPEDANCE AUDIOMETRY

An electroacoustic impedance meter with a headset attachment is used to administer impedance audiometry. The impedance test battery consists of three separate evaluative procedures: tympanometry, static compliance, and acoustic reflex thresholds.

Tympanometry is an objective measure of the mobility (or compliance) of the tympanic membrane as air pressure is varied in the external canal. The air pressure range is from +200 mm H_2O to −400 mm H_2O. The results of tympanometry are recorded on a graph called a "tympanogram." Air pressure changes are recorded on the horizontal axis, and changes in compliance on the vertical axis. Tympanograms are generally classified according to an "A-B-C" system described by Jerger (Fig. 38–3).[5]

Static compliance determines the compliance of the middle ear system while at rest. The normal range for static compliance is between 0.30 ml and 1.60 ml. The physical volume test (PVT) is a unique part of the static compliance test procedure. The PVT is a volume measurement taken when +200 mm H_2O is introduced into the external ear canal. This measurement value usually does not exceed 1.4 ml in an ear with an intact drum because the impedance

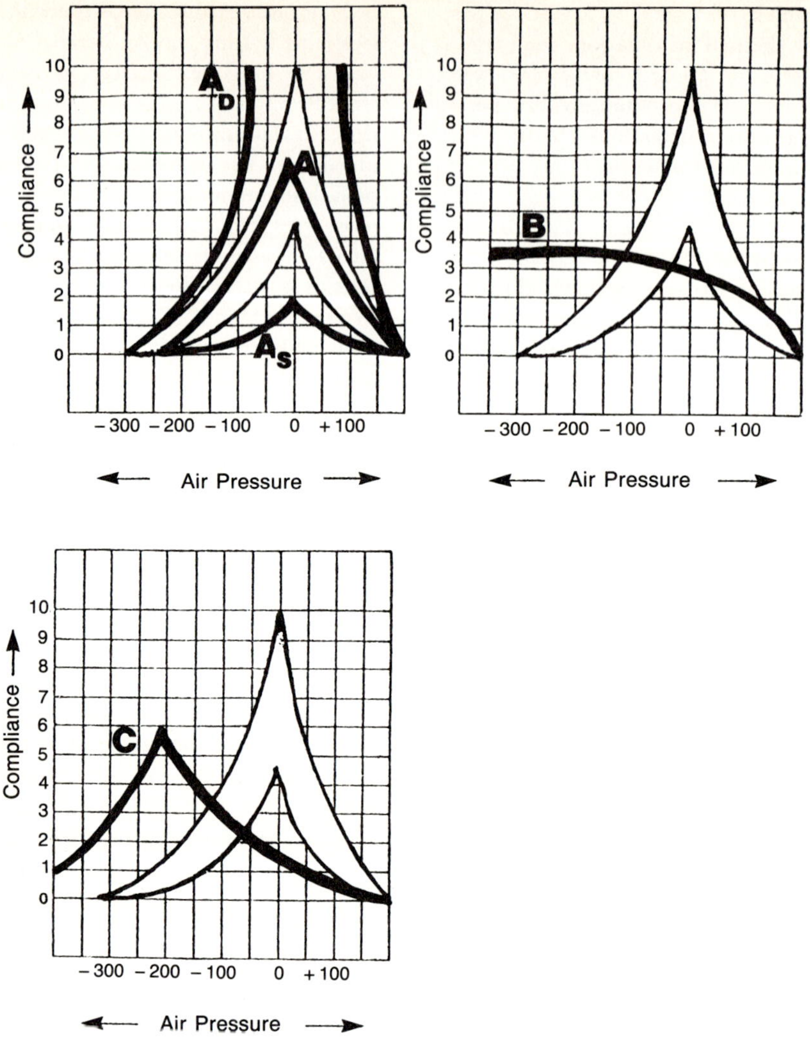

Figure 38–3 The tympanogram classification according to Jerger. Modified from Jerger J. Clinical experience with impedance audiometry. Arch Otolaryngol 1970; 92:311.

meter is measuring only the small cavity between the probe tip and the tympanic membrane. However, if a perforation or patent ventilation tube is present in the drum membrane, the impedance meter makes a volume measurement of a much larger cavity, that is, 4.0 to 5.0 ml, which includes the middle ear space.

The immittance meter, originally used to identify conductive hearing loss, is now being applied increasingly for the evaluation of inner ear, retrocochlear, and brain stem disorders. Interpretation of crossed and uncrossed (contralateral and ipsilateral) acoustic reflexes are especially valuable.

Cochlear Hearing Loss

An acoustic reflex in the presence of a moderate to severe sensorineural loss is an indirect measure of recruitment. The sensation level at which the acoustic reflex is obtained is inversely related to the degree of cochlear hearing loss. The acoustic reflex sensation level decreases from approximately 70 dB for patients with a 20-dB cochlear hearing loss to approximately 25 dB for patients with an 85-dB cochlear hearing loss.

Jerger and co-workers concluded that as long as the cochlear hearing loss is less than 60 dB, there is a 90 percent likelihood for the presence of the ipsilateral and crossed acoustic reflexes to be observed when the earphone is over the ear with the hearing loss.[6] As the sensorineural loss increases above 60 dB, chances of observing the acoustic reflex are reduced. At 85 dB, the chances are only 50 percent; if the hearing loss is 100 dB, 5 to 10 percent of patients have a reflex. Thus an acoustic reflex at a sensation level of 60 dB or less with a hearing loss of 85 dB or less provides a strong indication of a cochlear lesion. In patients with unilateral cochlear hearing loss of less than 85 dB, the clinician should be able to elicit the reflex bilaterally.

Conductive Hearing Loss

The crossed acoustic reflex can be obtained in patients with unilateral conductive hearing loss only when the loss is mild. When the loss exceeds 30 dB, however, the crossed acoustic reflex is obscured bilaterally. This fact is of sufficient clinical importance to warrant further explanation of the mechanisms involved. If the sound stimulus is presented to the ear with the conductive loss, the greater than 30-dB hearing loss prevents the signal from being perceived at a high enough sensation level to elicit the acoustic reflex in either ear. When the earphone is on the normal ear, the ipsilateral reflex is normal; however, because the contralateral probe is in the ear with the unilateral conductive loss, the mechanism causing the conductive loss prevents a change in compliance. Naturally, in a bilateral conductive loss, both the crossed and uncrossed reflexes are absent bilaterally. Jerger and co-workers reported that the presence of an air-bone gap of only 10 dB is sufficient to obscure the reflex to the probe ear nearly 80 percent of the time.[7] Conversely, if acoustic reflexes can be noted in the probe ear, with ipsilateral or contralateral stimulation, for a significant conductive hearing loss to exist in that ear is virtually impossible.

Retrocochlear Lesions

Careful interpretation of the acoustic reflexes can also supply diagnostic information about the presence of cerebellopontine angle tumors. The reflex in these patients is usually absent or decays with continued stimulation (acoustic reflex decay).

The acoustic reflex is absent 30 percent of the time in patients with tumors of the eighth cranial nerve who have normal pure-tone thresholds and in 70 percent when a 30-dB hearing loss is present. Therefore the absence of the acoustic reflex, with normal or near-normal hearing levels, suggests retrocochlear pathologic conditions (in the absence of middle ear abnormalities).

In recent years, the diagnostic value of comparing ipsilateral and contralateral acoustic reflexes has also been reported. Comparison of crossed and uncrossed reflexes appears to be most useful in differentiating intra-axial and extra-axial brain stem lesions.[8] Patients with disorders of the eighth nerve typically exhibit a reflex pattern characterized by absent, elevated, or decayed acoustic reflexes on the affected side (i.e., ipsilateral stimulation) and normal reflexes when stimulated from the unaffected side (i.e., contralateral stimulation). Patients with intra-axial lesions typically exhibit normal ipsilateral reflexes, but absent (or abnormal) contralateral reflexes.

CONDUCTIVE HEARING LOSS

There are numerous causes of conductive hearing impairment, most of which can be medically or surgically treated, thus resulting in partial or total alleviation of the conductive hearing loss.

EXTERNAL EAR

Cerumen Impaction

An overabundance of the waxy debris that partially or totally occludes the external ear canal is referred to as impacted cerumen or "ear wax." Cerumen impaction is the most common cause of conductive hearing loss involving the external ear. Located in the cartilaginous portion of the external auditory meatus are the glands responsible for secreting cerumen. When these glands produce an oversecretion, the ear may easily become occluded with cerumen.

Persons with impacted cerumen may complain of a "plugged" or "stuffy" feeling in their ears and/or a decrease in hearing sensitivity. Some persons also complain of tinnitus. Cerumen impaction results in a purely conductive hearing loss, that is, normal bone-conduction thresholds and depressed air-conduction thresholds. The degree of loss is variable and can range from a pure-tone average (PTA) of 25 dB in one patient to 45 dB in another. Speech discrimination scores generally remain unaffected. Hearing levels should return to normal when the cerumen is removed by a physician.

When an ear canal is totally occluded with cerumen, a type B ("flat") tympanogram with a very small physical volume is observed. A type B curve is obtained when the mass of cerumen completely occludes the ear canal and all of the sound pressure of the probe tone is reflected back to the pick-up microphone. The unusually small volume measurement is due to the fact that the cerumen is taking up space in the ear canal; thus the volume between the probe tip and tympanic membrane is decreased.

When an ear is not totally occluded with wax, but only a pinhole exists through the wax to the tympanic membrane, then the tympanogram could conceivably be a type A, indicating normal tympanic membrane mobility at normal atmospheric pressure. The presence or absence of acoustic reflex thresholds is, of course, dependent upon the degree of conductive hearing loss and upon whether or not the cerumen is completely blocking the eardrum. The impedance probe may easily become blocked with cerumen during the evaluation of such a problem.

If an ENG is performed on a normal patient with impacted cerumen, the caloric responses are, in most instances, reduced severely on the side of the impaction. Thus for every patient to have an otoscopic examination prior to administering an ENG is important; otherwise an erroneous unilateral weakness could occur. In the case of a patient with bilateral impaction, an erroneous bilateral weakness to calorics could result.

Otitis Externa

When there is an infection of the skin of the external ear, the conditon is called otitis externa. There are numerous causes of otitis externa that can be bacterial, fungal, or viral in nature. For a complete and detailed description of the causes of the condition, the interested reader is directed to English and Sargent's chapter (Chapter 46).

The most dramatic symptom of otitis externa is severe, sometimes excruciating, pain. The patient may also complain of drainage from the ear and a decrease in hearing. However, not all cases of otitis externa demonstrate concurrent hearing loss. A hearing loss due to otitis externa is purely conductive and is usually mild, with a PTA of 20 to 30 dB hearing threshold level. Typically, the patient is in such a state of discomfort that earphones must be hand-held during audiologic testing to prevent increased pressure on the pinna.

Impedance testing is not advisable if the patient is having considerable pain. However, in those cases where tympanometry and acoustic reflex testing can be accomplished, the results may vary from a type A tympanogram with normal acoustic reflex thresholds to a type B tympanogram with absent reflexes.

ENG is rarely, if ever, performed on patients with active external otitis media. If ENG is indicated, it is usually scheduled when the patient's infection has resolved.

Congenital Anomalies of the External Ear

Congenital anomalies affecting the external ear may be classified as minor or major. Minor anomalies include preauricular appendages, macrotia (abnormal enlargement of the pinna), and lop ears. These anomalies are not always associated with hearing loss. Major anomalies include microtia and atresia.

Microtia

The ear with congenital microtia can vary from a small, mildly deformed pinna to a totally absent pinna with no external auditory meatus to a complete atresia of the canal. Unilateral microtia occurs approximately six times more frequently than bilateral microtia, is more common in males than females, and affects the right ear more often than the left. Congenital microtia is usually associated with atresia of the external auditory canal and may involve one of several etiologic factors. The defect could be of first and second branchial arch origin, chromosomal defects, heredity, maternal thalidomide, or maternal rubella.[9]

When microtia is present in conjunction with complete atresia of the external auditory meatus, a maximum conductive hearing loss of 60 dB is present. On occasion, one also sees the conductive loss present in the opposite, supposedly normal ear as well. Audiologists should aways observe the condition of the external ear and canal of every patient he or she tests.

In the case of a microtic ear with a normal external ear canal, impedance can be easily performed. Tympanometric results are consistent with the condition of the tympanic membrane and middle ear.

Atresia

Although atresia usually occurs in conjunction with microtia, there are instances in which atresia occurs as an isolated anomaly. In such cases, the deep portion of the external auditory meatus is canalized, but the outer portion is filled with bone or fibrous tissue, or it may be occluded by a plate or a bone referred to as an atresia plate.

When atresia occurs with microtia, one can expect middle ear defects to be present. Examples of such defects include a sclerotic mastoid, fused ossicular chain, or fixation of the stapes in the oval window. There are also cases in which atresia and microtia with middle ear abnormalities also demonstrate impaired inner ear function. As with microtia, the causes of atresia range from unknown causes to heredity to chromosomal defects or maternal rubella.

A maximum conductive hearing loss of 60 dB is present in the completely atretic ear that has no inner ear involvement. In those cases of atresia with inner ear dysfunction as well, a mixed hearing loss is present, the degree being dependent upon the amount of inner ear involvement. Impedance audiometry cannot be carried out on an atretic ear because of the absence of an external auditory meatus.

Middle Ear

Otitis Media or Middle Ear Effusion

Oititis media is an inflammation of the middle ear that occurs most frequently during childhood and typically occurs bilaterally. Recently the term "middle ear effusion" has been defined to refer to otitis media. The two terms are used interchangeably. The nature of otitis media is often one of recurrent, transient episodes. Most children experience at least one episode of otitis during their first few years of life; however, some children have many recurrent bouts of the disease before their second birthday. These children have been termed "otitis-prone" owing to the fact that they have been plagued with six or more recurrent episodes of otitis media, the first of which occurred during the first year of life.[10]

The early detection of otitis media cannot be overemphasized. A considerable amount of literature deals with speech, language, educational, and medical complications, not to mention fluctuant hearing loss, resulting from undetected and/or untreated effusion[1,11] The detection, treatment, and management of this middle ear disease process continues to be a controversial subject. With the advent of impedance audiometry, many audiologists, otologists, and other associated health professionals have recognized the potential of utilizing this technique for screening large numbers of asymptomatic children for middle ear disease. However, the controversy remains, in part because the literature lacks an adequate body of sound research to support mass impedance screening and also in part because physicians vary considerably in their approach to the treatment and management of the disease.

Serous Otitis Media. Serous otitis media refers to an accumulation of fluid in the middle ear space. The most common cause of serous otitis media is eustachian tube dysfunction, which prohibits the middle ear space from being adequately ventilated. Serous otitis media is common in preschool and school-age children. Infants with serous otitis can remain asymptomatic for months, thus precluding early detection and treatment of the disease process. Refer to Chapter 46 for a detailed discussion of the medical aspects of all forms of otitis media.

The audiogram obtained from a patient with serous otitis media shows a purely conductive hearing loss, which could range from a PTA of 15 dB to a PTA of 30 to 40 dB, depending upon the thickness of the fluid, the amount of negative pressure, and the degree of eardrum retraction. Speech discrimination scores are good to excellent (84 to 100 percent), generally remaining unaffected by the conductive element. There is little correlation between the specific degree of hearing loss and the presence of middle ear fluid.

Tympanograms are either type B or type C, depending upon the stage of the disease process. In the initial stages of serous otitis, before fluid accumulates, a type C tympanogram is observed, indicating a significant amount of negative middle ear pressure. Recently, Orchik et al reported that the more negative the pressure observed with a type C curve, the higher the probability of finding a significant amount of fluid in the middle ear.[12]

A type B tympanogram may be obtained from an ear that is in the fluid accumulation stage of the disease. When the middle ear is completely filled with serous fluid, a type B almost always results. It is interesting to follow cases of serous otitis media with serial tympanograms over a 2- to 3-week period. One observes a type C tympanogram as negative pressure fills the middle ear cavity. Then the type C becomes a type B as the fluid accumulation begins. As the disease is resolving either spontaneously or with medical treatment, one sees a return of the type C curve, indicating a reversal of the disease, with a final observation of a normal type A tympanogram when eustachian tube function has returned to normal (Fig. 38–4).[9] Acoustic reflex thresholds are generally absent; however, this finding also varies depending upon the degree of hearing loss and the degree of disease present in the probe tip ear.

Acute Otitis Media. Acute otitis media is characterized by a middle ear filled with suppurative or purulent fluid. The patient with acute otitis media presents typically with moderate to severe ear pain. Infants who have acute otitis media often cry and pull and tug at their ears. If an infant, child, or adult is in considerable pain from the infection, whether they will tolerate earphones or an impedance probe tip is questionable.

As with serous otitis media, the hearing impairment in acute otitis media is also purely conductive in nature. The decrease in hearing could conceivably range from 15 dB to 30 to 40 dB. The configuration of the hearing loss can vary considerably. If, on the one hand, the hearing test is performed at a stage of the disease at which only negative pressure exists, then a "stiffness tilt" could be displayed on the audiogram; that is, the thresholds

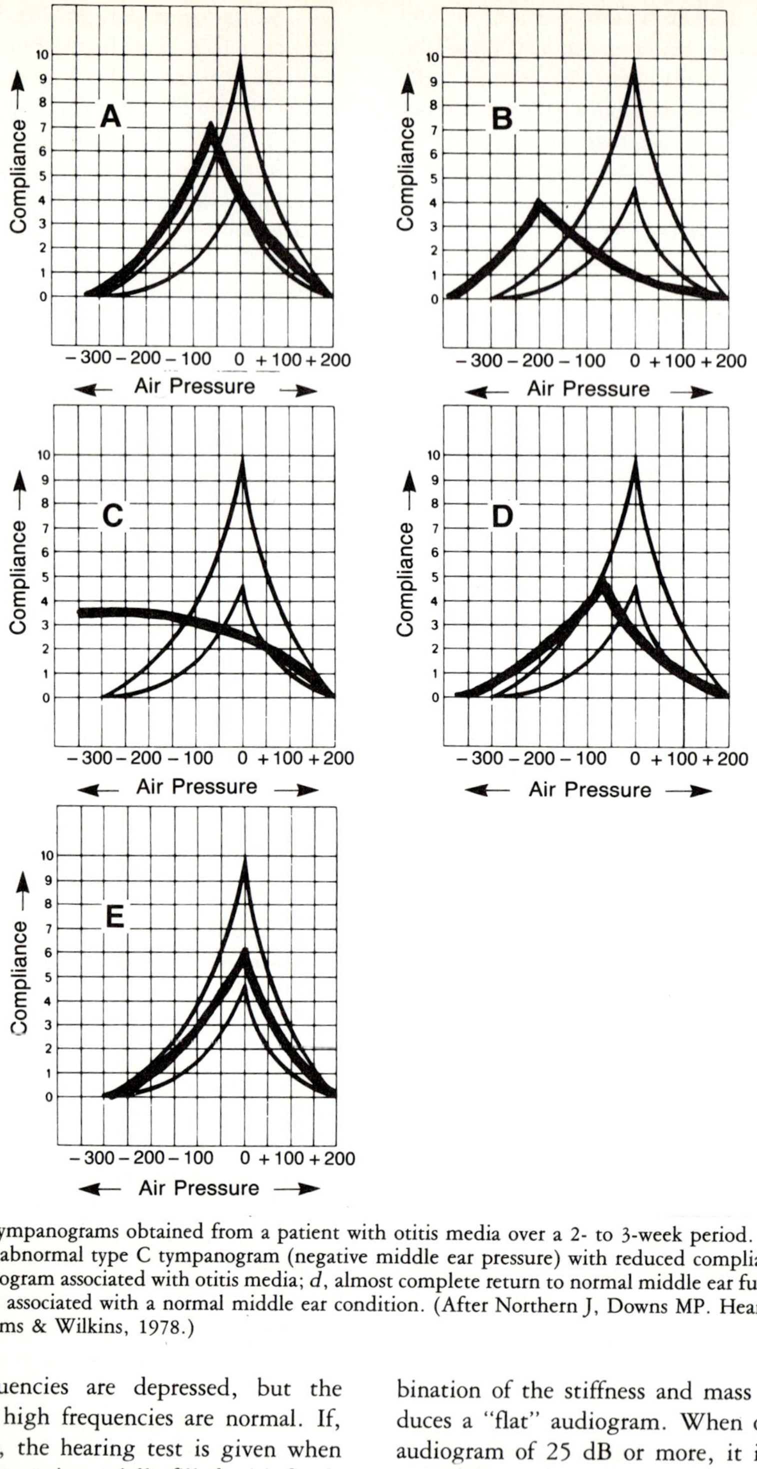

Figure 38-4 Serial tympanograms obtained from a patient with otitis media over a 2- to 3-week period. *a*, A Normal type A tympanogram; *b*, an abnormal type C tympanogram (negative middle ear pressure) with reduced compliance; *c*, an abnormal type B "flat" tympanogram associated with otitis media; *d*, almost complete return to normal middle ear function; *e*, completely normal tympanogram associated with a normal middle ear condition. (After Northern J, Downs MP. Hearing in children. 2nd ed. Baltimore: Williams & Wilkins, 1978.)

for the low frequencies are depressed, but the thresholds for the high frequencies are normal. If, on the other hand, the hearing test is given when the patient's middle ear is partially filled with fluid, then an audiogram with a "mass tilt" occurs because of the increased mass in the system caused by the fluid. A mass tilt is the opposite of the stiffness tilt; that is, thresholds are normal in the low frequencies and depressed on the high. Refer to Bess's chapter (Chapter 39) for a discussion of the effects of the mass and stiffness on the audiogram. The third type of configuration one might expect to see is a combination of the stiffness and mass tilts, which produces a "flat" audiogram. When one obtains a flat audiogram of 25 dB or more, it is evidence of increased mass and stiffness within the middle ear system. In the case of acute otitis media as well as serous otitis media, a flat audiogram is common, owing to the combination effects of negative pressure producing stiffness and fluid producing mass within the middle ear. Speech discrimination scores generally remain unaffected.

Tympanograms are either type B or type C, depending upon the accumulation of negative pressure and fluid in the middle ear cavity. Acoustic reflexes are either elevated or absent, depending upon the degree of conductive hearing loss, whether it is unilateral or bilateral, and the extent of the otitis media. As mentioned earlier, impedance audiometry may be unsuccessful if the patient's ears are hurting to any significant extent.

ENG conducted on a patient with either serous or acute otitis media may show adversely affected caloric responses. We have evaluated patients with serous and acute otitis media who have had depressed caloric responses, but normal responses on repeat testing when the disease had resolved.

Chronic Otitis Media. Chronic otitis media is characterized by a permanent perforation of the tympanic membrane. The types of perforations symptomatology, and treatment of chronic otitis media are discussed at length in Chapter 46.

In the early stages of chronic otitis media, a conductive loss is present. As with other forms of otitis media, the degree of impairment may range from mild to moderate. Speech discrimination scores remain good to excellent. If the disease is amenable to medical treatment, hearing levels will return to normal. Goin reports that perforations that involve less than 20 percent of the pars tensa cause a hearing impairment of 15 dB or less; larger perforations of the pars tensa produce a greater impairment; and a total perforation can cause a 30-dB loss.[13] If the ossicular chain is involved with the perforation, the loss may be as great as 45 dB.

There are reports that indicate that sensorineural hearing loss may develop in patients with severe, long-term chronic otitis media. English et al studied 404 patients with various types of otitis media.[14] They found a decline in bone-conduction thresholds as the severity and duration of the disease increased. The bone thresholds did not improve with treatment. Based on the findings of their study, English et al concluded that sensorineural hearing loss can be a natural consequence of chronic otitis media.

In a simple case of chronic otitis media, that is, one in which only a perforation exists with minimal drainage, a type B tympanogram with an accompanying large physical volume on the impedance test is obtained.

In other, more advanced cases of chronic otitis media, different impedance findings may result. For example, if a cholesteatoma evolved that closed the perforation of the drum as well as invaded the middle ear space, then to obtain a type A or a type C tympanogram would be possible. Acoustic reflexes are usually absent in these cases of chronic otitis as well.

ENG can be performed on patients with chronic otitis media; however, modifications and cautions must be exercised. If a water caloric stimulus is used, the ear must be cleaned by a physician following the procedure. Usually a system involving an air caloric stimulus is used with patients who have perforations. In either case, however, the caloric test results must be viewed with caution. The reason is that the two ears are not equal to begin with and do not receive equal stimulation. Thus one cannot definitively state the symmetry or asymmetry of the two ears when one of the ears has a perforation of the tympanic membrane.

Cholesteatoma

A cholesteatoma is the accumulation of the exfoliated keratin in the middle ear or mastoid, arising from keratinizing squamous epithelium (i.e., skin in the wrong place) that has grown from the external auditory canal.[15] Cholesteatomas may be congenital or acquired and usually occur in the middle ear and mastoid air cell system. Cholesteatomas can also arise in other areas of the termporal bone, but these are rare.

Persons with cholesteatoma demonstrate a variety of audiologic findings. The degree of hearing loss depends, to some extent, upon the severity and location of the cholesteatoma. In an attic cholesteatoma, the hearing may be relatively normal because the cholesteatoma has not affected the ossicular chain or inner ear. In cases in which the disease erodes the ossicles, the audiogram may show a 30- to 40-dB conductive hearing loss. Furthermore, there are cases of mixed and sensorineural hearing loss associated with the effects of recurrent middle ear infections and cholesteatoma.

Ears with cholesteatoma may present different tympanogram types, depending upon the type and extent of ossicular involvement. The type A tympanogram may be observed in those cases in which the cholesteatoma has not exerted any damage to the ossicles. In such cases, acoustic reflexes are usually slightly elevated. However, if a conductive loss of sufficient magnitude exists, reflexes may be absent bilaterally. In cases in which the cholesteatoma fills up most or all of the middle ear space, creating additional mass, then a type B curve with absent acoustic reflexes is seen. A type AD tympanogram with absent reflexes may be seen in those cases in which the cholesteatoma has eroded one or more of the ossicular joints, causing an ossicular disarticulation.

Mastoiditis

Mastoiditis refers to inflammation of the mastoid air cells. Because the mastoid air cell system communicates directly with the middle ear space, infectious fluids in the middle ear can easily spread to the mastoid area, resulting in mastoiditis.

Although the frequency with which mastoiditis occurs has not diminished since the 1940s,[16] the prognosis has changed dramatically. Prior to the advent of antibiotics, mastoiditis was a much feared disease, especially in children. Fear existed because of the life-threatening nature of the disease in which the infection of the mastoid system could easily spread to the meninges of the brain and cause meningitis. The potential for meningitis still exists today; however, the disease process is treated and managed earlier and more effectively than it was years ago.

As with other serious forms of middle ear disease, a significant conductive hearing loss results from mastoiditis. Sensorineural hearing loss may eventually be present as a sequel to the disease. Speech discrimination scores should remain unaffected as long as the impairment remains conductive or mildly mixed in nature.

Various impedance findings are possible with mastoiditis, which are dependent on the mechanical changes in the middle ear due to the disease. If the middle ear is filled with pus or cholesteatoma, a type B tympanogram with absent acoustic reflexes results. If a perforation is present, a type B tympanogram, large PVT measurement, and absent reflexes are found. If the mastoiditis is present with a cholesteatoma that has eroded portions of the ossicular chain, then a type AD curve with absent reflexes is present. Of course, it is also possible for a type A tympanogram to result if the middle ear spaces and structures are unaffected.

Otosclerosis

Otosclerosis is a disease that attacks the bony capsule of the inner ear by turning it into soft spongy bone. It causes a progressive hearing loss because of the increased fixation of the stapes footplate in the oval window. The audiogram reveals a conductive hearing loss. In the early stages of the disease, the air-conduction thresholds show a stiffness tilt because of the incomplete fixation of the stapes footplate. However, as the disease progresses and the stapes becomes completely immobilized, the mass increases and the effects are seen in the audiogram, which becomes flat across frequencies. Carhart's notch, which is a depression in bone-conduction thresholds from 500 Hz through 4,000 Hz, with 2,000 Hz demonstrating the greatest shift, may also be seen in otosclerosis.[17]

During the early stages of otosclerosis, the air-bone gap may be less than 30 dB. As the disease progresses and the anterior portion of the footplate is firmly fixed, a conductive loss of approximately 40 dB is seen. When the entire pheriphery of the oval window is involved, the conductive impairment may be 40 dB or more.[15] The maximum degree of conductive loss cannot exceed 60 dB, owing to the fact that sound begins to be transmitted to the cochlea via bone conduction at 60 dB. Patients with otosclerosis usually reveal a shallow type A tympanogram with absent acoustic reflexes bilaterally.

Ossicular Discontinuity

Ossicular discontinuity refers to a disruption of the ossicular chain, which can be caused by a number of different factors. Many cases of ossicular discontinuity are the end result of recurrent or chronic middle ear infections. Head trauma can also cause a disruption of the ossicular chain in spite of whether or not a temporal bone fracture was sustained. Ossicular damage from head trauma can affect one or all the ossicles and in a variety of ways. Damage could include fracture of the manubrium, the long process of the incus, or the stapedial crura or dislocation of the incus. However, discontinuity is more likely to occur from severe head trauma such as a temporal bone fracture as opposed to minimal head traumas.

Trauma to the tympanic membrane can also cause ossicular discontinuity. For example, if a diver hits the water with sufficient force on the side of his head, or a fighter is punched on the side of the head or face, or an obtusive object such as a Q-tip is inadvertently forced into the ear canal, the eardrum could spontaneously rip and strike one of the ossicles, resulting in a discontinuity.

Depending on the etiology of the ossicular disruption, a patient may present with a variety of symptoms. Pain is often present in trauma cases, and facial paralysis may be present in fracture cases. Almost without exception a maximum conductive hearing loss of 60 dB is evident. In cases in which otitis media coexists with the discontinuity, the hearing loss may not be as great due to some sound transmission via the fluid.[18]

The classic type AD tympanogram is obtained from an ear with disarticulation and an intact tympanic membrane. Acoustic reflexes are usually absent; however, there are exceptions. Even in view of a large conductive loss, if a connection exists between the stapedius tendon and that portion of the ossicular chain still attached to the tympanic membrane, a contraction can occur. This is seen when the break is in the anterior crus of the stapes.[19]

Temporal Bone Fracture

There are two types of temporal bone fracture: longitudinal and transverse. Clinically, the otologic effects of the two fracture types are quite different. The longitudinal type will be discussed next since it causes a conductive hearing loss. Transverse fractures will be discussed under the section Sensorineural Hearing Loss.

Longitudinal Temporal Bone Fracture. Longitudinal fractures are less destructive than transverse fractures. Hearing loss following a longitudinal fracture may be conductive, sensorineural, or mixed. The degree of loss may range from mild to severe. Although most patients reveal a conductive impairment, a considerable number of patients show a sensorineural hearing loss. The configuration of the sensorineural losses can vary from a loss in the high frequencies to a loss involving most of the frequencies. It is interesting to note that bone-conduction thresholds usually show improvement during the first few weeks following trauma, owing to recovery of the cochlea from that portion of hearing loss due to temporary threshold shift.[15]

Tympanogram types vary depending upon the condition of the tympanic membrane, middle ear space, and ossicles. If a tympanogram is obtained from an ear with a recent longitudinal fracture where there is still a perforation in the eardrum, a type B curve with an accompanying large volume is obtained, regardless of whether the ossicles have been disrupted. However, if tympanometry is performed after spontaneous healing of the drum, then a type A tympanogram results if the middle ear space is clear and the ossicles are intact. A type AD curve may result if the drum is intact, but ossicular disarticulation is present.

Results of acoustic reflex testing are also variable. Reflexes are usually absent in those ears with significant conductive or mixed hearing losses and abnormal tympanograms.

Vestibular symptoms vary considerably depending upon the type of temporal bone fracture sustained. Approximately 50 percent of patients with a longitudinal fracture reveal a positional nystagmus of the benign paroxysmal type, with the nystagmus beating toward the involved ear when it is the undermost ear. However, this finding is usually not evident on an ENG tracing since the nystagmus is typically rotatory in nature and is better determined by visual observation with or without Frenzel's glasses. Vestibular testing with ENG is usually normal with no spontaneous or postional nystagmus and with normal responses to caloric stimulation.[20]

SENSORINEURAL HEARING LOSS

The audiometric configurations of sensorineural hearing losses vary, but are characterized by depressed air- and bone-conduction thresholds, which are equal or with ± 10 dB of each other for all frequencies. Unlike conductive impairments, most sensorineural losses are permanent and irreversible. The degree, configuration, and laterality of sensorineural impairments are important considerations in a person's ability to communicate effectively. A person with a moderate to severe bilateral loss has a much greater difficulty in communicative situations than a person who has a unilateral profound loss with normal hearing in the contralateral ear.

Head Injuries

Transverse Temporal Bone Fracture

Transverse temporal bone fractures occur much less frequently than the longitudinal type, but are considerably more destructive and are often bilateral. Transverse fractures most often result in a "dead" ear; that is, there are no measurable responses to auditory stimuli.[15,20] In ears with a transverse fracture and a hemotympanum present, a type B tympanogram may be seen due to the mass of fluid in the middle ear space. Those ears with resolved hemotympanum probably demonstrate normal type A tympanograms. A "dead" ear has absent reflexes when the earphone is placed over it, but normal reflexes when the earphone is on the good ear with the probe tip in the bad ear (assuming that the "good" ear is relatively normal). In those cases in which facial paralysis accompanies a "dead" ear, acoustic reflexes are absent bilaterally.

In transverse fractures, a mild spontaneous nystagmus beating toward the uninvolved side may persist indefinitely and can be documented through ENG. In addition to a spontaneous nystagmus, the ENG recording shows an absent vestibular response to caloric stimulation on the involved side.[20]

Presbycusis

Sensorineural hearing loss due to the aging process had been termed "presbycusis." Although presbycusis affects an enormous number of aging persons in our society, it is a poorly understood disease process. A thorough discussion of aging and hearing impairment has recently been published by Roush.[21]

The exact etiology of presbycusis remains unknown. However, current etiologic research is focused on specific pathophysiologic processes in the aging ear. Most of the current literature discusses Schuknecht's classification of the four basic pathologic processes that lead to presbycusis.[22] These are (1) sensory, (2) neural, (3) metabolic, and (4) mechanical processes, and they are discussed by English and Sargent (Chapter 46).

Hearing loss due to presbycusis is sensorineural in nature and can be of a variable degree and configuration, depending upon the type of presbycusis manifested. Most patients with presbycusis complain of an inability to understand speech. Many patients exhibiting presbycusis improve their communication function through the use of properly fitted amplification.

Tympanograms are usually type A unless there is a conductive component to the sensorineural impairment. Acoustic reflex thresholds may be obtained at normal, reduced, or elevated sensation levels or may be absent, depending upon the degree of hearing loss and whether or not recruitment or a conductive component is present.

Dysequilibrium is a frequent complaint among the aged population. Schuknecht also describes four types of dysequilibrium associated with old age, three of which are manifested and differentiated clinically.[15] The fourth type has been pathologically documented and is termed "cupulolithiasis." Each of the four types will be described briefly.

Cupulolithiasis. Cupulolithiasis is characterized by severe, sudden episodes of vertigo that are brought about by certain head positions. Aging is not the only cause of cupulolithiasis; however, when the onset is in old age, the symptoms can be expected to endure the remainder of the person's life without significant improvement. Pathologic studies have indicated that the disorder is caused by deposits on the cupula of the posterior semicircular canal. Thus the problem is located in the vestibular endorgan.

Ampullary Dysequilibrium. This disorder is manifested by vertiginous attacks precipitated by angular head movements. For example, when the head is moved quickly from right to left, the person experiences a rotation sensation for several seconds. Although there is no pathologic explanation for this disorder, it is possibly caused by degenerative changes in the ampullae of the semicircular canals. This theory is supported in part by the decreased vestibular response to rotation and caloric stimulation as a normal function of aging.

Macular Dysequilibrium. This dysfunction is manifested by vertigo that is produced by changes in head position relative to gravity. For example, arising from bed in the morning may produce an attack. Caloric responses for persons demonstrating this disorder are generally normal for age. It is postulated that the symptoms arise from degenerative changes in the utricle and saccule.

Vestibular Ataxia. This problem is characterized by a constant feeling of dysequilibrium while walking. Unsteadiness does not occur when sitting or standing. Again, in this group, caloric responses are depressed, but are normal for age. Clinically, the symptoms suggest a loss of vestibular control over the lower limbs. The sites of lesion proposed are central in origin, such as the vestibular nuclei or the vestibulospinal tracts, and are not thought to involve the peripheral vestibular system.

Ototoxicity

Ototoxicity refers to damage of the auditory and/or vestibular portion of the inner ear brought about by the administration of certain drugs. Certain ototoxic drugs are predisposed to affecting the auditory portion of the inner ear, while the vestibular portion remains normal, and the reverse is also true. Furthermore, there are ototoxic drugs that dramatically affect both the auditory and vestibular systems of the inner ear. Variables such as drug dosage, renal status, general health, and history of previous ear disease play an important role in an individual's predisposition to ototoxicity.

Persons sustaining inner ear damage from ototoxic agents complain of either a decrease in hearing sensitivity or vestibular difficulties, and some individuals may complain of both. Ototoxicity results in a sensorineural hearing loss that is bilateral and symmetrical in most cases. However, there are instances in which the hearing loss is asymmetrical, and others in which the deficit is unilateral. The high frequencies appear to be affected first, and this correlates well with temporal bone studies documenting damage to the basal and middle portions of the cochlea. If the damage becomes more severe and widespread, hearing across all frequencies is depressed. The degree of hearing loss can range from mild to profound. Tinnitus usually accompanies the ototoxic hearing loss, regardless of whether it precedes the loss or occurs simultaneously.[23] Type A tympanograms are obtained unless a conductive component to the sensorineural loss occurs. Acoustic reflex thresholds are variable, depending upon the degree of hearing loss.

In patients with damage to the vestibular endorgan as a result of ototoxicity, the damage can often be documented clinically through the use of ENG. The most concrete finding would be bilaterally depressed responses to bithermal caloric stimulation. Some patients may also reveal a spontaneous or positional nystagmus following vestibular insult. The individual with vestibular damage usually compensates for the loss within a matter of months, but compensation is dependent upon the age of the patient as well as the condition of the visual and proprioceptive senses.

Rehabilitative measures of the patient suffering from hearing impairment caused by ototoxicity vary depending upon the degree and extent of the handicap. Some patients require a hearing aid in conjunction with speech reading therapy and counseling, whereas others, who perhaps sustain only a unilateral loss, required only minimal counseling concerning what communication difficulties to expect and how to conserve the hearing in the good ear through hearing conservation tactics.

NOISE-INDUCED HEARING LOSS

Although the auditory system is an extremely sensitive and resilient one, it is easily subject to decreased sensitivity as a result of exposure to loud noise. The auditory mechanism is simply not equipped to handle prolonged exposure to loud noise. In addition, the auditory mechanism is susceptible to acoustic trauma if exposed to a loud explosion or sudden blast, where the noise is brief in duration but extremely intense. Persons experiencing acoustic trauma may demonstrate severe otologic and audiologic manifestations and may require surgical intervention.

Unlike acute acoustic trauma or noise exposure, hearing loss resulting from chronic exposure to noise in an insidious mishap. A person can work in a noisy environment for years and years and remain relatively asymptomatic, perhaps experiencing only occasional tinnitus or slight temporary shifts in auditory sensitivity.

The terms "temporary threshold shift" and "permanent threshold shift" have become the descriptors used to differentiate between temporary and permanent auditory deficits. Temporary threshold shift occurs when a person is subject to loud noise for a short period of time. Immediately following the exposure, auditory thresholds may be depressed, but return to normal levels within a period of time. Permanent threshold shift refers to a permanent reduction in auditory thresholds as a result of a long history of chronic noise exposure.

The identification of early noise-induced hearing loss is extremely important to prevent the adverse effects of permanent threshold shift. Early identification can best be achieved through regular audiologic testing. In such an early stage, the person may not be aware of any decrease in hearing and does not have any problem with speech discrimination ability. The most common audiologic indicator of a noise-related hearing deficit is a drop or "notch" at 4,000 Hz. With continued exposure to noise, however, the 4,000 Hz notch may deepen and/or widen, and decreases in speech discrimination may be seen.

As the length of exposure to noise increases to years, the audiometric thresholds not only deepen at 4,000 Hz, but also begin to drop significantly at 1,000 Hz to 3,000 Hz with concurrent drops in speech intelligibility. As the exposure to noise continues even longer, the loss of auditory sensitivity progresses and can reach a point where not only are all frequency thresholds depressed, but there may be no measurable hearing for the high frequencies, with poor speech discrimination scores. Thus the effects of noise, although minimal at first, can have devastating effects upon auditory sensitivity. Equally disturbing is the fact that the effects of noise and the effects of presbycusis are additive; that is, the amount of auditory deprivation is the sum of the two independent sources of damage, namely, noise and old age.

One of the most disturbing symptoms of noise-induced hearing loss is the presence of tinnitus.[24] Tinnitus is the subjective perception of noise in the ear, which can be localized usually to one or both ears and is typically described as ringing, whistling, buzzing, whirring, chirping, roaring, or hissing. Although the literature on tinnitus diagnosis and treatment exceeds 200 journal articles published since 1900, little is really known about this distressing symptom. A thorough recent monograph on the management of the tinnitus patient is recommended for additional information.[25]

The physiologic mechanism that produces tinnitus is still under discussion. Two major viewpoints, currently under consideration, have been expressed by Davis[26] and Kiang et al.[27] The Davis theory is that mild tinnitus corresponds to spontaneous discharge of auditory nerve fibers and is essentially "normal." More hyperexcitability drives the nerve fiber(s) to a faster rate of spontaneous discharge and more severe tinnitus. The discharges of the more sensitive auditory nerve fibers are accelerated by even minute mechanical disturbances.

The Kiang group, studying ototoxic hearing loss in animals, noted the most striking effect of kanamycin on the spontaneous activity of the nerve fiber to be the elimination of activity in the nerve units. Since ototoxic hearing loss is nearly always accompanied by persistent tinnitus, Kiang offers the supposition that the absence of neural activity results in the subjective perception of sound.

Recently, however, procedures to relieve tinnitus have been described that have resulted in substantial success. Application of these techniques in the patient with tinnitus associated with noise-induced hearing loss seems worthwhile. Through biofeedback, the patient is taught to relax, which results in increased circulation. Biofeedback electromyographic devices work through sensors placed on the frontal muscle, and the patient views the electrical output on the frontal muscle by observing a voltmeter and listening to clicks presented by earphones. Another technique for relief of tinnitus involves the fitting of a "tinnitus masker." The tinnitus masker is an electronic device worn like an ear level hearing aid with a "tube fitting," which produces low-intensity broad-band noise shaped to emphasize the high-frequency spectrum, effectively masking the patient's tinnitus. Saltzman and Ersner recommended the use of a hearing aid to tinnitus sufferers so that amplification could mask the patient's head noises.[28] Vernon and his associates at the Kresge Hearing Research Laboratory in Portland have evaluated tinnitus in over 500 patients, of whom approximately 50 percent indicate a history of noise exposure.[29]

An interesting aside related to the work of Vernon and his associates is their discovery that when masking of tinnitus is effective, it produces a suppression of the tinnitus that extends beyond the duration of the masker. They have termed this phenomenon "residual inhibition." Although much is still to be learned about these techniques for relief of the tinnitus sufferer, it would appear that fitting the patient with amplification, recommending biofeedback therapy, or seeking evaluation with a tinnitus masker has merit for patients with noise-induced tinnitus.

The symptom of vertigo is uncommon in persons with noise-induced hearing loss. Typically, vertigo may be associated with acoustic trauma, but rarely as a result of chronic noise exposure. The effect of noise exposure on the vestibular system is an area that has been somewhat neglected. Few, if any, studies have been performed to determine the type and extent, if any, of vestibular damage following noise exposure.

Management of noise-induced hearing loss is difficult, at best. From the habilitative point of view, one must be concerned with prevention of exposure to excessive noise and with recommendation of hearing protectors for those who must work in noisy environments. Persons must be educated about the harmful effects of noise as well as how to prevent hearing loss from noise. Rehabilitative measures include the fitting of proper amplification for degree of hearing loss; speechreading sessions; scales of communication function to assess areas of communication difficulties; biofeedback techniques; and fitting of tinnitus maskers. Of course, not all of these methods benefit every person equally well. Considerable counseling is required, as well as trial periods, in order to determine what rehabilitative method best suits an individual.

LABYRINTHITIS

The term "labyrinthitis" denotes an infection of the inner ear labyrinth. A review of the literature reveals several different classification systems for differentiation among the types of labyrinthitis. Schuknecht divides his classification into four categories based on the pathogenesis (i.e., origin and development of a disease) of labyrinthitis: acute toxic labyrinthitis, acute suppurative labyrinthitis, chronic labyrinthitis, and labyrinthine sclerosis.[15] English reports four types of labyrinthitis differentiated on a clinical basis: circumscribed labyrinthitis, diffuse serous labyrinthitis, acute suppurative labyrinthitis, and chronic suppurative labyrinthitis.[30] The four types usually do not exist independently, but rather tend to blend with one another. Readers are referred to Chapter 46 for a complete discussion of labyrinthitis.

Viral Labyrinthitis

The diagnosis of viral labyrinthitis is made primarily on clinical findings. Many different types of viruses have been indicated as a cause of labyrinthitis. Among these are measles, mumps, common cold, chicken pox, and upper respiratory infection. The primary symptom of viral labyrinthitis is sensorineural hearing loss, either unilateral or bilateral. Since measles and mumps are probably the most common viral etiology of this type of hearing loss, both will be discussed next.

MENIERE'S DISEASE

A patient with Meniere's disease most often complains of whirling vertigo upon initial visit to an otologist's office. Of course, this vertigo varies depending upon the degree of hearing loss present, and for patients with Meniere's disease to notice a decrease in hearing before vestibular symptoms appear is not uncommon. Nevertheless, almost all patients with Meniere's disease report the classic symptoms of fluctuant hearing loss, episodic vertigo, and tinnitus.

The most common type of audiologic configuration is a flat or rising audiometric curve with predominant low-frequency involvement. Usually, as the disease progresses, the high frequencies are also affected.

Speech discrimination scores may be in agreement with the degree of hearing loss, but phonemic regression may also be seen in some patients. Phonemic regression refers to an abnormally low speech discrimination score, poorer than would be expected by the degree of hearing loss.

Impedance audiometry reveals normal type A tympanograms unless there is an accompanying middle ear problem. Acoustic reflexes are elicited at normal sensation levels when stimulating the good ear, assuming that the hearing is within normal limits in that ear. However, when the stimulation is applied to the involved ear, reflexes are frequently obtained at extremely reduced sensation levels, indicative of cochlear recruitment.

Vestibular testing with ENG is a useful adjunct in the differential diagnosis of Meniere's disease. ENG is most helpful in monitoring the progression of the disease. A positional nystagmus is usually present, particularly if the test is administered during or shortly following an attack of vertigo. As the disease progresses, the positional nystagmus may be evident at any time during an ENG test. Bithermal calorics typically show a reduced vestibular response (i.e., unilateral weakness or canal paresis) on the involved side. This reduction in vestibular function may be insignificant in the early stages of the disease, but will most likely emerge as the duration of the disease increases.

Measles and Sensorineural Hearing Impairment

The onset of hearing loss from measles is difficult to pinpoint, and it is usually not associated with any middle ear or CNS disease. What is known from histopathologic studies of temporal bones is that the virus does enter the labyrinth, causing degeneration of the organ of Corti and its related structures.

The degree of hearing loss from measles can vary. The classic audiometric configuration is a bilateral symmetrical high-frequency sensorineural hearing loss ranging from 40 to 60 dB. Measles virus is thought to be the causative agent in a large number of deaf children.[30]

Impedance audiometry should be consistent with the degree of hearing loss; that is, tympanograms should be normal unless concomitant middle ear disease occurs and acoustic reflexes are normal, elevated, or absent, depending upon the degree of loss as well as whether recruitment is present or not.

ENG usually demonstrates reduced or absent responses to calorics bilaterally. This reduction is an indication that the measles virus also entered the vestibular labyrinth and caused destruction of the vestibular end-organs.

Mumps and Sensorineural Hearing Impairment

Unlike measles-induced hearing loss, mumps-related hearing loss is usually sudden and unilateral. Similar to measles, the mumps virus also enters the labyrinth and causes severe degenerative changes of the organ of Corti and its surrounding structures. Vertigo with associated nausea and vomiting typically accompanies the sudden hearing loss. Often, the mumps virus is not linked with these symptoms until years later. Although it has been thought that the vestibular apparatus remains relatively unaffected, recent literature suggests that this may not be so. Males are more often affected by mumps than females.

A typical audiogram obtained from a child thought to have acquired the loss as a result of a mumps virus would show completely normal hearing in one ear and severely impaired hearing in the opposite ear. Children with this type of audiogram may have difficulty in school and should be provided with preferential seating so that their normal hearing ear is facing the teacher and/or class.

A recent study of vestibular symptoms in mumps deafness investigated vestibular function with ENG in 20 patients with unilateral deafness due to mumps.[31] Nine of the 20 subjects had vertigo at the time they became ill with the mumps. Five of those nine had normal caloric responses with ENG; three had reduced responses; and one had no response to calorics in the audiologically impaired ear. No definitive correlation between vertigo and permanent caloric impairment was found. However, an interesting finding in the study was that five of 11 subjects without a history of vertigo revealed reduced or absent responses to caloric stimulation. Overall, in the 20 subjects, 45 percent had impaired caloric responses. It is important to note that some of these subjects might have become "tumor suspect" patients had the connection between unilateral auditory and/or vestibular function returned to normal, as illustrated by a case reported by the investigators in which severe auditory and vestibular impairment returned to normal within 6 months.

ACOUSTIC TUMOR

The acoustic nerve tumor is a benign tumor that typically arises from the vestibular portion of the eighth cranial nerve. In most cases, the tumor begins to grow within the internal auditory meatus. As the tumor grows, pressure is put on the nerve fibers located in the internal auditory canal, including the facial nerve, the inferior and superior vestibular nerves, and the auditory (or cochlear) nerve. The increased pressure on these nerves may create specific symptoms, such as hearing loss, vertigo, tinnitus, and facial weakness, which assist the physician in making an accurate diagnosis of the tumor.[32]

Patients with acoustic tumors may have any variety of four general symptoms including sensorineural hearing loss, dizziness, tinnitus, and facial weakness. Diagnosis includes a wide variety of medical tests that may include computerized tomography scans, petrous pyramid polytomograms, magnetic resonance imaging, angiography, ENG, auditory evoked response measurement, and a complete battery of audiologic tests as described in Chapter 40 by Sanders.

Glasscock and Hays warn that an eighth nerve pathology pattern in the diagnostic audiologic test battery does not necessarily indicate the presence of an acoustic tumor.[33] Johnson reported audiometric results found in 500 patients with confirmed acoustic tumors and found that only 50 percent of these cases revealed "typical" audiometric results.[34] Johnson indicated that audiometric results are less accurate in patients with small tumors.

Vertigo is a common complaint of patients with acoustic tumor. ENG should be included in the differential diagnostic test battery. Evaluation of the vestibular response is commonly done with cold water caloric irrigations to identify unilateral vestibular weakness through observation of nystagmus, although bithermal calorics and ENG are better test procedures for vestibular function.

Linthicum and Churchill reported vestibular findings obtained from 200 patients with proved acoustic neuromas tested with minimal ice water caloric irrigations and ENG.[35] They found that 82 percent of the patients showed reduced caloric vestibular response on the affected ear. The incidence of positive response was found to be directly related to the size of the tumor.

SUMMARY

The purpose of this chapter was to provide useful information on the nature, etiologies, and the manifestations of various hearing disorders. Descriptions of typical audiometric configurations, impedance, and ENG findings associated with different types of ear disease have been provided. It is important to keep in mind that composite test results must be considered when identifying and classifying hearing disorders.

REFERENCES

1. Northern JL, ed. Communication disorders related to otitis media. Seminars in speech, language & hearing 1982; 3(4):281–356.
2. Bess FH, Tharpe AM. Unilateral hearing impairment in children. Pediatrics 1984; 74(2):206–216.
3. Norris TW. Electronystagmography. In: Northern JL, ed. Hearing disorders. Boston: Little, Brown, 1984:205.
4. Kileny P. Evaluation of vestibular function. In: Katz J, ed. Handbook of clinical audiology. 3rd ed. Baltimore: Williams & Wilkins, 1985:582.
5. Jerger J. Clinical experience with impedance audiometry. Arch Otolaryngol 1970; 92:311–324.
6. Jerger J, Jerger S, Mauldin L. Studies in impedance audiometry: I. Normal and sensorineural ears. Arch Otolaryngol 1972; 96:513–520.
7. Jerger J, Anthony L, Jerger S, et al. Studies in impedance audiometry: III. Middle ear disorders. Arch Otolaryngol 1974; 99:165–171.
8. Jerger S, Jerger J. Diagnostic value of crossed and uncrossed acoustic reflexes. Arch Otolaryngol 1977; 103:445–453.
9. Northern J, Downs MP. Hearing in children, 3rd ed. Baltimore: Williams & Wilkins, 1984.
10. Howie V. Acute and recurrent acute otitis media. In: Jaffe B, ed. Hearing loss in children. Baltimore: University Park Press, 1977:421.
11. Bluestone C, Klein JO, Paradise J, et al. Workshop on effects of otitis media on the child. Pediatrics 1983; 71(4):639–652.
12. Orchik DJ, Dunn JW, McNutt L. Tympanometry as a predictor of middle ear effusion. Arch Otolaryngol 1978; 104:4–7.
13. Goin DW. Chronic inflammatory diseases of the middle ear and mastoid. In: English G, ed. Otolaryngology—a textbook. Hagerstown, MD: Harper & Row, 1976:167.
14. English GM, Northern JL, Fria TJ. Chronic otitis media as a cause of sensorineural hearing loss. Arch Otolaryngol 1973; 98:18.
15. Schuknecht HF. Pathology of the ear. Cambridge, MA: Harvard University Press, 1974.
16. Gates GA, Meyerhoff WL. Tympanomastoidectomy. In: Jaffe B, ed. Hearing loss in children. Baltimore: University Park Press, 1977:555.
17. Carhart R. Effect of stapes fixation on bone conduction response. In: Schuknecht HF, ed. Otosclerosis. Boston: Little, Brown, 1962:175.
18. Linthicum F. Ossicular chain destruction. In: Jaffe B, ed. Hearing loss in children. Baltimore: University Park Press, 1977:452.
19. Northern JL. Impedence audiometry for otologic diagnosis. In: Shambaugh G, Shea J, eds. Shambaugh fifth international workshop on middle ear mircosurgery and fluctuant hearing loss. Huntsville, AL: Strode Publications, 1977:75. 82.
20. Barber HO. The diagnosis and treatment of auditory and vestibular disorders after head injury. Clin Neurosurg 1972; 10:355–370.
21. Roush J, ed. Aging and hearing impairment. Seminars in hearing 1985; 6(2):99–219.
22. Schuknecht HF. Further observations on the pathology of presbycusis. Arch Otolaryngol 1964; 80:369–382.
23. Bergstrom LB, Thompson P. Ototoxicity. In: Northern JL, ed. Hearing disorders. Boston: Little, Brown, 1984:119.
24. Northern JL, Zarnoch JM. Aural rehabilitation of noise in-

duced hearing loss. Otolaryngol Clin North Am 1979; 12(3):693–703.
25. Sweetow R, ed. Management of the tinnitus patient. Sem Hear 1987; 8(1):1–75.
26. Davis H. Abnormal hearing and deafness. In: Davis H, Silverman S, eds. Hearing and deafness. 4th ed. New York: Holt, Rinehart & Winston, 1978.
27. Kiang NYS, Moxon EC, Levine RA. Auditory-nerve activity in cats with normal and abnormal cochleas. In: Wolstenholme GE, Knight J, eds. Sensorineural hearing loss. London: J & A Churchill, 1970:241.
28. Saltzman M, Ersner MS. A hearing aid for relief of tinnitus aurium. Laryngoscope 1947; 57:358–366.
29. Vernon J. Tinnitus. In: Northern J, ed. Hearing disorders. 2nd ed. Boston: Little, Brown, 1984:291.
30. English GM. Inflammatory diseases of the inner ear. In: English G, ed. Otolaryngology—a textbook. Hagerstown, MD: Harper & Row, 1976:221.
31. Hyden D, Odkvist LM, Kylen P. Vestibular symptoms in mumps deafness. Arch Otolaryngol [Suppl] 1972; 360:182–183.
32. Weaver M, Staller S. The acoustic tumor. In: Northern J, ed. Hearing disorders. 2nd ed. Boston: Little, Brown, 1984:171.
33. Glasscock M, Hays J. Pitfalls in the diagnosis of acoustic and other cerebello-pontine angle tumors. Laryngoscope 1973; 83:1038–1045.
34. Johnson E. Auditory test results in 500 cases of acoustic neuroma. Arch Otolaryngol 1977; 103:152–158.
35. Linthicum FH, Churchill D. Vestibular test results in acoustic tumor cases. Arch Otolaryngol 1968; 88:604.

39

Basic Hearing Measurement

Fred H. Bess, Ph.D.

Forty-five years have now passed since Bunch published the classic text, *Clinical Audiometry.*[1] This book outlined the basic techniques available at that time for measuring auditory function. During this period, the primary audiometric tools used for the evaluation of the auditory system consisted only of tuning forks and vacuum tube audiometers. Essentially no mention was made of speech audiometry, and, of course, Metz's well-known monograph on acoustic impedance would not be published until 1946.[2]

It is almost superfluous to note that innumerable improvements have been made since that time in the attempts to evaluate the auditory system. This chapter concentrates on current knowledge related to the basic hearing evaluation. Specifically, there are three basic procedures commonly employed in the assessment of the auditory system. These include (1) pure tone measures, (2) speech measures, and (3) electroacoustic impedance measures. Pure tone and speech measures will be the focus of this discussion since the use of impedance is covered in Chapter 41. Since most introductory chapters of this sort give only incidental treatments to speech measures, this evaluation procedure receives somewhat greater emphasis.

PURE TONE MEASURES

For more than six decades, pure tone audiometry has played an important role in the assessment of hearing sensitivity. Pure tone measurements have been employed to (1) aid in the identification of different auditory lesions; (2) monitor hearing sensitivity following surgical or medical treatment; (3) serve as an excellent screening device in identification audiometry, especially for young children; (4) estimate the degree of handicap produced by the hearing impairment; and (5) assist in the identification of educational and social needs, as well as aid in the selection of appropriate rehabilitative procedures. These fundamental yet invaluable applications of pure tone audiometry have established this measurement technique as the central component of the basic hearing evaluation.

The Audiometer

The audiometer is an electronic instrument that is used by the audiologist to quantify hearing levels. Historically, the first audiometer can be traced to Hartmann's "acoumeter" in 1878.[1] In 1879, Hughes described an instrument called an "electric genometer,"[2a] which was designed to measure hearing ability and was christened "audiometer" by Richardson.[3] In that same year (1879), there is evidence to suggest that Alexander Graham Bell had developed a plan for an electrometer and audiometer.[4] However, it was actually the advent of vacuum tubes in the 1920s, that led to the more precise control of audio signals and made pure tone audiometry feasible.

The modern-day trend in solid-state electronics is reflected in the contemporary audiometer. Today's audiometer is capable of delivering a variety of audio signals (pure tones, noise, speech) via any of several possible transducers (earphones, speakers, bone vibrator). The basic components of an audiometer are as follows: (1) a frequency selector dial, which provides for the selection of different pure tone frequencies; (2) an interrupter switch, which is used to turn the tone "on" or "off"; and (3) a hearing level dial (attenuator), which controls the intensity of the signal. An output switch determines whether the signal is to be directed to the earphones (right or left) or to the bone vibrator. Basic audiometers also contain a noise generator so that masking of the contralateral ear can be employed when needed.

Reference Levels in Audiometry

The human ear does not perceive all frequencies at the same sound pressure level. It is therefore clinically expedient to calibrate audiometers in such a way as to compensate for the differential sensitivity of the auditory system to various frequencies. That is, at the zero reading on the hearing loss dial, the signal is automatically presented at a normative threshold level for each test frequency. Consequently, the setting of the hearing level dial provides a direct reflection of the amount of hearing loss.

Historically, several different standard reference levels have been used to represent the zero hearing level of pure tone audiometers. In 1933, Sivian and White conducted a classic experiment that was designed to determine threshold sensitivity under carefully controlled laboratory conditions.[5] The monaural hearing thresholds obtained by Sivian and White are illustrated in Figure 39–1. One can see that the hearing sensitivity under monaural listening conditions is maximal between 1,000 and 4,000 Hz, becoming less sensitive at both the higher and the lower frequencies.

In 1938, Beasley conducted a United States Health Survey on normal hearers that later became the first standard for the audiometric zero of pure tone audiometers.[6] Recall that the Sivian and White data were obtained under experimental laboratory conditions.[5] However, the hearing threshold data collected by Beasley were obtained in a clinical setting where the testing equipment and conditions were not carefully controlled.[6] As a result, the hearing levels were noted to be 15 to 20 dB higher than those levels obtained in the study by Sivian and White.[5] Nonetheless, the hearing threshold data generated from the Health Survey were adopted by the American Standards Association (ASA) in 1951 for the calibration of audiometers, and these data are also displayed in Figure 39–1.

It was noted during the period following the adoption of the ASA standard that the British standards varied from the American standard on the average of 10 dB across the frequency range. It seemed to be the consensus that these differences were due, at least in part, to the more exacting measurement procedures employed by the British. As a consequence of these discrepancies, the International Standards Organization (ISO) collected several available studies on hearing threshold sensitivity from throughout the world and selected 15 studies that fulfilled stringent experimental criteria. The data from these studies were combined and adopted as a recommended standard in 1964 (ISO-1964). Shortly thereafter the American National Standards Institute (ANSI-1969) adopted a standard that is similar to ISO-1964 and is the most commonly used standard in the United States. The ANSI-1969 data for TDH-39 earphones are also plotted in Figure 39–1. It is of interest to note how closely the present day standard agrees with the minimum audible pressure values established in 1933 by Sivian and White. Such a close similarity suggests that present-day clinical testing conditions have improved to the extent that they are now more closely approximating experimental conditions.

When considering reference levels for audiometry, two frequently used terms related to this

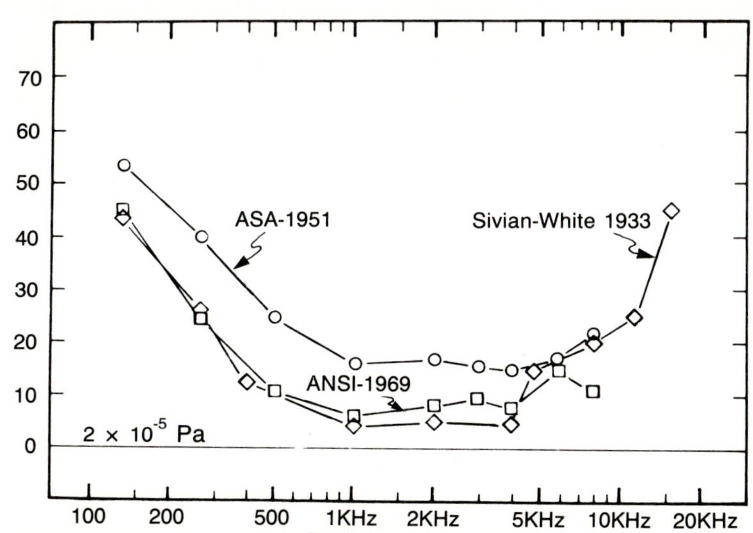

Figure 39–1 ASA-1951 and ANSI 1969 standard reference levels for representing zero hearing level on the pure tone audiometer. (Included is threshold sensitivity data [monaural] obtained by Sivian LJ, White SD. On minimum audible sound fields. J Acoust Soc Am 1933; 4:288.)

topic warrant clarification. First, hearing threshold level (HTL) is defined by ANSI-1969 as the amount of decibel loss for a given ear as it relates to a standard audiometric threshold. There is a growing trend toward using the term "hearing level" (HL),[7] instead of HTL.

Another term in need of definition is sensation level (SL). Sensation level refers to the number of decibels by which the intensity of a sound exceeds the threshold of a particular ear. Hence, if a signal were presented to the ear at 50 dB and if the threshold for that ear is 30 dB, the SL would be 20 dB. Both HL and SL will be used frequently throughout this chapter.

The Audiogram

The audiogram provides a means to display audiometric data and to classify an auditory impairment permanently. According to ANSI specifications for pure tone audiometers (ANSI S3.6–1969), the audiogram should be shown as a graticule with the frequencies (in Hz) displayed on the abscissa, using a logarithmic scale, and the hearing levels (in dB) shown on the ordinate, using a linear scale. They also recommend that the graticule be set up in such a way that one octave on the frequency scale be equivalent to 20 dB on the HL scale.

A rather controversial issue among audiologists relative to the audiogram is the choice of symbols used to convey audiometric information. Prior to 1974, there were no standards for audiometric symbols, and consequently audiologists used a variety of standardized symbol systems. Although the development of the recommended guidelines by the American Speech and Hearing Association (ASHA) helped to reduce much of the confusion and inconsistency associated with audiometric symbols, the chaos surrounding this issue remains unresolved. Some clinicians argue that the symbol system advocated by ASHA is too complex; that is, there are too many symbols, thus making it more difficult to discern audiometric patterns and air-bone relationships. In 1976, Jerger proposed what he considered to be a more lucid symbol system for use in scholarly publications.[7a] Jerger's recommended system simplified the process by reducing the number of audiometric symbols and by using separate audiograms for each ear. This two-graph system is popular among members of the medical community, especially otolaryngologists. By using a two-graph system, only two symbols are needed to display air conduction and bone conduction data, and the use of masking may be symbolized by merely filling in an open symbol. The stated advantages of this system are that (1) there is no need for color coding; (2) only two symbols are required; and (3) important audiometric information for the ear in question is not contaminated by symbols from the contralateral ear. These advantages are clearly indicated in Figure 39–2. The lower portion of this figure illustrates the way in which a case of bilateral conductive hearing loss is displayed by means of Jerger's proposed system. The top portion of this figure shows this same audiogram using the ASHA system. By comparison, the lucidity of Jerger's audiometric symbol is evident.

Classification of a Hearing Impairment

Several classification systems based on the pure tone audiogram have been developed in an attempt to estimate the extent of handicap produced by a hearing impairment. Such information has proven useful in planning rehabilitative strategies for a hearing impaired individual. A strong relationship is known to exist between those pure tone frequencies considered most important for speech recognition (500, 1,000, and 2,000 Hz) and the actual threshold for speech. Hence, the audiogram serves as an excellent means for predicting the degree of hearing loss for speech as well as estimating the subsequent handicap. An example of such a classification system is shown in Figure 39–3. This figure, adapted from several categorization schemes,[8-10] illustrates the various classes of hearing impairment and the terms commonly used to describe the magnitude of the hearing loss. In this particular scheme, the different classes of hearing loss ranging from normal to profound are based on the average hearing threshold at 500, 1,000, and 2,000 Hz. The probable effects of these different hearing loss categories on a person's ability to understand speech are also included on this figure. Note that within the classification of normal limits, which ranges from −10 to 26 dB, there should be no significant difficulty hearing and understanding faint speech. However, recent clinical evidence on children suggests that even a mild sensitivity loss (15 to 26 dB) can result in difficulty understanding faint speech. An investigation by Quigley and Thomure has inferred that even slight losses are capable of inducing an educational handicap.[11] Thirty-seven elementary school children with hearing thresholds in the better ear ranging from 15 to 26 dB lagged behind expected performance by approximately 1 year on a series of language subtests. Even children with unilateral sensorineural losses experience complications in auditory and psychoeducational tasks.[12,13] After observing some of the apparent handicapping effects produced by repeated episodes of chronic otitis me-

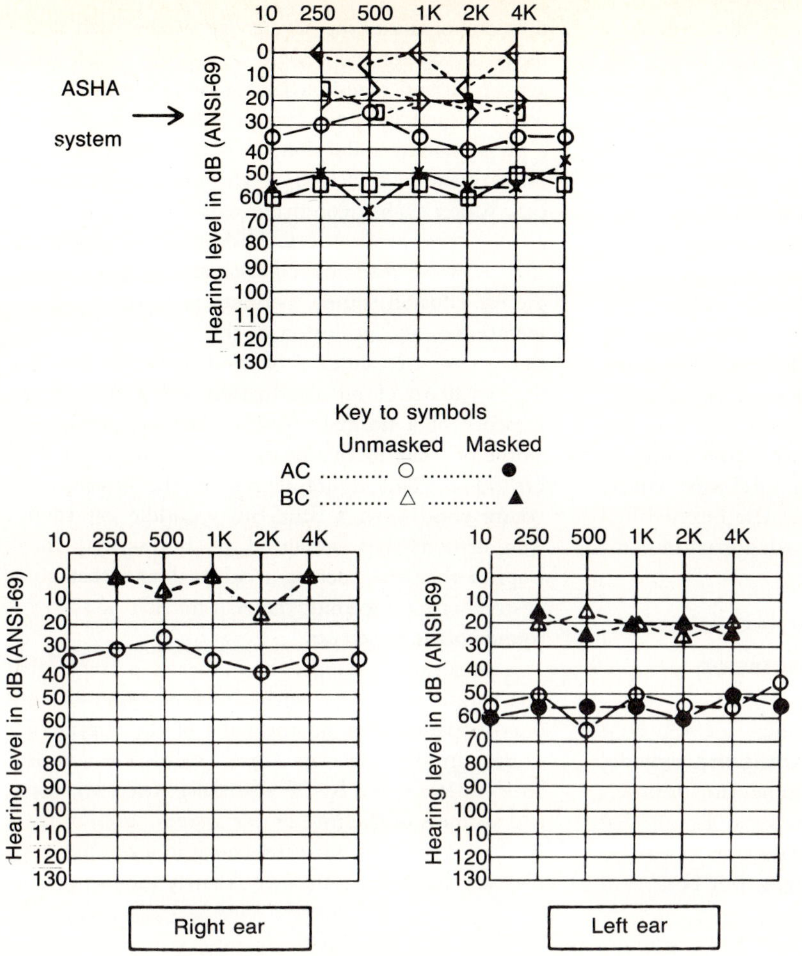

Figure 39–2 Audiograms and symbol system suggested by Jerger, lower portion. An exemplary case of bilateral conductive hearing loss is displayed using the Jerger symbol system. The top portion illustrates the way in which the same case is depicted using the ASHA system (From Jerger J. A proposed audiometric symbol system for scholarly publications. Arch Otolaryngol 1976; 102:33.)

dia, Downs has suggested that a hearing impairment occurs in children when an average hearing loss of 15 dB or worse is evident.[14] A similar low "fence" has also been advocated for adults.[15] Further, Kryter suggests using a 1,000, 2,000, and 3,000 Hz average for describing the impairment in subjects with high-frequency sensorineural hearing loss.[15] If one continues to observe impairments of communication and language in both children and adults as the result of only slight reductions in hearing sensitivity, it may be necessary to reconsider the limits of normal hearing in the classification system.[16]

Air and Bone Conduction Hearing

Pure tone audiometry in the basic hearing evaluation is composed of obtaining threshold measurements by means of the techniques of both air and bone conduction. Threshold is defined clinically herein as the minimum effective sound pressure that a listener can detect approximately 50 percent of the time. Clinical threshold measurement of hearing sensitivity by air conduction denotes a process whereby sound is transmitted via earphones through the external auditory meatus, across the middle ear mechanism, and to the cochlea and associated neural pathways to the brain. Hence a hearing loss by air conduction may reflect the presence of an auditory disorder anywhere along the conductive and sensorineural pathways. That is, the hearing deficit may be due to a middle ear complication, a lesion at the cochlea, or a disorder along the neural pathways to the cortex.

In the threshold measurement of bone conduction, audiofrequency vibrations are transduced by a vibrator applied to the skull and conducted directly to the cochlea. When the skull is set into vibration, sound energy is radiated into the external canal space via the canal walls and transmitted to the tympanic membrane. This form of response may be altered by the occlusion of the external canal, and it is commonly referred to as the "occlusion effect." The "occlusion effect" refers to the enhanced loudness of a bone-conducted signal following the occlusion of the ear canal. The effect is seen predominantly in the lower frequencies and reaches magnitudes of 20 to 25 dB. Tonndorf suggests that this phenomenon may be explained by a "high pass filter" effect.[17] When the skull is set into vibration, sound waves originating from the osseous and cartilaginous walls of the ear canal are radiated into the canal space. Although some of this acoustic energy reaches the tympanic membrane, much of the low-frequency sound is dissipated into the environment—hence the term "high pass filter." When the canal is occluded, the low-frequency energy is retained in the ear, and subsequently more of it is transmitted to the middle and inner ear. In addition to the occlusion effect, the bone conduction response may also be modified by ear canal resonance and by impedance at the tympanic membrane.[17,18]

Audiogram Interpretation

A comparison of the relationships between bone conduction and air conduction sensitivity provides the basis for differentiating middle ear disorders (conductive) from sensorineural lesions. Recall that air conduction audiometry is a reflection of the integrity of the entire auditory system, but bone conduction measures the sensitivity of the cochlea directly, bypassing the middle ear system. Thus, when air conduction thresholds are reduced in sensitivity or are normal and bone conduction has not exhibited a proportionate reduction, it would imply that the impairment was located at the external or middle ear. When such a condition exists, it is said to be a conductive hearing loss. Middle ear complications such as otosclerosis, ossicular chain disruption, middle ear effusion (fluid), perforation of the tympanic membrane, and occlusion of the ear canal, to mention a few, are examples of conditions that can produce deficits of air conduction sensitivity in the presence of a normal cochlea. An audiometric example of a conductive hearing loss is shown in Figure 39–4. This figure represents the hearing of a young child with a fluid-filled middle ear cavity. The air-bone gap evidenced at all test frequencies implies that the cochlea is normal and that some obstruction is impeding the transmission of air-borne sound to the inner ear.

Johansen developed audiometric patterns that one might anticipate with different types of conductive pathologies on the basis of the effects they exert on middle ear impedance.[19] Middle ear impedance is determined by the resistance (friction), mass, and stiffness of the middle ear system. Each of these components varies with frequency in a unique manner. For example, resistance is fairly independent of

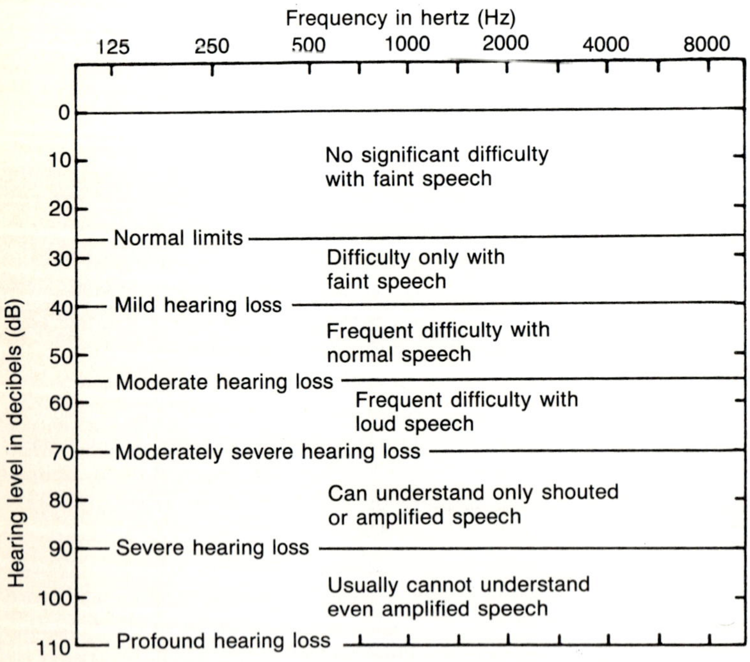

Figure 39–3 Audiometric illustration of a hearing loss classification scheme and terms used to describe the severity of hearing loss. The possible effects on speech understanding for each category are also provided.

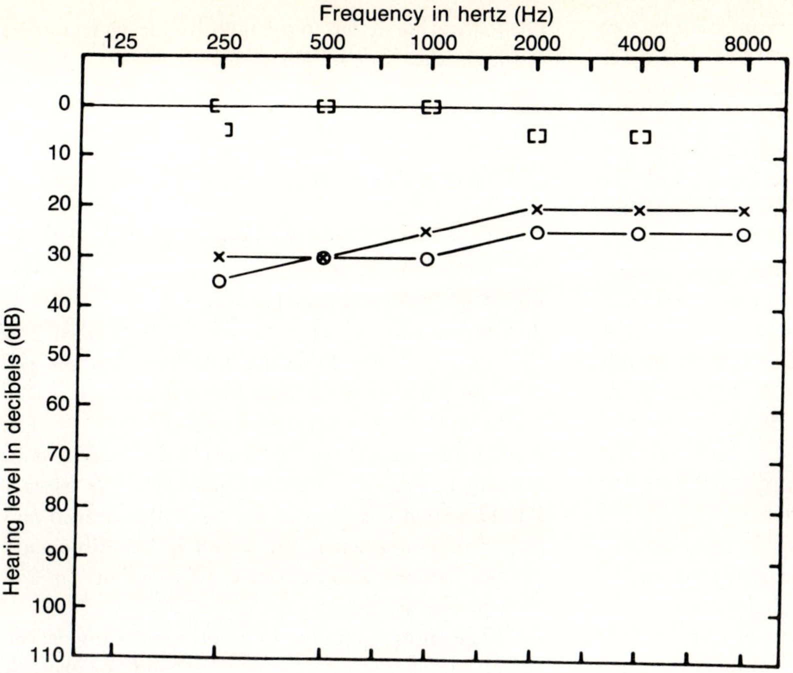

Figure 39–4 Audiometric example of a conductive hearing loss.

frequency, whereas reactance varies directly with frequency, and elastic reactance varies inversely with frequency. Figure 39–5 from Johansen depicts these features graphically in the form of audiometric configurations expected from various manipulations of the middle ear impedance.[19] Hence, if the mass of a system is increased, it is noted that the effect is to impair the transmission of high-frequency energy; but increased stiffness impairs the low frequencies; and increased friction is seen to affect all frequencies. It is possible, of course, to have an ear that manifests both mass and stiffness problems, in which case, ideally, threshold deficits would occur in the low and high frequencies but not the mid-frequency region. Examples of increased mass might be due to a growth in the external auditory meatus or to fluid resting behind the tympanic membrane. A stiffness component may be brought about by such middle

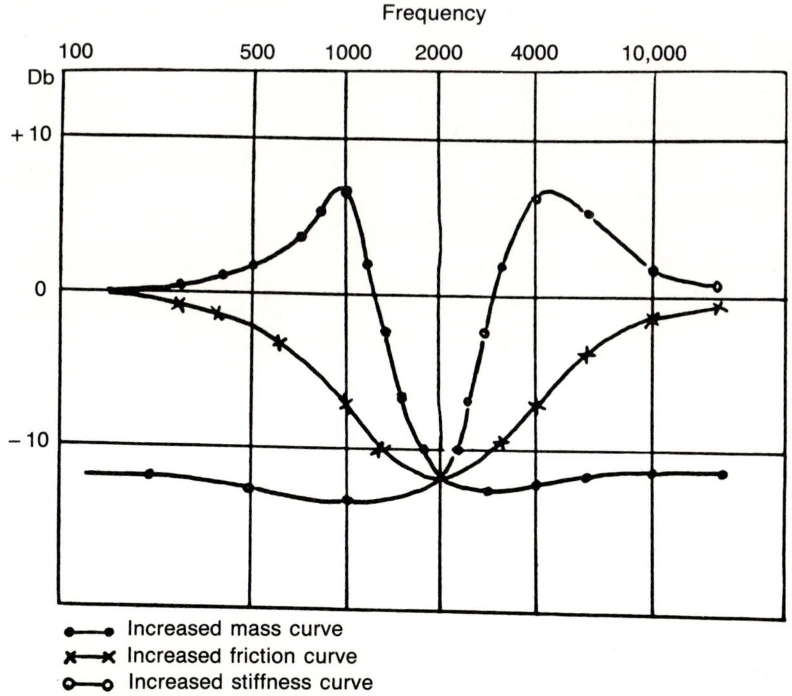

Figure 39–5 Graphic display of expected audiometric patterns in conductive pathologies by their influence on middle ear impedance. Note that increased mass affects high-frequency transmission; increased stiffness impairs low frequencies; and increased friction affects all frequencies. (From Shambaugh GE. Surgery of the ear. 2nd ed. Philadelphia: WB Saunders, 1967:388.)

ear complications as negative intratympanic pressure or fixation of any of the ossicular bones. Examples of friction changes on the middle ear system are not so easily identified.[20] Although some clinicians have suggested that Figure 39–5 is something of an oversimplification, it does provide a general guideline for expectant audiometric configurations in purely conductive pathologies.

When both air conduction and bone conduction thresholds are abnormal, but bone conduction is better than air conduction, the condition is classified as a mixed hearing loss. An example of this type of hearing problem is shown in Figure 39–6. The conductive loss is evidenced by the discrepancies between air and bone sensitivity, and the concomitant cochlear involvement is implied by the abnormal bone thresholds.

In a sensorineural hearing impairment, air conduction and bone conduction thresholds are nearly equivalent at all test frequencies. Numerous conditions are known to produce this type of impairment. Some of these include congenital complications such as heredity, viruses, ototoxic poisoning, and birth trauma, as well as acquired disorders such as inflammatory diseases (measles, mumps), noise, and presbycusis (hearing loss due to age). Those pathologic conditions known to produce conductive and sensorineural hearing loss are presented in detail in Chapter 38. An example of a sensorineural hearing loss due to the aging process is shown in Figure 39–7. One can see that both air and bone conduction thresholds are essentially compatible. Also note the greater hearing deficit in the high-frequency region—a result characteristic of sensorineural involvement.

Clinical Measurement of Threshold

Basic pure tone audiometry begins with air conduction measurements at octave intervals ranging from 250 to 8,000 Hz followed by bone conduction measurements at octave intervals from 250 to 4,000 Hz. The examiner first instructs the patient on the listening and response task at a language level that is appropriate to the listener. The instructions should specify that (1) the listener is to respond to even the softest signals, (2) the listener should respond as soon as the tone is perceived and stop responding when the sound is inaudible, and (3) the listener will be tested first in one ear and then in the other ear.

The most common form of responding is the raising and lowering of a finger, hand, or arm. If the listener reports any differences in hearing sensitivity between ears, it is recommended that the examiner begin testing the better ear first. The earphones are then placed carefully on the patient's head. The earphones should be attached with a fairly tight spring-tension headband that permits a firm yet comfortable fit.

Threshold determination in clinical audiometry incorporates a modification of the classic psychophysical method of limits.[21] In this technique, the

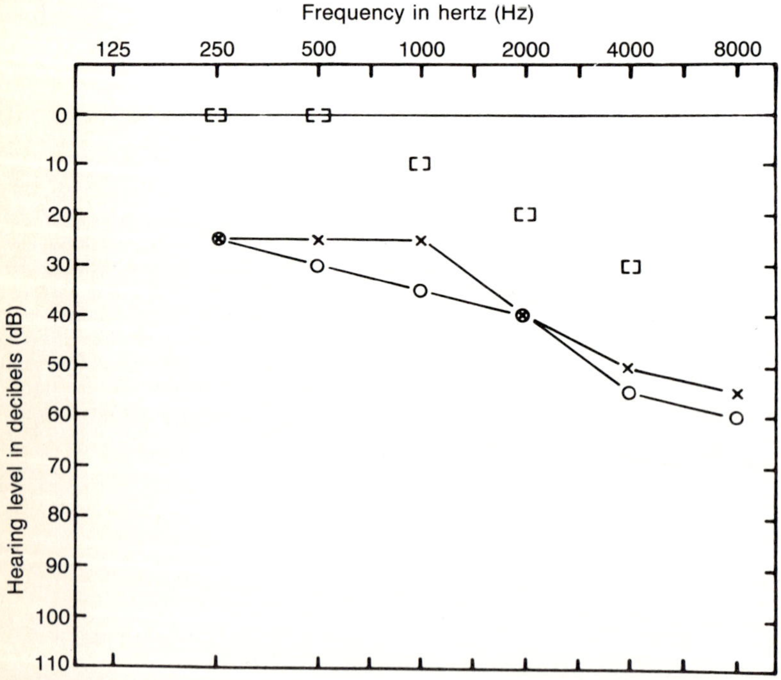

Figure 39–6 Audiometric example of a mixed-type hearing loss.

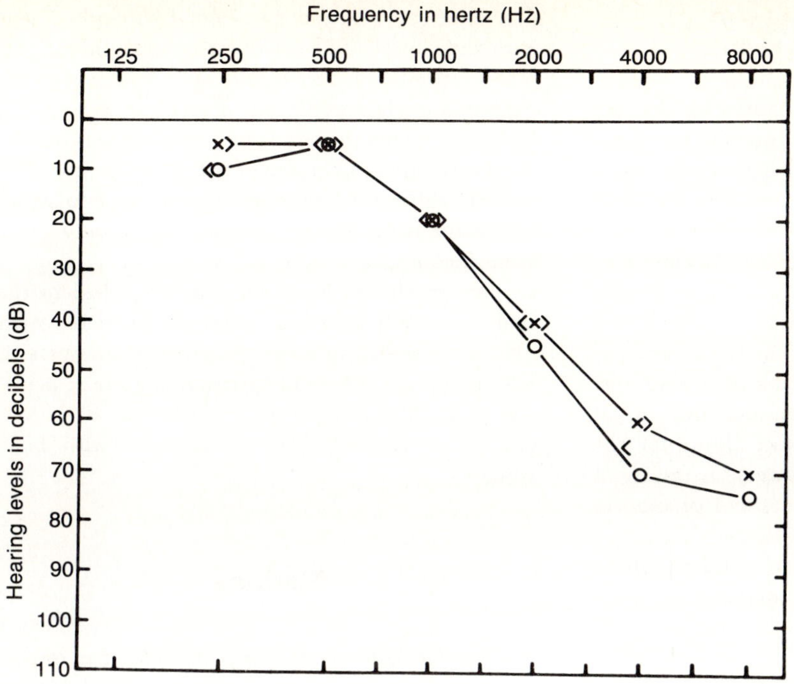

Figure 39–7 Audiometric example of a high-frequency sensorineural hearing loss.

experimenter usually controls the intensity of the signal and presents stimuli at levels both above and below the listener's threshold. There are two basic phases in the threshold determination process: a familiarization and exploration phase and a threshold-seeking phase.

Familiarization and Exploration Phase

1. Begin with 1,000 Hz in the better ear and introduce a pulsed (interrupted) signal at a hearing level of about 30-dB HL. If no response is elicited, increase the intensity by 20 dB and present the signal again. Continue to increase the intensity of the signal in 20-dB steps until a response is obtained.
2. With each response, decrease the intensity in 10-dB steps until a hearing level is reached that does not produce a response.

Threshold-Seeking Phase

1. Once the subject fails to respond to the signal, the threshold-seeking procedure begins using an ascending technique. Following a failure to obtain a response, the signal is increased in 5-dB increments until the patient signifies that the stimulus was perceived.
2. Following a patient response, the intensity of the tone is decreased by 10 dB, and another ascending series is begun.
3. Continue to increase in 5-dB steps with every failure to obtain a response and decrease in 10-dB steps with every positive response until an intensity is obtained at which the patient responds 50 percent of the time. This hearing level is then recorded as threshold.
4. After testing at 1,000 Hz, proceed to 2,000, 4,000, and 8,000 Hz, respectively. Next return to 1,000 Hz and retest the threshold for a reliability check before proceeding to frequencies 500 and 250. According to ASHA guidelines, if there is a difference of 20 dB or more between any adjacent frequencies from 500 to 8,000 Hz, additional measurements at intraoctaves should be made.[22]
5. After completing the test sequence for one ear, switch to the opposite ear and repeat the previous procedures.

Essentially, the same procedures are used in the threshold measurement of bone conduction at frequencies of 250 to 4,000 Hz. The bone vibrator is placed on the mastoid prominence of the test ear. To insure the best placement, it is sometimes helpful to introduce a pure tone (say 1,000 Hz) through the vibrator at a suprathreshold level and then vary the location of the vibrator on the mastoid until the subject notifies the examiner that the signal is loudest. It is particularly important not to place the vibrator against the auricle. Following the completion of the test sequence for one ear, the vibrator is moved to the opposite ear, and the threshold procedures described earlier are repeated.

Important Variables in Threshold Measurement

There are several imporatant variables that are known to influence directly the threshold measurement of both air conduction and bone conduction. Some of these factors important to consider are listed next.

Appropriate Calibration of the Audiometer. In order for the audiologist to be assured of reliable results, it is necessary to calibrate and maintain the audiometer at periodic intervals. The three basic parameters in need of calibration check on a pure tone audiometer are intensity, frequency, and time. ANSI has developed criteria and tolerance limits for the appropriate calibration of audiometers. A review of these specific calibration techniques and procedures is reported by Wilber.[23]

Test Environment. To insure valid threshold measures, the audiometric test environment must meet the noise-level criteria of ANSI. If noise levels within the test environment are in excess of allowable standards, the pure tone audio signals can be masked, and consequently hearing levels may be reported incorrectly.

Instructions to the Patients. Another important variable in threshold measurement concerns the instructions that the examiner provides the listener. For example, researchers know that thresholds in the higher frequencies (2,000 to 8,000 Hz) can vary by as much as 7 dB, depending on whether the criterion for response was the perception of a tonal quality or simply perception of sound.[24]

Other Variables in Threshold Measurement. Other rather obvious variables in threshold measurement include age, intelligence, and motivation of the listener; physiologic conditions of the test environment; astuteness and experience of the examiner; and the difficulty associated with the stimulus presentation technique.

In air conduction measurement, positioning of the earphones may also be a potential factor for producing threshold error. Variability in threshold can be introduced by even minor changes in the fit of the earphones. In fact, standard deviations in threshold as large as 5 to 7 dB were reported by Steinberg and Munson.[25] The audiologist must take care to insure that the tension-band provides a snug comfortable fit and that the earphone is well positioned over the ear canal opening.

There are several additional variables influencing threshold measurement that are unique to bone conduction. Two variables that can introduce sources of error in the threshold measurement are (1) *Placement of the bone vibrator.* In bone conduction testing, the oscillator may be placed on the mastoid process or the frontal bone. Frontal bone placement is thought to yield better test-retest reliability, improve intersubject variability, and reduce the participation of the middle ear in cochlear reception.[26] However, more intensity is required to reach threshold with frontal placement of the bone vibrator. The average difference between frontal and mastoid placement is 10 dB. (2) *Vibrator application force.* Bone conduction thresholds also vary depending on the force with which the vibrator is applied to the skull. Generally speaking, vibrators associated with most commercial audiometers produce pressures of 300 to 400 g. Threshold variation is greatest below 400 g. At present, 550 g (5.4 Newtons) is the recommended vibrator force to be used with bone vibrators.

Masking

In the determination of threshold it is important that the ear under test is not influenced directly by the auditory sensitivity of the nontest ear. However, recall from the discussion on bone conduction that the skull vibrates as a rigid body when forced into vibration. It should not be surprising to learn that when the bone vibrator is placed on one side of the head and a signal is presented, both cochleas are stimulated equally. Such a "cross over" phenomenon is also known to occur in air conduction audiometry, particularly in those subjects with unilateral or asymmetric hearing loss. When a signal presented to the impaired ear of those individuals reaches rather high intensities, it can "cross over" via the skull to the nontest ear. The loss of intensity that occurs as the signal is transmitted across the skull from one ear to the other is called interaural attenuation (IA). Essentially, IA quantifies the extent to which one ear is isolated from the other. IA for air conduction (supra-aural phones) may be conservatively estimated at 40 dB, but has been shown to range from approximately 40 to 80 dB. That is, if the air conduction signal in the test ear exceeds the bone conduction threshold of the nontest ear by 40 dB or more, cross over can occur. For bone conduction audiometry the IA is zero. Thus, under certain circumstances, nontest ear could potentially influence or participate in the threshold measurement of the test ear. When such a condition exists, it becomes necessary to introduce masking to the contralateral ear as a means of preventing the nontest ear from participating in the test.

Generally speaking, on the one hand, masking should be employed in air conduction audiometry whenever the level of the test tone minus the IA is equal to or exceeds the bone conduction threshold of the nontest ear. Stated otherwise, masking is needed whenever the signal presented to the test ear exceeds the bone conduction sensitivity in the nontest ear by more than 40 dB. On the other hand, masking for bone conduction should be employed whenever there is an air-bone gap in the test ear, since the IA is zero. Martin has suggested that because of the variability known to occur between air and bone conduction thresholds, smaller air-bone gaps such as 5 to 10 dB should be disregarded. Hence, according to Martin, masking should be employed whenever there is an air-bone gap of 10 dB or greater in the test ear.[27]

The two most common types of noise available on today's commercial audiometers are white noise, more commonly called broad-band noise, and narrow-band noise. Broad-band noise is composed of a wide spectrum of frequencies containing equal energy within each cycle. The frequency band of this noise cuts off at 6,000 Hz owing to the limited response characteristics of the earphones. By band-pass filtering broad-band noise, the production of a narrow band of noise is possible. It has long been recognized that a narrow band of noise centered on the frequency of a given pure tone is the most efficient masker of that tone.[28,29] The additional frequencies in a broad-band noise contribute primarily to the added loudness of the signal and minimally to the masking effect.

Most available diagnostic audiometers calibrate the masking noise in terms of effective masking. Effective masking refers to the amount of threshold shift (in dB) produced by a given amount of noise. Hence a noise that is capable of shifting an air conduction threshold in the masked ear by 45 dB is 45 dB of effective masking. Continuing with this concept, 35 dB of effective masking would mask out a 35-dB tone; however a 40-dB tone would be audible.

When masking the nontest ear, the audiologist must be careful not to use too much masking. If the masking noise in the nontest ear becomes too loud, it may cross over and be heard in the test ear. Thus to mask the ear under test is potentially possible. In order to avoid this problem, the presentation level of the masking noise of the nontest ear cannot exceed the bone conduction threshold in the test ear by more than 40 dB. In some situations, such as a large bilateral air-bone gap of 50 to 60 dB, it is impossible to obtain a sufficient amount of effective masking in the nontest ear without having crossover to the test ear. Such a condition has been described by Naunton as a "masking dilemma."[30]

Perhaps the most popular method of masking is the "plateau" technique developed by Hood.[31] Briefly, this technique involves the following steps:

1. Obtain an unmasked threshold.
2. Introduce masking to the nontest ear at a minimal level, typically 10 dB above the air conduction threshold of the nontest ear, and increase in 10-dB steps, redetermining threshold at each step.
3. Continue with step 2 until a threshold plateau is reached. A plateau is defined as that point at which no threshold change is observed with increased masking over a 20-dB range.
4. If the threshold remains stable with an increase in masking level, the threshold may be considered a valid result.

Clinical masking is an important and necessary practice in the determination of pure tone thresholds. The audiologist must develop the skills to recognize when to mask and to carry out quickly the appropriate procedures under clinical conditions. For a more detailed coverage of this topic the reader is referred to the work of Goldstein and Newman[32] and Sanders.[33]

SPEECH MEASURES

Although pure tone thresholds convey much information about the characteristics of the auditory system, they do not provide the audiologist with any precise measure of a person's ability to receive and code the speech message. Because of the limitations of pure tone measures in predicting functional efficiency for speech, supplemental clinical tests using various types of speech materials have long been a part of the basic hearing evaluation. Hence speech audiometry, a technique designed to assess a person's ability to hear and understand speech stimuli, has become a necessary tool in the overall assessment of a hearing handicap. Speech audiometry is useful in the validation check of pure tone data, in differential diagnosis, in evaluating the outcome of surgery, in the assessment of hearing aid use, and in quantifying functional changes in the pathologic process of the ear. My intent in this section is to review some of the applications of speech audiometry in the basic hearing evaluation. Specifically, this portion of the chapter is designed to familiarize the reader with clinical protocol in speech testing as well as to review some of the more common materials employed in the measurement techniques.

Speech Audiometer

Speech audiometry generally requires a two-room testing suite—a control room that contains the audiometric equipment and the audiologist and an evaluation room where the patient is located (Fig. 39–8). Most diagnostic audiometers include the appropriate circuitry for both pure tone measurement and speech audiometric evaluation. The speech circuitry portion of a diagnostic audiometer consists of a calibrated amplifying system having both variable inputs and outputs. Most commonly, the speech audiometer accommodates inputs for a microphone, tape recorder, and phonograph. Thus it is possible to conduct speech testing utilizing "live" speech (microphone) or prerecorded materials. A preamplifier, gain control, and volume unit (VU) meter follow the input and provide the audiologist with the capacity to monitor the speech signal to a predetermined level on the VU meter. The VU meter is followed by an attenuator calibrated in 1- or 2-dB steps over a range of at least 100 dB and connected to an amplifier. The output of the speech signal may be directed to earphones, a bone vibrator, or a loudspeaker situated in the test room. Speech audiometric testing can therefore be conducted in one ear (monaurally), in both ears (binaurally), or in a sound field environment. Many diagnostic audiometers employ a dual channel system that enables the examiner to incorporate two inputs at the same time and to direct these signals to any of the output modes.

In order to insure valid and reliable measurements, the circuitry of a speech audiometer must be calibrated regularly. As with the pure tone audiometer, linearity of attenuation, harmonic distortion, and acoustic output as measured through TDH-49 earphones all need to be carefully evaluated. The VU meter of the system should also be checked for stability. Furthermore, consideration must also be given to the calibration of loudspeakers. The audiologist must learn to examine the loudspeaker for its frequency response and harmonic distortion. Finally, the alternative input systems such as the phonograph and tape recorder are in need of calibration check semiannually if used with any degree of regularity. Specific procedures for calibrating various aspects of this equipment are reported elsewhere.[23,34]

The acoustic output of the speech audiometer is calibrated in dB for the normal hearing threshold. According to the most recent standards for speech audiometers, 0.0-dB HL is equivalent to 20-dB SPL (re 20 μPa) when measured through TDH-49 earphones. Because of the discrepancy (approximately 7.5 dB) between earphones (TDH-49 in MX41/AR cushions) and sound field measurements, the output from a loudspeaker is calibrated to approximately 12.5-dB SPL. This calculated difference in audiometric zero for earphones and loudspeakers makes it possible for one to obtain equivalent speech thresholds under these two conditions.

Assessment of Speech Reception Threshold

Speech reception threshold (SRT) is recognized as the intensity at which an individual is able to identify simple speech materials approximately 50 percent of the time. It is included in the basic hearing evaluation for two specific reasons. First, it serves as an excellent reliability check against the pure tone threshold data. That a strong correlation exists between the average of the pure tone thresholds obtained at the frequencies known to be important for speech (i.e., 500, 1,000, and 2,000 Hz) and the SRT is now well established. Large discrepancies between the SRT and this pure tone average may be suggestive of a functional disorder. A second important reason for including the SRT in the hearing evaluation is that it provides a reference for conducting speech discrimination tests. That is, once the degree of hearing loss for speech is determined it is possible to calculate the SL for evaluating how well an individual can understand comfortably loud speech (words). Another important application of the SRT, beyond that of the basic hearing evaluation,

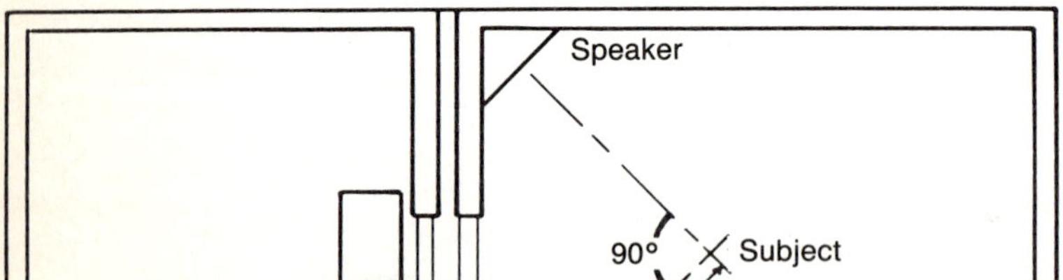

Figure 39–8 A typical two-room test set-up for conducting speech audiometry.

is the determination of functional gain in the hearing aid selection.

Speech Threshold Materials

Historically, Hughson and Thompson were the first to measure the SRT in a group of subjects with hearing impairment.[35] Using Bell Telephone sentences, Hughson and Thompson presented several sentences at successively lower intensity levels until the listener was able to understand only two-thirds of the spoken sentences; this became the speech reception threshold.

Hudgins and co-workers selected spondaic words (two-syllable words spoken with equal stress on each syllable) as their materials for measuring the SRT.[36] These words were developed on the basis of "familiarity, phonetic dissimilarity, normal sampling of English speech sounds and homogeneity with respect to audibility."[36] From these selected criteria, homogeneity was considered most important for threshold measurement because it enhances the precision with which the threshold could be calculated. Further, in the interest of saving time, it is desirable to determine the SRT with as few items as possible.[37]

It was on the basis of these criteria that the Harvard lists, known as PAL (Psychoacoustic Laboratory) Auditory Tests No. 9 and No. 14, evolved. These two spondee tests were composed of 42 disyllabic words, each of which are randomized five times and recorded on discs. The PAL No. 9 test was developed in such a way that a 4-dB attenuation rate was built into the recording following the presentation of six spondees. The PAL No. 14 test utilized the same words as PAL No. 9; however, all of the test items were recorded at the same level. The examiner then manually attenuated the signal following the presentation of the spondaic words.

Based on several years of clinical experience with the Harvard spondee lists (Nos. 9 and 14), Hirsh et al noted several limitations of these tests.[38] They proposed modifications of the PAL test that were designed to provide two improvements. First, the words from the Harvard lists were restricted to the more familiar spondees, and, second, considerable improvements were made in the quality of the recordings. By eliminating those words considered too difficult or too easy, the 84 spondees were reduced to 36 words recorded on a master tape and then randomized to provide six different scramblings of the original list. A carrier phrase, "say the word," preceded each stimulus item and was presented at an intensity of +10 dB relative to the words. Preliminary investigation of these modified lists revealed that some of the words differed considerably in difficulty despite the attempts to increase the homogeneity. Hence the more difficult words were increased by +2 dB, and the easier words were reduced by 2 dB on the final recordings. This modified version of the Harvard lists was referred to as the Central Institute for the Deaf (CID) Auditory Test W-1 or W-2, and the scramblings were designated as lists A, B, C, D, E, and F. In the W-1 version of this test, all of the words were recorded in one intensity; whereas with the W-2 recording, the intensity of the signal was attenuated on the disc by 3 dB following the presentation of every three words. A performance-intensity function of the W-1 version is shown in Figure 39–9. One can see that with a restricted intensity range, there is a marked increase in identification between 20 and 80 percent.

Since the development of the CID spondee lists, several attempts have been made to increase the homogeneity of these words.[39-43] In a comprehensive review of these studies, Olsen and Matkin concluded that the homogeneity of spondees could be improved significantly by limiting the selection of test items to only the less difficult spondees.[37]

Speech Threshold Procedures

Several different procedures have been advocated for determining the SRT utilizing spondee words. Although it is not the intent of this section to present all of the techniques available, some of the more popular and well-accepted methods will be explored. Any of these procedures may be employed, incorporating recorded materials or utilizing monitored live voice.

Hirsh and co-workers[38] modified a procedure advocated by Hudgins et al [36] for use with the W-2 lists. In the W-2 version of the CID lists, the intensity of the words is attenuated 3 dB following the presentation of every three words. Hence, the test covers an intensity range of 33 dB, and, on the average, each word represents 1 dB of attenuation. Threshold was determined by subtracting a decibel value corresponding to the number of words that the listener repeated correctly from the level at which the first group of three words was presented. A 1.5-dB constant is then subtracted from the threshold value.

The Committee on Audiometric Guidelines of ASHA also proposed a procedure using most of the 36 spondaic words from the CID W-1, W-2 lists.[44]

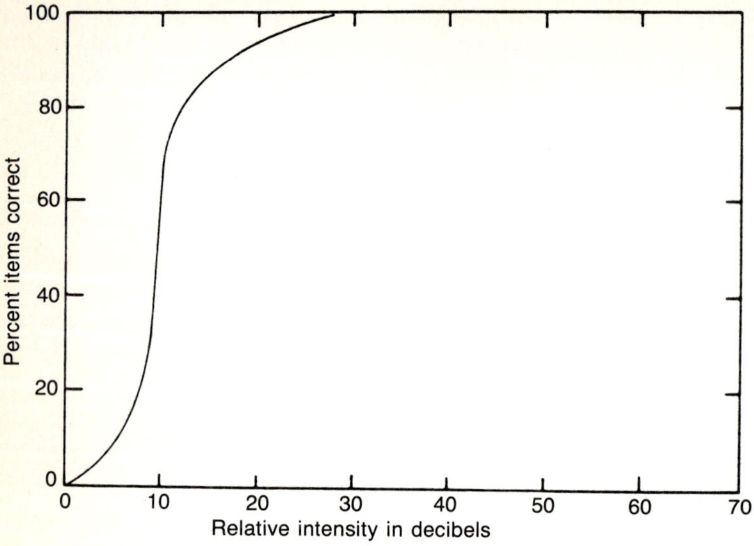

Figure 39-9 A performance-intensity function of spondaic materials based on the Central Institute for the Deaf (CID) Auditory Test W-1.

(Six of the words were replaced with spondees from the PAL list.) The procedure involves an ascending technique with blocks of four test items presented in 5-dB increments. The ascent is terminated when the listener responds correctly to three or more spondees in a set, and a new ascent is begun. Threshold is defined as the lowest level at which half or more of the spondaic words are repeated correctly. A minimum of two ascending series is required.

Tillman and Olsen have suggested a procedure that was adapted from the method developed by Hirsh and co-workers and has received wide acceptance.[45] Briefly, this technique consists of two essential phases, an exploration phase and a threshold-seeking phase. An outline of these follows. The first is the exploration phase:

1. Familiarize the listener with the test items.
2. Present one spondee at 30 to 40 dB above the estimated threshold.
3. If the listener responds correctly, attenuate the signal 10 dB and present another spondee.
4. Continue with step 3 until an incorrect response is obtained. Following an incorrect response, present a second spondee at the same intensity level.
5. If the second word is missed, increase the signal by 10 dB and begin to seek threshold. If the response to the second word is correct, attenuate the signal 10 dB; continue with step 3 until two consecutive words are missed.

The second is the threshold-seeking phase:

1. Begin at 10 dB above the level where two consecutive words are missed, and present two spondee words.
2. Attenuate by 2 dB, and present two more spondees. spondees.
3. Continue to present two spondees at each 2-dB interval until the listener misses at least five of the last six words presented.*
4. When five of the last six words are missed, the number of correct responses is tabulated, the total is decreased by one and subtracted from the hearing level setting at which the test began.

Jerger and Jerger developed an interesting procedure for estimating a speech threshold using information derived from the performance-intensity (PI) function for phonetically balanced (PB) monosyllabic words (PI-PB).[46] In an earlier work, Jerger and Jerger had shown that the PI-PB was most valuable in the differentiation of cochlear and retrocochlear disorders, and they consequently recommended this clinical technique as a standard procedure for all audiologic evaluations.[47] Performance-intensity functions were determined by presenting sets of 25 monosyllabic words at several successively higher suprathreshold levels, reaching a maximum intensity

* If less than five of six words are repeated correctly at the starting level, it is necessary to increase the level 4 to 6 dB and begin a new descent.

of 110-dB SPL. Baseline intensity levels were developed in a normal-hearing population for the 50 percent reference and for the 25 percent reference. Two reference norms were developed because a preliminary study had indicated that in those patients with maximum discrimination scores of more than 70 percent, the best predictor of the speech threshold was the intensity level yielding a 50 percent score. However, for those patients whose maximum discrimination scores were less than 70 percent the best estimation of pure tone sensitivity was the 25 percent reference. Threshold estimations were determined by taking the difference between the SPL, which provided either a 50 percent or 25 percent score, and the appropriate normal reference SPL (50 percent or 25 percent).

An example of how this procedure can be used with a typical patient is shown in Figure 39–10. This figure depicts the audiogram and performance-intensity functions of a subject exhibiting a mild unilateral hearing impairment in the left ear and relatively normal hearing sensitivity in the right ear. Maximum discrimination ability in the right ear was 100 percent, whereas the maximum intelligibility score in the left ear was 80 percent. The estimated speech threshold results for both ears are also seen to be almost equivalent to the pure tone averages.

Assessment of Speech Discrimination

Although the speech threshold provides the clinician with an index of the degree of hearing loss, it does not offer any information on a person's ability to make distinctions among the various acoustic cues in spoken language at conversational intensity levels. Unlike the situation with the SRT, attempts to calculate a person's ability to understand speech based on data from the pure tone audiogram have been unsuccessful. Hence various discrimination tests have been developed for the purpose of estimating a person's ability to understand conversational speech. Three of the more clinically accepted forms of discrimination testing include phonetically balanced word lists, multiple-choice tests, and sentence tests.

Phonetically Balanced Word Lists

The first word recognition test that incorporated the use of monosyllabic words was the material developed by Egan[48] at the Harvard Psychoacoustic Laboratories. The criteria used in the generation of these lists served as the basis for the development of future word discrimination tests. These criteria included (1) monosyllabic structure, (2) equal average difficulty, (3) equal range of difficulty, (4) equal composition of phonetic classes, (5) phonetic compositions representative of English speech, and (6) words in common usage. The phonetic composition was established using Dewey's frequency count of written English words found in newsprint.[49] That is, the frequency of each phonetic class in the initial, medial, and final positions was tabulated. Although Egan initially attempted to satisfy the phonetic balance criteria using only 25 words, he soon discovered that 50 words were necessary. The selected words that met the aforementioned criteria were grouped into 20 lists composed of 50 monosyllables each. These lists became known as the PAL PB-50s and continue even today to be used in the assessment of word recognition ability.

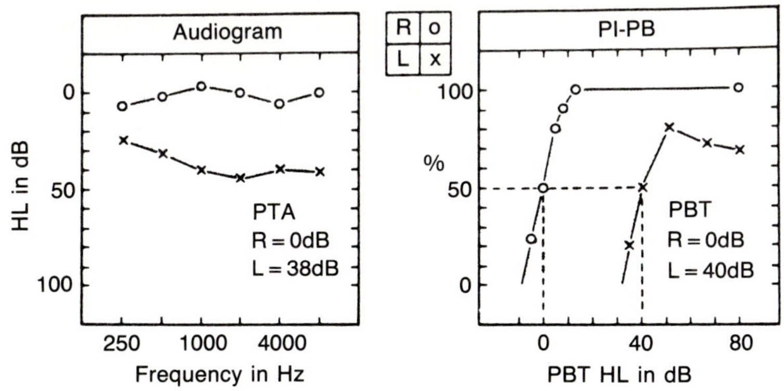

Figure 39-10 Case example of estimating a speech threshold from the performance-intensity (PI) function of phonetically balanced (PB) words. Note that the speech thresholds taken at the intensity level yielding a 50 percent score were in close agreement with the pure tone averages. (From Jerger S, Jerger J. Estimating speech threshold from the PI = PB function. Arch Otolaryngol 1976; 102:487.)

Following several years of widespread clinical usage, it became apparent that several limitations were associated with the PAL-50 tests. The primary criticism of the PAL lists was that the vocabulary was too difficult for many patients. In an attempt to improve on the PAL lists, Hirsh and co-workers restricted the vocabulary to those words considered more familiar to the general population and improved on the phonetic balance. In addition, they developed standardized recordings of the modified lists.[38] To achieve a better phonetic composition, a criterion of spoken rather than written English was employed. The lists were constructed in such a way as to reflect proportionately the same number of consonants and consonant compounds in the initial and final positions. The revised version of the PAL lists was composed of 200 words, which were grouped into four lists of 50 words each. These lists have become commonly known as the CID W-22s and are now recognized as the most popular speech discrimination test used by audiologists.[50]

Many clinicians were not completely satisfied with the tests developed by Egan[48] and Hirsh et al,[38] and consequently several alternative discrimination tests have been proposed. Foremost have been the clinical discrimination test that has evolved from the work of Lehiste and Peterson.[51] They proposed a set of lists using the concept of phonemic rather than phonetic balancing. Lehiste and Peterson contended that it is impossible to develop a true phonetic balance within a 50-word list because speech elements within a word are influenced directly by contiguous speech sounds. Test items developed by Lehiste and Peterson were selected on the following basis: (1) a high degree of familiarity, (2) carefully controlled phonemic balance, and (3) words of the consonant-nucleus-consonant (CNC) variety. Phonemic balancing was established by first determining the frequency of occurrence of each initial, medial, and final phoneme in a corpus of familiar words (N = 1263) taken from Thorndike and Lorge.[52] Ten lists of 50 monosyllabic words each were then constructed. The phonemic composition of each 50-word list was proportional to the total pool of words from which the items were selected. Peterson and Lehiste later revised these lists to reflect greater familiarity.[53]

Because there was limited information available regarding the reliability and interchangeability of the ten Lehiste and Peterson lists and because the lists contained imperfect phonemic balancing, Tillman et al developed two new lists known as the Northwestern University Auditory Test No. 4 (NU-4), using 1,263-word pool.[54] The original two lists were then expanded to four 50-word lists recognized as the now popular Northwestern University Auditory Test No. 6 (NU-6).[55] Each of these lists has been scrambled four times, thereby providing a total of 16 lists.

For comparison purposes, representative performance-intensity functions of these lists (Nos. 2, 3, 4, 5) (normal hearers) appear in Figure 39–11. Because of their widespread usage, lists from two different recordings of the CID W-22 lists are illustrated. One can readily observe that although the functions are similar, differences do exist between the tests. The most difficult tests among these monosyllabic materials are the Harvard PAL 50s. On the most linear portion of the curve (20 to 80 percent), identification increases at a rate of 3.8 percent per decibel. Conversely, the original version of the NU-6 materials[45] and the CID W-22 lists[56] exhibit steepness slopes of 5.6 percent per decibel and 5.0 percent per decibel, respectively. It is of interest to note the differences observed in the functions of the two recorded versions of the CID W-22s (Nos. 3 and 4). The more recent recording[57] exhibits a steepness slope of 4.6 percent per decibel, and the function is displaced to higher sensation levels than the original version. Such differences illustrate clearly that two different recordings of the same material can yield significantly different performance functions.

Multiple-Choice Tests

The several apparent limitations of the conventional open-set PB words led some clinicians to direct their attention to alternative formats for word discrimination testing. The closed-set format inherent with multiple-choice tests provides several advantages over other open-set word recognition tests. For example, the closed-set format limits the number of available items from which the subject must select the test word. Further, the closed-set format minimizes the length of listening time required to familiarize a subject with the test vocabulary and consequently reduces the potential for a practice effect. Other stated advantages of the closed-set format include elimination of examiner bias, ease of administration, and simplified scoring techniques.

The most widely recognized multiple-choice test, the Modified Rhyme Hearing Test (MRHT), was introduced in 1968 as a recorded clinical test of speech discrimination by a group from the Stanford Research Institute.[58] Historically, the MRHT evolved from the original rhyme test introduced by Fairbanks.[59] The rhyme test was composed of 250 monosyllabic words arranged into 50 groups of five

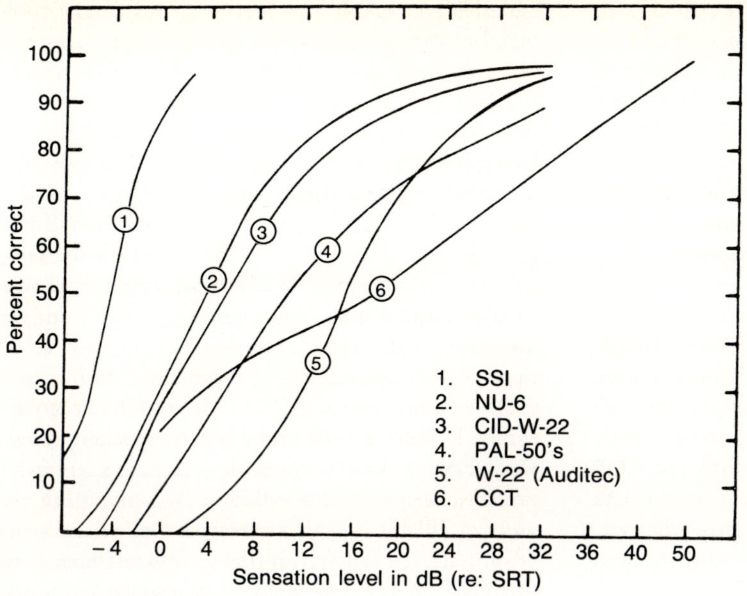

Figure 39–11 Performance-intensity functions of different discrimination tests. Functions 3 and 5 represent two different recordings of the W-22 material.

words each. Subjects were provided with the word stem in written form and given the task of completing the test word, (i.e.,—ot,—ay,—op). Thus the rhyme test was designed to assess a person's ability to differentiate initial consonant phonemes. The 18 consonants that composed the rhyme test approximated 90 percent of all consonants in the English language.

In 1965, a version of the rhyme test was developed by House and co-workers for the purpose of evaluating speech communication systems.[60] The House et al version was composed of 50 sets of six rhyming consonant-vowel-consonant (CVC) test items recorded at six different primary-to-secondary ratios (P:S).* The listener's task was to draw a line through the word perceived in the test ensemble.

Kruel et al developed the clinical version of the MRHT,[58] using essentially the same vocabulary as House et al.[60] A few of the original 300 monosyllables introduced by the latter investigators were changed because of repetition or because some of the words were considered objectionable. The clinical MRHT consisted of six 50-word lists, with each list composed of 50 six-word ensembles. Each ensemble of words varied relative to initial consonant or final consonant position, and the remainder of the word was held constant. A sample test ensemble is shown in Figure 39–12. In an effort to restrict wide variations in performance, noise levels were adjusted to the extent that normal hearers perceived the test items at a 96, 83, and 75 percent correct response performance level. Kruel et al recommended that the MRHT be administered clinically at a most comfortable loudness (MCL) level.[58]

Another multiple-choice test is the California Consonant Test (CCT)—a consonant identification test developed for and standardized on a hearing impaired population. Introduced by Owens and Schubert in 1977,[61] this test was developed on the basis that (1) there was a need for a test that allowed phoneme variation in only one position in any given

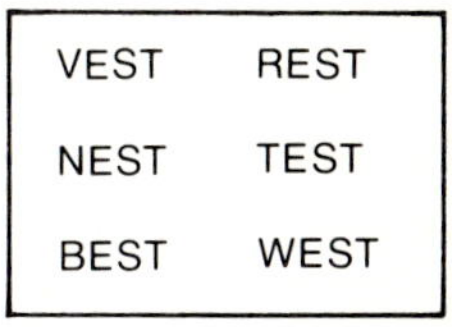

Figure 39–12 A typical test ensemble used in the Modified Rhyme Hearing Test (MRHT).

* P:S refers to the relationship between the speech signal and the competing noise. The primary signal represents the speech message, whereas the secondary signal refers to the background noise. Thus a primary-to-secondary ratio of +6 dB (P:S = +6) implies that the speech signal is 6 dB more intense than the noise.

item; (2) a test should employ an easily manageable number of foils; and (3) test format and standardization should be dictated by results of the clinical population for whom the test is intended. The CCT is composed of two different scramblings of 100 test items, each of which was arranged within an ensemble of four CVC monosyllabic words. For each item the words are assembled so that either the initial two phonemes are the same, with the final two varying, or, conversely, the final two phonemes are the same, with the initial phoneme varying. Of the 100 test items, 36 phonemes were located in the initial position, whereas 64 of the consonants were found in the final position. An example of four different test ensembles is shown in Figure 39–13. Since the test format and test items used with the CCT were developed through the careful analysis of data collected on patients with predominantly high-frequency hearing loss,[62] it is not surprising to find that the mean performance scores for this test are correlated to the degree of high-frequency sensorineural hearing loss. Additional multiple-choice tests have been developed over the years,[63-66] but at present have not yet received widespread clinical usage. On the one hand, when one compares these multiple-choice lists to other test materials, it is of interest to note that the performance-intensity function for the MRT (quiet) in normal hearers is similar to that of the CID W-22s.[67] On the other hand, the performance-intensity function for the CCT is displayed in Figure 39–11 along with several of the other tests. One can see that the function for the CCT is distinctively different from the other test materials. The slope of the function is almost linear, with identification increasing at a rate of only 1.6 percent per decibel. Further, it is noted with this gradual slope that the asymptote or maximum intelligibility is not reached until 50-dB SL.[68]

Another development in speech audiometry is the emergence of a closed-set response nonsense syllable test. Developed by Resnick, this test is composed of consonant-vowel and vowel-consonant syllables categorized into seven subtests of seven to nine syllables each.[69] These subtests differ in the following manner: (1) both voiced and voiceless consonants are represented; (2) the consonants occur in both the initial and final positions; and (3) the vowel context varies. The subject's response to a syllable within a given subtest is limited to syllables within the same subtest. An advantage of this test is that it is possible to analyze errors with respect to place and/or manner of articulation. The test is composed of 62 items, which includes one repeat item within each subtest (actual items = 55). The test has been recorded by both a male and a female speaker. A carrier phrase ("You will mark ________ please") precedes each stimulus syllable. By scrambling the order of syllables within subtests as well as the order of subtests, 16 different forms of this test have been produced. A cafeteria noise may also be employed to assess identification under adverse listening conditions. This test appears to have excellent potential and certainly merits further investigation.

BACK	______	GAVE	______
BAT	______	GAME	______
BATCH	______	GAZE	______
BATH	______	GAGE	______
THIN	______	LEASE	______
TIN	______	LEASH	______
SIN	______	LEAF	______
SHIN	______	LEAP	______

Figure 39–13 Examples of four different test ensembles used in the California Consonant Test (CCT).

Sentence Tests

In an attempt to approximate everyday speech more closely, several speech identification tests have been developed using sentences as the basic test item. A stated advantage of sentence material over other types of speech tests is that sentences approximate the spectral characteristics of connected discourse while controlling for sentence length and semantic content, thus increasing the test's face validity.

The first sentence test designed for the clinical purpose of assessing speech discrimination ability was developed and recorded at the Central Institute for the Deaf.[8,70] This discrimination test was prepared to represent everyday speech and vocabulary and is composed of 100 sentences divided into ten sets of ten sentences each. The sentence length varies from 2 to 12 words, and the responses are scored on the basis of 50 key words contained within each group of sentences. At present, however, there are no commercial recordings of these materials, and the clinical application of the CID sentences is somewhat limited.

In 1965, Speaks and Jerger developed a set of synthetic sentences for use in research.[71] The materials were designated as synthetic sentences because they did not represent "actual" sentences and because the sequence of words within each test item was constructed according to predetermined rules on the basis of conditional probabilities of word sequence. The lists are now commonly referred to as the synthetic sentence identification (SSI) test. Using the 1,000 most common words from Thorndike and Lorge,[52] first-order synthetic sentences were constructed by selecting each word at random from the word pool to create a "sentence" of specified length. An example of a first-order sentence is:

"Due his along such near nearly."

Thus each word had basically no meaningful relationship to any adjacent word in the synthetic sentence. Second-order approximation sentences were established in the following manner. First, a word was selected at random from the Thorndike and Lorge pool. Next an individual was asked to select a second word from the same pool, which might logically follow the first word in a declarative or imperative sentence. Without having knowledge of the first word, another person was requested to select a third word from the pool, which would reasonably follow the second word. An example of a second-order approximation is:

"Three came home on any woman can."

Third-order approximations were developed by randomly selecting a word pair from the second-order sentences and then adding a third word, selected from the pool, as a reasonable term to follow the word pair. The first word was then disregarded and another individual chose an appropriate word to complete the triplet. The following is a sample of a third-order approximation:

"Forward march said the boy had a."

Utilizing such a procedure, sentences that were equivalent in length could be developed as specified in level or order of sentence approximation. Hence different sets of ten sentences composed of varying orders of approximation were constructed by means of a closed-set format. After the presentation of a single sentence, the task of the listener was to identify which of the ten sentences was perceived. The most common means of response was for the subject to press a response button adjacent to the appropriate sentence or to call out the number of the sentence perceived.

A sample performance-intensity function for the SSI is displayed in Figure 39–11. It is readily seen that this test is much easier than other materials shown in this figure. In an effort to increase the difficulty of this test, a competing speech message was mixed with the sentences. For clinical evaluation purposes, it was recommended that the SSI be administered at a message-to-competition ratio (MCR) of 0.0 dB; that is, both the speech and the competition are delivered at the same intensity level. This amount of competition provided performance scores in normal hearers that were comparable to scores obtained with phonetically balanced materials in quiet.

A sentence identification test, referred to as the speech perception in noise (SPIN), has been proposed by Kalikow et al.[72] The eight available lists of the SPIN are each composed of 50 sentences that are generally five to eight words in length. The last word of each sentence is the test item. Twenty-five of the sentences contain test items that are classified as having "high predictability," which means that the word is readily predictable given the context of the sentence. Conversely, 25 sentences have test items with "low predictability." An example of a sentence containing "high predictability" is:

"The boat sailed across the *bay*."

whereas an example of a sentence with "low predictability" is:

"John was talking about the *bay*."

The recordings of these sentences also contain a background of babble-type competition, which is composed of 12 voices reading continually. This adverse competition can be mixed with the sentences at any desired P:S ratio.

Clinical Strategies in Speech Discrimination

The speech discrimination score can be influenced (sometimes to a large extent) by several variables, most of which are related to the procedures used in test administration. Because of their important implications for the audiologist, several of these variables are considered next.

Test Presentation

The audiologist needs to give thought to the details of test presentation. Speech discrimination scores can be affected dramatically by speaker differences, methods used in recording the test materials, and characteristics of the test equipment. When considering the protocol for presenting the test materials, there seem to be three issues that are of special concern to the clinician: (1) whether to use recorded materials or to employ a monitored live voice (MLV) presentation, (2) whether to utilize a carrier phrase, and (3) how to determine the appropriate intensity level at which to administer the test materials.[73]

Clinicians disagree over which mode of test

presentation, MLV or prerecorded, is the most appropriate. Those clinicians who are critics of MLV believe that unless standardized recorded materials are used, results between test conditions cannot be compared, primarily because of the speaker differences. However, advocates of MLV feel that live presentation affords greater clinical flexibility and argue even further that there is evidence of acceptable test-retest reliability with this technique.[74] However, there is recent evidence that does not support the use of MLV. Brandy demonstrated that recorded materials offered a greater reliability than MLV in normal hearers.[75] In another study, Penrod and Price noted marked variability in word discrimination scores among sensorineurally impaired hearers when listening to different audiologists (N = 4) who were accustomed to the MLV technique.[76] They observed that variability in performance increased as discrimination decreased, and they questioned the validity of MLV when used with persons having problems in understanding speech.

A common practice in the assessment of speech discrimination is to preface each test item with a carrier phrase such as "Say the word __________," "You will say __________," or "Write the word __________." Carrier phrases are used for two purposes. First, they prepare the listener for the upcoming stimulus item; second, they help the clinician monitor the intensity of the speech signal on the VU meter. Traditionally, the carrier phrase is monitored to a predetermined level on the VU meter and the stimulus item is then delivered naturally.

Some investigators have questioned whether the use of a carrier phrase is necessary.[77,78] In their study, Martin and co-workers observed that many of the subjects with sensorineural hearing loss specified a preference for having a carrier phrase precede the stimulus word.[77] Gladstone and Siegenthaler reported that slightly poorer discrimination scores are obtained when a carrier phrase is deleted.[79]

In the interest of reducing overall test time and for the purpose of improving test standardization, McLennan and Knox proposed a technique that provided for subject-controlled delivery of the speech signal.[78] This free operant system did not employ a carrier phrase since the self-initiating delivery was thought to suffice as a preparatory set. When this technique was compared to the conventional test presentation procedure that employed the carrier phrase, no difference in word discrimination scores was obtained. Further, most of the listeners in this study expressed a preference for the free operant technique. Such a technique appears to have clinical promise.

Another important consideration for the audiologist is determining what intensity level is most appropriate for administering a speech discrimination test. Of course, one's objective is to estimate the listener's maximum ability to understand speech—often referred to as the "PB-max" when phonetically balanced monosyllabic materials are used. The only true means of obtaining a best speech discrimination score is to administer a performance-intensity function. That is, several lists should be presented at successively higher intensity levels. However, such a procedure is clinically impractical, and clinicians instead attempt to estimate maximum discrimination ability from just one intensity level presentation, usually 40-dB SL for monosyllabic words. It is important to note that the intensity needed to yield a maximum discrimination score varies depending on the test material to be used. The variations in scores that may occur as a function of material are illustrated in Figure 39–11. For example, note that when using the CCT, an intensity presentation of 50-dB SL is required to achieve a maximum score,[68] whereas only a 25-dB SL is needed to reach a best score with the original recordings of W-22 materials.

Many audiologists favor using a MCL level for presenting speech discrimination tests. However, such a procedure does not generally yield a maximum speech discrimination score among hearing impaired listeners. Clemis and Carver were among the first to report that MCL did not guarantee a maximum discrimination score.[80] In a study using patients with Meniere's disease, the authors noted that none of the subjects received a PB-max at his or her reported comfortable loudness setting. In support of these findings, Ullrich and Grimm noted that only three of ten sensorineurally impaired listeners achieved maximum discrimination at an MCL level.[81] The remaining seven subjects yielded discrimination scores at the MCL setting that was 16 to 28 percent poorer than scores achieved at higher intensity. Needless to say, it is almost impossible to determine a maximum discrimination score if only one presentation level is employed.

Ideally, it is recommended that the clinician administer the discrimination test at two or three successively higher intensity levels if time permits. Understandably, however, such a practice is simply not always practical in the clinical milieu; and sometimes the clinician has to select one intensity level presentation for estimating the PB-max.

Auditor Bias

The most common practice of scoring the responses of a speech discrimination test is for the clinician to judge whether the listener's verbal response was correct or in error.[50] However, several investigators have reported that an auditor bias may be present if verbal responses are employed. For example, Merrell and Atkinson studied the effects of verbal versus written responses of a hearing impaired subject using a 25-member panel of normal hearers.[82] When using verbal responses, the range of discrimination scores based on the different auditors' perception of the words was from 14 to 21 percent. Further, the auditors definitely tended to err in favor of accepting incorrect verbal responses. Hence Merrell and Atkinson recommended obtaining a written response from the listener in an effort to obtain a more reliable speech discrimination score. Other investigations have since offered support for the findings of Merrell and Atkinson.[83,84] Disarno and McGinnis also reported numerous examiner errors when sound field discrimination testing was conducted in a background of competing noise.[85]

Thus it is apparent that auditor bias is a variable that can affect the result of the discrimination test significantly. If the subject is able and if time permits, a written response should be employed in an effort to minimize this effect.

Abbreviated Discrimination Tests

Several attempts have been made to shorten some of the present discrimination tests in an effort to reduce the overall evaluation time. Although the concept of abbreviating discrimination tests has been surrounded with controversy, some of the proposed modifications have gained widespread usage in the clinical setting.

Perhaps the most popular technique for abbreviating discrimination tests is the use of 25-word half lists rather than the customary 50-word full lists. According to the survey on audiometric practice by Martin and Forbis, it is common for clinicians to use only 25 words.[50] A review of the literature on split-half reliability with word discrimination tests suggests that half lists can be used for the measurement of speech discrimination in both normal hearers[74,86–90] and sensorineurally impaired listeners[89,91] with good assurance that the score does not differ significantly from the full-list score. Opposition to half-list testing has been made on the basis that spuriously high correlations occur since the subtest score is part of the whole list score.[92,93] Clinicians have also argued that the use of 25-word tests alters the phonetic balance of the list.[92,94] However, the justification for maintaining phonemic balancing has been contested.[95]

Several studies have questioned the validity of using half-list discrimination tests. Jirsa et al examined split-half reliability for the CID W-22 and NU-6 word discrimination tests in normal hearers and sensorineurally impaired listeners.[96] They concluded that the results did not support the use of 25-word lists.

Schwartz et al examined the use of half-lists for the NU-6 and the MRHT as a function of P:S ratio with broad-band noise (white) in normal hearing listeners.[97] Even though the statistical analysis supported half-list testing, it was noted that the wide dispersions among the individual data discouraged the use of half-list measures in the background of noise—at least for normal listeners. In their study, the authors noted that over one-third of the individual discrimination scores achieved between the first and second half lists exceeded 10 percent.

Finally, Edgerton et al examined the usefulness of half lists in the hearing aid selection process.[98] In support of Schwartz et al,[97] they found that for many subjects individual differences between half-list scores were 10 percent or more. They concluded that the practice of using half lists in the hearing aid selection was not justified.

In addition to the half-list testing, other attempts have been proffered for the express purpose of decreasing the evaluation time. In 1974, Rose developed a ten-word discrimination test that could be used as a screening tool in determining whether to administer the half or full list.[99] Briefly, ten words from the CID W-22 lists A and B were selected on the basis of the frequency of errors made by a large group of sensorineurally impaired subjects. According to Rose, if a subject failed to miss the first ten words, then there was no need to continue presenting the remaining words in the list. That is, if a listener was able to respond correctly to the ten most difficult words in the list, there was a high probability that the listener would experience no problems with the remaining easier words. If one or more of the ten words were missed, however, the examiner would continue with the remaining words in the half or full list. My experience with NU-6 materials would suggest that a ten-word test such as that described by Rose has merit as a screening tool in the clinic and can save valuable time.

Another approach to shortening the discrimination test procedure was proffered by Lynn.[100] In a pilot study, Lynn proposed pairing the words from the entire 50 words in the list, thus administering two words following each carrier phrase. Using only ten normal hearers and ten subjects with hearing impairment, Lynn noted that a paired-word presentation produced essentially the same score as a 50-word presentation.[100] Stach conducted a follow-up investigation of the paired-word presentation concept using NU-6 materials on both normal hearers and sensorineurally impaired listeners.[101] Preliminary data lend further support to the use of paired-word delivery in discrimination testing.

Because of the time involved in the delivery of 50-word stimulus items, efforts have been made to reduce or shorten the current tests. If it is necessary for the clinician to reduce evaluation time, it appears that the ten-word screening device or the paired-word delivery test has greater clinical merit than using 25-word lists. The clinician is cautioned, however, that test variability increases considerably as the number of test items is reduced.[102]

Adverse Listening Conditions

There are known limitations associated with the assessment of speech discrimination ability in a quiet environment. First, clinicians know that many of the available speech discrimination tests fail to differentiate among hearing impaired listeners when administered in a quiet test condition. That is, the tests simply do not appear difficult enough to identify the discrimination problems experienced by many listeners with hearing loss. Second, such a testing condition does not reflect adequately the typical environment usually encountered under everyday listening situations.

In an attempt to increase the difficulty of the identifying task and to simulate a more realistic listening environment, audiologists have turned to the use of various types of background noises and competing messages in the assessment of speech discrimination. In 1968, Carhart emphasized the need for clinicians to assess discrimination ability under conditions that more closely approximated typical listening situations.[103] Carhart's impressions on this subject can best be summarized by his statement: ". . . once we have developed good methods for measuring a patient's capacity to understand speech under adverse listening conditions we will possess the audiological tools for dealing much more insightfully with his everyday listening problems." Unfortunately, there are no standardized procedures, to date, for assessing discrimination under adverse listening conditions, even though there is an abundance of literature in this area.

I should mention at this point that the speech discrimination data to be discussed herein were all obtained under monaural earphone conditions. That is, the speech and the noise were presented simultaneously to one earphone. Although for audiologists to assess discriminative ability in a sound field setting is common practice, there is a significant dearth of literature dealing with this testing condition.

Although numerous types of background noise have been used in testing for speech discrimination, broad-band noise is probably employed most frequently in the clinical setting because white noise is a common stimulus readily available on most diagnostic audiometers. A review of the data obtained from some representative studies that have employed continuous broad-band noise (P:S = 0) in the presence of monosyllabic materials for normal hearers is summarized in Table 39–1.

It is evident from this table that there is marked variability within and between studies when examining similar materials. Such inconsistencies appear to be a major difficulty in measuring discrimination in the background of noise. The studies that appear in this table all reported large measures of dispersion.

In addition to the large variability seen with speech in noise, there appears to be evidence of a practical effect—at least when using white noise. Tobias noted significant improvements in speech discrimination scores following 25 minutes of practice in a background of white noise.[104] In support of this finding, Sever reported improvement in the retest scores for all noise conditions. Sever noted that some subjects demonstrated as much as 20 percent improvement on the retest condition.[105] More recently, however, Gengel and Miller failed to observe a practice effect when discrimination was assessed in the presence of broad-band noise.[106] Since it is a

TABLE 39–1 Word Recognition Scores in the Presence of White Noise (P:S = 0) From Several Studies

Author(s)	*Test Material*	*x̄ Word Discrimination (%)*	*Range (%)*
Egan[48]	PAL PB 50	40	—
Rupp and Phillips[140]	CID W-22	72	36–92
Keith and Talis[141]	CID W-22	82	(10)
Sever[105]	NU-6	48	30–66
Olsen et al[123]	NU-6	74	56–94

common procedure to use a P:S ratio in the hearing aid selection procedure, the existence of a practice effect could have serious clinical implications. If improvement is noted in word discrimination following the administration of several tests, it would be important to establish whether the improvement was due to the hearing aid or to the effect of practice.

Other types of background noises or competition have been used in speech discrimination tests, including filtered and shaped white noise, modulated white noise, cafeteria noise, and spoken messages (one talker and multitalkers). Although all such background signals are known to degrade the speech signal to various degrees, the problem of variability still exists.

The wide variability of speech performance produced by noise in normal hearers is also evident among sensorineurally impaired listeners—perhaps to an even greater extent. Even so, hearing impaired subjects appear to experience far greater difficulty in the presence of noise and competing messages than does the normal hearer. Hence, by measuring discrimination under adverse listening conditions, the clinician is able to assess more adequately the communicative handicap imposed by a sensorineural disorder.

Intuitively, the underlying basis for measuring discrimination in the presence of a background of competition appears logical. Unfortunately, however, clinicians have concentrated their efforts on testing in quiet conditions, and clinicians still do not have an accepted standardized procedure for measuring reception against competition. Toward this end, there is an important need to develop a standard means for assessing speech performance in the presence of competition that specifies the material, noise type, P:S ratio, and testing procedure.[73]

Hence the audiologist is faced with deciding which of these many clinical strategies are most appropriate in the assessment of speech discrimination. Further, it is important to emphasize that the clinical strategies employed must be considered when interpreting the speech discrimination findings.

For a review of speech materials designed especially for children, the reader is referred elsewhere.[37,73]

Clinical Utilization of Speech Discrimination Tests

Historically, the assessment of speech discrimination has been most commonly used for the purpose of predicting social adequacy, for differentiating among various types of auditory disorders, and for the use in the selection of hearing aids. Various attempts to predict the extent of a handicap from the speech discrimination data have met with limited success, and this topic will therefore not be discussed in this section. Those who wish to review some of the efforts to develop handicap scales are referred to the works of Davis,[107] High et al,[108] Niemeyer,[109] and Silverman et al.[110] Although prediction of social adequacy continues to be in its rudimentary stages, some rather general guidelines for evaluating discriminative ability have been suggested[111] and are shown in Table 39–2.

A more popular application of the speech discrimination tests is their use for differentiating among individuals with auditory pathology. Unfortunately, speech audiometry in its conventional form is limited in diagnostic value. That is, a speech discrimination test administered at only one suprathreshold intensity level does not aid in differentiating among various auditory lesions. This is because of the wide overlap in discrimination scores among different pathologic groups. The problem of overlap is exemplified by the discrimination data shown in Table 39–3. Although mean differences are apparent, the ranges in scores for each etiologic group is extremely large. Even though speech discrimination tests show considerable overlap in performance scores, they can provide a general index of suspicion for peripheral impairments. Some illustrative examples of performance-intensity functions using monosyllabic materials (W-22) typically seen in conductive impairments (2), sensorineural involvements (3 and 4), and retrocochlear lesions (5) are shown in Figure 39–14. A performance-intensity function for a normal hearer (1) is also provided for comparison. One can see that the function for a person with a conductive impairment is similar to that for normal listeners. When the test items are presented at intensities sufficient to overcome the conductive hearing loss, word identification increases at a rate similar to that of the normal hearer until a 100 percent correct level is reached. Subjects with conductive hearing loss generally exhibit word discrimination scores of 90 percent or better unless there is concomitant cochlear involvement. However, individuals with sensorineural

TABLE 39–2 General Guide for Evaluating Word Discrimination

Word Discrimination (%)	*Classification*
90–100	Normal
75–90	Slight difficulty
60–75	Moderate difficulty
50–60	Poor
≤50	Very poor

From Goetzinger CP. Word discrimination testing. In: Katz J, ed. Handbook of clinical audiology. 2nd ed. Baltimore; Williams & Wilkins, 1978: 149.

TABLE 39–3 Mean Word Recognition Scores (NU-6) Obtained in Four Different Etiologic Groups

Diagnosis	*N*	*Ears*	*x̄ Word Discrimination (%)*	*Range (%)*
Sudden deafness	19	19	32	0–100
Meniere's disease	112	136	78	8–100
Acoustic neuroma	71	73	55	0–100
Presbycusis	83	103	94	36–100

involvement frequently exhibit a reduction in the slope of the function such as that seen in Figure 39–14. In curve number 3, note that a PB-max was reached although it was reduced significantly from the PB-max of the normal or conductively impaired listener. Some subjects with sensorineural hearing loss may exhibit a slight decrease in word recognition with increasing intensity once a PB-max has been achieved. An example of this type of function is shown in curve number 4. Note that once the PB-max is reached at approximately 40-dB SL, the word discrimination score declines slightly. Possible explanations for this slight reduction in word discrimination include evidence of loudness recruitment,[112–114] the presence of harmonic distortion,[115] or upward spread of masking.[73]

As noted from curve number 5, considerably greater rollover effects are seen in retrocochlear disorders. In fact, the presence of this dramatic rollover in word discrimination ". . . raises the strong presumption of retrocochlear disorder."[47] Such a finding prompted Jerger and Jerger to advocate the use of PI-PB functions in differential diagnosis.[47] Research by Dirks and co-workers and Bess, Josey, and Humes has confirmed the diagnostic value of the rollover phenomenon in retrocochlear disorders.[116,117]

A criticism often made against the monosyllabic PB words is that they are simply too easy to differentiate effectively between normal and hearing impaired subjects. Such criticism has been made of both the CID W-22 lists[45,56,70,94] and the NU-6 test.[118,119] To illustrate this point, Carhart reported the cumulative distribution of word discrimination scores (W-22) obtained from 170 hearing impaired subjects (Fig. 39–15).[94] These data show that only 3.6 percent of the subjects did not score at least

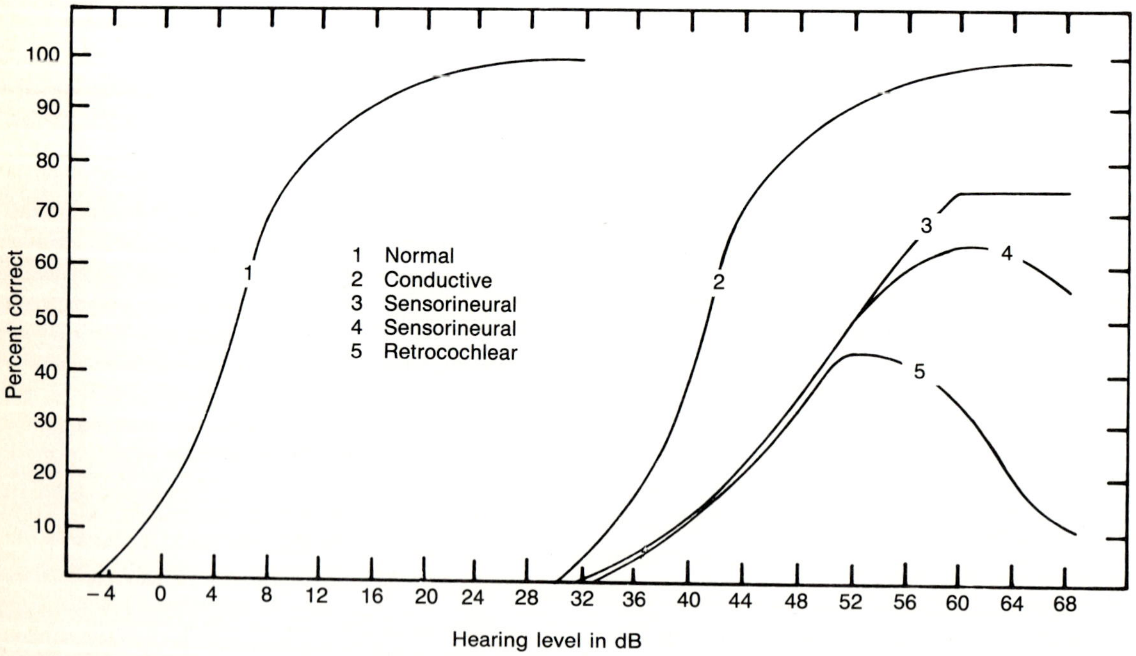

Figure 39–14 Illustrative examples of performance-intensity functions seen with normal hearing, conductive hearing losses, sensorineural impairments, and retrocochlear lesions.

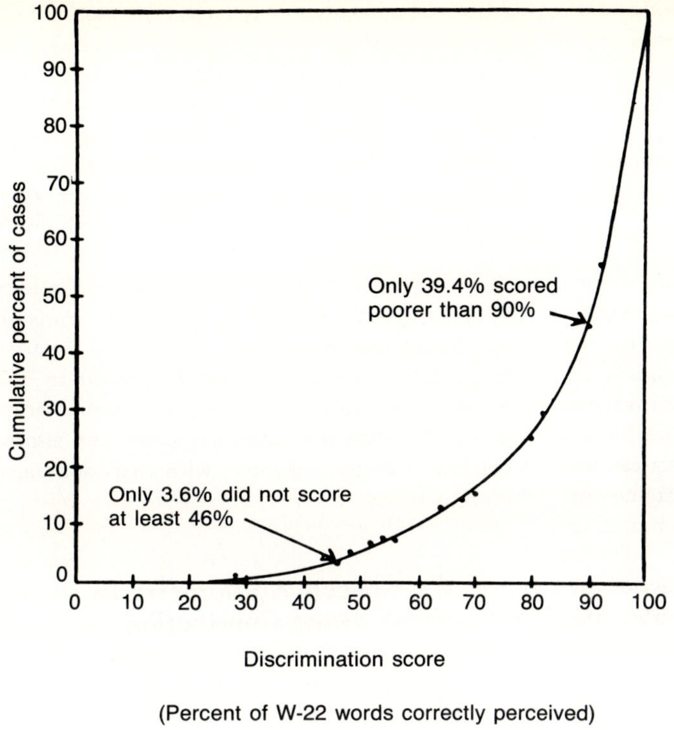

Figure 39-15 Cumulative distribution of word discrimination scores (W-22) obtained from 170 subjects with sensorineural hearing loss. (From Carhart R. Problems in the measurement of speech discrimination. Arch Otolaryngol 1965; 82:203.)

46 percent and that only 39.4 percent attained discrimination scores poorer than 90 percent. Similarly, Walden et al demonstrated the clinical insensitivity of the NU-6 test.[119] Three thousand subjects with high-frequency sensorineural hearing loss were found to yield an average word discrimination score of 97.5 percent. The clinical insensitivity of the NU-6 test has also been demonstrated with subjects displaying flat audiometric configurations.[120]

In an effort to improve the sensitivity of word discrimination tests, attempts have been made to incorporate a background of competing noise. Liden proposed the use of a low-pass filtered white noise, suggesting that it is a sensitive tool for differentiating among hearing impaired listeners.[121] A follow-up study confirmed the improved test sensitivity and also noted increased test-retest reliability.[122]

Olsen and co-workers examined the use of assessing word discrimination in the presence of white noise with various auditory disorders, and they noted that 62 percent of the subjects with retrocochlear lesions demonstrated a marked decrease in word intelligibility; however, 38 percent did not.[123]

Word discrimination tests have also been commonly used in the hearing aid evaluation process since first proposed by Carhart.[124] However, clinicians have strongly argued that speech discrimination tests lack the appropriate sensitivity and also exhibit too much variability to be useful in differentiating among hearing aids.[125,126] Nevertheless, the majority of clinicians continue to employ speech discrimination tests in the hearing aid evaluation procedure.

Masking

In speech audiometry, there exists the possibility of cross over from the test ear to the nontest ear just as it does in pure tone measurements. Consequently, when the level of the speech signal presented to the test ear exceeds the bone conduction threshold of the nontest ear, masking is necessary. Whereas word discrimination is presented at suprathreshold levels, the possibility of cross-level with these tests is even greater than with the SRT. Effective masking levels need to be established for the spoken message. Olsen and Matkin noted that the sound pressure level of broad-band noise must be roughly 20 dB greater than the intensity of the speech in order to mask speech awareness thresholds effectively.[37] Sanders suggested that the effective masking levels for speech be obtained by averaging the effective masking levels for pure tones at 500, 1,000, and 2,000 Hz.[33] Finally, effective levels may be calculated in normal hearers by establishing the level at which speech becomes inaudible for a given amount of noise. For testing the SRT, the plateau method of masking is recommended.[31] For word discrimination testing, Martin has suggested the following: "The effective masking level for the masked ear is equal to the HL at which the discrimination is performed, minus 40 dB for interaural attenuation, plus the largest air-bone gap in the masked ear."[27]

Pure Tone Sensitivity and Speech Test Results

There is a plethora of evidence that demonstrates a close relationship between pure tone information and the speech reception threshold. Several investigators have proposed formulas for relating the pure tone data to speech reception threshold.[127-129] Some of these techniques appear somewhat involved and therefore lack clinical utility. However, Carhart's most recent suggestion seems practical for clinical use.[127] This technique involves averaging the threshold at 500 Hz and 1,000 Hz and subtracting 2 dB.

Some clinicians question the usefulness of the speech reception threshold. As mentioned earlier, the greatest value to measuring the SRT is that it serves as an excellent reliability check for the pure tone test. If a discrepancy between the SRT and two-frequency (500, 1,000 Hz) or three-frequency (500 to 2,000 Hz) pure tone average exceeds 10 dB, there is cause to question the reliability of the test results. When such a condition exists, the possibility of examiner error or a functional hearing problem should be considered. The SRT also has value in the hearing assessment of young children. In some instances when pure tone threshold measurements cannot be performed successfully with younger children, simple speech threshold testing can be conducted. The speech tests can then be used to achieve a rough estimate of hearing sensitivity.

The technique of estimating speech thresholds from the PI-PB function also correlates well with the pure tone average.[46] Such close agreement between the speech threshold and pure tone data was found to be consistent in a large, diverse clinical population (N = 1,267). In those instances when the speech threshold and pure tone average did not agree, such as in sloping and rising configurations, estimated speech threshold was found to correlate with the high-frequency sensitivity levels. This technique of estimating the speech threshold from the performance-intensity function appears to have great clinical utility, particularly for those clinicians who frequently employ performance-intensity functions in their basic audiologic test battery.

Attempts to establish a uniform relationship between pure tone thresholds and speech intelligibility at suprathreshold levels have met with limited success. Hirsh described the situation most appropriately when he stated that "the relationship between the audiogram and discrimination loss is one of the greatest points of ignorance in contemporary audiology."[56] Young and Gibbons investigated the relationship between speech discrimination scores and threshold measurements in a hearing impaired population.[130] These investigators concluded that the relationship is insufficient between speech intelligibility and pure tone thresholds. Similar findings have been reported by Elliot[131] and Ross et al.[132] It also appears that the shape of the audiometric configuration has little to do with discrimination ability. Recall that Walden and co-workers reported a mean discrimination score of 97 percent in 3,000 subjects with high-frequency sensorineural hearing loss.[119] Excellent discrimination scores have also been observed among listeners with flat audiometric configurations.[120]

Speech Audiometry by Bone Conduction

There are several investigators who have advocated the use of bone conduction speech audiometry as part of the basic evaluation.[133–137] The delivery of speech signals through a bone vibrator have been reported to be useful in the assessment of speech thresholds and in testing speech discrimination. Proponents of this technique suggest that bone conducted speech offers several advantages. Assessment of speech by bone conduction is considered useful as a reliability check for the pure tone bone conduction thresholds, as a valuable tool in the evaluation of young children or other difficult-to-test patients, and as a predictor of cochlear reserve after middle ear surgery.

Recent evidence has revealed that the maximum output level of one of the more commonly used bone vibrators (Radioear B-70-A) is 65 to 70 dB HL and in order to keep total harmonic distortion below 10 percent the output limit should not exceed 55 dB HL.[138] Despite some evidence to the contrary, the usefulness of bone conduction speech discrimination seems rather limited when one considers the output capabilities of bone conduction vibrators. However, measurement of speech reception thresholds by bone conduction can be of value if the clinician is aware of and tests within the limits of the vibrator.

SUMMARY

Bunch could not have foreseen the tremendous growth that audiology would experience in the years following his seminal publication of *Clinical Audi-*

ometry.[1] A significant area of growth has been the refinement of old techniques and the development of new procedures for evaluating auditory function. This chapter has focused on those techniques most commonly employed in basic hearing measurement. Pure tone measurement continues to be the focal point of the hearing evaluation. This time-honored assessment procedure has multiple applications, as outlined in this chapter, and there is essentially no substitute for its use. The development of speech audiometry has proved to be a valuable adjunct to pure tone measures. Unfortunately, however, there are still numerous limitations in the present methods for measuring discrimination ability. Of particular concern is the clinical insensitivity of commonly used discrimination tests and the apparent wide variability produced by using a noise background. Thus there seems to be an important need to develop new methods for assessing a hearing impaired person's ability to understand speech. Two specific areas of need noted by Jerger are (1) defining in more detail the discrimination problems of the hearing impaired and (2) developing new appropriate instruments to identify these problems.[139]

REFERENCES

1. Bunch CC. Clinical audiometry. St. Louis: CV Mosby, 1943.
2. Metz O. The acoustic impedance measured on normal and pathological ears. Acta Otolaryngol 1946 (Suppl); 63:1–254.

2a. Hughes, DE. On an induction-current balance and experimental researches made therewith. Proc R Soc London 1879; 29:56–65.

3. Richardson RW. Some researches with Professor Hughes' new instrument for the measurement of hearing: the audiometer. Proc R Soc London 1879; 29:65–70.
4. Fellendorf GW. Bell's audiometer. Am Speech Hear Assoc 1976; 18:563–565.
5. Sivian LJ, White SD. On minimum audible sound fields. J Acoust Soc Am 1933; 4:288–321.
6. Beasley WC. National health survey hearing study series. Bulletin No. 5. Washington: United States Public Health Service, 1938.
7. Katz J. Handbook of Clinical Audiology, 3rd ed. Baltimore: Williams & Wilkins, 1985.

7a. Jerger J. A proposed audiometric symbol system for scholarly publications. Arch Otolaryngol 1976; 102:33–36.

8. Davis H, Silverman RS. Hearing and deafness, 3rd ed. New York: Holt, Rinehart & Winston, 1970.
9. Goodman A. Reference zero levels for pure-tone audiometer. Am Speech Hearing Assoc 1965; 7:262–263.
10. Kemker FJ. Classifications of auditory impairment. In: Glasscock ME, ed. Sensorineural hearing loss in children: early detection and intervention. Otolaryngol Clin North Am 1975; 8:3–17.
11. Quigley SP, Thomure FE. Some effects of hearing impairment upon school performance. Springfield, IL: Illinois Office of Education, 1968.
12. Bess FH, ed. Unilateral sensorineural hearing loss in children. Ear Hear 1986; 7.
13. Bess FH, Tharpe AM. Unilateral hearing impairment in children. Pediatrics 1984; 15:206–216.
14. Downs MP. The expanding imperatives of early identification. In: Bess FH, ed. Childhood deafness: causation, assessment and management. New York: Grune & Stratton, 1977: 95.
15. Kryter KD. Impairment to hearing from exposure to noise. J Acoust Soc Am 1973; 53:1211–1234.
16. Bess FH. The minimally hearing impaired child. Ear Hear 1985; 6:43–47.
17. Tonndorf J. Bone-conduction. In: Keidel WD, Neff WD, eds. Handbook of Sensory Physiology. Vol. VI. Part 3. New York: Karger, 1976: 37.
18. Dirks D. Bone-conduction testing. In: Katz J, ed. Handbook of Clinical Audiology. 3rd ed. Baltimore: Williams & Wilkins, 1985: 202.
19. Johansen H. Relation of audiograms to the impedance formula. Acta Otolaryngol 1948; Suppl 74.
20. Shambaugh GE. Surgery of the Ear. 2nd ed. Philadelphia: WB Saunders, 1967.
21. Carhart R, Jerger JF. Preferred method for clinical determination of pure-tone thresholds. J Speech Hear Disord 1959; 24:330–345.
22. American Speech and Hearing Association. Guidelines for manual pure-tone audiometry. Asha 1978; 20:297–301.
23. Wilber LA. Calibration, pure tone, speech and noise signals. In: Katz J, ed. Handbook of Clinical Audiology. 3rd ed. Baltimore: Williams & Wilkins, 1985: 116.
24. Pollack, T. The atonal interval. J Acoust Soc Am 1948; 20:146–149.
25. Steinberg JC, Munson WA. Deviations in the loudness judgements of 100 people. J Acoust Soc Am 1936; 8:71–80.
26. Dirks D. Bone-conduction measurements. In: Jerger J, ed. Modern developments in audiology. 2nd ed. New York: Academic Press, 1973: 1.
27. Martin FN. Introduction to audiology. Englewood Cliffs, NJ: Prentice-Hall, 1975.
28. Sanders JW, Rintelmann WF. Masking in audiometry; a clinical evaluation of three methods. Arch Otolaryngol 1964; 80:541–556.
29. Studebaker GA. On masking in bone-conduction testing. J Speech Hear Res 1962; 5:215–227.
30. Naunton RF. A masking dilemma in bilateral conduction deafness. Arch Otolaryngol 1960; 72:753–757.
31. Hood JD. Principles and practice of bone conduction audiometry. Laryngoscope 1960; 70:1211–1228.
32. Goldstein BA, Newman GW. Clinical masking: a decision-making process. In: Katz J, ed. Handbook of clinical audiology. 3rd ed. Baltimore: Williams & Wilkins, 1985: 170.
33. Sanders JW. Masking. In: Katz J, ed. Handbook of clinical audiology. 2nd ed. Baltimore: Williams & Wilkins, 1978: 124.
34. American Standards Association. American National Standards Specifications for audiometers. S3.6-1969. ANSI: New York, 1970.
35. Hughson W, Thompson EA. Correlation of hearing acuity for speech with discrete frequency audiograms. Arch Otolaryngol 1942; 36:526–540.
36. Hudgins CV, Hawkins JE Jr, Karlin JE, Stevens SS. The development of recorded auditory tests for measuring hearing loss for speech. Laryngoscope 1947; 57:57–89.
37. Olsen WO, Matkin ND. Speech audiometry. In: Rintelmann WF, ed. Hearing assessment. Baltimore: University Park Press, 1979.
38. Hirsh IJ, Davis H, Silverman SR, Reynolds EG, Eldert E, Bensen RW. Development of materials for speech audiometry. J Speech Hear Disord 1952; 17:321–337.
39. Beattie RC, Edgerton BJ, Svihovec DV. An investigation of the auditec of the St. Louis recordings of Central Institute for the Deaf spondees. J Am Aud Soc 1975; 1:97–101.
40. Bowling LS, Elpern BS. Relative intelligibility of items on CID Auditory Test W-1. J Aud Res 1961; 1:152–157.

41. Conn M, Dancer J, Ventry IM. A spondee list for determining speech reception threshold without prior familiarization. J Speech Hear Disord 1975; 40:388–396.
42. Curry ET, Cox BP. The relative intelligibility of spondees. J Aud Res 1966; 6:419–424.
43. McLauchlin RW, Rosenblatt R, Rupp RR. The relative intelligibility of an expanded list of spondaic words. Michigan Speech Hear J 1973; 7:43–49.
44. American Speech and Hearing Association Committee on Audiometric Evaluation. Guidelines for determining threshold level for speech. Asha 1977; 19:241–243.
45. Tillman TW, Olsen WO. Speech audiometry. In: Jerger J, ed. Modern developments in audiology. 2nd ed. New York: Academic Press, 1973: 37.
46. Jerger S, Jerger J. Estimating speech threshold from the PI-PB function. Arch Otolaryngol 1976; 102:487–496.
47. Jerger J, Jerger S. Diagnostic significance of PB word functions. Arch Otolaryngol 1971; 93:573–580.
48. Egan J. Articulation testing methods. Laryngoscope 1948; 58:955–991.
49. Dewey G. Relative frequency of English speech sounds. Cambridge: Harvard University Press, 1923.
50. Martin FN, Forbis NK. The present status of audiometric practice: a follow-up study. Asha 1978; 20:531–541.
51. Lehiste I, Peterson GE. Linguistic considerations in the study of speech intelligibility. J Acoust Soc Am 1959; 31:280–286.
52. Thorndike EL, Lorge I. The teacher's word book of 30,000 words. New York: Columbia University Press 1944, 1952.
53. Peterson GE, Lehiste I. Revised CNC lists for auditory tests. J Speech Hear Disord 1962; 27:62–70.
54. Tillman TW, Carhart R, Wilber L. A test for speech discrimination composed of CNC monosyllabic words. Northwestern University Auditory Test No. 4. Technical Documentary Report No. SAM-TDR-62-135, 1963, USAF School of Aerospace Medicine, Brooks Air Force Base, Texas.
55. Tillman TW, Carhart R. An expanded test for speech discrimination utilizing CNC monosyllabic words. Northwestern University Auditory Test No. 6. Technical Report No. SAM-TR-66-55, 1966, USAF School of Aerospace Medicine, Brooks Air Force Base, Texas.
56. Hirsh IJ. The measurement of hearing. New York: McGraw-Hill, 1952.
57. Beattie RC, Edgerton BJ, Svihovec DV. A comparison of the auditec of St. Louis cassette recordings of NU-6 and CID W-22 on a normal hearing population. J Speech Hear Disord 1977; 42:60–64.
58. Kruel EJ, Nixon JC, Kryter KD, Bell DW, Lang JS, Schubert ED. A proposed clinical test of speech discrimination. J Speech Hear Res 1968; 11:536–552.
59. Fairbanks G. Test of phonemic differentiation: the rhyme test. J Acoust Soc Am 1958; 30:596–600.
60. House AS, Williams CE, Hecker MHL, Kryter KD. Articulation testing methods. Consonantal differentiation in a closed-response set. J Acoust Soc Am 1965; 37:158–166.
61. Owens E, Schubert ED. Development of the California consonant test. J Speech Hear Res 1977; 20:463–474.
62. Schubert ED, Owens E. CVC words as test items. J Aud Res 1971; 11:88–100.
63. Black JW. Multiple-choice intelligibility tests. J Speech Hear Disord 1957; 22:213–235.
64. Griffiths JD. Rhyming minimal contrasts: a simplified diagnostic articulation test. J Acoust Soc Am 1967; 42:236–241.
65. Pederson OT, Studebaker GA. A new minimal contrasts closed-response-set speech test. J Aud Res 1972; 12:187–195.
66. Schultz MD, Schubert ED. A multiple choice discrimination test (MCDT). Laryngoscope 1969; 79:382–399.
67. Kopra LL, Blosser D, Waldron DL. Comparison of Fairbanks rhyme test and CID auditory test W-22 in normal and hearing-impaired listeners. J Speech Hear Res 1968; 11:735–739.
68. Schwartz DM, Surr R. Three experiments on the California consonant test. J Speech Hear Disord 1979; 44:61–72.
69. Levitt H, Resnick SB. Speech reception by the hearing impaired; methods of testing and the development of new tests. In: Ludzigsen C, Barfod J, eds. Sensorineural hearing impaired and hearing aids. Scand Audiol 1978; Suppl 6: 107–130.
70. Silverman SR, Hirsh IJ. Problems related to the use of speech in clinical audiometry. Ann Otol Rhinol Laryngol 1955; 64:1234–1244.
71. Speaks C, Jerger J. Method for measurement of speech identification. J Speech Hear Res 1965; 8:185–194.
72. Kalikow DN, Stevens KN, Elliot LL. Development of a test of speech intelligibility in noise using sentence materials with controlled word predictability. J Acoust Soc Am 1977; 61:1337–1351.
73. Bess FH. Clinical assessment of speech recognition. In: Konkle DF, Rintelmann WF, eds. Principles of speech audiometry. Baltimore: University Park Press, 1983: 127.
74. Resnick DM. Reliability of the twenty-five word phonetically balanced lists. J Aud Res 1962; 2:5–12.
75. Brandy WT. Reliability of voice tests of speech discrimination. J Speech Hear Res 1966; 9:461–465.
76. Penrod JP, Price LL. Variability of sensorineural impaired adults during clinical word discrimination testing. Paper presented at the Annual American Speech and Hearing Association Convention, Chicago, 1977.
77. Martin FN, Hawkins RR, Bailey HAT. The non-essentiality of the carrier phrase in phonetically balanced (PB) word testing. J Aud Res 1962; 2:319–322.
78. McLennan RO Jr, Knox AW. Patient controlled delivery of monosyllabic words in a test of auditory discrimination. J Speech Hear Disord 1975; 40:538–543.
79. Gladstone VS, Siegenthaler BM. Carrier phrase and speech intelligibility score. J Aud Res 1971; 11:101–103.
80. Clemis JD, Carver WF. Discrimination scores for speech in Menieres disease. Arch Otolaryngol 1967; 86:614–618.
81. Ullrich K, Grimm D. Most comfortable listening level presentation versus maximum discrimination for word discrimination material. Audiology 1976; 15:338–347.
82. Merrell HB, Atkinson CJ. The effect of selected variables upon discrimination scores. J Aud Res 1965; 5:285–292.
83. Lovrinic JH, Burgi EJ, Curry ET. A comparative evaluation of five speech discrimination measures. J Speech Hear Res 1968; 11:372–381.
84. Nelson DA, Chaiklin JB. Writedown versus talkback scoring and scoring bias in speech discrimination testing. J Speech Hear Res 1970; 13:645–654.
85. Disarno NJ, McGinnis MS. Variability of examiner error in speech discrimination testing in noise. Paper presented at the Annual American Speech and Hearing Association Convention, Chicago, 1977.
86. Burke KS, Shutts RE, King WP. Range of difficulty of four Harvard phonetically balanced word lists. Laryngoscope 1965; 75:289–296.
87. Elpern B. The relative stability of half list and full list discrimination tests. Laryngoscope 1961; 71:30–36.
88. Manning WH, Shaw CK, Maki JE, Beasley DS. Analysis of half-list scores on the PBK-50 as a function of time compression and age. J Am Aud Soc 1975; 3:109–111.
89. Rintelmann WF, Schumaier DR, Jetty AJ, Burchfield SA, Beasley DS, Mosher NA, Mosher RA, Penley ED. Six experiments on speech discrimination utilizing CNC monosyllables. J Aud Res 1974; 2(Suppl):1–30.
90. Shutts R, Burke K, Creston J. Derivation of twenty-five word PB lists. J Speech Hear Disord 1964; 29:442–477.

91. Campanelli PA. A measure of intra-list stability of four PAL word lists. J Aud Res 1962; 2:50–55.
92. Grubb, P. A phonemic analysis of half-list speech discrimination tests. J Speech Hear Res 1963; 6:271–276.
93. Grubb P. Some considerations in the use of half list speech discrimination tests. J Speech Hear Res 1963; 6:294–297.
94. Carhart R. Problems in the measurement of speech discrimination. Arch Otolaryngol 1965; 82:253–260.
95. Tobias J. On phonemic analysis of speech discrimination tests. J Speech Hear Res 1964; 7:95–102.
96. Jirsa RE, Hodgson WR, Goetzinger CP. Unreliability of half-list discrimination tests. J Am Aud Soc 1975; 2:47–49.
97. Schwartz DM, Bess FH, Larson VD. Split half reliability of two word discrimination tests as a function of primary-to-secondary ratio. J Speech Hear Disord 1979; 42:440–445.
98. Edgerton BJ, Klodd DA, Beattie RC. Half-list speech discrimination measures in hearing aid evaluations. Arch Otolaryngol 1978; 104:669–672.
99. Rose DE. A 10-word speech discrimination screening test. Paper presented at the Annual American Speech and Hearing Association Convention, Las Vegas, November 4–6, 1974.
100. Lynn G. Paired PB-50 discrimination test. A preliminary report. J Aud Res 1962; 2:34–36.
101. Stach B. Master's Thesis, Vanderbilt University, 1979.
102. Thornton AR, Raffin MJM. Speech-discrimination scores modeled as a binomial variable. J Speech Hear Res 1978; 21:507–518.
103. Carhart R. Future horizons in audiological diagnosis. Ann Otol Rhinol Laryngol 1968; 77:706–716.
104. Tobias JV. Effect of practice on intelligibility of masked speech. Paper presented at the 85th meeting of the Acoustical Society of America, Boston, 1973.
105. Sever J. Speech discrimination in normal hearing individuals under adverse listening conditions. Master's Thesis, Central Michigan University, 1973.
106. Gengel RW, Miller LS. A clinical pass/fail criteria for word discrimination in noise. Paper presented at the Annual American Speech and Hearing Association Convention, Houston, 1976.
107. Davis H. The articulation area and social adequacy index for hearing. Laryngoscope 1948; 58:761–778.
108. High WS, Fairbanks G, Glorig A. Scale for self-assessment of hearing handicap. J Speech Hear Disord 1964; 29:215–230.
109. Niemeyer W. Speech audiometry with phonetically balanced sentences. Int Aud 1965; 4:97–101.
110. Silverman SR, Thurlow WR, Walsh TE, Davis H. Improvement in the social adequacy index of hearing following the fenestration operation. Laryngoscope 1948; 58:607–631.
111. Goetzinger CP. Word discrimination testing. In: Katz J, ed. Handbook of clinical audiology. 2nd ed. Baltimore: Williams & Wilkins, 1978: 149.
112. Hedgecock LC. The measurement of auditory recruitment. Arch Otolaryngol 1955; 62:515–527.
113. Huizing HC, Reyntjes JA. Recruitment and speech discrimination loss. Laryngoscope 1952; 62:521–527.
114. Schultz MD, Streepy CS. The speech discrimination function in loudness recruiting ears. Laryngoscope 1967; 77:2114–2127.
115. Yantis PA, Millin JP, Shapiro I. Speech discrimination in sensorineural hearing loss: two experiments on the role of intensity. J Speech Hear Res 1966; 9:178–193.
116. Bess FH, Josey AF, Humes LE. Performance intensity functions in cochlear and eighth nerve disorders. Am J Otol 1979; 1:27–31.
117. Dirks DD, Kamm C, Bower D, Bettsworth A. Use of performance intensity functions for diagnosis. J Speech Hear Disord 1977; 42:408–415.
118. Edgerton BJ, Danhauer JL. Clinical implications of speech discrimination testing using nonsense stimuli. Baltimore: University Park Press, 1979.
119. Walden BE, Prosek RA, Worthington DW. The prevalence of hearing loss within selected vs. army branches. Final Report Interagency No. IAO 4757. U.S. Army Medical Research and Development Command, Washington, 1975.
120. Bess FH, Townsend TH. Word discrimination for listeners with flat sensorineural hearing losses. J Speech Hear Disord 1977; 42:232–237.
121. Liden G. Undistorted speech audiometry. In: Graham AB, ed. Sensorineural hearing processes and disorders. Boston: Little, Brown, 1967: 339.
122. Cohen RL, Keith RW. Use of low-pass noise in word recognition. J Speech Hear Res 1976; 19:48–54.
123. Olsen WO, Noffsinger D, Kurdziel S. Speech discrimination in quiet and in white noise by patients with peripheral and central lesions. Acta Otolaryngol 1975; 80:375–382.
124. Carhart R. Tests for selection of hearing aids. Laryngoscope 1946; 56:780–794.
125. Shore I, Bilger RC, Hirsh IJ. Hearing aid evaluation: reliability of repeat measurements. J Speech Hear Disord 1960; 25:152–170.
126. Schwartz DM, Walden BE. Speech audiometry and hearing aid assessment: a reappraisal of an old philosophy. In: Konkle DF, Rintlemann WF, eds. Principles of speech audiometry. Baltimore: University Park Press, 1983: 321.
127. Carhart R, Porter LS. Audiometric configuration and prediction of threshold for spondees. J Speech Hear Res 1971; 14:486–495.
128. Harris JD, Haines HL, Myers CK. A new formula for using the audiogram to predict speech hearing loss. Arch Otolaryngol 1956; 63:158–176, 64:477.
129. Quiggle RR, Glorig A, Delk JH, Summerfield AB. Predicting hearing loss for speech from pure tone audiograms. Laryngoscope 1957; 67:1–15.
130. Young MA, Gibbons EW. Speech discrimination scores and threshold measurements in a non-normal hearing population. J Aud Res 1962; 2:21–33.
131. Elliot LL. Prediction of speech discrimination scores from other test information. J Aud Res 1963; 3:35–45.
132. Ross M, Huntington DA, Newby HA, Nixon RF. Speech discrimination of hearing impaired individuals in noise: its relationship to other audiometric parameters. J Aud Res 1965; 5:47–72.
133. Goetzinger CP, Proud GO. Speech audiometry by bone conduction. Arch Otolaryngol 1955; 62:632–635.
134. Hahlbrock K. Bone conduction speech audiometry. J Int Audiol 1962; 1:186–188.
135. Hoople G, Bradley WA. A practical method for assessing cochlear reserve. Trans Am Acad Ophthalmol Otolaryngol 1964; 68:70–73.
136. Kasden SD, Robinson M. Bone conduction speech discrimination in different pathologies. J Aud Res 1973; 13:268–270.
137. Robinson M, Kasden S. Bone conduction speech audiometry: a calibrated method to predict post-stapedectomy discrimination scores. Ann Otol Rhinol Laryngol 1970; 79:818–824.
138. Barry SJ, Gaddis S. Physical and physiological constraints on the use of bone-conduction speech audiometry. J Speech Hear Disord 1978; 43:220–226.
138. Beasley WC. National health survey hearing study series. Bulletin No. 5. Washington: U.S. Public Health Service, 1938.
139. Jerger J. Research priorities in auditory science—the au-

diologist's view. Paper presented at the scientific dedication conference, Boys Town Institute for Communication Disorders in Children, Omaha, Nebraska, October 5 and 6, 1978.
140. Rupp RR, Phillips D. The effect of noise background on speech discrimination function in normal hearing individuals. J Aud Res 1969; 9:60–63.
141. Keith R, Talis H. The effects of white noise on PB scores of normal and hearing impaired listeners. Audiology 1972; 11:177–186.

40 Diagnostic Audiology

Jay W. Sanders, Ph.D.

Diagnostic audiology is the advanced psychoacoustic and electrophysiologic study of impaired auditory response. Of course, all audiometric assessments, from pure tone air conduction threshold measurement to electric response audiometry, can be viewed as diagnostic in that any and all audiometric responses can provide information of value in the determination of the nature and cause of an auditory disorder. Generally, however, the term "diagnostic audiology" has been reserved for specialized procedures beyond the conventional pure tone and speech tests used to quantify a hearing loss. The special tests used in diagnostic audiology are qualitative rather than quantitative; that is, emphasis is on the nature of the response rather than on the degree of hearing loss. One product of this advanced study of auditory function is a determination of the site of the lesion in the auditory system—valuable information to the physician in the diagnosis of the problem. The audiologist does not diagnose the disorder, since diagnosis of a medical problem is the province of the physician; rather the audiologist seeks to understand aberrant auditory behavior and in so doing is able to provide diagnostic information. Ideally, the physician and the audiologist study the hearing disorder together, each applying his or her expertise and each sharing findings with the other to achieve a more complete management of the complex problem of hearing loss.

Because diagnostic audiology includes assessment of the system from pinna to cortex, some delineation is necessary. Procedures for determination and evaluation of conductive hearing loss, including immittance study of the middle ear, are regarded as part of the basic hearing evaluation and are included in the chapters devoted to that aspect of auditory assessment (see Chapters 39 and 41). Audiologic methods for the evaluation of lesions in the central nervous system are also considered separately (see Chapter 44). This chapter on diagnostic audiology is confined to the study of sensorineural hearing loss resulting from impairment in the peripheral auditory system and thus is concerned with the effects on auditory response of lesions of the cochlea and the eighth cranial nerve.

THE CLASSIC DIAGNOSTIC TEST BATTERY

During the 1950s and early 1960s, largely through the work of James Jerger and his associates at Northwestern University and stemming from a landmark study of diagnostic audiology by Dix, Hallpike, and Hood in 1948,[1] a series of qualitative audiometric tests was developed, all directed toward distinguishing between cochlear and retrocochlear sites of lesions in sensorineural hearing impairment. The tests were designed to investigate auditory response in two areas—suprathreshold loudness and auditory adaptation. Through experimental study and clinical usage, the tests came to constitute a battery of diagnostic procedures, including tests for loudness recruitment, differential sensitivity for intensity, and abnormal auditory adaptation.

Loudness Recruitment

The concept of diagnostic auditory testing in patients with sensorineural hearing loss had its origin in the discovery of an auditory response that came to be called "loudness recruitment" and in the significance of the response in understanding the nature of sensorineural impairment. Further special tests that became part of the diagnostic battery were developed either as alternative methods of testing for recruitment or as supplements to the recruitment test.

Recruitment

Loudness recruitment is a particular kind of suprathreshold loudness response observed in certain ears with sensorineural hearing loss. It differs in nature from the response in certain other ears with sensorineural loss and in ears with normal hearing or conductive loss. The recruitment phenomenon was first described in 1924 by Pohlman and Kranz, who found that stimuli at suprathreshold levels appeared to have normal loudness in some impaired ears.[2] Four years later, Fowler noted that an experience of equal loudness in both ears at a suprathreshold level could be achieved by some patients with unilateral hearing loss, but with a greater sensation level in the normal ear.[3] On the basis of this observation, Fowler developed a direct test for the response in 1936,[4] and in 1937 he coined the term "recruitment" for what appeared to be a more rapid growth of loudness in the impaired ear.[5] Since that time the following definition of recruitment has evolved into a classic: "Recruitment is an abnormally rapid growth of loudness with an increase in intensity." Although the concept of recruitment as an abnormal loudness response has been questioned,[6] the definition has continued to be used widely.

Tests for Recruitment

Fowler's test for recruitment, developed in 1936, was the alternate binaural loudness balance test. Although subsequent studies have proposed various modifications and refinements in methodology,[7–9] the essential procedure remains unchanged. In order to permit a comparison of loudness growth between a normal ear and an impaired ear, a test frequency is selected at which the patient has hearing loss in one ear and normal hearing in the opposite ear. The stimulus is then presented alternately to the two ears. The intensity of the test tone is maintained at a constant level in one ear and varied in the other ear until the tones are at equal loudness in the two ears. A comparison is then made of the sensation levels required for equal loudness. In a nonrecruiting ear, equal loudness is achieved with equal sensation levels. Equal loudness with a significantly smaller sensation level to the impaired ear suggests that loudness has grown more rapidly with an intensity increase in that ear and so indicates the presence of loudness recruitment. Jerger proposed that the alternate binaural loudness balance test results be interpreted according to the following criteria:[8]

1. No recruitment: equal loudness at equal sensation levels plus or minus 10 dB.
2. Complete recruitment: equal loudness at equal hearing levels plus or minus 10 dB.
3. Partial recruitment: equal loudness at sensation levels between those for no recruitment and complete recruitment.

The range of plus or minus 10 dB around the ideal result was suggested as a margin for error of measurement.

A fourth possible result on the alternate binaural loudness balance test, not included in Jerger's descriptive categories of no recruitment, partial recruitment, and complete recruitment, was demonstrated in 1948 by Dix, Hallpike, and Hood.[1] That result has come to be known as "decruitment," an abnormally slow growth of loudness with an increase in intensity. Decruitment, found by Dix et al in a patient with an acoustic tumor, is shown on the alternate binaural loudness balance test when the sensation level in the poor ear is significantly greater than that in the good ear: the opposite of a recruitment result. In subsequent studies, decruitment has generally been found in some patients with impairment of the eighth nerve, and it suggests a transmission loss in the impaired nerve.[10–14]

A second loudness balance test for recruitment was described by Reger, also in 1936.[15] Fowler's binaural test is limited to patients with unilateral hearing loss since it requires loudness balancing between an impaired ear and a normal ear. Reger's test, a monaural procedure, uses the loudness balance method to compare loudness growth between two test frequencies in the same ear: one frequency at which hearing is impaired and one at which hearing is normal. Since sensorineural impairment often produces a bilaterally symmetrical high frequency loss with normal hearing in the lower frequencies, the Reger test extended loudness balance testing to many patients for whom the alternate binaural loudness balance test could not be used. The Reger test has come to be known as the monaural loudness balance or the monaural bifrequency loudness balance test.

The results of the loudness balance tests for recruitment are interpreted through a comparison of the sensation levels and hearing levels required in the two ears (alternate binaural loudness balance test) or at the two frequencies (monaural bifrequency loudness balance test) for equal loudness. These results can be shown graphically either on Fowler's laddergram[4] or on a loudness growth function described by Steinberg and Gardner.[16] Figure 40–1 illustrates the laddergram method in four cases. In each case, hearing was normal (0 dB hearing threshold level) in the left ear and impaired (45 dB hearing threshold level) in the right ear. The test signal was presented to the right ear at fixed sensation levels of 20, 40, and 60 dB and then varied in intensity in the left ear to achieve equal loudness. Case A in the figure illustrates no recruitment, in that equal loudness is achieved at equal sensation levels. Case B shows partial recruitment; case C shows complete recruitment; and case D shows decruitment. Figure

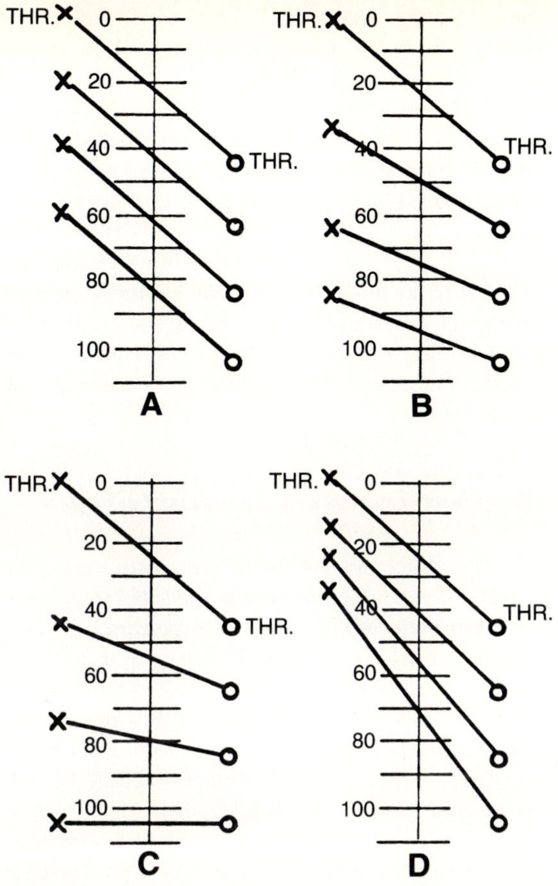

Figure 40–1 Alternate binaural loudness balance test results illustrating, *A*, no recruitment, *B*, partial recruitment, *C*, complete recruitment, and, *D*, decruitment.

40–2 illustrates the loudness growth function method of graphic representation. The solid line is the nonrecruitment result expected from a normal hearer with thresholds in both ears at a 0 dB hearing threshold level. The broken line is the function for the ear with complete recruitment, as shown in case C in Figure 40–1. The plotted points are hearing level in the good ear on the ordinate and hearing level in the impaired ear on the abscissa. Note that at a hearing level of 90 dB to the right ear, recruitment is complete.

Clinical Significance

Although recruitment was observed in 1924 and tests for the response were developed in 1936, the clinical significance of the phenomenon was not recognized until much later. Fowler's intent with the alternate binaural loudness balance test was to demonstrate early otosclerosis, based on the hypothesis that a partial stapedial fixation would result in a recruitment-like loudness growth in the impaired ear as higher intensities overcame the partial fixation. Unsuccessful in this intent, Fowler did point out that recruitment distinguished consistently between conductive and sensorineural impairment.[4,5] This distinction was already possible, of course, through the much simpler procedures of tuning fork tests and pure tone audiometry, and thus recruitment and recruitment testing generated little interest. Then, in a 1948 study of the alternate binaural loudness balance test in sensorineural impairment, Dix, Hallpike, and Hood demonstrated that recruitment was characteristically present in ears with Meniere's disease, but was absent in ears with a hearing loss resulting from an eighth nerve disorder.[1] This finding generated tremendous interest in recruitment, since the important distinction between cochlear and neural sites of lesions had not been possible previously through audiometric testing. Follow-up studies with loudness balance tests have confirmed the findings of Dix et al,[17–22] and recruitment has continued to be regarded as a direct result of cochlear pathology.

Differential Sensitivity to Intensity

The interest in recruitment generated by the 1948 report of Dix et al led to a renewed study of loudness balance testing, but it also led to efforts to find some alternative method of recruitment testing. Although the loudness balance methods are excellent procedures for demonstrating recruitment, they do have limitations. Special equipment is needed; the

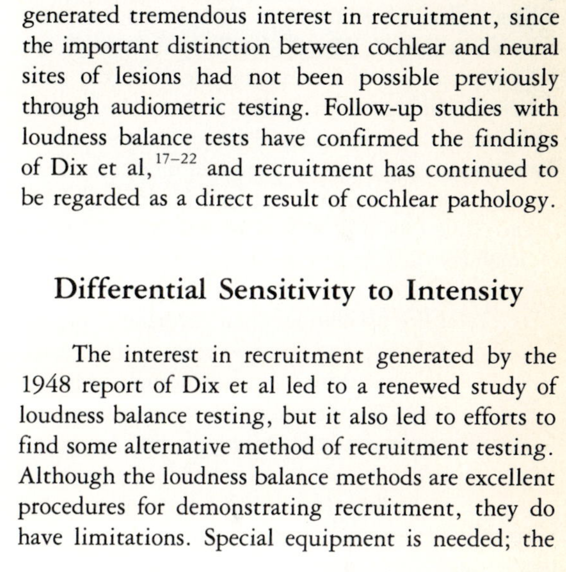

Figure 40–2 Alternate binaural loudness balance test results plotted as a function of sensation levels at equal loudness for a normal ear and for an ear with complete recruitment. HL = hearing level.

tests are time-consuming and tiring to the patient; and they require normal hearing, either in the opposite ear (alternate binaural loudness balance test) or at least at one frequency in the test ear (monaural bifrequency loudness balance test). These limitations led investigators to seek a simpler, quicker test for recruitment that would be applicable with any audiometric configuration.

Difference Limen for Intensity

The auditory response selected for study as an alternative measure of loudness recruitment was the difference limen for intensity. The rationale was that if loudness growth with an intensity increase is abnormally rapid in the recruiting ear, then the just-noticeable-difference in loudness must be abnormally small, and this reduced just-noticeable-difference would be indicated by a reduced difference limen for intensity. The earliest proposal of a reduced difference limen for intensity as an indirect indication of loudness recruitment was that of Békésy, who suggested in 1947 that a decrease in the amplitude of the intensity oscillations (pen excursions) on his automatic audiometer observed in some patients with sensorineural impairment resulted from a reduced difference limen for intensity and was equivalent to Fowler's recruitment test.[23] During the next few years, other investigators developed procedures for measurement of the difference limen for intensity at suprathreshold levels.[24–27] Although the methodology varied, each procedure was based on the expectation that the recruiting ear would have a reduced (smaller than normal) difference limen for intensity at and near the threshold of sensitivity. Clinical application of the various methods demonstrated that the difference limen for intensity test could distinguish successfully between cochlear and retrocochlear pathology. Concurrently, however, other investigators were comparing difference limen for intensity and loudness balance test results and finding sufficient disagreement to discredit the difference limen for intensity as a test of recruitment.[28,29]

In 1954 Hirsh, Palva, and Goodman concluded that the difference limen for intensity test does not distinguish between recruiting and nonrecruiting ears.[30] Their conclusion was supported in 1955 by Jerger, who also evidenced doubt that the difference limen for intensity tests were measures of recruitment.[26] As a result of these findings and conclusions, the tendency was to discard the difference limen for intensity method as a failure because it was not acceptable as an indirect test for recruitment. At that time the loudness balance test was so firmly entrenched that investigators did not consider the possibility that the disagreement between the difference limen for intensity and loudness balance test results might, at least in some instances, be the fault of the loudness balance test. Fortunately, the problems were resolved in 1961 when Jerger pointed out that regardless of whether the difference limen for intensity method tested for recruitment, it did distinguish between cochlear and retrocochlear pathology and thus provided a second audiologic procedure in addition, rather than as an alternative, to loudness balance testing for determining the site of lesions in sensorineural impairment. With this proposal, Jerger laid the foundation for the concept of a battery of diagnostic tests.

The Short Increment Sensitivity Index

The difference limen for intensity test that emerged from the confusion was the short increment sensitivity index (SISI), a test of suprathreshold differential sensitivity to intensity.[31] The SISI does not actually measure the difference limen for intensity, but rather evaluates the patient's ability to hear intensity differences of 1 dB at a sensation level of 20 dB. The 1 dB intensity difference was selected on the basis of previous research[26] as being easily heard by ears with cochlear loss but not by ears with normal hearing, conductive loss, or retrocochlear pathology.

The SISI uses the quantal method of psychophysics, in that the intensity differences are increments of short duration superimposed on a continuous carrier tone presented at a sensation level of 20 dB. The test consists of a series of 20 increments of 1 dB, and the patient's score on the test is the number of increments heard, stated as a percentage. Increments of 2 to 5 dB are used to orient the patient to the task before the test is begun and to reorient him if necessary during the test.

In their report of the SISI, Jerger et al found that ears with cochlear pathology yielded consistently high scores on the test—never less than 70 percent—whereas in ears with conductive or retrocochlear impairment, scores on the test were low—never greater than 15 percent.[31] They concluded that, in some manner, cochlear pathology renders an ear unusually sensitive to small changes in intensity, thereby permitting it to hear the 1 dB increment with ease. By implication, the 1 dB increment is not heard in the normal ear or in ears with conductive or retrocochlear pathology because, with normal cochleae, they are not endowed with increased sensitivity to intensity. Subsequent studies have confirmed the clinical findings of Jerger and his associates, and the strong tendency for scores to cluster in the very high or very low portion of the range[33,34] has led to a categorization of scores into diagnostic ranges: 0 to 30 percent—negative for cochlear pathology; 70 to 100 percent—positive for cochlear pathology; 35 to 65 percent is defined as "questionable." The tendency toward very high or very low scores has been so strong that Owens' proposal[35] to terminate the test after ten increments if response has been highly positive or highly negative has been widely accepted.[36]

Although since the initial report of Jerger et al[31] the SISI has shown something less than 100 percent accuracy in predicting the sites of lesions, it was found to be generally helpful as a diagnostic test supplementary to the loudness balance tests for recruitment and was accepted as part of what was to become a classic battery of special auditory tests. Also accepted was the concept that cochlear pathology in some unexplained manner renders the ear more sensitive to small changes in intensity.

Loudness Tests

In the early development of the diagnostic audiologic procedures based on loudness response at suprathreshold levels, the concept that developed as an explanation of the test results was that the presence of cochlear pathology, in some manner not clearly understood, renders the ear more sensitive to intensity. The presence of recruitment and positive scores on the SISI were attributed to this abnormally increased sensitivity brought about by cochlear pathology. This is not true, but the misconception of recruitment and positive SISI scores as abnormal, pathologic responses has persisted and is still held by many clinicians today.

Loudness Recruitment

The misconception of suprathreshold loudness test results developed naturally from the early demonstrations of recruitment with the alternate binaural loudness balance test in patients with unilateral hearing loss. Loudness growth in the impaired ear was found to differ from loudness growth in the normal ear and thus was assumed through simple logic to be abnormal—that is, different from normal must be abnormal. The later discovery by Dix et al that recruitment was limited to ears with cochlear pathology completed the concept,[1] and recruitment came to be regarded as an abnormal loudness response resulting from cochlear pathology. The absence of recruitment in the ear with sensorineural loss from eighth cranial nerve pathology was regarded as a normal response. It was assumed that with a normal cochlea the ear with an eighth nerve lesion is not endowed with increased sensitivity to intensity and thus is expected to give a "normal" loudness response, a response like that in the normal ear.

The Short Increment Sensitivity Index

With the concept established for recruitment, it was only natural for the same reasoning to be applied to differential sensitivity for intensity as employed by the short increment sensitivity index (SISI). A comparison of normal ears with those having cochlear pathology demonstrated a greater sensitivity to small changes in intensity in the ear with cochlear pathology, and once again different from normal was equated with abnormal. Positive scores on the SISI were regarded as a demonstration of an abnormal, pathologic sensitivity brought about by cochlear pathology, and negative SISI scores in the ear with eighth nerve pathology were considered to be the expected "normal" response from the ear with a normal cochlea.

A Second Look

The basic problem leading to the misconception was a failure to remember that the comparisons of loudness response in normal ears and ears with cochlear pathology that led to the definition of abnormality in the ears with cochlear impairment were made at equal sensation levels and thus at different sound pressure levels. The perception of loudness is initiated in the cochlea, regardless of the sensation level of the stimulus. In the normal ear and the ear with a conductive hearing loss, a signal presented at a sensation level of 20 dB reaches each cochlea at the same sound pressure level. In the normal ear and the ear with a cochlear hearing loss, however, a signal to each ear at a sensation level of 20 dB reaches the cochlea of the impaired ear at a much higher sound pressure level, and a loudness response to a stimulus at a 20 dB sensation level is a response to a signal of much greater intensity in the ear with cochlear pathology. As a result, the alternate binaural loudness balance test and the SISI compare the loudness response to a low-intensity signal in the normal ear with the response to a high-intensity stimulus in the ear with cochler pathology, and the differences in response are a result of differences in presentation level—not of an abnormal increase in sensitivity in the impaired ear. It is interesting to note that the difference in low- and high-intensity response was part of the earliest observation of what came to be called loudness recruitment. In 1924, Pohlman and Kranz noted that in certain instances a decreased acuity at threshold seemed to "disappear quite completely" at higher intensities.[2]

The differences in loudness responses at low and high intensities can be demonstrated simply through a comparison of normal ears. For example, an alternate binaural loudness balance test between a normal ear and a masked normal ear is a comparison of loudness growth at low and high intensities in normal ears, and it gives a complete recruitment result in the masked ear.[6] In the same vein, SISI scores in the normal ear are negative when the test is presented at a low sound pressure level, but when the test is done at a high intensity, the normal ear yields positive scores.[37–39] These results on the SISI are not unexpected when one recalls that the difference limen for intensity in the normal ear is much smaller (less than 1 dB) at high intensities than at low.[40,41]

The foregoing considerations suggest that loudness recruitment and positive SISI scores in the ear with cochlear pathology are normal loudness responses at the high intensity required for test presentation and not the pathologic result of abnormal sensitivity to intensity. However, completion of the concept requires an answer to a further question. If recruitment and positive SISI scores are a result of high-intensity presentation, why does the ear with eighth nerve pathology show no recruitment and negative scores on the SISI when the tests are presented at high intensity? The only plausible answer to the question is that a lesion of the eighth nerve produces a transmission loss in the impaired nerve. Some time ago, Jerger described the eighth nerve as a "bottleneck" for complex information in order to explain the severe breakdown in speech discrimination ability in patients with eighth nerve pathology.[42] It would appear that the eighth nerve is also a bottleneck for suprathreshold loudness information. The information is generated in the cochlea, but is affected in transmission by the neural pathology—a kind of neural conductive impairment. The complete concept, then, is that recruitment and positive SISI scores are normal loudness responses at high intensity and that the abnormal, pathologic results of loudness balance tests and the SISI are an *absence* of recruitment and *negative* SISI scores, both indicative of eighth nerve pathology.

This explanation of suprathreshold loudness response in ears with sensorineural hearing loss fits the facts of auditory behavior much more completely than did the original concept, in that it provides a rational basis for decruitment, a slower than normal growth of loudness with an increase in intensity. Further, it explains the poorer than normal response on the SISI in some patients with eighth nerve pathology who cannot hear SISI increments of 2 or even 3 dB. In the impaired eighth nerve, the transmission loss varies in magnitude with the severity of the lesion, presenting a continuum of effect from none to severe. Thus, in the ear with eighth nerve pathology, results on the alternate binaural loudness balance test can range from complete recruitment (no transmission loss) through no recruitment to decruitment (severe transmission loss), depending upon the effect of the pathology. Similarly, results on the SISI can range from positive scores to an inability to hear increments of 2 or 3 dB. The concept of a continuum of effect also makes it unnecessary to assume a concomitant cochlear lesion in ears with eighth nerve pathology that give cochlear results on tests of suprathreshold loudness response. In these ears, the neural lesion may be sufficient to produce a decreased sensitivity, but apparently is not imposing a significant effect on the transmission of suprathreshold loudness information. The normal cochlea generates a normal response at the high intensity occasioned by the threshold impairment. With the transmission of suprathreshold information unaffected, the result is a normal loudness response at high intensity—recruitment and positive SISI scores.

Clinical Interpretation

The clinical interpretation of recruitment and positive SISI scores is unchanged by viewing these results as normal loudness responses at high intensity. In the ear with sensorineural hearing loss, the results should still be regarded as indicative of cochlear pathology, but for a different reason: they are normal loudness responses at high intensity and thus inconsistent with eighth nerve pathology. The important difference is in the clinical interpretation of the absence of recruitment and negative scores on the SISI. Whereas these results may have been dismissed as "inconclusive" or even "normal," their occurrence should be viewed as the abnormal, pathologic effects of a transmission loss in an impaired eighth nerve.

Abnormal Auditory Adaptation

Auditory adaptation is generally defined as a decrease in auditory sensitivity during auditory stimulation as a result of the stimulation. Adaptation is sometimes referred to as perstimulatory fatigue to distinguish it from poststimulatory fatigue, the temporary threshold shift that is present following intense auditory stimulation. During the 1950s, concurrent with the development of tests for loudness recruitment and for differential sensitivity for intensity, investigators became interested in the diagnostic implications of abnormal auditory adaptation. Here again, however, initial interest was in the relationship of adaptation to loudness recruitment.

The Threshold Tone Decay Test

Although auditory adaptation, normal and abnormal, was demonstrated as early as 1882,[43] concentrated study and the development of clinical methods of assessment had their origin in the early 1950s. One of the early reports stimulating further study was that of Hallpike and Hood in 1951.[44] These investigators noted an abnormal adaptation, which they called "relapse," in patients with Meniere's disease and suggested that relapse, in addition to recruitment, was another manifestation of end-organ disease. In a further study reported in 1955, Hood again reported relapse in patients with a cochlear disorder.[45] On the basis of these findings, Carhart proposed the threshold tone decay test as a simple clinical test for abnormal auditory adaptation that might be used in addition to loudness balance tests to identify a cochlear lesion.[46] One of the advantages of the threshold tone decay test is that elaborate equipment is not required. The test stimulus is a continuous pure tone. The patient is instructed to signal when the tone is heard and to maintain the response as long as the tone is audible. The tone is presented at the patient's hearing threshold level, and the patient's response is timed. If the response is discontinued in less than 60 seconds, the stimulus intensity is immediately increased by 5 dB without interrupting the tone, and timing is restarted. The objective is to determine the least intensity at which the patient can maintain a response for 60 seconds. The difference in this level and the patient's hearing threshold level is the tone decay in decibels.

In describing the application of the threshold tone decay test in patients with sensorineural impairment, Carhart reported that results ranged from the expected to the "bizarre." In some patients with cochlear pathology, the expected tone decay of 20 to 30 dB was observed, but in a few patients with sensorineural loss of unknown origin, tone decay was greater than 50 to 60 dB; indeed, some patients were unable to maintain a response for 60 seconds at any intensity within the limits of the audiometer. In a follow-up study, Jerger, Carhart, and Lassman[47] took note of several earlier reports of excessive adaptation in patients with acoustic tumor.[48–50] Using the interrupted and continuous tones on Békésy's automatic audiometer in the sweep and fixed frequency modes, the Northwestern University group found a moderate abnormal adaptation in ears with cochlear pathology as expected, but they also found excessive adaptation in two ears with confirmed acoustic tumors. They concluded that, in agreement with Hallpike and Hood,[44] ears with cochlear pathology show abnormal adaptation, but only to a moderate degree. They concluded further that excessive adaptation indicates a lesion of the eighth nerve. Subsequent studies, using a variety of adaptation test methods, confirmed these conclusions,[51–56] and the Carhart tone decay test or some modification thereof became part of the classic diagnostic test battery.

Tone Decay Test Modifications

Although the effectiveness of the Carhart tone decay test in predicting the site of the lesion was unquestioned, it is time-consuming; and several investigators have proposed modifications of the procedure in an effort to decrease the time required for testing.

Rosenberg's proposal retained part of the Carhart procedure in that each time the patient indicates that he or she no longer hears the tone, the intensity is increased immediately by 5 dB, but timing of the response is not restarted.[54] Rather, decay from threshold is measured over a total time of 1 minute.

The modified tone decay test described by Green[51] employed Rosenberg's 1 minute test,[54] but it included specific instructions to the patient that the response must be to the original tonality of the stimulus. Green had observed that in some patients, stimulus quality changes subjectively from a pure tone to an atonal noise before it becomes inaudible and that response to the noise led to an inaccurate assessment of adaptation. Subsequent investigators have also noted this loss of tonality in some patients, and the instruction modification proposed by Green has become an important part of tone decay testing, whatever specific method is employed.

The tone decay test method of Owens measures decay only to a sensation level of 20 dB, but attention is given to the rate at which decay occurs.[52] Owens noted that in the ear with cochlear pathology, decay is progressively slower at higher sensation levels; whereas in the ear with a lesion of the eighth nerve, the rate of decay does not change or changes little with each 5 dB increase in intensity.

The modification described by Olsen and Noffsinger is only a slight departure from the original Carhart threshold tone decay test,[57] in that the Carhart procedure is retained in its entirety, but the test is begun at a sensation level of 20 dB rather than at threshold. The rationale was that in most ears having moderate or no abnormal adaptation, the test could be completed in 1 minute; whereas ears with excessive adaptation would be tested as carefully as with the Carhart threshold tone decay test.

Several studies have provided comparative evaluations of some of the procedures for testing auditory adaptation, including the use of interrupted and continuous tones at fixed frequencies on the Békésy audiometer.[57–59] Results of these studies agree on a clear superiority for the Carhart threshold tone decay test, beginning either at threshold or at a sensation level of 20 dB, as suggested by Olsen and Noffsinger.[57]

Békésy Audiometry

In the search for an effective method of demonstrating abnormal auditory adaptation, two basic approaches have emerged. One is the threshold shift method of Carhart using a conventional pure tone audiometer,[46] and the other is a threshold tracking method using the automatic audiometer developed by Békésy in 1947.[23] The Békésy audiometer permits patient control of the attenuator and provides a graphic write-out of threshold response to a single pure tone stimulus (fixed frequency) or to a pure tone that is constantly changing in frequency across the available range (sweep frequency). Because of the on effect, the interrupted tone of the Békésy audiometer does not produce adaptation; whereas adaptation does result from the constant pressure on the system produced by the continuous tone. The difference in hearing threshold level over time for the two stimuli, represented by the separation between the response tracings, is a direct measure of auditory adaptation.

Threshold tracking response to a fixed frequency stimulus was used in several of the earlier studies that demonstrated excessive adaptation in patients with a lesion of the eighth nerve[48–50] and in a study by Jerger et al in which both the fixed and sweep modes were used in distinguishing between the moderate abnormal adaptation in cochlear pathology and the excessive adaptation in a lesion in the eighth nerve.[47] In 1960, however, Jerger presented a much more detailed study of auditory adaptation measurement by the use of automatic audiometry through an analysis of threshold responses to interrupted and continuous tones, in fixed and sweep frequency modes, for 434 patients who represented a wide range of hearing loss and etiology.[60] These patients were all tested with a Grason-Stadler Békésy audiometer having an attenuation rate of 2.5 dB per second and a frequency change in sweep frequency mode of one octave per minute. The sweep frequency results permitted an evaluation of adaptation at every point on the frequency range, with a more intense examination at low, middle, and high frequencies through the fixed frequency responses. Jerger's analysis of the Békésy audiograms permitted him to divide them into four categories according to the degree of adaptation shown and the frequencies at which it occurred on the sweep frequency audiograms. The fixed frequency results were regarded as supplementary to and supportive of the sweep frequency patterns.

The audiograms categorized by Jerger as type I and type III were clear-cut and definitive. In the type I, hearing threshold levels were the same for the interrupted and continuous tones, and the response tracings were interweaving across the entire frequency range and at the fixed frequencies, thus indicating no adaptation at any frequency. The type I audiogram was obtained almost exclusively from normal hearers and patients with conductive loss, but it was also observed in a few ears with sensorineural impairment. In the type III pattern, hearing threshold levels for the interrupted tone were the same as those obtained by conventional audiometry, but response to the continuous tone showed an immediate breakaway from that for the interrupted tone, with no stabilization at any intensity to the limits of the audiometer: a response clearly indicative of rapid excessive abnormal adaptation. The type III was found in patients with retrocochlear pathology.

It was with the type II Békésy audiogram, obtained from ears with cochlear pathology, and the type IV, obtained from ears with retrocochlear pathology, that problems arose. These patterns presented by Jerger were sufficiently nondescript and similar to cause almost immediate confusion. In both, on a sweep frequency test, the continuous tone tracing breaks away from that for the interrupted tone, but it stabilizes at a higher hearing threshold level and parallels the interrupted tone tracing throughout the remainder of the frequency range. The original distinction was in the frequency at which the breakaway occurred, in that the type II showed a breakaway at about 1,000 Hz, whereas in the type IV, the breakaway was below 500 Hz. However, in a later report, Jerger indicated that the type II can also show a breakaway below 500 Hz, and he pointed out that the distinction between the two patterns is in the degree of the breakaway, with the type IV showing considerably more separation between interrupted and continuous tone tracings than that shown in the type II.[8] Later studies have continued to investigate the confusion between type II and type IV patterns, and in some instances have proposed solutions, including discarding the type IV category.[37,61,62]

One source of the confusion with type II and type IV Békésy audiograms in clinical application has been the apparent need on the part of some clinicians to force responses into one diagnostic category or another, discarding as unclassifiable and thus meaningless any that do not fit. This approach ignores the fact that Békésy audiometry is simply a specific method for testing threshold auditory adaptation, and the result is a measure of that phenomenon, regardless of whether it fits neatly into a predetermined pigeonhole. A Békésy audiogram with a separation of 20 to 30 dB between the interrupted and continuous tracings is perhaps neither type II nor type IV, and it does not have to be classified as either to have diagnostic significance. Rather, like a threshold shift of 30 to 35 dB on the Carhart tone decay test, it is a test result indicating abnormal auditory adaptation, somewhat greater than that usually seen in cochlear pathology, but less than that expected in eighth nerve disorder, and so it is not inconsistent with either lesion site.

In spite of the problems and confusion with Békésy audiometry, clinicians accepted the procedure with the diagnostic categories described by Jerger as another test of auditory adpatation. The addition of this procedure to those already available completed the classic special test battery.

The Test Battery Approach

With Jerger's description in 1960 of Békésy audiometry as a test for auditory adaptation,[60] the clinician had four different diagnostic test procedures for determining the site of a lesion in the peripheral auditory system. However, it remained for Jerger to propose using the tests in combination, with interpretation based on the pattern of results from several tests rather than on the outcome of any one test.[63] The results obtained by Jerger with 52 patients having well-defined sites of lesions are summarized in Table 40–1. As pointed out by Jerger, the predictive accuracy was less than perfect for each of the three tests used, but when the tests were combined, predictive accuracy improved to 79 to 98 percent for the various tests in pairs and to 100 percent when the results of all three tests were considered for each patient. Although there was not complete agreement with the test battery approach,[7] many clinicians concerned with diagnostic audiology adopted the concept, and the approach has continued to be used to the present.

A further addition to the special test battery was the diagnostic interpretation of the word recognition score. Following several earlier reports of speech discrimination loss out of proportion to the pure tone audiogram in patients with pathology of the eight nerve,[14,18,64,65] Jerger described the eighth nerve as a "bottleneck" in the transmission of a complex stimulus and suggested that a severe loss in speech discrimination ability indicated a lesion in this region of the auditory system.[42] Later reports of diagnostic audiometry in patients with sensorineural impairment have included word recognition scores along with the results of loudness balance tests, SISI, tone decay test, and Békésy audiometry in the determination of the sites of lesions.

Cochlear Pathology

Further studies of diagnostic audiometry have continued to show a reasonably good predictive accuracy for the various tests of the classic battery in ears with cochlear pathology. Table 40–2 summarizes the results from three later reports in comparison with the 1961 data of Jerger.[63] With the exception of the speech discrimination test, predictive accuracy of the various tests was better than 80 percent. These results demonstrate that the diagnostic tests developed during the 1950s have continued to yield a high probability of correct identification of the ear with cochlear pathology.

Eighth Nerve Pathology

Results with the classic special test battery over the years since its development have not been nearly as encouraging in ears with an eighth nerve lesion as in ears with cochlear pathology. Table 40–3 summarizes the predictive accuracy of the various tests in eight studies, beginning with the 1961 report of Jerger.[63] With the exception of the tone decay test, all of the procedures have shown a steady decline in accuracy to little better than chance. Interestingly, the tone decay test, not included by Jerger, has continued to be a reasonably good predictor, certainly better than any of the other procedures.

Accompanying the alarming decline in the predictive accuracy of the individual tests has been a decline in the accuracy of interpretation based on the pattern of results from the test battery. Clemis and Mastricola found test results consistent with eighth nerve pathology in only 39 percent of 121 patients with an eighth nerve lesion.[66] What were described as "mixed findings" were obtained in another 33 percent, however, and in some of these ears the pattern of results might have been interpreted as at least suggestive of eighth nerve pathology. Nevertheless,

TABLE 40–1 A Summary of Diagnostic Test Results in 52 Patients with Well-Defined Lesions

	Site of Lesion			
Test	*Conductive (n = 21)*	*Cochlear (n = 20)*	*Eighth Nerve (n = 11)*	*Predictive Accuracy* (%)*
Alternate Binaural Loudness Balance				
Complete	0	10	0	
Partial	0	5	2	
None	21	5	9	
Accuracy	100%	75%	82%	86
Békésy				
Type I	19	1	0	
Type II	2	19	0	
Type III	0	0	7	
Type IV	0	0	4	
Accuracy	90%	95%	100%	94
SISI				
Positive	2	20	0	
Questionable	4	0	1	
Negative	15	0	10	
Accuracy	71%	100%	91%	86

*Number of ears in percentages in which the test result is consistent with the site of the lesion.

From Jerger J. Recruitment and allied phenomena in differential diagnosis. J Aud Res 1961; 1:145.

TABLE 40–2 The Predictive Accuracy (Percent) of Diagnostic Tests in Ears with Cochlear Pathology in Four Reports*

Test	*1961 (n = 20)*	*1969 (n = 23)*	*1969 (n = 89)*	*1974 (n = 100)*
SD	—	83	83	71
ABLB	75	100	—	87
Békésy	95	100	83	93
SISI	100	91	92	88
TDT	—	96	—	82

* With the classic test battery.

Abbreviations: SD = speech discrimination; ABLB = alternate binaural loudness balance; SISI = short increment sensitivity index; TDT = threshold tone decay.

After Jerger J. Recruitment and allied phenomena in differential diagnosis. J Aud Res 1961; 1:145–151. Tillman TW. Special hearing tests in otoneurologic diagnosis. Arch Otolaryngol 1969; 89:25–30. Johnson EW. Clinical applications of special hearing tests. Arch Otolaryngol 1973; 97:92–95. Sanders JW, Josey AF, Glasscock ME. Audiologic evaluation in cochlear and eighth nerve disorders. Arch Otolaryngol 1974; 100:283.

TABLE 40–3 The Predictive Accuracy (Percent) of Diagnostic Tests in Ears with Eighth Nerve Pathology in Eight Reports*

Test	*1961 (n = 11)*	*1965 (n = 110)*	*1969 (n = 23)*	*1969 (n = 157)*	*1973 (n = 321)*	*1974 (n = 28)*	*1976 (n = 121)*	*1977 (n = 500)*
SD	—	71	57	66	55	44	50	56
Békésy	100	73	70	67	60	51	47	57
SISI	91	60	50	76	63	48	60	55
ABLB	82	60	52	—	—	67	57	50
TDT	—	76	80	—	—	69	77	78

* With the classic test battery.

Abbreviations: SD = speech discrimination; SISI = short increment sensitivity index; ABLB = alternate binaural loudness balance; TDT = threshold tone decay.

After Jerger J. Recruitment and allied phenomena in differential diagnosis. J Aud Res 1961; 1:145–151. Johnson EW. Auditory test results in 110 surgically confirmed retrocochlear lesions. J Speech Hear Disord 1965; 30:307–317. Tillman TW. Special hearing tests in otoneurologic diagnosis. Arch Otolaryngol 1969; 89:25–30. Johnson EW. Audiologic diagnosis of acoustic neuromas. Arch Otolaryngol 1969; 89:280–284. Johnson EW. Clinical applications of special hearing tests. Arch Otolaryngol 1973; 97:92–95. Sanders JW, Josey AF, Glasscock ME. Audiologic evaluation in cochlear and eighth nerve disorders. Arch Otolaryngol 1974; 100:283–289. Clemis JD, Mastricola PG. Special audiometric test battery in 121 proved acoustic tumors. Arch Otolaryngol 1976; 102:654–656. Johnson EW. Auditory test results in 500 cases of acoustic tumor. Arch Otolaryngol 1977; 103:152.

this still leaves a predictive accuracy considerably less than that reported by Jerger in 1961. In another of the studies included in Table 40–3, Johnson found consistent evidence from the test battery of eighth nerve pathology in less than half the 500 ears with acoustic tumors included in the series.[67] In still another of the reports, completely consistent results were found in only 18 percent of the ears with eighth nerve pathology.[59] However, a clinical interpretation of eighth nerve pathology, based on mixed findings that were regarded as at least suggestive of retrocochlear lesions, was made in another 64 percent of the ears, giving a test battery predictive accuracy of 82 percent. However, it should be pointed out that this study included three additional diagnostic tests (modified SISI, acoustic reflex, and brief tone audiometry) not shown here and not regarded as part of the classic special test battery.

The decline in predictive accuracy of the classic diagnostic audiometric tests, individually and in a battery, in ears with eighth nerve pathology is a direct result of the increasingly higher level of suspicion of that disorder, leading to study and diagnostic evaluation at a much earlier stage in the development of the problem. In ears with acoustic tumor, several studies have shown a relationship between the tumor size and the consistency of audiometric tests, with diagnostic audiometric testing considerably less accurate in ears with small tumors.[67–69] The inverse relationship between successful surgery and tumor size places a large premium upon the earliest possible diagnosis, and the classic diagnostic test battery is least efficient in the early stages of tumor development.

Comment

The results of the studies summarized in Tables 40–2 and 40–3 lead to the following generalizations concerning the classic test battery:

1. In ears with sensorineural hearing loss from cochlear pathology, there is a high probability that diagnostic test results will be consistent with the cochlear lesion.
2. In ears with eighth nerve pathology, classic retrocochlear test results should be regarded as strong evidence of that site of lesion. However, because of their poor sensitivity to retrocochlear pathology, negative results on one or more of the tests do not necessarily rule out eighth nerve pathology. A pattern of test results with two or even one indicative of an eighth nerve lesion should be a basis for suspicion.

The decreased accuracy of most of the tests constituting the classic special test battery to little better than chance in ears with eighth nerve pathology raises serious questions about the value of the tests in neuro-otologic diagnosis. The results of later studies of these procedures support the need, described by Clemis and Mastricola[66] and reiterated by Sanders and Bess,[70] for a revision of the test battery. Tests that are no longer effective in distinguishing cochlear and retrocochlear pathology should be discarded and replaced with new procedures that are more sensitive to minimal pathology.

ADDITIONAL TEST PROCEDURES

With the decline in the effectiveness of the classic special audiometric test battery in diagnostic audiometry, a number of different tests with improved sensitivity have been proposed as supplements to the battery or as replacements for some of the classic tests. In some instances, the additional procedures are simply modifications of existing tests, designed to examine the same auditory phenomena but in a different manner; whereas in other cases, the tests are completely different concepts of diagnostic audiology.

The Modified SISI

Almost from its introduction, clinicians began to experience problems with the SISI, in that ears with cochlear pathology with only mild to moderate hearing loss tended toward low scores, a result inconsistent with cochlear disorder. Owens encountered this problem with some of his subjects with cochlear pathology with mild hearing loss, but found that positive scores could be obtained in these subjects by presenting the test at a higher sensation level.[35] In addition, however, he found that normal ears also yielded positive scores at high sensation levels. With the test presented at increasingly higher levels, all of 27 untrained normal hearers had scores of 60 percent or higher at a sensation level of 75 dB. With five trained, normally hearing subjects, Young and Harbert found that all five obtained scores of 65 percent or higher by a presentation level of 45 dB sound pressure level.[39] In an earlier report of two patients with confirmed acoustic tumors but little or no hearing loss, Thompson found negative scores on the SISI at a high sensation level (75 dB) in the ears with tumors, even though in each case the opposite normal ear achieved a positive score at that presentation level.[71] On the basis of the results of SISI tests at successively higher hearing levels in 30 normal ears and 231 ears with cochlear pathology, Cooper and Owen recommended a 90 dB hearing level as a minimum presentation level for the SISI to insure a positive score in all ears with cochlear pathology regardless of the degree of hearing loss.[72] Their assumption was that even at this level the ear with retrocochlear pathology would continue to yield a negative score.

Our results have also demonstrated a stronger tendency toward positive scores in ears with cochlear pathology when the test is given at high-intensity levels.[73,74] Table 40–4 summarizes the results of the high-intensity SISI at four test frequencies in 67 ears with cochlear pathology. In all but one of the ears, the test was positive for cochlear pathology at one or more test frequencies, resulting in a predictive accuracy for the test of 98 percent. Table 40–5 is a comparison of results obtained with the standard SISI (20 dB sensation level) and the modified SISI (80 dB hearing level) in 26 ears with mild to moderate hearing loss from cochlear impairment. Modifying the SISI to have a presentation at a high intensity instead of the usual 20 dB sensation level brought about an increase in predictive accuracy in these patients from 19 to 88 percent. These results are not surprising when one recognizes that in normal and cochlear impaired ears, the SISI score is related to the intensity at which the test is presented rather than to the presence or absence of cochlear pathology. In the ear with only a mild to moderate cochlear hearing loss, the standard 20 dB sensation level is a low hearing level, and a negative score is not unexpected.

Negative SISI scores in the ear with retrocochlear pathology have been explained as a result of a transmission loss in the impaired eighth nerve. With the finding that in ears with normal hearing and with mild to moderate cochlear hearing loss, the SISI score can be changed from negative to positive by increasing the intensity at which the test is presented, the question arises whether the transmission loss in the ear with retrocochlear pathology will be overcome by increasing the test intensity level, thereby resulting in an undesired change from negative to positive scores in these ears. In our initial study of this question, we found that SISI presentation at increasingly higher hearing levels in 24 ears with acoustic tumors did indeed result in an increased number of ears with positive scores on the test.[73] Whereas only 17 percent of the group had positive scores at the standard 20 dB sensation level, positive scores were obtained by 49 percent when the test was given at a hearing level of 105 dB. Our later study reported SISI results at increasing hearing levels in 68 ears with acoustic tumors, all of which yielded negative scores on the test at the 20 dB sensation level.[74] The results, shown in Figure 40–3, indicate that although none of the ears changed from negative to positive scores at hearing levels of 70 or 75 dB, presentation at progressively higher hearing levels resulted in a steady increase in the number of ears with positive scores. At a hearing level of 90 dB, recommended as a minimum presentation level

TABLE 40–4 The Results of 89 Modified SISI Tests in 67 Ears with Cochlear Pathology*

	Test Frequency (Hz)			
Score	*500–1,000*	*2,000*	*4,000*	*Total*
Positive				
≥70%	9	25	47	81
Questionable				
35–65%	1	0	4	5
Negative				
≤30%	2	1	0	3

* The test was done at a minimum hearing level of 85 dB.

TABLE 40–5 Standard and Modified SISI Results in 26 Ears with Mild to Moderate Hearing Loss from Cochlear Pathology*

	Method			
	Standard		*Modified*	
Score	*(N)*	*(%)*	*(N)*	*(%)*
Positive				
≥70%	5	19	23	88
Questionable				
35–65%	5	19	2	8
Negative				
≤30%	16	62	1	4

* Test presentation at a hearing level of 80 dB.

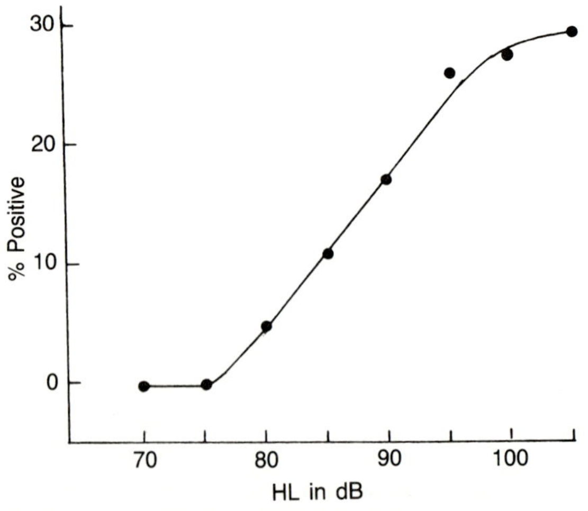

Figure 40–3 Number of ears (percentage) with positive short increment sensitivity index (SISI) scores at increasing hearing levels (HL) in 68 ears with eighth nerve pathology.

by Cooper and Owen,[72] 17 percent of the ears had changed from negative to positive scores. For this group of patients, this change is a 17 percent decrease in the predictive accuracy of the test, a decrease the clinician can ill afford.

The findings summarized here indicate that presentation of the SISI at a high intensity can bring about a considerable improvement in the predictive accuracy of the test in the ears with cochlear pathology, but that presentation at hearing levels greater than 70 to 75 dB can result in decreased predictive accuracy in ears with a retrocochlear lesion. Although the use of a hearing level of 75 dB for the modified SISI probably results in negative scores in a few ears with cochlear pathology with mild loss, it appears more desirable to avoid positive scores in ears with retrocochlear pathology, thereby leading to the recommendation of a hearing level of 75 dB for the modified SISI. The standard sensation level of 20 dB should be continued in ears with a hearing loss of 60 dB or greater.

Speech Audiometry

The earliest use of the word recognition test in diagnostic audiometry was simply an expectation of a severe reduction in word recognition ability in ears with eighth nerve pathology.[14,42,65] However, later reports have indicated a poor predictive accuracy for the word recognition score, especially in patients with eighth nerve pathology.[66,59]

The Performance-Intensity Word Recognition Function

Another approach to the word recognition test as a diagnostic procedure has been the use of the articulation function—the function obtained by determining word recognition scores across a range of sensation levels. As early as 1961, Jerger and Bucy noted a peculiarity in the articulation function in an ear with a confirmed acoustic tumor;[76] in 1971, Jerger and Jerger examined this concept further with speech test results for 41 ears with cochlear pathology and for 10 ears with confirmed acoustic tumors.[77] Word recognition scores were obtained with half-lists of the NDRC PB-50 word lists in sensation level steps of 10 to 20 dB to complete a performance-intensity (PI) function. But unlike the conventional procedure for determining an articulation function, testing did not cease with the attainment of a maximum score plateau, but was continued to presentation at a sound pressure level of 110 dB. Results indicated a strong tendency for scores in the ear with cochlear pathology to remain fairly stable at a maximum score plateau, even at high intensity. In ears with eighth nerve pathology, however, the scores at high intensity showed a distinct "rollover" effect: with initial increases in intensity, scores improved to a maximum score plateau, but with a further intensity increase, word recognition ability deteriorated, dramatically so in some cases. Because some degree of "rollover" may occur in ears with cochlear pathology, the significant result on the test is neither the presence nor the degree of "rollover," but rather the "rollover" relative to the maximum score. The "rollover" (best score minus the poorest score after "rollover") is divided by the best score ($PB_{max} - PB_{min}/PB_{max}$) to obtain a PI-PB index. Jerger and Jerger found that an index of 0.45 provided a complete separation of the cochlear and eighth nerve pathology ears, with indexes higher for the ears with an eighth nerve lesion and lower for the ears with cochlear pathology.[77] In a later study of the PI-PB function, Dirks and associates also found a distinct separation of cochlear and eighth nerve pathology ears with an index of 0.45.[78] In a still later study using different test materials, Bess, Josey, and Humes found the clearest separation with an index of 0.25.[79] In all three studies, however, the PI-PB function provided a sharp distinction between the two sites of lesions, with ears with an eighth nerve disorder tending strongly toward much higher indexes than those for ears with a cochlear lesion. For the three studies, the predictive accuracy for both sites of lesions was 90 to 100 percent.

The Synthetic Sentence Test

The PI-synthetic sentence identification (PI-SSI) function described by Jerger and Hayes[80] is a further diagnostic speech test that serves as a valuable adjunct to the PI-PB test. In the PI-SSI test, a function is obtained with the synthetic sentence material described by Speaks, Jerger, and Trammell.[81] The sentences are presented against a competing message of continuous discourse at a message to competition ratio of 0 dB at increasing sensation levels up to high intensity, providing a PI function. The PI-PB and PI-SSI function tests used in combination permit allowances to be made for the audiometric configuration, in that the PB test material is more affected by hearing loss in the high frequencies, whereas the synthetic sentences are more sensitive to loss in the low frequencies. The sentences are also more sensitive to central auditory system pathology, and the combination of PI-PB and PI-SSI may be helpful in distinguishing among cochlear, eighth nerve, and central pathology.

Békésy Audiometry

Békésy audiometry, as originally described by Jerger,[60] is a specialized test of auditory adaptation in which Békésy's automatic audiometer is used to record threshold responses to interrupted and continuous tones across a range of frequencies and at fixed frequencies. The results are categorized by site of lesion according to the relationship between the interrupted and continuous tone tracings. In later years, modifications of the test have been proposed in efforts to increase the sensitivity of the procedure in cases of retrocochlear pathology.

The Forward-Backward Discrepancy Test

This test is carried out in the same manner as the original Békésy test for auditory adaptation,[60] and the results are interpreted in the same way. But in addition, after the patient has traced responses to the interrupted and continuous tones across the frequency range from low to high, the audiometer is reversed and a response is obtained to the continuous tone backward, that is, from high to low frequency. The results of this additional procedure are interpreted in terms of the relationship between the forward and backward continuous tone tracings, and significant discrepancies between the tracings are regarded as suggestive of eighth nerve pathology. Jerger, Jerger, and Mauldin reported a predictive accuracy of 99 percent in 121 ears with cochlear pathology and 78 percent in 23 ears with retrocochlear lesions.[75] In a recent analysis of the accuracy and feasibility of several diagnostic tests, Musiek and associates recommended the inclusion of the Békésy forward-backward discrepancy test in the diagnostic test battery.[82]

The Békésy Comfortable Loudness Test

This modification of Békésy audiometry, proposed by Jerger and Jerger in 1974, grew out of their hypothesis that in the ear with eighth nerve pathology, the auditory signs in the early stages of the lesion are likely to be cochlear in nature, and that cochlear results are especially likely to occur in tests done at or near threshold.[83] They went on to suggest that the earliest signs of eighth nerve pathology appear at high intensity, with indications of eighth nerve disorder occurring near threshold levels only after progression of the neural lesion. On the basis of this hypothesis, Jerger and Jerger proposed obtaining Békésy tracings at the patient's most comfortable loudness levels rather than at threshold. The rationale was that the abnormal auditory adaptation in eighth nerve pathology is more likely to occur at the higher intensities required for a most-comfortable-loudness response. Analysis of the Békésy comfortable loudness test results for 164 ears supported the hypothesis. Jerger and Jerger described three patterns of interrupted and continuous tone tracings obtained at the higher intensity as "negative" for eighth nerve pathology but consistent with normal hearing, conductive loss, or cochlear pathology, and three response patterns as "positive" for eighth nerve lesions. The basic distinction between the negative and positive patterns is in the degree of auditory adaptation shown in the continuous tone response, with the positive patterns displaying excessive adaptation in a part of or all of the frequency range. As a further step in the test procedure, a negative pattern on the forward tracings is followed up with a backward tracing with the continuous tone, and analysis is of the forward-backward discrepancy. The results reported by Jerger and Jerger are summarized in Table 40–6. In a few instances, the results had to be described as "unclassifiable" because the patients traced responses to both the interrupted and continuous tones at the limits of the audiometer, maintaining that the sound never became uncomfortably loud. In most cases, however, positive and negative pattern responses showed good agreement with the actual site of the lesion. The predictive accuracy of the test was 69 percent in ears with retrocochlear pathology and 90 percent in ears without a retrocochlear lesion (normal, conductive, coch-

TABLE 40–6 Results of Békésy Comfortable Loudness (BCL) Audiometry in 164 Ears

	Test Results					
	*Negative**		*Positive**		*Unclassified*	
Subjects	*(N)*	*(%)*	*(N)*	*(%)*	*(N)*	*(%)*
Normal, conductive and cochlear	133	90	3	2	12	8
Retrocochlear	2	12	11	69	3	19

*For retrocochlear pathology.

From Jerger J, Jerger S. Diagnostic value of Békésy comfortable loudness tracings. Arch Otolaryngol 1974; 99:351.

lear). The false positive incidence was only 2 percent, and the false negative incidence, only 12 percent. These results represent a considerable improvement in diagnostic accuracy over threshold Békésy audiometry.

The Acoustic Reflex Test

The acoustic reflex test is a specialized measurement of the acoustic stapedial reflex threshold with an immittance bridge or meter as a diagnostic test in the ear with sensorineural impairment. Since concern is with the auditory response, the stimulated ear is the test ear. In present usage, the acoustic reflex test consists of two parts and evaluates two different aspects of auditory response: suprathreshold loudness and auditory adaptation.

The Metz Test

This part of the acoustic reflex test was proposed by Metz in 1952 as a direct test for loudness recruitment.[84] Although agreement has been incomplete,[32] the acoustic reflex has been regarded as a suprathreshold loudness response, with the acoustic reflex threshold occurring in the normal ear at sensation levels of 70 to 90 dB. Metz argued that because of the rapid growth of loudness at suprathreshold intensities, the acoustic reflex threshold in the recruiting ear occurs at the same hearing levels as in the normal ear; but because of the hearing loss in the impaired ear, the reflex thresholds are at reduced sensation levels. Later studies have generally agreed that reflex thresholds at sensation levels of less than 60 dB are consistent with loudness recruitment.[19,21,85] Further reports have also found the acoustic reflex threshold at reduced sensation levels in ears with cochlear pathology,[85a,86] and Northern has suggested a sensation level of 60 dB as a cutoff.[87] Table 40–7 summarizes the results of the Metz test in 105 ears with cochlear pathology.[88] As can be seen, seldom did the reflex occur at a reduced sensation level when the hearing threshold level was within normal limits at a given test frequency, whereas the acoustic reflex threshold was almost always at a reduced sensation level when the hearing threshold level was 30 dB or greater. For the 105 ears of the study, the predictive accuracy of the test was 99 percent, in that the reflex occurred at a reduced sensation level at one or more test frequencies in 99 percent of the ears.

Some may argue that the Metz test is not a test of loudness recruitment and that the reflex threshold at a reduced sensation level is not a result of the recruitment phenomenon. As pointed out by Jerger, however, the question is really of little consequence in the diagnostic application of the acoustic reflex test.[89] Whether the procedure demonstrates recruitment or not, the important consideration is the fact that an acoustic reflex at a reduced sensation level is highly consistent with the presence of cochlear pathology.

TABLE 40–7 Ears with Cochlear Pathology with a Reflex Threshold at 60 dB SL or Less re Hearing Threshold Level (N = 105)

	Test Frequency (Hz)			
HTL	*500 (%)*	*1000 (%)*	*2000 (%)*	*4000 (%)*
0 to 25 dB	17	26	11	0
30 dB or more	99	97	99	97

Abbreviations: SL = sensation level; HTL = hearing threshold level.

Reflex Decay and Hearing Level

A second application of the acoustic reflex test was provided when Anderson, Barr, and Wedenberg pointed out that the ear with eighth nerve pathology also gives an acoustic reflex response that differs from the response in the normal ear.[90] In 17 ears with tumors involving the eighth nerve, Anderson et al found the acoustic reflex threshold to be abnormally elevated to hearing levels beyond 100 dB. In seven patients, the reflex could not be obtained even with a stimulus at a hearing level of 120 dB. In the ten patients for whom reflexes were obtained, they found rapid decay (adaptation) of the reflex at all test frequencies during continuous stimulation at a level 10 dB above the reflex threshold. The procedure for the decay test was to determine the "half-life" of the reflex, that is, the time in seconds required for the reflex to decay to one-half its original amplitude during continuous stimulation. In all of their patients, the half-life was less than 5 seconds. They pointed out that the decay may occur in the normal ear at 2,000 and 4,000 Hz but not at 500 or 1,000 Hz, and they proposed the latter two frequencies for the reflex decay test.

Later studies have strongly supported the findings of Anderson et al, at least in the high probability of elevated reflex thresholds in ears with retrocochlear pathology.[67,85a,88,91,92] Table 40–8 summarizes the results of seven separate studies of the acoustic reflex test in ears with eighth nerve pathology, beginning with the 1970 report of Anderson, Barr, and Wedenberg.[90] Although the predictive accuracy of the test has decreased somewhat from

TABLE 40–8 Number and Percentage of Ears Positive for Eighth Nerve Pathology in Seven Reports of the Acoustic Reflex Test in Ears with Acoustic Tumor

Results	*1970 (n = 17)*	*1974 (n = 30)*	*1975 (n = 28)*	*1976 (n = 24)*	*1976 (n = 84)*	*1977 (n = 75)*	*1981 (n = 152)*
Positive for eighth nerve pathology							
Number	17	26	24	19	64	64	117
Percentage	100	87	86	79	76	85	77
Elevated reflex	17	22	19	11	55	39	106
Abnormal decay	10	4	6	8	9	25	17

After Anderson H, Barr B, Wedenberg E. Early diagnosis of VIIIth nerve tumors by acoustic reflex tests. Acta Otolaryngol [Suppl] (Stockh) 1970; 263:232–237. Jerger J, Harford E, Clemis J, Alford B. The acoustic reflex in eighth nerve disorders. Arch Otolaryngol 1974; 99:409–413. Olsen WO, Noffsinger D. Acoustic reflex and reflex decay. Arch Otolaryngol 1975; 101:622–625. Sheehy JL, Inzer BE. Acoustic reflex test in neuro-otologic diagnosis. Arch Otolaryngol 1976; 102:647–653. Sanders JW, Josey AF, Glasscock ME. The acoustic stapedial reflex test in cochlear and eighth nerve disorders. Paper presented at the Third International Symposium on Impedance Audiometry, American Electromedics Corporation, New York, 1976. Johnson EW. Auditory test results in 500 cases of acoustic tumor. Arch Otolaryngol 1977; 103:152–158. Sanders JW, Josey AF, Glasscock ME, Jackson CG. The acoustic reflex test in cochlear and eighth nerve pathology ears. Laryngoscope 1981; 91:787.

that of the original study, it is still high, especially in comparison with the diagnostic tests that constitute the classic special test battery. Further, it should not be concluded that a test result that was not positive for an eighth nerve lesion was necessarily negative. In some instances a result has to be considered inconclusive. For example, absence of a reflex in an ear with a hearing loss of 80 dB or greater cannot be regarded as either positive or negative. The results in the table also illustrate the fact that, since the original report of Anderson et al, the predominant indicator of eighth nerve pathology has been an elevation of the acoustic reflex threshold, with reflex decay an infrequent response.

In an effort to improve the diagnostic accuracy of clinical interpretation of test results, my colleagues and I have proposed a modification of the interpretation categories for the acoustic reflex test.[93] Whereas in previous studies results have been interpreted as either positive or negative for a given site of a lesion, we have suggested adding a third category of "questionable." The rationale for this category is that when the Metz test[84] is combined with the procedures of Anderson et al,[90] it is possible to obtain results that are in conflict. For example, the acoustic reflex threshold may be at a reduced sensation level but at an elevated hearing level, or the reflex threshold may be at a reduced sensation level and a normal hearing level, but show abnormal decay. In both of these possible test outcomes, one aspect of the results suggests cochlear pathology, whereas another indicates an eighth nerve lesion. According to our proposal, these results would be described as questionable—neither confirming nor ruling out a suspected site of a lesion. In an analysis of acoustic reflex test results in 152 ears with cochlear pathology and 152 ears with eighth nerve tumors, we found that adding the "questionable" category resulted in a marked improvement in the overall accuracy of the test in patients with eighth nerve pathology. Although the positive rate was reduced from 97 to 83 percent for cochlear lesions, the false negative rate in these ears continued to be low. In patients with eighth nerve tumors, the positive rate of 77 percent was unchanged, but, importantly, the false negative rate was reduced from 23 percent to only 9 percent.

The Ipsilateral Reflex Test

An instrumentation improvement permitting an ipsilateral observation of the acoustic reflex has been a valuable addition to the diagnostic application of the test. In this procedure, the stimulus is presented through the probe tube, and the reflex is observed in the stimulated ear. Measurement of the ipsilateral reflex may permit the clinician to rule out one or more possible causes for an abnormal response on the contralateral test. For example, if a stimulus to a right ear suspected of having eighth nerve pathology fails to elicit a reflex in the left ear on contralateral testing, any of the following could be the reason:

1. Middle ear impairment in the left ear.
2. Seventh cranial nerve lesion on the left side.
3. Brain stem lesion in the crossing pathways.
4. Eighth cranial nerve lesion in the right ear.

The presence of a reflex in the left ear on ipsilateral measurement in that ear would rule out the first two possibilities, strengthening the probability of eighth nerve pathology in the right ear.

The 90th Percentile Levels

As pointed out previously, a problem in combining the Metz[84] approach to the interpretation of the acoustic reflex test with that of Anderson, Barr, and Wedenberg[90] is the potential for conflicting results. In other words, the acoustic reflex threshold in an ear with cochlear pathology may be at a reduced senstion level, consistent with a cochlear lesion, but also at an elevated hearing level, suggesting retrocochlear pathology. As pointed out by Silman and Gelfand, the acoustic reflex threshold in the ear with cochlear pathology is at normal hearing levels only when the hearing loss at the test frequency is no greater than about 50 to 55 dB.[94] When hearing loss exceeds 55 dB, the acoustic reflex threshold is at increasingly higher hearing levels that may be regarded as abnormally elevated. In 544 ears with normal hearing or cochlear hearing loss, Silman and Gelfand found that the mean acoustic reflex threshold at 500, 1,000, and 2,000 Hz did not exceed a hearing level of 95 dB when hearing loss at the test frequency was 55 dB or less; whereas for greater hearing loss, the mean acoustic reflex threshold occurred at hearing levels of up to 115 dB. At the 90th percentiles of the distributions, the acoustic reflex threshold hearing level was 95 to 110 dB for hearing loss to 55 dB, but was increased to hearing levels as high as 125 dB for hearing loss greater than 55 dB. As a result of these findings, Silman and Gelfand proposed that a clinical interpretation of the acoustic reflex test should be based on the hearing level of the acoustic reflex threshold, ignoring the sensation level. An acoustic reflex threshold at or below the 90th percentile level of their report for the degree of hearing loss at the test frequency should be regarded as consistent with cochlear pathology.

In a follow-up study of the 90th percentile level approach to the interpretation of the acoustic reflex test, Olsen, Bauch, and Harner examined the acoustic reflex threshold in 30 ears with acoustic tumors and 30 ears with cochlear pathology, which were matched in hearing loss with the ears with tumors.[95] They found that the acoustic reflex threshold hearing level exceeded the 90th percentile levels of Silman and Gelfand[94] in 83 percent of the ears with tumors, but in only 3 percent of the ears with cochlear hearing loss, thus lending strong support to the proposal of Silman and Gelfand.

In a further follow-up study, I examined the 90th percentile levels approach to 133 ears with cochlear pathology and 129 ears with confirmed acoustic tumors.[96] Although no attempt was made to match the groups in hearing threshold levels, the degree of loss at the test frequencies ranged from 0 to 90 dB plus in each subject group. The results of the analysis with three different criteria are summarized in Table 40–9. With the 90th percentile levels, the site of the lesion was correctly identified in 92 percent of the ears with cochlear lesions. With these ears, the predictive accuracy of the diagnostic criteria of Metz[84] and of Anderson, Barr, and Wedenberg[90] was only 80 percent. Although the false negative incidence was only 1 percent, the results had to be regarded as questionable or inconclusive in 19 percent. For the ears with tumors, the predictive accuracy with the 90th percentile levels was 76 percent, but the false negative incidence was high at 24 percent. With the earlier criteria,[84,90] 72 percent of the ears with tumors were identified correctly, and the results were false negative in only 10 percent. For 17 percent, however, the results had to be regarded as questionable or inconclusive. When the results of the reflex decay test were combined with the 90th percentile levels determination, results were positive in 76 percent of the ears with tumors, the false negative incidence was reduced to 15 percent, and only 9 percent were questionable. For the ears with cochlear pathology, results with the 90th percentile levels and the decay test were positive in 89 percent, negative in 8 percent, and questionable in 3 percent. These results suggest that the 90th percentile levels approach of Silman and Gelfand,[94] combined with the results of the reflex decay test and adding the diagnostic category of "questionable," will provide a more accurate determination of the site of a lesion.

Quantification of the Acoustic Reflex

A further modification of the acoustic reflex test, proposed in several recent studies,[97–100] that demonstrates an even greater sensitivity of the test for eighth nerve pathology is the precise quantification of the various parameters of the reflex, such as the latency, rise-decay times, and amplitude. Quantification is accomplished by recording the reflex for off-line computer analysis[98] or by a direct measurement with a storage oscilloscope[97] or an averaging computer.[100,101] In a study of 21 patients, all suspect for acoustic tumors on the basis of previous tests, Mangham, Lindeman, and Dawson identified the ears with tumors with a predictive accuracy of 100 percent on the basis of the quantified acoustic reflex.[98] Although further data are needed, quantification shows great promise for the improvement of an already excellent diagnostic auditory test.

The Auditory Brain Stem Response

The auditory brain stem response has proved to be an extremely sensitive and accurate test for determining the site of a lesion in an ear with a sensorineural impairment. A number of studies have reported a predictive accuracy for the auditory brain

TABLE 40–9 Evaluation of Acoustic Reflex Test Results in Ears with Cochlear and Eighth Nerve Pathology Using Three Criteria.*

	Site of Lesion					
	*Criterion A**		*Criterion B**		*Criterion C**	
Test Results	*Cochlear*	*Eighth Nerve*	*Cochlear*	*Eighth Nerve*	*Cochlear*	*Eighth Nerve*
Cochlear	92%	24%	80%	10%	89%	15%
Eighth nerve	8	76	1	72	8	76
Questionable	—	—	3	12	3	9
Inconclusive	—	—	16	5	—	—

* Criterion A: 90th percentile levels of Silman and Gelfand;[94] Criterion B; Criteria of Mertz[84] and of Anderson et al;[90] Criterion C: 90th percentile levels plus the reflex decay test.[90]

stem response of 90 to 100 percent in patients with eighth nerve pathology,[71,102–108] and several have described the auditory brain stem response as the most sensitive audiologic indicator available for distinguishing between cochlear and eighth nerve pathology.[70,71,82]

The auditory brain stem response is an electrophysiologic procedure for recording the computer-averaged electrical activity generated in the eighth nerve and brain stem by an acoustic stimulus. The typical response in a normal system is a wave form consisting of a series of five to seven peaks, numbered sequentially according to the order of appearance or latency.[109] Because of its pominence and persistence, the fifth peak, wave V, has generally been given specific attention in a determination of abnormality. The indications of a retrocochlear lesion are a complete absence of wave V in response to a clearly audible signal or the presence of wave V at an abnormally prolonged latency. The latter may take the form of an abnormally increased absolute latency of wave V, increased interwave latency differences (I to III, III to V, I to V), and an increased interaural wave V latency difference.

In the diagnostic application of the auditory brain stem response one must remember, of course, that the procedure is not an acoustic tumor test; rather, it is an assessment of the integrity of the neural system from the cochlea through the brain stem. Just as a normal response can occur in an ear with neural pathology, so can an abnormal auditory brain stem response occur in the absence of an acoustic tumor. Such a response is not necessarily a false negative result, however, and care should be taken in assigning that label, since other neurologic disorders affecting the auditory pathways can result in abnormal auditory brain stem response results.[110–113]

When compared with other tests, new procedures, as well as the classic special tests, the auditory brain stem response does indeed appear to be the most sensitive and accurate diagnostic auditory test available for the qualitative assessment of sensorineural hearing loss.

A REVISED SPECIAL AUDITORY TEST BATTERY

The analysis of the predictive accuracy of the classic auditory test battery presented in this chapter demonstrates the inadequacy of most of the classic tests and indicates the need to replace these procedures with measures more sensitive to eighth nerve pathology in the early stages of its development. On the basis of information presently available, the following tests are recommended:

The Auditory Brain Stem Response. The auditory brain stem response has proved to be the most sensitive auditory measure presently available for determining the site of a lesion in sensorineural impairment. A major drawback is the cost of the equipment, and so the test does not have to be available in every clinic. However, it should be available to every patient suspected of having retrocochlear pathology, either directly or through referral.

The Acoustic Reflex Test. This test is also a highly sensitive procedure in distinguishing between cochlear and retrocohclear pathology. Further study of various modifications of this test, such as quantification of the reflex, may result in even greater sensitivity.

Special Speech Tests. The PI-PB and PI-SSI function tests, although perhaps not as sensitive as the auditory brain stem response and acoustic reflex tests, can provide valuable additional qualitative information in the assessment of sensorineural hearing loss.

The Tone Decay Test. This procedure is the only test from the classic special test battery that has continued to demonstrate an acceptable predictive accuracy, at least when it is done with the Carhart procedure or with the modification of the Carhart method proposed by Olsen and Noffsinger.

Supplementary Tests. The modified SISI and the Békésy comfortable loudness test can be used to supplement the four tests just described. The modified SISI tends strongly toward postive scores in ears with cochlear pathology, and although a positive score cannot be regarded as ruling out a retrocochlear lesion, negative scores should be considered as highly suspicious. Although data on the Békésy comfortable loudness test are somewhat limited, the available results suggest that the procedure may be a valuable supplement to other tests.

It may be noted that the recommendation continues to be for a battery of tests. Although some of the procedures developed to supplement or replace the classic test battery have demonstrated marked improvement in predictive accuracy, none is perfect, and accurate determination of the site of a lesion is still more likely if consideration is given to the pattern of results obtained from a combination of diagnostic tests.

Finally, it should be emphasized that these recommendations for a diagnostic test battery are based on information available at this time. Diagnostic audiology is a highly dynamic facet of the profession, with rapid developments and changes in concepts and procedures. The clinician must keep up with these developments and modify clinical procedures accordingly.

REFERENCES

1. Dix MR, Hallpike CS, Hood JD. Observations upon the loudness recruitment phenomenon, with especial reference to the differential diagnosis of disorders of the internal ear and VIIIth nerve. J Laryngol Otol 1948; 62:671–686.
2. Pohlman AG, Kranz FW. Binaural minimum audition in a subject with ranges of deficient acuity. Proc Soc Exp Biol Med 1924; 20:335–337.
3. Fowler EP. Marked deafened areas in normal ears. Arch Otolaryngol 1928; 8:151–155.
4. Fowler EP. A method for the early detection of otosclerosis. Arch Otolaryngol 1936; 24:731–741.
5. Fowler EP. The diagnosis of disease of the neural mechanism by the aid of sounds well above threshold. Trans Am Otol Soc 1937; 27:207–219.
6. Sanders JW. Recruitment. In: Rintelmann WF, ed. Hearing assessment. Baltimore: University Park Press, 1979: 261.
7. Hood JD. Basic audiological requirements in neuro-otology. J Laryngol Otol 1969; 83:695–711.
8. Jerger J. Hearing tests in otologic diagnosis. Asha 1962; 4:139–145.
9. Jerger J, Harford ER. Alternate and simultaneous binaural balancing of pure tones. J Speech Hear Res 1960; 3:15–30.
10. Davis H, Goodman AC. Subtractive hearing loss, loudness recruitment and decruitment. Ann Otol 1966; 75:87–94.
11. Dix MR, Hallpike CS. The otoneurologic diagnosis of tumours of the VIII nerve. Proc R Soc Med 1958; 51:889–892.
12. Fowler EP. Some attributes of "loudness recruitment" and "loudness decruitment." Trans Am Otol Soc 1965; 53:78–84.
13. Hallpike CA. The loudness recruitment phenomenon: its clinical significance and neurological basis. Proc R Soc Med 1965; 58:190–196.
14. Walsh TE, Goodman A. Speech discrimination in central auditory lesions. Laryngoscope 1955; 65:1–8.
15. Reger SN. Differences in loudness response of the normal and hard-of-hearing ear at intensity levels slightly above threshold. Ann Otol Rhinol Laryngol 1936; 45:1029–1039.
16. Steinberg JC, Gardner MB. The dependence of hearing impairment on sound intensity. J Acoust Soc Am 1937; 9:11–23.
17. Eby LG, Williams HL. Recruitment of loudness in the differential diagnosis of end-organ and nerve fiber deafness. Laryngoscope 1951; 61:400–413.
18. Goodman AC. Some relations between auditory function and intracranial lesions with particular reference to lesions of the cerebellopontine angle. Laryngoscope 1957; 67:987–1010.
19. Kristensen HK, Jepsen O. Recruitment in otoneurological diagnosis. Acta Otolaryngol 1952; 42:553–560.
20. Simonton KM. End-organ deafness. Arch Otolaryngol 1956; 63:262–269.
21. Thomsen KA. The Metz recruitment test and a comparison with the Fowler method. Acta Otolaryngol 1955; 45:544–552.
22. Yantis PA. Locus of the lesion in recruiting ears. Arch Otolaryngol 1955; 62:625–631.
23. Békésy G. A new audiometer. Acta Otolaryngol 1947; 35:411–422.
24. Denes P, Naunton RF. The clinical detection of auditory recruitment. J Laryngol Otol 1950; 64:375–398.
25. Jerger J. A difference limen recruitment test and its diagnostic significance. Laryngoscope 1952; 62:1316–1332.
26. Jerger J. Differential intensity sensitivity in the ear with loudness recruitment. J Speech Hear Disord 1955; 20:183–191.
27. Luscher E, Zwislocki J. A simple method for indirect monaural determination of the recruitment phenomenon (difference limen in intensity in different types of deafness). Acta Otolaryngol 1954; 78:156–168.
28. Liden G, Nilsson G. Differential audiometry. Acta Otolaryngol 1950; 38:521–527.
29. Lund-Iversen L. An investigation on the difference limen determined by the method of Luscher and Zwislocki in normal hearing and in various forms of deafness. Acta Otolaryngol 1952; 42:219–224.
30. Hirsh IJ, Palva T, Goodman AC. Difference limen and recruitment. Arch Otolaryngol 1954; 60:525–540.
31. Jerger J, Shedd JL, Harford ER. On the detection of extremely small changes in sound intensity. Arch Otolaryngol 1959; 69:200–211.
32. Scharf B. Acoustic reflex, loudness summation, and the critical band. J Acoustic Soc Amer 1976; 60:753–755.
33. Griffing TA, Tuck GA. Split-half reliability of the SISI. J Aud Res 1963; 3:159–164.
34. Yantis PA, Decker RL. On the short increment sensitivity index (SISI test). J Speech Hear Disord 1964; 29:231–246.
35. Owens E. The SISI test and VIIIth nerve versus cochlear involvement. J Speech Hear Disord 1965; 30:252–262.
36. Martin FN. The SISI test. In: Katz J, ed. Handbook of clinical audiology. 3rd ed. Baltimore: Williams and Wilkins, 1985:292.
37. Owens E. Békésy tracings and site of lesion. J Speech Hear Disord 1964; 29:456–468.
38. Owens E. Differential intensity discrimination. In: Rintelmann WF, ed. Hearing assessment. Baltimore: University Park Press, 1979:235.
39. Young IM, Harbert F. Significance of the SISI test. J Aud Res 1967; 7:303–311.
40. Riesz RR. Differential intensity sensitivity of the ear for pure tones. Phys Rev 1928; 31:867–875.
41. Swisher LP. Response to intensity change in cochlear pathology. Laryngoscope 1966; 76:1706–1713.
42. Jerger J. Audiological manifestations of lesions in the auditory nervous system. Laryngoscope 1960; 70:417–425.
43. Green DS. Tone decay. In: Katz J, ed. Handbook of clinical audiology. 3rd ed. Baltimore: Williams & Wilkins, 1985:304.

44. Hallpike CS, Hood JD. Some recent work on auditory adaptation and its relationships to the loudness recruitment phenomenon. J Acoust Soc Am 1951; 23:270–274.
45. Hood JD. Auditory fatigue and adaptation in the differential diagnosis of end-organ disease. Ann Otol Rhinol Laryngol 1955; 64:507–518.
46. Carhart R. Clinical determination of abnormal auditory adaptation. Arch Otolaryngol 1957; 65:32–39.
47. Jerger J, Carhart R, Lassman J. Clinical observations on excessive threshold adaptation. Arch Otolaryngol 1958; 68:617–623.
48. Kos CM. Auditory function as related to the complaint of dizziness. Laryngoscope 1955; 65:711–721.
49. Lierle DM, Reger SN. Experimentally induced temporary threshold shifts in ears with impaired hearing. Ann Otol Rhinol Laryngol 1955; 64:263–277.
50. Reger SN, Kos CM. Clinical measurements and implications of recruitment. Ann Otol Rhinol Laryngol 1952; 61:810–823.
51. Green DS. The modified tone decay test (MTDT) as a screening procedure for eighth nerve lesions. J Speech Hear Disord 1963; 28:31–36.
52. Owens E. Tone decay in eighth nerve and cochlear lesions. J Speech Hear Disord 1964; 29:14–22.
53. Owens E. Békésy tracings, tone decay and loudness recruitment. J Speech Hear Disord 1965; 30:50–57.
54. Rosenberg PE. Rapid clinical measurement of tone decay. Paper presented at the National Convention of the American Speech and Hearing Association, New York, 1958.
55. Sorensen H. Clinical application of continuous threshold recording. Acta Otolaryngol 1962; 54:403–422.
56. Yantis PA. Clinical applications of the temporary threshold shift. Arch Otolaryngol 1959; 70:779–787.
57. Olsen WO, Noffsinger D. Comparison of one new and three old tests of auditory adaptation. Arch Otolaryngol 1974; 99:94–99.
58. Parker W, Decker RL. Detection of abnormal auditory threshold adaptation. Arch Otolaryngol 1971; 94:1–7.
59. Sanders JW, Josey AF, Glasscock ME. Audiologic evaluation in cochlear and eighth nerve disorders. Arch Otolaryngol 1974; 100:283–289.
60. Jerger J. Békésy audiometry in analysis of auditory disorders. J Speech Hear Res 1960; 3:275–287.
61. Hopkinson NT. Modifications of the four types of Békésy audiograms. J Speech Hear Disord 1966; 31:79–81.
62. Hughes RL, Winegar WJ, Crabtree JA. Békésy audiometry: type 2 versus type 4 patterns. Arch Otolaryngol 1967; 86:424–430.
63. Jerger J. Recruitment and allied phenomena in differential diagnosis. J Aud Res 1961; 1:145–151.
64. Schuknecht H. Perceptive hearing loss. Laryngoscope 1958; 68:429–439.
65. Schuknecht H, Woellner RC. Hearing loss following partial section of the cochlear nerve. Laryngoscope 1953; 63:441–465.
66. Clemis JD, Mastricola PG. Special audiometric test battery in 121 proved acoustic tumors. Arch Otolaryngol 1976; 102:654–656.
67. Johnson EW. Auditory test results in 500 cases of acoustic tumor. Arch Otolaryngol 1977; 103:152–158.
67a. Johnson EW. Auditory test results in 110 surgically confirmed retrocochlear lesions. J Speech Hear Disord 1965; 30:307–317.
68. Jerger J, Waller J. Some observations on masking and the progression of auditory signs in acoustic neuroma. J Speech Hear Disord 1962; 27:140–143.
69. Johnson EW. Audiologic diagnosis of acoustic neuromas. Arch Otolaryngol 1969; 89:280–284.
70. Sanders JW, Bess FH. Special auditory testing: review and update. Am J Otol 1981; 3:172–176.
71. Thompson G. A modified SISI technique for selected cases with suspected acoustic neuroma. J Speech Hear Disord 1963; 28:299–302.
72. Cooper JC, Owen JH. In defense of SISI's. Arch Otolaryngol 1976; 102:396–399.
73. Sanders JW, Josey AF, Glasscock ME. The modified SISI in patients with VIIIth nerve tumor. Paper presented at the National Convention of the American Speech and Hearing Association, Washington, DC, 1975.
74. Sanders JW, Josey AF, Glasscock ME. The SISI at high intensity in eighth nerve pathology ears. Paper presented at the National Convention of the American Speech and Hearing Association, San Francisco, 1978.
75. Jerger J, Jerger S, Mauldin L. The forward-backward discrepancy in Békésy audiometry. Arch Otolaryngol 1972; 96:400–406.
76. Jerger J, Bucy PC. Audiological findings in an unusual case of VIIIth nerve lesion. J Aud Res 1961; 1:25–34.
77. Jerger J, Jerger S. Diagnostic significance of PB word functions. Arch Otolaryngol 1971; 93:573–580.
78. Dirks D, Kamm D, Bower D, Betsworth A. Use of performance-intensity functions for diagnosis. J Speech Hear Disord 1977; 42:408–415.
79. Bess F, Josey AF, Humes L. Performance intensity functions in cochlear and eighth nerve disorders. Am J Otol 1979; 1:27–31.
80. Jerger J, Hayes D. Diagnostic speech audiometry. Arch Otolaryngol 1977; 103:216–222.
81. Speaks C, Jerger J, Trammell J. Comparison of sentence identification and conventional speech discrimination scores. J Speech Hear Res 1970; 13:755–767.
82. Musiek FE, Mueller RJ, Kibbe KS, Rackliffe LM. Audiologic test selection in the detection of eighth nerve disorders. Am J Otol 1963; 4:281–287.
83. Jerger J, Jerger S. Diagnostic value of Békésy comfortable loudness tracings. Arch Otolaryngol 1974; 99:351–360.
84. Metz O. Threshold of reflex contraction of muscles of the middle ear and recruitment of loudness. Arch Otolaryngol 1952; 55:536–543.
85. Alberti P, Kristensen R. The clinical application of impedance audiometry. Laryngoscope 1970; 80:735–746.
85a. Olsen WO, Noffsinger D. Acoustic reflex and reflex decay. Arch Otolaryngol 1975; 101:622–625.
86. Jerger J, Jerger S, Mauldin L. Studies in impedance audiometry. I. Normal and sensorineural ears. Arch Otolaryngol 1972; 96:513–523.
87. Northern JL. Clinical management procedures. In: Jerger J, ed. Handbook of clinical impedance audiometry. Dobbs Ferry, NY: American Electromedics Corporation, 1975: 21.
88. Sanders JW, Josey AF, Glasscock ME. The acoustic stapedial reflex test in cochlear and eighth nerve disorders. Paper presented at the Third International Symposium on Impedance Audiometry, American Electromedics Corporation, New York, 1976.
89. Jerger J. Diagnostic use of impedance measures. In: Jerger J, ed. Handbook of clinical impedance audiometry. Dobbs Ferry, NY: American Electromedics Corporation, 1975: 149.
90. Anderson H, Barr B, Wedenberg E. Early diagnosis of VIIIth nerve tumors by acoustic reflex tests. Acta Otolaryngol [Suppl] 1970; 263:232–237.
91. Jerger J, Harford E, Clemis J, Alford B. The acoustic reflex in eighth nerve disorders. Arch Otolaryngol 1974; 99:409–413.
92. Sheehy JL, Inzer BE. Acoustic reflex test in neuro-otologic diagnosis. Arch Otolaryngol 1976; 102:647–653.
93. Sanders JW, Josey AF, Glasscock ME, Jackson CG. The acoustic reflex text in cochlear and eighth nerve pathology ears. Laryngoscope 1981; 91:787–793.
94. Silman S, Gelfand SA. The relationship between magnitude of hearing loss and acoustic reflex threshold levels. J Speech Hear Disord 1981; 46:312–316.
95. Olsen WO, Bauch CD, Harner SG. Application of Silman

and Gelfand (1981) 90th percentile levels for acoustic reflex thresholds. J Speech Hear Disord 1983; 48:330–332.
96. Sanders JW. Evaluation of the 90th percentile levels for acoustic reflex thresholds. Paper presented at the National Convention of the American Speech-Language-Hearing Association, San Francisco, 1984.
97. Clemis JD, Sarno CN. The acoustic reflex latency test: clinical application. Laryngoscope 1980; 90:601–611.
98. Mangham CA, Lindeman RC, Dawson WR. Stapedius reflex quantification in acoustic tumor patients. Laryngoscope 1980; 90:242–250.
99. McPherson DL, Thompson D. Quantification of the threshold and latency parameters of the acoustic reflex in humans. Acta Otolaryngol 1977; Suppl. 353:1–37.
100. Zito F, Roberts M. The acoustic reflex pattern studied by the averaging technique. Audiology 1980; 19:395–403.
101. Sanders JW, Humes L. A direct method for quantification of the acoustic reflex. Paper presented at the National Convention of the American Speech-Language-Hearing Association, Detroit, 1980.
102. Barrs DM, Brackmann DE, Olson JE, House WF. Changing concepts of acoustic neuroma diagnosis. Arch Otolaryngol 1985; 111:17–21.
103. Bauch CD, Rose DE, Harner SG. Auditory brainstem response results from 255 patients with suspected retrocochlear involvement. Ear Hear 1982; 3:83–86.
104. Bauch CD, Olsen WO, Harner SG. Auditory brainstem response and acoustic reflex test. Arch Otolaryngol 1983; 109:522–525.
105. Clemis JD, McGee T. Brain stem electric response audiometry and the differential diagnosis of acoustic tumors. Laryngoscope 1979; 89:31–42.
106. Glasscock ME, Jackson CG, Josey AF, Dickens J, Wiet R. Brainstem evoked response audiometry in clinical practice. Laryngoscope 1979; 89:1021–1034.
107. Josey AF, Jackson CG, Glasscock ME. Brain stem evoked response audiometry in confirmed eighth nerve tumors. Am J Otol 1980; 1:285–290.
108. Selters WA, Brackmann DE. Acoustic tumor detection with brain stem electric response audiometry. Arch Otolaryngol 1977; 103:181–197.
109. Jewett DW, Williston JS. Auditory evoked far fields averaged from the scalp of humans. Brain 1971; 94:681–696.
110. Gilroy J, Lynn GE. Computerized tomography and auditory-evoked potentials. Arch Neurol 1978; 35:143–147.
111. Starr A, Achor J. Auditory brain stem responses in neurological disease. Arch Neurol 1975; 32:761–768.
112. Stephens SD, Thornton ARD. Subjective and electrophysiologic tests in brain stem lesions. Arch Otolaryngol 1976; 102:608–613.
113. Stockard JJ, Rossiter VS. Clinical and pathologic correlates of brain stem auditory response abnormalities. Neurology 1977; 27:316–325.

41 Acoustic Immittance Measurements in Clinical Audiology

James W. Hall III, Ph.D.
James F. Jerger, Ph.D.

In 1946, Otto Metz systematically evaluated the acoustic immittance of normal and abnormal ears.[1] (Note that immittance is a generic term for describing the physical properties of the ear. It may be quantified as either ad*mittance,* (Y), or *im*pedance, (Z). Impedance is a measure of the opposition of energy flow into the middle ear. Admittance, the reciprocal quantity, is the ease of energy flow into the middle ear.) Metz described distinct changes in acoustic immittance associated with different middle ear disorders. In a 20-year period following Metz's classic work, his basic findings were confirmed and expanded by numerous investigators.[2–7] During the early 1970s, the remarkable value of immittance audiometry in the detection and description of auditory dysfunction was repeatedly demonstrated.[8,9] Immittance measurements were applied in screening of hearing,[10,11] differentiation of conductive versus sensorineural auditory dysfunction,[8,9,12–15] differentiation of cochlear versus retrocochlear auditory dysfunction,[14,16–19] identification and localization of central auditory disorder,[20–24] prediction of hearing level,[25–27] and hearing aid evaluation.[28–31]

With few exceptions, these studies were conducted with single-component, single-frequency acoustic immittance measurements. That is, one physical dimension of aural acoustic immittance was measured, the magnitude of acoustic impedance, with a fixed, low probe-tone frequency (226 Hz). Even though the clinical validity and value of this test protocol is beyond question, a host of investigators have, since 1975, clearly demonstrated that measurement of multiple components of aural acoustic immittance, such as susceptance and conductance concomitantly with admittance and the admittance phase angle, with multiple probe-tone frequencies, for example 226 Hz, 660 Hz, and 810 Hz, can contribute importantly to the clinical assessment of middle ear status.[32–39]

Immittance measurement offers unique clinical advantages, including objectivity, ease of administration, and versatility. Because of these advantages, it has assumed a major role in the audiometric test battery. In this chapter, we will present an overview of clinical immittance measurements, including a discussion of the basic instrumentation, a description of the three general immittance measures, and principles of test interpretation. For a comprehensive review of the history and physical principles of aural acoustic immittance, we highly recommend a recent American Speech-Language-Hearing Association monograph by Van Camp, Margolis, Wilson, Creten, and Shanks.[37] Shanks[35] and Hall[40] also present readable discussions of current principles of tympanometry.

INSTRUMENTATION

Early studies of aural acoustic immittance utilized mechanical measuring devices.[1,2,7] In general, the design and function of these instruments were not well suited for clinical application. In 1960, Terkildsen and Scott-Nielsen first described an electroacoustic immittance meter.[41] This instrument, a precursor of current acoustic immittance measuring devices, offered distinct clinical advantages.[42] Currently, there are over a dozen brands of clinical immittance meters, with over 30 models available commercially.

Most clinical immittance meters actually measure impedance and consist of three major components. The first component is the electrical circuit used in monitoring acoustic impedance either at the probe tip, for many commercial instruments, or more accurately corrected to the plane of the tympanic membrane. A pure-tone oscillator generates a tone, usually at 226 Hz, but optimally at one or more higher frequencies as well. The tone is delivered continuously to the ear through a small tube set within a probe. The "probe tube" is fitted with a soft rubber cuff, permitting an airtight seal with the external ear canal wall. The "probe tone" usually has a nominal intensity of 85 dB sound pressure level (SPL) measured in a rigid-walled 2-ml cavity. When the probe is sealed within the external ear canal, however, the exact SPL of the probe tone is proportional to the effects of the ear canal volume and the acoustic impedance of the middle ear vibratory system. With the influence of the ear canal volume accounted for, the greater the impedance of the middle ear mechanism, the greater the probe tone's intensity within the external ear canal, and vice versa. For most commercial instruments, the intensity of the probe tone within the sealed external ear canal is monitored continuously by a small pressure-sensitive microphone within the probe assembly. Two-component electroacoustic commercially available instruments, and specially designed devices that are likely to be available commercially soon,[33,43] permit the measurement of complex variables, including susceptance, conductance, and admittance phase angle. Impedance and admittance meter design is reviewed in greater detail in the recent monograph by Van Camp and colleagues (p 31).[37]

Traditionally, immittance of the middle ear system was reported as the volume of air (in cubic centimeters, cc or cm^3, or milliliters, ml), yielding equivalent compliance.[44] Technically, the quantity being measured was immittance vector magnitude. Since the normal ear and the ear with reduced mobility (e.g., an otosclerotic ear) is stiffness controlled at 226 Hz and, therefore, the principal factor influencing immittance is compliance, this factor alone has typically—and incorrectly—been the term used to express results of the immittance measurement procedure. Expressing immittance values in terms of equivalent volume of air in cubic centimeters or milliliters is not necessarily accurate for normal ears at higher probe-tone frequencies, for normal neonatal ears, nor for some types of middle ear pathology.

The second major component of the clinical immittance meter is an air pressure system consisting of a pump and manometer. This component permits precise manipulation of air pressure within the enclosed ear canal. The minimal capacity of the air pressure system is typically from +200 to −400 mm H_2O pressure or decapascal (daPa). One daPa equals 1.02 mm H_2O, and so the two units of pressure are practically equivalent.

The third component of the immittance meter generates acoustic signals used to elicit contraction of the stapedius muscle (the acoustic reflex). Signals usually include pure tones at octave frequencies of 250 or 500 Hz to 4,000 Hz and a broad-band or white noise signal. Many immittance meters also generate high-pass and low-pass noise band signals. Initially, clinical immittance devices permitted measurement of acoustic reflexes only in the contralateral or "crossed" mode. That is, the signal is presented to one ear by earphone while immittance change is measured with the probe assembly in the opposite ear. Currently, however, most clinical instruments permit measurement of acoustic reflexes in both the contralateral and ipsilateral or "uncrossed" modes. In the ipsilateral mode, the signal is delivered to the ear by a small transducer located with the probe assembly, and the acoustic immittance change is measured in the same ear.

TYMPANOMETRY

Tympanometry reflects a change in the physical properties of the middle ear system and tympanic membrane as air pressure in the external ear canal is varied. Tympanometry requires an airtight or hermetic seal between the immittance probe cuff and external ear canal walls.

Ear Canal Volume

Tympanometry begins with the introduction of relatively high (+200 daPa) or low (−400 daPa) pressure into the external ear canal. At these pressures, impedance of the middle ear and tympanic membrane is practically infinitely high and admittance is virtually zero. Therefore immittance is measured only for the volume of air enclosed within the ear canal between the probe tip and the tympanic membrane. Actually, the volume is measured most accurately by tympanometry at −400 daPa, whereas estimations at +200 daPa generate relatively large errors.[35] Ear canal volumes range from 0.50 to 1.00 ml in children and 0.65 to 1.75 ml in adults. Volumes may be somewhat smaller in females than in males.[45] Ear volume estimation is a routine component of tympanometry with commercially available instruments (Fig. 41–1). The immittance of air

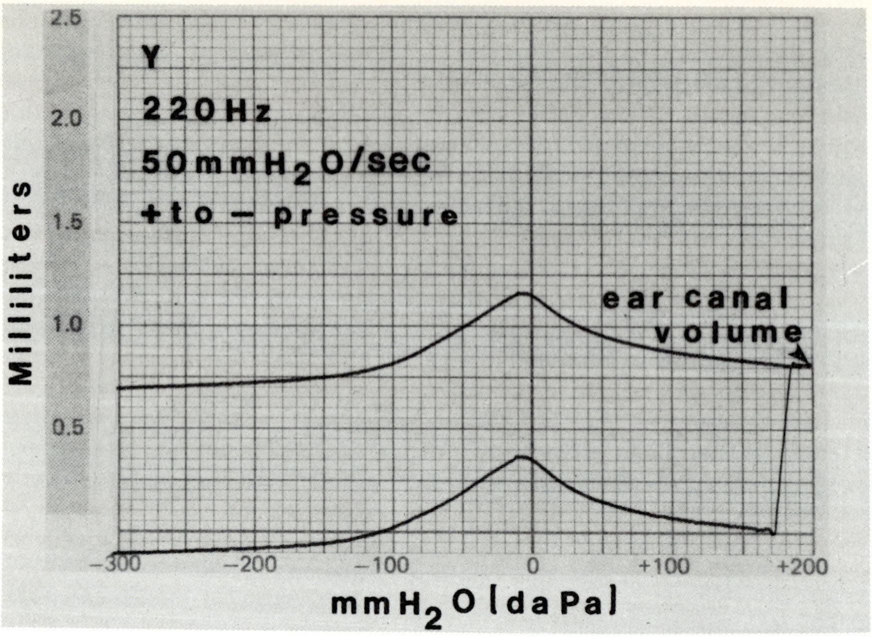

Figure 41–1 Normal admittance /*Y*/ tympanograms. Lower tympanogram was recorded in a baseline-correct mode. Automatic ear canal volume estimation is shown on the right.

within the enclosed ear canal consists of one dimension, compliance reactance, and does not change as a function of variations in air pressure.[35]

Single-Component Tympanometry

With single-component tympanometry, admittance (Y) (often referred to simply as compliance) of the middle ear system increases (impedance [Z] decreases) as ear canal pressure approaches approximately 0.0 daPa (see Fig. 41–1). At 0.0 daPa, or often at a slightly negative pressure, such as 0.0 to −25.0 (as reported by Jerger[9]), admittance is maximal (impedance is minimal). Then, with further variation in air pressure, the magnitude of these middle ear physical quantities approach their respective baseline values. Immittance values may differ for the positive versus negative pressure extremes, as illustrated in Figure 41–1. Immittance pressure functions may be recorded continuously on a strip-chart recorder or x-y plotter, or immittance values at different pressure readings may be plotted manually.

Tympanogram Classification

There are a variety of classification systems for single-component (admittance or impedance), low probe-tone frequency (226 Hz) tympanograms.[6,9,46–48] Jerger's system is simple and clinically popular. With this system, tympanograms are classified as type A, type B, or type C (Fig. 41–2).[9] The type A, or normal tympanogram, has a peak (point of maximum admittance or compliance) at or near normal atmospheric pressure, within the range of 0.0 to −100 daPa pressure. A type B tympanogram has no distinct point of maximum admittance. As pressure in the ear canal is varied, the admittance changes relatively little. In some cases, the type B tympanogram is virtually flat. However, the type B tympanogram may more closely resemble a "rounded" type A. And, in another variation of the type B tympanogram, the admittance gradually increases with a pressure change throughout the range of +200 to −400 daPa pressure without a peak. Tympanogram type C has a distinct point of maximum admittance. However, the peak occurs when air pressure in the ear canal exceeds −100 daPa relative to normal atmospheric pressure.

The three single-component tympanogram types described in Jerger's classification system adequately differentiate many middle ear pathologic entities.[9] However, variations of these types have been described. The type A tympanogram may be excessively deep (AD), reflecting a highly compliant middle ear system or a flaccid tympanic membrane.[9] A higher probe-tone frequency (e.g., 600 Hz or 800 Hz) may yield a W-shaped tympanogram or an undulating tympanogram, even in persons with unequivocally normal hearing.[49,50] These tympanograms are sometimes classified as type D[50] and type E.[51]

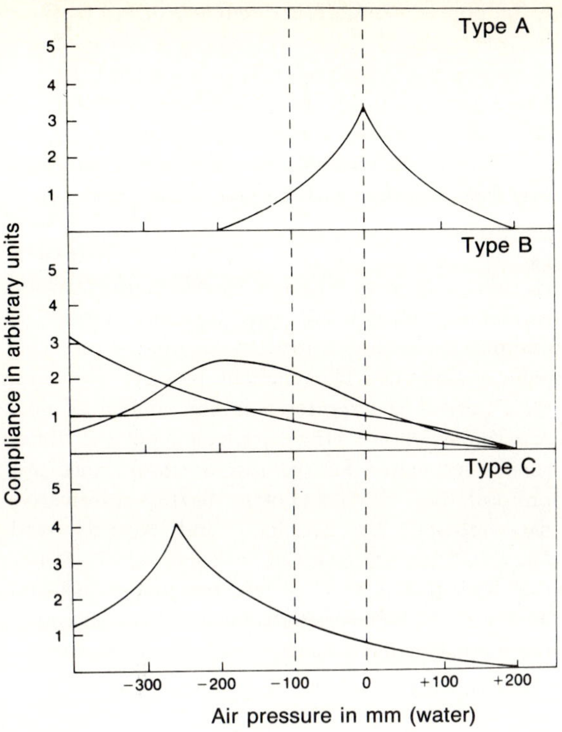

Figure 41–2 Tympanogram types according to the clinically popular classification system reported by Jerger.[9]

Static Immittance

Static immittance, often a component of tympanometry, is acoustic immittance of the middle ear at rest, that is, under normal atmospheric pressure. This static immittance is in contrast to the immittance pressure function (i.e., tympanogram), which is a dynamic measure of middle ear physical properties. Static immittance is best measured at 226 Hz for practical and scientific reasons (p 41).[37] Clinically, static immittance is determined by first estimating the physical volume of air in the external ear canal. This measurement is made at an air pressure extreme that produces minimal baseline admittance (maximal impedance) as noted before. Then static immittance of the middle ear system is calculated by subtracting the estimated ear canal volume from the peak immittance value from tympanometry. Such calculations, either manual or automatic, may be subject to error if only vector magnitude information is used (e.g., the admittance or the compliance quantities in single-component instruments) without regard to the quantity phase angle.[35] However, calculations based on a 226-Hz probe tone in normal ears probably produce clinically negligible error.

When measured at 226 Hz and described as compliance of an equivalent volume of air, normal static immittance values range from about 0.30 to 1.60 ml.[13] These values are influenced to some extent by the age and sex of the patient. Static admittance (compliance) tends to increase with chronologic age from 1 to 35 years.[13,45] The increase during this age range is greater for males than for females. Above 35 years of age, static admittance gradually decreases with age.[13,45] The average values above 70 years of age approach the lower limit of the normal range (0.30 ml). In general, static admittance is greater in males than in females.

As Van Camp and colleagues point out,[37] little unified normative data on static immittance in physical units exist, such as admittance in acoustic mmhos collected according to well-defined and clinically applicable methodology. Data reported by Koebsell and Margolis[52] and Wilson, Shanks, and Kaplan[39] and recommended by Van Camp et al (p 43)[37] are displayed in Table 41–1.

Static immittance can contribute to the identification and differentiation of middle ear disorders.[8,9,12] The most common middle ear disorders, fixation of the ossicular chain, middle ear fluid, and

TABLE 41–1 Admittance and Impedance Normative Data in Physical Units Recommended by Van Camp et al[37]

Population	*Index*	*Admittance (Y) (acoustic mmhos)†*	*Impedance (acoustic ohms)*
Children*	Lower limit	0.35	1100
	Median	0.53	1900
	Upper limit	0.90	2900
Adults	Lower limit	0.50	570
	Median	0.91	1100
	Upper limit	1.75	2000

Data were collected with a 226-Hz probe frequency at a slow air pump speed (50 daPa/sec for children and 25 daPa/sec for adults).

* Children were in the age range of 3 to 5 years; mean age for adults was 25.6 years.

† Under standard barometric conditions the admittance units are equivalent to volume units (cc or ml).

discontinuity of the ossicular chain, characteristically alter static immittance.

Interpretation of static immittance values is further confounded by a general but often unappreciated principle in impedance audiometry. Impedance findings reflect the function of the middle ear system; they do not define nor diagnose middle ear pathology.[15] For example, static compliance is sensitive to the reduced mobility of the ossicular chain that is associated with otosclerosis. Static compliance is altered by a mechanical effect. However, the mechanical effect—increased ossicular chain stiffness—is not invariably associated with otosclerosis; other clinical entities, for example, adhesive otitis media, may similarly restrict ossicular chain mobility. Interpretation of low static compliance values is further complicated by the possible influence of the patient's age. Above 35 years of age, static compliance tends to decrease with increasing age. In persons of 30 to 40 years, the average static compliance value usually differentiates the normal ear from the ear with diagnosed otosclerosis.[45] Above age 60, however, the normal ear and otosclerotic ear are indistinguishable by static compliance alone.[45]

It would appear from this discussion that, in view of the lack of normative data in physical units, the considerable overlap of normal and clinical expectations, and the methodologic factors affecting measurement,[37,39,53] static immittance is of little value in the identification and differentiation of middle ear disorders. Indeed, its usefulness, when evaluated alone, is limited. However, interpreted in conjunction with other audiometric tests, static immittance can assume a more valued role.

Tympanogram Gradient

In addition to measurement of ear canal volume, pressure for peak immittance, and static immittance, gradient has recently received renewed interest as a clinically useful tympanometric parameter.[47,52,54–56] A detailed discussion of gradient, a quantification of tympanogram shape, is beyond the scope of this chapter. An example of one measure of gradient, a computation of tympanogram admittance relative to a pressure range, is illustrated in Figure 41–3 (see Hall for a review of the gradient concept[40]). Briefly, a half-amplitude admittance (Y) point is determined on each side (positive and negative pressure directions) by dividing the total amplitude on each side by two

$$Yx - Yc\,\mathrm{pos}/2 = Yb$$

$$Yx - Yc\,\mathrm{neg}/2 = Ya$$

as in Figure 41–3. The difference in air pressure between each of these points on the slope of the tympanogram (pressure for Ya; Pa; pressure for Yb: Pb) is referred to as delta (difference) pressure, or ΔP, and is stated in decaPascals.

Each of the tympanograms shown in Figure 41–3 is from a subject with normal hearing sensitivity, including absence of an air-bone gap. However, subject JH reported that as a child he had numerous ear infections with frequent spontaneous tympanic membrane ruptures and myringotomies. Otoscopic examination indicated marked scarring of the tympanic membrane. The gradient pressure difference for a patient is interpreted in the context of normative data that is either available from the literature or generated for the specific immittance test protocol used in an audiology facility. Normative data reported by deJonge[55] and Koebsell and Margolis[52] are summarized in Table 41–2. Referring back to Figure 41–3, the tympanogram's gradient pressure difference for subject TH is well within the normal region (exactly at deJonge's fiftieth percentile), whereas JH has an abnormally small pressure difference.

The gradient pressure difference index is easy to calculate, which is a clinical asset, and, based on the findings of deJonge[55] and Koebsell and Margolis,[52] contributes information unavailable from the simple static immittance measures. Furthermore, these investigators speculate that the gradient pressure difference may have more desirable sensitivity and specificity characteristics for detection of high-impedance (low admittance) middle ear pathology. Although the technique is clinically attractive, it awaits documentation in patient populations. To provide meaningful data, optimal studies of this and other tympanometric measures should be carried out with real physical units of immittance (e.g., acoustic ohms for impedance or mmho for admittance).

Multiple-Frequency, Multiple-Component Tympanometry

Since their introduction in the early 1970s, clinical aural acoustic immittance measures have most often been made for a single-component, compliant reactance with a single probe frequency (usually 226 Hz). There are probably three major reasons for this trend. First, up until recently only one manufacturer (Grason Stadler) marketed an instrument with the capacity for more sophisticated measurements. Now several different brands are available commercially. Second, many otologic diseases increase middle ear impedance or stiffness (e.g., otitis media, eustachian tube dysfunction with tympanic membrane retrac-

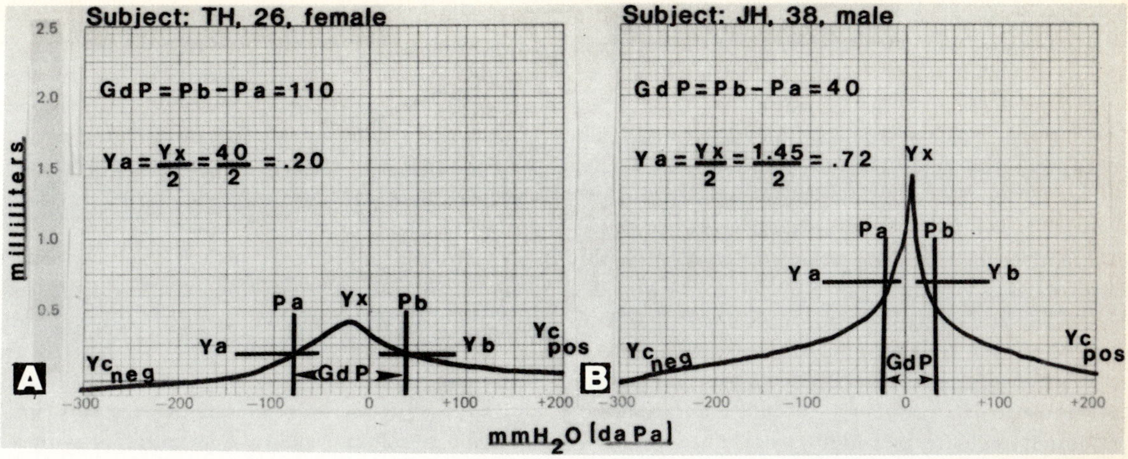

Figure 41-3 Example of calculation of tympanogram gradient for difference in pressure (GdP) for an ear with *A*, normal admittance (subject TH) and *B*, an ear with high admittance (subject JH).

tion), which in many cases is detected and adequately described with a low-frequency probe tone and acoustic compliance (the reciprocal of stiffness). Third, tympanograms generated for multiple components with higher frequencies tend to be more complex and, initially, less easy to categorize and interpret clinically, in contrast to the more familiar and simple bell-shaped tympanograms produced with traditional techniques. For example, reports of early studies of high-frequency tympanometry describing W-shaped tympanograms (referred to as type D and E) in apparently normal ears implied difficulty in differentiating normal from abnormal findings clinically[49,50,56] and associated the pattern with normal neonatal middle ear status.[57] Another concern was the occurrence of the W-shaped tympanogram in patients with a variety of different types of middle ear pathologies.[49]

TABLE 41-2 Normative Data for Children[52] and Adults[55] for Tympanometric Gradient (GdP) Based on the Difference in Pressure (dP) Between Half-Amplitude Points on Admittance Tympanogram

Population	*Index*	*GdP (daPa)*
Children*	Mean	133
	10th percentile	80
	90th percentile	200
Adults†	50th percentile	110
	5th percentile	63
	90th percentile	162

Data were collected with a 226-Hz probe frequency at a standard air pump speed of 50 daPa/sec. See text for details on the calculation of GdP.

* Data for 88 ears of 46 children between the ages of 3.7 and 5.8 years.

† Data for right ears of 83 college students with an average age of 22 years.

Colletti[23] and Vanhuyse, Creten, and Van Camp[38] first systematically and mathematically related the varied multipeaked tympanogram patterns (W-shaped tympanograms) to normal middle ear function versus otologic pathology. The overall clinical objective of multifrequency and multicomponent tympanometry is to identify and define specific middle ear dysfunctions associated with low-impedance abnormalities (different types and degrees of ossicular chain disruptions) and certain high-impedance abnormalities (various types and degrees of ossicle fixations). Single frequency and component tympanometry has inadequate sensitivity to these entities. Van Camp and colleagues present three arguments for adding high-frequency (they recommend either 660 or preferably 678 Hz, an integral multiple of 226 Hz) two-component tympanometry to the routine immittance test battery: (p 50)[37] (1) low-impedance abnormalities produce unique tympanogram shapes only for high probe frequencies, (2) contralateral acoustic reflex measurement in both adult and neonatal populations is possible with a higher-frequency probe tone because the 226-Hz probe tone is appropriate only for adults, but unsuitable for neonates, and (3) ipsilateral acoustic reflexes, which are useful clinically, are contaminated by artifacts at 226 Hz, but not at 660 Hz.[58]

There are a number of thorough descriptions of multifrequency, multicomponent tympanometric patterns and the rules used in their clinical application, including, of course, the differentiation of normal from pathologic ears.[32,33,35–37,40,53,59] What follows here is a review of some of the important factors in measurement and an outline of the terminology used in the categorization of multifrequency, multicomponent (susceptance, conductance, admittance) tympanometry with commercially available equipment. The reader is strongly encouraged to select among the references noted previously for additional information in his or her preparation for clinical application of this technique.

Interpretation of multifrequency, multicomponent tympanometry is essentially an exercise in pattern recognition. At this point, clinical conclusions are based primarily on qualitative rather than quantitative analysis. Terminology for description of complex tympanograms is noted in Figures 41–4 and 41–5. The complexity of tympanograms varies depending on the number of peaks, or extrema, for each component at each frequency. An extreme may be referred to as a maximum (increased admittance) or a minimum (decreased admittance). Therefore the simplest normal pattern has one peak for susceptance (B), one for conductance (G) and one for admittance (Y), or 1B1G1Y (see Figure 41–4). A bell-shaped tympanogram for each component is found for the majority of normal ears, but there are at least 5 other normal patterns, as displayed in Table 41–3. A pattern occurring in 4.5 percent of the normal population studied by Creten and colleagues,[53] a 3B3G3Y tympanogram, is illustrated in Figure 41–5. This middle ear is mass controlled at ambient ear canal pressure (0.0 daPa), and both susceptance and conductance tympanograms have a minimum peak in the center and a maximum on either side. This tympanogram pattern met two criteria for it to be classified as normal. First, the pressure interval between the two maximum peaks was greater for the susceptance than the conductance curve. And, second, in accordance with data of Van de Heyning et al,[60] for this 3B3G3Y tympanogram type (at 660 Hz), the two susceptance maxima were within a pressure range of no greater than 75 daPa.

This pattern schema includes an admittance phase angle quantity, $Y\phi$ since phase was reported in some of the basic studies of multifrequency, multicomponent tympanometry.[32,36,53,61,62] Phase angle measurement is not a standard feature on commercially available immittance instruments at this time.

For meaningful clinical application of tympanometry, importantly, one must recognize the influence of test variables, including, in addition to probe frequency and the admittance component measured, the direction (positive-to-negative versus negative-to-positive) and rate (e.g., 25, 50, or 100 daPa per second) of pressure change[49,63] and the number of successive tympanometry trials for a patient while the ear canal remains sealed.[63]

Restraint and caution in the clinical application of tympanometry are warranted. Diagnosis of middle ear pathology can rarely be made on the basis of tympanometry alone,[9,35,37] whereas routine otoscopic examination is sufficiently sensitive for differential

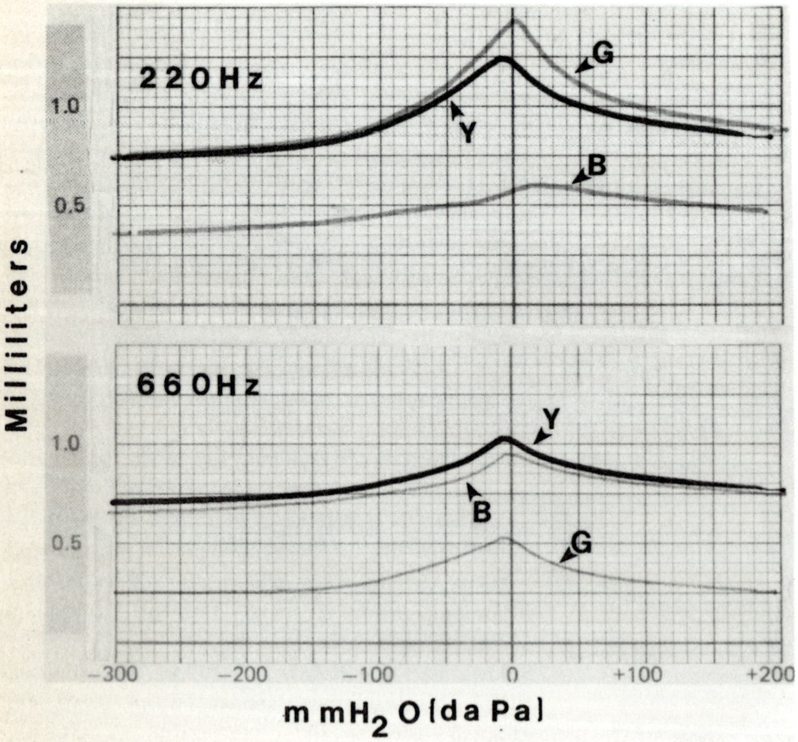

Figure 41–4 Bell-shaped, multi-probe-frequency, multicomponent admittance tympanograms for a normal ear. Abbreviations for components: Y = admittance; B = susceptance; G = conductance.

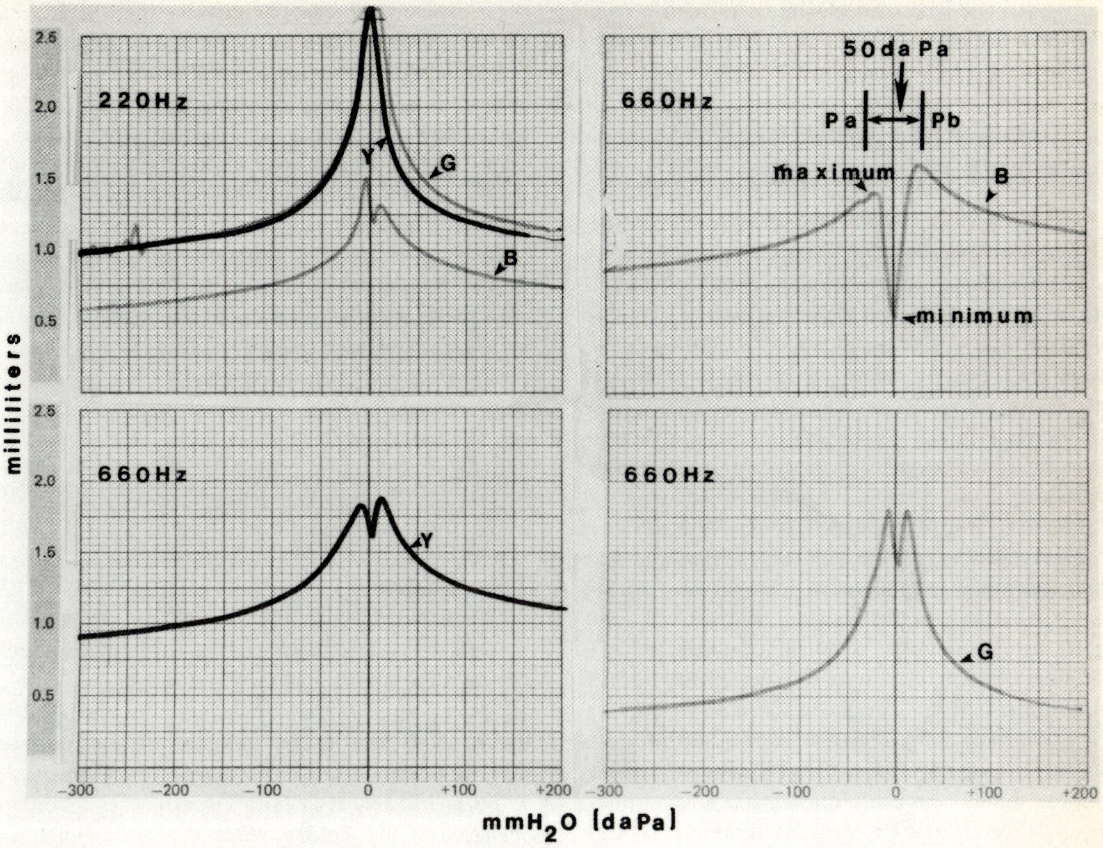

Figure 41–5 Multi-probe-frequency, multicomponent admittance tympanograms for an ear with a scarred tympanic membrane but normal hearing. *Pa* and *Pb* refer to the negative and positive pressure values, respectively, of the maximum admittance peaks. Tympanogram components are defined in the legend for Figure 41–4.

diagnosis of certain pathologies. As Van Camp et al point out, the sensitivity of tympanometry exceeds its specificity.[37] In other words, middle ear pathology is invariably detected by an abnormal tympanometric pattern (high sensitivity), but to record abnormal patterns in nonpathologic ears as well is not uncommon. Furthermore, inconsistencies among tympanometric patterns and types of pathologies are expected, such as mass-controlled tympanogram shapes in ears with otitis media (a stiffness abnormality). Yet one pathology, such as otosclerosis, may produce distinctly different tympanograms in different patients. These clinical problems are certainly not unique to tympanometry. Confirmation, or a cross-check of the results of a single test procedure, such as tympanometry, with independent measures of auditory function, for example, pure-tone audiometry, is always good clinical practice.[64]

TABLE 41–3 Proportion of Differen' Types of Normal Multicomponent Tympanograms with a 660-Hz Probe-Tone Frequency and an Air Pump Speed of 27 daPa/sec for 132 Young Adults

Tympanogram Type	*Subjects (%)*
1B 1G 1Y 1 ϕ	56.8
3B 1G 1Y 1 ϕ	25.8
3B 1G 3Y 1 ϕ	2.3
3B 3G 3Y 1 ϕ	4.5
3B 3G 3Y 3 ϕ	1.5
5B 3G 3Y 3 ϕ	9.1

Abbreviations: B = susceptance; G = conductance; Y = admittance; ϕ = Y phase angle. Numbers indicate the number of tympanogram peaks for the component.

From Creten WL, Van de Heyning PH, Van Camp KJ. Immittance audiometry. Normative data at 200 and 660 Hz. Scand Audiol 1985; 14:117.

Nonetheless, from the preceding review, it is clear that tympanometry has a secure role in clinical audiology. We concur heartily with Lilly that "the time is past for audiologists and manufacturers to debate the relative merits of low-frequency verus middle frequency probe tones" and "to debate the relative merits of acoustic impedance, acoustic admittance, magnitude, phase or SPL measurements in EAM (external auditory meatus)" (p 307)[33] The time has come for applying the combinations of instrumentation, techniques, and immittance quantities in clinical aural immittance measurement that are most effective for the description of middle ear function of a given patient.

ACOUSTIC STAPEDIAL REFLEX

Anatomy

A sufficiently intense sound, presented to the normal ear, produces reflex contraction of the stapedius muscle. The acoustic stapedial reflex is a bilateral brain stem–mediated reflex. That is, sound presented to either ear causes stapedius muscle contraction in both ears. Stapedius muscle contraction is the final step in the neuromuscular reflex. Hall recently reviewed current knowledge of acoustic reflex anatomy and physiology.[65] Briefly, the afferent or sensory portion consists of the cochlea and the eighth (acoustic) cranial nerve. The cochlea transduces the acoustic signal to a neural correlate. The eighth nerve transmits neural information to the central auditory nervous system. The central portion of the reflex consists of auditory and facial nerve nuclei in the brain stem. There are direct and indirect brain stem pathways. The direct pathways, which are most studied, probably consist of a 3- or 4-neuron arc; they include (1) neurons from the ventral cochlear nucleus, terminating in the region of the ipsilateral motor facial nerve nucleus and in the ipsilateral and contralateral medial superior olivary nucleus, (2) neurons from in and around the medial superior olivary nucleus, terminating on the ipsilateral or contralateral region near the motor nucleus of the facial nerve, and (3) motor neurons of the facial nerve, the efferent or motor portion of the arc, which originate from the area around the facial nerve motor nucleus and terminate on the ipsilateral stapedius muscle. The stapedial is the smallest skeletal muscle in mammals.[66]

An indirect acoustic reflex pathway has also been described. Although the anatomic details are not well defined, it appears to be slower, polysynaptic, and involves the reticular formation components.[20,67] Of clinical relevance is the contribution of this indirect pathway to the susceptability of the acoustic reflex to central nervous system depressants, such as barbiturates.[68] Cortical mediation of acoustic reflex activity has been suggested,[69,70] but not fully documented.

Therefore the acoustic reflex arc is both "crossed" and "uncrossed;" that is, sound presented to one ear produces stapedius muscle contraction in the opposite ear and in the ear stimulated. Contraction of the stapedius muscle tenses and stiffens the ossicular chain. The primary mechanical effect is decreased mobility of the ossicular chain. The increase in stiffness, and consequently acoustic impedance, reduces the efficiency of sound transmission by the middle ear mechanism. With stapedius muscle contraction, then, the middle ear system with its higher impedance (reduced admittance) accepts less energy than when at rest. Altered immittance of the middle ear system is easily detected at the plane of the tympanic membrane by commercially available immittance instruments. Stapedius muscle activity and, therefore, changes in middle ear immittance may be elicited by a variety of nonacoustic stimuli. In immittance audiometry, however, these changes are elicited by acoustic signals.

Response Parameters

Threshold

Stapedius muscle contraction in response to relatively high intensity sounds was demonstrated over 50 years ago.[1,71,72] In normal ears, as displayed in Figure 41–6, the acoustic reflex is elicited by pure-tone signals at 85 to 95 dB hearing level (HL) and by broad-band noise at 65 to 85 dB.[13,73–77] Standard deviation of the acoustic reflex threshold is approximately 5 dB for tonal stimuli and 10 dB for noise.[13,78] Acoustic reflex threshold, the response parameter most often applied clinically, is usually defined as the lowest sound intensity level producing a reliable change in middle ear immittance, as detected by visual monitoring of a meter or analysis of a graphic recording. To adhere to preferred behavioral pure-tone audiometric techniques in reflex threshold measurement is unnecessary, and no differences in thresholds obtained with ascending versus descending intensity protocols exist. Signal averaging techniques, similar to those employed in auditory evoked response recording, appear to enhance the sensitivity and accuracy of acoustic reflex measurement.[79] Three acoustic reflex parameters, in addition to threshold, are reported in the literature and are of clinical value.

Latency

Latency is the time interval between stimulus presentation and some measure of related immittance change. This statement is necessarily rather vague since precise and consistent definition of the onset of reflex activity is problematic. Minimal latency in normal human subjects is approximately 10 msec, as recorded by the direct myographic detection of action potentials in the contralateral sta-

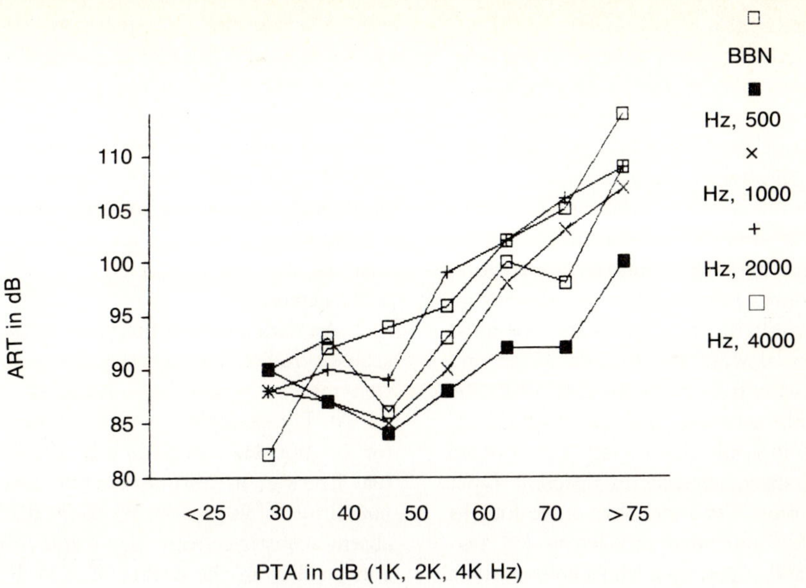

Figure 41-6 Contralateral acoustic reflex threshold (ART) for four tonal stimuli and a broad-band noise (BBN) stimulus as a function of a pure-tone average (PTA) for 671 subjects aged 1 to 20 years with normal hearing or sensorineural auditory impairment. Tone stimulus intensity is in dB hearing level; noise stimulus is in dB sound pressure level. (From Hall JW III, Weaver T. Impedance audiometery in a young population: effects of age, sex, and minor tympanogram abnormality. J Otolaryngol 1979; 8:210.)

pedius muscle elicited by tonal stimuli.[80] Latency values obtained clinically with commercially available equipment may be considerably greater (e.g., 100 msec) and inexact, because of inherent time constraints of the device and temporal distortion produced by filter components.[81–84] Clinical usefulness of acoustic reflex latency is further limited by interactions among stimulus intensity, frequency, and absolute reflex amplitude.[83,85,86] Jerger et al provide a concise current review of reported clinical applications and technical difficulties of acoustic reflex latency measurement.[83]

Decay

Since the clinical introduction of immittance measurements, acoustic reflex decay has held an important place in diagnostic audiometry.[16] In the acoustic reflex decay test, a pure-tone stimulus is presented continuously for 10 seconds at an intensity level of 10 dB above the threshold for the stimulus. The reflex-related immittance change is recorded graphically and examined for evidence of a decrease in amplitude of 50 percent or greater during the time course. Although slight decay is found in some normal ears and is common in patients with cochlear deficits,[63,87–89] significant decay (more than 50 percent) is a powerful sign of eighth nerve (retrocochlear) auditory dysfunction. Sensitivity of acoustic reflex decay in this population is approximately 85 percent.[16,90–93] Acoustic reflex decay may also be a sign of brain stem auditory pathology.[65,94]

Amplitude

Acoustic reflex growth, or an increase in amplitude (magnitude) as a function of increased stimulus intensity, was reported in early papers on immittance measurements[95] and has since been studied extensively and applied clinically.[20,96–104] Unlike latency, assessment of reflex amplitude is relatively straightforward and can be carried out with standard equipment. Factors such as age, middle ear status, stimulus frequency and bandwidth, static immittance, and sensorineural hearing impairment must be taken into account in the evaluation of eighth nerve or central nervous system auditory function with the amplitude parameter.[97–99]

Factors Influencing Acoustic Reflex Measurement

Each of the acoustic reflex characteristics noted before are, to varying extents, affected by instrumentation, stimulus parameters, subject factors, nonpathologic factors, such as drugs, and both peripheral and central auditory dysfunction. A complete discussion of these factors is beyond the scope of this chapter, but is offered by others.[65,89,105–108]

A broad range of stimulus parameters influence acoustic reflex threshold, decay, latency, and amplitude. Most important are mode of stimulus presentation (ipsilateral versus contralateral), frequency, bandwidth, and duration. Chronologic age and gender are the principal subject characteristics.

Middle ear and facial nerve status are important determinants in the application of acoustic reflexes in the identification and definition of sensorineural and central auditory impairment. In discussing acoustic reflex findings in abnormal ears, we must make a distinction between the stimulated ear and the ear with the probe tip, the probe ear. With the probe tip in an ear with middle ear dysfunction, acoustic reflexes are typically absent. Jerger et al noted the proportion of absent reflexes in different types of middle ear disorder.[12] In more than three-fourths of all patients with confirmed otosclerosis (77 percent), otitis media (91 percent), and cholesteatoma (82 percent), reflexes were absent for a 1,000-Hz signal. More than half of their patients with a tympanic membrane abnormality (55 percent) or discontinuity (53 percent) had absent reflexes. With the probe in the involved ear, there is a high likelihood of absent reflexes even if the air-bone gap is slight (e.g., 5 to 10 dB). Even minor middle ear aberrations in the probe ear, such as slight negative pressure of a highly compliant system, usually elevate the crossed acoustic reflex threshold in the opposite stimulated ear.[73,97–99]

When sound is presented to a conductive ear and immittance change is measured in the opposite normal ear (crossed reflex), there is a direct and predictable relationship between the reflex threshold level and the degree of conductive sensitivity loss, as indicated by the air-bone gap. Acoustic reflex threshold is elevated by the degree of sensitivity loss. For example, a 20-dB conductive loss would usually elevate the threshold by approximately 20 dB. Since the average acoustic reflex threshold is 85 dB HL for pure-tone signals, a conductive loss of 30 dB HL would elevate the threshold to 115 dB HL. Thus, with a maximum available stimulus intensity of 110 dB HL, acoustic reflexes would probably be immeasurable. According to Jerger et al, in an ear with a conductive loss with an air-bone gap of greater than 50 dB, the likelihood that reflexes are absent is 90 percent.[12]

As with tympanometry and static immittance, acoustic reflex findings that are evaluated in isolation may be ambiguous (Tables 41–4, 41–5, and 41–6). For example, a reflex threshold of 95 dB HL for a 1,000-Hz signal may be consistent with normal hearing, a mild conductive loss, or a sensorineural loss of as great as 65 to 70 dB HL. Similarly, absent acoustic reflexes may result from a middle ear abnormality in the probe, or recording ear, a facial nerve (seventh cranial nerve) abnormality on the probe side, a moderate conductive or a profound sensorineural loss in the stimulated ear, or any combination of these abnormalities. In general, then, the findings of any single immittance measure may be ambiguous in a substantial proportion of patients.

Finally, any drug acting on the central nervous system can potentially alter acoustic reflex activity.[68,108] The possible effects of alcohol, barbiturates, ketamine, and commonly used sedatives should always be considered in the clinical interpretation of acoustic reflex findings.

PATTERNS OF IMMITTANCE AUDIOMETRY FINDINGS

We have stressed that findings for a single immittance measurement—tympanometry, static im-

TABLE 41–4 Pattern of Aural Acoustic Immittance Findings in Three Types of Middle Ear Abnormalities

	Abnormality		
Immittance Finding	*Ossicular Fixation*	*Ossicular Disruption*	*Otitis Media*
Tympanogram	A or A-shallow	A or A-deep*	C or B
Static immittance	Low to normal	High	Low
Acoustic reflexes			
Crossed: signal in normal ear; probe in abnormal ear	Absent	Usually absent	Absent
Crossed: signal in abnormal ear; probe in normal ear	Absent	Absent	Elevated or absent
Uncrossed: signal and probe in abnormal ear	Absent	Usually absent	Absent

* Multi-component 660-Hz probe-tone frequency tympanogram has broad W-shape or multiple peaks.

TABLE 41–5 Pattern of Aural Acoustic Immittance Findings in Normal Hearing Versus Sensorineural Impairment

Immittance findings	*Normal*	*Sensorineural Impairment* *Cochlear*	*Sensorineural Impairment* *Eighth Nerve*
Tympanogram	Normal	Normal	Normal
Static immittance	Normal	Normal	Normal
Acoustic reflexes			
Signal in impaired ear; probe in normal ear			
Threshold	Normal	Normal	Elevated or absent
SPAR*	Normal	Loss	Loss
Decay	Normal	Slight	Abnormal

* Sensitivity prediction by the acoustic reflex.

mittance, or acoustic reflexes—have limited diagnostic value. For the most part, this limitation is due to the large overlap between normal expectations and findings for different clinical groups. Still, combined findings of the immittance test battery are usually effective in differentiating clinical otologic entities. The diagnostic effectiveness of immittance measurements depends on accurate interpretation of the pattern of results. Skill in immittance "pattern recognition" (p 149)[15] is required. We will now present an overview of immittance patterns that characterize some relatively common clinical otologic disorders. Detailed discussion of acoustic immittance pattern interpretation is available in the literature.[14,15,37,40,65]

Conductive Versus Sensorineural Abnormalities

A sensorineural abnormality is presumed if all immittance findings are normal (see Table 41–5). That is, tympanograms are normal (type A or one of the normal high-probe frequency, multicomponent types shown in Table 41–3), static immittance values are within normal limits, and both crossed and uncrossed acoustic reflexes are present at normal levels and at all test frequencies. If any of the three immittance findings are abnormal, however, a conductive auditory impairment must be suspected.[15] This is a fundamental rule in immittance test interpretation in the differentiation of conductive versus sensorineural abnormalities.

Conductive Abnormalities

The pattern of immittance findings most consistent with conductive abnormalities is (1) abnormal tympanogram, (2) abnormal static immittance values, and (3) elevated or absent acoustic reflexes.[9,14,15] However, this unequivocally conductive pattern often may be incomplete (see Table 41–4). Therefore, if any immittance findings are abnormal, a conductive abnormality must be considered. An accurate definition of the hearing loss then depends on careful interpretation of immittance findings in conjunction with other audiometric test results, such as air- and bone-conduction pure-tone audiometry and sensorineural acuity level. Keep in mind that immittance findings are not pathonomonic and their

TABLE 41–6 Pattern of Aural Acoustic Immittance Findings for Peripheral Versus Central (Brain Stem) Auditory Dysfunction

Immittance Finding	*Auditory Dysfunction* *Peripheral*	*Auditory Dysfunction* *Brain Stem*
Tympanogram	Normal	Normal
Static immittance	Normal	Normal
Acoustic reflexes		
Uncrossed		
Threshold	Normal	Normal
Amplitude	Normal	Normal
Crossed		
Threshold	Normal	Elevated or absent
Amplitude	Normal	Reduced

* Sensitivity prediction by the acoustic reflex.

accurate interpretation does not constitute an otologic diagnosis.

Otosclerosis. In patients with otosclerosis and related ossicular chain fixation, the admittance tympanogram for a 226-Hz probe tone is usually a shallow type A, static admittance is low, and the acoustic reflexes are usually absent in both ears (see Fig. 41–7 and Table 41–4). Fixation, the mechanical effect on the ossicular chain that usually results from otosclerosis, reduces the mobility of the middle ear system. As expected, average static compliance in otosclerotic patients tends to be lower (0.35 ml) than normal (0.67 ml).[12] However, the range of static compliance values for normal ears and fixed ears overlaps to some extent. Thus low static compliance does not invariably imply fixation, nor does normal static compliance routinely rule out the possibility of fixation. In fact, few otosclerotic ears can be identified by static compliance alone.[12]

Although tympanogram depth in otosclerotic ears may vary and static admittance may fall within the normal range, the finding of a type A tympanogram in an ear with conductive loss is a distinct sign of ossicular chain fixation. In some cases of early ossicular chain fixation, the acoustic reflex recorded with the probe in the conductive ear may be present at normal levels. Generally, however, the reflex appears rarely and is characterized by a negative deflection (decreased impedance) at both the onset and offset of the eliciting signal. A negative deflection at the onset of the reflex time course is common in normal ears. However, the negative deflections at both the onset and offset of the reflex time course invariably reflect early fixation of the ossicular chain.[15] Typically, both crossed and uncrossed acoustic reflexes recorded from the involved ear are similarly affected. In most cases of ossicular chain fixation, however, both crossed and uncrossed reflexes are absent.

Otitis Media. There are numerous reports of immittance findings in patients at various stages in the development of otitis media.[8,9,11,12,54,56,109,110] Usually a negative middle ear pressure develops secondary to insufficient eustachian tube function and inadequate ventilation of the middle ear space. The resultant retraction of the tympanic membrane pro-

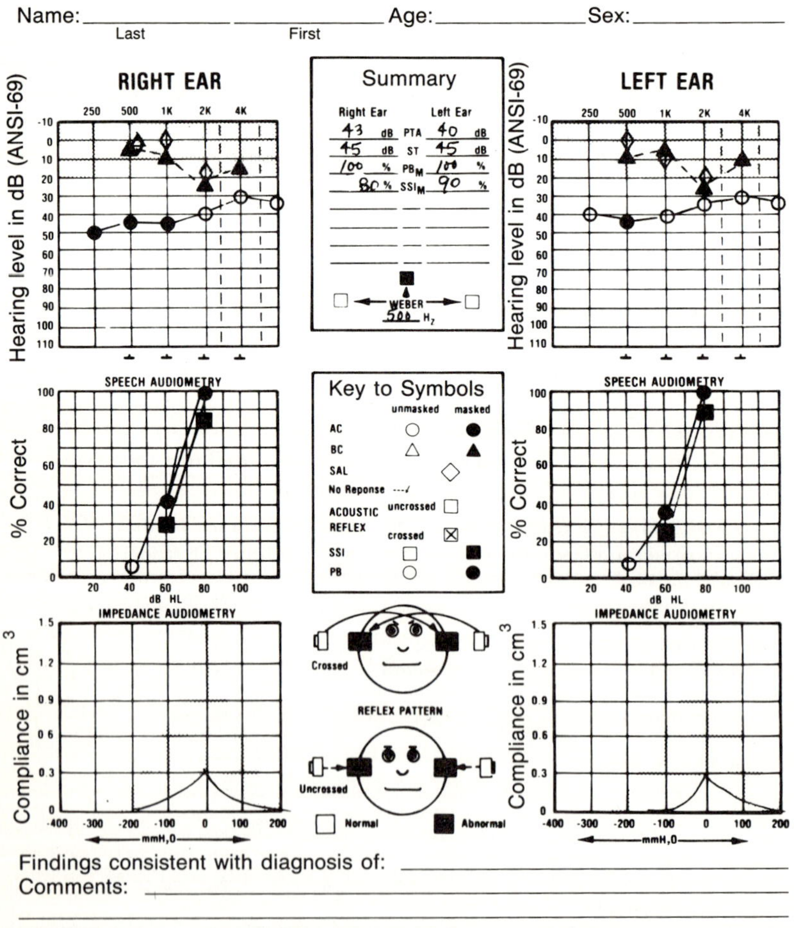

Figure 41–7 Pattern of pure-tone, speech, and immittance audiometry findings for an adult with bilateral otosclerosis.

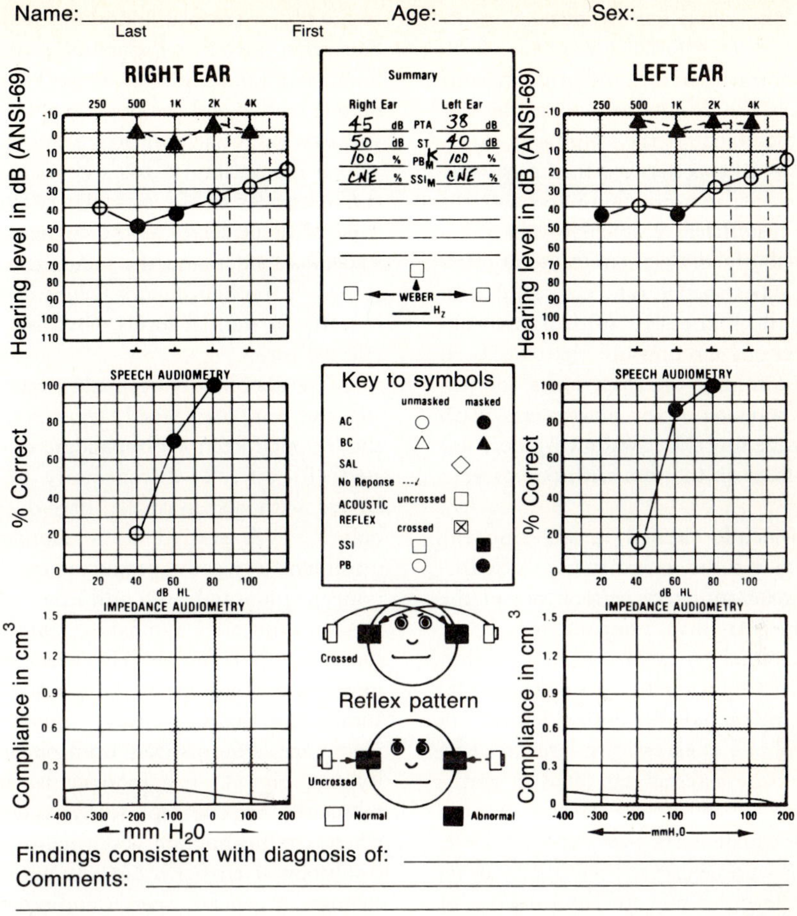

Figure 41–8 Pattern of pure-tone, speech, and immittance audiometry findings for a child with bilateral otitis media.

duces a type C tympanogram or a simple but abnormal multicomponent type. The tympanogram peak is displaced in a negative pressure direction by an amount that approximates negative pressure in the middle ear space. As exhaustion of air in the middle ear space continues, the peak is systematically displaced toward more negative pressure (see Fig. 41–2). At the extreme, the peak may actually lie beyond the negative pressure limits of the air pump and manometer scale of most clinical immittance meters, producing a gradually rising tympanogram. In the final stages of this process, there is effusion from the tissues lining the middle ear space. Fluid in the middle ear space is first reflected by a rounding of the tympanogram peak. Then, since increased fluid severely restricts the mobility of the ossicular chain, impedance increases. At the most extreme stage, the tympanogram shows virtually no change as air pressure is varied. During the development of otitis media, static immittance systematically decreases.

Fluid in the middle ear space markedly reduces static compliance. An average static compliance value of 0.29 ml is found in this population.[12] Although this value is well below the normal average (0.67 ml), overlap of static compliance for normal versus pathologic ears exists, as with otosclerosis, and static compliance alone has limited diagnostic value. In the early stages of otitis media, reflected in the type C tympanograms, both crossed and uncrossed acoustic reflexes may be recorded. However, in ears with negative pressure of greater than −200 daPa, there is little likelihood of recording either ipsilateral or contralateral reflexes (Fig. 41–8). Acoustic reflexes are rarely present when recorded in an ear with otitis media characterized by a type B tympanogram.

As a result of this documented sensitivity to mechanical alteration in middle ear function that is associated with the development of otitis media, immittance measures, particularly tympanometry, have assumed a primary role as a method for screening children for middle ear disorders.[10,11,111]

Tympanic Membrane Perforation. Ventilation tubes in the tympanic membrane are a popular therapy for otitis media. Static immittance is especially useful in the assessment of the patency of ventilation tubes in the tympanic membrane. Normally, the volume of the external ear canal is 0.50 to 1.50 ml. If a normal external ear canal volume (at +200 or −400 daPa) is obtained, then the ventilating tube is obstructed. If the volume is excessively larger than normal expectations, then it is likely that the tube is patent, permitting air to enter the middle ear space. Insufficient eustachian tube function was cited previously as a primary cause of otitis media. Eustachian tube function can be assessed with patent ventilation tubes in place. With normal eustachian tube function, air pressure that has been introduced into the middle ear space leaks out, especially during swallowing or jaw movement. With faulty eustachian tube function, swallowing does not relieve the air pressure in the ears with patent ventilation tubes.

Using the principle applied in assessing the function of ventilation tubes, one may use static immittance measurement to detect perforations of the tympanic membrane. An intact tympanic membrane is inferred if the external ear canal volume is within the normal range and bilaterally symmetrical. If, however, this volume exceeds the normal limits and especially if the volume is excessively large relative to that of the opposite external ear canal, a perforation of the tympanic membrane is expected. Often, in patients with adequate eustachian tube function, estimated ear canal volume exceeds the upper limits of the instrument (e.g., 5 ml). In the presence of an adequate coupling between the probe tip and the external ear canal walls (a hermetic seal), this finding is highly suggestive of a perforated tympanic membrane. For patients with a perforated tympanic membrane, the inability to build air pressure on the tympanic membrane precludes completion of tympanometry and static immittance measurement. Thus acoustic reflex measurement, normally made at the point of peak immittance, cannot be carried out.

Ossicular Discontinuity. The characteristic pattern of findings in ears with ossicular discontinuity is an abnormally deep (AD) admittance tympanogram at 226 Hz or with multifrequency, multicomponent measurements, a complex, broad regular W-pattern or irregular pattern with many peaks. Static immittance values exceed the normal range, and acoustic reflexes with the probe in the affected ear are not observed (see Table 41–4 and Fig. 41–9). However, inconsistencies in this pattern of results are common.[12] The tympanogram may not be excessively deep or may reflect multiple middle ear dysfunctions, and static immittance values may be within normal limits. In addition, in some cases, acoustic reflexes may be present at relatively normal levels even with the probe in an ear with ossicular discontinuity and a substantial air-bone gap.[15] These seemingly incompatible findings may be observed in two variations of ossicular discontinuity. In one, a functional connection exists between the stapedius muscle tendon and the portion of the ossicular chain still attached to the tympanic membrane. In the other, a total discontinuity exists between the stapes and the remainder of the ossicular chain, but a fibrous band of tissue serves as the connection between the stapedius tendon and the incus, the malleus, or the stapes. In both instances, acoustic reflexes may be observed at normal levels when the probe is in the affected ear.

The abnormally deep admittance tympanogram and the complex, broad, multipeaked susceptance and/or conductance tympanograms that are associated with ossicular discontinuity are also evident in an ear with an unusually flaccid tympanic membrane.[15,49] A scarred or a monomeric tympanic membrane typically produces an excessively deep tympanogram and high admittance values (see Fig. 41–5). Clinically, tympanic membrane abnormalities are more common. However, evaluation of the immittance findings in conjunction with pure-tone audiometry findings clearly differentiates tympanic membrane abnormalities from ossicular discontinuity (see Fig. 41–9). In ossicular discontinuity, a substantial air-bone gap usually occurs (30 to 50 dB), whereas tympanogram abnormalities rarely produce a substantial air-bone gap. As with conductive pathology in general, speech audiometry performance at high-stimulus intensity levels is characteristically good.

Sensorineural Abnormality

The diagnostic value of the immittance test battery in sensorineural abnormalities rivals its proven effectiveness in differentiation of middle ear disorders (Table 41–5).

Cochlear Loss. The expected immittance pattern in cochlear disorder is a normal type A tympanogram, static compliance within the normal range (0.30 to 1.60 ml), and acoustic reflex thresholds of 85 to 95 dB HL for pure-tone signals (see Table 41–5). On the one hand, as stressed previously in this chapter, an abnormality in any of these three measures suggests the possibility of a middle ear dysfunction. On the other hand, if immittance results do meet these three criteria for normality, the existence of a conductive abnormality is extremely unlikely. The diagnostic task, then, is verification and definition of the sensorineural impairment.

An immittance finding unique to cochlear auditory deficit is the presence of acoustic reflex thresholds in the 85 to 96 dB HL range. In cochlear

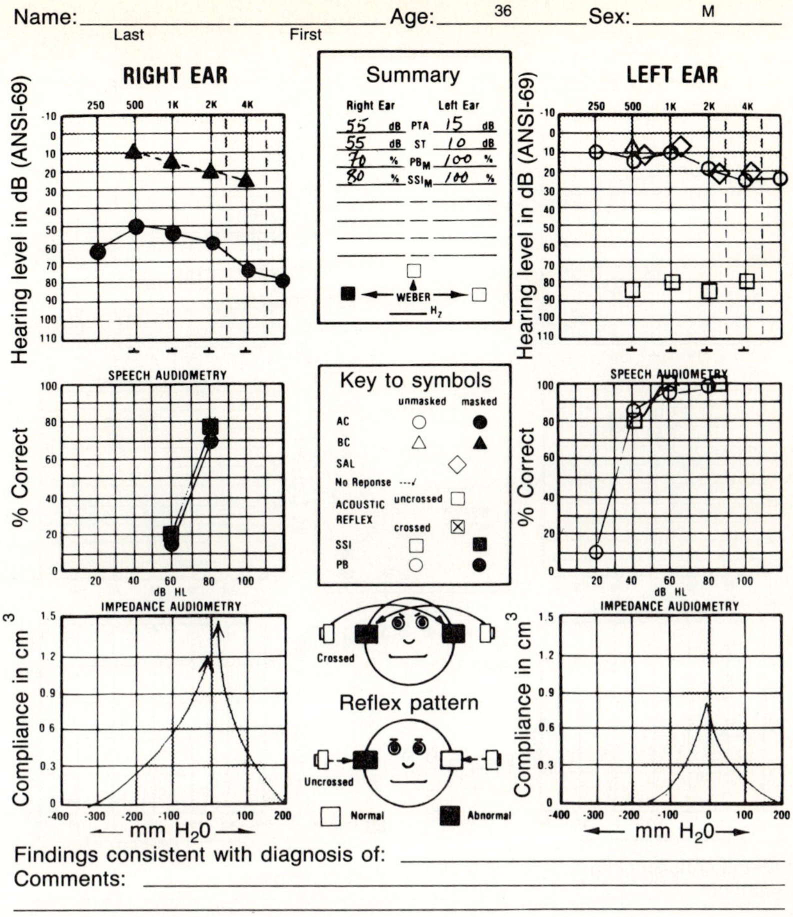

Figure 41–9 Pattern of pure-tone, speech, and immittance audiometry findings for an adult with trauma-related disruption of the ossicular chain on the right.

hearing impairment, the reflex may be elicited at reduced sensation levels. That is, whereas the sensation level for the acoustic reflex in the normal ear is usually 70 to 95 dB HL, the sensation level in the ear with purely cochlear hearing loss may be reduced to 20 to 50 dB HL (Fig. 41–10). The basis for this reduced reflex sensation level in cochlear impairment is unclear.[15] However, abnormally reduced sensation levels (less than 65 to 70 dB HL) for crossed and uncrossed reflex thresholds to pure-tone signals almost invariably reflect a cochlear sensitivity loss. Also shown in Figure 41–10 is diminished word recognition (phonetically balanced words) ability, even at high intensity levels, and reasonably good synthetic sentence identification performance associated with high-frequency sensorineural impairment.

In addition to identification of cochlear abnormalities, acoustic reflex thresholds may help to define the degree and configuration of the loss. In 1974, Niemeyer and Sesterhenn reported that sensorineural loss differentially affected reflex thresholds for pure tone versus noise signals.[27] Their findings were subsequently confirmed repeatedly in relatively large clinical populations.[105,112,113] In ears with cochlear

TABLE 41–7 SPAR Criteria for Estimation of Sensorineural Hearing Loss[74,112]

Tone-Noise Difference		*1,000 Hz ART**	*Noise ART*	*Prediction of Impairment*
≥20 dB	and	<95 dB	Anywhere	Normal
<20 dB	or	≥95 dB	≤95	Moderate
<20 dB	or	≥95 dB	>95	Severe

* ART = contralateral acoustic reflex threshold for 1,000-Hz tone or broad-band noise signal presented via TDH-49 earphones.

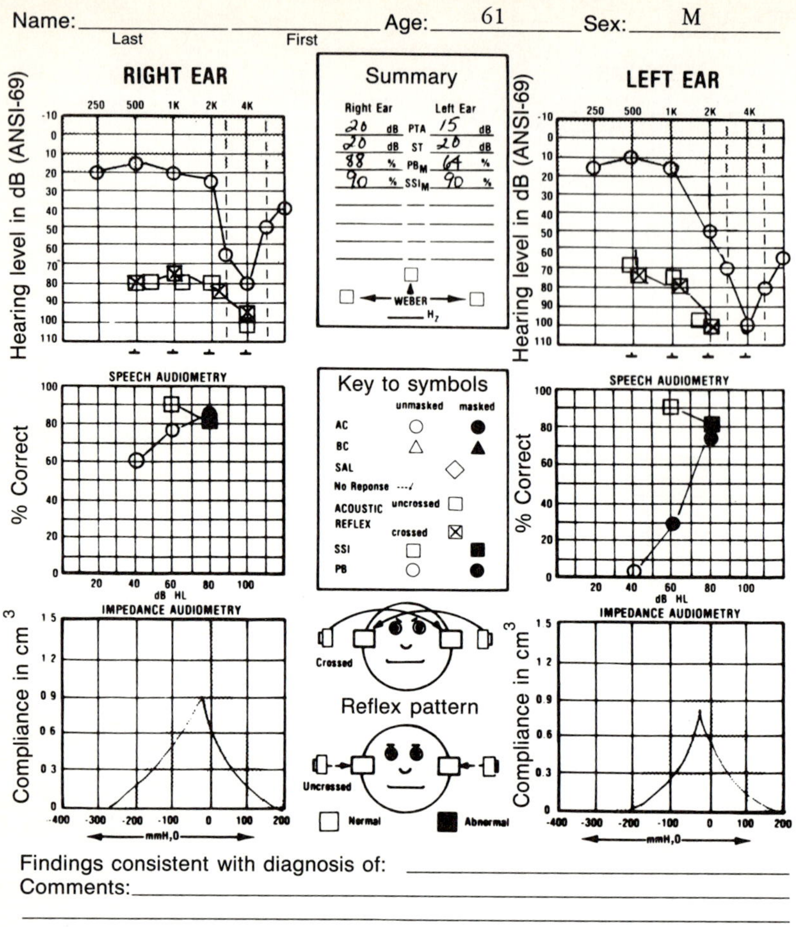

Figure 41–10 Pattern of pure-tone, speech, and immittance audiometry findings for an adult with a bilateral high-frequency sensorineural auditory deficit associated with chronic exposure to excessive noise levels.

hearing impairment, the hearing level of the acoustic reflex threshold for pure-tone signals remains constant or may actually improve slightly as hearing loss increases up to approximately 50 to 60 dB HL (see Fig. 41–6). However, the acoustic reflex threshold for noise signals systematically increases as cochlear sensitivity loss increases. In the normal ear, acoustic reflex thresholds for pure-tone signals are elicited at 85 to 95 dB HL, and reflex thresholds for broad-band noise signals are elicited at 75 to 85 dB SPL. Thus in normal ears, there is a noise-tone difference. Since in cochlear loss, acoustic reflex thresholds for broad-band noise signals systematically increase, while reflex thresholds for pure-tone signals remain essentially constant, the noise-tone difference tends to diminish with increased sensitivity loss. Comparison of the reflex thresholds for pure tone versus noise signals is the basis of hearing loss prediction by the acoustic reflex.

A variety of prediction methods have been developed.[25–27,114,115] The most widely used method clinically is the sensitivity prediction by the acoustic reflex (SPAR). The SPAR (Table 41–7) is especially useful in pediatric populations, both for identification of sensorineural loss[26,113] and for confirmation of behavioral audiometric test findings.[64] In patient populations for whom cooperation and, therefore, test time is severely limited, the acoustic reflex for a noise signal alone can help to identify patients with serious hearing impairments that will require more detailed assessment. We have found the guidelines in Table 41–8 useful in this regard.

Eighth Cranial Nerve Dysfunction. The expected immittance pattern in eighth cranial nerve dysfunction is a normal type A tympanogram, normal static immittance, and abnormal acoustic reflexes (see Table 41–5). Anderson et al first described the three acoustic reflex abnormalities associated with eighth nerve dysfunction: (1) absent acoustic reflexes, (2) elevated acoustic reflex thresholds, and (3) acoustic reflex decay.[16] Typically, acoustic reflexes are absent when the sound is presented to an ear with eighth nerve dysfunction, even if there is only a mild sensitivity loss.[16,17,116] In con-

TABLE 41–8 Guidelines for Identification of Serious Hearing Loss with Crossed Acoustic Reflex Threshold for a Broad-Band Noise (BBN) Signal

Acoustic Reflex Threshold for BBN in dB SPL	*(N)*	*Pure-Tone Average (500–2,000 Hz in dB)* *<35 (%)*	 *≥35 (%)*
65	(2)	100	0
70	(6)	100	0
75	(20)	100	0
80	(32)	100	0
85	(51)	69	31
90	(76)	76	24
95	(66)	55	45
100	(39)	28	72
105	(25)	16	84
110	(4)	0	100
115	(5)	0	100

Data are proportion of subjects with no serious hearing loss vs. those with serious hearing loss. Subjects were 326 patients aged 12 to 86 years.

From Hall JW III, Berry GA, Olsen K. Identification of serious hearing loss with acoustic reflex data: clinical experience with some new guidelines. Scand Audiol 1982; 11:251.

trast to the ear with cochlear hearing impairment, the sensation level of the acoustic reflex threshold is not reduced in ears with retrocochlear or eighth nerve hearing loss. Instead, the acoustic reflex threshold is elevated, usually by the amount of sensitivity loss. Since the normal acoustic reflex threshold is approximately 85 dB HL and the maximum signal intensity used in clinical acoustic reflex measurement is usually 110 dB HL, acoustic reflexes are unlikely to be observed in an ear with eighth nerve dysfunction having a sensitivity loss of greater than 25 to 30 dB HL. In contrast, again, acoustic reflexes are expected in cochlear loss of up to 65 or 70 dB HL. Acoustic reflexes are absent in approximately 63 percent of patients with confirmed eighth nerve dysfunction.[17] Therefore absence of reflexes in a patient with mild or moderate sensorineural loss raises the strong suspicion of a lesion of the eighth nerve.

In some patients with eighth nerve lesions, the acoustic reflex may be present but elevated. Acoustic reflexes observed only at relatively high-intensity levels (100 dB HL and above) in an ear with mild sensorineural loss is a sign of eighth nerve dysfunction. Furthermore, in these cases in which reflexes are present, reflex decay, reduced amplitude, and/or delayed latency may be observed.[16,17,86] Reflex decay correctly identifies over one-third of those subjects with confirmed eighth nerve dysfunction in whom acoustic reflexes are present.[26] In combination, abnormal reflex elevation and/or decay correctly identifies 85 percent of patients with confirmed eighth nerve lesions.[91]

Acoustic reflex measurements have documented diagnostic value in most patients with sensorineural abnormalities. In some cases, however, the results may be ambiguous. The degree of sensitivity loss is an important factor in the interpretation of acoustic reflex findings. For example, absent acoustic reflexes in a sensorineural loss are usually considered a sign of eighth nerve dysfunction. However, acoustic reflexes are probably absent in a purely cochlear impairment if hearing threshold levels exceed 60 dB HL. In fact, the signal may not ever reach sufficient "loudness" to elicit the reflex. In severe sensorineural impairments, then, absence of acoustic reflexes is ambiguous and does not contribute to the differentiation of cochlear versus eighth nerve site. However, this principle is not intransitive. That is, the presence of acoustic reflexes in severe sensorineural loss (greater than 60 dB HL) must be considered a cochlear sign.

In any patient with acoustic reflex abnormalities, the possibility of spurious middle ear abnormality must be ruled out. Elevation or absence of crossed acoustic reflexes with sound in one ear, and of uncrossed acoustic reflexes with sound in the opposite ear, suggests middle ear dysfunction in the "probe" ear. Probe effects, in which the common factor in reflex abnormalities is the probe ear, preclude valid interpretation of acoustic reflexes in differentiation of sensorineural impairments.[97–99]

Peripheral versus Central Auditory Dysfunction

The diagnostic usefulness of immittance measurements also includes differentiation of peripheral versus central auditory dysfunction (see Table 41–6). Griesen and Rasmussen first described discrepancies in crossed versus uncrossed acoustic reflex thresholds in patients with central auditory lesions at the brain stem.[24] In 1977, Jerger and Jerger confirmed their findings, reporting that in some patients with brain stem auditory disorder, crossed acoustic reflexes were absent; whereas uncrossed reflexes were present at normal levels.[117] Although this "horizontal pattern" of acoustic reflexes was observed in most of the patients with brain stem lesions, variations in the pattern were observed.[117] Recent studies have proven that the amplitude measurement is, in many cases, a more sensitive index of brain stem dysfunction than threshold.[65,99,100] This specific application of acoustic reflex measurements was recently reviewed by Hall.[65]

IMMITTANCE MEASUREMENT IN SPEECH PATHOLOGY

Immittance measurements are useful in persons with speech, voice, and language disorders.[64,82,113,118–127] In these populations, immittance measurement serves at least three functions.

First, hearing sensitivity can be predicted by the acoustic reflex in the person with communicative disorder. Hearing sensitivity is, of course, a critical factor in speech and language development. In the very young child and the neurologically impaired or emotionally impaired child, traditional behavioral audiometry is often ineffective. Methods for hearing sensitivity prediction by the acoustic reflex, for example the SPAR, are relatively independent of behavioral factors. These methods, then, permit reasonably accurate identification of hearing loss and objective confirmation of behavioral test results in difficult-to-test children.[64] Acoustic reflex measurements have been successfully applied in children with cerebral palsy,[122] mental retardation,[123,124,126,128,129] and autism.[127] In our experience, acoustic reflex measurement is similarly useful in neurologically impaired adults, such as aphasic adults.

Second, immittance measurements are used to assess and monitor middle ear function in clinical populations having a high incidence of middle ear pathology, for example, children with cleft palate[118–120] and mental retardation.[123,124,126]

Third, acoustic reflex measurements seem to have a potential value in the study of speech discrimination abilities[130–132] and peripheral versus central auditory function in learning disabilities, stuttering, spastic dysphonia, head injury, and neuromuscular diseases.[82,121,133–136]

SUMMARY

Acoustic immittance measurements include tympanometry, calculation of static immittance of the middle ear, and assessment of the acoustic reflex. For over 15 years, each of these measurements has played an important role in clinical audiology. Tympanometry is useful in the estimation of ear canal volume and the differentiation of middle ear pathologies. Recent papers have suggested that a special technique for tympanometric analysis, quantification of tympanogram gradient, may have clinical potential in immittance evaluation of middle ear disease. Although tympanometric data are often recorded with a single immittance component (e.g., impedance) and a single low probe-tone frequency (e.g., 226 Hz), multi-component (e.g., admittance, susceptance, conductance) and multi-probe-tone frequency (e.g. 226, 660, and 810 Hz) tympanometry offers distinct clinical advantages for identification and description of middle ear dysfunction associated with certain pathologic processes. Immittance meters for multi-component and multi-frequency tympanometric recordings are now commercially available from several manufacturers.

Static immittance measurements, interpreted in isolation, rarely permit confident identification of middle ear pathology. The two major limitations of static immittance are lack of adequate normative data, as reported in physical units, and the considerable overlap among data obtained from normal versus pathologic ears. Nevertheless, static immittance contributes importantly to the diagnostic value of patterns of immittance findings.

Acoustic reflex measurements have diverse and diagnostically-powerful clinical applications, including prediction of degree of sensorineural hearing impairment, differentiation among cochlear versus retrocochlear lesions, identification and localization of brain stem auditory pathology and noninvasive monitoring of facial nerve function. Computer-assisted recording and averaging of latency, amplitude, and decay parameters has enhanced the sensitivity and specificity of acoustic reflexes in clinical audiology.

In combination, the three major immittance measurements—tympanometry, static immittance, and the acoustic reflex—offer unique clinical advantages in evaluation of the auditory system. Each is an essential component of the basic audiologic test battery.

REFERENCES

1. Metz O. The acoustic impedance measured on normal and pathological ears. Acta Otolaryngol [Suppl] 1946; 63.
2. Feldman A. Impedance measurements at the ear drum as an aid to diagnosis. J Speech Hear Res 1963; 6:315–327.
3. Feldman A. Acoustic impedance measurements as a clinical procedure. Int Audiol 1964; 3:156–166.
4. Klockhoff I. Middle ear muscle reflexes in man. Acta Otolaryngol [Suppl] 1961; 164:1–91.

5. Lamb LE, Peterson J, Hanson S. Application of stapedius muscle reflex measures to diagnosis of auditory problems. Int Audiol 1968; 7:188–189.
6. Lidén G. Tests for stapes fixation. Arch Otolaryngol 1969; 89:215–219.
7. Zwislocki J. Some impedance measurements on normal and pathologic ears. J Acoustic Soc Am 1957; 29:1312–1317.
8. Alberti PW, Kristensen R. The clinical application of impedance audiometry. Laryngoscope 1970; 80:735–746.
9. Jerger J. Clinical experience with impedance audiometry. Arch Otolaryngol 1970; 92:311–324.
10. Harker LA, Van Wagoner R. Application of impedance audiometry as a screening instrument. Arch Otolaryngol 1974; 77:198–201.
11. Brooks DN. Impedance measurement in screening for auditory disorders in children. Hear Instr 1974; 36:20–21.
12. Jerger J, Anthony L, Jerger S, Mauldin L. Studies in impedance audiometry. III. Middle ear disorders. Arch Otolaryngol 1974; 99:165–171.
13. Jerger J, Jerger S, Mauldin L. Studies in impedance audiometry. I. Normal and sensori-neural ears. Arch Otolaryngol 1972; 96:513–523.
14. Jerger JF. Diagnostic audiometry. In: Jerger JF, ed: Modern developments in audiology. New York: Academic Press, 1973:75.
15. Jerger JF. Diagnostic use of impedance measures. In: Jerger JF, ed. Handbook of clinical impedance audiometry. New York: American Electromedics, 1975:149.
16. Anderson H, Barr B, Wedenberg E. Intra-aural reflexes in retrocochlear lesions. In: Hamberg C, Wesall J, eds. Nobel symposium 10: disorders of the skull base region. Stockholm: Almquist & Wiksell, 1969.
17. Jerger J, Harford E, Clemis J, Alford B. The acoustic reflex in eighth nerve disorders. Arch Otolaryngol 1974; 99:409–413.
18. Olsen WO, Noffsinger D, Kurdziel S. Acoustic reflex and reflex decay. Arch Otolaryngol 1975; 101:622–625.
19. Sanders JW, Josey AF, Glasscock ME III. Audiological evaluation in cochlear and eighth nerve disorders. Arch Otolaryngol 1974; 100:283–289.
20. Borg E. On the neuronal organization of the acoustic reflex. A physiological and anatomic study. Brain Res 1973; 49:101–123.
21. Bosatra A, Russolo M, Poli P. Oscilloscopic analysis of the stapedius muscle reflex in brain stem lesions. Arch Otolaryngol 1976; 102:284–285.
22. Colletti V. Some stapedius reflex abnormalities in normal and pathological conditions. J Laryngol Otol 1974; 88:127–137.
23. Colletti V. Stapedius reflex abnormalities in multiple sclerosis. Audiology 1975; 14:63–71.
24. Griesen O, Rasmussen PE. Stapedius muscle reflexes and otoneurological examinations in brain stem tumor. Acta Otolaryngol 1970; 70:366–370.
25. Baker SR, Lilly DJ. Prediction of hearing level from acoustic reflex data. Presented at the American Speech and Hearing Association Convention, Houston, November 20, 1976.
26. Jerger J, Burney P, Mauldin L, Crump B. Predicting hearing loss from the acoustic reflex. Arch Otolaryngol 1974; 99:11–22.
27. Niemeyer W, Sesterhenn G. Calculating the hearing threshold from the stapedius reflex threshold for different sound stimuli. Audiology 1974; 13:421–427.
28. McCandless G. Miller D. Loudness discomfort and hearing aids. Natl Hear Aid J 1972; 3:7,28,32.
29. McCandless GA. Future directions. In: Jerger JF, ed. Handbook of clinical impedance audiometry. New York: American Electromedics, 1975:176.
30. Rappaport B, Tait C. Acoustic reflex threshold measurement in hearing aid selection. Arch Otolaryngol 1976; 102:129–132.
31. Snow T, McCandless G. The use of impedance measures in hearing aid selection. Natl Hear Aid J 1976; 7:32–33.
32. Creten WL, Van Camp KJ, Maes MA, Vanpeperstraete PM. On the diagnostic value of phase-angle tympanograms. Audiology 1981; 20:1–11.
33. Lilly DJ. Multiple frequency, multiple component tympanometry: new approaches to an old diagnostic problem. Ear Hear 1984; 5:300–308.
34. Margolis RH, Van Camp KJ, Wilson RH, Creten WL. Multifrequency tympanometry in normal ears. Audiology 1985; 24:44–53.
35. Shanks JE. Tympanometry. Ear Hear 1984; 5:268–280.
36. Van Camp KJ, Creten WL, Van de Heyning PH, Decraemer WF, Vanpeperstraete PM. A search for the most suitable immittance components and probe tone frequency in tympanometry. Scand Audiol 1983; 12:27–34.
37. Van Camp KJ, Margolis RH, Wilson RH, Creten WL, Shanks JE. Principles of tympanometry. Rockville, MD: American Speech-Language Hearing Association, 1986.
38. Vanhuyse VJ, Creten WL, Van Camp KJ. On the W-notching of tympanograms. Scand Audiol 1975; 4:45–50.
39. Wilson RH, Shanks JE, Kaplan SK. Tympanometric changes at 226 Hz and 678 Hz across 10 trials and for two directions of ear canal pressure change. J Speech Hear Res 1984; 27:257–266.
40. Hall JW III. Contemporary tympanometry. Sem Hear 1987; 8:319–327.
41. Terkildsen K, Scott-Nielsen S. An electroacoustic impedance measuring bridge for clinical use. Arch Otolaryngol 1960; 72:339–346.
42. Lilly DJ. Measurement of acoustic impedance at the tympanic membrane. In: Jerger JF, ed. Modern developments in audiology. 2nd ed. New York: Academic Press, 1973:345.
43. Lilly DJ. Advances in instrumentation for the measurement of aural acoustic immittance. Personal communication.
44. Terkildsen K, Thomson K. The influence of pressure variations on the impedance of the human ear drum. J Laryngol Otol 1959; 73:409–418.
45. Hall JW III. Effects of age and sex on static compliance. Arch Otolaryngol 1979; 105:601–605.
46. Bluestone CD, Berry QC, Paradise JL. Audiometry and tympanometry in relation to middle ear effusions in children. Laryngoscope 1973; 83:594–604.
47. Cooper JC Jr, Hearne EM III, Gates GA. Normal tympanometric shape. Ear Hear 1982; 3(5):241–245.
48. Gersdorff MC. Personal results, trial of classification and standardization in clinical impedancemetry. J Otolaryngol [Suppl 5] 1977; 6:156–166.
49. Alberti PW, Jerger JF. Probe-tone frequency and the diagnostic value of tympanometry. Arch Otolaryngol 1974; 99:206–210.
50. Lidén G, Harford E, Hallen O. Tympanometry for the diagnosis of ossicular disruption. Arch Otolaryngol 1974; 99:23–29.
51. Harford RE. Tympanometry. In: Jerger JF, ed. Handbook of clinical impedance audiometry. New York: American Electromedics, 1975:47.
52. Koebsell KA, Margolis RH. Tympanometric gradient measured from normal preschool children. Audiology 1986; 25:149–157.
53. Creten WL, Van de Heyning PH, Van Camp KJ. Immittance audiometry. Normative data at 200 and 660 Hz. Scand Audiol 1985; 14:115–121.
54. Brooks DN. An objective method of detecting fluid in the middle ear. Int Audiol 1968; 7:11280–11286.
55. deJonge R. Normal tympanometric gradient: a comparison of three methods. Audiology 1986; 25:299–308.
56. Lidén G, Peterson JL, Bjorkman G. Tympanometry: a method for analysis of middle ear function. Acta Otolaryngol [Suppl] 1970; 263:218–224.

57. Keith RW. Impedance audiometry with neonates. Arch Otolaryngol 1973; 97:464–467.
58. Green KW, Margolis RH. Detection of hearing loss with ipsilateral acoustic reflex thresholds. Audiology 1983; 22:471–479.
59. Van Camp KJ, Vogeleer M. A tympanometric approach to otosclerosis. Scand Audiol 1986; 15:109–114.
60. Van de Heyning PH, Van Camp KJ, Creten WL, Vanpeperstraete PM. Incudo-stapedial joint pathology: a tympanometric approach. J Speech Hear Res 1982; 25:611–618.
61. Lutman ME. Phasor admittance measurements of the middle ear. I. Theoretical approach. Scand Audiol 1984; 13:253–264.
62. Lutman ME, McKenzie H, Swan IRC. Phasor admittance measurements of the middle ear. II. Normal phasor tympanograms and acoustic reflexes. Scand Audiol 1984; 13:265–274.
63. Wilson RH, McCullough JK, Lilly DJ. Acoustic-reflex adaptation: morphology and half-life data for subjects with normal hearing. J Speech Hear Res 1984; 27:586–595.
64. Jerger J, Hayes D. The cross-check principle in pediatric audiometry. Arch Otolaryngol 1976; 102:614–620.
65. Hall JW III. The acoustic reflex in central auditory dysfunction. In: Pinheiro ML, Musiek FE, eds. Assessment of central auditory dysfunction: foundations and clinical correlations. Baltimore: Williams & Wilkins, 1985:103.
66. Lyon MJ, Malmgren LT. A histochemical characterization of muscle fiber types in the middle ear muscles of the cat. Acta Otolaryngol 1982; 94:99–109.
67. Brodal LA. Neurological anatomy in relation to clinical medicine. New York: Oxford University Press, 1981.
68. Hall JW III. The effects of high-dose barbiturates on the acoustic reflex and auditory evoked responses. Acta Otolaryngol 1985; 100:387–398.
69. Downs DW, Crum MA. The hyperactive acoustic reflex: four case studies. Arch Otolaryngol 1980; 106:401–404.
70. Gelfand SA, Silman S. Acoustic reflex thresholds in brain-damaged patients. Ear Hear 1982; 3:93–95.
71. Jepson O. The threshold of the reflexes of the tympanic muscles in a normal material examined by means of the impedance method. Acta Otolaryngol 1951; 39:406–498.
72. Luscher E. Die Funktion des Musculus Stapedius beim Menschen. Z Hal-Nasen-U Ohrenheilk 1929; 23:105–132.
73. Hall JW III, Weaver T. Impedance audiometry in a young population: effects of age, sex, and minor tympanogram abnormality. J Otolaryngol 1979; 8:210–222.
74. Jerger J, Hayes D, Anthony L, Mauldin L. Factors influencing prediction of hearing level from the acoustic reflex. Monogr Contemp Audiol (Maico) 1978; 1:1–20.
75. Laukli E, Mair IWS. Ipsilateral and contralateral acoustic reflex thresholds. Audiology 1980; 19:469–479.
76. Lindgren F, Nilsson R, Axelsson A. The acoustic reflex threshold in relation to noise-induced hearing loss. Scand Audiol 1983; 12:49–55.
77. Moller AR. Acoustic reflex in man. J Acoust Soc Am 1962; 34:1524–1534.
78. Wilson R, McBride L. Threshold and growth of the acoustic reflex. J Acoust Soc Am 1978; 63:147–154.
79. Stach BA, Jerger JF. Acoustic reflex averaging. Ear Hear 1984; 5:289–296.
80. Perlman HB, Case TJ. Latent period of the crossed stapedius reflex in man. Ann Otol Rhinol Laryngol 1939; 48:663–675.
81. Church GT, Cudahy EA. The time course of the acoustic reflex. Ear Hear 1984; 5:235–241.
82. Hall JW, Jerger JF. Acoustic reflexes in spastic dysphonia. Arch Otolaryngol 1976; 102:411–415.
83. Jerger J, Oliver TA, Stach B. Problems in the clinical measurement of acoustic reflex latency. Scand Audiol 1986; 15:31–40.
84. Ruth R, Niswander P. Acoustic reflex latency as a function of frequency and intensity of eliciting stimulus. J Am Aud Soc 1976; 2:54–60.
85. Borg E. Time course of the human acoustic stapedius reflex. Scand Audiol 1982; 11:237–242.
86. Jerger J, Hayes D. Latency of the acoustic reflex in eighth-nerve tumor. Arch Otolaryngol 1983; 109:1–5.
87. Fowler CG, Wilson RH. Adaptation of the acoustic reflex. Ear Hear 1984; 5:281–288.
88. Oviatt DL, Kileny P. Normative characteristics of ipsilateral acoustic reflex adaptation. Ear Hear 1984; 5:145–152.
89. Sellari-Franceschini P, Bruschini P, Pardini L, Berrettini S. Quantification of the parameters of the acoustic reflex in normal ears. Audiology 1986; 25:165–175.
90. Hirsch A, Anderson H. Elevated stapedius reflex threshold and pathologic reflex decay. Acta Otolaryngol [Suppl] 1980; 368.
91. Jerger S, Jerger J. Evaluation of diagnostic audiometric tests. Audiology 1983; 22:144–161.
92. Mangham CA, Lindeman RC, Dawson WR. Stapedius reflex quantification in acoustic tumor patients. Laryngoscope 1980; 90:242–250.
93. Olsen W, Stach B, Kurdziel S. Acoustic reflex decay in 10 seconds and 5 seconds for Meniere's disease and for 8th nerve tumor patients. Ear Hear 1981; 2:180–181.
94. Jerger J, Neeley JG, Jerger S. Speech, impedance and auditory brainstem response audiometry in brain-stem tumors. Importance of a multiple test strategy. Arch Otolaryngol 1980; 106:218–223.
95. Metz O. Studies on the contraction of the tympanic muscles as indicated by changes in the impedance of the ear. Acta Otolaryngol 1951; 39:397–405.
96. Greenfield DG, Wiley TL, Block MG. Acoustic-reflex dynamics and the loudness-discomfort level. J Speech Hear Res 1985; 50:14–20.
97. Hall JW III. Acoustic reflex amplitude. I. Effect of age and sex. Audiology 1982; 21:294–309.
98. Hall JW III. Acoustic reflex amplitude. II. Effect of age-related auditory dysfunction. Audiology 1982; 21:386–399.
99. Hall JW III. Quantification of the relationship between crossed and uncrossed acoustic reflex amplitude. Ear Hear 1982c; 3:296–300.
100. Hayes D, Jerger J. Signal averaging of the acoustic reflex: diagnostic application of amplitude characteristics. Scand Audiol 1983; 17:31–36.
101. Ruth RA, Tucci DL, Nilo ER. Effects of ear canal pressure on threshold and growth of the acoustic reflex. Ear Hear 1982; 3:39–41.
102. Silman S, Gelfand SA. The relationship between magnitude of hearing loss and acoustic reflex threshold levels. J Speech Hear Disord 1981; 46:312–316.
103. Sprague BH, Wiley TL, Block MG. Dynamics of acoustic reflex growth. Arch Otolaryngol 1981; 20:15–40.
104. Wilson RH. The effects of aging on the magnitude of the acoustic reflex. J. Speech Hear Res 1981; 24:406–414.
105. Silman S. The acoustic reflex. New York: Academic Press, 1985.
106. Osterhammel D, Osterhammel P. Age and sex variations for the normal stapedial reflex thresholds and tympanometric compliance values. Scand Audiol 1979; 8:153–158.
107. Popelka GR. Acoustic immittance measures: terminology and instrumentation. Ear Hear 1984; 5:262–267.
108. Hodges A, Ruth RA. Subject related factors influencing the acoustic reflex. Semin Hear 1987; 8:339–357.
109. Brooks DN. The use of the electro-acoustic impedance bridge in the assessment of middle ear function. Int Audiol 1969; 8:563–569.
110. Harford ER, Bess FH, Bluestone CD, Klein JO. Impedance screening for middle ear disease in children. New York: Grune & Stratton, 1978.

111. Holte L, Margolis R. Screening tympanometry. Semin Hear 1987; 8:329–337.
112. Hall JW III. Predicting hearing level from the acoustic reflex. In: Jerger J, Acton MA, eds. Handbook of clinical impedance audiometry. New York: American Electromedics, 1980:141.
113. Hall JW III. Central auditory function in spastic dysphonia. Am J Otolaryngol 1981; 2:188–198.
114. Hall JW III. Predicting hearing level from the acoustic reflex: a comparison of three methods. Arch Otolaryngol 1978; 104:602–605.
115. Margolis RH, Fox C. A comparison of three methods for predicting hearing loss from acoustic reflex thresholds. J Speech Hear Res 1977; 20:241–253.
116. Hannley M, Jerger J. PB rollover and the acoustic reflex. Audiology 1981; 20:251–258.
117. Jerger S, Jerger J. Diagnostic value of crossed vs. uncrossed acoustic reflexes. Arch Otolaryngol 1977; 103:445–453.
118. Bess FH, Lewis HD, Cieliczka DJ. Acoustic impedance measurements in cleft palate children. J Speech Hear Disord 1975; 40:13–24.
119. Bess FH, Schwartz DM, Redfield NP. Audiometric, impedance, and otoscopic findings in children with cleft palates. Arch Otolaryngol 1976; 102:465–469.
120. Billings BL, Lowry LD. Tympanometry, impedance, and aural reflex testing in a cleft palate population. Cleft Palate J 1974; 11:21–27.
121. Hall JW III, Jerger JF. Central auditory function in stutterers. J Speech Hear Res 1978; 21:324–337.
122. Keith RW, Murphey KP, Martin F. Acoustic impedance measurement in the otological assessment of multiply handicapped in chilldren. Folia Phoniatr (Basel) 1977; 29:311–314.
123. Lamb LE, Norris TW. Acoustic impedance measurement. In: Fulton RT, Lloyd LL, eds. Audiometry for the retarded. Baltimore: Williams & Wilkins, 1969.
124. Lamb LE, Norris TW. Relative acoustic impedance measurement with mentally retarded children. Am J Ment Defic 1970; 75:51–56.
125. McCall G. Acoustic impedance measurement in the study of patients with spasmodic dysphonia. J Speech Hear Disord 1973; 38:250–255.
126. Niswander PS, Ruth RA. Prediction of hearing sensitivity from acoustic reflexes in mentally retarded persons. Am J Ment Defic 1977; 81:474–481.
127. Suria G, Serra-Raventos W. Acoustic impedance measurement and autistic children. Folia Phoniatr (Basel) 1975; 27:387–388.
128. Givens GD, Bronerwine L. Estimation of auditory sensitivity from the acoustic reflex with mentally deficient children. J Aud Res 1983; 23:109–117.
129. Poole PB, Sheeley EC, Hannah JE. Predicting hearing sensitivity and audiometric slope for mentally retarded persons. Ear Hear 1982; 3:77–82.
130. Chadwell DL, Greenberg HJ. Speech intelligibility in stapedectomized individuals. Am J Otol 1978; 1:103–108.
131. Dorman M, Cedar I, Hannley M, Lee M, Lindholm JM. Influence of the acoustic reflex on vowel recognition. J Speech Hear Res 1986; 29:420–424.
132. Mahoney T, Vernon J, Meikle M. Function of the acoustic reflex in discrimination of intense speech. Arch Otolaryngol 1979; 105:119–123.
133. Hall JW III, Huangfu F, Gennarelli TA. Auditory function in acute head injury. Laryngoscope 1982; 93:383–390.
134. Hall JW III, Huangfu M, Gennarelli TA, Dolinskas CA, Olson K, Berry GA. Auditory evoked response, impedance measures and diagnostic speech audiometry in severe head injury. Otolaryngol Head Neck Surg 1983; 91:50–60.
135. Thomas WG, McMurry G, Pillsbury HC. Acoustic reflex abnormalities in behaviorally disturbed and language delayed children. Laryngoscope 1985; 95:811–817.
136. Yamane M, Nomura Y. Analysis of stapedial reflex in neuromuscular diseases. ORL J Otorhinolaryngol Relat Spec 1984; 46:84–96.

42 Auditory Brain Stem Response and Electrocochleography

Steven J. Staller, Ph.D.
Laura K. McFarlane Lunde, M.A.

The proliferation of auditory evoked potentials over the last decade has had a significant effect on the diagnostic capabilities and the scope of the clinical audiologist. The Auditory Brain Stem Response (ABR) has become an indispensable component in the evaluation of hearing sensitivity in infants and in multiply handicapped children, as well as in the evaluation of neuropathology in both children and adults. In addition, interest in recording cochlear receptor potentials via extratympanic Electrocochleography (ECoG) has renewed in the past several years.

The history of evoked potentials has seen a variety of long latency responses that have been investigated and eventually abandoned. The major reason for the lack of clinical acceptance has centered around the variety of factors that affect these potentials. The ABR and ECoG are both short latency responses that are extremely resistent to subject and pharmacologic variables that plagued the longer latency potentials. Consequently, these tests demonstrate excellent reliability, which is essential to clinical application.

The scope of this chapter will be to provide an introduction and an overview of the clinical applications of ABR and ECoG. This overview will include a consideration of the relationship between physiologically based tests and the traditional behavioral test procedures.

AUDITORY BRAIN STEM RESPONSE

The ABR has become an indispensable component in the audiological assessment of infants, of multiply handicapped children, and of retrocochlear pathology in adults. The major clinical applications of the ABR include assessment of (1) hearing sensitivity in high-risk infants, in normal term newborns, and in difficult to test and multiply handicapped children, (2) neurologic status of high-risk newborns, (3) patients who are at risk for cerebellopontine angle tumors, (4) patients with suspected brain stem disease affecting the auditory brain stem pathways, and (5) patients with suspected functional hearing loss.

The ABR is a series of seven scalp positive electrical events (waves) that reflect the sequential activation of the eighth nerve and the ascending auditory pathways within the brain stem. Early attempts to localize the specific generators of each wave failed to account for the extremely complex and redundant pathways that conduct auditory information through the brain stem. More recently, the consensus holds that only the first wave is generated by a single source, the intracanalicular segment of the eighth nerve.[1,2] The remaining ABR waves appear to reflect the complex interaction of multiple neural generators from the proximal eighth nerve through the pons and caudal midbrain.[3,4,5] Therefore, the ability to localize pathology to a single site within the brain stem based on the alteration of an ABR wave is probably not possible. However, for clinical purposes, determination of the level of involvement is feasible and will be discussed in a later section.

NORMAL RESPONSE CHARACTERISTICS

The seven components of the ABR occur in the first 10 msec following the onset of a transient acoustic stimulus. The first five waves are adequately reliable to be clinically useful and, by convention, are labeled one through five. A classic ABR elicited by a high-intensity click stimulus is depicted in Figure 42–1. The ABR is considered to be a "far field" potential, since it is recorded from the surface of the scalp at a distance from the brain stem generators buried deep within the cranial cavity. Several fundamental aspects of the ABR are considered to be useful as diagnostic measures. The two most significant of these are latency and amplitude. Latency is the timing of the response and may be measured in absolute or in relative terms. Absolute, or peak, latency is the amount of time between the onset of the eliciting stimulus and the occurrence of a particular wave. Peak latency incorporates a variety of variables, including (1) the amount of time for the stimulus to travel between the headphone or speaker and the tympanic membrane, (2) transmission time through the middle ear and the cochlea, and (3) conduction velocity and synaptic transmission along the neural pathway. In contrast, interwave latency, which is the time between two ABR waves, reflects almost exclusively the function of the neural pathway between the generators of the two waves and is, therefore, a more sensitive index of neural pathology.

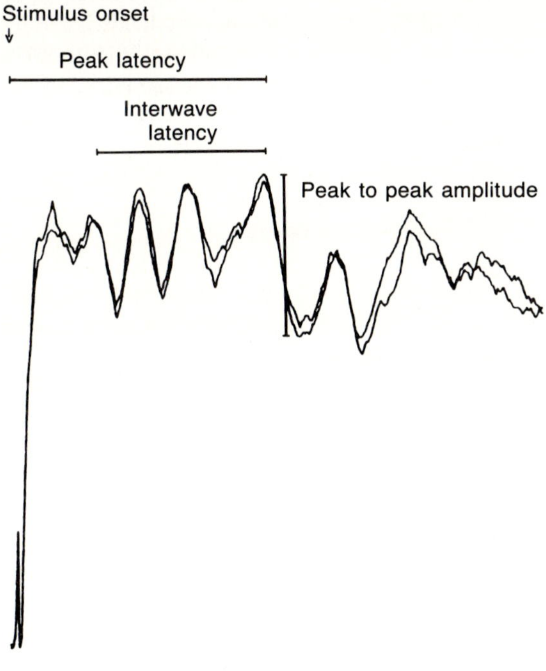

Figure 42–1 Diagnostic measures of ABR. Peak latency is the time between the stimulus and the occurrence of the peak. Interwave latency is the time between two peaks, and peak to peak amplitude is measured between the positive peak and the following negative trough.

Amplitude is a much more variable measure than latency. A variety of factors, including muscle artifact, electrical interference, and electrode impedance, can all have a significant effect on response amplitude. In an attempt to minimize the inherent variability of amplitude measures, a comparison of the amplitude relationship between two ABR waves may be calculated. This so called "amplitude ratio" minimizes extraneous variables that affect the amplitude of the entire ABR sequence and enhances pathologic influences that selectively reduce the amplitude of only one or two waves.

RECORDING VARIABLES

Because the ABR is a far field response, the precise placement of recording electrodes is less significant than with near field potentials (such as the later cortical potentials or the cochlear potentials recorded by ECoG). Two recording electrodes are used to accomodate the differential preamplifiers almost universally utilized in the current generation of evoked potential systems. Differential preamplifiers reduce extraneous electrical noise by amplifying the difference in voltage between an active (noninverting) and a reference (inverting) electrode. Electrical activity that originates from outside the cranium, such as electrical interference from fluorescent lights or from remote muscle activity, has the same phase and amplitude at both electrodes and, therefore, is rejected by the amplifier. In contrast, electrical energy originating between the two electrodes, as is the case for brain stem electrical activity, is seen at opposite polarities at the two electrode sites and therefore is amplified.

The active electrode can be placed anywhere in the vicinity of the cranial vertex (top of the skull). Many clinicians prefer using the top of the forehead just below the hairline as the active electrode site in order to facilitate the electrode application. The reference electrode is typically placed on the earlobe of the ear that is being stimulated in order to enhance the amplitude of Wave I that is generated by the ipsilateral eighth nerve. A third electrode (ground) is placed on the forehead or the contralateral earlobe.

Surface disk electrodes that are silver, silver coated with silver-chloride, or gold are typically used. Needle electrodes may also be used, but the disadvantages of patient discomfort and the reduced surface area of needles compared to disks make their use less common. An exception is the use of ABR during surgical procedures to monitor hearing or brain stem status. In this application, expediency and stability across time make needles more useful.

The use of the vertex electrode referenced to the ipsilateral earlobe is referred to as an ipsilateral ABR and yields the classic waveform morphology seen in Figure 42–2. A second electrode configuration (montage) using the contralateral earlobe as a reference electrode site is sometimes used in an attempt to enhance the definition of Wave V by separating the IV–V wave complex into two distinct peaks.[6,7] This contralateral ABR montage may be recorded simultaneously on a second amplifier channel (in two channel systems) and has been advocated to clarify waveform definition in cases where the IV–V complex is fused. The practice of comparing Wave I recorded ipsilaterally with Wave V recorded contralaterally should be used with caution, however, since the latency of both Waves III and V may be significantly altered.[6,7]

Filters are typically used to eliminate electrical or biologic noise that is not in the bandwidth of interest surrounding the ABR. Predominant ABR spectral energy is between 50 and 1,000 Hz.[8] In order to stabilize the electrical baseline, most clinical protocols utilize a bandpass from 100 Hz to 3,000 Hz. Narrowing the bandpass beyond this in an attempt to reduce extraneous muscle artifact from tense or restless patients can have a deleterious effect. Analogue filters cause phase shifting, which can alter the latency of ABR components if too narrow a bandpass is used.[9] An effective alternative that is being incorporated into some evoked potential systems is a digital filtering system that processes the response after averaging is completed. Digital filtering effectively removes artifact out of the frequency band of interest without introducing any phase shifting.[9,10]

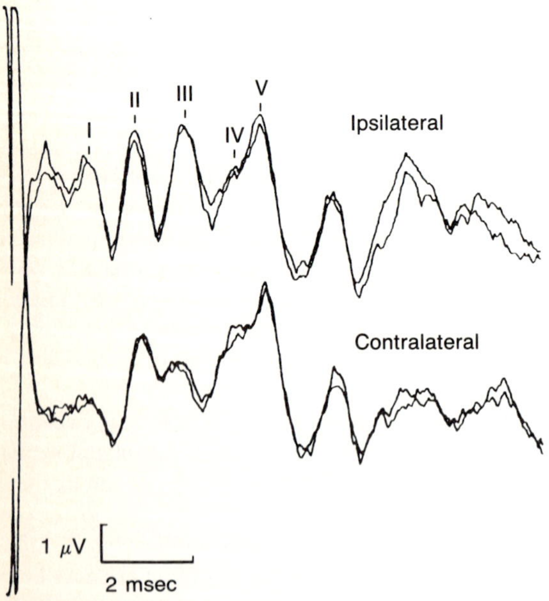

Figure 42–2 Normal ABR recorded with ipsilateral and contralateral electrode configurations. Note reduced amplitude of Wave I and increased prominance of Wave IV on the contralateral recording.

STIMULUS VARIABLES

In order to extract the extremely tiny electrical events of the auditory brain stem pathways from the high level of background biologic and electrical noise, stimuli that cause a large number of auditory neurons to discharge simultaneously must be used. The most efficient stimulus at eliciting this type of synchronous discharge is a short duration (100 μsec) square wave pulse. When this type of transient pulse is transduced by a typical headphone, a broad spectrum stimulus, known as a broad band click, is produced. Although a click is temporally precise, it does not provide frequency specific information, which is a major disadvantage when using ABR to assess hearing sensitivity. The correlation between click-induced ABR and audiometric thresholds is strongest between 1,000 Hz and 4,000 Hz.[11] This reflects the predominant frequency of the stimulus, as well as the more precise synchrony of the basal end of the cochlea.

Intensity

The effects of stimulus intensity on the ABR have been studied in detail.[6,11,12,13] A systematic increase in peak latency of all ABR waves occurs with a progressive decrease in stimulus intensity. Plotting changes in Wave V latency as a function of stimulus intensity creates an "intensity-latency function," which is depicted in Figure 42–3. The crosshatched area is the normal range for adults. The normal slope of the I-L function is between 28 and 40 μsec per decibel in subjects older than approximately 2 years of age.[13,14]

Although the latency of each ABR wave shifts significantly with intensity change, the interwave latencies remain relatively constant.[15] As stimulus intensity is increased progressively, more basal hair cells are stimulated, thereby shortening the mechanical transmission time within the coch-

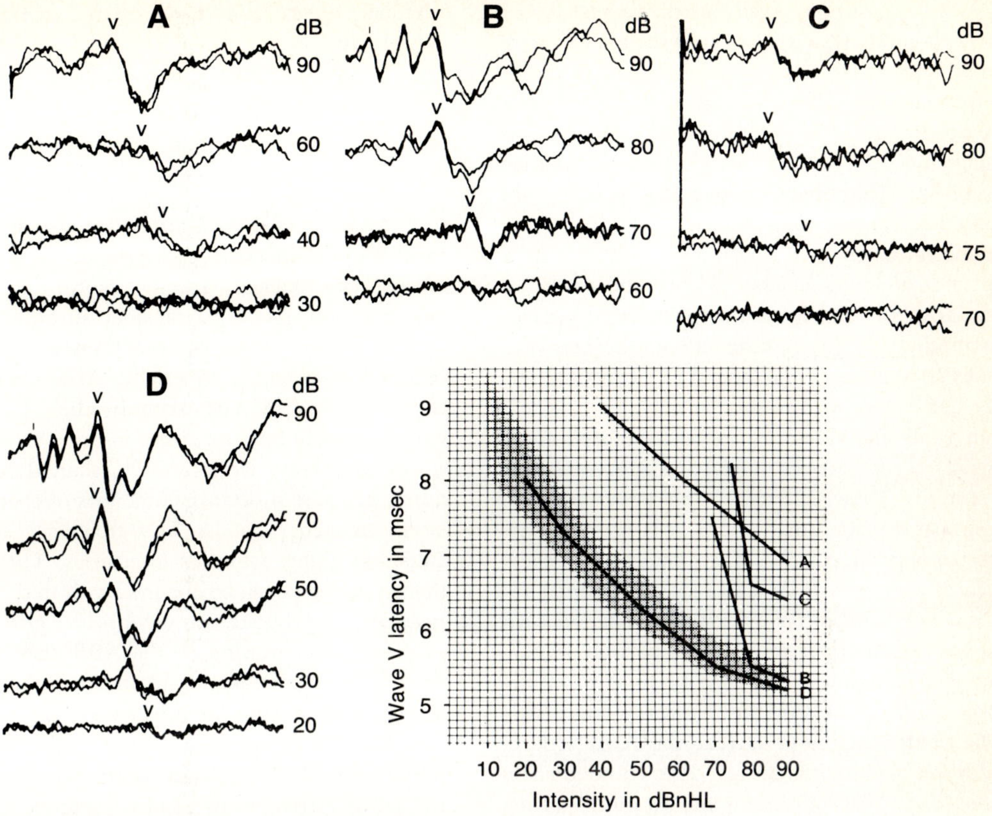

Figure 42–3 Intensity-latency function: the shaded area depicts the normal range of Wave V latency as a function of intensity. *A*, Mild conductive hearing loss. Note poor morphology of waveforms and gradual shift in latency of the Wave V. The I = L function is shifted in latency approximately the amount of the air-bone gap. *B*, Moderate sensorineural hearing loss. Note excellent waveform definition and normal latencies at high intensity with rapid deterioration and shift of latency near threshold. *C*, Severe precipitous high frequency sensorineural hearing loss. Note poor waveform definition and abnormal delay in Wave V at high intensity, with rapid deterioration and shift in latency near threshold. *D*, Normal hearing. Note excellent waveform definition at high intensity, with gradual deterioration of potentials and shift in latency as threshold is approached.

lea.[16,17] This fact has significant implications for frequency specificity, since a much broader segment of the cochlea responds to high intensity stimulation than responds to threshold stimulation.

Absolute Wave V threshold is the most common ABR measure used to estimate behavioral thresholds. In normal adults, the Wave V threshold is approximately 10 dB higher than the behavioral threshold for the same stimulus.

Rate

The rate of stimulus presentation also has a significant effect on the ABR waveform. Rates above approximately 30 stimuli per second tend to increase both peak latencies and interwave latencies.[5,18,19] Peak definition also tends to degrade above 30 stimuli per second. For clinical use, a compromise must be reached since, although faster stimulus rates decrease test time, they also degrade ABR response quality. Most clinical protocols utilize slower rates (between 10 and 20 stimuli per second) to enhance peak definition when assessing suspected neuropathology. Faster rates (around 30 stimuli per second) are used when assessing infants and children, when time is a more critical factor. Extremely fast rates (i.e., >70 stimuli per second) may be used to assess subtle neuropathology more critically by stressing the neural system.[20,21] Another factor in determining the rate of stimulation is the effect of electrical artifact on recording ABR responses. The presence of line current electrical artifact in ABR recordings is increased if stimulus rates equal to the line current frequency are used. Therefore, in the United States, repetition rates equal to 60 Hz line frequency or sub-harmonics of 60 Hz (i.e., 10, 20, 30 . . .) should be avoided.

Polarity

Polarity refers to the direction in which the headphone diaphragm moves at the onset of a stimulus. With the click typically used to elicit ABR, the headphone moves either toward the ear to create a condensation wave or away from the ear to create a rarefaction wave. The ABR can be generated by a single polarity series of stimuli, either condensation or rarefaction, or by clicks that alternate in polarity (Fig. 42–4). The effects of stimulus polarity are complex and remain controversial. Wave I appears to be the most sensitive to stimulus polarity. As a group, normal adults generate slightly shorter Wave I latencies and larger Wave I amplitudes to rarefaction stimuli.[22,23] This finding influences interwave latencies as well, since the later ABR waves are relatively unaffected by stimulus polarity.

In some individuals, significant morphologic differences occur between rarefaction and condensation stimuli. These differences can even yield responses that are abnormal to one polarity and normal to the opposite polarity. The significance of these differences continues to be debated. If abnormal responses are obtained to one polarity, stimulation with the opposite polarity is often useful as well. Alternating polarity stimuli may also be used to eliminate the influence of stimulus artifacts. The disadvantage of this technique is that the ABR reflects the addition of two different responses (condensation + rarefaction). This addition tends to round off individual waves and may create artificial phase cancellation.

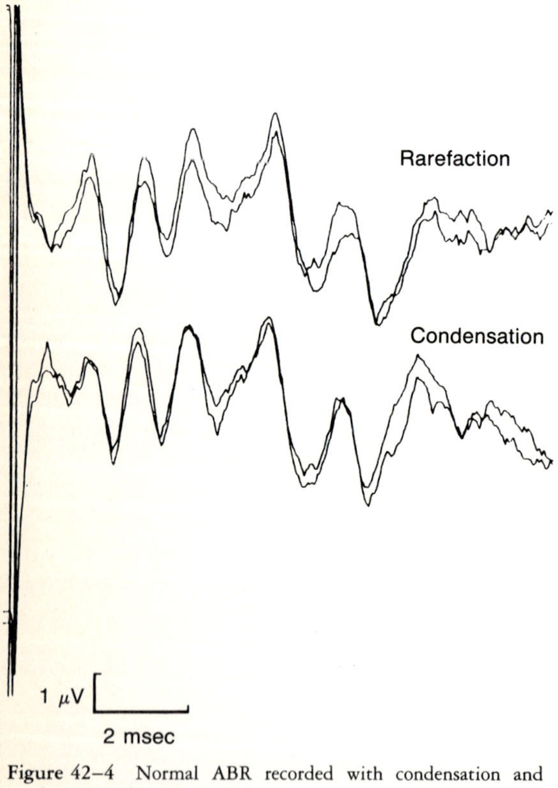

Figure 42–4 Normal ABR recorded with condensation and rarefaction click stimuli. In some patients with high-frequency hearing loss, significant waveform differences can be seen.

Frequency Specific Stimuli

A variety of investigators have attempted to use tonal stimuli to elicit the ABR in an attempt to obtain more frequency specific information.[24,25,26] As has been mentioned, a transient stimulus must be used in order to elicit the synchronous neural burst required to obtain a recordable ABR. When tonal bursts are used as ABR stimuli, these bursts must have extremely fast rise times in order to ensure adequate synchrony. Unfortunately, short duration tone bursts generate substantial amounts of energy in adjacent frequency bands. This frequency spread increases at higher stimulus intensities. Therefore, although responses can be obtained with mid- and high-frequency tone bursts, a much broader portion of the cochlea is contributing to the ABR than would be implied by the frequency of the stimulus, particularly at higher stimulus intensities.[27]

For clinical purposes, tone bursts below approximately lk Hz are not as effective for eliciting the ABR. Attempts to record responses at 500 Hz require the use of a filter bandpass that includes more low-frequency energy. A high-pass filter cutoff of 30 Hz can increase the amplitude of ABRs to lower frequency tone bursts. Attempts to improve the frequency specificity of both low- and high-frequency tone bursts involve either manipulation of the stimulus envelope or incorporation of a masking paradigm. Alteration of the shape of the tone burst stimulus envelope can optimize the concentration of energy to a narrow frequency band.[28,29] Mixing high-pass or notched masking noise with click or tonal stimuli has also been suggested as a means of isolating stimulation to a specific frequency region within the cochlea.[30,31] This method can be particularly effective with low- and mid-frequency tonal stimuli, since without masking they readily spread to the basal cochlea. Introduction of broad spectrum noise masking that is high-passed with a steep roll off filter (>90 dB per octave) prevents the basal end of the cochlea from responding to mid- and low-frequency tone burst stimuli. In the same way, notch filtered noise has a narrow band of energy removed that corresponds to the center frequency of a tone burst. This restricts the area along the cochlear partition that responds synchronously to the tone burst.

Suffice it to say that ABR is a high-frequency biased response and, at best, is not nearly as frequency specific as behavioral audiometric testing. Caution should be utilized whenever attempting to infer frequency specific behavioral thresholds from ABR, even when using masked tone burst stimuli.

SUBJECT VARIABLES

The primary advantage of ABR, in contrast to longer latency evoked potentials, is its extreme robustness. Although few nonpathologic subject variables significantly effect the ABR, those that do must be considered when clinically evaluating patients.

Age

Age is probably the most significant nonpathologic subject variable, particularly in infant and in geriatric populations. ABR potentials demonstrate significant maturation during the first 18 to 24 months of age.[32,33,34,35] Although the major ABR response components (I, III, & V) are generally present in normal term babies, peak latencies, interwave latencies, and general waveform morphology are quite different than a typical adult waveform (see Fig. 42–5). Both peak and interwave latencies are substantially longer in the infant. Wave I is often twice as large in the infant while Wave V is relatively smaller. Wave I systematically decreases in latency and in amplitude during the first 2 to 3 months of life. This maturation occurs more rapidly than the latency reduction and the amplitude increase of the later components, which typically take up to 18 months. This finding suggests that the maturation of the peripheral portion of the auditory system occurs more rapidly than maturation of the central auditory pathways within the brain stem. Peripheral maturation is thought to reflect primarily middle ear conductive function, while central development probably reflects synaptic efficiency and central myelinization.

Premature infants demonstrate additional developmental immaturity with peak and interwave latencies that progressively increase at younger gestational ages.[36] Application of pediatric norms adjusted by week of gestational age is critical for appropriate interpretation of clinical recordings in this population.

Subjects over the age of 50 years may also demonstrate subtle increases in ABR latency and, in some cases, a somewhat disorganized waveform morphology, compared to younger subjects.[37,38,39] These observations are not universally accepted because several studies have reported the lack of significant differences between young and old subjects.[40,41] The contradiction between studies may reflect the confounding effect of high-frequency hearing loss that has not been adequately controlled for in most studies.

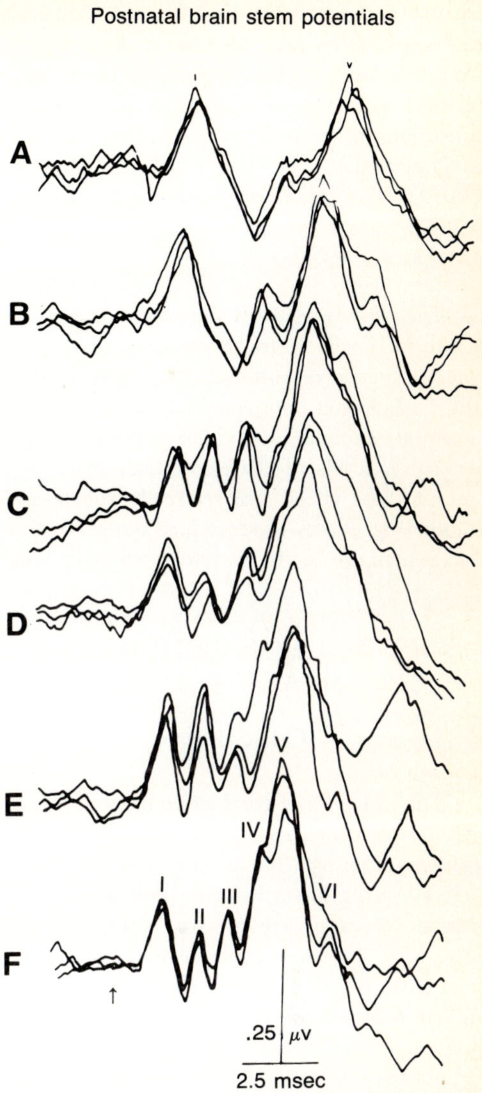

Figure 42–5 Maturation of the ABR. *A*, Newborn; *B*, 6 weeks; *C*, 3 months; *D*, 6 months, *E*, 1 year; *F*, adult. Note decrease in latency of Wave I and Wave V and better definition of intermediate peaks with maturation. (Reprinted with permission from Salamy A, McKean C. Postnatal development of the human brain stem potentials during the first year of life. Electroencephalogr Clin Neurophysiol 1976; 40:418.)

Gender

Small, but significant, differences have been noted between male and female subjects.[42] Females tend to demonstrate shorter latencies and larger amplitudes than males. These gender effects are more significant in the later response components creating interwave latencies, which are also slightly shorter in females.

Temperature

Significant changes in core temperature have

been shown to create prolongations in ABR peak and in interwave latencies.[7] This factor is not significant in most clinical diagnostic settings, but can come into play in comatose patients or in intraoperative applications where body temperature may be deliberately altered.

Pharmacologic Agents

The ABR is relatively resistant to changes caused by clinical levels of most sedatives and anesthetic agents.[43] Subtle response changes have been noted with barbiturates, intoxicating levels of alcohol, thiopental, cholinergic and serotonergic drugs, and therapeutic levels of diazepam (valium).[44,45,46,47,48] Most of these effects are relatively subtle and the confounding effects of secondary temperature alteration contribute to the waveform changes noted.

EFFECTS OF PERIPHERAL HEARING LOSS

Conductive

The influence of conductive hearing loss on the ABR relates primarily to the reduction of effective stimulus intensity that reaches the cochlea. Conductive hearing losses increase peak latencies by the amount of the conductive component present.[14,24,49,50] In other words, a 60-dB stimulus is attenuated to 40 dB by the presence of a 20-dB conductive component. Therefore, the peak latency obtained at 60 dB would be equal to that obtained by a normal ear at 40 dB. This deficit occurs at each intensity sampled, thus creating a conductive I-L function that parallels the normal I-L function, but that is increased in latency by the amount of the conductive loss. (See Fig. 42–3) Interwave latencies are not affected by the presence of conductive pathology. The early ABR peaks (I to III) may also be absent in large conductive losses. This absence may reflect temporal smearing of the transient stimulus due to the presence of the conductive pathology.

The ABR intensity-amplitude function can also be affected by the presence of conductive pathology. ABR amplitude growth at near threshold levels is often smaller in the presence of conductive pathology than with normal hearing or with cochlear pathology. The certainty of response detection at low suprathreshold levels is reduced when visual detection is used as the sole determinant of response presence. An artificially greater difference between ABR and behavioral threshold can be introduced.

The appearance of a conductive hearing loss can also be artificially created by collapsing a patient's ear canals with headphones. This collapse is more likely to occur during evoked potential evaluations because patients are typically in a reclining position. Care should be taken to ensure that ear canal collapse does not occur. Insert receivers are also commercially available with frequency response characteristics that are similar to TDH-39 headphones.[51] Inserts prevent the possibility of ear canal collapse and are particularly useful for intraoperative applications. Inserts do, however, introduce a temporal delay that varies as a function of the tubing length. This delay must be taken into account when calculating peak latencies. Separate norms should be determined if insert receivers are to be utilized.

Click stimuli delivered through a bone conduction oscillator may also be used to elicit the ABR. This technique allows direct quantification of the amount of air-bone gap by comparison of ABR thresholds to bone versus air conducted clicks.[52,53] Although bone conducted ABR is used clinically, there are a variety of methodological problems that must be taken into account. The frequency spectrum of most bone oscillators is significantly lower than typical audiometric headphones. A latency prolongation of about 0.5 msec is introduced compared with air conducted clicks.[53] The maximum stimulus intensity is also limited to approximately 50 dB nHL, thus restricting the magnitude of loss that can be assessed. Mastoid placement of the oscillator has the advantage of increasing the effective intensity that can be delivered to the cochlea, compared to forehead placement. However, mastoid placement may also introduce air conducted acoustic radiations. In spite of these methodological concerns, bone conducted ABR can be performed clinically if caution is taken to minimize the influence of extraneous variables. Normative data should be collected for both air and bone conduction stimuli on the same sample of subjects.

Cochlear

Cochlear pathology also has a significant effect on the ABR. Unlike conductive losses, the dynamic range for intensity is significantly reduced in patients with cochlear pathology. ABR waveforms in these patients demonstrate rapid amplitude growth at low sensation levels and normal latencies when stimuli exceed approximately 20 dB SL. (see Fig. 42–3)

As has been mentioned, ABR is high-frequency biased and depends, to a great extent, on the integrity of basal hair cells. Therefore, low-frequency cochlear hearing losses yield ABR responses to clicks that have essentially normal thresholds, latencies, and

I-L functions. On the other hand, steeply sloping high-frequency hearing losses have a dramatic effect on the ABR. ABRs from this type of hearing loss have peak latency delays and steeply sloping I-L functions that typically do not reach normal latencies, even at very high intensities.[11,15,44,54,55] Presumably, this fact reflects the additional time required for the traveling wave to reach viable mid-frequency hair cells. Waveform morphology in precipitous high-frequency losses is also affected, with Wave I often diminished in amplitude or absent. Interwave latencies typically remain normal, but in some cases, have been reported to decrease.[15,54] This latter phenomenon may reflect differential sensitivity of the various ABR peaks to frequency. Wave I appears to be generated more basally within the cochlea than Wave V. If so, high-frequency hearing losses should selectively delay Wave I more than Wave V, thereby creating a reduction in interpeak latency.

DIAGNOSTIC INTERPRETATION

Clinical appliciations of ABR break down into two general categories: (1) assessment of auditory sensitivity and (2) assessment of pathology affecting the auditory pathways from the eighth nerve through the brain stem. The two ABR measurements that are salient to the assessment of auditory sensitivity are threshold and I-L function. Both measurements are dependent on the presence of an intact neural pathway capable of generating synchronous electrical activity. In the absence of this condition, little can reliably be said about threshold sensitivity.

As has been mentioned, the relationship between ABR and behavioral threshold in the 1,000 Hz to 4,000 Hz frequency region is well established. Incorporation of suprathreshold measures and the construction of an I-L function allows inferences to be drawn regarding the etiology of any hearing loss that might be present. By the same token, suprathreshold measures alone cannot reliably predict behavioral thresholds, since cochlear hearing losses generate robust ABR waveforms with short peak latencies at near threshold stimulation levels.

NEUROPATHOLOGY

To assess neuropathology with ABR, moderately high stimulus intensities are typically used to ensure adequate visualization of all major response components and to override the influence of peripheral hearing loss. The salient ABR measures used to assess retrocochlear and/or neurologic pathology include (1) interwave latencies, (2) amplitude ratios, (3) rate functions, (4) absence of waves, and (5) interaural latency differences (ILD). The prolongation of interwave latencies, either unilaterally or bilaterally, is one of the most common manifestations of neuropathology. Interwave latencies are relatively insensitive to the effects of peripheral hearing loss (except in cases of high-frequency precipitous cochlear losses where interwave latencies may be reduced). Therefore, interwave latencies are excellent for the assessment of neural system integrity.

Amplitude ratio measures have also been suggested as indices of eighth nerve (Fig. 42–6) and brain stem pathology; however, the clinical utility of these measures remains controversial. As with all amplitude measures, amplitude ratio measures are influenced by a variety of methodological and subject variables. However, these measures may be of value in some cases of retrocochlear pathology.[56,57] The amplitude ratio is derived by dividing the peak to peak amplitude of Wave V by the same amplitudes of Wave I. Ratios of less than 1.0 have been cited as pathologic, although individual laboratory norms should be developed to account for potential methodological variables. Separate pediatric norms should also be determined, since normal amplitude ratios vary developmentally.

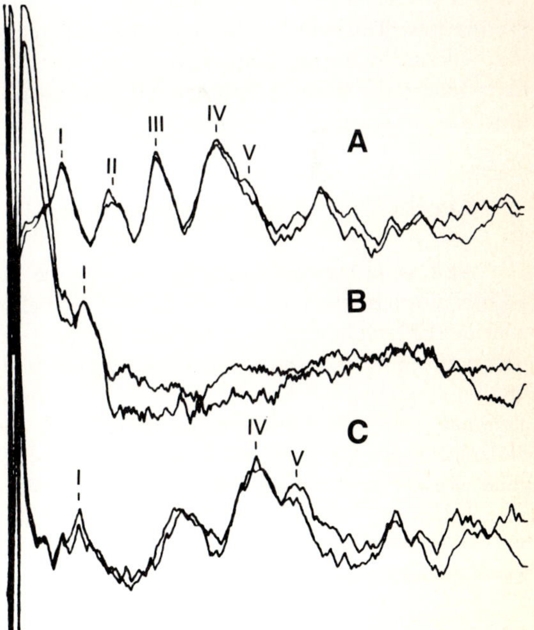

Figure 42–6 Effect of eighth nerve pathology on the ABR. *A*, Normal responses. *B*, Acoustic neuroma: Delay in Wave I, with absence of Waves II to V. *C*, Acoustic neuroma: normal latency Wave I, with delayed responses II to V.

Rate functions are a means of stressing the neural system by reducing the interstimulus interval and inducing pathologic fatigue. Faster stimulation rates cause a normal reduction in Wave V amplitude and a prolongation of peak latencies that is greater for the later ABR waves, thereby creating a concomitant increase in interwave latency. The physiologic basis for the latency shift is presumed to be the neural refractory period that, in pathologic neurons, is excessively prolonged under the stress of reduced interstimulus intervals. Agreement on the criterion for abnormal rate functions is not well established. Generally, Wave V latency shifts exceeding 0.30 msec per 20 stimuli per second increase are considered to be pathologic.[18,57,58]

The absence of later ABR components in the presence of early waves is probably one of the strongest indications of neural pathology. The presence of early waves confirms the integrity of the peripheral auditory mechanism and precludes the possibility of technical artifacts. The absence of later waves in the presence of neural pathology is presumed to reflect disruption of the synchronous neural volley at the point along the auditory pathway where the lesion occurs.

Interaural latency differences can be the most sensitive indices of pathology; however, these differences are confounded by the presence of unilateral hearing loss. This will be discussed in detail in the next section. Interaural comparisons of interwave latency reduce the effect of such hearing loss and improve the sensitivity of the measure.

Cerebellopontine Angle Lesions

ABR is an extremely sensitive test in the diagnosis of acoustic neuromas and of other cerebellopontine (CP) angle tumors. A variety of studies report between 90 and 98 percent positive ABR findings in confirmed CP angle tumors.[59–64] The most common effect of these tumors on the ABR is the unilateral prolongation or obliteration of waves beyond Wave I or II. Other ABR changes that have been noted include a delayed Wave V with no other waves present or a total absence of the entire ABR waveform. Relationships have not generally been found between tumor size and the amount of ABR latency prolongation, except in cases of extremely large tumors where contralateral prolongations of the III to V interval have been reported.[59] The poor correlation between tumor size and the extent of ABR abnormality relates to the influence of tumor location. Extremely small tumors in the internal auditory canal can exert significantly more pressure on the cochlear nerve than larger tumors that extend into the cerebellopontine angle.

Although ABR is extremely sensitive to the presence of CP angle lesions, this test is not without weaknesses. One of the most significant weaknesses is the confounding influence of peripheral hearing loss. This weakness becomes an acute problem when a patient presents with unilateral hearing loss and attempts are made to compare response latencies between the patient's two ears. This comparison is known as an interaural latency difference and has been found to be one of the most sensitive indices of retrocochlear pathology. An interaural latency difference for Wave V latency exceeding 0.2 msec was originally proposed as significant for the presence of unilateral cerebellopontine angle lesions. Unfortunately, unilateral high-frequency sloping cochlear hearing losses also yield peak latency delays that often exceed 0.2 msec, thereby creating an inordinately high false positive rate. Although peripheral hearing losses do not prolong interwave latencies, precipitous cochlear losses often obliterate Wave I, thus preventing the distinction of peripheral from neural latency delay. Several measures have been suggested to attempt to reduce ABR false positive rates including (1) an interaural latency difference criterion exceeding 0.3 msec as significant, (2) correction factors to reduce the influence of hearing loss on latency delays, and (3) use of an ECoG electrode in the ear canal to enhance the presence of Wave I.

Correction factors are based on the assumption that latency delays attributable to peripheral hearing loss can be subtracted out. Selters and Brackmann[59] suggested subtracting 0.1 msec for every 10 dB of hearing loss above 50 dB HL at 4 k Hz. However, correction factors must be utilized with caution, since the configuration (i.e., slope) of the loss may have as much of an effect on the latency of the ABR as the amount of loss at any one frequency. Attempting to address this concern, Jerger and Mauldin[11] proposed subtracting 0.2 msec for every 30 dB of threshold difference between 1 k Hz and 4 k Hz.

The use of an ECoG electrode in the ear canal as a reference is another means of minimizing the ambiguity introduced by the presence of significant hearing loss. These electrodes enhance the amplitude of Wave 1, thereby making it visible in some cases when surface electrodes on the earlobe cannot record the amplitude.[15] This enhancement allows measurement of interwave latencies that help discriminate between cochlear and neural pathology.

Another disadvantage of the ABR is its inability to distinguish tumors from nontumor lesions affecting the brain stem auditory pathways. Any lesions that delay or desynchronize the neural volley result in pathologic changes in the ABR. Conversely, lesions of the CP angle or brain stem that do not impinge on the auditory pathways yield normal ABRs in the presence of pathology. The sensitivity of ABR to other types of cerebellopontine angle tumors may also be lower than to the classic schwannoma or to acoustic neuroma.[64]

Intrinsic Brain Stem Lesions

ABR is also a valuable adjunct in the diagnosis of lesions that originate intrinsically or within the central nervous system tissue of the brain stem. Intrinsic brain stem lesions can include tumors, vascular lesions, or demyelinating diseases such as multiple sclerosis. The influence of these types of lesions on the ABR is predicated on the basis of their compromise of the brain stem auditory pathways. If damage is restricted to levels rostral to the midbrain or to neural tissue other than the auditory pathways, the ABR typically is normal.

ABR changes associated with intrinsic brain stem lesions include (1) prolongation of interwave latencies, (2) absence of later response components, (3) selective reduction of later wave amplitude, or (4) inordinately large amplitude early waves. Rate function abnormalities have also been cited, although the sensitivity of this measure is less clear. The ability to localize or to lateralize lesions within the brain stem is limited by the complex interaction of generators for each given response component. Lesions exclusively affecting Waves IV and V generally (although not universally) have been attributed to pathology of the rostral pons and the midbrain.[42,65] Low brain stem lesions of the caudal pons are thought to begin influencing the ABR at Waves II and III.

The correlation of ABR changes with the side of pathology has also remained somewhat ambiguous. Unlike the extrinsic cerebellopontine angle lesions, few intrinsic brain stem lesions reported in the literature have been documented to exclusively affect the auditory pathways unilaterally. Low brain stem lesions appear to correlate better with lateralized pathology than with lesions above the level of the caudal pons. These lesions primarily create ipsilateral ABR changes.[66,67] Lesions above this level may create ipsilateral, contralateral, or bilateral ABR changes, although a higher incidence of contralateral ABR changes have been noted.[65,68]

Tumors

Intrinsic brain stem tumors may involve cells originating within the supportive interstitial tissue (gliomas) or the meningial coverings of the central nervous system (meningiomas). The influence of these types of tumors on the ABR is dependent on the level of involvement and the extent of auditory pathway compromise. As has been mentioned, distinguishing tumor from nontumor lesions is not possible with ABR.

Multiple Sclerosis

Multiple sclerosis (MS) is characterized by multiple white matter lesions (plaques) that reflect the breakdown of myelin, which surrounds most neural axons. These plaques result in the disruption of impulse conduction along axonal pathways, thereby creating a variety of intermittent sensory and motor disturbances. MS is difficult to diagnose because of the capricious nature of the disease and because of the difficulty in identifying clinically silent lesions that often occur. ABR is a noninvasive means of documenting the presence of these plaques if they occur within the brain stem auditory pathways (Fig. 42–7). Reports of the incidence of ABR abnormalities in patients with confirmed MS range from approximately 50 to 70 percent.[66,69,70] In patients

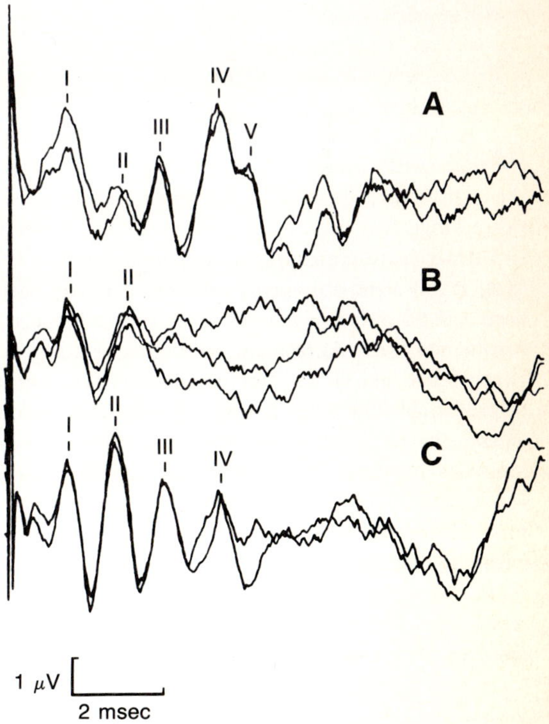

Figure 42–7 Effect of multiple sclerosis on the ABR. *A*, Normal responses. *B*, Waves I and II present, with successive peaks absent. *C*, Waves I through IV present with absent Wave V and abnormal V:I amplitude ratio.

without clinical brain stem symptomatology, ABR abnormality decreases to between 30 and 50 percent.[71] Because MS plaques occur more frequently in the visual and somatosensory pathways, evoked potentials utilizing visual (VEP) and somatosensory (SEP) stimuli demonstrate a higher incidence of abnormalities than does the ABR.[70,72] Combining all three modalities of evoked potentials increases the sensitivity to around 90 percent in definite MS patients.

ABR changes associated with an increased repetition rate have been reported to occur more frequently in MS patients than in other brain stem lesions. In addition, MS is one of the few pathologies that can result in poor intertrial replicability.

Vascular Lesions

Infarctions or hemorrhages that create primary or secondary damage to the auditory brain stem pathways affect the ABR. A variety of studies have demonstrated prolonged interwave latencies or later wave absence from vascular lesions within the pons or caudal midbrain.[42,67,73,74] Transient vascular events that do not result in permanent damage, such as transient ischemic attacks (TIA), are less often correlated with ABR abnormalities.[71]

Coma

A large number of studies have attempted to correlate ABR findings with the type and the severity of coma, along with attempting to prognosticate long-term neurologic outcome.[75,76,77] ABR is an attractive test for use in comatose patients because it can be reliably performed, even shortly postonset, and is relatively resistent to the influence of barbiturate level. Agreement on the relationship between ABR and coma remains controversial owing to procedural differences between studies (i.e., length of time between onset and the test, differences in normal criteria, and unknown amounts of hearing loss present) as well as to differences in patient samples. However, ABR does appear to correlate well with the patient's changing pathophysiologic status associated with anoxia, intracranial pressure, and cerebral perfusion pressure. The ability to prognosticate clinical outcome based on the ABR remains poor.

PEDIATRIC APPLICATIONS

The assessment of neurologic integrity and auditory sensitivity in high-risk or multiply handicapped pediatric populations is probably the most widely used application of ABR. The major pediatric applications of ABR include (1) the assessment of high-risk neonates in the neonatal intensive care unit (NICU), (2) the obtaining of more precise information about suspected hearing loss in multiply handicapped children, and (3) the evaluation of infants or of children who have failed other auditory screening procedures. Galambos[78] has recommended ABR assessment on (1) all NICU graduates, (2) all infants who fail a high-risk register, (3) infants who fail behavioral screening, or (4) infants considered to be suspect for hearing loss for any other reason.

NICU Screening

The incidence of significant hearing loss has been cited by the Joint Committee on Infant Hearing (1982) to occur in from 2.5 to 5 percent of NICU graduates. Hearing loss in this population was significantly under-identified prior to the use of ABR as a screening tool. Although ABR is extremely sensitive to neonatal hearing loss, considerable controversy remains over the incidence of false positive findings in this population. In reviewing a series of 10 studies citing initial ABR failure rate and the incidence of subsequent hearing loss on follow-up of NICU graduates, Stein[79] initially reported failure rates that were generally between 15 and 20 percent. The incidence of significant hearing loss on follow-up, however, ranged from only 1.5 to 5 percent of the population, thus reflecting a fairly high false positive rate. The range of initial failures reported was also extremely broad, with rates as high as 59 percent in one study.[80] The reasons for the wide range of ABR failure rates, as well as for the incidence of false positive findings, have been hotly debated during the past several years. Possible explanations include (1) inordinately stringent failure criteria, (2) the presence of transient conductive pathology that resolves prior to follow-up testing, (3) immaturity of the infants' auditory brain stem pathways, and (4) technical or methodological artifact. The extent of interaction between any of these factors and the incidence of false positive findings is difficult to infer, but there do appear to be some factors that are relevant. The age at which infants are tested and the rigor of the pass-fail criteria appear to be critical to the sensitivity and the specificity of ABR screening programs. Testing infants at graduation from the NICU allows more control over the testing environment, as does accessing the infants when they are physiologically more stable and older.

Establishing appropriate pass-fail criteria is probably one of the most critical aspects of any screening program. Although the thrust of screening programs must be to identify all children with hearing loss, appropriate pass-fail criteria should accomplish this goal with the least amount of inappropriate failures. Most ABR screening programs utilize a two stage pass-fail criteria. Two stimulus intensities are presented, typically at 60 dB nHL and at 25 to 40 dB nHL. In order to pass, responses must be present at both intensities and Wave V must occur at the appropriate age-adjusted latency at the higher intensity. This latter criteria allows the assessment of neurologic function in addition to the assessment of hearing sensitivity. Utilizing a lower intensity level than 30 dB nHL appears to contribute to higher false positive rates. Raising the level to 35 or 40 dB nHL may be appropriate.

The age at which the testing is performed can also have a significant effect on the results obtained. A significant number of the NICU population is premature. There is some evidence that infants younger than 36 weeks gestation have a higher incidence of transient ABR abnormalities, presumably attributable to central nervous system (CNS) immaturity. Many high-risk screening programs attempt to test the infants just prior to discharge in order to minimize this variable.

Although some concern has been expressed regarding the incidence of false positive findings, ABR has clearly been shown to sensitively identify hearing loss in the neonatal population. Prior to the application of ABR in this population, many pediatric hearing losses went unidentified for extended and critical periods of time. ABR allows ear specific assessment of high-risk infants at the earliest possible age. The disadvantage of over-identifying some normal infants must be weighed against not identifying some hearing impaired infants if ABR is not used.

Pediatric Neuropathology

ABR assessment of high-risk infant populations provides information regarding neurologic integrity as well as auditory sensitivity, as already described. As in the adult population, ABR correlates of neuropathology in pediatrics include (1) prolonged interwave latencies, (2) abnormal amplitude ratios, and (3) significant interwave latency shifts with increasing stimulation rates.

Many congenital, perinatal, and neonatal diseases and/or insults can cause significant neurologic sequellae that are often reflected in ABR abnormalities. Periventricular hemorrhage, asphyxia,[81] hyperbilirubinemia,[82] meningitis,[83] brain stem gliomas,[84] cytomegalic virus, and phenylketonuria[20] are some of the diseases that have documented ABR correlates. Although ABR can be helpful in the diagnosis and the management of these pediatric diseases, ABR's ability to prognose long-term neurologic outcome is much less secure.

A variety of transient neurologic disorders have been shown to create reversible ABR abnormalities. This finding strengthens the diagnostic relationship between ABR changes and acute neurologic status, but confounds the ability to prognose recovery. Hecox and Cone[81] cited several central ABR abnormalities associated with acute asphyxia in infants. Of these abnormalities, only the presence of abnormal Wave I to V amplitude ratios prognosed poor long-term neurologic outcome. Unfortunately, the absence of this abnormality did not insure positive neurologic outcome, nor was it applicable in premature infants. Clearly, caution should be exercised when interpreting any ABR characteristics in younger premature infants because of their reversibility. Conversely, the sensitivity of ABR to dynamic neurologic processes makes ABR an effective tool with which to monitor changes over time in neurologic status, as well as to evaluate the effects of treatment regimens.

Hearing Loss in Older Children

The third application of pediatric ABR is to assess hearing loss in older children who are difficult to test with conventional techniques or who have failed screening procedures. The focus of this application is to confirm the presence of hearing loss, as well as to provide information regarding the configuration, severity, and etiology of hearing loss. As with any diagnostic procedure, ABR should be considered one measure of a test battery and is used in conjunction with impedance and behavioral audiometric tests to provide a complete diagnostic picture.

Children older than approximately 1 year may require sedation in order to minimize extraneous muscle activity while recording the ABR. In our experience, the risks associated with sedation can be acceptably minimized if performed (1) under medical supervision, (2) in facilities equipped with emergency resuscitation equipment, (3) with appropriate protocols, and (4) with trained personnel. Chloral hydrate is the most commonly used sedative reported, although secobarbitol and a combination of demerol, phenergan, and thorazine have also been suggested.

As has been described, ABR to clicks provides information primarily about the 1,000 Hz to 4,000 Hz frequency region. Some form of tonal stimuli must be used in order to obtain information about mid- and low frequencies. Rapid onset tone bursts mixed with high-passed or notched masking noise appear to be the most efficient means of obtaining mid-frequency information. Our clinical experience has led us to utilize 1 kHz tone bursts with high-pass masking noise along with click stimuli in the assessment of these children. Shaping the stimulus envelope to minimize frequency spread can further improve the frequency specificity of the ABR.[28] Unfortunately, ABR provides less than optimal frequency specificity, even with these procedures. However, comparison of thresholds obtained from a 1 kHz tone burst in conjunction with a click provides information regarding the audiometric slope of hearing loss and prevents exclusively low-frequency hearing losses that do not affect click ABRs being missed.

Information obtained from stimuli below 1 kHz with ABR is much less reliable than that obtained from high-frequency tone bursts or from clicks. The significant phase shifting that occurs at the apical end of the cochlea is much less conducive to generating the synchronous bursts of electrical activity required to elicit ABR recordings. Although a variety of reports discuss low-frequency ABRs, clinical data should be interpreted with caution. Our clinical protocol incorporates the use of 500 Hz tone bursts with high-pass masking only if the child remains asleep and all other salient measures have been obtained. Reduction of the low-frequency filter to 30 Hz in order to improve the response detection has been suggested in recording 500 Hz responses.[85] Longer latency evoked potentials (SN-10, MLR, 40 Hz ERP) have been advocated as more appropriate indices of low-frequency hearing. However, their discussion is beyond the scope of this chapter. The use of longer latency potentials introduces additional subject variables, and their application in pediatrics remains a subject of much debate.

ELECTROCOCHLEOGRAPHY

The clinical use of electrocochleography (ECoG) has increased in the past few years, primarily owing to the prevalence of ABR averaging computers, the development of noninvasive electrodes,and interest in the differential diagnosis of cochlear pathology. ECoG is the recording of the electrical potentials of the cochlea and eighth nerve, through placement of an electrode in proximity to the middle ear. Many of the recording considerations for ECoG are the same as those for ABR and are described in detail in the previous section. The potentials recorded by ECoG include the cochlear microphonic (CM), the summating potential (SP), and the whole nerve action potential (AP) of the eighth nerve. The CM is a graded alternating current (AC) potential that directly reflects the frequency and the intensity of the eliciting stimulus and is generated primarily by the outer hair cells. The CM reflects the point by point vibration of the basilar membrane in the basal turn when recorded from outside the cochlea.

The SP is a complex, direct current (DC), cochlear receptor potential, also thought to be generated by the outer hair cells. The SP reflects a rectified DC version of the displacement pattern of the cochlear partition. The SP can have positive or negative components, depending on the intensity and the frequency of the stimulus and on the recording site[86,87]. The response is almost always negative when recorded extratympanically in man, and is seen on the leading edge of the action potential when elicited with a short duration click. Because the SP is thought to reflect the distortion characteristics of the basilar membrane, the SP appears to be sensitive to pathophysiologic conditions that influence the mechanical integrity of the cochlear partition, such as endolymphatic hydrops.

The action potential (AP) is the compound response of the eighth nerve, generated by the summation of a large number of synchronously firing individual auditory neurons. The AP is synonymous with Wave I of the ABR when recorded with surface electrodes from the scalp.

Initial clinical interest in these potentials centered around the physiologic assessment of hearing loss in infants in the early 1960s. In the United States, efforts were directed towards noninvasive recordings from the external auditory meatus.[88,89] These recordings proved to be relatively insensitive near threshold and were eventually abandoned with the clinical development of ABR. Not until 1981 and series of articles by Coats[90] assessing patients with Meniere's disease did ECoG came into relatively widespread use.

Recording Electrodes

With the exception of the active electrode and the filter bandpass, the instrumentation, recording, and stimulus parameters are similar to those of the ABR. The recording montage consists of an active electrode in the ear canal or on the promontory, a reference electrode on the contralateral earlobe, and a ground electrode on the forehead. The location of the active electrode is the most critical factor in recording the ECoG.[91]

Transtympanic technique involves the placement of a teflon insulated needle electrode through the tympanic membrane and onto the cochlear promontory. A major advantage of this technique is the extremely large response obtained owing to the proximity of the recording electrode to the cochlear generator site. However, at this distance small changes in placement can dramatically change the amplitude and polarity of the SP.[92,93] While transtympanic technique is widely used in Europe, its invasive nature, requiring local anesthesia and placement by a physician, has prevented acceptance in the United States.

Extratympanic ECoG has been gaining popularity because of the availability of several commercial electrodes. These electrodes provide smaller amplitude, but reliable responses, at suprathreshold levels. The most commonly used electrode is a small silver ball mounted on a plastic strip, designed by Coats and manufactured by Lifetech, Inc. (Houston, Texas). This "eartrode" is inserted into the ear canal to rest approximately 4 mm from the tympanic membrane in the posterior-inferior quadrant of the canal. (Fig. 42–8) The ear canal must be meticulously cleansed prior to electrode placement with sequential irrigation of 2 percent hydrogen peroxide, water, and isopropyl alcohol.[90] The eartrode can be placed with visualization from a head mirror or an operating microscope, and standard audiometric headphones can be used with little discomfort. Consistancy of placement, variability in canal shape, and degree of patient hearing loss can have significant effects on the quality of responses obtained with this electrode.

Placement of the eartrode near the tympanic membrane results in much larger responses than those obtained with disk electrodes on the earlobe or with electrodes placed distally in the cartilaginous portion of the canal.[91,94,95,95a] However, large differences in response amplitude reported across normative studies suggest that the eartrode may be sensitive to user and equipment differences. The issue of amplitude is a critical one, as the size of the SP-AP complex may affect the reliability of the recording. Smaller amplitude responses tend to have greater intertrial variability (Fig. 42–9), presumably owing to reduced signal to noise ratios.[93]

The impedance of the Life Tech electrode ranges from approximately 20 kohms to greater than 100k ohms. When referenced to traditional disk electrodes, this impedance mismatch presents problems when interfaced with typical differential preamplifiers used in clinical evoked potential systems. Unbalanced impedance results in higher baseline noise levels and decreased signal to noise ratios. This problem is further compounded in patients with moderate or severe hearing losses, in which the amplitude of the potential is reduced and the signal to noise ratio further decreased. Although the eartrode may be more effective than more distally placed electrodes, the sensitivity to placement and to canal characteristics, along with the inherently high impedance, makes the eartrode less than ideal with these patients.

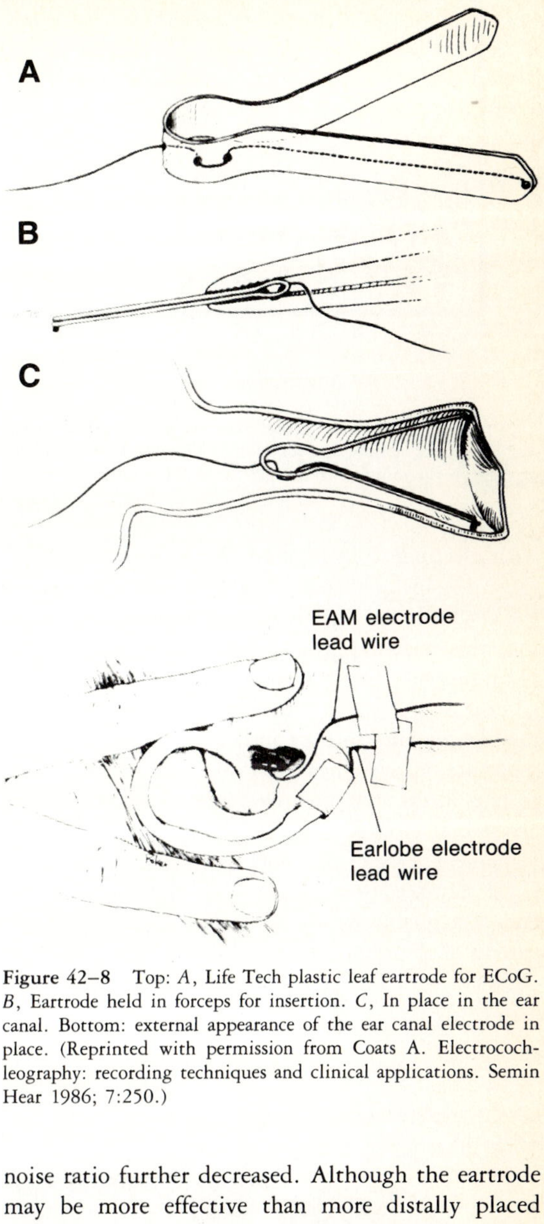

Figure 42–8 Top: *A*, Life Tech plastic leaf eartrode for ECoG. *B*, Eartrode held in forceps for insertion. *C*, In place in the ear canal. Bottom: external appearance of the ear canal electrode in place. (Reprinted with permission from Coats A. Electrocochleography: recording techniques and clinical applications. Semin Hear 1986; 7:250.)

Another commercial extratympanic electrode is the Axonics-3M disposable foam earplug electrode (currently manufactured by Nicolet Biomedical, Madison, WI). This electrode consists of a silver impregnated foam plug saturated with electrode gel, and is designed to sit within the cartilaginous portion of the ear canal in the manner of an impedance probe tip (Fig. 42–10). A headband module with a transducer accompanies the electrode and allows both recording and stimulus delivery. The position of the recording site in the distal portion of the canal produces smaller amplitude responses when compared

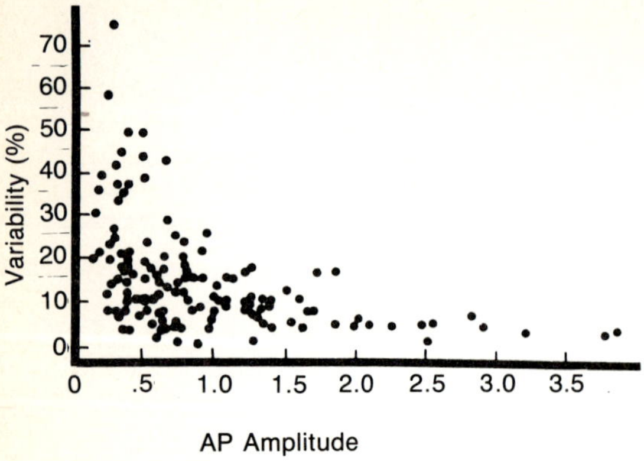

Figure 42–9 Maximum SP-AP ratio variability across trials within one test session, as a function of AP amplitude. Note the decrease in variability with an increase in AP amplitude.

with electrodes placed deep in the ear canal[91,93,95] (Fig. 42–11). However, the large surface areas of the electrode provides lower impedance, thus making this electrode more compatible with ABR preamplifiers. The tradeoff of low impedance and clinical ease of use is counterbalanced by lower amplitude responses that are inadequate in patients with moderate or severe hearing losses. The need for new designs in extratympanic electrodes is evident. There are several electrodes in the prototype stage of development. One of the more promising electrodes is a gel saturated small foam plug embedded in the end of a pliable plastic tube that rests against the surface of the tympanic membrane.[91] The responses obtained with this electrode are significantly larger than other extratympanic electrodes because of the proximity of the electrode to the cochlear generators. Although the impedance is extremely high, (> 100 kohms), the intertrial variability is reduced owing to the size of the responses obtained. While both electrode impedance and proximity to the generator site contribute to the size of the potentials recorded, proximity appears to outweigh the detrimental effects of high impedance. Both this electrode and the transtympanic needle electrode produce extremely large responses in spite of high impedances.[91]

Whitaker[96] has also reported another type of extratympanic ECoG electrode in development. This electrode consists of an open sleeve with a large silver surface that conforms to the wall of the ear canal. The large area of the electrode allows for low, stable impedance. The insertion is into the cartilaginous portion of the canal and allows for the use of standard audiometric headphones. The depth of placement appears comparable to the Axonics-3M and imparts the same characteristics as the other distally placed electrodes previously described. The ability to use a standard audiometric headphone precludes the purchase of the stimulus delivery system module required by the Axonics-3M.[96]

Recording Variables

Filter bandwidth and averager sweeptime are the only other significant methodological differences, other than the recording electrode, between ABR and ECoG. ECoG recordings have traditionally been

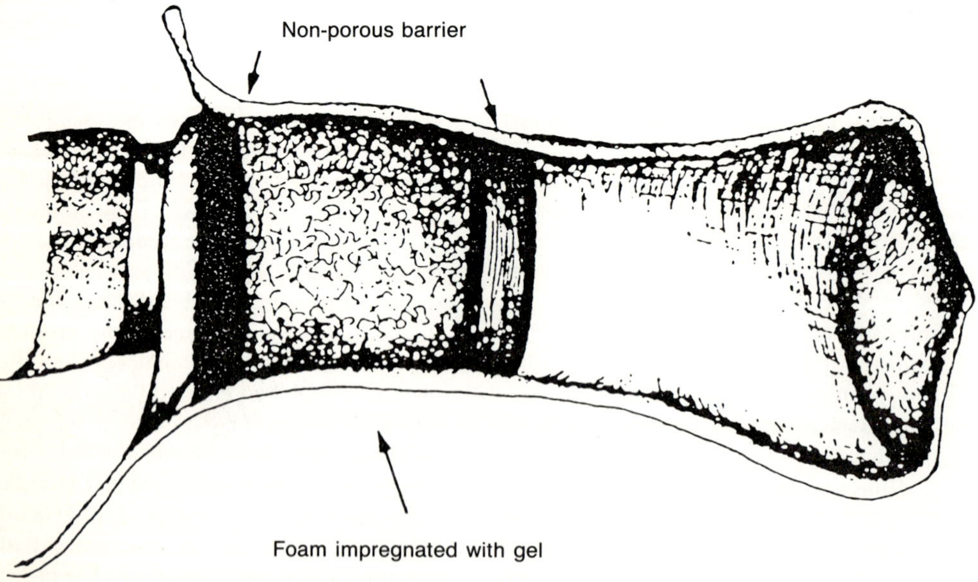

Figure 42–10 Schematic of Axonics-3M ear canal electrode in place. (Reprinted with permission from Ferraro J, Ruth R. Clinical electrocochleography. Hear J 1985; 38:51.)

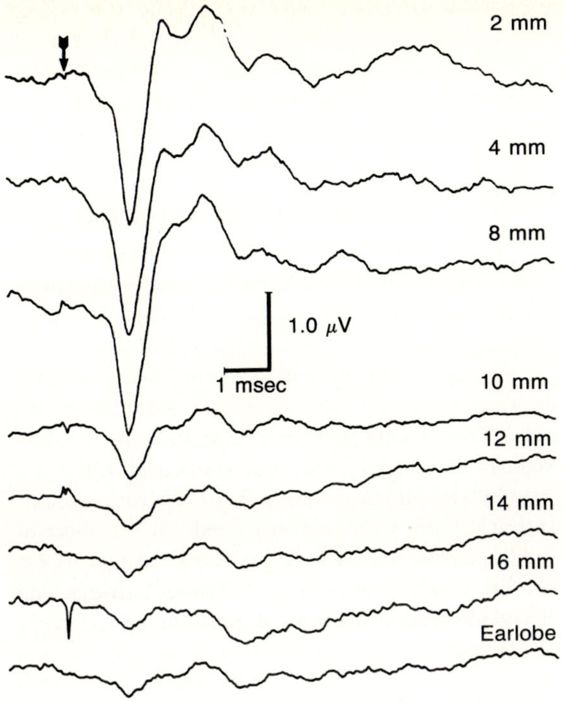

Figure 42–11 Extratympanic ECoG recordings taken from progressively increasing distances from the tympanic membrane. Note significant reduction in amplitude between 8 and 10 mm. The arrow indicates stimulus onset. (Reprinted with permission from Staller S. Electrocochleography in the diagnosis and management of Meniere's disease. Semin Hear 1986; 7:267.)

made with lower high-pass filter cutoffs to accomodate the DC nature of the SP. However, in response to transient clicks, the SP is also transient, with primarily high-frequency spectral energy. As such, AC amplifiers with bandwidths of 10 Hz to 3 kHz adequately process the response.

The response analysis, or "sweeptime," is also modified in many clinical ECoG protocols. The sweeptime may be reduced to 5 msec to provide greater resolution of the short latency responses, and the average sweeptime may begin prior to the onset of the stimulus, thus serving as a prestimulus baseline that may be used in the measurement of the SP and the AP amplitudes.[95] Other minor variations in the recording parameters include an increase in the number of averages recorded, depending on the amount of muscle or of electrical artifact. Stimulus rates typically vary from approximately eight to eleven per second. Occasionally, an extremely fast rate (> 100 per second) may be used to assess adaptation of the AP.[95] This techinque will be described in more detail in the following section. Like the ABR, the ECoG is elicited with a short duration, broad band click stimulus. Tonal stimuli, which may provide valuable diagnostic information, have largely been ignored with extratympanic techniques.

Response Characteristics

Recordings of the CM from the external auditory canal primarily reflect activity from the basal turn of the cochlea. Research to date has failed to show that the CM is sensitive to pathophysiologic changes in the cochlea, and because the CM is phase dependant, the use of alternating polarity stimuli cancels the response.

The AP appears as a sharp negative spike that occurs at approximately 1.5 msec poststimulus onset when generated with a high-intensity stimulus. The amplitude of the AP is affected by several factors, including (1) the magnitude and the type of hearing loss, (2) the integrity of the hair cell population in the cochlea, (3) the electrode placement, and (4) the impedance. In normal hearing ears, the amplitude of the AP increases slowly as the stimulus is raised from near threshold to moderate levels, then increases quickly as the stimulus is raised to high-intensity levels.[97] This steeply sloping portion of the AP amplitude-intensity function can be reduced or eliminated, depending on the magnitude, the slope, and the type of hearing loss.

The SP appears as a negative shoulder on the leading edge of the AP when recorded from the ear canal and elicited by a short duration broad band click. Absolute amplitude of the SP has been shown to be an extremely variable measure that reflects both physiologic and nonphysiologic variables.[96,98] SP amplitude decreases as a function of intensity, but since it is a receptor potential, SP amplitude does not demonstrate a refractory period and is, therefore, unaffected by stimulus rate increases.[99] Eggermont, in an attempt to reduce the inherent variability of the SP, proposed that SP amplitude be measured in proportion to the AP amplitude, as an SP-AP ratio.[100] Most clinical investigators have accepted this method of measurement and have reported that SP amplitude covaries as a function of AP amplitude.[90,95,98,101]

The method of measurement of the SP:AP amplitude ratio has varied among investigators (Fig. 42–12). The SP amplitude is determined by a measure from the prestimulus baseline to the most negative point of the SP prior to the AP following the stimulus. In an effort to reduce the affect of the AP on the SP amplitude, an alternative test technique has been proposed, based on the differential effects of rate on the SP as compared to the AP. Increased rate decreases the amplitude of the AP owing to normal neural adaptation, while the SP remains unaffected. Therefore, an average of the high rate and the low rate responses should reduce the influence of the AP on the SP amplitude.[95,102] Debate over the measurement of the AP has stemmed from ques-

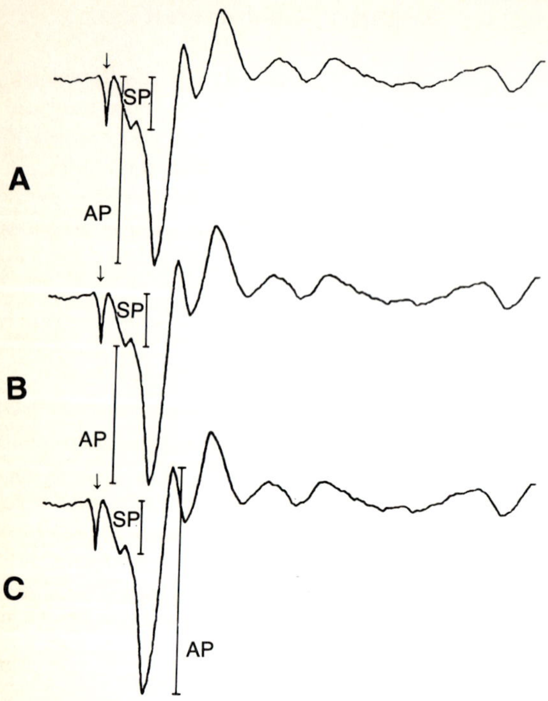

Figure 42–12 Differing methods of measurement of the SP-AP amplitude ratio. *A*, AP measured from the prestimulus baseline to the negative peak. *B*, AP measured from the base of the SP to the negative peak. *C*, AP measured from the negative peak to the positive trough between the AP and Wave II of the ABR.

tions of whether the amplitude of the AP measured from the prestimulus baseline is actually the sum of both the SP and the AP. Alternative methods have been proposed, including measurement from the base of the SP to the negative peak of the AP or from the positive trough between the AP and Wave II of the ABR to the negative peak of the AP. The most common method currently being used is the measurement of both the SP and the AP amplitudes from the prestimulus baseline.

ECoG IN MENIERE'S DISEASE

The major clinical application of ECoG is the diagnosis of Meniere's disease, a condition characterized by the presense of a quadrad of symptoms: (1) fluctuant hearing loss, (2) tinnitus, (3) aural pressure or fullness, and (4) episodic attacks of vertigo. This disease was first described by Prosper Meniere in 1861,[103] and was confirmed histologically by Hallpike and Cairns in 1938 with the demonstration of endolymphatic hydrops.[104] Electrocochleographic studies have correlated changes in the SP with a variety of indices of Meniere's disease and of endolymphatic hydrops. Significant SP:AP ratio enlargements have been reported in between 57 and 68 percent of patients with classic Meniere's disease[90,98,101,105,106,107] (Fig. 42–13). Abnormality of the SP-AP complex has been investigated using measures of both duration and amplitude. Recent studies, however, have failed to find duration to be a sensitive pathophysiologic index to hydrops, while amplitude is highly correlated.[98,101] Abnormal enlargement of the SP amplitude relative to the AP amplitude has been cited as a ratio of greater than 50 percent by some investigators, while others have reported that abnormal enlargement of the ratio varies as a function of AP amplitude[90,101] (Fig. 42–14).

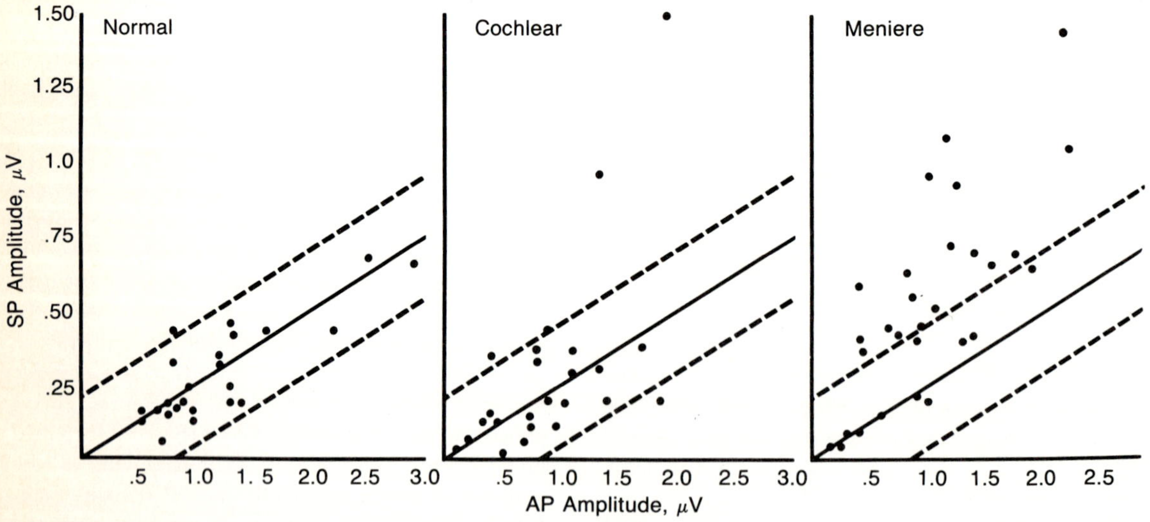

Figure 42–13 Scatter plot of SP versus AP amplitude from the otologically normal group, sensory hearing loss (non-Meniere's) subjects and the Meniere's group. Note 62 percent of the Meniere's group demonstrated significant enlargement ($p = 0.05$) of the SP-AP amplitude ratio. (Reprinted with permission from Goin D, Staller S, Asher D, Mischke R. Summating potential in Meniere's disease. Laryngoscope 1982; 92:1383.)

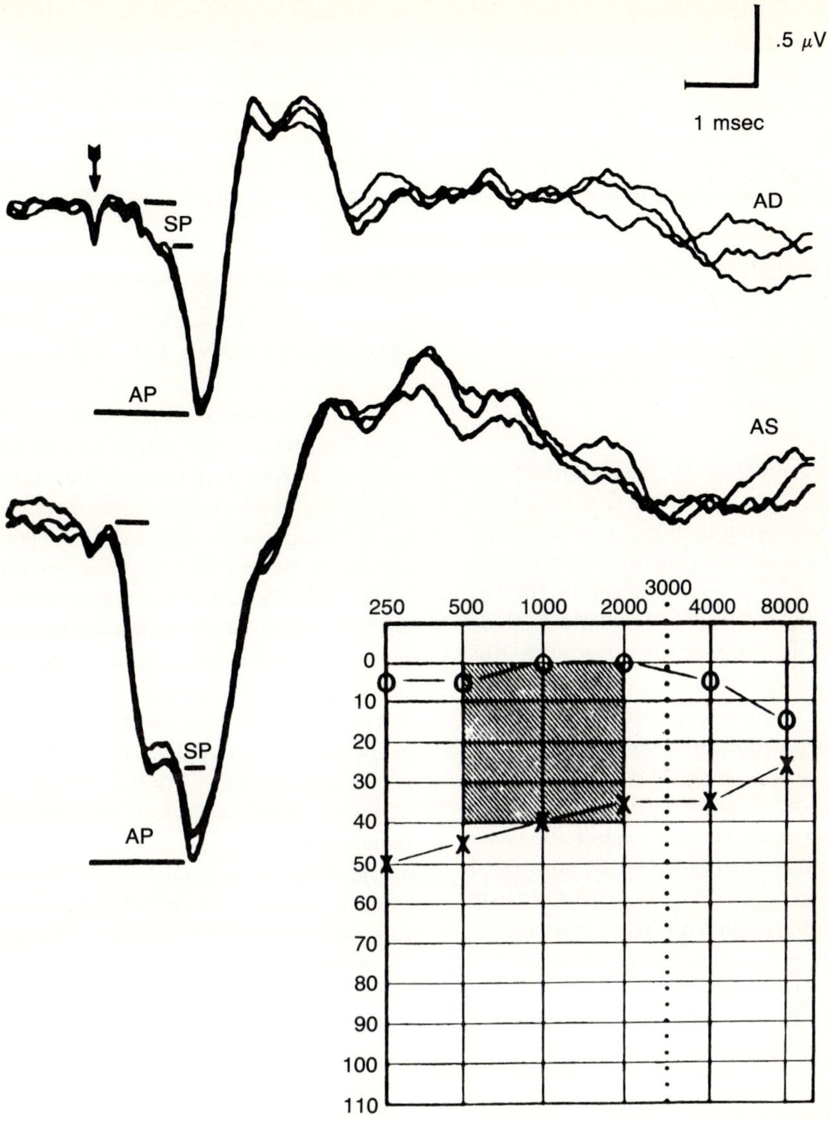

Figure 42–14 ECoG recordings from a patient with classic Meniere's disease in the left ear (As). Note significant enlargement of the SP-AP amplitude ratio in the involved ear.

The strength of the relationship between SP enlargement and Meniere's disease is increased by data suggesting that patients who are actively symptomatic at the time of the test are more likely to show abnormal amplitude ratios than patients who are not currently experiencing symptoms. The presense of hearing loss and of aural pressure is highly correlated with SP-AP enlargement.[108] Meniere's patients with hearing loss in the higher frequencies have also been found to have a higher incidence of positive ECoG test results.[109,110,111]

Another link between ECoG changes and Meniere's disease is the influence of glycerol. The effect of glycerol dehydration in patients with Meniere's disease has been well documented in the literature. Hearing thresholds improve as the osmolality gradient between serum and endolymph causes fluid to be withdrawn from the inner ear. Significant reductions in the SP have also been demonstrated following glyceral dehydration in 55 to 69 percent of Meniere's patients.[99,102,112,113] In addition, the glycerol test has been shown to agree with ECoG test results in 67 percent of patients with Meniere's disease.[101]

Changes in the SP of patients with Meniere's disease have been presumed to occur as a result of a shift in the basilar membrane caused by increased endolymphatic fluid pressure and/or volume.[114] However, these changes may result from some other aspect of Meniere's disease, such as biochemical abnormalities, endocochlear potential change, or altered circulation to the stria vascularis.

In an attempt to elucidate the mechanism of

SP changes, animal models have been developed. SP changes have been documented in guinea pigs with endolymphatic hydrops induced by obliterating the endolymphatic sac and by obstructing the endolymphatic duct.[101,105,115,116] Although these changes have consistently correlated with the presence of endolymphatic hydrops, several cases of minimal hydrops have resulted in rather striking SP changes.[105] This finding may suggest that SP changes may not exclusively reflect the influence of hydrops.

Surgical Management of Meniere's Disease

Surgical management of Meniere's Disease has been predicated on the assumption that endolymphatic pressure relief during hydropic attacks should relieve the otologic symptoms of Meniere's. Placement of a tube, valve, or silastic sheet in the endolymphatic sac with drainage to the mastoid or the subarachnoid space is designed to accomplish this relief. Several investigators have attempted to use ECoG as a means of improving patient selection and of prognosticating postoperative outcome. Postoperative, as well as intraoperative, ECoG changes have also been evaluated in an attempt to document the physiologic effects of shunt surgery. Significant short-term reductions in the SP have been demonstrated following shunt surgery.[101,111,117] These changes have correlated well with symptomatic relief and suggest a physiologic basis for postoperative improvement. Data on a limited number of patients has also suggested that patients with abnormal preoperative ECoGs tend to have better postoperative results.[117]

Specificity of ECoG to Meniere's Disease

A critical factor in determining the effectiveness of ECoG is its specificity to Meniere's disease. Both sudden hearing loss and perilymphatic fistulas have demonstrated SP enlargement in some cases.[99,102] Preliminary results obtained in our laboratory have shown abnormal SP:AP amplitude ratios in some patients with surgically comfirmed fistulas and subsequent improvement of the SP amplitude with surgical repair. ECoG studies performed on guinea pigs with experimentally-induced perilymphatic fistulas have supported our clinical findings.[118] Although the relationship between sudden hearing losses and ECoG changes questions the specificity of the SP to hydromechanical defects, the case of perilymphatic fistula may manifest changes in cochlear mechanics which are quite similar to hydrops. Fistulas may create the same type of pressure imbalance through reduced perilymph volume that occurs in endolymphatic hydrops through increased endolymph volume. While the specificity of ECoG to Meniere's may be less than ideal, the mechanism of hydrops may provide the link to abnormalities seen with other pathologies. Clearly, further investigation into these areas is needed.

SPECIAL AND FUTURE APPLICATIONS OF ABR AND ECoG

Unique information provided by ABR and ECoG regarding the status of the peripheral and the central auditory system have secured their role in the clinical arena. Development of new applications continues to broaden this role and to support its cost effectiveness. Several directions that are currently being investigated include (1) intraoperative monitoring of posterior fossa surgical procedures (ABR), (2) assessment of performance with a hearing aid (ABR), (3) comparison of binaural with monaural responses in children with auditory processing disorders (Binaural Interaction ABR), and (4) evaluation of suspected perilymphatic fistulas (ECoG).

Both ABR and ECoG are well suited for integration into the diagnostic repertoire of the clinical audiologist in a variety of settings. In addition to their strength in providing diagnostic information to augment behavioral procedures, the sensitivity of ABR and ECoG to underlying processes should provide avenues to improve our understanding of the mechanisms of pathology that underlie hearing loss.

REFERENCES

1. Moller A, Jannetta P, Moller M. Neural generators of brainstem evoked potentials: results from human intracranial recordings. Ann Otol Rhinol Laryngol 1981; 90:591–596.
2. Hashimoto I, Ishiyama Y, Yoshimoto T, Nemoto S. Brainstem auditory-evoked potentials recorded directly from human brain-stem and thalamus. Brain 1981; 104:841-859.
3. McPherson D, Hirasugi Y, Starr A. Auditory brain stem potentials recorded at different scalp locations in neonates and adults. Ann Otol Rhinol Laryngol 1985; 94:236–243.
4. Buchwald J, Huang C. Far-field acoustic response: origins in the cat. Science 1975; 189:382–384.
5. Picton T, Stapells D, Campbell K. Auditory evoked potentials from the human cochlea and brainstem. J Otolaryngol (Suppl 9)1981; 10 :1–41.
6. Stockard J, Stockard J, Westmoreland B, Corfits J. Brainstem auditory-evoked responses. Normal variations as a function of stimulus and subject characteristics. Arch Neurol 1979; 36:823–831.
7. Stockard J, Stockard J, Sharbrough F. Nonpathologic factors influencing brainstem auditory evoked potentials. Am J EEG Tech 1978; 18:177–209.

8. Elberling C. Auditory electrophysiology: Spectral analysis of cochlear and brainstem evoked potentials. Scand Audiol 1979; 8:57–64.
9. Boston J, Ainslie P. Effects of analog and digital filtering on brain stem auditory evoked potentials. Electroencephalogr Clin Neurophysiol 1980; 48:361–364.
10. Moller A. A digital filter for brain stem evoked responses. Am J Otolaryngol 1980; 1(5):372–377.
11. Jerger J, Mauldin L. Prediction of sensorineural hearing level from the brainstem evoked response. Arch Otolaryngol 1978; 104:456–461.
12. Worthington D, Peters J. Electrophysiologic audiometry. Ann Otol Rhinol Laryngol 1980; 74:59–62.
13. Pratt H, Sohmer H. Intensity and rate functions of cochlear and brainstem evoked responses to click stimulation in man. Arch Otorhinolaryngol 1976; 212:85–92.
14. Hecox K, Galambos R. Brainstem auditory evoked responses in human infants and adults. Arch Otolaryngol 1974; 99:30–33.
15. Coats A, Martin J. Human auditory nerve action potentials and brain stem evoked responses. Effects of audiogram shape and lesion location. Arch Otolaryngol 1977; 103:605–622.
16. Teas D, Eldridge D, Davis H. Cochlear responses to acoustic transients and interpretation of the whole nerve action potentials. J Acoust Soc Am 1962; 34:1438–1459.
17. Eggermont J. Electrocochleography. In: Keidel W, Neff W, eds. Handbook of sensory physiology. Vol. 3. Auditory system. Clinical & special topics. Heidelberg: Springer-Verlag, 1976.
18. Don M, Allen A, Starr A. Effect of click rate on the latency of auditory brain stem responses in humans. Ann Otol Rhinol Laryngol 1977; 86:186–196.
19. Fowler C, Noffsinger D. Effects of stimulus repetition rate and frequency on the auditory brainstem response in normal, cochlear-impaired, and 8th nerve/brainstem-impaired subjects. J Speech Hear Res 1983; 26:560–567.
20. Hecox K, Cone B, Blaw M. Brainstem auditory evoked response in the diagnosis of pediatric neurological diseases. Neurology 1981; 31:832–839.
21. Weber B, Fujikawa S. Brainstem evoked response (BER) audiometry at various stimulus presentation rates. J Am Audiol Soc 1977; 3:59–62.
22. Maurer K, Schafer E, Leitner H. The effects of varying stimulus polarity (rarefaction vs. condensation) on early auditory evoked potentials (EAEP's). Electroencephalogr Clin Neurophysiol 1980; 50:332–334.
23. Emerson R, Brooks E, Parker S, Chiappa K. Effects of click polarity on brainstem auditory evoked potentials in normal subjects and patients: Unexpected sensitivity of Wave V. Ann NY Acad Sci 1982; 388:710–721.
24. McGee T, Clemis J. The approximation of audiometric thresholds by auditory brain stem responses. Otolaryngol Head Neck Surg 1980; 88(3):295–303.
25. Stapells D, Picton T. Technical aspects of brainstem evoked audiometry using tones. Ear Hear 1981; 2:20–29.
26. Kileny P. The frequency specificity of tone-pip evoked auditory brain stem responses. Ear Hear 1981; 2(6):270–275.
27. Folsom R. Frequency specificity of human auditory brainstem responses as revealed by pure-tone masking profiles. J Acoust Soc Am 1984; 75:919–924.
28. Gorga M, Worthington D. Some issues relevant to the measurement of frequency-specific auditory brainstem responses. Semin Hear 1983; 4:353–362.
29. Wightman F. Detection of binaural tones as a function of masker bandwidth. J Acoust Soc Am 1971; 50:623–636.
30. Picton T, Ouelette J, Hamel G, Smith A. Brainstem evoked potentials to tonepips in notched noise. J Otolaryngol 1979; 8:289–314.
31. Don M, Eggermont J. Analysis of the click-evoked brainstem potentials in man using high-pass noise masking. J Acoust Soc Am 1978; 63:1084–1092.
32. Salamy A, McKean C. Postnatal development of the human brainstem potentials during the first year of life. Electroencephalogr Clin Neurophysiol 1976; 40:418–426.
33. Stockard J, Stockard J. Brainstem auditory evoked potentials in normal and otoneurologically impaired newborns and infants. In: Henry C, ed. Current clinical neurophysiology update on EEG and evoked potentials. New York: Elsevier North, 1980.
34. Salamy A, Mendelson T, Tooley W. Developmental profiles for the brainstem auditory evoked potential. Early Hum Dev 1982; 6:331–339.
35. Starr A, Amalie R, Martin KW, Sanders S. Development of auditory function in newborn infants revealed by auditory brainstem potentials. Pediatrics 1977; 60:831–839.
36. Schulman-Galambos C, Galambos R. Brain stem auditory-evoked responses in premature infants. J Speech Hear Res 1975; 18:456–465.
37. Rowe M. Normal variability of the brainstem auditory evoked response in young and old adult subjects. Electroencephalogr Clin Neurophysiol 1978; 44:459–470.
38. Thomsen J, Terkildsen K, Osterhammel P. Auditory brainstem responses in patients with acoustic neuromas. Scand Audiol 1978; 7:179–183.
39. Jerger J, Hall J. Effects of age and sex on the auditory brainstem response. Arch Otolaryngol 1980; 106:382–391.
40. Rosenhamer H, Lindstrom B, Lundborg T. On the use of click-evoked electric brainstem responses in audiological diagnosis. II. The influence of sex and age upon the normal response. Scand Audiol 1980; 9(2):93–100.
41. Beagley H, Sheldrake J. Differences in brain stem response latency with age and sex. Br J Audiol 1978; 12:69–77.
42. Stockard J, Rossiter V. Clinical and pathologic correlates of brain stem auditory response abnormalities. Neurology 1977; 27:316–325.
43. Stockard J, Sharbrough F. Unique contributions of short-latency auditory and somatosensory evoked potentials to neurologic diagnosis. Prog Clin Neurophysiol 1980; 7:231–263.
44. Rosenhamer H. The auditory evoked brainstem electric response (ABR) in cochlear hearing loss. Scand Audiol 1981; Suppl 13:83–93.
45. Schwartz D, Olsen K, Berry G, Murray B. Auditory evoked potentials in severe head injury. Paper presented at the Annual Convention of the American Speech-Language-Hearing Association. Cincinatti, OH, November, 1981.
46. Adams D, Watson D, McClelland R. The effects of diazepam on the auditory evoked brainstem potentials. Presented at the Second International Symposium on Evoked Potentials. Cleveland, OH, October, 1982.
47. Bobbin R, May J, Lemoine R. Effects of pentobarbital and ketamine on brain stem auditory potentials. Arch Otolaryngol 1979; 105:467–470.
48. Bhargava V, Salamy A, McKean C. Effect of cholinergic drugs on the brainstem auditory evoked response (far-field) in rats. Neuroscience 1978; 3:821–826.
49. Finitzo-Hieber T, Hecox K, Cone B. Brainstem auditory evoked potentials in patients with congenital atresia. Laryngoscope 1979: 89:1151–1158.
50. Fria T, Sabo D. Auditory brainstem responses in children with otitis media with effusion. Ann Otol Rhinol Laryngol 1980; 68:200–206.
51. Clemis J, Ballad W, Killion M. Clinical use of an insert earphone. Ann Otol Rhinol Laryngol 1986; 95:520–524.
52. Hooks JR, Weber B. Auditory brain stem responses to bone conduction stimuli in premature neonates: a feasibility study. Ear Hear 1984; 5:42–46.
53. Mauldin L, Jerger J. Auditory brain stem evoked responses to bone-conducted signals. Arch Otolaryngol 1979; 105:656–661.
54. Coats A. Human auditory nerve action potentials and brain stem evoked responses. Latency-intensity functions in detec-

tion of cochlear and retrocochlear abnormality. Arch Otolaryngol 1978; 104:709–717.

55. Yamada O, Kodera K, Yagi T. Cochlear processes affecting Wave V latency of the auditory evoked brainstem response: A study of patients with sensory hearing loss. Scand Audiol 1979; 8:67–70.
56. Musiek F, Kibbe K, Rackliffe L, Weider R. The ABR I-V amplitude ratio in normal, cochlear and retrocochlear ears. Ear Hear 1984; 5:52–55.
57. Musiek F. ABR in eighth nerve and brainstem disorders. Am J Otol 1982; 3:243–248.
58. Gerling I, Finitzo-Hieber T. Auditory brainstem response with high stimulus rates in normal and hearing impaired patient populations. Ann Otol Rhinol Laryngol 1983; 92:119–123.
59. Selters W, Brackmann D. Acoustic tumor detection with brainstem electric response audiometry. Arch Otolaryngol 1977; 103:181–187.
60. Bauch C, Rose D, Harner KKS. Brainstem responses to tone-pip and click stimuli. Ear Hear 1980; 1:181–184.
61. Clemis J, McGee T. Brainstem electric response audiometry and the differential diagnosis of acoustic tumors. Laryngoscope 1979; 89:31–42.
62. Josey A, Jackson C, Glasscock M. Brainstem evoked response audiometry in confirmed eighth nerve tumors. Am J Otolaryngol 1980; 1(4):285–290.
63. Eggermont J, Don M, Brackmann D. Electrocochleography and auditory brainstem electric responses in patients with pontine angle tumors. Ann Otol Rhinol Laryngol 1980; 89 (Suppl 75):1–19.
64. Staller S, Lunde L, Ernst T, Goin D, Mischke R. ABR in patients with von-Recklinghausen's disease. Paper presented at the annual convention of the American Speech-Language-Hearing Association. Detroit, MI, November, 1986.
65. Starr A, Hamilton A. Correlation between confirmed sites of neurological lesions and abnormalities of far-field auditory brainstem responses. Electroencephalogr Clin Neurophysiol 1976; 41:595–608.
66. Chiappa K, Harrison J, Brooks E, Young R. Brainstem auditory evoked responses in 200 patients with multiple sclerosis. Ann Neurol 1980; 7:135–143.
67. Brown R, Chiappa K, Brooks E. Brainstem auditory evoked responses in 22 patients with intrinsic brainstem lesions: implications for clinical interpretations. Electroencephalogr Clin Neurophysiol 1981; 51:38.
68. Epstein C, Stappenbeck R, Karp H. Brainstem auditory evoked responses in palatal myoclonus. Ann Neurol 1980; 7:592–596.
69. Robinson K, Rudge P. The use of the auditory evoked potential in the diagnosis of multiple sclerosis. J Neurol Sci 1980; 45:235–244.
70. Green J, Price R, Woodbury S. Short-latency somatosensory evoked potentials in multiple sclerosis. Comparison with auditory and visual evoked potentials. Arch Neurol 1980; 37:630–633.
71. Chiappa K. Evoked potentials in clinical medicine. New York: Raven Press, 1983.
72. Purves S, Low M, Galloway J, Reeves B. A comparison of visual, brainstem auditory, and somatosensory evoked potentials in multiple sclerosis. Can J Neurol Sci 1981; 8:15–19.
73. Hashimoto I, Ishiyama Y, Tozuka G. Bilaterally recorded brain stem auditory evoked responses. Their asymmetric abnormalities and lesions of the brain stem. Arch Neurol 1979; 36:161–167.
74. Green J, McLeod S. Short latency somatosensory evoked potentials in patients with neurological lesions. Arch Neurol 1979; 36:846–851.
75. Mjoen S, Nordby H, Torvik A. Auditory evoked brainstem responses (ABR) in coma due to severe head trauma. Acta Otolaryngol 1983; 95:131–138.
76. Sanders R, Smriga D, McCullough D, Duncan P. Auditory brainstem responses in patients with global cerebral insults. J Otolaryngol 1981; 10:52–58.
77. Greenberg R, Newlon P, Hyatt M, Harayan R, Becker D. Prognostic implication of early multimodality evoked potentials in severely head-injured patients. A prospective study. J Neurosurg 1981; 55:227–236.
78. Galambos R. Use of the auditory brainstem response (ABR) in infant hearing testing. In: Gerber S, Mencher G, eds. Early diagnosis of hearing loss. New York: Grune & Stratton, 1978.
79. Stein L. ABR screening and follow-up results with NICU infants. Presented at the 18th Annual Colorado/Audiology Workshop, Aspen, CO, March, 1984.
80. Roberts J, Davis H, Phon G, Reichert T, Sturtevant E, Marshall R. Auditory brainstem responses in pre-term neonates: maturation and follow-up. J Pediatr 1982; 101:257–263.
81. Hecox K, Cone B. Prognostic importance of brainstem auditory evoked responses after asphyxia. Neurology 1981; 31:1429–1433.
82. Kaga K, Kitazumi E, Kodama K. Auditory brain stem responses of kernicterus infants. Int J Pediatr Otorhinolaryngol 1979; 1:255–264.
83. Ozdamar O, Kraus N, Stein L. Auditory brainstem responses in infants recovering from bacterial meningitis. Arch Otolaryngol 1983; 109:13–18.
84. Nodar R, Hahn J, Levine H. Brain stem auditory evoked potentials in determining site of lesion of brain stem gliomas in children. Laryngoscope 1980; 90:258–266.
85. Davis H, Hirsh S. The audiometric utility of the brain stem response to low-frequency sounds. Audiology 1976; 15:151–195.
86. Dallos P. The auditory periphery: Biophysics and physiology. New York, NY: Academic Press, 1973.
87. Berlin C. Electrocochleography: an historic overview. Semin Hear 1986; 7:241–246.
88. Cullen J, Ellis M, Berlin C, Lousteau R. Human acoustic nerve action potential recordings from the tympanic membrane without anesthesia. Acta Otolaryngol 1972; 74:15–22.
89. Berlin C, Cullen J, Ellis M, Lousteau R, Yarbrough W, Lyons G. Clinical application of recording human 8th nerve action potentials from the tympanic membrane. Trans Am Acad Opthalmol Otolaryngol 1974; 78:401–410.
90. Coats A. The summating potential and Meniere's disease: summating potential amplitude in Meniere and non-Meniere ears. Arch Otolaryngol 1981; 107:199–208.
91. Stypulkowski P, Staller S. Clinical evaluation of a new ECoG recording electrode. Ear Hear 1987; 8(4):(in press).
92. Kanzaki J, Ouchi T, Yokobori H, Ino T. Electrocochleographic study of summating potentials in Meniere's disease. Audiology 1982; 21:409–424.
93. Staller S. Electrocochleography in the diagnosis and management of Meniere's disease. Semin Hear 1986; 7:267–277.
94. Ferraro J, Murphy G, Ruth R. A comparative study of primary electrodes used in extra-tympanic electrocochleography. Semin Hear 1986; 7:279–287.
95. Coats A. The normal summating potential recorded from the external ear canal. Arch Otolaryngol Head Neck Surg 1986; 112:759–768.
95a. Coats A. Electrocochleography: recording techniques and clinical applications. Semin Hear 1986; 7:247–266.
96. Whitaker S. Sequential electrocochleography and auditory dehydration testing in patients with Meniere's disease. Semin Hear 1986; 7:329–337.
97. Yoshie N. Diagnostic significance of the electrocochleogram in clinical audiometry. Audiol 1973; 12:504–539.
98. Gibson W, Prasher D, Kilkenny G. Diagnostic significance

of trans-tympanic electrocochleography in Meniere's disease. Ann Otol Rhinol Laryngol 1983; 92:155–159.

99. Morrison A, Moffat D, O'Connor A. Cliical usefulness of electrocochleography in Meniere's disease: An analysis of dehydrating agents. Otolaryngol Clin North Am 1980; 13:703–721.
100. Eggermont J. Summating potentials in electrocochleography: relation to hearing disorders. In: Rubin R, Elberling C, Salomon G, eds. Electrocochleography. Baltimore, MD: University Park Press, 1976:67.
101. Goin D, Staller S, Asher D, Mischke R. Summating potential in Meniere's disease. Laryngoscope 1982; 92:1383–1389.
102. Moffat D, Gibson W, Ramsden R, Morrison A, Booth J. Trans-tympanic electrocochleography during glycerol dehydration. Acta Otolaryngol 1978; 85:158–166.
103. Meniere P. Mémoire sur des lésions de l'oreille interne domnant lieu a des symptomes de congestion cérébrale apoplectiform. Gaz Med Paris 1861; 16:597–601.
104. Hallpike C, Cairns H. Observations on the pathology of Meniere's syndrome. J Laryngol Otol 1938; 53:625–665.
105. Kumagami H, Nishida H, Mariuchi H. Changes of the action potential, summating potential and cochlear microphonic in experimental endolymphatic hydrops. ORL 1981; 43:314–327.
106. Ferraro J, Best L, Arenberg I. The use of electrocochleography in the diagnosis, assessment and monitoring of endolymphatic hydrops. Otolaryngol Clin North Am 1983; 16:69–82.
107. Chatrian G, Wirch A, Edwards K, Turella G, Kaufman M, Snyder J. Cochlear summating potential to broadband clicks detected from the human external auditory meatus: a study of subjects with normal hearing. Ear Hear 1985; 6:130–138.
108. Ferraro J, Arenberg I, Hassanein R. Electrocochleography and symptoms of inner ear dysfunction. Arch Otolaryngol 1985; 111:71–74.
109. Kumagami H, Nishida H, Baba M. Electrocochleographic study of Meniere's disease. Arch Otolaryngol 1982; 108:284–288.
110. Gibson W, Prasher D. Electrocochleography and its role in the diagnosis and understanding of Meniere's disease. Otolaryngol Clin North Am 1983; 16:59–68.
111. Coats A, Jenkins H, Monroe B. Auditory evoked potentials: The cochlear summating potential in detection of endolymphatic hydrops. Am J Otolaryngol 1984; 5:443–446.
112. Coats A, Alford B. Meniere's disease and the summating potential. III: The effects of glycerol dehydration. Arch Otolaryngol 1981; 107:469–473.
113. Dauman R, Aran J, Portmann M. Summating potential and water balance in Meniere's disease. Ann Otol Rhinol Laryngol 1986; 95:389–395.
114. Durrant J, Dallos P. Modification of DIF summating potential components by stimulus biasing. J Acoust Soc Am 1974; 56:562–570.
115. Kitahara M, Takeda T, Yazawa Y, Matsubara H, Kitano H. Experimental study on Meniere's disease. Otolaryngol Head Neck Surg 1982; 90:470–481.
116. Kimura R. Experimental blockage of the endolymphatic duct and sac and its effect on the inner ear of the guinea pig. Ann Otol Rhinol Laryngol 1967; 76:664–687.
117. Gibson W, Moffat D, Ramsden R. Clinical electrocochleography in the diagnosis and management of Meniere's disease. Audiology 1977; 16:389–401.
118. Ackley S. Electrocochleographic and histopathological observation of experimental perilymphatic fistula in guinea pigs. Doctoral Dissertation, University of Colorado, 1985. orado, 1985.

43 Early Identification of Hearing Loss

Marion P. Downs, M.A., D.H.S.
Katherine Pike Gerkin, M.A.

THE NEED FOR EARLY IDENTIFICATION

How necessary is it to identify hearing losses at the earliest possible age? Various developmental theories have been proposed to answer that question: the empiricist theory, holding that the infant's mind is a blank slate on which is written that knowledge coming in from the senses; the rational-constructionist theory, claiming that a preexisting mental structure guides the selection of organized aspects of sensory experiences and that young children play an active role in seeking out the most helpful experiences; and the critical period theory, which postulates a preexisting language structure that must have optimal inputs at optimal times in order to develop to full potential. The latter two theories fit most closely the observable facts on development of hearing skills. The critical period theory, in particular, agrees most closely with what has been observed about hearing loss.

Are there such things as critical periods? If so, what are the discrete fundamental skills that precede speech, listening, and language and should be available at the proper time? These questions must be answered if clinicians are to know when it is essential to identify hearing loss.

Critical Period Theory

For a long time, only reports from anecdotal observations and animal research were available to buttress the critical period theory. The earliest recorded discussion concerned the wild boy of Aveyron in 1796, purportedly reared by wild animals until he was found by Dr. Itard.[1] Despite Itard's intensive attempts to teach him to speak, no intelligible language was ever elicited. Critical periods for learning speech and language had passed, if this historical report is to be credited.

A similar modern-day study has been reported concerning Genie, a child who was isolated in a closet for 11 years of her life.[2] When removed and given therapy, she responded well to speech and language training and has been cited as a "case of language acquisition beyond the critical period." However, in examining Genie's history, one finds that for the first 20 months of life she was exposed to the stimulation of family life like other children.

Genie's case thus actually demonstrates the importance of critical periods, showing that exposure in the first 2 years of life is indeed crucial to the effective acquisition of speech and language at any time later in life. A parallel example is the story of Helen Keller, who became deaf and blind at the age of 2 years after participation in a familial language environment of good quality during those 2 years. When the famous incident occurred in which tactile language was presented to her, she was able to tap into the store of basic language she had learned as an infant and rapidly recapture her childhood understanding through the new modality. Tactile language does not come as easily nor as effectively to the child born deaf and blind.

Often one hears of outstanding deaf individuals with an unusually high level of speech and language who are cited as examples of how well deaf people can achieve even if schooling is started later in childhood. When one examines carefully the case histories of these people, one often finds that normal hearing was, or could have been, present for the first year or two or three of life. A substrate of neurologic connections for speech and of conceptual connections for language has been laid down that facilitates the superior achievement.

The two areas where critical periods are most important are in cognitive competence and in auditory perception. Cognition, of course, is almost inseparable from language skills. Most tests of cognitive abilities involve language skills of some sort. And auditory perceiving is the avenue through which language has been learned in the course of evolution, although it is not the indispensable requisite, as is seen from the level of language that can be learned through manual signing and finger spelling.

CRITICAL PERIODS AND LANGUAGE LEARNING

The failure of Head Start programs to produce permanent gains in achievement has pointed up the importance of critical periods.[3,4] Guinagh and Jester noted the absence of long-term gains in intervention programs starting at age 3 years, showing that the only programs that have produced long-term treatment effects are those that focus on parents and start well before 3 years of age.[4] The reason for the failures, according to Hunt, is that the intervention has been too little and too late to overcome sufficiently the incompetence resulting from the first 3 or 4 years spent in disadvantaged homes.[5] Hunt calls this incompetance "a verbal analogue of disease," which could be wiped out by an early community intervention program analogous to smallpox inoculation.

Investigations on humans have attempted to pinpoint the crucial times when high-quality language must be available to the child if permanent deficits are to be avoided. McKay et al studied children from a low socioeconomic group to whom they applied a program of treatment beginning at 42 months and at older age periods.[6] The younger the children were when they entered the program, the greater was the effect of treatment. But despite intensive treatment, the gap did not close between the abilities of the experimental group and those of a control group of children from high socioeconomic levels. It was evident to the authors that "retardation is less amenable to modification with increasing age." Intervention at 42 months was shown to be too late to close the gap effectively.

In a study of adopted children, Dennis identified the age of 2 years as critical for exposure to good language stimulation. He compared children in a foundling home who were adopted at different ages.[7] The babies adopted from the home by 2 years of age eventually showed IQs 50 points higher than those adopted after 2 years of age. Dennis concluded that intervention should occur well before 2 years of age if it is to be successful.

The longitudinal study by Heber and Garber of ghetto children whose mothers had IQs in the 70s confirms the need for early intervention.[8] A previous long-term study had shown that such children had IQs of close to 100 at 2 years of age. But by the time they were 14 years old, their IQs had receded to scores in the 70s, similar to their mothers'. A language stimulation program beginning at birth with one group of these children resulted in mean IQs at 2 years of 127. A control group showed the usual 100 scores at 2 years of age, and by 4 years of age, these were tending to become even lower. But by 4 years of age, the intervention group's IQs were going upward, reaching a mean score of 130. No more telling report than this could be found on the value of early intervention to prevent the pseudoretardation of disadvantaged children. Other reports show that the slowing of development can be identified in such children by 11 to 13 months.[9,10]

The level of language development in hearing impaired children has been shown to relate directly to the age at which habilitation is begun. The Lexington School for the Deaf compared infants who had been admitted before 16 months of age with those admitted between 16 and 24 months.[11] At 40 months, the children admitted before 16 months had statistically higher scores in speech, language, and social interaction measures. Mother-infant communication was superior in the earlier admitted children—another factor that may have had an effect on the outcome. In any case, it was the early recognition of the hearing loss that permitted the optimal handling for better language skills.

ANIMAL STUDIES

Animals can be studied under more rigid control than can humans. Whenever investigations have been made using animal models, the results have shown that, as Hebb stated, "the organization of adult behavior is largely determined by the quality of infant experience and learning."[12] Hebb demonstrated that impaired early experience caused permanent changes in the structure of the central nervous system (CNS) in rats, primarily in the cerebral cortex.

Greenough further confirmed the neurologic deficits in rats that result from early experiential deprivation.[13] Rats that were reared in an environmentally complex condition showed more higher-order dendritic branching in all the CNS neurons examined than did rats reared in isolation. Similar results appear in trained versus untrained animals.

In the area of vision, Reisen showed that a chimpanzee raised in darkness for his or her first 3 months never acquired adequate vision.[14,15] But if chimpanzees are reared normally for 3 months and then subjected to darkness for 6 months, they quickly regain perfect vision when exposed again to light.

CRITICAL PERIODS AND EARLY AUDITORY DEPRIVATION

The research on early experiential deprivation has been distinct from that on early auditory deprivation. Yet the two are analogous, if not completely parallel. Language and its correlate, cognition, may be innate functions that are dependent on early experience, but the requisite experiences come largely through the sensory avenue of audition. In infancy, the auditory system is plastic and can be modified by variations in the reception of auditory stimuli.[16] Inadequate stimuli result in deviant development of the central auditory nervous pathways because the cortical afferent and peripheral efferent systems exert reciprocal control over each other. The central auditory system cannot develop fully unless it receives input from the inner ear. Researchers have shown that reduced auditory input results in central deficits in animals and most probably in humans. The resultant reduction in language and cognitive skills can also be termed a "central deficit." In the realm of the severely and profoundly deaf, the Lexington School report cited previously showed the benefit of early identification of deafness.

The improved speech and language skills of the earlier-identified group in the Lexington study may be due to the fact that language stimulation was available during critical periods or that a more optimal climate for learning was created by better mother-infant relationships. Either way, the necessary condition is early identification and training. The goal is to improve the low language levels of students in schools for the deaf and of those reported as equivalent to grade 4.3 at the very best.[17]

The language problems of the deaf are highlighted by Templin's studies comparing the language skills of the deaf with the skills of matched groups of normals.[18] In some areas, such as understanding of word meanings, sentence construction, and analogies, the deaf showed no systematic improvement beyond 11 years of age. The normals continued to improve their language skills up to the age of 14, which was the upper limit of the study. The deficits of the deaf reflect the fact that hardly any deafness was identified and habilitated before 2 or 3 years during the time period represented in the study.[19]

An explanation for the deficits has been undertaken by Menyuk, who points out that by 40 days of life infants can differentiate phonemic and intonation changes.[20] Therefore she says,

> the infant seems sensitive to certain acoustic, or speech parameters that will later play a crucial role in his comprehension and production of speech. Such aspects not only play a role in speech sound acquisition but also in grammar acquisition, since voice is used to mark number and tense differentially.

Intonation also plays an important role in language acquisition. In the babbling stage, around 3 to 4 months, she says, "the infant is sorting out the acoustic data in terms of speech production categories, later to be mapped into word production. These categorizations may be crucially important for later language development." Therefore "the term 'early' in early detection turns out to be early indeed."

The most telling evidence of the degree of language retardation caused by auditory deprivation during the first year is the economic record of the deaf population. Schein and Delk point out that those who were deaf at birth earn 18 percent less per year than those who became deaf at 6 years of age.[21] These differences may not seem immense, but when multiplied by the numbers involved they represent close to 2 billion dollars per year in manpower earnings lost to society. If identification of deafness could be made at birth and early language input given that would raise the language level of the congenitally deaf, some or all of those billions per year could be saved.

Severe or profound congenital hearing losses are not the only kind of deprivations causing problems. In recent years, a great many reports have appeared showing that mild conductive hearing losses, if incurred during the first 2 years of life, also result in some degree of language deficiency.

These reports are summarized in a comprehensive overview of the subject sponsored by the National Institute of Child Health and Development.[22] The consensus was that recurrent otitis media with effusion represents a hazard to the cognitive development of young children. The identification of children who are at risk for such delayed development forms an entirely new category of identification and will be handled separately.

In addition to mild conductive losses, another type of loss previously considered innocuous has now been shown to handicap children significantly—the unilateral hearing loss. A loss in one ear can no longer be overlooked by educators since a large study showed that many children suffer educational handicaps as a result of a hearing loss in one ear, even when the other ear is perfectly normal.[23] Bess and his associates studied 60 children 6 to 13 years old who had normal hearing in one ear, but sensorineural hearing losses of over 45 dB in the other ear. Although all of them had been given preferential seating in the classroom, 35 percent of them had failed one or more grades in school, and another 13 percent were in need of special resource assistance—a total of almost 50 percent with educational problems.

From animal studies, apparently any degree of hearing loss that is incurred during early life causes irreversible central auditory pathway effects. Webster and Webster have shown analogous CNS correlates due to auditory deprivation and have further pinpointed periods that are critical to adequate function.[24,25]

Webster and Webster first gave a group of mice conductive hearing losses for the first 45 days of their lives, then sacrificed them and examined their auditory nervous systems. A control group of normal mice were also examined at 45 days. The results showed that the mice with conductive loss had significant deficits in their auditory pathways as compared with the controls; the statistically significant results are as follows:

1. Smaller globular cells in the central cochlear nucleus and the smaller neurons in the medial nucleus of the trapezoid body.
2. Fewer neurons in the dorsal cochlear nucleus.

One question remained for these researchers—to determine whether or not the central deficiencies could be restituted if hearing was restored after 45 days. Accordingly, Webster and Webster repeated the experiment, but this time they restored the hearing of the experimental mice at 45 days and allowed them to live for another 45 days in normal environments. Upon sacrificing both groups, they found that the central auditory deficits of the experimental group had not been restituted. Evidently, these central auditory connections depended on early stimulation for their development, and later exposure did not accomplish restitution. When the time period of restoring hearing was manipulated in a further study, they pinpointed the critical period as one corresponding to age 0 to 3 years in humans.[26] Parallel findings have been reported in the visual field by Brattgard,[27] Cragg,[28] and Guillery and Kaas.[29,30]

There seems to be little doubt that auditory and visual processing must develop while the brain is still plastic, and, if any sensory deprivation occurs at this time, permanent and irreversible deficits will occur in the processing of the acoustic or visual signals. Clearly, the success of any program of prevention of the effects of sensory deficits rests upon the identification of the problem before critical periods have passed. Habilitation can be completely successful only if it is begun before these crucial times pass by. Identification programs are thus the key to the prevention of speech and language deficits caused by hearing loss.

METHODS OF IDENTIFICATION

Hearing screening has proved to be one of the most acceptable screening procedures in a multitude of health detection programs. For all periods of life, hearing screening techniques have been standardized so that higher yields and greater validity are obtained than in most other health-related identification procedures. Furthermore, when one applies criteria for what should be considered an acceptable screening program, hearing screening emerges with the highest of ratings.

The comparison of yields from various newborn screening programs in Table 43–1 illustrates the relative status of hearing screening.[31] Not only does hearing screening yield the highest returns among these diseases, but it is also more productive of results once the problem is identified. Clinicians know that when phenylketonuria is identified, intervention may not completely alleviate the retardation. And if a child is falsely identified as having phenylketonuria and treated, serious harm can result. Only in maple syrup urine disease and in hearing problems are the results certainly advantageous and the treatment harmless if applied properly.

In every other way, hearing screening at any age in life meets all the criteria that public health experts require of a successful screening program.[32] These are

1. Occurrence frequent enough or consequence serious enough to warrant mass screening.
2. Amenability to treatment or prevention that forestalls or changes the expected outcome.
3. Availability of facilities for diagnosis and treatment.
4. Cost of screening reasonably commensurate with benefits to the individual.

TABLE 43–1 Yield in Screening Tests

Disease Screened	*Yield*
Phenylketonuria	one in 15,000 births
Combined immunodeficiency disease	25 in 3 million births
Maple syrup urine disease	one in 30,000 births
Neonatal hyperthyroidism	one in 6,000 births
Neonatal hearing screening	one in 750 births
High-risk register	one in 50 to 100 births

5. A screening tool that validly differentiates the disease from nondisease.

6. Acceptance by the public.

Hearing screening at every age level meets these criteria, as we will demonstrate. But it also meets specific goals—goals that are different at each age level. The discussion of the various age-specific screening procedures that follows considers all these aspects.[33]

Newborn Screening

The main goal in newborn screening is to identify all hearing losses that are present at birth so that training can be instituted that allows the hearing impaired child to attain his or her best potential functioning.

The search must begin in the newborn nursery. Several alternative procedures that accomplish identification in the newborn nursery have been approved by various national groups. Any of these, or any combination of them, is an acceptable approach to a newborn identification program.

The High-Risk Register

Public health specialists have stated that to be effective a high-risk register must have a prevalence of the condition 14 times greater than that found in the general population.[34] Some of the programs described herein have found a prevalence of hearing loss of one in 40, as compared with one in 700 in the general population, easily 14 times greater. Thus the yield makes it statistically an acceptable approach. A typical yield from a high-risk program is shown in Table 43–2. This report shows that 11 percent of the infant population was found on the simplified register that is recommended. The yield from the register was one in 100, which means that 100 babies had to be tested in order to find one with a hearing impairment.

The high-risk concept assumes that one can identify a small group of children whose history or physical condition identifies them as possessing a high chance of having the handicap searched for. In the case of hearing loss, a large number of factors have been associated with the handicap. However, studies have shown that the greatest number of hearing impaired children fall into seven categories. These seven categories have been recommended by a national Joint Committee of Infant Hearing.[35] The seven categories are

1. A family history of childhood hearing impairment.
2. Congenital perinatal infection (e.g., cytomegalovirus, rubella, herpes, toxoplasmosis, syphilis).
3. Anatomic malformations involving the head or neck (e.g., craniofacial syndromal abnormalities, overt or submucous cleft palate, morphologic abnormalities of the pinna).
4. Birthweight less than 1,500 g.
5. Hyperbilirubinemia at a level exceeding indications for exchange transfusion.
6. Bacterial meningitis, especially *Haemophilus influenzae*.

TABLE 43–2 Confirmed Hearing Loss on High-Risk Register (January 1982 to December 1986)

High Risk Factor	*Number*	*Degree of Loss*	*Type of Loss*
Family history	4	Severe/profound (2) Moderate/severe (2)	Sensorineural Sensorineural
Defects of head & neck (syndromal abnormalities)	6	Severe/profound (1) Severe/profound (2) Moderate (2) Moderate/severe (1)	Sensorineural Mixed Conductive Mixed
Cytomegalovirus	1	Moderate/severe	Sensorineural
Low birthweight	1	Moderate	Sensorineural
Low apgar, hyperbilirubinemia	1	Severe/profound	Sensorineural
Low apgar, hyperbilirubinemia; family history of unilateral loss	1	Profound (unilateral)	Sensorineural

Total births: 12,739
High risk: 1,399 or 11 percent
Hearing loss requiring habilitation 14 or one in 100 of high-risk babies.

7. Severe asphyxia that may include infants with Apgar scores of 0 to 3 or who fail to institute spontaneous respiration by 10 minutes and those with hypotonia persisting to 2 hours of age.

The implementation of a high-risk register varies according to local situations. Several basic methods are in use, around which individual programs can be built in line with prevailing needs. These methods of implementation are as follows.

Through Trained Volunteers. Initially volunteers are trained by physicians and audiologists to gather information from the infants' charts and to present brief questionnaires to the mothers. When volunteers are used, it may be necessary for legal clearance to be obtained from the mothers, which will allow these nonprofessional people to examine the medical charts. The following is adequate: "I consent to authorize the hearing screening counselor to view the medical records of my newborn infant to assist in advising me and/or my infant's attending physician."

Once the high-risk information is obtained, a supervisor must take care of the follow-up of the infants found to be at risk. The Joint Committee specified that these babies must be tested in an audiologic facility within 2 months. Therefore the parents or the managing physician must be contacted and informed where they are to bring the infant for testing. It is important to select qualified audiologic centers to which to refer parents.

In order to secure the follow-up in such a program, the services of a one-third to one-half time supervisor are necessary. This person need not be a professional, and so the expense is not high. In order to defray the cost of materials and of the supervisor, each parent is charged a certain amount—usually $10.00 to $15.00 in such a program—as an equivalent to a laboratory fee.

Through a Public Health Agency. Some states have begun to conduct high-risk programs through their maternal and child health departments. For example, the Colorado program has enlisted private hospitals in the state to compile registers. Nurses in the newborn nurseries fill out the questionnaire and search the chart records for the high-risk categories. Regional audiologists are trained to do the follow-up testing of these infants, and parents are directed to bring the babies to these audiologic centers to be tested. The cost of the tests is borne by the public health facility. The services of a one-half to two-thirds time person are required to supervise the state program.

Through Private or Community Agencies. Facilities such as a speech and hearing center may conduct a high-risk program in local hospitals after securing the cooperation of the attending physicians, nurses, and hospital administrators. The compilation of the register may be done by audiologists or other employees of the center; the follow-up procedures may also be undertaken by the center.

Hearing Screening by Behavioral Testing

Screening through observations of behavioral responses to sound stimuli has not been accepted as a single method of screening for hearing at birth. However, it is advocated by many as a supplement to a high-risk register and as such has been approved by the Joint Committee.

The recommended procedure for behavioral screening is outlined in the report of an International Conference on Early Identification in Halifax, Nova Scotia, in 1974. The recommendations included the following salient points.[36]

1. The stimulus should be 90 dB (sound pressure level) in intensity and with a low frequency attenuation of greater than 30 dB per octave below 750 Hz.
2. The infant should be asleep, with eyes closed and no body movement, for at least 15 seconds before the stimulus is presented.
3. The only acceptable response is a generalized body movement involving more than one limb and accompanied by some form of eye movement.
4. Scoring should be done by two observers, independent of each other. Two (of eight maximum) stimulus responses should be positive to score as a pass, and failures should be retested at least once.

As can be seen from Table 42–2, when the entire nursery population was screened with a 90-dB stimulus, approximately 60 percent of the confirmed cases of hearing impairment were identified by behavioral observations. No hearing impairments were identified by the behavioral screening alone. All the severe losses were detected by the screening, but some of the mild and moderate losses were missed. This finding corroborates Mencher's statement that hearing losses less than the 75-dB average cannot be expected to be identified by a 90-dB screening stimulus.[37]

Crib-O-Gram Testing

An automated technique of behavioral screening has been developed by Simmons.[38] He utilizes a motion-sensitive transducer attached underneath the infants' bassinets, with a strip chart to record motion, an automatic timer, and a loudspeaker. A high-frequency signal of 92 dB is presented at scheduled intervals in the nursery, and movements of the infants in response to the stimulus are recorded on the chart. Eight cribs can be monitored simultaneously.

Simmons reports that the crib-o-gram has identified deafness in 12 of 1,000 in the intensive care nursery and in one in 1,000 in a regular nursery. The cost of the units is potentially low. This technique has been regarded as one that may receive general approval when data from field trials have been obtained. On the whole, newborn screening has become a viable procedure and will undoubtedly undergo general implementation in the next few years.

Auditory Brain Stem Response

This testing has become widely used in identification and is considered the method of choice among most clinicians involved in assessing the integrity of the auditory system in infants. These far-field potentials were first described by Jewitt and Willeston.[39] The response pattern is a series of waves that reflect activity from the eighth cranial nerve and ascending auditory pathways within the brain stem.

Although auditory brain stem response is a desirable technique for testing infants, the procedure is not without limitations; these recordings do not guarantee normal auditory perception.[40,41] In addition, an infant with a low-frequency hearing loss may exhibit normal auditory brain stem response thresholds.[42] Conversely, Jerger and Mauldin have shown that thresholds of infants with high-frequency losses may be overestimated with the brain stem response.[43] Finally, there are cases of auditory brain stem response failures who later exhibit measurable hearing. Worthington and Peters reported four patients with either absent auditory brain stem responses who actually had measurable hearing using behavioral methods or thresholds that were appropriate for audiometric configurations, for example, the patients had far better behavioral thresholds than an auditory brain stem response.[41] These inconsistencies in brain stem response recordings are brought to the readers' attention not as a deterrent to use it with infants, but as a cautionary note when employing it as a screening technique. There are many nonpathologic as well as pathologic factors that may alter the test.

If auditory brain stem response is the method chosen for infant screening, there is a plethora of instruments available from which to choose. These instruments range in price from approximately $7,000 for a limited screening device to $30,000 for a unit with multipurpose evoked potential capabilities.

Screening the Infant from Birth to 3 Years

Even when a newborn screening program is in use, further hearing screening is requisite for the older infant. At every routine health visit, a child's hearing should be checked in the well-baby clinic, a private physician's office, or a public health center. The goal is now not only to identify the severe hearing losses that might develop after birth, but also to detect ear conditions that may cause mild hearing losses. One might say that at this age level, one is looking for both deafness and ear disease. Both can be identified with the simple techniques that will be described.

The newly recognized urgency of identifying ear disease early in life has necessitated a new and dedicated approach to screening in infancy. The comprehensive review by Kavanagh has shown that children who have a history of recurrent otitis media that begins in the first 2 years of life are at a high risk of having auditory learning problems and reduced language skills.[22]

Detecting Hearing Loss

The new electrophysiologic testing and operant conditioning procedures that can be used clinically to estimate the degree of hearing loss an infant may have are described in Chapter 50. These techniques cannot yet be used for mass screening, and one must depend at present on the art of observing infants' behavioral responses to various sounds. Such observations are used routinely in programs throughout the world.[44,45] For example, Feinmesser and Tell describe screening at 5 to 7 months with noisemakers in the Israel State Child Clinics.[46] They state that such behavioral screening identified, before 1 year of age, 60 percent of the babies who were found by 3 years of age to have hearing loss. For the most part, the more severe losses were identified during the first year; others were found in later behavioral screening. Thus, although the technique is a relatively imperfect tool for screening, behavioral tests of responses to noisemakers are worth performing.

A procedure that attempts to use the best of the foreign techniques may utilize one or two persons.

Equipment. Five noisemakers are recommended: two with high-frequency sounds (a bell and a high-pitched rattle sound), two with low-frequency sounds (a squeeze toy and a clacker), and one loud sound from a horn or rattle covering most of the frequency range.

Technique. The child is seated on the mother's lap. If two persons are available, one distracts the child's attention with a simple toy held about 1 m in front of him or her. The other person makes a sound at the side and close to the floor, out of the peripheral vision of the child. (One tester modifies the technique by kneeling at a 45-degree angle to the side and front of the child with the distracting toy in one hand and the noisemaker out of sight in the other. While the child is distracted, the tester makes the sound in the hand held close to the floor, out of the peripheral vision of the child.)

If an orientation response is seen after one or two presentations, the alternate frequency noisemaker is then presented on the same side. After the observation, the tester goes on the other side and uses the other high- and low-frequency noisemakers.

The final test is to present the loud noisemaker close to the child's ears to see whether a startle or jump can be seen. This test confirms the validity of the earlier tests and eliminates the possibility that a deaf child may be so visually alert that this constant "scanning" behavior may look like a hearing response.

Expected Responses. The kinds of responses one looks for are age-specific, depending on the maturation of the infant. Therefore they are described in appropriate age intervals:

Birth To 4 Months. At this age, auditory responses are largely reflexive. In a quiet environment, one may see an eye blink or eye widening response to the softer noisemakers, but these responses are not standardized. The only reliable response is a startle or eyeblink to the loud noisemaker. At 3 or 4 months, the infant may begin to turn his or her head toward a sound, but this response again is not yet reliable.

Four To 7 Months. By 4 months, the infant begins to turn his or her head toward the sound source in a wobbly way, and by 7 months he or she turns his or her head directly toward the side. However, it is not a direct localization of the sound at the lower level, only a turn toward the side.

Seven To 9 Months. During this period, the infant begins to find the sound source on the lower level, locating it directly by 8 to 9 months. He or she does not yet look directly at a sound on a higher plane, above his or her eye level.

Nine To 13 Months. By the end of this period, the infant is able to localize directly sounds in any plane. Full maturation of the child's auditory development has been attained.

Thirteen To 36 Months. The same responses are seen in this period: localization in all planes. Other factors begin to enter into the testing in this period and must be considered. For example, a 2 to 3 year old may hear the sound, but inhibits his or her orienting to it because he or she is aware that the examiner is making the sound. Therefore the two-person technique is more reliable at an older age, provided one can outwit the child's curiosity and awareness of the testing situation.

The value of these observations is that they not only tell whether the child hears, but also give a rough assessment of auditory development. For example, if a 10-month-old child is unable to locate a sound source on a lower level, he or she is functioning at a lower developmental level than his or her age. Such a child should be referred for developmental testing, even if his or her hearing is normal.

At every age, a loud noisemaker should be presented 10 cm from the ear in order to see whether a startle reaction or eyeblink can be elicited. This presentation should conclude every test protocol for a child.

Children 4 months and older who fail to respond to two of the noisemaker signals should be referred for testing in an audiologic center. Up to 4 months, the failure to produce a startle or eyeblink to the loud sound constitutes a failure.

Questionnaires For Parents. It is useful to get some idea from the parents as to how the child is functioning. A communication questionnaire may bring out facts that are not evident in the hearing test findings. The questionnaire in Appendix 1 covers both auditory behavior and developmental milestones. If either is deficient, the child should be referred for appropriate evaluation.

Detecting Ear Disease

The use of acoustic impedance bridge is described in Chapter 41. Its application as a screening tool for infants and children is strongly recommended by the author(s), with the limitations that will be described. The accumulation of reports corroborating the validity and reliability of impedance testing (tympanometry) in identifying ear disease has confirmed beyond question its value is screening.[47] Its correspondence with good pneumatic otoscopy by qualified otolaryngologists has been reported as 96 percent in most of the studies.[48] In point of fact, the impedance test detects more subtle changes than can be seen in pneumatic otoscopy.

Two qualifications must be made to the validity of impedance testing and its use in screening. For infants under 7 months of age, tympanometry is of limited validity, according to Paradise.[49] These findings do not mean that tympanometry should never be done in infants under 7 months of age; they do mean that tympanometry can be depended on in 70 percent of the cases to be accurate at this age rather than in 96 percent, as in other instances. Furthermore, when flat type B curves are found, tympanometry can be depended on to be accurate in 83 percent of the cases. This means that there is still great virtue in carrying out tympanometry in infants under 7 months of age, provided one is aware of the degree of accuracy to be expected. Certainly one can feel confident about referring an infant when a type B curve is found.

Guidelines for tympanometry and acoustic reflex tests were recommended by an international task force that met in Nashville in 1978; a second set of impedance screening guidelines were published by the American Speech and Hearing Association in 1979.

Screening at 3 to 5 Years

At this age, the more severe congenital losses have been discovered, and what one is mainly concerned with are the conductive losses that are due to otitis media. Because such losses are mild, pure-tone screening should be done at soft levels of 15 dB or less. When such levels are used outside a sound room, to test frequencies lower than 1,000 Hz is not feasible because of the masking effect of ambient noise on those frequencies. The most important test for this age group is impedance testing, for it identifies ear conditions that may not be identified by hearing screening. However, pure-tone screening must be done in order to detect any sensorineural loss that might have developed.

Pure-Tone Screening

Play Conditioning Techniques. For 3 and 4 year olds, the best technique is to use play conditioning. Some motivational game is required, such as peg board and pegs, ring tower, blocks to build, or pennies and piggybank.

The procedure is as follows: With the earphones on the child's ears, the examiner takes his or her hand with a peg (or other toy) in it, places it up to his or her ear, and presents a 50-dB, 1,000-Hz tone. The examiner then guides his or her hand with the peg into the peg board and, finally, praises him or her. This procedure is repeated twice. Then the examiner gives the child the peg and tells the child to do it him- or herself. Then the 50-dB tone is presented. If the child places the peg correctly, he or she is given the peg, and the tone is presented at 15 dB. If the child puts the peg in, the examiner changes to the next frequency. (The order is 1,000, 2,000, and 4,000 in one ear and 4,000, 2,000, and 1,000 in the other ear). The child then switches to the other ear and starts at 4,000 Hz.

Criteria for Pass or Fail. A child who fails to respond at 15 dB to any one frequency in either ear fails the test and should be screened later the same day. If he or she still fails, he or she should be referred for medical examination and audiologic assessment.

THE IDENTIFICATION OF THE MILD HEARING LOSS OF OTITIS MEDIA

A policy statement of the American Academy of Pediatrics has stated that

> There is growing evidence demonstrating a correlation between middle ear disease with hearing impairment and delays in the development of speech, language and cognitive skills. . . When a child has frequently recurring acute otitis media and/or middle ear effusion persisting for longer than three months, hearing should be assessed and the development of communicative skills must be monitored.

Unfortunately, not all children are given ear examinations with pneumatic otoscopy at well-baby health visits, and 46 percent of all cases of otitis media are asymptomatic, and so not all middle ear problems are automatically identified.[50] Therefore it is necessary to actively search for those children who may be at risk for recurrence of this disease.

It is known that the average hearing loss from otitis media ranges from 26 to 31 dB.[51] This degree of loss is difficult to identify in the young child by means of the behavioral observations described previously; however, a study of 760 children from birth to 3 years reports that 50 percent of all the children who failed a tympanometry test had also failed noisemaker tests.[52] Therefore identifying those children who have the more severe losses from otitis media may be a useful procedure. Several programs have reported success with noisemaker screening of children younger than 3 years: the state of Tennessee has successfully utilized this technique in their state Public Health program,[53] and the countries of Israel, England, and Holland routinely employ noisemaker screening in their well-baby clinics or nursing programs.[54]

The most useful tool to identify middle ear disease is tympanometry, which was discussed previously. Objections have been voiced to tympanometry screening programs because of the large numbers of false-positives that are found, despite the prescribed rescreening of failures. However, physicians should be advised of the fact that 40 percent of children with significant conditions of serous otitis media have it on a fluctuating basis.[50] Therefore many children who are at risk for problems from serous otitis are free from symptoms part of the time; these children appear in the physician's office symptom-free despite the two abnormal tympanograms and an abnormal audiogram from a screening program. In such cases, the children should not be ignored, but should be considered at risk for recurrence and monitored carefully for at least 6 months until it is apparent they will not have further episodes.

The important question that must be answered, according to the Academy of Pediatrics' policy statement, is: Does the child who is found to have recurrent otitis media show any language delays that may have been caused by the disease? Fortunately, the clinician can effectively answer that question with new language screening tools that have been developed for the child from birth to 3 years old. The most widely used screening test for young children is the Early Language Milestone scale (ELM), developed by a pediatrician, Dr. James Coplan, and validated on a high-risk population.[55] The scale tests for receptive language, expressive language, and visual language skills and can be administered in 1 to 3 minutes. This type of screening is recommended as an integral part of any screening program that proposes to identify children with hearing losses from otitis media, since it completes and corroborates the identification of hearing losses that produce measurable handicap.

The solution for this problem lies, of course, in prevention. Prevention has three aspects: identification, medical treatment, and educational habilitation. Identification of hearing loss has been the major topic of this chapter.

The second avenue of prevention is medical treatment. It is absolutely mandatory that any child with a bout of otitis media be seen by his or her physician for consideration of medical treatment or surgery. The criteria for medical treatment or placement of polyethylene tubes are dependent upon the physician. Note that any child who has had three bouts of otitis media during the first year of life is at risk for language and cognitive problems.

The third type of prevention is educational habilitation. The first option available is a home language stimulation program. This type of program is already being given to children who are at developmental risk and is absolutely essential for any child who experiences recurrent otitis media. The second option for habilitation is the placement of hearing aids. Hearing aids can be used successfully in a number of cases, but the success depends on parents' involvement and their conviction that the hearing loss does exist, as well as upon the support of the physician who manages the child. When all these things are obtained, the results are gratifying, to say the least. For example, 5 years ago we identified a child who was 6 months old and had a series of bouts of otitis media. Medical treatment was instituted and myringotomy and tubes applied, but she continued to have recurrent bouts of serous otitis. At the age of 10 months, we decided to institute a home language intervention program and also to apply a mild hearing aid. At that time, her language development lagged approximately 4 months. At 14 months, she was still 5 months behind in language development. However, with the constant use of the hearing aid and a mother who cooperated in a home stimulation program, by 24 months of age her language level was at a 21-month level, and at 36 months her language level was accelerated 2 months beyond her chronologic age. By the age of 4 years, her language level was that of a 5 year old. By this time, she no longer needed to wear the hearing aid because medical intervention had been successful in treating her ears, and she now had normal hearing. Heroic treatment indeed, but the results were worth the effort expended.

SUMMARY

Whether an infant has a severe congenital hearing loss or a mild loss from serous otitis media, the problem should be detected in the early months of life and treated educationally and medically. Probably every month of sensory deprivation at an early age results in cumulative language deprivation. Fortunately, methods are available that are cost effective and valid. They should be employed universally.

APPENDIX 1

Questions to Ask Mother at the Well-Baby Examination

2 Months

Hearing

1. Have you had any worry about your child's hearing? YES NO
2. When your child is sleeping in a quiet room, does he or she move and begin to wake up when there is a loud sound? YES NO

Development and Communication

3. Does your child lift up his or her head when he or she is lying on his or her stomach? YES NO
4. Does your child smile at you when you smile at him or her? YES NO
5. Does your child move both hands together in the same way? YES NO
6. Does your child look at your face without your making gestures at him? YES NO

4 Months

Hearing

1. Have you had any worry about your child's hearing? YES NO
2. When your child is sleeping in a quiet room, does he or she move and begin to wake when there's a loud sound? YES NO
3. Does your child try to turn his or her head toward an interesting sound, or when his or her name is called? YES NO

Development and Communication

4. Does your child lift his or her head up to 90 degrees and look straight ahead? YES NO
5. Does your child touch his or her hands together and play with them? YES NO
6. Does your child laugh and giggle without being tickled or touched? YES NO
7. Does your child coo to him- or herself and make noises when he or she is alone? YES NO

6 Months

Hearing

1. Have you had any worry about your child's hearing? YES NO
2. When your child is sleeping in a quiet room, does he or she move and begin to wake up when there's a loud sound? YES NO
3. Does your child turn his or her head toward an interesting sound or when his or her name is called? YES NO

Development and Communication

4. Does your child lift up his or her head and chest with his or her arms? YES NO
5. Does your child keep his or her head steady when sitting? YES NO
6. Does your child roll over in his or her crib? YES NO
7. Does your child reach for objects within his or her reach and hold them? YES NO
8. Does your child see small objects like peas or raisins? YES NO

8 MONTHS

Hearing

1. Have you had any worry about your child's hearing? YES NO
2. When your child is sleeping in a quiet room, does he or she move and begin to wake up when there is a loud sound? YES NO
3. Does your child turn his or her head directly toward an interesting sound or when his or her name is called? YES NO
4. Does your child enjoy ringing a bell or shaking a rattle? YES NO

Development and Communication

5. Does your child support most of his or her weight on his or her legs? YES NO
6. Can your child sit alone unaided for 5 minutes? YES NO
7. Can your child sit and look for objects that have fallen out of sight? YES NO
8. Can your child pick up two objects, one in each hand? YES NO
9. Can your child transfer an object from one hand to the other? YES NO
10. Can your child feed him- or herself a cracker? YES NO
11. Does your child make a number of different sounds and change their pitch? YES NO
12. Does your child clap his or her hands in imitation and make noises at the same time? YES NO

10 Months

Hearing

1. Have you had any worry about your child's hearing? YES NO
2. When your child is sleeping in a quiet room, does he or she move and begin to wake up when there is a loud sound? YES NO
3. Does your child turn his or her head directly toward an interesting sound or when his or her name is called? YES NO
4. Does your child try to imitate you if you make his or her own sounds? YES NO

Development and Communication

5. Does your child play peek-a-boo with you? YES NO
6. Can your child stand for at least 5 seconds, holding onto the crib or chair? YES NO
7. Does your child try to hold onto a toy when it is pulled away? YES NO
8. Is your child shy or afraid of strangers? YES NO
9. Can your child pull him- or herself to standing position alone? YES NO

12 Months

Hearing

1. Have you had any worry about your child's hearing? YES NO
2. When your child is sleeping in a quiet room, does he or she move and begin to wake when there is a loud sound? YES NO
3. Does your child turn his or her head directly toward an interesting sound or when his or her name is called? YES NO
4. Is your child beginning to repeat some of the sounds that you make? YES NO

Development and Communication

5. Can your child pick up a raisin or a pea? YES NO
6. Can your child sit up without help? YES NO
7. Does your child wave bye-bye or play pat-a-cake when you tell him or her to? YES NO
8. Can your child say "mama" or "dada"? YES NO

REFERENCES

1. Lane H. The wild boy of Aveyron. Cambridge: Harvard University Press, 1977.
2. Fromkin V, Krashen S, Curtiss S, Rigler D, Rigler M. The development of language in Genie: A case of language acquisition beyond the "critical period." Brain Lang 1974; 1:81–107.
3. Edwards EP. Kindergarten is too late. Saturday Review 1968; 51:60–79.
4. Guinagh BJ, Jester RE. Long-term effects of infant stimulation programs. Adv Behav Pediatr 1981; 2:81–110..
5. Hunt J McV. Parent and child centers: their basis in the behavioral and educational sciences. Am J Orthopsychiatry 1971; 41:13–38.
6. McKay H, Sinisterra L, McKay A, Gomez H, Lloreda P. Improving cognitive ability in chronically deprived children. Science 1978; 200:270–278.
7. Dennis W. Children of the creche. Century Psychology Series. New York: Prentice-Hall, 1973.
8. Heber R, Garber H. An experiment in the prevention of cultural-familial retardation. Washington DC: United States Dept. of HEW, Office of Education, Resources Information Center, 1970.
9. Wachs U, Hunt J McV. Cognitive development in infants of different ages and from different environmental backgrounds. Merrill-Palmer Q Behav Devel 1971; 17:288–317.
10. Messer SB, Lewis M. Social class and sex differences in the attachment and play behavior of the year-old infant. Atlantic City, paper presented at the Easter Psycho Assn 1970.
11. Greenstein JM, Greenstein BB, McConville K, Stellini L. Mother-infant communication and language acquisition in deaf infants. New York: Lexington School for the Deaf, 1976.
12. Hebb DO. The effects of early experience on problem-solving at maturity. Am Psychol 1947; 2:306–307.
13. Greenough WT. Experiential modification of the developing brain. Am Sci 1975; 63:37–46.
14. Reisen AH. Effects of stimulus deprivation on the development and atrophy of the visual sensory system. Am J Orthopsychiatry 1960; 30:23–36.
15. Reisen AH. The development of visual perception in man and chimpanzee. Science 1947; 106:207–208.
16. Ruben RJ, Rapin I. Plasticity of the developing auditory system. Ann Otol Rhinol Laryngol 1980; 89:303–311.
17. Survey of Hearing Impaired Children and Youth. Washington, DC: Gallaudet College, Office of Demographic Studies, series D 1971:9.
18. Templin M. Vocabulary problems of the deaf child. Int Audiol 1966; 5:349.
19. Bergstrom L. Viruses that deafen. In: Bess FH, ed. Childhood deafness: causation, assessment and management. New York: Grune & Stratton, 1977:53.
20. Menyuk P. Effects of hearing loss on babbling in the language-acquisition stage. In: Jaffe B, ed. Hearing loss in children. Baltimore: University Park Press, 1977.
21. Schein JD, Delk MT. The deaf population of the United States. Silver Spring, MD: National Association of the Deaf, 1974.
22. Kavanagh JF, ed. Otitis media and child development. Parkton, MD: York Press, 1986.
23. Bess F, Thorpe AM. An introduction to unilateral sensorineural hearing loss in children. Ear Hear 1986; 7:3–13.
24. Webster DB, Webster M. Neonatal sound deprivation affects brain stem auditory nuclei. Arch Otolaryngol 1977; 103:392–396.
25. Webster DB, Webster M. Auditory brain stem sound deprivation and critical periods. Arch Otolaryngol 1979.
26. Webster DB, Webster M. Mouse brainstem auditory nuclei development. Ann Rhinol Laryngol 1980; 89 [Suppl. 68]:254–256.
27. Brattgard SO. The importance of adequate stimulation for the chemical composition of retinal ganglion cells during early postnatal development. Acta Radiol [Suppl.] 1952; 96:1–80.
28. Cragg B. The development of synapses in kitten visual cortex during visual deprivation. Expl Neurol 1975; 46:445–451.
29. Guillery R, Kaas J. The effects of monocular lid suture upon the development of lateral geniculate nucleus in squirrels. J Comp Neurol 1974; 154:433–442.
30. Guillery R, Kaas J. The effects of monocular lid suture upon the development of visual cortex in squirrels. J Comp Neurol 1974b; 154:443–452.
31. Downs MP. Expanding imperatives of early identification. In: Bess FH, ed. Childhood deafness: causation, assessment & management. New York: Grune & Stratton, 1977.
32. Frankenburg W. Evaluation of screening procedures. In: Gold EM, ed. Earlier recognition of handicapping conditions of childhood: proceedings of a regional institute. Berkeley:

University of California School of Public Health, 1971:42–51.
33. Downs MP. Auditory screening. Otolaryngol Clin North Am 1978; 11:611–629.
34. Richards IDG, Roberts CJ. The AT RISK infant. Lancet 1967; 2:711–714.
35. Joint Committee on Infant Hearing 1982 Statement. Asha 1982; 24:1017–1018.
36. Mencher GT, ed. Early identification of hearing loss. Basel, Switzerland: S Karger, 1975.
37. Mencher GT. A program for neonatal hearing screening. Audiology 1974; 13:495–500.
38. Simmons FB. Automated hearing screening test for newborns: the crib-o-gram. In: Mencher G, ed. Early identification of hearing loss. Basel, Switzerland: S Karger, 1975.
39. Jewitt DL, Willeston JS. Auditory-evoked far field averages from the scalp of humans. Brain 1971; 94:681–696.
40. Goldstein PJ, Krumholz A, Felix JK, Shannon D, Carr RF. Brainstem-evoked response in neonates. Am J Obstet Gynecol 1979; 135:622–628.
41. Worthington DW, Peters JF. Quantifiable hearing and no ABR: Paradox or error? Ear Hear 1980; 1:281–285.
42. Galambos R, Hecox KE. Clinical applications of the auditory brainstem response. Otolaryngol Clin North Am 1978; 11:709–722.
43. Jerger J, Mauldin L. Prediction of sensorineural hearing level from the brainstem evoked response. Arch Otolaryngol 1978; 104:456–461.
44. Borkowska-Gaertig D, Urbanska I, Sobieszczanska-Radoszewska L, Rzedowska Z, Rola-Janicki A. Evaluation of three-stage hearing testing programme for children in Poland. In: Mencher G, ed. Early identification of hearing loss. Basel, Switzerland: S Karger, 1975; 122–132.
45. Stensland-Junker K. BOEL—a child welfare program for early screening for communication abilities. In: Mencher G, ed. Early identification of hearing loss. Basel: S Karger, 1976.
46. Feinmesser M, Tell L. Evaluation of methods for detecting hearing impairment in infancy and early childhood. In: Mencher G, ed. Early identification of hearing loss. Basel: S Karger, 1976.
47. Northern JL. Clinical application of impedance audiometry. In: Northern JL, ed. Hearing disorders. Boston: Little, Brown, 1976.
48. Paradise JL, Smith CG, Bluestone CD. Tympanometric detection of middle ear effusion in infants and young children. Pediatrics 1976; 58:198–210.
49. Paradise JL. Management of middle ear effusions in infants with cleft palate. Ann Otol Rhinol Laryngol [Suppl. 25] 1976; 85:285–288.
50. Marchant C, Shurin PA, Tutihasi MA, Turczyk VA, Wasikowski DE, Feinstein, JC. Detection of asymptomatic otitis media in early infancy. In: Lim D, ed. Recent advances in otitis media with effusion. Philadelphia: BC Decker, 1984.
51. McDermott JC, Giebink GS, Le CT, Harford ER, Paparella MM. Children with persistent otitis media. Arch Otolaryngol 1983; 109:360–363.
52. Downs MP, Walker DD, Northern JL, Gugenheim S. Unpublished data from Screening for communication disorders in children, a study funded by the Robert Wood Johnson Foundation. Denver, 1987.
53. Cascarella-Buchanan JE. Finding ears that do not hear. Tennessee Med Assoc J 1986; January:39.
54. Audiology in Practice. Excerpta Medica 1986; 3(4):1–8.
55. Coplan J, Gleason JR, Ryan R, Burke MG, Williams ML. Validation of an early language milestone scale in a high-risk population. Pediatrics 1982; 70:677–683.

44

Hearing and Immittance Screening

Kathryn E. Bright, Ph.D.
Jackson Roush, Ph.D.

Screening for disease in children has long been regarded as an important and necessary component of pediatric health care. Screening for hearing loss has been routinely administered in most states for over 50 years. More recently, preschool and newborn hearing screening programs have become increasingly popular. The following review addresses the topic of identification audiometry in the preschool and school-age child. For a review of hearing screening procedures with the newborn, the interested reader is referred to Chapter 43 of this volume.

In 1966, the National Conference on Identification Audiometry specified that the major purpose of hearing screening is to "locate children who have even minimal hearing problems so they can be referred for medical treatment of active ear pathology discovered to be present, so that remedial educational procedures can be instituted at the earliest possible date."[1] Several studies have suggested that even a mild degree of hearing loss can have debilitating effects on a child's speech and language development, auditory processing capabilities, and academic performance.[2–11] Although other studies[12–17] have questioned this assertion, the possibility of a causal relationship should be seriously considered until more conclusive data are available. Many professionals believe that a critical period exists for learning speech and language,[18,19] and that the earlier a hearing loss is identified and remediated the better are the chances of preventing long-term disability. In addition, research on the effects of mild bilateral and unilateral sensory deprivation in animals has further emphasized the importance of early identification of hearing loss. There is evidence that even a mild hearing loss may result in maturational delays and neurophysiologic changes within the central auditory system.[20–25]

Sensorineural or conductive hearing loss frequently occurs in the absence of other disorders and may go unnoticed, or the hearing loss may be masked by or mistaken for other disorders. In addition, children are often incapable of reporting a hearing loss to parents or teachers. A further complication exists when children have fluctuating hearing loss or hearing loss with a delayed onset. These children may respond inconsistently to screening measures. Even children with identified sensorineural hearing loss may acquire a conductive overlay or may experience a progressive loss. It is therefore imperative that preschool and school-age children be screened for hearing loss at regular intervals and that no child suspected of or at risk for hearing loss be overlooked.

Exactly how many preschool and school-age children are hearing-impaired is not known. Figures regarding the prevalence of hearing loss in children vary depending on the criteria used and methods of assessment. (Prevalence refers to the total occurrence of a disorder within a population whereas incidence refers to the number of new occurrences of the disorder within a specified time period.)[26] Most investigators have reported that approximately 5 percent of children screened will be referred for additional testing.[27–29] In a review of 31 studies conducted between 1926 and 1960, Connor reported a prevalence of hearing loss ranging from 0.5 percent to 21 percent.[30] More recent reports of failure rates have ranged from 3.5 percent[31] to 26.7 percent.[32] Pass-fail criteria, tester experience, test environment, equipment, types of tests used, and seasonal variation all contribute to the number of children who fail the screening.[33] It is important to note that, while related, the screening failure rate is not synonymous with the prevalence of hearing loss. For example, if pass-fail criteria are stringent many more children will fail the screening than if the criteria are lax.

The prevalence of hearing loss and hence the screening failure rate, is also influenced by the characteristics of the population screened. For example, it has been reported that low socioeconomic status may be related to the incidence of hearing loss and ear disease.[32,34] Eskimos,[35,36] American Indians,[37-39] children with cleft palates,[40,41] and children with Down's syndrome[42] have a higher prevalence of conductive hearing loss and ear disease than other populations. Males aged 14 to 18 years have been noted to have a higher prevalence of high frequency sensorineural hearing loss than females in this age group.[43,44] Such factors need to be carefully considered when planning a screening program. A thorough summary of the literature regarding screening of special populations has been completed by Northern.[45]

It is important to emphasize that identification audiometry is only one component of a thorough hearing conservation program.[46] Identification procedures are not designed to determine how much or what type of hearing impairment exists. Once a possible disorder is identified, further audiologic, medical, or psychoeducational testing must be completed to determine the extent of the disorder and the appropriate course of treatment.

GENERAL CONSIDERATIONS REGARDING IDENTIFICATION AUDIOMETRY

Reliability and Validity

In order to apply and interpret screening tests appropriately, the reliability and validity of the tests should be known. Reliability refers to the consistency and stability of a measurement, or, stated differently, the degree to which the test results can be attributed to systematic sources of variance.[47,48] A correlation coefficient (a number between -1.0 and $+1.0$) is often used to express the consistency or agreement between two sets of scores.

Several types of reliability may be measured. Test-retest reliability is a correlation of scores from test administration on two different occasions; alternate-form reliability is a correlation of scores from two versions of the same test, split-half reliability is a correlation of the scores obtained from two halves of the same test, and interexaminer reliability is a correlation of results of a test administered by two different examiners. A fifth type, function reliability, refers to the stability of the function being measured.[19] For example, if the hearing ability of an individual changed during the testing period or between repeated tests, function reliability would be poor. When screening to determine the presence or absence of a disorder, function, test-retest, and interexaminer reliability are the types of reliability one is generally most concerned with.

Co-positivity and co-negativity of a test are also measures that provide information regarding the reliability of a test.[19,33] Results of a screening test administered by an inexperienced examiner may be compared to results obtained by an experienced tester. Co-positivity reflects the extent to which the two examiners are in agreement in detecting the presence of hearing loss, and co-negativity reflects the extent to which the examiners are in agreement in ruling out hearing loss. Figure 44–1 illustrates the manner in which co-positivity and co-negativity are calculated. The extent to which the two testers are not in agreement may also be calculated. The false negative rate reflects the percentage of time the tester fails to identify the presence of hearing loss, and the false positive rate reflects the percentage of time the tester identifies the presence of hearing loss incorrectly. The goal of an effective screening program is to maintain the lowest possible rate of false positive and false negative outcomes.

Validity refers to the accuracy and appropriateness of inferences that can be made from test results. In other words, estimates of validity determine the extent to which a test measures what it is supposed to measure.[47,48] It should be noted that validity is inferred, not measured. It is a judgment regarding whether or not the test is accurate, marginal, or unsatisfactory. As with reliability, several types of validity may be considered and all are interrelated. Two of these are criterion-related validity and content validity. A test has criterion-related validity when its results compare favorably to the results from another test, the criterion. A hearing screening test may be said to have criterion-related validity if it correctly identifies those individuals having hearing loss as demonstrated by a complete audiologic evaluation. Content validity of a test refers to how well the items on a test represent the performance which it is purported to measure. For example, a test utilizing speech stimuli might be considered to have poor content validity if the purpose of the test is to assess high frequency hearing loss.

Estimation of sensitivity and specificity are two methods of assessing the validity of tests.[19,33,49] Many

Inexperienced examiner	Experienced examiner: Positive (Fail–hearing loss)	Experienced examiner: Negative (Pass–no hearing loss)
Positive (fail)	A — Agreement in identifying positives (co-positivity)	B — False positive
Negative (pass)	C — False negative	D — Agreement in identifying negatives (co-negativity)

$$\text{Co-positivity} = \frac{A}{A + C} \times 100$$

$$\text{False negative rate} = \frac{C}{A + C} \times 100$$

$$\text{Co-negativity} = \frac{D}{B + D} \times 100$$

$$\text{False positive rate} = \frac{B}{B + D} \times 100$$

Figure 44–1 Calculation of co-positivity and co-negativity for two examiners.

auditory site-of-lesion tests have been evaluated in terms of sensitivity and specificity,[49] and hearing screening tests require similar scrutiny. Sensitivity refers to a test's ability to identify correctly the presence of a disorder. Specificity refers to a test's ability to identify correctly persons not having the disorder. Conversely, as mentioned previously, incorrect identification of the disorder is known as a false positive result, and failure to identify the disorder when it is present is a false negative result. These terms are illustrated in Figure 44–2 with the corresponding equations for determining the percent score for each factor. The ideal test would have high values for both sensitivity and specificity and low false-negative and false-positive values. In general, sensitivity and specificity are related in a complex manner. Figure 44–3 illustrates the inverse relationship between sensitivity and specificity. In most cases, as sensitivity increases, specificity must decrease.

The goal in designing a screening test is to achieve a balance between sensitivity, specificity, the false-positive rate, and the false-negative rate. Adjusting pass-fail criteria is one method of maintaining the proper balance. For example, if the pass-fail criteria are too stringent as indicated by the dotted line A in Figure 44–3, all of the individuals will fail and the test will have 100 percent sensitivity and a high false-positive rate. Conversely, if the pass-fail criteria are too lax, as indicated by line B, everyone will pass the screening test. In this case, there is 100 percent specificity and a high false-negative rate. Adjustment of the pass-fail criteria may be effective in bringing these measures into balance (see line C, Fig. 44–3).

Ideally, both reliability (co-positivity and co-negativity) and validity (sensitivity and specificity) should be evaluated for every screening program; however, for a variety of reasons, including added time and expense, such evaluations are seldom performed. It is hoped that additional research regarding the reliability and validity of screening tests will lead to more efficient and effective test procedures.

Types of Screening Tests

Speech Tests

Because young children generally respond more readily to speech than to tonal stimuli, several speech screening tests have been developed. The Fading Numbers Test,[50] developed in the 1920s, was one of the first screening tests to be utilized and was designed to evaluate groups of up to 40 children at a time.[50] The stimulus was a recording of a woman's voice repeating pairs of numbers. Each child was required to write down numbers between one and ten (except seven) as they were heard, and each set of numbers progressively decreased in level. One limitation of this test was that children too young to record numbers could not be evaluated.

The Bennett Test, described in 1951, used a closed set of four monosyllabic words that were phonetically similar.[51] Children were instructed to point to the appropriate picture in response to a recorded word. Spondaic words (two-syllable words, such as hotdog and cowboy) were recommended by Meyerson

Diagnostic test results

Screening test results	Disorder present	Disorder not present	
Positive (fail)	A Correct identification of abnormal subjects (sensitivity)	B	Positive identifications A + B
Negative (pass)	C	D Correct identification of normal subjects (specificity)	Negative identifications C + D
	Total disordered A + C	Total nondisordered B + D	Total tested A + B + C + D

$$\text{Sensitivity} = \frac{A}{A + C} \times 100$$

$$\text{Specificity} = \frac{D}{B + D} \times 100$$

Figure 44–2 Correct identification of abnormal subjects (sensitivity [Cell A]) and normal subjects (specificity [Cell D]) for a screening test.

for screening the hearing of children.[52] Again, the words were represented by pictures and each child was instructed to point to the appropriate picture. A version of the test in which the spondaic words were high pass filtered was also used in an attempt to identify children with hearing loss in the higher frequencies.

One of the most popular of the screening tests that use speech as stimuli has been the Verbal Auditory Screening for Children (VASC) test, a test

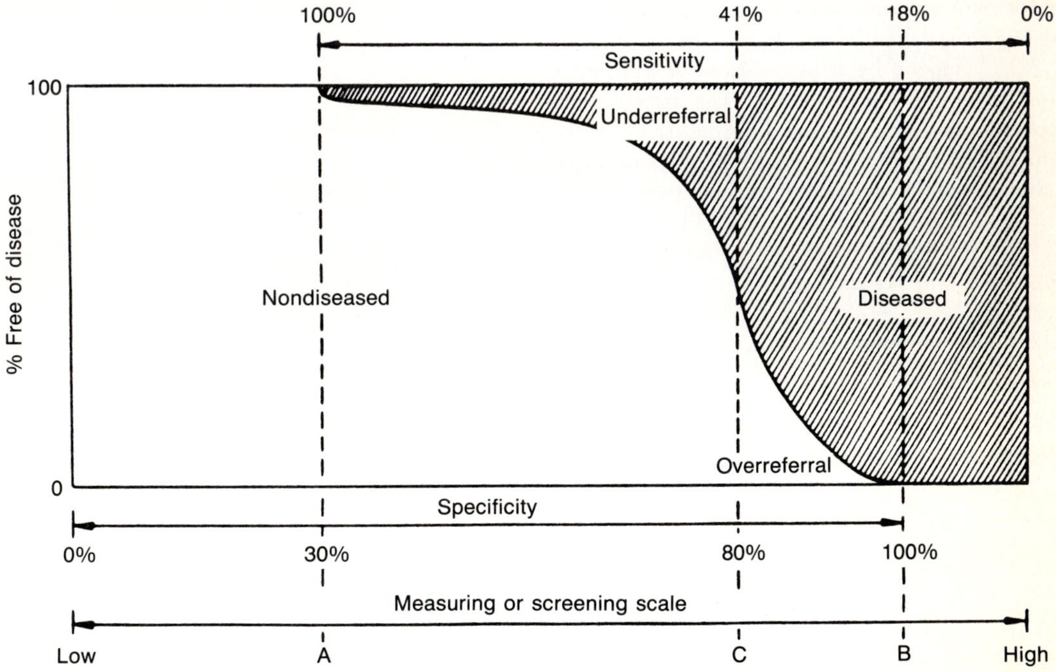

Figure 44–3 Relationship between sensitivity and specificity and overreferral and underreferral.

originally developed for screening preschoolers.[53] Taped lists of 12 spondaic words corresponding to pictures are presented to two children at a time. Each child is instructed to point to the appropriate picture and the levels of the word gradually decrease. An observer records the responses of each child. An advantage of the VASC test is that volunteers can be easily trained to administer the test.

Unfortunately, the use of speech stimuli for screening purposes has been shown to result in an excessive rate of false negatives. The reason for this is evident if the spectral characteristics of speech are considered. Since most of the energy in the speech signal is contained within the lower frequency regions of the spectrum, children with mild hearing losses or losses above 500 Hz are able to perform adequately on these measures by utilizing the low frequency cues of speech. This is especially true if the stimuli are presented in a closed-set format. False-negative rates as high as 58 percent have been reported for screening tests using speech stimuli[54] and, as a result, speech tests have fallen out of favor for identification purposes.

Pure Tone Tests

One of the first pure tone screening tests was described by Newhart in 1938[55] and the method, referred to as the sweep-check screening test, is still popular today. The sweep-check test consists of a series of pure tones at specific test frequencies presented at a constant intensity level. The child is instructed to respond by raising a hand or pushing a button when the tone is heard. The sweep-check procedure is recommended by the American Speech-Language-Hearing Association (ASHA) Committee on Audiometric Evaluation.[56] ASHA recommends screening at 1,000, 2,000, and 4,000 Hz, using levels of 20 dB Hearing Level (HL) (re: ANSI-1969) at 1,000 and 2,000 Hz and levels of 20 or 25 dB HL at 4,000 Hz (Table 44–1). In a comprehensive review of screening procedures published in 1961,[46] the sweep-check procedure was the method of choice, and the frequencies recommended for screening included 500 Hz (if the testing environment was quiet enough), 1,000, 2,000, 4,000 and 5,000 Hz. It was also recommended that screening be completed in a sound-treated booth. Screening at 500 Hz seems desirable if hearing losses secondary to middle ear disorders are to be identified; however, when a sound-treated test environment is unavailable, ASHA does not recommend screening at or below 500 Hz—this is based on several studies in which environmental noise was found to interfere to a significant degree. Likewise, screening at 6,000 Hz is not recommended because of the apparent variability of responses at this frequency.[56]

An evaluation of the procedures recommended by ASHA was completed in 1974 by Wilson and Walton using a group of more than 7,800 school children.[57] Rescreening of failures was included in the testing paradigm as recommended by ASHA. The procedure was found to be more than 95 percent accurate when compared with results of a threshold test.

Several authors have suggested screening at one or two frequencies in an effort to make the screening process more economical and efficient.[58–61] Considering the variety of possible audiometric configurations, however, screening at only one frequency could cause the sensitivity of the screening procedure to be unacceptably low. The available data regarding this issue have not supported the assertion that screening at one or two frequencies is an effective means of identification in children.[59,62]

Group Screening Tests

Several of the screening tests mentioned earlier were designed to test large groups of children at one time. The Fading Numbers Test[50] and the Bennett Test[51] are examples of group tests using speech as stimuli. Several pure tone screening tests were also developed for use with groups. Among these are the

TABLE 44–1 Summary of ASHA Recommendations for Pure-Tone Hearing Screening*

Test Frequencies	*Intensity Level*	*Pass-Fail Criteria*
1,000, 2,000, and 4,000 Hz	20 dB HL	Failure to respond at any frequency in either ear.

* If pure-tone screening is not performed in conjunction with acoustic immittance screening, 500 Hz should also be included.

Pulse Tone Test,[63] the Massachusetts Test,[64] the Modified Massachusetts Test,[65] and the Johnston Group Screening Test.[66] These test procedures may be used with groups of 10 to 40 children and all but the Johnston test require written responses.

Although group procedures appear to save time and money when large numbers of children must be screened, several factors must be considered when assessing the effectiveness of group screening.[67,68] Many of the group tests require a written response making them impractical for young children and special populations. In addition, there is the risk that children will copy responses from each other during a group test or will fail to attend adequately to the task. Difficulties also arise when attempting to find a room large enough and quiet enough for testing as many as 40 children at one time. Another problem is the extensive calibration and maintenance required for a large number of earphones. Additionally, the time required to set up and take down multiple listening stations and to score the response sheets makes the group procedure less efficient. Most audiologists believe that the problems inherent in group screening make it a less desirable technique than individual screening even with large numbers of children.

Acoustic Immittance Tests

When traditional hearing screening tests are used, mild hearing loss secondary to middle ear disease may go unidentified. Otitis media is the most common cause of ear disease in school-age children[69] and is one of the most common infectious diseases in children.[70] The disease is unpredictable and often transient, and the degree of hearing loss associated with it is highly variable, ranging from no measurable hearing loss to a moderate conductive impairment.[71]

The high prevalence of otitis media and associated conductive hearing loss in preschool and school-age children has motivated audiologists to seek a screening strategy that will assist in the identification of these disorders. Because the hearing loss associated with otitis media is often low frequency in nature, it has been recommended in the past that pure tone screening tests include frequencies below 1,000 Hz. As discussed previously, however, the testing environment is not usually quiet enough to allow inclusion of the lower frequencies. Immittance procedures, which became routinely available to audiologists in the 1970s, are believed by many to be a solution to this dilemma. (Immittance is the general term used to denote either acoustic impedance or acoustic admittance.)

Immittance screening generally involves obtaining a tympanogram and may also include acoustic reflex testing. The procedure is quick and relatively easy to complete with children and provides objective information regarding the status of the middle ear.[19] Background noise levels do not affect test results; therefore the problems associated with finding a quiet test environment do not apply. However, it should be remembered that immittance screening provides information about middle ear status; it does not provide information regarding auditory sensitivity. For this reason, it is generally recommended that immittance procedures be used as a supplement to traditional pure tone screening.[71]

Critics of immittance screening cite the transient nature of otitis media, and its tendency to resolve spontaneously in some cases, as evidence that the technique may result in an excessive false-positive rate. In addition, the treatments that are available for middle ear disease are controversial and sometimes ineffective. Before immittance screening can be performed, many professionals believe it is necessary to conduct an otoscopic inspection.[33] The combination of otoscopy and immittance procedures requires that testers have more extensive training than that involved with traditional screening techniques. The amount of training required and the extent of the information obtained from the immittance procedure have caused some to criticize the technique as being too complex for routine application.[72] Nevertheless, technological improvements have greatly simplified the instrumentation used in acoustic immittance screening, and the procedure is now accepted as a routine test procedure in many school systems.

Currently there are two sets of widely accepted guidelines for immittance screening. The ASHA Subcommittee on Impedance Measurement developed a set of guidelines for those who wish to design a screening program including immittance.[71] The guidelines are summarized in Table 44–2 and Figure 44–4. ASHA recommends a minimum air pressure range of +100 to −300 daPa and a probe tone frequency between 220 and 300 Hz. When the acoustic reflex is included, the recommended frequency is 1,000 Hz at levels of 100 dB HL for contralateral stimulation and 105 dB Sound Pressure Level (SPL) for ipsilateral stimulation. If the tympanometric peak pressure falls between −200 and +100 daPa and the acoustic reflex is present, the screening is passed and no further testing is necessary. If the tympanometric peak suggests mildly positive or negative pressure and the acoustic reflex is absent, rescreening is recommended. Finally, ASHA recommends that if middle ear pressure clearly falls outside the normal range and the acoustic reflex is

TABLE 44–2 Summary of ASHA Recommendations for Immittance Screening

Classification	*Initial Screen*	*Disposition*
I Pass	Tympanogram: Normal* or Mildly Positive/Negative† Acoustic Reflex: Present‡	Clear; no return
II At risk	Tympanogram: Abnormal§ and Acoustic Reflex: Present‡ OR Tympanogram: Normal* or Mildly Positive/Negative† Acoustic Reflex: Absent‡	Retest 3–5 weeks If results fall into Class I, pass If results fall into Class II, fail and refer
III Fail	Tympanogram: Abnormal§ Acoustic Reflex: Absent‡	Refer

* Peak at ±50 mm/H_2O
† +50 to +100 mm/H_2O or −50 to −200 mm/H_2O
‡ Contralateral tone 1,000 Hz at 100 dB HL or ipsilateral tone at 105 dB HL
§ Pressure peak more than +100 mm H_2O or more negative than −200 mm H_2O

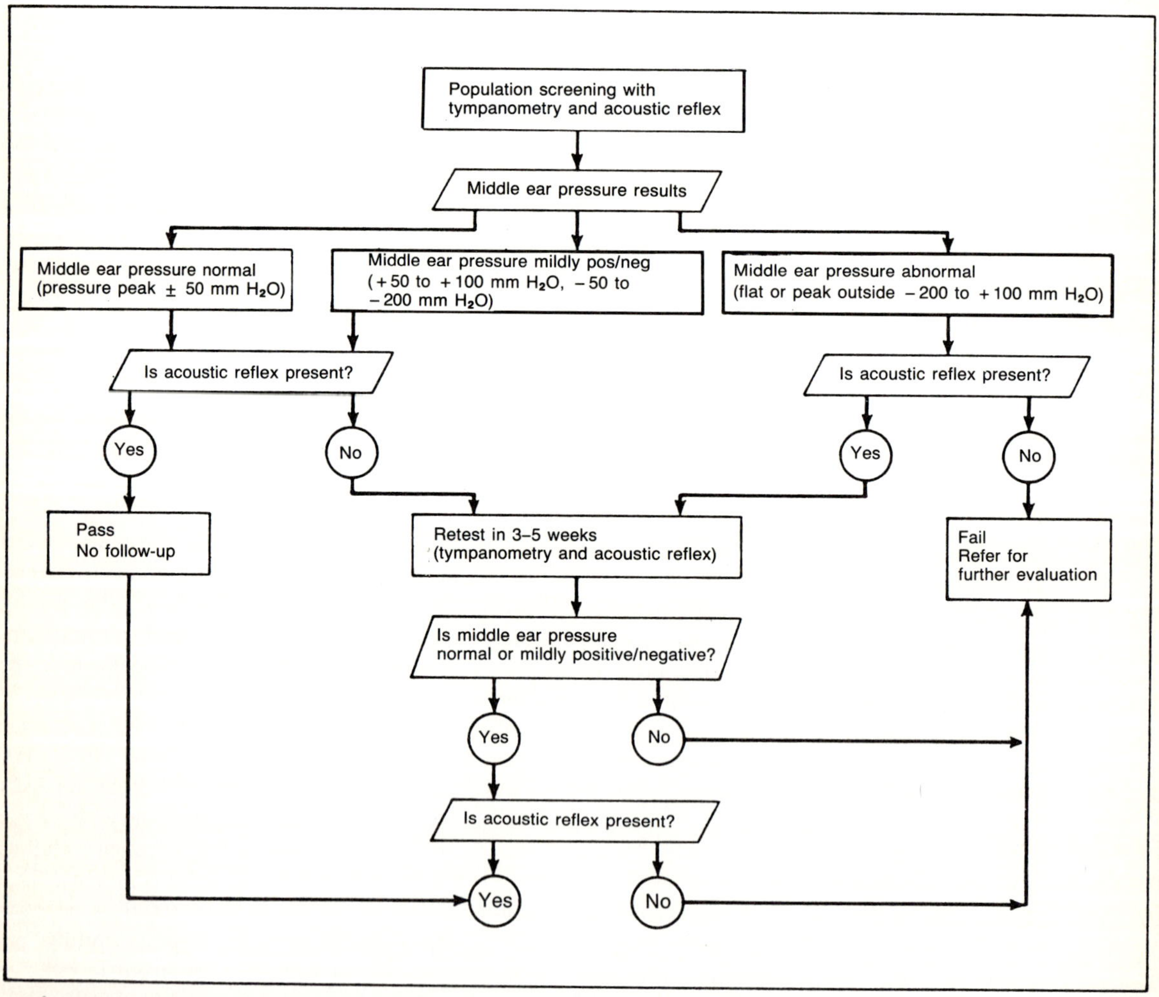

Figure 44–4 Flow chart depicting guidelines for impedance screening interpretation and pass-monitor-fail criteria. (Reproduced with permission from American Speech Language Hearing Association guidelines for acoustic immittance screening of middle ear function. Asha 1979; 2:287.)

TABLE 44–3 Summary of Nashville Symposium Guidelines for Impedance Screening

Classification	*Initial Screen*	*Retest*	*Subject Outcome*
1	Tympanogram: Normal* and Acoustic reflex: Present†	Not required	Cleared
2	Tympanogram: Abnormal‡ and/or Acoustic reflex: Absent†	Tympanogram: Abnormal‡ and/or Acoustic reflex: Absent†	Referred
3	Tympanogram: Abnormal‡ and/or Acoustic reflex: Absent†	Tympanogram: Normal* and/or Acoustic reflex: Present†	At risk—recheck at a later date

* Clear peak between +50 and −200 mm H_2O
† Contralateral or ipsilateral tone 1,000 Hz at 105 dB HL
‡ Flat or rounded, or negative pressure equivalent beyond −200 mm H_2O

absent, a referral for further evaluation is warranted.

The Nashville Task Force also recommended a set of guidelines for acoustic immittance screening which are summarized in Table 44–3.[72] The Task Force recommends using an air pressure range of −400 to +100 daPa and a 220 to 300 Hz probe tone for tympanometric testing. For the acoustic reflex test, a tone between 1,000 and 3,000 Hz at a level of 105 dB HL for contralateral stimulation and 105 dB SPL for ipsilateral stimulation, is recommended. When the tympanometric peak pressure is greater than or equal to −200 daPa and the acoustic reflex is present, the screening is passed. When the tympanometric configuration is flat or rounded or when peak tympanometric pressure is less than or equal to −200 daPa, the tympanogram is considered abnormal. If either the acoustic reflex is absent or the tympanogram is abnormal, a screening retest is recommended, and if the second screening is not passed, further testing is warranted.

The major difference between the two sets of guidelines lies in the referral criteria for further evaluation. ASHA recommends immediate referral if both the tympanogram and the acoustic reflex are abnormal. The Nashville guidelines, on the other hand, recommend rescreening 4 to 6 weeks after the initial test is failed. Several studies have attempted to evaluate the efficacy of these referral criteria. In general, when immittance measures are done concurrently with otoscopy, there appears to be reasonably good agreement between immittance results and medical findings. Schow et al applied ASHA's immittance screening protocol to a group of children seen for routine medical examinations in a pediatric office.[73] Their findings indicated an overall agreement of 73 percent with a false-positive rate of 16 percent and a false-negative rate of 5 percent. Other studies have shown that a lapse of several days between the screening and medical examination, as is often the case with school screening programs, may result in an excessive number of false-positive referrals, presumably due to spontaneous improvement during the interim. Using the ASHA guidelines, Lucker,[74] in a school-age population, and Roush and Tait,[75] in a preschool-age sample, predicted an overreferral rate in excess of 50 percent. Both studies predicted a substantial reduction in the number of false positives by employing a rescreening modification prior to medical referral. Specifically, children in ASHA's "fail" category were retested within 2 weeks of the initial screening, and children classified as being "at risk" were retested 4 to 6 weeks later. Queen et al, using a similar modification for screening a large group of school-age children, reported a reduction in referrals from approximately 17 percent to 6 percent by rescreening all children in the "fail" and "at risk" categories.[76] They further modified the ASHA criteria by eliminating the acoustic reflex except in cases showing "borderline" middle ear pressure, feeling that this procedure also tended to reduce specificity unnecessarily. Other investigators have found the acoustic reflex to be a useful supplement to tympanometric data.[73]

In summary, acoustic immittance screening appears to be an effective means of identifying middle ear disease in children. There is, however, a need for further research aimed at investigating the validity of existing protocols and their pass-fail criteria. A related need is the determination of whether tympanometric shape and acoustic reflex data should be included in these protocols. Some have advocated immediate referral of children displaying specific abnormalities in tympanometric configuration;[33,75] others have not found this practice useful in improving the agreement with medical findings.[73] There is similar lack of agreement with regard to the acoustic reflex; some have found the inclusion of this measure useful[73] whereas others have reported an increase in false-positive referrals.[76] Until more definitive conclusions can be reached, it seems advisable to rescreen all children prior to medical referral except for those who fail both the pure tone and acoustic immittance screenings. In such cases a direct medical referral is warranted. Those cleared on rescreening should still be considered "at risk" and followed periodically to identify any recurrence of middle ear disease.

IMPLEMENTATION OF THE SCREENING PROGRAM

Test Environment

The ideal test environment is a sound-treated booth that attenuates ambient noise at the frequencies to be tested. The allowable noise levels recommended by ANSI and the allowable ambient noise for screening according to the ASHA procedure are displayed in Table 44–4. If the ambient noise is above these levels, thresholds will be elevated and many will fail the screening inappropriately. The effect of ambient noise on threshold is greatest at the lower frequencies and is the primary reason ASHA recommends screening only at 1,000 Hz and above unless a sound-treated environment is available.[56]

When a test booth is not available, which is often the case when screening in schools, several alternatives may be considered. A mobile hearing screening unit may be purchased and moved from site to site. These units are specially constructed vans or trailers that house a sound-treated booth and audiometric equipment. However, they are costly and therefore not feasible for many school systems.

A less expensive alternative is to equip each screening audiometer with circumaural earphones. These earphones have large cushions that fit around the pinna and attenuate some ambient noise. When the test environment is fairly noisy, however, the amount of attenuation provided is usually inadequate. Furthermore, because of their bulkiness, circumaural earphones are impractical with small children.

When screening is to be done in a school, it is often possible to find a quiet area in the library or music room; however, it is important to determine how the ambient noise levels fluctuate during the day. A seemingly quiet environment may become quite noisy between class periods, at lunch time, or during recess. Other factors such as lighting, room size, visual distractions, air circulation, and location of electrical outlets must all be considered when selecting a screening site.

Test Equipment and Calibration

Pure tone audiometers are divided into three basic types: wide range, limited range, and narrow range.[77] All three types may be used for screening; however, narrow or limited range audiometers are typically designed for such use. For most applications, the screening audiometer need not be equipped to do bone conduction measurements, speech testing, or masking.

Audiometers used for screening should be sturdy and easily portable. Calibration is always critical but it becomes a particularly important consideration when an audiometer is moved frequently and exposed to a variety of environmental conditions. It is recommended that audiometers be checked annually for accuracy of frequency and temporal characteristics and that they be checked at least quarterly for accuracy of output levels.[78] A careful listening check should be completed at the beginning of each day, and a spare set of properly calibrated earphones should be readily available.

Portable acoustic immittance screening devices are also commercially available. Although some of the early models were difficult to use and prone to malfunction, most of the newer devices are easy to operate and reliable in performance. For screening purposes, a hand-held probe assembly is generally best. Most of the screening units can generate a hard copy and many are now equipped with a computer interface for automatic record keeping and retrieval.

TABLE 44–4 Allowable Ambient Noise Levels

Test Frequency *Octave Band Cutoff* *Frequencies*	*500* *300* *600*	*1,000* *600* *1,200*	*2,000* *1,200* *2,400*	*4,000* *2,400* *4,800*
Allowable ambient noise for threshold at Zero HL (re: ANSI-1969)[77]	26	30	38	51
Plus ASHA screening level re: ANSI-1969[77]	20	20	20	25
Resultant maximum ambient noise allowable for ASHA screening	46	50	58	76

Personnel

In many states, school screening programs are coordinated by the state department of health or education. These agencies may employ audiologists to screen children in rural areas or small school districts. Large districts often employ their own audiologists to conduct screening programs and to provide audiologic follow-up. The actual testing is often done by volunteers, school nurses, speech-language pathologists, or other school personnel. In these cases, an audiologist must be available to supervise the program and to train the examiners. It is imperative that each examiner be thoroughly trained in screening techniques, equipment maintenance, troubleshooting, interpretation of test results, and record keeping. Training should involve hands-on experience or field training. Table 44–5 contains a list of screening pitfalls that often encumber inexperienced examiners. Some states require examiners to participate regularly in a training course. It is recommended that all screening personnel participate in the training program so that the program's test procedures and philosophy are understood by all.

Counseling, Follow-up, and Record Keeping

When a child fails a screening test, the parents or guardians must be notified either by telephone or by mail. Direct mailing is preferable to sending the results home with the child or relying on school personnel to transmit the findings. The implications of hearing loss must be carefully explained to the parents; they should not be overly alarmed, but must be encouraged to seek appropriate follow-up. It is best to avoid using the term "failure" in reference to screening results. Instead, the parents and school personnel should be informed of a possible problem and the specific steps to be taken to follow up. Children suspected of having middle ear disease need a prompt medical examination, preferably by a physician specializing in diseases of the ear, nose, and throat (otolaryngologist). In such cases, it is generally advisable to have the parents consult with their pediatrician or family physician regarding the selection of an otolaryngologist. Children suspected of having a sensorineural hearing loss should be referred for a complete audiologic evaluation in conjunction with an otologic examination. If a permanent hearing loss is identified, ongoing audiologic management will be required and the parents will need careful counseling and guidance. Teachers should also be notified of the results as they can often provide valuable information with regard to daily classroom performance. Teachers can also assist in making appropriate changes in the child's listening environment while at school.

In school screening programs, careful records must be kept and audiologic or medical follow-up reports requested. Without information regarding

TABLE 44–5 Pitfalls to Avoid in Hearing and Immittance Screening

Pitfalls to Avoid in Hearing Screening	*Pitfalls to Avoid in Immittance Screening*
Child observing dials. This should be avoided at all times, because children will respond to the visual cues. The most appropriate position to seat the child is at an oblique angle, so the tester and audiometer are out of the child's peripheral vision.	Clogged probe and probe tip. The probe and probe tips must be kept free from earwax.
Examiner giving visual cues (facial expression, eye or head movements, etc.)	Probe tip too large or too small. Each ear canal is different and may require a different sized probe tip. Utilization of the correct size for each child will avoid possible errors.
Incorrect adjustment of the head band and earphone placement. Care must be taken to place the earphones carefully over the ears so that the protective screen mesh of the earphone diaphragm is directly over the entrance of the external auditory canal. Misplacement of the earphone by only one inch can cause as great as a 30–35 dB threshold shift.	Head movement, swallowing, or eye blinks. The child should be kept still during testing, as a sudden abnormal movement during testing may be interpreted as a reflex.
Vague instructions	Probe tip against ear canal wall. The probe tip must be inserted directly into the ear canal and when the canal is not straight, the tip must be kept away from the canal wall.
Noise in the test area	Debris in ear canal. The ear canal should be inspected before testing to ensure that it is clear.
Over-long test sessions. The screening should require only 3–5 minutes. If a child requires significantly more time than this, the routine screening should be discontinued and a short rest taken. If the child continues to be difficult to test, play conditioning should be used.	
Too long or too short a presentation of the test tone. The test stimulus should be presented for 1–2 sec. If the stimulus is for a shorter or longer time than this, inaccurate responses may be obtained.	

From Roser RJ, Northern JL. Screening for hearing loss and middle ear disorders. In: Roeser RJ, Downs MP, eds. Auditory disorders in school children. New York: Thieme-Stratton, 1981 with permission.

follow-up, effective educational planning and remediation cannot be accomplished and the success of a screening program cannot be evaluated. Examiners must ensure that records are well organized and up to date. Several forms for this purpose have been developed by Anderson[27] and by Barrett.[79] The use of a computerized data-base management system can be invaluable for record keeping and program evaluation.

Testing Strategies

Preschool Children

When screening preschool-age children, the goal is to identify a hearing loss that may have been previously overlooked or to identify the presence of a middle ear disorder. Because of the high incidence of otitis media in this age group, immittance screening is a particularly important component of the screening program. Pure tone screening tests should also be employed. Many of the older children may be able to respond using conventional pure tone testing methods. Younger children, however, require conditioning to play audiometry or localization to a sound source.

For screening children in the 1 to 3 year age range, portable speaker or tape recorder devices are available.[80,81] The child is seated on the parent's lap between two speakers situated at the child's ear level. The loudspeakers are connected to a cassette tape recorder that produces calibrated sound stimuli of varying frequency and intensity. The child is conditioned to turn his head toward the speaker from which the sound originated. A simpler version of this technique may be achieved by activating noisemakers such as rattles, bells, and squeeze toys; however, the loss of frequency specificity increases the potential for false-negative responses, especially in cases of high-frequency sensorineural loss.

For children in the 3 to 5 year age range, conditioned play audiometry is generally the technique of choice. A bucket and blocks or other small objects are assembled and the child is conditioned to place an object in the bucket whenever a tone is heard. Once the child is properly conditioned, the frequencies to be tested may be presented at 20 or 25 dB HL in each ear to complete the screening. Most children condition fairly easily to this procedure and it need not be time-consuming.

School-age Children

The goal in screening school-age children is to identify educationally-handicapping hearing losses. Even a very mild degree of hearing loss may interfere with a child's ability to develop the skills necessary to succeed academically. Immittance screening should be used as a means of identifying middle ear pathology, and traditional pure-tone screening testing should be used to identify hearing impairment.

It is recommended by ASHA that children through grade three be screened yearly. After grade three, the data available are not clear as to how often screening should be provided. After evaluating data from 14,800 high school students, Downs, Doster, and Weaver reported that the number of individuals with previously undetected hearing loss was minimal.[82] However, other studies have demonstrated that the incidence of high frequency hearing loss (4,000 to 6,000 Hz) increases in the upper grades, especially in males. Each program will need to evaluate the feasibility of screening beyond grade three based on its own experience and availability of resources.

ASHA recommends that certain populations be tested annually regardless of age. These include the following groups:

1. Students who repeat a grade
2. All students who are new to the school or district
3. Students who missed a previous screening test
4. Students with speech or language difficulties
5. Students returning to school after a serious illness
6. Students enrolled in remedial programs
7. Students referred by a teacher for hearing testing.

SUMMARY

The specific design of a screening program will require adaptation to each individual set of circumstances. However, there are some fundamental guidelines that should be considered when planning a program of identification audiometry. It is important to remember that pure tone and acoustic immittance tests differ significantly in their underlying purpose. Though pure tone screening is useful in identifying children with educationally significant hearing loss, it is largely ineffective as a means of identifying middle ear disease. Likewise, tympanometric measurements are unaffected by hearing sensitivity and are, therefore, of no value in detecting the presence of hearing loss. A comprehensive screening program includes both pure tone and acoustic immittance measures for children at the preschool and lower elementary levels. Immittance screening can be omitted in the upper grade levels where the incidence of middle ear disease is far lower.

Pure tone screening should be carried out in a relatively quiet environment, free from visual distractions and other disturbances. The test frequencies should include 1,000 and 2,000 Hz at a presentation level of 20 dB and 4,000 Hz at a level of 25 dB. Children who fail the pure tone screening at any frequency should be rescreened, preferably on the same day but within 2 weeks of the initial screening. Those who fail the rescreening should be referred to an audiologist for complete assessment, and if found to have a sensorineural hearing loss, referred also for otologic examination. Acoustic immittance should include tympanometric measurements from −300 to +200 daPa, and children exhibiting abnormal patterns should be rescreened in 2 to 4 weeks. Those exhibiting abnormal findings on rescreening should be referred for medical examination, preferably by an otologist. Individuals who fail the initial screening but pass the follow-up test should be monitored periodically to check for recurrence of middle ear disease. Direct medical referral without rescreening is advisable only if the child fails both the pure tone and acoustic immittance screening. Regardless of the outcome, written notice of the screening results should be provided for the child's parents and teacher.

The potentially serious implications of undetected hearing loss and middle ear disease affirm the importance of appropriate identification audiometry. With careful planning and implementation, a hearing and immittance screening program can be a highly rewarding and cost-effective endeavor.

REFERENCES

1. National Conference on Identification Audiometry. Baltimore, 1966. (Annotation made during opening speech).
2. Eisen NH. Some effects of early sensory deprivation on later behavior: the quondom hard-of-hearing child. J Abnorm Soc Psychol 1962; 65:338.
3. Holm VA, Kunze LH. Effect of chronic otitis media on language and speech development. Pediatrics 1969; 43:833–839.
4. Needleman H. Effect of hearing loss from early otitis media on speech and language development. In: Jaffe B, ed. Hearing loss in children. Baltimore: University Park Press, 1977.
5. Katz J. The effects of conductive hearing loss on auditory function Asha 1978; 20:879–886.
6. Zinkus PW, Gottlieb MI, Schapiro M. Developmental and psychoeducational sequelae of chronic otitis media. Am J Dis Child 1978; 132:1100–1104.
7. Mustain WD. Linguistic and educational implications of recurrent otitis media. Ear Nose Throat J 1979; 58:218–222.
8. Ruben RJ, Hanson DG. Summary of discussion and recommendations made during the workshop on otitis media and development. Ann Otol Rhinol Laryngol 1979; 88:107–111.
9. Downs MP. Identification of children at risk for middle ear effusion problems. Ann Otol Rhinol Laryngol 1980; 89:168–171.
10. Brandes PJ, Ehinger DM. The effects of early middle ear pathology on auditory perception and academic achievement. J Speech Hear Disord 1981; 46:301–307.
11. Welsh LW, Welsh JJ, Healy MP. Effect of sound deprivation on central hearing. Laryngoscope 1983; 93:1569–1575.
12. Rapin I. Conductive hearing loss effects on children's language and scholastic skills. A review of the literature. Ann Otol Rhinol Laryngol 1969; Suppl. 88:60.
13. Ventry IM. Effects of conductive hearing loss: fact or fiction. J Speech Hear Disord 1980; 45:143–156.
14. Menyuk P. Design factors in the assessment of language development in children with otitis media. Ann Otol Rhinol Laryngol 1979; 88:78–87.
15. Menyuk P. Effect of persistent otitis media on language development. Ann Otol Rhinol Laryngol 1980; 89:257–263.
16. Ayukawa H, Rudmin F. Letter to the editor: Does early middle ear pathology affect auditory perception skills and learning? Comment on Brandes and Ehinger. J Speech Hear Disord 1981; 48:222–223.
17. Allen DV, Robinson DO. Middle ear status and language development in preschool children. Asha 1984; 26:33–37.
18. Lenneberg EH. Biological foundations of language. New York: John Wiley & Sons, 1967.
19. Northern JL, Downs MP. Hearing in children. 3rd ed. Baltimore: Williams & Wilkins, 1984.
20. Tees RC. Effects of early auditory restriction in the rat on adult pattern discrimination. J Comp Physiol Psychol 1967; 63:389–393.
21. Batkin S, Groth H, Watson JR, et al. Effects of auditory deprivation in the development of auditory sensitivity in albino rats. Electroencephalogr Clin Neurophysiol 1970; 28:351–359.
22. Silverman MS, Clopton BM. Plasticity of binaural interaction. I. Effect of early auditory deprivation. J Neurophysiol 1977; 40(6):1266–1274.
23. Clopton BM, Silverman MS. Plasticity of binaural interaction. II. Clinical period and changes in midline response. J Neurophysiol 1977; 40(6):1275–1280.
24. Webster DM, Webster M. Neonatal sound deprivation affects brainstem auditory nuclei. Arch Otolaryngol 1977; 103:392–396.
25. Webster DM, Webster M. Effects of neonatal conductive hearing loss on brainstem auditory nuclei. Ann Otol Rhinol Laryngol 1979; 88:684–688.
26. Moscicki EK. The prevalence of "incidence" is too high. Asha 1984; 26:39–40.
27. Anderson CV. Conservation of hearing. In Katz J, ed. Handbook of clinical audiology. 2nd ed. Baltimore: Williams & Wilkins, 1978.
28. Silverman RS, Lane HS, Calvert DR. Early and elementary education. In: Silverman RS, Davis H, eds. Hearing and deafness. New York: Holt, Rinehart, & Winston, 1978.
29. Eagles EL, Wishik SM, Doerfler LG. Hearing sensitivity and ear disease in children: a prospective study. Laryngoscope 1967 (Monograph) :1–274.
30. Connor LE. Determining the prevalence of hearing impaired children. Except Child 1961; 27:337–344.
31. Robinson GC, Anderson DO, Mogohodam HK, et al. A survey of hearing loss in Vancouver school children: methodology and prevalence. Can Med Assoc J 1967; 97: 1199–1207.
32. Fay TH, Hochberg I, Smith CR, et al. Audiologic and otologic screening of disadvantaged children. In: Glorig A, Gerwin K, eds. Otitis media. Springfield, IL: CC Thomas, 1972.
33. Roeser RJ, Northern JL. Screening for hearing loss and middle ear disorders. In: Roeser RJ, Downs MP, eds. Auditory disorders in school children. New York: Thieme-Stratton, 1981.
34. Vinther B, Pederson CB, Elbrond O. Otitis media in childhood. Sociomedical aspects with special reference to day-care conditions. Clin Otolaryngol 1984; 9:3–8.
35. Kaplan GY, Fleshman JK, Bender TR, et al. Long-term effects of otitis media: a ten year cohort study of Alaskan Eskimo children. Pediatrics 1973; 52:577–585.

36. Van Wagoner RS, Chun TH. Hearing loss in Southeast Alaska. Alaska Med 1974; 16:61–63.
37. Lewis, C. The Montana otitis media project. Hear Instruments 1975; 26:21–22.
38. McCandless GA. Screening for middle ear disease on the Wind River Indian Reservation. Hear Instruments 1975; 26:19–20.
39. Johnson JS, Watrous BS. An acoustic impedance screening program with an American Indian population. In: Harford ER, Bess FH, Bluestone CD, et al. Impedance screening for middle ear disease in children. New York: Grune & Stratton, 1978.
40. Pannbacker M. Hearing loss and cleft palate. Cleft Palate J 1969; 6:50–56.
41. Yules RB. Hearing in cleft patients. Arch Otolaryngol 1970; 91:319–323.
42. Downs MP, ed. Communication disorders in Down's syndrome. Semin Speech Lang Hear 1980; 1:1.
43. Weber HJ, McGovern FJ, Fink D. An evaluation of 1,000 children with hearing loss. J Speech Hear Disord 1967; 32:343–354.
44. Hull FM, Meilke PW Jr, Timmons RJ, et al. The national speech and hearing survey: preliminary results. Asha 1971; 13:501-509.
45. Northern JL. Impedance screening in special populations: state of the art. In: Harford ER, Bess FH, Bluestone CD, et al. Impedance screening for middle ear disease in children. New York: Grune & Stratton, 1978.
46. Darley FL, ed. Identification audiometry. J Speech Hear Disord 1961:Monograph 9.
47. Standards for educational and psychological tests. Washington, DC: American Psychological Association, 1974.
48. Anastasi A. Psychological testing. 4th ed. New York: Macmillan, 1976.
49. Jerger S. Decision matrix and information theory analysis in the evaluation of neuroaudiological tests. Semin Hear 1983; 4:121–132.
50. Fowler FP, Fletcher H. Three million deafened school children: their detection and treatment. JAMA 1926; 87:1877–1882.
51. Bennett SM. A group test of hearing for six-year-old children. Br J Educ Psychol 1951:45-52.
52. Meyerson L. Hearing for speech in children: a verbal audiometric test. Acta Otolaryngol 1956; Suppl. 128:1–165.
53. Griffing CS, Simonton KM, Hedgecock LD. Verbal auditory screening for pre-school children. Trans Am Acad Opthalmology Otolaryngol 1967; 71:105–111.
54. Mencher GT, McCullock BF. Auditory screening of kindergarten children using the VASC. J Speech Hear Disord 1970; 35:241–247.
55. Newhart HA. A new pure tone audiometer for school use. Arch Otolaryngol 1938; 28:778–779.
56. ASHA committee on audiometric evaluation guidelines for identification audiometry. Asha 1975; 17:94–99.
57. Wilson WR, Walton WK. Identification audiometry accuracy: evaluation of a recommended program for school-age children. Lang Speech Hearing Serv Schools 1974; 5:8–12.
58. House HP, Glorig A. A new concept in auditory screening. Laryngoscope 1957; 67:661–668.
59. Siegenthaler BM, Sommers RK. Abbreviated sweep check procedures for school hearing testing. J Speech Hear Disord 1959; 24:249–257.
60. Maxwell WR, Davidson GD. Limited frequency screening and ear pathology. J Speech Hear Disord 1961; 26:122–125.
61. Norton MC, Lux E. Double frequency auditory screening in public schools. J Speech Hear Disord 1961; 26:293–299.
62. Stevens DA, Davidson GD. Screening tests of hearing. J Speech Hear Disord 1959; 24:258–261.
63. Reger SN, Newby HA. A group pure-tone hearing test. J Speech Hear Disord 1947; 12:61–66.
64. Johnston PW. The Massachusetts hearing test. J Acoust Soc Am 1948; 20:697–703.
65. DiCarlo LM, Gardner EF. The efficiency of the Massachusetts pure-tone screening test as adapted for a university testing program. J Speech Hear Disord 1953; 18:175–182.
66. Johnston PW. An efficient group screening test. J Speech Hear Disord 1952; 17:8–12.
67. Wilson WR, Walton WK. Public school audiometry. In: Martin FN, ed. Pediatric audiology. Englewood Cliffs, NJ: Prentice-Hall, 1978.
68. Bess FH, McConnell FE. Audiology, education, and the hearing impaired child. St. Louis: CV Mosby, 1981.
69. Simons MR. Acoustic impedance tests. In: Goodhill V, ed. Ear diseases, deafness, and dizziness. Hagerstown, MD: Harper & Row, 1979.
70. Klein JO. Epidemiology of otitis media. In: Harford ER, et al, eds. Impedance screening for middle ear disease in children. New York: Grune & Stratton, 1978.
71. American Speech Language Hearing Association guidelines for acoustic immittance screening of middle-ear function. Asha 1979; 21:283–288.
72. Harford ER, Bess FH, Bluestone CD, Klein JO. Impedance screening for middle ear disease in children. New York: Grune & Stratton, 1978.
73. Schow RL, Pederson JK, Nerbonne MA, Boe R. Comparison of ASHA's immittance guidelines and standard medical diagnostic procedures. Ear Hear 1981; 2(6):251–255.
74. Lucker JR. Application of pass-fail criteria to middle ear screening results. Asha 1980; 22:289.
75. Roush J, Tait C. Pure tone and acoustic immittance screening of preschool-age children: an examination of referral criteria. Ear Hear 1985; 6(5):245–249.
76. Queen S, Moses F, Wood S. The use of immittance screening by the Kansas City, Missouri Public School District. Semin Speech Lang Hear 1981; 2:119.
77. Specifications for audiometers. American National Standards Institute. Specifications for audiometers. ANSI S3.6. New York: ANSI, 1969.
78. Wilber LA. Calibration: puretone, speech and noise signals. In: Katz J, ed. Handbook of clinical audiology. 3rd ed. Baltimore: Williams & Wilkins, 1985.
79. Barrett K. Hearing and immittance screening of school-age children. In: Katz J, ed. Handbook of clinical audiology. 3rd ed. Baltimore: Williams & Wilkins, 1985.
80. Horton KB. Infant cassette screener. Nashville, TN: The Bill Wilkerson Speech and Hearing Center, 1972. (Bureau of Education for the Handicapped Outreach Project, Grant No. 900760441).
81. Weber H. Infant visual reinforcement unit. Denver: Colorado Hearing Systems Inc, 1985.
82. Downs MP, Doster ME, Weaver, M. Dilemmas in identification audiometry. J Speech Hear Disord 1965; 30:360–364.

45 Central Auditory Tests

Robert W. Keith, Ph.D.

Our purpose in this chapter is to provide a basic understanding of the principles that apply to the measurement of central auditory function when diagnosing lesions of the central auditory pathways or identifying auditory perceptual dysfunction. This chapter is intended to serve as a reference source for graduate students in the field of speech and hearing and for graduates who may not have had formal training in this interesting area. We have tried to keep in mind advice overheard in conversation between two people in an airport lobby that "when you write for students you are writing for the future—not for today's practitioner." Thus, we have included some basic information about the principles of central hearing tests that continues to be applicable. The chapter includes a discussion of anatomy, definitions of some terminology of auditory abilities, and some factors that influence central hearing test results. A few of the current tests of central auditory function are reviewed out of a need to discuss the state of the art. Some of these tests may fall into disuse in the future as better procedures are developed, but they will have served to point the way.

The final section is on auditory perceptual problems in children. This subject is still poorly understood. However, more professionals have become interested in this difficult area, and our understanding of auditory perceptual dysfunction is increasing. Provided that this trend continues, a revision of this section may soon be required.

Although the evaluation of the central auditory nervous system has been possible for many years, with original studies beginning during the 1950s, widespread interest in central hearing testing is just beginning to emerge in the mainstream practice of audiology. Central auditory testing began with a few individuals who had the insight and curiosity to develop new ideas and who were able to point the way for others. Unfortunately, some of the early investigators had too little vision. For example, Alajouanine et al[1] wrote that "an audiometric symptomatology of disorders at the level of cortical activity centers has to be considered impossible." That unfortunate epitaph should be remembered by any student who may feel that there are no frontiers remaining in audiology, because in that same year Bocca et al[2] demonstrated that temporal lobe tumors resulted in decreased performance to sensitized speech tests. Other authors have expressed greater expectation for the future of central hearing testing, including Matzker,[3] who stated that "the assessment of pathological changes within the central auditory pathways will gain more and more importance in the future."

Acceptance of the clinical importance of central hearing tests has come slowly. Carhart's[4] comment, that "tests for central auditory dysfunction . . . are often viewed as esoteric curiosities rather than as tools holding serious promise for improved diagnosis," holds as true now as it did in 1969. Nevertheless, the accumulating knowledge of central auditory processes and the results of tests using various audiologic batteries indicate that central hearing testing has an increasingly valuable role for identifying auditory pathway lesions, for describing auditory perceptual abilities, and for remediation.

NEUROANATOMY

Tests of central auditory function are best understood with knowledge of the anatomy and physiology of the central auditory nervous system (CANS). The reader is referred to Chapter 2 of this book for reviews of anatomy and physiology. In addition, the reader may wish to review other descriptions that have appeared recently.[5–8] Briefly, the CANS is a complex and diffuse system of interconnecting neural pathways with afferent and efferent connections between cochlea and cortex (Fig. 45–1). Electrical signals generated in the hair cells of the organ of Corti travel through the auditory portion of the eighth cranial nerve into the medulla of the

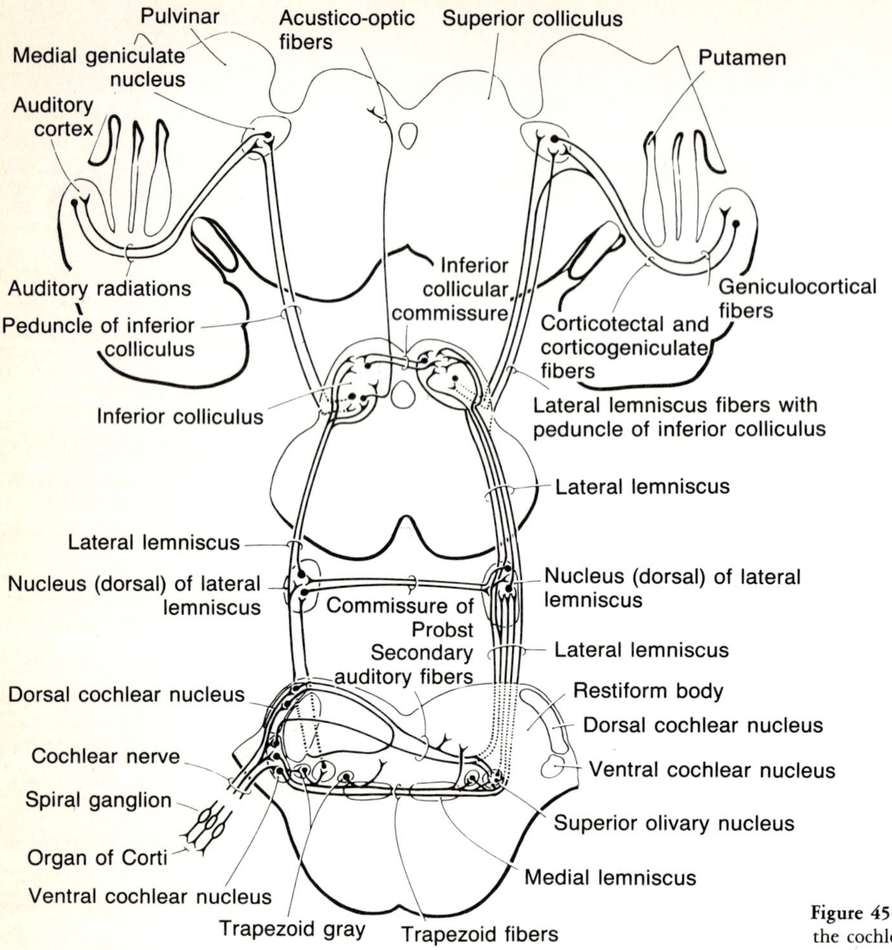

Figure 45–1 Auditory pathway from the cochlea to the cerebral cortex.

brain stem where most fibers terminate in one of the subdivisions of the cochlear nucleus complex. Some fibers of the auditory nerve ascend to the ipsilateral superior olivary complex. Three bundles of fibers arise from the cochlear nuclei; the trapezoid body, the striae (lines) of Manakow, and the striae of Held. A direct ascending pathway lies between the cochlear nuclei and the inferior colliculus on the contralateral side. Another ascending pathway goes from the cochlear nuclei, through the trapezoid body, to the contralateral superior olivary complex. Fibers from the cochlear nuclei project to the cerebellar vermis and the ipsilateral superior olive. Because the superior olivary complex receives innervation from both cochlear nuclei, it is the first place in the ascending auditory nervous system to receive acoustic information from both ears. Binaural interaction has been found to occur in individual neurons of the medial superior olive.[9]

The lateral lemniscus receives fibers from the contralateral cochlear nuclei and ipsilateral superior olive. Most of these fibers terminate in the inferior colliculus. The ascending pathway continues as the brachium of the inferior colliculus that terminates in the medial geniculate body. Some fibers cross the midline as the commissure of the inferior colliculus to join the two inferior colliculi.

The main afferent flow from the medial geniculate body forms the thalamocortical connections with primary termination in the temporal lobe of the cortex, specifically anterior, transverse, temporal gyri (Heschl's convolutions), which is area 41 of Brodmann. Other areas of the cortex are stimulated by auditory signals, but they may not be strictly auditory areas, because they are also activated by other sensory stimuli. The auditory reception areas of the two temporal cortices appear to be interconnected through neural pathways that lie in the splenium of the corpus callosum.

The afferent auditory system is structured in such a way that tonotopic organization is maintained at each level of the auditory system from cochlea to cortex. That is, the spatial frequency arrangement of high to low tones running from base to apex of the cochlear partition is maintained from cochlear nucleus to temporal cortex.

Tonotopic organization is only one of the many neural functions provided by the CANS in analyzing incoming sound. It appears that single neural units are individually tuned to provide a frequency selectivity of response. A neural unit not only has its best frequency of response, but also responds to other frequencies provided that they are at higher intensities. Analysis of sound also occurs in neurons that are sensitive to variations in interaural phase relations. Some neurons are activated by one ear yet are inhibited by the other ear, and inhibition of one stimulus may occur as a result of second stimulus. Some neural units respond more readily to tones that change in frequency than to steady tones, and some units respond to tones rising in frequency whereas others respond to a lowering in frequency. The rate of neural firing also changes with intensity. With continued high-intensity input, adaptation of response occurs.

An efferent auditory system also exists with descending pathways beginning as projections from the auditory cortex and continuing throughout the system. The efferent pathways include the colliculocochlear bundle, the olivocochlear bundle, and the recurrent fiber tract. They provide "marked efferent innervation of the organ of Corti" to both the inner and outer hair cells.[10] The presence of an efferent system suggests a feedback loop that may act as a regulatory system to aid in stimulus sorting.[11]

At least two auditory reflexes exist. One provides for turning of the head and eyes toward the source of sound. That reflex pathway originates from connections between the inferior and superior colliculi going to nuclei in the brain stem, which controls head and eye movement. A second reflex occurs between the superior olivary bodies and the motor nuclei of the trigeminal and facial nerves for contraction of the tensor tympani and stapedial muscles in the middle ear.

The functional significance of each substation of the CANS is only partially known. Studies on animals have shown that destruction of the auditory cortex does not substantially impair an animal's threshold for pure tones or its ability to localize the source of sound. Localization appears to result from analysis that occurs lower in the auditory system, probably at the level of the superior olivary complex, and binaural integration of incoming signals probably first occurs at that level. Interaction among auditory and other sensory inputs may occur at the level of the medial geniculate body, and other integrative functions are suggested by connections between the cochlear nuclei and cerebellum. In addition, an alerting or activating function is implied from connections with the reticular formation.

The auditory cortex is unquestionably involved in auditory perceptual processes, including the final analysis and interpretation of sound, and association of sound with meaning. Human language functions appear to be related primarily to the left hemisphere in most individuals, although the right hemisphere is also capable of interpreting speech. In some persons it is normal for the right hemisphere to be dominant for speech, especially when they are left-handed.

Clearly only the most brief details have been provided for a highly complex and beautifully organized sensory system. Although mysteries remain as to how auditory analysis is finally accomplished, the auditory system presents a complex interaction of neural signals at nearly all levels of the CANS, from the superior olivary complex to the auditory cortex. Moreover, the neural pathways are not simply passive conductors of an electrical signal, but analysis takes place at all levels of the auditory system from cochlea to cortex. Although the ascending auditory pathway is often regarded as a crossed pathway, with sound to one ear primarily stimulating the opposite temporal lobe, the opportunity for crossover of auditory information through several commissures creates some difficulty in localizing sites of auditory damage.

CENTRAL AUDITORY ABILITIES

When considering central auditory abilities, it is useful to differentiate results that occur from monaural versus binaural stimulation. The auditory system comprises two independent neurologic channels. Each channel can process speech adequately to achieve intelligibility, and the normal listener can listen selectively with one ear or the other. Binaural reception of incoming sound has distinct advantages over monaural reception, however, both for intelligibility of speech and for spatial orientation. In a discussion of binaural reception, Carhart[12] pointed out that binaural stimulation results in improved auditory thresholds through summation, yielding a steeper articulation gain function and improved speech discrimination of quiet sounds over monaural stimulation. Binaural stimulation also facilitates listening to speech in noise and results in a reduction in the disturbing subjective experience of background noise. When competing sounds are present, binaural hearing is necessary for the separation of sound sources. In fact, binaural hearing is necessary both for localizing the source of sound and for three-dimensional orientation in acoustic space.

Carhart pointed out that binaural reception does not increase the capacity of the listener to handle information, because the amount of auditory information that a listener can assimilate is limited. In a report of experiments on auditory perception,

Broadbent[13] stated that an individual can monitor sensory information from many sources simultaneously but, when informational content from one of the channels is either very high or very important, the organism attends to that and discards information that is, at the time of reception, irrelevant. The reader can identify with that concept by considering, for example, what it is like to take a final examination in college. In such a situation the information received visually on paper is so important that the student is generally unaware of either the environment or background sounds.

In audition, the listener who attends to a primary message may not be able to give back information about a distracting message, or the listener who listens intently with one ear is unable to specify what was presented to the opposite ear. The inability to attend selectively to one stimulus may create learning problems, a subject that will be discussed later in this chapter.

The specific auditory abilities that result from anatomic and physiologic characteristics of the auditory system are highly complex and interrelated. Unfortunately, authors define terms differently, and the lack of standardization of terminology leads to misunderstanding among workers in the field and to poor communication of test results.[14] Nevertheless, an analysis of auditory abilities is necessary to aid systematic thinking about higher auditory properties. Additional discussion of auditory abilities is included in Chapter 10 in this book.

The building blocks of audition are frequency, intensity, and time, and their psychological correlates are pitch, loudness, and duration. Assuming normal perception of these parameters and a normal peripheral auditory mechanism, it is possible to determine those auditory abilities that are central in nature. The following terms appear on many authors' lists of central auditory abilities.

Localization. The ability to locate auditorily the source of sound. This ability requires binaural hearing.

Binaural Synthesis. The ability to integrate centrally incomplete stimulus patterns presented simultaneously or alternately to opposite ears.

Figure Ground. The ability to identify a primary signal or message in the presence of competing sounds. This term was initially used in relation to vision. Auditorily, the task may be more difficult, because both the primary and competing sounds change their acoustic features continually over time. Auditory figure ground can be a monaural or a binaural task.

Binaural Separation. The ability to listen with one ear while ignoring stimulation of the opposite ear. Dichotic listening, as a binaural separation task requires the listener to attend to, and report back, different signals presented simultaneously to two ears.

Memory. The ability to store and to recall auditory stimuli, including the ability to recall the length or number of auditory stimuli; and sequential memory, or the ability to recall the exact order of auditory stimuli presented.

Blending. The ability to form words out of separately articulated phonemes.

Discrimination. The ability to determine whether two acoustic stimuli are the same or different. In speech, auditory discrimination is the ability to recognize fine differences that exist among phonemes.

Closure. The ability to perceive the whole (word or message) when parts are omitted.

Attention. The ability to persist in listening over a reasonable period.

Association. The ability to establish a correspondence between a nonlinguistic sound and its source.

Cognition. The ability to establish a correspondence between a linguistic sound and its meaning. Cognition is the highest level of auditory perception and results from a summation of all auditory (and all sensory) tasks.

This list is intended to include those central auditory abilities that are most frequently measured by tests of central auditory function. It is not intended to be complete, because various authors have identified subskills of auditory abilities, and perhaps even subskills of subskills.

CONSIDERATIONS BEFORE ADMINISTRATION OF CENTRAL HEARING TESTS

Any discussion of central hearing tests is complicated by a need to define the terminology being used, the population to whom the test is to be administered, and finally, the purpose for which the tests are intended. The process of definition is an exclusive one, because the concept of central processing is so inclusive. One current problem with the use of the term "central auditory dysfunction" is that its understanding depends upon who uses the label. Butler* pointed out that "audiologists," "speech language pathologists," and "teachers" each have a perspective. The audiologists' past "anatomic" perspective has differed from the speech language pathologists' "cognitive" perspective that stresses information-processing strategies. Special education and

---

* Butler K, personal communication.

learning disability teachers talk about auditory processing disorders and often do not engage in the debate about the centrality of the disorder they are observing. Thus, they look at auditory processing disorders in terms such as difficulty in following oral directions and failure to comprehend academic instructions. Another problem with definitions is that many auditory abilities are so highly correlated that it is nearly impossible to test one ability in isolation. Also the lack of an agreed definition of auditory perceptual disorders means that no one can publish valid data on the prevalence of auditory perceptual problems in adults, and so the rate of false positive identification of a central lesion is unknown. Finally, the strong emphasis on assessing auditory processing abilities in children for educational purposes has, until the introduction of the Pediatric Speech Intelligibility Test,[15] overshadowed the question of identifying auditory pathway lesions in that age group. When to counsel parents to seek a medical opinion regarding possible lesions, and when to advise that the child's problem is primarily educational is a difficult clinical problem. The sensitive clinician should be aware of these issues and find the balance between unnecessarily alarming parents that auditory processing difficulties imply that a dangerous lesion exists and failing to recognize the potential significance of deteriorating symptoms. Children with progressive neurological symptoms or deterioration of auditory processing abilities should be referred to an appropriate physician for diagnostic evaluation.

Another problem arises when attempts are made to isolate auditory skills as already defined. Witkin et al[16] point out that auditory processing tasks are, by nature, complex and overlapping. Given the high intercorrelation among auditory perceptual tasks, it is virtually impossible to test auditory skills independently.

Wiig and Semel[17] listed questions to ask when selecting a comprehensive test battery.

Content Validity. Does the test measure the specific skill that the examiner wishes to probe?

Reliability. Is the test consistent on retest? Is it internally consistent with high split-half reliability? Do items from any two halves of a test, when scored independently, yield equivalent results?

Efficiency. Does the test provide for economy of time in administration and scoring?

Task Analysis. Does the test require a cross-modality response, for example, between visual and auditory modes? If so, which modality is actually being tested? Does the task involve recognition, memory, linguistic processing, etc.?

Age Level. Is the age range from which the test was designed appropriate for the person being tested?

We propose some additions to Wiig and Semel's list.

Sensitivity. Does the test correctly identify those people who have central auditory dysfunction? Sensitivity is defined as the percent of individuals with a certain problem who are so specified by the test. It is designated in percent as a ratio of true-positive over the sum of true-positive plus false-negative identifications (Table 45–1).

Specificity. Does the test correctly identify those people who have normal auditory function? Specificity is defined as the percent of individuals who do not have a certain problem and who are so specified by the test, and is designated in percent as a ratio of true-negative over the sum of true-negative plus false-positive identifications (see Table 45–1).

Normative Data. Were norms developed on random samples of adequate size? Are normative data available for subjects of both sexes and various age and socioeconomic levels? Use of norms should be restricted to subjects represented in the normative population.

PRINCIPLES OF DIAGNOSTIC TESTING

A majority of speech measures that assess the CANS are based on the principle of redundancy expressed by Bocca et al.[18] That principle, as reviewed by Teatini,[19] is shown in Table 45–2. According to the model shown in this table, the acoustic properties of speech are redundant, because there is normally a broader range of frequencies, greater amplitude, longer duration, and more favorable speech-to-noise ratio (S:N) than is minimally required for understanding speech. Redundancies of speech can be reduced a number of ways including filtering, interrupting, or time-compressing the message, and lowering S:N.

Similarly, following "the principle of physiologic safety,"[19] the intrinsic or neuroanatomic pathways are usually redundant. Table 45–2 could be expanded to show that when extrinsic redundancy is normal but the intrinsic redundancy of the subject is reduced, speech intelligibility is again rather good. By implication nondistorted speech is unable to detect lesions of the CANS. Therefore, sensitized speech tests (i.e., those with reduced redundancy) are required for diagnostic testing.

Two additional concepts are helpful when considering central hearing tests; the "subtlety" and the "bottleneck" principles.[20,21] The first of these states that the subtlety of the auditory manifestation increases as the site of lesion progresses from periph-

TABLE 45–1 Evaluating the Accuracy of a Test or Diagnostic Examination: Sensitivity and Specificity

	Population	
Test Results	*With Problem*	*Without Problem*
Positive	Have Problem Have Positive Test = True (TP)	No Problem but Have Positive Results = False Positives (FP)
Negative	Have Problem but Have Negative Test = False (FN)	No Problem Have Negative Test = True Negatives (TN)
	Sensitivity (in %) = $\frac{TP}{TP + FN} \times 100$	Specificity (in %) = $\frac{TN}{TN + FP} \times 100$

eral to central. At a peripheral level the presence of a lesion may be demonstrated with relatively simple tests such as a pure tone threshold measure. At more central sites the presence of a lesion can be demonstrated only by means of considerably more subtle auditory tasks, such as sensitized speech tests.

The bottleneck principle states that a complex auditory stimulus, such as speech, encounters a point of neural congestion at the eighth nerve and brain stem. Although lesions at those sites markedly reduce the ability to understand speech, lesions more peripheral or central have relatively less effect on speech discrimination ability. The subtlety and bottleneck principles were suggested by Jerger[20,21] several years ago to serve as "guideposts for further research," and their general applicability has not changed.

FACTORS AFFECTING CENTRAL AUDITORY TEST RESULTS

Several auditory and nonauditory factors can affect the results of central auditory tests. If misinterpreted, these factors can lead to a false impression of central auditory dysfunction. In a review of these factors, Davis et al[22] include peripheral hearing loss, age, intelligence, use of prescribed drugs, and the subject's linguistic background. To that list could be added poor motivation and poor confidence to guess.

TABLE 45–2 Diagnostic Principles of Intrinsic and Extrinsic Redundancy

Extrinsic		*Intrinsic*		
Redundancy of Message	→	Redundancy of Subject	→	Intelligibility
Normal		Normal		Good
Reduced		Normal		Rather good
Reduced		Reduced		Poor

Regarding peripheral hearing loss, Davis et al stated that the effect of a conductive loss can generally be counteracted by increasing the intensity at which tests are administered.[22] Katz,[23] however, has reported that a substantial number of reversals can occur on the Staggered Spondaic Word (SSW) test when a conductive loss is present, leading to the impression of a central auditory dysfunction.

Sensorineural hearing impairments have significant effects on central auditory tests, and often compromise the interpretation of the results.[24–26] According to Lynn and Gilroy,[27] the presence of a sensorineural hearing loss must be considered when attempting to attach significance to an abnormal central test score, and at times the status of the central auditory system cannot be accurately assessed because of peripheral contamination. In addition, the Jergers* state that they have not been very successful when administering central tests in the face of asymmetrical peripheral hearing sensitivity. While the SSW test manual provides instruction for correction of raw scores to reduce the effects of cochlear-based word discrimination errors on central test findings, that correction has been disputed by some clinicians.[27] In 1983, Fifer et al[28] published a dichotic sentence identification test designed for use with hearing impaired adults. Mueller et al[29] found that

* Jerger S. Personal communication. 13 April 1977.

this test is less sensitive than other dichotic speech materials for identifying subjects with known cortical lesions. They note that the test is unique because it was designed specifically for use with the hearing impaired.

Age has a dramatic effect on results of central hearing testing, both in the young subject and in the elderly. The normative data of nearly every test of central auditory function show increasing auditory abilities in the young until approximately the age of 11 years.[30–33] Persons over the age of 60 show lowered scores for sensitized speech tests even when peripheral hearing sensitivity is normal, as a result of neural degeneration.[34] With these findings, care must be taken to use age-appropriate normative values in evaluating results of central auditory tests.

The effect of intelligence on central test findings is less well documented than other factors. Bocca[35] reported that results of sensitized speech are increasingly poor as IQs fall below 100. Performance scores on the Goldman-Fristoe-Woodcock Test of Auditory Discrimination[30] indicate that scores obtained on educable mentally retarded children fall far below the scores obtained on a general population and trainable mentally retarded children are essentially unable to perform the task. Katz[36] reviewed some early attempts to modify central auditory tests for use with mentally retarded children but reported few systematic data. On the other end of the intelligence scale, Bocca[35] found no increase in speech intelligibility of filtered and time-compressed speech for IQs up to 141, although he did report a positive relationship between intelligibility of interrupted speech and IQ. Until additional data are available, the clinician will have to analyze the task and the age for which the test was designed, and adjust normative data before interpreting test scores obtained on a retarded person.

Drugs are known to reduce performance on central tests if they are CNS depressants.[37] Amphetamine-like drugs that stimulate the CNS have been shown to improve sensitized speech scores in some patients.[22,36] Children who are on Ritalin or a similar drug for hyperactivity may have improved central hearing test scores because their behavior is improved. Before administering central hearing tests, a careful history should be taken to determine whether the person is on antidepressant, anticonvulsant, or other behavior-modifying drugs.

When people are administered sensitized speech tests in a language other than their native language, the results usually fall below the normal values for each individual. Davis et al[22] found this effect on a high-pass filtered speech test, Gat and Keith[38] on a speech in noise task, Rawizer[39] on the SSW test, and Keith et al[40] on the SSW and dichotic consonant-vowel (CV) test. Keith et al found that the dichotic CV test had less linguistic bias for some speakers of English as a second language (e.g., Hindis). However, some languages do not have the same phonetic content as English (e.g., Arabic) and listeners have difficulty hearing those speech sounds even when they are proficient in the second language and have used it for many years. These results show that even dichotic CV tests are not free of linguistic bias. Examiners must be aware of the consequences on test results of subjects who are tested in a second or foreign language. This bias is especially important (in the United States of America for example) when attempting to describe central auditory abilities for purposes of determining educational placement for children from nonEnglish-speaking homes.

TESTING FOR LESIONS OF THE CENTRAL AUDITORY PATHWAYS

Physiologic Measures

Two important procedures for assessing the central auditory system and especially the brain stem pathways include stapedial reflex tests and recording of the auditory brain stem response.

The presence of an eighth nerve lesion has marked effects on the stapedial reflex including elevated or absent thresholds and reflex decay. Stapedial reflex decay with eighth nerve lesions was first reported by Anderson et al[41] and has been observed by many authors since then. Johnson[42] reported that abnormal stapedial reflex findings were obtained in 88 percent of confirmed acoustic neuromas.

Intra-axial lesions of the brain stem can be differentiated from eighth nerve lesions by comparing results of contralateral (reflex-eliciting sound and measuring probe in opposite ears) and ipsilateral (sound and probe in same ear) stapedial reflexes.[43] When an eighth nerve lesion is present, the contralateral and ipsilateral stapedial reflexes are absent with sound presented to the affected ear. When a brain stem lesion affects the decussating neural pathways, the contralateral stapedial reflexes are absent while the ipsilateral reflex remains intact. A third pattern of response emerges when a lesion extends out of the axis of the brain stem and involves the eighth nerve. In this case, the only uninterrupted neural pathway would be on the unaffected ear, and the ipsilateral stapedial reflex should be present on that side. Finally, Thomas et al[44] reported preliminary data that showed acoustic reflex abnormalities in 32 percent of behaviorally disturbed and language delayed children. They simply presented their data as interesting evidence of possible brain stem involvement in their sample population. Additional discussion of stapedial reflex testing can be found in Chapter 41 of this text.

Electrophysiologic assessment of the auditory system is done by measuring neuroelectric potentials using scalp electrodes. These electrical potentials are of small amplitude, and require amplification of up to 200,000 times. Responses to multiple-stimulus presentations are averaged using computer techniques. The latencies of response are stable in the time domain with the various components of the response, or "waves," generated at different neuroanatomic sites in the central auditory system.[45] Figure 45–2 shows a proposed correlation between each of the first seven waves and its anatomic site in the auditory nerve and brain stem.[46] Disruption of the auditory pathway at different locations from the eighth nerve to the inferior colliculus results in delay in latency of corresponding waveforms or loss of components.[47] Recently, the measurement of middle and late cortical-evoked potentials including the P-300 and slow (expectancy) wave are being used to study cognitive aspects of information procession. Additional discussion of recording of the auditory-evoked potentials can be found in Chapter 51 of this text.

Behavioral Measures

Auditory tests that require an overt response by the subject are defined in this chapter as behavioral measures. These tests can be classified according to the manner of stimulus presentation. In monotic tests a single stimulus is presented to one ear at a time. In diotic tests the same stimulus is applied to the two ears; in dichotic tests two different stimuli are presented simultaneously to both ears; and in binaural fusion tests portions of an incomplete and unintelligible speech message are presented simultaneously to opposite ears.

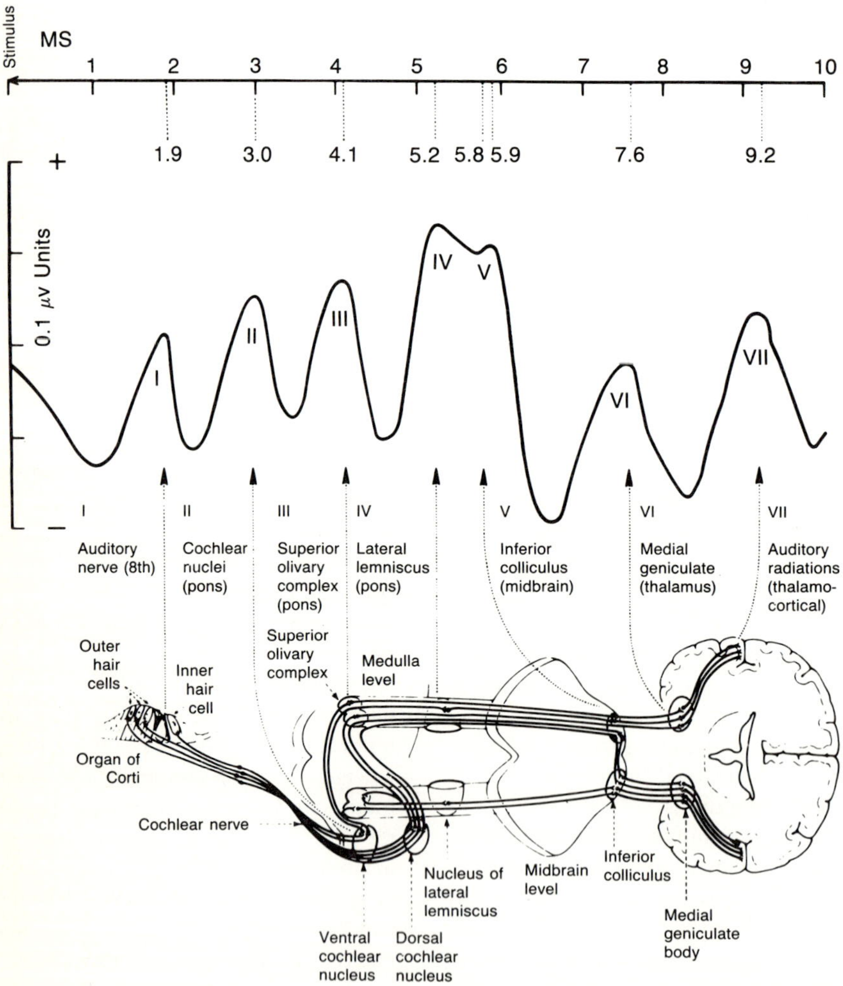

Figure 45–2 Anatomical correlation of components of short latency auditory evoked response.

Sensitized Speech Tests

Monotic sensitized speech tests include filtered, time-compressed, and interrupted speech originally studied by Bocca et al,[18] Bocca and Calearo,[48] and Korsan-Bengsten,[49,50] speech-in-noise testing,[51] and Synthetic Sentence Identification (SSI) tests when done in the presence of an ipsilateral competing message (ICM).[52]

Filtered Speech. Although various low-pass filtered conditions have been used, a cut-off frequency of 500 Hz and a rejection rate of about 17 dB per octave has been used almost exclusively for diagnostic purposes with adults. Some authors use a fixed sensation level of presentation; for example, Lynn and Gilroy[53] use 50 dB sensation level (SL), whereas others appear to prefer to run a performance intensity function using the filtered stimuli.[54] Bocca and Calearo[48] stated that there is no substantial difference in results whether the stimuli are phonetically balanced word lists or sentence material. The essential finding in filtered speech tests is that the speech intelligibility score is reduced in the ear contralateral to a temporal lobe lesion (Fig. 45–3). The difference between ears should be greater than 20 percent to be significant.[55] According to Korsan-Bengsten,[49] the filtered speech test is the most sensitive of the distorted speech measures for testing cortical auditory function.

Time-Compressed Speech. Time compression is accomplished by electronic means that result in a reduction in the total duration of a speech message without a substantial change in the fundamental frequency or pitch of the voice. Results of testing on normal listeners indicate that speech intelligibility decreases gradually from 30 to 60 percent time compression and falls dramatically at 70 percent compression.[56] They also found that intelligibility scores increase as a function of intensity with little improvement above 32 dB SL. Both Calearo and Antonelli[54] and Korsan-Bengsten[50] found that results of time-compressed speech are similar to filtered speech when a temporal lobe lesion is present. Kurdziel et al[57] found marked reduction of intelligibility scores in the contralateral ear for patients with diffuse temporal lobe lesions. They found little reduction in scores on patients with discrete lesions (following anterior temporal lobe surgery) that did not appear to have involved the primary auditory areas of the brain.

Interrupted Speech. These tests are done by using an electronic switch to interrupt speech at various rates from 1 to 20 interruptions per second (ips), and at various on times including 33, 50, and 67 percent.[48,58] The optimal interruption rate is probably 10 ips with 50 percent on time. Results are interpreted similar to those obtained with filtered speech, with 15 to 25 percent reduction in intelligibility of scores found on the ear contralateral to a temporal lobe lesion.[55]

Synthetic Sentence Identification with Competing Message. This unique approach to diagnostic speech audiometry was first suggested by Speaks and Jerger[59] and applied clinically in 1968.[52] In this test, 10 synthetic sentences are presented to the subject at 50 dB SL under various signal-to-noise conditions of ipsilateral (ICM) and contralateral competing message (CCM). The competing message consists of a single speaker reading a narrative tale on the life of Davey Crockett.

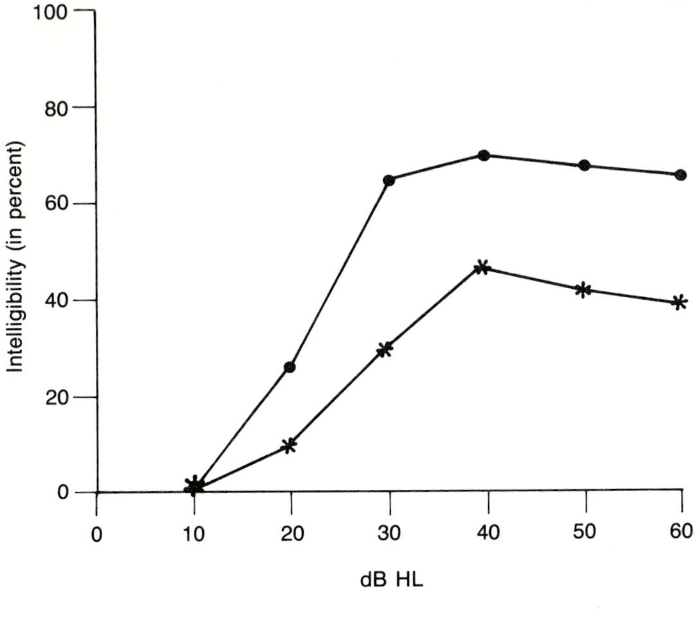

Figure 45–3 Performance intensity function for filtered speech in cases of right temporal lobe lesions. A 20 to 40 percent loss in the contralateral ear must be noted.

The advantage of synthetic sentences is that they provide a closed set of stimulus materials that are controlled for informational content with limited opportunity for prediction through linguistic rules. Examples of three synthetic sentences are shown in Table 45–3.

Generally, the results of the SSI testing are interpreted in the following way.[60] Eighth nerve lesions are characterized by poor performance on the ear ipsilateral to the lesion with the ICM and CCM tasks.

Brain stem lesions are characterized by poor performance with ICM and relatively good performance with CCM. The ICM deficits are observed on the ear contralateral to the lesion unless the lesion extends across the midline, in which case ICM performance is depressed bilaterally.

Temporal lobe lesions are characterized by poor performance with ICM and CCM. ICM deficits are observed on both ears or the ear contralateral to the lesion, and the CCM deficit is observed on the ear contralateral to the affected temporal lobe. The overriding principle in these patients is that they have relatively more difficulty with the CCM tasks than with ICM tasks.

Summary of Sensitized Speech Tests. Sensitized speech tests show no dominance effect in adults, and normal patients have equivalent scores for both ears. When a lesion of the auditory cortex is present, sensitized speech tests yield mild to moderately reduced intelligibility scores in the ear contralateral to the lesion. Brain stem lesions affect the sensitized speech scores to a greater extent than cortical lesions. The reduced intelligibility occurs on either the same or the opposite side of the brain stem lesion, depending on the neural pathways involved. Scores are often reduced bilaterally when the lesion crosses the midline or through secondary effects of pressure, even from remote lesions.

Dichotic Speech Tests

Dichotic listening tests are done by presenting different stimuli simultaneously to the two ears. These tests have been used extensively to study central auditory function and hemisphere dominance, in addition to being used for diagnostic purposes. Speech ranging from nonsense syllables to sentences are used

TABLE 45–3 Examples of Seven-Word Synthetic Sentences

A small boat with picture has become
Built the Government with a force almost
Go change your car color is red

From Jerger J, Speaks C, Trammel J. A new approach to speech audiometry. J Speech Hear Disord 1968; 33:318.

as stimuli. They include dichotic consonant vowels,[61] digits,[62] words,[33] spondees,[23] and sentences.[32]

Dichotic CV Test. Berlin et al[61] developed dichotic test materials in which six stop-vowel syllables /pa/, /ba/, /ta/, /da/, /ka/, and /ga/ served as consonant-vowel (CV) syllables. Audiotapes are prepared using a male voice to record a random series of the 15 possible dichotic pairs, each pair occurring twice, for a total of 30 trials. The stimuli were taped using computer techniques to obtain precise delays between onset times of the CV pairs.

The time delays were 0 (no delay), 90 msec, 120 msec, and 180 msec. Taped materials are presented to the listener at 70 to 80 dB sound pressure level (SPL), once with the right ear leading and once with the left ear leading for all conditions. A visual display of the test paradigm is shown in Table 45–4.

Using this test paradigm Berlin et al[61] found that (1) right ears generally yield higher scores than the left ears with 0 msec lag; and (2) time staggering dichotically enhances the lagging syllable at 30 and 90 msec with closure between 180 and 250 msec, although the right ear performance is better when summed over all time conditions.[63] Normative data obtained on 12 subjects are shown on Figure 45–4.[64] Investigation of test-retest reliability on dichotic CV tests yields correlation coefficients of +0.66 to +0.80.[65–67] In addition, Speaks and Niccum[67] found "large" trial-to-trial variability for individual normal listeners, and a "large" number of listeners who failed to show a right-ear advantage. The results of the Speaks and Niccum study should not be interpreted as indicating that the dichotic CV tests are more or less reliable than other audiologic tests, because the question of reliability of all clinical-diagnostic tests has been generally ignored.

One additional factor in dichotic CV testing is the instruction given to listeners. Free recall instructions require the listener to report any CV stimulus heard. Directed ear listening conditions require the subject to respond to what was heard from the right ear during a series of CV stimulus pairs, and then from the left ear for a second series. Using a free recall technique several investigators have found no maturation effect among listeners ranging from 3 years to college age.[61,68,69] This finding differs from dichotic listening tasks that use stimuli with greater linguistic content. There is, however, a marked maturation effect when directed ear listening techniques are used. For example, studies by Obrzut et al[68] and Hynd et al[70] found a right ear advantage in normal children, whether attention was directed to the right or left ear. The amount of between ear differences in normal children ranged from 9 to 11 percent in favor of the right ear. Keith et al[71] stud-

TABLE 45-4 Dichotic CV Test

	Right Ear Lag					*Left Ear Lag*	
(R) Ear	ga	ta	ba	ba	ba	ka	ta
(L) Ear	ba	ga	ga	ka	ta	pa	da
	180	120	90	0	90	120	180
				TIME (msec)			
	Left Ear Lead			*Simultaneous*		*Right Ear Lead*	

ied directed ear listening tasks in normal adults and found that subjects showed right ear advantage on directed right listening and left ear advantages on directed left listening conditions. The ear advantage averaged 35 percent on directed right and 21 percent on directed left. These results showed a previously unreported maturational effect on dichotic CV testing.

When a temporal lobe lesion is present, (1) there is a severe loss of dichotic speech information in the ear contralateral to the lesion, and (2) the normal advantage of the lagging message is lost.[72–74] Speaks et al[75] found that monotic scores for CV materials were higher than dichotic scores in the better ear of patients with damaged temporal lobes. These findings suggest that dichotic test scores in the better ear are lowered by the presence of speech in the poorer ear, and that factor should be accounted for in testing patients. Mueller et al,[29] on the other hand, reported without comment that the mean right ear score for individuals with right posterior temporal lobe damage showed group performance that was better than their normals.

Staggered Spondaic Word Test (SSW). Katz[23,76–78] designed the Staggered Spondaic Word (SSW) test, a 40-item test of spondee words that contains two non-competing and one competing condition (Table 45–5). Presentation levels are 50 dB above speech reception threshold (SRT) for each ear. The test is scored by computing the percentage of error for each test condition; right noncompeting (RNC), right competing (RC), left competing (LC), and left noncompeting (LNC). According to Katz, raw SSW scores (R-SSW) are corrected (C-SSW) by the amount of the W-22 percentage error to reduce the effects of peripheral loss on central test findings. Lynn and Gilroy[27] felt that one cannot parcel out the peripheral from the central component in word discrimination scores and used only the uncorrected SSW scores. Arnst and Doyle[79] studied this problem and reported that cochlear hearing loss with a pure-tone average less than 50 dB HL did not affect the corrected SSW result. With greater hearing loss the effect of the peripheral lesion was to shift the listener's score to a poorer performance category, creating the impression of a central auditory disorder when none was present.

Results of normal adults indicate essentially no error under any test condition. A lesion of the central auditory reception area generally shows a high percentage of errors in the competing condition of the ear contralateral to the lesion. An example of

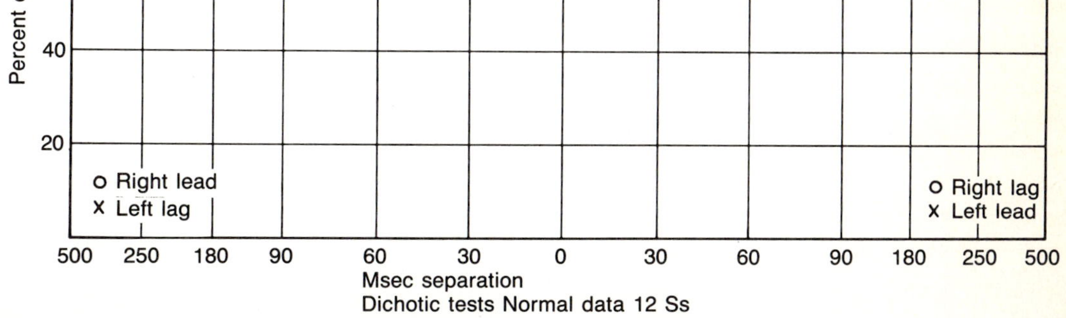

Figure 45–4 Dichotic normal lead-lag data: experiment 1, 0 to 90 msec (N = 12); experiment 2, 90 to 500 msec (N = 12).

TABLE 45-5 SSW Test Time Sequence

	No. 1	No. 2	No. 3
(R) Ear	UP	STAIRS	
(L) Ear		DOWN	TOWN
	Non-competing (RNC)	*Competing (RC, LC)*	*Non-competing (LNC)*

normal SSW test findings is shown in Figure 45–5, along with results of a patient with a left temporal lobe lesion. These results show decreased performance in the right ear in the competing condition. Although they are not well understood, response bias errors indicate possible dysfunction in nonauditory reception areas of the brain.

Competing Sentence Test. The competing sentence test is one of four subtests included in a battery developed by Willeford.[32,80,81] Ten sentence pairs are presented simultaneously with the primary message at 35 dB SL and the competing message at 50 dB SL. Although Willeford's original interest was in assessment of auditory behavior in children, the battery has been used in evaluation of adult patients with neurologic disorders. Generally, the results indicate the expected contralateral ear effect with decreased competing sentence scores on the ear opposite a temporal or parietal lobe lesion.[27,82]

Summary of the Dichotic Speech Testing Model. The dichotic speech model states that auditory performance will be poorer on the ear opposite a temporal lobe lesion. Most reports in the literature confirm this finding. After reviewing results

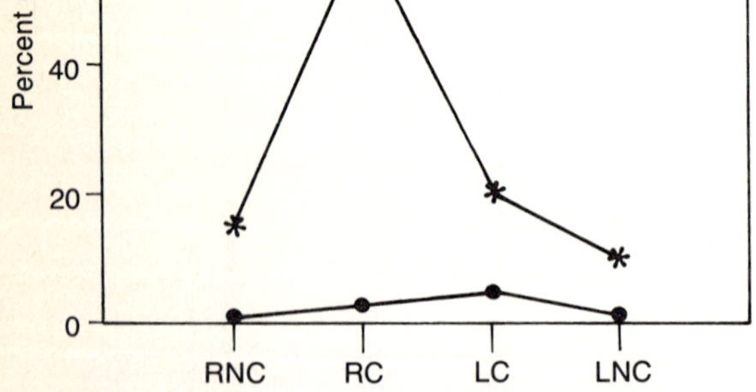

Figure 45–5 R-SSW results obtained on subjects with normal performance (lower line) and a subject with a left-sided temporal lobe lesion (upper line).

of 40 patients with right and left temporal lobe lesions, however, Olsen[74] warned that

> ... inferences should not be made relative to site or site of involvement exclusively from dichotic test results. The (auditory) system is too complex to allow a single pattern of results to be associated with involvement of one side or another. . . . While subtle auditory dysfunction at the level of the temporal cortex cannot be determined, tests as difficult as the dichotic CV are necessary to identify subtle auditory dysfunction at the level of the temporal cortex.

In addition, Collard et al[83] reported results of pre- and postoperative dichotic testing on a group of patients with epileptogenic lesions. They found no clear relationship to the side of the lesion. They hypothesized that there may be differences between patients with epileptogenic foci and those with tumors or stroke. More importantly, their data show that, as a group, auditory processing capacity was unchanged by temporal lobectomy. In fact, the study of auditory processing abilities in patient populations may be a more significant future contribution to patient care than the identification of specific lesions. For example, Mueller et al[29] stated that results of central auditory testing are useful in detecting injury to the auditory areas of the brain stem or cortex and "can be used to monitor recovery of auditory processing skills and provide a framework for counseling the patient (and the patient's family) concerning their communication capabilities." That application has been addressed in the literature by Grimes et al,[84] who studied patients with Alzheimer's disease, and Bergman et al,[85] who studied patients with head injury and stroke to determine "functional disorders of communication."

Binaural Fusion

Patients with brain stem lesions present several complex problems that make it difficult to develop a large clinical sample. Some patients are severely ill, which makes it hard to do behavioral tests, and many have peripheral hearing loss or are elderly, which makes interpretation of results difficult.

Development of clinical patterns of audiometric test results that reflect typical brain stem pathology is difficult, and different authors have published what appear to be contradicting brain stem patterns. According to Antonelli,[34] a collection of homogeneous data in lesions at the brain stem level is more difficult than in lesions of the temporal lobe because of the complicated crowding of neural circuitries in a limited space. Small lesions can affect large portions of the auditory tract, and small variations in the extent of lesions can produce wide variations in auditory disorders.

Despite these limitations, tests that assess the patient's ability to fuse incomplete messages presented binaurally appear to be sensitive to lesions of the brain stem. Those tests in current use include the Matzker Test of Binaural Fusion and the Rapidly Alternating Speech Perception (RASP) test. A special test of brain stem function is the test of masking level difference (MLD).

Matzker Test of Binaural Fusion. Binaural resynthesis of filtered speech was described as early as 1929 by Fletcher. Subsequently, Matzker[3] described a binaural fusion test in which a low-frequency band from 500 to 800 Hz and a high-frequency band from 1815 to 2500 Hz were presented to opposite ears. Neither pass band was intelligible by itself, but, for persons with normal hearing, integration of the binaural signals resulted in scores approaching those of nondistorted speech. Matzker considered that the integration took place at the level of the brain stem where the auditory pathways from the two ears are interconnected, and results of histologic section of deceased patients who did poorly on his test showed changes "particularly within the olivary region." His initial data also show reduction in binaural fusion scores resulting from cortical lesions remote from the brain stem, though affecting it by "vascular reflexes." Matzker's original findings and impressions have been supported by Smith and Resnick[24] and Palva and Jokinen.[86]

Smith and Resnick[24] used filtered consonant nucleus consonant (CNC) word lists presented at 30 dB SL. Two dichotic conditions were tested with the low- and high-pass bands presented alternately to opposite ears, and one diotic condition in which both noise bands are presented simultaneously to both ears. Palva and Jokinen[86] presented word lists at 50 dB SL under two monotic conditions with both noise bands presented to one ear at a time and one dichotic condition in which the noise bands were presented simultaneously to opposite ears. Willeford's[32] test battery included a binaural fusion test. Unfortunately he did not recommend a dichotic-diotic comparison in his procedures. Rather, he assigns the test ear to the ear receiving the low-pass band speech.

Results of binaural fusion tests are especially affected by peripheral hearing loss and aging. A temporal lobe lesion affecting the auditory reception areas results in lower diotic scores in the contralateral ear as found on other sensitized speech tests. Palva and Jokinen[86] considered greater than 15 percent difference in monaural scores to be significant for indicating a temporal lobe lesion. They reported that binaural fusion scores are well preserved in cases of unilateral temporal lobe lesions, which indicates that the fused signal is represented in both hemispheres, with the normal test score resulting from the noninvolved hemisphere.

The presence of a brain stem lesion results in poor discrimination scores because of inability to fuse the two pass bands. Smith and Resnick[24] considered the binaural fusion task to be positive for brain stem problems when diotic enhancement is 18 to 34 percent over at least one of the dichotic conditions. Palva and Jokinen[86] found the binaural test to be positive when the binaural discrimination score was more than 10 percent worse than the poorer monaural score. Willeford[32] considered any binaural fusion score poorer than 75 percent to be positive. No author has attempted to specify the exact site of lesion within the brain stem based on binaural fusion scores alone.

Rapidly Alternating Speech Perception. The RASP test is another binaural test that is sensitive to the presence of brain stem dysfunction. The test stimuli comprise sentence material presented at 30 dB SL and alternated between ears every 300 msec.[32] Usually, monaural scores are below 10 percent and binaural listening conditions are above 95 percent.[27] The presence of a temporal lobe lesion, especially on the left side, can reduce RASP test scores slightly—for example, to 80 percent—whereas brain stem lesions reduce scores to a greater degree through an inability to fuse the alternating message. Lynn and Gilroy[27] reported RASP data on small groups of subjects with normal hearing and patients with eighth nerve, low pons and cerebellopontine (CP) angle, upper brain stem, and unilateral lesions. All groups yielded mean RASP scores greater than 80 percent, except for the low pons and CP angle groups, which yielded mean scores of less than 40 percent.

Masking Level Differences. A masking phenomenon known as the masking level difference (MLD) or binaural release from masking occurs when a binaurally presented stimulus, either a signal or masker, is interaurally out of phase with itself when the other stimulus is in phase. The result of this stimulus presentation is a decrease in the effective masking of the noise over listening conditions when both signal and masker are either in phase or out of phase. The greatest MLD effect occurs when the signal is out of phase by 180 degrees at the ears while the noise is in phase bilaterally.[87] For example, when a binaural signal, such as speech, is in phase, it is heard at the center of the listener's head. If it is out of phase, it is heard at the listener's ear. The same is true for a masking noise. Therefore, if speech is presented out of phase at the same time that noise is presented in phase bilaterally, the speech is heard at the listener's ear and the noise is heard in the center of the head. The amount of release from masking under these listening conditions is reported to range from 8 dB to 14 dB for normal subjects.[26,87,88] MLDs are thought to result from binaural interaction at the level of the trapezoid body and the olivary bodies.[64]

Results of studies indicate that MLDs are reduced below normal values when a brain stem lesion is present,[26,87] although they are relatively unaffected by the presence of temporal lobe damage.[89] Unfortunately, mean data indicate that the effects of brain stem lesions on the magnitude of the MLD are small and may be difficult to interpret in individual cases, although at least one case report showed marked effects on the MLD from the lateromedial inferior pontine syndrome.[90] In addition, all investigators have reported that the test is susceptible to peripheral hearing loss requiring relatively normal hearing for the test to have diagnostic value in detecting lesions of the central auditory nervous system. In spite of these difficulties, the student should keep an open mind to the future usefulness of this interesting test.

Summary

These and other behavioral and physiologic tests can be used in an audiologic test battery to aid in the identification of lesions of the CANS. Which test is most sensitive is difficult to determine, because surgical confirmation verifying site of lesion is not always available. In one of few such reports, Lynn and Gilroy[27] compared results of undistorted speech tests, low-pass filtered tests, SSW, and competing sentence tests on patients with temporal and parietal lobe lesions. They reported raw SSW scores as alternate-binaural (Alt-Bin) for the SSW non competing conditions, and simultaneous-binaural (Sim-Bin) as the SSW competing conditions (Fig. 45–6). This figure indicates that the competing conditions of the SSW and low-pass filtered tests appear to be the most sensitive for identifying temporal lobe lesions. Many more studies of this kind are required to sort out relative advantages of the various tests that are available.

Figure 45–6 resulted from a retrospective analysis of patient data. Lynn and Gilroy[27] pointed out that, prospectively, attempts to interpret test data are complicated by many factors. For example, hemispheric dominance, involvement of auditory pathways in the corpus callosum, secondary effects from infiltration or pressure of a mass lesion, and the depth of the lesion are some factors that confound interpretation of results. Therefore, it may not be possible to indicate with precision the site of lesion in the CANS. Nevertheless, the audiologic battery can be helpful in determining that a central auditory pathway lesion is present, and can describe

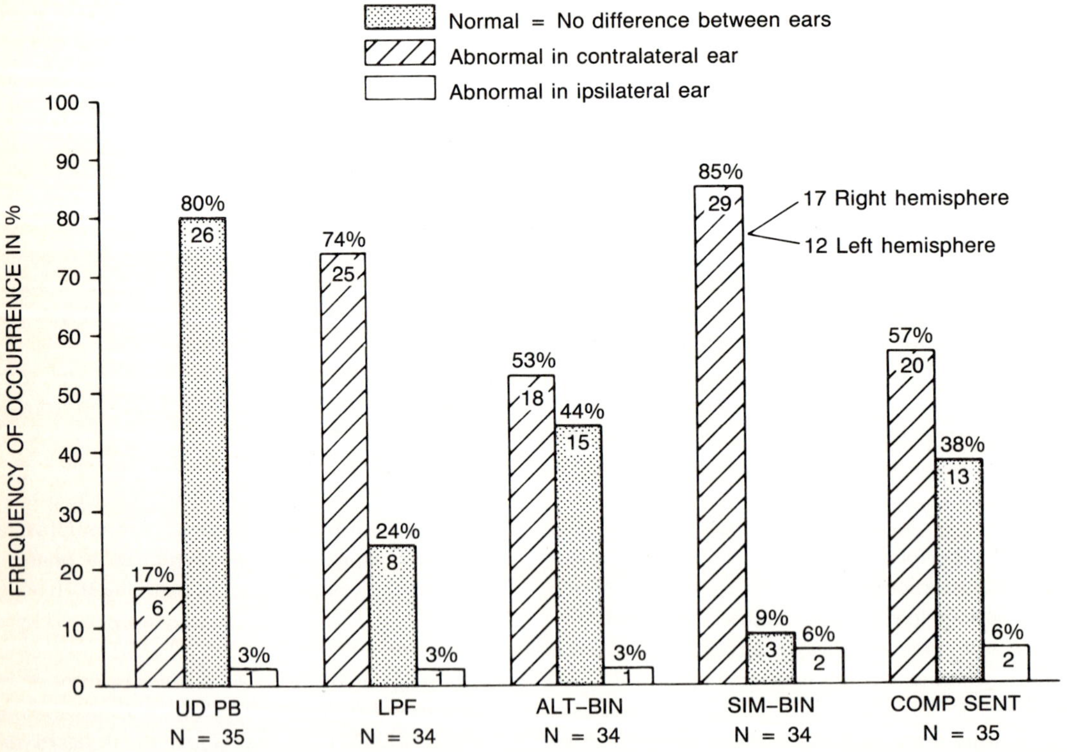

Figure 45–6 Frequency with which normal and abnormal speech discrimination scores occurred with the central auditory test battery in 35 patients with confirmed temporal lobe lesions. (From Lynn GE, Gilroy J. Evaluation of central auditory dysfunction in patients with neurological disorders. In: Keith RW, ed. Central auditory dysfunction. New York: Grune & Stratton, 1977:204.)

auditory processing skills for the purposes of determining functional disorders of communication.

CENTRAL HEARING TESTING WITH CHILDREN

The use of central hearing tests in the assessment of auditory perceptual skills has taken on added importance with the recent educational emphasis on children with learning disabilities. That emphasis has come into greater focus with the enactment of the *Education for All Handicapped Children Act* (PL94-142).[91] That document lists as one of the handicapping conditions "children with specific learning disabilities." The definition of learning disabilities includes "disorders in one or more of the basic psychological processes involved in understanding or in using language, spoken or written, which disorder may manifest itself in imperfect ability to listen . . ." The classification does not include children with learning problems resulting primarily from a hearing loss. The general need posed by PL94-142 is to find ways to identify and manage problems with auditory processing and language that contribute to a child's educational problems. Specifically, audiologists, speech language pathologists, and others need to examine models that clarify the relationship between auditory processing and language disorders. They need to develop valid and reliable tests that specify problems in "listening" that relate to learning problems, and they need to develop and verify approaches to remediation that will result in enhanced learning.

Auditory Tests Used With Children

A large number of procedures are available that attempt to measure central auditory abilities in children. Some of the tests can be categorized according to the primary auditory ability that they attempt to measure. For example, Table 45–6 includes the list of auditory abilities listed earlier in this chapter and several tests that attempt to measure that ability. The list of tests is not nearly complete, and in some cases only one or two subtests of a test battery are listed.

Several problems are encountered when categorizing auditory abilities and tests as shown in Table 45–6. One is that a high correlation exists among various auditory perceptual abilities and, as Witkin[92] stated, "tasks used in studies which attempt to isolate one or another aspect of auditory perception may really be testing one or more ability." A second problem exists in the lack of agreement on definitions of terminology regarding auditory abilities, and, given a certain task, the lack of agreement on what that task is measuring. For example, in reviewing the Goldman-Fristoe-Woodcock Test of Auditory

TABLE 45–6 Examples of Tests That Attempt to Measure Certain Auditory Abilities

Auditory Abilities	*Test*
Localization	Sound field localization
Binaural synthesis	Rapid alternating speech perception
	Binaural fusion test
Figure ground	GFW test of auditory discrimination
	SCAN auditory figure ground subtest
Binaural separation	Dichotic consonant vowel tests
	Dichotic digits
	Dichotic word subtest of SCAN
	Staggered spondee word test
	Willeford competing sentence test
Memory	ITPA auditory sequential memory
	Koppitz visual auditory digit span
	Wepman auditory memory span and sequential memory tests
	GFW auditory memory test
	Token test for children
Blending	ITPA sound blending subtest
	GFW test of sound blending
	Roswell-Phall auditory blending test
Discrimination	Wepman auditory discrimination test, revised
	GFW auditory discrimination test
	Lindamood auditory conceptualization test
Closure	Time-compressed speech
	ITPA test of auditory closure
	Low-pass filtered word tests
Association	Competing environmental sound test
Cognition	Carrow test of auditory comprehension of language
	Wechsler intelligence scale for children, revised (WISC-R)

TABLE 45–7 Central Auditory Processing (CAP) Test Norms Competing Sentence Norms (Percent)

		Expected Result			*Mean*			*SD*			*Range*		
Age	*N*	*Weak Ear*	–	*Strong* Ear*	*Weak Ear*	–	*Strong* Ear*	*Weak Ear*	–	*Strong* Ear*	*Weak Ear*	–	*Strong* Ear*
5	25	20	–	90/100	24.8	–	94.0	35.9	–	4.4	0/80	–	90/100
6	40	60	–	90/100	59.5	–	96.5	33.2	–	4.0	0/100	–	90/100
7	40	70	–	100	67.8	–	97.5	31.2	–	3.6	0/100	–	90/100
8	40	80	–	100	83.0	–	98.0	22.2	–	3.2	10/100	–	90/100
9	40	90	–	100	93.0	–	98.8	9.8	–	2.6	70/100	–	90/100
10	40	100	–	100	98.4	–	99.2	3.6	–	2.6	90/100	–	90/100
5/10	225	70	–	100	71.6	–	95.9	22.7	–	3.5	0/100	–	90/100

* Strong ears were predominantly right ears. Left ears were the strong ears in only 13 of the 225 subjects.

Discrimination, Bannatyne[93] reported that "The one major problem I have with this test is that it is a test of auditory closure and not, as the authors believe, a test of auditory discrimination." Numerous similar examples exist in the literature.

Many other tests are difficult to categorize in terms of the auditory ability that is measured. These tests include, for example, the Pinheiro test of pitch pattern recognition,[94] masking level differences,[95] and the Wichita tests of auditory fusion developed by McCroskey.[95a] Tests like these can further describe children's central auditory processing abilities. Other tests, for example, the Pediatric Speech Intelligibility test (PSI),[15] have been used specifically for identification of central auditory lesions in children although they can also be used to describe functional auditory abilities. The SCAN test,[33] developed by this author, is a screening test used to identify auditory processing disorders in children.

The value of these tests is that they appear to indicate whether a child's auditory abilities are "normal" or "disordered," although exactly how the test results relate to functional behavior in the classroom is not always clear. Many children who do poorly on these tests also have a deficit in language, reading, or learning. However, some children who score poorly on auditory perceptual tasks achieve normally in other skill areas. One of the major problems in central auditory testing is that many of the available tests are poorly normed, and there are too few data on mean performance and variability on a task, and standard scores and confidence intervals are not available.

Auditory Abilities in Children

Results of sensitized speech and dichotic listening tests on normal children indicate that auditory perceptual skills continue to mature until about the age of 12 years, at which time scores are comparable to those of adult listeners.[31,32,96,97] The normal data are characterized by large standard deviations around the mean for younger children (5 and 6 years old), with variability decreasing with advancing age. In addition, a strong dominance effect usually is shown on results of tests on younger children with the right ear yielding substantially better scores than the left. The ear difference gradually disappears by the age of 10 years. Examples of the normal maturation effects, variability of results, and ear effects are shown in Tables 45–7 and 45–8.[98] The implications are that results of tests on an individual child must be carefully interpreted according to relevant normative data, and, if none are available, that interpretation is difficult at best.

Results of auditory perceptual testing obtained on children with language, reading, or learning disabilities indicate that they score poorer than normal children on most auditory subtests. For example scores

TABLE 45–8 Filtered Speech Norms (Percent)

		Mean			*Average Ear*	*SD*			*Range*		
Age	*N*	*LE*	–	*RE*	*Difference**	*LE*	–	*RE*	*LE*	–	*RE*
5	Insufficient at present										
6	40	60.6	–	60.9	5.4	9.8	–	9.7	42/84	–	44/82
7	40	64.7	–	64.6	6.3	8.8	–	7.5	52/86	–	52/86
8	40	65.8	–	65.7	6.7	7.9	–	8.4	52/86	–	56/92
9	40	68.2	–	67.9	5.4	9.4	–	9.2	56/92	–	56/92
10	40	71.2	–	72.7	5.3	6.2	–	6.2	66/84	–	64/82
6/10	200	66.1	–	66.4	5.8	8.4	–	8.2	42/92	–	44/92

* Only 18 of the 200 subjects had ear differences which exceeded 10 percent. The greatest difference in any subject was 16 percent.

on tests of auditory figure ground are reported by several authors to be poorer for learning disabled (LD) children than for normal children.[30,99–103] Similar results were obtained for filtered speech tests,[104] SSW tests,[105] and tests for masking level differences.[95] Auditory memory is often reported as being poor in children with learning disabilities[17,106–109] as is auditory discrimination.[110] Manning et al[111] reported that children who "displayed learning difficulties" did more poorly under 60 percent time compression of speech, although there was a great deal of variability in their results. Sommers and Taylor,[112] using a dichotic listening task, reported that children with language disorders had differences in ear preference, using the left ear more than normal children. Willeford[32,113] also reported cases of children with learning disabilities who did poorly on one or more subtests of his sensitized speech battery.

Occasionally, a report can be found in which differences between groups of normal and LD children are not as clear. Welsh et al[114] studied these two groups using a battery of tests that included Goldman-Fristue-Woodcock (GFW) auditory discrimination and Illinois Test of Psycholinguistic Abilities (ITPA) sound blending, auditory closure, and auditory sequential memory tests. Significant differences between groups were found only on the test of auditory sequential memory. Pinheiro[94] reported data on the Willeford battery, the SSW, and pitch pattern recognition tests. Summary results of cases reported are not abnormal when compared to SSW and to Willeford's 1978 norms, although individual cases showed deficiencies on different subtests. Larsen et al[115] administered the auditory and visual sequential memory and sound blending subtests of the ITPA, the Wepman Auditory Discrimination test, and the Bender Visual-Motor Gestalt test to normal and LD children, and found significant differences between groups only on the Bender test.

The purpose of reviewing articles showing both relationships and nonrelationships between auditory processing skills and learning disabilities is to demonstrate that there is not a consensus on these issues. That differences in opinion exist is not surprising in view of the wide range of auditory skills that fall under the umbrella of auditory perception and lack of agreement on definitions of both "auditory perception" and "learning disability."

Remediation

Any discussion of central auditory dysfunction in children leads inevitably to the problem of remediation. When the diagnostic evaluation is completed, the parent, the teacher, the speech and language pathologist, and the audiologist must ask, "Now what do I do?" The answer to that question, like so many others, is not simple. The assessment of central auditory abilities for both diagnostic and remediation purposes promises to remain a controversial issue for some time to come. At the heart of the issue is a disagreement among professionals concerning whether disorders of auditory perception cause speech and language, reading, or learning disabilities or whether they are just highly correlated.

This disparity of views is exemplified by the following statements. Bannatyne[106] wrote that "the vast majority of reading disability cases have a fundamental problem with auditory processing. . . ." By contrast, Rees[116] wrote that "while correlational studies examining the auditory skills of children with reading disorders show that these children do significantly more poorly . . . there is no good argument to support the conclusion that this association is a causal one." The problem goes beyond a disagreement about cause and effect relationships, however, and there is general disagreement and poor documentation to substantiate whether auditory perceptual deficits can be remediated and, if so, whether remediation of specific isolated auditory skills is of any value in improving overall educational or language performance.

If there were a generally accepted auditory perceptual deficit hypothesis, it would state that auditory perception is fundamental to learning language and that auditory processing deficits cause disorders in area of language, reading, and learning;[117] that auditory perception can be readily broken down into specific deficits that are amenable to training;[17,118] that a hierarchy of auditory perceptual skills exists with processes moving from simple to complex and that remediation should follow the same order.[17,107,119–121]

These and other authors have suggested techniques for designing remediation programs, and a number of commercial programs that approach remediation on a systematic basis are available.[122] The purposes and expectations of auditory perceptual remediation include facilitation of auditory-perceptual processing abilities,[17] improvement in reading,[119] learning to listen as a prerequisite to the understanding of spoken language,[123,124] and improving general academic success.[125]

Opponents of a perceptual deficit hypothesis claim that while auditory perceptual disorders are related to disorders of language, reading and learning, they are not the cause of those problems. Rees[116,126] has presented data supporting the philosophy that there is little foundation for the notion that most children with reading, speech, and language disorders have a fundamental problem of auditory perception of speech. She recognizes the correlational studies between these abilities but feels that available data do not support the conclusion that the association is a causal one. In a speech to the California Speech and Hearing Association, Rees[127] stated that auditory perceptual skills are "the result of having learned one's language." That is, a language disorder results in an auditory perceptual dysfunction in that insufficient linguistic, semantic, and cognitive skills are available to enable the child to develop strategies for dealing with the auditory perceptual task. Vellutino et al[128] claim that the relationship between perceptual and conceptual functioning is probably reciprocal rather than sequential. When discussing visual perceptual deficit theories of reading disability, Vellutino et al suggest that disorders of visual abilities can be interpreted as "secondary manifestations of verbal-mediation difficulties that are Visual-Verbal deficits rather than Visual-Perceptual deficits.

Marquardt and Saxmann[129] also note that the relationship between perception and production of language is not clearly defined, even in children with normal linguistic abilities. Their study showed that children with underdeveloped articulation skills also showed depressed scores on auditory tests of language comprehension and tests of auditory sound discrimination. Marquardt and Saxman comment, however, that their data are best explained by a general developmental lag, and that the importance of subskills to speech and language acquisition remains to be demonstrated.

In a review of the literature concerned with relationships of auditory-perceptual skills to reading ability, Lyon[130] concluded that the available data do not support the view that intact auditory-perceptual skills are necessary for the adequate development of reading ability. A number of investigations cited by Lyon indicated that poor readers manifest difficulties in auditory perception. An equal number of studies found good readers who demonstrated deficits in auditory skills and poor readers who demonstrated adequate auditory-perceptual abilities. Lyon cautions that correlational studies relating poor auditory-perceptual abilities and reading should be interpreted with care.

This writer believes that language and auditory perception develop simultaneously, although it is unlikely that they develop independently. Some basic auditory-perceptual skills (e.g., appreciation of frequency, intensity, and duration) serve as building blocks of audition leading to language development through imitation. As language skills are acquired, children acquire other linguistically dependent auditory-perceptual skills, such as memory, discrimination, closure, and blending. In addition, as the child's neuroanatomic pathways mature, the ability to cope with dichotic listening tasks, binaural release from masking (MLD), and other nonlinguistically based listening skills begin to improve.

What then about remediation? Some authors have insisted that success in remediation occurs either because the child is being trained to the test because the child's attention to the task is improved. In fact, one author claims that the entire problem of learning disability can be attritubed to a disorder of attention.[131] Even Wepman[108–110] stated that success in training memory span, sequential memory, and auditory discrimination has not been proven empirically. Willeford[132,133] reported that most traditional therapy techniques did not dramatically improve the child's ability to perceive and integrate auditory information.

Taylor[134] suggested that many "auditory processing difficulties" are really problems in listening. He claimed that since research is not available to show that auditory processing training has any benefit, all children with these problems should be first entered into programs that teach listening. Children who do not benefit from that approach could then be given more serious attention.

There is no easy answer to when and how to approach remediation. It is clear from our present knowledge that recommendations for remediation must evolve from an interdisciplinary approach to the assessment of a child's learning problem.[135] Suggestions for classroom management combined with direct intervention in therapy should enable many children to improve their educational situation. In addition, professionals can use perceptual areas of relative strength to improve auditory-perceptual deficits and assist children to develop "strategies for coping."[136]

SUMMARY

In this chapter we make three main points: (1) there is poor agreement on definition of terminology relating to auditory perceptual deficits; (2) there is poor agreement on the cause and effect relationship of auditory-perceptual deficits and language, reading, or learning disorders; and (3) there is poor agreement on whether auditory-perceptual deficits can be remediated.

The student and working clinician who are looking for answers will undoubtedly find this chapter frustrating to read. However, its purpose is not to provide pat solutions to difficult problems, but to heighten awareness of existing differences of opinion, to make students and clinicians uncomfortable with accepting simplistic explanations or approaches, and to show some of the opportunities for future investigation.

In this complex subject, the following are some questions that need to be addressed in the near future.

1. What is the cause and effect relationship between auditory-perceptual skills and language abilities? Are auditory-perceptual skills fundamental to learning language, or is language fundamental to auditory perception?

2. Which of the auditory-perceptual skills are required for imitation to learn language, and which of the auditory-perceptual skills require linguistic, semantic, and cognitive skills?

3. What is the prevalence and implication of auditory-perceptual disorders in a normally achieving population of children?

4. What is normal behavior on tests of auditory-perceptual abilities for children of different ages and cultural and linguistic backgrounds?

5. To what degree can auditory-perceptual deficits be remediated, and what degree of improvement in social interaction, language, reading, or learning disabilities can be expected?

In conclusion, the temptation to use labels gives a false sense of security and confidence that a problem has been described adequately. Unfortunately, labels such as "auditory-perceptual dysfunction" fail to reveal anything about the nature of the problem and what parents, teachers, and speech and language pathologists can and should do about it. The first thing that can be done to avoid problems in labeling is to describe both the auditory ability that is considered deficient, and the task used to measure that ability. Following an adequate description, it may be easier to determine how that deficit may be related to other problems and what strategy should be used in coping with it.

REFERENCES

1. Alajouanine T, Aubry M, Pialoux P. Les grande activitiés du lobe temporal. Paris: Masson, 203. Quoted in Bocca E, Calearo C. Central hearing processes. In: Jerger J, ed. Modern developments in audiology. New York: Academic Press, 1963.
2. Bocca E, Calearo C, Migliavacca F, Cassinari V. Testing "cortical" hearing in temporal lobe tumours. Acta Otolaryngol (Stockh) 1955; 45:282–304.
3. Matzker J. Two new methods for the assessment of central auditory function in cases of brain disease. Ann Otol Rhinol Laryngol 1959; 68:1185–1197.
4. Carhart R. Special hearing tests for otoneurological diagnosis. Arch Otolaryngol (Stockh) 1969; 89:38–41.
5. Cummings CW, Fredrickson JM, Harker LA, Krause CJ, Schuller DE. Otolaryngology-head and neck surgery, IV: ear and skull base, part 1. St Louis: CV Mosby, 1976:2555.
6. Musiek FE, Baran JE. Neuroanatomy, neurophysiology, and central auditory assessment. Part I: brain stem. Ear Hear 1986; 7:206–219.
7. Musiek FE. Neuroanatomy, neurophysiology, and central auditory assessment. Part II: the cerebrum. Ear Hear 1986; 7:283–294.
8. Musiek FE. Neuroanatomy, neurophysiology, and central auditory assessment. Part III: corpus callosum and efferent pathways. Ear Hear 1986; 7:349–358.
9. Morest DK. Structural organization of the auditory pathways. In: Tower D, ed. Human communication and its disorders. 3: The nervous system. New York: Raven Press, 1975.
10. Diamond IT, Feldman M, Galambos R, et al. Neuroanatomy of the auditory system. Arch Otolaryngol (Stockh) 1973; 98:397–413.
11. Glattke T. Elements of auditory physiology. In: Minifie F, Hixon T, Williams F, eds. Normal aspects of speech, hearing and language. Englewood Cliffs, NJ: Prentice-Hall, 1973.
12. Carhart R. Binaural reception of meaningful material. In: Grahm AB, ed. Sensorineural hearing processes and disorders. Boston: Little, Brown, 1967.
13. Broadbent DE. Perception and communication. Oxford: Pergamon Press, 1958.
14. Keith RW. Central auditory testing: some ongoing questions. Hum Commun Can 1985; 9:145–150.
15. Jerger S, Jerger J. Pediatric speech intelligibility test: performance-intensity characteristics. Ear Hear 1982; 3:325–334.
16. Witkin BR, Butler KG, Whalen TE. Auditory processing in children: two studies of component factors. Lang Speech Hear Serv School 1977; 3:140–154.
17. Wiig E, Semel EM. Language disabilities in children and adolescents. Columbus, OH: C Merritt, 1976.
18. Bocca E, Calearo C, Cassinari V. A new method for testing hearing in temporal lobe tumours. Acta Otolaryngol (Stockh) 1954; 44:219–221.
19. Teatini GP. Sensitized speech tests: results in normal subjects. In: Rojskjaer C, ed. Speech audiometry. Second Danavox Symp, Odense, Denmark, 1970:37.
20. Jerger J. Audiological manifestations of lesions in the auditory nervous system. Laryngoscope 1960; 70:417–425.
21. Jerger J. Observations on auditory behavior in lesions of the central auditory pathways. Arch Otolaryngol (Stockh) 1960; 71:797–806.
22. Davis RJ, Kastelanski W, Stephens SDG. Some factors influencing the results of speech tests of central auditory function. Scand Audiol 1976; 5:179–186.
23. Katz J. The staggered spondaic word test. In: Keith RW, ed. Central auditory dysfunction. New York: Grune and Stratton, 1977.
24. Smith B, Resnick D. An auditory test for assessing brain stem integrity: a preliminary report. Laryngoscope 1972; 82:414–424.
25. Beasley D, Freeman BS. Time altered speech as a measure of central auditory processing. In: Keith RW, ed. Central auditory dysfunction. New York: Grune & Stratton, 1977.
26. Quaranta A, Cassano P, Cervellera G. Clinical value of the tonal masking level difference. Audiology 1978; 17:232–238.
27. Lynn GE, Gilroy J. Evaluation of central auditory dysfunction in patients with neurological disorders. In: Keith RW, ed. Central auditory dysfunction. New York: Grune and Stratton, 1977.
28. Fifer RJ, Jerger JF, Berlin C, Tobey EA, Campbell JC. Development of a dichotic sentence identification test for hearing impaired adults. Ear Hear 1983; 4:300–305.
29. Mueller HG, Sedge RK, Salazar AM. Auditory assessment of neural trauma. In Miner M, Wagner K, eds. Neuro-

trauma: treatment rehabilitation and related issues. Stoneham, MA: Butterworths, 1985.
30. Goldman-Fristoe-Woodcock test of auditory discrimination. Circle Pines, Minn: American Guidance Service, 1970.
31. Katz J, Illmer R. Auditory perception in children with learning disabilities. In: Katz J, ed. Handbook of clinical audiology. Baltimore: Williams and Wilkins, 1972.
32. Willeford J. Assessing central auditory behavior in children: a test battery approach. In: Keith RW, ed. Central auditory dysfunction. New York: Grune and Stratton, 1977.
33. Keith RW. SCAN, a screening test for auditory processing disorders. San Antonio: Psychological Corporation, 1986.
34. Antonelli AR. Sensitized speech tests in aged people. In: Rojskajaer C, ed. Speech audiometry. Odense, Denmark: Second Danavox Symposium, 1970.
35. Bocca E. Distorted speech tests. In: Grahm AB, ed. Sensorineural hearing processes and disorders. Boston: Little, Brown, 1967.
36. Katz J. Differential diagnosis of auditory impairments. In: Fulton RT, Lloyd LL, eds. Audiometry for the retarded: with implications for the difficult-to-test. Baltimore: Williams & Wilkins, 1969.
37. Calearo C, Antonelli AR. Audiometric findings in brain stem lesions. Acta Otolaryngol (Stockh) 1968; 66:305.
38. Gat I, Keith RW. An effect of linguistic experience on auditory word discrimination by native and non-native speakers of English. Audiology 1978; 17:339–345.
39. Rawizer SJ. Performance of non-native English speakers on the staggered spondaic word test. In: Arnst D, Katz J, eds. Central auditory assessment: the SSW test development and clinical uses. San Diego: College Hill Press, 1982.
40. Keith RW, Katbamna R, Tawfik S, Smolak L. The effect of linguistic background on staggered spondaic word and dichotic consonant vowel scores. Brit J Audiol 1987; 21:21–26.
41. Anderson H, Barr B, Wedenberg E. Early diagnosis of VIII N. tumours by acoustic reflex tests. Acta Otolaryngol [Suppl] (Stockh) 1970; 263:232–237.
42. Johnson EW. Auditory test results in 500 cases of acoustic neuroma. Arch Otolaryngol (Stockh) 1977; 103:152–158.
43. Jerger S, Jerger J. Diagnostic value of crossed versus uncrossed acoustic reflexes. Arch Otolaryngol (Stockh) 1977; 103:445–453.
44. Thomas WG, McMurry G, Pillsbury H. Acoustic reflex abnormalities in behaviorally disturbed and language delayed children. Laryngoscope 1985; 96:811–817.
45. Buchwald J, Huang C. Far-field acoustic response: origins in the cat. Science 1975; 189:382–384.
46. Moller AR. Physiology of the ascending auditory pathway with special reference to the auditory brainstem response (ABR). In: Pinheiro ML, Musiek FE, eds. Assessment of central auditory dysfunction. Baltimore: Williams and Wilkins, 1985.
47. Keith RW, Jacobson J. Demyelinating disease. In: Jacobson J, ed. The auditory brainstem response. San Diego: College-Hill Press, 1984.
48. Bocca E, Calearo C. Central hearing processes. In: Jerger J, ed. Modern developments in audiology. New York: Academic Press, 1963.
49. Korsan-Bengsten M. Speech audiometry. Rojskjaer C, ed. Second Danavox Symp, Odense, Denmark: 1970.
50. Korsan-Bengsten M. Distorted speech audiometry. Acta Otolaryngol (Stockh) 1973; [Suppl]:310.
51. Heilman KM, Hammer LC, Wilder BJ. An audiometric defect in temporal lobe dysfunction. Neurology 1973; 23:384–386.
52. Jerger J, Speaks C, Trammel J. A new approach to speech audiometry. J Speech Hear Disord 1968; 33:318–328.
53. Lynn GE, Gilroy J. Neuro-audiological abnormalities in patients with temporal lobe tumors. J Neurol Sci 1972; 17:167–184.
54. Calearo C, Antonelli AR. Disorders of the central auditory nervous system. In: Paparella M, Shumrick DA, eds. Otolaryngology 2: Ear. Philadelphia: WB Saunders, 1973.
55. Calearo C, Antonelli AR. "Cortical" hearing tests and cerebral dominance. Acta Otolaryngol (Stockh) 1963; 56:17–26.
56. Beasley D, Schwimmer S, Rintelman W. Intelligibility of time compressed CNC monosyllables. J Speech Hear Res 1972; 15:340–350.
57. Kurdziel S, Noffsinger D, Olsen W. Performance by cortical lesion patients on 40% and 60% time compressed materials. J Am Audiol Soc 1976; 2:3–7.
58. Jerger J. Diagnostic significance of the SSI test procedures: Retrocochlear site. Paper presented Second Danavox Symp, Odense, Denmark: 1970; 29–30.
59. Speaks C, Jerger J. A method for measurement of speech identification. J Speech Hear Res 1965; 8:185–194.
60. Keith RW. Synthetic sentence identification. In: Keith RW, ed. Central auditory dysfunction. New York: Grune and Stratton, 1977.
61. Berlin CI, Porter RJ, Lowe-Bell SS, Berlin H, et al. Dichotic signs of the recognition of speech elements in normals, temporal lobectomees, and hemispherectomees. IEEE Trans Audio Electroacoust AU 1973; 21:189–195.
62. Musiek FE. Assessment of central auditory function: the dichotic digit test revisited. Ear Hear 1983; 4:79–83.
63. Berlin CI, Lowe SS, Cullen JK, et al. Central auditory dysfunction. Paper presented Ann Conv Am Speech Hearing Assoc, New York City, 1970.
64. Berlin CI, Lowe SS. Differential diagnostic evalution: central auditory function. In: Katz J, ed. Handbook of clinical audiology. Baltimore: Williams & Wilkins, 1972.
65. Ryan W, McNeil M. Listener reliability for a dichotic task. J Acoust Soc Am 1974; 56:922–1023.
66. Blumstein S, Goodglass H, Tarter V. The reliability of ear advantage in dichotic listening. Brain Lang 1975; 2:226–236.
67. Speaks C, Niccum N. Variability of the ear advantage in dichotic listening. J Am Audiol Soc 1977; 3:52–57.
68. Obrzut J, Hynd G, Obrzut A, Pirozzolo F. Effects of directed attention on cerebral asymetry in normal and learning disabled children. Dev Psychol 1981; 17:118–125.
69. Schulman-Galambos C. Dichotic listening performance in elementary and college students. Neuropsychologia 1977; 15:577–584.
70. Hynd G, Cohen M, Obrzut, J. Dichotic consonant-vowel (CV) testing in the diagnosis of learning disabilities in children. Ear Hear 1983; 4:283–286.
71. Keith RE, Tawfik S, Katbamna, B. Performance of adults on directed listening tasks using a dichotic CV test. Ear Hear 1985; 6:270–273.
72. Berlin CI, Lowe-Bell SS, Jennetta PJ, et al. Central auditory defects after temporal lobectomy. Arch Otolaryngol 1972; 96:4–10.
73. Brown HP. Performance on a dichotic speech test by patients with cortical lesion. Paper presented Ann Conv Am Speech Hearing Assoc, Las Vegas: 1974.
74. Olsen W. Performance of temporal lobectomy patients with dichotic CV test materials. Paper presented Ann Conv Am Speech Hearing Assoc, Chicago, 1977.
75. Speaks C, Gray T, Miller J, Rubens A. Central auditory deficits and temporal lobe lesions. J Speech Hear Disord 1975; 40:192–205.
76. Katz J. The use of staggered spondaic words for assessing the integrity of the central auditory nervous system. J Auditory Res 1962; 2:327–337.
77. Katz J. The SSW test: an interim report. J Speech Hear Disord 1968; 33:132–146.
78. Brunt MA. The staggered spondaic word test. In: Katz J, ed. Handbook of clinical audiology. Baltimore: Williams and Wilkins, 1972.
79. Arnst DJ, Doyle PC. Verification of the corrected staggered spondiac word score in adults with cochlear hearing loss.

Ear Hear 1983; 4:243–246.
80. Willeford J. Central auditory function in children with learning disabilities. Paper presented Ann Conv Am Speech Hearing Assoc, Las Vegas, 1974.
81. Willeford J. Sentence tests of central auditory function. In: Katz J, ed. Handbook of clinical audiology. 2nd ed. Baltimore: Williams & Wilkins, 1978.
82. Lynn GE, Gilroy J. Central aspects of audition. In: Northern JL, ed. Hearing Disorders. Boston: Little, Brown, 1976.
83. Collard ME, Lesser RP, Luders J, Dinner DS, et al. Four dichotic speech tests before and after temporal lobectomy. Ear Hear 1987; 7:363–369.
84. Grimes AM, Grady CL, Foster NL, Sunderland T, Patronas N. Central auditory function in Alzheimer's disease. Neurology 1985; 3:352–358.
85. Bergman M, Hirsch S, Solzi PO, Mankowitz Z. Interhemispheric suppression: a new test of central auditory function. Ear Hear 1987; 8:147–150.
86. Palva A, Jokinen K. The role of the binaural test in filtered speech audiometry. Acta Otolaryngol (Stockh) 1975; 79:310–314.
87. Olsen W, Noffsinger D. Masking level differences for cochlear and brain stem lesions. Ann Otol Rhinol Laryngol 1976; 85:820–826.
88. McFadden D. Masking and the binaural system. In: Tower D, ed. Human communication and its disorders. 3: The Nervous System. New York: Raven Press, 1975.
89. Cullen JK, Thompson CL. Masking release for speech in subjects with temporal lobe resections. Arch Otolaryngol (Stockh) 1974; 100:113–116.
90. Noffsinger D, Kurdziel S, Applebaum EL. Value of special auditory tests in the latero-medial inferior pontine syndrome. Ann Otol Rhinol Laryngol 1975; 84:384–391.
91. Roeser RJ, Downs JP. Auditory Disorders in School Children. 2nd ed. New York: Thieme-Stratton 1987.
92. Witkin BR. Auditory perception: implications for language development. Lang Speech Hear Serv 1971; 4:31–52.
93. Bannatyne A. Programs, materials and techniques: GFW test of auditory discrimination. J Learn Disabil 1975; 8:130–132.
94. Pinheiro M. Tests of central auditory function in children with learning disabilities. In: Keith RW, ed. Central auditory dysfunction. New York: Grune & Stratton, 1977.
95. Sweetow RW, Reddell RC. Masking level differences for children with auditory perceptual problems. Paper presented Ann Conv Am Speech Hearing Assoc, Chicago, 1977.
95a. McCroskey R. Witchita auditory processing test. Tulsa, OK: Modern Education Corp, 1986.
96. Berlin CI, Hughes L, Lowe-Bell SS, Berlin H. Dichotic right ear advantage in children 5 to 13. Cortex 1973; 9:393–401.
97. White E. Children's performance on the SSW test and Willeford battery: interim clinical data. In: Keith RW, ed. Central Auditory Dysfunction. New York: Grune and Stratton, 1977.
98. Willeford JA. Assessment of central auditory disorders in children. In Pinheiro ML, Musiek FE, eds. Assessment of central auditory dysfunction. Baltimore: Williams and Wilkins, 1985.
99. Lasky E, Tobin H. Linguistic and non-linguistic competing message effects. J Learn Disabil 1973; 6:243–250.
100. Marsh DH. Auditory figure-ground ability in children. Am J Occup Ther 1973; 27:218–225.
101. Carlin M, Kasten R. Listening skills of children in regular and learning disability classrooms. Paper presented Ann Conv Am Speech Hearing Assoc Chicago, 1977.
102. Hand JB, McGroskey RL. Auditory figure ground among dysphasic children. J Kansas Speech Hear Assoc 1977; 17:49–57.
103. Palanker S. A study of the effects of a competing message on normal and learning disabled children. Master's Thesis, Cincinnati, OH: Univ Cincinnati, 1978.
104. Farrer S. An experimental design for a filtered word test to identify auditory learning-disabled children. Master's Thesis. Univ Cincinnati. Cincinnati, OH: 1977.
105. Stubblefield J, Young C. Central auditory dysfunction in learning-disabled children. J Learn Disabil 1975; 8:89–94.
106. Bannatyne A. Language, reading and learning disabilities. Springfield, IL: CC Thomas, 1971.
107. Kirk S, Kirk W. Psycholinguistic learning disabilities: diagnosis and remediation. Urbana, IL: Univ Illinois Press, 1971.
108. Wepman J, Morency A. Manual of the audito-sequential memory test. Los Angeles: Western Psychological Services, 1973.
109. Wepman J, Morency A. Manual of the audito-memory span test. Los Angeles: Western Psychological Services, 1973.
110. Wepman J. Manual of the auditory discrimination test. Los Angeles: Western Psychological Services, 1973.
111. Manning W, Johnston K, Beasley D. The performance of children with auditory perceptual disorders on a time compressed speech discrimination measure. J Speech Hear Disord 1977; 42:77–84.
112. Sommers R, Taylor M. Cerebral speech dominance in language-disordered and normal children. Cortex 1972; 7:224–232.
113. Willeford J. Central auditory function in children with learning disabilities. Audiol Hear Ed February/March, 1976; 12–20.
114. Welsh MW, Allison RB, Dahle A. Psychometric differences in learning disordered and normal children. J Develop Disabil 1975; 1:17–24.
115. Larsen S, Rogers D, Sowell V. The use of selected perceptual tests in differentiating between normal and learning-disabled children. J Learn Disabil 1976; 9:32–37.
116. Rees N. The speech pathologist and the reading process. Asha 1974; 16:255–258.
117. Rampp D. Proceeding of the Memphis State University First Annual Symposium on Auditory Processing and Learning Disabilities, 1972.
118. Butler KG. Auditory perceptual processing and dysfunction. 16th Int Cong Logopedics Phoniatrics. Interlaken, 1974. Basel: Karger, 1976:65–69.
119. Lindamood CH, Lindamood PC. The A. D. D. program: auditory discrimination in depth. Boston: Teaching Resources Corp, 1969.
120. Butler KG. Auditory perceptual training. Acta Symbol 1972; 3:123–125.
121. Lasky E. An approach to auditory processing. Acta Symbol 1973; 4:51–62.
122. Rupp D, Olsen D, Saxman S, Shapiro E, Doyle K. Auditory perception and processing skills: commercially available resources for assessment and remediation. Program in Special Education. Speech and Hearing Sciences. Univ Michigan. Revised, April 1978.
123. Semel E. Sound order sense: a development program in auditory perception. Chicago: Follette Publishing, 1970.
124. Witkin BR. Auditory perceptual training program. Hayward, CA: Alameda County Schools, 1973.
125. Willette R, Jackson B, Plekins I. Auditory perceptual training. Niles, IL: Developmental Learning Materials, 1970.
126. Rees N. Auditory processing factors in learning disorders: a view from Procrustes' bed. J Speech Hear Disord 1973; 38:304–315.
127. Rees N. When is an auditory processing disorder not an auditory processing disorder. Paper presented California Speech Hearing Assoc, Palo Alto, California, April 1976.
128. Vellutino F, Steger B, Moyer S, et al. Has the perceptual deficit hypothesis led us astray? J Learn Disabil 1977; 10:375–385.
129. Marquardt T, Saxman J. Language comprehension and au-

ditory discrimination in articulation deficient kindergarten children. J Speech Hear Res 1972; 15:382–389.
130. Lyon R. Auditory perceptual training: the state of the art. J Learn Disabil 1977; 10:564–572.
131. Russ AO. Psychological aspects of learning disabilities and reading disorders. New York: McGraw-Hill, 1976.
132. Willeford J. Central auditory processing test norms. Unpublished data, March, 1978.
133. Willeford J, Billger J. Auditory perception in children with learning disabilities. In: Katz J, ed. Handbook of clinical audiology. 2nd ed. Baltimore: Williams and Wilkins, 1978.
134. Taylor K. People hearing without listening: problems of auditory processing in the classroom. Res Teach English 1978; 12:61–75.
135. Keith RW, Stromberg E. An interdisciplinary approach to the identification and assessment of auditory processing disorders. J Childhood Comm Disord 1985; IX:15–30.
136. Youkilis D. Comment made at a meeting of the Southwestern Ohio Speech Hearing Assoc, Cincinnati, Ohio, February 1977.

46 Medical and Surgical Treatment of Hearing Loss

Gerald M. English, M.D., F.A.C.S.
Ruth S. Sargent, M.A.

This chapter contains discussions of the medical and surgical treatment of diseases and disorders that cause hearing impairment. A complex variety of defects, diseases, and disorders can cause hearing loss of varying degrees. These are classified as congenital, inflammatory, traumatic, neoplastic, and miscellaneous disorders.

Often medical and surgical treatments are integrated during the course of a disease, and one therapy does not necessarily exclude the other. A complete description of treatment is not possible in a text of this type, but an attempt has been made to include as much information as possible. There are disease entities in which controversy exists as to the preferred method of treatment, and in each of these instances, the reader is referred to other sources of information. A discussion of the complications of treatment is included when a hearing impairment or vestibular disturbance results from the treatment. Some disorders that do not have associated hearing loss and are not amenable to treatment have also been omitted.

The treatment of a specific disease is not always the same. Many factors influence the physician's decisions. Age, sex, occupation, social status, and the patient's general health, including concomitant disorders, are factors that the physician evaluates when choosing and recommending therapy. The medical and surgical treatment of most diseases is continually evolving, with the formation of new concepts and revision of older ideas. This text should be used as a guide; it is not intended to be an exclusive source of information.

CONGENITAL AND HEREDITARY DISEASES

There is an important distinction between congenital and hereditary diseases. Congenital diseases are those entities that are present at birth. Many such diseases and disorders are acquired, including maternal rubella (measles) and lues (syphilis). Hereditary diseases are those that are transmitted genetically from the parents to the child, such as otosclerosis. Hearing losses are associated with many of these disorders, and although the diseases are quite different they are discussed together.

External Ear

Microtia, Anotia, and Atresia. Anomalies of the external ear are usually associated with a hearing loss. The most common abnormalities consist of faulty development of the auricle and external auditory canal (Fig. 46–1). Microtia, anotia, and atresia of the ear canal arise from abnormal development of the external ear.[1] These may be associated with a conductive hearing loss (40 to 60 dB air-bone gap) even when the canal is patent.[2] An obstructed ear canal with anomalies of the middle ear and ossicular chain produces a severe hearing impairment. In some patients, there is a sensorineural hearing loss caused by a concomitant inner ear anomaly. An x-ray examination is necessary to determine the extent of the abnormality and the advisability of surgical treatment. Surgery to restore hearing should be consid-

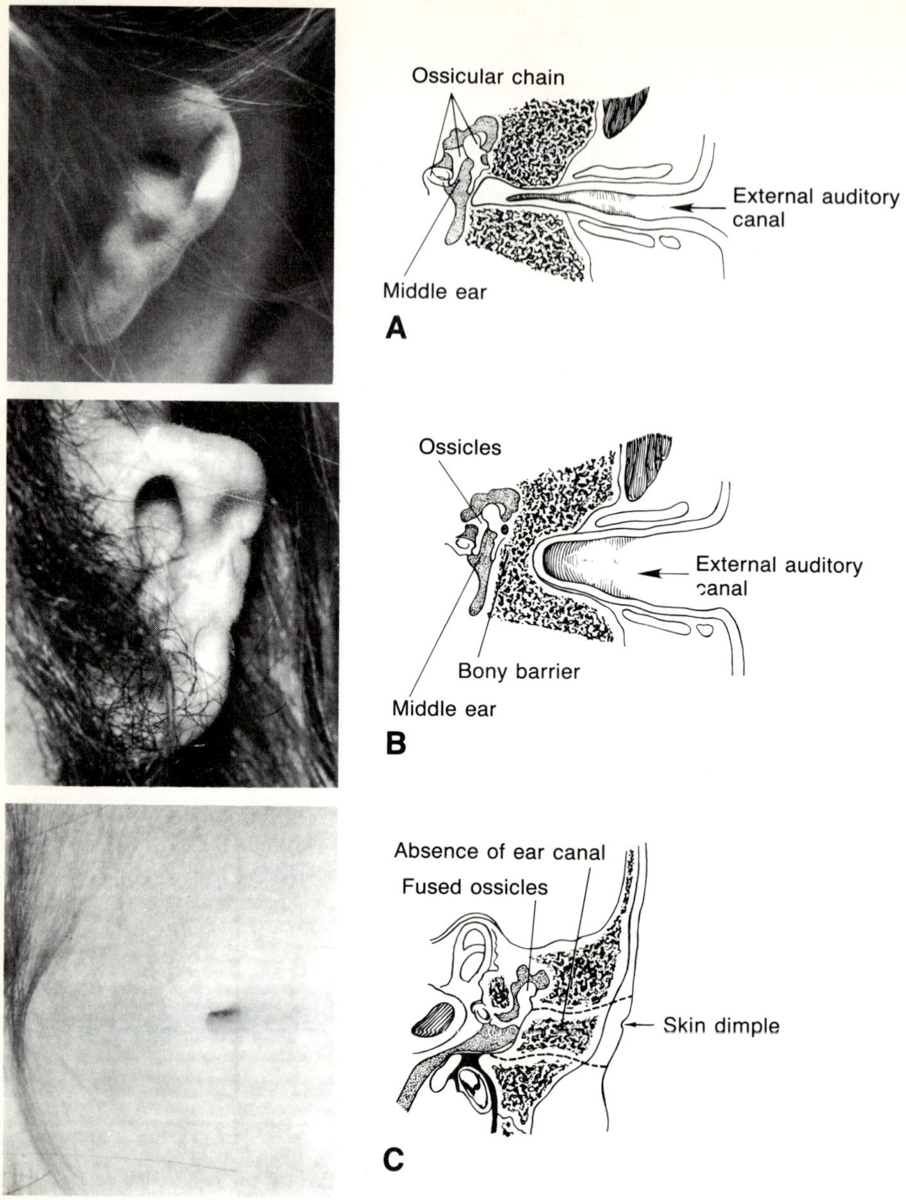

Figure 46–1 Photos and drawings of microtia and atresia. *A*, 11-year-old white female with auricular deformity and tiny, incomplete external auditory canal. *B*, 24-year-old white male with auricular deformity and atresia of external auditory canal. *C*, 12-year-old white female with absence of auricle and tiny skin dimple that corresponds to the location of the external auditory canal.

ered only after the patient has been fully evaluated. In many patients, a two-stage operation is necessary (Fig. 46–2). The surgeon must choose and design the operation that exactly fits the needs of the particular patient's abnormality.[3] In some patients, the best treatment is not to operate. There is no single surgical procedure that is suitable for all the patients. Dead ears, facial nerve paralysis, and chronic otorrhea can result from an unnecessary or inappropriate operation. When surgery is not possible or when it fails to restore the hearing, amplification, preferential seating in school, and speech therapy should be instituted.

There are three basic groups of patients with these anomalies, classified by degree of anatomic involvement from mild to severe.

Patients in the first group have fixed stapes footplates and otherwise relatively normal external and middle ears. Several methods of surgical treatment are available, including stapes mobilization,

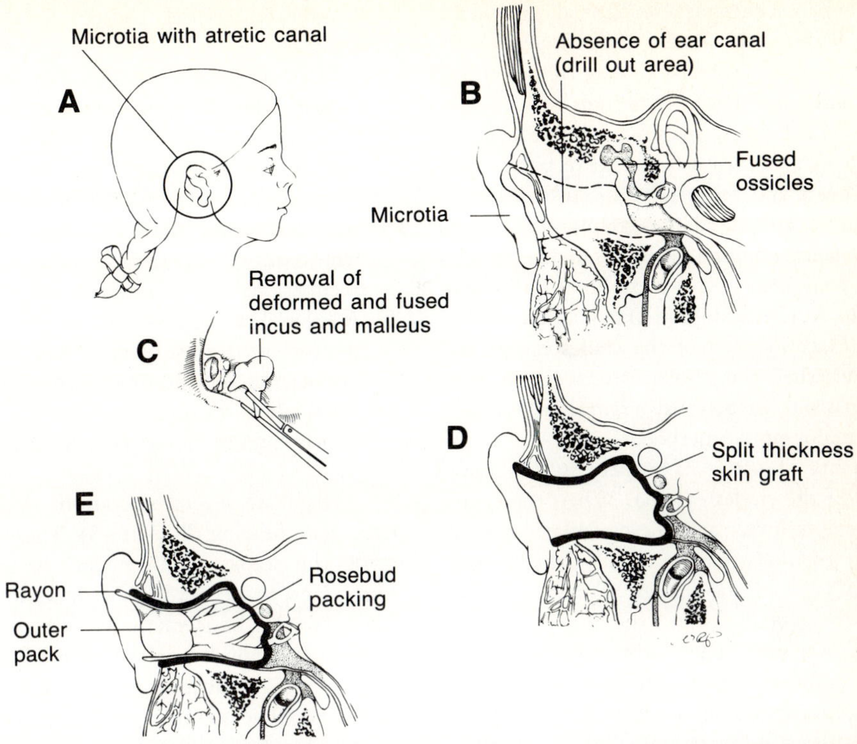

Figure 46–2 Drawings of repair of atresia. *A*, Microtia with an atretic external auditory canal. *B*, Absence of the ear canal and fused ossicles. The drill-out area is shown by the dotted line. *C*, The deformed incus and malleus are removed. *D*, An external auditory canal has been created by removing the atretic plate of bones. A split thickness skin graft has been inserted. *E*, The skin graft is securely packed in position. This graft is positioned to make contact with the capitulum of the stapes.

stapedectomy, and drill-out of the oval window. Mobilization offers the advantage of at least partial closure of the air-bone gap in hearing with less likelihood of postoperative complications, such as sensorineural hearing loss. Stapedectomy and drill-out procedures result in more complete closure of the air-bone gap, with a slight increase in possibility of postoperative complications, such as perilymph leak, meningitis, facial paralysis, or a "dead" ear.

Patients in the second group include more severe anatomic abnormalities, including absence of the external meatus and tympanic membrane and malformation of the stapes. The mastoid air cell system is usually intact, but surgery is less likely to be successful than for the first group of patients. If one ear is normal, it is usually better not to operate on the abnormal ear.

The third group includes individuals without an external meatus and tympanic membrane who have stapedial deformities plus poor or absent pneumatization of the mastoid air cell system. These patients are poor surgical candidates. Those with unilateral abnormalities should not have surgery because the results are poor. Also, the risks of an injury to the facial nerve from the surgery reduce the acceptability of the operation.[4]

Middle Ear

Stapes Footplate Fixation. Stapes footplate fixation, fusion of the ossicles, and absence of the ossicles are commonly associated with atresia of the external auditory canal. Some of these entities have been discussed in the previous section.

Vascular Anomalies. Congenital vascular anomalies include the anomalous carotid artery and prominent jugular bulb. The anomalous carotid artery is usually unilateral. These patients may complain of a pulsating tinnitus in the involved ear, and usually a bruit (noise) can be heard in the external auditory canal by the examiner. There may be a conductive or mixed hearing loss, and a vascular mass can be seen in the inferior portion of the ear behind the tympanic membrane. There are usually no other associated anomalies.

Eustachian Tube Atresia. Eustachian tube atresia is most common in the third group of patients who have an associated absence of the mastoid air cell system. These patients are poor candidates for surgery because the middle ear cleft is small or atretic.

Congenital Cholesteatoma. Congenital cholesteatoma of the middle ear and mastoid are dysplasias that have a characteristic clinical presentation.[5] These lesions are usually associated with a conductive hearing loss. There is a white colored mass within the middle ear space behind an intact tympanic membrane. Petrous pyramid cholesteatomas are usually associated with a facial nerve palsy that is gradual in onset and progressive in nature. Polytome radiography, computed tomography (CT), and magnetic resonance imaging (MRI) scans are much better than a conventional x-ray examination in determining the exact location and extent of any bony erosion. The exact location of the cholesteatoma is important. Whether the cholesteatoma is in the middle ear, mastoid, or petrous pyramid is best determined by radiographic methods.

The primary objective of surgery is the complete excision of the cholesteatoma. When the tympanic membrane is intact and the ossicular chain is not disrupted, good hearing can usually be obtained by surgical excision of the disease. When there is disruption of the ossicular chain, the hearing results are less satisfactory. An "open" operation in which the posterior auditory canal is removed (modified radical mastoidectomy or radical mastoidectomy) gives poorer but occasionally satisfactory hearing results. These patients often require periodic cleaning of the mastoid cavity and usually must avoid situations in which water enters the cavity.

Otosclerosis. Otosclerosis is a hereditary disorder that is thought to be due to an autosomal dominant gene.[6] It occurs in about 1:500 people in the United States. The hearing loss usually begins between the ages of 20 and 25 and is often exacerbated by pregnancy. The prevalence is 1:8 in adult white females and 1:15 in adult white males. Otosclerosis is much less common in Orientals and Negroes. Both ears are affected in most patients. The sites of predilection are the oval and round window areas. The physical examination is usually normal, but a pink mass may be seen on the promontory of the middle ear (Schwartze's sign) during the active stages of the disease.

Patients who are candidates for a stapedectomy should have the following before surgery:

1. The Rinne tuning fork test should be negative. This indicates an air-bone gap of 20 dB or more.
2. Those patients with a bilateral hearing loss are better candidates for stapedectomy than those with normal hearing in one ear. However, there are some patients with unilateral hearing loss who need binaural hearing in their occupations. An operation is indicated in these patients.
3. Most patients with otosclerosis have good discrimination and will benefit from a hearing aid. This should always be discussed with the patient before surgery is chosen as the method of treatment.
4. The stapedectomy operation is an elective procedure, and the risks and morbidity should be discussed fully before the patient makes a decision to have the operation. The surgery should be performed at a convenient time when the patient has ample time to recover. Those patients who require exceptionally good balance in their occupations should probably forego surgery.
5. A severe hearing loss does not necessarily exempt the patient from surgery. When there is a mixed loss with a significant sensorineural component, a stapedectomy may improve the hearing sufficiently for a more satisfactory hearing aid fitting.

There are several operations that give the patient good hearing (Fig. 46–3). These operations include the stapes mobilization, an anterior crurotomy, and stapedectomy with various prostheses. There are two basic methods of stapes surgery. The first group includes partial or total removal of the stapes with the introduction of a metal or plastic prosthesis. The second group of procedures consists of the use of an autogenous tissue graft or repositioning of parts of the patient's stapes. This latter technique avoids the use of artificial materials in the middle ear. A closure of the air-bone gap to 10 dB or better can be achieved in 80 to 90 percent of patients. A sensorineural hearing loss with an associated loss of speech discrimination (30 percent or more) occurs in 1 to 3 percent of patients. A decrease in speech discrimination of 10 to 30 percent has been encountered in about 6 percent of patients. A hearing aid may be needed in some patients after stapes surgery, but the timing is important.[7]

There are several possible complications of stapes surgery. Injury to the chorda tympani nerve causes a loss of taste in the anterior two-thirds of the tongue on the operated side. A dry mouth from a decrease in the secretory function of the submandibular and sublingual glands may occur when the chorda tympani nerve is injured. These symptoms usually subside within a few weeks.

A perilymph fistula occurs when the prosthesis perforates the oval window membrane or an inadequate membrane is formed. A sudden or rapid change in atmospheric pressure that occurs when flying in an unpressurized aircraft, scuba diving, or traveling at high altitudes in the mountains can produce a perilymph leak about the prosthesis.[8] A sharply pointed stapes prosthesis is more apt to cause a leak than the stainless steel wire or platinum loop. These patients usually experience a sudden loss of hearing and a discrimination score that is poorer than the pure tone configuration would indicate. The hearing

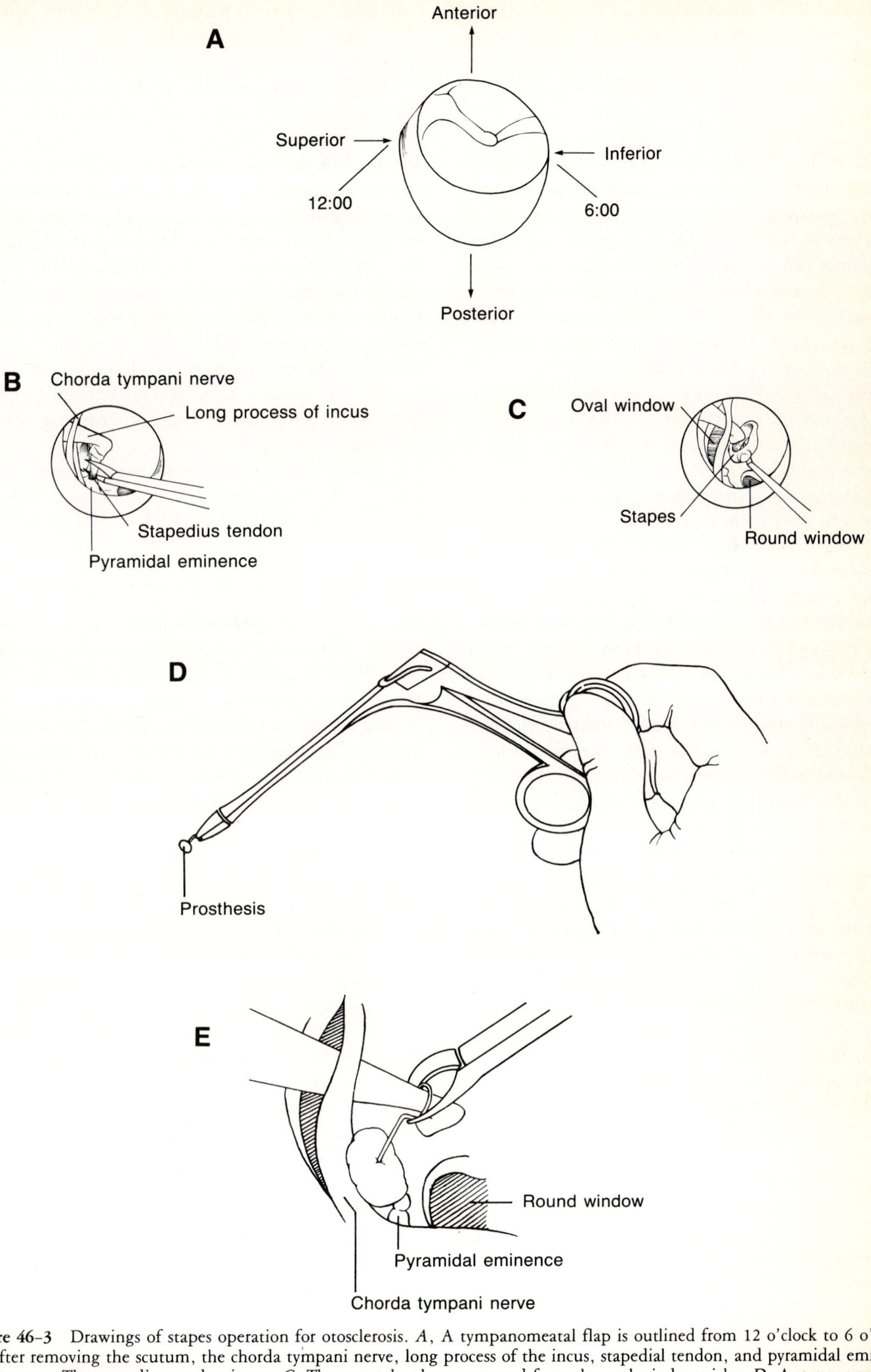

Figure 46–3 Drawings of stapes operation for otosclerosis. *A*, A tympanomeatal flap is outlined from 12 o'clock to 6 o'clock. *B*, After removing the scutum, the chorda tympani nerve, long process of the incus, stapedial tendon, and pyramidal eminence can be seen. The stapedius tendon is cut. *C*, The stapes has been removed from the oval window niche. *D*, A stapes prosthesis is prepared for insertion into the middle ear. *E*, The stapes prosthesis is placed into the middle ear and attached to the long process of the incus. The tympanomeatal flap is then returned to its normal anatomic position and the procedure is completed.

impairment may fluctuate from mild to severe. There is an associated dysequilibrium. A prompt surgical exploration of the ear with closure of the fistula is the only satisfactory means of treatment. A tissue graft is the best method of closing the fistula.

Sudden sensorineural hearing loss may occur months or years after stapedecomy. This is more common after a traumatic operation or following a revision operation.

There are several problems that produce recurrence of the conductive hearing loss after stapes surgery. A regrowth of otosclerotic bone, resorption of the long process of the incus, ankylosis of the malleus and incus, or displacement of the prosthesis will cause a gradual or sudden conductive hearing loss. Foreign bodies and adhesions in the vestibule of the inner ear may cause a sensorineural hearing loss and vertigo when the patient is exposed to loud sounds (Tullio phenomenon).

Osteogenesis Imperfecta. The syndrome of blue sclerae (blue-colored whites of the eyes), fragile bones, and deafness was first described by van der Hoeve and de Kleijn. The hearing loss found in these patients is indistinguishable from otosclerotic deafness. A theory has been advanced that osteogenesis imperfecta and otosclerosis are based upon a common genetic abnormality and that otosclerosis occurring alone is a local manifestation of osteogenesis imperfecta.[9,10] This theory is supported by the fact that many patients with otosclerosis have blue sclerae but no evidence of fragile bones. In addition to the bony lesion that fixes the stapes footplate, many of these patients have an associated atrophy of the stapes crural arches. The hearing loss begins shortly after puberty when the fractures of the long bones become less frequent. It is a gradually progressive loss. The incidence of a concomitant sensorineural hearing loss is greater in osteogenesis imperfecta than in otosclerosis.

The types of treatment, the hearing results, and the complications of the treatment are almost identical to those obtained in otosclerosis.

Osteopetrosis (Albers-Schönberg Disease). This disease of bone may involve the temporal bone. It can produce a conductive or a sensorineural hearing loss. The conductive hearing loss is due to fixation of the ossicular chain by the osteopetrotic bone. The cause of the sensorineural hearing loss is not clear. These patients often have a recurrent facial paralysis on one or both sides.

Inner Ear

Hereditary Deafness. A wide variety of congenital and hereditary inner ear diseases have been described. About 90 percent of hereditary sensorineural hearing loss is recessive and 10 percent is dominant.

In dominant disorders, if one parent carries the affected gene, the incidence of the disorder is about 50 percent in the offspring of that union. Penetrance and sex linkage will modify that incidence.

In recessive hereditary traits, both parents must be carriers of the defective gene to produce the abnormality in an offspring. According to Mendelian law, only 25 percent of the offspring will be affected. For this reason, there is often no family history of deafness, and this makes it difficult to establish the hereditary nature of the deafness. Excessive hearing losses are common in consanguineous marriages. The recessive sensorineural hearing loss may be static or progressive, and both ears are usually involved.

These patients are usually treated with rehabilitative measures, such as amplification, lipreading, and, when the deafness is total, manual signing.

CONGENITAL ACQUIRED DEAFNESS

Birth Injuries. Birth injuries have not been clearly demonstrated as a cause of deafness. Several factors, including prematurity, prolonged gestation, prolonged or difficult labor, Caesarean delivery, breech deliveries, placenta previa, toxemia of pregnancy, drugs, and asphyxia neonatorum are suspected as causing deafness. The treatment of the deafness should be instituted as early as possible, but surgery for the hearing loss should be delayed until the child is old enough to have a careful audiometric assessment and can cooperate adequately.

Viral Infections. Maternal rubella (measles) may cause many congenital defects, including deafness, cataracts, cardiovascular defects, microcephaly, dental defects, and general stunting of growth and development. These problems are more apt to occur when the rubella occurs during the first and second trimesters of pregnancy. There is a sensorineural hearing loss in most patients. Anomalies of the middle ear are much less common.

Drugs. Drugs, such as thalidomide, have a teratogenic effect. In addition to ectromelia (small bones of one or more limbs), intestinal, genitourinary and cardiovascular defects, there are often severe deformities of the ears. Malformations of the auricle, external auditory canals, middle ear, and inner ear have been reported. There may be a mild to a complete loss of hearing. Livingston found that 75 percent of patients with ear deformities from thalidomide were satisfactory candidates for surgery.[11]

Quinine, when used for malarial therapy in a pregnant woman, may cause profound deafness in the newborn child. The hearing impairment is a severe bilateral sensorineural hearing loss. These children require amplification and special auditory training at an early age.

RH Disease. Hyperbilirubinemia (erythroblastosis fetalis) occurs from an Rh incompatibility (mother Rh negative and child Rh positive). The affected children have a hemolytic anemia, jaundice, encephalopathy, and deafness. Mental retardation, emotional instability, and convulsions also occur. The hearing losses are bilateral, sensorineural, and most severe in the high frequencies. Methods of prophylaxis and improved management of neonatal hyperbilirubinemia have almost eliminated this disorder as a cause of deafness. The hearing losses are usually treated with amplification, lipreading, preferential seating in school, and a hearing conservation program.

Hypothyroidism. Cretinism is a condition that is found among people who live in specific geographic areas. It includes delayed growth, mental retardation, and a combined conductive and sensorineural hearing loss. The deafness does not arise from hypothyroidism after birth, but from maternal hypothyroidism. This maternal metabolic problem produces abnormalities in the developing ear. A conductive hearing loss is usually due to ankylosis or fixation of the stapes, and can usually be corrected by a stapes mobilization operation. The sensorineural hearing loss is due to degeneration of the organ of Corti and cochlear neurons.

INFLAMMATORY DISEASES

External Ear

There are several varieties of inflammation of the external ear that cause a conductive hearing loss. The mechanism of this hearing loss is usually from an obstruction or occlusion of the ear canal. The severity of the conductive hearing loss is proportional to the degree of obstruction. These conditions must be treated by an otologist to avoid scarring or stenosis of the ear canal. Hairpins, Q-tips, and paper clips should not be used to clean the canal.

External otitis is a common disease of the ear. The usual symptoms are pain, swelling, hearing loss, and drainage from the ear. Swimming and the trauma from attempts to clean the ear contribute to this problem. This condition is seen more often in warm, humid climates and during the summer months. The degree of hearing loss is quite variable.

The basic treatment consists of cleaning the ear canal with suction or irrigation. The swelling and pain make cleaning difficult, but it should be as complete as possible. A specimen of pus should be obtained for culture and sensitivity tests. A "wick" placed in the ear canal can be moistened with antibiotic drops several times each day. This reduces the swelling and inflammation of the canal and allows a more thorough cleansing later. When there is fever, cellulitis, or swollen lymph nodes, a systemic antibiotic is required. Those patients who have recurrent external otitis should avoid water in the ears.

Chronic External Otitis

Chronic external otitis consists of the complications of an untreated or poorly treated acute infection. The two most common complications of external otitis are stenosis of the external canal and perichondritis. A stenotic canal occurs when chronically inflamed skin or scar tissue blocks the external canal. These patients have continuous symptoms of drainage, hearing loss, and sometimes pain. To treat this problem, the stenotic segment of the ear canal is excised and the canal enlarged. This area is then lined with a skin graft.

Perichondritis and Chondritis

Perichondritis or chondritis of the auricle occurs when trauma or an infection causes a separation between the cartilage and its perichondrial layer. This reduces the blood supply to the cartilage, and the cartilage rapidly melts away. The ear is red, painful, swollen, and tender (Fig. 46–4). Large doses of in-

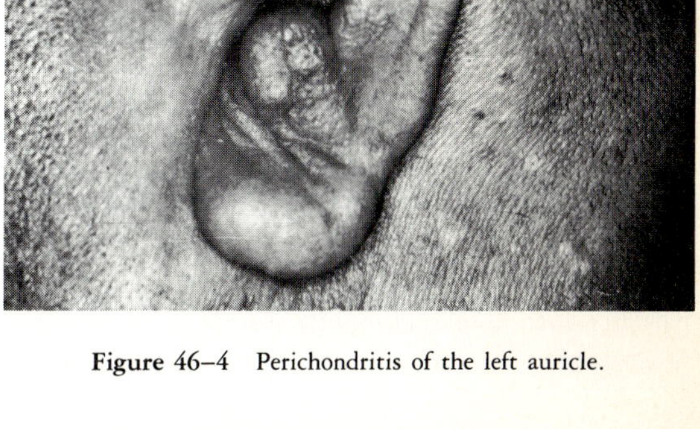

Figure 46–4 Perichondritis of the left auricle.

travenous antibiotics and complete surgical excision of devitalized cartilage are the essentials of treatment.

Tympanic Membrane, Middle Ear, and Mastoid

Myringitis

Myringitis is an inflammation of the tympanic membrane that usually occurs with infections of the middle ear or external auditory canal. It may arise as an isolated infection. The tympanic membrane is thicker than normal but when there is infection of the middle ear with an accumulation of pus, the membrane may bulge into the external auditory canal. With necrosis of the tympanic membrane, a perforation and drainage will ensue. Virulent hemolytic streptococcal infections can produce a total necrosis of the membrane. This is a rare occurrence because antibiotics are effective in controlling the growth of this organism.

Bullous myringitis is an inflammation of the tympanic membrane and adjacent skin of the external auditory canal that is associated with influenza epidemics. Hemorrhagic bullous myringitis may occur with meningoencephalitis and is thought to have a viral etiology. There are blebs of serum and blood within the tympanic membrane. Surprisingly, there is only a minimal hearing loss. The bullae may become infected with bacteria, and this disease can be confused with acute otitis media. The treatment consists of analgesics for pain, antibiotics for the infection, and incision and drainage of the bullae.

Tympanosclerosis. Tympanosclerosis is a term that is applied to various forms of scar tissue that form in the tympanic membrane, middle ear, eustachian tube, or mastoid. This occurs most often in patients who have had serous or acute otitis media, rather than chronic otitis media. It is the consequence of the healing processes of these inflammatory diseases. Surgical excision of this tissue from around the ossicles can be technically very difficult and the tissue tends to recur even after a thorough removal.

Replacement membranes (monomeric membranes) result from the healing of a perforation. Thin areas occur when the fibrous layers of the tympanic membrane fail to proliferate and the new tympanic membrane consists of the external epithelium and mucosa from the middle ear. These areas are almost transparent and may simulate a perforation. Some patients with thin membranes have a perforation in the tympanic membrane when there are changes in atmospheric pressure. These individuals may benefit from a surgical repair (grafting) to strengthen the area. Thick areas occur when there is a proliferation of dense collagenous fibrous tissue in the intermediate layer of the tympanic membrane. This may be the initial phase of tympanosclerosis.

Acute Otitis Media

This is one of the more common ear diseases encountered in clinical practice, and it is more common in children than in adults. Although it is no longer a life-threatening disease, there is a considerable morbidity. It is an illness that incapacitates the patient for some time.

These patients have pain, fever, hearing loss, and vertigo. There is redness and swelling of the tympanic membrane and as the pressure within the middle ear increases, bulging of the tympanic membrane becomes apparent. If a perforation occurs from necrosis of the tympanic membrane, the patient usually experiences a sudden relief of pain. A bloody purulent material flows from the ear (otorrhea), and the temperature usually falls. When the purulent material is aspirated from the ear canal, a thickened tympanic membrane and perforation are apparent.

Medical treatment consists of antibiotics, decongestants, and analgesics. These agents reduce swelling and congestion about the eustachian tube and provide better drainage of the middle ear via that route. Acetominophen every four hours reduces fever and pain. Dry local heat may also help to relieve the pain. Occasionally, analgesic ear drops will be useful for this problem.

Myringotomy is used for specific clinical situations: intense pain, an impending complication or perforation, and a persistent conductive hearing loss are the usual indications for the operation (Fig. 46–5). A local anesthetic is usually sufficient for the procedure, although small children may require a general anesthetic. A myringotomy can give an immediate relief of pain, and the drainage initiates recovery from the disease. The myringotomy incision heals spontaneously and the hearing returns to normal within a short period of time in most patients.

Serous Otitis Media

Serous otitis media refers to an accumulation of fluid in the middle ear space. It may follow an inadequately treated acute otitis media or arise from a noninfectious etiology. The character of the fluids varies greatly. It may be thick and almost gluelike, or thin and watery. There are several synonyms for

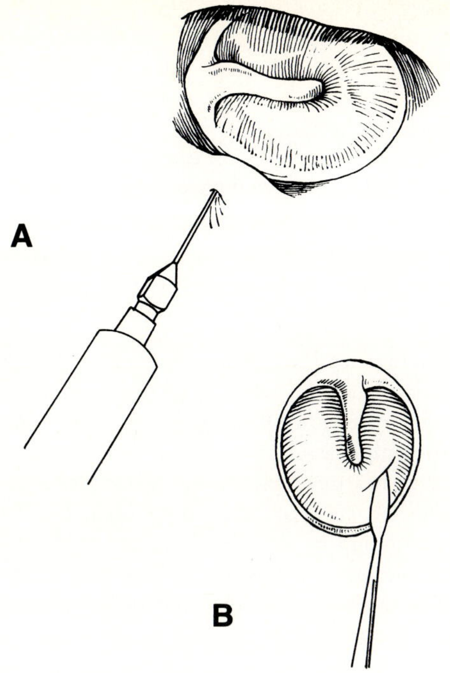

Figure 46–5 Myringotomy. *A*, Myringotomy can be performed with local anesthesia. The solution is injected into the external auditory canal. *B*, An incision is made in the anterior-inferior quadrant of the tympanic membrane.

this condition, including otitic salpingitis, middle ear effusion, glue-ear, or obstructive middle ear disease. It occurs most often in young children in the preschool and elementary school age groups. It is much less common after adolescence or in adults.

The eustachian tube is a principal factor in the etiology of this disease. Obstruction of the eustachian tube impairs ventilation, and a negative pressure occurs in the middle ear and mastoid air cells. Fluid is then drawn into these spaces. This fluid will drain through the eustachian tube if the obstruction is relieved, but when the obstruction is prolonged, a chronic condition ensues. Patients with cleft palate, enlarged adenoids, nasopharyngeal tumors, allergic upper respiratory disease, and poorly formed eustachian tubes are more apt to have this condition. Bacteria and viruses often migrate through the eustachian tube and cause infection and a typical clinical picture of acute otitis media.

These patients have a sense of fullness in the ear, a conductive hearing loss, and "cracking" sounds in the ear. Children with this problem often perform poorly in school, and the condition may contribute to behavioral problems in the family and classroom. The tympanic membrane is retracted and the manubrium of the malleus appears to be shorter than normal. In some patients, an air fluid level or bubbles can be clearly seen through the tympanic membrane. A Siegle pneumatic otoscope will reveal that the tympanic membrane has decreased mobility. Audiometry and tympanometry have diagnostic and prognostic value in these patients.[12]

The treatment is designed to reventilate the middle ear. Both medical and surgical treatment can be used. Decongestants help reduce the edema about the eustachian tube orifice. Antibiotics are required for patients in whom an infection of the nose, nasopharynx, or paranasal sinuses is thought to be present. A Valsalva maneuver (forcing air into the middle ear cavity via the eustachian tube) performed four to six times per day will sometimes relieve the obstruction of the eustachian tube. This medical program successfully relieves the middle ear effusion in many patients. Those patients who do not respond to medical treatment should have surgery. Only 15 to 20 percent of patients require surgical treatment of the middle ear effusion. Tympanotomy, aspiration of the fluid, and insertion of a ventilating tube through the tympanic membrane provides continuing ventilation of the middle ear (Fig. 46–6). This prevents further accumulations of fluid. There are several advantages to this form of treatment. It immediately restores hearing. The tubes prevent further accumulations of fluid for the period of time they are in place. It is not unusual for the tubes to remain in the ear for several weeks or months. They are then spontaneously extruded. The inflammation in the middle ear usually subsides when the fluid is removed and air enters the middle ear. In most patients, the perforation of the tympanic membrane heals spontaneously after the tube extrudes. If the

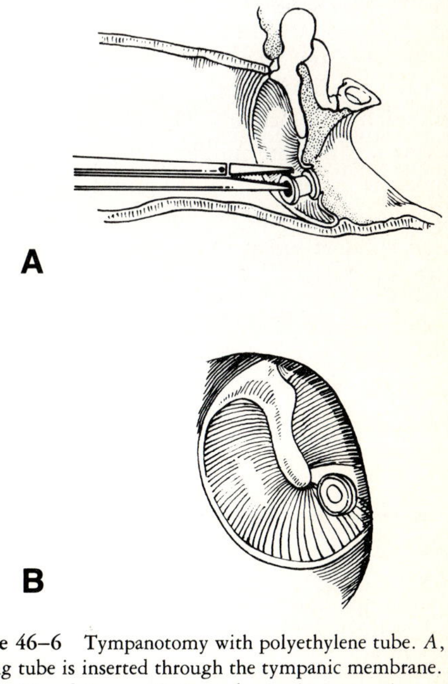

Figure 46–6 Tympanotomy with polyethylene tube. *A*, A ventilating tube is inserted through the tympanic membrane. *B*, The relationship of the ventilating tube to the tympanic membrane, malleus, and middle ear.

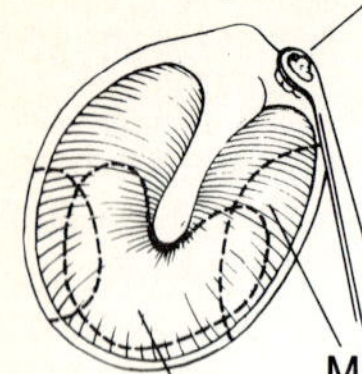

Figure 46–7 Three types of perforations of tympanic membrane.

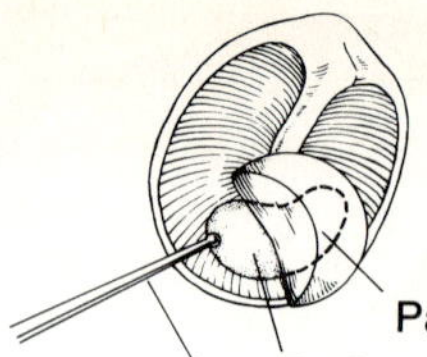

Figure 46–8 Cauterization and patching of tympanic membrane.

condition recurs, there are special tubes that resist extrusion that should be used. The adenoids should be removed if they are the cause of the eustachian tube obstruction.

Chronic Otitis Media

Chronic otitis media is a disease that is characterized by a permanent perforation of the tympanic membrane with or without associated middle ear or mastoid disease. There are three types of perforations: central, marginal, and attic (Fig. 46–7). The first two types involve the pars tensa and the latter the pars flaccida of the tympanic membrane. The marginal and attic perforations are more often associated with cholesteatoma than the central type. There are some diseases, such as tuberculosis, and burns of the tympanic membrane when hot sparks enter the ear, that produce multiple perforations.

Small central perforations cause a conductive hearing loss of 15 dB or less. Larger perforations can produce a 30 dB hearing loss. Ossicular damage greatly increases the conductive hearing loss (30 to 45 dB loss). A sensorineural hearing loss may result from chronic otitis media.[13] The severity of the inflammation within the middle ear and its duration are important factors in the magnitude of the sensorineural loss. Paparella and Brady hypothesize that the round window membrane is semipermeable and that toxic products enter the perilymph and endolymph.[14] These toxins gradually destroy the organ of Corti.

A persistent, painless drainage from the ear is not uncommon in these patients. It is usually a thin, watery, foul-smelling drainage. Pain is not a common complaint and when it occurs, a complication is usually present. Dizziness is the symptom of a serious complication.

The treatment of chronic otitis media is both medical and surgical, depending upon the type of perforation and its size and duration. Medical treatment is necessary to reduce the infection within the ear. The ears should be dry and free of infection for several months before surgery is performed. Aural hygiene consists of keeping water from the external auditory canal. These patients should avoid swimming and water contamination of the ear during showering or shampooing. Small central perforations can be cauterized with trichloroacetic acid and a small patch applied over the perforation. Many small perforations heal with this form of treatment (Fig. 46–8). Medical treatment can also increase the success of surgical treatment.

There are several operations that can be used for chronic otitis media. These vary from simple myringoplasty to tympanomastoidectomy. Mastoid surgery is reserved for those patients with cholesteatoma or mastoid infections. The types of operations and relative indications for each are presented in Table 46–1.

Surgery (Fig. 46–9) is successful in 85 to 90 percent of patients when tympanic membrane grafting is the procedure. There is usually a 30 dB or smaller hearing loss. The other types of tympanoplasty are successful in restoring hearing to less than a 30 dB loss in 75 percent of patients. When the entire ossicular chain is destroyed, only 50 percent of patients gain and maintain a hearing level of 30 dB or less.

TABLE 46–1 Types of Surgery for Chronic Otitis Media

Operation	*Perforation*	*Complications*	*Hearing Loss*
Myringoplasty, type I	Central	None	15–20 dB
Tympanoplasty, type II	Central or marginal	Ossicular necrosis	30–45 dB
Tympanoplasty, type III	Central or marginal	Ossicular necrosis	45 dB
Tympanoplasty, type IV	Central or marginal	Ossicular necrosis: mastoid infections	45+ dB

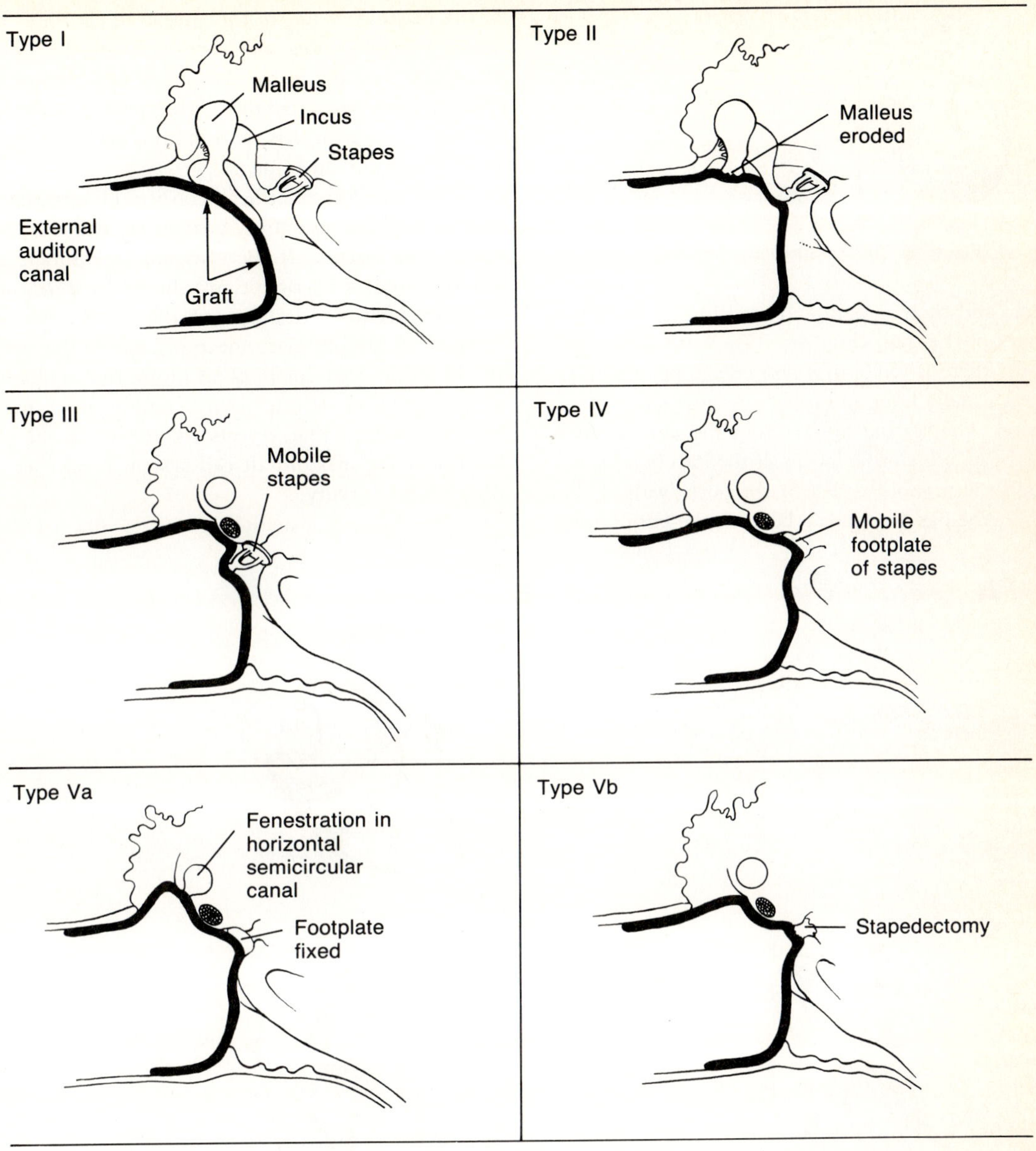

Figure 46–9 Types of tympanoplasty. *Type I*, The graft is placed on the tympanic membrane. *Type II*, The graft is draped onto a remnant of malleus and incus. *Type III*, The graft is placed onto the capitulum of the stapes. *Type IV*, The graft is placed onto a mobile stapes footplate. *Type Va*, A graft is placed over a fenestration opening into the horizontal semicircular canal when the stapes footplate is fixed. *Type Vb*, The graft is placed over the oval window niche after the stapes has been removed.

Cholesteatoma (Keratoma)

This disease consists of an epithelial lined space containing an accumulation of desquamated skin cells within the mastoid or middle ear spaces. Cholesteatomas are sometimes congenital in origin, or they may arise from attic and marginal perforations (Fig. 46–10). They may be very destructive and occasionally lethal.[15]

These patients usually complain of low intensity pain and otorrhea. The hearing loss is greater when the ossicular chain is involved. Infections within the cholesteatoma often cause an osteitis with absorption of surrounding bone. The otorrhea from this disease is usually thicker, greenish in color, and foul smelling. Coexistent infections must be treated before and after surgery is performed. The operations for these problems are shown in Figure 46–11.

Acute Mastoiditis

Acute mastoiditis occurs in conjunction with acute otitis media. The symptoms of otitis media are

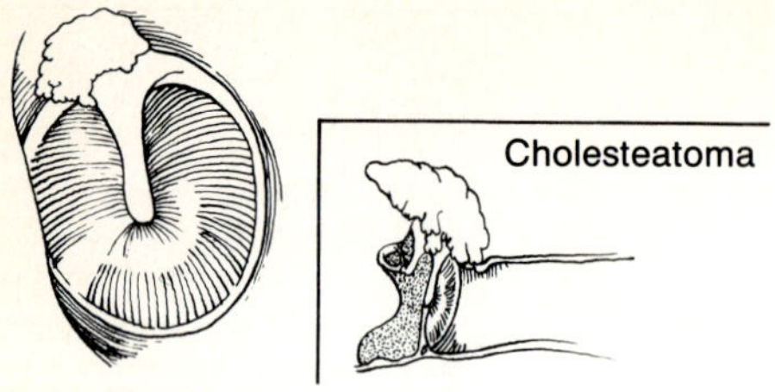

Figure 46–10 An attic cholesteatoma.

present, and there is pain and swelling in the mastoid area of the skull (Fig. 46–12). With severe infections, there is tenderness and edema of this area. There is usually fever and other systemic signs of an infection. The hearing loss is about the same as that caused by an acute otitis media. If the infection breaks through the mastoid cortex or the outer wall of the mastoid, the pus may spread beneath the periosteum of the mastoid or its tip into the neck (Bezold's abscess). These infections can also extend into the middle or posterior cranial fossae. Several complications, including facial nerve paralysis, thrombosis of the lateral sinus, labyrinthitis, and brain abscess can occur from a mastoid infection.

The medical treatment consists of intravenous antibiotics, decongestants, analgesics, bed rest, and careful observation. If the tympanic membrane has not ruptured, a myringotomy should be performed to allow adequate drainage of the middle ear and mastoid. A simple mastoidectomy is required when the infection does not respond promptly, or there is an indication of an impending complication. An x-ray examination that reveals resorption of the trabeculae of the mastoid air cell system is another indication for surgery.

The hearing usually returns to normal after

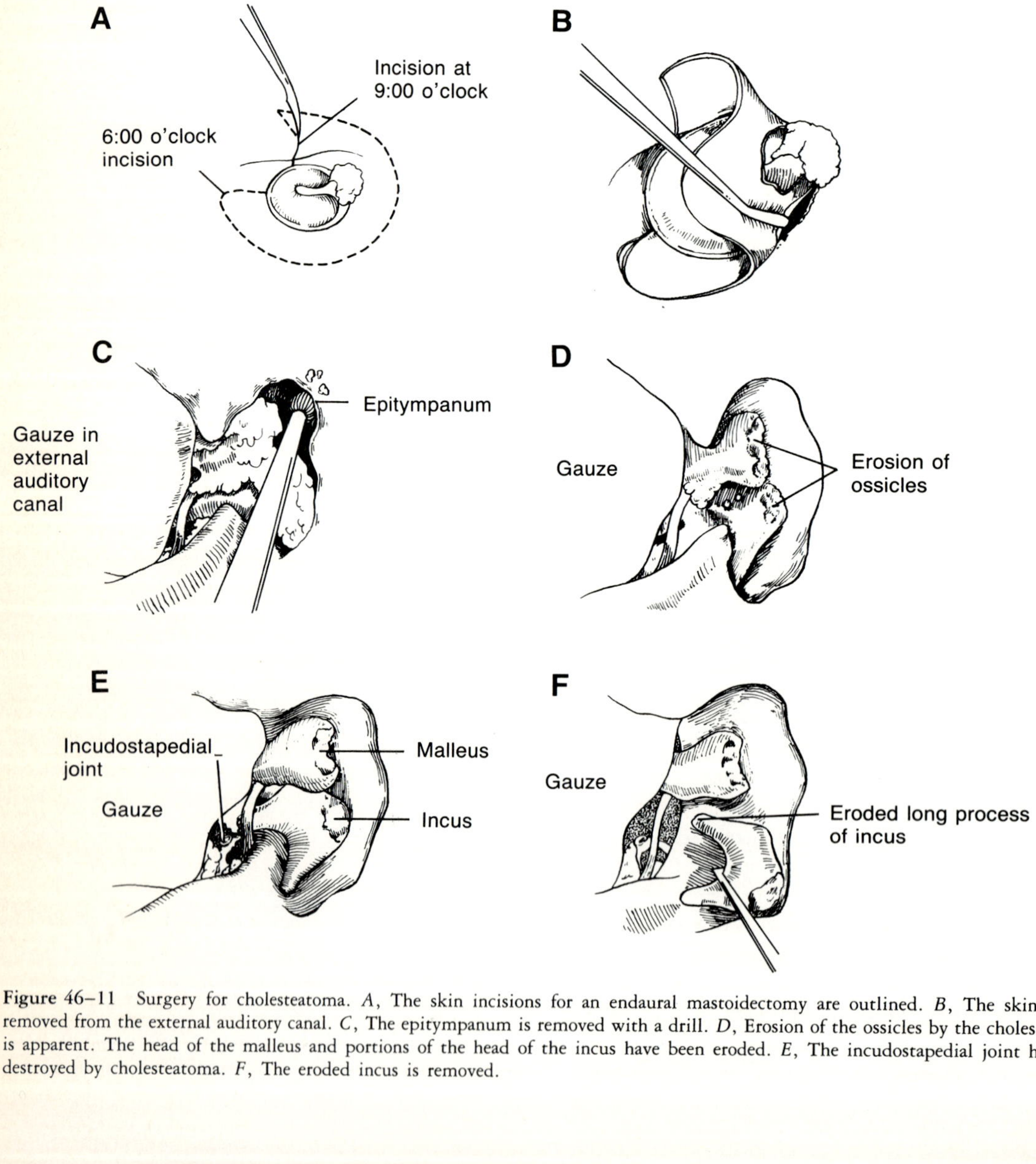

Figure 46–11 Surgery for cholesteatoma. *A*, The skin incisions for an endaural mastoidectomy are outlined. *B*, The skin flap is removed from the external auditory canal. *C*, The epitympanum is removed with a drill. *D*, Erosion of the ossicles by the cholesteatoma is apparent. The head of the malleus and portions of the head of the incus have been eroded. *E*, The incudostapedial joint has been destroyed by cholesteatoma. *F*, The eroded incus is removed.

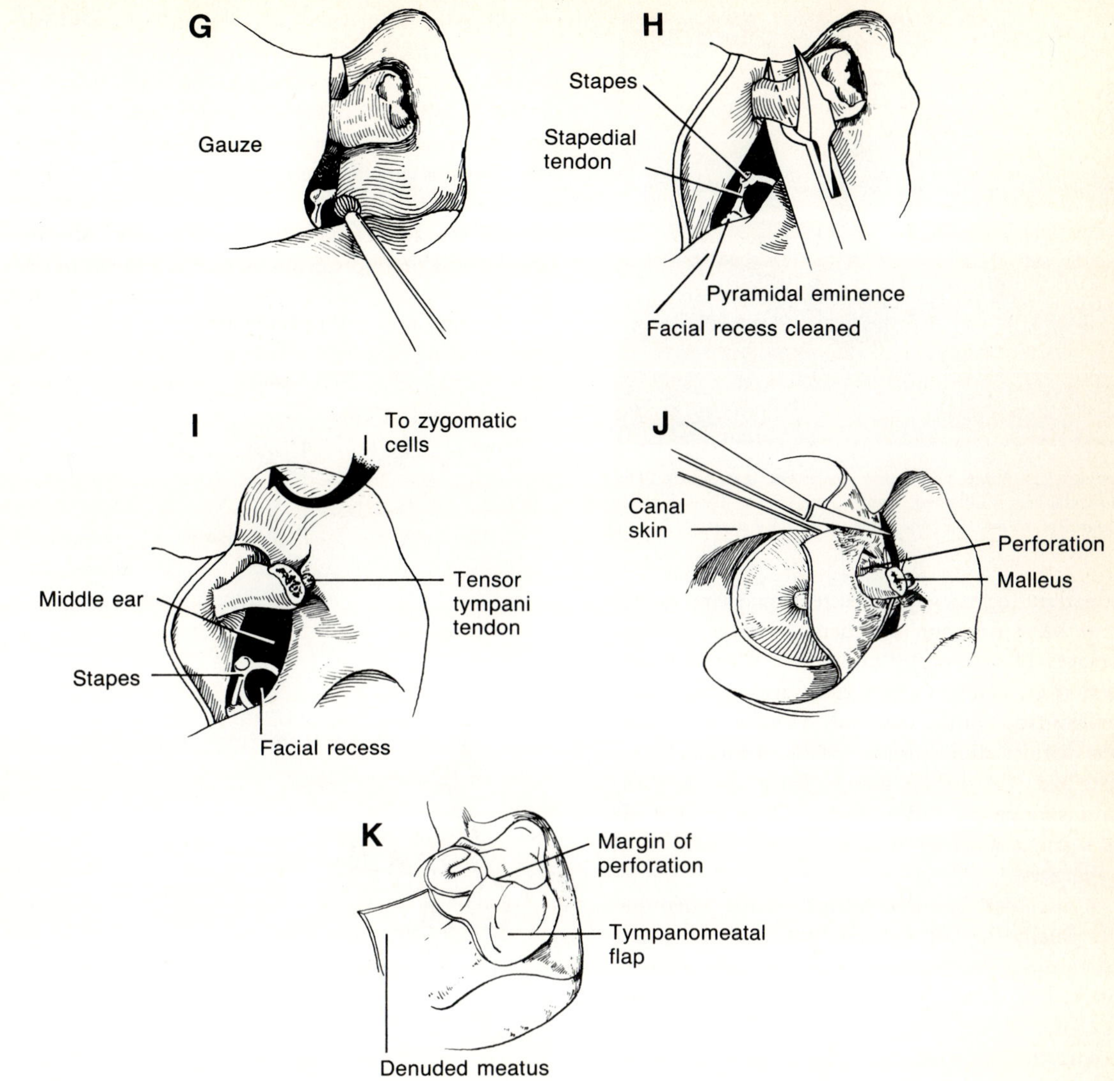

Figure 46–11 Continued *G*, The stapes and oval window niche are exposed by drilling into the facial recess area. *H*, The head of the eroded malleus is removed. *I*, The middle ear and mastoid cavity have been exposed and all the cholesteatoma removed. *J*, Canal skin is incised and repositioned about the long process of the malleus. *K*, The canal skin is draped into the mastoid cavity to serve as a graft for the cavity.

treatment if there has not been damage to the ossicular chain or labyrinth. The acute infection, however, often causes a mild sensorineural hearing loss. This is most pronounced in the high frequencies and it often persists after the infection has subsided. This is presumably caused by the effect of the bacterial toxins on the basal turn of the cochlea.

Chronic Mastoiditis

Chronic infections of the middle ear and mastoid are often associated with damage to the ossicles, otic capsule, and mastoid bone. Cholesteatomas are the most common cause of these problems, but chronic osteitis may also damage these structures. When the otic capsule is damaged, a perilymph fistula can result and cause a severe sensorineural hearing loss and vertigo. Any progressive osteitis is an indication for vigorous medical and surgical therapy. When the inflammation is controlled, there may be partial or complete obstruction of the eustachian tube. Without aeration, the tympanic membrane collapses. This process is referred to as atelectasis of the middle ear.

Acute Labyrinthitis

Labyrinthitis results from agents that are transmitted to the inner ear from the middle ear or mastoid (tympanogenic), meninges (meningogenic), and

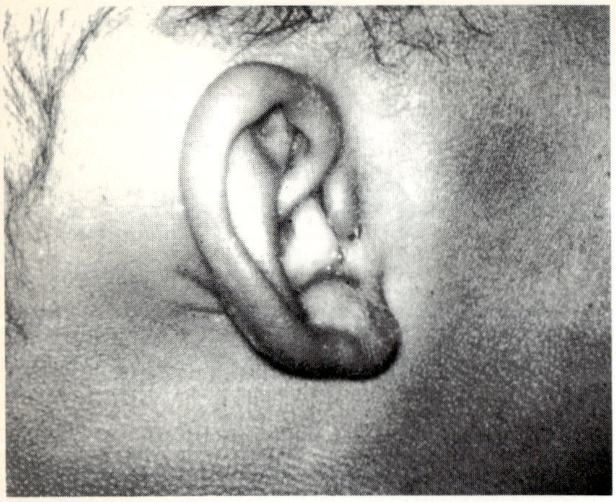

Figure 46–12 Acute suppurative coalescent mastoiditis. The postauricular area is inflamed, swollen, and tender. There is thick mucopurulent secretion in the external auditory meatus.

blood stream (hematogenic). Bacterial and viral agents are the most common offenders; however, foreign substances placed in the middle ear during stapes surgery (i.e., gelfoam and various drugs) may cause an inflammation of the inner ear. There are four more or less distinct clinical types of labyrinthitis: (1) circumscribed, (2) diffuse serous, (3) acute, and (4) chronic suppurative labyrinthitis. These are not always distinct entities; they sometimes blend with one another.

A circumscribed labyrinthitis occurs when one canal, usually the lateral horizontal canal, is eroded and a localized inflammation occurs. Surgery, chronic otitis media, and cholesteatomas are the most common causes of this process. If the inflammation is not controlled and eradicated, the process spreads to involve the entire inner ear, and a diffuse labyrinthitis occurs. These patients have recurrent dizziness that is increased with movements of the head and body. There is usually a sensorineural hearing loss that becomes progressively more severe.

A suppurative infection of the inner ear produces a complete sensorineural hearing loss, severe vertigo, tinnitus, nausea, vomiting, and ataxia. The acute stage lasts for 2 to 6 weeks, and when the inflammation reaches the chronic phase (10 weeks) the symptoms usually subside. In about 6 months, the labyrinthine spaces are partially or completely filled with new bone (labyrinthitis ossificans). There is complete deafness, mild vertigo, and a spontaneous nystagmus toward the good ear. The early stages of this infection respond well to antibiotic therapy. If the infection is not controlled with antibiotics, meningitis or a brain abscess may ensue. A labyrinthectomy may be required to control the infection in some of these patients (Figs. 46–13 and 46–14).

Viral labyrinthitis occurs from mumps, measles, chicken pox, influenza, the common cold, and poliomyelitis. Measles labyrinthitis creates a significant number of deaf children. These patients have a 40 to 50 dB high-frequency sensorineural hearing loss and about half of the patients will be totally deaf. There is no effective medical treatment for those with a total hearing loss, although the less severely affected can be helped with hearing aids. Mumps labyrinthitis produces deafness that is sudden in on-

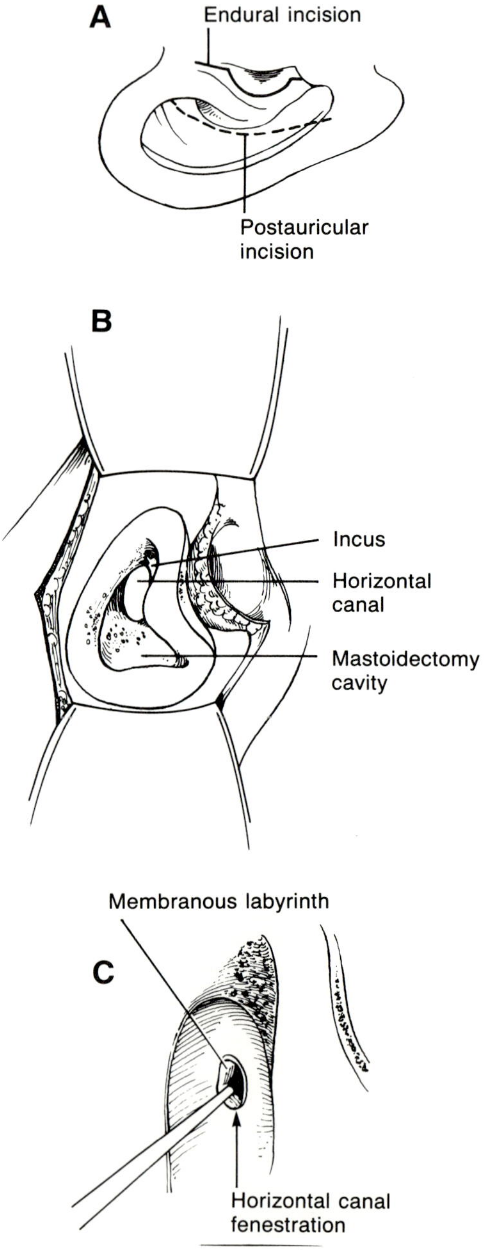

Figure 46–13 Transmastoid labyrinthectomy. *A*, A postauricular incision is made and the mastoid cortex exposed. *B*, A complete mastoidectomy has been performed. The horizontal canal and incus have been exposed. *C*, The horizontal canal has been fenestrated and the membranous labyrinth removed with a right angle pick.

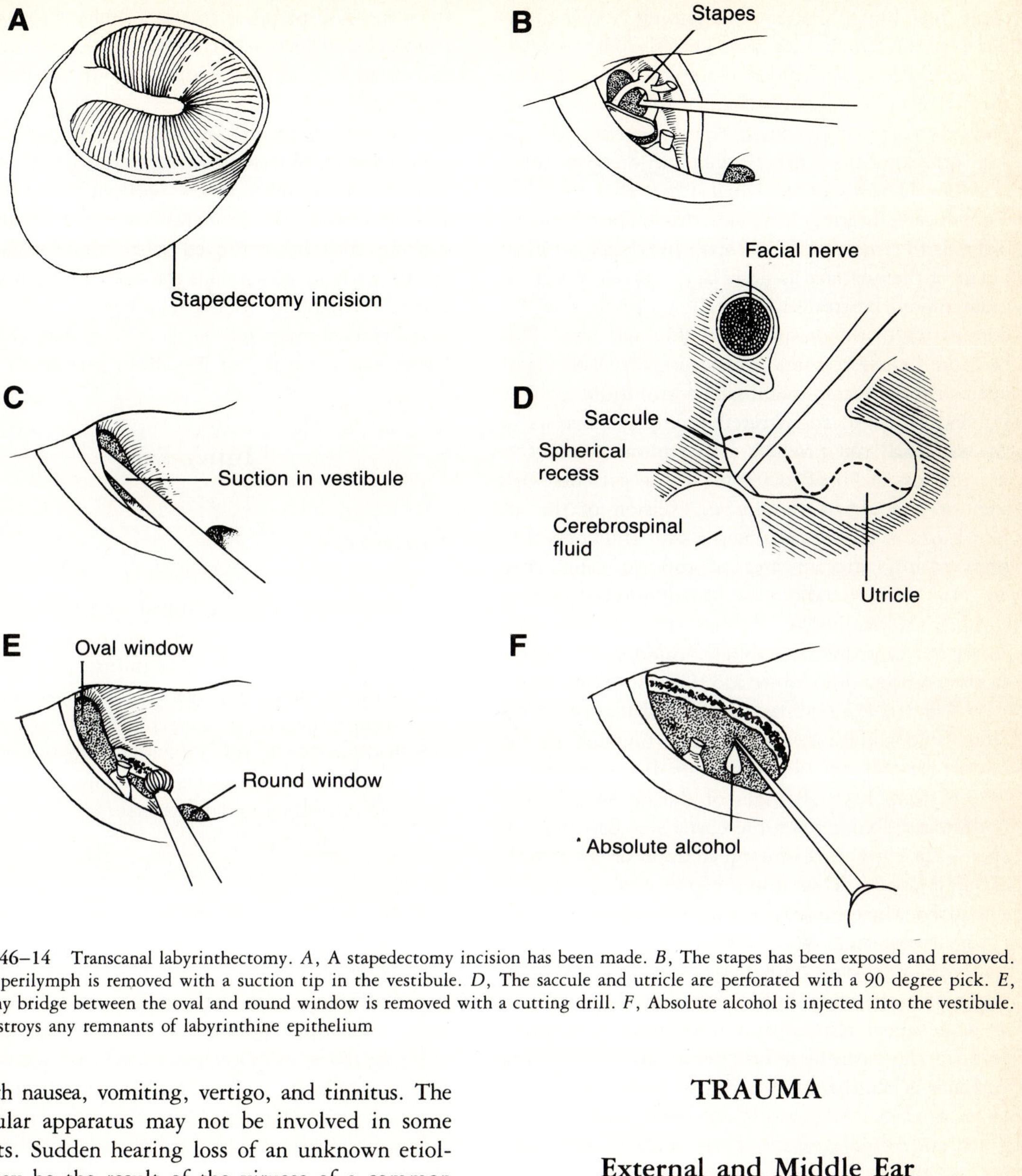

Figure 46–14 Transcanal labyrinthectomy. *A*, A stapedectomy incision has been made. *B*, The stapes has been exposed and removed. *C*, The perilymph is removed with a suction tip in the vestibule. *D*, The saccule and utricle are perforated with a 90 degree pick. *E*, The bony bridge between the oval and round window is removed with a cutting drill. *F*, Absolute alcohol is injected into the vestibule. This destroys any remnants of labyrinthine epithelium

set with nausea, vomiting, vertigo, and tinnitus. The vestibular apparatus may not be involved in some patients. Sudden hearing loss of an unknown etiology may be the result of the viruses of a common cold or influenza.

Syphilis

Syphilis of the temporal bone is rare, except in congenital infections or neurosyphilis. There is a sudden sensorineural hearing loss that increases rapidly over a period of a few months or years. It nearly always becomes quite severe. There is vertigo that tends to subside as the hearing loss increases.[16] Intravenous penicillin and corticosteroids appear to give either permanent or temporary improvement in the auditory thresholds of patients with congenital syphilis.

TRAUMA

External and Middle Ear

Several forms of trauma cause injuries to the auricle and external auditory canal.[17] The most common injuries occur from accidents, wrestling, boxing, burns, and frostbite. There is not an associated hearing loss unless the external auditory canal is involved, the tympanic membrane perforated, or the ossicles dislocated. A patient who has an injury to the external ear should be tested to determine if there is a hearing impairment. The severity of the hearing loss is dependent upon the type and extent of the injury to the tympanic membrane and middle ear. There may be very little evidence of an external injury with a blow to the auricle, but a 15 to 20 dB hearing loss may result from perforation of the tympanic membrane. Patients sustaining avulsion injuries of the auricle may have entirely normal hearing after debris and blood clots are removed from the ear canal. A surgical repair of the ear canal that prevents narrowing, constriction (stenosis), or closure (atresia) of the canal is important. Stenosis causes retention of wax and epithelial debris that produces a conductive hearing loss, and this material can be difficult to remove. When a stenosis occurs, surgical repair of the ear canal is necessary. Atresia of the ear canal should be treated surgically to prevent an accumulation of the desquamated skin and wax. This "acquired cholesteatoma" can cause extensive damage to the tympanic membrane and middle ear if it is not recognized and treated promptly. Atresia of the ear canal can produce a maximum conductive hearing loss of 50 dB or more. Those patients with stenosis and atresia require an excision of the affected area of the ear canal and a split thickness skin graft to the affected area of the ear canal (Fig. 46–15). These operations are usually successful in returning the hearing to within normal limits. Any associated tympanic membrane, middle ear, or ossicular problem will require additional surgical repair.

Barotitis is a traumatic disorder that occurs most often from sudden severe negative pressure in the middle ear and mastoid air system. It occurs during descent from high altitudes or during ascent from underwater diving when the eustachian tube fails to open sufficiently to permit equalization of the middle ear air pressure. This failure of the eustachian tube to equalize the tympanic pressures may be caused by (1) poor eustachian tube function from congenital, anatomic, or chronic pathologic conditions; (2) acute changes in the eustachian tube from the edema of an acute upper respiratory infection; and (3) failure to open the eustachian tube while sleeping during descent. When there is a large enough difference between atmospheric pressure on the tympanic membrane and middle ear pressure, several changes in the middle ear and mastoid occur. The tympanic membrane will be retracted or displaced into the external auditory canal. If the tympanic membrane is thin (monomeric) a perforation may result. Fluid or blood may develop in the middle ear. The mucosa becomes hyperemic, edematous, and ecchymotic. The middle ear is then filled with a transudate that may become bloody in character. There is severe pain during the acute phase that slowly subsides over a period of a few hours. When the eustachian tube function improves, the middle ear effusion gradually resolves over a period of 2 to 6 weeks. This problem rarely occurs in patients who fly in pressurized aircraft. However, individuals who fly with head colds are more apt to develop barotitis. Repeated Valsalva maneuvers and nasal decongestant agents may reduce the susceptibility to this problem. Postponing flying trips when there is severe nasal airway congestion from a "cold" also reduces the incidence of this problem.

Severe sensorineural hearing loss has been associated with barotrauma due to rupture of the oval and round windows. These perilymph fistulae may heal spontaneously or require surgical repair. The hearing may be improved when the fistula is repaired with an autogenous tissue graft. Simmons reported 15 patients with a sensorineural hearing loss from barotrauma, and he theorizes that these patients had a rupture of Reissner's membrane.[18]

Inner Ear

Fractures

Disturbances of vestibular and auditory function are the largest group of objectively demonstrable complications from a head injury. Alexander and Scholl found that 15 percent of 551 patients with head injuries had signs of cerebral injury and 33 percent had hearing losses, probably from the injury.[19]

There are two varieties of temporal bone fractures: longitudinal and transverse.

Longitudinal Fractures

Longitudinal fractures occur most often from blows to the parietal and frontal areas of the skull. The longitudinal fracture is a linear break through the floor of the middle cranial fossa that extends parallel and adjacent to the anterior margin of the petrous pyramid (Fig. 46–16). These patients have a laceration of the tympanic membrane, bleeding from the external auditory canal, a "step-like" deformity of the external auditory canal, a facial weakness or paralysis (25 percent), cerebrospinal fluid otorrhea, and dislocation of the ossicles. The lacerated tympanic membrane, hemotympanum, and ossicular dislocations cause a conductive hearing loss. Tympanic membrane lacerations usually heal spontaneously, but when the ossicles have been dislocated there is a variable conductive hearing loss that may be permanent unless corrected by reconstruction of the ossicular chain. Many of these patients have a sensorineural hearing loss that varies from a high tone loss to a wide frequency impairment. Some improvement can be expected during the first 3 weeks after injury as the cochlea recovers from the temporary threshold shift.

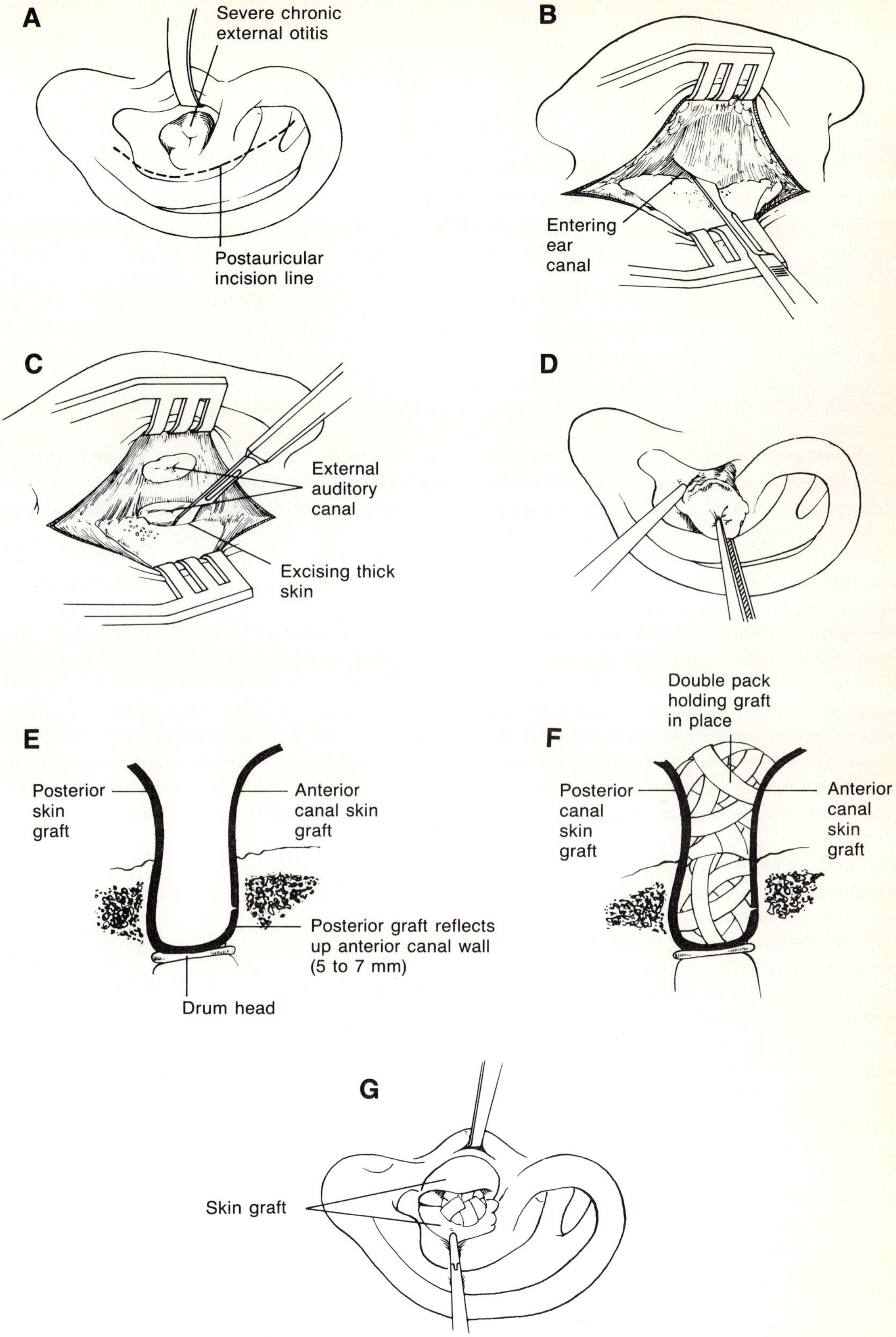

Figure 46–15 Surgery for external auditory canal stenosis. *A*, A postauricular incision is made. *B*, The external auditory canal is entered. *C* and *D*, The thick skin of the external auditory canal is excised. *E*, A skin graft is then placed into the external auditory canal. *F*, The graft is packed securely in position. *G*, The skin graft is pulled through the external auditory meatus and positioned to provide covering for the entire external auditory canal.

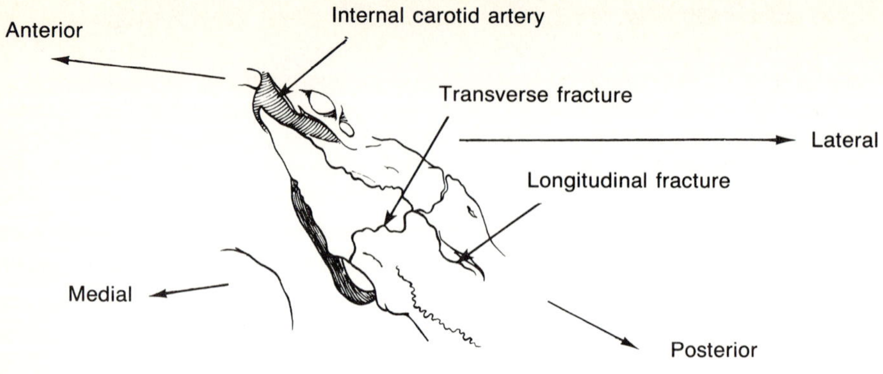

Figure 46–16 Fractures of the temporal bone.

Transverse Fractures

A transverse fracture occurs perpendicular to the long axis of the petrous bone (Fig. 46–16). It results from blows to the occiput. In about 50 percent of cases, the facial nerve is lacerated, and there is a facial paralysis that is permanent unless immediate repair is performed. Bleeding from the ear canal is uncommon, but a hemotympanum is a frequent finding with a dark blue tympanic membrane that later becomes light blue, then red in color before complete resolution occurs in two to four weeks. Cerebrospinal fluid may continue to leak from the ear canal or eustachian tube after the blood is absorbed. In these individuals the blood may drain via the eustachian tube into the nasopharynx, rather than from the ear canal. These fractures are associated with extensive damage to the membranous labyrinth of the inner ear, and there is a complete loss of cochlear and vestibular function. This results in a permanent, complete loss of hearing, severe tinnitus, and vertigo. The tinnitus may subside over a period of several weeks or months. The vertigo is associated with nausea and vomiting. These symptoms subside slowly over a period of 2 to 4 weeks, although there is unsteadiness and a tendency to fall toward the affected side that lasts for many months. A mild spontaneous nystagmus can be seen, with the quick component to the opposite side for many months or years after the injury. After 6 months or more, the quick phase may change direction toward the affected side. This is usually demonstrated by electronystagmography with the eyes closed.

Surgical treatment is designed to repair the facial nerve and close any defects in the middle ear or mastoid through which cerebrospinal fluid is leaking into the middle ear. Occasionally, a craniotomy is necessary to stop the cerebrospinal fluid leak. A labyrinthectomy is required for some patients who have persisting episodes of vertigo.

Surgical Trauma

Probably the most common injury to the inner ear occurs during mastoid surgery. This consists of a fistulization of the horizontal semicircular canal. The horizontal canal lies in a prominent position in the mastoid antrum. When the bone of the canal is removed without tearing the membranous labyrinth, the result is a mild sensorineural hearing loss and a moderate loss of vestibular function. When the membranous labyrinth is injured, the result is a profound sensorineural hearing loss and a severe loss of vestibular function. Accidental dislocation or fracture of the incus and stapes may occur during mastoid or middle ear surgery. A surgically induced (stimulation) hearing loss may result from contact of the drilling burr with an intact ossicular chain.

Noise Deafness

The loss of hearing that occurs from exposure to high intensity noise may be temporary or permanent. A transient sensorineural hearing loss from overuse of radio cassette head phones has been reported.[20] Similar losses have occurred from portable telephones.

There is no specific medical or surgical treatment for noise-induced hearing loss. Prevention is the only successful method of avoiding these problems. There are several protective devices that are effective. Severe impact noise can rupture the tympanic membrane or the round window membrane or dislocate the ossicular chain. These problems often require surgical intervention.

Labyrinthine Concussion

A blow to the head may cause deafness and dysequilibrium.[21,22] These symptoms may result from a combined injury to the central nervous system and the labyrinth. Labyrinthine concussion ordinarily arises from blows that are severe enough to cause a loss of consciousness. Moderate blows have been associated with a permanent sensorineural loss when the blow was delivered to the occiput. Presumably, a blow to the head creates a pressure wave in the skull which is transmitted through the bone to the cochlea. The injury to the membranous labyrinth arises from this intense physical (acoustic) stimulation. Another possible mechanism is the sudden acceleration or deceleration of the head. This creates movement of the stapes footplate with a corresponding inertia of the tympanic membrane, malleus, and incus.

Ototoxicity

There are several drugs that affect the inner ear and create either temporary or permanent alterations of auditory or vestibular function.[23] Several factors correlate with the degree of ototoxicity. These factors may predispose the patient to the risk of a hearing loss.

Serum levels of the ototoxic agent are extremely important. The blood stream is the principal means by which drugs reach the inner ear, and the higher the blood level, the more likely it is to injure the inner ear.

Synergism means that the combination of ototoxic drugs has a greater effect than would be expected from a single drug. Because synergism occurs, the total combined doses of concurrently administered drugs cannot be used as an indicator of their safety. Ototoxic drugs remain in the inner ear system longer than in the serum, and they may accumulate to unpredictably higher levels.

Kidney function is an important factor in ototoxicity. The kidney is responsible for filtering ototoxic drugs from the blood stream and excreting them from the body. With acute or chronic renal disease, this filtering mechanism is less efficient and the drugs remain longer and accumulate to higher levels in both the blood stream and the inner ear. Nephrotoxicity is a common problem with the aminoglycoside antibiotics, such as streptomycin, dihydrostreptomycin, neomycin, kanamycin, gentamycin, and vancomycin.[24] This toxic action may be temporary and reversible, but a temporary decrease in kidney function increases the potential risk to the inner ear. A preexisting sensorineural hearing loss predisposes the patient to an ototoxic effect. Age is another factor in ototoxicity. The very young and old have renal function that predisposes them to an ototoxic effect. There are some individuals who may have an unpredictable or atypical response to a drug. There are no clues that these individuals have an increased risk of ototoxicity. High frequency audiometry is a useful technique for monitoring and detecting an early hearing loss in patients who receive ototoxic drugs.[25]

Congenital ototoxic hearing loss occurs when the mother is administered an ototoxic drug during pregnancy. Many drugs cross the placental barrier and damage the developing inner ear. Any of the ototoxic drugs may be responsible for this type of hearing loss. Quinine and chloroquine are examples of drugs that can cause a congenital hearing loss. Ototoxic drugs administered during neonatal or infant life may also cause a hearing loss. In the differential diagnosis of neonatal deafness, the possibility of an ototoxic hearing loss should always be considered.

Aspirin (acetylsalicylic acid) may have an ototoxic effect when used in high doses (i.e., the treatment of arthritis). The hearing loss is sensorineural with a characteristic temporary threshold shift that is reversed when the drug is discontinued. The loss is in the high frequencies, is bilateral, symmetrical, and usually preceded by tinnitus. Occasionally patients will have a permanent loss.

Quinine and chloroquine phosphate are used to treat malaria. Congenital permanent hearing loss has been reported with the use of these drugs during pregnancy.

PROFOUND NERVE DEAFNESS

There are only a few medical or surgical treatments for patients with profound sensorineural hearing losses. A powerful hearing aid may be useful; however, there are some patients who do not benefit from that method of treatment. For these individuals, the cochlear implant may be indicated.[26,27,28,29]

Before an implant is recommended, patients should be thoroughly evaluated. The guidelines for patient selection are presented in Table 46–2.

There are a few surgical complications from a cochlear implant, as well as problems associated with

TABLE 46–2 Guidelines for Patient Selection

The patient must be age 18 or older
A profound postlingual hearing loss
Little or no benefit from amplification
Psychological stability
A normal otologic examination
A normal cochlea on CT scan examination
Absent responses to evoked potential tests
A positive response to electrical stimulation of the promontory
No contraindications to surgery

the mastoidectomy. These include infection, trauma and facial nerve paralysis or stimulation. However, these have not been a major problem.

Not all the patients who receive an implant enjoy the same degree of benefit. Some patients have been reported to achieve excellent results with good speech discrimination; whereas, others do not improve beyond the level that was achieved with amplification.

The hearing results from cochlear implants depend upon the intelligence of the recipient, the patient's motivation, and any complications from the operation. Most patients have at least an improved ability to appreciate sounds and better speech recognition, especially when combined with lipreading. An occasional patient has some ability for interactive conversation without the use of lipreading.

NEOPLASMS

External Ear

Benign Neoplasms

There are several benign neoplasms of the auricle and external auditory canal. Most of these tumors do not cause a hearing loss unless there is an occlusion of the ear canal. This produces a conductive hearing loss that may be an indication for surgical excision of the tumor. These tumors may interfere with the extrusion of cerumen and epithelial debris. Periodic cleansing of this material may be necessary to avoid infections of the ear canal. There are benign epithelial, neurogenic, cartilaginous, glandular, vascular, and bony tumors.

Malignant Neoplasms

Epidermoid carcinomas are common malignant neoplasms of the external ear (Fig. 46–17). The most common symptoms are the presence of the tumor mass, otorrhea, pain, and hearing loss. The hearing loss is usually a conductive hearing loss. Treatment consists of surgery alone or in combination with preoperative or postoperative irradiation.

Malignant melanomas are very aggressive epithelial tumors that require aggressive and radical surgical excision. They have a poor prognosis because local, regional, and distant metastasis cannot always be controlled by surgery.

Middle Ear

Benign Neoplasms

Tumors that arise from paraganglionic bodies or tissue in the middle ear are referred to as glomus jugulare and glomus tympanicum tumors. They usually occur in middle age and are more common in females than males. The initial symptom is a hearing loss in 90 percent of the patients with this problem. This impairment may be a conductive, sensorineural, or mixed hearing loss. A pulsating tinnitus occurs in about 50 percent of patients and pain in about 25 percent. Vertigo arises from invasion of the inner ear and is present in about 25 percent of patients. The tumor may involve the mastoid, petrous apex, external ear canal, and jugular foramen. When the tumor invades the jugular foramen, it may involve the ninth, tenth, eleventh, and twelfth cranial nerves. At least one cranial nerve was involved in 44 percent of patients reported by McCabe and Fletcher.[30] Otologic examination typically reveals a reddish blue, pulsating mass behind the inferior portion of the tympanic membrane. Special diagnostic x-ray examinations (retrograde jugulography and carotid arteriography) are necessary to determine the extent of these tumors.

Malignant Neoplasms

Epidermoid carcinomas can arise in the middle ear or invade the middle ear from the external auditory canal. About three-fourths of the widely invasive tumors that occur in the ear canal, middle ear, and mastoid are squamous cell carcinomas, and about 11 percent of the patients have a tumor that has spread to the neck nodes by the time they seek medical treatment.[31]

The most common symptoms are bloody otorrhea, hearing loss, pain, facial paralysis, mastoid swelling, and vertigo. In many patients (50 percent), there has been a chronic otorrhea with the onset earlier in childhood. The hearing loss may be conductive, sensorineural, or mixed. Vertigo and sensorineural hearing loss occur from tumor invading the labyrinth.

The treatment of these tumors is usually a radical operation, such as temporal bone resection, which includes a combined extracranial and intracranial resection (Fig. 46–18). Cryosurgery has been used to palliate those patients who have recurrent tumors. Lewis reports a 28 percent, 5-year cure rate for 100 cases.[31]

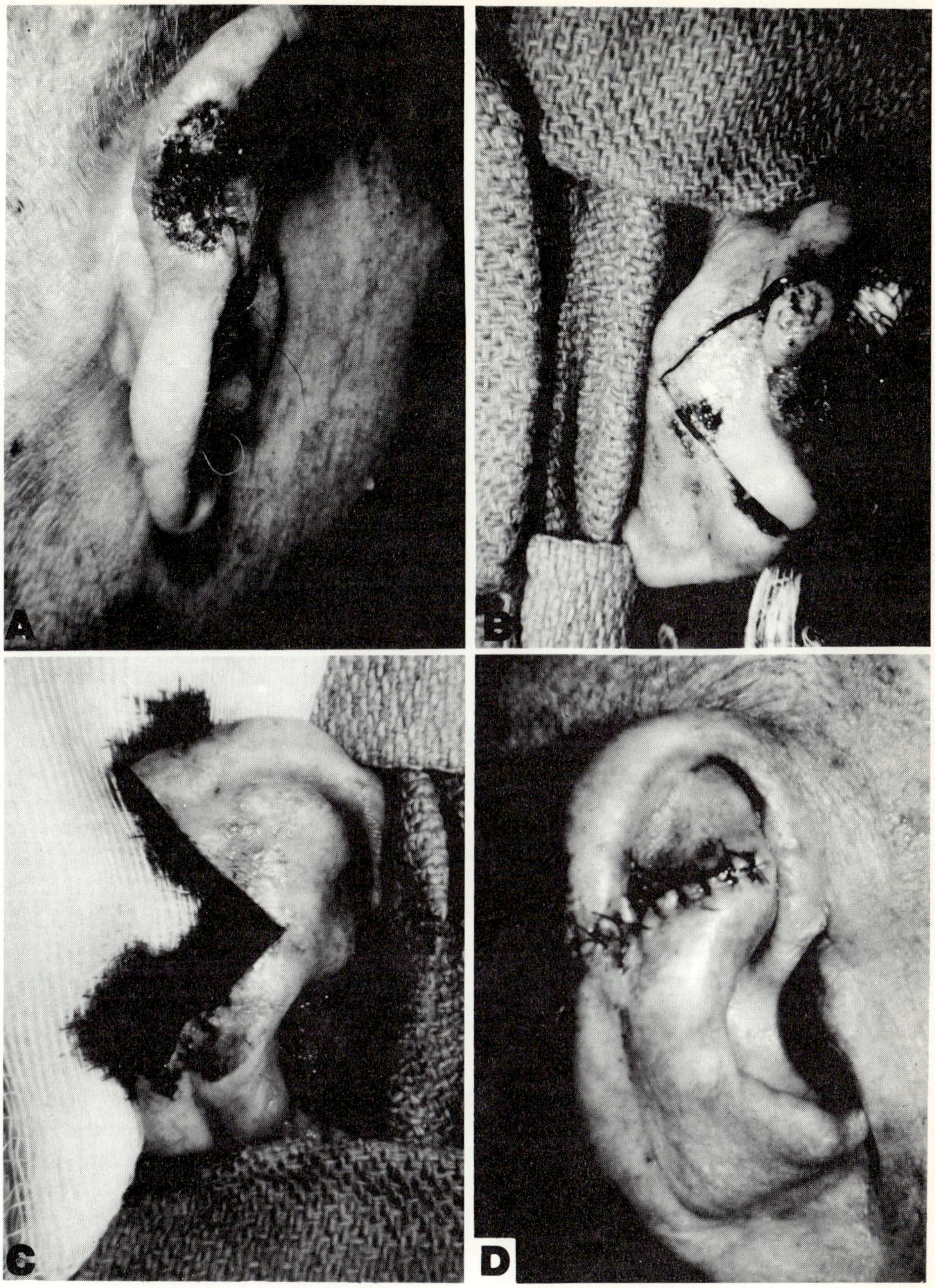

Figure 46–17 Surgery for carcinoma of the external ear. *A*, An ulceration of the lateral margin of the helix that is consistent with a squamous cell carcinoma. *B*, Postauricular incisions. *C*, Completed wedge resection of the tumor. *D*, Closure of surgical defect.

Sarcoma

There are two types of sarcomas that occur in the middle ear and mastoid. Each type is discussed as a separate entity.

Rhabdomyosarcoma is almost exclusively a disease of children. It is nearly always fatal. The tumor occurs during the first 10 years of life, mostly during the first 5 years. The initial symptoms are bloody otorrhea and facial paralysis. The hearing loss initially is conductive but later a sensorineural component occurs from invasion of the labyrinth. Vertigo occurs when the tumor reaches the inner ear. Most attempts to remove the tumor with a mastoidectomy are unsuccessful. Radiation therapy has been of some value.

Chondrosarcomas are malignant neoplasms that arise from cartilage. They occur predominantly in

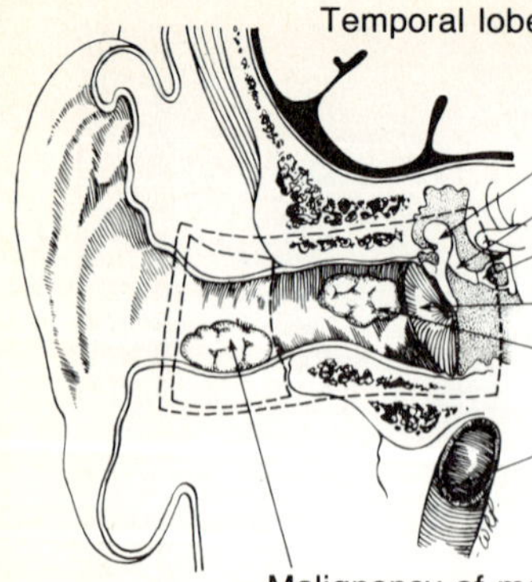

Figure 46–18 Carcinoma of the external canal. The limits of the resection (dotted line) are indicated for tumors in the membranous and bony external auditory canal.

adults between the ages of 20 and 50 years. These tumors arise in the apex of the temporal bone. The symptoms are hearing loss, pain, otorrhea, and an enlarging mass. The hearing impairment is usually sensorineural. Occasionally, they involve the middle ear and cause a conductive hearing loss. Radical surgical excision is the treatment for these progressive tumors.

Metastatic Neoplasms

Tumors may extend into the middle ear and mastoid via the eustachian tube, tympanic membrane from the external auditory canal, or directly into the mastoid bone from the overlying skin. The most common route of extension is through the tympanic membrane. Squamous cell carcinoma, lymphoma, and adenocarcinomas can migrate from the nasopharynx along the eustachian tube into the middle ear and mastoid. These patients usually have a middle ear effusion and conductive hearing loss due to poor ventilation of the middle ear. A careful nasopharyngeal examination is essential in any adult with a unilateral conductive hearing loss from middle ear effusion. A tympanotomy and ventilating tube will relieve the hearing impairment, but when the primary nasopharyngeal carcinoma is not diagnosed the middle ear effusion persists and becomes more profuse. A biopsy of the nasopharynx will make the diagnosis and must be repeated until cause of the middle ear effusion is established. The treatment of nasopharyngeal carcinoma is beyond the scope of this chapter.

Inner Ear

Benign Neoplasms

Acoustic neuromas, neurilemmomas, and neurofibromas are more properly called schwannomas. These tumors arise from the Schwann cells of the sheaths of cranial and spinal nerve roots and peripheral nerves. Most of the tumors that arise in the internal auditory canal arise from the vestibular nerves. They rarely arise from the seventh (facial) nerve or auditory branch of the eighth nerve. Many are entirely asymptomatic. Hardy and Crowe discovered six minute vestibular schwannomas in a histologic study of 250 temporal bones removed at autopsy.[32] Later, Leonard and Talbot described four asymptomatic schwannomas in 883 temporal bones.[33]

These tumors cause vestibular and auditory dysfunction, summarized in Table 46–3. Either the hearing loss or vestibular dysfunction may be the first symptom to appear. The auditory symptoms may be present for many years. The principal vestibular complaint is unsteadiness with occasional episodes of vertigo and associated nausea.

Headaches occur with larger tumors. This pain is located in the occiput and frontal areas of the skull. The headaches are increased with stooping, straining, or sneezing. A tumor that grows into the cerebellopontine angle will, in time, exert pressure on the adjacent pons or cerebellar hemispheres. This causes incoordination of movement and nystagmus. The incoordination occurs in the lower extremities first and later involves the upper extremities. The patient tends to fall toward the side with the tumor.

TABLE 46–3 Auditory and Vestibular Complaints from Eighth Nerve Tumors

Balance disturbance Hearing loss Tinnitus	70%
Balance disturbance Hearing loss	11%
Tinnitus Hearing loss	7%
Tinnitus Balance disturbance	4%
Hearing loss only	7%

Adapted from Sanders JW, Josey F, Glasscock ME. Audiologic evaluation in cochlear and eighth nerve disorders. Arch Otolaryngol 1974; 100: 284.

Nystagmus is horizontal, with the quick component away from the side of the lesion.

In addition to the eighth cranial nerve (auditory), the fifth (trigeminal) and seventh (facial) nerves are the most often involved. Compression of the trigeminal nerve may result in a stabbing pain with numbness and paresthesia of the face. Corneal anesthesia occurs on the side of the tumor in as many as 75 percent of patients. The facial (seventh) nerve is less often affected than the trigeminal (fifth) nerve. Symptoms of facial nerve involvement are spasms of the facial muscles and partial or complete paralysis. The other cranial nerves (four, nine, and ten) are involved late in the disease. The sixth cranial nerve causes diplopia due to paralysis of the lateral rectus muscle of the eye. When the ninth and tenth cranial nerves are involved, there is a loss of the pharyngeal reflexes and a laryngeal paralysis resulting in dysphagia and dysphonia.

As the tumor enlarges, it may obstruct the outflow of cerebrospinal fluid, causing an internal hydrocephalus. This produces headache, diplopia, papilledema, vomiting, and eventually cerebellar and respiratory crisis with death.

A common auditory manifestation is a loss of speech discrimination that is out of proportion to the pure tone thresholds. Schuknecht and Woellner reported that 75 percent of nerve fibers can be lost without creating a pure tone loss if the organ of Corti is intact.[34] This implies that a few fibers can transmit pure tone stimuli of threshold magnitude, whereas many fibers are needed to carry the complex neural patterns of speech.

Many sophisticated procedures are available for the diagnosis of these tumors. Polytomography, posterior fossa CT scans, and MRI scans are the x-ray examinations most often used to diagnose these tumors (Fig. 46–19).

The treatment of the tumor depends upon several factors. The age of the patient, the size of the tumor, and associated health problems are the most important factors. A system of operations has been devised for tumors of each size and stage of development. The middle cranial fossa operation is used for tumors confined to the internal auditory canal.[35] The translabyrinthine approach is used for tumors that extend beyond the internal auditory canal but are not associated with an increase of cerebrospinal fluid pressure. The combined suboccipital petrosal operation is reserved for large tumors with an increase of cerebrospinal fluid pressure. These operations have greatly reduced the morbidity and mortality of treating these tumors and it may be possible to conserve the hearing in some patients[36] (Figs.46–20 and 46–21).

Von Recklinghausen's disease (neurofibromatosis) is associated with bilateral, vestibular schwannomas in about 5 percent of the patients with the disease. This disease is more common in females than in males. The clinical manifestations, diagnosis, and treatment are much the same as those in patients with vestibular schwannomas. A young person with a unilateral vestibular schwannoma and neurofibromatosis has a great probability of eventually developing a bilateral tumor.

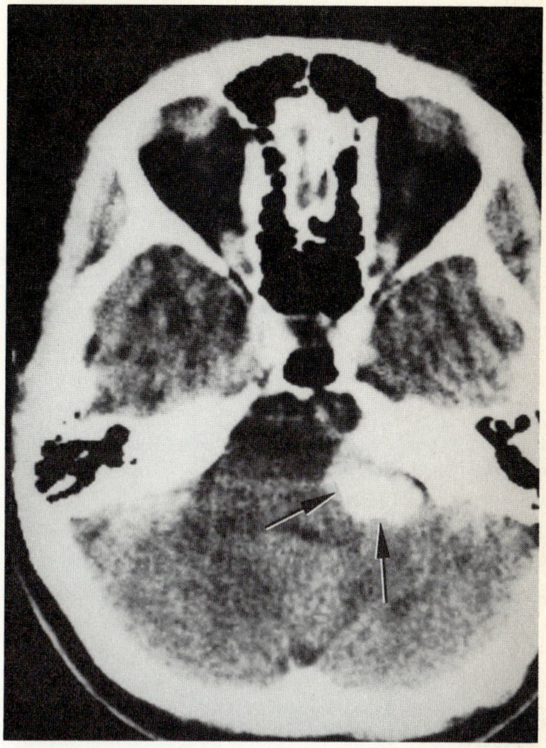

Figure 46–19 A CT scan of an acoustic neuroma (arrows).

Other central nervous system tumors may arise in the cerebellopontine angle. Gliomas of the pons, astrocytomas, medulloblastomas, ependymomas, and glioblastomas can occur in this area. Meningiomas arise from the arachnoid villi. They are much rarer than schwannomas of the vestibular nerve, occurring in a 1:12 ratio.

These tumors produce symptoms that are quite similar to those caused by schwannomas. Because they extend to the cerebellopontine angle and arise from the central nervous system, a neurosurgical operation is usually required to successfully remove them.

Metastatic Neoplasms

Tumors metastasize to the temporal bone most often via hematogenous spread. The order of frequency for the primary carcinoma is breast, kidney, stomach, larynx, prostate, and thyroid gland. The temporal bone metastasis may be the first indicator of a malignant disease, but more often the temporal

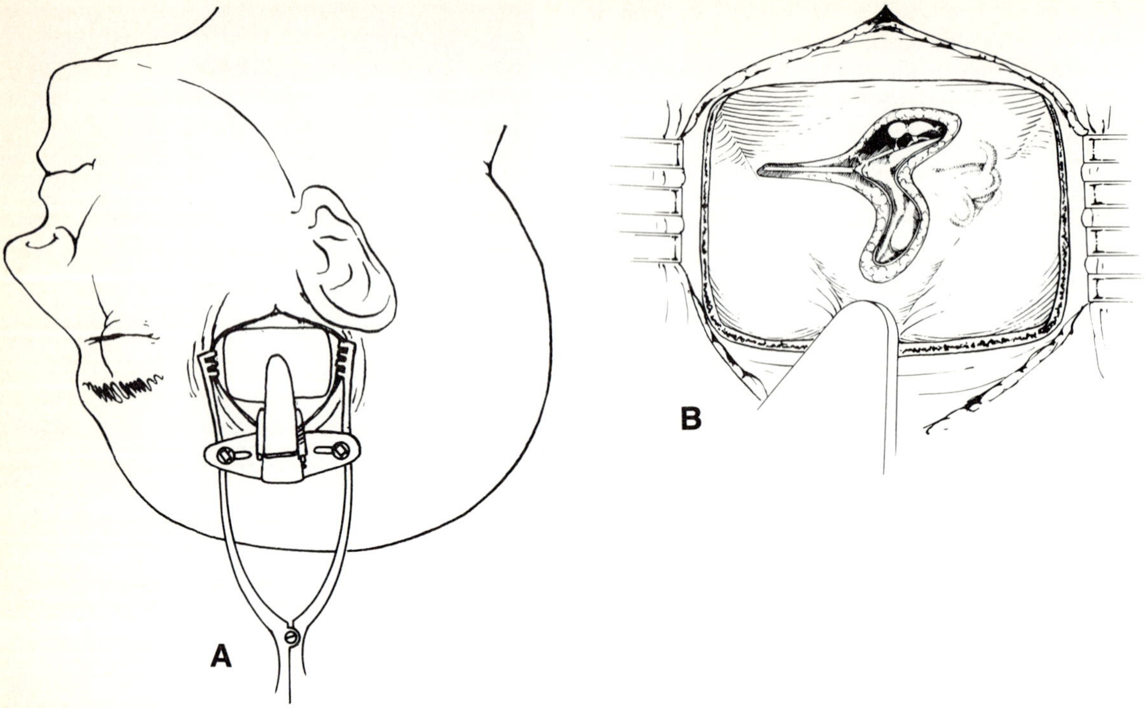

Figure 46–20 Middle fossa surgery for acoustic neuroma. *A*, Incision and temporal craniotomy. *B*, Exposure of the internal auditory canal.

bone involvement occurs late in the course of the disease and the otologic symptoms are overshadowed by the primary tumor or other metastasis.

The symptoms depend upon the location and size of the metastasis. When the external auditory canal, middle ear, mastoid, or eustachian tube is involved, the patient has a conductive hearing loss and pain. If the metastasis lodges in the petrous bone or internal auditory canal, a sensorineural hearing loss, vertigo, or facial paralysis is the clinical presentation.

Leukemia may involve the temporal bone in two forms: (1) leukemic infiltration, and (2) hemorrhage. The infiltration of leukemic cells occurs in the tympanic membrane and mucous membrane of the middle ear and mastoid. The infiltrates are also seen in the perilymphatic spaces of the inner ear. A lowered resistance often leads to a bacterial infection of the middle ear and mastoid. Hemorrhages are common and may consist of small isolated hemorrhages or massive bleeding. Bleeding into the middle ear may result in sudden hearing loss or dysequilibrium. A hearing loss has been reported in patients with leukemia, and there are patients with a sensorineural hearing loss.

Multiple Myelomas

This is a distinct malignant disease of the skeletal system. The majority of patients are between 40 and 60 years of age and the disease is more common in males. The disease has a variable rate of progression, with an average survival of about 2 years. Eventually nearly every bone in the body is affected, including the skull. The temporal bone is involved in the terminal stages of the disease. There are myeloma cells in the marrow spaces and an infiltrate in the mucous membranes. There are punched out lesions of the bone. The symptoms caused by the tumor within the temporal bone are overshadowed by the manifestations of the skeletal disease.

VESTIBULAR DISORDERS

There are relatively few vestibular diseases that have an associated hearing loss, although many otologic diseases have a hearing impairment with associated vertigo. The two symptoms are obviously interrelated, but this discussion includes only those problems in which vertigo or a vestibular symptom is the primary complaint.

Meniere's Disease

The cause of this disease is unknown in about 65 percent of patients. A more or less specific etiology has been detected in the other 35 percent, including food allergy (14 percent), syphilis (7 percent), adrenal or pituitary insufficiency, hyperthyroidism stenosis of the internal auditory canal, and physical and acoustic trauma.

The triad of symptoms from this disease was first described in 1861 by Prosper Meniere. These patients complain of episodic vertigo that lasts for several minutes or hours. They have an illusion of motion that may be associated with nausea, vomiting, tachycardia, palpitation, weakness, sweating, and prostration. When the attack of vertigo subsides, the patients often remain free of symptoms for weeks, months, or even years. There is often a low frequency fluctuating hearing loss in one ear. When the attack subsides, the hearing usually returns to normal; however, when the disease has been present for some time, the hearing does not return to normal, and there is a gradual decline in hearing acuity. Tinnitus is the third part of the symptom complex. It is often described as a low-pitched, unilateral sound that also disappears or subsides to a less intense level when the attack subsides. There may be a sensation of fullness or pressure in the affected ear. Noise or sound intolerance and disharmonic diplacusis are sometimes described by patients with this disease.

There are four subvarieties of Meniere's disease—Lermoyez syndrome, Tumarcinn's otolithic crisis, cochlear hydrops, and vestibular hydrops—and each has a different clinical presentation. The disease is nearly always unilateral, but in 10 to 15 percent of patients, the disease affects both ears. Audiology and vestibular tests are helpful in diagnosing Meniere's disease. There are two basic methods of treatment. Medical therapy is indicated for patients with relatively mild attacks early in the course of the disease. Most patients respond to medical therapy.

A wide variety of medications have been used with success. In addition, psychotherapy is effective in those patients who have anxiety, apprehension, guilt feelings, or problems adapting to social situations. There are also a number of general measures that help relieve the patient's symptoms. These are summarized in Table 46–4.

Central nervous system sedatives or hypnotic compounds help relieve the anxiety, apprehension, and stresses that sometimes precipitate the attacks. Parasympatholytic and anticholinergic (atropine SO_4 and Benadryl) medications sometimes reduce the ex-

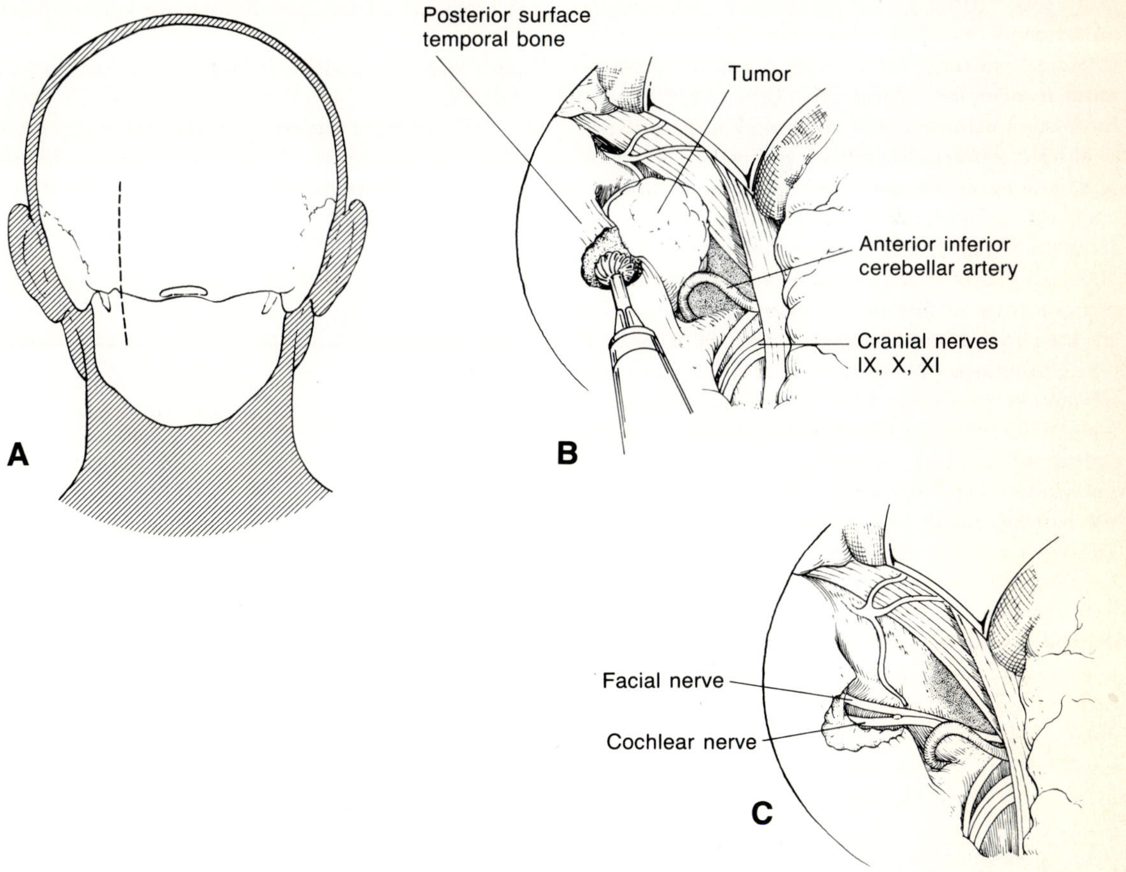

Figure 46–21 Posterior fossa surgery for acoustic neuroma. *A*, Posterior craniotomy incision. *B*, An acoustic neuroma in the cerebellopontine angle that extends into the internal auditory canal. *C*, Completed resection of an acoustic neuroma.

TABLE 46–4 General Treatment Measures for Meniere's Disease

Avoid tension and stressful situations
Avoid alcohol
Discontinue all but life-supporting medications, especially:
- Barbiturates
- Tranquilizers
- Birth control pills
- Ototoxic drugs: ASA, quinine, etc.

Make certain that necessary medications are being used properly.
- Digitalis
- Insulin
- Thyroid
- Steroids

Get plenty of rest; e.g., 7 to 8 hours of sleep per day
Have a good, well-balanced diet; avoid excessive eating
Exercise regularly
- Walking
- Jogging
- Bicycling
- Swimming

From English GM, ed. Otolaryngology—A Textbook. Hagerstown, MD: Harper & Row, 1976:104.

citability of the vestibular system. These are most useful when given early in the course of the disease. Vasodilator therapy has been advocated and used for many years. Although its use is based upon empirical evidence, this method of treatment is successful for some patients. Intravenous histamine diphosphate is given for 3 consecutive days. After the intravenous treatments, histamine diphosphate is administered subcutaneously twice each week. Nicotinic acid is administered twice each day in a flushing dose. An antihistamine (Benadryl), bioflavonoids, ataractics (Atarax), and a low sodium diet (less than 800 milligrams of sodium) are often used in conjunction with the histamine therapy. Corticosteroids are used to reduce inflammation and the effects of certain allergens. They are ordinarily administered for short periods of time and in carefully controlled doses. Diuretics are used to reduce the excessive intralabyrinthine fluid pressure that is characteristic of the disease. They sometimes give dramatic relief of the patient's symptoms, although it has not been demonstrated that they affect the fluid pressure of the inner ear.

There are about 10 to 20 percent of patients with Meniere's disease who do not respond to medical therapy. Some of these patients become candidates for surgery. The operation used will depend upon (1) the patient's clinical progress; (2) the hearing levels in the affected ear; (3) the hearing levels in the unaffected ear; (4) the degree of incapacity produced by the patient's disease; and (5) the patient's general health.

There are nondestructive (shunting and drainage) operations and destructive procedures. The indications for these two types of operations are shown in Table 46–5. Most patients respond to a nondestructive operation. These patients have a unilateral loss that is fluctuating, and there is usually fairly good discrimination. Distortion of sound is noted during the attacks, but this subsides during quiescent phases of the disease. The saculotomy and "tack" operations are the simplest techniques, and they control the symptoms of vertigo in about 65 percent of patients. About 25 percent have diminished hearing and fullness in the ear after the operation. Tinnitus recurs in many patients who have had the operation.

The endolymphatic sac decompression and shunt operations give the following results: improvement or relief of vertigo in about 65 percent; fullness and pressure reduced in 75 percent; tinnitus diminished in 65 percent; hearing improved in 7 percent and decreased in about 40 percent.

The destructive operations are performed on patients who have a more disabling form of Meniere's disease. These procedures are designed to destroy the cochlear and vestibular function in the affected ear. Depending upon the patient's particular problem, there may be an increase in the symptoms of vertigo, tinnitus, and fullness for a short period of time after surgery. These problems usually subside, and the patient is able to resume normal activities.

There are a variety of vestibular problems in which the hearing is ordinarily not affected. Benign paroxysmal positional vertigo, vestibular neuronitis, and cervical vertigo are examples of these problems.

TABLE 46–5 Indications for Surgery for Meniere's Disease

Operations	*Clinical Picture*
Nondestructive	Vertigo, poor medical control with some incapacitation Vertigo does not respond or responds poorly to medical treatment Fluctuating hearing loss Good discrimination (75% or better)
Destructive	Vertigo uncontrolled and severe incapacitation Permanent, nonfluctuating unilateral sensorineural hearing loss Poor discrimination (60% or less) Failure to respond to a nondestructive operation

DISORDERS OF AGING AND METABOLISM

Presbycusis

Presbycusis implies a hearing loss caused by the degenerative changes of aging. These losses are usually symmetrical and slowly progressive. The onset and progression vary widely depending upon genetic factors, physical stress, and environmental factors such as climate and diet.

Schuknecht describes four types of presbycusis that result from the selective deterioration of different morphologic structures within the cochlea.[37] These structures may be involved individually or in combination. When these types appear in a pure form, they have a characteristic functional pattern that can be identified by history, otologic examination, and the audiogram.

Sensory Presbycusis. This is characterized by degeneration or atrophy of the organ of Corti in the basal end of the cochlea. The audiogram reveals an abrupt, high-frequency loss. The speech discrimination is usually quite good.

Neural Presbycusis. Neural presbycusis occurs from a degeneration of cochlear neurons. It can begin at any age but has little effect on hearing until late in life. At this time, there is a progressive loss of speech discrimination which is relatively more severe than the pure tone loss. This has been called phonemic regression. These patients often have other indicators of degenerative changes in the central nervous system. Motor weakness, lack of coordination, tremor, irritability, loss of memory, and intellectual deterioration are examples of the effects of such degeneration.

Strial Presbycusis. Strial presbycusis is vascular in origin. An atrophy of the stria vascularis causes metabolic changes in the cochlea. The hearing loss is typically insidious in onset between the third and sixth decades of life. It progresses slowly. These patients exhibit a flat audiometric curve with an excellent discrimination score. They do not complain of discomfort for loud sounds (recruitment) or distortions of sound (diplacusis).

Cochlear Conductive Presbycusis. This appears to be a mechanical problem that results from stiffness of the basilar membrane. This is not a pathologically proven entity. This form of presbycusis usually becomes evident in middle age and the audiogram exhibits bilateral symmetrical losses with a straight line descending audiometric pattern. The speech discrimination score is inversely related to the steepness of the threshold curve. The greatest losses are for the high frequencies, which are derived from the basal end of the cochlear area where the basilar membrane is thicker and shorter. The least losses are in the low frequencies, which are located in the apical area where the membrane is thinner and wider.

There is no satisfactory surgical treatment for presbycusis. Medical treatment consists of counseling the patient, the family, and associates regarding the hearing impairment and the patient's need for visual clues during conversation. Formal speech reading lessons may assist the patient a great deal. Amplification is helpful in those patients with an adequate discrimination score and dynamic listening range. Avoiding excessive noise and the use of properly fitted ear protectors will help prevent further injury to the cochlea.

Hypothyroidism

There is a general impression that decreased thyroid function is associated with a hearing loss, but there is not a clear causal relationship between the thyroid function and hearing loss. Apparently almost half of the patients with hypothyroidism have an improvement in hearing when they are treated with thyroid hormone. These losses may be conductive or sensorineural or both.

Diabetes Mellitus

Vascular changes are common in patients with diabetes mellitus. It is reasonable to expect that these changes would involve the inner ear. It is difficult, however, to determine a more precise relationship between the diabetes and the degree and type of hearing loss. Some patients have exhibited vascular changes in the vessels of the inner ear (stria vascularis). However, there is no convincing evidence that patients with diabetes mellitus have an increased incidence of hearing loss.

Hypoglycemia

This has been correlated with hearing loss. Weille found 42 percent of patients with Meniere's disease had hypoglycemia at some point during a glucose tolerance test.[38] By contrast, there is only a 15 percent incidence of hypoglycemia in patients with a diagnosis other than Meniere's disease.

SUMMARY

This chapter is not intended to make medical diagnosticians out of speech pathologists and audiologists. As members of a professional team primarily concerned with the best possible medical and therapeutic care of each individual patient, speech and hearing professionals should have a clear understanding of problems that can be treated either medically or surgically.

Often a speech pathologist or audiologist is contacted regarding ear problems. It is hoped that this chapter will provide some familiarity with medical and surgical treatment so that appropriate referrals will be made. Also, an understanding of the skills of the speech pathologist and audiologist enables the otologist to use their skills in the total care of his patients. The ultimate benefit to each patient from the resources of the entire team cannot be denied.

REFERENCES

1. Jahrsdoerfer RA, Hall JW III. Congenital malformations of the ear. Am J Otol 1986; 7:267–269.
2. Phillips SC, Miyamoto RT. Congenital conductive hearing loss in Apert syndrome. Otolaryngol Head Neck Surg 1986; 95:429–433.
3. Colman BH. Surgical techniques and results in congenital malformations. Proceedings of the fifth international workshop on middle ear microsurgery and fluctuant hearing loss. Huntsville, AL: Strode Inc, 1977: 202.
4. Mattox DE, Fisch U. Surgical correction of congenital atresia of the ear. Otolaryngol Head Neck Surg 1986; 94(5):574–577.
5. Lipkin AF, Cocker NJ, Jenkins HA. Hereditary congenital cholesteatoma: a variant of branchio-oto dysplasia. Arch Otolaryngol Head Neck Surg 1986; 112(10):1097–1100.
6. Morrison AW, Bundey SE. The inheritance of otosclerosis. J Laryngol Otol 1970; 84:921–932.
7. Smyth GDL, Hassard TH. Hearing aids post-stapedectomy: incidence and timing. Laryngoscope 1986; 96(4):385–388.
8. Hemenway WG, Hildyard VH, Black FO. Post-stapedectomy perilymph fistulas in the Rocky Mountain area: the importance of nystagmography and audiometry in diagnosis and early tympanotomy in prognosis. Laryngoscope 1968; 78:1687–1715.
9. Wullstein H, Olgivie R, Hall I. Van der Hoeve's syndrome in mothers and daughters. J Laryngol Otol 1960; 74:67–83.
10. Olgilvie R, Hall I. On the etiology of otosclerosis. J Laryngol Otol 1962; 76:841–896.
11. Livingstone G. Congenital ear anomalies due to thalidomide. Proc Roy Soc Med 1965; 58:493–497.
12. Gates GA, Avery C, Cooper JC, Hearne EM, Holt GR. Predictive value of tympanometry in middle ear effusion. Ann Otol Rhinol Laryngol 1986; 95(1): 46–50.
13. English GM, Northern JL, Fria TJ. Chronic otitis media as a cause of sensorineural hearing loss. Arch Otolaryngol 1973; 98:18–22.
14. Paparella MM, Brady DR, Hoel R. Sensorineural hearing loss in chronic otitis media and mastoiditis. Trans Amer Acad Ophthal Otolaryngol 1970; 74:108–115.
15. Jahrsdoerfer RA, Gardner G, Yeakley JW, Karam CR. Lethal cholesteatoma. Otolaryngol Head Neck Surg 1986; 95:507–510.
16. Karmody CS, Schuknecht HF. Deafness in congenital syphilis. Arch Otolaryngol 1966; 83:18–26.
17. English GM. Common injuries to the ear. Primary Care 1976; 3:507–520.
18. Simmons FB. Theory of membrane breaks in sudden hearing loss. Arch Otolaryngol 1968; 88:41–48.
19. Alexander A, Scholl R. Beschwerden und Störungen in Hör und Gleichgewichtsorgan bei der Nachuntersuchung Schädelverletzter. Mschr Ohren Heilk 1938; 72:1021–1058.
20. Lee PC, Sanders CW, Gantz BJ, Otto SR. Transient sensorineural hearing loss after overuse of portable headphone cassette radios. Otolaryngol Head Neck Surg 1985; 93(5) 622–625.
21. Dix M, Hallpike C. The pathology, symptomatology and diagnosis of certain common disorders of the vestibular system. Proc Roy Soc Med 1952; 45:341–352.
22. Igarashi M, Schuknecht HF, Myers E. Cochlear pathology in humans with stimulation deafness. J Laryngol 1964; 78:115–123.
23. Bergstrom L, Thompson P. Ototoxicity. In: Northern J, ed. Hearing disorders. Boston: Little, Brown, 1976:136.
24. Matz GJ. Aminolycoside ototoxicity. J Otolaryngol 1986; 7(2):117–119.
25. Tange RA, Dreschler WA, van der Hulst RJAM. The importance of high-tone audiometry in monitoring for ototoxicity. Arch Otorhinolaryngol 1985; 242(1):77–81.
26. Gantz B, McCabe B, Tyler R, Preece J. Evaluation of four cochlear implant designs. Presented at the International Cochlear Symposium & Workshop. Melbourne, Australia, August 1985.
27. Schindler R, Kesler D, Rebscher S, Yanda J, Jackler R. The UCSF/Storz multi-channel cochlear implant: patient results. Laryngoscope 1986; 96:597–603.
28. Parkin JL, Eddington DK, Orth JL, Brachmann DE. Speech recognition experience with multi-channel cochlear implants. Otolaryngol Head Neck Surg 1985; 93(5):639–645.
29. Hough J, Vernon J, Johnson B, Dorman K, Himelick T. Experiences with implantable hearing devices and a presentation of a new device. Ann Otol Rhinol Laryngol 1986; 95(1): 60–65.
30. McCabe B, Fletcher M. Selection of therapy of glomus jugulare tumors. Arch Otolaryngol 1969; 89:156–159.
31. Lewis J. Temporal bone resection in treatment of tumor. In: English GM, ed. Otolaryngology. Philadelphia: Harper & Row, 1987.
32. Hardy M, Crowe S. Early asymptomatic acoustic tumors: report of six cases. Arch Surg 1936; 32:292–301.
33. Leonard J, Talbot M. Asymptomatic neurilemmoma. Arch Otolaryngol 1970; 91:117–124.
34. Schuknecht HF, Woellner R. An experimental and clinical study of deafness from partial section of the cochlear nerve. J Laryngol Otol 1955; 69:75–97.
35. Glasscock ME III, Kveton JF, Jackson CG, Levine SC, McKennan KX. A systematic approach to the surgical management of acoustic neuroma. Laryngoscope 1986; 96:1088–1094.
36. Smith MFW. Conservation of hearing in acoustic schwannoma surgery. Am J Otol [Suppl] 1985; (Nov):161–163.
37. Schuknecht HF. Further observations on the pathology of presbycusis. Arch Otolaryngol 1964; 80:369–382.
38. Weille F. Hypoglycemia in Meniere's disease. Arch Otolaryngol 1968; 87:555–557.

Rehabilitation of the Hearing Impaired

47 Education of the Hearing Impaired Learner

Donald G. Ferguson, Ed.D.
Doin E. Hicks, Ed.D.
Glenn S. Pfau, Ph.D.

Formal education of individuals with hearing impairment has had a varied and uneven development during its history in the United States. Some misunderstandings outside of and within the field persist regarding the educational implications of a hearing loss. It is hoped that over the years these differences have become fewer in number and smaller in magnitude. In this chapter, our intent is to summarize the current state of affairs and to deal with some of the most significant points of contention and congruence within the field of education of the hearing impaired. The primary audience is the student of speech and hearing who has not had extensive experience and training with educational problems facing hearing impaired persons. In general terms, objectives are twofold: (1) to provide a discussion of several major educational needs and concerns and (2) to demonstrate that solutions to educational problems of hearing impaired persons are complex, requiring an extensive range of remediation techniques, with the individual always being the point of focus.

A POINT OF DEPARTURE

Despite the low incidence of hearing impaired young people in special schools (an estimated 69,000 nationally), there is great heterogeneity in the types of programs offered by the approximately 1,000 different special school settings in the country, not considering the wide variance in programming in the hundreds of regular classrooms in which many hearing handicapped pupils are placed. The often used term "*the* education of *the* deaf" can be misleading if, for instance, an inference is made that "the deaf" are some sort of homogeneous group exhibiting uniform, predictable characteristics and that a single, unique approach to teaching is applicable to all members of such a group. The fact is that there is much variation within this select population, and thus the approach, methodology, curricula, and techniques of their education must also vary.

Much difference of opinion persists about the appropriate terminology and definitions; our intention here is not to propose a resolution of the matter. The term "hearing impaired" is used throughout this chapter to include all learners with a hearing loss who are handicapped to such an extent that some form of special education is required for optimal learning to take place. Included, therefore, are deaf persons, who, according to the definition accepted by the Conference of Executives of American Schools for the Deaf, have a loss of 70 dB or greater in their better ear, and hard-of-hearing persons, who have a loss of 35 to 69 dB in their better ear.

Despite the mentioned heterogeneity, certain similarities exist among hearing impaired persons in learning characteristics and in the type of schooling indicated. Also present are many similarities to the academic program designed for the normally hearing, nonhandicapped population. Northcott cautions against perceiving exceptional and nonexceptional groups as discrete and against making "corresponding assumptions about sharp distinctions in the basic nature and learning styles between each."[1] She goes on to state that "these latter two fall instead along a continuum of uniqueness." The more severe the handicap, the more specialized and individualized becomes the educational approach.

Consequently, one can say that education of hearing impaired learners is characterized by diversity in both substance and form. Then, too, education for these learners is not the singular province of the classroom teacher, any more than it is for any other learner. Schooling can be a powerful influence in human development, but, as Garretson points out, typical schooling, at least quantitatively, influences the lives of most learners less than television, the home, and the broader community.[2] He states that of the total of 8,760 hours in a year, 720 are spent in classrooms, as contrasted with as much as 2,600 hours spent viewing television! No understanding of how these young people learn can be complete without also focusing on life outside the school. Particular reference is made later in this chapter to the crucial role of parents in the educational process, from infancy through emancipation.

For over a century, the field of education of hearing impaired learners in the United States has experienced continuing controversy over methodology. Should learners be taught by means of oral methods only or through manual communication? Is some combination of these preferable? Should audition and speech be the primary modalities in the teaching of language or do congenitally deaf persons conceptualize and learn language in a totally different way from normally hearing children? Professionals in the field have viewed these as anything but purely academic considerations; indeed, these issues are real and intense and have sometimes produced polarization in the profession possibly unparalleled by anything in regular education. As a consequence, the field has been victimized by the pitfalls of dichotomous thinking with the accompanying misfortune of a single methodologic issue frequently obscuring the equal (or greater) importance of other educational and curricular considerations.

The current movement is more toward conciliation and avoidance of unilateral approaches. In the first place, the field is, or should be, sobered by the reality that no research basis exists for certitude about the optimal schooling for hearing impaired young people. School achievement levels of this population are alarmingly low when compared with those of nonexceptional children and youth. Rather than espousing methodologic absolutes, professionals should exhibit humility in light of the relatively low level of academic success experienced by the majority of students who have a profound and congenital hearing loss.

As Moores puts it,

> Given the present state of knowledge, educators making decisions regarding methodology must do so in the face of great uncertainty. In thinking through the problem, they must be aware that if their orientation is wrong, their decision will have lasting detrimental effects on children . . . Research should not necessarily be for the "best" method for all children, but rather the preferred method for a particular child at a particular stage of development.[3]

A combined position statement by three influential organizations in the field of education of the hearing impaired is worthy of note. The statement has the agreement of the Alexander Graham Bell Association for the Deaf, the Convention of American Instructors of the Deaf, and the Conference of Executives of American Schools for the Deaf: ". . . No single method of instruction and/or communication (oral or total communication) or educational setting can best serve the needs of all hearing impaired children (deaf and hard of hearing) of school age."[3a]

COMMUNICATION MODALITIES

The methods mentioned herein refer to receptive and expressive language modes used by and for hearing impaired people in communication. There are several described next. As noted, different terms are used to label these modalities.

Oral Method

Used as a primary means of learning language, this mode, also known as the oral-aural method, places reliance on a combination of residual hearing and speechreading (lipreading). Expressive language is solely through speech, the notion being that reliance on gestures and other manual ways of communication reduces reliance upon speech and impairs its normal development. A basic assumption is that deaf and hard-of-hearing people must develop means of communicating effectively in a hearing world, and to do so they also must adapt to the communicative modality of the majority culture.

Unisensory Method

Unlike the oral method, the unisensory method places no emphasis on the acquisition of language through visual means. Therefore speechreading is not taught. It is also referred to as the auditory method or the acoupedic method. The mode derives its various names because of its singular attention to residual hearing, even in the cases of children with profound losses.

Rochester Method

This approach incorporates a form of manual communication—finger spelling—in conjunction with reliance upon speechreading and residual hearing. No use of signs is made for instruction, but rapid finger spelling is used concurrently with speech. The name of this method is associated with the school where it was first employed, The Rochester School for the Deaf, Rochester, New York.

Total Communication

This combined method makes use of all modes of communication, including speechreading, speech, audition, finger spelling, natural gestures, facial expressions, and manual sign language. Whereas finger spelling is the one-hand form of communication to indicate letters of the alphabet, signing involves both hands and the body in conveying whole concepts within a single movement. Various modes are used simultaneously.

Despite the methodologic differences that have characterized the field of deafness, there are several points of agreement. Broadly speaking, we can safely say that all educators of hearing impaired learners want their students, upon final commencement from school, to be economically efficient and independent, socially responsive, fully actualized persons with self-esteem on a level comparable to that of any other person. There is agreement, too, as Reynolds and Birch point out,[4] that despite great difficulty for some hearing impaired students, the following assets are worthy of all educational effort:

1. Knowledge of one's native language.
2. Clear oral speech.
3. Understanding of the oral speech of others.
4. Ability to read with speed and comprehension.
5. Ability to understand abstract concepts.

Reynolds and Birch also point out several conditions that influence education and result in different forms of specialized intervention.[4] The first of these is the nature of the defect. In their words, "The more the sounds and the speech range are blocked out by the hearing impairment, the more serious the special education problem." Second, the degree of loss has gradations of influence, with greater demands on the special education program as the impairment becomes more severe. Age of onset is a third consideration. The earlier in childhood the deficit was experienced, the more serious the educational problem. Children born with the handicap and those who become deaf during infancy (prelingually deaf) require different and more elaborate educational intervention than those who become impaired later in life, in particular after the acquisition of language (postlingually deaf). A fourth consideration is the cognitive level at which the child functions. The more intelligent the hearing impaired child, the more effective he or she tends to be in acquiring knowledge and skills necessary for more normal functioning in society. An important point is that extreme patience and caution must be exercised in determining the intellectual level of the child. Too often, hearing impaired children have been inappropriately labelled mentally retarded and instructed as such. Fifth, the nature and amount of sensory and intellectual stimulation are crucial factors. So that educational intervention can have constructive impact, it should be presented in an orderly manner with regularity and should occur as early as possible. Educational programming in recent years has begun to take more into account the crucial factor of timing.

EARLY INTERVENTION

From several vantage points, and in the opinion of many writers in the field, the most fruitful period to acquire and develop language is in infancy and during the preschool years. As Reynolds and Birch state, "The teaching of a language system in the earliest childhood years is of overriding importance." This notion has long been recognized, and some efforts have been made toward systematic educational intervention in the lives of very young hearing impaired learners. However, anything approaching comprehensive educational programming for the infant and preschool population has been a recent development. Improved diagnostic and assessment procedures have been conducive to this goal.

In the past, one major impediment to dealing with this group was undetected hearing losses in infants and very young children. Changes began to take place approximately a quarter of a century ago. Calvert points out that

> ... the growth of early education is reflected in the annual reports of programs and classes for children under six years of age published in the *American Annals of the Deaf.* In the two decades from 1951 to 1971 the number of programs accepting children under three years of age rose from 109 to 369, while programs accepting children in the first year of life, absent from the 1951 report, numbered 65 by 1971.[5]

To date, 18 states provide financial support for educatio[illegible] programs beginning at birth for the hearin[illegible]ed.

Despite recent developments and the relatively high value placed on early childhood education, programming for this age group clearly has a long way to go. Added impetus has been given to states through their public schools by recent federal legislation to provide full educational services to handicapped children, including those in early childhood. The most significant legislation is known as the Education for All Handicapped Children Act of 1975.

Moores observes that additional impetus for early childhood education for the hearing impaired came from experience nationally in Head Start programs funded by the federal government for children from economically disadvantaged families.[3] At least in broad strokes, the Head Start program had a significant influence on education of the deaf, despite disappointing research results regarding the effect on the general population of nonhandicapped learners. The rubella epidemic of the mid-1960s, which resulted in a comparatively high incidence of deaf infants, also had a significant impact on the development of early childhood programs. This epidemic occurred at a time when the trend to move education downward had begun.

A persistent and nagging concern to professionals has long been the reality of low scores on achievement tests by school-age hearing impaired children. Early intervention programs have been seen as a long-sought boon to help minimize this problem.

Research results, although inconclusive, have influenced educational programming for the young child. For example, Guralnick states that findings support the involvement of hearing impaired preschoolers with more advanced hearing peers who can serve as valuable instructional resources and as models for "appropriate social, play, and communicative behavior." Many studies have pointed out the constructive influence of modeling or imitative behavior among young children, which is impeded if any child remains out of contact with children of other ages. Such is the case with many hearing impaired children who are isolated from appropriate educational programs and who come from families unaware of the importance of such involvement. Even though there is an absence of hard data, according to Calvert there are "frequent school reports of those who are started on amplification and auditory training very early making superior use of their hearing."[5]

Program Emphases in Early Childhood

All infant and preschool programs place considerable emphasis on utilization of whatever residual hearing the child possesses. Programs designed around amplified hearing as the sole mode for language development gradually follow the unisensory method described earlier. Many are not purely acoupedic in nature, but place preferential reliance on the ear rather than on visual or tactile senses for learning. According to this emphasis, primary effort is directed toward encouraging the infant to develop a listening attitude and what Mavilya calls a "hearing personality."[7] She describes the Infant Center at the Lexington School for the Deaf in New York City where mobiles spin or clown faces light up as hearing impaired babies change the pitch or loudness of their voices; thereby "the infant experiments vocally and acquires language in the same manner as a hearing child."

Connor stresses the importance of such programs: "The fortunate deaf babies who start their auditory, cognitive, speech and social activities before six months of age are capable of avoiding the mute period which plagues deaf children in the latter half of their first year."[8] Research has indicated that hearing impaired infants without specialized training cease to babble as early as 24 to 26 weeks of age. Mavilya observes that "babbling is essential for later speech development, so it is reasserted often through amplification."[7] Teachers and parents of deaf infants are urged to provide constant vocal stimulation in the home and later in preschool to develop a "posture of hearing." Physical stimulation is likewise crucial since motor activity and vocalization are related. In other words, maximal physical or motor activity leads to greater oral production.

Calvert and Silverman are proponents of an approach they call the "auditory global method," which also places primary emphasis on the auditory channel.[9] Nevertheless they point out that it may not be a satisfactory approach for all children, and so they recommend periodic reassessment in the event alternate approaches are indicated.

Alternative methods include, of course, combined emphasis on visual along with oral and aural channels. Currently the use of both finger spelling and signing are common in early childhood educational programs.[10]

Meadow cautions against too much stress on early intervention; such emphasis could lead to excessive expectations for verbal achievement.[11] She feels that too much attention can be given to oral progress with an "accompanying reduction in the relaxed, playful, creative, happy interaction that may be necessary for normal growth and development." Mavilya similarly urges teachers to see and treat hearing impaired infants and young children as small human beings rather than merely as "two big ears."[7] She also recommends a middle-of-the-road approach that "includes all manner of activities geared towards stimulating a child's growth in speech, language, listening, and cognition with plenty of time for free play as well as the opportunity for structured individual and group activities."

According to Moores, the following four factors in combination have contributed to recent improvement in early childhood education for hearing impaired children:[3]

1. Cognitive and academic training.
2. Use of combined oral and manual communication.
3. Improved utilization of residual hearing.
4. More parental involvement.

Parental Involvement

The most constant and influential teacher of any child—preschool or otherwise—is the parent. Some parents of hearing impaired children are not in a position to spend as much time or effort as others in their difficult role as home educators; then, too, some parents understand more easily than others the implications of hearing impairment. Therefore, statements about the role of parents in educational programs and their general involvement in the life of their hearing impaired child apply unevenly. Nevertheless, all parents are primary influences in shaping the total development of their children.

Educators in the field realize how imperative it is to work with parents in the home in order for the benefits of school to be maximized. In both institutions, key emphasis must be on individuality and flexibility, an acceptance of the child as he or she is, and a willingness to shift instruction among alternatives until the most comfortable and efficient learning style of each child is identified. Teachers endeavor to reach parents on a one-to-one basis and/or in small group sessions to help them utilize and reinforce techniques for language acquisition. They cooperate with the home to help develop an awareness of what a hearing loss means socially and emotionally to the child. Such an awareness is important for all peers and adults who touch the lives of the hearing impaired.

It is essential for parents to guard against development of overdependency through a highly protective, solicitous relationship. Such an environment not only impedes the healthy growth of the hearing impaired child, but could also aggravate the home situation by causing sibling resentment. Therefore, parent education needs to concentrate on what the hearing impaired child is capable of doing now and what he or she can be expected to do in the future. This optimism should not deny the frustrations and other realities of the handicap. But dwelling on the deficit is counterproductive when such attention leads to defeatism and guilt by either the child or the parent. It is depressing for the child to feel that he or she is never going to live up to parental expectations (because of cruel comparisons with siblings or other peers) in such areas as speech, reading rate and comprehension, social graces, or any other dimension.

Professionals working with parents can do them a great service by reducing the potential frustration they face when selecting a school for their child. Parents need to understand the variety of approaches available and what role is played in education by special service personnel, such as the audiologist, speech therapist, school nurse, resource teacher, psychologist, and others. Parents should also be helped to recognize biases on the part of anybody giving them advice. Anyone to whom they turn who favors a given system of instruction for all children to the categorical exclusion of other options should be held suspect. Then, too, physicians should be relied upon for their area of expertise, but they may venture outside that realm by urging parents to be patient and allow nature somehow to take its course when educational action should be taken.

Time is a crucial factor. Although we do not recommend that a hearing impaired child be changed constantly or capriciously from one educational situation to another, options and considerable variety among special and regular schools are available. Parents and children should be free to exercise those options, dependent to some degree, of course, on the economic status of the home.

SCHOOL PLACEMENT

Mention throughout this chapter has been made of the diversity of educational settings that exist for the schooling of hearing impaired children. These options are grouped according to the following types. Data used were derived from 1977 and 1978 publications of the Office of Demographic Studies, Gallaudet University.

Residential Schools

As the name implies, children enrolled in this type of school typically live away from home, although 15 to 20 percent of the residential school enrollment are students who attend only during the day. In other words, they live off campus, generally with their parents. There are 79 residential schools in the country—public or private—developed solely to serve hearing impaired children. Approximately 32 percent of the hearing impaired children in the country attend residential schools. At one time over 75 percent were enrolled in this type of setting. (Enrollment data are reported annually in the Directory issue of the *American Annals of the Deaf.*)

Day Schools

As the name implies, these special schools have no overnight accommodations. No children are in residence, but the school, which is housed in a separate building, is entirely geared to a special purpose—instruction for hearing impaired young people. There are approximately 89 of these institutions, usually located in large population centers. Also, there are 84 programs classified as schools for the multi-handicapped that serve hearing impaired students with additional handicaps. Some of these programs are residential in nature and others are day school programs.[12]

Full-Time Classes

In this type of setting, sometimes referred to as "day programs," learners spend essentially all of their time "in a class consisting only of hearing impaired children, the class itself being located in a local school which is not limited to hearing impaired children."[13] Approximately 20 percent of the nation's school-age children with hearing impairment are placed in a full-time special education class of this nature.

Integrated

In these settings, the hearing impaired child spends all or part of the school day in regular classrooms with hearing children. "Mainstreaming" is the term most frequently used to denote this group. The hearing impaired child may be involved in a special class part of the day with other hearing impaired children and the remainder of the time with normally hearing children, or in a resource room for special education for a portion of each week, or in tutorial arrangements with a visiting (itinerant) teacher. In 1974 to 1975, 436 school districts reported offering integrated part-time classes and services for hearing impaired learners,[12] a figure that has risen and will continue to do so with the spread of mainstreaming (integration).

Two-thirds of the children in residential schools are profoundly deaf (i.e., 91 dB or greater loss in the better ear), whereas less than one-fifth of the enrollees in integrated programs have this degree of loss. Karchmer and Trybus point out that "as the severity of the hearing loss increases, the proportion enrolled in integrated programs declines rapidly."[13] Then, too, integrated programs tend to enroll two to three times as many postlingually hearing impaired children as do other programs.

MAINSTREAMING

A further word on integration and mainstreaming is in order because of the central attention this type of educational placement is currently receiving. No greater boon to this development could be imagined than that which comes from the following language of Public Law 94–142 (Education of All Handicapped Children Act of 1975). In order for a state to be eligible for funds under this Act, procedures must be established

> . . . to assure that, to the maximum extent appropriate, handicapped children, including children in public or private institutions or other care facilities, are educated with children who are not handicapped, and that special classes, separate schooling, or other removal of handicapped children from the regular education environment occurs only when the nature of severity of the handicap is such that education in regular classes with the use of supplementary aids and services cannot be achieved satisfactorily.

Public Law 94–142 sets forth many other provisions for dealing with handicapped children, including heavy emphasis on the place of parents in educational decisionmaking about their child and the need for intensive individualization. For each handicapped learner, an individualized educational program must be developed regardless of the type of school or class attended—regular or special. This measure can become a highly constructive influence in moving schools to act on the intention to meet individual pupil needs. A hard-of-hearing or deaf child in a regular school setting clearly has the right to such action. Along this line, Healey states that "The future in regular education for the child with hearing impairment has and will continue to depend, in great measure, on the educational establishment's success in finally addressing the needs of the individual learner."[14]

In addition to the legal argument for mainstreaming handicapped children, many other ideas are advanced in defense of this type of placement. For example, Bricker outlines a rationale drawn from socioethical and psychological literature along with legislative arguments.[15] She points to integration as a means of eliminating the deleterious effects of segregation and the stigma often attached to "the less successful" student. Society at large is afforded an opportunity to become more aware of the handicapped child through integrative approaches and can thereby make a more positive and enlightened response toward the different child. (The opposite response also is a possibility. One may become more negative and prejudiced because of the psychological threat to wholeness when faced with others' handicaps.) Psychologically, integration creates a more demanding environment to which the handicapped child must react and one which is rich in opportunities to learn by imitation.

Here again, however, the field of education of the hearing impaired faces the danger of wallowing in another unneeded argument. Care must be exercised so that professionals and parents do not perceive mainstreaming as "the only way to go"; with such thinking, special classes and schools end up on a blacklist to be eradicated at the earliest possible time. Unless care is taken as the pendulum swings toward mainstreaming, parents, educators, and children associated with special schools may incur the damaging stigma of their schools' being "second class" or, worse, places of last resort. In truth, there is no reason to believe that special schools, including residential schools for the deaf, should not remain a part of our educational system and pridefully so.

One need only look at intelligent precautions about mainstreaming by organizations and authors who highly favor the concept to realize that it is simplistic and erroneous to make a dichotomy of the matter. The Council for Exceptional Children sets forth the following statement about what mainstreaming is *not:*

1. Wholesale return of all exceptional children in special classes to regular classes.
2. Permitting children with special needs to remain in regular classes without the support services they need.
3. Ignoring the need of some children for a special program that can be provided in the general education program.
4. Less costly than serving children in special contained classrooms.

Reynolds and Birch, who highly endorse mainstreaming, state that "not all [the] hearing impaired are best served by full mainstreaming. Some profit most from partial mainstreaming. Some, at least for a time, are best separated completely for intensified special teaching."[4] They point to the new role the residential school can play as a resource center in training and research. Indeed, the accumulated experience in these institutions can be valuable sources of assistance to mainstreamed students and their teachers, to day classes, and to day schools in addition to the provision of direct services to hearing impaired students with complex, demanding educational problems that cannot be solved elsewhere.

Birch, in an earlier publication, set forth the following five key arrangements that must be made when integrating hearing impaired children:[16]

1. Regular class teachers are assigned hearing impaired pupils only with the teachers' prior knowledge and consent.
2. In-service instruction is made readily available for all faculty and staff before mainstreaming is started.
3. The hearing impaired pupils who attend regular schools have skills and achievements comparable to those found in the rest of the class.
4. The regular teachers and pupils are oriented and assisted sufficiently regarding communication with the hearing impaired pupil so that it does not constitute a major problem.
5. Both continuing and emergency assistance is available.

Cost savings is often advanced as an argument and incentive for mainstreaming. As Healey observes, "such generalizations are premature."[14] Among other items, he lists the following as undesirable results of lowered costs: (1) no support services (e.g., vocational, audiologic); (2) heavy class or case loads for teachers and clinicians; (3) inadequate in-service education; (4) limited or no parent counseling; and (5) no necessary materials or equipment purchased. Some of these same weaknesses were found years ago in studies of inadequately supported special schools for the hearing impaired.[17,18] The times hardly call for a return to past ills in the name of progress.

CURRICULUM PLANNING

Regardless of the setting in which hearing impaired students are placed, substantive questions about what they should be able to accomplish in school must be raised and answered. The scope and sequence of learning experiences selected and organized for them constitute vital curriculum decisions. Some of the decisions about hearing impaired learners are necessarily unique to them because of their handicap; many others are essentially the same as those decisions made for normally hearing children and youth. Concepts of time and space, cognitive factors such as moving from the simple to the complex, from the concrete to the abstract, and other similar considerations have basically the same curricular implications for hearing impaired learners as for the nonhandicapped.

There are few specialized, written curriculum guides available on a large scale for teachers of hearing impaired students. The exceptions, of course, are the many helpful materials printed on the subject of language arts instruction. From time to time, curriculum plans in special schools have been developed in most of the content areas, but these have been more local in nature, less elaborate, and few in number by comparison with the whole field of language. One assumption about the paucity of materials in the other subject matter fields is that hearing impaired learners can master arithmetic, science, history, geography, and other school subjects in the same way as any other learner. Consequently, according to this view, curricula designed for use by general public schools are deemed applicable for the hearing impaired enrollment as well, after some modification.

An opposing view is that the handicap of deafness calls for many types of curriculum plans developed specifically for the population in question; therefore it is deemed unfortunate that professionals in this field do not have more curriculum guidelines of a specialized nature at their disposal. Content should be presented in smaller increments, and vocabulary in all subject matter areas developed differently; consequently, curriculum plans developed for regular learners, even after making major adaptations, generally do not suffice. Courses of study in algebra and biology, for instance, have been developed for hearing impaired high school students at the Model Secondary School for the Deaf on the Gallaudet University campus. When it existed, the Bureau of Education for the Handicapped of the Department of Health, Education, and Welfare was instrumental in sponsoring the production and dissemination of instructional guides for use in classrooms for the deaf.

Regardless of the view held about written curriculum plans, perception of education for the hearing impaired as being highly esoteric or having a mystique all its own can be counterproductive, especially in an era when more regular classroom teachers are being asked to participate on at least a partially integrated basis in this type of education. The field can ill-afford continued insularism.

If the school curriculum for all children is perceived as a moving wheel, hearing impaired students take their natural place in the journey alongside of others. According to Brameld, who proposes such a model, the rim of this wheel represents humankind's predicaments and aspirations.[19] These are the ultimate ends of education. The hub becomes the point of focus for study, shifting even daily or weekly among such topics as the community, electricity, the Westward Movement, the space age, population control, the first Thanksgiving, and so on. The spokes in this model are subject matter fields—the basic skills and content areas.

Although this curriculum model holds generally in education for hearing impaired students, one spoke has been decidedly out of proportion to the others and always will be—the area of language. As mentioned before, other curricular modifications are also wisely made. A few of these are discussed briefly later on in this section, but first a word about language instruction.

Language

In making decisions about curricular programs for the hearing impaired, little disagreement occurs over the need for a heavy emphasis on the teaching of language. As pointed out in the section on early intervention, an emphasis on language acquisition should begin at birth. In hearing children, this type of learning comes naturally, almost like breathing. One of the human's most distinguishing characteristics, therefore, is acquired with great ease by them. For hearing impaired children, especially those profoundly deaf from infancy, the acquisition of standard English becomes one of the most arduous tasks imposed on any human being. In school, it becomes every teacher's challenge to assist hearing impaired children and youth in this endeavor. And regardless of the hub of the curricular wheel, the specter of the language problem looms large and is ever present, and so this skill area has to be out of proportion to some of the others. How to help these learners acquire adequate command of standard English is an educational undercurrent in every classroom—from academic to vocational and from physical education to art.

There are two schools of thought on the accomplishment of this task; neither philosophy has been implemented in pure form except in a few situations. One approach takes off directly from the natural way in which hearing children acquire language. It is sometimes known as the informal approach. Children are taught language spontaneously as the need for it arises in play and other natural, social situations. Whether through speech-reading, residual hearing, signing, finger spelling, or a combination of all these communicative modes, the informal way of teaching language withholds systematic explanations of language as such until later in school life. In other words analyses of sentence structure are not provided.

The formal approach stresses grammatic principles early in school and throughout all the grades, using the process of memorization and various symbols to represent parts of the sentence. Several systems for teaching sentence structure have been devised over the years for use in classrooms for hearing impaired learners. The most common of the approaches, still in use today in many schools, is what is known as the Fitzgerald Key, named after its originator, Edith Fitzgerald (a hearing impaired person herself who taught at the North Carolina School for the Deaf). This key can be used to unlock a sentence by breaking it down into WHO, WHAT, and WHERE components with correlative use being made of six symbols to identify verbs, infinitives, participles, connectives, pronouns, and adjectives. This scheme employs considerable teacher direction with much use of a chalkboard or transparencies; workbook exercises are provided to each learner for practice purposes.

The artificiality of instruction, as opposed to the "natural," in any of the formal approaches to language is like that associated with grammar lessons taught to normally hearing students. Examples of these are diagramming sentences and performing other analytic tasks in which rules and drill and practice are stressed. The similarity does not end there. Formal grammar *understood* by any student—normally hearing or deaf—does not invariably lead to the implementation of standard English in daily life. For all the emphasis placed on language instruction, results are many times disappointing, whether the approach has been formal, informal, or the usual combinations of both. Typically, achievement test scores for hearing impaired students, regardless of the school setting or instructional approach used, tend to be as much as 6 or more years below their hearing counterparts at the age of high school graduation. This means that graduating seniors on a grade-equivalency basis are at about the level that average hearing students achieve when concluding elementary school (sixth grade).

Many precautions must be exercised, however, in the interpretation of test scores. Paper and pencil results do not reveal the sum total of linguistic ability or achievement. Some highly verbal children, for instance, do not always do well on written tests of expressive or receptive skills. Then, too, many students can score well on tests of reading ability, for example, but seldom use a library.

Little satisfaction is derived by special teachers of the hearing impaired from the fact that normally hearing students are also often found to be lacking in the language arts. And so the search for the elusive language break-through continues in education of hearing impaired students.

Visualization

In Caccamise's view, hearing impaired pupils have three kinds of learning problems that are peculiar to them and call for special educational modifications: (1) learning language, (2) learning to communicate, and (3) learning to use vision and other senses to help overcome the hearing handicap.[20] Much has already been stated about his first two points in this chapter. The exemplary classroom for the hearing impaired, among other modifications, contains and uses many multimedia materials, acceding to the fact that compensations for a hearing deficit can derive from the other sensory avenues for learning, especially the visual modality.

A tremendous impetus for the more enlightened use of all forms of instructional media has come to the field over the past two decades from the Captioned Films and Telecommunications Branch (formerly called Captioned Films for the Deaf, then Media Services and Captioned Films), administered by the United States Department of Education. Since 1958, the federal government has acquired, captioned, and distributed thousands of films for both entertainment and educational purposes in order to enhance the lives of hearing impaired children and adults. In addition, it has provided literally millions of media items either by permanent placement or on a loan basis to classrooms for the deaf; these have been in the form of filmstrips, instructional kits, overhead projectors, transparencies, and other media-related materials. Teachers have also been directly assisted through workshops that focus on the proper utilization of instructional media.

The captioned films program has also sponsored considerable research on the impact of multisensory approaches to learning. One of its many specialized activities, Project LIFE (Language Improvement to Facilitate Education of hearing impaired children) yielded many audiovisual materials, all of which were designed according to a programmed instructional model and which likewise involved classroom teachers in utilization workshops.

Efforts in schools for hearing impaired children to provide comprehensive ways for them to experience the world vicariously through visuals of all sorts are augmented on an even higher plane through actual experiences out of the classroom within the community. Again, impetus has come at least in part from the federal government for this type of education. Many federal and state agencies have encouraged schools to offer their deaf students meaningful experiences away from the four walls of the classroom and out within the community. These experiences are not necessarily vocationally oriented, nor must community-based education in general focus merely on the world of work. Such inroads to life outside the schools give children enrolled in elementary and secondary education a view, a feel, indeed a smell of community life in its totality—economics, politics, history, and so on. For some children, such an effort may involve them in their first trip into a large department store or specialty shop. At the other extreme, it may mean a protracted involvement in a set of work and study experiences within the health professions over a period of a year or longer.

Formal education of all children and youth has frequently been castigated for its heavy orientation toward printed matter as a medium for learning. It is even more reprehensible when that is all that is offered to the hearing impaired for whom the printed page frequently poses a set of frustrating and discouraging problems.

Individualization

Broadly conceived, curriculum plans are written fundamentally with "common learnings" in mind. Slavishly implemented, they produce an intellectual conformism in which individual uniqueness is obscured. Of course, such a result is unintended. In proposing the moving wheel as a curriculum model, Brameld pointed out that plans set forth must allow individuals to develop and explore their own capabilities.[19] In his words, a desirable curriculum is one that serves "each individual's own time and concerns." Therefore it is important to keep track of each individual learner's progress in relation to any larger scheme of things based on societal expectations and handled in group learning situations.

As noted earlier, Public Law 94–142 makes it clear that regardless of whatever else may be available in the form of written curriculum plans, each child with special needs will have an individual educational program. On this matter, the law reads as follows:

> The term individualized education program means a written statement for each handicapped child developed in any meeting by a representative of the local educational agency or an intermediate educational unit who shall be qualified to provide, or supervise the provision of, specially designed instruction to meet the unique needs of handicapped children, the teacher, the parents or guardian of such child, and, wherever appropriate, such child, which statement shall include (a) a statement of the present level of educational performance of such child, (b) a statement of annual goals, including short-term instructional objectives, (c) a statement of the specific educational services to be provided to such child, and the extent to which such child will be able to participate in regular educational programs, (d) the projected date for initiation and anticipated duration of such services, and appropriate objective criteria and evaluation procedures and schedules for determining, on at least an annual basis, whether instructional objectives are being achieved.

As a result, curriculum planning for individual hearing impaired children is likely to take place with greater precision than ever before and in light of more exacting, comprehensive diagnoses than previously employed. At the Kendall Demonstration Elementary School on the Gallaudet University campus, for instance, the assessment plan, coupled with each child's individual educational program includes frequent diagnoses in each of the following areas: medical, audiologic, perceptual-motor, socioemotional, communication and language, and educational (the latter including achievement testing that has been standardized on a hearing impaired pupil population).

Individual curriculum plans by their very nature must account for the fact that besides differences in intellectual functioning, children learn at different rates, their cognitive styles vary, social situations affect learning differently, and learners have preferences among various media and vary greatly in their degree of dependence and/or independence.

Traditional education has been seriously examined in recent years both in regular and special schools, making way for more open approaches to learning. Individualization is a central idea behind this movement. Openness implies fewer pressures and less predetermination from outside the learner. Consequently, more student-initiated activities are encouraged within classrooms. Interest centers are in evidence, games are prevalent, and small group and individual presentations are more frequent than learning experiences by the group as a whole. Where whole schools are committed to this way of teaching and learning, many of the trappings of tradition have come down, including walls, and the atmosphere has become a more pleasant, flexible place in which to move about, inquire, and learn. In his endorsement of open education, Craig makes the following statements:

> In addition to the flexibility provided in the selection of subject matter the organization of this material can be tailored to provide an individualized approach to learning. Both the content and the process of education can be readily adapted for individual students. Perhaps one of the major benefits, however, results from the independence the deaf child can demonstrate in the open classroom setting, if one of the educational goals for deaf children is to reduce dependence and encourage self-sufficiency. This approach to learning should have significant benefits.[21]

POSTSECONDARY EDUCATION

In a technologically oriented society, it is understandable that an elementary and secondary education for hearing impaired students or any others does not suffice in helping them become employable in highly skilled, technical positions. Consequently, considerable growth has occurred of postsecondary programs for the hearing impaired nationally in recent years. Many of these programs are geared toward technical and vocational training and are associated with established institutions for hearing students. According to the most recent survey of college and career opportunities for the hearing impaired, 60 programs were available in 30 different states (along with five in Canada), all of which tended to serve regional rather than merely local needs.[22] (Regions least served were in the South and Northeast.)

Special services provided by institutions offering such programs include at least interpreting (manual communication), along with tutorial and note-taking services. In addition, some institutions provide special class sections for hearing impaired enrollees only, special vocational and personal counseling, adapted sociocultural activities, and supervised housing. In all, 3,700 students enrolled in these 60 programs for the hearing impaired, with none of the programs having fewer than 10 students.[22] The mean enrollment for the programs, exluding Gallaudet and the National Technical Institute for the Deaf, was 37.

Every year, several hearing impaired students enroll in colleges and universities for the hearing which offer no specialized programs or services for persons with a hearing loss. The exact number of these students is difficult to determine because there is no national reporting procedures for this population. However, according to the *Volta Review* (which annually reports figures on this type of enrollment), each year during the last decade, fewer than 100 hard-of-hearing or deaf students were in attendance at institutions offering no special services for persons with hearing impairment.

Over half of all the postsecondary enrollment in programs for the hearing impaired attend two institutions that are national and/or international in scope and service. The first of these is Gallaudet University in Washington, D.C., the only liberal arts college in the world for hearing impaired students and primarily limited to them at the undergraduate level. Founded in 1864, Gallaudet University is geared to a broad, liberal education as well as occupational preparation and graduate study.

Slightly more than a century after the founding of Gallaudet University, the National Technical Institute for the Deaf (NTID) was created in 1965. It is affiliated with the Rochester Institute of Technology in Rochester, New York. As the name implies, this institution focuses on technical education offering 46 curricular options, some of which are of a year's duration for the student, others leading to baccalaureate and master's degrees. Both Gallaudet University and NTID have been substantially financed by the federal government, as have three model two-year institutions that offer regional, comprehensive postsecondary programs for the hearing impaired. These are the St. Paul Technical Vocational Institute in Minnesota, Delgado Junior College in New Orleans, Louisiana, and Seattle Community College in Seattle, Washington. Within the group receiving federal assistance also is California State University at Northridge, which offers both undergraduate and graduate programs to hearing impaired students. Each of these programs enrolls approximately 50 to 160 hearing impaired students annually.

SUMMARY

The education of hearing impaired persons is not without major problems and controversy on the one hand, and an air of optimism on the other. Perhaps the most objective and comprehensive look at education of hearing impaired persons was taken in 1965 by a blue ribbon committee appointed by the Secretary of Health, Education, and Welfare. This now classic study (referred to as the "Babbidge Report," so named for the Committee Chairman, Dr. Homer D. Babbidge Jr.) provides great insight into the successes, failures, struggles, and sheer determination that characterize the efforts to bring quality education to hearing impaired youth. The summary of this report speaks of a need and concern that remains relevant:

> The American people have no reason to be satisfied with their limited success in educating deaf children and preparing them for full participation in our society . . . This unsatisfactory state of education of the deaf cannot be attributed to any lack of dedication to those who teach and work with the deaf. The basic explanation lies in our failure to launch an aggressive assault on some of the basic problems of language learning of the deaf through experience or well-planned and adequately supported research, and in our failure to develop more systematic and adequate programs for educating the deaf at all levels.[23]

The authors have attempted to highlight those areas that are most pressing to educators of the hearing impaired and that, to the student, might be most useful both as an introduction to and as a motivation for delving further into this challenging field of study.

Language and communication remain the major nemeses for hearing impaired persons and the central professional concern of those who would help them acquire these skills. Though inseparable in many respects, language is a prerequisite to achieving communication skill, regardless of the modality used. Language sophistication is a singular achievement of humans. Without intensive educational intervention, the hearing impaired person is likely to be deprived of this most basic tool. Helen Keller viewed deafness as the greater of her two major handicaps and did so precisely because of the language problems imposed by deafness. She says of the human voice: ". . . it brings language, sets thoughts astir, and keeps us in the intellectual company of man."[24]

Levine has drawn a compelling characterization of the potential plight of those affected by early severe deafness in the following description: "for here is found the closest modern equivalent to the linguistic state of preverbal man. To be born without the ability to hear is to be born without the natural ability to acquire language; without verbal language, normal human development is blocked."[25]

Owing to space constraints, difficult decisions were made with regard to topics for inclusion in this chapter and those to omit entirely or to mention only in passing. In the final analysis, the major criterion for the inclusion of topics was to treat those closest to the learning process itself, since all factors influencing the educational enterprise could not be explored.

Descriptions of major approaches in communication for hearing impaired students are described without any attempt to make judgements about a preferred modality beyond the caution for openness and objectivity.

Early intervention and parental involvement are suggested as particularly crucial to all areas of development for the hearing impaired child. Aside from the obvious need to begin communication and language training early, the total dimension of development is enhanced by early, positive success in the habilitation process.

School placement is discussed within the context of a diversity of options. Particular attention is drawn to the current trends to integrate or mainstream handicapped children within regular classroom settings. Arguments for and against this approach are provided, and the reader is cautioned to regard all currently available placement options as viable and necessary. As with other aspects of programming, the child's needs are the dominant consideration, and placement should not be viewed as a static element; thus placement mobility is desirable so long as it relates to a comprehensive plan.

The curriculum for hearing impaired learners derives its primary uniqueness from problems associated with learning language. Specialized curricula as well as adaptations of general curriculum materials usually are concerned with accommodating language deficits experienced by most hearing impaired persons. As well, within this context, attempts are made to use the visual avenue for learning insofar as possible. This attempt implies extensive use of visual media, including multimedia formats within presentation modes.

Finally, the concept of individualization is strongly supported as it relates to curricular considerations for hearing impaired students. Recent legislation mandating such an approach is seen as potentially positive.

Numerous additional and important topics are left for the serious reader to pursue in other ways. Administration, including program and personnel management, staffing, preservice and in-service training, certification, finance, community and/or parent relations, legislation, and a host of other areas are not included. Similarly, within program considerations, no attempt has been made to exhaust such issues as assessment, after-school programs, residence-hall programs, parent education, or even curricular considerations.

The reader is encouraged to utilize the chapter's list of references to seek other such resources in an effort to explore broadly one of the most exciting and challenging areas within the education profession.

REFERENCES

1. Northcott WH. Integrating the preprimary hearing impaired child: an examination of the process, product, and rationale. In: Guralnick MJ, ed. Early intervention and the integration of handicapped and nonhandicapped children. Baltimore: University Park Press, 1978:207.
2. Garretson MD. The residential school. Deaf Am 1977; 29:19–22.
3. Moores DF. Educating the deaf; psychology, principles, and practices. Boston: Houghton Mifflin, 1978.

3a. Educational Programming for the Hearing Impaired (Deaf and Hard of Hearing) Resolution passed by the Council of Educators of the Deaf, Executive Board, Boston, MA, June 23, 1976.

4. Reynolds MC, Birch JW. Teaching exceptional children in all America's schools. Revised ed. Reston, VA: Council for Exceptional Children, 1982.
5. Calvert DR. Communication practices: aural/oral and visual/oral. In: Frisina DR, ed. A bicentennial monograph on hearing impairment: trends in the U.S.A. Washington DC: The Alexander Graham Bell Association for the Deaf, 1976:76.
6. Guralnick MJ. Integrated preschools as educational and therapeutic environments: concepts, design, and analysis. In: Guralnick MJ, ed. Early intervention and the integration of handicapped and nonhandicapped children. Baltimore: University Park Press, 1978:115.
7. Mavilya MP, Mignone BR. Educational strategies for the youngest hearing impaired children (0 to 5 years of age).

Jackson Heights, NY: The Lexington School for the Deaf, 1977.

8. Connor L. In: Foreword to Mavilya MP, Mignone BR. Educational strategies for the youngest hearing impaired children (0 to 5 years of age). Jackson Heights, NY: The Lexington School for the Deaf, 1977.
9. Calvert DR, Silverman R. Speech and deafness. Washington, DC. Alexander Graham Bell Association for the Deaf, 1975.
10. Jordan IK, Gustason G, Rosen R. Current communication trends at programs for the deaf. Am Ann Deaf 1976; 121:527–532.
11. Meadow K. Self image, family climate and deafness. Soc Forces 1969; 47:428–438.
12. Rawlings B, Trybus R. Personnel, facilities and services available in schools and classes for hearing impaired children in the United States. Am Ann Deaf 1978; 123:99–114.
13. Karchmer MA, Trybus RJ. Who are the deaf children in "mainstream" programs? Series R, Number 4. Washington, DC; Office of Demographic Studies: Gallaudet University Press, 1977.
14. Healey WC. Integrated education. In: Frisina DR, ed. A bicentennial monograph on hearing impairment: trends in the U.S.A. Washington, DC: Alexander Graham Bell Association for the Deaf, 1976.
15. Bricker DD. A rationale for the integration of handicapped and nonhandicapped preschool children. In: Guralnick MJ, ed. Early intervention and the integration of handicapped and nonhandicapped children. Baltimore: University Park Press, 1978.
16. Birch JW. Hearing impaired pupils in the mainstream. Washington, DC: Leadership Training Institute/Special Education, University of Minnesota, Exceptional Child Program, Bureau of Adult and Occupational Education, U.S. Office of Education, Dept. of HEW, 1975.
17. Brill R, Merrill E, Frisina DR. Recommended organizational policies in the education of the deaf. Washington DC: Conference of Executives of American Schools for the Deaf, 1973.
18. Mulholland A, Fellendorf G, eds. National research conference on day programs for hearing impaired children. Washington, DC: Alexander Graham Bell Association for the Deaf, 1968.
19. Brameld T. A cross-cutting approach to the curriculum: the moving wheel. Phi Delta Kappan 1970; 51:346–348.
20. Caccamise F. "Musts" for hearing people. Am Ann Deaf 1974; 119:296–297.
21. Craig WN. Curriculum: its perspectives and prospects. In: Frisina DR, ed. A bicentennial monograph on hearing impairment: trends in the U.S.A. Washington, DC: Alexander Graham Bell Association for the Deaf, 1976.
22. Rawlings B, Trybus R, Biser J. A guide to college/career programs for deaf students. Washington, DC: Gallaudet University Press, 1978.
23. Babbidge HD, ed.. Education of the deaf: a report to the secretary of health, education and welfare. Report by the HEW advisory committee on the education of the deaf. Washington, DC: U.S. Government Printing Office, 1965.
24. Keller H. Helen Keller in Scotland. London: Methuen, 1933:68.
25. Levin ES. The psychology of deafness. New York: Columbia University Press, 1960:27.

Suggested Reading

Birch JW, Reynolds MC. Special education as a profession: where we came from and where we are going. Excep Ed Q 1982; 2:1–10.

Brill RG. Education of the deaf. Wahington, DC: Gallaudet University Press, 1974.

Jacobs LM. A deaf adult speaks out. Washington, DC: Gallaudet University Press, 1980.

Lowenbraun S, Appleman K, Callahan J. Teaching the hearing-impaired. Columbus, OH: Charles E. Merrill, 1980.

Meadow K. Deafness and child development. Berkeley: University of California Press, 1980.

Morsink CV. Teaching special needs students in regular classrooms. Boston: Little, Brown, 1984:48.

Ross M, Noble LW, eds. Educating hard of hearing children. In: Special education in transition. Reston, VA: The Council for Exceptional Children, 1981.

Schultz JB, Turnbull AP. Mainstreaming handicapped students. 2nd ed. Boston: Allyn & Bacon, 1984:32.

48 Aural Rehabilitation in the Adult

Raymond H. Hull, Ph.D.

The purpose of this chapter is to provide its readers with information on one of the most fascinating aspects of the field of audiology: the process of aural rehabilitation. Its emphasis and direction focus on giving students a taste of what the process is all about. Rather than dwelling upon past research in the area, which can be found in almost every other text written on this topic, I have attempted to summarize what audiologists now know about the processes involved in serving adults who are hearing impaired, and then present information on what the process is and procedures for the administration of aural rehabilitation services.

Audiologists are attempting to serve a very special clientele—adults who perhaps were, for all practical purposes, normally functioning people prior to the acquisition of a frustrating and, in many instances, debilitating hearing impairment. They may be more or less socially inclined; may be the provider for a family; may enjoy watching television or attending the theater or concerts; may enjoy traveling; and may desire to meet new people, talk to their friends, and enjoy other aspects of human existence that are enhanced by, or have as their requisite, the ability to communicate efficiently with others. As a result of decreased auditory acuity, however, many adults find previously enjoyable and/or necessary aspects of their life difficult or perhaps even impossible. A job may be in jeopardy because efficient communication is a prerequisite. Or withdrawal from previous social contacts may be deemed the only alternative since missed messages; inappropriate responses to questions; and resulting frustration, anger, and embarrassment over an inability to understand what others are saying occurs with greater frequency.

A hearing impairment, no matter what the cause, can result in dramatic changes in the lives of adults, changes that can alter the course of their existence. An example of the type of client I am discussing comes to mind. When this 29-year-old client was first seen in this clinic, he was still somewhat stunned because of all that had happened to him. He had sustained multiple gunshot wounds to the head received during an oil well brawl in Texas. A severe meningeal infection occurred secondary to the head wounds, and large doses of ototoxic drugs were administered to save his life. As the result of those two assaults on his auditory mechanism, he sustained a significant hearing loss bilaterally. To add insult to injury, because of the resulting communication problems and therefore social and economic deficits, his wife divorced him, leaving him very much alone. He was seen in this clinic as a severely hearing impaired young man who was understandably distressed and concerned about what the future held for him. Aural rehabilitation services were administered in conjunction with efforts by the District Vocational Rehabilitation office and the involvement of his parents. Two initial areas of aural rehabilitation services were concentrated upon: communication training for vocational placement and social communication. Efforts toward increased social activity were stressed equally with successful vocational placement to combat the depression he was experiencing. Much counseling was involved, with self-actualization and development of coping behavior as primary goals. He is now succeeding in achieving as normal a function as is possible in spite of all that has happened to him.

Other adult clients seen by the audiologist may have acquired hearing loss as the result of noise exposure and are simply experiencing difficulty in social functioning. Their hearing impairment may be causing them frustration, but the service aspect, in most instances, is not as comprehensive as that necessary for the client cited previously.

No matter what the severity of the hearing disorder, these adults require aural rehabilitation services by the audiologist. They range in age from teenagers to, and including, the elderly. And they come in many shapes and sizes, abilities and disabilities. However, they are no different than other people except that they have sustained a sometimes debilitating loss of hearing.

The field of aural rehabilitation that serves these people is as challenging as it is rewarding. The professional audiologists who coordinate and provide these services are challenged by the personal commitment that is involved and the breadth of knowledge that is required. For those who are willing to accept the privilege and challenges involved in serving people who possess one of the most frustrating of all handicaps—hearing impairment—and in helping them achieve their potential in maintaining or regaining communicative function, the satisfactions abound.

WHAT IS AURAL REHABILITATION?

Approaches to the process of aural rehabilitation for the adult are almost as numerous as the number of professional audiologists who provide the service. The term ''aural rehabilitation'' implies many facets of a process, which in its totality manifests itself as helping people who possess impaired hearing. Probably because the field of audiology is still in its youth, however, the search for consistent and descriptive terminology for what audiologists do continues. The descriptions currently used by groups of audiologists across the United States include such terms as "rehabilitative audiology," "aural rehabilitation," and "habilitative audiology." The Committee on Rehabilitative Audiology of the American Speech and Hearing Association (1977) has recommended the use of the term "audiologic rehabilitation" to identify the audiologist as the provider of those services. For consistency, however, I will use in this chapter "aural rehabilitation," a term still generally accepted at this time. Since the term "habilitation" refers to the learning of skills that did not develop because of some interference with the developmental process, but the term "rehabilitation" refers to the restoration of skills that have become impaired, the term "aural rehabilitation" to refer to the restoration of communication skills that have become impaired because of a deficit in auditory function seems to be an accurate descriptor.

The facets of the process of aural rehabilitation will be discussed in this chapter. But before that task is undertaken, let us look at this aspect of the field of audiology through a basic definition. What is aural rehabilitation? In its broadest sense, it encompasses a philosophy that a handicapped person has the right to be helped to become a "complete" person and not only to be restored as much as possible to usefulness and dignity, but also to be aided in reaching his or her own highest potential.[1] However, that definition can apply to most other helping professions who engage in rehabilitative services for handicapped people. The term "aural," which precedes rehabilitation in this discussion, narrows the field considerably. Thus the definition implies helping people with impaired hearing to reach their maximum potential in their communicative needs, whether those needs be vocational, educational, social, or personal. Further, our definition incorporates a broad spectrum of ages, from the vocational age of 16 years to, and including, the elderly adult. This topic, then, becomes a formidable one in terms of its breadth.

What Does Aural Rehabilitation for the Adult Involve?

Approaches to the process of aural rehabilitation vary from professional to professional, as do their philosophies. Even though philosophies vary, however, they all seem to center on several important points; those are to provide services that, in the end, (1) facilitate emotional adjustment to the frustrations and anxieties that accompany depressed hearing; (2) assist hearing impaired people to learn to use their residual hearing as efficiently as possible in environments that previously hindered communication; (3) evaluate and fit hearing aids and other assistive listening devices on behalf of hearing impaired adults; (4) assist hearing impaired people to learn to utilize supplemental visual clues in environments where depressed hearing interferes with efficient communicative function; and (5) facilitate adjustment among family members and peers to the communicative difficulties the hearing impaired person faces and to the resulting concerns and frustrations of both parties.

No matter what approach is taken in the provision of aural rehabilitation services, the aforementioned goals generally remain the same. They may be prioritized differently, and other terms may be used, but the intent is constant. In other words, the process of aural rehabilitation usually refers to (1) counseling to facilitate adjustment to acquired hearing loss, both for the person who possesses the impairment and others who are closely involved in that person's life, and (2) provision of services that aid in the facilitation of more efficient use of the person's residual hearing and the use of supplemental visual clues. The aspects referred to under (2) have been generally referred to as evaluation and fitting of hearing aids, auditory training, and speechreading. As procedures involved in aural rehabilitation services become more sophisticated, however, professionals are involving more than those terms imply when strictly defined.

PROCEDURES OF AURAL REHABILITATION

Lipreading

The old schools of lipreading generally stressed the definitive use of vision to supplant impaired auditory function. Those traditionally included, for example, the approach by Martha Bruhn who, in 1902, introduced the Mueller-Walle method of lipreading to this country.[2] It was a strictly analytic approach, which stressed development of lipreading skills through kinesthetic awareness of the movements involved in speech production, the imitation of visible speech, and rhythmic analytic drill.

The Jena method, supported and taught by Anna Bunger (in 1932), also stressed an analytic approach to the teaching of lipreading.[3] The client was taught to become kinesthetically aware of the patterns of movement for speech sounds. Vowel and consonant charts were used to familiarize the client with the formation of the phonemes of speech. The remainder of the sequence of lessons stressed the factors of kinesthesis, imitation, and rhythm.

The approach introduced by Nitchie in 1903 broke away from the more analytic approaches and advocated a "whole thought" concept. It stressed a working relationship between mind and eye and made way for a phychological-synthetic basis for lipreading. Emphasis was placed on grasping the "whole" of a message when not all could be heard rather than working with the analytic "pieces," as advocated by Bruhn and Bunger. Elizabeth Nitchie, Edward Nitchie's wife, revised the approach and added lesson materials, but Edward's original wholistic philosophy remained.[4] Ordman and Ralli[5] developed additional materials with input from Elizabeth Nitchie and others. Their objective was to create lifelike material for lessons in lipreading.

The Kinzie sisters developed lipreading materials that combined both the Mueller-Walle and Nitchie approaches.[6] Their method involves a graded sequence of lipreading lessons for children and adults, geared for varying levels of lipreading ability. Their approach was more structured than, for example, the Nitchie approach.

Although the aforementioned methods were stringently adhered to by those who advocated and used them, their effectiveness is questioned. Strict methods of "lipreading," which are presented as a structured sequence of lessons, are generally felt to be unsatisfactory for two basic reasons:

1. After the sequence has been completed, clients generally emerge as good or as poor in their ability to communicate with others as they were when they began.
2. Those approaches do not lend themselves to a basic need in the process of aural rehabilitation, which involves addressing communicative difficulties that clients face daily and assisting them in learning strategies that may facilitate more efficient communicative function in spite of their auditory deficit.

The strict approaches discussed previously, and others like them, are based on the assumption that the lessons, if adhered to and learned, assist hearing impaired people to identify the visual aspects of speech. And so advocates of lipreading felt that hearing impaired people should be able to communicate better in their individual "real worlds." Although that assumption appeared rational and realistic to those who promoted the use of those relatively unalterable approaches, in the end, it was generally not a valid one.

Further, results of studies on the strength of vision in speech perception have not supported its efficiency when used alone. For example, early investigations by Heider and Heider,[7] Utley,[8] DiCarlo and Kataja,[9] Woodward and Barber,[10] Brannon,[11] Hutton,[12] O'Neill,[13] Erber,[14] Binnie et al,[15] and myself[16] all evaluate vision alone as contributing only approximately 50 percent to speech intelligibility when no auditory information is available. However, among the authors cited above, DiCarlo and Kataja found that both experienced and inexperienced lipreaders could identify only about 19 percent of the items on the Utley test, "How well do you read lips?" as a visual-only task.[9] Yet Erber has confirmed that for essentially inaudible speech, intelligibility scores remain at approximately 50 percent.[14] I also found that among young adults who possessed normal language function, a visual-only presentation of sentence materials resulted in only approximately 50 percent of words identified correctly.[16] However, less than 30 percent of the sentences were identified relative to their content when subjects were forced to depend only on vision. Over 28 years ago, Hutton wisely concluded that visual-only presentation of speech materials does not provide sufficient clues for efficient communication.[12]

The reason for the lack of definitiveness in the solely visual reception of speech is probably the result of (1) the similarity of some phonemes, (2) the difficulty in identifying some phonemes because they are not visible by observing the lips, and (3) the general lack of redundancy of the visemes of speech relative to the comprehension of verbal messages. Audition, even at minimal levels, adds greatly to the synthesis and closure required to comprehend speech.

Speechreading and Auditory Training

For those who possess any level of usable residual hearing, the combined use of visual and auditory clues to enhance communication has been found to be a viable approach in the process of aural rehabilitation. Since there are few hearing impaired persons who do not possess at least some usable hearing and since there are few communicative circumstances in which audition would not be beneficial, the combined use of vision and audition with or without amplification is stressed by most professionals who provide aural rehabilitation services.

Numerous studies have been conducted to sift through the sensory modalities used to perceive speech in an attempt to determine which, singly or in combination, serve to enhance speech perception. In all respects, the positive influence of audition on vision, and vice versa, has been supported even in the poorest listening conditions. Early studies conducted by O'Neill,[13] Sumby and Pollack,[17] Miller and Nicely,[18] Prall[13] Hutton et al,[20] Van Uden,[21] Duffy,[22] Ewertsen et al,[23] Erber,[24-26] Binnie et al,[15] and myself[16] have all confirmed that the complement of vision to audition and of audition to vision is real and is an important factor in speech intelligibility. Even in the poorest listening environments or with filtering to simulate the communicative impact of hearing impairment, the complement still exists.

Although the clinician should make hearing impaired clients aware of the fact that certain phonemes of speech look alike on the lips—for example, /b/, /p/, /m/; /f/, /v/; /t/, /d/; and others—and so may cause word confusions, the complement of audition and vision should be stressed whether individual clients can gain significant benefit from amplification or not. When impaired hearing is interfering with communication, the clinician must make the client aware of the benefits of the use of visual clues. But during practice sessions, the clinician should make auditory clues available in order for the complement of the two to become evident and the sessions more realistic with regard to the client's "real world" experiences. Further, other aspects relative to the benefits of visual clues should also be stressed. These include, for example, the "body language" of the speaker—facial expressions, gestures, expressions of the eyes, posture, and general attitude or communicative mode of the speaker. Additional emphasis can be placed on the auditory system during therapy sessions, thus simulating the world of the client and providing practice in the tolerance of degraded speech, for example, and in the use of visual clues when noise compounds the client's impaired hearing. This practice involves the use of environmental noise, either taped or live.

In other words, the combined use of vision and audition in the process of aural rehabilitation provides much more than the traditional mode of therapy, which involved training in "lipreading" only. Since there are few persons who do not possess at least some usable hearing and since there are few communicative environments in which residual hearing cannot be used to some extent, the inclusion of audition in therapy with hearing impaired adults is a logical approach.

Aural Rehabilitation

A total client-oriented approach to the process of aural rehabilitation involves more than speechreading and/or auditory training. Those aspects are certainly a part of the process in most instances, but still only a part.

The most critical aspect to consider when confronted with an adult client (or any client) is the client him- or herself. In failing to do so, many of the earlier approaches to aural rehabilitation lost their validity. They appeared to view each client as being just like every other and began aural rehabilitation treatment on page one of a therapy manual. When the final lesson was completed, clients, ready or not, were expected to have improved in their ability to communicate with others. Although the majority of problems encountered by hearing impaired adults involve a decreased ability to communicate with others, especially in adverse listening environments, each client also faces unique and special problems as a result of his or her auditory deficit. In order for aural rehabilitation treatment to be appropriate and meaningful for clients, the approach must also relate to their individual problems and communicative needs.

Group Involvement

In that light, the audiologist may, for example, feel that group involvement is appropriate for general discussions of (1) hearing impairment, its causes, and resulting handicapping effects on communication; (2) the increased difficulties noted when a hearing impaired person finds him- or herself in environmentally distracting situations, such as in noise; (3) general training in listening skills and use of supplemental visual clues; (4) general group sharing of the frustrations of attempting to cope with impaired hearing; and (5) problem solving: to address specific communicative environments of people that may be causing individuals difficulty. The latter area lends itself especially well to group discussion. The sharing among and between members of thoughts, frustrations, and experiences provides insights and a sense of awareness that "I am not alone." Individual treatment may not provide for such an emotional release. A skilled audiologist working with a small group of hearing impaired adults can help provide a stimulating, and in all respects, a powerful source of strength for those clients through the use of group interaction.

Beyond Speechreading and Auditory Training

Through the previous discussions, something beyond speechreading and auditory training occurs. And what occurs is an important part of the process of aural rehabilitation. It involves the development of an understanding and an awareness on the part of individual clients of what the hearing impairment is, why communication is more difficult, why amplification has in all probability not brought hearing back to normal, why more difficulty is experienced in noisy environments, and, perhaps more importantly, that the anger, frustrations, and concerns being experienced are normal reactions and that others are also experiencing them. For rehabilitation to have a chance of occurring, these questions and concerns must be aired. I have observed aural rehabilitation programs in which those discussions were not encouraged, and those programs were doomed to failure from the start. This interaction is called, for lack of a better term, "counseling." The process of counseling will be discussed in more detail later in this chapter, particularly as it is woven throughout the process of aural rehabilitation.

The Remaining Aspects

What else does the process of aural rehabilitation involve? The following are other critical elements:

Hearing Aid Orientation. For those clients who can benefit from amplification, careful orientation and adjustment to their particular device and/or to a hearing aid per se are extremely important for success in other aspects of the aural rehabilitation program. Further, an introduction to other assistive listening devices for home, office, or church use is important here.

Program Design. Designing a program for increased communicative efficiency must be based upon individual clients' prioritized needs. In all probability, this involves continued counseling, adjustments in the use of amplification, problem solving relative to specific communicative environments, becoming aware of visual components of speech that facilitate communication, learning to cope with adverse listening environments, and others.

Continued Group and/or Individual Counseling. Counseling can occur with great success on a group basis. But, for those with special needs, it must also occur on an individual basis.

Assessment of Communicative Gains. Communicative gains, or lack of them, must be assessed as per clients' prioritized communicative needs.

This approach is a logical one that is, for reasons of its comprehensive nature, not called "speechreading and/or auditory training," but those aspects are certainly included if needed for individual clients. For some, the process of aural rehabilitation may involve a session or two to provide a client with suggestions on more efficient communication in his or her most frequented environment, and perhaps several more brief contacts to follow up on the client's success. Other contacts with that client may be for hearing aid reevaluations and/or annual checks of auditory function. Other persons may require a full program of counseling and therapy, but again the process depends upon individual needs.

The following is a description of a suggested process of aural rehabilitation for adult clients, utilizing the four areas presented previously.

The Process of Aural Rehabilitation

The following approaches to aural rehabilitation treatment appear to be effective for both younger and elderly clients simply because they focus on the client's own communicative problems resulting from the auditory deficit and his or her specific and prioritized communicative needs. For the young adult, problems and needs may involve primarily job and social environments. A confined elderly client's prioritized problems and communicative needs may be concerned with efficient social communication in his or her environment and may, for example, include a simple rearrangement of furniture for greater ease in talking with family and friends.

In other words, this discussion on the process of aural rehabilitation is problem oriented and centers on the needs of individual clients. Whereas audiologists who utilize structured, "speechreading manual"–oriented programs observe their hearing impaired adult clients excuse themselves from attending "speechreading groups" with greater frequency as the weeks go by, audiologists who use "needs-oriented" programs, such as described here, generally experience an influx of clients who have specific communicative goals in mind and desire the audiologist's services.

AURAL REHABILITATION TREATMENT PROGRAM

The following are the components of a viable aural rehabilitation program.

Counseling

The process of counseling, in any manner of speaking, is incorporated into all aspects of the aural rehabilitation treatment program. It is sometimes called facilitating adjustment to an unwanted auditory deficit and the frustrations faced by the person who possesses the deficit. It is also occasionally called "motivation counseling," in order to encourage and stimulate a desire to become involved in a program of aural rehabilitation. It is sometimes called "assertiveness training," in order to encourage clients who may have withdrawn from important social situations because they have given up or feel that others must not want them to be involved, since the normally hearing people are apparently unwilling to make adjustments in their manner of speaking or in the communicative environment. However, the normally hearing people may not be aware of adjustments that may facilitate communication for the hearing impaired person. A little positive assertiveness on the part of the hearing impaired client may be all that is necessary to permit participation once again in environments heretofore avoided because of their difficulty.

The process of counseling is also sometimes referred to in the context of developing coping behaviors or enhancing a natural trait in humans and other animals to adjust to their environments; in other words, clients learn to make otherwise difficult circumstances tolerable. For example, noisy or other distracting environments are frustrating to most persons who possess a sensorineural hearing impairment. These environments may make them upset or even angry. The anger can further interfere with communication that may have taken place in that specific environment. Learning to cope, to understand the reason for the added difficulty resulting from the noise of a party or an office complex, can help to ease the frustration and facilitate the adjustments that may need to be made to aid the hearing impaired adult to function with greater efficiency.

No matter what descriptive terms are used, it remains that the process involves counseling: the verbal and emotional interaction between the provider of services and the client. The process centers on (1) the provision of information that facilitates an understanding of the whys (the reasons) for the difficulties and frustrations the client is experiencing; (2) the airing of concerns, and even anger, on the part of the client before a professional he or she has grown to trust and respect; (3) the development on the part of the client of an understanding of ways in which he or she can cope within and even manipulate an otherwise intolerable communicative environment so that it is less intolerable or in which he or she can manipulate in a positive way the person who is speaking so that he or she can be more easily understood; and, in the end, (4) the facilitation of adjustment on the part of hearing impaired clients to an otherwise frustrating and debilitating hearing impairment and adjustment to what may be to them a sign or symbol of disability, an "artificial" device—a hearing aid.

Planning the Treatment Program

It is essential that each client's aural rehabilitation treatment program be organized and designed around the client's communicative needs; the client must become an integral part of the planning process. His or her priorities and/or immediate needs must be considered, and realistic goals established. These clients, as adults, are usually cognizant of the difficulties that are encountered in their most frequented environments; thus they are also generally realistic, not only of what they expect of themselves relative to their capabilities for improvement, but also of those communicative and/or environmental aspects that they may not be able to change. Therefore, they should be involved in the planning of their treatment program and also in the determination of whether improvements in communicative function have occurred.

The following is an example of the planning process.

1. Adult clients, no matter what their chronological age, are asked to write or, if writing is difficult, to verbally list situations in which they experience the greatest communicative difficulties. It should be stressed that clients should include only those situations or environments that they typically face or that they expect to face, such as a new job or a trip to visit relatives. Vague or unrealistic situations are not to be included.

2. Clients are then asked to consider the importance of these situations or environments and to prioritize them in accordance with their immediate or long-term importance. Further, they are requested to choose the important situation or environment in which they would, if given a choice, most desire to improve first, then second, then third, and so on until their choices have been exhausted. Then the reasons why the prioritized communicative difficulties and needs were selected by the client, their immediate or long-term importance, and expected outcomes as they are realistically predicted at that point in time are discussed.

3. From that information, each client's treatment program is designed. After discussing the prioritized communicative situations or environments that are apparently the most difficult for individual clients, slight alterations in their choices are occasionally made. Generally speaking, however, their priorities remain the same and are, in most instances, realistic about the possibility for attaining positive change in their communicative behavior.

Treatment

After the priorities have been established by the client and jointly determined to be realistic by the client and audiologist, treatment begins. However, remember that the treatment was actually initiated at the onset of the client and audiologist contact. The following are steps in the process.

Effect of Hearing Impairment on Auditory Function

Even though an explanation of the audiometric results of each client's hearing loss is conducted at the time of the initial evaluation, further discussion of the effect of the shape and degree of hearing impairment on auditory function is important. This discussion should stress the client's ability to understand the speech of others and the compounding effects of the listening environment. Diagrams of the ear and blackboard drawings of audiograms are used. In order not to demean adult clients, technical terminology is always used, but with immediate explanatory definitions. This holds true for all ages of adult clients, from the younger one to the more elderly. Discussion is open for questions and clarification. Questions often center around the ''whys'' of misinterpretation of verbal messages: *why* certain sounds of speech are heard more clearly than others, *why* hearing impairment has occurred, *why* hearing aids do not help in all communicative environments, and other questions and concerns, including why normally hearing persons frequently do not make the necessary adjustments to facilitate communication with hearing impaired persons. Is it lack of knowledge or an unwillingness to help?

Fears and frustrations are generally aired during these discussions if the client or clients have grown to trust the audiologist. In group treatment sessions, the airing of such concerns can facilitate a greater understanding (perhaps in some for the first time) that others have experienced similar difficulties, anger, or frustration, and they are, indeed, not alone with their disability. A lasting camaraderie sometimes develops within groups of clients. However, it must be stressed again that numbers of clients possess specific communicative needs or less common auditory disorders for which treatment is best provided individually. For example, it is unrealistic for a person who possesses a severe speech discrimination problem to be subjected to further frustration in a group discussion in which he or she is able to understand little or nothing of what is said. This unnecessary exposure may only strengthen his or her conviction that the auditory problems are beyond treatment and so further increases a sense of isolation and defeat. The knowledgeable audiologist wisely places persons who cannot yet function in a group treatment environment into an individual setting. In that sense, it may be best, except for such aforementioned discussions, to place all new clients in individual treatment before introducing them to a group setting.

Prioritized Communicative Situations

After the discussion of the function of the auditory mechanism, the causes of hearing impairment, and their impact on communication has been at least initially completed (which may require one or even two 1-hour sessions wherein clients' questions and discussions are aired), the sessions then center on each client's prioritized communicative situations or environments. Assignments are made that require them to bring descriptions of experiences they have faced within that highly prioritized area. Instances and circumstances in which they have experienced difficulty within that environment, the speaking habits of those within that environment, and lighting and physical characteristics of the environment are written down, drawn, and illustrated in any other way by clients and brought to treatment sessions for discussion. Solutions to those problem situations are discussed. In group sessions, the other clients are involved in the discussions. Not only do their insights prove important since some may have encountered a similar situation at some previous time, but also the group sharing provides alternatives and solutions that may also be beneficial to the others at some time in the future. During individual sessions, of course, the discussions involve only the client and the audiologist. The client or the audiologist redraws the diagrammed communicative environment on the blackboard. The client's usual position in that environment, for example, his or her usual chair or desk, is drawn into the diagram, attempting to maintain the sense of space found in the actual setting and including the position of those persons with whom the client communicates.

The client is first asked how he or she perceives that environment and what previous attempts have been made to alter the environment or the other people for greater efficiency in communications. If attempts have been made, they are reviewed using the blackboard diagram. After that review, the discussion on other alternatives or ideas or manipulation of the environment or the people within it begins.

As the discussion of the client's prioritized difficult situations is taking place and alternatives are presented and diagrammed, the apparently relevant or feasible suggestions are given to him or her as assignments for trial in those environments. Successes or failures are reported back during the following session, or when the client has experimented with the suggestion, to determine if greater ease of communication was noted.

Development of Assertive Behaviors

During the sessions that revolve around client's prioritized communication difficulties, other aspects involved in developing coping behaviors are discussed. Paramount in those discussions is, for lack of a better term, development of assertive behaviors. Clients are told that in too many instances, persons who possess auditory impairment have felt defeat in attempts at efficient communication frequently enough that they, out of self-defense, become increasingly submissive. Prior to the acquisition of their hearing loss, they probably blamed the listening environment and/or a poor speaker when they experienced difficulty understanding what was said on occasion. And, in most instances, they were probably correct. However, many adults who have acquired hearing impairment eventually begin to blame their inability to cope in various environments on themselves or the majority of difficulties in communication on their hearing impairment alone. Clients are told that in some instances in which their hearing or their ability to function communicatively is blamed, impaired hearing may not actually have been totally at fault. However, when impaired hearing has caused innumerable difficulties in, for example, auditorily distracting environments, and defeat has become commonplace, their concept of the path of least resistance may be simply to place all blame on their impaired hearing. With that attitude, however, withdrawal from most environments may become the only alternative for those hearing impaired persons.

Discussions focus on the fact that in a number of environments where communication takes place, impaired hearing indeed interferes, particularly in understanding what is said (speech discrimination). In many instances, however, a share of the blame must also be placed on the listening environment, the speaker, or both. It must be understood that difficulties in communication are not always the fault of impaired hearing, and that adjustments within the environments can be made, or adjustments that the speaker can make may facilitate greater efficiency in communicating. There are occasions when the client must take the initiative in facilitating those adjustments. In some instances, the client must advise others that changes in their physical position or patterns of speech within that environment must be made so that he or she can communicate more efficiently. Some clients tell me that they simply do not have the courage to confront the person with whom they are speaking or to suggest changes in the listening environment. But, in most instances, they would very much like to do so. A spark of desire, then, is noted. This spark is generally most noticeable in group treatment where clients remember, discuss, and together become angry at the apparent lack of consideration of some speakers in, and designers of, meeting rooms, offices, churches, and other environments in which they find themselves.

Suggestions on tactful but direct ways of advising others on how they might change their patterns of speech or the listening environment are presented to the clients. However, the clients must also be instructed on what "clear speech" consists of. The audiologist may want to refer to the study by Picheny,

Durlach, and Braida for further information on that topic.[27] Clients practice these suggestions and attempt to determine how they might react to them if they were the one being asked to make those adjustments. In a group treatment environment, clients practice these strategies on one another.

Clues on Content of Verbal Messages

Another important aspect of treatment encompasses important parts of communication that provide clients with clues as to the content of verbal messages. Those include (1) the predictability and redundancy of the American English language (linguistic redundancy); (2) the predictability and redundancy in the content of conversations, particularly if the client is familiar with the speaker (content redundancy); (3) information on the predictability and the redundancies of the content of verbal messages in certain environments (environmental redundancy); (4) the development of skills in making closure, that is, to grasp the meaning of verbal messages when not all information is available (cloze technique); (5) developing skills in the use of visual clues along with residual hearing in conjunction with the above (vision and audition with closure); (6) developing communicative skills and coping behaviors in noisy or otherwise distracting environments.

The sessions, which progress from (1) through (6) consist of general information and practice, which appear to be of common benefit for most clients. During the first part of each of these sessions, discussions of difficulties that individual clients faced during the period since the last session and the results of suggested steps toward enhanced communication that were tried by clients continue. The six areas listed previously are presented as progressive formal sessions after these discussions and are designed to serve as the most structured portion of the aural rehabilitation treatment program. Not all clients require this aspect. Some appear to benefit most from the prioritizations and the group or individual discussions of difficult listening environments and learning to cope with them. Others may require only a thorough hearing aid orientation program with suggestions on how to manipulate their communicative environments to their best advantage.

For the present discussion, however, the following more thoroughly describes the content of each step of the more formal treatment sessions.

Linguistic Redundancy. The American English language is fairly redundant in regard to the position of various parts of speech within sentences. That is to say, the position of principal words such as nouns, pronouns, and direct objects are constant in general usage, as are function words, descriptors such as adjectives and adverbs, and action words such as verbs. Although the technical names for various parts of speech are not stressed to any degree, the importance of those words within verbal messages are stressed, particularly as they relate to their position and deriving the meaning of those messages. This aspect of the treatment program capitalizes on the fact that the majority of adult hearing impaired clients possess normal or near normal language function. It stresses the fact that as people listen to others, they consciously or unconsciously key in on those words within conversations that allow them to derive the content and meaning of statement. In noisy or otherwise distracting environments, listeners depend even more on this capability. Less of the message may be "heard," but still the listener can, in most instances, keep track of the content of the message. Occasionally, however, the listener may have to ask the speaker to repeat what appeared to be a key word that was missed because of the poor listening environment. However, the reason the listener was able to determine that the missed word was an important one was his or her almost innate knowledge of the English language. And the listener suspected that without knowing the word, the probability of following the conversation accurately may be jeopardized.

The treatment session or sessions which stress this important component of efficient listening and use of visual clues are designed to bring that functional language ability to a more conscious level once again. Some clients have become so depressed over their impaired hearing and encountered listening difficulties that such skills become repressed unless brought to a conscious level. Others may have forgotten that such instantaneous adjustments were made during conversation in difficult listening environments prior to the acquisition of their hearing loss.

The blackboard is used extensively during these sessions to demonstrate the general position of important parts of speech within conversations and, if a word is missed, its probable degree of importance. For example, a missed noun, when knowledge of the previous discussion is unavailable, will in all probability require a request for repetition of that word. On the one hand, the probability of correctly guessing a noun, when for example, the sentence was something about "A ______ was seen sitting in front of Bobby's dog house the other night," is very low. On the other hand, if the word "sitting" within that sentence was not heard, missing that verb within the sentence leaves less chance for content error, and the hearing impaired listener may be able to continue to follow the conversation with accuracy.

This aspect may be covered in one to three sessions, but is stressed continually throughout all other aspects of the treatment program as difficult conversations or words within them are faced.

Content Redundancy. It has been said that the same people generally say the same things on similar occasions. If, for example, you and another person have been friends for some time, if you think about it, you are almost able to predict what the other person is going to say within a given circumstance. Further, if you have planned to attend a lecture on a given topic, the lecture is usually more clearly understood if you are already familiar with the content or have taken it upon yourself to prepare by reading on the topic prior to the lecture. Again, some hearing impaired adults are experiencing such concern over the difficulties they face that this common but positive influence on efficient communication and skill in listening is somehow suppressed. For some clients, it is only necessary to bring it to their attention. For other clients, however, examples and experiments must be used to help them take advantage of these aspects of listening that permit greater ease of communication.

An example of an experiment that brings this phenomenon to light involves asking individual clients to think about a friend or family member with whom they communicate regularly. They are then asked to write down that person's interest areas (family, a child, a pet, television, or others). They are further asked to write down the most frequent topics of conversation, including frequently used phrases or words. They are then asked to study them and think about those lists prior to the time the client is with his or her friend. After being with the friend, the client is asked to check the lists and note which topics, interest areas, and familiar phrases and words were used. Clients are generally surprised when they find that they were able to predict, with some accuracy, the topics of conversation. If they complete the same exercise in relation to others with whom they find themselves communicating, they generally find that they can listen and participate in conversations with greater ease. Further, the clients are asked to complete the same lists when they meet new people and talk with them. The more one knows and remembers about a person, the more communication is facilitated. Clients are also advised to prepare for lectures, plays, movies, or meetings by reading and otherwise investigating topics, people's manner of speaking, and the listening environment prior to attending.

Environmental Redundancy. Not only do the same people generally say the same things on similar occasions, but they also say them in similar places. A conversation during a sidewalk chance meeting generally contains similar comments, but depends upon (1) who it is: your minister, an old friend, a former school teacher, your spouse's best friend, or the salesperson who has been trying to sell you a new car; (2) what the weather is like on that day (beautiful, hot, snowing badly, or looks as though it might rain); and other such variables. In other words, depending upon who the person is and other environmental factors, if the hearing impaired person is aware of those influences in that environment, a conversation can usually be predicted with reasonable accuracy.

Sessions centered on this topic of redundancy involve predicting conversations in various physical environments. The client(s) and audiologist design environments that he or she frequents. For example, if a client has as one of his or her prioritized difficult communicative environments the yearly Thanksgiving dinner that alternates between cousin Lucille's and Aunt Genevieve's house, with the knowledge previously acquired regarding content redundancy, the content and environmental redundancies can be discussed for those environments. Included in that session should be a discussion of those persons who are usually there (barring the unforeseen appearance of a male friend whom a niece brings to meet the family on that day). With the client's knowledge of the people who will probably be there on Thanksgiving Day, and the "usual" conversations of those people, their interests, and what conversations generally center on during dinner and after dinner, the conversations can probably be plotted and outlined with a fair degree of accuracy. A realization of the redundancies that are found within given environments are sometimes surprising to hearing impaired clients, but that realization can also facilitate increased efficiency in communication within them.

Closure. Being cognizant of the redundancies that exist within verbal and nonverbal communication (linguistic, content, and environmental), the ability to make closure is enhanced. However, some practice in a treatment setting is usually necessary not only to increase the client's skill in making closure, but also to enhance the client's confidence that it can be done with some efficiency.

These treatment sessions involve providing the client(s) with knowledge of (1) the speaker and (2) the physical environment. With that information at hand, and possibly including the content of the conversation up to that point, the client is presented with a series of blanks drawn on the blackboard that represent the words within that conversation. As can be seen in Figure 48–1, a word is given by the clinician in its correct position within that sentence of the conversation. The client is then asked to make closure and predict the sentence content.

If the client hesitates, or does not want to ven-

1. How	___	___	___	___	___	___	?
2. How	___	it	___	___	___	___	?
3. How	___	it	___	going	___	___	?
4. How	___	it	___	going	this	___	?
5. How	has	it	___	going	this	___	?
6. How	has	it	___	going	this	year	?
7. How	has	it	been	going	this	year	?

Figure 48–1 Example of sequence of word presentation for exercises in closure.

ture a guess, he or she is asked to guess. "Given the physical location of the conversation, your knowledge of the speaker and the content of the conversation up to this time, and the word that you heard within the sentence, what do you think he or she said?" The client then usually ventures some guesses. If the client is not able to make closure with only one word, another is added in another part of the sentence, as is seen under "Trial number 2" in Figure 48–1. The client is again asked to venture an opinion as to the content of the sentence. If, again, the client is not able to make closure, words are added one at a time, as can be seen under Trials 3, 4, 5, 6, and 7 in Figure 48–1, until closure is made.

In most instances, after confidence is gained and the linguistic, content, and environmental redundancy concepts are reemphasized, along with knowledge of the speaker and the prior content of the conversations, clients, including elderly clients, are frequently able to correctly predict the content of those messages with as few as one or two words available out of an average eight-word sentence. Confidence on the part of the client that closure can be made after bringing the other components learned up to that time to a high level of awareness is probably most important in terms of carry-over into the client's real world.

A word of caution is warranted here. Too much confidence can be as detrimental as too little confidence when it comes to communication. The hearing impaired adult must also be instructed to be cautious (not reckless) when attending to the speech of others. What one thinks he or she hears should not be interpreted as always being correct. Caution can prevent embarrassment[28,29]

Vision and Audition with Closure. Throughout all aspects of the aural rehabilitation treatment program, emphasis is placed on, for lack of a better phrase, grasping for every bit of auditory and visual information from all possible communicative settings and speaker and listener interactions. If clients usually wear hearing aids, they should be requested to wear them during treatment sessions. Treatment also provides an ideal setting for hearing orientation for those who have purchased a new aid. The benefits of supplemental visual clues, practice in using them, attending to behaviors, and instruction on the use of important visual, including confusing phonemes, are stressed throughout the treatment program. However, sessions on identifying individual phonemes of speech have not been considered viable approaches for hearing impaired adults except for those who are profoundly hearing impaired.

Visual clues are stressed during the treatment sessions on closure. For example, when an individual word is placed in its appropriate place within a series of word "blanks" (see Fig. 48–1), the client is asked to make closure and identify the content of the sentence within that conversation. When the client has given his or her opinions as to the content of the sentence, the audiologist then presents the sentence in its entirety to the client(s), requiring that the client(s) attend closely to visual clues (the face of the audiologist). As the sentences are being presented, the audiologist also uses voice as close to the client's speech reception threshold as is possible. Clients are, then, being provided instruction to develop skills in (1) knowledge about the linguistic, content, and environmental redundancies in language and (2) the efficient use of vision with minimal auditory clues. Again, not only is skill in communication being developed, but also confidence that greater efficiency in communication can be a reality.

Developing Coping Behavior in Noisy Environments. Common among hearing impaired adults who possess sensorineural impairments are their complaints of a reduced ability to hear and, more importantly, to understand speech when they find themselves in noisy environments. Physiologically and acoustically, the interference is as real as their hearing impairment. The additive factors involved in attempting to hear the phonemic elements of speech while listening through ears that possess a high-frequency hearing impairment in a noisy environment made up of rather low-frequency sounds of high intensity make speech discrimination difficult. Further, in a generally corresponding manner, as the listening environment becomes less favorable, the hearing impaired listener's frustration also becomes greater. This frustration, in turn, generally reduces the listening efficiency that a person may have developed to aid his or her communicative function in such an environment. Frustration and resulting anxiety and possible anger, then, generally result in a reduction of communicative efficiency. The result may be a further increase of frustration and anger, until either the hearing impaired listener leaves the environment in frustration or attempts to calm him- or herself and then to try again (the latter is the less common response).

The negative response of hearing impaired people to noisy environments is common, but that response tends to further reduce those persons' ability to function communicatively. With reduced hearing interfering so greatly with efficient communication in a noisy environment, further reduction in function due to a lack of an ability to cope emotionally in that environment can leave one unable to communicate in or tolerate the environment.

Treatment sessions in noise should at least initially center on the development of *coping* behavior rather than on developing specific skills in speech discrimination. Once positive coping behavior has been established, treatment based on enhanced speech discrimination can follow.

Environmental noise that is the same as or similar to that experienced by clients is first of all listened to in a treatment session and discussed. Questions such as "What does it sound like to you?" and "How does it make you feel?" are brought before the client(s). Those questions and others are asked as the intensity of the noise is gradually increased. This aspect of treatment should be conducted in a "typical" room environment with stereophonic reproduction equipment for the greatest realism. A small tape recorder is generally not adequate for these sessions.

Clients discuss the noise, generally without hesitation. They say, "It sounds just like noise!" "It frustrates me," "It makes me angry sometimes," "I just want to get away," and other similar statements. It is incumbent upon the audiologist to also enter the conversation. He or she can truthfully say that "It frustrates me too when I find myself in a noisy place. It sometimes makes me angry, and sometimes when it bothers me enough, I feel like leaving that place." Empathy during this discussion is important, but the audiologist, if his or her hearing is normal, must never suggest that his or her frustrations have the same basis as those of the hearing impaired clients. However, it is important to permit and encourage a free discussion among clients relative to their feelings about the environmental noise. Venting their feelings is the first step toward developing coping behavior.

Treatment sessions in noise occur as one of the last phases of the aural rehabilitation program. They may include, after the discussions are exhausted, sessions on closure as discussed earlier, but in ever increasing levels of noise. Simulated social conversation or office conversations have been found to facilitate further analysis of noisy environments and coping behavior. If during the practice sessions clients begin to become overtly frustrated and the beginnings of anger or withdrawal are evident as the result of an increased noise level, it is appropriate to cease the noise at a logical point in the activity and to encourage them to talk again about their feelings. Never, under *any* circumstances, should the noise obviously be stopped because someone appears frustrated. If the client feels that you are concerned enough about him or her to turn off the noise, then fears about his or her ability to eventually learn to cope in that environment are further increased.

As discussion is held during that short break, further questions about feelings are appropriate. During these sessions, however, it is generally best to allow the clients to initiate the discussion and vent their frustrations. Again, empathy is important.

The development of coping behavior involves more than building tolerance or a "thicker skin" to interfering noise; it also involves discussions about the practice in manipulating the environment and/or the person(s) with whom the client may be speaking. For example, if the environment becomes intolerable and it is one within which the client must attempt to cope frequently and if the assertiveness and ideas on manipulating the listening environment spoken about earlier have made an impact, some decisions can be made. For example, if the environment is an office or meeting room, some suggestions by the hearing impaired person on how the situation can change positively are important. If the client's most difficult listening environment involves social gatherings, then in treatment suggestions and activities are appropriate if they encourage him or her to request, for example, that the person with whom he or she is speaking move to a quieter place—a hallway or a quieter and less distracting corner of the room, which permits talking with greater ease. Again, many clients state that they do not feel that they possess the courage to assert themselves in such a manner. Sessions that provide suggestions on ways in which positive change can be made, and support in gaining the courage and self-reliance that permit the changes to be made, are critically important.

Increasing tolerance to noise, enhancing communicative abilities through selective listening and use of visual clues, providing instruction on ways in which noisy environments can be altered or personal adjustments made within them, and acquiring the courage to follow through are the bases for this important aspect of aural rehabilitation treatment.

EVALUATION OF SUCCESSES IN TREATMENT

Early Attempts

Numerous attempts at the development of formal procedures that would determine improvements in hearing impaired adults' ability to communicate have been made throughout the past four decades. Filmed tests of lipreading, for example, were developed in the 1940s as an attempt to both assess and teach lipreading. Mason introduced a series of 30 silent films for purposes of lipreading instruction.[30] Morkovin developed films that depicted "real life" situations for lipreading therapy called the "Morkovin Life Situation" films.[31] The situations for lipreading advocated a theme approach. The films were interesting to watch, but were difficult to use for either therapy or assessment. Further, the films quickly became dated because of the actors' clothing styles and a few of the themes. They were also generally not suited for adults.

The filmed test for lipreading that received the most attention by researchers was developed by Utley.[8] The test contains three parts. Part I utilizes single words, and part II contains sentences. Both parts I and II were filmed in black and white. Part III consists of a five-part story test filmed in color.

The Mason, Morkovin, and Utley tests have been assessed for both reliability and validity. Scores for subject responses between the tests have appeared to demonstrate generally positive correlations. However, DiCarlo and Kataja felt that the tests, particularly the Utley and Morkovin films, primarily assessed the persistence and frustration tolerances of the viewers.[9] Simmons has concluded that the Utley and Mason films appear to measure something related to lipreading ability, but whatever it is, it can only be related to part of the ability of hearing impaired people to communicate in spite of their hearing impairment.[32] Thus the validity of these tests was questioned, and those same questions continue today. Those tests are also not generally used today. While such tests of lipreading may have provided some information on a person's ability to identify words while using visual clues, it is questionable whether a general correlation exists between the test scores and a hearing impaired person's ability to communicate daily.

Other attempts at developing assessment procedures included a filmed multiple choice test developed by Taaffe and Wong at the John Tracy Clinic,[33] the use of panels of judges and interview methods to assess improvements or lack of them in lipreading,[32] and self-administered multiple-choice procedures.[34] They too have generally not been accepted as valid procedures for determining how well a hearing impaired adult may be able to function communicatively in his or her educational, occupational, or social environments.

Even though attempts have been made over the years to assess skills that lead to enhanced communicative abilities, the question of how those abilities are best assessed remains unanswered. However, audiologists may now be headed in the right direction. That direction is focused on clients' opinions of their difficulties in communication and their feelings of self-adequacy in their frequented communicative environments. The philosophy of self-evaluation appears to be most important when working with hearing impaired adults, including both younger and older populations.

One viable approach in attempting to assess the handicap of hearing impairment and subsequent changes that may occur as the result of aural rehabilitation services is through the use of self-rating scales of communicative function. The most useful appear to be those that can stress clients' most difficult communicative environments and/or their prioritized communicative needs. Such scales include (1) the Hearing Handicap Scale (HHS) developed by High et al,[35] (2) the Denver Scale of Communication Function,[36] (3) the Hearing Measurement Scale,[37] and (4) the Profile Questionnaire for Rating Communicative Performance.[38] The profiles by Sanders relate to specific communicative environments, including the home environment, work environment, and social environment.[38] All three may be applicable for the younger hearing impaired adult, but the profiles for home and social environments may be most appropriate for many elderly adults.

A scale developed specifically for institutionalized older adults is the Denver Scale of Communication Function for Senior Citizens Living in Retirement Centers.[39] This scale is an outgrowth of the Denver Scale of Communication Function. Variables such as writing skills and inappropriate responses are provided for. The test is divided into seven major categories, including

1. Family
2. Emotional

3. Other persons
4. General communication
5. Self-concept
6. Group situations
7. Rehabilitation

Responses are based on yes and no answers. The only drawback at present is the scoring procedure, a semantic differential scale that is confusing to some elderly persons.

It must be stressed that the most valuable format for the assessment of progress in communicative abilities must take into consideration the client him- or herself and the client's communicative priorities and feelings of self-adequacy. This format is particularly true for adult and elderly clients. For example, if improvements are noted by the client in communication within a highly prioritized environment, then that aspect of the aural rehabilitation program has been successful. A scale that takes into account the client's decisions about communicative environments in which he or she has the greatest difficulty, and allows the client to prioritize them in relation to their importance is the UNC Communicative Appraisal and Priorities Scale. Since adult clients are generally aware of those situations in which they have the most difficulty, they are usually also aware of improvements that may be taking place. This awareness is particularly true if the aural rehabilitation program per se is based on those specific prioritized communicative environments. If baselines of communicative behavior have been established at the time treatment is begun, then progress can be plotted. Such documentation can not only support the audiologist's efforts in determining the validity of his or her chosen treatment procedures, but can also serve to encourage clients that progress is indeed being made. The early approaches to the testing of "lipreading" skills did not possess that capability.

The following approaches to assessment appear to be reasonable. They are[40]

1. Observing the results of the case history relative to the possible causes of the auditory deficit, its duration, and the current social and environmental status of the elderly client.

2. Utilizing the audiometric results, particulary the type, degree, and configuration of the hearing loss, and importantly the results of speech discrimination assessment.

3. Assessing the results of a hearing aid evaluation, determining the possible benefits of amplification, and fitting the instrument if warranted.

4. Assessment of the client's ability to utilize visual clues with minimal audition, which may include monosyllabic words, sentences, and everyday conversation. Recommended sentence lists include the Denver Scale Quick Test of Lipreading,[41] the CID Everyday Sentences,[42] and the UNC Sentence Test of Speechreading.[43]

5. Assessment of the impact of the hearing impairment by the use of one of the scales or profiles of communication function. Those recommended include the Denver Scale of Communication Function, the Denver Scale of Communication Function for Senior Citizens, the Profile Questionnaire (Home and Social) by Sanders, and the Communicative Appraisal and Priorities Scale.[38]

6. Plans for aural rehabilitation treatment and post-treatment assessment should be based only upon the clients' communicative needs and priorities. Only then will the audiologist be adding validity to his or her treatment goals.

SUMMARY

The intention of this discussion of aspects of aural rehabilitation and aural rehabilitation treatment is not the presentation of an approach, but rather avenues for treatment that are useful for those who are providing or intend to provide services on behalf of adult clients. They are strategies for young or elderly adult clients who have specific needs and communicative goals in mind. Most of all, clinicians must be continually cognizant of the fact that they are working with adults, no matter what their age. They are adults who are searching for help to function more efficiently in a human's most human interaction—communication.

REFERENCES

1. Braceland FJ. The restoration of man. Donald Dabelstein Memorial Lecture, presented at the Annual Conference of the National Rehabilitation Association, 1963.
2. Bruhn MD. The Mueller-Walle method of lipreading. Washington, DC: The Volta Bureau, 1949.
3. Bunger AM. Speech-reading—Jena method. Danville, IL: The Interstate Printers and Publishers, 1961.
4. Nitchie EH. New lessons in lipreading. Philadelphia: JB Lippincott, 1950.
5. Ordman AO, Ralli MP. What people say. Washington, DC: Alexander Graham Bell Association for the Deaf, 1957
6. Kinzie CE, Kinzie R. Lipreading for the deafened adult. Philadelphia: John C. Winston, 1931.
7. Heider FK, Heider GM. A comparison of sentence structure of deaf and hearing children. Psychol Monogr 1940;52:42–103.
8. Utley J. Factors involved in the teaching and testing of lipreading ability through the use of motion pictures. Volta Rev 1946;38:657–659m.
9. DiCarlo LM, Kataja R. An analysis of the Utley lipreading test. J Speech Hear Disord 1951;16:226–240.
10. Woodward MF, Barber CG. Phoneme perception in lipreading. J Speech Hear Res 1960;3:212–222.

11. Brannon JB. Speechreading of various speech materials. J Speech Hear Disord 1961; 26:348–353.
12. Hutton C. Combining auditory and visual stimuli in aural rehabilitation. Volta Rev 1959;56:316–319.
13. O'Neill JJ. Contributions of the visual components of oral symbols to speech comprehension. J Speech Hear Disord 1954;19:429–439.
14. Erber NP. Interaction of audition and vision in the recognition of oral speech stimuli. J Speech Hear Res 1969;12:423–425.
15. Binnie CA, Montgomery AA, Jackson PL. Auditory and visual contributions to the perception of selected English consonants. J Speech Hear Res 1974;17:619–630.
16. Hull RH. The effect of syntactic word variations on the predictability of sentence content in speechreading. J Acad Rehabil Audiol 1976;9:42–56.
17. Sumby WH, Pollack I. Visual contributions to speech intelligibility in noise. J Acoust Soc Am 1954;26:212–215.
18. Miller GA, Nicely PE. An analysis of perceptual confusions among some English consonants. J Acoust Soc Am 1955;27: 338–352.
19. Prall J. Lipreading and hearing aids combine for better comprehension. Volta Rev 1957;59:64–65.
20. Hutton C, Curry ET, Armstrong MB. Semidiagnostic test materials for aural rehabilitation. J Speech Hear Disord 1959;24:318–329.
21. Van Uden A. A sound-perceptive method. In: Ewing AWG, ed. The modern educational treatment of deafness. Washington, DC: Volta Bureau, 1960:3.
22. Duffy JK. Audio-visual speech audiometry and a new audio and audiovisual speech preception index. Maico Audiol Library Series 1967;5:(9).
23. Ewertsen HW, Nielsen BH, Nielsen SS. A comparative analysis of the audiovisual, auditive, and visual perception of speech. Acta Otolaryngol [Suppl] (Stockh) 1970;263:299–230.
24. Erber NP. Auditory and audiovisual reception of words in low-frequency noise by children with normal hearing and by children with impaired hearing. J Speech Hear Res 1971;14:496–512.
25. Erber NP. Speech-envelope cues as an acoustic aid to lipreading for profoundly deaf children. J Acoust Soc Am 1972;51:1224–1227.
26. Erber NP. Auditory, visual and auditory-visual recognition of consonants by children with normal and impaired hearing. J Speech Hear Res 1972;15:413–422.
27. Picheny MA, Durlach NI, Braida LD. Speaking clearly for the hard of hearing II: acoustic characteristics of clear and conversational speech. J Speech Hear Res 1986;29:434–446.
28. Gordon-Salant S. Effects of aging on response criteria in speech-recognition tasks. J Speech Hear Res 1986;29:155–162.
29. Marshall L. Auditory processing in aging listeners. J Speech Hear Disord 1981;24:226–237.
30. Mason JK. A cinematic technique for testing visual speech comprehension. J Speech Disord 1943;8:271–278.
31. Morkovin BS. Life-situation speechreading through the cooperation of the senses. Los Angeles: University of Southern California, 1948.
32. Simmons AA. Factors related to lipreading. J Speech Hear Res 1959;2:340–352.
33. Taaffe G, Wong W. Study of variables in lipreading stimulus materials. John Tracy Clinic research papers III. Los Angeles: The John Tracy Clinic, 1957.
34. Black JW, O'Reilly PO, Peck L. Self-administered training in lipreading. J Speech Hear Disord 1963;28:183–186.
35. High WS, Fairbanks G, Glorig A. Scale for self-assessment of hearing handicap. J Speech Hear Disord 1964;29:215–230.
36. Alpiner JG, Chevrette W, Glascoe G, Metz M, Olsen B. The Denver scale of communication function. In: Alpiner JG, ed. Handbook of adult rehabilitative audiology. Baltimore: Williams & Wilkins, 1978:53.
37. Nobel WG, Atherley GRC. The hearing measurement scale: a questionnaire for the assessment of auditory disability. J Aud Res 1970;10:229–250.
38. Sanders DA. Profile questionnaire for rating communicative performance. In: Pollack MC, ed. Amplification for the hearing impaired. New York: Grune & Stratton, 1975:363.

Zarnoch JM, Alpiner JG. The Denver scale of communication function for senior citizens living in retirement centers. In: Alpiner JG, ed. Handbook of adult rehabilitative audiology. Baltimore: Williams & Wilkins, 1978:166.

Hull RH. Rehabilitative audiology, Part I—the adult, and part II—the elderly client. New York: Grune & Stratton, 1982.

39. Zarnoch JM, Alpiner JG. The Denver scale of communication function for senior citizens living in retirement centers. In: Alpiner JG, ed. Handbook of adult rehabilitative audiology. Baltimore: Williams & Wilkins, 1978:166.
40. Hull RH. Rehabilitative audiology, Part I—the adult, and part II—the elderly client. New York: Grune & Stratton, 1982.
41. Alpiner JG. Evaluation of communication function. Denver scale quick test. In: Alpiner JG, ed. Handbook of adult rehabilitative audiology. Baltimore: Williams & Wilkins, 1978:36.
42. Central Institute for the Deaf. CID everyday sentences. In: Davis H, Silverman SR, eds. Hearing and deafness. Philadelphia: Holt, Rinehart & Winston, 1965:549.
43. Hull RH. UNC sentence test of speech reading. In: Hull RH, ed. Rehabilitative audiology. New York: Grune & Stratton, 1982:511.

49 Hearing Aids

James R. Curran, M.S.

The history of the electronic hearing aid can best be summarized as an evolutionary process of ever greater miniaturization and refinement. Early instruments utilized component parts of the telephone system, and later hearing aids were built with radio components and public address system equipment.[1] In 1937, Knudsen and Jones described an ideal hearing aid, which was composed of a "very good" microphone, a "first class" amplifier, and a "laboratory receiver,"[2] and concluded:

> As to portability, it would be very difficult at the present time to compress this equipment into a bulk of much less than one half cubic foot, and to reduce its weight below twenty-five pounds.

But wearable hearing aids of much less weight and smaller size were already beginning to be manufactured at that time. Subsequently, rapid progress in miniaturization continued to occur so that in 1966 Lybarger was able to report a reduction in size averaging 11 percent per year over a period of approximately 28 years.[3] The trend toward reduction in size and weight has continued since then but at a somewhat slower pace. In 1974, Lybarger reported that the average weight for body-worn instruments was 57.2 g[4]; for eyeglass aids, 11.4 g; for behind-the-ear aids, 8.6 g; and for in-the-ear aids, 4.0 g. These figures remain representative of current hearing aid weights.

Although the size reduction that is practical would appear to have a lower limit because controls, switches, and batteries must be large enough to be easily manipulated by the geriatric user, each decade has nevertheless provided further breakthroughs in miniaturization that were unforeseen years earlier. More importantly, it would appear that each significant iteration in size reduction has been accompanied by greater consumer acceptance and a concomitant increase in sales. Witness the explosive growth of sales in the middle 1980s in North America as the in-the-canal hearing aid was introduced and the ascendance of in-the-ear hearing aids in percentage of units dispensed (70 percent) as compared with behind-the-ear hearing aids (28 percent).[5] In the United States, it has been fairly well accepted that the impetus for reducing the dimensions of the hearing aid is the perception that the consumer is reluctant to call attention to hearing impairment. This reluctance has necessitated devising methods for either concealing the aid's presence (incorporating the hearing aid in an eyeglass temple is the obvious example) or making the aid smaller.

One is tempted to predict that with the present in-the-canal aid the ultimate refinement in size has been reached, but such statements are usually proven wrong as soon as they are made.[6] Rather history suggests that improvements in size reduction are incremental in nature and continuously flow from various sources. Evolutionary change is characteristic of hearing aid development, and one can expect continuing gradual reduction in gross size of hearing aids to occur as a result of further, although modest, miniaturization of transducers, internal switches and controls, amplifier components and assemblies, and improvements in the methods of transducer mounting and suspension.

Size versus Performance

Prior to 1968, the trend toward miniaturization had some adverse effects on certain aspects of hearing aid performance. In recent years, however, performance degradation related to size reduction has no longer been apparent. In fact, the introduction of miniature electret condenser microphones in the early 1970s provided significantly wider bandwidth capability than was previously available with substantially larger microphones. With the microphones, receivers, and modern amplifier assemblies now in common use, any systematic relationship between reduced size and inadequate performance no longer appears to exist. In many respects, some large body type instruments of just a few years ago fail to match the performance of most currently available head-worn aids.

From the designers' point of view, improvements in modern hearing aids have entered another phase in which miniaturization, although essential and important, is not entirely the prime moving force in development of new instrumentation, which it has been ever since the development of the first electric hearing aid. Rather attention has shifted to efforts at gaining a better, more refined insight into such issues as to how electroacoustic performance and sophisticated component and amplifier design affect subject performance,[7,8] the influence of the coupling of the hearing aid to the ear on performance, the development of special fitting applications,[9] and improvement in overall hearing aid durability.

TYPES OF HEARING AIDS

Modern hearing aids are available in five basic configurations, according to the place where each is worn: behind-the-ear, in-the-ear, in-the-canal, eyeglass, and on-the-body types. At the time of this writing, behind-the-ear aids account for approximately 28 percent of the total volume sales in the United States; in-the-ear instruments, including in-the-canal aids, 70 percent; eyeglass aids, 1 percent; and body aids, 1 percent.[5] The statistics reflect a rather recent and drastic change in the distribution of hearing aids by model. Eight years earlier, in 1978, the annual sales breakdown was reported as follows (rounded off): behind-the-ear, 56 percent; eyeglass, 10 percent; body aids, 1 percent; and in-the-ear aids, 30 percent.[10] The most obvious changes are the dramatic increase reported for in-the-ear hearing aid sales and the corresponding substantial decrease in sales of all other types of aids.

Behind-The-Ear Type

Until recently, the behind-the-ear hearing aid was the most popular type of instrument incorporating a microphone, amplifier, receiver, and battery with associated controls into a curved case that rests behind the pinna. Amplified sound is conducted to the ear canal through an earhook, translucent polyvinyl tubing, and earmold. Modern behind-the-ear instruments vary widely in size, generally, but not always, in relationship to the power output capability. The maximum power output (saturation sound pressure level 90, SSPL90) may be as little as 100 dB and as high as 130 dB SPL, and acoustic gain (the amount of amplification provided by the hearing aid specified in decibels) may vary from as little as 15 to 20 dB (high frequency average–Full on Gain, HFA-FOG) to as high as 70 dB. Recent improvements in mechanical isolation and acoustic sealing of transducers have made it possible to provide extremely high-gain, high-output behind-the-ear instruments that have extended bandwidth with minimal problems caused by internal acoustic or mechanical feedback.

There has been a marked trend in recent years to incorporate multiple miniature, externally accessed trimmer controls in behind-the-ear aids. These trimmer controls are used by dispensers to modify the output, gain, high or low portions of the frequency response, threshold of compression, and other hearing aid performance parameters. Manufacturers offer an exceptionally wide variety of different response options, and they tend to combine many frequency response variations into one instrument. Models are available that have, as standard or optional features, a magnetic induction coil to assist in telephone usage, patient-operated external switches for reducing the low-frequency portion of the instrument's response, and electrical sockets for connection of the hearing aid amplifier to auditory trainers and other assistive listening devices. The behind-the-ear hearing aid offers the dispenser great latitude in response and fitting modifications. For this reason, it appears to be the instrument of choice when fitting children, and it is useful in cases where complex or experimental amplifier or tranducer assemblies that require large amounts of space are to be installed such as multichannel compression circuits, digital microprocessor chips, or directional microphones.

In-The-Ear Type

Virtually ignored as a viable amplification alternative 15 years ago, the in-the-ear instrument has grown enormously in popularity in North America since then. Two distinct types of in-the-ear aids are available: the custom instrument, in which the components of the instrument are individually assembled in a molded acrylic shell obtained from the patient's ear impression, and the modular type, in which the hearing aid components are preassembled in a small standard case, which attaches to a custom earmold by means of screws or a snap assembly. However, the latter type of in-the-ear aid has not met with substantial acceptance in North America and accounts for less than 1 percent of total sales.[5] At one time accounting for 10 percent of total sales at its height of popularity in the early 1960s, the modular in-the-ear instrument diminished in sales when the custom in-the-ear aid was introduced. Limitations of the modular version include feedback problems due to difficulty in securing proper earmold and instrument fit, lack of space for adequate venting, and limited performance options.

The custom in-the-ear aid is a good example of the continuing search for improvement and refinement of a promising concept. When first introduced in the mid-1960s, transducers and circuits were oversized and lacked important performance characteristics, making these aids marginally effective. Little gain or power could be delivered, consistent venting was difficult to accomplish, and sophisticated assembly techniques had not been developed. With time, these limitations have been overcome or radically improved, making today's in-the-ear aid capable of providing amplification from very low gain (10 to 15 dB) and low output (90 to 100 dB SSPL90), up to approximately 65 dB gain and 130 dB SSPL90. By extending or shortening the canal of the custom mold so that the cavity between the tip of the mold and the eardrum is enlarged or reduced, the output of these instruments can be further increased or reduced.[11] Some manufacturers offer two or three controls for frequency response, gain, and output alteration, plus they offer telephone switches, CROS-BiCROS variations, and other modifications to facilitate fitting special needs.

At first glance, the success of the in-the-ear instrument may appear to be primarily related to the fact that it is less conspicious and more convenient to use than the behind-the-ear aid. However it is more likely that its acceptance is based on other determining factors. First, the microphone, placed as it is at the concha plane, more closely simulates the natural reception function of the ear and affords approximately 4 to 10 dB more amplification in the high frequencies when compared to a behind-the-ear microphone location.[12] Second, the tubing-associated resonance that is present at approximately 1,000 Hz in all behind-the-ear hearing aids is eliminated, which results in the primary resonance of the in-the-ear system to fall in the vicinity of 2,000 Hz. Therefore the frequency of resonance of the in-the-ear aid approximates that of the unoccluded ear, a condition of amplification considered to be more acceptable to the average user.[13] Clinicians also believe that elimination of the tubing-associated resonance at 1,000 Hz is beneficial because the presence of peaks in the amplified response results in less overall energy being delivered when the instrument has been set at the most comfortable listening level.[14]

The manufacturer normally selects and installs the specific performance in a given custom in-the-ear (or in-the-canal) instrument based upon audiometric, master hearing aid, or other test results provided by the dispenser. Just as clinicians differ in their opinions as to what particular model aid may work best in a specific instance, manufacturers do not agree unanimously as to what constitutes the best custom in-the-ear performance for a particular individual. Unless otherwise specified by the clinician, the dispenser is provided with an instrument from the manufacturer believed to be appropriate, and the performance installed in it is based upon experience accrued by the manufacturer with that type of hearing loss. If the choice of performance parameters is inappropriate, these can usually be altered somewhat by the use of trimmer controls, venting, and other minor earmold adjustments. If these dispenser modifications do not provide appropriate amplification, the instrument may be returned to the manufacturer for further changes in the electroacoustic performance.

Obviously, it is in the best interest of the manufacturer to develop a reliable, consistent protocol for installation of appropriate hearing aid performance in in-the-ear aids, one that leaves as little margin for error as possible. The nature of competition in the marketplace is such that consistently inappropriate selection of gain, SSPL90, and frequency response by the manufacturer causes the dispenser to seek a new supplier. However, the manufacturer does have an advantage over the individual dispenser in knowing whether the performance selected for a given loss may be appropriate, because the manufacturer can monitor returns of hearing aids for modification, remake, or credit over periods of time; this type of feedback triggers ongoing changes in the performance selection protocol whenever circumstances warrant.

In-The-Canal Type

Introduced on an occasional experimental basis in 1982 and 1983, the in-the-canal aid, a further refinement of the in-the-ear aid, accounted for approximately 15 percent of the total hearing aids sold in North America in 1986.[5] With the advent of the smaller transducers, amplifiers, and controls developed for in-the-ear aids, it became possible in selected instances to package these components in earshells that are confined to the external canal portion of the ear only. As with any development of this type, deficiencies in the early models were encountered, which are now gradually being overcome. Initially, problems with feedback, lack of performance range, lack of trimmer controls and venting, as well as limitations caused by canal size were noted. As one might expect, consumer demand has resulted in a focusing of resources by manufacturers on the resolution of these problems; as a result, the range of possible fittings has increased markedly with a concomitant reduction of tendency to acoustic feedback. Problems caused by insufficient canal size have diminished because of improved techniques in manufacturing, which provide increased room for venting and installation of trimmer controls. At this writing, considerably more refinement of the in-the-canal hearing aid can be expected, and like in-the-ear aids, growth in unit sales will increase substantially as the problems are further resolved.[15,16]

Eyeglass Type

Between 1959 and 1962, eyeglass instruments were the most popular of all hearing aid styles.[17] Today, their use has diminished to less than 1 percent of the total dispensed, and they have virtually disappeared from the catalogues of all but a few European manufacturers. At one time, eyeglass instruments featured the same range of performance, features, and options that were available in the behind-the-ear models. The components were built into the eyeglass temple, and the amplified sound was delivered to the ear through a tube or earmold assembly.

Eyeglass aids are somewhat less sturdy than behind-the-ear aids because of their long, slender shape. Further limitations include the lack of variety of different hinge types for attachment to modern high-fashion eyeglass frames, the difficulty sometimes encountered in obtaining a comfortable "no-slip" fit, and the fact that when the patient removes his or her glasses, the aid is also removed. When an eyeglass instrument is in need of repair, especially in cases of CROS or Bi-CROS, the need for a spare pair of glasses may become a serious inconvenience.

Body Type

Also called conventional or pocket hearing aids, the body aid contains a microphone, battery, and amplifier in a package separate from the receiver. The main chassis is worn either in a pocket, attached to undergarments, or in a special carrier on the chest. A flexible wire cord connects the main case to a button type external receiver that, in turn, snaps into a custom earmold. The amount of gain may vary from as little as 35 dB to as much as 85 dB, and maximum power output (SSPL90) may range from 110 dB to 150 dB SPL. Multiple trimmer controls and switches, often cleverly concealed and used in conjunction with receiver options, provide a wide range of performance changes. Although body instruments afford the greatest amount of overall power for use with severe to profound losses, body aids with significantly less power and gain are also available for less severe problems.

At one time, body aids were the only aids considered for recommendation for children, and they still remain popular with some clinicians for the extremely young. But the current trend has been away from body aids to ear level instruments for children whenever possible for three reasons: (1) to take advantage of the improved performance provided by the microphone located at ear level rather than on the chest (body-baffle effects that build up low frequencies are a particularly negative concomitant of body aid amplification); (2) to minimize resistance by the child to wearing a hearing aid, which may occur as he or she becomes older; and (3) to facilitate the fitting of binaural amplification. Heretofore, the body aid was viewed as having the greatest ability to sustain the most punishment, thus offering the most durability; because of its size, the body aid has been characterized as having the ability to process speech signals with the highest fidelity. However, these attributes become significantly less true as more sophisticated, rugged transducers, improved amplifiers, and advanced assembly techniques have come into common use in ear-level aids. The popularity of body aids has decreased steadily, comprising less than 1 percent of the aids dispensed, but there may always be a need for the special advantages that they afford.

COMPONENTS

Over the past 15 years, progress in miniature transducer technology probably has improved hearing aid performance more significantly than any other single development. Wider bandwidth, improved ability to withstand shock, and ever decreasing size without sacrifice of sensitivity or power handling capabilities are representative characteristics of the new generation of microphones and receivers.

Microphones

Three types of miniature microphones have been used in hearing aids: magnetic, ceramic, and electret. Although once used extensively, the magnetic (or dynamic) microphone is rarely seen today. Magnetic microphones operate on the principle of variable electromagnetic reluctance, in which movement of the diaphragm causes changes in a magnetic field, which in turn induce an electrical current in a small coil. Because of their balanced armature construction, magnetic microphones do not have good ability to withstand the stresses of shock. An important design consideration in early hearing aids using magnetic transducers was the specification of proper shock mounting and vibration isolation. To minimize mechanical feedback tendencies, the magnetic microphone and receiver diaphragm were generally oriented at right angles to each other, and the response of the instrument electrically rolled off in the extreme high and low frequencies.[18] Consequently, the need for transducers that could resist shock and vibration without sacrificing bandwidth led to the development of the ceramic and then the electret condenser microphone.

Ceramic Microphones

Introduced in 1968, the ceramic microphone operates on the piezoelectric principle. The diaphragm is mechanically connected to a cantilever mounted bar of piezoelectric ceramic material; when bent, this material produces minute voltage variations proportional to the small movements of the diaphragm. The primary advantages of the ceramic microphone over its magnetic counterpart are excellent frequency response, particularly in the low frequencies, and a reduction in mass by approximately one-half, thus reducing the microphone's susceptibility to vibration and shock. However, the ceramic microphone is sensitive to externally generated vibrations at extremely low frequencies, and as a result, subjects wearing these microphones have occasionally reported hearing a thumping noise caused by head movement accompanying brisk walking.

Because of the overall improvement in the frequency response of the ceramic microphone, which was especially apparent at the low frequencies, hearing aids began to be designed with greatly emphasized low-frequency responses. It was suggested that improved low frequencies added a more "natural" sound to the hearing aid, and this effect was quite apparent to the normal hearing listener. But subsequent experience has shown that excessive low-frequency amplification may actually reduce discrimination performance for many hearing impaired adult listeners regardless of the threshold configuration of the hearing loss, probably because of the effects of upward spread of masking and temporal masking.[19–26]

Electret Condenser Microphones

Within a few years after the introduction of the ceramic microphone, the now widely used electret condenser microphone became available for use in head-worn hearing aids.[27] In addition to sensitivity comparable to that of a ceramic microphone and the broad flat-frequency response, the electret's most exciting characteristic is its inherently low-vibration sensitivity, made possible by the extremely low mass of the diaphragm. This low mass and the fact that the low mass diaphragm is the only moving part reduce susceptibility of electret microphones to shock, stress, and damage. Even though the electret condenser principle has been known for a long time, new electret materials and methods of charging these materials have made the electret condenser microphone resistant to long-term changes in sensitivity produced by high humidity and temperature.[28,29]

The prime determinants of the overall frequency response in any given hearing aid are the individual response shapes of the microphone and receiver and the response of the amplifier. Electret microphones are commonly utilized to shape the low-frequency portion of the frequency response because they are available with a standard essentially flat-response shape and also with low-cut responses; for example, they have either a −6 dB per octave or a −12 dB per octave cut below 1,600 Hz. The availability of these additional responses in microphones is an important factor in producing instruments that have substantial low-frequency roll offs (i.e., high-frequency emphasis) on the order of 18 to 24 dB gain per octave from 500 Hz to 1,000 Hz.

The newest generation of electret microphones are characterized by their even greater low-vibration sensitivity, that is, the use of a thinner electret diaphragm to reduce mechanical inertia. As a consequence, these microphones appear to provide an improved ability to withstand mechanical feedback oscillations, a consequential benefit in modern in-the-ear and in-the-canal aids where ever higher levels of useful gain and output are an important objective.

An important contribution to microphone technology is the stepped response microphone, which incorporates a desirable frequency response for the fitting of high-frequency losses. Based on the work of Skinner,[30] it combines a reduced level of low-frequency amplification with a smooth increase in high-frequency emphasis, and it appears to provide more satisfactory high-frequency amplification in canal aids where there is often the need for some amount of minimal low-frequency amplification to add a perception of improved signal quality (Fig. 49–1)

Directional Microphones

Most microphones used in hearing aids have equal sensitivity to sound from all (360 degree) an-

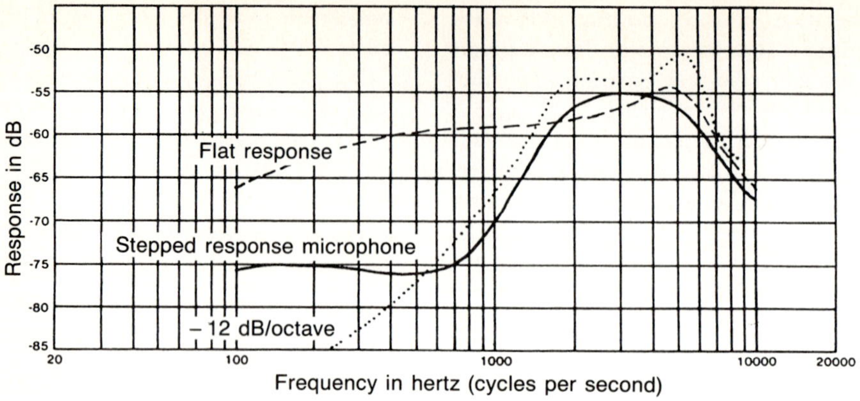

Figure 49–1 The response of three microphone types commonly utilized in hearing aids. Different slopes assist the manufacturer to shape the frequency response as desired. (From Knowles Advance Information Release, No. 107, July, 1984).

gles of incidence. That is, they are omnidirectional. If an omnidirectional microphone (also referred to as a pressure microphone) is suspended in an anechoic space, the resultant polar diagram (a plotting of the output of the microphone for all angles of incidence) would look like a circle, thus showing uniform sensitivity in all directions. Yet the directional microphone does not have uniform sensitivity for all angles of sound incidence, but rather it is less sensitive to signals that emanate from the rear, or 180 degrees. Over a limited range of frequencies, the difference between front (0 degrees) and back (180 degrees) sensitivity may be as much as 20 dB. This "sound cancelling" property of the directional microphone is the result of the microphone's having two sound inlets rather than just one, as in a pressure microphone. Each sound inlet (or port) leads to an opposite side of the microphone diaphragm. The rear inlet is further modified with an acoustic "filter" that produces a time delay to all signals entering this inlet. The transmission of signals to the "rear" of the diaphragm is delayed with respect to signals that enter the front inlet and reach the opposite side of the diaphragm. Signals entering the front inlet first are processed with no delay or loss of sensitivity, but signals entering the rear inlet are delayed by approximately the same amount of time it takes for a sound wave to travel the distance between the two microphone inlets. Therefore, when sound emanates from 180 degrees, the signals reaching the diaphragm from each inlet are delayed by the same amount and the sound waves that impinge on each side of the diaphragm are of approximately equal and opposite force, resulting in little or no diaphragm movement. (See Lentz,[31] Mueller et al,[32] and Hawkins and Yacullo[33] for information concerning subjects' performance with directional microphone hearing aids).

An important variation of the standard cardioid directional microphone is the so-called ultracardioid (or supercardioid) response pattern. Preves pointed out that the ultracardioid response pattern produces more signal rejection from the rear hemisphere than does the cardioid response pattern when standard measures of comparative performance (developed by the inventors of directional microphones in the 1930s to assess the amount of directivity present in a microphone),[34] are used.

Receivers

Modern magnetic air conduction receivers operate on the balanced armature principle and can be divided into two basic types. Internal receivers (the most common) are used inside the case of the aid, and external receivers are remote from the aid and connected to the main chassis of the aid by a cord.

The output sensitivity and frequency range of internal receivers present an interesting relationship. A general rule results: the wider the bandwidth of the receiver, the less overall sensitivity available; and conversely, the more sensitive the receiver (which results in achieving potentially greater gain and output levels), the narrower its bandwidth. Accompanying this bandwidth and sensitivity trade-off is the consideration of physical size of receivers. Based on hard-won experience, industry tends to believe that "adequately small" hearing aid size is an important marketing consideration. Any component that takes up an inordinate amount of volume in an instrument puts undesirable restrictions on other parts in the design. The need for power, which usually requires a larger size, must be balanced against the requirements for acceptable bandwidth and response, and the necessity to effectively control overall size. Fortunately, the size of receivers continues to diminish steadily, and receiver responses are becoming ever broader, extending into higher frequencies.

Amplifier Assemblies

Electronic amplifiers in modern hearing aids operate from a single cell battery supply (1.30 to 1.55 volts) with the exception of a few body aids, which require two battery cells. The design and method of manufacture of these miniature electronic circuit assemblies varies widely from manufacturer to manufacturer. Few manufacturers still build their amplifiers from discrete (singly packaged) transistors, resistors, and capacitors; most use complex monolithic integrated circuits or custom designed hybrid circuits. Hearing aid circuit assemblies generally are configured to utilize all available space around the geometrically shaped microphone, receiver, battery, and volume control. The circuit's function is to amplify the small signal produced by the microphone 1 million times or more and transmit this power to the receiver. Amplifiers may be broadly categorized as class A, class B (or push-pull), AGC (or compression), diode or soft peak clipping (or curvilinear compression), or hard peak clipping. Several manufacturers have introduced amplifiers that have been termed "automatic signal processors" (ASP),[35–37] but that are usually, but not always, special forms of AGC. In the most common variation, an automatic low-cut is activated by high-intensity, low-frequency input signals, which results in freeing the listener from some of the deleterious effects of low-frequency background noise. For more information about hearing aid design and circuitry, see Krebs,[38] Curran and Ely,[39] Heide,[40] Hogg,[41] Staab,[42] Braida et al,[43] Sandlin,[44] Libby,[45] Smriga,[46] and Buerkli-Halevy.[47]

The movement towards the incorporation of digital amplifier assemblies into hearing aids has been slow and cautious. Although holding great promise for resolving some of the most difficult fitting problems, these assemblies have significant drawbacks relating to size, battery consumption, and internal noise that have held back development.[48–51] More than likely, initial forms of digital amplifiers in hearing aids will involve hybrid applications, with combinations of analogue and digital circuitry joined together to perform separate amplification functions.[52,53] (For a survey of current microprocessor technology in amplification, see Curran and Preves.[54])

Volume Control

The hearing aid volume control is a key component in a well-designed, well-built instrument. It must be capable of approximately 15,000 operations over the life of a hearing aid and must faithfully control the amplifier signal level. It will be exposed to a veritable flood of chemicals, water, and salt and rough mechanical manipulation. The actual resistance element in a conventional hearing aid volume control is a semicircular arc with a length of no more than 10 mm. In this short distance, it must control 40 to 50 dB of amplifier gain range. Factors such as resistance taper, total angular rotation, torque, rotational noise, wiper tension, moisture seal, lubrication, electrical termination, and mounting are all important elements in these miniature controls. The volume control continues to remain a critical wear part within the hearing aid, and its life is affected not only by its design, but especially by the care it is given by the patient as well.

At the time of this writing, development of digital type volume controls is underway, wherein digital logic increases and decreases gain in preset increments, responding to a slight touch or, alternatively to movement of a rotary or toggle switch. These volume controls have the distinct advantage of no moving parts, which should reduce the chances of mechanical breakdown. But they are dependent upon a small amount of current drain being available from the battery in order to maintain memory, which may increase levels of battery consumption.

MEASUREMENT AND PERFORMANCE

The methods and procedures used to measure the electroacoustic performance of a hearing aid strongly affect one's understanding of its capabilities and help one form opinions as to its appropriateness. Since the hearing aid is meant to be the principal ingredient in the solution of a rehabilitative or habilitative problem, how its performance is understood and conceptualized has direct bearing on its successful application. Therefore it is important to examine various factors that together affect the perception and interpretation of an aid's operation. This is a significant consideration, for the same aid may appear to be acceptable under one method of measurement, but may appear unacceptable when another procedure is employed or conditions of measurement change or are not well controlled. It is necessary to develop an appreciation and an understanding of the factors that may be responsible for producing changes in measurements.

Measurement Equipment

The environment in which the hearing aid is placed during the measurement procedure is a critical factor. Optimized measurement conditions would require the use of an anechoic chamber to minimize standing waves and reflections at the signal source and thus produce a free-field test environment. However, this condition is not practical for most facilities, and therefore nonanechoic pressure type hearing aid test boxes of considerably smaller dimensions are used. The insides of the boxes are usually lined with soft absorbent material to minimize reflections and may or may not utilize compressor microphones to hold the level of the input signal constant. Even with precautions, these test systems fall far short of providing an error-free anechoic measurement environment and can be a source of significant measurement differences.

Measurement Standards

Standardized measurement and specification of hearing aid performance characteristics have evolved from an early position of voluntary usage by individual manufacturers[55–57] to a position today of mandatory participation. Although a standardized measurement procedure has existed since 1960,[58–61] it was not until the promulgation of ANSI standard S3.22[62] (Specification of Hearing Aid Characteristics) that the hearing aid industry began to measure and express hearing aid performance according to one set of rules and tolerances. This standard was incorporated into a federal regulation (Hearing Aid Devices: Professional and Patient Labeling and Conditions for Sale) and put into effect by the Food and Drug Administration on August 25, 1977. It requires that technical data useful in checking and describing the performance of a hearing aid must accompany the delivery of each hearing aid. Subsequently, the standard was revised primarily to include clarification of the text, but no fundamental changes in procedures were made.[63]

When the gain or the maximum power output (SSPL90) of a hearing aid is measured, a sinusoidal input signal of a known constant SPL value is impressed on the diaphragm of the microphone of the hearing aid. The output of the hearing aid is delivered through a standard connector to a hard-walled 2-cm^3 cavity of specific dimension. A high quality condenser microphone detects the sound pressure generated in the hard-walled cavity. This signal is amplified by a microphone amplifier, and a graphic readout of the SPL is provided for each frequency.

Information about the acoustic performance of an individual hearing aid is often expressed on a strip chart graph. A common form is shown in Figure 49–2, where the gain and power output curves of a moderate power in-the-ear instrument are shown.

Although the 2-cm^3 coupler is an attempt to simulate the properties of the average normal human ear with an earmold in place, the actual space between the tip of the earmold and the eardrum varies from person to person. Additionally, middle ear impedance values vary across subjects and across frequency. Pinna-, head-, and body-baffle effects plus resonances of the individual ear canal are also absent from the measurement system when the 2-cm^3 coupler is used.[64–66] Therefore curves obtained on the

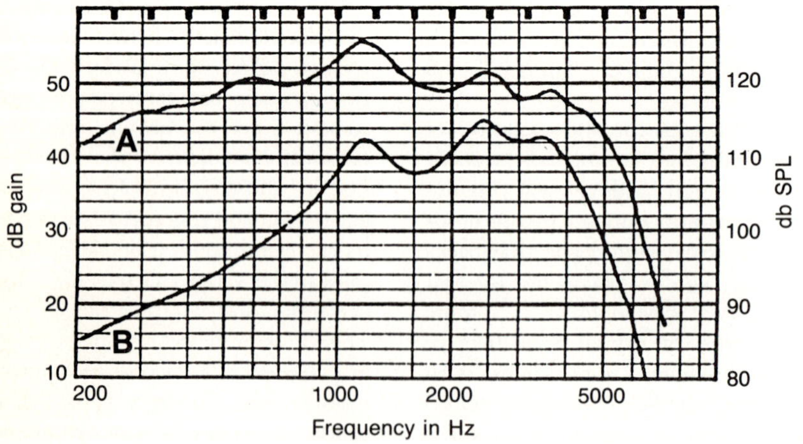

Figure 49–2 Curve A depicts the SSPL90, or power output curve across frequency, of a typical hearing aid as measured on a 2cm^3 coupler, 90 db SPL pure tone input. The output levels are shown on the right of the graph. Curve B shows the response of the same aid to a 60 db SPL swept pure tone input signal; gain values are at left.

2-cm^3 coupler are not a totally accurate reflection of the performance of an aid in a real ear. This particular fact continues to be a source of some difficulty for clinicians and dispensers when preselecting aids for evaluation on the basis of data that has been gathered on the 2-cm^3 coupler and reported in technical specification sheets. It is useful to understand that, in actual use, each hearing aid's performance varies according to the size, shape, and impedance of the cavity into which it is connected, the manner in which it is coupled to the cavity, the setting of the volume control, the level of the input signal, and the position of the microphone. Measurements performed according to ANSI standard S3.22[63] are merely reflections of the aid's performance under specific, controlled, arbitrarily selected conditions, and as such, they are better viewed as a method for ensuring baseline performance and product uniformity, not necessarily for purposes of selecting and fitting a hearing aid.

Parenthetically, it is not always well understood that significant intramodel electroacoustic performance variations exist that can affect fittings if instruments are recommended or selected for use from inspection of manufacturer specification sheets. The specification sheet response curves and other electroacoustic data provided by the manufacturer are an average of the performance of many samples of the same model. As such, the data do not describe the performance of the specific instrument under consideration, unless it is an in-the-ear or in-the-canal instrument that is furnished with its own performance curves. Response curve tolerances permitted by the ANSI standard S3.22[63] are fairly wide, approaching 4 to 5 dB for some measurements. This tolerance range literally means that the curve for instrument A can be at least 4 to 5 dB different than that for instrument B of the same model at various portions of the spectrum and still be within tolerance.

Gain and Output Relationships

Full-on gain is usually measured with a 60 dB input with volume control full on. In real life, the hearing aid is exposed to any number of input values of different levels and frequencies when it is being worn. The soft sound of a whisper, perhaps 30 to 40 dB SPL, to the peak sound of a door slam, perhaps as much as 110 to 120 dB SPL, are sounds that every hearing aid user may be exposed to in his or her environment. How does the hearing aid respond to all of the various levels of signals that impinge on the microphone? The next few sections deal briefly with this interesting and important interaction.

Here it is useful to state three interrelated concepts that are important to better understand hearing aid amplification. Incidentally, this discussion is limited to linear aids (noncompression aids) because, although they function to a degree in a similar manner, compression aids incorporate nonlinear properties that materially affect the simple relationships explained next.

First, the volume control should be viewed as a controller of gain. As the volume control is turned up, gain increases; as it is turned down, gain decreases. Second, input level plus gain equals output level. Use of this simple equation is fundamental to an understanding of the function of hearing aids. Third, the hearing aid cannot amplify beyond SSPL90, no matter how high the input level becomes.

Assuming that a given hearing aid has a 40 dB full-on gain and an SSPL90 of 120 dB SPL, a 60 dB SPL input signal would produce a 100 dB SPL output level (60 + 40 = 100). Here "output" is defined simply as the sum of the input plus the gain and is distinguished from the maximum power output (MPO) or SSPL90. Therefore the output (input plus gain) of this hearing aid would be 100 dB SPL or 20 dB below the SSPL90 (MPO) of the instrument. When the volume control is turned down half way (assuming that the taper of the volume control is linear), the same input level (60 dB SPL) would provide an output of 80 dB SPL. If one wishes to assume that most normal speech at a distance of 3 feet is approximately 70 dB SPL, then the output of the hearing aid with a speech input signal now becomes 90 dB SPL (70 dB SPL input plus one-half gain [20 dB] equals 90 dB SPL). If the speech input signal is raised to 80 dB SPL, the output correspondingly becomes 100 dB SPL; if the signal is raised to 90 dB SPL, the output becomes 110 dB SPL; and so on, until the SSPL90 of the hearing aid is reached. At that point, further increases in input do not result in further increases in output, for the aid has been forced into saturation and cannot amplify beyond that level. If the input should become 110 dB SPL, as when a door slams, the gain (by definition) can be no more than 10 dB since the SSPL90, that is, the point beyond which the aid cannot amplify, remains at 120 dB SPL, and the rule states that input level plus gain equals output.

Although the patient is able to rotate the volume control up and down, and thereby change the gain of the hearing aid, he or she is unable to protect him- or herself from being exposed to extraordinarily loud sounds solely by turning the volume control down. At the moment that an intense abrupt signal occurs in the patient's environment, its level is added to the gain level established by the volume control setting. The sum of the level of the high-input signal plus the level of the gain may force the instrument to reach SSPL90. If the SSPL90 of the hearing aid exceeds the level that the subject can tolerate, this highly amplified signal may cause the subject severe discomfort. For this reason, adjusting the SSPL90 (MPO) to a level at or below the uncomfortable level (UCL, TD) is one of the most critically important considerations in properly fitting a patient, because he or she has little or no direct control over the level of input signals that he or she is exposed to during daily activities.[67–73]

Distortion

Distortion products can be measured in the output signal of hearing aids, especially when forced into saturation. Some researchers have suggested that there is a causal relationship between the amount of distortion present in a given hearing aid and the intelligibility and quality of the speech signal that it process.[74] The usual presumption is that, if distortion is present in the signal, the clarity of the amplified speech signal is necessarily reduced to a certain degree. As a result, researchers have made numerous attempts to relate performance on standardized speech discrimination tests to the amount of harmonic distortion present.

The exact correlation, if one exists, between intelligibility, quality, and distortion in hearing aids is very difficult to analyze;[75–77] it is hard to tease out the precise nature of the systematic relationship that is presumed to exist.[78] Consider that harmonic distortion is only one of the many forms of distortion that exists and can be quantified in hearing aids.[79,80] In addition to harmonic distortion, which is the expression of the amount of nonlinearity present in the instantaneous transfer function (the input versus output of any amplifying system), the other types of distortion present in hearing instruments include intermodulation distortion (which is really only a special case of nonlinearity), phase distortion, frequency distortion, transient distortion, and distortion due to noise in the circuit.[81] It is safe to say that no one is certain at what exact level each type of distortion begins to affect the amplified signal so as to cause deterioration of a subject's performance. There are no unequivocally definitive studies showing the nature of the interaction between the various types of distortion and their relative impact on performance. Nevertheless, *harmonic* distortion measurements have become the single measurement most people refer to when they speak of "distortion" in a hearing aid.[82] The other forms of distortion are often overlooked, perhaps only because it is easier to measure harmonic distortion or because total harmonic distortion is usually the only distortion measurement reported by the manufacturer.

As well, an individual harmonic distortion score itself is not an absolute, uncontaminated value. Depending on which method of measurement is used, harmonic distortion values may actually vary as the conditions of measurement change.[83] For example, (1) a different score may be obtained each time a different fundamental frequency is selected for measurement; (2) more than one formula for the calculation of total harmonic distortion scores can be used, and each may produce a different score; (3) as input is increased, the score generally increases as the output of the instrument approaches its SSPL90 at any given frequency; (4) unless precautions are taken, the harmonic distortion score can be artificially inflated by the presence of noise in the measurement environment, noise in the instrument itself, or noise in the measuring equipment; (5) additionally, certain frequency response configurations can result in producing a score containing a measurement artifact;[84] and (6) harmonic distortion scores may be variously expressed as either total harmonic distortion or second or third harmonic distortion, and each score may differ from the other.

For these reasons and more, it is misleading to assign a single figure of merit, such as 10 percent, as the criterion of acceptability for a hearing aid simply because so many different factors tend to influence the level of the obtained score.[85]

The many complicating factors that influence a subject's performance, such as the instrument's frequency response, the speech materials used, the SSPL90 of the aid, and the manner of coupling to the ear, make it nearly impossible to treat harmonic distortion as an independent variable uncontaminated by other uncontrolled factors.[86–88]

Schweitzer et al[89] felt, on the basis of their results, that using total harmonic distortion scores as a means of ranking hearing aids from more acceptable to less acceptable is probably an undependable procedure. They suggested that the source of the difficulty is the irregular transfer function, that is, the built-in frequency distortion that is characteristic of hearing aids. Other investigators have actually found a reverse relationship in their studies in which best performance by subjects correlated most highly with instruments having greatest amounts of harmonic distortion, and worst performance was related to the least distorted aids.[90,91]

What can be concluded from the foregoing? Perhaps the safest course to follow is to ensure that the aids one fits and recommends meet the criteria for total harmonic distortion specified by the manufacturer. When an aid appreciably surpasses these levels, it is clearly not functioning as intended and therefore requires service. Above all, one should always keep in mind that the presence of low harmonic distortion values in an aid is no guarantee that the patient will experience success when fitted with that aid.

KEMAR Measurements

Until the introduction of KEMAR, a realistic manikin incorporating median adult anthropomorphic values,[92] the conventional method for measuring hearing aid performance has been by using the 2-cm^3 coupler in a test box or anechoic space. The KEMAR manikin incorporates a different coupler, the Zwislocki coupler, more correctly referred to as the occluded ear simulator.[93,94] This coupler more accurately simulates the acoustic behavior of the ear canal than does the hard-walled 2-cm^3 coupler. It incorporates the acoustic impedance at the eardrum of a median adult ear over the frequency range from 100 to 10,000 kHz.[95]

Therefore the occluded ear simulator coupler resembles the typical behavior of the average normal adult ear; when used in KEMAR, it allows hearing aid performance measurements that approximate that of the instrument when worn in real life under simulated conditions of use.[96–98] Figure 49–3 is a comparison of full-on gain curves obtained on a 2-cm^3 coupler as opposed to those obtained on KEMAR in an anechoic chamber by means of the occluded ear simulator.

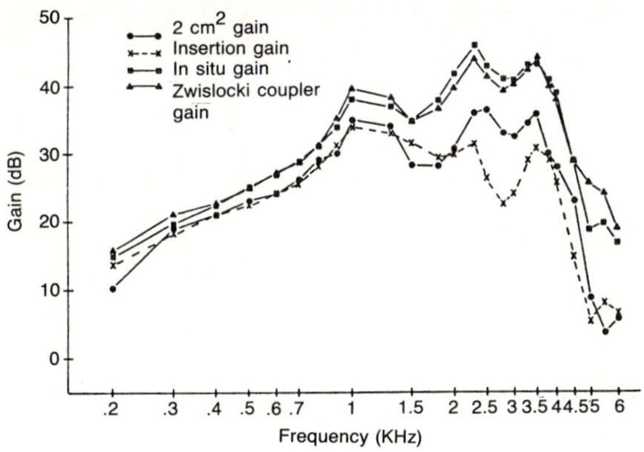

Figure 49-3 The in situ gain is obtained with the hearing aid connected to the occluded ear simulator, which is mounted in KEMAR; the input level is subtracted from the output. When the instrument is measured on the Zwislocki coupler (occluded ear simulator), the coupler is not mounted on KEMAR. The insertion gain response is obtained on KEMAR with occluded ear simulator; it is simply the subtraction of the unoccluded external ear effects (canal resonance plus pinna, head and body baffle properties) from the in situ response. This condition occurs when the ear is occluded by an earmold or earshell since it removes the external ear effects. The insertion gain therefore is seen as a valid measure of the actual gain provided by the instrument while worn. All four curves were obtained using one aid in an anechoic chamber, 0° azimuth. (From Hawkins DB, Schum DJ. Relationships between various measures of hearing and gain. J Speech Hear Disord 1984; 49:94.)

The Speech Signal

The speech signal is transformed significantly by the hearing aid and the earmold as it traverses from its origin in a free field to the tympanic membrane. The spectrum of spoken speech, as measured in a free field, contains greater intensity at the low frequencies than at the high.[99,100] The familiar long-term average speech spectrum shows a maximum at the lower frequencies, between 300 and 700 Hz, and a reduction in intensity across frequency at the rate of approximately 6 to 10 dB per octave above that point. Although this is the long-term average spectrum of the speech signal at its point of origin, if the same speech signal is measured at the tympanic membrane (with no aid or earmold), a characteristic increase in amplitude is seen in the region of 2,500 to 3,000 Hz on the order of 5 to 15 dB. This increase in intensity in the higher frequencies is due to the resonant effects of the unoccluded ear canal plus head and pinna diffraction effects.[101–103] Therefore the average normal listener in a sound field, with unoccluded ear canal, receives a unique two-humped speech signal (see Fig. 49–4), one hump at the lower frequencies, below 1,000 Hz, and one slightly above 2,500 Hz.[104,105]

Alterations to the Speech Signal

It is important to realize that, when the hearing aid is fitted to the patient, it is more properly viewed as a total *system,* which includes not the only the hearing aid proper, but also the method by which the aid is connected to the ear and the acoustic load into which the aid delivers its signal. These and other factors markedly influence the distribution of energy at the eardrum. Figure 49–5 shows the results of probe tube measurements of five subjects, each wearing an identical aid and similar earmold at an identical setting.[106] From the frequency response as measured by IEC and ANSI standards, notice the substantial variation especially at the high frequencies and the large range of variability between individuals. Here, although attempts were made to duplicate exactly as far as possible the earmold and coupling system used by each subject, the minute differences in coupling and the contribution of other influencing factors across subjects produced substantial variations in the frequency response of the in-

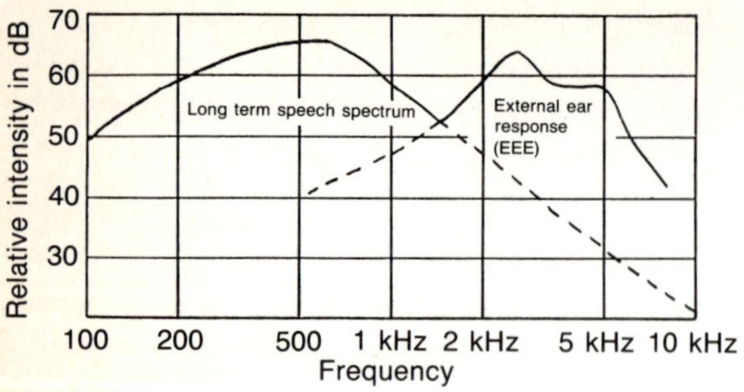

Figure 49–4 Solid line is approximate representation of the long-term average speech spectrum measured at the tympanic membrane. Curve is constructed by combining the long-term speech spectrum as measured in a sound field (approximately 1 meter from the speaker's mouth) with the eardrum pressure response (EEE) of KEMAR. (After Pascoe DP. An approach to hearing aid selection. Hear Instr 1978; 29(6):12–16, 38, and Killion MC, Monser EL. CORFIG: coupler response for flat insertion gain. In: Studebacker GA, Hochberg I, eds. Acoustical factors affecting hearing aid performance. Baltimore: University Park Press, 1980:149.)

strument when worn. Some of the sources that determine or modify the amplified signal as it is transmitted through the hearing aid system in the individual subject are listed next.

Microphone Position Influences

Gross differences are possible when the microphone is located at body level as opposed to ear level;[107–110] it is not generally appreciated that, even with two or more behind-the-ear instruments of the same shape, small differences in microphone positioning may cause variations in response.[111] The same aid worn on two different subjects also produces minor deviations in response, especially in the higher frequencies, due to head and pinna configuration differences.[112] Subtle variations in frequency response also accrue as the microphone position is changed within an in-the-ear aid,[113] or when microphone position in a behind-the-ear aid is compared to position in an in-the-ear aid, or similarly, when an in-the-canal aid microphone location is compared to that of an in-the-ear aid.[12,65]

Ear Hook and Tubing Properties

In the behind-the-ear aid, the length of tubing and its internal diameter when the aid is fitted is not always identical to the conditions of measurement in the 2-cm^3 coupler. The incorporation of filters or other modifications to the hook or tubing directly influence the response.[114] Unless these modifications are performed in the identical manner to that specified by the manufacturer, there are considerable differences.[115] In the in-the-ear or canal aid, tubing length and internal diameter are chosen by the manufacturer and are reflected in the instrument's response chart provided by the factory at the time of manufacture.

Earmold Configuration

Possibly the greatest contribution to variation in the instrument's response is contributed by the coupling apparatus. Much could be said about the differences in response produced by the unique geometry of the individual earmold or shell of the custom in-the-canal or in-the-ear aid.[116–118] The gross effects have been well documented in the literature (e.g., Courtois and Berland,[119,120] Lyregaard,[121] and Dillon[122]). However, the slight variations attributable to modest individual differences in structure and form are virtually impossible to predict a priori. The foregoing is true of all types of earmolds (or in the in-the-canal or in-the-ear aids, the custom shell configuration), but may be most strikingly apparent when the open (unoccluded) condition is considered. The response changes that accrue as the coupling varies, for example, from a tube to a CROS mold, to a free field mold, or to an acoustic modifier with various venting systems, again are known only in the general sense. Specifically little can be predicted about how much of the unamplified speech signal enters into the external ear through the various venting arrangements or about the part that the resonance of the middle ear plays in contributing to the overall spectrum in each individual case and the subsequent influence on performance.[123] (See Mynders,[124] and Microsonics,[125] for descriptions of earmold types and shapes.)

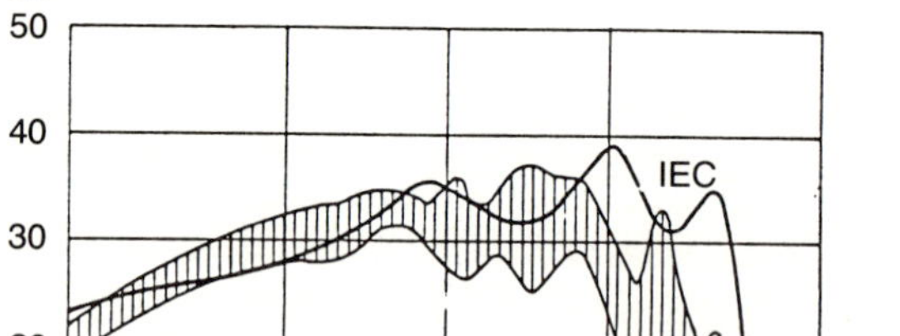

Figure 49–5 Solid line represents a BTE hearing aid measured in 2 cm^3 coupler. Shaded area shows insertion gain of same aid (with earmold) on 5 subjects, revealing substantial variation in response range, especially in higher frequencies. (From Dalsgaard SC. On insertion gain. In: Burkhard M, ed. Manikin measurements. Elk Grove, IL: Knowles Electronics, 1978:19.)

Earmold Circumference Leak

An unspecified amount of amplified acoustic signal emanates from the space between the tip of the earmold and the eardrum to the outside environment around the circumference of the earmold. This "slit" leak has the effect of producing an acoustic resistance damping, shunting the vent resonance and so primarily affects the mid and low frequencies, but is not confined to these regions alone.[117,126,127] Since the fit of the earmold or the in-the-ear and in-the-canal shell is only casually under the control of the clinician, the resultant amount of leak and its impact on the gain and frequency response is virtually unknown before the fitting is made.

Space Between the Tip of the Earmold and the Tympanic Membrane

It is well known that the volume to which the hearing aid is coupled appreciably determines the overall SPL levels that are generated.[128] The average enclosed ear canal cavity for adults varies from 1.0 to 1.4 ml and is less for children.[129,130] As the volume of any given cavity becomes smaller, the SPL increases proportionately. In fact, if the volume of a cavity is reduced in size by one-half, the expected increase in sound pressure is 6 dB, which represents a doubling of sound pressure. Unless the effect of the volume of the ear canal-eardrum cavity to which the aid is connected is accurately assessed beforehand, both the resultant gain and output (SSPL90) can be significantly greater or less than intended in a specific instance. Prior to the fitting in the average clinical setting, predicting the depth of insertion of the individual mold into the ear, except in the most general way, is virtually impossible. Since the acoustic load to which the hearing aid is connected affects the output of the instrument, and differences in the intracanal volume result in variations in load impedance, as such, SPL levels at the eardrum may be affected in a singular and unexpected way.

Impedance of the Middle Ear System

The middle ear impedance has been shown to affect sound transmission to the cochlea significantly.[131] For example, changes in mass in the middle ear would probably affect high-frequency transmission. However, although elaborate research instrumentation has been introduced recently, routine high-frequency impedance testing is generally not feasible to perform in the clinic.[132,133] Ears that exhibit abnormal middle ear functioning produce an undetermined effect on the transmission of energy through the middle ear unless, as suggested, the impedence across frequencies is well established prior to the fitting.[134]

Interactions Between Receiver Impedance and Load Impedance

This factor can be considered a subset of the preceding two. Even in the average normal ear, there may be a mismatch to a greater or lesser degree between the impedance of the receiver system used in the instrument and the impedance of the external or middle ear system, which could result in an unpredictable increase or decrease in the ease of energy transfer.[135,136]

Although the individual contribution of each of these seven factors is unknown with reference to their ultimate influence on the distribution of sound pressure at the eardrum prior to the initial fitting, each to a differing degree helps determine the eventual shape of the frequency response and the eventual transmission of the amplified signal to the cochlea when the aid is fitted. These factors can be controlled in a general way by the clinician, but their cumulative effect on the response is extremely difficult at this time to accurately anticipate in the average clinical setting.[137]

Thus the spectrum of the unamplified signal may undergo considerable transformation from its source, during its journey through the hearing aid system, until it reaches the cochlea. The additive effects of earmold, position of the hearing aid microphone, acoustic load, and other factors account for the change in shape. Of course, changes to the speech signal are additionally precipitated by the particular amplifying characteristics of the hearing aid.

EVALUATION AND FITTING

Predictive Versus Adaptive Fitting Strategies

Since the early Carhart papers,[138–141] which described methods developed essentially in the Armed Forces rehabilitation hospitals during World War II, hearing aid evaluation and fitting has focused mainly on *selecting* the best instrument from among many choices for the individual. Most of the resultant procedures that have been developed since then usually involve some type of *predictive* protocol. That is, the initial evaluation or measurement attempts to forecast the likelihood of success the subject will experience with a given aid or with one that incorporates a specified set of electroacoustic characteristics. That the different procedures have fallen short of their goal is well documented. In audiology, the proper method of hearing aid selection involves more unresolved issues, controversies, and differences of opinion than almost any other subject.[78,142–153]

Upon close examination, no one current method of selecting or fitting hearing aids withstands serious scrutiny.[154] Some excellent methods require great amounts of time to complete, resulting in fatigue in the subject, casting doubt on the validity or reliability of the results, or are time inefficient in active clinical or dispensing settings.[152,155] Others that may be time efficient appear to rely more on the experience and clinical insight of the clinician rather than on objective selection criteria.[156] One of the most popular methods for hearing aid selection—that is, estimating the gain, frequency response, and SSPL90 by means of formulas based partially or wholly on pure tone and other thresholds—fails to take into account individual differences or the effects of the coupling configuration (except in the most general average way), and each formula produces different results. Additionally, in an attempt to be highly objective in establishing aided efficacy, the procedures typically make no provision for aided speech discrimination performance.[13,153,157–164] Some of the most enlightened and progressive research of the last decade has been performed using variations of the master hearing aid;[165–170] nevertheless, the use of a master hearing aid can be criticized because it does not afford absolute correspondence between the test conditions and the eventual instrument(s) fitted.[171–174] Large numbers of clinicians routinely perform some type of speech testing to estimate the ultimate effectiveness of the fitting or to select between instruments, yet that comparative aided evaluations using speech stimuli are totally unreliable is well documented.[175] Probe microphone measurements of aided performance have substantive merit, for they allow visualization of the shape of the amplified signal at the tympanic membrane. However, that these measurements tell us nothing about the subject's perception of the aided speech signal is not well understood.

Yet audiologists are dispensing and fitting hearing aids successfully in ever growing numbers, and are increasingly incorporating hearing aid dispensing as an integral part of their clinical activities. Why the disparity between the lack of predictive efficiency of the methods and procedures that are in use or that are taught, and the obvious success in fitting that is testified to and apparent upon examination of the clinical activities of many dispensing professionals? It is inconceivable that the entire corps of dispensing audiologists is engaged in misrepresenting their success in dispensing. The answer to this contradiction is apparent when one analyzes the typical steps that are followed as an aid is dispensed.

The Typical Evaluation and Fitting Protocol

First, a careful patient history is obtained, and a hearing evaluation is performed. These provide a current estimate of the subject's hearing status, a perspective concerning previous hearing problems, and indications as to what the subject might require to hear better in the future. Unless the actual threshold information is used as part of the initial selection procedure, the primary and most important reason for the first step is to establish a baseline measurement of hearing and listening efficiency against which future changes can be compared. Additionally, it serves as a screening tool for ruling out possible medical or other contraindications to wearing a hearing aid. The first step of the hearing aid evaluation then is the foundation of the entire fitting process, but can be used only in a gross, preliminary way to assist in the selection of the hearing aid.

The second step is the selection for use one of the many methods that are available to preselect or order an instrument or, more appropriately, instruments for use by the patient. (See Mueller[176] for a current discussion of binaural amplification.) Since none of the existing methods provide a precise prediction of appropriate performance and acceptability, but rather since each reveal flaws in their methodology,[154] there is little to suggest that one procedure is intrinsically superior to another. The choice of which method or procedure to use is left up to the judgement of the individual clinician and the particular circumstances of the individual clinical setting. Some methods preferred by certain clinicians result in satisfactory fittings; the same methods in the hands of other clinicians may not be as successful. The goal of any selection procedure that is used and the criteria by which it should be evaluated should be to recommend or provide instrumentation with a minimum of difficulty or valuable time expended. The instruments should lend themselves easily to the myriad adaptive postfitting procedures that are surely needed after the initial fitting is recommended.

The third step of the process comprises the *core* act of hearing aid fitting. It takes place after the original selection or recommendation has been effected and after the aid has been initially fitted to the subject. Only after practice with the aid(s) does the patient learn to be a significantly informed listener. Usually, the subject's ability to discriminate between different signals and ignore unwanted noise improves, expectations and demands become modified, and the subject's ability to recognize when he or she is hearing well or not improves markedly in relation to the initial amplified experience. A unique interaction between patient and the hearing aid takes place, and only at this point can the patient and the fitter mutually decide what subsequent changes and modifications to the fitting are required in order to improve and *adapt* it if required. To do this step presupposes that the patient can communicate his or her experiences to the dispenser, and that the dispenser can interpret the patient's report about what is being heard. The third step, most importantly, also requires familiarity with the techniques and procedures that are necessary to effect electrical and acoustic performance changes in the hearing aid and coupling system (e.g., Orton[177,178]).

The foregoing suggests that 40 years of preoccupation with devising a valid and reliable *predictive* selection procedure may possibly have produced a sort of myopia with reference to the real world of hearing aid fitting and dispensing. Hearing aids are being well fitted by the thousands daily in professional private practices and retail offices in North America, and, in effect, the emphasis in these offices has been perforce on the modification and the adaptation of the product to the needs of the patient *after* the initial fitting has been accomplished.

Until recently, few audiologists received satisfactory exposure to the skills and techniques that are emphasized and necessary in an *adaptive* fitting regimen. The reasons are varied and many, not the least of which is that audiologists must deal with the problem of amplification in the pediatric population; in these cases, there is often no opportunity for qualitative subjective feedback from the patient. To clinicians who are faced with the pressing problem of recommending appropriate amplification in infants and children, it certainly appears eminently reasonable and desirable that a reliable, objective, *predictive* fitting procedure be devised.[179,180] Nevertheless, adult candidates for amplification make up the bulk of most audiologic dispensing practices, and therefore emphasis on postfitting adjustment, care, and counseling should receive far more attention than they do in present day training programs.

The Overlooked Contribution of CROS

CROS is an acronym for Contralateral Routing of Signals and is a particular hearing aid configuration in which the instrument's receiver and amplifier are worn on one ear, connected by a cord to the microphone that is placed on the opposite ear. The CROS hearing aid was originally introduced to overcome problems associated with the head shadow effect in a unilaterally impaired subject. By placing the microphone on the more impaired side, sound is picked up and then routed through a cord behind the head or through an eyeglass frame to the opposite side and into the better ear.[181–183] Almost overlooked in the literature describing CROS was the significance of the unique manner of coupling, wherein sound is delivered into the better ear through a tubing inserted in the ear canal rather than by means of full earmold. By using a tubing only, substantial filtering of low-frequency sounds occurs so that only higher frequencies reach the eardrum. This important development led to a better appreciation of the role that the high frequencies play in providing improved intelligibility in hearing aid amplification.[20,24]

Parenthetically, that the best candidates for CROS are subjects with some high-frequency hearing loss in the aided ear soon became apparent.[184] Subjects with normal hearing in the aided ear are less likely to be successful with CROS, usually because the amplification they receive, even through the tubing, is slightly more than is needed or that can be tolerated.

In the late 1960s and early 1970s, CROS hearing aids became the instrument of choice for patients with bilateral high-frequency impairment. The obvious advantage of providing high-frequency amplification with no low-frequency amplification, coupled with the fact that the subject was able to hear low-frequency sounds normally (assuming his or her hearing was good in the low frequencies), proved to be a beneficial development. These hearing aids were accompanied by few or no problems with acoustic feedback because of the separation of the microphone and the receiver. Immediately, the very subjects who had previously caused the most difficulty—those with high-frequency sensorineural loss—often became the best candidates for amplification and were routinely fitted successfully.[185–187] Familiarity with open canal fittings led to the more convenient IROS (Ipsilateral Routing of Signals) fittings, that is, monaural or preferably binaural ear level instruments employing some form of open, unoccluded coupling.

Experience with CROS, then, in its many variations (Bi-CROS, Hi-Bi-CROS, Mini-CROS, Focal-CROS, Hi-CROS, and Uni-CROS are some of the other members of the CROS family) led to a growing awareness of the tremendous influence that hearing aid coupling has on altering the response of the instrument.[188] (For a more complete description of the CROS family, see Harford and Dodds[189] and Pollack.[190]) The incidence of recommendations for CROS-type instruments has fallen dramatically in recent years, primarily because their application to high-frequency losses has been supplanted by the more appropriate IROS-type fittings.

The Acoustic Coupling

As pointed out previously, the nature and type of the connecting apparatus that couples the hearing aid to the external auditory meatus play critically important roles in modifying the acoustic performance of the hearing aid. In fact, the response of any given instrument typically can be made to vary substantially merely by altering certain dimensions of the earmold and its associated tubing systematically. Although an improved understanding of the capacity of the earmold to affect performance has come about in recent years, the early literature, with a few exceptions,[191] tended to overlook and neglect its importance. It is difficult to believe at first glance that such a small, almost insignificant, element in the hearing aid chain can produce dramatic differences in hearing aid and listening performance. Earlier, clinicians and dispensers had tended to minimize the overall impact of minor changes in the interior diameter of the tubing, changes in type and size of the vent, and differences in depth of insertion of the earmold or tubing into the canal. But the literature of the last 15 years is replete with examples of how alterations in electroacoustic performance occur as a result of particular forms of earmold modification,[192–200] and with examples of changes in listener performance that appear to be related to changes in earmold configuration.[129,201–208]

Sullivan Acoustic Coupling Classification System

Table 49–1 shows a summary of Sullivan's system for hearing aid fittings based on the configuration of acoustic coupling of the hearing aid to the ear.[209,210] A pragmatic categorization of hearing aid fittings, it recognizes the profound influence that the characteristic shape of the earmold or earshell has on the amplified spectrum. This systematic arrangement of important information relative to the acoustic effect of the earmold assists in understanding better a crucial aspect of hearing aid fitting.

The class I fitting, essentially for mild and high-frequency losses, combines amplification from the instrument with direct transmission of the unamplified signal to the eardrum through a maximum size vent. The external ear effects (open ear canal resonance plus pinna-, head-, and body-baffle effects) are largely retained because the ear canal remains essentially unoccluded. Examples of class I fittings would include tube fittings and free field or CROS and similar molds or ITE "helix" or free field shell configurations (see Microsonic).[125]

Class II fittings (partially occluded, partially unoccluded) are used with mild to moderate losses, and employ couplings that utilize somewhat smaller venting than class I. As a result, there is some modification to the external ear effects, but amplification is still a combination of the hearing aid amplified signal plus the unamplified vent-transmitted signal. The typical class II fitting employs some variation of the acoustic modifier earmold (short or medium canal length, medium to large venting).[211]

Class III and IV fittings are reserved for moderately severe to profound losses. They are essentially identical, save that class IV fittings for severe to profound losses are hermetically sealed (resulting in a substantial elimination of an inadvertent leak around the circumference or through the mold or shell), whereas class III fittings for moderately severe to severe losses incorporate a minimum vent or some degree of slit leak and are not hermetically sealed. In both cases, a deeply inserted mold is utilized, and amplification is delivered virtually entirely by means of the hearing aid itself. Obviously, ear canal resonance is lost because the ear canal is occluded, but some of the pinna-, head-, and body-baffle effects

TABLE 49–1 Sullivan Acoustic Coupling-Based Classification For Hearing Aid Fittings

		Maximum Usable		*Direct Acoustic Input*							
Class	*PTA/SRT Range in HL*	*HFA Gain*	*In Situ Output (SPL)*	*Mixed With Aided Input*	*Transmission Loss*	*External Ear Effects (EEE)*	*Vent Effects*	*Resonance Type*	*Residual Canal Volume (V3)*	*Hermetic Seal*	*Probe Insertion Method*
I	15–40 dB	10–25 dB	75–90 dB	Both	None	Essentially unchanged	Maximum acoustic	$^{1}/_{4}$ wave resonance	Maximum	None	Periphery of mold/shell
II	25–55 dB	20–35 dB	80–100 dB	Both	Mild high cut	Modified	Minimum acoustic	Helmholtz resonator		None	Periphery of mold/shell
III	40–90 dB	30–55 dB	95–115 dB	Aided greater than direct	Low pass; < 750–1K Hz	Absent	Essentially slit leak or small vent	$^{1}/_{2}$ wave resonance		Relatively tight	Periphery, but probe tube vent suggested
IV	70–90+dB	50–65+dB	110–135+dB	Aided only	All frequencies	Absent	None	½ wave resonance	Minimum	Complete as possible	Probe tube vent essential

may be retained depending upon the position of the microphone.

Real Ear Measurements

It has become routinely feasible to measure and compare the level and shape of the unamplified and amplified signal at the eardrum because of the recent availability of convenient real ear measurement systems.[13,163,164,212] Each instrument utilizes a thin flexible tubing that can be easily inserted into the ear canal through or around the ear mold or ear shell. A sensitive miniature microphone is connected to the tubing, and a microprocessor helps maintain desired signal levels at the point of measurement and stores and treats results. Various input signals are employed, including warble tone, shaped noise, clicks, and so on, and the results are displayed on a screen or printed out as desired. Open canal measurements of external ear effects are obtained and subtracted from the amplified signal (in situ response), and the difference is termed "insertion response," (or insertion gain), the actual amount of gain provided by the hearing aid. (see Fig. 49–6).[96,213,214]

There is some evidence that insertion gain may be equivalent to functional gain measurements.[215–217] Accordingly, because of the length of time that is required to obtain functional gain thresholds and because of artifacts that accompany the functional gain procedure,[218] probe tube insertion gain measurements have been recommended as an alternative, more time efficient procedure.[164] Additionally, the effects of postfitting modifications and changes in the hearing aid's performance parameters can be easily measured and recorded, and the spectral changes can be compared to performance on standardized tests and inventories or to reports by the patient about his or her listening experience. This comparison can provide an important source of feedback about fitting techniques and procedures and so improve individual clinical skills and judgement. Real ear measurements hold great promise for hearing aid fitting in children, especially evaluating the SSPL90 levels being generated in the pediatric ear canal,[219] for being smaller than the average adult canal, the potential is present for producing excessively high output levels.[220]

As a method of providing a more reliable or valid hearing aid *selection* procedure or as a *predictor* of aided success, the probe microphone measurement method as it is presently configured may prove to have less utility. First, some estimate of aided speech recognition efficiency has traditionally been considered an important element in assessing appropriateness of the fitting, but probe microphone systems utilize nonspeech stimuli. Second it appears impossible to be able to predict speech recognition behavior from an analysis of the level and shape of the spectrum at the tympanic membrane, except in a general, hypothetical way. Further, many of the instruments incorporate methodology wherein pure tone threshold levels are entered, and the microprocessor then calculates the amount of insertion gain across frequency required to correct the hearing loss, according to algorithms stored in the instrument. The actual insertion gain provided by the hearing aid as it is worn is then compared to the values specified by the formula. It is left to the clinician to decide which of the formulas is the more valid or reliable for use; each provides dissimilar insertion gains, and there is little evidence to support the superiority of one over the other.

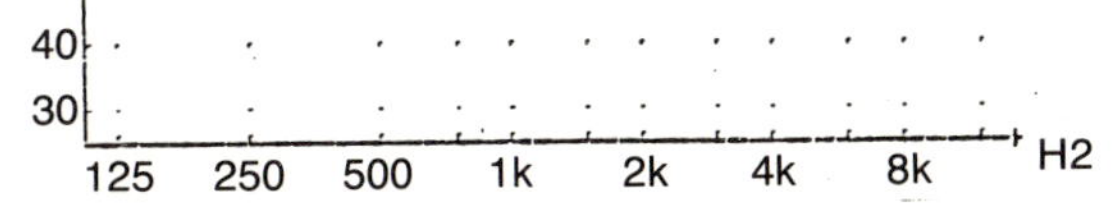

Figure 49–6 The in situ gain response shows the distribution of sound pressure in the ear canal produced by the aid as it is worn. The insertion gain is merely the difference between the unoccluded external ear resonance and the in situ response. The insertion loss is the amount of transmission loss produced by the insertion of the earmold/shell into the ear (aid off). (From Libby ER. The shift towards real ear measurements. Hear Instr 1986; 37(1):7.)

SUMMARY

At one time, subjects who had (a) poor speech discrimination, (b) sensorineural impairment, (c) thresholds better than a certain level on the audiogram, and either (d) unilateral or (e) minimal high frequency loss were automatically disqualified as candidates for hearing aids.

Currently, it is felt that few individuals who have the desire for amplification are automatically disqualified on the basis of the audiometric workup; most are candidates at least for a trial. Obviously, there are situations that invite caution; these include patients who exhibit marked sequelae to cerebral vascular episodes and geriatric patients or others with significant central findings. But simply stated, any hearing impaired individual willing to try amplification ought to be afforded the opportunity. Even further, the clinician or dispenser may be called upon to adopt a stance of positive active advocacy. The patient, as often as not, approaches amplification with caution, doubtful of success, often unwilling to admit the need for amplification. It is important to appreciate that motivating individuals to try amplification when the need is clearly apparent is a key aspect of the rehabilitative process.

REFERENCES

1. Lybarger SF. An early auditory training system. J Audio Eng Soc 1987; 35(4):270–275.
2. Knudsen VO, Jones IH. Artificial hearing aids. In: Studies of the VIII nerve. St Louis: The Laryngoscope Press, 1937:268.
3. Lybarger SF. A discussion of hearing aid trends. Int Audiol 1966; 5(3):376.
4. Lybarger SF. The acoustical engineer's viewpoint of hearing aid design. Bull NY Acad Med 1974; 15:8.
5. Hearing Industries Association. Statistical report, 4th Quarter, 1986. Washington, DC: HIA 1987; February.
6. Curran JR. Aspects of contemporary hearing aids. In: Lass NJ, McReynolds LV, Northern JL, Yoder DE, eds. Speech, Language, and Hearing. Vol. III. Philadelphia: WB Saunders, 1982:1108.
7. Szozda ME. Active filtering for hearing aids. Hear J 1987; 40(4).
8. Grosspietsch JK. The Zeta noise blocker: a basic reintroduction. Hear J 1987; 40(5).
9. Wolf HP, Powers TA. Remote control: the invisible touch. Hear J 1986; 39(10):18–20.
10. 28th annual facts and figures. Hear Aid J 1978; November.
11. Jirsa R, Norris T. Relationship of performance characteristics in hearing aids to cavity volume. Paper presented at the Annual Convention of the American Auditory Society, Las Vegas, 1977.
12. Preves D, Curran JR. Basic hearing science. In: Sandlin R, ed. Hearing instrument science and fitting practices. Livonia, MI: National Institute for Hearing Instruments Studies, 1985.
13. Libby ER. The 1/3–2/3 insertion gain hearing aid selection guide. Hear Instr 1986; 37(3):27–28.
14. Byrne D, Christen R, Dillon H. Effects of peaks in hearing aid frequency response on comfortable listening levels of normal hearing subjects. Aust J Aud 1981; 3(2):42–46.
15. Goldstein DP, Gleitman R. Experiences in dispensing in-the-canal hearing aids. Hear J 1986; 39(8):18–22.
16. Johnson EW. An analysis of 500 intra canal hearing aid fittings. Hear Instr 1985; 36(10):16–19.
17. Hearing Aid Industry Conference, Report of annual sales, 1959.
18. Maxwell RJ, Burkhard MD. Vibration isolation design. Franklin Park, IL: Knowles Electronics, 1969.
19. Sung GS, Sung RJ, Angelleli RM. Effect of frequency-response characteristics of hearing aids on speech intelligibility in noise. J Audiol Res 1971; 11:318–321.
20. Harrison A. The use of high frequency response hearing aids with moderate to severe hearing losses. Audecibel 1974; 23:137–144.
21. Danaher EM, Pickett JM. Some masking effects produced by low-frequency vowel formants in persons with sensorineural hearing loss. J Speech Hear Res 1975; 18:261–271.
22. Sweetow R. Masking effects of extended low frequency amplification. Doctoral dissertation, Northwestern University, 1976.
23. Franks JR, Staton R. Word discrimination performance using variable frequency response hearing aids. Hear Aid J 1977; 30:37–39.
24. Harford E, Fox J. The use of high-pass amplification for broad-frequency sensorineural hearing loss. Audiology 1978; 17:10–26.
25. Danaher EM, Wilson MP, Pickett JM. Backward and forward masking in listeners with severe sensorineural hearing loss. Audiology 1978; 17:324–338.
26. Trees DE, Turner CW. Spread of masking in normal subjects and in subjects with high frequency hearing loss. Audiology 1986; 25:70–83.
27. Fraim FW, Murphy PV. Miniature electret microphones. J Audiol Eng Soc 1970; 18:511–517.
28. Fraim FW, Murphy PV, Ferran RJ. Electrets in miniature microphones. J Acoust Soc Am 1973; 53:1601–1608.
29. Killion MC, Carlson EV. A sub-miniature electret condenser microphone of new design. J Audiol Eng Soc 1974; 22:237–243.
30. Skinner MW. Speech intelligibility in noise induced hearing loss: effects of high-frequency compensation. J Acoust Soc Am 1980; 67:306–317.
31. Lentz WE. A summary of research using directional and omnidirectional hearing aids. J Audiol Tech 1974; 13:44–65.
32. Mueller HG, Grimes AM, Erdman SA. Subjective ratings of directional amplification. Hear Instr 1983; 34(2):14–16; 47.
33. Hawkins DB, Yacullo WS. Signal-to-noise ratio advantage of binaural hearing aids and directional microphones under different levels of reverberations. J Speech Hear Disord 1984; 49:278–286.
34. Preves DA. Selecting the best directivity pattern for undirectional noise suppressing hearing aids. Hear Instr 1975; 26(10):18.
35. Griffing TS, Heide J. Automatic signal processor aids, part I: by definition. Hear Instr 1983;34(4):36–38.
36. Griffing TS, Heide J. Automatic signal processor aids, part II: fitting guidelines. Hear Instr 1983; 34(6):28.
37. Sigelman J, Preves DA. Field trials of a new adaptive signal processor hearing aid circuit. Hear J 1987; 40(4):24–29.
38. Krebs D. Output limiting and relative harmonic distortion. Oticongress 1972; 2:3–10.
39. Curran JR, Ely WG. Clearing the compression jungle. Hear Instr 1973; 24:17.
40. Heide J. Output limitation. Hear Instr 1974; 25(5):26–28.
41. Hogg DC. Putting compression into perspective. Hear Aid J 1976; 29(7):11.
42. Staab WJ. Hearing aid handbook. Blue Ridge Summit, PA: Tab Books, 1978.
43. Braida L, Durlach N, Lippman R, Hicks B, Rabinowitz W, Reed C. Hearing aids—a review of past research on linear amplification, amplitude compression and frequency lowering. ASHA Monogr No. 19, Rockville, MD, ASHA, 1979.
44. Sandlin RE. Advances in hearing aid technology. In: Jerger J, ed. Hearing disorders in adults. San Diego: College-Hill Press, 1984:118.
45. Libby ER. Hearing instrument systems technology and performance standards. In: Sandlin R, ed. Hearing instrument science and fitting practices. Livonia, MI: National Institute for Hearing Instruments Studies, 1985:201.
46. Smriga D. Modern compression technology-developments and applications. Hear J 1985; 38(6):28–32.
47. Buerkli-Halevy O. Hearing aid design parameters affecting performance in noise. Hear J 1986; 39(2):18–22.
48. Cole WA. Prospects for the application of high technology to hearing aids. Hear Instr 1983; 34(1):6–12.
49. Schneuwly D. Digital technology; the hearing aid and computer fittings. Hear Instr 1985; 36(1):16–17.

50. Staab WJ. Digital hearing aids. Hear Instr 1985; 36(11):14–24.
51. Nielsen B. Digital hearing aids: where are they? Hear Instr 1986; 37(2):6,45.
52. Mangold S, Leijon A. A programmable hearing aid with multichannel compression. Scand Audiol 1979; 8:121–126.
53. Mangold S, Leijon A. Multichannel compression in a portable programmable hearing aid. Hear Aid J 1981; 34(6):6,29–32.
54. Curran JR, Preves D. Microcomputers and hearing aids. In: Northern JL, ed. The personal computer for speech, language and hearing professionals. Boston: Little, Brown, 1986:209.
55. Romanow FF. Methods for measuring the performance of hearing aids. J Acoust Soc Am 1942; 13:294–304.
56. Kranz FW. Tentative code for measurement of performance of hearing aids. J Acoust Soc Am 1945; 17:144–150.
57. Mundel AB, Carlisle RS. Broadened criteria of hearing aid performance. J Acoust Soc Am 1947; 19:639–644.
58. American National Standards Institute. Electroacoustical characteristics of hearing aids. New York: ANSI 1960; standard S3.3.
59. Lybarger SF. A new HAIC standard method of expressing hearing aid performance. Hear Instr 1961; 11:16.
60. Lybarger SF. Performance measurements on ear-level hearing aids. J Audiol 1966; 5(3):376.
61. American National Standards Institute. Methods of expressing hearing aid performance. New York: ANSI 1976; standard S.322.
62. American National Standards Institute. Specification of hearing aid characteristics. New York: ANSI 1976; Standard S.322.
63. American National Standards Institute. Specification of hearing aid characteristics. New York: ANSI 1982; standard S.322.
64. Lybarger SF. Selective amplification—a review and evaluation. J Am Aud Soc 1978; 3(6):258–266.
65. Killion MC, Monser EL. CORFIG: coupler response for flat insertion gain. In: Studebaker GA, Hochberg I, eds. Acoustical factors affecting hearing aid performance. Baltimore: University Park Press, 1980:149.
66. Lybarger SF, Teder H. 2cc coupler curves to insertion gain curves: calculated and experimental results. Hear Instr 1986; 37(11):36–40.
67. Berger KS. The use of uncomfortable loudness level in hearing aid fitting. Maico Audiol Libr Series 1976; 15(2).
68. Dirks D, Kamm C. Psychometric functions for loudness discomfort and most comfortable loudness levels. J Speech Hear Res 1976; 19:613–627.
69. Dillon H, Macrae J. Derivation of design specifications for hearing aids. National Acoustic Laboratories. Commonwealth Dept. of Health, NAL Report No. 102, October, 1984.
70. Dillon H, Chew R, Deans M. Loudness discomfort level measurements and their implications for the design and fitting of hearing aids. Aust J Audiol 1984; 6(2):73–79.
71. Hawkins DB. Selection of a critical electroacoustic characteristic: SSPL90. Hear Instr 1984; 35(11):28–30.
72. Hawkins DB, Walden BE, Montgomery A, Prosek RA. Description and validation of an LDL procedure designed to select SSPL 90. Ear Hear 1987; 8(3):162–169.
73. Walker G, Dillon H, Byrne D, Christen R. The use of loudness discomfort levels for selecting the maximum output of hearing aids. Aust J Audiol 1984; 6:23–32.
74. Lotterman SH, Kasten RN. The influence of gain control rotation of nonlinear distortion in hearing aids. J Speech Hear Res 1967; 10:593–599.
75. Jerger JF, Speaks C, Malmquist C. Hearing aid performance and hearing aid selection. J Speech Hear Res 1966; 9:136–149.
76. Jerger JF, Malmquist C, Speaks C. Comparison of some speech intelligibility tests in the evaluation of hearing aid performance. J Speech Hear Res 1966; 9:253–258.
77. Jirsa RE, Hodgson WR. Effects of harmonic distortion in hearing aids on speech intelligibility for normals and hypacusics. J Audiol Res 1970; 10:213–217.
78. Jerger JF. Behavioral correlates of hearing aid performance. Bull Prosthet Res 1967; 10:62–75.
79. Witter HL, Goldstein DP. Quality judgments of hearing aid transduced speech. J Speech Hear Res 1971; 14:312–322.
80. Briskey RJ, Wruk K. Acoustic influence of insert vents. Hear Instr 1974; 25:12–14.
81. Ely WG. A primer in distortion in hearing aids. Hear Aid J 1974; 27(8):10–11,34.
82. Burnett ED. A new method for the measurement of nonlinear distortion using a random noise test signal. Bull Prosthet Res 1967; 10:79–92.
83. Olson WO. The influence of harmonic and intermodulation distortion of speech intelligibility. Scand Audiol 1971; 1:109–125.
84. Curran JR. Harmonic distortion and intelligibility. Hear Aid J 1974; 27(8):12,39.
85. Schweitzer HC, Causey CD, Bowling LS, Howard MT. The influence of hearing aid nonlinear distortion on two auditory tasks. J Am Audiol Soc 1979; 4:132–140.
86. Harris JD, Haines HL, Kelsey PA, Clack TD. The relation between speech intelligibility and the electroacoustic characteristics of low frequency circuitry. J Audiol Res 1961; 1:357–381.
87. Bode DL, Kasten RN. Hearing aid distortion and consonant identification. J Speech Hear Res 1971; 14:323–331.
88. Chial MR, Hayes CS. Hearing aid evaluation methods: some underlying assumptions. J Speech Hear Disord 1974; 39:270–279.
89. Schweitzer HC, Causey GD, Tolton MC. Nonlinear distortion in hearing aids: the need for reevaluation of measurement philosophy and technique. J Am Audiol Soc 1977; 2:132–141.
90. Olson WO, Carhart R. Development of test procedures for evaluation of binaural hearing aids. Bull Prosthet Res 1967; 10:22–49.
91. Jerger J, Thelin J. Effects of electric acoustic characteristics of hearing aids on speech understanding. Bull Prosthet Res 1968; 10:159–197.
92. Burkhard MD, Sachs RM. Anthropometric manikin for acoustic research. J Acoust Soc Am 1975; 58:214–222.
93. Zwislocki JJ. An acoustic coupler for earphone calibration. Rep. LSC-S-7, Lab Sensory Communication, Syracuse University, 1970.
94. Zwislocki JJ. An ear-like coupler for earphone calibration. Rep. LSC-S-9, Lab Sensory Communication, Syracuse University, 1971.
95. American National Standards Institute. For an occluded ear simulator. New York: ANSI 1979; standard S3.25.
96. American National Standards Institute. Methods of measurement of performance characteristics of hearing aids under simulated in-situ working conditions. New York: ANSI 1985; standard S3.35.
97. Beck LB, Causey GD. A comparison of orthotelephonic and substitution measurement methods on KEMAR. Paper presented at the Annual Convention of the American Speech and Hearing Association, Chicago, 1977.
98. Kuhn GF, Burnett ED. The acoustic pressure field alongside a manikin's head with a view towards in-situ hearing aid tests. J Acoust Soc Am 1977; 17:144–150.
99. Dunn HK, White SD. Statistical measurements on conversational speech. J Acoust Soc Am 1940; 11:278–288.
100. Stephens SS, Egan JP, Miller GA. Methods of measuring speech spectra. J Acoust Soc Am 1947; 19:771–780.
101. Wiener F, Ross D. The pressure distribution in the audi-

tory canal in a progressive sound field. J Acoust Soc Am 1946; 18:401–408.
102. Berland O, Nielson TE. Sound pressure generated in the human external ear canal by a free sound field. Sound 1969; 3:78–81.
103. Shaw EAG. Transformation of sound pressure for the free field to the eardrum in the horizontal plan. J Acoust Soc Am 1974; 56:1848–1861.
104. Niemoller AF, McCormick L, Miller JD. On the spectrum of spoken English. J Acoust Soc Am 1974; 55:461(A).
105. Pascoe DP. An approach to hearing aid selection. Hear Instr 1978; 29(6):12–16,38.
106. Dalsgaard SC. On insertion gain. In: Burkhaurd M, ed. Manikin measurements. Elk Grove, IL: Knowles Electronics, 1978.
107. Byrne DJ. Some implications of body-baffle for hearing aid selection. Sound 1972; 6:86–91.
108. Erber NP. Body-baffle and real ear effects in the selection of hearing-aid units for deaf children. J Speech Hear Disord 1973; 38:224–231.
109. Lybarger SF, Barron FE. Head baffle effect for different hearing aid microphone locations. J Acoust Soc Am 1965; 38:922(A).
110. Randolph K, Gierala V, Ross M. Hearing aid microphone location and speech discrimination: hearing impaired adults. Paper presented at the Annual Convention of the American Speech and Hearing Association, Chicago, 1977.
111. Kuhn GF, Guernsey RM. Sound pressure distribution about the human head and torso. J Acoust Soc Am 1983; 73(1):95–105.
112. Kuhn GF. The pressure transformation from a diffuse sound field to the external ear and to the body and head surface. J Acoust Soc Am 1979; 65(4):991–1000.
113. Hoke ML. Improving speech discrimination in noise. Hear Instr 1976; 27(8).
114. Killion MC, Wilson DL. Response modifying earhooks for special fitting problems. Audecibel 1985; 24(4):28–30.
115. Goldstein BA. Effect of discrimin/indiscriminate placement of sintered hearing aid filters. Paper presented at ASHA Annual Convention, Atlanta, 1979.
116. McDonald FD, Studebaker GA. Earmold alteration effects as measured in the human auditory meatus. J Acoust Soc Am 1970; 48:1366–1372.
117. Cox R. Acoustic aspects of hearing aid-earmold coupling. Monogr Contemp Audiol 1979; 1(3).
118. Lybarger SF. Earmold venting as an acoustical control factor. In: Studebaker GA, Hochberg I, eds. Acoustical factors affecting hearing aid performance. Baltimore: University Park Press, 1980:197.
119. Courtois J, Berland O. No-mold fittings. Audecibel 1972; 21:171–181.
120. Courtois J, Berland O. No-mold fittings. Audecibel 1973; 22:28–29.
121. Lyregaard PE. Improvement of the high frequency performance of BTE hearing aids. Hear Instr 1982; 33(2):38–43,62.
122. Dillon H. Earmolds and high frequency response modification. Hear Instr 1985; 36(12):8–12.
123. Surr RK, Scherr CK, Williams BS. Earmold selection for high frequency hearing loss. Hear Instr 1984; 35(11):17–21.
124. Mynders JM. Human acoustic couplers. In: Sandlin R, ed. Hearing instrument science and fitting practices. Livonia, MI: National Institute for Hearing Instruments Studies, 1985.
125. Microsonic Custom Earmold Manual. Revised 4th Ed. Ambridge, PA, 1986.
126. Studebaker GA, Cox RM, Wark DJ. Earmold modification effects measured by coupler, threshold and probe techniques. Audiology 1978; 17:173–185.
127. Macrae J. Acoustic modification of hearing aids. Hear Instr 1985; 36(12):13–15.
128. Ely WG. Electroacoustic modification of hearing aids. In: Bess F, Freeman B, Sinclair J, eds. Amplification in education. Washington: AG Bell, 1981.
129. Northern JL, Downs MP. Hearing in children. 3rd ed. Baltimore: Williams & Wilkins, 1984:289.
130. Bratt GW, Sander JW, Larson VD. Occluded ear canal volume and SPL in children. Paper presented at ASHA Annual Convention, Detroit, 1980.
131. Gilman S, Dirks DP, Stern R. The effect of occluded ear impedances on the eardrum SPL produced by hearing aids. J Acoust Soc Am 1981; 70(2):370–386.
132. Hudde H. Measurement of the eardrum impedance of human ears. J Acoust Soc Am 1983; 73(1):242–243.
133. Rabinowitz W. Measurement of the acoustic input immittance of the human ear. J Acoust Soc Am 1981; 70(4):1025–1035.
134. Egolf DP, Feth LL, Cooper WA, Franks JR. Effects of normal and pathologic eardrum impedance on sound pressure in the aided ear canal: a computer simulation. J Acoust Soc Am 1985; 78(4):1281–1285.
135. Preves DA, Orton JF. Use of acoustic impedance measures in hearing aid fitting. Hear Instr 1978; 29(6):22–24,34.
136. Navarro MR. Hearing aid fitting as an impedance matching process. Hear Instr, 1982; 33(2):28.
137. Cox RM. Functional correlates of electroacoustic performance data. In: Studebaker GA, Bess FH, eds. The Vanderbilt hearing aid report. Philadelphia: Monogr Contem Audiol, 1982.
138. Carhart R. The selection of hearing aids. Arch Otolaryngol 1946; 44:1–18.
139. Carhart R. Tests for the selection of hearing aids. Laryngoscope 1946; 56:780–794.
140. Carhart R. Hearing aid selection by university clinics. J Speech Hear Disord 1950; 15:105–113.
141. Carhart R. Hearing aid selection by university clinics. J Speech Hear Disord 1950; 15:105–113.
142. McConnell F, Silber EF, McDonald D. Test-retest consistency of clinical hearing aid tests. J Speech Hear Disord 1960; 25:273–280.
143. Shore I, Bilger RC, Hirsh I. Hearing aid evaluation: reliability of repeated measurements. J Speech Hear Disord 1960; 25:152–170.
144. Zerlin S. A new approach to hearing aid selection. J Speech Hear Res 1962; 5:370–376.
145. Resnick DM, Becker M. Hearing aid evaluation . . . a new approach. Asha 1963; 5:695–699.
146. Jeffers J, Smith CR. On hearing aid selection—in part a reply to Resnick and Becker. Asha 1964; 6:504–506.
147. Reddell RC, Calvert DR. Selecting a hearing aid by interpreting audiogram data. J Audiol Res 1966; 6:445–452.
148. Thompson G, Lassman F. Listener preferences for selective vs. flat amplification for a high-frequency hearing loss population. J Speech Hear Res 1970; 13:670–672.
149. Millin JP. Practical and philosophical consideration. In: Pollack M, ed. Amplification for the hearing impaired. New York: Grune & Stratton, 1975.
150. Shapiro I. Hearing aid fitting by prescription. Audiology 1976; 15:164–173.
151. Collins MJ, Levitt H. Comparison of methods for predicting optimum fractional gain. In: Studebaker GA, Hochberg I, eds. Acoustical factors affecting hearing aid performance. Baltimore: University Park Press, 1980.
152. Cox RM. A structured approach to hearing aid selection. Ear Hear 1985; 6(5):226–239.
153. Byrne D, Dillon H. The National Acoustic Laboratories (NAL) new procedure for selecting the gain and frequency response of a hearing aid. Ear Hear 1986; 7(4):257–265.
154. Schwartz DM. Hearing aid selection methods: an enigma.

In: Studebaker GA, Bess FH, eds. The Vanderbilt hearing aid report. Upper Darby, PA: Monogr Contem Audiol, 1982.

155. Skinner MW, Pascoe DP, Miller JD, Popelka GR. Measurements to determine the optimal placement for speech energy within the listener's auditory area: a basis for selecting amplification characteristics. In: Studebaker GA, Bess FH, eds. The Vanderbilt hearing aid report. Upper Darby, PA: Monogr Contemp Audiol, 1982.
156. Schachterle BD. Hearing aid selection: one dispenser's point of view. In: Curran J, guest ed. Patterns in private practice dispensing. Seminars in hearing. New York: Thieme, 1986:7(2):199.
157. Seiler J. A formula for fitting hearing aids. Hear Dealer 1971; 22(3):18–19,30.
158. Berger KW. Prescription of hearing aids: a rationale. J Am Aud Soc 1976; 2(3): 71–78.
159. Byrne DJ, Tonisson W. Selecting the gain of hearing aids for persons with sensorineural hearing impairment. Scand Audiol 1976; 5:51–59.
160. Berger KW, Hagberg EN, Rane RL. Prescription of hearing aids: rationale, procedures and results. Kent, OH: Herold Publishing House, 1977.
161. Berger KW, Hagberg EN, Rane RL. A method of hearing aid prescription. Hear Instr 1978; 29(6):12–13.
162. McCandless GA, Lyregaard PE. Prescription of gain/output (POGO) for hearing aids. Hear Instr 1983; 34(1):16–21.
163. Libby ER. The shift towards real ear measurements. Hear Instr 1986; 37(1):6–7,50.
164. Libby ER, Northern JL, Sullivan RF. Clinical application of probe microphone real ear measurements. Audiol Acoust 1986; 25(2):42–53.
165. Pascoe DP. Frequency responses of hearing aids and their effects on the speech perception of hearing impaired subjects. Am J Otol Rhinol Laryngol [Suppl] 1975; 84(23).
166. Lawrence DW, Blackledge V. Protocol for evaluation of the effect of hearing aid electroacoustic parameters on the perception of amplified speech. J Am Aud Soc 1977; 2:197–201.
167. Lawrence DW, Halladay H, Blackledge VO. Listener performance as a criteria for setting frequency selection parameters of hearing instruments, part I. Audiol Hear Educ 1977; 3(2):26.
168. Lawrence DW, Halladay H, Blackledge VO. Listener performance as a criteria for setting frequency selection parameters of hearing instruments, part II. Audiol Hear Educ 1977; 3(3):18.
169. Levitt H, Collins MJ. An experimental proticol for the prescriptive fitting of a wearable master hearing aid. In: Studebaker GA, Hochberg I, eds. Acoustical factors affecting hearing aid performance. Baltimore: University Park Press, 1980.
170. Miller JD, Niemoeller AF, Pascoe D, Skinner MW. Integration of the electroacoustic description of hearing aids with the audiologic description of clients. In: Studebaker GA, Hochberg I, eds. Acoustical factors affecting hearing aid performance. Baltimore: University Park Press, 1980.
171. Franks JR. The master hearing aid. In: Yanick P, Freifeld S, eds. The application of signal processing concepts to hearing aids. New York: Grune & Stratton, 1978:85.
172. Zelnick E. Review of suggested hearing aid procedures. In: Zelnick E, ed. Hearing instrument selection and evaluation. Livonia, MI: National Institute for Hearing Instrument Studies, 1987:25.
173. Voroba B. Perspectives on the state of hearing aid fitting practices. Audecibel 1982; 31:12–16.
174. Voroba B. A tool for the optimization of hearing aid fittings. Hear Instr 1984; 35(1):12–16.
175. Schwartz DM, Walden BE. Speech audiometry and hearing aid assessment: a reappraisal of an old philosophy. In: Konkle D, Rintelman W, eds. Principles of speech audiometry. Baltimore: University Park Press, 1983:321.
176. Mueller HG, guest ed. Binaural amplification special issue. Hear J 1986; 39(11).
177. Orton JF. Acoustic modification for custom in-the-ear aids, earmolds, current practice and technology, 1984. Br Soc Audiol 1984.
178. Orton JF. Perfecting your craft; the fine art of in-office ITE modification. Hear J 1984; 37(10):7–15.
179. Schwartz DM, Larson VD. Hearing aid selection and evaluation procedures for young children. In: Bess FN, ed. Childhood deafness: causation, assessment and management, New York: Grune & Stratton, 1977:217.
180. Seewald RC, Ross M, Spiro MK. Selecting amplification characteristics for young hearing impaired children. Ear Hear 1985; 6(1):48–53.
181. Wullstein HL, Wigand ME. A hearing aid for binaural hearing for single ear deafness and its requirements. Acta Otolaryngol (Stockh) 1962; 54:136–142.
182. Harford E. Innovations in the use of modern hearing aids. Int Audiol 1967; 6:311–321.
183. Dodds E, Harford E. Modified earpieces and CROS for high frequency hearing losses. J Speech Hear Res 1968; 11:204–218.
184. Dodds E, Harford E. Follow-up report on modified earpieces and CROS for high frequency hearing losses. J Speech Hear Res 1970; 13:41–43.
185. Dunlavy AR. CROS: the new miracle worker. Audecibel 1970; 19:141–148.
186. Curran JR. Understanding and using CROS fittings and open-canal amplification. Hear Instr 1971; 22(8):22–26,40.
187. Schuneman JR, Viscomi GJ. Open canal amplification. Trans Am Acad Ophthalmol Otolaryngol 1974; 78:256–260.
188. Green DS, Ross M. The effect of a conventional versus a nonoccluding (CROS-type) earmold upon the frequency response of a hearing aid. J Speech Hear Res 1968; 11:638–647.
189. Harford E, Dodds E. Versions of the CROS Hearing aid. Arch Otolaryngol 1974; 100:50–58.
190. Pollack M. Special applications of amplification. In: Pollack M, ed. Amplification for the hearing impaired. New York: Grune & Stratton. 1975:243.
191. DeMers V. The open mold application in difficult fits. Hear Aid J 1950; 3:20.
192. Lybarger SF. Earmold acoustics. Audecibel 1967: 16:9–19.
193. Studebaker GA. The acoustical effect of various factors on the frequency response of hearing aid receiver. J Audiol Eng Soc 1974; 22:329–334.
194. Studebaker GA, Cox RM. Side branch and parallel effects of real ears and in acoustical and electrical models. J Am Audiol Soc 1977; 3:108–117.
195. Sung RJ, Sung GS, Hodgson WR. Acoustic influence of select-a-vent earmold and tone tube modifications on hearing aid performance. J Am Audiol Soc 1975; 1:15–20.
196. Killion MC. Problems in the application of broadband hearing aid earphones. In: Studebaker GA, Hochberg I, eds. Acoustical factors affecting hearing aid performance. Baltimore: University Park Press, 1980.
197. Macrae J. A new kind of earmold vent-the high-cut cavity vent. Hear Instr 1981; 32(10):18, 64.
198. Macrae J. Venting without feedback-further developments of the high-cut cavity vent. Hear Instr 1983; 33(4):12–14, 42.
199. Mueller HG, Schwartz DM, Surr RK. The use of the exponential horn in an open mold configuration. Hear Instr 1981; 32(10):16–18, 64.
200. Killion MC. Recent earmolds for wideband BTE and ITE hearing aids. Hear J 1984; 37(8):15–22.
201. McClellan ME. Aided speech discrimination in noise with

vented and unvented earmolds. J Audiol Res 1967; 7:93–100.
202. Green DS. Nonoccluding earmolds with CROS and IROS hearing aids. Arch Otolaryngal 1969; 89:96–102.
203. Weatherton MA, Goetzinger CP. The effects of various modified earmolds on hearing sensitivity. J Audiol Res 1970; 25–32.
204. Frank TA, Karlovich RS. Ear canal frequency response and speech discrimination performance as a function of hearing aid earmold type. J Audiol Res 1973; 13:124–129.
205. Konkle DF, Bess FH. Custom made vs. stock earmolds in hearing aid evaluations. Arch Otolaryngol 1974; 99:140–144.
206. Hodgson WR, Murdock C. Effect of the earmold on speech intelligibility in hearing aid use. J Speech Hear Res 1970; 13:290–297.
207. Jetty AJ, Rintleman WF. Acoustic coupler effects on speech audiometric scores using a CROS hearing aid. J Speech Hear Res 1970; 13:101–114.
208. Libby ER. Achieving a transparent, smooth, wideband hearing aid response. Hear Instr 1981; 32(10):9–12.
209. Sullivan RF. Part I: an acoustic coupling-based classification system for hearing aid fittings. Hear Instr 1985; 36(9):25–28.
210. Sullivan RF. Parts II and III: an acoustic coupling-based classification system for hearing aid fittings. Hear Instr 1985; 36(12):16–23.
211. Plotkin W. Report on the use of modified earmolds in the selection of hearing aids. Paper presented at Annual Convention of ASHA, 1962.
212. Mueller HG, Sweetow RW. A clinical comparison of probe microphone measurements systems. Hear Instr 1987; 38(6):20–21, 57.
213. Hawkins DB, Schum DJ. Relationships between various measures of hearing aid gain. J Speech Hear Disord, 1984; 49:94–111.
214. Madsen PB. Insertion gain optimization. Hear Instr 1986; 37(1):28–32.
215. Zemplenyi J, Dirks D, Gilman D. Probe-determined hearing aid gains compared to functional and coupler gains. J Speech Hear Disord 1985; 28:394–404.
216. Mason D, Popelka GR. Comparison of hearing aid gain using functional, coupler and probe-tube measurements. J Speech Hear Disord 1986; 29:218–226.
217. Hawkins DB, Montgomery AA, Prosek RA, Walden BE. Examination of two issues concerning functional gain measurements. J Speech Hear Disord 1987; 52:56–63.
218. Macrae J. Invalid aided thresholds. Hear Instr 1982; 33(9):20–22.
219. Harford E, Leijon A, Liden G, Ringdahl A, Dahlberg AK. A simplified real ear technique for verifying the maximum output of a hearing aid. Ear Hear 1983; 4(3).
220. Gabbard SA, Northern J. Real ear hearing instruments measurements in children. Hear Instr 1987; 38(9):11–13, 67.

50 Pediatric Audiology

Allan O. Diefendorf, Ph.D.

Pediatric audiology is entering its fifth decade as a specialized area of auditory assessment and educational management. Consistent with the nature of growth, certain milestones were achieved that have been pivotal in the development of this specialty area.

From the early work of Ewing and Ewing,[1] Hardy, Pauls, and Bordley,[2] and Myklebust,[3] the inception of pediatric audiology was seen when it became obvious that some segment of the health care community must be responsible for the identification and management of hearing impaired children. Subsequently, the importance of pediatric audiology was established when it became unquestionably clear that unidentified hearing loss can have dramatic effects on early speech and language acquisition; and with delayed or impaired communication capabilities, a child may also be delayed cognitively, socially, and emotionally.[4] Pediatric audiology grew significantly when the prevalence of hearing loss was determined (one of every 1,000 to 2,000 live births and significantly greater than that among certain high-risk neonates).[5] These data pointed out that hearing loss should be a high-priority disorder in need of screening as early as birth.

The past decade in pediatric audiology has matured rather significantly by broadening its focus from deafness to hearing. Peripheral and central hearing disorders are being investigated with greater precision, and test procedures coupled with a better understanding of auditory behavior are resulting in more accurate assessment of hearing loss. Unilateral hearing losses, mild hearing losses, high-frequency hearing losses, severe to profound hearing losses, and central hearing skills are being identified earlier.

The need for appropriate intervention and management of these children certainly appears to be the major thrust of pediatric audiology today. However, early educational management for hearing loss can be provided only if assessment is effective and accurate. Thus auditory assessment continues to be a major component of pediatric audiology. This chapter is intended to highlight the important developments in pediatric audiology and focus on the significant advances made in pediatric hearing assessment over the past two decades. A philosophy that must prevail in this chapter is that auditory assessment is only the first step in providing a comprehensive management plan.

Although different investigators have indicated that the suspicion of hearing impairment occurs early in the first year of life, few children are actually diagnosed within their first year.[6–8] However, of greater concern than the number of hearing impaired children who are diagnosed late is the additional suggestion from these data that amplification assessment and habilitative planning are not initiated until the child is almost $2^1/_2$ years of age. Therefore this chapter is written on the following presumption: early assessment of hearing impairment must be followed up with a comprehensive plan of educational management, and, without such a plan, any program of screening and assessment for hearing impairment is, by itself, incomplete.

IDENTIFICATION OF AUDITORY PROBLEMS

Neonatal Screening

The desirability of early detection of hearing loss in infants led to experimentation with mass auditory screening of neonates. Large scale efforts to detect hearing loss through neonatal audiometric screening, often referred to as identification audiometry, got underway in the 1960s. Marion Downs and her associates pioneered these efforts;[9–11] however, many of the programs were probably not as well controlled nor executed as well as the Downs' program, and most were not successful.

Subsequently, in 1970, the United States Joint

Committee on Infant Hearing Screening was formed with representatives from the American Academy of Ophthalmology and Otolaryngology, the American Academy of Pediatrics, and the American Speech-Language-Hearing Association. The Joint Committee addressed itself to the use of behavioral tests of screening (monitoring of changes in the infant's state following presentation of high-intensity signals) in the newborn nursery, which had been previously proposed. Generally, the Joint Committee agreed that screening programs were not identifying deaf infants successfully and that the large number of false-positives were not only time and cost ineffective, but were also causing unnecessary parental anxiety. Following this review, the Joint Committee issued a statement that did not recommend mass behavioral screening, although it urged increased research efforts.

By inspecting unfavorable genetic histories and prenatal and perinatal health problems, it soon became apparent that certain aspects of the medical history could be used for identifying infants at risk for hearing loss. A report by Feinmesser and Tell provided strong evidence for using "risk factors for deafness" as a screening tool instead of behavioral screening.[12] These investigators saw a total of 17,731 newborns over a period of 3 years. At birth, the infants were given behavioral screening and were also subjected to a high-risk categorization. Twenty-three deaf children were identified by the end of the program; 17 of them had been on the high-risk register (26 percent false-negative rate), and only six had been identified by behavioral screening (74 percent false-negative rate). Their high-risk register included the following items:

1. Familial deafness.
2. Rubella during pregnancy.
3. Birth weight of 1,500 grams (3.3 pounds) or less.
4. Congenital craniofacial malformations.
5. Apgar score of 1 to 4.[12a,12b]
6. Hyperbilirubinemia: 20 mg per 100 ml and over.
7. Severe infections (neonatal).

The Joint Committee seriously considered the outcome of the Feinmesser and Tell study and, in a supplementary statement in 1973, recommended the use of a high-risk register to identify neonates in whom the probability of hearing loss could be expected to be higher than normal. The high-risk register is not really a register since children are not registered per se, except, of course, in those states where the program is so structured or mandated by law. The list of guidelines (the items on the register) includes those factors most likely to cause hearing loss; thus the register offers a pool from which the largest number of hearing impaired children is likely to be found. Mencher has suggested that the accuracy of the high-risk register (the theoretical maximum detection rate by a five-point register) is on the order of 66 percent.[13]

In 1982 the Joint Committee expanded and clarified the 1972 criteria (Table 50–1). The Joint Committee also recommended that infants identified by the high-risk register receive follow-up screening by no later than 3 months of age and that periodic reevaluation be performed if necessary to determine the status of the infants' hearing. In addition, the Joint Committee recommended that the diagnostic process be completed in infants suspected of having hearing loss and that habilitation be initiated by the age of 6 months. This recommendation reflects the widely accepted view that early identification and intervention is crucial for the language, cognitive, emotional, and social development of the hearing impaired child.

In a retrospective study by Stein, Clark, and Kraus, 25 to 30 percent of their hearing impaired children ($N = 108$) did not manifest any of the risk factors proposed in the 1982 Position Statement.[8] Further, Pappas studied 109 hearing impaired children retrospectively and found that only 46 percent would have routinely appeared among those infants with high-risk factors had the 1982 registry alone been used.[14] These studies point out the limitations of the high-risk register and indicate the need to use the high-risk register in conjunction with other screening techniques and follow-up procedures. The four procedures available for use in conjunction with the high-risk screening are behavioral observation audiometry, crib-o-gram, the auditory brain stem response, and immittance audiometry.

Behavioral Screening

Historical precedent has favored the approach of behavioral observation procedures, termed "be-

TABLE 50–1 1982 Joint Committee Expanded High-Risk Criteria

Family history of childhood hearing impairment
Congenital perinatal infection (e.g., cytomegalovirus, rubella, herpes, toxoplasmosis, syphilis)
Anatomic malformations involving the head or neck (e.g., dysmorphic appearance including syndromal and nonsyndromal abnormalities, overt or submucous cleft palate, morphologic abnormalities of the pinna)
Birth weight <1,500 g
Hyperbilirubinemia at level exceeding indications for exchange transfusion
Bacterial meningitis, especially *Haemophilus influenzae*
Severe asphyxia, which may include infants with Apgar scores of 0 to 3 or who fail to institute spontaneous respiration by 10 minutes and those with hypertonia persisting to 2 hours of age

havioral observation audiometry." Here, although the response is active, the infant is viewed as being passively involved with his or her environment. A typical method would be the introduction of measured noises into an adequate sound room where the infant is in a light sleep, or at least quiet, and the observation of various overt responses from the infant.

The controversy over newborn hearing screening using behavioral screening procedures (behavioral observation audiometry) can be examined by comparing the Feinmesser and Tell[12,15] investigations with investigations completed by Mencher[16] and Downs.[17] The high number of false-positives (307) and false-negatives (17) indicated that Feinmesser and Tell's behavioral screening procedures (motor responses from *awake* infants) were inefficient and invalid.

However, Mencher detected hearing loss in neonates through a combination of a high-risk register and a behavioral screening procedure.[16] Initially, 10,000 infants were seen, and 80 percent were followed up for a period of 2 years. The follow-up evaluations confirmed nine babies having auditory impairment. Of the nine babies, seven would have been identified by screening only (use of narrow-band noise to arouse the infant from light sleep), and five would have been detected by the high-risk register. Two babies had passed both the behavioral screening and a high-risk classification. Mencher concluded that both behavioral screening and a high-risk register are necessary for neonatal screening.

Moreover, Downs reported results that demonstrated impressive agreement for detecting hearing loss in neonates through a combination of behavioral screening and a high-risk register.[17] Of 3,681 infants screened, five were found to have auditory impairment. Those five were identified by both behavioral screening and the high-risk register. Downs used the register proposed by the Joint Committee on Infant Hearing Screening[18] and an arousal response from a light sleep. Although the possibility of false-negatives was not followed, Downs' data revealed only 18 false-positives in her population (<0.5 percent).

It appears from Downs' study, and the report by Mencher,[16] that an arousal response from a light sleep is a more valid response than reflexive behavior from awake infants and that the use of this criterion results in fewer false-positives when identifying hearing loss in neonates. When motor responses are observed from awake infants, the false-positive rate is increased tremendously, and behavioral screening becomes inefficient as a screening procedure.[12] Hodgson concluded from a review of the literature that behavioral screening of neonates is valid and efficient only when the babies are tested in a quiet room and arousal from light sleep is the criterion response.[19] Still, among the criticisms levied against behavioral observation techniques are observer and response pattern variables, stimulus variables, preinformation bias, contamination of environmental factors, and logistical complication; all of which can lead to high false-positive rates and unacceptable false-negative rates.

The Nova Scotia Conference on early identification of hearing loss recommended procedural approaches that may reduce or remove the effects of these several types of bias.[20] However, one difficulty that remains is the fact that the signal levels used in behavioral observation audiometry testing with neonates would, at best, identify only those infants with severe to profound losses. However, as pointed out by Downs, "in order to secure hearing tests on all infants by the age of six months, we must compromise with our highest expectations and return to some of the older basics of testing, at least for the immediately foreseeable future" (p 148)[21] With the data available from Stein et al[8] and Pappas,[14] clearly screening hearing beyond the high-risk register is necessary in the newborn nursery.

If behavioral observation audiometry is elected as a screening procedure for moderately severe to profound hearing loss, the recommendations of the Nova Scotia Conference should be followed.[20] The conference recommended that the infant be asleep prior to testing. Further, the test stimulus recommended is a predominately high-frequency complex signal with a sharp rise time, a maximum sound pressure level (SPL) of 90 dB, and a duration of one-half to 2 seconds. The "arousal response" stipulated can be any generalized body movement that involves more than one limb and is accompanied by some form of eye movement. They suggested one of two scoring criteria: that the observer not know when a signal is presented or that two observers score the infant's response independently. Finally, the conference recommended that two or more responses out of eight stimuli be a passing score. An acceptable ambient noise level was not recommended by this conference; however, the noise level should probably not exceed 60-dB SPL, as recommended by Northern and Downs.[22,23]

Jacobson and Morehouse[24] evaluated the behavioral procedure recommended by the Nova Scotia Conference and adopted by the Joint Committee[25] for screening hearing in the newborn nursery, using the auditory brain stem response as the standard. Based on their referral criteria, 349 infants received both assessment techniques. With the behavioral observation audiometry procedure, 60.2 percent of the infants failed compared to 13.7 percent of the infants when tested by the auditory brain stem response. Further, only 39.7 percent of the infants passed the behavioral observation audiometry screening, whereas 86.3 percent passed the auditory brain stem response testing. Of the 43 infants who failed the initial auditory brain stem response testing, 14 passed a subsequent test and 27 failed. Nineteen infants had mild conductive abnormalities in at least one ear, whereas the remaining eight had confirmed sensorineural hearing losses.

Two measures designed to describe test validity are sensitivity (the ability to correctly identify infants with hearing loss) and specificity (the ability to correctly identify normal hearing infants; see Fig. 50–1). On the basis of the initial auditory brain stem response test outcome, the sensitivity and specificity values for the behavioral screen were 87.5 percent and 13.4 percent respectively. From the findings of Jacobson and Morehouse, sensitivity performance was gained at the expense of the specificity measure.[24] The high rate of false-positives in this comparison resulted in a poor efficiency value for the behavioral screen.

Crib-O-Gram

Simmons and Russ[26] and Simmons[27] developed an automated procedure, the crib-o-gram for neonatal screening. The crib-o-gram monitors relatively diffuse respiratory and/or motor movements without requiring physical attachment to the infant. The technique involves a motion sensitive transducer placed beneath or in an infant's crib that is capable of detecting virtually any motor activity stronger than an eye blink or facial grimace.

The crib-o-gram is a timed, self-cycling system that turns on and shuts off following each complete stimulus presentation and response measurement interval. The current version of the crib-o-gram is a microprocessor unit, which performs the test and scores and interprets the results. Twenty times in a 24-hour period, the recorder is activated for approximately 17 seconds. Each cycle consists of recording baseline motor activity (12 seconds), presentation of a 92-dB, narrow-band (2,000 to 4,000 Hz) noise (1 second), and motion monitoring continuing for another 4 seconds before stopping. The cycle includes built-in control periods during which recordings are made, but actual presentation of the signal does not occur. Auditory response is determined by a comparison of movements recorded before and after the test signal. Responses in the form of baby movement (or lack of responses) are relayed to the microprocessor, which automatically determines whether or not the neonate has met the criteria required to pass the screening.

The crib-o-gram can be multichanneled to monitor multiple cribs or used in single units for special high-risk newborns. Both the individual and group test systems are extremely sensitive in detecting motor activity from the infant. Since both stimulus presentation and analysis of the response are controlled by the microprocessor, a nurse can perform the screening without the presence of an audiologist.

Simmons, McFarland, and Jones[28] and Sim-

POPULATION

	With hearing loss	**Without hearing loss**
Postive test results	Have hearing loss Have positive test = True positives (TP)	No hearing loss Have positive results = False positives (FP)
Negative test results	Have hearing loss Have negative test = False negatives (FN)	No hearing loss Have negative test = True negatives (TN)

Sensitivity (in %)

$$\frac{TP}{TP + FN} \times 100$$

Specificity (in %)

$$\frac{TN}{TN + FP} \times 100$$

Figure 50–1 Evaluating the accuracy of an assessment procedure: sensitivity and specificity.

mons[29] have reported data on more than 12,000 babies tested with the crib-o-gram, detecting and establishing firm diagnosis of hearing loss in 42 babies—an incidence of 1:1,000 in the well baby nursery (WBN) and 1:52 in the intensive care nursery (ICN). Of the 42 deaf babies, Simmons considers only two to be screening failures (false-negatives) that were identified at a later date. The data from the Stanford group suggest a false-positive rate of approximately 8 percent for the well babies and 20 percent for the intensive care babies. McFarland, Simmons, and Jones report sensitivity rates (percentage of hearing impaired babies detected) and specificity rates (percentage of normal hearing children who pass the screen) for the crib-o-gram.[28] Sensitivity for the WBN was 91 percent and the ICN was 82 percent. Specificity for the WBN was 92 percent and for the ICN 79 percent. McFarland et al concluded that the poor specificity in the ICN is likely due to the fact that ICN babies are generally less responsive to all external stimuli because of their poor health and weakened condition.[28]

Durieux-Smith, Picton, Edwards, Goodman, and MacMurray evaluated the crib-o-gram as a screening test for hearing loss in the ICN, using the auditory brain stem response as the standard.[30] With regard to false-positives and false-negatives, the results of this study indicated that approximately one-third of infants with auditory brain stem response levels of 30 dB hearing level (HL) failed the crib-o-gram screening (false-positives), whereas some of the infants with hearing losses that require medical or audiologic management were not identified by the crib-o-gram (false-negatives). Sensitivity reached 100 percent when a pass criterion of 50 dB HL was used for the auditory brain stem response. Further, because of the high rate of failures in the ICN, Duriuex-Smith et al suggested that the reliability of the crib-o-gram is better for infants of 38 weeks gestation and older.[30]

Simmons et al[28] and Simmons[31] have concluded that the crib-o-gram offers considerable promise as an automated newborn hearing screening system, effective in detecting not just severe to profound hearing loss, but moderate hearing loss as well. The research data would support this conclusion. Simmons and his associates continue to update their statistics and have cautioned that at least 100,000 infants must be screened and followed to establish firm confidence levels with the technique.

The Auditory Brain Stem Response

During the later part of the 1970s, two international conferences on newborn screening were convened: one in Nova Scotia[20] and the other in Saskatoon.[32] The conferees resolved that the auditory brain stem response was a viable screening test for the high-risk newborn population. As stated earlier, in its 1982 statement, the Joint Committee on Infant Hearing subsequently endorsed the "audiologic testing" of high-risk newborns because of the 2.5 to 5.0 percent associated incidence of moderate to profound hearing loss and suggested that the initial screening of these newborns should include the observation of behavioral or electrophysiologic responses to sound.

The ability to assess accurately infant peripheral auditory and neurologic function has been enhanced greatly by the introduction of auditory brain stem response audiometry. Normal results of an auditory brain stem response test consist of five to seven waves that occur in the first 10 msec following presentation of an abrupt acoustic stimulus (click). However, the infant auditory brain stem response differs in virtually all measurement parameters from the adult response. The waveform morphology of a typical infant consists of three vertex or forehead positive peaks in comparison to the six or seven seen in the adult.[33] The absolute and interpeak latencies of these waves are longer than adult waves, and the absolute and relative amplitudes are markedly different from those of the adult. Nevertheless, evidence suggests that waves I through V of the auditory brain stem response represent activity in or around the eighth cranial nerve, cochlear nucleus, superior olivary complex, lateral lemniscus, and inferior colliculus.[34]

With the early reports of Hecox and Galambos,[35] Schulman-Galambos and Galambos,[36,37] and Salamy and associates,[38,39] which demonstrated the apparent ease with which the auditory brain stem response could be recorded in young infants, came the motivation for subsequent attempts to use the electrophysiologic response in newborn screening. Since that time, arguments for and against screening with the auditory brain stem response have appeared in the literature. Some have emphasized that it inherently involves the use of expensive equipment, preferably skilled personnel, and the test itself can be time-consuming and yield results for which a straightforward interpretation is lacking.[33]

Conversely, Galambos has suggested that nearly every newborn with hearing impairment could be identified by administering an auditory brain stem response screening test to babies who (1) are graduates of the newborn intensive care unit (NICU), (2) appear on the high-risk register, (3) fail behavioral screening, and (4) are considered suspect for whatever reason.[40]

Unfiltered clicks offer an acceptable stimulus

for infant auditory brain stem response testing. As a transient, they provide the optimum stimuli for eliciting synchronized neural activity. In addition to reflecting the high-frequency resonance characteristics of the transducer under test, unfiltered clicks are also influenced by the middle and inner ear mechanics. Consequently, auditory brain stem response recordings represent a wide-band frequency spectrum and lack the specificity of pure tone audiologic assessment. Gorga, Worthington, Reiland, Beauchaine, and Goldgar suggest that click-evoked auditory brain stem response thresholds are related most closely to the audiometric thresholds at 2,000 and 4,000 Hz, with relatively poor agreement at either 1,000 or 8,000 Hz.[41] If more frequency-specific information is required, the use of filtered clicks, tone bursts, or tone pips are possible alternatives.[42]

Establishing the normality or abnormality of auditory brain stem responses is based on comparisons to what is considered typical for the subject being tested. Full-term neonates and older infants need norms that reflect their age. However, precise determination of age at birth is difficult, and so the norms must reflect approximate rather than exact ages. Each audiologic facility must obtain exclusive normative data. Because of the number of factors that influence the auditory brain stem response (equipment, ambient noise, stimulus frequency, intensity, rise-fall, duration), norms obtained from one test location cannot be used at another.

The preterm infant population presents a difficult group from which to obtain norms. A major problem arises from the fact that an infant born prematurely is abnormal.[43] Furthermore, a considerable number of risk factors (hyperbilirubinemia, hypoxia, respiratory distress, acidosis, aminoglycoside therapy) that occur in the preterm population may affect the auditory brain stem response.[43] However, one possible approach to establishing norms in this population is to obtain mean data from preterm infants who are healthy and free from as many risk factors as possible.

Although it has been shown that the auditory brain stem response is relatively resistant to pharmacologic insult,[44] attention,[45] or the state of consciousness,[46] apparently little procedural rationale exists for the use of sedation on infants. Personal experience has been that infants under the age of 12 months can be tested without sedation, providing that the infant undergoes some degree of sleep deprivation and is fed prior to testing.

The auditory brain stem response should not be conducted when the newborn is acutely ill. Newborns who are acutely ill are often the smallest and youngest and are simply too immature to yield consistent results. Additionally, they are usually attached to monitoring equipment that can be a source of excessive electrical artifact. It is advantageous to conduct the test when the infant is in the graduated care section of the ICU, is breathing room air, and is at least 35 weeks postconception (gestational age plus chronological age).

The majority of clinical decisions are based on the measurement of response latency and to a smaller degree response amplitude. It is wise to avoid the overuse of interwave latencies in the ICN. Due to a combination of maturation and a host of pathologic influences, interwave latencies are far too variable at this age.

In any diagnostic procedure that requires a decision process, procedural strategies and screening criteria must be resolved before the establishment of follow-up guidelines. Further, the operating characteristics of a test and the "cutoff score" (a decision of pass versus fail based on performance)[15] must be considered prior to the first screening test of auditory brain stem response.

The auditory brain stem response can serve as a valuable tool in programs aimed at screening newborns for congenital hearing loss. However, it is merely part of the program, and its use must be preceded by discriminating and realistic deliberation.

Immittance Audiometry

Jerger and Hayes have stressed the importance of employing an objective procedure as a "cross-check" in the use of behavioral audiometry with children.[47] The two procedures they suggested are auditory brain stem response and immittance audiometry.

The concept of hearing loss prediction by the acoustic reflex was introduced by Niemeyer and Sesterhenn.[48,49] They noted that the acoustic reflex threshold for white noise was lower than the acoustic reflex threshold for pure tones and that the difference in decibels between the two thresholds is related to the degree of sensorineural hearing impairment. Subsequently, Jerger, Burney, Mauldin, and Crump reported extensive clinical experience with the sensitivity prediction by the acoustic reflex (SPAR) method.[50] Based on acoustic reflex findings for 1,156 ears, Jerger et al concluded that with the SPAR method, hearing loss was predicted with reasonable accuracy.[50]

The success of the SPAR procedure has inspired a number of innovative approaches to predict hearing loss with acoustic reflex measurements. These approaches may be divided into three general categories—SPAR, regression equations,[51,52] and the bivariate plot system.[53] In general, all depend on the noise and tone difference in the acoustic reflex thresholds.

Hearing loss prediction by the acoustic reflex is influenced by a variety of factors, including degree of hearing loss,[54] central auditory dysfunction,[55] subject age, and minor middle ear dysfunction.[56] Of these factors, age and minor middle ear dysfunction have been associated specifically with a reduction in predictive accuracy for the SPAR method.

The clinical utility of acoustic reflex measurements in neonates remains uncertain, in turn rendering hearing loss identification and estimation from the acoustic reflex uncertain. For example, different investigators have reported a wide range of observable acoustic reflexes in neonates. At the extremes, Keith and Bench observed acoustic reflexes in only 5.4 percent of their newborns,[57] whereas Himelfarb, Shannon, Popelka, and Margolis reported acoustic reflexes in 88 percent of their sample.[58] These results fail to provide a clear picture describing the presence of or the ability to measure reflexes in neonates. Such factors as probe frequency, reflex-eliciting stimuli, instrumentation, criteria for determining the presence of an acoustic reflex, and other procedural differences need further investigation to establish clinical protocols that will increase the probability of obtaining accurate acoustic reflex measures on this population.[59]

In general, the SPAR methods, regression equations, and the bivariate plot system all appear to estimate, or identify, hearing loss with accuracy rates that usually exceed 60 percent. However, none of the methods invariably predict hearing loss without error. The SPAR methods, for example, are more successful in young children (ages 0 to 10 years) and becomes less accurate in older children and adults. In the Jerger et al study, 100 percent of the children predicted to have normal hearing did indeed show normal audiograms.[56] Severe hearing loss was accurately predicted in children 85 percent of the time. The prediction of moderate sensorineural hearing losses was accurate in 54 percent of the children. The SPAR methods are also characterized by false-positive errors ranging from 25 to 45 percent.[60,61] The Lilly regression equation tends to yield false-negative errors, at least in patients with moderate to severe sensitivity loss.[62] Further, degree of loss is often underestimated. According to Margolis and Fox, the false-positive error rate with the bivariate plot may be comparatively low (6 percent).[55]

In varied clinical populations, no method is without error. While the SPAR procedures developed by Jerger and his colleagues appear to be the most popular clinical methods, the bivariate plotting procedure of Popelka may be somewhat more accurate in predicting hearing loss.[63] Regardless of which method one employs to predict hearing level from the acoustic reflex, two important factors must be considered when utilizing the acoustic reflex data with the pediatric population: age and middle ear status; each may significantly influence predictive accuracy. Further, the clinical value of hearing loss prediction by the acoustic reflex, even with current methods, is probably enhanced by aligning the strengths of a particular method with clinical needs.

ASSESSMENT OF AUDITORY ABILITIES

Two General Approaches

Behavioral assessment of auditory function is based on the observation of overt responses to controlled auditory signals. The two general approaches that have been employed clinically may be differentiated by whether or not reinforcement is employed.

When no reinforcement is used, the procedure is usually called behavior observation audiometry; in the nonreinforced paradigm, the stimulus elicits the response, which is then prone to habituation. Beyond the newborn period, a number of sources have described the application of procedures of behavior observation audiometry to the developing infant. The procedures are generally discussed in terms of the factors that influence response behavior. In behavior observation audiometry, the probability of a response is dependent on the state of the infant, the nature of the auditory stimulus, the definition of the response, and the background ambient noise levels.

A second approach has evolved, which demonstrates that the behavioral assessment of infants can be accomplished through an operant conditioning paradigm. Applying the operant paradigm is not merely presenting an auditory stimulus, observing a response, and reinforcing that response. The stimulus does not "elicit" the response. In the operant paradigm, the auditory stimulus is introduced as a contingency to indicate the interval during which time an appropriate response has a consequence—that is, reinforcement. Subsequently, the response is strengthened by reinforcement. This approach recognizes a view of infants as active receptors of auditory information, who, if given the chance, interact with their auditory environment.

Although the assessment of auditory function utilizing procedures without reinforcement can be implemented at birth, procedures utilizing reinforcement cannot be implemented until the infant

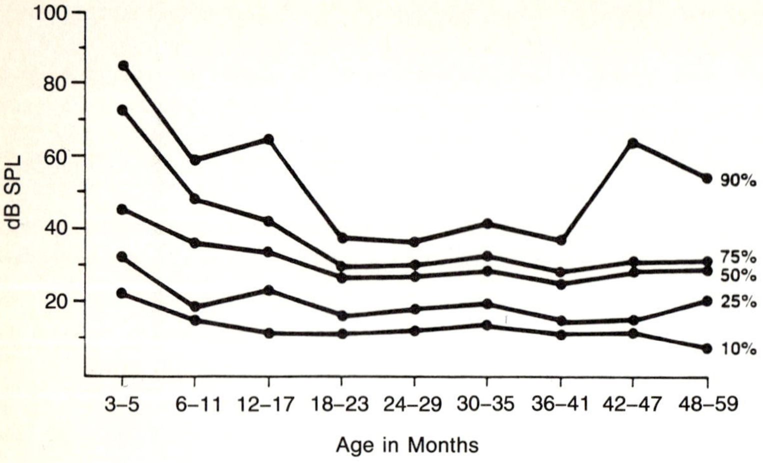

Figure 50–2 Intersubject variability in behavioral observation audiometry as a function of age. SPL = sound pressure level. (From Thompson G, Weber B. Responses of infants and young children to behavioral observation audiometry (BOA). J Speech Hear Disord 1974; 39:144.

reaches approximately 6 months of age. The age factor highlights developmental differences: specifically, when normal developing children can consistently demonstrate a specifically defined motor response.

Behavioral Observation Audiometry

The results of behavioral observation audiometry on infants and children have not been totally satisfying. For example, different investigators, using similar behavioral approaches without reinforcement, have reported dissimilar threshold results for infants of the same age.[22,23,64] These disparities are also reported in the literature for speech thresholds.

A second restriction with behavioral observation audiometry relates to the fact that thresholds show a wide range in normals. For example, Thompson and Weber looked at the intersubject variability in children ranging in age from 3 months to 4 years.[65] They found a range of 24 dB (24- through 29-month-old children) on the low end to 65 dB at the high end (3- to 5-month-old children) for responses between the tenth and ninetieth percentiles (Fig. 50–2). Others have reported similar dispersions, a fact that makes interpretation of test results difficult for other than severe losses.

A final problem with the behavioral observation audiometry approach is the need to select the auditory stimulus based on what is most novel to the youngster, and not necessarily on what stimulus might be needed for assessment purposes. For example, identification of high-frequency hearing losses could pose a problem since a number of investigators have shown that high-frequency signals are not effective with young children in a behavioral observation audiometry procedure.[66,67] Figure 50–3 shows the percentage of responses to five different stimuli across four different intensity levels.[67] These data show clearly the interaction of different stimuli at different levels on responses observed from a behavior observation audiometry procedure.

The restrictions imposed by stimulus factors and response factors on the validity and reliability of behavioral procedures with older infants and young children are clear: suprathreshold stimulation is required to elicit reflexive responses, and the probability of obtaining a response is dependent on the nature of the stimulus, the state of the child,[17,68] examiner bias,[69,70] and the ambient noise levels of the test environment. Even though behavior observation audiometry lacks precision in the determination of the exact hearing status of a child, it is still an alternative for children who are mentally im-

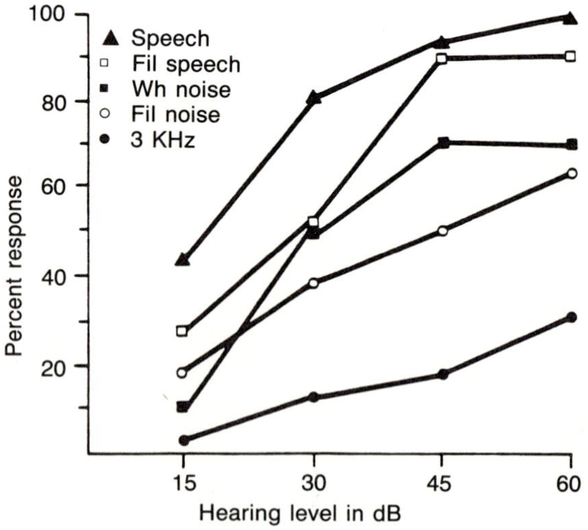

Figure 50–3 Percent response to five stimuli as a function of hearing level in infants 7 to 12 months of age. (From Thompson M, Thompson G. Response of infants and young children as a functioning of auditory stimuli and test method. J Speech Hear Res 1972; 15:705.)

paired or are severely developmentally delayed and for those youngsters who cannot be conditioned.

Procedures Utilizing Systematic Reinforcement

In order to overcome the restrictions imposed by behavioral observation audiometry, it is possible to approach the behavioral assessment of hearing in children through an operant conditioning procedure, specifically through an operant discrimination procedure. In an operant discrimination procedure, the stimulus is used to cue the child that a response results in reinforcement. Reinforcement is utilized to strengthen an easily monitored single response and to keep the infant in an aroused or motivated state. Maintaining motivation and a high response probability through the use of reinforcement allows one to investigate over time an infant's or a young child's auditory response behavior. This, then, allows more precise estimation of ability and reduces the habituation found in behavioral observation audiometry by allowing the infant to interact actively with his or her environment.

Operant Behavior

Operant behavior is frequently spoken of as willful or purposeful behavior. A behavioral response elicited by a stimulus is controlled by the consequence of the behavior. Operant behavior is increased or decreased in frequency by the changes that it brings about in the organism's environment. The events in an environment may be classified as positive reinforcers, negative reinforcers, and neutral events. Neutral events have little or no specific effect on behavior. Depending on the application of negative reinforcement or positive reinforcement, the probability of the response's effect can be either increased or decreased.

It is possible to increase the rate of response if a positive reinforcer is determined and applied. Since audible signals of the type used in assessing auditory function are known to have little reinforcing value to children,[71,72] the use of a test procedure in which the signal and reinforcer are separate and the signal serves only to cue the youngster that a correct response results in reinforcement is beneficial.

Within the operant discrimination paradigm used for hearing assessment, the use of different response modes has been explored; among several are the head turn and button press response. Likewise, different forms of reinforcement (positive) have been used—visual and tangible.

Historical Perspective of Visual Reinforcement

Dix and Hallpike introduced the "peep show" procedure, which reinforced a button press response to pure tone signals by presenting an illuminated picture.[73] Statten and Wishart maintained the concept of visual reinforcement with miniature scenes.[74] An elaborate doll house was constructed, and the doorbell button of the doll house was the response button. This procedure reinforced correct responses to auditory signals by the presentation of slides. Miller[75] and Lloyd[76] also used slides as reinforcing events. However, Miller recommended slide sets that tell a story as opposed to unrelated pictures.[75] Both of these procedures required a button press response.

Suzuki and Ogiba utilized visual reinforcement following a reflexive orientation response, and they called the procedure "conditioned orientation reflex" audiometry.[77,78] In this method, the signal is presented through speakers mounted at approximately 45-degree angles on both sides of the subject. Mechanical dolls located immediately below the speakers are activated following a localization response.

Liden and Kankkunen used slides as visual reinforcement and were the first investigators to call their procedure "visual reinforcement audiometry."[79] Rather than using a button press or reflexive orientation response, however, they listed four responses, any one resulting in reinforcement. The responses included: "reflexive behavior," "investigating responses," "spontaneous responses," and "head turning."

Historical Perspective of Tangible Reinforcement

Tangible reinforcers have also been used with the operant discrimination paradigm. Edible items, such as cereal, popcorn, crackers, candy, and various fluids, as well as nonedible objects such as miniature toys or tokens, have been used as material for tangible reinforcement in operant conditioning audiometry. Knox described a simple method of presenting small toys to young children who pressed a response switch when a pure tone was presented.[80] Meyerson and Michael reported using a tangible reinforcer in operant conditioning audiometry that involved two responses.[81,82] When there was no auditory signal present, pressing one button was reinforced on a partial schedule. When the signal was present, pushing a second button was reinforced on a similar schedule.

Several investigators reported that a single response system, which reinforced pressing the button only when the auditory signal was present, was the most efficient for clinical testing.[83–85] They used a 100 percent reinforcement schedule with the single response system. This operant procedure using tangible reinforcement is similar to the operant discrimination paradigm using visual reinforcers. The primary difference is in the reinforcement used.

Although several different operant approaches to the hearing assessment of infants and young children have been explored, two procedures have been refined with a supportive data base in the past decade. The first procedure involves the head turn response with visual reinforcement—called "visual reinforcement audiometry." Visual reinforcement audiometry has been chosen over conditioned orientation reflex audiometry since visual reinforcement audiometry specifies an operant head turn response and conditioned orientation reflex implies a nonspecific reflexive orientation behavior to sound (Figs. 50–4 and 50–5). The second procedure involves the bar press response with either edible or visual reinforcement (Figs. 50–6, 50–7, and 50–8). When edibles (or other tangibles) are used as reinforcers, the procedure has been called "tangible reinforcement operant conditioning audiometry" (TROCA); when a visual reinforcer has been used, it is called "visual reinforcement operant conditioning audiometry" (VROCA).[86]

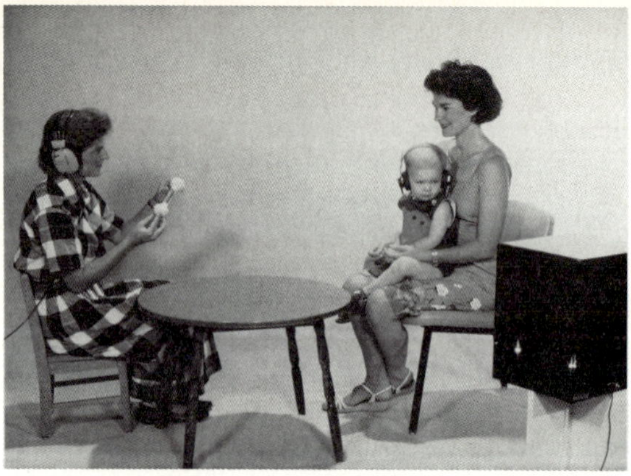

Figure 50–5 Visual reinforcement audiometry procedure. Infant demonstrating a head turn response.

Visual Reinforcement Audiometry

In addition to Suzuki and Ogiba[77,78] and Liden and Kankkunen,[79] several additional investigators have reported on the use of visual reinforcement audiometry procedures for assessment of hearing sensitivity in infants and young children.[87-91] These reports have highlighted the usefulness of visual reinforcement audiometry and have served to strengthen its use as an audiologic procedure today.

Visual reinforcement audiometry has emerged as a successful assessment procedure for infants and young children, 6 months through 2 years of age.[72] In visual reinforcement audiometry, conditioned head turns toward a sound source (localization in a sound field and a conditioned behavior under earphones) are reinforced by an attractive three-dimensional animated toy.[71] The success of visual reinforcement audiometry is certainly related to the fact that the response (head turn) and reinforcer (animated toy) are well suited to the developmental level of the children between these ages.

Visual reinforcement audiometry is based on the premise that the discrimination of a change in the child's auditory environment results in reinforcement. For example, if a child responds to the presence of sound from a background of silence, a discrimination has been made. Through operant conditioning, the child learns that a head turn to-

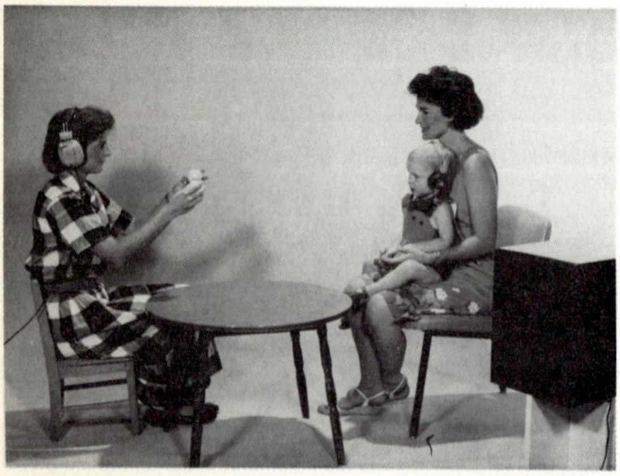

Figure 50–4 Visual reinforcement audiometry procedure. Infant in midline position.

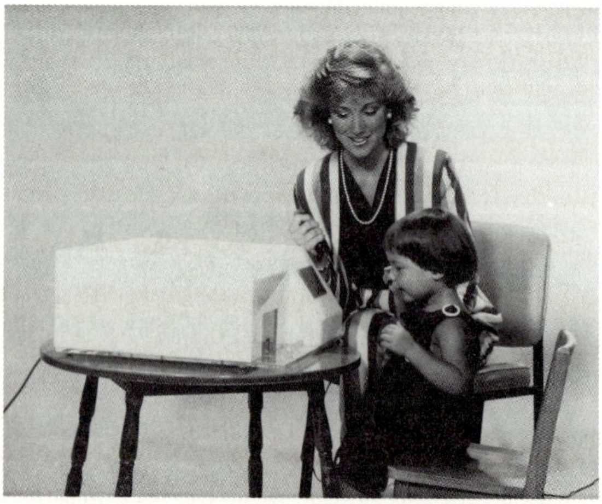

Figure 50–6 Tangible reinforcement operant conditioning audiometry procedure. Child conditioned to listen.

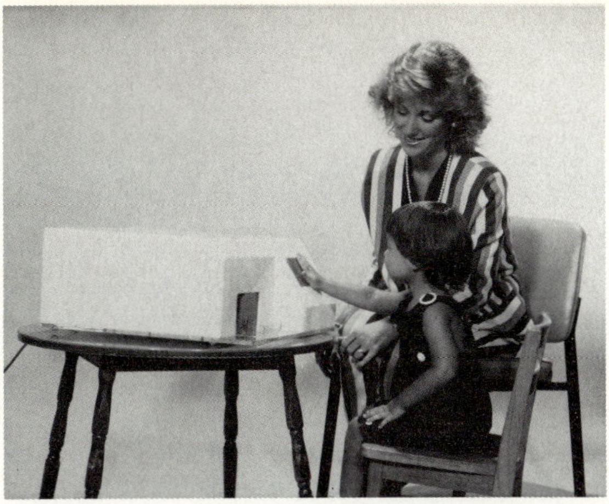

Figure 50–7 Tangible reinforcement operant conditioning audiometry procedure. Bar press response.

wards the reinforcer following the detection or discrimination of a change results in reinforcement.

The test room arrangement used in the visual reinforcement audiometry procedure is shown in Figure 50–9. The examiner in the control room activates the auditory stimulus and visual reinforcer and has full view of the testing situation. The test room is arranged with the parent and infant located behind a table in the center of the room. A loudspeaker is positioned at a 45-degree azimuth to the right or left of the infant's midline of vision. The visual reinforcer, housed in a dark plexiglass enclosure, is located at eye level. A second examiner, seated to the infant's side, encourages the child to observe passively or play with colorful, quiet toys in order to maintain the infant's head in a midline position. The auditory stimulus is not presented if the infant is looking at the assistant or loudspeaker, vocalizing, crying, or moving excessively.

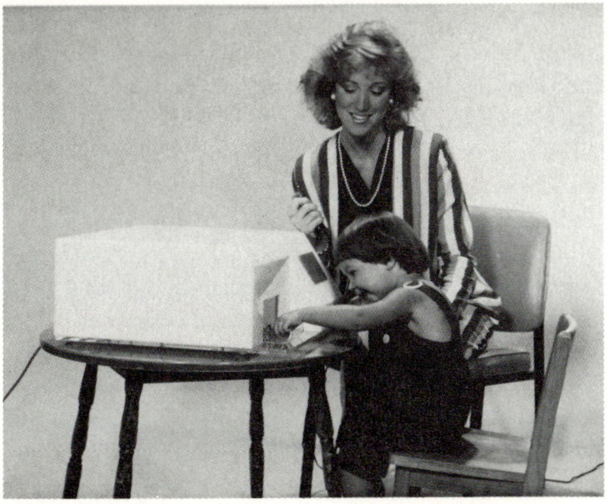

Figure 50–8 Tangible reinforcement operant conditioning audiometry procedure. Food reinforcement and the child completing the task.

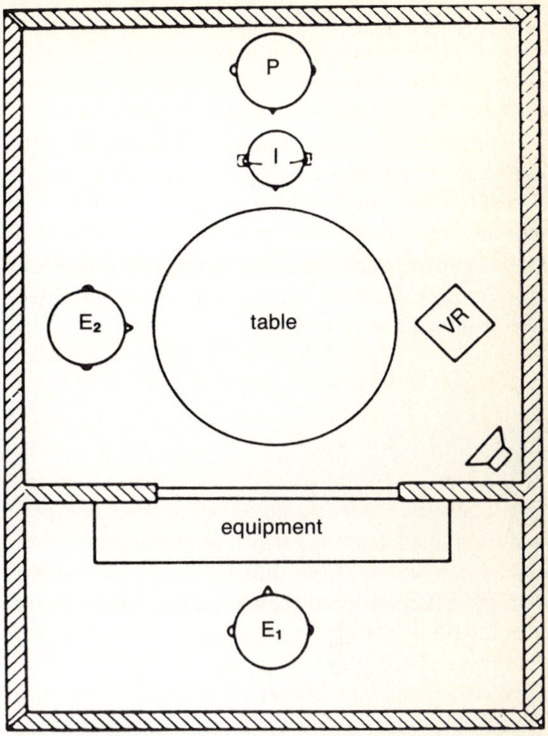

Figure 50–9 Test room arrangement. Abbreviations: E1 = examiner; E2 = test-room examiner; P = parent; I = infant; VR = visual reinforcer.

Test Room Examiner

The role of the individual in the room with the parent and child is crucial to the success of visual reinforcement audiometry. When limitations exist regarding personnel and two examiners cannot be utilized, a microprocessing computer can be implemented to control the activation and signal intensity of the auditory stimulus. In visual reinforcement audiometry, the test room examiner has two primary responsibilities: entertaining the child at the midline position (facing forward) with colorful, quiet toys and judging responses. If the youngster under test shows too much interest in the colorful toys, the potential exists for no response during a signal trial or for elevated minimum response levels.* On the other hand, if the youngster under test shows no interest or is bored with the colorful toys, false responses may occur regularly. The test room examiner must have a continuum of toys available and be

* Since "auditory threshold" represents a minimum auditory response level dependent upon the choice of psychophysical method and measurement step size, and therefore not one absolute level, and since auditory response levels may improve slightly with age due to attention and motivation, it may be more appropriate to use the term "minimum response level" rather than "auditory threshold."[92]

astute at judging when a toy change in either direction (more entertaining or less entertaining) may be necessary to maintain the child's midline position and optimum response state.

Since the test room examiner is required to judge responses, knowledge of signal trials versus control trials could possibly result in tester bias in the visual reinforcement audiometry test procedure. Therefore the test room examiner wears headphones and can be alerted by a signal (tone or light) that an observation interval is occurring.

Conditioning

There are currently no recommended test procedures for conducting visual reinforcement audiometry. However, if one adheres to the philosophy that reliable measurements are a direct result of the test instrument and the development of auditory stimulus and response control through conditioning, then the interaction between the subject, the test procedure, and the examiner in achieving precise results is an important part of that process.

Thompson and Folsom compared the effects of two conditioning procedures in the use of visual reinforcement audiometry with 1- and 2-year-old children.[93] One conditioning procedure used an initial stimulus presentation level (30-dB HL) and only two conditioning trials prior to the exploration of minimum response levels. The second procedure used a 60-dB HL initial presentation level and five conditioning trials prior to the exploration of minimum response levels. The data from the Thompson and Folsom study indicated no significant differences between the two conditioning procedures in regard to obtained minimum response levels or the number of false-positive responses observed during control trials.[93]

If a child fails to respond in visual reinforcement audiometry, the examiner can quickly introduce hearing level increments until a spontaneous response is observed. However, one must also recognize that for some hearing impaired children, localization to a sound source may not be a realistic response task.

If there is a reason to believe, based on case history information or initial testing trials, that a child may not condition well to the visual reinforcement audiometry procedure, it would be clinically advantageous to consider a test strategy that begins at a relatively soft level, so that if habituation occurs after a few trials, the opportunity to observe spontaneous responses at a soft level is available. This rationale would support the use of the 30-dB conditioning level in cases where there is doubt about the visual reinforcement audiometry procedure.

Minimum Response Levels

The information obtained from the Moore et al studies,[71,72] provided the necessary foundation for Wilson, Moore, and Thompson to investigate the minimum response levels of infants utilizing the visual reinforcement audiometry technique.[94] Ninety infants between 5 and 18 months of age were divided into groups of 15 according to age. Measurement of minimum response levels by means of a complex-noise signal involved starting a 0.0 dB SPL and ascending in 20-dB steps until the first response occurred. After a second positive response, sampling of minimum response levels began, using a protocol of attenuating the signal 20 dB after each response and increasing it 10 dB after each failure to respond. Minimum response level was defined as the lowest presentation level at which the infant responded at least three times out of six presentations. Figure 50–10 presents the minimum response levels obtained by visual reinforcement audiometry and provides comparative data from behavioral observation audiometry procedures.[65] The data from visual reinforcement audiometry indicate that the mean response levels improved slightly with age, ranging from about 30-dB SPL for 5 month olds to about 20-dB SPL for 7 to 18 month olds. For comparative purposes, the median response of ten normal hearing adults was 20-dB SPL under the same signal and measurement step conditions. The tenth and ninetieth percentile points were 20 and 40-dB SPL for 5 month olds and 20 to 30-dB SPL for 6 through 18 month olds.

Notice in comparing the minimum response levels for visual reinforcement audiometry to those for behavioral observation audiometry for the same ages, the difference favored the technique utilizing reinforcement. Even more importantly for infants 6 months of age and older, the range between the tenth and ninetieth percentile is reduced from the 45 to 50 dB reported for behavioral observation audiometry to 10 dB for visual reinforcement audiometry used in this study. Certainly for the audiologist desiring to assess mild hearing losses, the substantially tighter dispersion data obtained with the visual reinforcement paradigm would be desirable.

The implications from this study are substantial. The results demonstrate that (1) the minimum response levels obtained from infants for complex noise are close to those obtained from adults in the same situation and (2) the range of minimum response levels

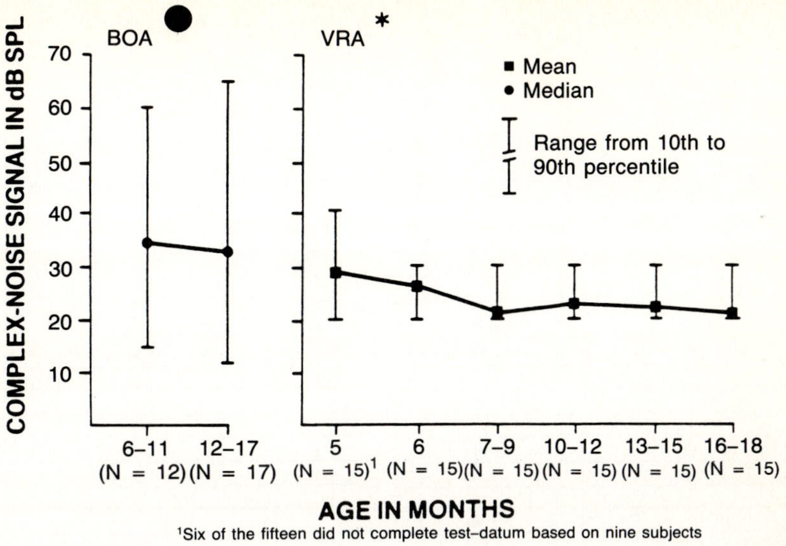

Figure 50–10 Auditory thresholds of infants as obtained by behavioral observation audiometry (BOA) and visual reinforcement audiometry (VRA) methods. Abbreviation: SPL = sound pressure level. (*From Wilson WR, Moore JM, Thompson G. Sound field auditory threshold of infants utilizing visual reinforcement audiometry (VRA). Paper presented at the American Speech and Hearing Association Annual Convention Houston, 1976. •From Thompson G, Weber B. Responses of infants and young children to behavioral observation audiometry (BOA). J Speech Hear Disord 1974; 39:145.)

for the population of presumed normal hearing infants is small.

Different studies using the protocol and precision suggested by Wilson and Moore have reported similar sound field minimum response levels for visual reinforcement audiometry.[95–97] In each report, minimum response levels are within a conservative definition of normal hearing (<20 dB HL) and only slightly elevated from adult comparisons. These data support the accuracy of visual reinforcement audiometry test procedures in correctly identifying normal hearing (good specificity). More important however, is the indication from these data that the visual reinforcement audiometry test procedure yields a tight grouping of minimum response levels for a normal population, thereby resulting in a wide range available for defining abnormal minimum response levels. Therefore visual reinforcement audiometry can meet the goals of identifying mild and moderate degrees of hearing loss as well as hearing losses with varying configurations. As is evident in Figure 50–11, the test-retest reliability of visual reinforcement audiometry (using conditioned play audiometry as the standard) is excellent with children who demonstrate different degrees and configurations of hearing loss. These three clinical cases from the files of these studies serve to support the sensitivity of the visual reinforcement audiometry test procedure.

Results of earphone assessment are also provided by Wilson and Moore.[94,97] Although earphone to pinna attachments in their study may have resulted in sound pressure leakage, thus causing elevated low-frequency minimum response levels, the results provided strong evidence supporting the use and success of earphone assessment with infants by means of visual reinforcement audiometry. As a final note, with an appropriate headband arrangement (and cooperation from the youngster under test), bone conduction measurements can be successfully made by means of visual reinforcement audiometry.

Sound Field Cautions

Sound field assessment is often the only alternative available to a clinician evaluating the pediatric patient. Warble tones and narrow bands of noise both appear to be in common clinical use. However, many questions remain about the specific parameters of each of these signals; wide-band stimuli have been good for maintaining uniform sound fields, but are not good stimuli for identifying frequency-specific hearing losses,[98] and adequate modulation rate of frequency modulated (FM) tones in the sound field for normal hearing individuals may be inadequate for accurately assessing hearing impaired individuals. In addition to questions concerning the choice and standards of stimuli to use in sound field assessment, there are questions about other aspects of sound field assessment that must be addressed in order to improve the precision of this means of assessment—namely, the patient's position relative to the loudspeaker, the physical environment, and calibrations considerations.

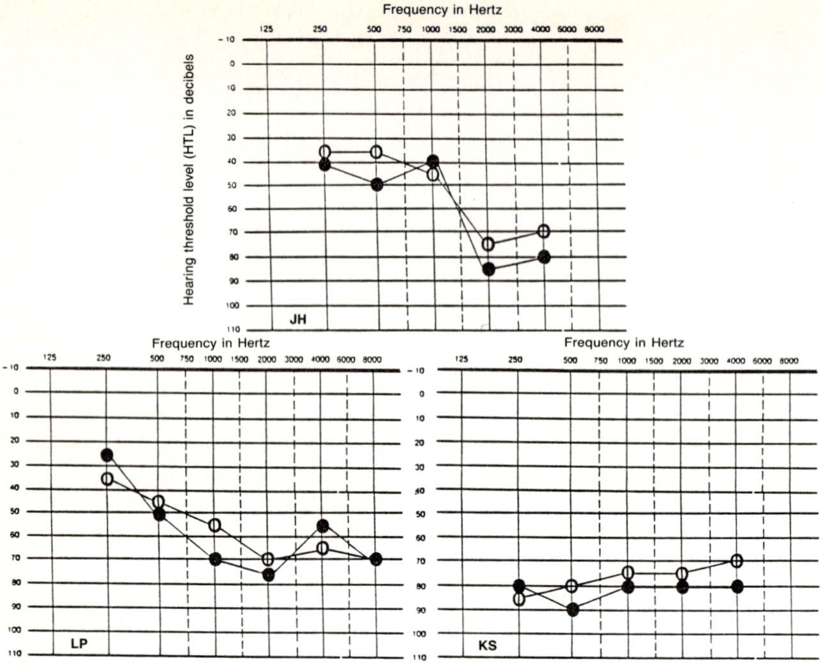

Figure 50–11 Longitudinal results of assessment: visual reinforcement audiometry (VRA)• and conditioned play audiometry (CPA)° (sound field). VRA before 18 months and CPA after 4 years.

In an excellent article by Walker, Dillon, and Bryne, these concerns are addressed with subsequent recommendations made.[99] This report suggests that the limitations of certain types of stimuli may not apply when the stimuli have optimal characteristics. Further, the authors state that if the recommendations and techniques described are utilized in sound field assessment, it is possible to achieve the same degree of precision and reliability that is achieved in audiometric measurements made under earphones.

Summary

The past decade of infant research has demonstrated that the head turn response is a natural and appropriate response for infants between 6 months and 2 years. Further, reinforcement significantly increases the response rate of infants. Thus visual reinforcement audiometry provides the following advantages over behavioral observation audiometry in clinical practice: (1) reduction of dispersion in estimates of minimum response levels; (2) high success rate; (3) test-retest reliability; (4) minimum response levels close to adult norms; and (5) time efficiency.

Tangible or Visual Reinforcement Operant Conditioning Audiometry

The basic paradigm used in the TROCA or VROCA procedure involves a bar press response coupled with either tangible or visual reinforcement. Lloyd et al were among the early pioneers in developing this procedure for difficult-to-test individuals.[83] The procedure uses principles and terminology associated with operant conditioning. TROCA or VROCA has been shown to be most effective with children between 2 and 4 years of age developmentally, but it is also effective with younger children as well as many difficult-to-test persons including those with mental impairment. Additionally, TROCA or VROCA can be used successfully as a drop back procedure when preschoolers have lost interest in play audiometry, but further audiometric information is necessary.

The TROCA or VROCA procedure uses positive reinforcement for appropriate responses and a mild punishment (timeout) for false responses. The child's behavior is conditoned until he or she pushes a response button whenever a sound is detected. With most children, it has been found that a secondary social reinforcement enhances auditory stimulus and response control.

For TROCA, the response and reinforcement delivery box (Fig. 50–12) encloses a Davis universal feeder that delivers reinforcement into a plexiglass reinforcement tray. The tray is lighted for approximately 2 seconds when reinforcement is delivered. To the right of the reinforcement tray is a plexiglass response button. For VROCA, visual reinforcement (animated toy animal) is the reward for appropriate responses.

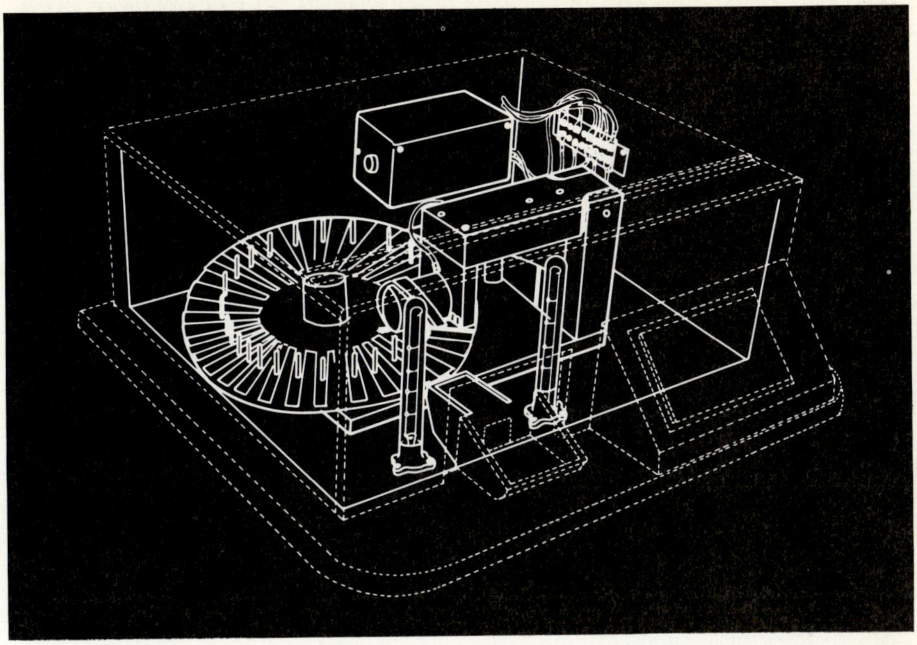

Figure 50–12 Response and reinforcement delivery box for tangible reinforcement operant conditioning audiometry (TROCA).

Lloyd et al employed continuous reinforcement in their initial study of TROCA.[83] Variable reinforcement schedules have also been investigated,[100] but there have been no reported studies determining which reinforcement schedule best maintains conditioning.

Minimum Response Levels

Utilizing the TROCA or VROCA procedures, several investigators have reported minimum response levels for young children.[101,102] Each of these investigators demonstrated that minimum response levels were tightly grouped and within normal ranges for their subjects, who ranged in age from 12 months to 2 years, suggesting good specificity with this procedure.

These studies demonstrated that auditory sensitivity measures can be obtained from young children by means of the TROCA technique. However, there is also agreement that conditioning time and therefore total testing time is extended with the TROCA or VROCA procedure. Just as important is the suggestion that once an infant or a young child is brought under stimulus and response control and demonstrates the ability to detect any acoustic change in his or her auditory environment, additional auditory testing may be implemented. For example, these acoustic changes may include special auditory tests such as speech and sound discrimination, the short increment sensitivity index (SISI), threshold tone decay, difference limen for intensity,[102a] and difference limen for frequency.

It appears that the success rate with these procedures may be related to age. For example, below 12 months of age, TROCA is less successful than visual reinforcement audiometry. However, TROCA may be more successful than visual reinforcement audiometry for children 24 to 30 months of age and older. At approximately 3 years of age, TROCA becomes less effective, and play audiometry then becomes a more appropriate test technique.

Conditioned Play Audiometry

Conditioned play audiometry is probably the most common procedure used in the assessment of young children. Through conditioning the child learns to engage in some activity—putting rings on a spindle, dropping or stacking blocks—each time he or she hears the signal (Figs. 50–13 and 50–14). These activities are assumed to be interesting to the child and to reinforce his or her responding. However, Fulton has pointed out that if the play activity is the consequenting event (reinforcement), what is the response?[101] Conversely, if the play activity is the response, what is the consequenting event? Because conditioned play audiometry does not follow a strict model of auditory Stimulus → Response → Reinforcer, the procedural arrangement can lead to confusion for the youngster, which may result in noncontingent random playing. In children for whom conditioned play audiometry is appropriate, sepa-

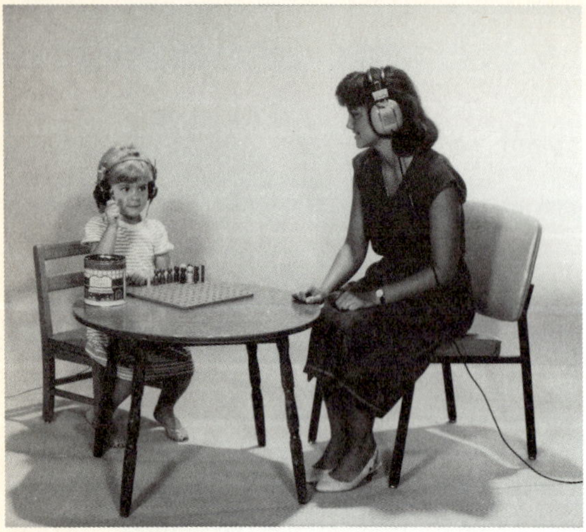

Figure 50–13 Conditioned play audiometry. Child conditioned to listen.

ration of response from reinforcement and adherence to the principles of the operant paradigm may improve this procedure's validity and reliability.

The pediatric literature clearly suggests that conditoned play audiometry is widely accepted among clinicians who interact with young children. Barr tested 135 children between the ages of 2 and 6 years with this procedure and found that the percentage of success was directly related to age.[103] Moreover, Thompson and Weber concluded that the rate of success in obtaining detailed information with conditioned play audiometry is limited for children under the age of 30 months.[65]

Minimum Response Levels

Experience with conditioned play audiometry indicates that minimum response levels can be obtained reliably when auditory stimulus and response control has been established and response criteria are maintained. Results from a clinical study of 40 preschoolers, age 30 to 48 months, revealed minimum response levels at a level of 10 dB or better.[104] These findings were in close agreement with other 4-year-old children, 32 with deviations of less than 5 dB.[104a]

When a child with either known or suspected hearing loss is assessed by means of any operant procedure it is likely that several paired conditioning trials (with a visual reinforcer demonstrating the bar press response, or completing the motor activity) at suprathreshold levels will be required to condition the response prior to exploration of minimum response levels. Obviously, the auditory signal must be audible if conditioning is to be established.

ASSESSMENT OF SUPRATHRESHOLD DISCRIMINATION ABILITIES

The primary focus of this chapter has been on the assessment of auditory minimum response levels with infants and young children. However, it is also important to present some information on suprathreshold auditory assessment. To view threshold assessment as the single objective in pediatric auditory assessment would be shortsighted.

Suprathreshold auditory assessment for infants and young children needs to include speech discrimination testing and assessment (when appropriate) of central auditory processing skills. With approaches that assess central auditory function, it may be possible to begin testing the auditory skills of infants and young children suspected of learning disabilities.

The Young Child

Over the past decade, studies on the perception of speech by infants have led to the conclusion that infants are able to perceive a variety of speech sounds at a very early age.[105–107] Although the primary focus of this work, to date, has been on theoretic issues in the area of infant speech perception, the application of infant assessment procedures to clinical populations holds great promise for investigating speech sound discrimination.

To address the issue of developmental changes in speech sound discrimination skills, Eilers et al modified visual reinforcement audiometry to overcome the limitations of the heart rate and high amplitude sucking paradigms and to achieve the fol-

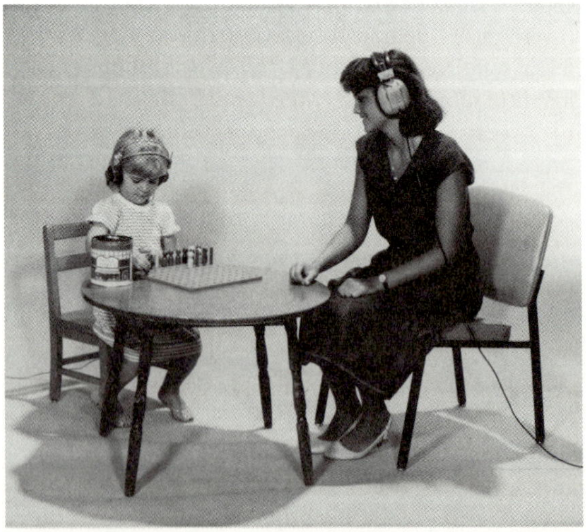

Figure 50–14 Conditioned play audiometry. Child completing motor activity.

TABLE 50–2 Discrimination Trial Structure

	Repeating Background Stimulus					*Target Stimulus*			*Repeating Background Stimulus*		
Time in seconds	1	2	3	4	5	6	7	8	9	10	11
Change trial	/sa/	/sa/	/sa/	/sa/	/sa/	/va/	/va/	/va/	/sa/	/sa/	/sa/
Control trial	/sa/	/sa/	/sa/	/sa/	/sa/	/sa/	/sa/	/sa/	/sa/	/sa/	/sa/

lowing goals for visual reinforcement audiometry: (1) to be applicable to a large proportion of infants tested, (2) to be time efficient, (3) to be capable of testing a single child's discrimination, (4) to be capable of evaluating multiple speech contrasts for each infant tested, (5) to be applicable across a wide age range, and (6) to employ a reinforcer that is independent from the stimuli to be discriminated.[106] In the visually reinforced infant speech discrimination paradigm (VRISD), infants are presented with one member of a contrastive stimulus pair at the rate of one syllable per second at a 50-dB sound pressure level. While the infant is entertained at midline, the speech sound is changed during a 4-second interval (Table 50–2). The infant is reinforced for a head turn at the change in signal by the visual reinforcer. Initially, the target stimulus is presented at a higher intensity than the background stimulus. Once the infant has demonstrated responses to the intensity and/or speech signal differences, the intensities are equated. Table 50–3 provides results from this study for the 6- to 8-month-old infants; Table 50–4 provides results for the 12- to 14-month-old infant.

The results of this study have shown that a high percentage of infants 6 to 14 months of age can be tested for discrimination of subtle speech contrasts. Additionally, the study has demonstrated that the VRISD paradigm can provide data repeatedly on individual infants in order to obtain information concerning discrimination of a variety of speech sound contrasts over time.

With the available research data base and with continued research in this area, particularly on optimum sensation levels, it is possible to implement clinical discrimination testing with infants.[108] The possibilities here are exciting for further assessment of infants' auditory abilities, and certainly one application of the VRISD paradigm is for more detailed assessment of hearing aid amplification in the young infant.

Utilizing the "same-different" speech sound discrimination approach with older infants is also possible by utilizing the TROCA paradigm. Now, rather than a head turn response to indicate the discrimination of a constrastive speech pair, the bar press response followed by reinforcement signifies the correct discrimination of a speech sound pair.

Even with conditioned play audiometry, the "same-different" speech sound discrimination approach is possible. However, by the time a child reaches the age at which conditioned play audiometry is the appropriate test technique, the child's receptive vocabulary could be at a level where more traditional approaches to speech discrimination can be implemented.

Speech audiometry is recognized as an essential part of a comprehensive audiological evaluation of the young child. Pure tone or noise band thresholds convey information about characteristics of the auditory system, but do not provide the audiologist with precise measure of a person's ability to receive and respond to the speech message. The audiometric threshold configuration is not always a good indication of an individual's ability to understand speech. Thus, determination of the degree of impairment may also be assisted by speech audiometry. However, when

TABLE 50–3 Perception of Speech Contrasts by 6- to 8-Month-Old Infants

	*Speech Contrast**									
Subject	*va-sa*	*sa-sa*	*sa-za*	*as-a:z*	*a:s-a:z*	*at-a:d*	*a:t-a:d*	*a:t-at*	*fa-θa*	*fi-θi*
1	S	S	S	S	S	S	NS	NS	NS	NS
2	S	S	S	S	S	S	NS	NS	NS	NS
3	S	S	S	S	S	S	NS	NS	NS	NS
4	S	S	S	S	S	S	NS	NS	NS	NS
5	S	S	S	S	S	S	NS	NS	NS	NS
6	S	S	S	S	S	S	NS	NS	NS	NS
7	S	S	S	S	S	NS	NS	NS	NS	S
8	S	S	S	S	S	S	NS	NS	NS	NS
9	S	S	S	S	S	S	S	S	NS	NS

* S = significant evidence of discrimination ($p < 0.05$); NS = evidence of discrimination was not obtained.

From Eilers RE, Wilson WR, Moore JM. Developmental changes in speech discrimination in infants. J Speech Hear Res 1977; 20:766 780.

TABLE 50–4 Perception of Speech Contrasts by 12- to 14-Month-Old Infants

Subject	Speech Contrast*									
	va-sa	*sa-sa*	*sa-za*	*as-a:z*	*a:s-a:z*	*at-a:d*	*a:t-a:d*	*a:t-at*	*fa-θa*	*fi-θi*
1	S	S	S	S	S	S	NS	NS	NS	S
2	S	S	S	S	S	NS	NS	NS	NS	S
3	S	S	S	S	S	S	NS	S	NS	S
4	S	S	S	S	S	S	NS	S	NS	S
5	S	S	S	S	S	S	S	S	NS	S
6	S	S	S	S	S	S	S	S	NS	S
7	S	S	S	NS	S	S	S	NS	S	S
8	S	NS	S	S	S	S	S	NS	NS	NS

* S =significant evidence of discrimination ($p < 0.05$); NS = evidence of discrimination was not obtained.
From Eilers RE, Wilson WR, Moore JM. Developmental changes in speech discrimination in infants. J Speech Hear Res 1977; 20:766.

using speech audiometry with young children, numerous variables can influence the outcome of test results that must be taken into consideration as follows: (1) selection of test material within the child's receptive vocabulary; (2) use of a nonverbal response task; (3) use of a test that is rapid and has sufficient appeal to keep the child's attention; and (4) use of reinforcement.

If a young child has a hearing loss or some other developmental disability, receptive vocabulary may be depressed. Thus chronological age has little, if anything, to do with the determination of the appropriate speech discrimination method. Every attempt must be made to select materials that fall within the child's receptive vocabulary. Otherwise the test outcome not only reflects limitations in auditory discrimination and recognition abilities, but also the language delay imposed by the hearing loss. Therefore clinicians must take a cautious approach and refrain from using inappropriate discrimination materials that contain unfamiliar words to a child sustaining a significant bilateral hearing impairment and accompanying language deficit. Furthermore, the response must be nonverbal due to the expressive language problems frequently exhibited by the hearing-impaired. Therefore, considering the factors of age and hearing-impairment, test instruments appropriate for children must be used to measure accurately speech discrimination.

THE OLDER CHILD

Haskins developed phonetically balanced lists composed of monosyllabic words selected from the spoken vocabulary of kindergarteners.[109] The phonetically balanced kindergarten lists of 50 words each have been used widely in work with children. Yet the receptive vocabulary level of the particular child under audiologic study is often unascertained before administration of these materials. Consequently, the phonetically balanced kindergarten-50 scores may be depressed in that they reflect language deficits as well as problems in auditory discrimination. Based on the research findings of Sanderson-Leepa and Rintelmann, which indicated that normal hearing preschoolers at $3^1/_2$ years of age yielded scores substantially lower than did older children, it is recommended that the clinician exercise caution in administering this test unless there is a relatively good assurance that the receptive vocabulary age of the youngster approaches at least that of a normal hearing kindergartener.[110]

No commercial version of this test has been recorded, and so each clinician performing this test must do so using monitored live voice. The drawbacks of monitored live voice when testing speech discrimination must be recognized, as they are with adults, particularly when testing children over time with different speakers.

Written responses on discrimination tests are essentially out of the question for most young children. Verbal responses may be limited not only by a language disorder or a vocabulary deficit, but also by an articulation problem or lack of motivation. To bypass these problems and still test discrimination ability with young children, picture discrimination tests may be used. Such tests include those reported by Ross and Lerman[111] entitled the Word Intelligibility by Picture Identification (WIPI) test and Siegenthaler and Haspiel's Discrimination by the Identification of Pictures test.[112]

The data provided by Sanderson-Leepa and Rintelmann demonstrated that normal hearing children at age $3^1/_2$ manifest a significant number of errors because the lists contain words not in their recognition vocabulary.[110] Thus, the use of WIPI test materials is appropriate for those children with receptive ages of 4 years and greater.

There are differences between the phonetically balanced words and the WIPI type approach to auditory discrimination testing besides the fact that the latter is pictorially represented. Phonetically balanced words represent an open response paradigm in which the child is forced to select an answer from an unlimited set of possibilities, whereas the WIPI test is a closed response set with the child's response being a forced choice.

Hodgson investigated the relationship between the WIPI test words used as an open-set and as a closed-set test for normal hearing children.[113] In the open-set condition, subjects repeated the WIPI test words. The closed-set response required the usual picture identification task. Subjects also repeated the words of a phonetically balanced kindergarten list administered in a conventional open-set fashion. Although there was no difference in the intelligibility of the WIPI test and phonetically balanced kindergarten words, use of the WIPI test as a closed-set test improved the discrimination scores by about 10 percent. Therefore it is advisable that the audiologic record include not only the scores obtained, but also the particular test materials used.

Siegenthaler and Haspiel developed a word recognition test that incorporates a closed-set response task: the Discrimination by the Identification of Pictures test.[112] This measure was designed for young children, with pictures selected for easy recognition by preschoolers. The stimuli consist of 48 pairs of familiar monosyllabic words that differ in distinctive features. A major drawback with this test is that only two illustrations are pictured on each response plate; thus there is a 50-50 probability for a correct chance response.

The Northwestern University-Children's Perception of Speech (NU-CHIPS) test by Elliott and Katz (1980) was developed as a speech discrimination test appropriate for children having a language age as young as 3 years. The stimuli consist of 50 monosyllabic words, which were arranged into four lists. The test was designed to be similar to other speech discrimination test procedures used when utilizing a closed-set, picture-pointing response task.[113a]

The development of a pediatric speech intelligibility (PSI) test by Jerger et al, characterizes the most recent construction of a discrimination test for children.[114] The PSI test was developed for children as young as 3 years of age for evaluating both peripheral and central components of auditory disorders.

In the development of the PSI test, the effect of receptive language skills was investigated thoroughly, and the outcome is a test that minimizes the contaminating influence of receptive language skills. Ten sentences and 20 words have been selected for the PSI test. The responses of a large group of normal children ranging in age from 3 to 7 years, for the 20 words, did not differ as a function of chronological age, vocabulary skill, or receptive language ability.[115] However, consistent differences in vocabulary and receptive language skills between children ranging in age from 3 to 6 years resulted in the development of two different sets of PSI sentence test materials.

In order to determine the validity of a test, or the extent to which the test actually measures what it purports to measure, its sensitivity and specificity must be known. The goal for any test is to maintain a balance between these factors.

Three speech discrimination tests (Word Intelligibility by Picture Identification, Pediatric Speech Intelligibility, and Northwestern University-Children's Perception of Speech) were compared in a study conducted by Dehart.[115a] The tests were administered in this study at three different intensity levels (20, 30, and 40 dB sensation level) to two groups of children who ranged in age from 4 years to 7 years. One group consisted of six normally hearing children, the second of six hearing impaired children with a sensorineural loss that ranged from moderate to severe.

The data obtained in this study were analyzed using a three factor analysis of variance. The results suggest that, overall, the optimal level for administration of these tests is 30 dB sensation level. In addition, the results also indicate that whereas the Pediatric Speech Intelligibility test has excellent specificity for the normally-hearing group, it has only poor sensitivity in the identification of the hearing-impaired group's discrimination difficulty. Both the Word Intelligibility by Picture Identification and Northwestern University-Children's Perception of Speech tests demonstrated excellent specificity and greater sensitivity than the Pediatric Speech Intelligibility test.

Jerger et al state that the slope of the performance-intensity functions for Northwestern University-Children's Perception of Speech test were more gradual than the slope of the Pediatric Speech Intelligibility test, which indicates that the test material of Northwestern University-Children's Perception of Speech is more difficult than the material of the Pediatric Speech Intelligibility.[115] The results of this study support the conclusion that the Pediatric Speech Intelligibility test was found to be the least sensitive and least difficult of the three tests. In addition, the results of this study suggest that the Word Intelligibility by Picture Identification test is more sensitive and more difficult than either the Pediatric Speech Intelligibility or the Northwestern University-Children's Perception of Speech tests.

The test stimuli used in this study were either restricted (Pediatric Speech Intelligibility) or unrestricted (Word Intelligibility by Picture Identification and Northwestern University-Children's Perception of Speech). The stimuli are considered restricted when each target item is specified, but foil items are not included. The words in a restricted set are not phonemically similar. Unrestricted refers to target items embedded among foil items, which may represent selected phonemic confusions. In attempting to minimize the influence of receptive language skills on test performance, the authors of the Pediatric Speech Intelligibility test used test materials representing the actual responses of children, with a restricted set of stimuli. Some clinicians criticize a restricted set, since it may not require phonemic discrimination. The child may more easily select the correct response in a restricted set since he may choose on the basis of an isolated consonant or vowel segment. The unrestricted set may be more difficult since the child must discriminate between slight phonemic differences (for example, mouse vs. mouth). The results of this study support the suggestion that an unrestricted set may be more difficult. The Word Intelligibility by Picture Identification and Northwestern University-Children's Perception of Speech, which both use unrestricted test stimuli, were found to be more difficult than the Pediatric Speech Intelligibility, which uses a restricted set of stimuli.

It must be noted that the results of this study are limited to the population of hearing impaired subjects studied. Different degrees of hearing impairment, as well as different configurations of loss, may alter the results of this study. However, it is clear that further research in the area of pediatric speech discrimination is warranted to allow understanding the relationship between specificity and sensitivity and discrimination ability.

To minimize and attempt to control for the effect of language and vocabulary on the discrimination score, Matkin recommended selecting the discrimination test on the basis of established or estimated receptive vocabulary age.[92] Information on the receptive vocabulary age may be obtained by the use of appropriate materials such as the Peabody Picture Vocabulary Test. Additionally, receptive language ability can be defined by the Northwestern Syntax Screening Test (NSST receptive). Matkin recommends the phonetically balanced kindergarten lists for children with a receptive vocabulary age of between 6 and 12 years and the use of the WIPI test if the receptive vocabulary age is between 4 and 6 years.

CENTRAL AUDITORY ASSESSMENT

The relatively recent focus on central auditory processing and its possible effect on language and learning has resulted in parents and school personnel referring their language impaired children to audiology clinics at earlier ages. Many of these children are found to have fluctuant conductive hearing losses or high-frequency losses. However, many demonstrate normal hearing for pure tones or noiseband stimuli and speech. Too often an audiologic evaluation of these children stops after a determination of normal or near-normal hearing levels. To view auditory function as being tied predominantly to sensitivity is totally inappropriate. The literature in this area clearly indicate that central lesions of the auditory system do not manifest themselves in changes in peripheral hearing sensitivity. Investigators and clinicians now agree that diagnosis of abnormalities in the central auditory system requires more than the routine test battery.

It has been found necessary to develop new speech tests and refine testing methodologies to evaluate the central auditory pathways. For example, complex speech materials, such as sentences, may be more sensitive to the presence of auditory processing disorders. According to Hodgson, the following five effects may be observed in the presence of pathology of the central auditory system: (1) pure tone thresholds are essentially normal in both ears; (2) suprathreshold pure tone tests are essentially normal in both ears; (3) speech discrimination scores may be reduced in the ear contralateral to the damaged portion of the brain, which becomes more evident if the speech is distorted; (4) dichotic listening tasks are more difficult than for persons with intact central auditory nervous systems; and (5) when speech is presented to one ear and a competing signal to the other ear, poor discrimination may be evident contralateral to the lesion.[116]

The focus on central auditory processing with infants is along three major lines in audiology today: (1) interest evolving around basic developmental questions; (2) localizing disorders of the auditory pathway; and (3) determining if a relationship exists between central auditory function and language learning impairments.

Behavioral research on central auditory processing abilities in infants is limited. However, infants as young as 6 months of age are demonstrating signs of central auditory processing in that they are developing sound localization abilities.[22,23] This ability indicates that 6-month-old infants are making use of auditory information arriving at both ears and are processing information in the central auditory system.

The utilization of the VRISD paradigm appears to allow for the investigation of the central auditory system in the infant and young child populations. Utilizing the VRISD paradigm, Wilson and I demonstrated that 6- to 8-month-old infants demonstrate a binaural resynthesis (fusion) ability.[117] In our research, two formant speechlike vowels (/i/) (/ɛ/) were presented in a diotic and dichotic mode. The results of this study indicated that the infants were able to fuse binaurally the dichotic vowel sounds, categorize the fused percept to be similar to the diotic presentation of the same vowel sound, and discriminate the one particular vowel sound from the other vowel sound.

The literature reports that binaural fusion has been utilized as a test of central auditory function with children as young as 5 years of age.[118] Additionally, Willeford suggested that this ability seems to be related to age, showing a "maturational pattern" from age 5 to 9 years. The mean scores on Willeford's norms do improve with age; however, the range of individual performance is so wide that differentiation of age by performance is difficult. The wide dispersion of scores at any single age raises questions about task variables as contrasted to developmental or maturational factors in binaural fusion. The data from Wilson and I would suggest that binaural fusion may not be strongly related to age, since infants at 6 months of age demonstrated success on a binaural resynthesis (fusion) task.[117]

Variables, such as language and vocabulary, instructions, memory, and response task, can influence a binaural fusion task. Perhaps these variables explain in part why such wide ranges of normal have been reported in the literature. Additionally, these variables may account for at least some of the reported improvement in performance with age. When these variables are controlled or eliminated, perhaps a closer estimate of the binaural fusion ability can be developed. Additionally, if these variables are controlled, other tests of central auditory function can be developed by means of the VRISD paradigm. For example, speech discrimination with either an ipsilateral or contralateral competing message may allow for further investigation of the brain stem and the temporal lobe regions. Although the work in this area is still in the experimental stages, the possibility of applying this information to disordered populations may become a clinical reality in the near future.

Another example of measuring central auditory processing skills in young infants has been demonstrated by Nozza.[119] Utilizing the head turn response, estimates of the masking level difference for both a 500 Hz pure tone and a speech sound (/ba/) were obtained. Infants demonstrated a release from masking for both signals, but their masking level differences were significantly smaller than those of adult controls. These data point out the remarkable ability of infants, and as important, the methodologic approaches that may be used to investigate the central auditory system in very young children.

Jerger et al indicate that a motivation for developing the PSI test was to construct a procedure for evaluating both peripheral and central components of auditory disorders in children.[115] These investigators, in an attempt to establish the validity of the PSI test as a means of detecting central auditory disorders, tested a series of children with documented central nervous systems (CNS) lesions.

Four children, three with surgically or roentgenographically confirmed brain stem or temporal lobe disorder and one with a nonauditory CNS disorder, were evaluated audiologically. The PSI central test battery (performance for words versus that for sentences, in quiet versus competition, and in ipsilateral versus contralateral competing modes) was administered. Preliminary results in children with CNS disorders suggest that the PSI test does not yield false-positive results in children without central auditory dysfunction and does yield abnormal results in children with confirmed central auditory disorder. In the three children with confirmed brain stem or temporal lobe disorder, abnormalities include rollover of the performance-intensity function in competition, abnormally poor maximum intelligibility scores in competition, and unusually slow rise to maximum performance in competition.

This early work in central auditory processing with infants and young children, utilizing the head turning paradigm for young children and the PSI test for older children, may lead to more detailed assessment of the entire auditory system in young children. If clinicians are to understand the total auditory system in children, they must include direct assessment of central auditory function in order to determine possible sites of medical pathology and/or possible causes of language learning disorders.

SUMMARY

This chapter has focused on the audiologic assessment of the pediatric population. From the progress in assessment techniques that has been made over the past decade, the pediatric population should no longer be considered a difficult-to-test population.

Because the focus has been on behavioral procedures, the topic of immittance measurement, specifically tympanometry, static compliance, and reflex measurements, has not been developed. A literature base does exist for the pediatric population, and the immittance procedures are fully applicable to neonates and infants (see Chapter 41). Although some caution needs to be placed on tympanometric interpretation for young infants, immittance measurement should be used routinely to supplement behavioral testing.

Finally, a test battery approach consisting of behavioral testing and immittance measures is recommended for pediatric assessment. When the results from this approach are inconclusive, or supplemental information is needed, electrophysiologic measures such as the auditory brain stem response and the 40-Hz middle latency response can be called upon.

REFERENCES

1. Ewing IR, Ewing AWG. The ascertainment of deafness in infancy and early childhood. J Laryngol Otol 1944; 59:309–333.
2. Hardy W, Pauls M, Bordley JE. Modern concepts of rehabilitation of young children with severe hearing impairment. Acta Otolaryngol (Stockh) 1951; 40:80.
3. Myklebust H. Auditory disorders in children. New York: Grune & Stratton, 1954.
4. Silverman SR. Hard-of-hearing children. In: Davis H, ed. Hearing and deafness—a guide for laymen. New York: Rinehart and Company, 1956:352.
5. Downs MP. Testing hearing in infancy and early childhood. In: McConnell F, Ward PH, eds. Deafness in childhood. Nashville: Vanderbilt University Press, 1966: 25.
6. Bergstrom L. Congenital deafness. In: Northern JL. Hearing disorders. 2nd ed. Boston: Little, Brown, 1984:171.
7. Liden G, Harford ER. The pediatric audiologist. From magician to clinician. Ear Hear 1985; 6:6–9.
8. Stein L, Clark S, Kraus N. The hearing-impaired infant: patterns of identification and habilitation. Ear Hear 1983; 4:232–236.
9. Downs MP, Sterritt GM. Identification audiometry for neonates: a preliminary report. J Aud Res 1964; 4:69–80.
10. Downs MP, Sterritt GM. A guide to newborn and infant hearing screening programs. Arch Otolaryngol 1967; 85:15–22.
11. Downs MP, Hemenway WG. Report on the hearing screening of 17,000 neonates. Int Audiol 1969; 8:72–76.
12. Feinmesser M, Tell L. Evaluation of methods for detecting hearing-impairment in infancy and early childhood. In: Conference on newborn hearing screening, proceedings summary and recommendations. San Francisco: United States Public Health Service and California State Department of Public Health, 1971: 119.

12a. Apgar V. A proposal for a new method of evaluation of the newborn infant. Anesth Analg 1953; 32:260.

12b. Apgar V, James L. Further observations on the newborn scoring system. Am J Dis Child 1962; 104:419.

13. Mencher GT. Infant hearing screening: the state of the art. Maico Audio Libr Series 1974; 12:7.
14. Pappas DG. A study of the high-risk registry for sensorineural hearing impairment. Head Neck Surg 1983; 91:41–44.
15. Feinmesser M, Tell L. Evaluation of methods for detecting hearing impairment in infancy and early childhood. In: Mencher G, ed. Proceedings of the Nova Scotia Conference on early identification of hearing loss. Basel: S Karger, 1976:355.
16. Mencher GT. Program for neonatal hearing screening. Audiology 1974; 13:495–500.
17. Downs M. Early identification of hearing loss: Where are we? Where do we go from here? In: Mencher G, ed. Proceedings of the Nova Scotia Conference on early identification of hearing loss. Basel: S Karger, 1976.
18. Joint Committee on Infant Hearing Screening. Supplementary statement on infant hearing screening. Asha 1972; 16:160.
19. Hodgson WR. Tests of hearing—birth through one year. In: Martin F, ed. Pediatric audiology. Englewood Cliffs, NJ: Prentice-Hall, 1978:174.
20. Mencher G, ed. Proceedings of the Nova Scotia Conference on early detection of hearing loss. Basel: S Karger, 1976.
21. Downs MP. Return to the basics of infant screening. In: Gerber SE, Mencher GT, eds. Early diagnosis of hearing loss. New York: Grune & Stratton, 1978:129.
22. Northern JL, Downs MP. Hearing in children. Baltimore: Williams & Wilkins, 1974.
23. Northern JL, Downs MP. Hearing in children. Baltimore: Williams & Wilkins, 1978.
24. Jacobson JT, Morehouse CR. A comparison of auditory brainstem response and behavioral screening in high risk and normal newborn infants. Ear Hear 1984; 5(4):247–253.
25. Joint Committee on Infant Hearing Screening. Ear Hear 1983; 4:3–4.
26. Simmons FB, Russ FN. Automated newborn hearing screening, the crib-o-gram. Arch Otolaryngol 1974; 100: 1–7.
27. Simmons FB. Automated hearing screening test for newborns: the crib-o-gram. In: Mencher G, ed. Proceedings of the Nova Scotia Conference on early identification of hearing loss. Basel: S Karger, 1976:180.
28. Simmons FB, McFarland WH, Jones FR. An automated hearing screening technique for newborns. Acta Otolaryngol (Stockh) 1979; 87:1–8.
29. Simmons FB. Patterns of deafness in newborns. Laryngoscope 1980; 90:448.
30. Durieux-Smith A, Picton T, Edwards C, Goodman JT, MacMurray B. The crib-o-gram in the NICU: an evaluation based on brain stem electric response audiometry. Ear Hear 1985; 6:20–24.
31. Simmons FB. Comment on hearing loss in graduates of a tertiary intensive care nursery. Ear Hear 1982; 3:188.
32. Gerber SE, Mencher GT. Proceedings of Saskatchewan Conference on early diagnosis of hearing loss. New York: Grune & Stratton, 1978.
33. Jacobson JT, Seitz MR, Mencher GT, Parrott V. Auditory brainstem response: a contribution to infant assessment and management. In: Mencher GT, Gerber SE, eds. Early management of hearing loss. New York: Grune & Stratton, 1981:151.
34. Fria TJ, Sabo DL. Auditory brainstem responses in children with otitis media with effusion. Ann Otol Rhinol Laryngol 1980; 68:200–206.
35. Hecox K, Galambos R. Brain stem auditory evoked responses in human infants and adults. Arch Otolaryngol 1974; 99:30–33.
36. Schulman-Galambos C, Galambos H. Brainstem auditory evoked responses in premature infants. J Speech Hear Res 1975; 8:456–465.
37. Schulman-Galambos C, Galambos R. Brainstem evoked response audiometry in newborn hearing screening. Arch Otolaryngol 1979; 105:86–90.
38. Salamy A, McKean CM, Buda FB. Maturational changes in auditory transmission as reflected in human brainstem potentials. Brain Res 1975; 96:361–366.
39. Salamy A, McKean CM. Postnatal development of the human brainstem potentials during the first year of life. Electroencephalogr Clin Neurophysiol 1976; 40:418–426.
40. Galambos R. Use of the auditory brainstem response (ABR) in infant hearing testing. In: Gerber SE, Mencher GT, eds. Early diagnosis of hearing loss. New York: Grune & Stratton, 1978:245.
41. Gorga MP, Worthington DW, Reiland JK, Beauchaine KA, Goldgar DE. Some comparisons between auditory brain stem response thresholds, latencies, and the pure-tone audiogram. Ear Hear 1985; 6:105–112.
42. Davis H. Principles of electric response audiometry. Ann Otol Rhinol Laryngol [Suppl] 1976; 28:1–96.
43. Cox LC, Hack M, Metz DA. Brainstem-evoked response

audiometry in the premature infant population. Int J Pediatr Otorhinolaryngol 1981; 3:213–244.
44. Sanders RA, Duncan PG, McCullough DW. Clinical experience with brain stem audiometry performed under general anesthesia. J Otolaryngol 1979; 8:24–32.
45. Picton TW, Hillyard SA. Human auditory evoked potentials: effects of attention. Electroencephalogr Clin Neurophysiol 1974; 36:191–200.
46. Sohmer H, Gafni M, Chisin R. Auditory nerve and brainstem responses: comparison in awake and unconscious subjects. Arch Neurol 1978; 35:228–230.
47. Jerger J, Hayes D. The crosscheck principle in pediatric audiometry. Arch Otolaryngol 1976; 102:614–620.
48. Niemeyer W, Sesterhenn G. Calculating the hearing threshold from the stapedius reflex threshold for different sound stimuli. Paper presented at the 11th International Congress of Audiology, Budapest, 1972.
49. Niemeyer W, Sesterhenn G. Calculating the hearing threshold from the stapedius reflex threshold for different stimuli. Audiology 1974; 13:421–427.
50. Jerger J, Burney P, Mauldin L, Crump B. Predicting hearing loss from the acoustic reflex. J Speech Hear Disord 1974; 39:11–22.
51. Baker SR, Lilly DJ. Prediction of hearing level from acoustic reflex data. Paper presented at the American Speech and Hearing Association Convention, Houston, Texas, 1976.
52. Rizzo S Jr., Greenberg HJ. Predicting hearing loss from the acoustic reflex. Paper presented at the 50th Meeting of the Acoustical Society of America, Boston, 1979.
53. Popelka GR, Margolis RH, Wiley TL. Effect of activating signal bandwidth on acoustic reflex thresholds. J Acoust Soc Am 1976; 59:153–159.
54. Jerger J, Hayes D, Anthony L, Mauldin L. Factors influencing prediction of hearing level from the acoustic reflex. Monogr Contempor Audiol 1978; 1:1–20.
55. Margolis RH, Fox CM. A comparison of three methods for predicting hearing loss from acoustic reflex thresholds. J Speech Hear Res 1977; 20:241–253.
56. Jerger J, Hayes D, Anthony L. Effect of age on prediction of sensori-neural hearing level from the acoustic reflex. Arch Otolaryngol 1978; 194:393–394.
57. Keith RW, Bench RJ. Stapedial reflexes in neonates. Scand Audiol 1978; 7:187–191.
58. Himelfarb M, Shannon E, Popelka G, Margolis R. Acoustic reflex evaluation in neonates. In: Gerber SE, Mencher GT, eds. Early diagnosis of hearing loss. New York: Grune & Stratton, 1978:109.
59. Johnson DE, Diefendorf AO. Acoustic-reflex testing with neonates. Hear J 1983; 36:26–29.
60. Keith RW. An evaluation of predicting hearing loss from the acoustic reflex. Arch Otolaryngol 1977; 103:419–424.
61. Hall JW. Predicting hearing loss from the acoustic reflex. In: Jerger J, Northern J, eds. Clinical impedance audiometry. 2nd ed. Acton, MA: American Electromedics, 1980:141.
62. Hall JW, Bleakney ME. Hearing loss prediction by the acoustic reflex: comparison of seven methods. Ear Hear 1981; 2:156–164.
63. Hall JW, Koval CB. Accuracy of hearing prediction by the acoustic reflex. Laryngoscope 1982; 92:140–149.
64. Murphy KP. Development of hearing in babies. Hear News 1961; 29:9–11.
65. Thompson G, Weber B. Responses of infants and young children to behavioral observation audiometry (BOA). J Speech Hear Disord 1974; 39:140–147.
66. Hoversten G, Moncur J. Stimuli and intensity factors in testing infants. J Speech Hear Res 1969; 12:687–702.
67. Thompson M, Thompson G. Response of infants and young children as a functioning of auditory stimuli and test method. J Speech Hear Res 1972; 15:699–707.
68. Eisenberg RB. Auditory behavior in the human neonate: functional properties of sound and their ontogenetic implications. Int Audiol 1969; 8:34–45.
69. Mencher GT, McCullouch B, Derbyshire AJ, Dethlefs R. Observer bias as a factor in neonatal hearing screening. J Speech Hear Res 1977; 20:27–34.
70. Weber BA. Validation of observer judgements in behavioral observation audiometry. J Speech Hear Disord 1969; 34:350–355.
71. Moore JM, Thompson G, Thompson M. Auditory localization of infants as a function of reinforcement conditions. J Speech Hear Disord 1975; 40:29–34.
72. Moore JM, Wilson WR, Thompson G. Visual reinforcement of head-turn responses in infants under 12 months of age. J Speech Hear Disord 1977; 42:328–334.
73. Dix MR, Hallpike CS. The peep show: a new technique for pure-tone audiometry in young children. Br Med J 1947; 2:719–723.
74. Statten P, Wishart DES. Pure-tone audiometry in young children: psychogalvanic-skin-resistance and peep-show. Ann Otol Rhinol Laryngol 1956; 65:511–534.
75. Miller AL. The use of slide projectors in pure-tone audiometric testing. J Speech Hear Disord 1963; 28:94–96.
76. Lloyd LL. Use of the slide show audiometric technique with mentally retarded children. Except Child 1965; 32:93–98.
77. Suzuki T, Ogiba Y. A technique of pure-tone audiometry for children under three years of age: conditioned orientation reflex (COR) audiometry. Rev Laryngol Otol Rhinol (Bord) 1960; 81:33–45.
78. Suzuki T, Ogiba Y. Conditioned orientation audiometry. Arch Otolaryngol 1960; 74:192–198.
79. Liden G, Kankkunen A. Visual reinforcement audiometry. Acta Otolaryngol (Stockh) 1969; 67:281–292.
80. Knox EC. A method of obtaining pure-tone audiograms in young children. J Laryngol Otol 1960; 74:475–479.
81. Meyerson L, Michael JL. The measurement of sensory thresholds in exceptional children: an experimental approach to some problems of differential diagnosis and education with special reference to hearing. Cooperative Research Project No. 418. Houston: United States Office of Education, Department of Health, Education, and Welfare, University of Houston, 1960.
82. Meyerson L, Michael JL. Assessment of hearing by operant conditioning procedures. Report of the proceedings of the International Congress on Education of the Deaf. Washington, DC: Gallaudett College, June 22–28, 1963. United States Government Printing Office, Senate Document #106, 88th Congress, 2nd Session, 1964.
83. Lloyd LL, Spradlin JE, Reid MJ. An operant audiometric procedure for difficult-to-test patients. J Speech Hear Disord 1968; 33:236–245.
84. Spradlin JE, Lloyd LL. Operant conditioning audiometry (OCA) with low level retardates: a preliminary report. In: Lloyd LL, Frisina DR, eds. The audiologic assessment of the mentally retarded: proceedings of a national conference. Parsons, KS: State Hospital and Training Center, 1965:45.
85. Spradlin JE, Lloyd LL, Hom GL, Reid MJ. Establishing tone control and evaluating the hearing of severely retarded children. In: Jervis GA, ed. Expanding concepts in mental retardation: a symposium from the Joseph P. Kennedy Jr. Foundation. Springfield, IL: CC Thomas, 1968:170.
86. Lloyd LL. Behavioral audiometry viewed as an operant procedure. J Speech Hear Disord 1966; 31:128–139.
87. Redell RC, Calvert DR. Factors in screening hearing of the newborn. J Aud Res 1969; 3:278–289.
88. Haug O, Baccarro P, Guilford F. A pure-tone audiogram on the infant: the PIWI technique. Arch Otolaryngol 1967; 86:101–106.
89. Tyberghein J, Forrez G. Objective (E.R.A.) and subjec-

tive (C.O.R.) audiometry in the infant. Acta Otolaryngol (Stockh) 1971; 71:249–252.

90. Warren VG. A comparative study of the auditory responses of normal and "at-risk" infants from twelve to twenty-four months of age using COR audiometry. Doctoral Dissertation, University of Southern California, Los Angeles, 1972.
91. Matkin ND, Thomas J. A longitudinal study of visual reinforcement audiometry. Paper presented at ASHA Convention, Las Vegas, 1974.
92. Matkin N. Hearing aids for children. In: Hodgson W, Skinner P, eds. Hearing aid assessment and use in audiologic habilitation. Baltimore: Williams & Wilkins, 1977:145.
93. Thompson G, Folsom RC. A comparison of two conditioning procedures in the use of visual reinforcement audiometry (VRA). J Speech Hear Disord 1984; 49:241–245.
94. Wilson WR, Moore JM, Thompson G. Sound field auditory thresholds of infants utilizing visual reinforcement audiometry (VRA). Paper presented at The American Speech and Hearing Association Annual Convention, Houston, 1976.
95. Diefendorf AO, Jennings S. Stimulus response comparisons between visual reinforcement audiometry (VRA) and behavioral observation audiometry (BOA). Paper presented at the American Speech-Language-Hearing Association Annual Convention, Cincinnati, 1983.
96. Goldman TM. Response of infants to warble-tone signals presented in soundfield using visual reinforcement audiometry. Masters Thesis, University of Cincinnati, 1979.
97. Wilson WR, Moore JM. Pure-tone earphone thresholds of infants utilizing visual reinforcement audiometry (VRA). Paper presented at The American Speech-Language-Hearing Association Convention, San Francisco, 1978.
98. Stephens MM, Rintelmann WF. The influence of audiometric configuration on pure-tone, warbled-tone and narrow-band noise thresholds of adults with sensorineural hearing losses. J Am Aud Soc 1978; 3:221–226.
99. Walker G, Dillon H, Bryne D. Sound field audiometry: recommended stimuli and procedures. Ear Hear 1984; 5:13–21.
100. Bricker DD, Bricker WA. A programmed approach to operant audiometry for low-functioning children. J Speech Hear Disord 1969; 34:312–320.
101. Fulton RT. Pure-tone tests of hearing—age one year through five years. In: Martin FN, ed. Pediatric audiology. Englewood Cliffs, NJ: Prentice-Hall, 1978:174.
102. Wilson WR, Decker NT. Auditory thresholds of infants using operant audiometry with tangible and/or visual reinforcement. Unpublished research, University of Washington, 1977.
102a. Fainberg J, Diefendorf A. Auditory intensity discrimination in normally-hearing infants. Paper presented at The American Speech-Language-Hearing Association Annual Convention, Los Angeles, 1984.
103. Barr B. Pure tone audiometry for pre-school children. Acta Otolaryngol [Suppl] (Stockh) 1955:121.
104. Diefendorf AO. The effect of a pre-play period on play audiometry. Paper presented at the Tennessee Speech-Language-Hearing Association Annual Convention, Memphis, 1981.
104a. Glorig A. Pure tone sweepcheck as an indicator of the pure tone threshold test. In: Gerwin KS, Glorig A, eds. Detection of hearing loss and ear disease in children. Springfield, IL: CC Thomas, 1974:149.
105. Aslin RN, Pisoni DB, Jusczyk PW. Auditory development and speech perception in infancy. In: Haith MM, Campos JJ, eds. Infancy and the biology of development. New York: John Wiley & Sons, 1983:573.
106. Eilers RE, Wilson WR, Moore JM. Developmental changes in speech discrimination in infants. J Speech Hear Res 1977; 20:766–780.
107. Eimas PD. Auditory and linguistic processing of cues for place of articulation by infants. Percept Psychophys 1974; 16:513–521.
108. Wilson WR, Widen JL, Diefendorf AO, Nozza R. Speech-sound discrimination testing of infants—a clinical reality. Presented at the Society for Ear, Nose, and Throat Advances in Children, Cincinnati, 1979.
109. Haskins H. A phonetically balanced test of speech discrimination for children. Masters thesis, Northwestern University, Evanston, Illinois, 1949.
110. Sanderson-Leepa ME, Rintelmann WF. Articulation function and test-retest performance of normal-hearing children on three speech discrimination tests: WIPI, PBK 50, and NU auditory test no. 6. J Speech Hear Disord 1976; 41:503–519.
111. Ross M, Lerman J. Picture identification test for hearing-impaired children. J Speech Hear Res 1970; 13:44–53.
112. Siegenthaler B, Haspiel G. Development of two standardized measures of hearing for speech by children. Cooperative research program, project #2372, United States Office of Education, 1966.
113. Hodgson W. A comparison of WIPI and PB-K discrimination test scores. Paper presented at the ASHA Convention, Detroit, 1973.
113a. Elliot LL, Katz DR. Northwestern University children's perception of speech. St. Louis: Auditec of St. Louis, 1980.
114. Jerger S, Lewis S, Hawkins J, Jerger J. Pediatric speech intellgibility test 1: generation of test materials. Int J Pediatr Otorhinolaryngol 1980; 2:217–230.
115. Jerger S, Jerger J, Abrams S. Speech audiometry in the young child. Ear Hear 1983; 4:56–66.
115a. Dehart NN. Comparing normally-hearing and hearing-impaired children's performance on the word intelligibility by picture identification, pediatric speech intelligibility, and Northwestern University children's perception of speech tests. Masters Thesis, University of Tennessee, Knoxville, Tennessee 1987.
116. Hodgson WR. Testing infants and young children. In: Katz J, ed. Handbook of clinical audiology. Baltimore: Williams & Wilkins, 1972:498.
117. Diefendorf AO, Wilson WR. Auditory fusion in infants: one aspect of central auditory function. Paper presented at ASHA Convention, Detroit, 1980.
118. Willeford J. Assessing central auditory behavior in children. In: Keith RW, ed. Central auditory dysfunction. New York: Grune & Stratton, 1977:43.
119. Nozza R. Infant binaural analysis: masking level difference for 500 Hz tone and for speech. Paper presented at The American Speech-Language-Hearing Association Annual Convention, Detroit, 1986.

51 Industrial Hearing Conservation

Wayne G. Bodenhemier, Ph.D.

The birth of industrial audiology as a distinct discipline and the beginning of interest and activity in industrial hearing conservation can be traced to the early 1970s. Despite the fact that the earliest attempt at federal regulation of occupational noise exposure took place in 1936 under the authority of the Walsh-Healy Public Contracts Act and despite the fact that the first monetary compensation for occupational hearing loss as an industrial disease was made in 1948, not until 1970 did the issue of noise exposure in the workplace come to a head. Two things happened: first, the passage of the Williams-Steiger Occupational Safety and Health Act (OSH Act) late in 1970 and second, the official acceptance of the notion that hearing loss caused by workplace noise exposure is preventable and that damages (in the form of worker's compensation) should be awarded to any worker whose employer fails to prevent its occurrence.

An estimate of the magnitude of the problem of work-related hearing loss was recently offered by Tempest when he wrote that "noise is almost certainly the most widespread hazard in the modern industrial environment."[1] He cited evidence indicating that slightly more than 20 percent of workers in industry in the United States are exposed to noise levels in excess of 90 dBA as a function of the daily equivalent continuous noise level. (Measurements made with the A-scale weighting network on a sound level meter have been found to simulate accurately the sensitivity of the human ear at low sound pressure levels. In occupational environments, the scale is the most widely used frequency response function for noise measurement. As opposed to the B- and C-scales, also found on many sound level meters, the A-weighting response is most useful for describing and for characterizing most environmental sounds from the standpoint of hearing damage risk.) Aram Glorig was perhaps more to the point when he observed that, of the more than 20 million Americans who are exposed to hazardous noise both on and off the job, more than 16 million have some degree of sensorineural hearing loss caused by occupational exposure alone.[2]

In this chapter, an attempt will be made to familiarize the reader with the broad spectrum of considerations and activities in which the audiologist is involved in the field of industrial hearing conservation.

WHY INDUSTRIAL HEARING CONSERVATION?

In addition to the large numbers of working men and women who have some degree of permanent hearing damage caused by exposure to workplace noise as mentioned earlier, and considering the large numbers of workers who are exposed to hazardous noise, there are at least two other reasons why industrial hearing conservation and industrial hearing conservation programs should be of the utmost interest and concern to the audiologist. First is the fact that federal and many state regulations are in existence that govern occupational noise exposure and actually require that employers provide hearing conservation programs for employees deemed at risk of workplace-induced permanent hearing loss. Second, and perhaps of even greater urgency, is the spectre of worker's compensation claims and the huge potential economic liability for industry and for society in general.

In my opinion, even though federal regulation of occupational hearing loss is not, nor should be, the most compelling reason to become involved in or to initiate an occupational hearing conservation program, understanding the government's involvement in order to gain an historical perspective of the problem is important. In addition, the current federal standard relative to industrial hearing conservation offers, I think, a sound structure upon which to build an effective program.

THE HISTORY OF FEDERAL REGULATION OF NOISE

Federal regulation of occupational noise exposure in the United States began in 1936 with the promulgation of the Walsh-Healey Public Contracts Act, which generally required that noise exposure in the workplace be reasonably controlled in order to minimize employee fatigue, thus reducing the probability of accidents. That was the good news! The bad news was that the Act was ignored for the next 34 years because of lack of enforcement, and industry did little, if anything, to respond to the need for hearing conservation measures among its employees.

Late 1970 brought about the passage of the Williams-Steiger OSH Act, and the entire picture of industrial hearing conservation changed significantly. Although the wording of this Act was identical to that of the earlier legislation, it specified that compliance with its requirements was mandatory and that, therefore, violation of the regulation would constitute violation of the Act itself. The noise-related portions of this legislation were designed to actively monitor and update noise exposure in the workplace. The Act required that, in all cases where sound levels exceeded certain predetermined levels, "a continuing, effective hearing conservation program shall be administered." Unfortunately, because of this rather vague wording, large differences of opinion arose as to the interpretation of the regulation. Many employers felt that the only method of compliance was to utilize engineering controls in an effort to reduce the workplace noise at its source. Others felt that an effective, acceptable hearing conservation program meant merely dispensing personal hearing protection devices to exposed workers. Still others felt that, in spite of the fact that periodic hearing testing was not identified specifically in the OSH Act as an element of a "continuing, effective" hearing conservation program, any attempts to reduce noise at the source or to protect the workers' hearing are futile unless they are monitored through a hearing testing program.

In 1974, the Occupational Safety and Health Administration (OSHA) published proposed requirements and procedures governing occupational noise exposure as mandated by the OSH Act of 1970.[3] This set of guidelines and recommendations was intended to settle the controversy surrounding appropriate compliance with the 1970 regulations, which aimed to achieve reduction of noise in the workplace primarily through engineering and/or administrative types of controls. The 1974 proposed requirements recognized that, until this reduction could be achieved realistically, other interim measures had to be relied upon in order to protect the hearing of the workers. These other measures included the wearing of personal hearing protection devices and periodic testing of hearing. For the next 7 years, heated exchanges between labor unions and management (what does management require and what will the union allow?), as well as between governmental agencies (for instance, OSHA and the Enviromental Protection Agency could not agree on the level of noise exposure necessary to begin hearing conservation), prevented any substantive progress toward the adoption of a final noise regulation.

In early 1981, and drafted during the final days of the Carter administration, OSHA published a hearing conservation amendment that was to become effective on April 15, 1981.[4] The Agency, now under the influence of the Reagan administration, received an overwhelming number of requests to reconsider as well as petitions to stay the proposed amendment. This response was based, in large measure, on charges that the proposed requirements were much too specification oriented and that many of the provisions were, in fact, not supported by substantial evidence. As a result, the effective date of the amendment was delayed several times. Finally, in August 1981, OSHA lifted the administrative stay on major portions of the amendment while continuing the administrative stay and reopening the public record for further comment on a number of other provisions.[5] The next year and a half or so was marked by public comment and administrative review of all submitted documents and evidence.

March 8, 1983, marked the publication of what was then thought to be the *final* hearing conservation amendment to the OSHA noise standard.[6] This rule became effective on April 7, 1983, and accomplished several things. First, it revoked many of the previously stayed provisions of the August 1981 amendment, thus striking them from the law. Second, it lifted the stay previously imposed on certain other portions of the amendment. Thirdly, it made certain technical changes and corrections to the noise standard. At this time, the majority of those responsible for hearing conservation in the workplace (the employer, hearing conservationists, state occupational safety and worker's compensation authorities) started implementing new programs or modifying existing programs to comply with a noise standard that was judged by most to be "acceptable and workable."

In April of 1984, the United States Fourth Circuit Court of Appeals first heard the case of Forging Industries Association and National Arborist Association versus Secretary of Labor. In this case, the plaintiffs contended that hearing loss is an "effect or result" and not a "hazard," and therefore not possibly regulated by OSHA. In addition, they alleged that the hearing conservation amendment requires action by employers when the cause of the hearing loss may not have been the workplace. On November 8, 1984, the Fourth Circuit Court issued a ruling that vacated the entire 1983 noise standard. The court (only three of nine judges participated in this decision) noted that an OSHA standard "is invalid if it requires an employer to take actions in regard to hazards existing outside the workplace . . . (and) under the hearing conservation amendment, employers may be subject to requirements, and penalties may be imposed, as a result of non-workplace hazards." They went further to say that "it is obvious that such a hearing loss can result from non-occupational noise exposure . . . yet the amendment makes the distinction between hearing loss caused by workplace sources and loss caused by non-workplace sources . . . and the rule contains no requirement that there be a determination of work-relatedness."

As a result of the Fourth Circuit Court decision, on December 28, 1984, the United States Department of Labor petitioned on behalf of the Secretary of Labor for a rehearing and suggested that it occur en bloc (before all 14 judges in the Fourth Circuit). In the interim, much correspondence in favor of the hearing conservation amendment was directed to OSHA and also to President Reagan, and OSHA sent a memorandum to all regional administrators dealing with the subject of interim guidance for the Hearing Conservation Amendment, which directed compliance officers to encourage employers to continue with hearing conservation programs already in existence. In addition, enforcement of the pre-1983 noise standard was emphasized. This meant that employers were again required to reduce noise exposure to the worker to or below the 90-dB 8-hour time-weighted average level through the use of engineering and/or administrative controls. Table 51–1 lists some of the more common types of engineering and administrative controls that might be implemented. If these types of control were determined to not be economically feasible, then providing adequate hearing protection to all employees exposed at or above that level was allowed. For all intents and purposes, the employer was again required to provide a "continuing, effective hearing conservation program," but the specific requirements of such a program were a debatable issue!

The rehearing of the Hearing Conservation Amendment by the entire United States Fourth Circuit Court of Appeals began on June 3, 1985, and on September 25, 1985, the unanimous decision to uphold the noise amendment *in its entirety* was handed down. This simply meant that the March 8, 1983, finalized federal noise regulation was officially "back in business" in its complete form. Table 51–2 presents a synopsis of the federal involvement with occupational hearing conservation, beginning with the Walsh-Healy Public Contracts Act.

HEARING CONSERVATION AMENDMENT: OCCUPATIONAL NOISE EXPOSURE

The finalized hearing conservation amendment to the OSHA noise standard, which became effective on April 7, 1983, specifies regulations and procedures in five separate and distinct areas. These areas are noise monitoring, audiometric testing, hearing protection, training, and recordkeeping. The requirements in each of these areas will be discussed in some detail because it is felt that knowledge of, and general adherence to, these requirements go a long way toward assuring an effective hearing conservation program in industry.

Noise Monitoring

Although the OSHA noise regulation has quite a bit of latitude concerning *how* noise monitoring information is obtained, it does require that the employer have a record of the employees' exposure to noise. OSHA's permissible exposure level is an 8-hour time-weighted average exposure of 90 dBA. The time-weighted average is obtained by measuring the amounts of time an employee spends in different noise levels throughout the workday and computing an "average" noise exposure according to a criterion level of 90 dB and a criterion time duration of 8 hours. Table 51–3 presents an abbreviated version of the OSHA permissible exposure levels and reference durations for steady-state noise. For any employee exposed above 90 dBA for 8 hours, annual audiometric testing and personal hearing protection are mandatory. In addition, economically and technologically feasible engineering and administrative controls must be used to reduce exposures at and above the 90 dBA level.

TABLE 51-1 Some Engineering and Administrative Noise Control Measures Used in Industrial Hearing Conservation Program

Engineering Controls	*Administrative Controls*
Assure proper maintenance of equipment and machinery; includes replacement/adjustment of parts as needed, regular lubrication	Arrange employee work schedules so that the 8-hour time-weighted average of 90 dBA is not exceeded
Substitute larger, slower machines for smaller, faster ones when economically feasible; specify hydraulic presses over mechanical presses and belt driven equipment over gear drives	Arrange for employees who have reached the upper limit of exposure duration for a particular noise to work the remainder of their shifts in an environment with a noise level well below 90 dBA
Substitute quiet processes for noisy ones when possible; use welding instead of riveting, pressing instead of rolling or forging	Divide noisy jobs among employees in order to keep individual noise exposure within permissible time limits
Dampen vibration; use rubber or plastic bumpers and/or cushions where feasible	If a noisy machine is needed less than full time, operate it a part of each day rather than all day for part of the week
Isolate noise sources; enclose unusually noisy machines; use baffles; confine noisiest machines to an isolated room	Arrange for occasional high-level noisy operations to be conducted at night, on weekends, or at other times when the fewest number of employees will be exposed
Isolated operator; provide an insulated enclosure for the operator of one or more machines	

The OSHA hearing conservation amendment created an "action level," which is a concept different from the permissible exposure level. The "action level" is defined as a time-weighted average exposure of 85 dBA. All employees exposed to a time-weighted average of between 85 dBA and 90 dBA must be included in a hearing conservation program, which includes annual audiometric testing and annual training *as a minimum.* These employees must also have personal hearing protection devices made

TABLE 51–2 Federal Regulation of Workplace Exposure to Noise and Occupational Hearing Conservation

Date	*Involvement*	*Comment*
1936	Walsh-Healy Public Contracts Act	Very little, if any, enforcement
1970	Williams-Steiger OSH Act	Compliance was mandatory; broad interpretation due to vague wording; required "continuing, effective" hearing conservation program
1974	Proposed requirements and guidelines governing occupational noise exposure	Required by OSH Act of 1970; intended to clarify OSH Act; did not settle compliance controversies
January 1981	Hearing Conservation Amendment (to become effective April 15, 1981)	Effective date delayed by Reagan administration; many provisions placed on administrative "stay"
August 1981	Administrative "stay" lifted on many portions of amendment	Public record reopened for provisions still on "stay"
March 8, 1983	"Final" Hearing Conservation Amendment published (became effective April 7, 1983)	Revoked many previously "stayed" provisions; lifted "stay" on other provisions; made changes and corrections of a technical nature
April 1984	Forging Industries Association and National Arborist Association versus Secretary of Labor	Case heard by United States Fourth Circuit Court of Appeals
November 8, 1984	Entire 1983 amendment vacated by Fourth Circuit Court	Enforcement of 1970 OSH Act was again emphasized
December 28, 1984	United States Department of Labor petitioned Fourth Circuit Court for a rehearing en bloc	Rehearing began on June 3, 1985
September 25, 1985	Unanimous decision by Fourth Circuit Court to uphold the March 8, 1983 noise amendment in its entirety	Generally accepted as a workable law

TABLE 51–3 OSHA Permissible Exposure Level for Steady-State Noise

Duration/Day (hours)	*TWA (dBA)*
1/4	115
1/2	110
3/4	107
1	105
1 1/2	102
2	100
3	97
4	95
6	92
8	90

Abbreviation: TWA = time-weighted average.

available to them, although the wearing of such devices is not mandatory in this category unless annual audiometric testing exhibits a standard threshold shift (defined as a change in hearing threshold relative to the baseline of an average of 10 dB or more at 2,000, 3,000, and 4,000 Hz in either ear) relative to the baseline hearing test.

OSHA allows that either "area" or "personal" noise monitoring can be used, but that the method chosen must be designed to identify all those employees requiring inclusion in the hearing conservation program (85 dBA time-weighted average or greater) and to ensure the proper selection of hearing protection devices. Although OSHA has made it clear that either "area" or "personal" noise monitoring can be used, it should be pointed out that the noise standard suggests that "area" type monitoring is generally not appropriate in circumstances of high worker mobility, in large noise level fluctuations, or in situations where impulse noise is present. In this regard, two issues must be taken into consideration by the audiologist involved in noise measurement. First, what type of noise is to be measured? And second, what type of instrumentation and measurement techniques need to be employed? These two questions are dealt with in a clear and comprehensive manner by both Goldstein[7] and Tempest[8], and it is suggested that these two sources be consulted before any attempt be made whatsoever at meaningful noise measurement. In fact, unless the audiologist has had extensive training and practical experience in this highly technical skill, it is recommended that these measurements be conducted by, or at least under the close scrutiny of, a person more qualified such as an acoustical engineer or perhaps an industrial hygienist. Heggie and Miller[9] emphasize the importance of clearly establishing the *reason* for making noise measurements, then selecting the procedures to suit the purpose, and finally selecting the appropriate instrumentation. They reiterate the fact that "documented evidence of daily noise dose is the basis for all subsequent action on compliance with the noise standard, the requirement for hearing conservation and the potential liability for work-related injury."

Two final requirements are stipulated by the OSHA hearing conservation amendment for noise monitoring. First, in order to ease some of the financial and administrative burden placed on the employer, the requirements call for remonitoring of noise exposure only when a change in production, process, equipment, or controls either potentially increases noise exposure or potentially increases the number of employees who need to be included in the hearing conservation program. And second, with respect to right-to-know legislation, the employer is responsible for notifying each employee exposed at an 8-hour time-weighted average of 85 dBA or more of the results of the noise monitoring.

It is important to remember that there are several good reasons why valid and reliable data on noise monitoring for employees is necessary. First, based on this data, decisions are made as to which employees are to be included in the hearing conservation program and which can be safely excluded. Second, critical decisions concerning personal hearing protection devices are dependent on the data. And third, OSHA requires it. In the case of an OSHA inspection, the OSHA Compliance Officer decides whether or not acceptable information is available that characterizes employees' noise exposure accurately.

Audiometric Testing

Audiometric testing is the cornerstone of any industrial hearing conservation program. Careful review and analysis of baseline and annual follow-up hearing tests provides invaluable information relative to the overall hearing conservation effort. For instance, judgements on the effectiveness of all hearing conservation components—such as personal hearing protection, engineering controls aimed at reducing noise at the source, and/or administrative controls whose purpose is to reduce the employees' time of exposure to potentially hazardous noise—revolve around a comparison of hearing test results from year to year. In other words, how else do you know that employees are wearing properly fitted and maintained hearing protection devices unless the annual hearing test results indicate that hearing sensitivity is not deteriorating? How do you know that implemented engineering controls were well advised unless you can demonstrate that exposed employees are not losing their hearing? Yet what if audiogram review reveals a significant number of hearing sensitivity changes related to noise? Obviously, this fact should trigger an immediate review of all hearing conservation measures, with appropriate modifications and adjustments where necessary.

The area of audiometric testing in an industrial hearing conservation program is obviously the one to which the audiologist brings the greatest amount of knowledge and expertise. It is incumbent upon him or her to bring together all of his or her academic training and practical experience along with a thorough understanding of the current OSHA noise regulations and any applicable state regulations so that the overall hearing conservation effort can be successful. This requirement is true regardless of whether the audiologist is serving as a consultant to industry and simply overseeing the audiometric program or is actually responsible for conducting the testing, review, and follow-up.

The 1983 OSHA hearing conservation amendment required that baseline audiograms must have been completed on all exposed employees by March 1, 1984. And so those companies that have not yet instituted an audiometric testing program as part of hearing conservation are *already* in violation of the law. Baseline hearing tests must now be completed within 6 months of any employee's first exposure at or above an 8-hour time weighted average of 85 dBA with one exception: for those companies utilizing mobile testing services, the baseline hearing test must be completed within 1 year of the first exposure at or above an 8-hour time-weighted average of 85 dBA; however, those employees *must* wear hearing protection devices for any period exceeding 6 months after the first exposure until the baseline hearing test is accomplished.

The baseline hearing test required by OSHA for an industrial hearing conservation program is a pure tone air conduction threshold audiogram at the test frequencies of 500, 1,000, 2,000, 3,000, 4,000, and 6,000 Hz. Many would argue that the test frequency of 8,000 Hz should be included because of the invaluable information that can be gained from it, particularly in cases of relatively early noise-induced hearing loss. This baseline hearing test becomes the point of reference against which the results of all future hearing tests are compared when judging the overall success or failure of the hearing conservation effort. Obviously, it is absolutely critical that a valid and reliable baseline test is obtained for each and every employee exposed to noise levels at 85 dBA or greater, and along these lines several issues must be given particular consideration. These issues revolve around concern for temporary threshold shift, a stable test environment, instrumentation and calibration, and tester competence.

Avoiding Temporary Threshold Shift

The baseline hearing test must be an accurate representation of true organic hearing levels at the required test frequencies. Therefore, care must be taken that each employee is tested at a time when no risk of falsely elevated thresholds exist as a result of a temporary threshold shift. With this in mind, the ideal time to administer baseline hearing tests is at the beginning of each work shift *before* the employee has the opportunity to be exposed to workplace noise that might cause a temporary threshold shift. This approach can be effective for smaller companies or for those that maintain an "inhouse" testing program; but for larger companies or those that rely on mobile testing services, it is not practical. Realizing the logistic and economic problems created for some companies by requiring 14 hours without exposure to workplace noise prior to the baseline hearing test, OSHA has specified that adequate and effective personal hearing protection devices may be used as a substitute for the 14-hour requirement. Along these same lines, and recognizing the potential contribution of nonoccupational noise exposure to temporary threshold shift, OSHA has placed on the employer the responsibility for notifying each employee of the need to avoid high levels of nonoccupational noise exposure for at least 14 hours prior to the baseline hearing test.

Test Environment

Valid and reliable threshold audiometry depends on an acceptably quiet test environment. Whether a commercially available, prefabricated, sound-treated booth is used or not, having the ambient noise levels in the immediate hearing testing vicinity measured and documented on a regular basis is vital to the success of any industrial hearing conservation program. OSHA has determined that all hearing tests administered as a part of any industrial hearing conservation program must take place in a room meeting the requirements listed in Table 51–4 and discussed in Appendix D (Audiometric Test Rooms) of the OSHA hearing conservation amendment. The sound pressure levels must be measured by means of a sound level meter that conforms to the requirements of the American National Standards Institute (ANSI) S1.4–1971 (R1976) for a type 1 or type 2 instrument and a frequency analyzer that meets the ANSI S1.11–1971 (R1976) requirements. Regular measurement and documentation of the ambient noise in the test room are recommended, that is, at the beginning, in the middle, and at the end of each test session or at any time that a noticeable subjective change in noise level occurs or if employee complaints about noisy test conditions become frequent. At any time that the ambient noise levels exceed those listed in Table 51–4, testing should be interrupted, cancelled, or delayed until such time that at least minimum OSHA standards are met. Current regulations mandate that the test environment's compliance with the levels listed in Table 51–4 be noted on each employee's audiogram or that the professional reviewing the hearing tests at least be informed of this compliance.

It should be routine procedure to locate the hearing testing facility away from the high-noise areas. Do not assume that the medical, first-aid, or safety departments are the best places to conduct hearing tests. Because of high ambient noise levels in adjacent manufacturing areas or because of the high-traffic nature of these locations, they often do not provide the best location for the testing. Careful analysis of ambient noise prior to locating the testing facility is required, and measurements should be made both during transient and high-noise periods rather than during periods of relative quiet.

One final comment concerning test environments needs to be made. More and more industrial hearing testing is being accomplished in mobile testing vans. The mobile units are often somewhat more susceptible to increased ambient background noise because of their locations, internal noise caused by frequent transport from location to location ("squeaks and creaks"), and induced vibration caused by internal and/or external movement. Recognizing this fact, the Council for Accreditation in Occupational Hearing Conservation (CAOHC) has published a list of minimum guidelines for mobile testing units.[10] Although these requirements are not part of the current OSHA noise regulation, awareness of them and adherence to them would probably be prudent policy when mobile hearing testing units are used.

TABLE 51–4 Maximum Allowable Background Octave Band Sound Pressure Levels for Audiometric Test Rooms

Center Frequency of Octave band (Hz)	*Maximum Sound Pressure Level (dB)*
500	40
1,000	40
2,000	47
4,000	57
8,000	62

Audiometers and Audiometer Calibration

Several types of audiometers can be used appropriately to accomplish the pure tone air conduction threshold hearing tests required by an industrial hearing conservation program—manual audiometers, self-recording or automatic audiometers, and the more recent microprocessor-controlled audiometers. The type chosen for any particular program or testing service depends on several factors including cost, number of tests to be administered, time restrictions, and tester training and competence. The advantages and disadvantages of the manual and self-recording audiometers in industrial hearing conservation programs have been thoroughly reported by Rintleman[11] and Harford,[12] and their efforts will not be repeated here. In addition, I have discussed the operation of the microprocessor-controlled audiometer and many of the perceived pros and cons of its use for industrial testing.[13] Only after careful consideration of each type of audiometer available can an informed decision be made as to which type or types are most appropriate for a particular application. Regardless of the type of audiometer used for industrial hearing conservation, the OSHA hearing conservation amendment clearly specifies the calibration requirements that must be satisfied. These requirements revolve around three distinct types of audiometer calibration: biologic, electroacoustic, and exhaustive.

The first type of calibration, biologic, involves a two step process that must be accomplished prior to each day's use. These two steps are (1) a threshold test and (2) a listening or performance check. The threshold test should be done on an individual with known, stable audiology thresholds, and each day's thresholds are compared with that person's baseline results. This type of situation works best for "in-house" hearing conservation programs when the same person or persons are almost always going to be available for the daily threshold test. However, for mobile testing services and for situations where the same person is not or cannot be available, this scenario is not practical. To cover this possibility, OSHA allows that a relatively inexpensive bioacoustic simulator can be substituted for a human subject in checking the output of the audiometer during the threshold test portion of biologic calibration.

If the threshold test portion of biologic calibration reveals deviations of 10 dB or greater at any one or more of the six required test frequencies, the standard requires that an acoustic calibration be performed. With human subjects, such deviation is likely to occur occasionally, and it is suggested that, if this procedure is used for threshold testing, three to five persons with known, stable thresholds should be available in order to check the deviating frequency(ies) before submitting the audiometer to an acoustic calibration. The bioacoustic simulator avoids this problem of human variability and error.

The listening check portion of biologic calibration is also performed prior to each day's use and involves the technician (to be discussed in the next section) or audiologist placing the audiometer earphones on his or her own ears and listening for any unusual or unexpected variations in tone pitch and loudness while sweeping through the frequency settings and the attenuator settings of the audiometer. In addition, careful attention is paid to any extraneous noise such as clicks or static that might be created when depressing the tone presentation switch or turning the frequency or intensity controls. During this listening check, the earphone cords should be examined closely for signs of wear and should also be manipulated while wearing the earphones in order to listen for any noises or tone interruption that would signal a defective or broken cord in need of replacement. It is important to emphasize at this point that the daily biologic calibration threshold data and the daily records of listening checks must be carefully recorded and maintained on an ongoing basis. Figures 51–1 and 51–2 are suggested sample forms that may be of some use in accomplishing this recordkeeping requirement.

The second type of calibration required by OSHA is electroacoustic calibration. This calibration is required at least annually or at any time that a consistent deviation of 10 dB or more is discovered during biologic calibration, and it involves the measurement of sound pressure output levels at the various test frequencies, the measurement of attenuator linearity, a frequency count, and finally a listening and visual check identical to that described earlier. This type of calibration can be easily and conveniently performed by an audiologist utilizing a type 1 or type 2 sound level meter, a type A coupler with appropriate accessories, and a frequency counter and timer. This collection of instrumentation allows the sound level meter to be converted into an "artificial ear" so that audiometer performance can be measured and compared to the tolerances permitted by ANSI S3.6–1969 (R1973). If the number of audiometers used in a hearing conservation program does not justify the expense of calibration equipment or if the calibration cannot be performed by an individual who is properly trained and familiar with the calibration process, the audiometer(s) can be sent to an outside calibration service company for annual calibration. Over a period of time, this approach can cost time and money.

The third and final type of audiometer calibration required by OSHA is the exhaustive calibration. This calibration is required at least every 2 years or at any time a change of 15 dB or greater is detected at any of the test frequencies during electroacoustic calibration. In addition to the functions that are checked and measured during the annual electroacoustic calibration, exhaustive calibration includes the measurement of harmonic distortion, tone envelope characteristics including rise and fall times,

Biologic Calibration

Checked by: ____________________ Audiometer: ____________________
Date: ____________________ Serial No.: ____________________

Gross Physical Check
- Check earphone cords and cushions for cracks or worn insulation ________
- Check for loose or out-of-line dials ________
- Straighten twisted cords and dust machine ________

Auditory Check: Listen Through Earphones
- With tone continuously on, twist cords and move wires near earphones; listen for static or intermittent tone R ____ L ____
- Turn tone on loudly; is tone steady and clear? R ____ L ____
- Listen for uniform increase in loudness as HL dial is turned from 0.0 dB to maximum ________
- Listen for clicks or static when HL dial, frequency dial, and interrupter switch are moved ________
- Disconnect R phone; set selector switch to R.; turn HL dial to 50 dB and frequency selector to 1,000 Hz; listen to L phone for tone ("cross-talk"); reverse procedure ________

Testing of Person with Known and Stable Hearing

	250	500	1K	2K	3K	4K	6K	8K
R								
L								

Name:
Date:
Tested by:
Has this audiometer been returned for recalibration in the past year?

Figure 51–1 An example of a form to assist in performing biologic calibration of audiometer.

Date	*Serial #*	*Make & Model*	*Jacks Seated*	*Cords OK*	*Headband Tension OK*	*Phone Cushions OK*	*Volume Increases, Decreases*	*Pitch OK*	*Tone On-off OK*	*Tone Presenter Inaudible*	*No Static*	*No Crosstalk*	*Tester Signature*

Figure 51–2 An example of a self-listening test of audiometer function.

overshoot and "off time", cross-talk between earphones, and any unwanted signals in the earphones. Ideally, audiometers that are in either very heavy use or very light use as part of an industrial hearing conservation program should be subjected to exhaustive calibration annually rather than every 2 years. Most usually, this type of calibration is performed by an outside service company or by the audiometer manufacturer.

Finally, if pulsed tone, self-recording (automatic), or microprocessor audiometers are used in an industrial hearing conservation program, they are required to meet more specifications in addition to those just outlined. These additional specifications can be found in Appendix C of the OSHA hearing conservation amendment and include such things as pulsed tone "on time," pentracing width requirements, and slewing rate for self-recording audiometers.

Tester Competence

The OSHA hearing conservation amendment requires that "audiometric tests shall be administered by a certified audiometric technician or an individual with equivalent training and experience." In most cases it is impractical and economically unfeasible for a fully certified audiologist to administer the pure tone air conduction threshold hearing tests required of an industrial hearing conservation program. He or she is more likely to be involved in the overall administration of the program and in the testing of employees who are difficult to test or who present other special problems. Therefore, the basic testing can be the responsibility of an appropriately trained and supervised audiometric technician. The training requirement of the OSHA regulations are best met by an accredited course offered under the direction of a person certified as a Course Director by CAOHC. The Course Director is most often an audiologist, but may also be a physician, industrial hygienist, industrial nurse, or any other individual interested in industrial hearing conservation. A minimum course study of 20 hours is required. The course concentrates on how to obtain valid and reliable pure tone air conduction threshold audiograms. Eight-hour refresher courses are required of both Course Directors and technicians every 5 years.

Hearing Protection

Prior to the March 1983 finalized OSHA hearing conservation amendment, the use of personal hearing protection devices was viewed as a last resort option; this was after economically and technologically feasible engineering and administrative controls failed to lower employee noise exposure to the permissible level of 90 dBA. However, in response to a decision rendered by the Ninth United States Circuit Court of Appeals, OSHA issued a set of guidelines that became effective in November 1983, which "allow greater flexibility in the use of personal protective equipment in lieu of engineering and/or administrative controls."[14] These guidelines indicate that hearing protection will be allowed if the protection can be demonstrated to lower the workers' exposure levels to the 90-dBA level. However, when the noise level exposure approaches the 100-dBA point, OSHA recognizes that the use of hearing protectors may not protect the worker adequately, and, at this level, feasible engineering and administrative controls are required. The new guidelines indicate that an OSHA inspector may issue a citation when engineering and/or administrative controls are both technically and economically feasible and (1) exposure levels are so high that hearing protectors alone may not reliably protect the worker and (2) the costs of engineering and/or administrative controls are less than the cost of an effective hearing conservation program. Further, if a hearing conservation program exists and annual hearing testing shows that employees are adequately protected, a control is considered to be unnecessary.

The requirements of the OSHA hearing conservation amendment are fairly specific as to the use, fitting, and attenuation of personal hearing protection devices and are summarized as follows:

1. Hearing protection devices must be made *available* to all employees exposed to an 8-hour time-weighted average of 85 dBA or greater.
2. The use of hearing protection devices is mandatory for all employees exposed to an 8-hour time-weighted average of 90 dBA or greater or for those employees exposed to an 8-hour time-weighted average of 85 through 89 dBA if a comparison of current annual hearing test results with the baseline results reveals a standard threshold shift.
3. The employees must be given several types of hearing protection devices from which to choose.
4. Proper initial fitting and supervision of hearing protection devices must be provided, and all employees must receive training in the use and care of them.
5. The effectiveness of the hearing protection devices must be evaluated to insure an attenuation to at least a time-weighted average of 90 dBA or 85 dB if an employee has experienced a significant threshold shift.
6. The adequacy of hearing protection devices must be reevaluated with changes in noise exposure.
7. Hearing protection devices are mandatory for those employees who are exposed to an 8-hour time-weighted average of 85 dBA or greater if a baseline hearing test has not been accomplished within 6 months of the first exposure at or above this level.

Personal hearing protection devices for the most part can be classified into two major types: inserts (most commonly referred to as earplugs) and earmuffs. Whereas earmuffs are basically the same from manufacturer to manufacturer with just some variability of certain features to accommodate particular individual preferences or needs, earplugs are available in three broad categories or classifications: premolded, moldable or formable, and custom molded. Harford[12] and Swift[15] provide comprehensive reviews of the types of personal hearing protection devices available as well as discussions on the advantages and disadvantages of each and on the factors that contribute to their successful use. In addition, Edwards et al[16] and Flugrath and Wolfe[17] offer detailed discussions of the effectiveness of earplugs and earmuffs, respectively, as worn in the workplace.

Evaluation of Personal Hearing Protection Device Attenuation

As indicated in the previously enumerated OSHA requirements for hearing protection devices, the adequacy of those devices must often be evaluated. Appendix B of the OSHA final hearing conservation amendment describes four methods of assessing the attenuation of hearing protection devices by the use of noise reduction rating. In addition, Appendix B also lists three additional methods described by National Institutes for Occupational Safety and Health (NIOSH), which can be used to measure the adequacy of hearing protection devices. The noise reduction rating is a single number description of any noise reduction by the hearing protection devices and represents the difference between the overall C-weighted sound level of a pink (flat) noise spectrum and the resulting A-weighted noise levels under the protector. The noise reduction rating uses the measured laboratory attenuation of various hearing protection devices, minus two standard deviations, in an attempt to assure that the attenuation values used in the calculation are actually obtainable by the majority of workers who are conscientious about using their protectors and wear them correctly. Furthermore, 3-dB correction factor is used to account for the uncertainty of using a flat spectrum noise in the initial calculation. Determination of the noise reduction rating then becomes

NNR = (Overall C-weighted sound level)
—(Overall A-weighted sound level under the protector [—2 SD])
—3 dB

where NRR is noise reduction rating and SD is standard deviation. The noise reduction rating is most often printed on each package containing hearing protection devices or is generally readily available from the manufacturer.

Making a determination of the attenuation of hearing protection devices for a particular noise environment is most likely easier and more convenient using one of the four noise reduction rating procedures described in Appendix B of the OSHA hearing conservation amendment rather than one of the three additional methods offered by NIOSH. The noise reduction rating procedures involve only the use of a dosimeter or a sound level meter with either C-weighted or A-weighted measurement potential. If C-weighted data are available, then the noise reduction rating is simply subtracted from this measurement in order to obtain an estimated A-weighted time-weighted average. Therefore,

$$\text{Effective exposure (dBA)} = \text{noise level (dBC)} - \text{NRR}$$

If only A-weighted data are available, a correction factor of 7 dB is subtracted from the noise reduction rating to correct for the spectrum differences between the C- and A-weighted networks. The procedure for determining the attenuation of hearing protection devices then becomes

$$\text{Effective exposure (dBA)} = \text{noise level (dBA)} - \text{NRR} - 7\ \text{dB}$$

If a dosimeter is used, Table A–1 of Appendix A of the OSHA hearing conservation amendment should be used to convert the readings in percent noise exposure (dose) to a time-weighted average in dBA. For example, if the dosimeter reading is 130 percent and the noise reduction rating of the hearing protection device being considered is 28, the following effective exposure would be calculated:

$$\begin{aligned}\text{Effective exposure (dBA)} &= 91.9\ \text{dBA} - 28 + 7 \\ &= 70.9\ \text{dBA}\end{aligned}$$

since 130 percent from Table A–1 is 91.9 dBA time-weighted average. Appendix A of the OSHA hearing conservation amendment provides a formula to calculate the time-weighted average in cases where the dose as read on the dosimeter is less than or greater than the values found in Table A–1.

In lieu of estimating effective exposure (dBA) under hearing protection devices with the noise reduction rating, NIOSH methods No. 1, No. 2, or No. 3 can also be used. In general, methods No. 1 and No. 2 are more complex than any of the noise reduction rating methods and require additional calculations. Method No. 1 seems to be the most accurate, but requires octave band noise data at the frequencies from 125 Hz to 8,000 Hz and detailed calculations (Q values) for each hearing protection device to noise spectrum combination. Method No. 2 is similar to the noise reduction rating and also requires the Q values of various protectors and the difference between the measured dBC and dBA levels. It also uses an adjustment of −3 dB for spectrum uncertainty, since actual octave band levels are not required. NIOSH method No. 3 is the simplest yet least precise since only the Q values for various hearing protection devices are needed. Caution must be exercised, however, when using this method in situations of widely varying noise spectrum levels.

The actual attenuation provided by any hearing protection device is known to be significantly less than the laboratory data provided by the manufacturer for reasons involving training, motivation, and utilization between employees exposed to noise and laboratory subjects. The OSHA hearing conservation amendment recognizes this disparity with a short statement in Appendix B, which reads:

> The employer must remember that calculated attenuation values reflect realistic values only to the extent that the protectors are properly fitted and worn.

Berger points out that this is a crucial statement, since the proper fitting and wearing of hearing protection devices by employees exposed to noise is probably the most difficult part of a hearing conservation program to implement.[18] He emphasizes that success in this endeavor "requires not only education, training, and the selection of comfortable and effective hearing protection devices, but perhaps more importantly, motivation, enforcement, and responsiveness to the needs of the hearing protected employees."

Training

Few would argue against the importance of training and education in obtaining the greatest amount of cooperation from employees who are included in the hearing conservation program (all employees exposed to an 8-hour time-weighted average of 85 dBA or greater). Therefore the training provisions in the OSHA hearing conservation amendment require employers to conduct annual training for all such employees. This training must include—at a minimum—information about the effects of noise on hearing; the purpose of hearing protection devices; the advantages and disadvantages of various types of hearing protection devices; instructions in the selection, fitting, use, and care of hearing protection devices; and the purposes and procedures of audiometric testing. The training program should be updated each year to include new information relative to changes in hearing protection devices and changes in specific work processes that might have an effect on individual noise exposure.

OSHA does not require, nor necessarily intend, that employee training be accomplished in one session, and any one or all of several formats can be used. For example, an explanation of audiometric tests and procedures might best be discussed immediately prior to the annual hearing testing, whereas detailed instructions on the use of hearing protection devices might be most effective at the time of initial fitting. Some employers prefer that annual training occur in one session with small groups of employees. Different parts of the training program may be conducted by different individuals as long as the required topics are covered and the topics can be presented orally, through the use of preprepared materials such as pamphlets or films, slide and/or tape shows. The OSHA training requirements are such that employees must be reminded at least each year that noise is hazardous to hearing and that they can prevent damage by wearing hearing protection devices where indicated, and by participating in audiometric testing. Many employers may find it useful and to their advantage to include other topics of discussion in the annual training program in addition to those required by OSHA. For instance, a discussion of the OSHA noise standard itself and the company's hearing conservation program, identification of specific machinery on the job site that could produce hazardous noise exposures, and the role of engineering and/or administrative controls in the reduction of noise exposure all might be useful additions to the training program in certain instances. OSHA encourages the employer or the professional administering the hearing conservation program to use his or her best judgement when deciding what to add to the basics of the required training program.

In the view of many, the OSHA requirements for an annual training program come just one step short of being an effective educational tool to help ensure the success of the hearing conservation program. Whereas the OSHA requirements apply only to those *employees* who must be included in the program, they do not apply to management and supervisors as well. For any hearing conservation program to be truly successful, it must be understood and fully supported by the entire company, from top levels of management on down. Therefore managers and supervisors should be included in the annual training and education program whether they are directly involved in the hearing conservation program or not. If management's committment to the hearing conservation program is strong, educational efforts will be more readily accepted by the employees, thus making the chances much better of having a successful program.

Recordkeeping

The fifth, and final, area in which the OSHA hearing conservation amendment approved finalized regulations was in recordkeeping. As dictated by a growing number of lawsuits and by the increasing number of worker's compensation claims (to be discussed later), the key word in any hearing conservation program is *documentation*.

Audiometric test records must include the name and job classification of the employee, the test date, the examiner's name, the date of acoustic or exhaustive calibration, measurements of the background sound pressure levels in the audiometric test room, and the employee's most recent noise exposure measurement. OSHA did not intend that all of the previously mentioned information be required to be recorded on the face of the audiograms. Rather, this information can be kept *with* the audiometric records if necessary so that the employer may maintain the information in a separate document(s) that is kept or filed with the audiometric test results.

Accurate records of all employee noise exposure measurements must be maintained and must be *retained* for 2 years. In the case of hearing test results, records must be retained for the duration of the affected employee's employment. However, because of firsthand experience in cases where hefty compensation settlements were granted years *after* an employee's termination of employment, I suggest that all records, including hearing test results, be kept *indefinitely*.

EFFECTIVE INDUSTRIAL HEARING CONSERVATION

Basic adherence to the OSHA finalized regulations in the five separate areas of noise monitoring, audiometric testing, hearing protection devices, training, and recordkeeping forms the basis of an effective industrial hearing conservation program whether or not compliance with OSHA is the main motivation for beginning or maintaining a program.

Most authorities in the field of industrial hearing conservation agree that an effective program is comprised of at least five core components. These components are (1) noise measurement and monitoring, (2) noise control (engineering and/or administrative controls), (3) hearing protection, (4) education and training, and (5) audiometric testing.

Of these five components, that of audiometric testing forms the cornerstone of the entire hearing conservation program. The evaluation of overall program effectiveness can be accomplished only by careful monitoring and analysis of the hearing test data obtained from the population exposed to noise. Without an evaluation of the hearing sensitivities of employees exposed to noise, how else can it be determined whether or not engineering and/or administrative noise controls that have been implemented are effective or need to be changed or modified? And how else can a judgement be made concerning the overall effectiveness of the personal hearing protection device effort? It would appear obvious that the absence of hearing changes in the population exposed to noise would indicate that the hearing conservation program is working, regardless of the presence and/or effectiveness of any one aspect of the program. Under these circumstances, the approach can be taken that "if it ain't broke, don't fix it!" On the other hand, the continued presence of unusual hearing changes would signal an ineffective program and the need for close review and modification of the noise control and/or hearing protection efforts.

In order that some judgement concerning hearing conservation program effectiveness can be made, a criterion must be established concerning the number of employees exposed to noise that exhibit hearing changes when annual hearing test results are compared with the baseline results. Must 100 percent of the employees tested show no change in hearing sensitivity before a program is considered to be "effective?" Obviously, such a requirement would be impractical as well as impossible given that some employees have hearing changes totally unrelated to occupational noise exposure and given that wide individual susceptibility to noise suggests that some people experience threshold shifts *regardless* of control measures and the diligent use of appropriate personal hearing protection devices. Also, published reports by Lilley et al,[19] Royster et al,[20] and others suggest that the evaluation of hearing conservation program effectiveness is further complicated by data that indicate different degrees of noise-induced hearing loss as a function of sex and race. With these complicating factors in mind, however, some standard must be used in order to judge the effectiveness of the hearing conservation program. General experience seems to indicate that a "good" program is one in which no more than 4 to 8 percent of the total employees show significant hearing change or require follow-up per year. Where 6 to 10 percent of those tested exhibit hearing changes, a review of the program components (hearing protection devices, for instance) and appropriate modification where necessary might be indicated. Programs showing greater than 10 percent of employees requiring annual follow-up should be considered to be ineffective and unacceptable, and major changes and modifications are required.

Previous mention of standard threshold shift and follow-up procedures leads naturally into a discussion of what OSHA requires when an employee with a standard threshold shift is identified. Under these circumstances, the employer is responsible for ensuring that certain procedures are accomplished *unless* a physician determines that the shift is *not* work related *nor* aggravated by workplace noise exposure. These follow-up procedures are as follows:

1. The employee must be informed *in writing* within 21 days of the determination of a standard threshold shift (*not* 21 days from the testing date, but rather 21 days from the time the employer is informed of the shift).
2. Those employees not using hearing protection must be fitted and trained in the use of hearing protection devices.
3. Those employees already using hearing protection devices shall be refitted or retrained and/or given a device offering greater attenuation.
4. The employee should be referred for clinical audiological evaluation and otological examination, as appropriate, if additional testing is necessary or if medical pathology of the ear is suspected.

OSHA does allow that the employer *may* obtain a retest within 30 days and consider those results as the annual audiogram in those cases where the annual test indicates a standard threshold shift. If the retest indicates no such shift, follow-up procedures are not required. In addition, allowance *may* be made for the contribution of aging on the annual hearing test *prior* to determining if a standard threshold shift has occurred. Appendix F of the finalized OSHA hearing conservation amendment outlines the procedures along with age correction tables for males and females for the determination of the contribution of aging to the change in hearing level.

The review and evaluation of a hearing test conducted as part of an industrial hearing conservation program and the identification of a standard threshold shift as defined by OSHA are relatively simple processes for the experienced audiologist. Furthermore, the follow-up procedures required by OSHA when a standard threshold shift is identified are straightforward and should present no serious problems. However, many would argue that only evaluating standard threshold shift and making recommendations and referrals based on its presence or absence puts the professional reviewing the hearing tests and/or the employer at great potential risk by not informing an employee of a medically significant condition related to his ears or hearing, even if it is totally unrelated to his employment. Feldman and Grimes[21] and Feldman[22] have recognized this problem and have made recommendations concerning the appropriate follow-up of threshold shifts over and above OSHA guidelines and a procedure for the appropriate review of industrial hearing tests. Cluff[23] also stresses this professional quandary and recommends that the American Council of Otolaryngology (ACO) referral criteria[24] be used by companies whose hearing conservation programs are not directed by physicians.

The previous discussion has focused on the necessary components of any industrial hearing conservation program, the evaluation of program effectiveness, and on follow-up procedures. The last section of this chapter focuses on the purposes and importance of these programs.

THE IMPACT OF INDUSTRIAL HEARING CONSERVATION

In spite of the fact that OSHA requires that all companies having employees exposed to an 8-hour time-weighted average 85 dBA or greater institute a hearing conservation program, compliance with OSHA is not the only, nor even perhaps the most important, reason to have such a program. Although I have stressed in this chapter that general adherence to OSHA guidelines goes a long way toward ensuring a comprehensive and effective program, more attention needs to be given to the threat that noise poses to the hearing of literally millions of men and women in this country and to the potential huge cost of worker's compensaion claims than to mere compliance with a Federal statute. Industrial hearing conservation should be "sold" to the employer and the employee as being a part of the overall employee health benefit package with the purpose of preserving a vital biologic function. The employer must be convinced that an effective program will help him to comply with OSHA, but, more importantly, help to ensure a healthier, happier, and therefore more productive workforce. The employee must be convinced that involved and active participation in the program will help to prevent irreversible hearing loss that can interfere with their earning power as well as with their enjoyment of life both during and following their wage-earning years.

What I have previously referred to as the growing spectre of worker's compensation for occupation hearing loss probably is, or should be, the biggest motivating force inducing employers to initiate and/or maintain comprehensive, effective industrial hearing conservation programs. Briefly, worker's compensation laws hold that industrial employers should be responsible for the costs of workplace disabilities without regard to any fault. The resulting economic losses are considered costs of production that are chargeable, to the greatest extent possible, as a price factor. These laws serve to relieve employers of liability from common-law suits involving negligence. Since 1911, when the first worker's compensation laws were enacted in the United States, each of the 50 states has followed suit and enacted similar legislation. Not until the late 1940s were the first claims for occupational hearing loss filed and not until the 1950s did New York, Wisconsin, and Missouri enact legislation that recognized occupational noise-induced hearing loss as a compensable disease. Currently, almost every state recognizes this type of hearing impairment as a workplace hazard with monetary awards based upon the degree of loss. However, it is important to recognize that a wide range of variability among the state compensation statutes exists, and anyone dealing with these issues should become totally familiar with the laws of the state(s) he or she is involved in. Some of the areas where the state laws differ are (1) whether or not a claimant is required to show "inability to work," "disablement," "inability to earn normal wages," or some other description of economic disability; (2) the formula used to determine hearing impairment; (3) waiting periods required prior to filing; (4) whether a deduction is made or not for the effects of presbycusis; (5) time limits for filing; and (6) whether or not willful failure to use hearing protection devices voids the right to file for compensation.

In addition to the various state worker's compensation laws, federal worker's compensation laws have also been enacted to protect civilian employees of the Federal government, for example, the District of Columbia Workmen's Compensation Act, the Federal Employees' Compensation Act (FECA), and the Longshoremen's and Harbor Workers' Compensation Act (providing for private or public employees in nationwide maritime work).

The damaging effects of workplace noise exposure have been recognized for many years. However, the awarding of major compensation for occupationally induced hearing loss is relatively new. An Environmental Protection Agency report in 1979 indicated that state and federal programs paid approximately 8,395 claims totalling $31 million for occupational hearing loss in 1977 alone.[25] This report went further to estimate that for the period of 1977 to 1987 the potential costs of state worker's compensation claims for occupational hearing loss would reach $365 million. More recently, Berger[26] estimated the potential compensation costs for occupational hearing loss to be $62 million in 1984 rising to $112 million in 1993 for a 10-year projected cumulative total of $871 million!

It has been estimated that approximately 1.7 million workers in the United States between the ages of 50 and 59 years have enough noise-induced hearing loss to be awarded compensation. According to a 1986 report by the United States Chamber of Commerce[27] the awards for occupationally induced hearing impairment in one ear in the various states range from $2,940 to $27,500 and from $11,676 to $96,250 for binaural impairment. If only 10 percent (a very conservative number) of the workers in this restricted age category were to file claims, based on an estimated current average claim on $3,500, the cost would approach $600 million alone!

Worker's compensation settlements in the government are even costlier than for private industry. In 1983 alone, FECA paid more than $25 million for 5,535 hearing loss claims and the Veterans' Administration (VA), which pays for claims filed by the military, paid $155 million for nearly 62,500 claims. Assuming a modest increase in claims activity of 7 percent each year for the next 10 years, the cumulative cost projections for FECA and the VA are estimated to be $339 million and $2.2 *billion,* respectively. In my own personal experience of the past 3 years as a consultant for the United States Department of Labor reviewing hearing loss claims of civilians employed by the Federal government (covered by FECA), I have seen an increase in the number of claims of 313 percent from 1984 to 1986.

The large current costs and the overwhelming potential costs of worker's compensation claims for occupational noise-induced hearing loss are painfully clear. An obvious and comparatively inexpensive alternative to these constantly spiraling costs is for the private employer and the government (i.e., the taxpayer) to protect themselves by implementing comprehensive and effective hearing conservation programs. As a result, worker's compensation claims for hearing loss will moderate, and insurance losses will be brought under control. As a bonus, the employee receives a more acceptable environment in which to work with the potential for better morale and increased productivity for the employer.

SUMMARY

The impact and implication of noise exposure on hearing in the workforce is staggering. The responsibilities of the audiologist in an industrial hearing conservation program are equally staggering and demand a broad range of knowledge and technical expertise. Whereas slight differences of opinion and philosophies can and do exist concerning the fine detail of an effective program, there is little argument that the audiologist must be thoroughly trained and well-versed in the areas of noise monitoring, audiometric testing, personal hearing protection, training and education, and recordkeeping.

Although the history of Federal regulation of workplace noise exposure has been long and sometimes arduous, the current OSHA noise standard provides a sound structure upon which to build an effective hearing conservation program that includes clearly-defined follow-up procedures and objective methods of evaluating effectiveness. If audiologists are going to make a significant contribution toward minimizing noise-induced hearing loss in the working population, a thorough understanding of these basic components of industrial hearing conservation programs is mandatory.

REFERENCES

1. Tempest W. Noise in industry. In: Tempest W, ed. The noise handbook. Orlando: Academic Press, 1985:180.
2. Glorig A. Noise: past, present, future. Ear Hear 1980; 1:4–18.
3. Federal Register. October 24, 1974; 39 (207):37773–37778.
4. Federal Register. January 16, 1981; 46 (11):4078–4179.
5. Federal Register. August 21, 1981; 46 (162):42622–42633.
6. Federal Register. March 8, 1983; 48 (46):9738.
7. Goldstein J. Fundamental concepts in sound measurement. In: Lipscomb DM, ed. Noise and audiology. Baltimore: University Park Press, 1978:3.
8. Tempest W. Noise measurement. In: Tempest W, ed. The noise handbook. Orlando: Academic Press, 1985:3.
9. Heggie SA, Miller TD. Monitoring employee noise exposure. Sound Vibr 1983; 10(1):17–19.
10. Council for accreditation in occupational hearing conservation. Haddon Heights, NJ: CAOHC Update, 1981:No. 7.
11. Rintleman WF. Manual and automatic audiometry. In: Olishifski JB, Harford ER, eds. Industrial noise and hearing conservation. Chicago: National Safety Council, 1975:625.
12. Harford ER. Industrial audiology. In: Lipscomb DM, ed. Noise and audiology. Baltimore: University Park Press, 1978:299.
13. Bodenhemier WG. Recent considerations in industrial hearing conservation. Semin Hear 1984; 5 (2):143–155.
14. Noise control report. November 21, 1983; 12 (24):184.
15. Swift RL. Personal hearing-protective devices. In: Olishifski JB, Harford ER, eds. Industrial noise and hearing conservation. Chicago: National Safety Council, 1975:526.
16. Edwards RG, Hauser WP, Moiseev NA, Broderson AB, Green WW. Effectiveness of earplugs as worn in the workplace. Sound Vibr 1978; 12(1):12–22.
17. Flugrath JM, Wolfe BN Jr. The effectiveness of selected earmuff-type hearing protectors. Sound Vibr 1971; 5(1):25–27.
18. Berger EH. The hearing conservation amendment (Part II). E.A.RLOG #12. Indianapolis: E-A-R Division, Cabor Corporation, 1983.
19. Lilley DT, Royster LH, Thomas WG. Evaluation techniques for industrial hearing conservation programs. J Acoust Soc Am 1977; 61(1,S77).

20. Royster LH, Thomas WG, Rosyter JD, Lilley DT. Potential hearing compensation cost by race and sex. J Occup Med 1978; 20(12):801–806.
21. Feldman AS, Grimes CT. Review and referral of industrial audiograms: a professional dilemma. Asha 1977; 19:231–234.
22. Feldman AS. Industrial audiogram review: the professional's dilemma. Hear Aid J 1982; 35(7):18–20.
23. Cluff GL. After the hearing test—what then? Occup Health Saf 1983; March:14–21.
24. Head and neck surgery: otologic referral criteria for occupational hearing conservation programs. Washington, D.C.: American Council of Otolaryngology, 1981.
25. Workers' compensation under state and federal programs. Environmental Protection Agency. 1979:EPA–550/9–79-101.
26. Berger EH. Workers' compensation for occupational hearing loss. E.A.RLOG #15. Indianapolis: E-A-R Division, Cabot Corporation, 1984.
27. Analysis of workers' compensation laws. Washington, D.C.: U.S. Chamber of Commerce, 1986.

52 Cochlear Implants

Dianne J. Mecklenburg, Ph.D.
Jon K. Shallop, Ph.D.

The capacity for sensory systems to receive direct information about the external world is directly related to the ability of their transducers to detect and convert external events into neural signals.[1] In the peripheral auditory system, the hair cells within the cochlea (the sense organ) are the transducers that receive and convert biomechanical information into biochemical and bioelectrical signals.[2] That is, in order for the perception of sound to take place, sound vibrations are translated into biomechanical activity, transduced into biochemical and bioelectrical signals, and transmitted along the central nervous system to the cortical areas of the brain for interpretation (Fig. 52–1). Cochlear hair cells are the most important link between the acoustic environment and the perception of that environment as a pattern of sound sensations. A severely impaired or totally nonfunctioning cochlea prevents the effective transmission of sound-related signals along the central auditory pathways even though the pathways may be completely intact. An auditory system can be impaired in its capacity to transfer mechanical energy (conductive hearing loss), transduce mechanical to electrochemical signals (sensory hearing loss), or transmit neuroelectrical signals (neural hearing loss).

HEARING AND SENSORY AIDS

Sensory aids are designed to provide information normally transmitted through audition to alternative sensory systems such as touch or vision.[3] Those stimulating the sense of touch, referred to as tactile aids, translate patterns of sound, either vibratory or electrical to the skin. Visual displays of sound have been developed to translate acoustic events into visual patterns or symbols that represent speech.

Generally, "hearing" aids may be any acoustic or electronic device that provides a means through which the normal central auditory system can receive auditory information. Acoustic hearing aids, as well as implantable middle ear prostheses, usually refer to devices that are designed to overcome the inability of the auditory system to transfer acoustic vibrations through the sense organ; a functioning cochlea (at some level) and a central auditory system are essential. Figure 52–2 illustrates the differences between these two types of hearing devices. At the input stage, hearing aids and cochlear implants are functionally identical. However, at the output stage, they differ because a hearing aid stimulates the cochlear sensory cells mechanically. A cochlear implant is designed to bypass a pathologic cochlea by transducing acoustic events directly into electrical signals. A functioning central auditory system (including the eighth cranial nerve) is essential, but a functioning cochlea is not. A cochlear implant obviates the need for biomechanical transmission of sound vibrations, whereas a hearing aid enhances biomechanical activity.

Clearly, hearing aids and sensory aids differ in their basic premise: hearing aids aim to supplement a partially intact auditory system, whereas sensory aids aim to bypass it by utilizing a replacement for the defective or absent sensory system, as demonstrated in Figure 52–3.

DEVELOPMENT OF COCHLEAR IMPLANTS

Cochlear implants are devices that are placed in close proximity to the auditory nerve and do not rely on viable sensory functioning of the cochlea. These devices consist of several components that simulate the normal conduction, transfer, and transformation functions of an intact outer, middle, and inner ear system. The underlying principle supporting the development of cochlear implants is that the auditory system is the most ideally organized sen-

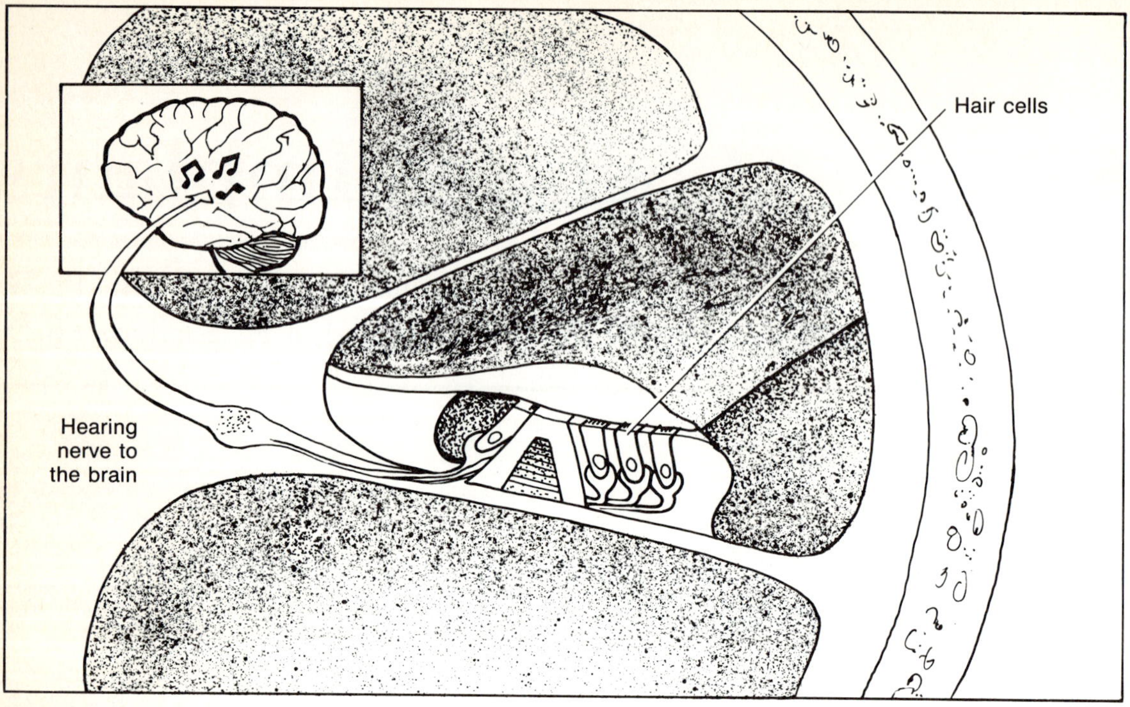

Figure 52–1 A cross-sectional view of the cochlea is depicted, which schematically shows the auditory pathway from the sensory hair cells to the auditory cortex.

sory system to receive and process meaningful sound. Thus the goal of cochlear implantation is to provide an electrical analogue or code of sound to a functioning auditory nerve that would otherwise be deprived because of sensory pathology.

The earliest experiment that suggested that direct stimulation of the eighth cranial nerve could elicit a percept of sound is credited to Djurno and Eyries.[4] During a surgical procedure for the removal of a cholesteatoma, a patient reported hearing sound when the auditory nerve was exposed and stimulated electrically. Since that time, interest in providing more sophisticated information to an intact neural system has been undertaken. The most direct approach was initiated by Simmons who imbedded electrodes in the modiolus of the cochlea.[5] Others chose to place electrodes in the scala tympani of the cochlea where the perilymph would serve as an efficient volume conductor of electrical stimuli and transmit to neural elements proximal to nonfunctional hair cells. Research in the 1960s leading to both single- and multisited stimulation within the cochlea of human subjects was conducted by House and his colleagues[6] and Michelson.[7] To date, over

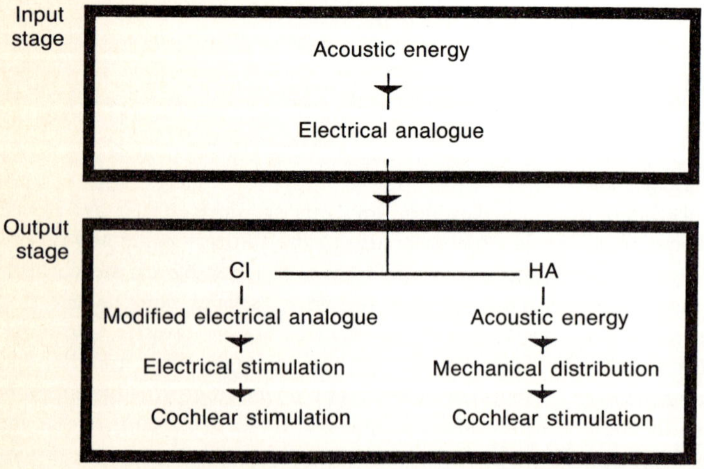

Figure 52–2 A comparison between conventional hearing aids and cochlear implants shows how they are similar from the input stage of the ear through to the sensory processing in the cochlea. Abbreviations: CI = cochlear implant; HA = hearing aid.

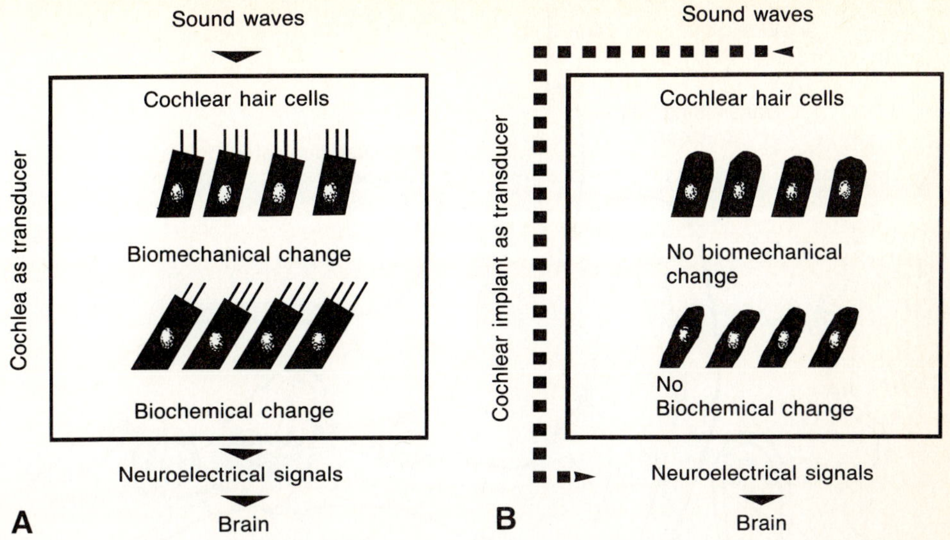

Figure 52–3 *A*, In the normal ear, sound is transduced by the cochlear hair cells into a neuroelectrical signal (code) that is transmitted to the brain. *B*, In the illustrated pathologic cochlea, the hair cells are nonfunctional, and the cochlear implant stimulates the auditory nerve directly.

25 cochlear implant designs have been implanted in thousands of subjects worldwide.

In the United States, an estimated 90,000 to 200,000 individuals have significant hearing loss that prevents the effective transformation of acoustic information into auditory sensations.[8] Although speechreading and/or tactile information may assist such individuals with speech understanding, they are unable to understand speech through the auditory system. Cochlear implants provide the opportunity to bypass a pathologic auditory system and to stimulate auditory nerve fibers.

Variations in the features of cochlear implants are, in the main, related to philosophical differences between the designers. However, they all share the common need of collecting sounds from the environment, converting them into electrical signals, and providing a means by which the processed signals can be transmitted to the intact neural elements of the auditory system. To accomplish this, there are both external (body worn) and internal (implanted) elements, as shown in Figure 52–4. Sound is picked up by a microphone, sent to a processing unit that manipulates the sound impulses in some manner, and sent directly through or across the skin to the electrode(s).

External Components

The directional electret microphone most often used in hearing aids is also the most commonly chosen type for cochlear implant systems, although some systems utilize omnidirectional microphones. The selection of the microphone is important in that it can have a major impact on the signal-to-noise ratio of the collected sounds.[9] The receiving microphone picks up the acoustic signal from the environment and transforms it into an electrical signal for input to a speech processing unit. The microphone changes mechanical sound sensations into electrical signals in the same manner as a hearing aid microphone. The microphone is usually located at ear level, as it would be in a behind-the-ear hearing aid. In some cases, however, the microphone is separate and can be placed in varying locations including the lapel, on the clothes, or in the processing unit itself.

The sounds from the environment are sent via a cable (or wire) to the processing unit where they are coded into a signal that causes neural elements of the auditory system to be stimulated. The processing units vary in size from approximately the size of a cigarette box[10] to that of a medium-sized portable tape player.[11,12] Most units have either a control that alters the sensitivity of the processing unit itself (Nucleus), an intensity potentiometer (House/3M), or both (Symbion). Some processing units provide external input sockets for directly connecting a second microphone, an FM auditory training unit, radio, television, and so forth. Batteries are housed within the processor. Once the signal has been coded, it is sent from the speech processor for transmission to the internal components via a cable.

The speech processor manipulates the acoustic

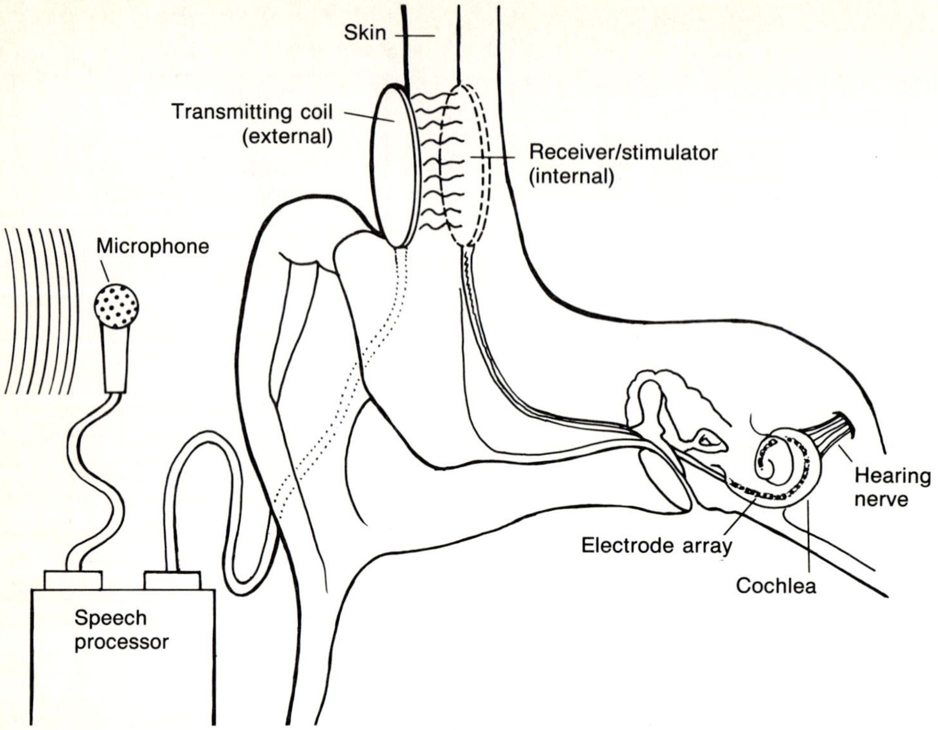

Figure 52–4 The components of a cochlear implant system include the pick-up microphone, speech processor, external transmitting coil, internal receiving coil, stimulator electronics for active devices, and the electrode array. Transmission from external to internal components in this illustration is transcutaneous.

signal in some fashion, either through filtering or extracting sound information, and transforms it into electrical signals that are coded for the auditory nerve. For example, the input signal can be divided into banks of filtered signals, or features can be extracted from the signal for transmission to the electrode array. One device provides little alteration of the original signal by providing an electrical analogue of the signal, transmitting it as a whole via a carrier frequency to the electrode array. Thus most cochlear implant systems can be divided into one of three systems: filter bank, full frequency, or feature extraction.

There are differences in the manner in which the coded signal is transmitted to an internal electrode array among the more than 20 devices that have been designed throughout the world. In some cases, there is a transmitting and receiving coil coupled with an internal electronics package (Fig. 52–5). In others, there is a passive receiver or a direct connector that transmits signals directly to the electrodes. In all systems, however, the transformed electrical signals are sent to electrodes that lie in close proximity to residual fibers of the acoustic nerve.

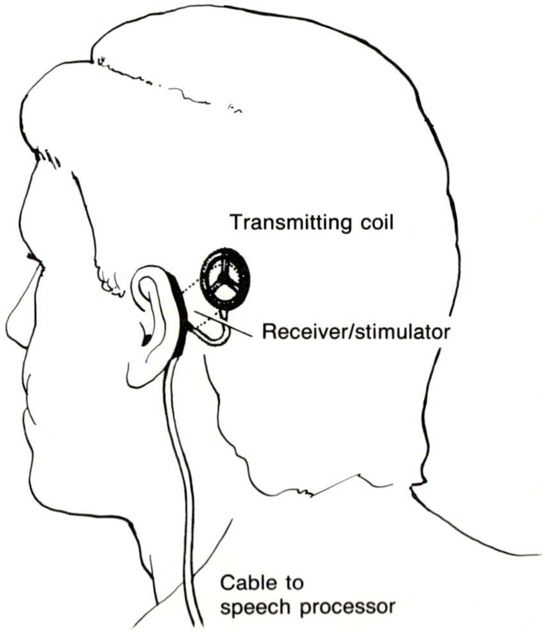

Figure 52–5 The signal from the speech processor passes along a conducting cable to the external transmitter (antenna). A radio frequency carrier can be used to transmit power and data to active internal components (receiver/stimulator).

Internal Components

The internal components of a cochlear implant include the receiving components and the electrode array (see Fig. 52–4). The receiving components are either active or inactive. Inactive simply means that the transmission may be to a coil that receives the signal by magnetic induction and is connected to an electrode array. These internal components are typical of single-channel cochlear implants such as the House/3M device.

If the internal components are active, power and data are transmitted to an internal receiver from the external speech processor. The internal receiver is active because the power "activates" circuitry within the receiver, which in turn initiates the stimulation signal to the electrode array, as illustrated in Figure 51–4. This type of system is typical of more complex multichannel feature extraction systems such as the Nucleus device.

Electrodes

Figure 52–6 illustrates two common types of electrodes used in cochlear implants: single-sited and multisited electrodes. Multisited electrodes are a necessity for multichannel cochlear implants because they enable the delivery of stimulation to several locations within the cochlea, which makes it possible to utilize the tonotopic characteristics of the residual fibers of the eighth cranial nerve. The single-sited electrode is one active electrode usually placed a short distance in the basal turn of the scala tympani. This type might then use an extracochlear "remote" ground electrode in the middle ear. A monopolar electrode array is typical of single-channel cochlear implants.

If the ground electrode for a single-sited electrode is remote, as in Figure 52–7, the electrode array is monopolar. However, if the ground electrode is in close proximity to the active electrode, then the stimulation mode is called bipolar. An example of a multisited electrode is shown in Figure 52–8. Bipolar stimulation enables the localized stimulation of nerve fibers because current flow is restricted to a small area between and near the active and ground (reference) electrodes.

Multichannel and Single-Channel Devices

Single-channel speech processing is illustrated in the upper portion of Figure 52–9. The sound input is coded by the single-channel processor, and all output information from the device is transmitted to the single, active electrode and its remote ground.

A multichannel device is also schematically illustrated in Figure 52–9. In this instance, the sound input is processed into multiple channels of information, which then must be transmitted to multiple electrodes. Typically, these electrodes are within the cochlea[13–15] or they can be placed on the medial wall of the middle ear.[11] These multichannel devices can have either monopolar[11,16] or bipolar[17,18] electrode arrays.

CODING STRATEGIES

Coding strategies have been developed for cochlear implant systems with the hope of providing information that will lead to the consistent recognition of speech and environmental sounds.[19,20] Several aspects of coding are relevant, including how

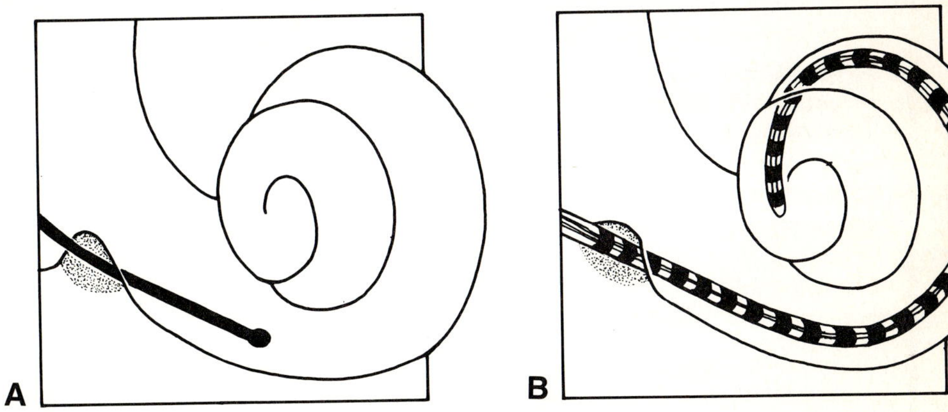

Figure 52–6 The electrode array for a cochlear implant is *A*, single-sited or *B*, multisited. In both cases, the electrode is shown to pass through the round window into the scala tympani.

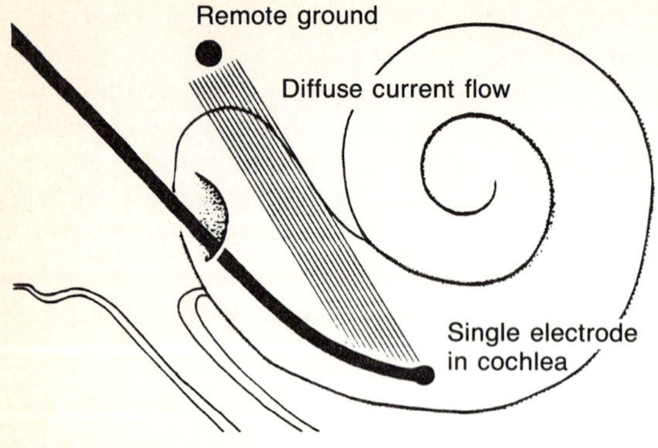

Figure 52–7 A monopolar electrode is shown with a remote ground in the middle ear. This electrode is typical for single-channel cochlear implants.

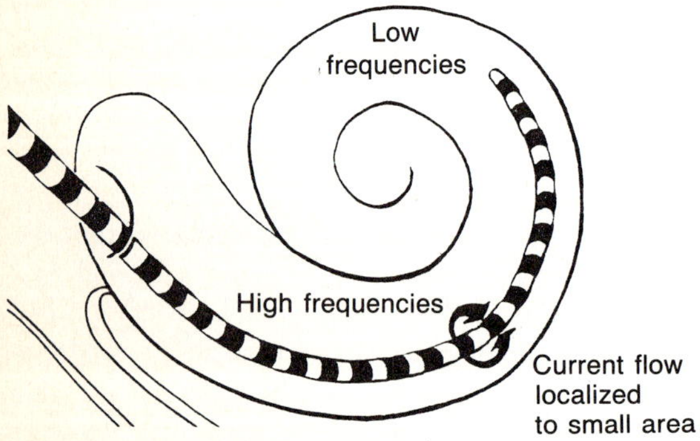

Figure 52–8 Bipolar stimulation is achieved by passing small amounts of current between two electrodes in close proximity. This type of electrode is typical for multichannel cochlear implants.

the signal is filtered or extracted. For example, sound might be processed as an analogue or digital signal; it can be sent to single or multiple electrodes; and if the system is multichannel, the coded signal can be transmitted serially or in parallel (simultaneously). Simultaneous data transmission means that a speech processor can transmit data to multiple electrodes at the same time. Such a coding method is typical of an analogue system using a filter-bank strategy. Sequential transmission means that the processed data are transmitted in a rapid sequence from the processor to the internal receiving package. This method is typical of a system that codes signals digitally or a system that transmits a rapidly multiplexed signal. Simultaneous and sequential processing and transmission may have the same perceptual effect due to the fact that the auditory system cannot resolve small temporal differences at the rapid coding rates of some cochlear implant systems.[4] Sequential and simultaneous coding of signals are used in multiple electrode systems.[21]

Acoustic Features of Speech

The major acoustic features of speech that should be analyzed and coded for transmission in a cochlear implant device are summarized in Figure 52–10. The fundamental frequency of a voice enables a listener to identify speaker age and sex, intonation of speech, prosody, and voicing. Additional information is provided by vowel formants and formant transitions. Specific vowels are identifiable from formant patterns and specific consonants are cued by transitions into and from the vowel nucleus. A simple cochlear implant system may select only a single acoustic feature such as fundamental frequency, whereas the more complex devices code several features of speech in order to facilitate recognition.

The fundamental frequency (F_0) of the human voice results from the vibratory cycle of the vocal folds. The vowel formants represent the acoustic resonances of the back (F_1) and front (F_2) cavities of the vocal tract as illustrated in Figure 52–11. If the vo-

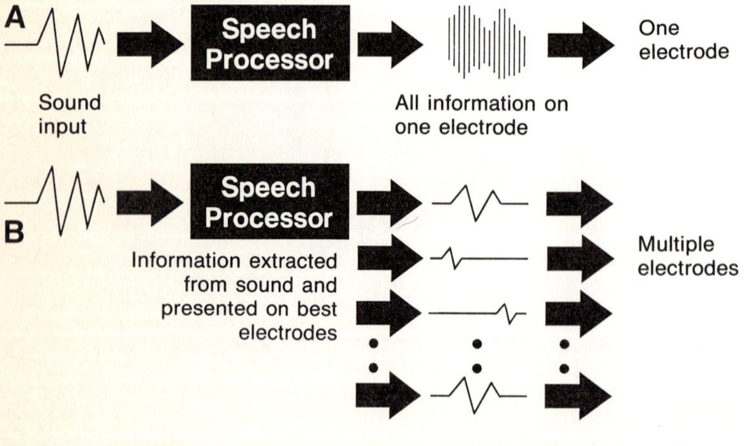

Figure 52–9 *A*, Single-channel and *B*, multichannel cochlear implant devices are illustrated, demonstrating how the multichannel system divides the signal into multiple signals for transmission to the multiple electrodes. A single channel device transmits all of the processed signal to one electrode.

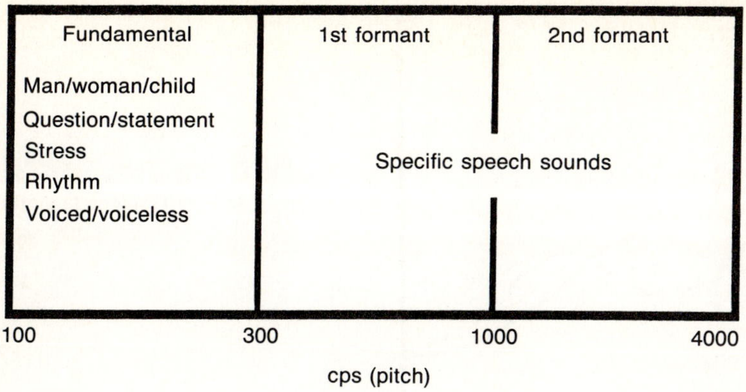

Figure 52–10 A model for speech coding explains how the fundamental frequency (F_0 and vowel formants (F_1 and F_2) provide various suprasegmental and segmental cues for speech perception. These are the primary acoustic features of speech that any cochlear implant system must code for optimal speech recognition.

cal tract is shaped for the specific vowels /i/ and /a/, then the vowel formant patterns differ, as illustrated in Figure 52–12. This figure also shows a difference in the fundamental frequency for /a/, which is higher than the fundamental frequency for /i/, as voiced by a female and male speaker, respectively. One might speculate that a cochlear implant with a multichannel coding strategy and multisited electrodes would be more capable (i.e., provide better speech recognition) of coding the acoustic features of speech in comparison to a single-channel device with a single-sited electrode.

Band-Filtering Strategy

One method of selecting frequency information is by dividing the speech frequencies (usually in the approximate range of 50 to 4,000 Hz) into a number of frequency bands and transmitting them as an electrical analogue representation of the speech signal. This method is often referred to as filter-bank coding. In this case, there is little direct manipulation of the signal, although different frequency bands may be emphasized by increasing their amplitude. Standard hearing aids use this principle. After the

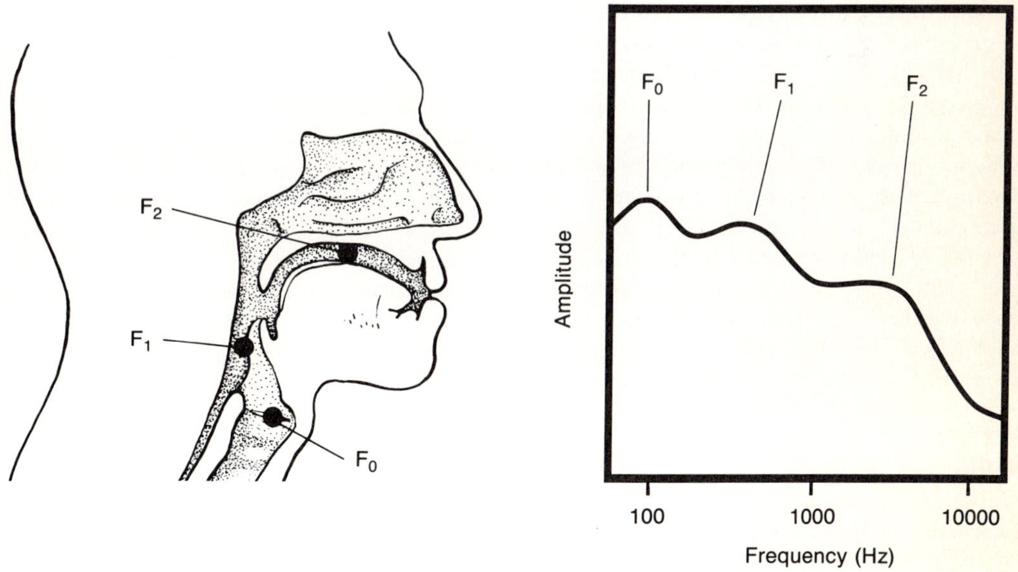

Figure 52–11 The human vocal tract at the level of the glottis is the source for the F_0, which is acoustically modified by the back (F_1) and front (F_2) cavity resonances. A spectrum of the output of the vocal tract is also shown with spectral peaks that correspond to the resonances of the vocal tract.

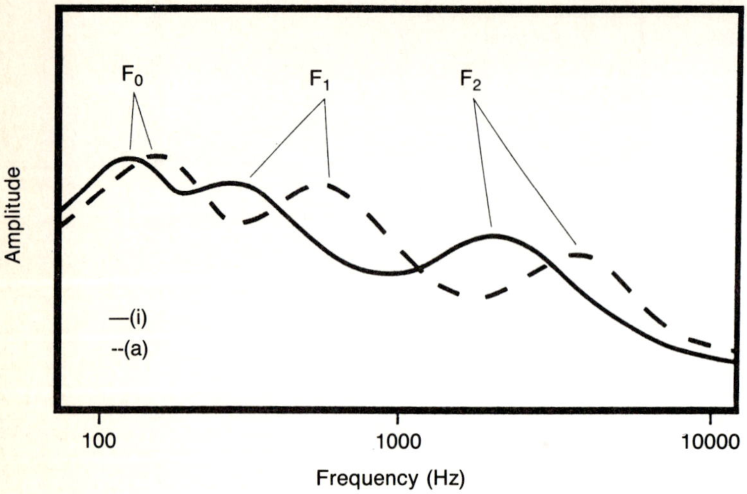

Figure 52–12 Spectra of the two English vowels /i/ and /a/ as spoken by a male and a female speaker, respectively.

filter-bank coding strategy divides the signal into a number of frequency bands, it transmits the analogue of the input signal received from the microphone to multiple electrodes.[17,22]

Full-Frequency Strategy

The speech processor with a full-frequency coding strategy receives the input electrical signal from the microphone and typically mixes the speech signal with a high-frequency carrier. The mixed signal is then sent directly to an electrode array, which usually consists of a single active electrode and remote ground electrode.[23,24] The single active and ground electrodes for such systems are typically monopolar in order to stimulate as many residual nerve fibers as possible. The speech processor in these devices simply outputs the analogue voltage on the carrier frequency,[24] or the signal may be band filtered, equalized, and output to a single active electrode.[25,26] One device that uses this method of frequency equalization, sometimes referred to as "multifrequency" coding, is the one developed in Austria by the Hochmair group. The full bandwidth of speech is split into four bands by the speech processor. Then the bands are independently balanced for loudness and recombined into a single signal. The output of the processor is sent to the paired single-channel electrodes via induction coils. This strategy of multifrequency coding is used for both the intra- and the extracochlear devices.

The House/3M cochlear implant is the most commonly used single-channel cochlear implant in the United States. The speech signal is processed by the amplitude modulation of a 16 kHz carrier frequency. The modulating signal is the output analogue voltage of the acoustic input. This output is transmitted via external and internal induction coils to the active and ground electrodes. This amplitude-modulated signal represents the temporal and amplitude characteristics of any input sound to the processor. Specific place-pitch information is not coded with this device.[27]

Feature-Extraction Strategy

Feature extraction is the most complicated coding strategy of present-day devices and requires sophisticated electronics to code the original speech signal. It codes characteristics of speech that are considered most important for recognition and comprehension and is based on speech perception research that has identified the major acoustic cues that contribute to speech recognition.[28,29] For vowels, formant patterns were found to provide significant information. Most importantly, listeners could identify the majority of vowels when the voicing frequency (the fundamental frequency) and as few as two formants (the first and second formants) were provided.[28] Indeed, when this type of information was provided to human subjects with a multichannel cochlear implant, "vowel labels could be assigned to the sensations produced by individual electrodes" (p 264).[30] Based on such perceptual studies, feature extraction for cochlear implant coding provided information representing the fundamental frequency, the maximum spectral peaks of selected formants, and the relative amplitudes of selected formants.[31,32] A model for this coding strategy is presented in Figure 52–13. The cochlear implant device that uses this strategy is manufactured in Australia by Nucleus Ltd. and marketed in the United States by Cochlear Corporation. This multichannel cochlear implant uses

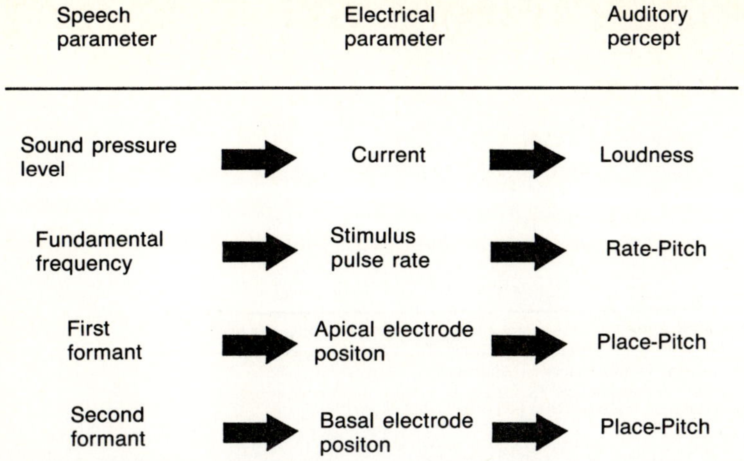

Figure 52–13 A model for feature extraction shows that the acoustic features of F_0, F_1, and F_2 are digitally coded in the Nucleus (Cochlear Corporation) device. The speech parameters are coded and transmitted to bipolar electrode pairs.

an active internal receiver-stimulator package, the heart of which is a small integrated CMOS electronic "chip."[33] A schema of the device in Figure 52–14 shows how the microphone input is processed for output to the cochlear implant recipient. The input is controlled first by an automatic gain control circuit and then the acoustic features—the fundamental frequency and the first and second formants—are extracted for digital coding. The digital codes are referenced to specific individual threshold and maximum comfort responses on each of 22 electrodes and then encoded for radio frequency transmission to the internal receiver-stimulator package that is attached to the electrode array. The transmitted signal is decoded by the active internal components, and discrete information is presented to bipolar electrodes in the sequence second formant followed by first formant at the pulse rate of the fundamental frequency. This sequencing simulates the cochlear travelling wave.

To illustrate how vowels are coded in the Nucleus feature-extraction system, first refer to Table 52–1, which describes some of the major acoustic features of nine English vowels. These features include only the first formant, the second formant, and the vowel duration. They provide the basic perceptual data for each vowel illustrated by a keyword ("heed, hid, head . . ."). The vowels are arranged in Table 52–1 in the order of decreasing second formant frequency, starting with the high front vowel /i/ at 2,290 Hz through the back vowel /ɔ/ at 870 Hz.

A simulation of how the nine English vowels in Table 52–1 are coded to a multisited electrode array is shown in Figure 52–15. In some instances, only the second formant is needed to differentiate the vowels across the electrode array. Obviously, the addition of the fundamental frequency, the first formant, and the vowel duration would provide more perceptual cues to enhance speech recognition.

The primary focus of the aforementioned feature-extraction strategy illustrates the ability of the

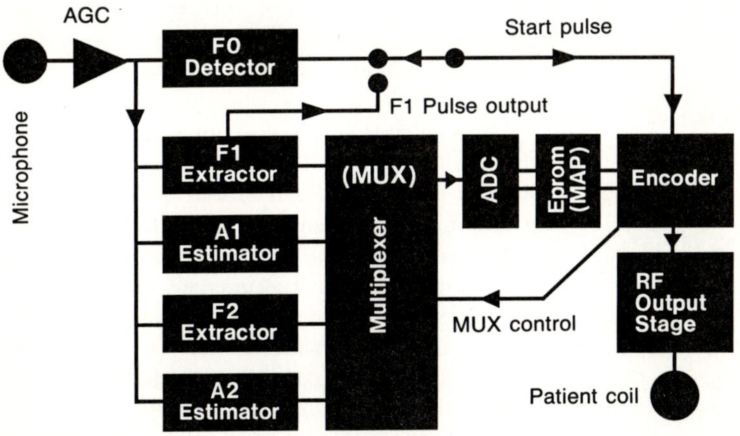

Figure 52–14 Details of the Nucleus (Cochlear Corporation) speech processor show how the device digitally codes speech acoustic features and transmits them to the implanted listener.

TABLE 52–1 Nine English Vowels Are Listed With a Keyword

Vowel	*Keyword*	F_1 *(Hz)*	F_2 *(Hz)*	*Duration*
/i/	Heed	270	2290	long
/ɪ/	Hid	390	1990	short
/ɛ/	Head	530	1840	long
/æ/	Had	660	1720	long
/ɝ/	Heard	490	1350	long
/ʌ/	Hud	640	1190	short
/ʊ/	Hood	440	1020	short
/u/	Who'd	300	870	long
/ɔ/	Hawed	570	840	long

Some of the more important acoustic features of each vowel are also described including the first formant (F_1), second formant (F_2), and duration (long versus short). The formant frequency information used in this table represents the formant values for adult males.
After Peterson GE, Barney HL. Control methods used in a study of the identification of vowels. J Acoust Soc Am 1952; 24:175.

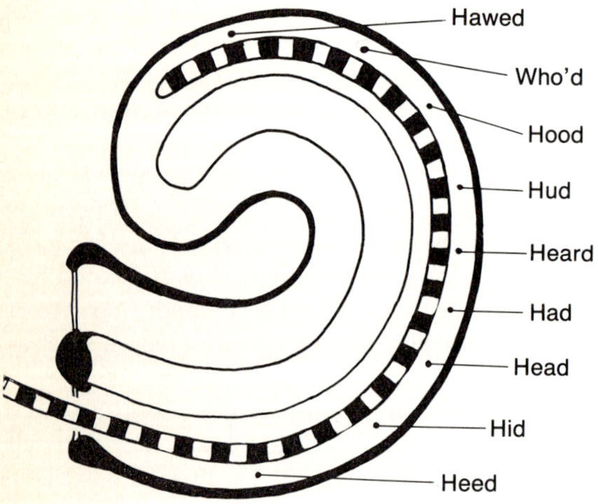

Figure 52–15 The nine English vowels listed in Table 52–1 are shown to stimulate auditory nerve fibers in the order of F_2 frequency from the basal (Heed) to apical (Hawed) turns of the cochlea.

Nucleus device to code vowels. However, this strategy also attempts to code consonants by rapidly tracking and coding the consonant-to-vowel and vowel-to-consonant formant transitions. The first and second formant transitions, coupled with the onset timing of voicing, provide the essential cues for place and manner of consonant production. Consonant voicing is cued by the presence or absence of the fundamental frequency before and during the articulation of consonants. For additional information, the reader should consult the excellent summary of the acoustic cues needed for the perception of speech by Borden and Harris.[34]

SIGNAL TRANSMISSION

Once the signal has been shaped by a particular coding strategy, it can either be sent directly through the skin via a percutaneous plug or transmitted across the skin by means of transcutaneous transmission, usually either by electromagnetic induction or by radio frequency signals (see Fig. 52–5). However, the simplest method of transmitting the coded signal from the speech processor to the electrode array is via direct wires. A primary advantage of such a transmission method is that it allows flexibility in the manipulation of stimulus parameters. Some of the first single- and multichannel cochlear implants used this method.[6] While the subject was present and "hardwired" directly to the stimulus generating system, the speech processor or laboratory computer could be "fine tuned." This fine tuning enabled many possibilities for the manipulation and control of stimulation parameters and allowed for experimentation relating to different coding strategies. A major disadvantage of such devices is that they were generally not wearable.

There are currently two wearable "hardwired" systems in clinical use that utilize a percutaneous plug.[11,13] Each system allows for flexibility because the electrodes can be connected directly to various experimental or prototype systems. They can also be connected to wearable speech processors for clinical evaluation. The use of a percutaneous connector may be restricted to adults because of the risk of infection at the site of the plug.[35]

It is possible to transmit the signal across the skin via electromagnetic induction. Small induction coil(s) on the external skin surface are connected to the speech processor, and the coil(s) transmit to the internal receiving coil(s), which are surgically placed just beneath the skin. The internal coil(s) are connected to the electrode array. If the internal device (receiver-stimulator) is active, power must also be transmitted with the coded data to provide energy to operate the internal electronics.

Data and power can be transmitted on a radio

frequency carrier to an internal active device. In this instance, the electrical power is used to activate the internal unit and decode the transmitted signal for stimulation of the electrode array. If the internal device is "passive," no further internal "decoding" or signal processing occurs.

Table 52–2 summarizes the coding strategies of the six cochlear implant systems, which have at least investigational status (clinical trials) within the United States. Note that both the House/3M and the Australia/Cochlear (Nucleus) systems have also received market approval from the United States Food and Drug Administration (FDA) for use in adults and are therefore no longer considered investigational devices. However, both remain investigational for use with children under the age of 18 years. All of the devices use intracochlear electrodes except for one version of the Vienna/3M device that utilizes a round window electrode. The Australia/Cochlear device (Nucleus) is the only one listed in Table 52–2 that uses a feature-extraction coding strategy.

PATIENT RESULTS

A cochlear implant should have the capability to encode environmental sounds and speech in a way that enables the recipient of the cochlear implant to interpret electrical signals in a manner similar to how a hearing person would interpret acoustic energy. If this encoding is accomplished effectively, the individual derives the maximum benefit from the cochlear implant and should experience an "improved quality of life." Improved "hearing" should be manifested by better sound detection, sound and speech discrimination (same versus different), speech identification, and speech recognition. Some comparative speech recognition results obtained from patients with single or multichannel implants will be described. The results are presented for closed-set and open-set subtests of the recorded Minimal Auditory Capabilities (MAC) test battery.[36–38]

Closed-Set Results

Closed-set tasks require the listener to identify the "correct" item from a choice of two or more.[39] Typically, such tasks limit the number of choices to five or fewer items. Examples of closed-set results for multichannel versus single-channel patients are shown in Figure 52–16. The multichannel patients achieved higher scores on all of the closed-set tasks in this study.[40] Closed-set results for the single-channel Vienna/3M device have been described by Rose et al.[41] Their findings demonstrated wide variability among their patients with single-channel devices, and, in general, the results of their study demonstrated closed-set performance scores that are poorer than typical results from patients with multichannel devices.

Open-Set Results

Open-set tasks require the listener to recognize words from a theoretically infinite set of choices. The

TABLE 52–2 Description of Six of the More Common Cochlear Implant Devices in the United States with Reference to Some of the Major Design and Coding Features

Name of Device	*Electrode Location/Depth*		*Analogue Digital*	*Coding Strategy*	*#CH*	*CP*
Australia/Cochlear†	Intra	25	Digital	Features $F_0/F_1/F_2$	1–22	RF
House/3M†	Intra	3–6	Analogue	Filtered AM 16 kHz	1	IN
UCSF/Storz*	Intra	12–24	Analogue	Band filtered	1–4	IN
Utah/Symbion*	Intra	12–22	Analogue	Filtered	1–4	PC
Vienna/3M*	Extra	0	Analogue	Band filtered	1	IN
Vienna/3M*	Intra	6	Analogue	Band filtered	1	IN

* = United States FDA approval as an investigational device for use with adults only.
† = United States FDA approval as an investigational device for use with children and market approval for use with adults.
Abbreviations:
#CH = number of stimulation channels available;
CP = coupling from processor to electrode array;
F_0 = fundamental frequency of voice;
F_1 = first formant of vowel(s);
F_2 = second formant of vowel(s);
AM = amplitude modulation of carrier frequency or analogue signal;
IN = induction coupling via small coil(s);
PC = percutaneous plug;
RF = radio-frequency transmission of data and power.

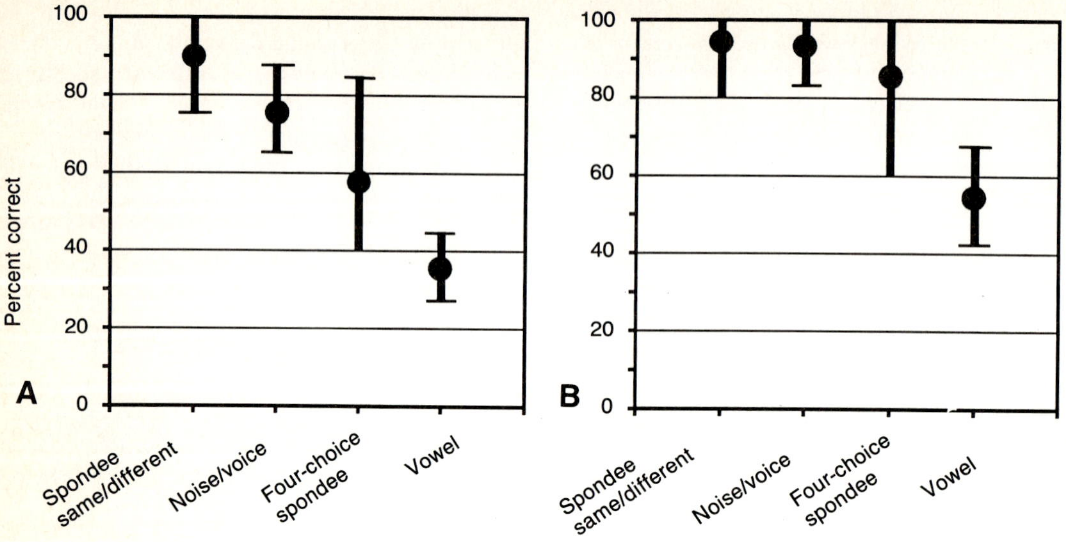

Figure 52–16 Closed-set speech perception results (mean and range) are shown for *A*, single and *B*, multichannel patients. (From Brimacombe J, Danhauer J, Mecklenburg D, Prietto A, Dowell R. Single-channel and multichannel cochlear implant users' performance on the MAC battery. Amer J Otol, in press.)

probability of correct responses for open-set tasks can be influenced by the nature of the task. For example, sentence recognition takes advantage of the predictability of word sequences in language, and so the task may be influenced by context. The results in Figure 52–17 demonstrate better performance for the patients with multichannel devices on the open-set subtests of the MAC battery.[40] They reported that patients with single-channel devices did not have the ability to recognize monosyllabic words, whereas a few patients with multichannel devices utilizing only fundamental frequency and second formant information achieved word recognition scores of greater than 20 percent on this subtest of the MAC battery. Similar results were reported by Lindeman et al. for one patient who had a single-channel device replaced with a multichannel device.[42] His CID sentence score improved from 1 percent with a single-channel device to 31 percent with the multichannel device.

The aforementioned results suggest that mul-

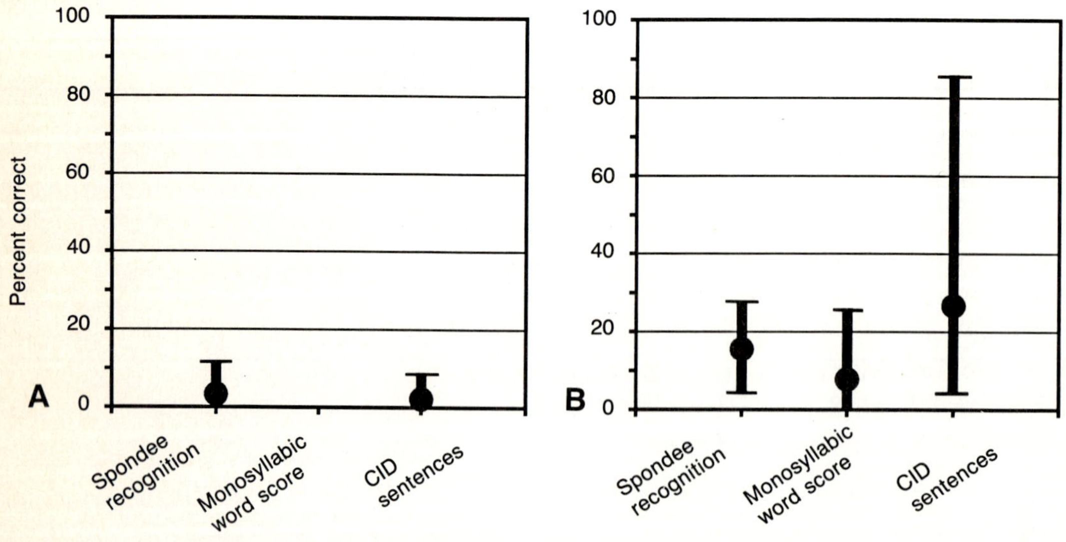

Figure 52–17 Open-set speech perception results (mean and range) are shown for *A*, single and *B*, multichannel patients. (From Brimacombe J, Danhauer J, Mecklenburg D, Prietto A, Dowell R. Single-channel and multichannel cochlear implant users' performance on the MAC battery. Amer J Otol, in press.)

tichannel cochlear implants, with multi-sited stimulation, achieve more frequency-specific information relating to the high-frequency components of speech. The recognition of speech without lipreading has been reported in the literature more frequently for multisited stimulation, although the proportion of single- to multisited cochlear implants is at least three to one. There are several references the reader might wish to consult about this matter.[16,17,38,42–48]

SUMMARY

Cochlear implants have evolved from single-ball electrode designs to multiple-electrode arrays that serve as the stimulation outputs for complex multichannel coding strategies. Present-day speech coding strategies are capable of presenting an electrical signal to residual eighth cranial nerve fibers, enabling those fibers to transmit the signal to the brain. For some patients, this signal can be interpreted as recognizable speech without lipreading. Speech processors have been reduced in size to a point where they are feasible to wear comfortably daily.

Among the six cochlear implant devices described in Table 52–2, four require greater than 10 mm for electrode insertion into the scala tympani, one of the devices can utilize an extracochlear electrode, three are multichannel, and five utilize filtered-analogue coding strategies. Thus, to date, the trend for cochlear implant designs seems to have been for intracochlear, filtered analogue, multichannel devices.

REFERENCES

1. Held R, Richards W. Perception: mechanisms and models. San Francisco: WH Freeman, 1972.
2. Zenner HP. Molecular structure of hair cells. In: Altschuler RA, Bobbin RP, Hoffman DW, eds. Neurobiology of hearing: the cochlea. New York: Raven Press, 1986:1–21.
3. Levitt H, Pickett JM, Houde R, eds. Sensory aids for the hearing-impaired. New York: IEEE Press, 1980.
4. Parkins CW. Cochlear prostheses. In: Altschuler RA, Bobbin RP, Hoffman DW, eds. Neurobiology of hearing: the cochlea. New York: Raven Press, 1986:455–473.
5. Simmons FB. Electrical stimulation of the auditory nerve in man. Arch Otolaryngol 1966; 84:2–54.
6. Luxford WM, Brackman DE. The history of cochlear implants. In: Gray RF, ed. Cochlear implants. San Diego: College-Hill Press, 1985:1–26.
7. Michelson RP. Electrical stimulation of the human cochlea. Arch Otolaryngol 1971; 93:317–323.
8. Ries, PW. The demography of hearing loss. In: Orlans H, ed. Adjustment to adult hearing loss. San Diego: College-Hill Press, 1985:3–21.
9. Clark GM, Tong YC. The engineering of future cochlear implants. In: Gray RF, ed. Cochlear implants. San Diego: College-Hill Press, 1985:211–228.
10. Fretz R, Fravel R. Design and function: a physical and electrical description of the 3M House cochlear implant system. Ear Hear 1985; 6(3) Suppl:14S–19S.
11. Banfai P, Hortmann G, Karczag A, Kubik S, Wustrow F. Results with eight-channel cochlear implants. In: Keidel WD, Finkenzeller P, eds. Cochlear implants in clinical use. Advances in audiology. Vol. 2. New York: S Karger, 1984:1–18.
12. Chouard C-H, Fugain C, Meyer B, Lacombe H. Long-term results of the multichannel cochlear implant. Ann NY Acad Sci 1983; 405:387–411.
13. McCandless G, Dankowski K, Smith L. Symbion cochlear implant device and program results. Am J Otol; in press.
14. Merzenich M, Kessler DK, Rebscher MS, Schindler RA. Progress in development and application of the University of California at San Francisco/Storz multichannel cochlear implant. Ann Otol Rhinol Laryngol 1987; 96(1) Suppl. 128:122–125.
15. Patrick JF, MacFarlane JC. Characteristics of mechanical properties of single electrodes and multielectrodes. Ann Otol Rhinol Laryngol 1987; 96(1) Suppl. 128:46–48.
16. Eddington DK. Speech recognition in deaf subjects with multichannel intracochlear electrodes. Ann NY Acad Sci 1983; 405:241–258.
17. Merzenich M. Coding of sound in a cochlear prosthesis: some theoretical and practical considerations. Ann NY Acad Sci 1983; 405:502–508.
18. Patrick JF, Crosby PA, Hirshorn MS, Kuzma JA, Money DK, Ridler J, Seligman PM. Australian multi-channel implantable hearing prosthesis. In: Schindler RA, Merzenich MM, eds. Cochlear implants. New York, Raven Press, 1985:93–100.
19. Evans EF. How to provide speech through an implant device. Dimensions of the problem: an overview. In: Schindler RA, Merzenich MM, eds. Cochlear implants. New York: Raven Press, 1985:167–183.
20. Moore BCJ. Speech coding for cochlear implants. In: Gray RF, ed. Cochlear implants. San Diego: College-Hill Press, 1985:163–179.
21. McDermott H. Cochlear implant for simultaneous multichannel stimulation. Ann Otol Rhinol Laryngol 1987; 96(1) Suppl. 128:67–69.
22. Eddington DK, Dobelle WH, Brackmann DE, Mladejovsky MG, Parkin JL. Auditory prosthesis research with multiple channel intracochlear stimulation in man. Ann Otol Rhinol Laryngol 1978; 87 Suppl. 53:5–39.
23. Hochmair ES, Hochmair-Desoyer IJ. An implanted auditory eight-channel stimulator for the deaf. Med Biol Eng Comp 1981; 19:141–148.
24. House WF, Berliner KI, Crary WG, Graham M, Luckey R, Norton N, Selters W, Tobin H, Urban J, Wexler M. Cochlear implants. Ann Otol Rhinol Laryngol 1976; 85 Suppl. 27:1–93.
25. Hochmair-Desoyer IJ, Hochmair ES, Burian K, Stiglbrunner HK. Percepts from the Vienna cochlear prosthesis. Ann NY Acad Sci 1983; 405:295–306.
26. Hochmair ES, Hochmair-Desoyer IJ. Aspects of sound signal processing using the Vienna intra- and extracochlear implants. In: Schindler RA, Merzenich MM, eds. Cochlear Implants. New York: Raven Press, 1985:101–110.
27. House WF. The cochlear implant: performance of deaf patients. Hearing Instruments 1981; 32(9):13–18.
28. Liberman A, Harris KF, Hoffman HS, Griffith EC. The discrimination of speech sounds within and across phoneme boundaries. J Exp Psych 1957; 54:358–368.
29. Tong YC, Blamey PJ, Dowell RC, Clark GM. Psychophysical studies evaluating the feasibility of a speech processing strategy for a multiple-channel cochlear implant. J Acoust Soc Amer 1983; 74:73–80.
30. Tong TC, Clark GM. Percepts from scala tympani stimulation. Ann NY Acad Sci 1983; 405:264–267.

31. Dowell RC, Seligman BE, Blamey PJ, Clark GM. Evaluation of a two-formant speech-processing strategy for a multichannel cochlear prosthesis. Ann Otol Rhinol Laryngol 1987; 96(1) Suppl. 128:132–134.
32. Seligman PM, Patrick JF, Tong YC, Clark GM, Dowell RC, Crosby PA. A signal processor for a multiple-electrode hearing prosthesis. Acta Otolaryngol (Stockh) [Suppl] 1984; 411:135–139.
33. Mecklenburg DJ, Brimacombe JA. An overview of the nucleus cochlear implant program. Semin Hear 1985; 6:41–51.
34. Borden GJ, Harris KS. Speech science primer: physiology, acoustics, and perception of speech. Baltimore: William & Wilkins, 1980.
35. Mangham CA, Luxford WM. Cochlear prosthesis surgery in children. Semin Hear 1986; 7(4):361–369.
36. Owens E, Kessler D, Tellen C, Schubert ED. The Minimal Auditory Capabilities Battery. St. Louis: Auditec, 1981.
37. Owens E, Kessler D, Tellen C, Schubert ED. The Minimal Auditory Capabilities Battery. St. Louis: Auditec, 1985.
38. Owens E, Kessler D, Raggio M. Results for some patients with cochlear implants on the Minimal Auditory Capabilities (MAC) Battery. Ann NY Acad Sci 1983; 405:443–450.
39. Bochner J, Garrison W, Palmer L. A closed-set sentence protocol for assessing speech discrimination in deaf individuals: the speech sound pattern discrimination test. Ear Hear 1986; 7(6):370–376.
40. Brimacombe J, Danhauer J, Mecklenburg D, Prietto A, Dowell R. Single-channel and multichannel cochlear implant users' performance on the MAC battery. Amer J Otol, in press.
41. Rose DE, Facer GW, King AM, Fabry DA. Results using 3M/Vienna extracochlear implant in five patients Ann Otol Rhinol Laryngol 1987; 96(1) Suppl. 128:114–117.
42. Lindeman RC, Mangham CA, Kuprenas SV. Comparison of performance with a single and multichannel cochlear prosthesis in the same reimplanted patient. Ann Otol Rhinol Laryngol 1987; 96(1) Suppl. 128:150–151.
43. Burian K, Eisenwort B, Hochmair ES, Hochmair-Desoyer IJ. Clinical experiences with 'Vienna cochlear implant'. Adv Audio 1984; 1:19–29.
44. Eddington DK. Speech discrimination in deaf patients with cochlear implants. J Acoust Soc Am 1980; 68:885–891.
45. Gantz BJ, McCabe BF, Tyler RS, Preece JP. Evaluation of four cochlear implant designs. Ann Otol Rhinol Laryngol 1987; 96(1) Suppl. 128:145–147.
46. Parkin JL, Dankowski MK. Speech performance by patients with multichannel cochlear implants. Otolaryngol Head Neck Surg 1986; 95(2):205–209.
47. Sachs MB, Miller MI. Pitch coding in the auditory nerve: possible mechanisms of pitch sensation with cochlear implants. In: Schindler RA, Merzenich MM, eds. Cochlear implants. New York: Raven Press, 1985:185–194.
48. Shallop JK, Beiter AL, Brackmann DE, Kienle ML, Miyamoto RT. Auditory performance in a patient with a single vs. a multi-channel cochlear implant. Paper presented at ASHA annual convention, Detroit, November 21, 1986.

E

I

J

K

L

N

O